David C. Sabiston, Jr., M.D.

James B. Duke Professor of Surgery
Chairman of the Department of Surgery
Duke University Medical Center
Durham, North Carolina

Margaret Q. Meyers
Beeper # 6090
382-1042

Sabiston's Essentials of Surgery

1987
W.B. Saunders
Company

Harcourt Brace
Jovanovich, Inc.

Philadelphia
London
Toronto
Montreal
Sydney
Tokyo

D1399130

13-emo
Heart
40-4

W. B. Saunders Company: West Washington Square
Philadelphia, PA   19105

Library of Congress Cataloging-in-Publication Data

Essentials of surgery.

1. Surgery.   I. Sabiston, David C., 1924–
   [DNLM: 1. Surgery. WO 100 E785]

RD31.E785   1987   617   86–26146

Editor: Dean Manke
Designer: Terri Siegel
Production Manager: Carolyn Naylor
Manuscript Editor: Carol J. Wolf
Illustration Coordinator: Lisa Lambert
Indexer: Dennis Dolan

Essentials of Surgery   ISBN: 0-7216-7874-2

Last digit is the print number: 9   8   7   6   5   4   3   2   1

This text is dedicated to medical students everywhere, who continually stimulate their teachers with incisive questions and dialogue, and who engender in them the enthusiasm necessary to remain abreast of the field.

THE EDITOR

CONTRIBUTORS

JOSEPH F. AMARAL, M.D.

Assistant Instructor, Department of Surgery, Brown University, Division of Biology and Medicine, Providence, Rhode Island. Surgical Fellow, Rhode Island Hospital, Providence.

Fluid and Electrolyte Management

DANA K. ANDERSEN, M.D.

Associate Professor of Medicine and Surgery, State University of New York, Health Science Center at Brooklyn. Attending Surgeon, State University Hospital and Kings County Hospital Center, Brooklyn. Consultant in Surgery, Veterans Administration Medical Center, Brooklyn.

The Pancreas

BRADLEY AUST, M.D., Ph.D.

Professor and Chairman, Department of Surgery, The University of Texas Health Science Center at San Antonio. Chief of Surgery, Bexar County Hospital District Hospitals. Consultant, Brooke Army Medical Center, Fort Sam Houston; Methodist Hospital, Veterans Administration Hospital, San Antonio State Chest Hospital, Humana Hospital San Antonio and Metropolitan.

Surgical Disorders of the Small Intestine

ERLE H. AUSTIN, M.D.

Associate Professor, Section Head, Pediatric Cardiac Surgery, Division of Cardiac Surgery, Department of Surgery, East Carolina University School of Medicine, Greenville, North Carolina. Attending Physician, Cardiothoracic Surgery, Pitt County Memorial Hospital, Greenville.

Disorders of Pulmonary Venous Return: Total Anomalous Pulmonary Venous Connection

ROBERT W. BARNES, M.D.

Professor and Chairman, Department of Surgery, University of Arkansas for Medical Sciences, Little Rock. Staff Surgeon, University of Arkansas, McClellan Memorial Veterans Administration Hospital, and Arkansas Children's Hospital, Little Rock.

The Arterial System

DOUGLAS M. BEHRENDT, M.D.

Professor of Surgery, University of Michigan Medical School, Ann Arbor. Staff, Section of Thoracic Surgery, University of Michigan Medical Center, Ann Arbor.

Transplantation

KIRBY I. BLAND, M.D.

Professor and Associate Chairman, Department of Surgery, University of Florida College of Medicine, Gainesville, Florida. Staff, Shands Hospital, Gaines-

ville Veterans Administration Medical Center, and Lake City Veterans Administration Medical Center.

The Breast

DANI P. BOLOGNESI, Ph.D.

James B. Duke Professor of Experimental Surgery, Department of Surgery; Director, Surgical Virology Laboratory, Duke University Medical Center, Durham, North Carolina.

Surgical Aspects of Viral Hepatitis and the Acquired Immune Deficiency Syndrome (AIDS)

MURRAY F. BRENNAN, M.D.

Professor of Surgery, Cornell University Medical College, New York, New York. Alfred P. Sloan Professor of Surgery, Chairman, Department of Surgery, Memorial–Sloan-Kettering Cancer Center, New York.

Nutrition and Metabolism in Surgical Patients

DENNIS E. BULLARD, M.D.

Assistant Professor of Neurosurgery and Pathology, Duke University Medical Center, Durham, North Carolina.

Neurosurgery

JOHN L. CAMERON, M.D.

Professor and Chairman, Section of Surgical Sciences, The Johns Hopkins University School of Medicine, Baltimore, Maryland. Chief of Surgery, The Johns Hopkins Hospital, Baltimore.

The Biliary System

DARRELL A. CAMPBELL, Jr., M.D.

Associate Professor of Surgery, University of Michigan Medical School, Ann Arbor. Director of Transplantation, Section of General Surgery, University of Michigan Medical Center, Ann Arbor.

Transplantation

W. RANDOLPH CHITWOOD, Jr., M.D.

Professor, Division of Cardiac Surgery, East Carolina University School of Medicine, Greenville, North Carolina. Chief of Cardiac Surgery, Pitt County Memorial Hospital, Greenville.

The Diagnosis and Management of Myasthenia Gravis

ORLO H. CLARK, M.D.

Professor of Surgery, University of California Medical Center, San Francisco. Staff, Veterans Administration Medical Center, University of California Medical Center, and Letterman General Hospital, San Francisco, and David Grant Medical Center, Travis, California.

The Pituitary and Adrenal Glands

JOHN J. COLEMAN III, M.D.

Associate Professor of Surgery, Emory University School of Medicine, Atlanta, Georgia. Chief of Plastic Surgery, Atlanta Veterans Administration Medical Center. Wadley R. Glenn Chair of Surgery, Emory University, Atlanta.

The Head and Neck

REX B. CONN, M.D.

Professor of Pathology and Laboratory Medicine, School of Medicine, Emory University, Atlanta, Georgia. Director, Clinical Pathology Laboratories, Emory University Hospital, Atlanta.

Normal Values

EDWARD M. COPELAND III, M.D.

The Edward R. Woodward Professor and Chairman, Department of Surgery, University of Florida College of Medicine, Gainesville, Florida. Chief of Surgery, Shands Hospital at the University of Florida, Gainesville.

The Breast

ROBERT J. CORRY, M.D.

Professor and Head, Department of Surgery, The University of Iowa College of Medicine, Iowa City. Chief of Surgery, University of Iowa Hospitals and Clinics. Consultant, Surgical Services, Iowa City Veterans Administration Medical Center.

Surgical Complications

PETER J. E. CRUSE, M.B., CH. B., F.R.C.S. (E&C)

Professor and Head, University of Calgary, Alberta, Canada, Head, Department of Surgery, Foothills Hospital, Calgary.

Wound Healing and Management

P. WILLIAM CURRERI, M.D.

Professor and Chairman, Department of Surgery, University of South Alabama College of Medicine, Mobile. Chief of Surgery, University of South Alabama Medical Center, Mobile.

Management of the Acutely Injured Person

DONALD C. DAFOE, M.D.

Assistant Professor of Surgery, University of Michigan Medical School, Ann Arbor. Staff, Section of General Surgery, University of Michigan Medical Center, Ann Arbor.

Transplantation

RALPH J. DAMIANO, M.D.

Chief Assistant Resident in Surgery, Duke University Medical Center, Durham, North Carolina.

Cardiac Neoplasms

R. DUANE DAVIS, Jr., M.D.

Research Fellow in Surgery, Duke University Medical Center, Durham, North Carolina.

Primary Mediastinal Cysts and Neoplasms

ANDRÉ DURANCEAU, M.D.

Professor of Surgery, Université de Montréal, School of Medicine, Montréal, Canada. Chief, Thoracic Surgery Service, Hôtel-Dieu de Montréal Hospital.

The Esophagus

LENNART FAGRAEUS, M.D., Ph.D.

Professor and Chairman, Department of Anesthesiology, College of Medicine, University of Oklahoma, Oklahoma City.

Anesthesia

JOSEPH C. FARMER, Jr., M.D.

Associate Professor, Division of Otolaryngology, Department of Surgery, Duke University School of Medicine, Durham, North Carolina. Staff, Otolaryngology, Duke University Medical Center, and Durham Veterans Administration Regional Medical Center. Consultant, Durham County General Hospital.

Otolaryngology

JOHN R. FARNDON, B.S., M.B., F.R.C.S.

Senior Lecturer in Surgery, University of Newcastle upon Tyne, United Kingdom. Consultant Surgeon, Royal Victoria Infirmary, Newcastle upon Tyne, United Kingdom.

The Thyroid

T. BRUCE FERGUSON, Jr., M.D.

Teaching Scholar in Surgery, Department of Surgery, Duke University Medical Center, Durham, North Carolina.

Management of the Surgical Patient with Cardiac Disease

ROBERT D. FITCH, M.D.

Assistant Professor, Orthopaedic Surgery, Duke University, Durham, North Carolina. Staff Orthopedic Surgeon, Duke University Hospital. Consultant Orthopedist, Lennox Baker Children's Hospital, Durham.

Fractures of the Upper Extremity; Introduction to Pediatric Orthopedics

DONALD S. GANN, M.D.

J. Murray Beardsley Professor of Surgery and Chairman, Department of Surgery, Brown University, Division of Biology and Medicine, Providence, Rhode Island. Surgeon-in-Chief, Rhode Island Hospital, Providence.

Fluid and Electrolyte Management

J. WILLIAM GAYNOR, M.D.

Senior Resident in Surgery, Duke University Medical Center, Durham, North Carolina.

Patent Ductus Arteriosus, Coarctation of the Aorta, Aortopulmonary Window, and Anomalies of the Aortic Arch

GREGORY S. GEORGIADE, M.D.

Associate Professor, General and Plastic Surgery, Duke University Medical Center, Durham, North

CONTRIBUTORS

Carolina. Assistant Director, Trauma Service. Unit Physician, Burn Unit, and S.I.C.U. Physician, Medical Central Officer for Duke Hospital Helicopter Air Transport Service, Duke University Medical Center, Durham.

Burns

LAWRENCE D. GERMAN, M.D.

Assistant Professor of Medicine, Duke University, Durham, North Carolina.

Cardiac Pacemakers

IAN R. GOUGH, M.B., B.S., F.R.A.C.S.

Associate Professor of Surgery, University of Queensland, Brisbane, Australia. Consultant Surgeon, Royal Brisbane Hospital, Brisbane.

The Parathyroid Glands

WILLIAM P. GRAHAM III, M.D.

Clinical Professor of Surgery, Hershey Medical Center, Pennsylvania State University College of Medicine, Hershey, Pennsylvania. Active Staff, Carlisle Hospital, Carlisle; Holy Spirit Hospital, Camp Hill; Harrisburg Hospital and Polyclinic Medical Center, Harrisburg; and Seidle Memorial Hospital, Mechanicsburg.

Surgical Disorders of the Skin

CHARLES S. GREENBERG, M.D.

Assistant Professor of Medicine and Pathology, Duke University, Durham, North Carolina. Director, Coagulation Laboratory, Duke University Medical Center, Durham.

Hemostasis: Pathophysiology and Management of Clinical Disorders

A. F. HANEY, M.D.

Associate Professor and Director, Division of Reproductive Endocrinology and Infertility, Department of Obstetrics and Gynecology, Duke University Medical Center, Durham, North Carolina.

Gynecologic Surgery

JOHN M. HARRELSON, M.D.

Associate Professor of Orthopaedic Surgery and Assistant Professor of Pathology, Duke University Medical Center, Durham, North Carolina. Chief, Orthopaedic Surgery, Durham Veterans Administration Medical Center, Durham.

Musculoskeletal Trauma: General Principles; Pelvic and Lower Extremity Fractures; General Orthopedics

RONALD C. HILL, M.D.

Assistant Professor of Surgery, West Virginia University School of Medicine, Morgantown. Consultant, Veterans Administration Hospital, Clarksburg, West Virginia.

Lung Abscess and Fungal Infections; Disorders of the Pleura and Empyema; Bronchiectasis

WILLIAM L. HOLMAN, M.D.

Teaching Scholar in Cardiac Surgery, Duke University Medical Center, Durham, North Carolina.

Thoracic Outlet Syndrome

E. CARMACK HOLMES, M.D.

Professor of Surgery, University of California School of Medicine at Los Angeles.

Principles of Surgical Oncology

STEFANIE S. JEFFREY, M.D.

Assistant Clinical Professor of Surgery, University of California Medical Center, San Francisco. Staff, Pacific Presbyterian Medical Center, San Francisco.

The Pituitary and Adrenal Glands

ROBERT N. JONES, M.D.

Assistant Professor, Department of Thoracic and Cardiovascular Surgery, Loyola University Medical Center, and Hines Veterans Administration Hospital, Maywood, Illinois.

Ebstein's Anomaly

M. J. JURKIEWICZ, M.D.

Professor of Surgery, Emory University School of Medicine, Atlanta, Georgia. Chief, Division of Plastic Surgery, Emory Affiliated Hospitals, Atlanta.

The Head and Neck

MARVIN M. KIRSH, M.D.

Professor of Surgery, University of Michigan Medical School, Ann Arbor. Staff, Section of Thoracic Surgery, University of Michigan Medical Center, Ann Arbor.

Transplantation

WARREN J. KORTZ, M.D.

Chief Resident, General Surgery, Duke University Medical Center, Durham, North Carolina.

Hernias

EDWIN LAFONTAINE, M.D.

Assistant Professor of Surgery, Université de Montréal School of Medicine, Montréal, Canada. Hôtel-Dieu de Montréal Hospital.

The Esophagus

BARRY A. LEVINE, M.D.

Professor, The University of Texas Health Science Center, San Antonio. Attending Physician, Medical Center Hospital and Audie L. Murphy Memorial Veterans Administration Hospital, San Antonio.

Surgical Disorders of the Small Intestine

W. MARSTON LINEHAN, M.D.

Assistant Professor of Urologic Surgery, Uniformed Services University of the Health Sciences, Bethesda, Maryland. Head, Urologic Oncology Section, Surgery Branch, National Cancer Institute, Bethesda.

The Urogenital System

GARY K. LOFLAND, M.D.

Assistant Professor of Surgery, State University of New York at Buffalo. Chief, Pediatric Cardiac Surgery, Buffalo Children's Hospital, Buffalo, New York.

Atrial Septal Defect, Ostium Primum Defect, and Atrioventricular Canal; Ventricular Septal Defects

JAMES E. LOWE, M.D.

Associate Professor of Surgery and Assistant Professor of Pathology, Duke University, Durham, North Carolina. Director, Surgical Electrophysiology Service, Duke University Medical Center, Durham.

Surgical Treatment of Cardiac Arrhythmias; Cardiac Pacemakers

H. KIM LYERLY, M.D.

Senior Resident in Surgery, Department of Surgery, Duke University Medical Center, Durham, North Carolina.

Surgical Aspects of Viral Hepatitis and the Acquired Immune Deficiency Syndrome (AIDS); Pulmonary Embolism; Arteriovenous Fistulas

BARRY D. MANN, M.D.

Assistant Clinical Professor, University of California, School of Medicine at Los Angeles.

Principles of Surgical Oncology

WILLIAM H. MARKS, M.D., Ph.D.

Assistant Professor of Surgery and Biochemistry, Stritch School of Medicine, Loyola University of Chicago, Chicago, Illinois. Staff, Loyola University Medical Center, Section of General Surgery, Maywood, Illinois.

Transplantation

TERUO MATSUMOTO, M.D., Ph.D.

Professor and Chairman, Department of Surgery, Hahnemann University, Philadelphia, Pennsylvania. Chief of Surgery, Hahnemann University Hospital. Attending Surgeon, St. Agnes Medical Center, Philadelphia.

The Spleen

RICHARD L. McCANN, M.D.

Assistant Professor of Surgery, Duke University Medical School, Durham, North Carolina. Attending Staff, Duke University Medical Center. Consultant, Durham Veterans Administration Medical Center, Durham.

The Lymphatic System

DONALD C. McILRATH, M.D.

Professor of Surgery, Mayo Medical School; Chairman, Department of Surgery, Mayo Clinic, Rochester, Minnesota.

Surgical Disorders of the Vermiform Appendix and Meckel's Diverticulum

JOSEPH S. McLAUGHLIN, M.D.

Professor of Surgery, Head, Division of Thoracic and Cardiovascular Surgery, University of Maryland School of Medicine, College Park, Maryland. Staff, University Hospital, College Park.

Surgical Disorders of the Pericardium

N. TAIT McPHEDRAN, M.D., F.R.C.S.C.

Professor, Department of Surgery, Faculty of Medicine, University of Calgary, Alberta, Canada. Senior Surgeon, Foothills Hospital, Calgary.

Wound Healing and Management

JON F. MORAN, M.D.

Associate Professor and Chairman, Department of Thoracic and Cardiovascular Surgery, University of Kansas Medical Center, Kansas City.

The Surgical Treatment of Pulmonary Tuberculosis

JOHN A. MORRIS, JR., M.D.

Assistant Professor of Surgery, Vanderbilt University School of Medicine, Nashville, Tennessee. Director, Division of Trauma, Vanderbilt University Hospital, Nashville.

The Acute Abdomen

RONALD LEE NICHOLS, M.D.

Henderson Professor and Vice-Chairman, Department of Surgery; Professor of Microbiology and Immunology, Tulane University School of Medicine, New Orleans, Louisiana. Attending Surgeon, Tulane Medical Center Hospital and Charity Hospital of Louisiana at New Orleans.

Surgical Infections and Choice of Antibiotics

P. MICHAEL OLMSTEAD, M.D.

Assistant Professor, The Pennsylvania State University School of Medicine, Hershey, Pennsylvania. Assistant Professor, Hershey Medical Center.

Surgical Disorders of the Skin

CRAIG O. OLSEN, M.D.

Instructor, Harvard Medical School, Boston, Massachusetts. Attending Physician, Department of Surgery, New England Deaconess Hospital, Boston.

Cardiopulmonary Bypass for Cardiac Surgery

W. CHRISTOPHER PEDERSON, M.D.

Assistant Professor of Surgery, Division of Plastic and Reconstructive Surgery, Duke University Medical Center, Durham, North Carolina.

Burns

ALICE R. PEREZ, M.D.

Fellow, Gastrointestinal Research, Department of Surgery, Temple University School of Medicine, Philadelphia, Pennsylvania.

Stomach and Duodenum: Surgical Anatomy, Physiology, and Pathology

MORTON H. PERLMAN, M.D.

Professor and Director, Division of Surgical Education, Department of Surgery, Hahnemann University, Philadelphia, Pennsylvania.

The Spleen

ROBERT B. PEYTON, M.D.

Assistant Professor of Surgery, New York Hospital, Cornell Medical Center, New York City, New York.

Ventricular Aneurysm

KENNETH P. RAMMING, M.D.

Professor of Surgery, Division of Oncology and Cardiothoracic Surgery. University of California School of Medicine, Los Angeles.

Diseases of the Colon and Rectum

J. SCOTT RANKIN, M.D.

Associate Professor, Department of Surgery, Duke University Medical Center, Durham, North Carolina.

Cardiopulmonary Resuscitation; The Coronary Circulation: Physiologic Determinants of Coronary Blood Flow, Cardiac Metabolism, and Intraoperative Myocardial Protection

DOUGLAS S. REINTGEN, M.D.

Chief Resident in Surgery, Duke University Medical Center, Durham, North Carolina.

The Liver

WALLACE R. RITCHIE, Jr., M.D., Ph.D.

Professor and Chairman, Department of Surgery, Temple University School of Medicine, Philadelphia, Pennsylvania. Chairman, Department of Surgery, Temple University Medical Center, Philadelphia.

Stomach and Duodenum: Surgical Anatomy, Physiology, and Pathology

BENJAMIN F. RUSH, Jr., M.D.

Professor and Chairman, Department of Surgery, University of Medicine and Dentistry of New Jersey/New Jersey Medical School, Newark. Surgeon-in-Chief, University Hospital, Newark.

Principles of Operative Surgery: Antisepsis, Asepsis, Technique, Sutures, and Drains

DAVID C. SABISTON, Jr., M.D.

James B. Duke Professor and Chairman, Department of Surgery, Duke University School of Medicine, Durham, North Carolina.

Milestones in Surgery; Preoperative Preparations of the Surgical Patient; Surgical Management of Morbid Obesity; The Liver; Hernias; Pulmonary Embolism; The Lungs and Chest Wall: Physiologic Aspects of Respiratory Function and Management of Respiratory Insufficiency in Surgical Patients; Bronchoscopy; Lung Abscess and Fungal Infections; Disorders of the Pleura and Empyema; Bronchiectasis; Carcinoma of the Lung; Thoracic Outlet Syndrome; Disorders of the Chest Wall; The Mediastinum: Primary Mediastinal Cysts and Neoplasms; The Heart: Patent Ductus Arteriosus, Coarctation of the Aorta, Aortopulmonary Window, and Anomalies of the Aortic Arch; Atrial Septal Defect, Ostium Primum Defect, and Atrioventricular Canal; Disorders of Pulmonary Venous Return: Total Anomalous Pulmonary Venous Connection; Ventricular Septal Defects; The Tetralogy of Fallot; Double Outlet Right Ventricle; Tricuspid Atresia; Truncus Arteriosus; Transposition of the Great Arteries; Congenital Aortic Stenosis; The Coronary Circulation: Physiological Determinants of Coronary Blood Flow, Cardiac Metabolism, and Intraoperative Myocardial Protection; Ventricular Aneurysm; Cardiac Transplantation: The Total Artificial Heart; Congenital Lesions of the Coronary Arteries; Acquired Diseases of the Aortic Valve; Acquired Mitral and Tricuspid Disease; Ebstein's Anomaly; Cardiac Neoplasms; Management of the Surgical Patient with Cardiac Disease; Cardiopulmonary Bypass for Cardiac Surgery

MICHAEL G. SARR, M.D.

Assistant Professor of Surgery, Mayo Medical School, Rochester, Minnesota.

The Biliary System

JOHN L. SAWYERS, M.D.

John Clinton Foshee Distinguished Professor and Chairman of Surgery, Vanderbilt University, Nashville, Tennessee. Surgeon-in-Chief, Vanderbilt University Hospital, Nashville.

The Acute Abdomen

WORTHINGTON G. SCHENK III, M.D.

Assistant Professor of Surgery, University of Virginia, Charlottesville. Attending Physician, University of Virginia Hospitals, Charlottesville. Consulting Physician, Veterans Administration Hospital, Salem, Virginia.

Surgical Disorders of the Veins

BRUCE D. SCHIRMER, M.D.

Assistant Professor of Surgery, University of Virginia, Charlottesville. Assistant Professor of Surgery, University of Virginia Hospitals, Charlottesville.

Preoperative Preparation of the Surgical Patient

JAMES A. SCHULAK, M.D.

Associate Professor of Surgery, Case Western Reserve University, School of Medicine, Cleveland, Ohio. Director of Transplantation, University Hospitals of Cleveland.

Surgical Complications

WILLIAM SCHUMER, M.D.

Professor and Chairman, Department of Surgery, and Professor, Department of Biochemistry, University of Health Sciences/The Chicago Medical School, North Chicago, Illinois. Attending Physician, Surgical Service, Veterans Administration North Chicago Medical Center. Chief, University Surgical Service, Saint Mary of Nazareth Hospital Center, Chicago. Visiting Faculty, Naval Hospital, Great Lakes, Illinois.

Homeostasis and Shock

JAMES H. F. SHAW, M.B., Ch.B.

Senior Lecturer in Surgery, Auckland University, New Zealand. Consultant, Surgeon, Auckland Hospital.

Nutrition and Metabolism in Surgical Patients

JAMES D. SINK, M.D.

Assistant Professor of Surgery, Emory University School of Medicine, Atlanta, Georgia. Staff, The Henrietta Egleston Hospital for Children, Emory University Hospital, Crawford W. Long Hospital, Atlanta.

Tricuspid Atresia; Truncus Arteriosus; Transposition of the Great Arteries

PETER K. SMITH, M.D.

Assistant Professor of Surgery, Duke University Medical Center, Durham, North Carolina.

Physiologic Aspects of Respiratory Function and Management of Respiratory Insufficiency in Surgical Patients

JAMES L. TALBERT, M.D.

Professor and Chief of Children's Surgery, University of Florida College of Medicine, Gainesville. Chief of Pediatric Surgery, Shands Hospital at the University of Florida, Gainesville, and University Hospital of Jacksonville, Florida.

Pediatric Surgery

NORMAN W. THOMPSON, M.D.

Professor of Surgery, University of Michigan, Ann Arbor. Chief, Division of Endocrine Surgery, University of Michigan Hospitals, Ann Arbor.

The Parathyroid Glands

JEREMIAH G. TURCOTTE, M.D.

F.A. Coller Professor of Surgery, University of Michigan, Ann Arbor. Chairman of the Department of Surgery, University of Michigan Medical Center, Ann Arbor.

Transplantation

ROSS M. UNGERLEIDER, M.D.

Assistant Professor of Surgery, Duke University, Durham, North Carolina. Chief, Pediatric Cardiac Surgery, Duke University Medical Center, Durham.

Bronchoscopy; Double Outlet Right Ventricle; Congenital Aortic Stenosis

JAMES R. URBANIAK, M.D.

Professor of Orthopaedic Surgery and Chief, Division of Orthopaedic Surgery, Duke University Medical Center, Durham, North Carolina.

The Musculoskeletal System; The Hand and Wrist; Fractures of the Spinal Column

PETER VAN TRIGT, M.D.

Assistant Professor of Surgery, Duke University Medical Center, Durham, North Carolina.

Acquired Mitral and Tricuspid Valvular Disease

KENT J. WEINHOLD, Ph.D.

Assistant Medical Research Professor, Department of Surgery, Duke University Medical Center, Durham, North Carolina.

Surgical Aspects of Viral Hepatitis and the Acquired Immune Deficiency Syndrome (AIDS)

J. MARK WILLIAMS, M.D.

Assistant Professor of Surgery, East Carolina University School of Medicine, Greenville, North Carolina. Staff, Pitt County Memorial Hospital, Greenville.

Acquired Diseases of the Aortic Valve

PREFACE

For some time, the publisher has urged that a more concise textbook for medical students be developed based upon the established standards of the *Textbook of Surgery: The Biological Basis for Modern Surgical Practice.* Following an extensive survey conducted among medical students and faculties in the United States and abroad, the need for a more *compact* text was unequivocally demonstrated. Although the respondents emphasized that a concise text was needed, a mandatory requisite was that the text represent a thorough work with in-depth coverage of surgical fundamentals, concepts, and adequate descriptive detail. For these reasons, the preparation of *Essentials of Surgery* was initiated and a group of prominent contributors assembled. The subjects presented are included in the standard text; however, primary attention has been placed upon surgical principles, with emphasis upon inclusion of all information regarded as *essential* for all medical students regardless of career choice. With these guidelines, a text approximately half the size of the standard edition has been developed with the intent to cover the subjects generally expected to be understood by all medical students. The surgical specialties including cardiothoracic surgery, neurosurgery, plastic and maxillofacial surgery, orthopaedics, otolaryngology, and urology are each presented as is gynecology.

The previously established policy of obtaining the most authoritative contributors continues as a paramount objective, and the participants in this edition are recognized figures in their respective fields. A brief description of the historical development of the subject is systematically presented in each section, with inclusion of only pertinent data required for a thorough understanding of the subject. The basic concept of the text is presentation in an orderly manner of the anatomic, pathologic, physiologic, pharmacologic, biochemical, and immunologic aspects of disease. Experience during the past several decades has continued to emphasize the increasing relationship between the basic sciences in medicine and their clinical counterparts in understanding the basis of the diagnosis and management of disease.

With the firm conviction that appropriate illustrations clarify even the most complex problems, this text bears the hallmark of its larger version with selections of the very best illustrations available in the literature. A pertinent bibliography is provided for each section, and, in addition, *selected references* are cited with a short description of the contents in order that the student may recognize the more important contributions in the literature.

In summary, *Essentials of Surgery* has been prepared with the specific goal of assembling that information expected to be acquired by medical students prior to graduation. The Editor is grateful for the opportunity provided by this challenge and trusts the goal has been achieved.

DAVID C. SABISTON, JR.

ACKNOWLEDGMENTS

The Editor is deeply indebted to each contributor to this first edition of *Essentials of Surgery*. The willingness of the participants to adhere to a standard format of presentation in order to achieve a uniform style and facilitate comprehension of the text, especially for medical students, is gratefully acknowledged. The painstaking revisions and responses to suggestions for appropriate additions have also been important features of this edition.

High tribute is due those members of the W. B. Saunders staff responsible for publication. Mr. Dean Manke provided strong support in the preparation of all aspects of this work, and his encouragement and enthusiasm have been key factors in making it a reality. He has consistently endorsed the concept of uncompromising quality and has afforded the support necessary to achieve excellence in the development of this text. Mr. Carroll C. Cann was of much assistance in the planning of this venture, and the contributions of Ms. Carolyn Naylor, who has been involved in all aspects of this work with an impressive commitment to detail, are gratefully acknowledged. Appreciation is also expressed to Terri Siegel, who designed the cover; to Carol J. Wolf, the very effective copy editor; to Lisa Lambert, who skillfully processed the illustrations; and to Dennis Dolan, who prepared the thorough index. Each of these is deserving of sincere thanks, as is Barbara Kindred of our editorial staff.

To my Residents in Surgery and the Research Fellows, I owe much for their encouragement and stimulation as well as their specific contributions. Special recognition is due Dr. H. Kim Lyerly, who contributed several chapters and, very importantly, reviewed the text with emphasis on the medical student's viewpoint. His tireless efforts led to many suggestions and revisions that were included in the final edition and have immeasurably improved the clarity and impact of this work.

Finally, a thoroughly dedicated colleague, Ms. Kathryn Slaughter, has brought her many talents in editorial preparation to the compilation of this book. Her critical and assiduous review of every chapter has been extraordinary, and her commitment, attention to detail, and excitement in developing this text have been a prime stimulus deserving of the highest praise.

DAVID C. SABISTON, JR.

CONTENTS

1

MILESTONES IN SURGERY 1
DAVID C. SABISTON, JR.

2

HOMEOSTASIS AND SHOCK... 10
WILLIAM SCHUMER

3

FLUID AND ELECTROLYTE MANAGEMENT 29
DONALD S. GANN AND JOSEPH F. AMARAL

4

PREOPERATIVE PREPARATION OF THE SURGICAL PATIENT 62
BRUCE D. SCHIRMER AND DAVID C. SABISTON, JR.

5

HEMOSTASIS: PATHOPHYSIOLOGY AND MANAGEMENT OF CLINICAL
DISORDERS 79
CHARLES S. GREENBERG

6

NUTRITION AND METABOLISM IN SURGICAL PATIENTS................... 96
MURRAY F. BRENNAN AND JAMES H. F. SHAW

7

ANESTHESIA.. 109
LENNART FAGRAEUS

8

WOUND HEALING AND MANAGEMENT 117
PETER J. E. CRUSE AND N. TAIT McPHEDRAN

9

BURNS... 122
GREGORY S. GEORGIADE AND W. CHRISTOPHER PEDERSON

10

PRINCIPLES OF OPERATIVE SURGERY: ANTISEPSIS, ASEPSIS,
TECHNIQUE, SUTURES, AND DRAINS 132
BENJAMIN F. RUSH, JR.

11

SURGICAL INFECTIONS AND CHOICE OF ANTIBIOTICS 141
RONALD LEE NICHOLS

12
SURGICAL ASPECTS OF VIRAL HEPATITIS AND THE ACQUIRED
IMMUNE DEFICIENCY SYNDROME (AIDS) 169
H. KIM LYERLY, KENT J. WEINHOLD, AND DANI P. BOLOGNESI

13
MANAGEMENT OF THE ACUTELY INJURED PERSON 180
P. WILLIAM CURRERI

14
SURGICAL COMPLICATIONS 201
JAMES A. SCHULAK AND ROBERT J. CORRY

15
TRANSPLANTATION 224
JEREMIAH G. TURCOTTE, DARRELL A. CAMPBELL, JR.,
DONALD C. DAFOE, DOUGLAS M. BEHRENDT,
MARVIN M. KIRSH, AND WILLIAM H. MARKS

16
PRINCIPLES OF SURGICAL ONCOLOGY 268
E. CARMACK HOLMES AND BARRY D. MANN

17
THE BREAST 288
EDWARD M. COPELAND III AND KIRBY I. BLAND

18
THE THYROID 327
JOHN R. FARNDON

19
THE PARATHYROID GLANDS 340
NORMAN W. THOMPSON AND IAN R. GOUGH

20
THE PITUITARY AND ADRENAL GLANDS 350
STEFANIE S. JEFFREY AND ORLO H. CLARK

21
THE ESOPHAGUS 363
ANDRÉ DURANCEAU AND EDWIN LAFONTAINE

22
THE ACUTE ABDOMEN 388
JOHN A. MORRIS, JR., AND JOHN L. SAWYERS

23
STOMACH AND DUODENUM 406

    I. Surgical Anatomy, Physiology, and Pathology 406
        WALLACE P. RITCHIE, JR., AND ALICE R. PEREZ

    II. Surgical Management of Morbid Obesity 427
        DAVID C. SABISTON, JR.

24
SURGICAL DISORDERS OF THE SMALL INTESTINE 429
    BARRY A. LEVINE AND J. BRADLEY AUST

25
SURGICAL DISORDERS OF THE VERMIFORM APPENDIX AND
MECKEL'S DIVERTICULUM 461
    DONALD C. McILRATH

26
DISEASES OF THE COLON AND RECTUM 471
    KENNETH P. RAMMING

27
THE LIVER 513
    DOUGLAS S. REINTGEN AND DAVID C. SABISTON, JR.

28
THE BILIARY SYSTEM 551
    MICHAEL G. SARR AND JOHN L. CAMERON

29
THE PANCREAS 587
    DANA K. ANDERSON

30
THE SPLEEN 615
    TERUO MATSUMOTO AND MORTON H. PERLMAN

31
THE LYMPHATIC SYSTEM 634
    RICHARD L. McCANN

32
HERNIAS 639
    WARREN J. KORTZ AND DAVID C. SABISTON, JR.

33
PEDIATRIC SURGERY 655
    JAMES L. TALBERT

34
OTOLARYNGOLOGY... 686
JOSEPH C. FARMER, JR.

35
THE HEAD AND NECK 706
JOHN J. COLEMAN III AND M. J. JURKIEWICZ

36
THE MUSCULOSKELETAL SYSTEM.............................. 736
JAMES R. URBANIAK

I. The Hand and Wrist 737
JAMES R. URBANIAK

II. Musculoskeletal Trauma: General Principles 755
JOHN M. HARRELSON

III. Fractures of the Upper Extremity........................... 758
ROBERT D. FITCH

IV. Pelvic and Lower Extremity Fractures 762
JOHN M. HARRELSON

V. Fractures of the Spinal Column........................... 768
JAMES R. URBANIAK

VI. Introduction to Pediatric Orthopedics 772
ROBERT D. FITCH

1. Scoliosis 772

2. Congenital Dislocation of the Hip 775

3. Legg-Calvé-Perthes Disease 778

4. Slipped Capital Femoral Epiphysis 780

5. Clubfoot 781

6. Torsional Deformities of the Lower Limbs 783

VII. General Orthopedics 785
JOHN M. HARRELSON

37
SURGICAL DISORDERS OF THE SKIN......................... 791
P. MICHAEL OLMSTEAD AND WILLIAM P. GRAHAM III

38
GYNECOLOGIC SURGERY 802
A. F. HANEY

39
THE UROGENITAL SYSTEM 826
W. MARSTON LINEHAN

Contents

40

NEUROSURGERY 856

DENNIS E. BULLARD

41

THE ARTERIAL SYSTEM 887

ROBERT W. BARNES

42

SURGICAL DISORDERS OF THE VEINS 933

WORTHINGTON G. SCHENK III

43

PULMONARY EMBOLISM 945

H. KIM LYERLY AND DAVID C. SABISTON, JR.

  I. Overview 945

  II. Chronic Pulmonary Embolism 956

44

THE LUNGS AND CHEST WALL 969

PETER K. SMITH AND DAVID C. SABISTON, JR.

  I. Physiologic Aspects of Respiratory Function and Management of
    Respiratory Insufficiency in Surgical Patients 969
    PETER K. SMITH AND DAVID C. SABISTON, JR.

  II. Bronchoscopy 980
    ROSS M. UNGERLEIDER AND DAVID C. SABISTON, JR.

  III. Lung Abscess and Fungal Infections 984
    RONALD C. HILL AND DAVID C. SABISTON, JR.

  IV. Disorders of the Pleura and Empyema 988
    RONALD C. HILL AND DAVID C. SABISTON, JR.

  V. Bronchiectasis 992
    RONALD C. HILL AND DAVID C. SABISTON, JR.

  VI. The Surgical Treatment of Pulmonary Tuberculosis 994
    JON F. MORAN

  VII. Carcinoma of the Lung 998
    DAVID C. SABISTON, JR.

  VIII. Thoracic Outlet Syndrome 1010
    WILLIAM L. HOLMAN AND DAVID C. SABISTON, JR.

  IX. Disorders of the Chest Wall 1012
    DAVID C. SABISTON, JR.

45

THE MEDIASTINUM 1020

  I. Primary Mediastinal Cysts and Neoplasms 1020
    R. DUANE DAVIS, JR., AND DAVID C. SABISTON, JR.

II. The Diagnosis and Management of Myasthenia Gravis 1036
W. RANDOLPH CHITWOOD, JR.

46
SURGICAL DISORDERS OF THE PERICARDIUM 1045
JOSEPH S. McLAUGHLIN

47
THE HEART 1054

I. Cardiopulmonary Resuscitation 1054
J. SCOTT RANKIN

II. Patent Ductus Arteriosus, Coarctation of the Aorta,
Aortopulmonary Window, and Anomalies of the
Aortic Arch 1061
J. WILLIAM GAYNOR AND DAVID C. SABISTON, JR.

III. Atrial Septal Defect, Ostium Primum Defect, and
Atrioventricular Canal 1076
GARY K. LOFLAND AND DAVID C. SABISTON, JR.

IV. Disorders of Pulmonary Venous Return: Total Anomalous
Pulmonary Venous Connection 1082
ERLE H. AUSTIN AND DAVID C. SABISTON, JR.

V. Ventricular Septal Defects 1085
GARY K. LOFLAND AND DAVID C. SABISTON, JR.

VI. The Tetralogy of Fallot 1089
DAVID C. SABISTON, JR.

VII. Double Outlet Right Ventricle 1095
ROSS M. UNGERLEIDER AND DAVID C. SABISTON, JR.

VIII. Tricuspid Atresia 1098
JAMES D. SINK AND DAVID C. SABISTON, JR.

IX. Truncus Arteriosus 1100
JAMES D. SINK AND DAVID C. SABISTON, JR.

X. Transposition of the Great Arteries 1102
JAMES D. SINK AND DAVID C. SABISTON, JR.

XI. Congenital Aortic Stenosis 1109
ROSS M. UNGERLEIDER AND DAVID C. SABISTON, JR.

XII. The Coronary Circulation 1114

1. Physiologic Determinants of Coronary Blood Flow, Cardiac
Metabolism, and Intraoperative Myocardial Protection 1114
David C. Sabiston, Jr., and J. Scott Rankin

2. Ventricular Aneurysm 1124
Robert B. Peyton and David C. Sabiston, Jr.

3. Cardiac Transplantation: The Total Artificial Heart 1127
David C. Sabiston, Jr.

XIII. Congenital Lesions of the Coronary Arteries 1128
      DAVID C. SABISTON, JR.

 XIV. Acquired Diseases of the Aortic Valve 1137
      J. MARK WILLIAMS AND DAVID C. SABISTON, JR.

  XV. Acquired Mitral and Tricuspid Valvular Disease 1142
      PETER VAN TRIGT AND DAVID C. SABISTON, JR.

 XVI. Ebstein's Anomaly 1153
      ROBERT N. JONES AND DAVID C. SABISTON, JR.

XVII. Surgical Treatment of Cardiac Arrhythmias........................... 1156
      JAMES E. LOWE

XVIII. Cardiac Neoplasms.. 1163
      RALPH J. DAMIANO, JR., AND DAVID C. SABISTON, JR.

 XIX. Cardiac Pacemakers... 1169
      JAMES E. LOWE AND LAWRENCE D. GERMAN

  XX. Management of the Surgical Patient with Cardiac Disease 1179
      T. BRUCE FERGUSON, JR., AND DAVID C. SABISTON, JR.

 XXI. Cardiopulmonary Bypass for Cardiac Surgery........................ 1185
      CRAIG O. OLSEN AND DAVID C. SABISTON, JR.

XXII. Arteriovenous Fistulas.. 1191
      H. KIM LYERLY AND DAVID C. SABISTON, JR.

48
NORMAL VALUES 1195
      REX B. CONN

INDEX 1209

MILESTONES IN SURGERY

DAVID C. SABISTON, JR., M.D.

The history of medicine is, in fact, the history of humanity itself, with its ups and downs, its brave aspirations after truth and finality, its pathetic failures. The subject may be treated variously as a pageant, an array of books, a procession of characters, a succession of theories, an expansion of human ineptitudes or as the very bone and marrow of cultural history.

Fielding H. Garrison

1

A knowledge of the development of surgery is of much significance in understanding its art and science as practiced today. The reason is straightforward, since surgical history provides a basis for an appreciation of the evolution of this increasingly important field in the medical sciences. Only the more significant and landmark achievements considered to be necessary for all medical students will be reviewed. Although ancient medicine holds much interest for historians and archeologists as evidenced by the earliest of known medical writings, these are seldom directly associated with the contemporary practice of clinical surgery. However, there were some notable descriptions of disease in the ancient writings including the definition of inflammation by Celsus, the Roman medical encyclopedist of the first century A.D. In defining inflammation, he said: "Now the characteristics of inflammation are four: redness and swelling, with heat and pain." In the second century, the works of Galen attracted much attention, as did his doctrine that disease is controlled by the "four humors." Surprisingly, this concept was accepted for centuries but became outmoded and was discarded during the Middle Ages.

PIONEERS IN SURGERY

All of medical science, in particular the field of surgery, is indebted to the first of the scientific anatomists, Andreas Vesalius (Fig. 1). He began detailed and accurate dissections of human anatomy while a medical student, and his careful descriptions and realistic illustrations completely changed the former emphasis on Galenical anatomy, which was based primarily on animal dissections. The day following his graduation as a doctor of medicine at the University of Padua, Vesalius was made a full Professor on the basis of his scholarly work in anatomic dissection. Within 4 months, his first atlas of anatomy, *De Humani Corporis Fabrica*, was published and became widely used. With this single work, he corrected many errors that had been passed on for a thousand years in Galen's anatomic reproductions.

A discovery that was to greatly affect the thinking on the subject of physiology was that of William Harvey (Fig. 2), who established the principles of the circulation. He demonstrated that when the heart contracts in systole, blood from the right ventricle flows through the pulmonary artery and into the lung. The blood then passes into the left atrium and ventricle to the systemic circulation. Al-

though he could not demonstrate the capillaries, Harvey proposed that anastomoses must be present between the arteries and veins to make possible his concept of a complete circulation.

The noted medical historian Fielding H. Garrison selected three surgeons whom he considered the greatest of all time. These included Ambroise Paré, John Hunter, and Joseph Lister (Fig. 3). Paré was a French military surgeon who had a keen observing mind and who reintroduced the ancient use of the ligature to control hemorrhage. He is also known for a classic controlled clinical experiment when, during the Battle of Denonvilliers (1552), he treated two injured soldiers with similar wounds as they lay side by side in a tent near the field of battle. The first soldier's wound was managed by the standard method of the day, that is, routine cauterization with boiling oil. The second soldier was managed by débridement, cleansing, and the application of a clean dressing. Paré later commented that he spent a restless night, being convinced that the second

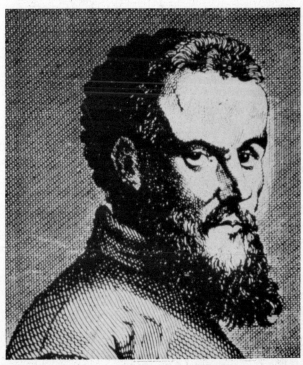

Figure 1. Andreas Vesalius (1514–1564).

1

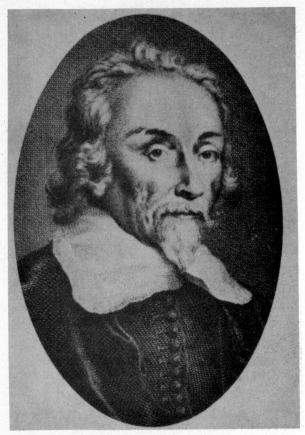

Figure 2. William Harvey (1578–1657).

patient would do very poorly. However, his wisdom was demonstrated the following morning when he found the second patient to be essentially without systemic symptoms, whereas the former had a high fever, tachycardia, and disorientation. When this new method became known, Paré was congratulated on the first successful case. He very humbly replied: *"Je le pansay, Dieu le guarit"* ("I dressed him, God healed him"). This quotation can be found today inscribed on Paré's statue in Paris.

John Hunter was a brilliant teacher of anatomy and surgery who will be remembered for his introduction of the *experimental method*. He systematically used animals to develop surgical techniques prior to their use in humans. A very thoughtful surgeon, and among the first to be scientifically oriented, his philosophy and practice are best

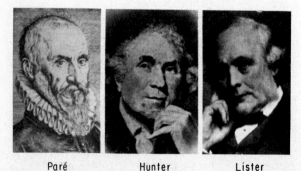

Paré   Hunter   Lister

Figure 3. Ambroise Paré (1510–1590), John Hunter (1728–1793), and Joseph Lister (1827–1912).

summarized in his response to a question from his friend and colleague, Edward Jenner, the discoverer of the small-pox vaccination. When the latter was speculating with ideas concerning hibernation in hedgehogs, Hunter simply said, "I think your solution is just, but why think? Why not try the experiment?" Hunter devised a number of operations and was particularly interested in arterial aneurysms. Following a life filled with contributions to anatomy, physiology, surgical pathology as well as clinical surgery, there is little wonder that Garrison said of him: "With the advent of John Hunter, surgery ceased to be regarded as a mere technical mode of treatment, and began to take its place as a branch of scientific medicine, firmly grounded in physiology and pathology."

Throughout the advances in medicine, the basic sciences frequently have been the source of discoveries and principles subsequently applied to clinical problems. A brilliant example is the work of Louis Pasteur (1822–1895), the originator of the germ theory of disease. In the mid-19th century, Pasteur was the first to show that fermentation and putrefaction were caused by living organisms, and he reasoned that the formation of pus in infected wounds had a similar pathogenesis. In 1867, Lister published the first of a series of papers introducing the concept of *antiseptic surgery*. The principles were based upon destruction of all living organisms, primarily bacteria which might come into contact with the patient's tissues during the surgical procedure. Careful cleansing of the skin of the patient and surgeon's hands alike and the use of sterile drapes surrounding the operative field and sterilized instruments formed the basis of antiseptic surgery. Lister's concepts and practice spread throughout the world. It is to Lister, more than any other, to whom primary credit should be given for the ultimate expansion in the great number and types of operations. When these procedures became safe for the patient with a sharp reduction in postoperative infection, the surgical management of a host of disorders became widely adopted.

THE DEVELOPMENT OF ANESTHESIA

The development of *anesthesia* was a major achievement that created the potential for many new, difficult, and much needed surgical procedures. As a medical student in 1799, Humphrey Davy prepared and inhaled large quantities of nitrous oxide and noted its analgesic effect. In experiments upon himself, he noted that headache and toothache "always diminished after the first four or five inspirations." He then summarized his findings saying, "As nitrous oxide in its extensive effects appears capable of destroying physical pain, it may be probably used with advantage during surgical operations."

In 1842, Crawford W. Long of Georgia was the first to use ether as an inhalation anesthetic in a planned surgical procedure in the excision of a lipoma of the neck. He used this technique in eight subsequent operations and carefully recorded them in his journal, but unfortunately did not publish these observations at the time.

In 1846, William T. G. Morton (Fig. 4) administered an ether anesthetic in Boston for surgeon John Collins Warren, which proved such a dramatic success that it was immediately published. It was this contribution that prompted Warren to say at the end of the procedure to those present: "Gentlemen, this is no humbug!" Shortly thereafter, use of ether anesthesia spread rapidly around the world. The impact of general anesthesia is clearly

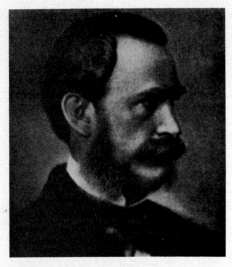

Figure 4. William T. G. Morton (1819–1868).

demonstrated by the use of chloroform soon thereafter for Queen Victoria during childbirth, giving rise to the term "chloroform a la reine" (for the Queen).

ROENTGENOGRAPHY

A monumental discovery was that of Röntgen (Fig. 5) with the introduction of the x-ray in 1895. From that time forth, refinements in radiography, including the use of contrast agents in the gastrointestinal tract and in arteriography, have greatly expanded the diagnostic potentials in this field. In addition, roentgen-guided radiography for needle biopsy, dilatation of vascular obstructions, and drainage of abscesses have been equally impressive.

DEVELOPMENT OF SURGICAL TRAINING PROGRAMS

Following the introduction of scientific principles to the discipline of surgery, emphasis began to be placed on the proper *training* of surgeons. The original patterns of

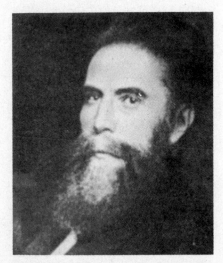

Figure 5. Wilhelm K. Röntgen (1845–1923).

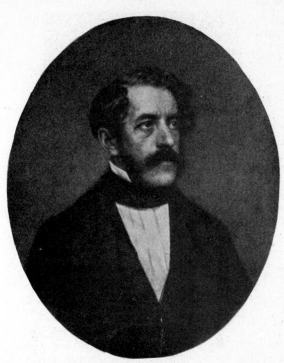

Figure 6. Bernhard von Langenbeck (1810–1887).

surgical training programs were established in Europe during the latter half of the 19th century, particularly in the university clinics of Germany, Switzerland, and Austria.[3] It was there that the surgical giants, all powerful in their respective fields, established the principle of progressive training over a period of years culminating in the position of Chief Resident. Most agree that the father of modern surgical training programs was Bernhard von Langenbeck (Fig. 6), an exceedingly gifted and skillful clinical surgeon. He was also a master teacher who surrounded himself with a group of bright young men and trained them with exceeding thoroughness. He was Chief of Surgery at the famed teaching institution, the Charité, affiliated with the University of Berlin. When Langenbeck's pupils completed his training program, they were called to other major universities and clinics throughout Europe to assume chairs of their own. Among the more notable of his trainees were Theodor Billroth (Fig. 7), who became Professor of Surgery at the University of Zurich and later at the University of Vienna, where he was Chief Surgeon to the world renowned Allegemeines Krankenhaus; Theodor Kocher (Fig. 8) left Berlin to become Professor at the University of Berne at the youthful age of 31, and Trendelenburg (Fig. 9) was appointed to the Chair in Leipzig. Many other notable figures from Langenbeck's training program followed in this tradition, and his fame in the production of leading clinical and academic surgeons of the day became firmly established.

The development of the surgical residency training programs in the United States is clearly related to the Langenbeck-Billroth school, since William S. Halsted (Fig. 10), the Professor at the newly opened Johns Hopkins University School of Medicine and Hospital, had been deeply impressed during his travels to Germany, Switzerland, and Austria by the Langenbeck plan just prior to his appointment in Baltimore. Halsted, generally regarded as the most outstanding surgeon in North America, regularly visited the major European clinics in the latter half of the 19th century. He became deeply impressed with the pro-

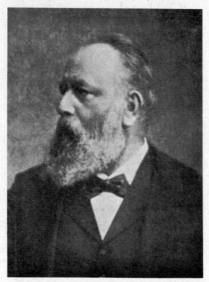

Figure 7. Theodor Billroth (1829–1894).

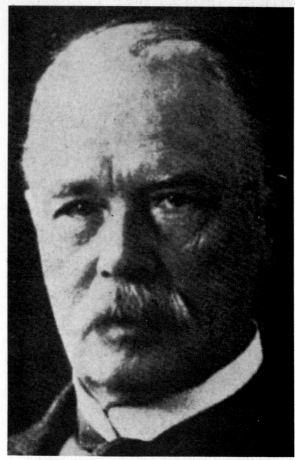

Figure 9. Friedrich Trendelenburg (1844–1924).

gressive system of surgical training and was completely devoted to the concept that highly selected, bright young trainees should begin as interns and gradually progress through the residency with increasing responsibility. He agreed with Langenbeck that upon completion of the Chief Residency the trainee should have essentially the same abilities as the teachers in the program. Thus, many of Halsted's trainees were appointed directly to prestigious academic chairs immediately upon completion of their surgical residency program.

Halsted's specific concepts of surgical training appear in his essay on "The Training of a Surgeon."[2] He said:

It was our intention originally to adopt as closely as feasible the German plan, which in the main, is the same for all principal clinics . . . every facility and the greatest encouragement is given each member of the staff to do work in *research*.

In this address delivered at Yale in 1904, Halsted stressed:

The assistants are expected in addition to their ward and operating duties to prosecute original investigations and to keep in close touch with the work in surgical pathology, bacteriology, and so far as possible physiology . . . Young men contemplating the study of surgery should early in life seek to acquire knowledge of the subjects fundamental to the study of their profession.

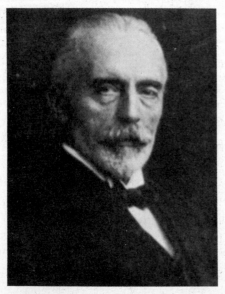

Figure 8. Theodor Kocher (1841–1917).

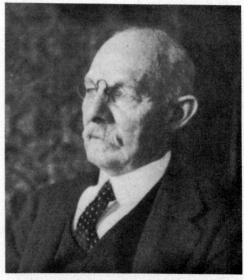

Figure 10. William S. Halsted (1852–1922).

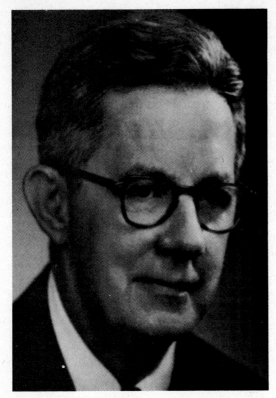

Figure 11. Alfred Blalock (1899–1964).

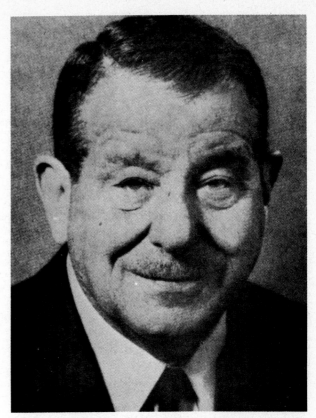

Figure 13. Isador S. Ravdin (1894–1972).

It was in this address that he also said:

We need a system, and we shall surely have it, which will produce not only surgeons but surgeons of the highest type, men who will stimulate the youths of our country to study surgery and devote their energies and their lives to raising the standard of surgical science.

Halsted's astonishing success in the training of surgeons was later duplicated by others including Blalock (Fig. 11), who was subsequently appointed to Halsted's post at Johns Hopkins. Other master teachers of many academic surgeons were Wangensteen (Fig. 12) at the University of Minnesota,

and Ravdin (Fig. 13) and Rhoads (Fig. 14) at the University of Pennsylvania. These gifted teachers produced many trainees who subsequently became Professors of Surgery and Chairmen of Departments.

In his Presidential Address to the American Surgical Association in 1956, Blalock emphasized his views on the significance of research in saying:

The only way an interested person can determine whether or not he has an aptitude in research is to give it a trial . . . My point is that he should not shy away from it because of a misconception and fear that he does not have originality. As a medical student, I felt pity for the investigator, but later this changed to admiration and envy.[1]

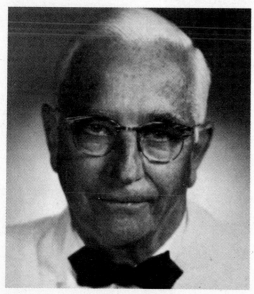

Figure 12. Owen H. Wangensteen (1898–   ).

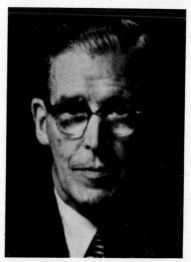

Figure 14. Jonathan Rhoads (1907–   ).

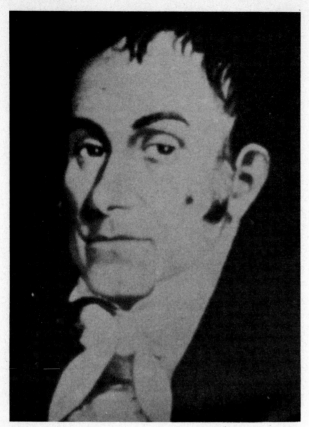

Figure 15. Ephraim McDowell (1771–1830).

MAJOR DEVELOPMENTS IN GENERAL SURGERY

The first successful laparotomy was performed in rural Kentucky on Christmas Day 1809 by Ephraim McDowell (Fig. 15). He had trained in Edinburgh under some of the finest teachers of the time. McDowell removed a huge ovarian tumor in a patient who recovered uneventfully and lived for many years thereafter. He later removed eleven other ovarian tumors with only one death.[4] Another major advance in abdominal surgery was made by Billroth of Vienna, who, in 1881, was the first to successfully perform a gastric resection. In a patient with an obstructing carcinoma of the pylorus, he removed the involved part of the stomach and re-established continuity by a gastroduodenostomy. The first cholecystectomy was performed in 1882 by Karl Langenbuch in a 43-year-old male who had had biliary colic for 16 years. In 1886, Reginald Fitts of Boston described the clinical findings and symptoms of acute appendicitis, and shortly thereafter McBurney of New York and others developed the appropriate surgical techniques to safely remove the inflamed appendix.

Hernia has been described through the centuries, and it is remarkable that surgical correction became achievable only a century ago. While a number of procedures were attempted during the 19th century, it remained for Bassini (Fig. 16) and Halsted to simultaneously but independently devise an anatomically designed operation that was at the time termed "the radical cure of inguinal hernia." These two surgical pioneers contributed greatly to marked improvement in long-term results following their procedures, and the principles of their operations remain in practice to this day.

Development of surgery of the thyroid gland was pioneered by Theodor Kocher. This master surgeon perfected the operation of thyroidectomy and in 1895 described 1000 thyroidectomies for goiter. At the time of his death in 1917, he had performed 5000 thyroidectomies in his clinic in Berne with a mortality of but 0.11 per cent. He also noted that following total thyroidectomy hypothyroidism was frequent and that administration of thyroid extract to these patients was followed by a return of normal metabolism. For his contributions to surgery of the thyroid gland and to management of hypothyroidism, Kocher became the first surgeon to be awarded the Nobel Prize in 1909.

The development of surgical procedures on the parathyroid glands was initiated by Mandl of Vienna in 1925 when he removed the first parathyroid tumor in a patient with advanced osteitis fibrosus cystica.

Following these landmark achievements, many other dates became significant as new procedures were successfully performed. These events are shown in Table 1.

Many specific contributions to surgery have had an extraordinary impact upon the field, and some of these will be considered individually. Concepts of fluid and electrolyte balance have their scientific origin in the early observations of Claude Bernard of Paris who, in 1859, published a series of lectures entitled "Liquids of the Organism." In these major contributions, he emphasized the significance of the *milieu intérieur*, which he proposed was the physiologic state that allowed an organism to exist independently. These concepts were furthered in subsequent years, primarily by Cannon, who introduced the term "homeostasis." *The Metabolic Care of the Surgical Patient*, a monograph by Francis D. Moore, remains the standard reference in this important field. Another major contribution made in the 1960s was the introduction of total parenteral alimentation following the notable experimental and clinical work of Dudrick and Rhoads. They showed experimentally that in paired canine littermates, one receiving normal alimentation by mouth and the other receiving its total caloric intake intravenously, both animals developed normally and

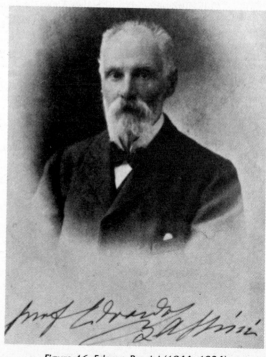

Figure 16. Edoaro Bassini (1844–1924).

TABLE 1. *Calendar of Major Contributions to Surgery*

1543	Vesalius publishes first accurate text of anatomy, *De Humani Corporis Fabrica*
1552	Paré treats wounded soldier by débridement and dressings at battle of Denonvilliers
1628	Harvey publishes *De Motu Cordis,* describing normal circulation of blood
1710	Anel operates for aneurysm by ligating artery above the sac
1727	Cheselden performs lateral operation for bladder stone
1759	Mestivier describes and operates for localized appendicitis
1809	McDowell performs ovariotomy
1817	Astley Cooper ligates abdominal aorta
1822	Sauter performs hysterectomy
1867	Lister introduces antiseptic surgery
	Bobbs performs cholecystostomy
1870	Thomas performs vaginal ovariotomy
1873	Billroth excises the larynx
1881	Billroth resects the stomach with gastroduodenostomy
	Wolfler introduces gastroenterostomy
1882	Langenbuch excises the gallbladder
	Winiwarter performs cholecystenterostomy
1884	Billroth excises pancreas for cancer
1885	H. Kummell performs choledochostomy
1886	Fitz describes acute appendicitis
1895	Röntgen discovers x-rays
1906	Landsteiner discovers blood types
1925	Mandl excises first parathyroid adenoma
1935	First sulfonamide by Domagk
1938	First successful closure of patent ductus arteriosus by Gross
1944	Penicillin in supply by Florey and Chain
	First successful closure of coarctation of aorta by Crafoord
	First successful subclavian-pulmonary anastomosis for tetralogy of Fallot by Blalock
1945	Portacaval shunt by Whipple
1951	First resection of abdominal aortic aneurysm by Dubost
	First closure of cardiac defect (atrial septal defect) by Gibbon, using extracorporeal circulation
1954	First successful renal transplant (long-term) by Murray
1958	First implantable cardiac pacemaker by Elmquist and Senning
1960	First artificial prosthetic cardiac valve (mitral) by Starr
1962	First saphenous vein to coronary artery anastomosis by Sabiston
1963	First successful liver transplant by Starzl
1964	First lung transplant by Hardy
1966	First pancreatic transplant by Najarian
1967	First successful heart transplant by Barnard
1982	First heart-lung transplant by Reitz

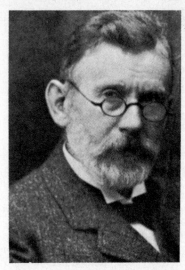

Figure 17. Paul Ehrlich (1854–1915).

noted the antibacterial properties of certain molds, especially *Penicillium notatum.* Florey and Chain found methods to produce penicillin in adequate amounts for clinical use in 1944. For this monumental achievement, these three workers were awarded the Nobel Prize in 1945.

The *hormonal* control of neoplastic disease was demonstrated by Huggins (Fig. 18) in 1940 when he showed that antiandrogenic treatment, consisting of orchiectomy or the administration of estrogen, could produce regression of advanced disseminated carcinoma of the prostate. For this work, as well as studies of serum enzymes and protein chemistry and the role of the adrenal gland in controlling metastases from neoplastic disease, Huggins was awarded the Nobel Prize in 1966.

In 1900, Karl Landsteiner first detected the presence of agglutinins and isoagglutinins in blood and found that blood could be typed into four groups. Although blood transfusions had been previously administered, success had

had similar weights when grown. This extraordinary contribution greatly altered the management and future course of many patients with severe nutritional problems, particularly those with enteric fistulas who had losses of large amounts of fluids and nutritive elements with a high morbidity and mortality rate.

The introduction of *chemotherapy* and *antibiotics* has greatly altered the course of many surgical procedures. Ehrlich (Fig. 17) is due initial credit for introducing a chemotherapeutic agent, *Salvarsan* ("606"), in the management of syphilis. In 1935, Domagk introduced *Prontosil*, a sulfonamide, and for the first time an agent was available that immediately attacked bacteria with dramatic clinical results for susceptible organisms. In 1929, Fleming had

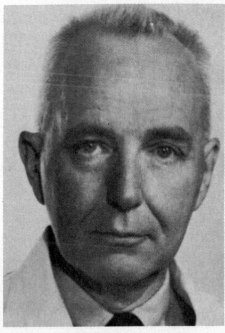

Figure 18. Charles B. Huggins (1901–   ).

been marred by many fatal reactions. When the ability to type blood was demonstrated, its use gradually became widespread and made possible many extensive surgical procedures not previously feasible. For his notable work, Landsteiner was awarded the Nobel Prize.

DEVELOPMENT OF VASCULAR AND CARDIOTHORACIC SURGERY

The field of vascular surgery became a reality when Alexis Carrel (Fig. 19) of Lyons demonstrated that it was possible to join the two ends of a divided blood vessel with careful surgical technique, fine needles, and carefully selected suture materials. This contribution led to primary healing of vessels without infection or thrombosis. Prior to his experimental and clinical work, there had not been a successful vascular anastomosis, attempts having ended in either thrombosis or infection. Carrel was also the first to transplant tissues and organs using his careful suturing techniques. He clearly predicted the scientific basis for the forthcoming field of transplantation, and for all of these landmark achievements he was awarded the Nobel Prize in physiology and medicine in 1912.

The first use of a saphenous vein to replace an artery was by Goyannes in Madrid in 1906. After correction of a popliteal arterial aneurysm, he restored vascular continuity using the patient's saphenous vein. Subsequent workers, especially DeBakey, demonstrated the feasibility of using *plastic arterial substitutes* with prolonged durability and consistent clinical success.

In the 1896 edition of Paget's *Surgery of the Chest,* one finds the following statement:

Surgery of the heart has probably reached the limits set by Nature to all surgery: no new method, and no new discovery, can overcome the natural difficulties that attend a wound to the heart. It is true that "heart suture" has been vaguely proposed as a possible procedure, and has been done on animals; but I cannot find that it has ever been attempted in practice.

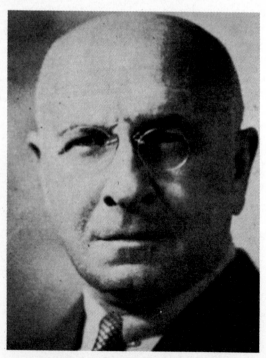

Figure 19. Alexis Carrel (1873–1944).

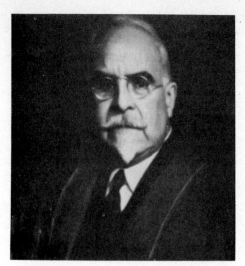

Figure 20. Rudolph Matas (1860–1957).

For this reason it is of special interest that in the same year, 1896, Ludwig Rehn first successfully closed a stab wound to the heart in a 22-year-old male who had been unconscious for a period of 3 hours prior to operation. Rehn controlled hemorrhage from a wound in the right ventricle with three silk sutures. This historic patient recovered, and the event marked the beginning of cardiac surgery.

Rudolph Matas (Fig. 20) was another surgical pioneer and, while Professor of Surgery at Tulane, first described his innovative endoaneurysmorrhaphy in the treatment of arterial aneurysms. This represented the first definitive management of aneurysms with restoration of the circulation and was received with much enthusiasm.

In 1925, Souttar of London was the first to introduce a finger into the left atrial appendage, accomplishing digital splitting of the stenotic mitral valve in a patient with rheumatic valvar disease. Unfortunately, this was not repeated until 1946, when Bailey and then Harken began the procedure again with much success. Closure of a patent ductus arteriosus was first successfully achieved by Gross in 1938. Strieder had closed a ductus a year earlier, but the patient succumbed. Coarctation of the aorta was corrected with end-to-end anastomosis by Crafoord in 1944.

Another remarkable achievement that has had a tremendous impact on the field of cardiovascular surgery was the introduction of cardiac catheterization by Forssmann in 1929. This pioneering work later became a routine diagnostic procedure when Cournand and Richards demonstrated its usefulness in the diagnosis of many forms of heart disease. These workers were awarded the Nobel Prize in 1956.

The treatment of congenital cyanotic heart disease was greatly augmented by Blalock in 1944, when he performed the first successful procedure for the tetralogy of Fallot. The subclavian artery was anastomosed to the pulmonary artery to improve blood flow to the lungs in patients with obstructive lesions in the pulmonary arterial circuit. The use of hypothermia in cardiac surgery permitted temporary interruption of the circulation, an approach stimulated by the early work of Bigelow, who showed in the experimental animal that the circulation could be safely interrupted for a period of 10 minutes or more at reduced temperatures without the damaging effects of cerebral hypoxia. This technique was applied successfully in the closure of an atrial septal defect by Lewis and Varco in 1952. The next notable achievement in this field was that of Gibbon, who developed extracorporeal circulation. This monumental advance began with laboratory experiments in 1931 and was systematically pursued by this dedicated investigator and his wife until 1953, when the heart-lung machine was first successfully employed in the closure of an atrial septal defect using the pump oxygenator to substitute for the heart and lungs while the defect was being corrected. Shortly thereafter and using this technique, Lillehei and also Kirklin successfully corrected ventricular septal defects, the tetralogy of Fallot, and many other congenital cardiac defects.

An abdominal aortic aneurysm was first corrected surgically by DuBost in Paris in 1951. In the same year, the first plastic arterial grafts were introduced experimentally by Voorhees and Blakemore. The first successful implantation of a prosthetic cardiac valve was achieved by Starr in 1960.

The surgical management of myocardial ischemia is now widespread. The first use of the saphenous vein bypass graft to the coronary circulation was in 1962. It was the application of this technique in a series of patients by Favaloro and Johnson that demonstrated its usefulness, and the procedure has now become the most common cardiac surgical procedure performed in the United States. It has been responsible for complete relief of anginal pain as well as a significant extension of the life span of many patients.

TRANSPLANTATION

The original experimental work establishing the feasibility of transplantation of tissues and organs was done by Carrel and associates at the turn of the century. The first successful long-term renal transplant was achieved by Murray in 1954. In 1963, Starzl successfully implanted a liver, and in 1964 the first lung transplant was made by Hardy. Najarian achieved a pancreatic transplant in 1966, and this entire field has now become a very important one throughout the world. The long-term survival of organ transplants has been significantly advanced with the introduction of agents to suppress rejection, including Imuran, steroids, anti-lymphocyte globulin, and more recently cyclosporine. Barnard, in 1967, was the first to successfully transplant the human heart, and this is now an everyday procedure. A combination heart-lung transplant was performed by Reitz in 1982, and this feat represents another distinctive advance in an ever-increasing field.

SUMMARY

It becomes clear in retrospect that many advances in surgery have been dependent upon previous discoveries. While the recent leaders in the field have expanded its horizons in ways previously not thought possible, much yet remains for the future. It is certain that the incorporation of fundamental biologic principles in the future, as in the past, will bring significant advances to this ever-expanding area of medicine. It should be constantly borne in mind that familiarity with achievements of the past is essential.

As Billroth stated so succinctly: "Only the man w[ho is] familiar with the art and science of the past is comp[etent] to aid in its progress in the future."

Finally, the student should continuously recall the fact that intellect and new ideas alone are not enough; rather, they must be combined with a committed and productive effort. The words of Sir William Osler, Regius Professor of Medicine at Oxford, speak brilliantly to this point. In replying to the medical students of the day who asked him to give them the reason for his extraordinary success in medicine, Osler simply replied:

It seems a bounden duty on such an occasion to be honest and frank, so I propose to tell you the secret of life as I have seen the game played, and as I have tried to play it myself. . . This I propose to give you in the hope, yes, in the full assurance that some of you at least will lay hold upon it to your profit. Though a little one, the master-word looms large in meaning. [WORK] It is the open sesame to every portal, the great equalizer in the world, the true philosopher's stone, which transmutes all the base metal of humanity into gold. The stupid man among you it will make bright, the bright man brilliant, and the brilliant student steady. With the magic word in your heart all things are possible, and without it all study is vanity and vexation. The miracles of life are with it . . . to the youth it brings hope, to the middle-aged confidence, to the aged repose. . . . It is directly responsible for all advances in medicine during the past twenty-five centuries.

SELECTED REFERENCES

Majno, G.: The Healing Hand: Man and Wound in the Ancient World. Boston, Harvard University Press, 1975.
For the student interested in the ancient medicine in China, India, Egypt, and Greece, this is a detailed reference source by an outstanding author.

Meade, R. H.: An Introduction to the History of General Surgery. Philadelphia, W. B. Saunders Company, 1986.
A thorough review of major contributions in the field of general surgery with extensive references.

Ravitch, M. M.: A Century of Surgery: The History of the American Surgical Association, Vols. 1 and 2. Philadelphia, J. B. Lippincott Company, 1981.
The papers presented at the annual meetings of the American Surgical Association, founded over a century ago, reflect most of the more recent important contributions to surgery. These are reviewed in these two volumes by a skillfull author.

Wangensteen, O. H., and Wangensteen, S. D.: The Rise of Surgery From Empiric Craft to Scientific Discipline. Minneapolis, University of Minnesota Press, 1978.
A fascinating volume with excellent references reviewing the history of surgery from its beginning to modern times. It is a very scholarly work and one that provides fascinating reading.

REFERENCES

1. Blalock, A.: The Nature of Discovery. Presidential address to the American Surgical Association. Ann. Surg., *144*:3, 1956.
2. Halsted, W. S.: The training of the surgeon. Bull. Johns Hopkins Hosp., *15*:267, 1904.
3. Sabiston, D. C., Jr.: A continuum in surgical education: Presidential address to the Society of University Surgeons. Surgery, *66*:1, 1969.
4. Sabiston, D. C., Jr.: Major contributions to surgery from the South. Presidential address to the Southern Surgical Association. Ann. Surg., *181*:5, 1975.

HOMEOSTASIS AND SHOCK

WILLIAM SCHUMER, M.D.

2

HOMEOSTASIS

In 1859, Darwin described the concept of "survival of the fittest," postulating the genetic changes that occur in animal differentiation for existence.[8] He did not describe the physiologic or metabolic adjustments that were necessary for man to attain dominance. This was pursued by Claude Bernard, who developed the concept of the constancy of the *milieu intérieur* and the physiochemical methods needed to define the mechanisms by which the organism maintains homeostasis.[3] Cannon, in 1918, introduced the term *homeostasis* after studying the neuroendocrine autoadjustments for maintaining physiologic stability.[6] In 1913, Henderson's *The Fitness of the Environment* described the correlative relations necessary for the organism to adjust to the environment. He later proposed the concept of *functional reserve*, which is defined as the reservoir of organ functional capacity that may be used to adapt to its milieu.[12] The scientific data base produced by these pioneers helped Selye in 1966 to describe the overreaction of these neuroendocrine adaptations to stress of acute and chronic disease as the "stress syndrome." He measured various endocrine and metabolic processes characterizing the overcompensation of these adaptation mechanisms producing disease.[30] Moore, in 1959 and 1963, in his two classics, *Metabolic Care of the Surgical Patient* and *The Body Cell Mass and Its Supporting Environment,* compiled and added radioisotopic studies to more clearly define man's response to surgical injury and disease.[19, 20] These studies inspired others to characterize the specific physiologic and biochemical alterations occurring after surgical stress.[2, 10, 15, 31, 33, 34]

Visualize prehistoric man being attacked by a carnivorous animal, with the anterior portion of the thigh lacerated. The quadriceps muscle is laid open and bleeding from arteries, veins, and capillaries. How did he respond to his injury in order to survive? First, the wound injury causes the nerve endings to release the catecholamine norepinephrine, which stimulates the hypothalamus. The hypothalamus secretes the corticotropin-releasing factor (CRF), which releases the hormones, adrenocorticotropic hormone (ACTH), vasopressin, and vasoactive intestinal peptide (VIP) from the anterior pituitary gland. ACTH promotes the production of glucocorticoids, mineralocorticoids, and androgenic and estrogenic steroids in the adrenal cortex.

Glucocorticoids also stimulate the synthesis of epinephrine in the adrenal medulla and act as a negative feedback control on pituitary ACTH release. In contrast, epinephrine and norepinephrine increase pituitary ACTH. Mineralocorticoids can be released from the adrenal cortex secondary to ACTH secretion, but they are produced primarily as a result of the *renin-angiotensin cycle*. Renin originates in the juxtaglomerular apparatus near the afferent arteriole in the glomeruli of the kidney. Renin acts on glycoprotein in the liver to produce angiotensin I, which is converted to angiotensin II. Angiotensin II stimulates the zona glomerulosa of the adrenal cortex to produce aldosterone.

Other anterior pituitary hormones released secondary to hypothalamic-promoting factors are growth hormone (GH), pituitary gonadotropin hormones, and thyroid-stimulating hormone (TSH). Endorphins and enkephalins are also secreted and have analgesic potencies 18 to 30 times stronger than morphine and play an important role in endogenous control of pain. These peptides also have a hypotensive effect in hypovolemic and septic shock. The specific effect of endorphins and enkephalins to stress is unknown. Growth hormone increases in stress and produces glycogenolysis and lipolysis with consequent hyperglycemia and hyperlipidemia. This furnishes the substrate necessary for energy production. Later, GH mobilizes amino acids for collagen synthesis and wound healing. Gonadotropic hormone function is depressed during stress. This probably causes menstrual aberrations after surgical stress. Testosterone, an anabolic hormone, has a nitrogen-retaining effect, and its effect in the recovery from stress is now being studied. The physiologic function of TSH in surgical stress is decreased, and apparently the increased oxygen consumption does not result from thyroxine release. Concomitantly, the posterior pituitary gland is secreting antidiuretic hormone (ADH). The stimuli for ADH secretion is the neural activation of the supraoptic nuclei in the hypothalamus. These nuclei also are sensitive to blood osmolality and blood volume. Osmoreceptor cells in the supraoptic nuclei are sensitive to the loss of water and total blood volume (Fig. 1).

The neuroendocrine response to injury is directly proportional to the severity of stress. How does the neuroendocrine metabolic response function in surgical stress? As an example, an injured man immediately secretes catecholamines for two reasons: first, to constrict precapillary sphincters to decrease volume loss and decrease vascular space to compensate for low blood volume, and, second, to initiate the hypothalamic pituitary adrenal reaction. The posterior pituitary secretes ADH to further decrease volume loss through urine excretion and to help maintain

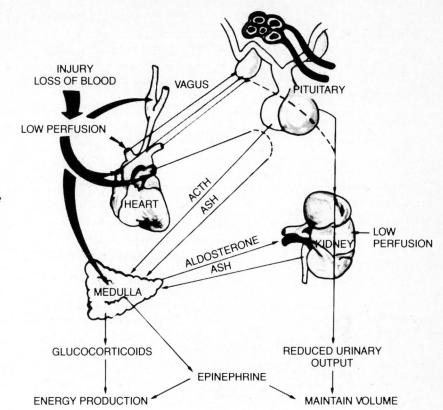

Figure 1. Neuroendocrine mechanism in the metabolic response to shock.

blood volume. Associated with the ADH effect is aldosterone production by the *juxtaglomerular renin complex*. Aldosterone causes renal retention of sodium and water and excretion of serum potassium derived from degenerating cells. This action augments the maintenance of blood volume, by retaining hydrophilic sodium, and electrolyte balance, by excreting potassium. The pituitary adrenocortical effect, i.e., release of corticosteroids, induces the metabolic effect. These steroids plus glucagon induce glucose production. Although catecholamines support the breakdown of glycogen in the liver and muscle to produce glucose (glycogenolysis), this storage molecule is insufficient for the energy needs of the stressed organism. Glucose-producing sugars, amino acids, and fats are necessary for glucose production. Glucocorticoids and glucagon potentiation catabolize muscle for the release of lactic acid, alanine, branched chain amino acids (leucine, isoleucine, valine), and fat to produce glycerol, which enters the liver for conversion to glucose (gluconeogenesis).[4] Man also utilizes fatty acids for direct conversion to energy by the oxidative Krebs and electron transport cycles. Catalytic glucose degradation by the glycolytic and oxidative cycles produces 38 moles of energy molecule adenosine triphosphate (ATP), which are used to fuel protein biosynthesis. Protein biosynthesis supports the molecules necessary for phagocytosis and the production of immunoglobulin, complement factors, and collagen (wound healing). ATP also fuels cell membrane function. The homeostasis of intracellular and extracellular electrolytes and water balance is dependent on Na/K ATPase function. These enzymes keep potassium within the cell and inhibit sodium and water from entering the cell.

Therefore, the neuroendocrine metabolic response to stress protects man from excessive loss of circulating volume and induces ATP production to combat infection and support wound healing. However, because this scheme evolved around the "survival of the fittest" principle, it did not protect the weak or the elderly. On the contrary, this response produces detrimental effects on debilitated patients who have little enzyme reserve. The catabolic phase (muscle and fat breakdown) further depletes substrate reserve and causes water retention, which taxes heart and kidney function in these patients. Therefore, overreaction to this neuroendocrine metabolic response must be prevented.

SHOCK

Circulatory shock is considered one of the most severe stimuli of the pituitary adrenal axis, therefore causing profound physiologic and metabolic sequelae. It is defined as inadequate circulating blood volume producing decreased perfusion, first to nonvital tissues (skin, connective tissue, bone, and muscle) and subsequently to vital organs (brain, heart, lungs, liver, and kidney). Decreased perfusion of nonvital tissues results in anaerobic metabolism because the nonvital tissue cell mass is significantly larger than the vital tissue cell mass. As circulating blood volume decreases, catecholamines and angiotensin are secreted; this increases peripheral resistance, thus producing low flow in the periphery. Later, baroreceptors in the atria and carotid and aortic bodies stimulate the vasomotor center in the medulla oblongata via the sympathetic nerves. The vasomotor center compounds sympathetic vasoconstriction further, increasing peripheral resistance (Fig. 2).

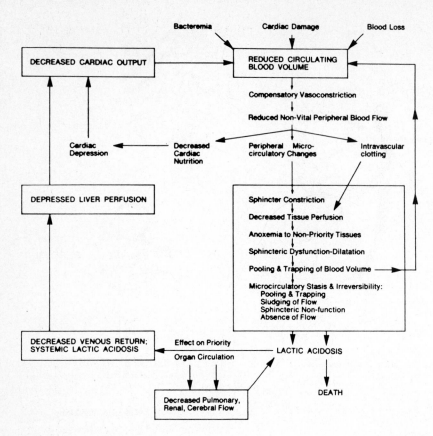

Figure 2. Feedback hemodynamic sequences in the progression of shock.

Classification

Circulatory shock can be classified as follows:

I. Cardiogenic
    1. Myocardial infarction
    2. Cardiac failure
II. Hypovolemic
    A. Exogenous
       1. Oligemic shock
       2. Plasma and electrolyte loss
          a. Burn shock
          b. Gastrointestinal losses
    B. Endogenous
       1. Septic shock
       2. Anaphylactic shock
III. Distributive
    1. Neurogenic
    2. Vasogenic

This classification is based on the causes for ineffective circulating blood volume. Since blood volume flow is a product of cardiac output and mean arterial pressure, any decrease in cardiac output due to infarction of the ventricle will decrease circulation of blood volume. Embarrassment of ventricular function by surgical resection or tamponade similarly reduces cardiac output and produces cardiogenic shock.

Any decrease in blood volume will produce inadequate circulation. Blood volume can be lost exogenously or endogenously (externally or internally). Hemorrhage causes total blood volume losses (red cell mass plus plasma volume). Burns and diarrhea cause plasma and electrolyte losses. Blood volume loss outside the body is referred to as exogenous shock. Blood volume loss internally ("leaking capillary syndrome") or interstitially, as in septic or anaphylactic shock, is referred to as endogenous shock.

The classification distributive shock is based on the discrepancy between total blood volume and vascular space. Normal blood volume is 73 ml. per kg., or approximately 5 liters of blood for a person weighing 70 kg. The vascular space, specifically the venous capacitance system, can absorb three times the normal volume. The mechanism that allows the organism to maintain normal flow and pressure is called the *Loven reflex*. This is a reflex adjustment of the caliber of the blood vessels in response to nutritional needs without causing significant disturbances of the general blood pressure or flow. Dilatation of one vascular bed is compensated by a vasoconstriction of other vascular beds. If due to paralysis of the neural or vasogenic factors, the splanchnic capillary bed or the venous capacitance system dilates excessively, effective circulating volume decreases, and shock ensues.

Cellular Metabolic Response to Shock

The crucial factor and common denominator of all types of shock is cellular hypoperfusion (Fig. 3*A*,*B*). This occurs first in the nonvital tissues of the gastrointestinal tract, muscle, connective tissue, and skin, and subsequently in the vital tissues of the brain, heart, lung, liver, and kidney. The result is cellular anoxia and starvation. Under these conditions, the minimal amounts of substrates available for passage through the cell membrane into the energy pathways are blocked by anoxia. For example, in septic shock, endotoxemia damages the membrane and later hypovolemia may compound this cellular injury. Endotoxin, enterotoxin, and exotoxin disrupt membrane receptor sites, impairing intracellular glycolysis and electron transport. Consequently, it is in the cell's energy pathways that the most profound metabolic effects of shock occur (Fig. 4).

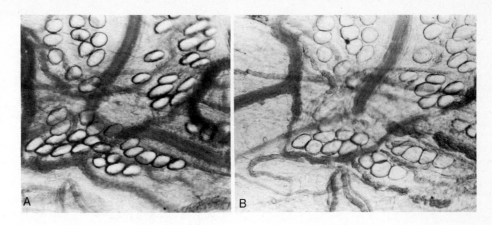

Figure 3. Dog omentum. A, Control. Microcirculation before bleeding. (Magnification, 450 ×) B, Microcirculation at 55 per cent of volume bled (pre-irreversibility). (Magnification, 450 ×)

Energy-Producing Pathways

Ordinarily, substrates such as glucose, glucogenic α-amino acids (alanine), and glycerol are actively transported into the liver cell by a transfer system requiring adenosine nucleotides. Energized adenosine nucleotides can be derived either anaerobically through glycolysis or aerobically through the citric acid cycle and electron transport system. The aerobic transfer is more efficient, but the anaerobic substrate level production of ATP can be effective in promoting substrate infusion into the cell. These substrates—glucose, amino acids, fatty acids, lactic acid, and glycerol—either can be metabolized to produce ATP or can be stored in the liver and muscle as glycogen via gluconeogenesis.

During shock, adequate perfusion of the cellular capillary bed is crucial. The cells of the peripheral tissues—skin, connective tissue, muscle, and gastrointestinal tract—react to the inadequate perfusion of decreased circulating volume by shifting to anaerobiosis. Immediately, the following deleterious series of events occur at the cellular level:

Substrate transport is impaired; there is a decrease in ATP and ADP production with subsequent derangement of the energy-dependent ATPase molecule; membrane dysfunction occurs; sodium and water enter and potassium exudes through the membrane; cellular swelling ensues; the glycolytic cycle is blocked at the mitochondrial entranceway (pyruvate-acetyl coenzyme A[CoA] step); finally, only 2 moles of ATP are produced from 1 mole of glucose. An adequately functioning citric cycle produces 38 moles of ATP; thus, anaerobic circulatory collapse reduces energy production by 95 per cent. Since the peripheral cellular mass is 75 per cent of the total body mass, any energy deficit in this area has myriad effects on the entire organism (Fig. 5).

A review of the changes occurring on specific peripheral tissues during shock is helpful in the elucidation of cellular metabolic dysfunction in shock.

NONVITAL ORGAN ENERGY METABOLISM

Skeletal Muscle Cell

Skeletal muscle adapts itself to anaerobiosis by rapidly increasing its energy output via various ATP-producing anaerobic mechanisms. These are phosphocreatine decomposition, myokinase reaction, and utilization of glycogen stores. However, during severe anaerobiosis these mechanisms are rapidly utilized and lactic acid formation accelerates. Muscle mass is one of the largest producers of lactic acid in shock, and during severe circulatory deficiency, muscle protein is consumed as one of the main sources of stored energy and acute catabolism of muscle mass occurs. Muscle branched chain amino acids and ketones are utilized for substrate when the muscle becomes glucose-deficient. The muscle oxidizes leucine to carbon dioxide and converts the carbon skeletons of aspartate, arginine, glutamine, isoleucine, and valine into Krebs cycle intermediates. During hypovolemic shock of any etiology, muscle increasingly releases branched chain amino acids and increases their serum concentration tenfold. Large concentrations of alanine and lactate are released and transported to the liver for conversion into glucose via gluconeogenesis, and glucose is then returned to the muscle. These cycles are called the *glucose-alanine cycle* and the *Cori (lactate) cycle.*

Gastrointestinal Cell

Curtailment of ATP production during shock profoundly affects gastrointestinal tract absorption of glucose and amino acids. The lack of perfusion through the gastrointestinal tract impairs mobilization of glucose, fatty acids, and also monoacylglycerol because of decreased lymphatic flow. Active transport is the mechanism for glucose and amino acid absorption, and the transport defect is probably due to the energy deficit. Active glucose transport is ATP-dependent and is associated with an ATPase

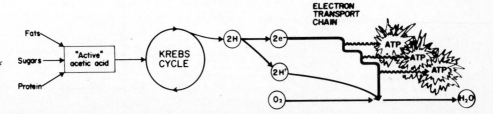

Figure 4. Biochemical anatomy of a cell.

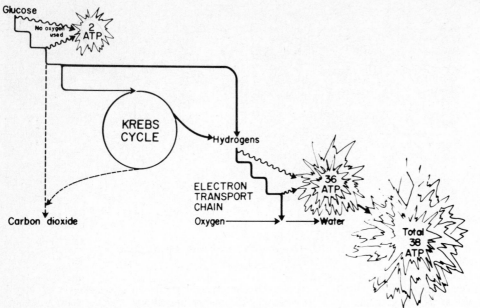

Figure 5. Production of adenosine triphosphate (ATP).

enzyme. This is evidenced by the fact that ouabain, an ATPase inhibitor, and phlorhizin, a competitive inhibitor, interfere with glucose absorption. Amino acid absorption is also ATP-dependent, as demonstrated by the fact that 2,4-dinitrophenol, an electron transport inhibitor, impedes the concentration of L-amino acids in the gastrointestinal mucosal cells. In hemorrhagic shock, specific gastrointestinal tract metabolic functions are impaired because of membrane energy dysfunction. Proton fluxes were measured in rabbit antral pouches with a sensitive microelectrode inserted into the mucosa.[1] The relative impermeability of rabbit antral muosa to H$^+$ apparently protected it against acute ulceration. When the rate of H$^+$ back diffusion was artificially increased to a level that was ulcerogenic in fundic mucosa by introducing hydrochloric acid into the pouches, ulceration also occurred in the antrum. Their findings also indicated that mucosal carbonic anhydrase had a protective function by contributing to the maintenance of normal intracellular acid-base balance in the epithelial cells and that acetazolamide, a potent inhibitor of anion transport that blocks chloride and bicarbonate exchange, disturbed this balance. Thus, the energy deficit of low-perfusion states can produce gastric ulceration. However, the most profound effect is a markedly increased cellular anaerobiosis producing large serum lactic acid concentrations. Experimental hemorrhagic shock studies show that of all the peripheral tissues the gastrointestinal tract is the largest producer of lactate (Fig. 6).[24]

Skin and Connective Tissue Cell

Skin and connective tissue, comprising 14 per cent of the total body cell mass, may produce marked anaerobiosis when inadequately perfused. Since connective tissue is the transitional area of inflammatory reaction, energy deficiency severely impairs its immune response to injury and wound healing by the following mechanisms:

Polymorphonuclear cells and other macrophages involved in the energy-requiring function of phagocytosis and opsonization are unable to clear the wound of foreign bodies; ground substance cannot be produced, and fibroblasts cannot synthesize procollagen; ATP-deficient collagen synthesis is inhibited in the messenger ribonucleic acid (MRNA) and transfer RNA (tRNA) processes;

and there is interference with the translational function on the fibroblast endoplasmic reticulum ribosome.

Thus, low-perfusion states interfere with host defense against infection and wound healing.

VITAL ORGAN ENERGY METABOLISM

Kidney Cell

After the patient has decompensated hemodynamically, vital organs become affected, with the kidney showing

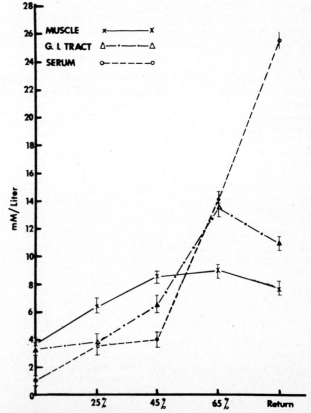

Figure 6. Lactic acid concentrations in muscle, gastrointestinal tract, and plasma in the dog.

the first involvement. In decompensated hypovolemic shock in experimental animals, there is a proportional decrease between renal pressure and flow. The following are the renal ultrastructural alterations in human shock of various etiologies:

1. Minimal to mild changes in glomeruli.

2. Focal necrosis of tubular epithelium with an increase in the number of secondary lysosomes or residual bodies.

3. Predominantly distal tubular casts accompanied by flattening of the tubular epithelium.

The highly metabolic tubular cell function is dependent on glomerular and tubular perfusion. Energy produced by the kidney's oxidative and decarboxylating reactions is used for active reabsorption of sodium and water. It is estimated that one oxygen molecule is needed for reabsorption of 20 to 30 sodium ions. Thus, the hypoxia of depressed perfusion decreases oxygen uptake and ATP production and increases water and sodium losses. This is present in septic shock, which originally produces polyuria and marked sodium loss; when these effects are negated by marked hypovolemia, decreased glomerular filtration occurs. Sodium potassium–activated ATPase is localized in the basolateral cell membrane of the proximal and distal nephrons. The luminal brush border of the proximal tubular cells is associated with a nonmitochondrial ATPase stimulated by bicarbonate and alkaline phosphatase. There is indirect evidence that ATPase is connected with either H^+ secretion or bicarbonate reabsorption. Calcium-activated ATPase is localized in the basolateral membranes of the proximal and distal nephrons. The lack of both ADP and renal cellular ATP deranges ATPase function, which interferes with sodium and hydrogen ion secretion and excretion and, consequently, with acid-base balance reparation. In profound hypovolemia, anaerobic metabolism produces metabolic acidosis, negating distal tubular function. Glutaminase I, a phosphate-dependent enzyme located in the renal tubular cell mitochondrion, increases its activity during metabolic acidosis by catalyzing ammonia formation via glutamine deamination and excreting H^+ as an ammonium salt. This oxygen-requiring enzyme is linked to the citric acid cycle because glutamine becomes glutamate so that it can ultimately enter the Krebs cycle and be converted to glucose.

The net synthesis of glucose is not a requirement for ammonia production, but the transport of malate and possibly oxaloacetate across the mitochondrial membrane, with subsequent conversion to phosphoenolpyruvate (PEP) by the PEP carboxykinase reaction, must be closely linked to the rate at which ammonia is being formed from glutamine with the mitochondria. Obviously, the lack of substrate, the diminished ATP production, and the overwhelming metabolic acidosis impair the kidney's compensatory ability and result in intracellular edema of the proximal and distal tubules, with release of lysosomal enzymes and functional failure. If uncorrected, tubular failure and necrosis lead to persisting renal insufficiency.

The Lung

Biochemically, the lung serves as a membrane exchanging oxygen for carbon dioxide, with these gases diffusing across the alveolar membrane into the red blood cells for transport to the tissues. Thus, the lung is primarily a gas exchanger passively equilibrating gases between the alveolar and red blood cells according to the ideal gas law. Minimal energy is expended in this process, and the lung functions without difficulty in shock states except in the presence of an alveolovascular membrane injury with accompanying edema and hyalinization. Hemoglobin transports the oxygen by a reversible molecular combination. Dissociation of hemoglobin and oxygen at the tissue level is represented by the hemoglobin-oxygen dissociation curve. In shock, this curve moves to the right, which decreases the affinity of hemoglobin for oxygen through four mechanisms:

1. Increased H^+ acidity (blood pH decrease).

2. Increased carbon dioxide tension.

3. Increased erythrocyte concentration of 2,3-diphosphoglycerate (2,3-DPG).

4. Increased body temperature.

The *Bohr effect*, increased carbon dioxide tension caused by increased hydrogen ion concentration secondary to peripheral metabolic acidosis of anaerobic metabolism, is probably due to increased carbonic acid generation and increased dissociation as expressed in the following formula:

$$H_2CO_3 \xrightleftharpoons[\text{anhydrase}]{\text{carbonic}} H^+ + HCO_3^-$$

2,3-DPG is a metabolic cofactor in the Embden-Meyerhof glycolytic pathway. In the erythrocyte, one 2,3-DPG molecule binds noncovalently to the α-amino group of the N-terminal valine residue of the 2β-chain of deoxyhemoglobin. Thus, 2,3-DPG pulls the equilibrium between oxyhemoglobin and deoxyhemoglobin plus oxygen to the right, favoring the deoxygenated state of hemoglobin, as shown in the following formula (dissociation of oxygen from hemoglobin catalyzed by 2,3-DPG):

$$Hb\,O_2 \xrightarrow{\text{DPG}} Hb \cdot DPG + O_2$$

In shock, erythrocytic 2,3-DPG significantly increases. Thus, when volume is replaced in shock patients, it should be noted that the decreased 2,3-DPG content of old stored blood may yield high oxygen affinity hemoglobin that could interfere with the erythrocytic delivery of oxygen at the tissue level. Finally, elevated temperature changes in septic shock patients also move the dissociation curve to the right and increase oxygen release.

The alveolar apparatus is composed of macrophages and Type I and II pneumocytes. Oxygen diffusion occurs across the membranous Type I pneumocytes, while Type II pneumocytes produce *surfactant*, a lipoprotein complex containing mainly L-dipalmitoyl phosphatidylcholine. The half-life of this saturated pulmonary lecithin is 14 hours, which suggests that active synthesis is required. Inclusion bodies in Type II alveolar cells show an uptake of 14C palmitate, which is indirect evidence of their synthesis in these cells. Surfactant is considered to be the substance maintaining the integrity of thin-walled alveoli by preventing the collapse and coaptation of alveolar cells. This is apparently accomplished by the dipolar effect of the fatty acid in surfactant—the negative charges repel each other, thus keeping the alveoli open. Because of their high metabolic rate, Type II cells are dependent on ATP for surfactant synthesis. In shock, dysfunction in Type I pneumocytes may cause a membranous leak, which fills the alveoli and produces a surfactant washout, compounding the atelectasis of adult respiratory distress syndrome. The pulmonary alveolar macrophage is a glucose and oxygen-utilizing phagocyte. It produces hydrogen peroxide (H_2O_2) but no hydroxyl radicals, a mechanism that apparently protects the alveolar space wherein the macrophage resides. Oxygen radicals produced intracellularly or released extracellularly may be important to the macrophage in its bactericidal activity, but they may also expose the cell to self-destruction by oxidant injury. The soluble sulfhydryl system in erythrocytes has been shown to protect the polymorphonuclear leukocyte and macrophage cell from oxidant injury by reducing hydrogen peroxide. The hexose monophosphate pathway works to regenerate reduced nicotine adenine phosphonucleotide (NADPH) so that reduced glutathione may be replenished. Any nascent oxygen (O^-)-releasing effect by the alveolar macrophage may damage Type I pneumocytes and may cause fluid to leak into the alveolus and depress surfactant production by Type II pneumocytes.

The Liver

Studies on the oxygen metabolism of the liver reveal increased oxygen uptake by this organ during endotoxin shock. Mitochondrial metabolism shows uncoupling of oxidative phosphorylation,[23] and this oxygen waste without energy accumulation is a continuous process associated with changes in the character of the mitochondria. This uncoupling process produces an increase of inorganic phosphates in the liver and a decrease in the concentration of both high-energy organic phosphates, ATP and ADP.

Liver cells have numerous metabolic functions, including (1) bile and cholesterol excretion, (2) gluconeogenesis, (3) detoxification, and (4) protein synthesis. Depressed perfusion secondary to all types of shock profoundly affects these functions.

Bile and Cholesterol Excretion. Studies on bile solubilization and excretion during shock indicate a marked decrease in bile formation and excretion. It has been noted that bile secretion is suppressed in patients after biliary tract operations with external drainage. This may be attributable to the oxygen or NAD dependence on the bilirubin-solubilizing reaction of glucuronide conjugation to bilirubin. In shock or low-flow states, a mild jaundice of 1.0 to 2.0 mg. per 100 ml. is usually present. Cholesterol either is taken up or is synthesized by the liver and is either excreted in the bile or is converted to bile acids.

Gluconeogenesis. The liver glycolytic intermediate pattern in sepsis arises from a block in an enzymatic step between fructose-1,6-diphosphate (FDP) and fructose-6-phosphate (F6P). Either fructose diphosphatase is inhibited, conserving the FDP supply, or phosphofructokinase is activated and more FDP accumulates in the metabolic pool. By a regulatory "feed-forward" control, the elevated FDP activates pyruvate kinase, depleting PEP, and thus explains the lowered concentration of this substrate in perfused or intact septic livers. A fall in glucose-6-phosphate (G6P) then results because of increased conversion into F6P and FDP. The net effect of these reactions is to route carbohydrate moieties away from gluconeogenesis. When glycogen is exhausted, the hypoglycemia of terminal sepsis and endotoxemia usually appears (Fig. 7).[34]

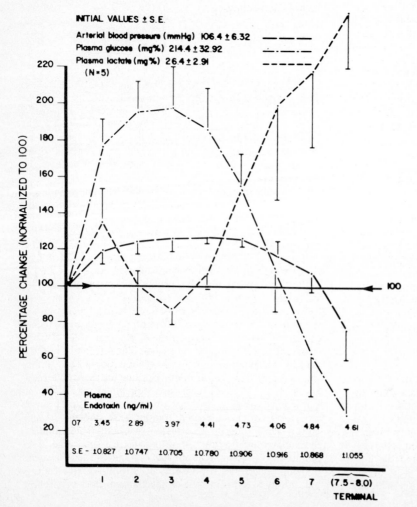

Figure 7. Metabolic and hemodynamic response to plasma endotoxin in rat peritonitis after cecal incision.

Detoxification. The liver is unable to detoxify because the allosteric enzymes, glucuronidases, sulfatases, and hydroxylases are NAD^+-dependent. This inhibits the detoxification and solubilization of various intermediate metabolites such as serotonin, histamine, and various steroids. There are oxidative reactions in the liver that act to metabolize certain inert hydrocarbons. This hydroxylation occurs in the endoplasmic reticulum of the hepatic cells. Hydroxyl compounds may be further oxidized to ketones or aldehydes by the action of the enzyme alcoholic dehydrogenases. The detoxifying function in the reticuloendothelial system of the liver may play a significant role in the neutralization of bacterial exotoxins and endotoxins.

Protein Synthesis. Decreased urea nitrogen in the blood of shock patients is not surprising because the deaminating and transaminating amino acid enzymes in the liver need ATP to produce glucose or substrates that enter into the citric acid cycle. These oxidative enzymes depend on cofactors for normal function. Thus, severe shock may produce liver failure with an attendant hyperammonemia. The total effect of these molecular changes is reflected in deranged ultramicroscopic anatomy (Fig. 8A,B).

The Heart

The cardiac muscle cell with its abundant mitochondria must produce high concentrations of ATP. These cells extract lactate, glucose, and fatty acids, and they convert these substrates to ATP. During severe hypotension, however, anaerobic metabolism produces rather than consumes lactic acid, indicating a dependence on anaerobic glycolysis for energy. Some of the capacity of the cardiac mitochondrial citric acid cycle and electron transport system is not restored to normal function after transfusion, as evidenced by persistently low levels of ATP in hemorrhagic shock. This translates into depressed left ventricular work, coronary flow, and ventricular oxygen consumption in postshock states. Blood levels of pyruvate and lactate remain significantly elevated during this same period. Lefer and Barenholz[17] described a myocardial depressant factor that appeared to be a vasoactive peptide produced by the pancreas during hemorrhagic shock. The marked decrease

in uptake and oxidation of free fatty acids greatly impairs myocardial energy metabolism. Concomitantly, lactate becomes a significant energy source. Thus, glycolytic metabolism may help protect the heart against anoxic injury. Furthermore, since fatty acid oxidation requires Krebs cycle intermediates, carbohydrate oxidation can be rate-limiting. Glucose transport and phosphorylation increase with anoxia, the latter because G6P inhibition of hexokinase is released as the glycolytic flux increases and G6P concentration falls. Glycolytic flux increases and phosphofructokinase (PFK) is released from inhibition by declining citrate and ATP, and PFK is activated by rising phosphate. Glycogen stores are rapidly depleted during anoxia since β-phosphorylase is stimulated by phosphate and released from inhibition by G6P and because epinephrine induces transformation of phosphorylase β to α.

Under severely hypoxic conditions, anaerobic metabolism cannot maintain the heart's high-energy phosphate stores. Consequently, first creatine phosphate and later ATP stores are diminished. Lactate production and glycolytic flux increase more than 20-fold. If anoxic conditions continue, acidosis produces a PFK inhibition that is rate-limiting, and thus hexokinase is inhibited by the increase in G6P. If ATP falls below the 2 mM. per gm., glycolytic flux will cease because there is insufficient ATP to phosphorylate F6P. The effects of shock on heart metabolism appear to be due to the anoxic defects because the results are the same as seen in the anoxic heart.

The Brain

The average oxygen utilization of the human brain ranges from 3.3 to 3.9 ml. per 100 gm. per minute (mean: 3.6 ml. per 100 gm. per minute). Rate increases in oxygen consumption can occur during convulsions but apparently not during mental activity. The intact brain's main substrate source of energy is glucose, which is metabolized in the glycolytic and Krebs cycles and hexose monophosphate shunt. Under ordinary conditions the lactate yield is low, 6 mM. per gm. wet weight per hour, but under adverse conditions it may increase to 400 mM. per gm. wet weight per hour. Normally, phosphocreatine and ATP concentrations are about 3 mM. per gm. wet weight, but hypoxia

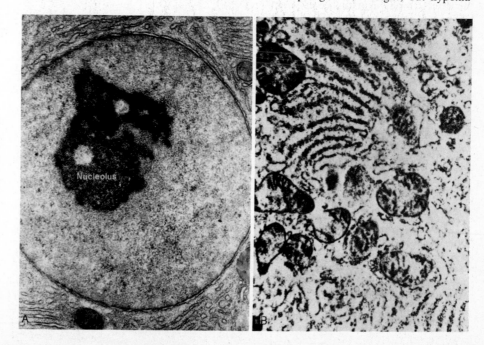

Figure 8. Hepatic cells. A, Electron microscopy of normal liver cell. Note normal endoplasmic reticulum and mitochondria. (Magnification, 45,000 ×) B, Electron microscopy of liver cell after hypovolemic shock. Note abnormal endoplasmic reticulum, disrupted mitochondria, and cytoplasmic edema. (Magnification, 45,000 ×)

causes a marked decrease of these compounds. Thus, the general requirements of brain cells for ATP production are similar to those of any other organ. The interdependence between the membrane potential and ionic concentrations is important for the nerve cell. In low-flow and anoxic states, ATP deficiency affects the sodium/potassium ATPase molecule along the membrane and, consequently, decreases impulse propagation.

Apparently, glutamic acid is the only amino acid metabolized in brain tissue. It participates in the brain's uptake of ammonia and combines with ammonia to form glutamine, which is then excreted in the plasma for liver metabolism. Glutamic acid is formed by the transamination of *ketoglutarate* formed in the Krebs cycle from the metabolism of glucose to produce pyruvate and then oxaloacetate. This is the brain's defense against anoxia, the ammonia of low perfusion and a hypoperfused liver. During shock, the brain is the last organ to be underperfused. It is protected from anaerobiosis by an "autonomic cerebral metabolism"; however, because of its metabolic complexity, it will not withstand prolonged hypoperfusion. Anoxia produces metabolic acidosis, enzyme dysfunction, cellular membrane leakage causing edema, attendant convulsion, coma, and, finally, death.[29]

Cardiogenic Shock

Cardiogenic shock results from cardiac failure, producing progressive circulatory collapse and death. It can be caused by pericardial, myocardial, or valvular factors, but occurs mainly by coronary occlusion or myocardial infarction. Cardiogenic shock after myocardial infarction is a state in which the systolic arterial pressure is less than 90 torr or 30 torr below previous level. Urinary output is less than 20 ml. per hour, and mentation is impaired. Peripheral vasoconstriction is evidenced by cold, clammy skin.

A myocardial depression factor has been reported and characterized in all types of experimental shock, making it difficult at times to differentiate between cardiogenic and other types of cardiac depression in the various types of shock.[17] Hemodynamic values do not differentiate between the two, since the decreased cardiac output and normal or increased peripheral resistance of cardiogenic shock are not different from those of the hypovolemic or the hypodynamic stage of septic shock. Therefore, a careful physical examination is mandatory to exclude valvular and pericardial disease. Chest x-ray, electrocardiogram, echocardiogram and noninvasive imaging studies, i.e., nuclear magnetic resonance and nuclide imaging, aid in differentiating pericardial tamponade and myocardial infarction.

Once the etiology of cardiogenic shock is determined, the hemodynamic defect should be ascertained by measuring cardiac output, stroke work, end-diastolic pulmonary artery pressure, and peripheral resistance. Cardiac performance is assessed by measuring (1) preload, (2) contractility, (3) afterload, (4) synergy of contraction, and (5) heart rate.

CARDIAC PERFORMANCE

Preload refers to the ventricle's end-diastolic circumferential fiber length and is therefore a function of end-diastolic volume and passive intramyocardial wall stress. Preload is measured by left ventricular end-diastolic pressure or pulmonary artery wedge pressure (PAWP). Normal wedge pressure is 12 torr and is measured through a flow-directed balloon tip catheter, the tip of which lies in a small pulmonary artery.

Contractility is a function of preload, peripheral resistance (afterload), and the force of the myocardial fiber, and, consequently, it is difficult to measure directly. The product of contractility is *stroke volume*, and since stroke volume times heart rate equals cardiac output, the measurement of cardiac output denotes the contractile force of the myocardial fiber.

Afterload is inversely related to stroke volume. It is the tension developed by the left ventricle to open the aortic valve and is related to the pressure in the aorta (aortic diastolic pressure) and the distal pressure in the systemic system (peripheral resistance). As peripheral resistance increases, the afterload also increases.

Synergy of contraction is related to an orderly distribution of myocardial contractile force. Disorder occurs in infarction of the myocardial wall with consequent *hypokinesis* (inward movement), *akinesis* (absent movement), *dyskinesis* (paradoxical movement), or *asynchrony* (asynchronous movement).

Cardiogenic shock reflects alterations of preload, contractility, and afterload. The objectives of therapy are to manipulate these determinants so as to improve cardiac output, decrease cardiac work, and maintain coronary blood flow (Table 1). A useful therapeutic regimen is as follows:

I. Preload
   A. Volume expansion monitored by PAWP
II. Contractility
   A. Drugs
      1. Norepinephrine
      2. Digitalis with or without glucagon
      3. Dopamine
      4. Dobutamine
   B. Counterpulsation
III. Afterload—nitroprusside
IV. Rate
   A. Drugs
      1. Lidocaine
      2. Digitalis
      3. Propranolol (beta-blockers)
V. Coronary perfusion
   A. Drugs—nitrates
   B. Counterpulsation

TABLE 1. *Normal Resting Hemodynamic Values*

Hemodynamic Parameters	Normal Values	
Right atrium	0–7	torr
Right ventricle		
Systolic	15–30	torr
Diastolic	0–8	torr
Pulmonary artery		
Systolic	15–25	torr
Diastolic	8–15	torr
Pulmonary artery wedge and left atrium	6–12	torr
Left ventricle		
Systolic	100–140	torr
End diastolic	3–12	torr
Systemic arteries		
Systolic	100–140	torr
Diastolic	60–90	torr
Oxygen consumption index	110–150	mL./min./m.^{2}
Arteriovenous oxygen difference	30–50	mL./L.
Cardiac index	2.5–4.0	L./min./m.^{2}
Resistances		
Pulmonary vascular	20–150	dynes/sec./cm.$^{-5}$
Systemic vascular	770–1500	dynes/sec./cm.$^{-5}$

TREATMENT

The treatment of cardiogenic shock is replenishment of volume by infusing saline or colloid via peripheral venous catheters at 10-minute intervals using the following criteria:

Pulmonary artery wedge pressure (PAWP)

If PAWP is 12 torr, infuse:	200 ml. slowly
If PAWP is 12 to 16 torr, infuse:	100 ml. slowly
If PAWP is 16 torr, infuse:	50 ml. slowly

Thereafter, continue to monitor PAWP and adjust infusion rate to maintain PAWP at 20 torr. Serum lactate, arterial pressure, and urinary output should return to normal levels. If there is no improvement after volume resuscitation, pharmacologic manipulation of afterload should be attempted by infusing nitroprusside at a dose of 20 μg. per minute. Contractility should be supported by judicious use of norepinephrine or digitalization with glucagon. Finally, if there is no response to support of preload, contractility, and afterload, counterpulsation should be instituted. Despite this rational therapeutic regimen, the mortality rate for cardiogenic shock is very high (70 per cent).

Hypovolemic Shock

A 65-year-old man is admitted to the emergency department with a 2-day history of melena associated with dizziness and light-headedness. The skin is pale, cold, and clammy. The radial pulse is weak, and the rate is 130 per minute. The patient is dyspneic with a respiratory rate of 24 breaths per minute, and the blood pressure (BP) is 110/60 torr. As the examination progresses, the patient becomes agitated and circumoral cyanosis appears. The mucous membranes become dry, the BP decreases to 80/40 torr, and the pulse rate increases to 150 per minute. A nasogastric tube is inserted, and bright red blood is aspirated.

PATHOPHYSIOLOGY

This is a description of hypovolemic or *hemorrhagic shock*, probably secondary to upper gastrointestinal hemorrhage. The volume loss from a bleeding gastric or duodenal ulcer stimulates pressure receptors in the aorta, heart, and carotid artery to release epinephrine, aldosterone, and antidiuretic hormones. These hormones in turn augment the heart rate and force of contraction, induce vasoconstriction, and decrease volume loss from the kidney. The increased cardiac output helps the remaining blood volume to meet the needs of the tissues for oxygenation. Peripheral vasoconstriction secondary to epinephrine and norepinephrine shunts blood to the vital tissues, decreasing blood flow to nonvital organs. When this occurs, although the BP is normal or almost normal in the systemic or large arteries, shock is occurring in the nonvital tissue microcirculation. Microcirculatory flow impairment causes a decrease in the transport of oxygen to these cells, which have a larger cell mass than the vital tissues. Without oxygen, the cells cannot metabolize glucose completely and must switch to anaerobic metabolism, which produces metabolic acids (specifically, lactic acid). The accumulation of these metabolic acids leads to metabolic acidosis.

This patient is in shock, and despite a BP of 110/60 torr, he is undergoing sympathetic or adrenergic stimulation with typical signs of peripheral constriction: pallor; sweating; cold, clammy skin; and fast, thready pulse. As bleeding

continues, despite the tachycardia and shunting, there is insufficient blood volume for vital organ perfusion. Blood pressure decreases, and the pulse rate increases. Inadequate blood flow to the brain produces anoxia and irritability. The circumoral cyanosis is a late sign of severe cellular anoxia in the face and head. Mucous membrane dryness indicates cellular dehydration. Cellular anoxia induces profound metabolic acidosis because large concentrations of lactic acid are being released owing to anaerobic metabolism. Concomitantly, each cell is releasing approximately 15 to 20 per cent of its water in an attempt to replenish vascular volume, which results in cellular dehydration.

The vital organs also react to decreased blood volume. The kidney glomerular filtration rate decreases, reducing urinary output. The liver's ability to produce new glucose is impaired. Certain lung areas become atelectatic because of inadequate perfusion. The heart and brain are not affected until the last stages of shock, when they deteriorate functionally.

MANAGEMENT

An appreciation of the appropriate pathophysiologic view of hypovolemic shock allows a rational approach to treatment. The first objective is to reduce or stop blood loss. If this is not possible, lost volume must be replaced fast enough to keep the vital and nonvital tissues perfused. Lost volume ideally should be replaced with packed red cells. However, because cross-matching requires 1 to 2 hours, the temporary use of balanced salt solutions is acceptable. These solutions include normal saline, Ringer's lactate, and Ringer's bicarbonate. Ringer's bicarbonate solution is generally preferred, since it remains uncertain whether the underperfused liver can metabolize lactate into carbon dioxide and water. If lactate is not metabolized, it is excreted by the kidney with sodium and potassium, which alters acid-base balance.

The preferred method for determining the patient's fluid status and estimating the volume of fluid to be administered involves placing a pulmonary artery pressure (PAP) catheter in a small branch of the pulmonary artery to measure pulmonary wedge pressure. Central venous pressure (CVP) should be monitored in young patients or in those with moderate hypovolemic shock. Before action is taken on measurements obtained via the CVP catheter, however, it should be recognized that it is deficient in three ways. First, it does not indicate the amount of volume needed; instead, it monitors cardiac competency by measuring the amount of volume the left myocardium can manage without failing. Second, it requires almost 24 hours for events occurring in the left side of the heart to propagate through the lung into the right ventricle, auricle, and superior vena cava. Third, any pathologic change in the pulmonary vasculature may produce venous hypertension. Therefore, the use of a PAP catheter is recommended in patients with shock who are critically ill, who are older than 50 years of age, or who have heart disease.

Kidney function is monitored by an indwelling catheter, and urinary output should be 30 to 70 ml. per hour. If it falls below 30 ml. per hour, fluid administration is increased and 25 gm. of mannitol may be given intravenously. If there is no improvement, furosemide is added and administered either continuously or in divided doses until a level of 2000 mg. is reached. If this is not beneficial, consideration should be given to treating the patient for established renal failure by peritoneal or renal dialysis. Blood pressure is preferably monitored by radial arterial cannulation. Another advantage of arterial cannulation is the ability to measure pH and blood gases.

The pH, P_{CO_2}, and P_{O_2} measurements are observed because they indicate the amount of oxygen the cells receive. The excessive acid produced by anaerobic metabolism can be treated with volume replacement and sodium bicarbonate. The indicated antacid dosage depends on the pH and P_{CO_2} measurements and their consequent base deficit. Sodium bicarbonate is administered on a milliequivalent-per-milliequivalent basis. Respiratory alkalosis may develop in some patients while compensating for the underlying acidosis. Other patients exhibit metabolic alkalosis secondary to the aldosterone effect of the kidney or to the iatrogenic overreplenishment of bicarbonate. Thus, the pH must be monitored carefully.

Monitoring of serum lactic acid is considered a valuable aid because lactic acid is the end metabolite of anaerobic metabolism, and a high serum lactate indicates that the cells are not being oxygenated or perfused. Contrariwise, a low serum lactate indicates that the cells are being perfused and that the patient's condition is improved.[5]

The P_{O_2} must also be observed carefully because, after resuscitation, confluent atelectasis may develop throughout both lung fields, associated with a P_{O_2} level of less than 60 torr, which remains unchanged after breathing 100 per cent oxygen. This may ultimately result in the adult respiratory distress syndrome.

The vasoconstrictors norepinephrine and metaraminol bitartrate are contraindicated in the treatment of hypovolemic shock because they overconstrict the peripheral arterioles and thus increase anaerobic metabolism and its consequence, acidosis. However, in patients who arrive in the emergency department with a markedly decreased BP, vital organ perfusion pressure must be maintained until enough volume has been administered for resuscitation. A phenylephrine hydrochloride solution (2 mg. per 100 ml.) may be given intravenously to keep the systolic BP at 80 torr. Dopamine in dosages of 10 to 20 µg. per kg. per hour can also be infused. The vasodilator phentolamine, in dosages of 5 mg. per hour, is useful in patients who remain overconstricted with cold, clammy skin and depressed urinary output after adequate fluid resuscitation.

In summary, hypovolemic shock is curable and best treated by reducing the loss of volume, then replacing the lost volume and correcting acid-base imbalance.[27]

Septic Shock

A 42-year-old woman is admitted complaining of epigastric pain of 5 days' duration that is radiating to the lower quadrant and is associated with nausea, vomiting, and constipation. The pain, originally severe, relents after 24 hours and then becomes generalized throughout the abdomen and is associated with chills and fever. On examination, the findings include rigidity, tenderness, rebound tenderness, and a tender mass in the right lower quadrant; rectal examination shows peritoneal bogginess with notable right lower quadrant tenderness.

At the time of admission, the patient complains of chills and the temperature is 39.4°C. The skin is flushed and warm. The BP is 120/80 torr. A course of antibiotics is begun. Later, the BP increases to 160/70 torr, and the pulse rate and urinary output decrease. The skin becomes cold and clammy, the BP decreases to 60/0 torr, and the pulse rate increases to 150 beats per minute.

PATHOPHYSIOLOGY

The sequence of events leading to septic shock begins with a bacterial invasion in the presence of a major septic process, such as pneumonitis, subacute bacterial endocarditis, ruptured viscus peritonitis, and abdominal abscess. The precipitating agents, gram-negative and gram-positive bacteria, are opsonized and phagocytosed, releasing into the bloodstream fragments that contain either exotoxin, the intracellular content of bacteria, or endotoxin, a lipoprotein-polysaccharide (LPS) macromolecule of the cell membrane. This occurs because the phagocytic phagolysosomes degrade the cytoplasmic and membranous portions of the bacterial cell. When released in the blood, endotoxin initiates antibody formation and complement interactions, which promote opsonization of the endotoxin fragments so that the reticuloendothelial (RES) cells can absorb them for detoxification. However, if the infection is overwhelming, the RES cells are inundated with LPS, their function is depressed, and the serum complement endotoxin reaction is accelerated.

Anaphylotoxins created by this interaction release histamine and heparin from mast cells, the phagocytosis factor releases lysosomal enzymes and superoxide radicals from polymorphonuclear leukocytes and the myeloperoxidase system and the immune adherence factor releases serotonin and histamine from platelets. These substances produce endothelial cell damage and marked capillary permeability, resulting in severe loss of plasma volume to the interstitial space throughout the capillary system. Loss of effective circulating blood volume produces circulatory collapse and shock.

The hemodynamic pattern during this immunologic reaction is a hyperdynamic phase characterized by decreased peripheral resistance secondary to the release of histamine and serotonin and an increase in cardiac output. With the loss of plasma volume, the circulatory response becomes similar to that of hypovolemic shock. There is release of epinephrine and norepinephrine, producing increased peripheral resistance and cardiac rate. Cardiac output is depressed because of decreased blood volume and venous return to the heart. This represents the *hypodynamic* phase of septic shock. Depressed perfusion of nonvital tissues produces deranged cellular metabolism. The lack of oxygen results in the anaerobic metabolism of glucose with increased production of lactic acid, the main cause of metabolic acidosis in the hypodynamic phase of septic shock. Impaired function of the Krebs cycle depresses ATP, or energy production. This energy deficit causes decreased membrane ATP and function, allowing further loss of fluid through endothelial cells and resulting in the intracellular edema of shock.

Recent work indicates that endotoxemia interferes with the production of new glucose from alanine, glycerol, and lactic acid. Apparently, this is caused by depression of rate-limiting enzymes, specifically phosphoenolpyruvate kinase and fructose diphosphatase, as well as an energy defect, since ATP is necessary for converting gluconeogenic precursors into glucose. Depressed gluconeogenesis may also cause the increase in lactic acid, since it is not being used by the liver for new glucose production.

New and important therapeutic concepts have been derived from studies of the immunology and molecular pathology of septic shock. *In vitro* studies of corticosteroids have shown that these agents have an anticomplementary effect. When administered *in vivo*, they decrease the serum histamine and serotonin levels secondary to complement reaction. They also aid in the induction of gluconeogenic enzymes. Studies of the hypoglycemia secondary to gluconeogenic inhibition show the need for an exogenous source of glucose. Therefore, glucose, insulin, and potassium solutions are now advocated as adjunctive resuscitative fluids. Although these studies were supported by good basic data, further investigation is needed for the improvement of present therapeutic concepts and techniques to counteract the devastating effects of the complement reaction, the gluconeogenic block, and the membrane injury of sepsis.[23, 26]

DIAGNOSIS

Septic shock can be diagnosed by a history of generalized or localized sepsis characterized by a hyperdynamic phase coinciding with the immunologic reaction to endotoxin. During this phase, there are notable increases in cardiac output, BP, and pulse rate as well as a decrease in urinary output, peripheral resistance, and arterial venous oxygen difference. Respiratory and metabolic alkalosis is often present. When this combination of symptoms is present, septic shock must be considered because the prognosis is more favorable than when treatment is delayed until the hypodynamic phase. In the hypodynamic phase, endothelial cell permeability ensues, there is loss of circulating blood volume, and, consequently, cardiac output and BP decrease, pulse rate and peripheral resistance increase, and the skin becomes cold and clammy. Metabolic acidosis is usually present. At this critical point, a provisional diagnosis of septic shock must be made and therapy must be begun. Waiting for confirmatory blood culture jeopardizes the patient's life.

TREATMENT

There are four principal objectives in the treatment of septic shock: (1) treatment of sepsis, (2) management of the hypovolemic state, (3) reparation of the metabolic acid-base imbalance, and (4) correction of the nutritional deficit. The treatment must be rendered concomitantly and rapidly. It is essential that the septic and hypovolemic processes be treated concomitantly, since preventing the complexing of antigen-antibody and complement will deter vascular permeability and its consequent hypovolemia. Prompt and adequate treatment of hypovolemia prevents the development of attendant cellular metabolic derangements.

All patients in septic shock should be managed on an intensive care unit. Septic shock is one of the most critical medical emergencies requiring specialized care by medical and paramedical staff trained in intensive care and supported by appropriate monitoring equipment. The following is an outline for treatment.

1. Treat the underlying cause of sepsis. Drain abscesses.
2. Provide respiratory care: if the patient is not dyspneic or cyanotic, administer 8 to 10 liters per minute of FIO_2 0.4 by a mask. If there has been injury to the chest or if there is dyspnea or cyanosis, insert an endotracheal tube and attach to a ventilator.
   a. If acute respiratory failure is present, attach the endotracheal tube to a ventilator and treat as follows: The mechanical ventilator should promote increased tidal volume driving pressure. Apply positive end-expiratory pressure to increase alveolar oxygen pressure and prevent alveolar collapse.
   b. Administer a diuretic such as furosemide in 50-mg. doses every 4 hours to maintain pulmonary artery pressure (PAP) at low normal levels.
   c. Administer albumin if measured colloid osmotic pressure is below normal range.
   d. Administer cardiotonic drugs to improve cardiac output if PAP or PAWP shows an abnormal increase.
   e. Administer antibiotics if the sputum culture is positive. The choice of antibiotic is dependent on culture and sensitivity.
3. Give 30 mg. per kg. body weight of methylprednisolone sodium succinate or 3 mg. per kg. body weight of dexamethasone sodium phosphate in a single bolus as soon as septic shock is diagnosed, and repeat after 4 hours if there is no beneficial response. Unless the septic shock is episodic, do not repeat.
   a. Infuse tobramycin, 5.0 mg. per kg. body weight per day, and clindamycin, 35 mg. per kg. body weight per day.
   b. Add ampicillin if Enterococcus is present.
4. Obtain three sets of blood cultures, including anaerobic ones. Monitor antibiotic levels with serial serum determinations, and determine sensitivities to antibiotics with Kirby-Bauer and bactericidal assays (Table 2).
5. Replace lost volume. Place an intravenous cannula, preferably 14 gauge, in a peripheral vein.
   a. Place a PAP or CVP catheter.
   b. Treat the hypovolemic phase of septic shock as hypovolemic shock, using balanced salt solution.
   c. Maintain blood pressure without increasing PAWP. If PAWP increases abnormally, cardiotonics must be given to maintain cardiac output: 500 μg. digitalis given immediately and followed by 250 μg. every 6 hours glucagon at a rate of 3 to 5 mg. per hour. The cardiotonic chosen may be 1.0 to 4 μg. per minute of solution of isoproterenol given to maintain systolic pressure above 80 torr or dopamine at a rate of 5 to 10 μg. per minute per kg. body weight for no longer than 8 hours or dobutamine at a rate of 10 μg. per minute per kg. body weight.
   d. Give blood as soon as it is available, keeping the hematocrit at 30 per cent or above.
6. Monitor the vital functions.
   a. Maintain and measure pulmonary artery pressure through the PAP catheter.
   b. Measure urinary output every hour. Maintain a urine output of 50 to 75 ml. per hour. If the urine output falls below 30 ml. per hour and there is no response to an increased infusion of Ringer's bicarbonate solution, infuse 12.5 gm. of mannitol over a period of 5 minutes. If mannitol fails to produce diuresis, give 50 mg. of furosemide intravenously. If diuresis does not occur, infuse furosemide continuously up to dose of 1 gm. If there is no improvement in urinary output, treat as established renal failure. Start infusions of Ringer's solution (preferably) containing 44 mMol./l. of sodium bicarbonate in both catheters (Table 3).
   c. Monitor blood pressure by cuff or, if warranted, by arterial catheter.
   d. Measure pH, Pco_2, and Pao_2 by either femoral or radial artery cannula.
   e. Determine levels of lactic acid and serum glucose every 2 hours until resuscitation is complete.

TABLE 2. Mortality Rate According to Bacterial Etiology in the Prospective Study

Bacterial Species	Per Cent Total	With Steroid*	Without Steroid*
Escherichia coli	20	1/18	4/17
Klebsiella-Aerobacter	22	3/21	7/15
Proteus	13	1/10	4/12
Pseudomonas	20	3/17	7/18
Paracolon	3	0/2	1/3
Bacteroides fragilis	13	2/10	4/12
Staphylococcus	5	0/5	2/3
Streptococcus	3	0/2	2/3
Mixed culture	2	0/1	2/2
TOTALS	100%	9/86	33/86
Total mortality rate		10.4%	38.4%

*Expressed in number of deaths among patients.

TABLE 3. Intravenous Infusion Other Than Blood or Plasma Used to Treat Shock

Name	Composition (mMol./liter)			
	Sodium	Potassium	Calcium	HCO₃
Ringer's injection	147	4.1	2.24	0
Ringer's bicarbonate*	191	4.1	2.24	44

*This is prepared as follows: 100 cc. Ringer's injection plus 44 mEq. NaHCO₃.

7. Position the patient either with head and feet both at 30 degrees or supine.
8. Keep the patient's temperature under 39°C. by use of a rectal thermistor-controlled water blanket.
9. Vasodilators, such as phentolamine, should be given at a constant infusion rate of 0.5 mg. per minute if the patient is unresponsive to general therapy, if there are clinical signs of sympathetic overactivity, or if the measured peripheral resistance has increased.
10. After resuscitation has begun, infuse hyperalimentation fluids every 8 hours through a PAP catheter. The formula should contain 1000 ml. of 20 per cent glucose, 44 mMol. of potassium chloride, 250 mg. of thiamine hydrochloride, 50 mg. of riboflavin, 1.0 gm. of ascorbic acid, 1.25 gm. of nicotinamide, 50 mg. of pyridoxine hydrochloride, and 500 mg. of sodium panothenate. Intralipid 10 per cent should be added after 2 days of sepsis. Branched chain amino acid infusion prevents septic catabolism and should be considered after resuscitation.

MONITORING

Monitoring of the patient in a state of septic shock requires continuous evaluation of the status of the following: (1) clinical signs, (2) peripheral perfusion, (3) vital organ function, and (4) volume requirements.

Clinical Signs

The two most important aspects in clinical monitoring are observation of the skin and of the sensorium. When the blood volume of the patient in septic shock is repleted and adequately perfuses the peripheral tissues, the skin becomes warm and dry and the color changes from grayish white to pink. During the hyperdynamic phase of septic shock, the skin may become reddened and moist, but this is easily differentiated from the warm, pink skin characteristic of a well-perfused periphery. Although the brain is the last vital organ to receive reduced circulating blood volume, the effect on the sensorium is demonstrated early in the shock state by the patient's irritability and restlessness. If the volume is not promptly replenished, coma may ensue.

Peripheral Perfusion

If shock is to be overcome, peripheral tissue perfusion must be constantly monitored. Skin color and temperature should be observed. Peripheral resistance, which is indicative of the status of the perfusion rate, can be measured. A high peripheral resistance indicates shunting, whereas a normal peripheral resistance indicates adequate perfusion. Another means of determining peripheral perfusion rate is to measure either the concentration of lactate or the lactate:pyruvate ratio. High concentrations of lactate indicate increased anaerobiosis produced by decreased perfusion; low concentrations signify improved or normal perfusion.

It is important to monitor peripheral cell function by measuring the arteriovenous oxygen difference ($C[a-v]O_2$) because the ability of the peripheral tissues to extract oxygen from the blood indicates their viability and also identifies the phase of septic shock. Once cell death occurs, oxygen extraction decreases. In the hyperdynamic phase of septic shock, it is difficult for the peripheral cells to extract oxygen because of the mitochondrial injury secondary to sepsis or endotoxemia. Later in the hypodynamic phase, oxygen extraction elevates the ($C[a-v]O_2$), which is similar to what occurs in hypovolemic shock. Measurement of pH and $PaCO_2$ monitors the acid-base alterations occurring secondary to anaerobic metabolism. These are indirect measurements, because the main component of anaerobic metabolic acidosis is lactic acid. Thus, lactic acid measurements are more current and direct methods of monitoring peripheral perfusion. However, pH and $PaCO_2$ determinations monitor the acid-base compensations of blood buffer, respiration, and kidney. A low pH and $PaCO_2$ (metabolic acidosis) indicate severe metabolic alterations secondary to peripheral cell anaerobiosis. In contrast, reparation of acid-base imbalance indicates improved perfusion.

Vital Organ Function

Heart. To monitor the heart, cardiac output and either CVP or PAWP should be measured through a CVP or PAP catheter.

Lung. Measurement of PaO_2 and $PaCO_2$ differentiates the type of extent of injury inflicted by the shock state on the alveolar-vascular membrane. For example, low PaO_2 measurement may indicate adult respiratory distress syndrome (ARDS), and high $PaCO_2$ and low pH measurements may indicate respiratory acidosis, probably representing an underlying massive atelectasis or ventilatory diffusion problems.

Liver. Serum glucose and lactate measurements (glucose:lactate ratio) determine the status of liver function. A glucose:lactate ratio of 10 or more indicates adequate liver function (gluconeogenesis and glycolysis); less than 10 falling to reversal of ratio indicates inadequate liver function due to depressed perfusion and possible hepatocellular damage.

Kidney. Renal function is monitored by measuring urinary output, normally 30 to 70 ml. per hour with urine osmolality of 600 mOsmol. per liter. The kidney responds to depressed circulating volume by retaining water, which increases urine osmolality (ADH effect). The glomerular filtration rate is also depressed, causing oliguria; as hypoperfusion progresses, nephron cell damage, inability to retain water, and finally a salt-losing nephritis ensue. This effect is reflected in urinary water and salt losses.

Volume Requirements

Volume is monitored by measuring PAP. The blood volume of the pulmonary vascular system is proportional to PAP: As PAP decreases, so does volume. Determination of CVP can be used to monitor young patients or those with moderate hypovolemic shock. However, it should be noted that the CVP catheter is capable of monitoring blood volume changes as long as the left myocardium is functioning normally, as long as there is no pulmonary hypertension, and as long as there is no severe shunting. Volume, being directly proportional to either urinary output or mean arterial pressure (MAP), can be indirectly monitored by measuring these two parameters. The pulse rate is inversely proportional to volume. Hematocrit, after transcapillary filling has occurred, is directly proportional to volume.

Mortality from septic shock has been estimated by various investigators to range within 10 to 70 per cent. It is the most difficult type of shock to treat. Unless early diagnosis is made and aggressive treatment is instituted immediately, based on the metabolic and immunologic pathologic alterations, optimal results will not be achieved.

Distributive Shock

Distributive shock can occur under the following conditions:

1. During spinal anesthesia; anesthetic drugs paralyze the neurogenic control of the precapillary sphincters and depress venomotor tone.

2. Use of vasodilator drugs such as nitrates.

3. Sudden release of a distended viscus; gastric dilatation or an obstructed intestine suddenly opening the capillary space to trap circulating volume.

4. Vasodilatation caused by unexplained reflex mechanisms, producing ineffective circulating volume and syncope, such as extreme pain, emotional stress, and fright.

The symptoms of distributive shock are little different from the other types of shock, and differentiation can be difficult. However, the history is usually quite helpful. The basic concept in treating distributive shock is to give vasopressors, such as phenylephrine and ephedrine, in order to decrease the vascular bed either by constricting precapillary sphincters or capacitance veins to force out stagnant blood volume. These vasopressors act quickly, and the effects are of short duration. If volume needs to be replaced, the amount should be monitored by either CVP or PAP catheters.

Most cases of distributive shock are self-limiting, and usually postural changes such as Trendelenburg or prone positions will be sufficient to return stagnant volume into the right side of the heart and maintain circulating volume.

Nutritional Requirements in Shock

Since shock is an energy-deficient disease, the need for substrates for energy production is paramount. Glucose is the principal molecule for energy formation. The cytosol, or cell sap, contains enzymes that catalyze the anaerobic metabolism of glucose intermediates; the mitochondria contain enzymes that complete the aerobic metabolism of glucose. Adenosine triphosphate, the energy molecule, is produced in the mitochondria by the electron transport system. This molecule stores the energy released by the oxidation of glucose as potential chemical energy and fuels the molecular reactions that form proteins and maintain the integrity of the cellular membrane.

Glucose can be stored in glycogen molecules in liver and muscle; however, during stress with surgical procedures, these stores are rapidly dissipated. Other molecules are needed that can be converted either to glucose or to intermediates of the energy cycles, and these are available as fats and proteins. Fats are oxidized to fatty acids and converted to the intermediates of the energy cycles, glycerol and acetyl coenzyme-A. Proteins are catabolized to glycogenic amino acids, which can also be converted to energy-cycle intermediates (Figs. 9 and 10).

There are many examples of the effect of stress on gluconeogenesis. Bacterial endotoxin administered parenterally has been shown to induce marked disturbances in carbohydrate metabolism. These disturbances appear as rapid depletion of hepatic glycogen, hypoglycemia, and an inability of the liver to synthesize glycogen and sugar from glucogenic amino and fatty acids. Endotoxemia depresses the activity of the liver enzymes responsible for gluconeogenesis. Endotoxin poisoning reduces the rate of glucose production in the liver.[16] Endotoxemia depresses lactate metabolism in the liver. Lactate is one of the main precursors of sugar production in the hepatic Cori cycle. Thus,

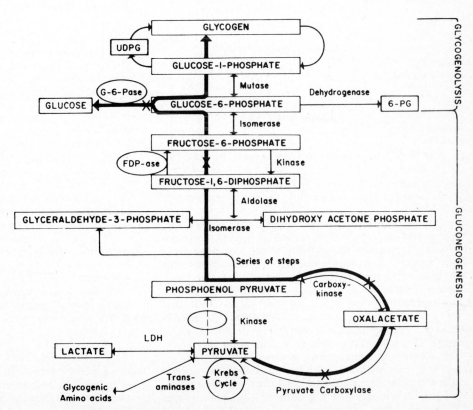

Figure 9. Normal gluconeogenic and glycogenic flux.

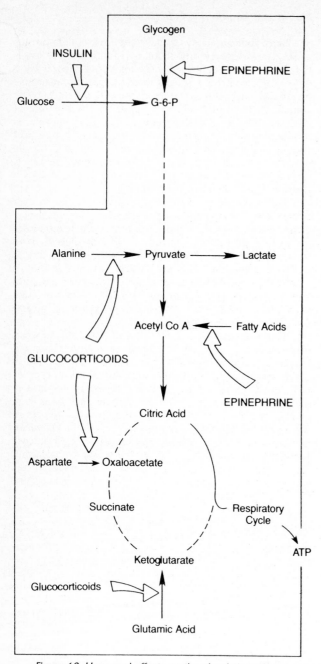

Figure 10. Hormonal effects on the glycolytic pathway.

these alterations reflect endotoxin induced changes in the level of blood glucose necessary for peripheral cellular metabolism.

Studies of Pearce et al.[21] indicate that the hypovolemic animal also undergoes a depression of hepatic gluconeogenesis. Apparently, this inability to produce sugar from gluconeogenic precursors is an essential disturbance of liver glucose metabolism in the hypovolemic and the septic animal. Thus, when the glycogen stores of liver and muscle are insufficient to supply the long-term glucose needs and the process of gluconeogenesis is inhibited, the shock-stressed organism needs an exogenous source of sugar, glycogenic amino acids, glycerol, ketones, and fatty acids. The efficacy of administering glucose as a substrate in traumatic and hypovolemic shock has been shown experimentally. Glucose protects the anoxic bowel segment, especially its mucosal function. When highly concentrated

glucose is administered to hypovolemic and traumatic shock patients, the function of vital organs, especially the heart and kidney, is improved.[9] Infusion of glucose-insulin-potassium (GIK) solution beneficially affects the anoxic and ischemic myocardium by preserving mechanical function, structure, and histology as well as ionic balance.[22] Infusing 1.5 ml. per kg. body weight per hour of GIK for a total of 48 hours alters substrate availability of glucose and changes the metabolic state from lipid to carbohydrate. The administration of ATP–magnesium chloride (ATP–MgCl$_2$) protects the animal in shock and also reinforces the concept that glucose administration is necessary to fulfill the energy requirements of the stressed organism.[2]

The beneficial effects of ATP–MgCl$_2$ infusion in experimental shock are now being studied in the human. Hirasawa et al.[13] showed some positive results with ATP–MgCl$_2$ in renal failure and sepsis in humans.[25]

Parenteral alimentation has a protein-sparing effect on the total organism. The infusion of glucose and amino acids obviates the need for endogenous protein and fat stores, resulting in decreased catabolism, more positive nitrogen balance, and less weight loss. The conservation of muscle protein allows the patient increased activity. Studies on clinical sepsis indicate that the synthesis of both acute phase and immunologic proteins decreases, and in late sepsis skin test hypersensitivity is reduced to a point of complete anergy.[18] Hyperalimentation decreases the energy deficit, increases protein synthesis, and promotes wound healing. Moreover, hyperosmotic parenteral solutions may act as osmotic diuretics during the antidiuretic phase of trauma, protecting the kidney against acute insufficiency. Fundamental defects in intermediary metabolism and energy production should be treated by nutritional support measures that address the specific biochemical defects of septic multiple organ failure.[32]

Substrates for Hyperalimentation Solutions

Glucose

There are many kinds of energy-producing molecules, but the most important component is glucose. A 6-carbon molecule, it yields a significant amount of energy when systematically oxidized. One molecular weight (1 mol.) completely degraded yields 288,800 calories (or 288.8 kcal.) to promote essential biochemical reactions. Glucose is the main energy source, but any molecule that can be transformed into the intermediates of the energy pathway is capable of producing ATP. For example, fructose, mannitol, or xylitol can be used as a glucose substitute. Not all tissues, however, can utilize these substrates. The brain does not metabolize fructose or mannitol, and the liver reacts adversely to xylitol. Glucose, therefore, remains the most desirable energy molecule.

Glucose in high concentrations requires insulin to be completely metabolized. In muscle, adipose tissue, and liver, insulin facilitates the intracellular transport of glucose and amino acids, a function that requires phosphate and potassium ions. Therefore, most hyperalimentation formulas include insulin and potassium, according to the patient's individual needs.

Amino Acids

Another component of the hyperalimentation formula is amino acid, which yields 4 calories per gram. There are two types of amino acid: (1) *nonessential*, which can be synthesized, and (2) *essential*, which cannot be synthesized in the human tissue cell. Essential amino acids include tryptophan, phenylalanine, lysine, threonine, valine, methionine, leucine, and isoleucine. Their natural structures are primarily L-forms; that is, the amine (NH_2) radical is in the levo (left) configuration. Not all amino acids can be changed into energy-cycle intermediates. Those that can be converted are referred to as *glycogenic amino acids*. This designation cannot be attributed to any particular configuration of their structure, but, interestingly, all glycogenic amino acids are of the essential type.

Of the *nonglycogenic amino acids,* histidine is usually included in amino acid infusions because after numerous reactions it can be converted to pyruvic or glutamic acid, both of which are intermediates of the energy cycles. Some essential amino acids such as leucine are *ketogenic*, since they can be converted to fatty acid structures. They contribute to the glyconeogenic scheme by augmenting the conversion of fatty acids to energy intermediates. Thus, amino acid solution provides the patient with the essential amino acids for tissue repair and adds calories for direct energy formation.

The septic process elicits mediator(s), such as glucagon, cortisol, and insulin, which induce muscle proteolysis. This increases production of branched chain amino acids (valine, leucine, and isoleucine), and aromatic amino acids (phenylalanine and tyrosine) as well as proline and sulfur amino acids. Muscle converts branched chain amino acids to their respective ketoacids for entrance into the citric acid cycle flow of substrates, where they are oxidized. The same occurs in the kidney, where alanine and glycine are used for gluconeogenesis. The protective effect of infused branched chain amino acids on muscle proteolysis is presently being studied.

VITAMINS

The third component of the hyperalimentation formula is vitamins. The vitamin B complex is essential for the proper functioning of energy pathways. The coenzyme thiamine plays an integral role in the conversion of the energy pathways from anaerobic to aerobic function. Riboflavin and nicotinic acid are integrates of the two main components of the electron transport system. Pantothenic acid in coenzyme-A is involved in the conversion of fatty acids into energy-cycle intermediates. Pyridoxine is a component of the coenzyme that either deaminates or transaminates amino acids to glucose skeletons for entrance into the energy pathways. Lipoic acid participates in the specific oxidation of pyruvate and succinate in the aerobic energy cycle. Vitamin B_{12}, or cyanocobalamin, is vital for the maturation of red blood cells and yields hydrogen ions, which are important in the formation of the specific amino acids required for the production of hemoglobin. Its deficiency results in the formation of immature red blood cells.

The role of vitamin C is unknown, but it apparently supplies both the hydrogen ions essential in the production of mature collagen and the OH^- radicals necessary for the hydroxylation of proline into hydroxyproline, an integral amino acid in collagen.

MINERALS

Several minerals are necessary for the proper functioning of the energy cycles. Potassium supports the enzymatic activity needed for protein synthesis as well as the transport of glucose across the cellular membrane. Magnesium is the catalyst for the enzymes of the glycolytic energy cycles.

Sodium and probably chloride are important ions in the maintenance of osmolarity. The trace elements copper, cobalt, manganese, zinc, and iodine are associated with important enzyme functions.[25]

Complications of Shock

The complications of shock include (1) ARDS, (2) acute renal insufficiency, and (3) disseminated intravascular coagulation (DIC).

ADULT RESPIRATORY DISTRESS SYNDROME

Adult respiratory distress syndrome can occur in any type of low-flow state and is primarily a "leaky capillary syndrome" of the pulmonary vasculature. There are two main causes of this permeability. First, excessive volume resuscitation increases hydrostatic pressure in the vasculature and forces plasma into the alveolar vascular membrane which thereby interferes with oxygen diffusion. Second, the capillary permeability may be produced by complement-induced reaction to the endotoxin in septicemia. Hypovolemia is thought to produce alveolar vascular injury resulting from cellular anoxia. Other causes of this injury include inhaled toxins such as oxygen, smoke, and erosive chemicals (ammonia, phosphogene, chlorine).[2] In addition, fat emboli and hematologic disorders, including DIC, massive blood transfusion, and prolonged cardiopulmonary bypass can produce alveolar injury.

The diagnosis of ARDS is based on a history of circulatory collapse and inadequate response of plasma oxygen tension (Po_2) to increased inspired oxygen administration (FIO_2). A Po_2 of less than 50 torr with administration of 40 per cent oxygen (FIO$_2$ 40) indicates a severe diffusion problem. The chest roentgenogram reveals confluent atelectasis, resulting from the fluid in the alveolus and inadequate surfactant production by injured Type II alveolar cells (Fig. 11*A,B*). This atelectasis and the alveolar vascular membrane edema or hyalinization produce a shunt of blood away from the collapsed alveoli and hyalinized membranes, which represents anatomic shunting (Fig. 12). A physiologic shunt occurs because perfusion of ineffective alveoli does not produce oxygen diffusion to the red cells. The direct measurement of the shunt or the use of a nomogram substantiates the diagnosis (Fig. 13). The following therapy is then instituted:

1. Insert an endotracheal tube and attach to a ventilator.
2. The ventilator should promote increased tidal volume and driving pressure to utilize non-atelectatic alveoli and promote oxygen diffusion.
3. Administer positive end-expiratory pressure or continuous positive end-expiratory pressure of 5 to 10 torr to maintain expansion of the alveoli and prevent coaptation of the alveolar walls due to the lack of surfactant.
4. Administer diuretics to maintain pulmonary wedge pressure at normal levels.
5. Infuse albumin if the colloid osmotic pressure is abnormally low.
6. Administer cardiotonics (dopamine or dobutamine) to increase cardiac output and maintain wedge pressure.
7. Administer antibiotics if sputum culture is positive.

ACUTE RENAL FAILURE

Acute renal failure results from hypovolemia (low flow in the glomeruli), which produces anoxia to the nephric

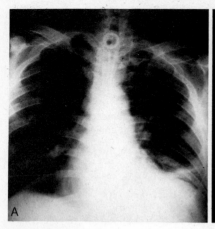
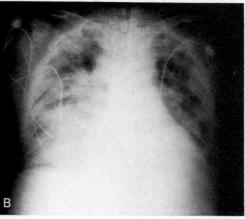

Figure 11. Chest roentgenogram in adult respiratory distress syndrome (ARDS). A, Before ARDS, B, After ARDS.

tubules and deranges the nephron cells. The insult may be endotoxic (septic shock), myoglobic (traumatized muscle), or acidotic. Aminoglycoside antibiotics and fluorine anesthetics are nephrotoxins that may cause acute renal insufficiency.

The recognition of early renal failure is based on decreased glomerular filtration rate producing oliguria. Urinary volume less than 350 ml. per day with a history of low-flow state should alert the observer to impending renal insufficiency. Further urine studies confirm the diagnosis. Urine sediment shows tubular, granular, or red cell casts. The most important diagnostic finding is the inability of the tubular cells to concentrate or dilute urine. The ratio of urine osmolality to plasma osmolality is normally 3, but in acute renal insufficiency it is less than 1.1. Creatinine clearance normally is 125 ml. per minute, but in acute renal failure it is less than 30 ml. per minute and can be as low as 2 ml. per minute. As the pathologic process continues, acidosis, hyperkalemia, and uremia ensue.

Treatment consists of both prophylactic and active phases. In the prophylactic phase, urinary output is measured hourly by a urinary catheter and should be maintained at 50 to 75 ml. per hour. If the urinary output falls below 30 ml. per hour, 500 ml. of Ringer's solution is infused because most acute renal insufficiency of circulatory shock is prerenal as a result of hypovolemia. If there is no increase in urinary output, 12.5 gm. of mannitol is infused. Thereafter, furosemide, up to a total of 2 gm., is infused, either in divided doses or continuously. If still no salutary effect is noted, a diagnosis of renal failure is established and the active treatment of renal failure is instituted. The treatment

consists of peritoneal dialysis or hemodialysis, renal hyperalimentation, and water administration, depending on the urinary output. Hyperkalemia and acidosis are controlled by potassium-absorbing resins and hemodialysis.

DISSEMINATED INTRAVASCULAR COAGULATION

Disseminated intravascular coagulation is a pathologic syndrome occurring as a complication of all types of circulatory shock. The syndrome can be classified into three phases: (1) consumption coagulopathy, (2) primary fibrinolysin coagulopathy, and (3) dilutional coagulopathy.

The pathophysiology of DIC is an abnormal reaction of the fibrinolytic system that controls the clotting of blood. When bleeding is excessive, the production of thrombin is markedly increased and thrombin potentiates the coagulation cascade. Most of these coagulation proteins and also thrombin are synthesized in the liver. If liver function is depressed, as it is in circulatory shock, the production of these clotting proteins cannot keep pace with consumption, and this results in consumption coagulopathy.

In addition to thrombin excess, the fibrinolytic cascade also is abnormally stimulated. The Hageman factor is markedly activated by endotoxin in septic shock, resulting in the conversion of plasminogen to plasmin, a potent

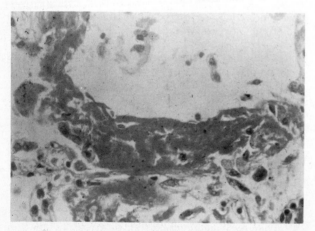

Figure 12. Hyalinization of the alveolar membrane.

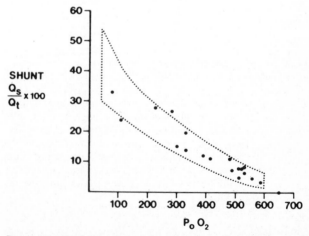

Figure 13. Shunt fraction versus oxygenation on 100 per cent oxygen. (Adapted from Moore, F. D.: Homeostasis: Bodily changes in trauma and surgery: The responses to injury in man as the basis for clinical management. In Sabiston, D. C., Jr. (Ed.): Davis-Christopher Textbook of Surgery. Philadelphia, W. B. Saunders Company, 1981, p. 40.)

TABLE 4. Treatment of Disseminated Intravascular Coagulation

	Platelets 6 U/M²	Vit K 5–10 mg. IV	FFP 10–15 ml./kg.	CryoPPT 4 U/10 kg.	Heparin 100 U/kg. q 4 hr. IV
Normotensive	±	±	±	0	0
Hypotensive					
Blood pressure restorable	±	±	±	±	0
Blood pressure not restorable	±	±	+	+	+
Bleeding	+	±	+	+	+
Not bleeding	0	±	0	0	±

Abbreviations: FFP = Fresh frozen plasma; IV = intravenous; CryoPPT = cryoprecipitate; + = recommended; 0 = not recommended; ± = dependent on platelet count or fibrinogen levels.

proteolytic enzyme capable of catabolizing fibrin. This lysing of fibrin produces further bleeding.

Another type of DIC resulting from the use of packed cells without plasma in resuscitation during hemorrhagic hypovolemic shock is dilutional coagulopathy. Platelets, clotting proteins, and calcium are not being replaced and are markedly decreased. Packed red cell transfusions utilizing balanced salt solutions as the vehicle further dilute platelets and clotting proteins. The syndrome may also be the result of sensitivity to heparin.

Diagnosis of DIC is based on findings of abnormal prothrombin time, thrombocytopenia, and fibrinogenopenia. Confirmatory tests include increased fibrin split products, increased thrombin time in 60 per cent of the cases, and decreased antithrombin III.

The pathologic effects of DIC are multisystemic, i.e., renal cortical necrosis, pulmonary edema, pancreatitis, myositis, gastrointestinal hemorrhage, hepatic failure, and cerebral manifestations (seizures). Treatment includes the judicious use of platelets, fibrinogen, and heparin to counteract thrombin activation of the clotting cascade and fresh frozen plasma to replace clotting factors. Aminocaproic acid is not effective as a plasmin inhibitor in clinical DIC (Table 4).

SELECTED REFERENCES

Axelrod, J., and Reisine, T. D.: Stress hormones: Their interaction and regulation. Science, *224*:452, 1984.
Stress stimulates several adaptive hormonal responses. Prominent among these responses are the secretion of catecholamines from the adrenal medulla, corticosteroids from the adrenal cortex, and adrenocorticotropin from the anterior pituitary. A number of complex interactions are involved in the regulation of these hormones. Glucocorticoids regulate catecholamine biosynthesis in the adrenal medulla and catecholamines stimulate adrenocorticotropin release from the anterior pituitary. In addition, other hormones, including corticotropin-releasing factor, vasoactive intestinal peptide, and arginine vasopressin stimulate, whereas the corticosteroids and somatostatin inhibit adrenocorticotropin secretion. Together, these agents appear to determine the complex physiologic responses to a variety of stressors.

Baue, A. E., and Chaudry, I. H.: Prevention of multiple systems failure. Surg. Clin. North Am., *60*:1167, 1980.
This classic paper describes the multiple systems failure syndrome and the proper treatment for its prevention.

Green, H. D., Bond, R. F., Rapela, C. E., Schmid, H. E., Manley, E., and Farrar, D. J.: Competition Between Intrinsic and Extrinsic Controls of Resistance Vessels of Major Vascular Beds During Hemorrhagic Hypotension and Shock. *In* Lefer, K. M., Saba, T. M., and Mela, L. M. (Eds.): Advances in Shock Research, Vol. 3. New York, Alan R. Liss, Inc., 1980, p. 77.
Systemic hemorrhagic hypotension activates extrinsic constrictor mechanisms that intensify the passive increase in vascular resistance in skin and overpower the intrinsic autoregulatory vasodilation in all active beds except those of the brain and heart, which are effectively protected from extrinsic control. This extrinsic constriction appears to be mediated principally by circulating catecholamine constrictor substances in skin, but probably involves both humoral and neural control mechanisms in the renal, mesenteric, hepatic and skeletal muscle beds. The neural mechanisms appear to be predominant in skeletal muscle.

MacLean, L. D., Duff, J. H., Scott, H. M., and Peretz, D. I.: Treatment of shock in man based on hemodynamic diagnosis. Surg. Gynecol. Obstet., *120*:1, 1965.
This report presents detailed hemodynamic studies from 20 patients with various types of shock. Two patterns were recognized: (1) hypovolemic shock, with low cardiac output, low central venous pressure, low blood pressure, and elevated arterial blood lactate that responded to inotropic and chronotropic stimulation of the heart by isoproterenol, and (2) septic shock. Emphasis is placed on establishing a hemodynamic diagnosis in all patients in shock before treatment is initiated.

Moore, F. D.: The effects of hemorrhage on body composition. N. Engl. J. Med., *273*:567, 1965.
A classic description of changes in body composition in man with venous hemorrhage of 500 to 1000 ml. Concepts and quantitation of plasma volume refill are introduced. Simultaneous movement of salt and water out of the circulation and albumin into the circulation in response to infusion of saline is noted, and its significance is discussed in terms of the microcirculation and therapy.

Schuler, J. J., Erve, P. R., and Schumer, W.: Glucocorticoid effect on hepatic carbohydrate metabolism in the endotoxin-shocked monkey. Ann. Surg., *183*:345, 1976.
This study describes the effect of glucocorticoid treatment on survival, on hepatic carbohydrate metabolism, and on levels of hepatic adenine nucleotides in the endotoxin-shocked monkey. Dexamethasone sodium phosphate (DMP) administered either at the time of endotoxin challenge or up to 90 minutes afterward significantly increased the survival rate. Endotoxin administered alone caused profound hypoglycemia and lacticacidemia, which were alleviated by the administration of DMP. Endotoxin administered alone significantly decreased the hepatic levels of glucose-6-phosphate (G6P), fructose-6-phosphate (F6P), phosphoenolpyruvate (PEP), adenosine triphosphate (ATP), adenosine diphosphate (ADP), and glycogen; and it significantly increased the hepatic levels of fructose-1,6-diphosphate, lactate, and adenosine monophosphate (AMP). The administration of DMP at the time of endotoxin challenge maintained the levels of all these metabolites at or near the control levels.

Shires, G. T., Carrico, C. J., and Canizaro, P. C.: Shock. Philadelphia, W. B. Saunders Company, 1973.
In this monograph, the clinical manifestations of shock, the physiologic responses, especially of fluid and electrolyte shifts, and pulmonary and kidney function are reviewed. The cellular response to shock with direct measurements of changes in active transport of ions, which has been the basis for the use of larger quantities of crystalloid solution for resuscitation, is herein carefully documented.

Skillman, J. J., Lauler, D. P., Hickler, R. B., Lyone, J. H., Olson, J. E., Ball, M. R., and Moore, F. D.: Hemorrhage in normal man: Effect on renin, cortisol, aldosterone, and urine composition. Ann. Surg., *166*:865, 1967.
The effect of hemorrhage on the stimulation of aldosterone, renin, and cortisol has been recorded in 11 normal healthy male volunteers. Hemodynamic changes have been correlated with the changes in hormone production, and individual variations have been noted.

REFERENCES

1. Barzilai, A. H., Schiessel, R., Kivilaakso, E., and Silen, W.: Ulceration of rabbit antral mucosa. Surg. Forum, *30*:9, 1979.
2. Baue, A. E., and Chaudry, I. H.: Prevention of multiple system failure. Surg. Clin. North Am., *60*:1167, 1980.
3. Bernard, C.: An Introduction to the Study of Experimental Medicine. New York, The Macmillan Company, 1927.

4. Bessey, P. Q., Watters, J. M., Aoki, T. T., and Wilmore, D. W.: Combined hormonal infusion simulates the metabolic response to injury. Ann. Surg., *200*:264, 1984.

5. Broder, G., and Weil, M. H.: Excess lactate: An index of reversibility of shock in human patients. Science, *143*:1457, 1964.

6. Cannon, W. B.: A consideration of the nature of wound shock. J.A.M.A., *70*:611, 1918.

7. Clowes, G. H. A., Jr.: Pulmonary abnormalities in sepsis. Surg. Clin. North Am., *54*:993, 1974.

8. Darwin, C.: On the Origin of the Species by Means of Natural Selection, or, the Preservation of Favoured Races in the Struggle for Life. London, John Murray, 1859.

9. Drucker, M. R., Pindyck, F., Brown, R. S., Elwyn, D. H., and Shoemaker, W. C.: The interaction of glucagon and glucose on cardiorespiratory variables in the critically ill patient. Surgery, *75*:487, 1974.

10. Dudrick, S. J., Steiger, E., and Long, J. M.: Renal failure in surgical patients: Treatment with intravenous essential amino acids and hypertonic glucose. Surgery, *68*:180, 1979.

11. Green, H. D., Bond, R. F., Rapela, C. E., Schmid, H. E., Manley, E., and Farrar, D. J.: Competition between intrinsic and extrinsic controls of resistance vessels of major vascular beds during hemorrhagic hypotension and shock. *In* Lefer, A. M., Saba, T. M., and Mela, L. M. (Eds.): Advances in Shock Research, vol. 3. New York, Alan R. Liss, Inc., 1980, p. 77.

12. Henderson, L. J.: Blood: A Study in General Physiology. New Haven, Conn., Yale University, 1928.

13. Hirasawa, H., Kobayashi, H., Tabata, Y., Soeda, K., Ohtake, Y., Oda, S., Kobayashi, S., Murotani, N., Odaka, M., and Sato, H: Effect of ATP-MgCl$_2$ administration on renal function and renal cellular metabolism following renal ischemia. Circ. Shock, *11*:141, 1983.

14. Hunter, J.: A Treatise on the Blood, Inflammation, and Gun-shot Wounds. London, John Richardson, 1974, p. 6.

15. Kinney, J. M.: A consideration of energy exchange in human trauma. Bull. N.Y. Acad. Med., *36*:617, 1960.

16. LaNoue, K. F., Mason, A. D., Jr., and Daniels, J. P.: The impairment of gluconeogenesis by gram-negative infection. Metabolism, *17*:606, 1968.

17. Lefer, A. M., and Barenholz, Y.: Pancreatic hydrolases and the formation of a myocardial depressant factor in shock. Am. J. Physiol., *233*:1103, 1972.

18. McLean, A. P. H., and Meakins, J. L.: Nutritional support in sepsis. Surg. Clin. North Am., *61*:681, 1981.

19. Moore, F. D.: Metabolic Care of the Surgical Patient. Philadelphia, W. B. Saunders Company, 1959.

20. Moore, F. D., Olesen, K. H., McMurrey, J. D., Parker, H. V., Ball, M. R., and Boyden, C. M. (Eds.): The Body Cell Mass and Its Supporting Environment: Body Composition in Health and Disease. Philadelphia, W. B. Saunders Company, 1963.

21. Pearce, F. J., Weiss, P. R., Miller, J. R., and Drucker, W. R.: Effect of hemorrhage and anoxia on hepatic gluconeogenesis and potassium balance in the rat. J. Trauma, *23*:312, 1983.

22. Rackley, C. E., Russel, R. O., Rogers, W. J., Mantle, J. A., McDaniel, H. G., and Papapietro, S. E.: Glucose-insulin-potassium administration in acute myocardial infarction. *In* Greger, W. P., Coggins, C. H., Hancock, E. W. (Eds.): Annual Review of Medicine, vol. 33. Palo Alto, Calif., Annual Reviews, Inc., 1982, p. 375.

23. Schuler, J. J., Erve, P. R, and Schumer, W.: Glucocorticoid effect on hepatic carbohydrate metabolism in the endotoxin-shocked monkey. Ann. Surg., *183*:345, 1976.

24. Schumer, W.: Lactic acid as a factor in the production of irreversibility in oligohaemic shock. Nature, *212*:1210, 1966.

25. Schumer, W., and Nyhus, L. M.: Nutritional requirements in shock: Liver metabolism. *In* Schumer, W., and Nyhus, L. M. (Eds.): Treatment of Shock. Philadelphia, Lea & Febiger, 1974.

26. Schumer, W.: Steroids in the treatment of clinical septic shock. Ann. Surg., *184*:333, 1976.

27. Schumer, W.: Hypovolemic Shock. J.A.M.A., *241*:615, 1979.

28. Schumer, W.: Septic shock. J.A.M.A., *242*:1906, 1979.

29. Schumer, W.: Overall cell metabolism. *In* Lefer, A. M., and Schumer, W. (Eds.): Molecular and Cellular Aspects of Shock and Trauma: Progress in Clinical and Biological Research. New York, Alan R. Liss, Inc., 1983, p. 472.

30. Selye, H.: Thrombohemorrhagic Phenomena. Springfield, Ill., Charles C Thomas, 1966, p. 9.

31. Shires, G. T., Canizaro, P. C., and Carrico, J.: Shock. *In* Schwartz, S. I., Shires, G. T., Spencer, F. C., and Storer, E. H. (Eds.): Principles of Surgery, 3rd ed. New York, McGraw-Hill, 1979, p. 135.

32. Siegel, J. H.: Relations between circulatory and metabolic changes in sepsis. *In* Greger, W. P., Coggins, C. H., and Hancock, E. W. (Eds.): Annual Review of Medicine, vol 32. Palo Alto, Calif., Annual Reviews, Inc., 1981, p. 175.

33. Skillman, J. J., Lauler, D. P., Hickler, R. B., et al.: Hemorrhage in normal man: Effect on renin, cortisol, aldosterone, and urine composition. Ann. Surg., *166*:865, 1967.

34. Yates, A. J. P., Schumer, W., Holtzman, S. F., and Kuttner, R. E.: Endotoxin role in peritonitis septic shock in rats. *In* Schumer, W., Spitzer, J. J., and Marshall, B. E. (Eds.): Advances in Shock Research, vol. 4. New York, Alan R. Liss, Inc., 1980, p. 63.

FLUID AND ELECTROLYTE MANAGEMENT

DONALD S. GANN, M.D. • JOSEPH F. AMARAL, M.D.

3

PHYSIOLOGY OF FLUIDS AND ELECTROLYTES

With its unique and complex physical properties, water is essential to almost all physiologic processes. The physicochemical characteristics that make water extremely important include its extensive hydrogen-bonding capacity, high dipole moment, highly organized structure, high boiling and freezing points, and high specific heat.[15] These properties derive from the distribution of electrons in a water molecule, the hydrogen ions having a slightly positive charge and the oxygen ion, with its lone pair of electrons, having a negative charge. This polarity allows extensive hydrogen bonding and a high dipole moment. In addition, this electron structure makes water weakly dissociable into hydrogen and hydroxyl ions.

The extensive hydrogen-bonding capacity of water molecules allows orientation in a highly organized structure similar to that of ice.[15] Because a large amount of heat is required to raise the temperature of water by 1°C. (specific heat), a considerable amount of energy is lost as water evaporates (perspiration). Thus, the extensive hydrogen bonding allows water to exert a major role in temperature regulation. It also renders water important in establishing the tertiary structure of macromolecules (such as proteins and nucleic acids) and in organizing amphoteric molecules with polar and nonpolar ends (such as lipids) into micelles.

The high dipole moment of water molecules causes orientation in an external electric field in such a way that they act as an electric buffer.[15] When ionic substances are placed in water, the water molecules form a hydrational shell around the individual ions and thereby reduce the electrochemical attraction between ions.[15] Therefore, water keeps electrolytes in solution and allows them independent motion. In addition, this property is important in nutrient transport and in partitioning substances in the various tissue compartments.

Distribution of Body Fluids

The total body water in man is divisible into two main components: the *extracellular water* (ECW) space, com-

posed of all water that is outside of cells, and the *intracellular water* (ICW) space, composed of all water that is inside cells. These compartments are separated by cell membranes with varying permeabilities. This separation results in differing ionic compositions within each compartment and also makes the measurement of component spaces of body water possible. The measurement of the size of the body fluid compartments can be determined by the *dilution principle*. This principle is based upon the concept that a substance that distributes itself equally and exclusively within a given fluid compartment can be used to determine the volume of that compartment (Fig. 1). Because

$$\text{Concentration} = \text{amount/volume} \qquad (1)$$

if a known amount of a substance not normally present in the body is injected into the blood, its concentration at steady state will be related to the volume of the compartment by the relationship:

$$\text{Volume} = (\text{amount injected} - \text{amount excreted})/ \atop \text{concentration at steady state} \qquad (2)$$

Since the amount excreted is usually negligible,

$$\text{Volume} = \text{amount injected/steady state concentration} \qquad (3)$$

A variety of substances that allow measurement of the various fluid compartments using the dilution technique have been recognized (Fig. 2). Of all the compartments, total body water (TBW) is the most accurately measured. In contrast, the intracellular water cannot be measured using these techniques directly because no substance is known to exclusively distribute itself in the intracellular space. As a result, intracellular water is estimated as the difference between total body water and extracellular water.

TOTAL BODY WATER

All fluid compartments in the body vary with age, sex, body build, physical activity, disease, and state of hydration. Total body water is measured using deuterium oxide or tritiated water. In the healthy adult male, TBW occupies 60 per cent of the body weight; in a healthy adult female,

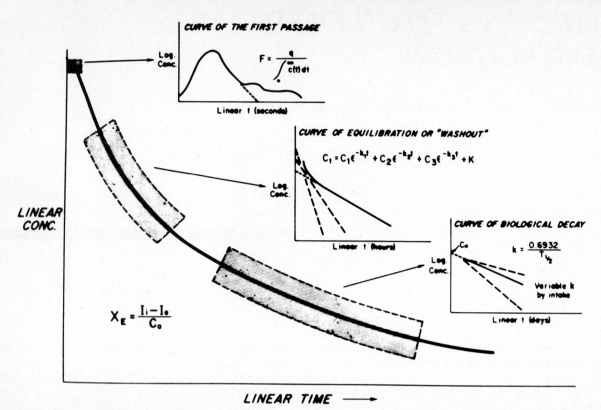

Figure 1. The isotope dilution principle. A stylized curve is shown for the dilution of an ion in body water components followed over time. The curve is divided into three approximate portions. The first is the "first pass" through heart and lungs and represents the formulation used for cardiac output measurements. The second declining slope (of variable pitch according to the element) represents the sum of a series of slopes, determined by rate-limiting membranes and flux rates. The final portion of the curve is a single exponential representing the biologic half-time of the element in the body. Mathematical formulations are shown for each portion of the curve. (From Moore, F. D.: J. Parenteral Enteral Nutrition, 4:227, 1980.)

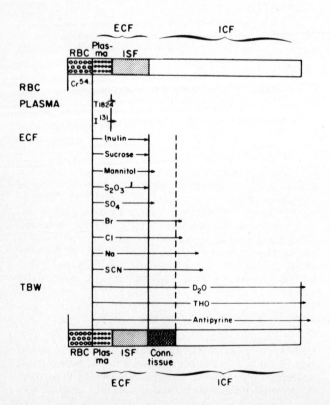

Figure 2. Substances used to measure the body fluid compartments. (From Winters, R. W.: Regulation of normal water and electrolyte metabolism. In The Body Fluids in Pediatrics. Boston, Little, Brown and Company, 1973, p. 97.)

TABLE 1. Total Body Water as a Function of Age and Sex*

| Age | Body Water (% Body Weight) | |
	Male	Female
0–1 day	79	
1–30 days	75.7	
1–12 months	64.5	
1–10 years	61.7	
10–16 years	58.9	57.3
17–39 years	60.6	50.2
40–59 years	54.7	46.7
60+ years	51.5	45.5

*Data obtained from Edelman, I. S., and Leibman, J.: Am. J. Med., 27:256, 1959; and Friis-Hansen, B.: Pediatrics, 28:169, 1961.

it occupies 50 per cent (Table 1). Adipose tissue contains very little intracellular water, whereas skeletal muscle has one of the largest water contents of all tissues (Table 2). Consequently, females with a larger adipose mass and smaller muscle mass than males have less TBW. Similarly, the TBW of athletic individuals is greater than that of nonathletic individuals, the TBW of the young is greater than that of the elderly, and the TBW of lean individuals is greater than that of obese individuals (Fig. 3). These changes also hold true for the ECW and the ICW compartments.

Total body water as a percentage of body weight decreases steadily with age (Table 1). Newborn infants have the highest percentage of water, with 75 to 80 per cent of body weight representing water. During the first few months after birth, this percentage decreases in both males and females to 65 per cent. The percentage of total body water remains at 65 per cent in both boys and girls until puberty, when adult patterns emerge. During advancing age, TBW decreases to 52 per cent in males and 47 per cent in females. This results from a decrease in intracellular water that is associated with a decrease in muscle mass.

EXTRACELLULAR WATER

Many substances are available to measure the volume of the extracellular water, and the calculated size of this compartment depends in part upon the method of determination used. Measurement of the ECW with *large* molecules such as insulin, mannitol, or sucrose appears to underestimate the size of the ECW compartment because of the slower diffusion of large molecules into noncellular

TABLE 2. Distribution of Water in the Tissues of a 70-kg. Man*

	Water (%)	Body Weight (%)	Liters of Water in 70 kg.
Skin	72	18	9.07
Muscle	72.6	41.7	22.10
Skeleton	22	15.9	2.45
Brain	74.8	2.0	1.05
Liver	68.3	2.3	1.03
Heart	79.2	0.5	0.28
Lungs	79.0	0.7	0.39
Kidneys	82.7	0.4	0.25
Spleen	75.8	0.2	0.10
Blood	83.0	8.0	4.65
Intestine	74.5	1.0	0.94
Adipose tissue	10.0	±10.0	0.70

*From Skeleton, H.: Arch. Intern. Med., 40:140, 1927.

spaces. Extracellular water space of 15 to 17 per cent of body weight is usually reported with these methods.[15] Measurement of the ECW with small molecules such as $^{35}SO_4$, ^{82}BR, and ^{24}Na appears to overestimate the ECW compartment because of the ability of these molecules to diffuse into cells. An extracellular water space of 21 to 27 per cent of body weight is usually reported when these methods are used.[15] In general, ECW is considered to occupy 20 per cent of the body weight and 40 per cent of the TBW.

The extracellular water is divisible into *plasma* and *interstitial fluid* (ISF). The plasma volume (PV) can be measured by using Evan's blue dye or radioiodinated albumin. It occupies approximately 5 to 6 per cent of the body weight and 20 per cent of the extracellular fluid volume. The plasma volume is not equivalent to the blood volume, which is the sum of the plasma volume and the red cell mass (RCM). The red cell mass can be determined by using chromium-, iron-, and phosphorus-labeled red blood cells (RBC). It comprises approximately 3 per cent of the body weight in males and 2 per cent in females. The total blood volume (TBV) may be calculated either by adding the independently determined RBC mass and plasma volume or by measuring the venous hematocrit (VH) and one of the two components of blood volume.

$$TBV = \frac{RCM}{VH} \times 100 = \frac{PV}{100 - VH} \times 100 \qquad (4)$$

The blood volume comprises approximately 8 per cent of the body weight in males and 7 per cent in females.

The ISF compartment comprises approximately 15 per cent of the body weight and 80 per cent of the ECW. It is composed of a rapidly equilibrating functional space between cells and capillary membranes, and of a slowly or

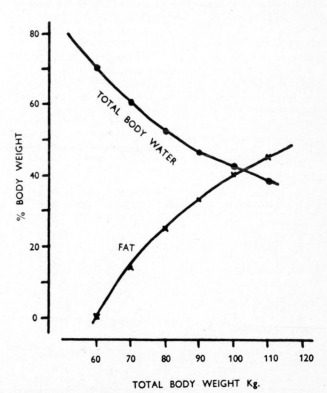

Figure 3. The inverse relationship between total body water and total body fat. (From Wilkinson, A. W.: Body Fluids in Surgery, 4th ed. New York, Churchill Livingstone, 1973, p. 5.)

non-equilibrating space made up of epithelial secretions, connective tissue water, joint space fluids, and cerebrospinal fluids (CSF), the "transcellular fluids." It should be noted that the transcellular space is not equivalent to the "third space." (See "Fluid and Electrolyte Balance: Intake Equals Output" later in this chapter.) The functional ISF comprises 90 per cent of the total ISF, and the transcellular space accounts for 10 per cent of the total ISF.

Intracellular Water

Since intracellular water can be estimated only as the difference between TBW and ECW, the ICW is the least accurately measured space. In normal adults, it constitutes approximately 30 to 40 per cent of the body weight (BW) and 55 to 60 per cent of the TBW. As noted previously, the greater the amount of adipose tissue, the smaller the size of the ICW.

In summary, the TBW in a 70-kg. adult male represents about 42 liters of water (60 per cent BW). The ECW consists of 14 liters (20 per cent BW) and the ICW of 28 liters (40 per cent BW). The total blood volume is equivalent to 6 liters (8 per cent BW) of which 2.0 liters is red cell mass (3 per cent BW) and 4 liters is plasma volume (5 per cent BW). The ISF volume is equivalent to 10.5 liters (15 per cent BW), of which 9.5 liters is functional and 1 liter is transcellular.

Electrolyte Composition of Fluid Compartments

The electrolytes in the body vary from the simple inorganic salts of sodium, potassium, calcium, and magnesium to complex organic molecules. Like water, these substances dissociate into negatively charged ions (anions) and positively charged ions (cations). The major cations are *sodium* and *potassium*, and the major anions are *chloride* and *bicarbonate*. Although the absolute amount of a particular ion in the body can be measured only by analysis of cadavers, the total exchangeable amount of an ion can be measured by using the dilution principle. The total exchangeable amount of an ion represents that portion of the total amount that is available for exchange and equilibration with a labeled form of the compound. With

sodium, total exchangeable sodium is not equivalent to total body sodium because a large amount, approximately 1000 mEq., is present in a non-exchangeable form. In contrast, total exchangeable potassium and total body potassium are equivalent because nearly all of the body potassium is exchangeable (less than 0.5 per cent is non-exchangeable).

With the variation in the permeabilities and active transport mechanisms present in the cell membranes that separate the fluid compartments, the various fluid spaces have differing ionic compositions. Sodium is the major *extracellular cation*, and potassium is the major *intracellular cation* (Table 3). Similarly, chloride and bicarbonate are the major *extracellular anions*, whereas inorganic and organic phosphates and proteins are the major *intracellular anions*. Because of these dominant relationships, the ECW is related directly to the total body sodium (or exchangeable sodium, Na_e), the ICW is related directly to the total body potassium (or exchangeable potassium, K_e), and the total body water is related directly to the sum of the total body sodium and the total body potassium.

$$\frac{Na_e}{ECW} = \frac{K_e}{ICW} \qquad (5)$$

Within a specific fluid compartment, the sum of the cations must equal the sum of the anions (the principle of *electrical neutrality*). In addition to easily measured ions, such as sodium, potassium, and chloride, the contribution of proteins must also be considered. At physiologic pH, proteins exist as anions. With plasma, proteins contribute 10 mEq. of anions per liter of plasma. Consequently, in plasma, the sum of chloride and bicarbonate plus 10 is equal to sodium ± 3 mEq. per liter. (The contributions of potassium, magnesium, and calcium are small enough that they need not be considered.)

In contrast, the concentrations of a particular ion, across two fluid compartments, need not be the same and electrical neutrality need not be maintained. This results from the differing permeabilities in cell membranes. In the case of the ISF and plasma, electrical neutrality is maintained across the capillary membranes but the concentrations of ions on either side of the capillary membranes are different. This occurs because the capillary membrane is

TABLE 3. *Electrolyte Composition of Body Fluid Compartments**

Electrolytes	Serum (mEq./liter)	Serum Water (mEq./liter)	Interstitial Fluid (mEq./liter)	Intracellular Fluid (Muscle) (mEq./liter kg. H_2O)	Total Body Content (mEq./kg.)	Total Exchangeable (mEq./kg.)
Cations						
Sodium (Na^+)	142	152.7	145	± 10	58	41.0
Potassium (K^+)	4	4.3	4	156	53.8	52.8
Calcium (Ca^{2+})	5	5.4		3.3	900	
Magnesium (Mg^{2+})	2	2.2		26	30.0	10
Total cations	153	165	149	195		
Anions						
Chloride (Cl^-)	102	109.7	114	± 2	33	33
Bicarbonate (HCO_3)	26	28	31	± 8	12.7	12.7
Phosphate (HPO_4)	2	2.2		95	576	
Sulfate (SO_4)	1	1.1		20		
Organic acids	6	6.5				
Protein	16	17.2		55		
Total anions	153	165	145	180+		

*Adapted from: Maxwell, M. H., Kleeman, C. R. Clinical Disorders of Fluid and Electrolyte Metabolism, 3rd ed. New York, McGraw-Hill, 1980, Chapters 1 and 8; Ruch, T. C., and Patton, H. D. Physiology and Biophysics, vol 2. Philadelphia, W. B. Saunders Company, 1974, p. 460; and Edelman, I. S., and Leibman, J.: Am. J. Med., 27:259, 1959.

INITIAL　　**EQUILIBRIUM**

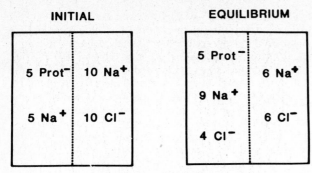

Figure 4. Gibbs-Donnan equilibrium.

freely permeable to all ions except proteins. Since proteins cannot enter the interstitial space from the plasma, more nonprotein anions must be present in the ISF than in the plasma. This creates a concentration gradient fostering the movement of diffusible anions out of the interstitium. Because cations must follow, the rise in plasma cation concentration fosters the movements of cations back into the interstitium along with diffusible anions. Eventually, an equilibrium is reached (*Gibbs-Donnan equilibrium*) in which the concentrations of cations in the plasma are increased and the concentrations of diffusible anions in the plasma are decreased (Fig. 4).

The status across cell membranes is more complex because a large differential in ionic composition is generated by the selective permeabilities and transport properties of these membranes. Although electrical neutrality is maintained within the ISF and within the ICW, an electrical potential difference is generated across cell membranes. In skeletal muscle cells, the membrane potential is approximately −90 millivolts (mV); in nerve cells, it is approximately −79 mV; and in liver cells, it is approximately −50 mV.[14] The electrical potential generated fosters the movement of cations into, and anions out of, the cell. In contrast, the concentration gradients foster movement of sodium and chloride into the cell and movement of potassium out of the cell. Since movement of chloride and potassium across cell membranes is faster than the movement of sodium, and since the major diffusible anions in the cell are chloride and sodium bicarbonate, sodium increases in the cell and potassium decreases. To maintain electrical neutrality within the cell, sodium must be pumped out of the cell and potassium into the cell. This is accomplished through the plasma membrane–bound, magnesium-dependent Na⁺–K⁺ ATPases that pump three sodium ions out in exchange for two potassium ions.[15]

Movement of Water between Intracellular and Extracellular Water: Osmosis

Cell membranes are freely permeable to water, so that the amount of water in a given compartment is determined by the number of osmotically active particles restricted to that compartment. Since osmotic forces move water from the area of lower *osmolality* to the area of higher osmolality, extracellular osmolality and intracellular osmolality must be equal (Fig. 5). Accordingly, *osmosis* is the major force establishing the water volume of the intracellular compartment. Thus, when the osmolality of the ECW decreases (e.g., loss of sodium), water moves into cells. Eventually, a new equilibrium is attained in which the osmolality is decreased and equal across all fluid compartments. The converse is also true for increases in the osmolality of a

specific compartment. It is important to realize that the osmolality between the ECW and the ICW is equalized by the movement of *water* and not by the movement of *solute*, since the cell membranes are impermeable to osmotically active solutes. Thus, if sodium without water is added to the ECW, the osmolality of both the ECW and ICW increases as water moves from the ICW to the ECW because the cell membrane is relatively impermeable to sodium. In contrast, solute can pass freely across the capillary membranes. Thus, the osmolality of the plasma and the osmolality of the ISF are equalized by the movement of both solute and water.

The *osmolarity* of a solution is the number of particles present per liter of water (mOsm. per liter). However, only 93 per cent of the plasma volume is water.[15] In addition, all of the solutes in the plasma may not be dissociated completely. Therefore, the osmolarity of a solution does not equal the effective solute or osmolality. The plasma osmolality is expressed as mOsm. per kg. of water and is measured by freezing point depression. The plasma osmolality can also be estimated from the concentration of the individual solutes in plasma. The main osmotic agents in the plasma are salts, glucose, and urea. Sodium chloride dissociates into 1.75 osmotically active particles in plasma water. Since plasma is 93 per cent water, the concentration of sodium salts to plasma osmolality is:

$$(1.75/0.93) \times [Na^+]p = 1.88[Na^+]p \qquad (6)$$

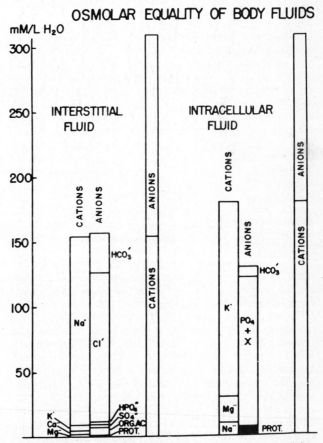

Figure 5. Gamblegram comparing the intracellular and extracellular osmolalities. As a result of the Gibbs-Donan equilibrium, the total amounts of cations and anions are different in each compartment and the total amounts of ions are the same in each compartment as a result of osmotic equilibrium. (From Gamble, J. L.: Chemical Anatomy, Physiology, and Pathology of Extracellular Fluid. Cambridge, Mass., Harvard University Press, 1964.)

The osmolal contribution of all the other salts in plasma is approximately 17 mOsm. per kg., which fortuitously equals $0.12[Na^+]p$.[24] Thus:

$$\text{Osmolality of plasma salts} = 1.88\,[Na^+]p + 0.12[Na^+]p = 2[Na^+]p \qquad (7)$$

Since glucose normally accounts for less than 5 mOsm. per kg. and urea is an ineffective osmotic solute because it readily diffuses across cell membranes, the effective plasma osmolality is closely approximated by the osmolality of plasma salts, i.e., $2[N2^+]p$. However, during hyperglycemia or uremia the contribution of glucose and urea to the effective plasma osmolality must also be considered. Glucose and urea are nondissociable molecules. Therefore, their osmotic contribution is equivalent to their molarity. Since both solutes are usually reported as milligrams per deciliter, they must first be converted to milligrams per liter. The total plasma osmolality is:

$$\text{Plasma osmolality} = 2[Na^+]p + \frac{[\text{glucose}]p \times 10}{180} + \frac{BUN \times 10}{28} \qquad (8)$$

$$= 2[Na^+]p + \frac{[\text{glucose}]p}{18} + \frac{BUN}{2.8} \qquad (9)$$

where BUN = blood urea nitrogen.

The osmolality of body fluids is well regulated by the neuroendocrine system and kidney (described later) within the range of 275 to 290 mOsm. per kg. A high osmolality implies either retention of sodium or loss of free water. Conversely, a low osmolality implies either retention of free water or loss of sodium. A loss of potassium can also lead to hypo-osmolality. As plasma concentrations of potassium decrease, a concentration gradient occurs, favoring the movement of potassium out of cells in exchange for sodium (electrical neutrality must be maintained within each compartment). Thus, hyponatremia and hypo-osmolality ensue. However, an excessive intake of potassium, even in the absence of potassium excretion, cannot lead to hyperosmolality because elevated potassium concentrations are toxic to cells and result in death before a significant alteration in osmolality occurs.[24]

Movement of Water and Solutes from the Plasma to Cells: Hydrostatic and Oncotic Pressure

Water movement between the plasma and the ISF occurs primarily through hydrostatic pressure and through colloid osmotic pressure. Plasma proteins cannot pass through the capillary membrane and, therefore, are very effective osmotic agents. The mean colloid osmotic, or *oncotic*, pressure for protein in the plasma is 28 mm. Hg and that for the interstitium is 5 mm. Hg.[14] Thus, the net colloid osmotic pressure of 23 mm. Hg moves the water from the interstitium to the plasma. It should be emphasized that the colloid osmotic pressure of the plasma proteins is greater than that predicted on the basis of the number of protein particles present in plasma. This difference is the result of the large number of cations that are attracted to proteins as the result of the Gibbs-Donnan equilibrium.

The plasma is at a considerably higher hydrostatic pressure than the interstitium. The mean capillary hydrostatic pressure is 17 mm. Hg, and the mean interstitial hydrostatic pressure is -6.3 mm. Hg.[14] Thus, the net hydrostatic pressure of 23.3 mm. Hg moves water from the plasma to the interstitium. However, there is a gradient of

hydrostatic pressure within the capillary such that the hydrostatic pressure at the arterial end of the capillary is 10 to 15 mm. Hg greater than at the venous end of the capillary (25 mm. Hg vs. 10 mm. Hg). Thus, the net hydrostatic pressure at the arterial end is 31.3 mm. Hg (25 + 6.3) and at the venous end is 16.3 mm. Hg (10 + 6.3).[14]

Since the net movement of water depends on the difference between the opposing forces generated by the net colloid oncotic pressure and the net hydrostatic pressure, it is apparent that at the arterial capillary end water moves from the plasma to the interstitium (filtration). The net pressure favoring filtration at the arterial capillary end is 8.3 mm. Hg (31.3 − 23). At the venous end of the capillary, the net pressure favors the reabsorption of water from the interstitium to the plasma by 6.7 mm. Hg (23 − 16.3). The overall effect of the hydrostatic pressure gradient results in a slight net filtration of fluid at the capillary bed. Because the mean capillary hydrostatic pressure is 17 mm. Hg, the net pressure favoring filtration is 0.3 mm. Hg,[14] i.e., (17−(−6.3)) − (28 − 5) (Fig. 6). However, fluid does not accumulate in the interstitium under normal conditions because the net filtered fluid returns to the circulation through the lymphatics.

The *Starling hypothesis* of capillary exchange expresses the relationships among the forces favoring filtration or reabsorption in the capillaries. According to this hypothesis, the direction of fluid movement across the capillary bed is determined by three factors: (1) capillary (Pc) and interstitial (Pi) *hydrostatic pressure*; (2) capillary (πc) and interstitial (πi) *colloid oncotic pressure*; and (3) the *permeability* (k) and *area* (A) of the capillary membranes. Since the forces causing fluid movement out of the capillaries are Pc and πi and the forces causing fluid movement into the

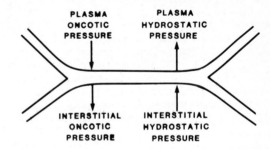

ARTERIAL END (mmHg)	FORCES OUT	VENOUS END (mmHg)
	FORCES OUT	
25	PLASMA HYDROSTATIC PRESSURE	10
5	INTERSTITIAL ONCOTIC PRESSURE	5
30		15
	FORCES IN	
28	PLASMA ONCOTIC PRESSURE	28
−6.3	INTERSTITIAL HYDROSTATIC PRESSURE	−6.3
21.7		22.3
8.3	**NET MOVEMENT**	−7.3

Figure 6. Starling equilibrium. (Data from: Guyton, A. C.: Textbook of Medical Physiology, Philadelphia, W. B. Saunders Company, 1976.)

capillaries are Pi and πc, net fluid flux is described by the equation:

$$F = kA[(Pc - Pi) - (πc - πi) =$$
$$kA (Pc + πi) - (Pi + πc)] \qquad (10)$$

When F is positive, the pressure favors filtration; when F is negative, the pressure favors reabsorption.

REGULATION OF FLUIDS AND ELECTROLYTES

Fluid and Electrolyte Balance: Intake Equals Output

So that fluid and electrolyte balance can be maintained, the output of water and electrolytes must match the intake. When intake exceeds output, accumulation of water or electrolytes is termed *positive balance*. Conversely, when output exceeds intake, the resultant reduction in water or electrolytes is termed *negative balance*. Under most circumstances, the intake and output are balanced by the interactions of the neuroendocrine system, the circulatory system, and the kidney.

Approximately two thirds of the oral intake of water is in the form of liquids, and a third is in the form of solids (Table 4). A small amount of water (5 to 15 per cent) is also synthesized daily in the body through the oxidation of foodstuffs. For example, approximately one liter of water is produced per kilogram of lipid metabolized.

The normal routes of water loss include *sensible* (measurable) losses through the urine, feces, and sweat, and *insensible* (nonmeasurable) losses through the evaporation of water through the lungs and the diffusion of water through the skin (Table 4). Although the insensible water losses are relatively fixed, the amount of water lost daily through the sensible routes varies with body temperature, ambient temperature, activity, and daily fluid intake. For example, under normal ambient conditions and normal activity, only 100 ml. of water is lost daily through sweat; with heavy exercise or high ambient temperature, however, these losses may increase to 1500 ml. Among the various routes of water loss, only that through the kidney can be controlled sufficiently to compensate for excessive intake or excessive loss of water. Under conditions of reduced water intake or excessive extrarenal loss, the renal excretion of water can be reduced to 300 ml. per day. In contrast, during excessive water intake or minimal extrarenal loss,

the renal excretion of water can be increased to 1500 ml. of water per hour.

The average American consumes approximately 6 to 15 gm. of salt (NaCl) per day. Since 58 mg. of NaCl are equivalent to 1 mEq. of Na^+ and 1 mEq. of Cl^-, the daily intake of sodium varies from 100 to 260 mEq. per day. If the use of salt at the table is omitted, the intake of sodium chloride can be reduced to 4 gm., or 70 mEq. of Na^+ per day. If the use of salt in cooking is also eliminated, the intake of sodium chloride can be reduced further to 3 gm. per day, or 50 mEq. of Na^+ per day. Finally, a therapeutic 2-gm. sodium chloride diet reduces the intake of sodium to 35 mEq. per day.[27]

To maintain balance, all ingested sodium must be excreted. The insensible losses of water via the lungs and skin are free of salt. Thus, the only important routes for sodium loss under normal circumstances are the intestinal fluids, urine, and sweat (Table 4). Under normal conditions, only 20 mEq. of sodium is lost by the intestine. However, this amount may decrease to zero with obstruction or may increase to 200 mEq. per hr. with severe diarrhea. Similarly, the loss of sodium through sweat in acclimatized individuals is approximately 15 mEq. per liter, but in the unacclimatized this loss may increase to 60 mEq. per liter. Since the loss of sodium under normal conditions through intestinal fluids and sweat is small, the control of sodium balance rests primarily upon the kidney. Under conditions of reduced intake or excessive extrarenal losses (negative sodium balance), renal excretion of sodium can be reduced nearly to zero.

Among surgical patients, an additional source of water and electrolyte loss must be considered: the *third space*. The third space results from injury, inflammation, or ischemia and represents sequestered extracellular fluid. Its size is proportional to the severity of the injury. Because the fluid and electrolytes in the third space are derived from the functional extracellular fluid, the increase in the size of the third space reduces the functional extracellular volume. In addition, the fluid that accumulates in the third space is equivalent in electrolyte composition to the extracellular fluid. Thus, for each liter of third space fluid sequestered, approximately 150 mEq. of sodium, 112 mEq. of chloride, and 4.6 mEq. of potassium are lost from the functional extracellular fluid. Since the volume of the third space is directly proportional to the severity of injury, minor operative procedures, such as an appendectomy, are associated with considerably less fluid sequestration than are major operative procedures such as extensive abdominal and retroperitoneal dissections. The most extensive third space losses are those that follow extensive burns and generalized sepsis.

Neuroendocrine Control of Renal Function

Changes in fluid and electrolyte balance and renal function occur after any acute injury, with most disease processes, and as a result of daily variations in intake and output. After injury and with disease, the degree of alteration depends, in part, on the severity of the illness or injury, on the quality and quantity of fluid replaced, on the age of the patient, on pre-existent illnesses, on concurrent medications, and on the anesthetic agents used. Both the volume and the composition of body fluids are sensed in specific receptor areas, and signals from these receptors are transduced by the effectors of the neuroendocrine system into changes in the renal handling of water and of electrolytes.

TABLE 4. Water, Sodium, and Potassium Balance in an Average 70-kg. Man

	Water (ml./day)	Sodium (mEq./day)	Potassium (mEq./day)
Intake			
Liquids	800–1500	50–100	50–80
Solids	500–700		
Oxidation	150–250		
Output			
Sensible			
Urine	800–1500	10–90	50–80
Intestine	0–250	0–20	Trace
Sweat	0–100	10–60	0–10
Insensible			
Lungs	250–350	0	0
Skin	250–350	0	0

STIMULI AND RESPONSE

The extracellular fluid volume itself is not monitored by the body. Instead, the effective circulating volume is monitored by arterial and renal baroreceptors and by atrial stretch receptors.[12] For *arterial baroreceptors*, the initiating signals are the arterial pressure and its rate of change. For *atrial stretch receptors*, the initiating signals are the atrial volume and its rate of change.

Although the effective circulating volume is usually related directly to the extracellular water, the circulating volume is effective only to the extent that it is sensed by these receptors. Pump failure (congestive heart failure) or sequestration of part of the circulating volume behind an obstruction (tension pneumothorax, cardiac tamponade, cirrhosis) leads to an effective circulating volume that is less than the total circulating volume. Because of the equilibrium described in the Starling hypothesis, the total circulating volume—and therefore the effective circulating volume—is reduced when there is a loss of plasma protein. In cirrhosis, the concentration of plasma protein is reduced as a result of decreased albumin synthesis, and in the nephrotic syndrome it is reduced as a result of the loss of albumin. In the latter, the effective circulating volume is reduced even though the total extracellular water is increased. Similarly, alterations in the permeabilities of capillaries will alter the equilibrium across the capillary bed. In the third space formation (tissue injury and sepsis), fluid is sequestered in tissues, and even though the extracellular volume is the same or increased, the effective circulating volume is decreased.

The afferent signals from high-pressure baroreceptors in the carotid arteries and aorta, and from low-pressure stretch receptors in the atria, exert a tonic inhibition over the release of many hormones and the activities of the central nervous system (CNS) and the autonomic nervous system.[12] When the effective circulating volume decreases, baroreceptors and stretch receptor activities decrease, thus releasing the tonic inhibition of the neuroendocrine system. This results in the increased secretion of adrenocorticotropic hormone (ACTH), vasopressin, beta-endorphin, and growth hormones through central pathways and in the increased secretion of epinephrine, renin, and glucagon through peripheral autonomic neural pathways. This response brings about further neuroendocrine changes, including (1) the stimulation of the formation of angiotensin by renin, (2) the stimulation of the secretion of aldosterone by angiotensin II and ACTH, (3) the stimulation of the secretion of cortisol by ACTH, and (4) the inhibition of the secretion of insulin by epinephrine.

Changes in the effective circulating volume are also sensed by stretch receptors in the juxtaglomerular complexes of the kidney. Activation of these stretch receptors by a decrease in the circulating volume stimulates the secretion of renin and therefore the formation of angiotensin and the secretion of aldosterone.

Since the extracellular fluid volume is proportional to the total body sodium, decreases in total body sodium are associated with decreases in the extracellular fluid. Conversely, increases in total body sodium are associated with increases in the extracellular fluid. Notable exceptions include the ingestion of salt in excess of free water and the excretion of free water in excess of sodium. Thus, the monitoring of total body sodium is an additional mechanism through which the extracellular fluid volume may be regulated. However, total body sodium itself is not measured. Instead, the concentration of sodium (chloride) in renal tubular fluid is evaluated by the macula densa of the

juxtaglomerular apparatus of the kidney.[9] When the amount of sodium (or chloride) delivered to the macula densa decreases, the macula densa is activated, thereby leading to the release of renin and ultimately to the formation of angiotensin and to the secretion of aldosterone. The delivery of sodium chloride to the macula densa can be reduced under several conditions, including (1) a decreased plasma concentration of sodium and chloride, (2) a reduced glomerular filtration rate, and (3) an increase in proximal tubular reabsorption of filtrate. However, these conditions may occur simultaneously in such a manner that one offsets the others. For example, during overhydration with hypotonic salt solutions, the reduction in the plasma concentration of sodium is offset by an increase in glomerular filtration and a decrease in the proximal reabsorption of filtrate.

Of equal importance in the regulation of extracellular fluid volume and serum sodium concentration is the monitoring of plasma osmolality. Changes in osmolality are sensed by osmoreceptors in the CNS (near the hypothalamic ventricles)[4] and by the extracerebral osmoreceptors in the liver.[25] The central osmoreceptors are sensitive to sodium concentration but not directly to tonicity. The extracerebral osmoreceptors appear to be sensitive to glucose and possibly other solutes. An increase in osmolality activates these receptors resulting in the secretion of vasopressin and in the stimulation of thirst.

Thirst is an extremely important mechanism through which hyperosmolality is prevented. (See the section on dehydration and hypernatremia later in this chapter.) Thirst is activated by at least two separate neuroendocrine mechanisms. One of these appears to sense changes in intracellular volume and therefore plasma osmolality. The other senses reductions in the effective circulating volume and is stimulated by angiotensin II.

Changes in total body potassium are also not monitored directly. Instead, the plasma potassium concentration is evaluated by the adrenal cortex. When the plasma potassium concentration increases, cells in the adrenal zona glomerulosa are directly activated, resulting in the secretion of aldosterone. Conversely, a decrease in the plasma potassium concentration inhibits the secretion of aldosterone by these cells.

The secretion of potassium by tubular cells occurs primarily by a passive process in the distal tubules. It is stimulated by an increase in the electronegativity of the tubular fluid, which may occur via an increase in distal sodium reabsorption, via an increase in the distal concentration of anions, or via an increase in the intracellular potassium concentration. Thus, the total body potassium is also monitored indirectly by the concentration of potassium present in renal tubular cells and by the electronegativity of the tubular fluid.

Under some circumstances, the plasma concentration of potassium varies directly with the intracellular potassium concentration. A decrease in intracellular potassium is associated with a decrease in plasma potassium as potassium moves into cells, and an increase in intracellular potassium is associated with an increase in plasma potassium as potassium moves out of cells. However, cell membranes are not freely permeable to potassium and the volume of plasma is considerably less than that of cells (5 liters vs. 28 liters). Therefore, changes in plasma and intracellular potassium concentrations are neither equal nor proportional. When potassium intake increases, both plasma and intracellular potassium concentrations increase. However, even though the absolute amount of potassium is greater in cells, the proportional increase is less than in plasma. Conversely, when potassium is lost, the proportional decrease is greater in the plasma than in cells, even though the total amount lost is greater in cells. This dissociation of relative concentrations of intracellular and extracellular potassium is important in determining the excitability of nerves and of muscle.

Furthermore, under many circumstances the plasma concentration of potassium does not vary directly with the intracellular stores. Changes in plasma pH, changes in insulin and catecholamine secretion, the breakdown of cells, and chronic disease all induce changes in the plasma concentration of potassium that may be in the opposite direction to the intracellular potassium stores. In fact, the concentration of hydrogen ions and the secretion of insulin are prime determinants of the plasma potassium concentration and both function irrespective of the intracellular potassium stores. Clearly, this is a hazardous situation because potassium may be lost in the urine despite a low intracellular concentration or retained in the body despite a high intracellular concentration.

When the concentration of hydrogen ions in the plasma increases acutely (*acidosis*), hydrogen ions enter cells and potassium ions leave cells.[7] Conversely, when the concentration of hydrogen ions decreases acutely (*alkalosis*), hydrogen ions leave cells and potassium ions enter cells.[7] However, this is not the result of a direct exchange of hydrogen ions for potassium ions. The concentration of hydrogen is too small (10^{-7}) to have any impact on the movement of potassium ions (10^{-3}) by direct exchange. Instead, the movement of potassium into or out of the cells is more likely to be the result of changes induced in the activity of Na-K ATPases by acidosis or alkalosis. Therefore, changes in the pH of plasma and cells result in alterations in the internal distribution of potassium such that the plasma concentration of potassium is not reflective of the intracellular concentration. In general, for each 0.1 unit change in pH, there is a *reciprocal change* in the potassium concentration of approximately 0.6 mEq. per liter.[24]

Changes in the secretion of insulin alter the intracellular to plasma potassium ratio because insulin moves glucose into cells and potassium follows. In fact, insulin may exert an important role in internal potassium homeostasis, since the secretion of insulin is stimulated by hyperkalemia and inhibited by hypokalemia.[24] Catecholamines also alter the internal distribution of potassium. Beta-adrenergic stimulation *increases* the uptake of potassium by cells, and beta-adrenergic blockade *decreases* the uptake of potassium.[8] However, the physiologic significance of these effects is unknown.

Any process that increases cell breakdown will also increase the extracellular potassium concentration because of the release of large amounts of potassium present normally in cells. In the crush syndrome or in deep burns, hyperkalemia may become a life-threatening problem because of the large release of potassium from damaged or irreversibly injured cells.

In conclusion, it is apparent that the plasma potassium concentration is a poor indicator of total body potassium because hyperkalemia or hypokalemia may exist with an increased, decreased, or normal content of potassium in the body. Therefore, therapeutic decisions to withdraw or give potassium must not be based on the plasma potassium concentration alone.

NEUROENDOCRINE EFFECTORS

Most of the known hormonal agents exert some influence on fluid and electrolyte balance. For example, gluca-gon decreases serum sodium by increasing serum glucose concentration as water moves from cells to balance the increase in the number of osmotically active particles (glucose) in plasma. Insulin, by moving glucose into cells, decreases serum potassium. Catecholamines, by increasing systemic vascular resistance and cardiac output, may deactivate baroreceptors. However, the primary effectors of fluid and electrolyte balance are aldosterone, angiotensin, vasopressin, and cortisol.

Aldosterone

Aldosterone[3, 8] is secreted by cells of the adrenal zona glomerulosa. The synthesis and release of aldosterone are controlled by at least four mechanisms. *Angiotensin II* is a potent stimulator of aldosterone secretion that acts via a calcium-dependent, cyclic adenosine monophosphate (cAMP)-independent pathway. The second stimulatory mechanism is through *ACTH*. Unlike angiotensin II, the action of ACTH is mediated by both calcium and cAMP. A third stimulatory pathway is via *potassium*. An increase in the concentration of potassium in the plasma leads to the stimulation of aldosterone secretion via a calcium-dependent, cAMP-independent pathway.

On a molar basis, ACTH is the most potent stimulator of aldosterone production. Accordingly, stress-induced elevations in plasma aldosterone are probably mediated primarily by ACTH. However, the stimulatory ability of ACTH is short-lived. The short-lived potency of ACTH and the normal response of ACTH deficient individuals to sodium restriction suggest that ACTH may play a minor role in the overall control of aldosterone secretion in chronic states. In chronic conditions, angiotensin II is probably the most potent stimulator of aldosterone secretion.

The fourth mechanism is an *inhibitory pathway* that blocks the later stages of aldosterone synthesis. Present evidence suggests that this pathway involves a tonic inhibition of aldosterone secretion by dopamine. This pathway may be the mechanism through which changes in extracellular sodium and extracellular volume act to alter aldosterone secretion.

The mechanism of action of aldosterone is similar to that of other steroid hormones. Aldosterone binds to cystolic receptors and is then transferred to the nucleus, where it binds to nuclear chromatin and increases the transcription of messenger ribonucleic acid (mRNA). The primary action of aldosterone is to promote the reabsorption of sodium and the secretion of potassium and hydrogen ions in the distal convoluted tubules and early collecting ducts of the kidney. Although this process has been described classically as an obligatory one-to-one exchange of sodium for potassium ions and of sodium for hydrogen ions, there is no evidence to support such a process. Furthermore, the amount of sodium reabsorbed exceeds greatly the amount of potassium or hydrogen secreted. Instead, the secretion of potassium and hydrogen appears to result from an increase in the electronegativity of the luminal tubular fluid as sodium reabsorption is stimulated by aldosterone. Aldosterone also increases sodium and chloride reabsorption in the early distal tubule.

Renin-Angiotensin[9, 17, 22]

Renin exists in an inactive form, *prorenin*, in myoepithelial juxtaglomerular cells of renal afferent arterioles. Renin secretion is under the control of three intrarenal receptors and several hormones and ions. The macula densa receptor of the renal juxtaglomerular apparatus responds to tubular fluid passing through the distal nephron. Both tubular sodium and chloride have been suggested to be the solutes sensed at the macula densa. The second intrarenal receptor is the neurogenic receptor on the juxtaglomerular cell membrane, which responds to beta-adrenergic stimulation by increasing renin secretion. The third intrarenal receptor is the vascular stretch receptor that is thought to be the juxtaglomerular cell itself. Other factors that modulate renin release include: ACTH, vasopressin, glucagon, prostaglandins, calcium, magnesium, and potassium.

After proteolytic cleavage of the renin zymogen, renin is released into the afferent arteriole, where it converts renin substrate (produced by the liver) to *angiotensin I.* Angiotensin I is a decapeptide that originally was thought to be an inactive precursor of angiotensin II. Recent evidence suggests that angiotensin I potentiates the release of epinephrine from the adrenal medulla and decreases blood flow to the juxtamedullary area of the kidney by selective renal vasoconstriction. However, angiotensin I functions primarily as a precursor of angiotensin II. In the pulmonary circulation, and to a lesser extent in the kidney, angiotensin I is converted by angiotensin-converting enzyme to angiotensin II. This enzyme is a carboxypeptidase that is identical to the kinase II that inactivates bradykinin.

Angiotensin II vasoconstricts arterioles and stimulates the secretion of aldosterone. Its importance in blood pressure control in normal and pathologic conditions is well documented. In addition, angiotensin II has direct chronotropic and inotropic actions on the myocardium, increases the secretion of vasopressin and ACTH, potentiates the action of ACTH on the adrenal cortex and the release of epinephrine from the adrenal medulla, increases sympathetic neurotransmission, and increases thirst.

Angiotensin III is the only active breakdown product of angiotensin II. It stimulates the secretion of aldosterone but has none of the vasoconstricting effects of angiotensin II. However, its physiologic significance remains unknown.

Arginine Vasopressin

Arginine vasopressin[4, 17, 23] is a nonapeptide that is released from the neurohypophysis primarily in response to an increase in plasma osmolality and a decrease in the effective circulating volume. Vasopressin has four principal actions. Of these, the best known action is the stimulation of the reabsorption of solute-free water in the distal tubules and collecting ducts of the kidney by increasing the tubular permeability. The promotion of water retention and the reduction of free water clearance is mediated by cAMP. Vasopressin also increases peripheral vasoconstriction, especially in the splanchnic bed. As a result of this action, it has been implicated in the pathogenesis of mesenteric infarction. Finally, vasopressin stimulates hepatic glycogenolysis and hepatic gluconeogenesis through a calcium-dependent, cAMP-independent mechanism.

ACTH-Cortisol

The secretion of ACTH and cortisol[3, 12] increases after any injury or stress. ACTH is released by chromophobe cells of the anterior pituitary gland and acts on cells of the adrenal zona fasciculata, stimulating cortisol production and release. This process involves a cAMP-mediated enhancement of the conversion of cholesterol to pregnenolone. ACTH itself is under the control of cortisol and corticotropin-releasing factor (CRF).

Cortisol produces a variety of metabolic effects, including (1) the stimulation of hepatic gluconeogenesis and amino acid transport; (2) the inhibition of hepatic glycolysis and of the hepatic action of insulin; (3) the potentiation of the hepatic action of glucagon and of epinephrine; (4) the inhibition of peripheral amino acid uptake; (5) the inhibition of the action of insulin on glucose uptake in peripheral tissues (insulin resistance); and (6) the facilitation of lipolysis, stimulated by lipolytic hormones in peripheral tissues. These actions result in the increased production of glucose and other solutes and a decrease in their utilization by peripheral tissues that appear to be important in the physiologic restitution of the effective circulating volume. Cortisol also is important in stabilizing cell membranes.

RENAL STRUCTURE AND FUNCTION: GLOMERULAR FILTRATION RATE AND TUBULAR REABSORPTION AND SECRETION

The basic functional unit of the kidney is the *nephron,* of which there are approximately one million in each kidney. Each nephron is composed of a glomerulus, proximal tubule, loop of Henle, distal tubule, and collecting duct (Fig. 7). The collecting ducts of each nephron join and eventually form the renal calyces. Each glomerulus is composed of a tuft of capillaries surrounded by *Bowman's capsule.* Here an ultrafiltrate of plasma is formed under the forces described in the Starling hypothesis (Fig. 8). This ultrafiltrate then enters the renal tubules, where, through the processes of reabsorption and secretion, the tubular fluid is modified on its way to the collecting ducts and ultimately the pelvic calyxes.

Eighty-five per cent of the glomeruli are located in the superficial areas of the renal cortex (superficial cortical

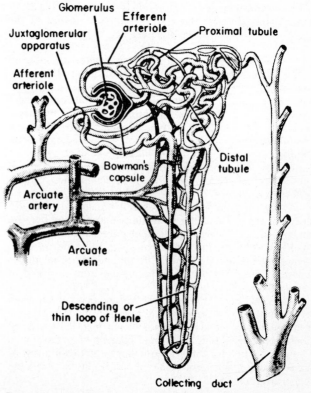

Figure 7. Anatomy of the nephron. (From Smith, H. W.: The Kidney: Structure and Function in Health and Disease. New York, Oxford University Press, 1951.)

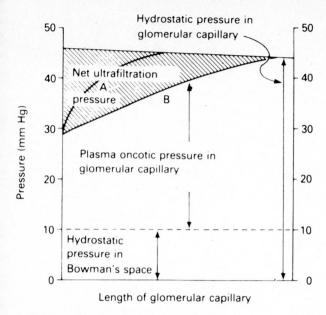

Balance of Mean Values

Hydrostatic pressure in glomerular capillary	45 mm Hg
Hydrostatic pressure in Bowman's space	10
Plasma oncotic pressure in glomerular capillary	27
Oncotic pressure of fluid in Bowman's space	0*
Net ultrafiltration pressure	8 mm Hg

Figure 8. Starling forces involved in the formation of the glomerular ultrafiltrate. (From Valtin, H.: Renal Function: Mechanisms Preserving Fluid and Solute Balance in Health. Boston, Little, Brown and Co., 1983.)

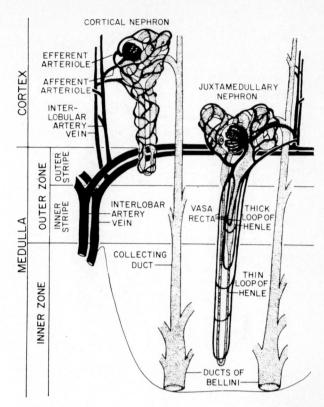

Figure 9. Blood supply to cortical and juxtamedullary nephrons. Note the longer loops of Henle of juxtamedullary nephrons compared with cortical nephrons. (From Pitts, R. F.: Physiology of the Kidney and Body Fluids. Chicago, Year Book Medical Publishers, 1974, p. 8.)

nephrons), and 15 per cent are located in the deeper cortical layers near the corticomedullary junction (juxtamedullary nephrons).[27] Whereas the superficial cortical nephrons have short loops of Henle, the juxtamedullary nephrons have long loops of Henle extending deep into the renal medulla (Fig. 9). Each of the nephrons is surrounded by a rich and complex network of peritubular capillaries that are involved in the delivery of nutrients to the tubular epithelial cells, the delivery of solutes to the tubular cells that are to be secreted, and the removal of materials that have been reabsorbed by the tubular cells (Fig. 9).

Approximately 25 per cent of the cardiac output flows to the kidneys. This results in the filtration into the renal tubules of approximately 180 liters of plasma water per day from the 1584 liters of blood that pass through the kidneys. (The normal renal blood flow is 1100 ml. per minute, and the normal renal plasma flow is 625 ml. per minute.[24, 27]) Because the tubular fluid, as it leaves the glomerulus, is an ultrafiltrate of plasma, it contains approximately 150 mEq. per liter of sodium; 112 mEq. per liter of chloride; 4.6 mEq. per liter of potassium; 26 mEq. per liter of bicarbonate; a variety of other anions, cations, and solutes; and little protein. Thus, as noted in Table 5, the tubules must reabsorb almost all of the solutes in the glomerular filtrate to maintain fluid and electrolyte balance.

Sodium reabsorption in the early proximal tubule involves isosmotic active transport of sodium that is preferentially cotransported with bicarbonate, divalent cations, and organic solutes (glucose, amino acids, lactate, phosphate) instead of chloride. This results in a chloride concentration gradient in the late proximal tubule that produces

passive transport of sodium. In addition, active transport of sodium also occurs in the late proximal tubule and is linked to chloride movement. In both regions of the proximal tubule, water follows passively. The resulting tubular fluid is isosmotic to plasma as it enters the loop of Henle.

In the loop of Henle, differing permeability and transport properties of the descending and ascending loops establish a hypotonic tubular fluid and a medullary osmotic gradient. The descending loop of Henle is permeable to water but relatively impermeable to NaCl. In contrast, the ascending thin and thick limbs of the loop of Henle are impermeable to water but transport chloride actively into the interstitium with sodium following passively. The medullary osmotic gradient that results regulates the urine osmolarity from 50 to 1200 mOsm. by the *countercurrent mechanism* (Fig. 10).[24, 27]

Since the reabsorption of sodium in the proximal tubule and the loop of Henle is coupled primarily with chloride,

TABLE 5. *Daily Reabsorption of Solutes by the Kidneys*

	Filtered	Excreted	Per Cent
Water	180 liters	0.5–3.0 liters	98–99
Na+	25,000 mEq.	50–200 mEq.	99+
Cl−	19,500 mEq.	50–200 mEq.	99+
HCO₃	4,500 mEq.	0	100
K+	720 mEq.	40–120 mEq.	80–95
Urea	54 gm.	27–32 gm.	40–50
Glucose	800 mm.	0.5 mm.	99.9

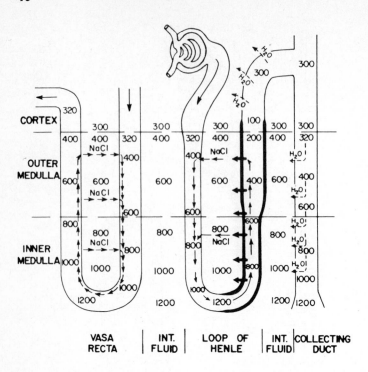

Figure 10. The "countercurrent" mechanism for concentrating urine. (From Guyton, A. C.: Textbook of Medical Physiology. Philadelphia, W. B. Saunders Company, 1976.)

if the reabsorption of chloride is complete, approximately 38 mEq. per liter of sodium will be presented to the distal tubule (Na − Cl = 150 − 112 = 38 mEq. per liter). Sodium reabsorption in the distal tubule is also active. Early in the distal tubule it is associated with passive chloride transport. In the distal portion of the distal tubule and the proximal portion of the collecting duct, sodium is reabsorbed and potassium and hydrogen ions are secreted. Both processes are controlled by aldosterone. The distal collecting ducts are relatively impermeable to water, sodium chloride, and urea in the absence of vasopressin. In the presence of vasopressin, the permeability of the distal tubules and distal collecting ducts to water increases and the permeability of the collecting ducts to urea increases.

Almost all of the potassium filtered by the glomerulus is reabsorbed in the proximal tubule and loop of Henle, leaving less than 1 mEq. of potassium per liter of tubular fluid in the distal tubule. In the distal tubule and the early collecting duct, potassium is secreted passively into the tubular lumen as the intracellular concentrations of potassium increase or the electronegativity of the tubular fluid decreases. This process is augmented by aldosterone. A low concentration of potassium in the distal tubular fluid also favors the passive secretion of potassium down a concentration gradient. Because of these processes, nearly all of the potassium excreted by the kidney is secreted into the urine.

Thus, the maintenance of fluid and electrolyte balance is dependent upon the formation of a large quantity of glomerular filtrate that is almost completely reabsorbed by the renal tubules prior to excretion. Variations in daily intake or nonrenal losses are compensated for by the amount secreted. For example, when sodium intake is in excess, less of the filtered load is reabsorbed and more is excreted. Conversely, when sodium intake is reduced or extrarenal losses are great, sodium reabsorption increases so that less than 1 mEq. per day of sodium is excreted.

PRACTICAL APPROACH TO THE DAILY MANAGEMENT OF FLUID AND ELECTROLYTES

The management of surgical patients frequently requires that nothing be taken orally. This may be necessary in order to keep the stomach empty prior to surgery and thus avoid aspiration, or it may be the result of postsurgical or traumatic ileus in which the ingestion of food and water results in cramps and vomiting. Patients with intestinal pathology such as Crohn's disease, ulcerative colitis and bowel obstruction benefit from the avoidance of oral intake, i.e., putting the bowel at rest, and comatose or anesthetized individuals are clearly unable to eat or drink. Under these circumstances, it is apparent that daily obligatory losses of fluids and electrolytes must be replaced parenterally or fluid and electrolyte imbalance will result. Thus, the practical approach to fluid and electrolyte management is to calculate the amount of fluid and electrolytes that are required by any individual as a result of obligatory losses (baseline requirements) and to add to this quantity any abnormal internal or external losses of fluids and electrolytes.

Baseline Requirements for Normal and Injured Man

In the absence of surgical procedures, injury, or illness, the daily baseline requirements in a 70-kg. man must account for the insensible loss of 750 ml. of essentially pure water through the skin and lungs and the sensible loss of hypotonic fluid equalling 100 ml. in sweat (under normal ambient conditions) and 250 ml. in stool. In addition, a normal individual must excrete approximately 600 mOsm. per day via the urine to maintain constant body composition. The volume of urine necessary for the excretion of this solute load depends upon the state of concentrating and diluting mechanisms in the kidney. If the urine is diluted maximally (40 mOsm. per kg. water), 15 liters of urine is required. If the urine is isotonic to plasma (300 mOsm. per kg. water), 2 liters of urine is required. If the urine is concentrated maximally (1200 mOsm. per kg. water), 400 to 500 ml. of urine is required. Therefore, *a normal 70-kg. man requires* 1600 ml. of fluid per day or approximately *20 ml. per kg. body weight per day*. This results in a urinary output of approximately 20 ml. per hour.

However, in the presence of surgery, injury or illness, the concentrating ability of the kidney is almost always impaired. (See the section on hypovolemia and hypotension later in this chapter.) Under these circumstances, the urine can be concentrated only to 850 mOsm. per liter of water and 700 to 1000 ml. of urine must be excreted to eliminate the solute load. Consequently, a *70-kg. surgical patient* requires approximately 2100 ml. of fluid per day or approximately *30 ml. per kg. body weight per day*. This results in a urinary output of 30 to 40 ml. per hour.

Since intracellular and extracellular fluid volumes vary as a function of body weight, *a rule of thumb is to estimate the daily baseline fluid requirements of injured and postoperative patients as 30 ml. per kg. body weight per day*. However, it should be remembered that obese individuals have proportionately less body water than do non-obese individuals. As a result, the daily fluid requirements of obese persons are more on the order of 20 to 25 ml. per kg. body weight per day. Similarly, females and elderly have a greater quantity of body fat than men and their fluid requirements are also closer to 25 ml. per kg. per day. It should also be noted that in the presence of normal renal, neuroendocrine, and cardiac function, it is always better to overestimate rather than underestimate fluid requirements. Excess water is usually excreted easily, and, if necessary, the excess can be aided by the use of diuretics. Similarly, congestive heart failure can usually be corrected with diuretics and digitalis. However, when renal failure ensues, it cannot be reversed by the clinician.

Although human beings can conserve sodium almost absolutely, they do so at the expense of potassium wasting, secondary to avid sodium retention and increased aldosterone secretion. In normal man, sodium intakes of 60 to 100 mEq. per day are adequate to prevent this. Therefore, as a rule of thumb, the administration of *1 mEq. of Na+ per kg. per day to normal and injured man will replace all the sodium normally lost*, allow sodium balance to be main-

tained, and prevent potassium wasting. If this is administered in the form of NaCl, chloride requirements will also be fulfilled. Under these conditions, the urinary losses of potassium will be reduced to approximately 30 to 60 mEq. per day or one-half mEq. per kg. per day. As a general rule, *approximately 30 to 40 mEq. per day* replaces adequately the daily losses of potassium.

Thus, a 70-kg. surgical patient requires 30 ml. per kg. per day of water (2100 ml.), 1 mEq. Na+ per kg. per day (70 mEq.) and 40 mEq. of K+ per day. Inspection of the commercially available solutions noted in Table 6 reveals that the water and sodium requirements of a 70-kg. man can be met by the parenteral administration of 2 liters of 0.2 per cent saline of D5 0.2 per cent saline (68 mEq. Na+ + 2000 ml. H₂O). The use of dextrose will decrease the amount of nitrogenous wastes that need to be excreted. However, immediately after operation the administration of dextrose frequently leads to hyperglycemia because of the impairment of glucose utilization that accompanies injury. Consequently, when dextrose solutions are used in the immediate postoperative period, they should be administered slowly. In addition to 2 liters of D5 0.2 per cent saline, 40 mEq. potassium chloride (KCl) per day, or 20 mEq. KCl per liter, should be given. If all this fluid is given in a bolus, the kidneys will rapidly excrete the excess fluid to maintain fluid balance. Since these daily losses are incurred over the course of 24 hours, baseline requirements should also be given over 24 hours. Thus, the daily baseline requirements of a 70-kg. surgical patient are met by the administration of D5 0.2 per cent saline with 20 mEq. KCl per liter at 80 ml. per hour.

Replacement of Abnormal Fluid Losses

Any abnormal losses must be added to the daily fluid and electrolyte requirements. Almost all of these losses are transcellular fluids that have an extremely varied ionic composition (Table 7). Even within a given class of transcellular fluids, e.g., gastrointestinal secretions, the ionic compositions vary significantly. However, the importance of these fluids in the management of fluid and electrolyte balance cannot be overstated. An abnormally high secretion and loss of any of these fluids (particularly gastrointestinal secretions) is a major cause of both fluid and electrolyte imbalance in surgical and nonsurgical patients. *Therefore, it is imperative that the volume and electrolyte composition*

TABLE 6. *Electrolyte Composition of Commercially Available Intravenous Solutions*

	Na+ (mEq./liter)	Cl− (mEq./liter)	K+ (mEq./liter)	HCO₃− (mEq./liter)	Ca+2 (mEq./liter)	Osmolality (mOsm/kg. water)	Calories
0.9% Sodium chloride	154	154				292	
0.9% Sodium chloride with 5% dextrose	154	154				565	200
0.45% Sodium chloride	77	77				146	
0.45% Sodium chloride with 5% dextrose	77	77				420	200
0.2% Sodium chloride with 5% dextrose	34	34				330	200
5% Dextrose in water						274	200
10% Dextrose in water						548	400
Ringer's lactate	130	109	4	(28)	3	277	
0.9% Ammonium chloride		168				338	
0.6m Sodium lactate	167			(167)		334	
3% Sodium chloride	513	513				960	
5% Sodium chloride	864	864				1617	

TABLE 7. *Approximate Electrolyte Composition of the Transcellular Fluids*

	Na^+ (mEq./liter)	K^+ (mEq./liter)	Cl^- (mEq./liter)	HCO_3^- (mEq./liter)	Volume (liters/day)
Saliva	30	20	35	15	1.0–1.5
Gastric juice, pH <4.0	60	10	90	–	2.5
Gastric juice, pH >4.0	100	10	100	–	2.0
Bile	145	5	110	40	1.5
Duodenum	140	5	80	50	–
Pancreas	140	5	75	90	0.7–1.0
Ileum	130	10	110	30	3.5
Cecum	80	20	50	20	–
Colon	60	30	40	20	–
Sweat	50	5	55	–	0–3.0
New ileostomy	130	20	110	30	0.5–2.0
Adapted ileostomy	50	5	30	25	0.4
Colostomy	50	10	40	20	0.3

of any transcellular fluid that is secreted in large quantities be measured so that daily requirements can be met. However, when this is not possible, the composition of these fluids can be approximated from Table 7 and the volume loss estimated.

GASTRIC LOSSES

Gastric juice is lost either through vomiting, nasogastric suction, or drainage of external gastric fistulas. Since gastric juice, on the average, contains 70 mEq. Na^+, 100 mEq. Cl^-, and 20 mEq. K^+, the best replacement of gastric juice in the absence of metabolic alkalosis is with D5 0.45 per cent saline with 20 mEq. KCl per liter. For example, if 1 liter of gastric fluid is lost, the daily fluid and electrolyte requirement would be:

$$2 \text{ liters D5 0.2 per cent saline } + 20 \text{ mEq. per liter KCl}$$
and
$$1 \text{ liter 0.45 per cent saline } + 20 \text{ mEq. per liter KCl} \quad (11)$$

In order for this to be received over 24 hours, all the fluid would have to be administered at 125 ml. per hour. (Since normal renal function will usually tolerate small increases in water and sodium, the daily requirements can be approximated by D5 0.45 per cent saline with 20 mEq. KCl per liter at 125 ml. per hour.) However, the administration of 0.45 per cent saline underreplaces the chloride lost and will prevent the correction of metabolic alkalosis. (See the discussion on the therapeutic approach to hypokalemia and hyperkalemia later in this chapter.) Therefore, in the presence of metabolic alkalosis, the best replacement solution for gastric juice is 0.9 per cent saline (normal saline). However, it should be remembered that this solution overreplaces the sodium lost.

Administration of Ringer's lactate closely approximates the chloride loss, but it overreplaces the sodium requirement and underreplaces the potassium loss. In addition, Ringer's lactate contains 28 mEq. of base (lactate is converted to bicarbonate in the liver). Since acid is already being lost in the gastric juice, the administration of Ringer's lactate may aggravate a potential alkalosis, and its use for replacement of gastric losses should be avoided.

BILIARY AND PANCREATIC LOSSES

Bile and pancreatic juice are very similar in composition, the major difference between them being the considerably higher concentration of bicarbonate in pancreatic juice (90 versus 40 mEq. per liter) (Table 7). The sodium, chloride, and potassium concentrations of both these solutions are approximated closely by Ringer's lactate. In addition, the loss of bicarbonate in biliary fluid is approximated closely by Ringer's lactate, but additional bicarbonate may be needed for pancreatic losses. Since 1 ampule of sodium bicarbonate contains 44 mEq. of sodium as well as bicarbonate in 50 ml. of water, volume overload may ensue.

ILEOSTOMY DRAINAGE AND SMALL BOWEL DIARRHEA

The composition of ileostomy fluid varies with the diet and the disease process present. Generally, it is equivalent to plasma. Thus, it is best replaced with Ringer's lactate. Similarly, diarrhea arising from the small bowel usually has a composition similar to that of plasma.

COLOSTOMY DRAINAGE AND LARGE BOWEL DIARRHEA

In the presence of normal colonic absorptive function, stool has approximately 60 mEq. Na^+, 30 mEq. K^+, and 40 mEq. HCO_3^-. However, with colonic diarrhea or excessive colostomy output, the absorptive function is usually disrupted. Thus, these abnormal secretions often have large quantities of potassium and bicarbonate. As a general rule, it is safe to use Ringer's lactate, but because of the significant variation present, measurement of the actual loss is best.

THIRD SPACE LOSSES

Third space losses of fluids and electrolytes are the most difficult to estimate. Although their composition is similar to that of extracellular fluid, their volume can only be approximated. *As a general rule, a useful estimate is that 1 liter of extracellular fluid is sequestered in each of the four abdominal quadrants that are traumatized or inflamed and 1 liter in each of the chest cavities.* Thus, the third space fluid formed by an uncomplicated cholecystectomy is on the order of 1000 ml., whereas the fluid formed after the extensive retroperitoneal dissection involved in an abdominal aortic aneurysm resection may be in excess of 2 liters. This fluid should be replaced with normal saline.

SWEAT AND FEVER

Sweat is a hypotonic solution that contains approximately 50 mEq. of Na^+ per liter, 55 mEq. Cl^- per liter, and 5 mEq. K^+ per liter in an unacclimatized individual. It is best replaced with 0.45 per cent saline. Usually, it is impossible to determine the amount of fluid lost by sweating and an estimate must be made from the clinical signs and symptoms of volume deficiency present. The general rule for fever is that for *each degree* of centrigrade temperature elevation, the daily fluid requirement increases by *250 ml. per day*. Since this loss is pure water, it can be replaced with D5W (or D5 0.2 per cent saline).

Assessment of the Adequacy of Fluid Replacement: Hemodynamics, Daily Body Weight, and Urinary Output

Once the patient begins to receive parenteral fluids, it cannot be assumed that fluid and electrolyte balance is being maintained. Furthermore, it cannot be assumed that the guidelines presented previously will be correct in a given patient. The fluids and electrolytes administered may be overestimated or underestimated; losses may increase; renal, circulatory, or endocrine function may become impaired; or new losses may ensue. Thus, it is important to monitor fluid and electrolyte status frequently in all patients who are receiving parenteral fluids. The adequacy of fluid replacement is assessed through (1) hemodynamics, (2) skin perfusion, (3) sensorium, (4) daily weight measurements, and (5) urinary output.

HEMODYNAMIC ASSESSMENT

When the effective circulating volume is decreased, venous return decreases. Since cardiac output is the product of the stroke volume and the heart rate, the heart rate must increase in order to maintain cardiac output, blood pressure, and, ultimately, tissue perfusion. Thus, tachycardia and a low central venous pressure are the first hemodynamic signs of hypovolemia. Arterial pressure is maintained until 10 to 20 per cent of the effective circulating volume is depleted, at which point orthostatic hypotension ensues. Further reductions in the intravascular volume are accompanied by hypotension, even in the supine position. It should be noted that postoperative tachycardia may also be the result of pain, anemia, anxiety, fever, hypoxia, cardiac arrhythmia, or endocrine disease (e.g., pheochromocytoma, thyroid storm). In addition, in patients who are taking beta-blocking agents such as propranolol, it may not be possible to increase the heart rate in response to a decrease in venous return.

In contrast to hypovolemia, overhydration is characterized hemodynamically by an elevation of peripheral and central venous pressure. Both neck veins and peripheral veins become distended. The concomitant increase in venous return increases stroke volume and, therefore, cardiac output (Starling's law of the heart). The increase in stroke volume and cardiac output is reflected by a bounding pulse, a wide pulse pressure, loud heart sounds, and mild to moderate hypertension. If cardiac function or renal reserve is marginal, congestive heart failure and pulmonary edema may ensue. At this point, extra heart sounds (S_3, S_4) and moist rales in the lung fields may be auscultated. Arterial pressure and effective circulating volume may actually decrease as a result of ineffective cardiac function. A radiograph of the chest prior to pulmonary edema may reveal distended pulmonary vessels and a slightly enlarged heart. After pulmonary edema ensues, peribronchial fluid cuffing of fluid and the characteristic butterfly pattern of alveolar edema may be seen.

SKIN PERFUSION

The maintenance of normal intravascular volume is reflected in the color, temperature, and moisture of the skin. When blood volume is adequate, the skin is warm, pink, and moist. As volume decreases, sympathetic tone increases and peripheral vasoconstriction ensues. This results in cool, pale, and dry extremities and dry mucous membranes. The reduction in effective circulating volume is accompanied by a reduction in interstitial fluid. Thus, skin turgor is poor. Intraocular pressure is also reduced and becomes perceptible at approximately 10 per cent dehydration as soft globes. In contrast, overhydration is associated with puffy, warm, pink edematous skin and the pooling of fluid in dependent areas, such as the sacrum and ankles (pitting edema). A major exception to this is sepsis. As a result of vasomotor dysfunction and a generalized capillary leak, extremities are warm, pink, and edematous despite a reduction in the effective circulating volume.

SENSORIUM

Although not specific for alterations in fluid balance, an alteration in mental status and CNS function often accompanies hypovolemia. These alterations include drowsiness, apathy, slow responses, and cessation of usual activity. If hypovolemia worsens, stupor and coma may ensue. These derangements in CNS function arise presumably from the loss of water from brain cells and eventually from a reduction in cerebral perfusion pressure. In contrast, hypervolemia does not usually alter CNS function. However, if hypervolemia becomes severe, brain cells may swell, leading to increased intracranial pressure, coma, and death.

BODY WEIGHT

Whereas alterations in hemodynamics, skin perfusion, urinary output, and the sensorium are very useful in assessing acute and large changes in fluid balance, they are not usually able to determine gradual and small changes. This is best assessed by the daily body weight. Rapid weight loss or weight gain is reflective of changes in total body water rather than in body mass. For example, an increase in body weight of 1 kg. in one day arises from the retention of 1 liter of water. Furthermore, patients who are not taking anything orally are catabolic and can gain weight only by the retention of water. Therefore, all patients who are receiving parenteral fluids should be weighed daily.

URINARY OUTPUT

Under most circumstances, daily and hourly urinary outputs are accurate measures of fluid balance. A decrease in urine output to less than 30 ml. per hour usually implies hypovolemia; an increase in urinary output to greater than 125 ml. per hour is usually reflective of hypervolemia. However, under some circumstances urinary output may be increased despite hypovolemia. Conversely, under some circumstances urinary output may be decreased despite hypervolemia. Therefore, when using this guide, one must be careful to exclude these paradoxical situations.

Polyuria

Polyuria is usually defined as a urinary output greater than 125 ml. per hour or 3 liters per day. However, it is apparent that even 50 ml. per hour may represent polyuria when the effective circulating volume is reduced, and urine formation should be minimal. The most common cause of polyuria is overhydration. This may be the result of over-zealous oral intake of fluids, of excessive parenteral administration of fluids or of mobilization of the third space. Polyuria may also be the result of osmotic diuresis, drug-induced diuresis, postobstructive diuresis, diabetes insipidus (DI), and high-output renal failure. All these conditions result in hypovolemia and ultimately renal failure if fluid intake does not parallel losses. Thus, it is imperative that all these processes be excluded before polyuria is attributed to hypervolemia and fluid intake is reduced. This can usually be established from the clinical history and a careful physical assessment of the patient.

In surgical patients, osmotic diuresis occurs most frequently as a result of glycosuria. The two factors that give rise to hyperglycemia and glucosuria in the surgical and injured patient are the intolerance to glucose uptake by peripheral tissues (insulin resistance) and the administration of glucose more rapidly than the patient can metabolize it. Other common etiologies include the previous administration of osmotic diuretics, such as mannitol, and the previous administration of intravenous contrast agents. The primary site of action of osmotic agents is at the proximal tubule, where they decrease sodium reabsorption through an increase in tubular osmolality. In addition, the increased volume in the nondistensible renal tubules increases the tubular flow rate, leading to a further decrease in sodium reabsorption. These result in the presentation of a large volume of NaCl and water to the distal tubules and collecting ducts. Since the distal tubules can increase NaCl reabsorption only to a limited degree, and since the action of vasopressin (and therefore water reabsorption) is impaired by a washout of the medullary osmotic gradient, an obligatory diuresis ensues. The site of action of non-osmotic diuretics, such as furosemide and thiazide, depends upon the specific agent. Nonetheless, the net result is an obligatory diuresis of salt and water. A postobstructive diuresis is occasionally seen in urologic patients in whom an obstruction of the urinary tract has been relieved. This involves a combination of salt wasting and a concentrating defect resulting from medullary washout.

The polyuria of diabetes insipidus is the result of either an absence of vasopressin secretion by the neurohypophysis (central DI) or an inability of vasopressin to stimulate water reabsorption in the collecting ducts (nephrogenic DI).[26] It is also possible to have a combination of central and nephrogenic DI (e.g., lithium intoxication). In the presence of DI, the urine osmolality is low, urine electrolyte concentrations are low, and the urine volume is high despite a normal or elevated plasma osmolality and normal or elevated electrolyte concentrations. If fluid intake is stopped, the high urinary output persists.

Polyuria may also be the result of high-output renal failure, chronic renal failure, or the resolution phase of oliguric renal failure. In all these processes, the kidney loses its ability to concentrate urine because of the loss of the medullary osmotic gradient that arises from the persistence of blood flow during a period when the delivery of sodium and chloride to the ascending limb of the loop of Henle and of urea to the collecting ducts is limited.[1, 19] This reduces the maximal concentrating ability to 350 mOsm. of solute per kg. of urine. In addition, there is a variable loss of tubular function that is reflected in an elevation of the plasma blood urea nitrogen (BUN) and plasma creatinine concentrations, and in abnormalities of renal tubular function tests such as the fractional excretion of sodium and the renal failure index (see section on oliguria next).

Although DI and polyuric renal failure are both associated with large volumes of hypo-osmolar urine in the presence of hypo-osmolar plasma, DI is associated only with tubular abnormalities in water reabsorption. Thus, polyuric renal failure can be differentiated from DI by the presence of tubular abnormalities other than those involving water.

Oliguria and Anuria

Oliguria is defined as the production of 50 to 400 ml. of urine per day, and anuria is defined as the production of less than 50 ml. of urine per day. The etiology of oliguria (and anuria) may be prerenal, postrenal, or intrinsic to the kidney (acute oliguric renal failure). Although the most frequent cause of oliguria is hypovolemia (prerenal), other causes must be excluded. These other etiologies are usually associated with normovolemia or hypervolemia.

The most common cause of postrenal obstruction is bladder neck or urethral obstruction. This occurs frequently in surgical patients as a result of prostatic hypertrophy or of blood clots in the bladder. It can easily be determined by the passage of a Foley catheter or by the irrigation of an existing catheter. *Therefore, the first step in the assessment of oliguria or anuria should be placement or irrigation of a Foley catheter.* Not only does this exclude bladder neck or urethral obstruction; it also allows for close monitoring of hourly urinary flow rates. Other causes of postrenal obstruction are less common. These include bilateral ureteral or ureteropelvic obstruction and unilateral ureteral or ureteropelvic obstruction in patients with only one kidney. These possibilities can be assessed by an ultrasound study of the kidneys.

Prerenal azotemia can result from insufficient blood volume (e.g., true hypovolemia), insufficient cardiac output (e.g., congestive heart failure), or insufficient renal flow (e.g., renal vein thrombosis). In most cases of prerenal azotemia, central baroreceptors and stretch receptors are inhibited through a reduction in the effective circulating volume. Similarly, the renal stretch receptors (juxtaglomerular apparatus) and the sodium and chloride receptors (macula densa) are activated. This results in enhanced sodium reabsorption, in enhanced water reabsorption, and in the formation of a small volume of urine that is high in nitrogenous wastes. Consequently, the urine is appropriately concentrated (specific gravity >1.020), the urine osmolality is greater than the plasma osmolality (Uosm >400 mOsm. per kg. and U per pOsm. >1.5), and the urine sodium is low (<20 mEq. per liter). Because urea reabsorption is coupled to sodium reabsorption in the early proximal tubule, the enhanced sodium reabsorption in prerenal azotemia increases urea reabsorption. In contrast, creatinine is neither secreted nor reabsorbed and its elimination depends only on the glomerular filtration rate (GFR). As long as the GFR remains near normal, serum creatinine remains normal. Therefore, in prerenal azotemia the plasma BUN:creatinine (Cr) ratio increases from the normal value of 10:1 to ratios of 20:1 or greater.[24]

In contrast to prerenal azotemia, acute renal failure is associated with a marked reduction in the GFR, with nonfunctional renal tubules, and with the accumulation of nitrogenous wastes. Since any urine that is formed is primarily an unmodified ultrafiltrate of plasma, the urine-specific gravity is similar to plasma (approximately 1.010), the urine osmolality is similar to plasma (Uosm <400 mOsm. per kg. and U/P ratio <1.1), and the urine sodium is high (>30 mEq. per liter). Because the GFR is reduced, creatinine is not excreted and serum creatinine (Cr) rises by 2 to 3 mg. per 100 ml. of plasma per day. The BUN also rises by 25 to 35 mg. per 100 ml. (60 to 90 mg. per 100 ml. in hypercatabolic patients), thus maintaining the plasma BUN:Cr ratio near normal (approximately 10:1).

The preceding differentiation of acute renal failure from prerenal azotemia is based on the urine indices of "classic cases." Unfortunately, many patients do not fit clearly into either pattern. For example, a patient with a reduction in GFR and hypovolemia will have indices that suggest both prerenal azotemia and acute renal failure. (See discussion on salt and water conservation later in this chapter.) As a result, numerous clinical indices have been developed to help differentiate acute renal failure from prerenal azotemia (Table 8). Among these, the fractional excretion of sodium (FE$_{NA}$) and the renal failure index (RFI) are most useful. Eighty-five to 95 per cent of all patients with prerenal azotemia have indices of less than 1, whereas less than 5 per cent of patients with acute renal failure have similar ratios.[20] During the time in which a definitive diagnosis is being made, it is imperative that cardiac output be maximized. This is not only therapeutic; it is also diagnostic. Prerenal failure will respond to these measures, but acute renal failure will not. In order to maximize cardiac output, a central venous or pulmonary artery catheter is necessary. Unless capillary wedge pressures are high (>20 mm. Hg) or there are overt signs of clinical cardiac failure, the first choice should always be fluids and not diuretics. If cardiac output is maximized and fluids have been of no benefit, renal failure is likely. In this situation, a trial of diuretics (furosemide or mannitol) is indicated because there is some evidence to suggest that these agents may convert oliguric renal failure to the more manageable nonoliguric form.

A similar diagnostic problem, frequently encountered in postoperative oliguric patients, is differentiating true hypovolemia from prerenal azotemia caused by an inadequate cardiac output (congestive heart failure). In the immediate postoperative period, the most frequent cause is true hypovolemia. In the absence of overt clinical cardiac failure, a fluid challenge of 250 to 500 ml. of normal saline or Ringer's lactate should be administered over 30 minutes. Most hypovolemic patients will respond with an improvement in urinary output. If there is no improvement or if the patient has a strong cardiac history, central venous pressure should be monitored.

Assessment of Serum Electrolytes

As a result of the ease and speed with which serum electrolytes are determined, clinical skills in the assessment of electrolyte disturbances have diminished. However, it is apparent that an understanding of the signs and symptoms of electrolyte abnormalities is necessary in order to avoid overlooking abnormalities.

SODIUM

The primary clinical signs and symptoms of hyponatremia (serum Na <130 mEq. per liter) and hypernatremia (serum Na >155 mEq. per liter) occur in the central nervous system. Mild to moderate hyponatremia (Na = 120 to 130 mEq. per liter) is manifested by lethargy, apathy, anorexia, hyperactive tendon reflexes, and muscle twitching. These result from swelling of cerebral cells as water moves into them to balance serum osmolality. However, unless the fall

TABLE 8. Diagnostic Indices in the Oliguric Patient*

	Prerenal Failure	Renal Failure
Uosm. (mOsm/kg. H$_2$O)	>500	<350
U specific gravity	>1.020	<1.010
U$_{NA}$ (mEq./l)	<20	>40
U$_K$ (mEq./l)	>40	<40
U/P urea nitrogen	>8	<3
U/P osmolality	>1.3	<1.1
U/P creatinine	>40	<20
Proteinuria	Negative/trace	Positive
Renal failure index (U$_{NA}$/Ucr/Pcr)	<1	>1
Fractional excretion sodium (U$_{NA}$/P$_{NA}$)/(Ucr/Pcr)	<1	>1
Blood BUN/Cr	>40:1	<20:1

*Adapted from Danielson, R. A.: Surg. Clin. North Am., 55:697, 1975; and Miller, T. R., et al.: Ann. Intern. Med., 89:47, 1978.

Abbreviations: U = Urine; U/P = urine-plasma ratio; U$_K$ = urokinase; BUN = blood urea nitrogen; Cr = creatinine; P$_{NA}$ = plasma sodium; U$_{NA}$ = urine sodium; Ucr = urine creatinine; Pcr = plasma creatinine.

in serum sodium is rapid, many patients exhibit no signs or symptoms until the serum sodium is 120 mEq. per liter or less. At that concentration, seizures, coma, loss of reflexes, and death may ensue if the hyponatremia is not treated. In contrast, hypernatremia is associated with restlessness, weakness, and dry, sticky mucous membranes. In addition, since hyponatremia is usually associated with fluid overload and hypernatremia with fluid deficit, the signs and symptoms of water imbalance discussed previously may also be present.

POTASSIUM

The signs and symptoms of potassium abnormalities are related primarily to the cardiovascular, gastrointestinal, and musculoskeletal systems. This derives from the important role potassium exerts on excitation-contraction coupling in muscle cells. Signs and symptoms of hypokalemia do not usually occur until the serum potassium concentration falls below 3.0 to 2.5 mEq. per liter. Among the signs and symptoms noted in Table 9, the most characteristic are the electrocardiographic (ECG) changes. These normally occur at a serum potassium of 3.0 mEq. per liter or less. However, patients with hypercalcemia or alkalosis, those with a rapid fall in serum potassium, or those taking digitalis preparations may manifest ECG changes at higher potassium concentrations.

Similarly, ECG changes are the most characteristic findings of hyperkalemia (K$^+$ 5.0 mEq. per liter). They do not usually occur until the serum potassium is greater than 6 mEq. per liter, but the appearance of these changes can be enhanced by hypocalcemia, acidosis, or a rapid elevation of serum potassium. Consequently, to avoid cardiac toxicity, intravenous potassium administration should not exceed 20 mEq. per liter and should be given only during careful monitoring of the patient's cardiac status. Furthermore, potassium must never be administered until an adequate urinary output is established.

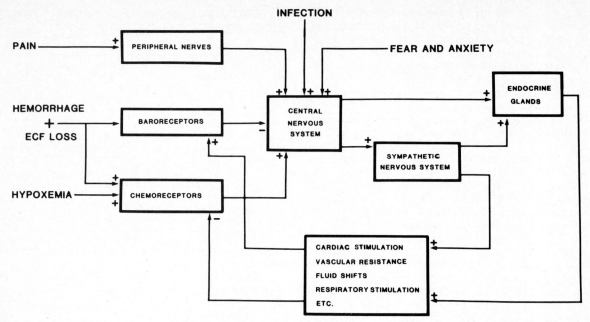

Figure 11. Overview of the neuroendocrine reflexes induced by injury and shock. (From Gann, D. S., and Amaral, J. F.: The pathophysiology of shock and trauma. In Zuidema, G. D., Rutherford, R. B., and Ballinger, W. F.: The Management of Trauma, 4th ed. Philadelphia, W. B. Saunders Company, 1985.)

THE PATHOPHYSIOLOGY OF FLUID AND ELECTROLYTE IMBALANCE

Reduction of the Effective Circulating Volume: Hypovolemia and Hypotension

A reduction in the effective circulating volume occurs commonly in surgical patients. It may be the result of loss of blood, as in hemorrhage; sequestration of fluids in third spaces that occur with injury, inflammation, and obstruction; loss of vascular tone, as in sepsis; pump failure, as in cardiogenic shock; inadequate oral intake, as in coma; or excessive unreplaced extrarenal losses, as in diarrhea, vomiting, and the drainage of fistulae. All of these insults activate the neuroendocrine system (Fig. 11). This leads to hemodynamic compensatory mechanisms to improve cardiac output and perfusion pressure, renal compensatory mechanisms to improve salt and water conservation, and elevations of plasma osmolality and plasma protein aimed toward the restitution of blood volume.

SALT AND WATER CONSERVATION

Since the formation of tubular fluid at the glomerulus is dependent upon the forces described in the Starling hypothesis of capillary equilibrium, it is apparent that the quantity of filtrate formed is dependent upon the renal perfusion pressure of the glomerulus. (See the discussion on hydrostatic and oncotic pressure earlier.) However, despite a reduction in renal perfusion pressure to 80 mm. Hg, renal blood flow (RBF) and GFR remain unchanged[2] (Fig. 12). The process by which RBF and GFR remain unchanged is intrinsic autoregulation. Although the exact mechanisms are unknown, it is postulated that tubuloglomerular feedback is involved.[21] This feedback is thought to involve individual nephrons sensing tubular fluid flow rate (chloride or sodium at the macula densa) and altering

glomerular capillary pressure primarily at the efferent arteriole. By increasing efferent arteriolar resistance, the fraction of peritubular blood that is filtered is increased, thereby allowing the maintenance of the total GFR.[2]

The increase in filtration fraction produces an increase in the oncotic pressure of peritubular capillary blood perfusing the proximal tubule. This results from the impermeability of glomerular basement membranes to protein. The increase in peritubular oncotic pressure produces an increased net transfer of water, NaCl, and $NaHCO_3$ from the proximal tubular filtrate to the peritubular blood. In addition, sympathetic nervous system activity may directly increase proximal tubular sodium transport and suppress the release of natriuretic hormone (cerebral) and of atrial natriuretic factor.

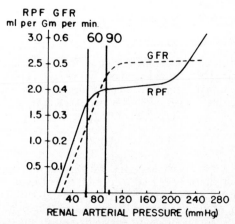

Figure 12. Autoregulation of renal blood flow. Despite a reduction in renal arterial pressure to 90 mm. Hg, renal blood flow and glomerular filtration rate (GFR) are maintained. RPF = Renal plasma flow. (Adapted from Ochwadt, B.: Prog. Cardiovasc. Dis., 3:501, 1961.)

The net result of these alterations is a decreased delivery of sodium, chloride, and filtered fluid to the loop of Henle. This produces a fall in medullary hyperosmolarity from which a defect in urine concentrating ability may develop.[28, 29] The latter results in the necessity to excrete a greater amount of urine (increased free water clearance) to eliminate the same amount of solute. This paradoxical increase in free water clearance has been called *polyuric prerenal failure*[19] and may be involved in the genesis of acute renal failure, particularly non-oliguric renal failure.[1]

Concomitant with the aforementioned compensatory mechanisms to enhance sodium reabsorption, there is a redistribution of blood flow from the superficial cortical glomeruli to the juxtamedullary glomeruli.[27] This increases sodium reabsorption by shifting blood flow to the juxta-medullary nephrons that have long loops of Henle. Various hormonal mediators have been implicated in the redistribution of renal blood flow, including catecholamines, angiotensin II, angiotensin I, prostaglandin E_2 (PGE_2), and vasopressin.[2] Present evidence supports the concept that the redistribution of intrarenal blood flow involves a balance mechanism between PGE_2-mediated medullary vasodilation and angiotensin-mediated medullary vasoconstriction.[2]

The maintenance of the normal medullary osmotic gradient requires the adequate delivery of sodium and chloride to the loop of Henle. Since hypovolemia and injury stimulate proximal reabsorption of sodium and chloride, the delivery of solute to the loop of Henle is decreased.[10] Therefore, the medullary osmotic gradient is washed out and a concentrating defect is seen in surgical patients.

Since sodium reabsorption in the ascending limb of the loop of Henle follows chloride passively, sodium delivery to the distal tubules is increased when chloride delivery to the loop is inadequate. This produces potassium wasting and metabolic alkalosis and is augmented by the secretion of aldosterone that accompanies hypovolemia and injury. Conversely, if sodium delivery to the distal tubules is inadequate, potassium will not be excreted, even in the presence of aldosterone, and hyperkalemia and metabolic acidosis may ensue.

During hypotension and injury, vasopressin secretion is stimulated by osmotic and non-osmotic (baroreceptor) pathways and results in water retention. However, when the countercurrent mechanism is disrupted by a fall in medullary osmolality, the action of arginine vasopressin (AVP) is impaired, resulting in the loss of free water.[28] Consequently, a normal or increased urinary output in a hypotensive or injured patient does not necessarily reflect adequate blood volume.

All the mechanisms for renal conservation of salt and water are directed to the prevention of further losses of circulating volume. In this regard, it is important to note that no increase in volume can occur even in the complete absence of renal excretion. Blood volume must be restored in order for the effective circulating volume, the cardiac output, and the vascular resistance to return to normal during hypovolemia.[5]

BLOOD VOLUME RESTITUTION

The restitution of blood volume can be achieved by the administration of exogenous fluids. If fluids are given intravenously, the increase in blood volume is direct. If these fluids are given orally, the increase in blood volume is through intestinal absorption, a process that, in part, is mediated by glucagon. In the absence of the administration of exogenous fluids, the blood volume must be restored from fluids present in the interstitial fluid and in the cells. This process may be thought of as occurring in two overlapping phases: the transcapillary refill phase and the plasma protein restitution phase (Fig. 13).

In the transcapillary refill phase, there is a net movement of protein-free fluid from the interstitium to the vascular space that is mediated by a fall in capillary pressure. The decrease in capillary pressure is initiated by hypotension and augmented by reflex sympathetic vasoconstriction.[11] According to the current concept of the Starling hypothesis of capillary equilibrium, as capillary hydrostatic pressure decreases during hypovolemic shock, the steady state flux of fluid is changed resulting in the net movement of the fluid into the capillary bed. (See section on hydro-

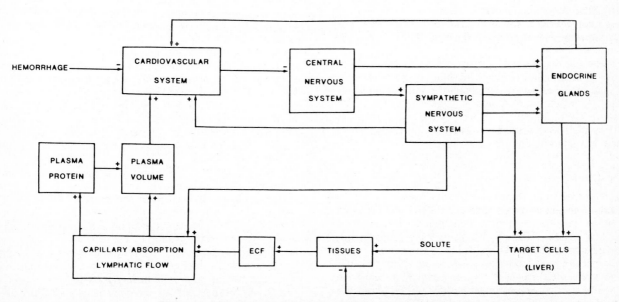

Figure 13. Schematic diagram of the restitution of blood volume.

static and oncotic pressure earlier.) This results in the restoration of 20 to 50 per cent of the blood volume loss.[5] Since this fluid is protein-free, interstitial colloid oncotic pressure and capillary hydrostatic pressure increase whereas capillary colloid oncotic pressure and interstitial hydrostatic pressure decrease. This results in the establishment of a new steady state in which further blood volume restitution is impossible.

Complete restitution of blood volume depends on the second phase, which is associated with the restitution of plasma protein and a shift of fluid from cells via the interstitial space to the capillary bed.[13] This movement of water appears to be mediated by a hormonally induced increase in extracellular osmolality. The protein involved in this process is primarily in the form of albumin. Since albumin synthesis takes at least 48 hours, the increase in plasma albumin must derive from the interstitium itself. Two mechanisms exist for the movement of protein from the interstitium to the capillary space, the lymphatics and the fenestrae of the capillary membrane. For either to be effective, interstitial pressure must increase. Because the compliance of the interstitium is fixed, an increase in volume leads to an increase in interstitial pressure. Since the plasma water is decreased in hypotension, an increase in interstitial volume must come from cells. Fluid will move out of cells only down an osmotic gradient. Therefore, this implies that an osmotic gradient exists between the intracellular and the extracellular space during hypotension and hypovolemia.

The osmotic gradient is produced transiently by a complex set of mechanisms that clearly depend upon the neuroendocrine response. An increase in cortisol is necessary but not sufficient to produce the increase in osmolality. In addition, an adrenal factor (catecholamines), a pituitary factor (probably vasopressin), and glucagon are required.[13] The source of solute production is the viscera, primarily the liver. These solutes, including glucose, phosphate, lactate, and pyruvate, are then delivered to the peripheral tissues, primarily muscle, where they increase the interstitial osmolality. Since the constituent molecules are relatively impermeable to cell membranes, an osmotic gradient is established and fluid moves from cells to the interstitium. In turn, the increase in interstitial osmolality leads to the movement of water from cells to the interstitium. The increase in interstitial volume results in an increase in interstitial pressure, which opens the capillary fenestrae, thus allowing protein to move through the capillary membrane.

The rise in osmolality also appears to contribute to the phase of transcapillary refill. The solute is delivered to the peripheral tissues, where it mediates the movement of water from cells to the interstitium, as is the case in the plasma protein restitution phase. Thus, by an increase in the interstitial pressures, the hyperosmolality also augments the transcapillary refill phase.[13]

Therapeutic Approach

The treatment of hypovolemia is directed to the correction of the underlying source of fluid loss and to replacement of the fluid loss. With hemorrhage, the source of bleeding must be identified and stopped. Concurrently, fluid resuscitation should be instituted with normal saline while packed red blood cells or whole blood are obtained. If packed RBCs are used for replacement, it should be remembered that approximately a liter of crystalloid fluid should be administered for each unit of RBCs given. The crystalloid fluid replaces not only the blood volume but also the interstitial volume, thereby allowing for the continued movement of protein into plasma. If the source of hypovolemia is from excessive third space losses or extrarenal losses, crystalloid replacement with fluid of appropriate electrolyte composition should be administered. In all instances of hypovolemia, fluid should be administered in quantities greater than those required for daily fluid maintenance until normovolemia is demonstrated clinically by the return of urinary output, skin perfusion, sensorium, and hemodynamic variables to normal.

During massive fluid replacement, plasma electrolytes should be carefully monitored. As noted previously, hypovolemia stimulates the retention of salt and water. As a result, the administration of hypotonic solutions leads to hyponatremia and the administration of hypertonic solutions leads to hypernatremia. Invariably hyponatremia in the surgical patient is the result of the administration of hypotonic fluid to postoperative or post-traumatic patients. In addition to abnormalities in serum sodium, abnormalities in serum potassium are also frequent. As a result of the high aldosterone secretion and increased delivery of sodium to the distal tubules associated with hypovolemia, potassium is secreted in the urine. This potassium wasting occurs even in the presence of a low total body potassium. Furthermore, the serum potassium concentration during hypovolemia is often not reflective of total body potassium because of concurrent metabolic acidosis. Thus, it is important to administer potassium during fluid resuscitation in hypovolemia. However, potassium replacement should not be instituted until urinary output is established because of the risks of hyperkalemia in renal failure.

Hyponatremia: Reduction of Serum Sodium

A measured serum sodium concentration of less than 135 mEq. per liter is indicative of hyponatremia. In most circumstances, the low concentration reflects the dilution of sodium ions by water. However, when the concentrations of either proteins or lipids in plasma are increased, a low serum sodium reflects not a dilution of sodium but, rather, a reduced volume of water per milliliter of plasma. The measurement of the serum sodium concentration is calculated from the amount of sodium present in the serum obtained from 1 ml. of plasma. During this calculation, it is assumed that 1 ml. of plasma is 93 per cent water and the actual amount is not measured. Although this is adequate under most circumstances, in the presence of hyperlipidemia or hyperproteinemia, 1 ml. of plasma contains less water because of the increased volume occupied by protein or lipid. Therefore, even though the ratio of water to sodium is unchanged, when the actual amount of sodium present in this plasma is compared with normal plasma, it is less. Although this suggests hyponatremia, it is actually pseudohyponatremia.

Since sodium is the primary determinant of plasma osmolality, hyponatremia is almost always reflective of hypo-osmolality. However, in the presence of hyperglycemia, a low serum sodium is usually not reflective of hypoosmolality. The increase in the number of glucose molecules in the plasma causes water to move from the cells and interstitium to the plasma. Therefore, although the sodium ions are diluted by water and hyponatremia is present, the plasma osmolality is normal or increased.

In the absence of an increase in osmotically active solutes such as glucose or of an increase in plasma proteins or lipids, hyponatremia occurs through two major mechanisms. Either vasopressin secretion is increased, or the diluting ability of the kidney is impaired. The increased secretion of vasopressin may be classified further as appropriate or inappropriate, depending upon whether or not stimuli for vasopressin secretion are present or absent. In all these situations, there is an accumulation of water in excess of salt. However, total body salt itself may be increased, decreased, or normal.

HYPONATREMIA ASSOCIATED WITH APPROPRIATE VASOPRESSIN SECRETION

Other than an increase in osmolality, most stimuli that increase vasopressin secretion also increase the secretion of aldosterone. For example, hypovolemia, hypoxia, pain, and anxiety increase the secretion of both vasopressin and aldosterone, thereby leading to increased reabsorption of salt and water. Under these conditions, hyponatremia can result by only two mechanisms. Either hypotonic fluids must be concurrently administered, or salt reabsorption must be impaired. Otherwise, both salt and water are reabsorbed in proportional quantities and a normal serum sodium concentration is maintained.

The most common mechanism for hyponatremia in surgical patients is the administration of hypotonic fluids. These may be in the form of intravenous fluids, enteral feedings, oral liquids, or food. Since there is more water available than salt in these solutions, water is reabsorbed in excess of salt in the presence of vasopressin and aldosterone, and hyponatremia ensues. In this setting, the urine sodium is decreased (U_{Na} <30 mEq. per liter) and the total body sodium is normal, decreased, or increased slightly.

An impairment in salt reabsorption may result from inadequate aldosterone production (Addison's disease, selective hypoaldosteronism, hyporeninemia), from salt-losing nephropathies (renal tubular acidosis), or from diuretic abuse. In all cases, sodium is wasted by the kidneys, total body sodium decreases, and hypovolemia ensues. The latter stimulates both water and salt reabsorption, but because of the impairment in salt reabsorption, water is reabsorbed in excess of salt and hyponatremia results. In Addison's disease there also appears to be stimulation of vasopressinergic neurons in the CNS that increases the secretion of vasopressin. In the presence of these conditions, the urinary sodium is increased (U_{Na} >40 mEq. per liter).

HYPONATREMIA ASSOCIATED WITH INAPPROPRIATE SECRETION OF VASOPRESSIN

Vasopressin secretion is considered inappropriate when physiologic stimuli known to increase vasopressin secretion are not present. The inappropriate secretion of vasopressin, or the syndrome of inappropriate antidiuretic hormone (SIADH), may be central or ectopic. Central SIADH occurs in association with disorders of the CNS (head trauma, brain tumor, infection, cerebrovascular accidents); with severe pulmonary infection; with drugs (opiates, chlorpropamide, tolbutamide, barbituates, nicotine, vincristine, carbamazepine, acetoaminophen, indomethacin); and with miscellaneous disorders (burns, alcohol, porphyria). Ectopic vasopressin secretion occurs usually from malignant tumors (lung, duodenum, pancreas, prostate). An SIADH-like syndrome is also associated with severe hypothyroidism, but in this situation it responds to appropriate hormonal replacement.

In all cases of SIADH, the urine is inappropriately concentrated (U_{osm}>p_{osm}), the urine osmolality fails to fall when a free water challenge is administered; renal function is otherwise normal; urinary sodium is increased U_{Na}>30 mEq. per liter) and matches dietary intake; adrenal and pituitary function is normal and the plasma osmolality increases during severe water restriction. A similar situation is *reset osmostat*, or *essential hyponatremia*, in which the inhibition of vasopressin secretion occurs at a lower plasma osmolality than normal. In contrast to SIADH, patients with essential hyponatremia respond to a water challenge with a decrease in urine osmolality and, as a result, rarely require specific therapy.

HYPONATREMIA RESULTING FROM AN IMPAIRED ABILITY OF THE KIDNEYS TO DILUTE URINE

In the absence of vasopressin secretion, the impaired ability of the kidneys to dilute urine results either from renal failure or from an increase in the proximal reabsorption of solute and water. In acute renal failure, the kidneys are limited in their ability to excrete water or sodium. Because water is normally ingested in excess of sodium, hyponatremia results. Furthermore, the increase in total body water and total body salt leads to extracellular fluid expansion and to edema.

An increase in the proximal reabsorption of solute and water occurs during cirrhosis, congestive heart failure, malignant ascites, and the nephrotic syndrome. Although the exact mechanism is unclear, the increase in proximal reabsorption in these edematous conditions probably results from a reduction in the effective circulating volume.[27] In turn, the increase in proximal reabsorption results in decreased delivery of sodium and chloride to the loop of Henle and to the distal tubule, sites where the selective reabsorption of these solutes normally produces a dilute urine. In these cases, osmotic diuresis, which limits proximal reabsorption, will correct the defect in the excretion of free water.

THERAPEUTIC APPROACH

The first step in the treatment of hyponatremia is to determine the etiology. This is best done on the basis of the patient's volume status and urinary electrolytes. If the extracellular volume is significantly increased and edema is present, the usual cause of hyponatremia is impaired renal diluting capacity. If the extravascular volume is decreased and hypovolemia is present, the usual cause is the appropriate secretion of vasopressin with hypotonic fluid replacement or with impaired sodium reabsorption. However, when the extravascular volume is normal or slightly increased, either the appropriate or inappropriate secretion of vasopressin may be responsible. A low urinary sodium in this setting suggests appropriate ADH with hypotonic fluid administration. A high urine sodium suggests either SIADH or salt wasting. These can be differentiated on the basis of a normal saline challenge. Patients with appropriate vasopressin secretion and impaired salt reabsorption will respond with an improvement in serum sodium, whereas patients with SIADH will not. Furthermore, fluid restriction will not improve the serum sodium concentration in patients with impaired salt reabsorption, but it will in patients with SIADH.

The treatment of hyponatremia in edematous conditions is the restriction of salt and water intake. Patients with renal failure should also undergo dialysis. In addition, vigorous attempts should be made to correct the underlying cause because these situations are usually refractory to any treatment directed to correcting the hyponatremia itself.[24, 27] In congestive heart failure, improvement of cardiac function with digitalis, diuretics, and fluid and salt restriction will often eliminate the excess water and sodium. In conditions with a low oncotic pressure, intravenous albumin may be of value, and in malignant ascites and cirrhosis, spironalactone, an anti-aldosterone agent, may aid in the reduction of ascites. However, because of the limited response of these illnesses to these treatment modalities, usually no specific measures other than fluid and electrolyte restriction are instituted until the serum sodium is less than 130 mEq. per liter or until symptoms develop. However, if symptoms do develop, mannitol may be of benefit by impairing the proximal reabsorption of solutes and water.

Hyponatremia secondary to appropriate vasopressin secretion is treated by the elimination of hypotonic fluids and by the administration of normal saline. Usually, this is sufficient in both forms to correct the hyponatremia gradually. In addition, it may be possible to increase water loss. For example, in the intubated patient one may increase the respiratory rate and volume and decrease the dead space and the hydration of the inspired air. Treatment with hypertonic saline is rarely, if ever, required.

The treatment of hyponatremia in SIADH is strict fluid restriction to 500 ml. per day or less. Lithium carbonate has been used to treat SIADH because it interferes with the action and inhibits the secretion of vasopressin. Similarly, demeclocycline has been used. However, both of these agents are potentially toxic and should be used only in patients who fail to respond to fluid restriction.

Hypernatremia: Elevation of Serum Sodium

By definition, hypernatremia (serum Na>150 mEq. per liter) results from an increase in the ratio of plasma sodium to plasma water. Since the plasma sodium is the prime solute contributing to plasma osmolality, hypernatremia is always associated with plasma hyperosmolality. However, hyperosmolality may exist without hypernatremia, as in hyperosmolar nonketotic coma or with the rapid administration of parenteral alimentation.

Hypernatremia results from either the loss of water in excess of salt (pure water or hypotonic water) or from the retention of salt in excess of water. Common to all forms of hypernatremia and hyperosmolality is the osmotic movement of water from cells to the ECW leading to the shrinkage of cells. The shrinkage of cells is greatest when the hypernatremia results from the loss of pure water or the addition of salt, and it is least when it results from the loss of hypotonic fluid. For example, when 1 liter of pure water is lost from the ECW, the increase in the osmolality of the ECW will be balanced by the movement of water from the intracellular space and the redistribution of solute within the ECW. Since the ICW space is two times as large as the ECW space, two thirds of the solute will be balanced by the movement of water from the ICW and one third by the redistribution of solute in the ECW. In contrast, if the fluid that is lost has one-half the tonicity of plasma, 2 liters of fluid must be lost to incur the same degree of cell shrinkage because 1 liter of the fluid lost is isotonic to plasma and, consequently, will not change the osmolality of the extracellular fluid.

Etiology

The most common cause of hypernatremia is the loss of water in excess of salt (pure water or hypotonic fluid), and it may result from nonrenal or renal sources. Under normal circumstances, an increase in serum sodium or osmolality is accompanied by thirst, an increase in the ingestion of water, an increase in the secretion of vasopressin, and an increase in the renal conservation of water. Therefore, in order for hypernatremia to worsen in the face of ongoing losses of water, a defect must also exist in one of these four regulatory mechanisms. However, in patients with absent vasopressin secretion (central DI) or with impaired vasopressin action on the kidney (nephrogenic DI) fluid balance is maintained near normal (150 to 155 mEq. Na+ per liter) through thirst and the increased ingestion of water. In contrast, patients with diminished thirst (hypodipsia) or with decreased access to water are unable to maintain fluid balance during periods of excessive loss even in the presence of maximal vasopressin secretion and action. Thus, it is apparent that severe hypernatremia occurs only in patients with hypodipsia (e.g., hypothalamic tumor), or in patients with a diminished access to water, such as in comatose and disoriented individuals, infants, and patients who cannot drink because of gastrointestinal disease or a surgical procedure.

Fever is a frequent cause of hypernatremia as a result of the loss of hypotonic fluid in sweat. In contrast, granulating wounds and burns result in hypernatremia primarily through the loss of free water. The loss of free water may also occur through the lungs in patients in whom ventilation is occurring through a tracheostomy tube with nonhumidified air. Hypernatremia may also be the result of the obligatory loss of hypotonic fluid during osmotic diuresis or of the inability to retain free water produced by central or nephrogenic DI. However, excessive gastrointestinal losses, such as those that occur in severe diarrhea or vomiting, do not usually produce hypernatremia because these fluids are isotonic.

Therapeutic Approach

Hypernatremia and hyperosmolality resulting from the loss of water rapidly produce cell shrinkage and eventually hypovolemia. If the condition remains uncorrected, coma and death ensue. Therefore, it is essential that these conditions be reversed by the administration of D5W when they result from the loss of pure water, 0.2 per cent saline when they result from the loss of water with small amounts of salt (<40 mEq. per liter), or 0.45 per cent saline when they result from the loss of water with moderate amounts of salt (<80 mEq. per liter). Unless symptoms are life-threatening, this should be done slowly because the rapid correction of hyperosmolality and hypernatremia can lead to cerebral edema, coma, and death. During hyperosmolar conditions, the brain accumulates osmolar solutes in excess of plasma solutes in an apparent attempt to maintain cell volume. If hypotonic solutions are administered rapidly at this time, the increased osmolality of neurons results in the accumulation of intracellular water and cerebral edema. Thus, the water deficit should be corrected slowly. In addition, if hypotension is also present, the contracted extracellular fluid (ECF) volume should be replaced with normal saline before correction of tonicity is attempted. Under these circumstances, the use of normal saline will still be hypotonic to body fluids and will avoid the risk of cerebral edema. Once hypovolemia is corrected, hypernatremia may be corrected gradually with D5W or 0.2 per cent saline.

The water deficit can be calculated from the patient's current body weight and plasma sodium (P_{NA}) concentration if it is assumed that no salt has been lost during the formation of hypernatremia. Under these circumstances:

$$(\text{Normal TBW}) (\text{normal } P_{NA}) = (\text{current TBW}) (\text{current } P_{NA})$$

and

$$\text{Water deficit} = \text{current TBW} - \text{normal TBW} \qquad (12)$$

Since P_{NA} equals 140 mEq. per liter:

$$\text{Normal TBW} = \frac{\text{current TBW (current } P_{NA})}{140} \qquad (13)$$

$$\text{Water deficit} = \text{current TBW} \frac{(\text{current } P_{NA} - 1)}{140} \qquad (14)$$

$$= 0.6 \times \text{body weight in kg.} \frac{(\text{current } P_{NA} - 1)}{140} \qquad (15)$$

It must be noted that this formula is an approximation based on the assumptions that salt has not been lost, that water is lost uniformly throughout all cells, and that the percentage of body weight represented by TBW in dehydrated males is 60 per cent (50 per cent in females). Although under most clinical circumstances these assumptions are frequently incorrect, this formula allows a rough estimation of the water deficit upon which fluid replacement can be based. In order to avoid rapid administration, half of the calculated fluid deficit should be administered during the first 12 hours and the remainder over the next 24 to 48 hours. In addition, the plasma sodium concentration should not fall by more than 15 mEq. per liter during a 6-hour period.[24]

INTAKE OF SALT IN EXCESS OF WATER: SALT INTOXICATION

Etiology

The intake of salt in significant excess of water is almost always accidental or iatrogenic (e.g., 3 per cent of NaCl instead of 0.9 per cent NaCl). The acute increase in the sodium concentration of the ECF causes water to leave cells by osmosis. In turn, the expansion of the ECF volume produces a brisk diuresis. However, the kidneys can excrete maximally only about 300 mm. of salt per kg. of urine. Thus, a net gain of salt and a net loss of intracellular water may occur.

Therapeutic Approach

The increase in total body sodium can be approximated from the plasma sodium concentration.

$$\text{Sodium gain} = (\text{current } P_{NA} - \text{normal } P_{NA}) \times \text{TBW} \qquad (16)$$

$$= (0.6) (\text{body weight in kg.}) (140 - \text{current } P_{NA}) \qquad (17)$$

From this the water deficit can be calculated as:

$$\text{Water deficit} = \frac{\text{sodium gained}}{140} \qquad (18)$$

or alternatively,

$$\text{Water deficit} = \text{current TBW} \frac{(\text{current } P_{NA} - 1)}{140} \qquad (19)$$

The water deficit should be administered very slowly in the form of D5W. In addition to the possibility of cerebral edema, the rapid administration of free water in this setting may lead to acute extracellular volume expansion. If symptoms of pulmonary edema develop, diuretics should be administered. Otherwise, diuretics should not be used routinely because the loss of hypotonic urine produced by diuretics may worsen the hypernatremia.

Alterations in Plasma Potassium: Hypokalemia and Hyperkalemia

As noted previously, the plasma potassium concentration is a poor indicator of total body potassium content, since hyperkalemia or hypokalemia may exist with either an increased, decreased, or normal content of potassium in the body. As a result, therapeutic decisions to withhold or give potassium should not be based solely on the plasma potassium concentration. Consideration must also be given to the volume, acid-base, and glucose status of the patient; to the possible existence of significant cellular breakdown; and to the presence of chronic disease.

HYPOKALEMIA: REDUCTION OF PLASMA POTASSIUM TO <3.5 MEQ. PER LITER

Etiology

Although under normal circumstances, the nonrenal losses of potassium are small and virtually all the potassium filtered by the kidneys is reabsorbed, prolonged starvation and poor nutrient intake (e.g., in alcoholism, anorexia nervosa) eventually lead to potassium depletion and hypokalemia. In addition, hypokalemia may result from increased renal excretion of potassium, increased nonrenal losses, or the movement of potassium into cells (e.g., in alkalosis, hyperinsulinism).

An increase in the secretion of potassium by the kidneys occurs either by an increase in the secretion of aldosterone or by an increase in the delivery of sodium to the distal tubules and proximal collecting ducts. In both cases, distal sodium reabsorption is increased and kaliuresis ensues as the transepithelial potential across the tubular cells increases. The secretion of aldosterone may be increased by physiologic stimuli such as volume or salt depletion, or it may be increased as a result of pathologic conditions such as primary hyperaldosteronism, *Bartter's syndrome* (hypersecretion of renin), licorice intoxication, glucocorticoid excess, or certain forms of congenital adrenal hyperplasia. An increase in the distal delivery of sodium results from volume expansion, from diuretics that block proximal tubular reabsorption of sodium (acetazolamide), from diuretics that block the reabsorption of sodium in the loop of Henle (thiazides and furosemide), and from diuretics that block both processes (osmotic diuretics). The presence of nonreabsorbable anions (carbenicillin) increases the

TABLE 9. Signs and Symptoms of Hypokalemia and Hyperkalemia

	Hypokalemia		Hyperkalemia		
	Moderate	*Severe*	*Moderate*	*Severe*	
Gastrointestinal		Ileus Anorexia Vomiting Constipation		Nausea Anorexia Vomiting Diarrhea	
Neuromuscular	Lethargy Weakness Cramps Hyporeflexia	Confusion Paralysis	Lethargy Weakness	Paralysis	
Cardiovascular	Low voltage Flat T waves Depression of ST-T segment Prominent U waves (>3.0 mEq./liter)	Increased P waves Prolonged P-R interval Widening of QRS complex (>2.0 mEq./liter)	Peaked T waves Shortening QT interval (6–7 mEq./l)	QRS Widening Depressed ST segments (7– 8 Widening Depressed ST segments (7– 8 mEq./liter)	Loss of T waves Heart block Diastolic asys- tole (<8 mEq./liter)
Aggravating factors	Hypercalcemia Digitalis Alkalosis Rapid decrease		Hypocalcemia Hyponatremia Acidosis Rapid increases		

delivery of sodium distally because electrical neutrality must be maintained in tubular fluid, and cation exchange occurs only in the distal tubules and collecting ducts. An increase in plasma bicarbonate (alkalosis) will increase the delivery of sodium (bicarbonate) distally because the proximal reabsorption of bicarbonate cannot increase actively. In renal tubular acidosis and other salt-wasting nephropathies, proximal reabsorption is impaired and distal delivery of sodium is increased. Finally, a decrease in serum chloride or magnesium also increases the delivery of sodium distally. Since the chloride concentration of tubular filtrate is reduced, most of the chloride in the filtrate is reabsorbed proximally with sodium and little is delivered to the loop of Henle. The marked reduction in the active transport of chloride in the ascending limb (and therefore the passive transport of sodium) results in the delivery of large amounts of sodium to the distal tubules.

The primary route for the nonrenal loss of potassium is the gastrointestinal tract (Table 9). Vomiting, diarrhea (especially the watery-diarrhea syndrome), laxative abuse, and villous adenoma of the colon are associated with significant losses of potassium and can lead to potassium depletion and hypokalemia. The loss of potassium in these conditions is via both the gastrointestinal tract and the kidney. The latter results from the significant losses of water, sodium, and chloride that accompany hypovolemia.

Treatment

The treatment of hypokalemia requires correction of the underlying cause and administration of potassium because it is almost always associated with a reduction in total body stores. Even during alkalosis, in which potassium moves into cells, the total body potassium is usually reduced because of the concomitant kaliuresis induced by alkalosis. If, in addition to alkalosis, volume depletion is present, the depletion of total body potassium is a virtual certainty because the distal reabsorption of sodium and the secretion of potassium is stimulated further. A classic example of this is the hypokalemic, hypochloremic metabolic alkalosis induced by protracted vomiting from pyloric obstruction or

hypertrophic pyloric stenosis. In this process, the obstruction of gastric outflow causes distention of the fundus and antrum, which leads to the production of acid and further distention. Vomiting ensues, and the process is reinitiated. The loss of large volumes of water, sodium, chloride, and acid lead to hypochloremic metabolic alkalosis. Although significant amounts of potassium are lost in the vomitus and may themselves lead to hypokalemia, the severe potassium depletion that occurs is also the result of the marked kaliuresis that accompanies volume depletion, alkalosis, and hypochloremia. In addition, the increase in the transepithelial electrical potential that is brought about by the increased delivery of sodium appears to stimulate hydrogen ion secretion distally, thus leading to a paradoxically acidic urine. If only potassium is replaced, the process will continue. Therefore, in order to correct the hypokalemia and alkalosis, it is imperative that chloride be given so that the persistent increased distal delivery of sodium can be reduced.

The preferred route for potassium replacement is oral and is usually adequate in patients who have mild to moderate hypokalemia. For more severe hypokalemia or for patients who are unable to take anything by mouth, the intravenous route can be used. However, it is imperative that the potassium not be administered rapidly, even in severely depleted patients, because of the risk of hyperkalemia and death. Therefore, rates of greater than 20 mEq. per hour should not be used.

HYPERKALEMIA: INCREASE OF PLASMA POTASSIUM TO >5.5 mEq. PER LITER

Etiology

Under normal conditions, an increased intake of potassium rarely results in hyperkalemia. The defense against hyperkalemia involves the movement of potassium into cells and the excretion of excess potassium by the kidneys. Most of the potassium administered, either orally or intravenously, moves rapidly into cells so that the rise in the plasma potassium concentration is minimized. This process is aided by the secretion of insulin. The small rise in plasma potassium stimulates the secretion of aldosterone, thereby leading to the excretion of excess potassium by the kidney. Approximately 30 per cent of the excess potassium is eliminated by the kidneys within 2 hours and approximately 80 per cent is eliminated within 6 hours.[24] However, if large amounts of potassium are ingested or administered rapidly, or if insulin deficiency is present, the cells may be unable to absorb sufficient quantities of potassium rapidly enough to avoid hyperkalemia. Furthermore, in the presence of potassium-sparing diuretics (spironolactone), of impaired renal function (acute or chronic renal failure), of impaired aldosterone secretion (Addison's disease, selective hypoaldosteronism, hyporeninemia), or impaired aldosterone action (lupus erythematosus, diabetes mellitus, sickle cell disease, renal transplant), even small amounts of excess potassium may lead to hyperkalemia. In all these situations, hyperkalemia is associated with an increase in total body potassium.

Equally frequent is the occurrence of hyperkalemia in the presence of normal or decreased potassium stores. This results from the movement of intracellular potassium into the extracellular space. Although this may be induced by the breakdown of cells, drugs (digitalis, succinyl choline), or insulin deficiency, it most commonly arises during acute acidosis.[7] As noted previously, the acute increase in the intracellular and extracellular potassium concentration leads to the movement of potassium out of cells. However, this is not true for chronic acidosis.[7] Both chronic respiratory and chronic metabolic acidoses are associated with little movement of potassium from cells, with kaliuresis, with a reduction in total body potassium, and with hypokalemia or normokalemia. Therefore, hyperkalemia in the presence of chronic respiratory or chronic metabolic acidosis should not be attributed to acidosis until other etiologies have been excluded.

Therapeutic Approach

The first step in the management of hyperkalemia is to make certain that true hyperkalemia is present. The potassium concentration measured by laboratories is the concentration in the serum and not that in the plasma *per se*. Since small amounts of potassium are released by leukocytes and platelets during the clotting of blood, the measured potassium concentration may be spuriously elevated. This may be accentuated further by the release of large amounts of potassium from RBCs during hemolysis. Therefore, whenever the serum potassium concentration is elevated, blood should be obtained with as little mechanical trauma as possible into a heparinized tube. Since pseudohyperkalemia is not associated with any symptoms, a clue to its presence is the absence of symptoms, the absence of ECG changes, and the absence of apparent cause. (See the section on potassium under "Assessment of Serum Electrolytes" earlier.)

Once true hyperkalemia is established, therapy should be directed to correcting the hyperkalemia and reversing the underlying cause. The plasma potassium concentration must be reduced regardless of the total body potassium stores because hyperkalemia itself is a potentially lethal situation. This can be accomplished acutely by administering glucose and insulin, by correcting any acute acidosis that is coexistent, and by administering bicarbonate. All these measures will move potassium into cells, thereby reducing the plasma potassium concentration. In nondiabetic patients, a 10 per cent solution of glucose may be

sufficient. However, in patients with severe hyperkalemia, a 50-gm. dose of glucose with 10 units of regular insulin may be administered intravenously.

Acutely, the untoward effects of hyperkalemia may be minimized by the administration of calcium. This is usually given *slowly* (over 5 minutes) in the form of a 10 per cent calcium gluconate solution (10 ml.). The calcium acts to lower the threshold potential required for electrical excitation, thereby improving muscle contraction and cardiac activity. However, because of its potentially lethal effects, calcium should be used only in severe hyperkalemia, and then only with the greatest care (including monitoring of the ECG).

Finally, the excess potassium must be eliminated. In patients with normal adrenal and renal function, correction of acidosis, reduction of potassium intake, and movement of potassium into cells may be sufficient. However, in patients with impaired renal, circulatory, or adrenal function, additional measures are necessary. The renal excretion of potassium can be increased by the administration of diuretics that increase the delivery of sodium to the distal tubules. When this is done, normal saline should be administered to avoid volume depletion. In patients with renal failure, dialysis will be necessary. The intake of potassium also must be reduced. Potassium should be removed from the diet and intravenous solutions. Any drugs that exist as the potassium salt (e.g., penicillin) should be avoided. The intake of potassium may also be reduced by cation-exchange resins, such as sodium polystyrene sulfonate (kayexalate). When these resins are given orally (20 gm. every 4 to 6 hours), 100 ml. of 10 per cent sorbitol should also be given to avoid constipation. When given by enema, 50 gm. (every 3 to 4 hours) should be mixed with 50 ml. of 70 per cent sorbitol and 100 to 150 ml. of tap water.

ACID-BASE BALANCE

Physiology

The pH of body fluids is maintained under normal conditions within the narrow range of 7.37 to 7.42. This range is necessary for the normal activity of enzymes and of muscles. The regulation of pH must occur in the face of a large daily production of organic and inorganic acids by metabolism. As such, it is apparent that a system for buffering and eliminating these acids is necessary to maintain the pH within this narrow range. Essentially, these processes are divisible into the rapid buffering of acids by the salts of weak acids, the rapid elimination of acids (as CO_2) through the lungs, and the slow excretion of acids by the kidneys.

An *acid* is defined as a substance that *donates protons* or as one that *increases* the hydrogen ion concentration when added to a solution. A *base* is defined as a substance that *accepts protons* or one that *decreases* the hydrogen ion concentration when added to a solution. It is clear from these definitions that the proton need not come from the acid itself, nor does it need to be taken up specifically by the base. For example, CO_2 is an acid, even though the molecule itself has no proton to donate. However, in solution, CO_2 is in equilibrium with carbonic acid which, in turn, is in equilibrium with bicarbonate:

$$CO_2 + H_2O \rightleftharpoons H_2CO_3 + H^+ + HCO_3^- \qquad (20)$$

Thus, the proton is derived from the dissociation of water and not from carbon dioxide itself.

Substances that dissociate into charged particles (ions) in solution are termed *electrolytes* and are classified as strong or weak. Strong electrolytes dissociate completely into ions when placed into solution, whereas weak electrolytes dissociate only partially. Therefore, NaCl is a strong electrolyte because it dissociates nearly completely when placed in solution into Na^+ and Cl^-. If in the process of dissociation the concentration of hydrogen ions in the solution increases, the electrolyte is an acid; if the concentration of hydrogen ions decreases, the electrolyte is a base. According to these definitions, HCl is a strong acid and CO_2 is a weak acid. Similarly, sodium hydroxide is a strong base and ammonia is a weak base.

A buffer is a mixture of a weak acid and its salt (conjugate base) or a mixture of a weak base and its salt (conjugate acid). As such, buffer systems are able to take up or release hydrogen ions, thereby helping to prevent large changes in the hydrogen ion concentration. However, it is important to note that buffers do not completely eliminate the changes in hydrogen ion concentration but only minimize them. When a strong acid is added to a solution containing a weak acid and its salt, we think of the conjugate base of the weak acid accepting a hydrogen ion from a strong acid to form a weak acid and the strong acid accepting a strong cation to form a neutral salt. For example:

$$HCl \quad + \quad NaHCO_3 \rightleftharpoons H_2CO_3 \quad + \quad NaCl \quad (21)$$
strong acid   buffer salt   weak acid   neutral salt

However, as noted previously, strong acids and strong electrolytes are dissociated completely in solution. Therefore, when a strong acid is added to a solution containing a buffer, the strong acid actually dissociates into strong anions and hydrogen ions. This in turn alters the equilibrium between weak acid and its salt such that the salt liberates its strong cation and associates with the hydrogen ion. That is:

$$H^+ + Cl^- + H_2CO_3 + Na^+ + HCO_3^1 \rightleftharpoons$$
$$H_2CO_3 + HCO_3^1 + Na^+ + Cl^- + H^+ \quad (22)$$
more   less

Therefore, it is the *difference* between the strong cations and the strong anions, the so-called *strong ion difference*, that is the primary determinant of the hydrogen ion concentration. As a result, in clinical practice the electrolyte concentrations can be used to predict the acid-base status. A strong anion gap, i.e., serum sodium>serum chloride, is associated with acidosis, whereas a strong cation gap, i.e., serum sodium<serum chloride, is associated with alkalosis.

In biologic systems, the major extracellular fluid buffer is bicarbonate and the major intracellular buffers are proteins and phosphates. In addition, there are many other buffers present, albeit in much smaller quantities, that have greater buffering capacity than bicarbonate. In extracellular fluid, a specific amount of inorganic phosphate can buffer more hydrogen ions than can the same amount of bicarbonate. Therefore, the hydrogen ion concentration is determined secondarily by the total weak acid buffers present and not by a single buffer, such as bicarbonate. However, under physiologic conditions, a single buffer pair can predict the acid-base status. According to the isohydric principle, when several buffers exist in a common solution, the buffer pairs are in equilibrium with the same concentration of hydrogen ions. Thus,

$$[H^+] = K_1 \times \frac{[H_2CO_3]}{[HCO_3^-]} = K_2 \times \frac{[H_2PO_4]}{[HPO_4^-]}$$
$$= K_3 \times \frac{[H\text{-protein}]}{[protein^-]} \quad (23)$$

Therefore, the hydrogen ion concentration can be determined in a common solution if the concentrations of only one buffer pair are known. Plasma is a homogenous solution to which the isohydric principle can be applied without error. In contrast, application of the isohydric principle to other fluid compartments is inaccurate because these compartments do not have a homogenous distribution of buffers between them. Nevertheless, it does allow one to determine qualitative changes.

The bicarbonate buffer system has been chosen in clinical practice for three main reasons. First, it is easily measured and is distributed primarily in the extracellular fluid. Second, although other buffers have a greater buffer capacity, bicarbonate is present in much greater quantities and is readily available from metabolic processes either as CO_2 or as bicarbonate itself. As a result, even though each increment of bicarbonate may buffer less hydrogen ions than other buffers, the total amount buffered by bicarbonate is greater. Third and most important, bicarbonate is a uniquely effective buffer because its concentration is controlled by the renal formation of bicarbonate, by the renal reabsorption of bicarbonate, and by ventilation. As noted in equation No. 20, the amount of bicarbonate present is a function of carbonic acid which, in turn, is a function of the dissolved CO_2. Since the dissolved CO_2 is proportional to Pco_2 by a solubility factor of 0.03, bicarbonate is dependent upon the Pco_2 and, therefore, on ventilation. These relationships become apparent when equation 20 is expressed by mass action:

$$[H^+] = Ka \times \frac{[H_2CO_3] + [CO_2]}{[HCO_3^-]}$$
$$= ka \frac{[H_2CO_3] + (Pco_2 \times 0.03)}{[HCO_3^-]} \quad (24)$$

Since at the temperature and ionic composition of body fluids, almost all carbonic acid in solution is present as dissolved CO_2, the negligible amount of H_2CO_3 present can be disregarded. Substituting 800 nmol. per liter for the dissociation constant of bicarbonate at 37°C., equation 24 reduces to:

$$[H^+] = 800 \times \frac{Pco_2 \times 0.03}{[HCO_3]} = 24 \times \frac{Pco_2}{[HCO_3^-]} \quad (25)$$

This equation is a simplification of the familiar Henderson-Hasselbach equation (equation 26) in which the relationship of pH to the bicarbonate buffer system is described:

$$pH = \log pka + \log \frac{[HCO^-_3]}{[H_2CO_3]} \quad (26)$$

Therefore, although the acid-base status is *determined* by the strong ion difference, the total weak acid buffers present and the partial pressure of carbon dioxide, that status can be estimated by the concentration of bicarbonate and the partial pressure of carbon dioxide.

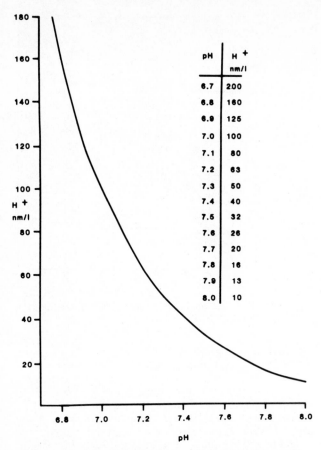

pH	H + nm/l
6.7	200
6.8	160
6.9	125
7.0	100
7.1	80
7.2	63
7.3	50
7.4	40
7.5	32
7.6	26
7.7	20
7.8	16
7.9	13
8.0	10

Figure 14. Relationship of hydrogen ion concentration to pH.

Equation 25 is considerably more useful in the practical management of acid-base disorders than equation 26. Although the pH is the negative logarithm of the hydrogen ion concentration (Fig. 14), a useful rule to remember when using equation 25 is that *at pH 7.40 the concentration of hydrogen ions is 40 nmol. per liter and within the pH range of 7.2 to 7.6, each 0.01 unit change in pH is approximated by a reciprocal change in the hydrogen ion concentration of 1 nmol. per liter.* For example, if the Pco_2 increases from the normal of 40 mm. Hg to 60 mm. Hg:

$$[H^+] = 24 \times \frac{60}{24} \times 60 \text{ nmol. per liter} \qquad (27)$$
$$\text{and pH} = 7.20$$

Similarly, if the bicarbonate concentration decreases from its normal value of 24 mEq. per liter to 18 mEq per liter:

$$[H^+] = 24 \times \frac{40}{18} = 60 \text{ nmol. per liter} \qquad (28)$$
$$\text{and pH} = 7.20$$

However, outside the range of 7.2 to 7.6, a small change in pH is accompanied by a much larger change in hydrogen ion concentration. For example, a change in pH from 7.1 to 7.0 represents a change in hydrogen ion concentration of 79 nmol. per liter to 100 nmol. per liter.

It is apparent from equation 25 that acidosis (an increase in $[H^+]$) can result from a decrease in bicarbonate (metabolic alkalosis), an increase in Pco_2 (respiratory acidosis), or a combination of these two processes (mixed metabolic-respiratory acidosis). Conversely, alkalosis (a

decrease in $[H^+]$) can result from an increase in bicarbonate (metabolic alkalosis), a decrease in Pco_2 (respiratory alkalosis) or a combination of these two processes (mixed metabolic-respiratory alkalosis). It is also apparent from equation 25 that an increase or decrease in bicarbonate can compensate for a primary increase or decrease in Pco_2 (metabolic compensation) and that an increase or decrease in Pco_2 can compensate for an increase or decrease in bicarbonate (respiratory compensation). It should be stressed that compensatory responses to acid-base disorders involve the system opposite the one that caused the primary disturbance and that these responses return the hydrogen ion concentration toward but not completely to normal.

In general, respiratory compensation occurs rapidly (within minutes) as a result of alterations in ventilation. Changes in the concentration of hydrogen ions are sensed by arterial chemoreceptors located in the carotid and aortic bodies and by neurons in the respiratory center of the medulla. Afferent signals from the chemoreceptors terminate in the respiratory center. An increase in the concentration of hydrogen ions directly and indirectly (via chemoreceptors) stimulates the respiratory center which, in turn, increases the activity of efferent pathways to the lung, thereby increasing alveolar ventilation. Conversely, a decrease in the hydrogen ion concentration inhibits the respiratory center, thereby decreasing alveolar ventilation. As noted in Figure 15, the response of alveolar ventilation to an increase in hydrogen ion concentration is greater than that to a decrease. As a result, metabolic acidosis is associated with a greater compensatory respiratory response than is metabolic alkalosis. In general, the respiratory compensation for metabolic acidosis is approximately a 1.2 mm. Hg decrease in Pco_2 for each 1.0 mEq. per liter decrease in the bicarbonate concentration, and for metabolic alkalosis it is a 0.6 mm. Hg increase in Pco_2 for each 1.0 mEq. per liter increase in bicarbonate. However, the response to metabolic acidosis is limited, since at a pH of

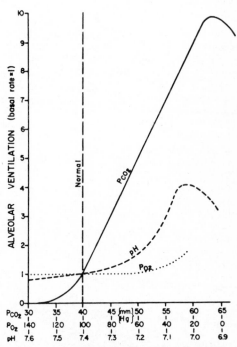

Figure 15. Effects of changes in Pco_2, pH, and Po_2 on alveolar ventilation. (From Guyton, A. C.: Textbook of Medical Physiology. Philadelphia, W. B. Saunders Company, 1976.)

7.0 or less the concomitant decrease in P_{CO_2} inhibits the respiratory center and the concomitant increase in P_{O_2} inhibits the chemoreceptors.

In contrast to the rapid compensation of the lungs, the metabolic compensation of primary respiratory acid-base disorders through the kidneys is slow, requiring hours to days before significant compensation is achieved. Under normal circumstances, the kidney maintains hydrogen balance by excreting the hydrogen ions that are formed from the daily production of fixed acids as ammonium ions (NH_4) and by excreting the acids themselves. In addition, the kidneys maintain the bicarbonate concentration by reabsorbing virtually all the bicarbonate that is filtered and by forming bicarbonate in the renal tubular cells. It should be noted that the renal handling of hydrogen and bicarbonate is not an independent process. The formation of bicarbonate from CO_2 in the presence of carbonic anhydrase generates free hydrogen ions. These hydrogen ions are then exchanged for sodium ions or secreted into the tubular fluid in conjunction with ammonia that is formed in renal tubular cells. Since the bicarbonate formed in the renal tubules is derived from CO_2, an increase in P_{CO_2} will stimulate bicarbonate formation. In addition, proximal tubular reabsorption of bicarbonate is enhanced when the P_{CO_2} increases, as noted in Fig. 16. Conversely, a decrease in P_{CO_2} decreases bicarbonate formation and diminishes bicarbonate reabsorption.

As a result of the slow renal compensation to primary respiratory acid-base disorders, acute and chronic disorders can be differentiated (Table 10 and Fig. 17). The only compensation that occurs during acute respiratory disorders is by the extracellular and intracellular buffers. During acute respiratory acidosis, the increase in P_{CO_2} produces an increase in dissolved CO_2. When CO_2 enters red blood cells, the carbonic acid formed is buffered by hemoglobin (Hb), resulting in the formation of bicarbonate.

$$Hb^- + H_2O + CO_2 \ H_2CO_3 + Hb^- \ H\ Hb + HCO_3^- \quad (29)$$

The bicarbonate that is formed in RBCs then diffuses out in exchange for chloride, thereby producing a small increase in the plasma bicarbonate concentration. In contrast, during chronic respiratory acidosis, increased renal reabsorption and formation of bicarbonate produces a large increase in

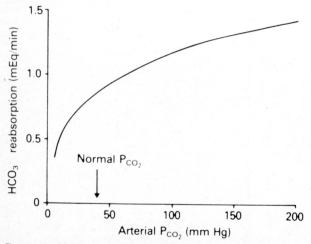

Figure 16. Relationship of the arterial P_{CO_2} to renal bicarbonate reabsorption. (From Valtin, H.: Renal function: Mechanisms Preserving Fluid and Balance in Health. Boston, Little, Brown and Co., 1983.)

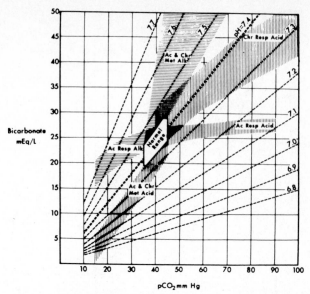

Figure 17. Acid-base nomogram. (From Arbus, G. S.: Can. Med. Assoc. J., 109:291, 1973.)

the plasma bicarbonate concentration. In general, during acute respiratory acidosis, the plasma bicarbonate concentration increases by 1.0 mEq. per liter for each 10 mm. Hg increase in P_{CO_2}, whereas during chronic respiratory acidosis the plasma bicarbonate increases by 3.5 mEq. per liter for each 10 mm. Hg increase in P_{CO_2}. Similarly, during acute respiratory alkalosis the bicarbonate concentration decreases by 2.0 mEq. per liter for each 10 mm. Hg decrease in P_{CO_2}, whereas during chronic respiratory alkalosis the plasma bicarbonate decreases by 5.0 mEq. per liter for each 10 mm. Hg decrease in P_{CO_2} (Table 10).

To assess the acid-base status of a patient, at least two of the three variables noted in equation 26 must be measured. Usually, the hydrogen ion concentration (as pH) and the P_{CO_2} are determined from the arterial blood gases and the plasma bicarbonate is calculated. Parenthetically, it should be noted that the plasma bicarbonate concentration is not equivalent to the total CO_2.

$$\text{Total } CO_2 = [HCO_3^-] + [\text{dissolved } CO_2] + [H_2CO_3] \quad (30)$$

Since H_2CO_3 is negligible in plasma:

$$\text{Total } CO_2 = [HCO_3^-] + [\text{dissolved } CO_2] = [HCO_3^-] + (P_{CO_2} \times 0.03) \quad (31)$$

Thus, an elevated total CO_2 indicates alkalosis but does not allow differentiation between a primary metabolic alkalosis and compensatory metabolic alkalosis.

When the plasma hydrogen ion and bicarbonate concentrations and the P_{CO_2} have been determined, the acid-base status can be defined. Straightforward disorders rarely present any diagnostic difficulties. For example, a pH of 7.46 with a P_{CO_2} of 44 mm. Hg and a bicarbonate of 30 mEq. per liter represents a definite metabolic alkalosis with respiratory compensation. It is apparent that the elevated P_{CO_2} is not primary; if it were, the patient would be acidotic not alkalotic. However, a pH of 7.50 with a P_{CO_2} of 40 mm. Hg and a bicarbonate of 30 mEq. per liter does not represent a pure metabolic alkalosis because there is no respiratory compensation. The absence of the rapid respiratory compensation suggests that there is a concomitant respiratory alkalosis. Thus, this patient has a mixed meta-

TABLE 10. Approximate Compensatory Responses for Acid-Base Disorders

Primary Disorder

Respiratory acidosis	$P_{CO_2} \geq 45$	$pH \leq 7.35$
Respiratory alkalosis	$P_{CO_2} \leq 35$	$pH \geq 7.45$
Metabolic acidosis	$HCO_3^- \leq 21$	$pH \leq 7.35$
Metabolic alkalosis	$HCO_3^- \geq 27$	$pH \geq 7.45$

Compensatory Responses

Acute respiratory acidosis	— 1.0 mEq. increase in HCO_3^- for each 10 mm. Hg increase in P_{CO_2}
Chronic respiratory acidosis	— 3.5 mEq. increase in HCO_3^- for each 10 mm. Hg increase in P_{CO_2}
Acute respiratory alkalosis	— 2.0 mEq. decrease in HCO_3^- for each 10 mm. Hg decrease in P_{CO_2}
Chronic respiratory alkalosis	— 5.0 mEq. decrease in HCO_3^- for each 10 mm. Hg decrease in P_{CO_2}
Acute metabolic alkalosis	— 0.6 mm. Hg increase in P_{CO_2} for each 1.0 mEq. increase in HCO_3
Chronic metabolic alkalosis	
Acute metabolic acidosis	— 1.2 mm. Hg decrease in P_{CO_2} for each 1.0 mEq. decrease in HCO_3
Chronic metabolic acidosis	

Pulmonary and Renal Compensatory Responses to Acid-Base Disorders

Acute respiratory acidosis
$$\frac{H}{P_{CO_2}} = -0.8$$

Chronic respiratory acidosis
$$\frac{H}{P_{CO_2}} = -0.03$$

Acute respiratory alkalosis
$$\frac{H}{P_{CO_2}} = +0.8$$

Chronic respiratory alkalosis
$$\frac{H}{P_{CO_2}} = +0.17$$

Acute on chronic respiratory acidosis
$$\frac{H}{P_{CO_2}} = (-0.4) - (-0.5)$$

Acute on chronic respiratory alkalosis
$$\frac{H}{P_{CO_2}} = +0.6 - 0.7$$

bolic-respiratory alkalosis. Conversely, although a pH of 7.40 with a P_{CO_2} of 50 mm. Hg and a bicarbonate of 30 mEq. per liter might be interpreted as complete respiratory compensation for a metabolic alkalosis, complete compensation rarely if ever occurs. Therefore, this patient has a mixed metabolic alkalosis-respiratory acidosis. In this regard, the most difficult acid-base disorders to interpret are superimposed acute respiratory disorders on chronic disorders. For example, a pH of 7.34 with P_{CO_2} of 60 mm. Hg and a bicarbonate of 31 mEq. per liter clearly represents

TABLE 11. Etiology of Respiratory Alkalosis

Hypoxia
  Ventilation-perfusion mismatch
    Adult respiratory distress syndrome
    Pulmonary embolism
  Anemia
  High altitude
  Congestive heart failure
Hypotension
Atelectasis
Excessive mechanical ventilation
Hypermetabolic states
  Fever
  Anemia
  Thyrotoxicosis
Central nervous system disorders
  Tumor
  Hemorrhage
  Infection
Pain
Psychogenic origin
Cirrhosis
Salicylate toxicity

a chronic respiratory acidosis. However, a pH of 7.28 with a P_{CO_2} of 70 mm. Hg and a bicarbonate of 32 mEq. per liter is difficult to interpret. If it were an acute respiratory acidosis with a P_{CO_2} of 70 mm. Hg according to Table 10, the bicarbonate would be only 27 mEq. per liter and the pH would be approximately 7.20. If it were a fully compensated respiratory acidosis, the bicarbonate would be 35 mEq. per liter and the pH would be 7.32. Therefore, this patient has either a mixed chronic respiratory acidosis with a metabolic alkalosis, a mixed acute respiratory acidosis with a metabolic alkalosis, or an acute respiratory acidosis on a chronic respiratory acidosis with appropriate metabolic compensation. These possibilities can be distinguished by evaluation of the clinical setting and by use of a nomogram such as shown in Figure 17. Alternatively, this differentiation can be made by evaluating the clinical setting and the change in hydrogen ion concentration and in P_{CO_2} from normal. Acute on chronic respiratory acidosis is associated with a $(\Delta[H^+]/\Delta P_{CO_2})$ equal to -0.5 (Table 11). In the present example, it equals -0.42. Therefore, this patient is likely to have an acute on chronic respiratory acidosis.

Alkalosis

Alkalosis is the most frequently observed acid-base disorder in traumatized, postoperative, and critically ill patients who have not deteriorated to serious renal, circulatory, or pulmonary dysfunction.[18] In a series of alkalotic patients, a mixed metabolic-respiratory alkalosis was most common, and of the two, respiratory alkalosis predominated. Although alkalosis is generally considered to be less harmful than acidosis, both respiratory and metabolic alkalosis are associated with numerous adverse effects that can be life-threatening. Alkalosis produces electrolyte abnormalities, including hypokalemia, hypocalcemia, and hypophosphatemia. These electrolyte disorders may result in myocardial irritability, particularly in the postoperative and digitalized patient, and in neuromuscular abnormalities. Alkalosis also hinders oxygen delivery by increasing the affinity of hemoglobin for oxygen, decreases arterial oxygen pressure by blunting the hypoxic drive and decreasing chemoreceptor sensitivity and increases oxygen consumption.[13]

Alkalosis also produces vasomotor abnormalities. Respiratory alkalosis produces cerebral vasoconstriction. Although hyperventilation is used in the management of elevated intracranial pressure, the attendant reduction in cerebral perfusion pressure may increase the risk of stroke, particularly in the elderly postoperative patient. Respiratory alkalosis also induces coronary vasoconstriction, thereby increasing the risk of angina in patients with coronary artery disease. In contrast, metabolic alkalosis produces coronary vasodilation.

RESPIRATORY ALKALOSIS

Respiratory alkalosis may follow hypoxic or hypotensive stimulation of aortic and carotid chemoreceptors leading to stimulation of the respiratory center and hyperventilation. In addition, psychogenic factors and hypermetabolic states, such as fever and thyrotoxicosis, stimulate the respiratory center, thereby producing respiratory alkalosis. Atelectasis produces respiratory alkalosis either through arteriovenous shunting and hypoxia or through direct nonhypoxic stimulation of the *Hering-Breuer reflex*. Similarly, pulmonary embolism may produce respiratory alkalosis either through hypoxic stimulation of the respiratory center or through nonhypoxic stimulation of the respiratory center that is mediated by vascular receptors in the pulmonary vasculature. Among the other etiologies listed in Table 11, excessive mechanical ventilation is of note, since it occurs frequently in surgical patients.

The signs and symptoms of respiratory alkalosis are related primarily to the central and peripheral nervous systems and are proportional to the severity of the alkalosis.[24] As such, symptoms are more prominent in acute than in chronic respiratory alkalosis. These symptoms include lightheadedness, altered consciousness, paresthesias, circumoral numbness, cramps, and carpopedal spasm (tetany). These symptoms are due to a decrease in ionized calcium that results from the decrease in hydrogen ion concentration.

Treatment of respiratory alkalosis is directed to correction of the underlying cause. If symptoms are severe, rebreathing of expired CO_2 will correct the hypocarbia. However, this should be done cautiously and slowly, since rapid reversal of respiratory alkalosis, especially when chronic, may lead to metabolic acidosis. As noted previously, renal compensation occurs slowly and involves the accumulation of acids such as lactic acid. If the P_{CO_2} is increased rapidly under these circumstances, the kidneys will be unable to excrete the acid load fast enough to avoid an accumulation of acids. Thus, metabolic acidosis ensues. It should also be noted that the administration of acid to improve respiratory alkalosis is never indicated because the primary solution is a reduction in carbon dioxide and not in acid *per se*.

METABOLIC ALKALOSIS

Metabolic alkalosis results from the inability of the kidneys to excrete a bicarbonate load. As such, metabolic alkalosis may result from enhanced proximal tubular reabsorption of bicarbonate, from enhanced distal tubular reabsorption of sodium, from a reduction in glomerular filtration, or from a combination of these processes (Table 12). Hypovolemia and injury stimulate all three mechanisms through a reduction in the effective circulating volume. Hypochloremia also stimulates all three mechanisms. As a result of the reduction of chloride in the glomerular filtrate, more bicarbonate must be reabsorbed with sodium than under normal circumstances. However, proximal tubular reabsorption of sodium is not complete when hypochloremia is present and more sodium is delivered distally. This then increases the distal tubular reabsorption of sodium and the regeneration of bicarbonate. In addition, hypochloremia appears to reduce the rate of glomerular filtration.[6] Hypokalemia also acts through multiple mechanisms to produce metabolic alkalosis. Although it does not directly enhance distal tubular reabsorption of sodium, it does increase the fraction of sodium that is reabsorbed in exchange for hydrogen, thereby increasing bicarbonate formation. In addition, hypokalemia may reduce directly glomerular filtration.[6]

Metabolic alkalosis also can be produced by the administration of bicarbonate, especially when the mechanisms noted above are operative. The bicarbonate load may be increased by the overzealous administration of sodium bicarbonate (indirectly as Ringer's lactate), or by blood transfusions. The latter increases the bicarbonate load through the metabolism of citrate. However, approximately 135 mEq. of citrate (8 units of blood) are required before a discernible alkalosis occurs. Metabolic alkalosis may also develop rarely in individuals who are ingesting excessive amounts of antacids, the milk-alkali syndrome.

The signs and symptoms of metabolic alkalosis are primarily those produced by the underlying cause. Unlike respiratory alkalosis, metabolic alkalosis itself produces few if any symptoms. This may result because bicarbonate is relatively impermeable to the blood-brain barrier, whereas carbon dioxide is freely permeable.

Treatment of metabolic alkalosis is directed toward stimulating renal excretion of bicarbonate. Therefore, the

TABLE 12. *Etiology of Metabolic Alkalosis*

Enhanced Proximal Reabsorption of Bicarbonate
Hypovolemia
Injury
Hypochloremia
Hypoparathyroidism
Diuretics
Enhanced Distal Tubular Reabsorption of Sodium
Hypovolemia
Injury
Hypochloremia
Hypokalemia
Diuretics
Corticosteroid excess
Hyperreninemia
Congenital adrenal hyperplasia
Licorice intoxication
Reduced Glomerular Filtration
Hypovolemia
Injury
Hypochloremia
Hypokalemia
Administration of Bicarbonate
Ringer's lactate
Sodium bicarbonate
Blood
Milk-alkali syndrome

mainstays of therapy are expansion of the effective circulating volume, replacement of chloride, and correction of hypokalemia. This is best achieved through the administration of normal saline with potassium chloride. It cannot be overemphasized that as long as one of these three entities remains uncorrected, metabolic alkalosis will persist. (See the discussion of hyperkalemia earlier.) Under rare circumstances, the use of arginine hydrochloride or ammonium chloride may be necessary to correct the alkalosis. These acids are used to supply chloride in a concentrated form and not to provide acid *per se*. As such, they may be indicated in severely alkalotic patients who require rapid correction of the alkalosis in preparation for emergency surgery. However, these agents are contraindicated in patients with hepatic or renal dysfunction because they will increase the blood urea and ammonia concentrations.

Acidosis

Acidosis is the most frequently encountered acid-base disorder in severely injured and critically ill patients who have suffered renal, pulmonary, or circulatory dysfunction.[18] The adverse effects of acidosis include a decrease in myocardial contractility, a decrease in sensitivity to catecholamines, an increase in the secretion of catecholamines, an increase in the serum potassium concentration, and a predisposition to cardiac arrhythmias. Metabolic acidosis reduces coronary blood flow and may lead to myocardial ischemia, whereas respiratory acidosis increases coronary blood flow. Respiratory acidosis also increases cerebral blood flow and may lead to cerebral edema and obtundation. Blood becomes more coagulable during acidosis, and the risk of capillary thrombosis is increased. Despite these impairments in cardiac function and blood flow, oxygen delivery during acidosis may be enhanced by a decrease in the affinity of hemoglobin for oxygen and by an increase in the sensitivity of chemoreceptors to hypoxia.

RESPIRATORY ACIDOSIS

Respiratory acidosis occurs by one of three mechanisms. It may result from inadequate excretion of CO_2, from loss of central respiratory control, or from increased CO_2 production[16] (Table 13). Inadequate excretion of CO_2 is synonymous with hypoventilation. Hypoventilation may result from ventilation-perfusion mismatch; from increased dead space; or from a reduction in tidal volume that is brought about by (1) airway obstruction, (2) impairment of respiratory muscles, or (3) injury of the chest wall. The loss of central respiratory control also leads to hypoventilation, and this may result from drugs, spinal cord injury, head injury, or cardiac arrest. Finally, during conditions when respiratory function is marginal, an increase in CO_2 production may produce hypercarbia. This usually occurs with a high-carbohydrate diet, particularly when given intravenously.

Most patients with respiratory acidosis will eventually become hypoxic if they continue to breathe room air. According to the alveolar gas equation:

$$PAO_2 = PO_2 - \frac{PaCO_2}{0.8} \qquad (32)$$

where PAO_2 = alveolar PO_2, PIO_2 = inspired PO_2, $PaCO_2$ = arterial PCO_2, and 0.8 = respiratory quotient.

At a barometric pressure of 760 mm. Hg (atmospheric), inspired room air at sea level has 47 mm. Hg of

TABLE 13. Etiology of Respiratory Acidosis

I. Impairment of Pulmonary Excretion of CO_2
  A. Ventilation-Perfusion Mismatch
    1. Pulmonary edema
    2. Severe pneumonia
    3. Asthma
    4. Chronic bronchitis
    5. Emphysema
  B. Increased Dead Space
    1. Pulmonary embolism
    2. During mechanical ventilation
  C. Insufficient Tidal Volume
    1. Airway obstruction
      a. foreign body
      b. mucous plug
      c. laryngospasm
      d. bronchitis
    2. Impairment of respiratory muscles
      a. myasthemia gravis
      b. poliomyelitis
      c. obesity—pickwickian
    3. Chest wall injury
      a. flail chest
      b. pneumothorax
    4. Disconnected respirator
II. Loss of Central Respiratory Control
  A. Drugs
    1. Anesthetics
    2. Opiates
    3. Barbiturates
    4. Oxygen in chronic respiratory acidosis
  B. Cardiac Arrest
  C. Spinal Cord and Head Injury
III. Increased CO_2 production

water vapor pressure, 563 mm. Hg of nitrogen pressure, and 150 mm. Hg of oxygen pressure. Thus,

$$PAO_2 = 150 - 1.25 \, PaCO_2 \qquad (33)$$

Not all the oxygen in the alveolus enters the blood. Normally, there is a 5- to 10-mm. Hg alveolar-arterial (A-a) oxygen gradient that increases with age. Thus, it is apparent from equation 33 that as $PaCO_2$ increases, PAO_2 and PaO_2 (arterial PO_2) decrease and patients become hypoxic. Furthermore, as a result of the increase in $PaCO_2$, the respiratory center becomes less sensitive to carbon dioxide and functions primarily as a result of hypoxic drive. In this setting, the correction of the hypoxia by the administration of oxygen may shut off the hypoxic drive, increase hypoventilation, and lead to respiratory arrest. As a result, oxygen must be given with extreme caution to patients with respiratory acidosis, particularly when it is chronic.

The symptoms of respiratory acidosis and hypercarbia include headache, blurred vision, fatigue, and weakness. If it progresses, tremors, asterixis, delirium, and somnolence become manifest as so-called *carbon dioxide narcosis*. These symptoms are thought to be the result of an increase in the pH of the CSF.[24]

The treatment of acute respiratory acidosis is aimed toward improving alveolar ventilation and depends on the underlying cause. For example, hypercarbia secondary to airway obstruction will be reversed rapidly by removing the airway obstruction and hypercarbia secondary to a pneumothorax will be corrected by a closed thoracostomy. In contrast, hypercarbia resulting from severe pneumonia or acute pulmonary edema may require endotracheal intubation and mechanical ventilation while the underlying cause is treated.

Chronic respiratory acidosis does not usually require any specific therapy directed at correcting the pH because renal compensation is usually effective in returning the pH toward normal. When it is necessary to correct the P_{CO_2} after renal compensation has occurred, an elevated bicarbonate in the CSF and metabolic alkalosis may ensue.

METABOLIC ACIDOSIS

Metabolic acidosis results either from an inability to retain bicarbonate or from an inability to excrete acids. The former may result from excessive renal losses or excessive gastrointestinal losses. In surgical patients, loss of bicarbonate through the gastrointestinal tract predominates (Table 14). The inability to excrete an acid load may result from impaired renal excretion of acids or from an overproduction of acids in the presence of normal renal function (Table 14). Whereas an impairment of acid excretion usually leads to the accumulation of both inorganic and organic acids, the overproduction of acids always leads to the accumulation of organic acids, most frequently lactate. Lactic acidosis may result from ischemic stimulation of lactate production (hypoxia, hypoperfusion), from impaired hepatic metabolism or from impaired glucose metabolism that arises in untreated diabetes mellitus.

Shock is the most common cause of lactic acidosis. The reduction in tissue perfusion leads to ischemia and thus to anaerobic metabolism and the production of lactate. Shock also leads to the release of catecholamines, angiotensin, and vasopressin. As a result, tissue perfusion may decrease further with a concomitant increase in lactate production. Serum lactate may be augmented by arteriovenous shunting and impaired hepatic metabolism of lactate. Excess lactate is a good prognosticator of survival. However, it is important to recognize that the elevated concentration of lactate is the result of hypoperfusion and not the cause of it.

Metabolic acidosis may be differentiated by the presence of a normal or increased anion gap (Table 14). The anions in plasma that are usually measured are chloride

and bicarbonate, and the sum of the chloride and bicarbonate concentrations is normally 8 ±4 mEq. per liter less than the sodium concentration.[24, 27] This normal anion gap arises because anions such as phosphates, sulfates, and proteins are not considered and it is similar to the strong ion difference noted previously. When metabolic acidosis results from the loss of bicarbonate in the urine or gastrointestinal fluids, the decrease in bicarbonate requires greater amounts of chloride to be reabsorbed with sodium. Thus, the anion gap remains normal and hyperchloremia ensues. When acidosis arises from the accumulation of an organic acid (e.g., lactic acid), electrical neutrality must be maintained, primarily by an increase in the reabsorption of sodium. Therefore, the anion gap increases and serum chloride remains relatively normal. A similar process occurs with inorganic acid accumulation, as in renal failure. However, when the accumulation of inorganic acids is the result of the administration of acid, the cation is usually neutralized by chloride. As a result, a hyperchloremic metabolic acidosis with a normal anion gap is usually present.

Prominent signs and symptoms of metabolic alkalosis include an increased incidence of cardiac arrhythmias, impaired cardiac function, and hyperkalemia. In addition, neurologic manifestations ranging from lethargy to coma are seen and appear to arise from an increase in the pH of cerebrospinal fluid.

Treatment of metabolic acidosis is directed first to correction of the underlying cause. In most situations, especially those associated with the overproduction of organic acids, this will be sufficient. However, if the pH is less than 7.2 or if the acidosis is the result of excessive losses of bicarbonate, bicarbonate should be administered. The total bicarbonate deficit can be calculated as:

$$\text{Bicarbonate deficit} = (\text{body weight in kg.}) (0.4) \atop (\text{normal} - \text{observed HCO}_3) \qquad (34)$$

Only half of this deficit should be replaced during a 3- to 4-hour period, and it should be done only in conjunction with careful monitoring of the patient's acid-base and electrolyte status. Severe hypokalemia, hypocalcemia, hypomagnesemia, and fluid overload may follow the administration of bicarbonate and a rebound metabolic alkalosis may ensue.

TABLE 14. *Etiology of Metabolic Acidosis*

Increased Organic Acids—Increased Anion Gap
 Uremia: renal failure
 Lactic acidosis: hyperfusion, hypoxia, diabetes
 Ketoacidosis: diabetes; starvation
 Drugs
  Ethylene glycol
  Salicylates
  Methanol
  Paraldehyde
Increased Inorganic Acids—Normal Anion Gap with
  Hyperchloremia
 Inability to excrete acid
  Renal failure
  Distal renal tubular acidosis
  Addison's disease
  Hypoaldosteronism
 Excessive loss of bicarbonate
  Gastrointestinal fistula
  Diarrhea
  Proximal renal tubular acidosis
  Ureterosigmoidostomy
  Early renal failure
 Administration of acid
  Blood transfusions—citrate
  Ammonium chloride
  Arginine hydrochloride

SELECTED REFERENCES

Beck, L. H.: Body fluid and electrolyte disorders. Med. Clin. North Am., 65:24, 1981.
  A recent monograph devoted to fluid and electrolyte disorders with emphasis on practical diagnosis and management.

Dunn, M. J.: Renal Endocrinology. Baltimore, Williams & Wilkins, 1983.
  A complete review of the endocrine actions of the kidneys and the effects of the endocrine system on renal failure.

Kurtzman, W. A., and Batelle, D. C.: Acid-base disorders. Med. Clin. North Am., 67:751, 1983.
  A recent monograph devoted to acid-base imbalance with emphasis on pathophysiology and management.

Leaf, A., and Cotran, R.: Renal Pathophysiology. New York, Oxford University Press, 1976.
  A concise and easily understood discussion of the pathophysiology of fluid, electrolyte, and acid-base disorders.

Maxwell, R. H., and Kleeman, C. R.: Clinical Disorders of Fluid and Electrolyte Balance, 3rd ed. New York, McGraw-Hill, 1980.
  An authoritative medical text of fluid and electrolyte physiology and disorders, including a detailed discussion on the fluid and electrolyte status in numerous diseases.

Moore, F. D.: Energy and the maintenance of the body cell mass. J. Parenteral Enteral Nutrition, 4:227, 1980.
  A summary of a great surgical investigator's extensive work in body

composition and energy maintenance, including formulas for estimating the fluid and electrolyte compartments according to age, sex, and body weight.

Stewart, P. A.: How to Understand Acid-base. New York, Elsevier, 1981.
A mathematical description of acid-base physiology presenting the classic approach based on pH, P_{CO_2} and HCO_3^- as well as the new approach based on the strong ion difference and total anion-buffers as developed by the author.

Winters, R. W.: The Body Fluids in Pediatrics. Boston, Little, Brown and Co., 1973.
The standard text on the pathophysiology and management of fluid and electrolytes in pediatric patients.

REFERENCES

1. Anderson, R. J., Linas, S. L., Berns, A. S., Henrich, W. L., Miller, T. R., Gabow, P. A., and Schrier, R. W.: Non-oliguric renal failure. N. Engl. J. Med., *296*:1134, 1977.
2. Baer, P. G., and McGiff, J. C.: Hormonal systems and renal hemodynamics. Ann. Rev. Physiol., *42*:589, 1980.
3. Baxter, J. D., and Tyrrell, J. B.: The Adrenal Cortex. *In* Felig, P., Baxter, J. D., Broaders, A. E., and Frohman, C. A. (Eds.): Endocrinology and Metabolism. New York, McGraw-Hill, 1981, p. 385.
4. Bie, P.: Osmoreceptors, vasopressin and control of water excretion. Physiol. Rev., *60*:961, 1980.
5. Byrnes, G. J., Pirkle, J. C., and Gann, D. S.: Cardiovascular stabilization after hemorrhage depends upon restitution of blood volume. J. Trauma, *18*:623, 1978.
6. Cogan, M. G., Liu, F. U., Berger, B. E., Sebastian, A., and Rector, F. C., Jr.: Metabolic alkalosis. Med. Clin. North Am., *67*:903, 1983.
7. Cox, M.: Potassium homeostasis. Surg. Clin. North Am., *65*:363, 1981.
8. Dunn, J. M.: Renal Endocrinology. Baltimore, Williams & Wilkins, 1983.
9. Fray, J. C. S., Lush, D. J., and Valentine, A. N. D.: Cellular mechanisms of renin secretion. Fed. Proc., *42*:3150, 1983.
10. Gann, D. S., and Wright, H. K.: Increased renal sodium reabsorption after depletion of the extracellular or intravascular fluid volumes. J. Surg. Res., *6*:196, 1966.
11. Gann, D. S.: Endocrine control of plasma protein and volume. Surg. Clin. North Am., *56*:1135, 1976.
12. Gann, D. S., Ward, D.G., and Carlson, D. E.: Neural control of

ACTH: A homeostatic reflex. Recent Prog. Horm. Res., *35*:357, 1978.
13. Gann, D. S., and Amaral, J. F.: The pathophysiology of trauma and shock. *In* Zuidema, G. D., Rutherford, R. B., and Ballinger, W. F., II (Eds.): The Management of Trauma. Philadelphia, W. B. Saunders Company, 1985.
14. Guyton, A. C.: Textbook of Medical Physiology. Philadelphia, W. B. Saunders Company, 1976.
15. Hays, R. M.: Dynamics of body water and electrolytes. *In* Maxwell, R. H., and Kleeman, C. R. (Eds.): Clinical Disorders of Fluid and Electrolyte Balance, 3rd. ed. New York, McGraw-Hill, 1980.
16. Kaehny, W.: Respiratory acid-base disorders. Med. Clin. North Am., *67*:914, 1983.
17. Krams-Freidmann, N.: Hormonal regulation of hepatic gluconeogenesis. Physiol. Rev., *64*:170, 1984.
18. Lyons, J. H., and Moore, F. D.: Post-traumatic alkalosis: Incidence and pathophysiology of alkalosis in surgery. Surgery, *60*:93, 1966.
19. Miller, P. D., Krebs, R. A., Neal, B. J., and McIntyre, D. P.: Polyuric prerenal failure. Arch. Intern. Med., *140*:907, 1980.
20. Miller, T. R., Anderson, R. J., Linas, S. L., et al.: Urinary diagnostic indices in acute renal failure: A prospective study. Ann. Intern. Med., *89*:47, 1978.
21. Navar, A. G., Ploth, D. W., and Bull, P. D.: Distal tubular feedback control of renal hemodynamics and autoregulation. Ann. Rev. Physiol., *42*:557, 1980.
22. Peach, M. J.: Renin-angiotensin system: Biochemistry and mechanisms of action. Physiol. Rev., *57*:313, 1977.
23. Robertson, G. L.: Diseases of the anterior pituitary. *In* Felig, P., Baxter, J. D., Broadus, A. E., and Friedman, G. A.: Endocrinology and Metabolism. New York, McGraw-Hill, 1981, p. 251.
24. Rose, D. B.: Clinical Physiology of Acid Base and Electrolyte Disturbances. New York, McGraw-Hill, 1977.
25. Sawhenko, P. E., and Friedman, M. I.: Sensory functions of the liver—a review. Am. J. Physiol., *236*:R5, 1979.
26. Singer, I.: Differential diagnosis of polyuria and diabetes insipidus. Med. Clin. North Am., *65*:303, 1981.
27. Valtin, H.: Renal function: Mechanisms preserving fluid and solute balance in health. *In* Renal Dysfunction: Mechanisms involved in fluid and solute imbalance. Boston, Little, Brown and Company, 1983.
28. Wright, H. K., and Gann, D. S.: Correction of defect in free water excretion in postoperative patients by extracellular fluid volume expansion. Surgery, *158*:70, 1963.
29. Wright, H. K., and Gann, D. S.: A defect in urinary concentrating ability during postoperative antidiuresis. Surg. Gynecol. Obstet., *121*:47, 1965.

PREOPERATIVE PREPARATION OF THE SURGICAL PATIENT

BRUCE D. SCHIRMER, M.D. • DAVID C. SABISTON, JR., M.D.

4

The most important aspects of the practice of surgery involve acquiring the decision-making process necessary to evaluate the indications for and the urgency of a surgical procedure. Equally important is the acquisition of the appropriate technical skills necessary for performing the procedures. Although descriptions of the latter can be found in many atlases and illustrated texts, nevertheless years of training and practical experience in a well-supervised residency program are necessary to acquire these skills. Experience is the primary factor in developing the clinical decision-making skills of the surgeon in planning the preoperative phase of the patient's care. The goal of this chapter is to set forth certain commonly held principles concerning the general preoperative evaluation and preparation of the surgical patient that, once learned, allow more emphasis on the detail of each clinical problem.

PREOPERATIVE COMMUNICATION

The doctor-patient relationship is best established by thorough communication. It is essential to devote the effort necessary to establish an appropriate relationship preoperatively that makes certain the patient completely understands the problem and is reassured about the reason for the operation and the results expected. In addition, consideration of the patient's family and their concerns is another prime responsibility of the surgeon. Legal suits are more likely to occur in situations in which these relationships and concerns have not been addressed. Appointed times for preoperative discussions with both the patient and, as indicated or desired, the patient's family are essential elements in preoperative preparation. Discussion should terminate only when the physician is confident the patient and family understand the indications for the operation, the essential features of the procedure, and the attendant risks of the proposed operation. All questions must be thoroughly answered so as to convey the important information, allay anxiety from fear of the unknown, and minimize unnecessary worry over problems unlikely to occur.

In discussions of the details of an operation, the terminology used should be made completely understandable to the patient. Aspects of all operations that should be discussed include the site of the incision, the required

monitoring equipment and intravenous lines, possible use of nasogastric tubes, use of drains, and special nursing care procedures in which patient cooperation will be necessary postoperatively. The need for and approximate estimates of length of stay in the recovery or intensive care areas should be explained. Procedures that inherently greatly alter bodily image or function, such as tracheostomy or colostomy, must be explained with respect to their immediate and long-term effects.

Pertinent potential complications related to each operation should be explained, but only emphasized in detail if their likelihood is great or their consequences grave. The operative mortality must also be discussed. This discussion is best handled by the responsible surgeon rather than an assistant. Documentation of the preoperative discussion in the chart as well as the signed operative permit is a standard procedure.

Preoperative communication is also essential between the surgeon and other members of the team. In particular, communication with referring physicians regarding indications and plans for operation is appropriate and courteous. Assisting members of the operating team must be informed of anticipated procedures so that their skills are coordinated in the most helpful fashion.

Care should be taken to avoid having a number of the members of the team discuss the planned operation with the patient or his family. Despite presentation of the same information, the interpretation from two different conversations may be perceived as conflicting, and such instances create unnecessary confusion.

ASSESSING OPERATIVE RISK

Realistic estimates of operative risk can be accurate only if they are applied toward similar groups of patients undergoing the same procedure. Factors considered in assessing perioperative risk include those related to the patient, the disease, the overall body condition, and the proposed operation. The Physical Status Scale of the American Society of Anesthesiologists is shown in Table 1.[4] Postoperative and anesthesia-related mortality has been shown to correlate well with these classifications.[68, 90, 99, 153] Death rates range from 0.01 per cent (category 1) to 18 per cent (category 4).[68] The addition of the emergency

TABLE 1. Classification of Physical Status*

1. A normal healthy patient   ●01% most
2. A patient with mild systemic disease
3. A patient with severe systemic disease that limits activity but is not incapacitating
4. A patient with incapacitating systemic disease that is a   18% most constant threat to life
5. A moribund patient not expected to survive 24 hours with or without operation.

In event of emergency operation, precede the number with an E.

*From American Society of Anesthesiologists: Anesthesiology 24:111, 1963.[4]

TABLE 2. Electrolyte Composition of Intravenous Fluids

Solution	Na+	K+	Ca++	Cl−	HCO3−
Normal saline, 0.9 NaCl	154			154	
Ringer's lactate	130	4	3	109	28
Half-normal saline, 0.45 NaCl	78			78	
Quarter-normal saline, 0.25 NaCl	39			39	

classification causes estimated anesthetic and surgical mortalities to double for categories 1, 2, and 3. Patients in categories 4 and 5 have no increased risk for the addition of the emergency setting.[75]

The operative procedure itself is associated with an important risk that must be considered in assessing perioperative risks. Open heart surgery, craniotomy, major abdominal surgery, and operations for major trauma are each associated with relatively high procedure-related risks. Mortality rates for specific procedures vary from institution to institution based on expertise and volume.[92]

The decision to perform an operation and its urgency must be related to the therapeutic benefit likely to be obtained versus the operative risk. Knowledge of the *natural history* of a disease is extremely helpful. If such data are known, such as the study by Estes for patients with abdominal aortic aneurysm,[51] the decision rests on firmer scientific grounds. Similarly, the timing of an operation can often be important in influencing the ultimate outcome. Cardiac valve replacement prior to myocardial deterioration from valvular heart disease is an example, it being preferable to operate before the ventricle is too badly affected by the valvular disease. Massive hemorrhage and trauma obviously require emergent intervention, but even in these settings optimal survival will be achieved only if concomitant attention is given to appropriate physiologic support.

FLUIDS AND ELECTROLYTES

Optimization of intravascular volume to ensure adequate tissue perfusion as well as correction of any acid-base or electrolyte disturbances present is always a paramount consideration even in the most emergent operative settings. Only efforts to maintain circulation and ventilation have greater priority in preparing the patient for operation.

The most common preoperative disorder of fluid imbalance is *intravascular volume depletion*. This usually is a result of disease process, such as from hemorrhage, vomiting, or diarrhea. Tachycardia, hypotension, oliguria, increased urinary osmolality, decreased urine sodium concentration, and absence of significant edema confirm the diagnosis. Hydration with fluid appropriate to replace the loss is indicated. In general, transfusion of blood products is necesssary for replacement of blood loss whereas isotonic saline solutions are given for less severe hypotension and volume depletion.

In the setting of emergent resuscitation from hypovolemic shock, the immediate infusion of 2 liters of Ringer's lactate solution is recommended as both a resuscitative measure and a means of roughly estimating intravascular blood loss. The electrolyte composition of Ringer's lactate

is similar to that of plasma (Table 2). Its isotonicity is matched only by normal saline (0.9 per cent NaCl), but the latter's high chloride composition can lead to hyperchloremic metabolic acidosis if administered in large quantities.

Replacement of fluid from known sources of loss, such as vomiting or fistulas, is accomplished by administration of fluid similar in composition to that of the source. The average electrolyte composition of gastrointestinal secretions is shown in Table 3. The composition of fluid lost with diarrhea varies widely, but it usually is high in sodium, potassium, and basic ions, and its loss leads to hyperchloremic acidosis.

Adequate hydration is achieved when there is sufficient intravascular volume to assure good organ perfusion. Urinary output of more than 30 ml. per hour in the adult or 1 ml. per kg. per hour in the child usually ensures adequate renal perfusion. However, the use of osmotic and loop diuretics may lead to adequate urinary output despite poor perfusion. Therefore, measurement of central venous or pulmonary capillary wedge pressure is often required to monitor optimal levels of hydration. Signs of overhydration are manifested by pulmonary and peripheral edema.

When peripheral edema is present with hypotension, intravascular volume depletion may be a result of abnormal fluid shifts into the extracellular fluid space. These may be stimulated by hypoalbuminemia, which may be present from a variety of causes such as hepatocellular dysfunction, malnutrition, burns, or sepsis. Treatment of the underlying disorder leading to hypoalbuminemia is usually necessary before replacement therapy becomes totally effective.

Disorders of excessive intravascular volume are characterized by pulmonary edema. These conditions, unless quite acute, are accompanied by overexpansion of the extracellular component of body fluid as well. The most common causes include renal failure, congestive heart failure, and cirrhosis. In renal failure, the intravascular and extracellular compartments are equilibrated and total body water and sodium overload are present. Careful monitoring of intake and output and daily weights usually suffice in the preoperative preparation of patients in renal failure. Careful attention to volume status and electrolyte disorders by maintaining the dialysis schedule is necessary to provide optimal preoperative management.

TABLE 3. Approximate Electrolyte Composition (mEq./100 ml.) of Gastrointestinal Secretions*

	Na+	K+	Cl	HCO3−
Saliva	60	20	16	50
Gastric	59	9.3	89	0–1
Duodenal	105	5.1	99	10
Bile	145	5.2	100	50
Pancreas	142	4.6	77	70

*Adapted from Randall, H. T.: Surg. Clin. North Am., 56:1019, 1976.

The decrease in cardiac output associated with *congestive heart failure* results in increased hydrostatic pressure within capillaries leading to a net shift of water to the interstitial space and an effective loss of intravascular volume. Resulting decreased perfusion is interpreted by the kidneys as a condition requiring retention of excess sodium and water. Therapy consists of salt and water restriction and the use of potent loop diuretics such as furosemide.

Cirrhosis also represents a condition of excess body retention of sodium and water in the extracellular space. Increased portal pressure secondary to increased splanchnic blood volume leads to transudation of water and sodium into the peritoneal cavity as ascites. Diuresis in patients with cirrhosis must be a gradual process because only between one half to 1 liter per day of ascites can effectively be mobilized into the intravascular space. Hypokalemia should be avoided because this may induce increased renal ammonia production and resultant hepatic coma. Therefore, restriction of free water and gentle diuresis with potassium-sparing diuretics such as spironolactone are used to treat fluid overload in cirrhotic patients.

ELECTROLYTE ABNORMALITIES

Hyponatremia

The serum sodium content is usually the initial marker used to detect abnormalities of sodium and water metabolism. Relative hyponatremia is often a manifestation of water balance excess rather than a sodium deficit. Hyponatremia and accompanying decreased total body sodium and hypotonicity can occur when losses of sodium via gastrointestinal, renal, or other causes exceeds the water deficit. Treatment is repletion of intravascular volume with isotonic saline.

Hyponatremia and hypotonicity more commonly occur as a result of disorders that increase total body water to a greater extent than total body sodium. Urinary sodium content is less than 10 mEq per liter.[93] Congestive heart failure, cirrhosis, and renal failure may all cause such hyponatremia. Severe hyponatremia and hypotonicity may be life-threatening as a result of accompanying cerebral edema. In symptomatic patients, administration of small amounts of hypertonic saline along with potent diuretics is indicated.

Patients with hyponatremia but normal total body sodium content have accompanying hypotonicity as a result of increased total body water. Edema is absent. The syndrome of inappropriate antidiuretic hormone (SIADH) secretion most commonly causes this condition. Patients with this syndrome have an excess of total body water and a high urine sodium concentration and osmolality. They should be treated by water restriction.[55]

Hypernatremia

Hypernatremia may be present in the settings of normal, decreased, or, rarely, increased total body sodium. Diabetes insipidus is an example of hypernatremia with normal total body sodium. Impairment of the renal concentrating mechanism caused by lack of ADH and accompanying polydipsia, polyuria, and hypotonic urine suggests the diagnosis. Treatment consists of administration of vasopressin.

Hypotonic fluid loss can result in hypernatremia and hypertonicity with decreased total body sodium. Since gastric and intestinal secretions are hypotonic, prolonged nasogastric suction or severe vomiting may cause these findings. Therapy is directed to restoration of intravascular volume followed by gradual restoration of water and sodium deficits.

Hypokalemia

Hypokalemia is usually associated with decreased total body potassium. By far, the most common cause is the chronic use of diuretics, and in this setting the relative plasma hypokalemia may reflect a large total body potassium deficit. Other common causes for hypokalemia include gastrointestinal losses, as from vomiting or diarrhea, and renal losses, as from renal tubular acidosis. It is especially important to correct hypokalemia preoperatively in patients with a history of cardiac disease or in those undergoing cardiac or pulmonary procedures. The incidence of postoperative cardiac arrhythmias, particularly atrial fibrillation, is higher following these procedures and will be further increased in the setting of hypokalemia. Hypokalemia also exacerbates arrhythmias in patients on digitalis therapy.

Potassium chloride is the electrolyte of choice for correcting metabolic alkalosis and hypokalemia from diuretic use or gastrointestinal losses. If renal potassium wasting has led to metabolic acidosis, potassium bicarbonate is effective. Oral administration safely allows intake of the large quantities of potassium necessary to correct the deficit. For example, if serum potassium is 2.5 mEq. per liter, the estimated potassium deficit is 300 to 400 mEq. Should intravenous supplementation be necessary, the sclerosing effect of potassium solutions on veins usually makes central venous access necessary and slow injection is important. The safe limit of administration via this route is 20 mEq. of potassium per hour.

Hyperkalemia

Serum potassium can be elevated as a result of increased potassium intake, decreased renal excretion, cell death and potassium release, and conditions producing hypoaldosteronism. The most important clinical condition involving hyperkalemia is acute renal failure (ARF). It is unwise to proceed to operation unless potassium can first be effectively removed. Hemodialysis or peritoneal dialysis is the best option; the former is normally indicated in the acute setting. Should preoperative hyperkalemia be present in the emergent situation, serum potassium levels determine the therapy. If potassium levels are 6.5 mEq. per liter or less, simple measures to remove potassium, such as potassium-binding ion exchange (Kayexelate) resins are recommended. Hydration and concurrent administration of furosemide may decrease potassium levels.

If the serum potassium is greater than 6.5 mEq. per liter, a *serious* condition exists requiring emergent therapy. The most rapid treatment for reversing the cardiac manifestations of hyperkalemia is intravenous calcium gluconate. Sodium bicarbonate or glucose and insulin temporarily lower plasma potassium content by shifting potassium ions to the intracellular space. Therapy to shift potassium ions into the intracellular space alone is only temporary and should be followed with measures to remove potassium.[142]

Hypercalcemia

Diseases of the parathyroid glands, parathormone metabolism, and metastatic malignant tumors with accompanying bony destruction may all be preoperative causes of hypercalcemia. Usually, only the latter may cause life-threatening hypercalcemia with the appearance of neurologic and neuromuscular symptoms. Treatment consists of high-volume intravenous administration of isotonic saline along with furosemide to essentially dilute the ion's effects. Addressing the focus of the problem, such as radiation therapy for areas of bony metastases, provides palliation.

ACID-BASE DISTURBANCES

Metabolic Alkalosis

Causes of metabolic alkalosis include conditions leading to an increase in alkali or loss of acid. Intravenous sodium bicarbonate, lactated Ringer's solution, citrate from banked blood, or acetate from intravenous hyperalimentation all contain alkali. Nasogastric suction and vomiting as well as renal mineralocorticoid excess seen in hyperaldosteronism lead to acid loss.

Treatment of metabolic alkalosis begins by ensuring that the kidney can excrete an adequate bicarbonate load. Replacement of intravascular and extracellular volume counteracts "contraction" alkalosis. Other requirements of the nephron for excretion of bicarbonate include adequate available chloride and potassium for exchange. After adequate expansion of extracellular fluid volume, the next treatment of choice for simple metabolic alkalosis is potassium chloride (KCl) administration. If this proves inadequate, in severe cases acid administration using 0.1N HCl in 5 per cent D5W may be given up to 0.2 mEq. per kg. per hour via a central vein.[157]

Metabolic Acidosis

Metabolic acidosis is defined as a decline in the serum pH and serum bicarbonate concentrations. For purposes of classification, metabolic acidosis is usually divided into conditions in which a normal "anion gap" (where Na $-[(Cl) + (HCO_3)] <4$) is present and those associated with an increased anion gap. Normal anion gap causes of metaboic acidosis include renal disease leading to bicarbonate loss (renal tubular acidosis), certain drugs (acetazolamide), ileal loop with stasis, diarrhea, or a pancreatic fistula. High anion gap causes include diabetic ketoacidosis, lactic acidosis, toxins (salicylate, methanol), and uremia.

Treatment of normal anion gap acidosis is conservative and involves the etiologic agent when possible. High anion gap acidosis also requires treatment of the offending condition. Dialysis may be required to remove drugs or to correct uremia. Diabetic ketoacidosis is discussed later. Lactic acidosis is often fatal if associated with shock and tissue hypoperfusion, and the latter must be treated if the condition is to be reversed. Sodium bicarbonate therapy may be necessary in an emergent situation (cardiopulmonary arrest). The goal should be maintenance of serum pH in the 7.15 to 7.25 range to avoid the cardiac complications seen at lower pH levels and also to avoid rebound alkalosis when the condition leading to the acidosis is corrected.[66]

BLEEDING DISORDERS AND TRANSFUSIONS

The best screening procedure for bleeding disorders is a careful history. Patients with a history of prolonged

bleeding following dental procedures, hematoma formation and intra-articular bleeding after trauma, or easy bruising all warrant screening laboratory evaluation for surgical bleeding disorders. Screening laboratory tests are not efficacious for routine, uncomplicated procedures in those without a bleeding history. However, prior to major vascular procedures in which substantial blood loss is expected, or for procedures involving percutaneous puncture of vascular structures such as an arteriogram, coagulation studies are normally obtained.

The *prothrombin time* (PT) is an evaluation of the extrinsic coagulation sequence, and *activated partial thromboplastin time* (PTT) is an evaluation of the intrinsic coagulation sequence. The *platelet count* and *bleeding time* quantitate the amount of platelets available and measure their function. These four screening tests are sufficiently sensitive to identify significant surgical bleeding disorders in over 95 per cent of patients with bleeding abnormalities. Nevertheless, they should not be used routinely as screening procedures because a careful history has been shown to be effective in predicting prolongation of any one single test in a high percentage of patients.[49]

A history of aspirin ingestion is of concern preoperatively, since it causes irreversible effects on platelet aggregation for the life of the affected platelets (7 to 10 days). Therefore, the bleeding time will be prolonged in patients with platelet dysfunction caused by aspirin.

Hemophilia may be suggested by family history. If factor VIII (hemophilia A) or factor IX (hemophilia B) levels are present at less than 25 per cent of normal, this disease can present with intraoperative or postoperative surgical bleeding. Prophylaxis for hemophiliacs consists of the administration of cryoprecipitate containing factor VIII to raise levels to 80 per cent of normal or obtain an VIII:C ratio of 80 to 100 (U per 100 ml.). The cryoprecipitate is normally given beginning 2 hours prior to operation as a loading dose and continued in maintenance doses every 12 hours for 1 to 2 weeks following major procedures.[81]

Liver disease, especially Laennec's cirrhosis, is the most common cause of prolonged PT. Patients with disorders of malabsorption of vitamin K may also manifest a prolonged PT. Such patients should be prepared preoperatively with parenteral administration of 10 mg. of vitamin K as well as transfusion immediately preoperatively with fresh frozen plasma if necessary.

Patients requiring anticoagulants, either heparin or Coumadin, warrant special consideration preoperatively. Since anticoagulation will again be required in the postoperative period in order to avoid exposing these patients to the dangers of thromboembolic events, it is best not to fully reverse anticoagulation for long periods of time. Operations on the central nervous system (CNS), liver, and eye require full anticoagulant reversal at the time of surgery.[50] For other major procedures, titrating the anticoagulation to the lower end of the therapeutic range may be sufficient. This is facilitated by switching to heparin in those patients who have been taking Coumadin, since adjustments in anticoagulation from heparin are made more rapidly. Parenteral vitamin K or the infusion of fresh frozen plasma is recommended to reverse anticoagulation from Coumadin or heparin preoperatively.

Patients with Underlying Blood Disorders

Patients with underlying blood disorders such as anemia, thrombocytopenia, leukemia, and polycythemia require special preoperative consideration. Anemia increases the risk of surgery and anesthesia in patients with hemoglobin levels less than 10 gm. per 100 ml.[94] by compromising the ability of maximal oxygen delivery to the tissues during periods of surgical stress. Therefore, preoperative transfusions may be indicated in some anemic patients.

When the decision has been made to transfuse a patient, it is best to administer blood at least 24 hours prior to operation and with a recommended maximum of 2 units of blood per day. This allows adequate time for the body to reaccumulate normal levels of 2,3-diphosphoglycerate (DPG) as well as avoiding volume overload.[14]

Sickle cell anemia is a disease associated with significant surgical morbidity. Conditions that precipitate sickle cell crisis, such as hypothermia, infections, acidosis, and dehydration, are to be avoided. Administration of oxygen for 24 hours prior to operation is recommended, as is preoperative exchange transfusion to lower the hemoglobin S level to less than 30 per cent.[77]

Patients with polycythemia vera have an increased risk of perioperative complications from hemorrhage. It is recommended that phlebotomy and myelosuppressive agents be used to maintain the hematocrit less than 52 per cent in these patients for several months prior to elective surgery.[160]

Patients with leukemia and granulocytopenia of less than 1000 per mm³ have an increased risk of surgical infection.[16] Antibiotics are indicated prophylactically in such patients. In patients with leukemia and platelet counts below 50,000, supplementation is given with immediate preoperative transfusion of platelets to minimize bleeding.[15]

Transfusions

The availability of an adequate supply of cross-matched blood is a prerequisite for any elective surgical procedure. In the very emergent situation, transfusion may proceed with type-specific or even O-negative blood, depending on the urgency of the situation. Such emergent transfusions are usually limited to emergency rooms of large trauma centers or military settings, and have the increased risk of immediate minor compatibility transfusion reactions and delayed major incompatibility reactions with subsequent transfusion.[137] The amount of blood required for intraoperative transfusion depends on the extent of the surgical procedure. Experience is the best guideline for quantitating such preparation. However, mention should be made that the number of units of blood ordered prior to many elective procedures often exceeds the number actually used. Having a sample of the patient's blood available in the blood bank under a "type and hold" situation may often be a sufficient margin of safety for procedures in which the blood loss will not normally be excessive or rapid.

PROPHYLAXIS OF POSTOPERATIVE DEEP VEIN THROMBOSIS

Postoperative deep venous thrombosis and thromboembolism may lead to a potentially fatal postoperative complication from ensuing pulmonary embolus. An estimated 2.5 million cases of deep vein thrombosis occur annually, with more than 600,000 episodes of pulmonary embolism and 200,000 deaths.[17, 67] Approximately 15 per cent of all deaths in acute care hospitals result from pulmonary embolism.[38] It is the most common fatal event following the more usual surgical procedures such as herniorrhaphy and cholecystectomy.[11]

Routine prophylaxis for deep venous thrombosis is unnecessary in patients at low risk for this problem. The latter group includes patients younger than 40 years old who are of normal weight and have no venous disease. In this group, the risk of complications from therapy exceeds the risk of pulmonary embolism. Demonstrated risk factors for postoperative thromboembolism include cardiac disease (especially atrial fibrillation and congestive heart failure); carcinoma of the lung, gastrointestinal, or genitourinary tract; paraplegia; trauma; age over 40, and venous disease of a lower extremity.[120]

Prophylactic techniques for prevention of deep vein thrombosis include both mechanical and chemical techniques. The position recommended for prophylaxis of deep vein thrombosis and pulmonary embolism is shown in Figure 1. Trials comparing leg elevation with elastic stockings and aspirin have shown that simple leg elevation is as efficacious as either of these measures in reducing the incidence of deep vein thrombosis.[129] Elastic stockings alone generally have been found not to be of significant benefit in decreasing the incidence of deep vein thrombosis.[20] External pneumatic compression (EPC) has thus far proved to be the most beneficial of mechanical techniques used in the perioperative period,[23, 33, 39, 102, 114, 136] but it is cumbersome and seldom necessary. Studies in which chemical prophylactic techniques have been combined with EPC have failed to show any consistent augmentive decrease in the incidence of venous thrombosis and pulmonary embolism.[125]

Heparin given in a dose of 5000 units subcutaneously 2 hours preoperatively and then at 8- to 12-hour intervals postoperatively has been shown in over 27 trials to be effective in decreasing the incidence of postoperative deep vein thrombosis.[3, 63, 120, 122] The incidence of pulmonary embolism was reported reduced from 6 to 0.6 per cent in one study.[83] However, the most convincing data seem to show that although low-dose heparin may reduce the incidence of calf vein thrombosis, it does not appear to significantly decrease the incidence of iliac and femoral vein thrombosis and pulmonary embolism.[78] Complications of low-dose heparin therapy have been significant and include an increased incidence of wound hematoma.[109] Most failures of low-dose heparin therapy occur (1) following operations that greatly stimulate thrombosis, such as hip replacement, (2) in patients with an active thrombotic process, or (3) when poor absorption or clearance of heparin results in inadequate therapeutic levels.

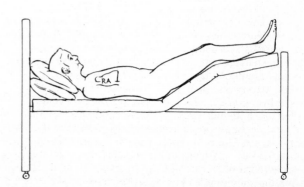

Figure 1. Correct position for lower extremities in prophylaxis of pulmonary embolism. Note the additional break at the knee. It is important that the level of the veins in the lower extremities be above the mean level of the right atrium (RA). (From Sabiston, D. C., Jr. (Ed.): In Textbook of Surgery, 13th ed. Philadelphia, W. B. Saunders Company, 1986, p. 1742.)

Dextran indirectly decreases platelet adhesiveness and alters the ability of plasminogen to degrade fibrin polymers. Some clinical trials with dextran have shown less impressive results in preventing postoperative deep vein thrombosis than trials with heparin. Other trials involving patients undergoing total hip and knee operations have shown dextran to be more beneficial than heparin.[12, 123] Aspirin has been found to have only mixed results[31, 56] and is generally not recommended. Combined chemotherapeutic or mechanical techniques have been used in several trials and, in general, have failed to show much substantial additive effect.[120] Further studies are needed to determine the best therapeutic regimen that combines good efficacy of prophylaxis against deep venous thrombosis with the safety of a low incidence of bleeding complications. Probably some combination of mechanical techniques and heparin or dextran chemoprophylaxis will be the solution.

PREOPERATIVE NUTRITION

Patient Status

The nutritional status of the patient is an important preoperative consideration. It is estimated that one fourth of hospitalized patients suffer from combined protein-calorie malnutrition.[24] This may be a result of the patient's underlying disease. However, at times it may simply be the failure of appropriate adequate dietary intake for the patient. Consideration of sufficient nutritional support is often delayed until a state of severe depletion exists.

Patients may be classified generally into three categories regarding status and requirements[138]:

1. Those with little if any starvation (weight loss <10 per cent body weight),

2. Those with starvation from disease processes (such as obstructing carcinomas) in whom current caloric needs based on basal metabolic rate are below normal.

3. Patients with hypermetabolic states, such as burns or sepsis, who require above average caloric intake to meet daily energy requirements.

The goals of nutritional support differ with respect to each of these groups. Patients in good nutritional status without excess metabolic demands can tolerate several days of intravenous glucose as their only caloric source without adverse effects in terms of operative morbidity or mortality. However, patients with excessive preoperative weight loss may be unable to tolerate the demands of surgery. For such patients, weight gain through the achievement of an anabolic state may be the preoperative goal. In the hypermetabolic, septic, traumatized, or otherwise stressed patient, actual weight gain may prove to be an overly difficult goal during the course of the acute disease process. Instead, the goal is maintenance of visceral proteins, body weight, and prevention of an overly catabolic state until the time of recovery when weight gain becomes feasible again.

Various parameters have been used to confirm the suspicion of advanced malnutrition. Weight loss is one important predictor of nutritional status, as are clinical impressions of severely malnourished patients. For patients with less obvious clinical findings, quantitative criteria such as nitrogen balance and biochemical, immunologic, and anthropometric parameters are useful. When nutritional deficiency is confirmed, however, none of these parameters alone has proved an effective monitor of nutritional support. The clinical picture combined with data from several of these criteria is most accurate in assessing the need for and progress of nutritional support.[65]

Malnutrition has many adverse effects on the body's ability to withstand the stresses of the perioperative period. The negative nitrogen balance of severely hypermetabolic patients may be as high as 50 to 60 gm. of protein per day.[138] This rapidly depletes visceral organ mass and strength. Deep breathing and movement of the chest are lessened and lead to possible atelectasis, pneumonia, and pulmonary insufficiency. Decreased energy from poor caloric intake results in more inactivity postoperatively and predisposes the patient to complications such as deep venous thrombosis and decubitus ulcers. Chronic depletion of serum proteins can result in postoperative sodium and water retention with resulting edema, poor wound healing, and exacerbation of any underlying congestive heart failure. Malnutrition lessens the body's immune competence[89, 139] suggesting malnourished patients are at a greater risk for postoperative infectious complications.

Several studies have attempted to define that group of patients whose preoperative poor nutritional status places them at a significantly increased risk for perioperative complications or death. Buzby and associates[25] have developed a Prognostic Nutritional Index (PNI), which they propose accurately predicts patients in this category. A Scandinavian group used other preoperative nutritional criteria to predict differences in complications during hospitalization.[159] Other studies have questioned the accuracy of the PNI.[48, 121] Turner and associates found that 15 criteria of preoperative nutritional parameters could clarify patients into categories of high or low chance for complications only with very low specificity.[151] Controversy continues concerning the best method of performing meaningful preoperative nutritional assessment.

Preoperative nutritional supplementation for at least 5 days in certain subsets of nutritionally depleted patients can significantly lessen postoperative complications.[117] This has been demonstrated in patients with esophageal[42] and other gastrointestinal cancer.[105] Extensively burned patients also require vigorous nutritional support before survival is achieved with some regularity.[22] The immune status of traumatized and septic patients can also be improved with adequate nutritional support.[139]

Considerations in Nutritional Support

Enteric feeding is the preferred route of nutritional support if the gastrointestinal tract is functioning normally. Enteral feedings avoid the risk of intravenous catheter–related problems such as sepsis or thrombosis, and the cost per day is substantially less than when parenteral nutrition is used. Furthermore, unless a patient has a specific intestinal disorder preventing digestion and absorption of lipids, complex carbohydrates, or protein, non-elemental liquid enteral formulas are better tolerated and show equal nutritional benefit compared with more expensive elemental enteral feedings.[52]

Total parenteral nutrition, first popularized by Dudrick,[46] is indicated in the perioperative setting in which a nonfunctional gastrointestinal tract prevents adequate enteral nutritional intake. Central venous access is essential because the hypertonicity of the solution requires a high-volume venous flow to prevent phlebitis. The subclavian route is generally preferred, and meticulous care of the catheter site is essential; low institutional infection rates have been achieved through the use of specially trained parenteral support personnel to supervise and perform catheter care and dressing changes.[127] Formulas are modified to an individual patient's requirements. Standard formulas usually begin with 50 ml. of 8.5 per cent amino acid solution and 500 ml. of 50 per cent dextrose per liter, with vitamins, heparin, insulin, albumin, and electrolytes added as indicated. Essential fatty acid requirements are met through an at least twice weekly administration of 500 ml. of isotonic fat solution.

INFECTIOUS COMPLICATIONS

Wound infection and postoperative sepsis are primarily related to the risk factors for infection present at the time of operation. These factors include the host's defense mechanisms, the environment in which infection occurs, and the microorganisms producing the infection.[103] Host-defense mechanisms are governed in part by nutritional competence. Measures that improve or normalize host-defense mechanisms, limit the environmental exposure to highly pathogenic organisms, and limit the degree of tissue contamination with such viable organisms all serve to decrease the incidence of postoperative infection.

Delayed hypersensitivity skin testing is one measure of immune competence. Anergy is associated with a much higher than otherwise predicted incidence of postoperative sepsis and death.[95] Conditions associated with anergy include advanced age, sepsis, trauma, shock, malnutrition, and hemorrhage. Causes of anergy that can be corrected preoperatively should be treated to improve the patient's ability to fight subsequent infectious challenges. Thus far, no specific immune stimulatory agent for improving host-defense mechanisms has proved widely efficacious preoperatively.

Meticulous sterile technique in the operating room as well as proper attention to the surgical principles of gentle tissue handling, hemostasis, wound irrigation, and appropriate wound closure will eliminate the causes of most surgical wound infections. Skin preparation can influence the infection rate in clean surgical cases.[2, 41] Depilatory hair removal or abstinence from razor shaving is preferable to razor shaving, particularly if the latter is done hours in advance of the operation.[53, 133]

PROPHYLACTIC ANTIBIOTICS

Prophylactic antibiotics are indicated (1) when the risk of morbidity from infection at operation outweighs the possible adverse problems of drug reaction, drug cost, and emergence of resistant bacteria or (2) when a wound infection would be life-threatening. The choice of antibiotic to be administered depends on the type of contaminating organism most likely to be encountered in a given procedure. The drug must be effective against the majority of bacteria found such that the total bacterial count can be decreased sufficiently for the host to clear the remaining organisms.

The timing of administration of prophylactic antibiotics is important. Overwhelmingly, studies have shown that if prophylactic antibiotics are to be most effective, they must be administered preoperatively to produce adequate tissue and blood levels of the drug at the time of operation.[21, 107] Parenteral, usually intravenous, administration is recommended just prior to the start of a procedure.[35] A single dose may be sufficient,[143] but the duration of antimicrobial prophylaxis should not exceed 48 to 72 hours by most guidelines.[5, 34, 35, 107, 143, 156] Prolonged drug administration has

shown no added benefit in reducing infection rates and only increases the risk of bacterial superinfection or drug toxicity.

The ideal properties for a prophylactic agent include specificity for the likely pathogens, low toxicity, bactericidal activity, and low cost. Serum concentrations should reach therapeutic levels soon after administration and remain elevated sufficiently long to avoid repeated intraoperative doses of the drug. Cephalosporins have emerged as the agents of choice in prophylaxis for most common surgical procedures.[5] When gram-positive organisms such as *Staphylococcus aureus* are of major concern, penicillinase-resistant penicillins are used with good success.

Antibiotic prophylaxis has shown some modest benefit with surgical procedures on the biliary tract,[28, 86] and antibiotics are indicated in high-risk gastroduodenal procedures in which obstruction or bleeding is present.[87] Adequate antibiotic prophylaxis can be achieved with a single dose of cephalosporin preoperatively in elective vaginal hysterectomy,[74] and a course of antibiotics for 24 to 48 hours preoperatively to sterilize the urine in patients prior to urologic procedures is also beneficial.[13]

Preoperative attention to decreasing the contamination present from bowel flora at the time of colorectal procedures consists of three aspects: (1) mechanical intestinal cleansing, (2) oral antibiotics to decrease the bacterial count in the colon, and (3) systemic prophylactic antibiotics for maximal protection. Mechanical cleansing normally includes the use of a liquid or low-residue diet for several days prior to the procedure. In addition, cathartics and enemas or purgatives, such as a polyethylene-glycol based liquid (Go-Lytely)[1] or lactated Ringer's solution,[108] can be administered orally or via nasogastric tube in large volumes.

Oral antibiotics that are poorly absorbed and remain in the gastrointestinal tract are given between 8 and 24 hours prior to operation.[158] Postoperative wound infection rates decrease from 30 to 40 per cent in patients with only mechanical bowel preparation to 8 to 10 per cent in patients receiving both mechanical and oral antibiotic bowel preparation.[32, 155]

Parenteral antibiotics (cephalosporins) are effective in reducing the incidence of wound infections in patients undergoing colorectal procedures to about 25 per cent of the incidence seen in patients receiving only mechanical bowel preparation.[144] One cooperative study suggests that as an adjunct to mechanical bowel preparation parenteral cephalosporin is not as effective in preventing wound infection as is an oral antibiotic regimen of neomycin and erythromycin.[36] Whether parenteral antibiotics along with oral antibiotics lead to a further decrease in infectious complications of colorectal surgery has yet to be determined.

PREOPERATIVE CONSIDERATIONS BY ORGAN SYSTEMS

Cardiovascular System

Perioperative myocardial infarction or cardiac complications such as congestive heart failure or arrhythmias are major causes of operative morbidity and mortality. Perioperative myocardial infarction is the leading cause of operative mortality for most thoracic, aortic, and abdominal operations. Therefore, preoperative identification of patients with a high risk for cardiac complications and subsequent appropriate management is important in minimizing the rate of such complications. The incidence of cardiovascular complications in the general population undergoing general anesthesia, however, is only 0.2 per cent.[148]

The most important factors in preoperatively predicting cardiac risks and complications from noncardiac procedures can be estimated from a thorough history, physical examination, and electrocardiogram (ECG).[148] The single most important factor in the history is documentation of a myocardial infarction occurring within the previous 6 months. Recurrent myocardial infarction occurs in as many as 30 per cent of patients undergoing surgical procedures within 3 months of a myocardial infarction and in 15 per cent of patients whose operation is 3 to 6 months after an infarction.[58, 59, 140, 148] The incidence remains about 5 per cent for operations performed 6 months or longer after a previous myocardial infarction.

Preoperative congestive heart failure is also a significant risk factor, as are other factors summarized in Table 4.[59] In the study depicted in Table 4, the authors derived a multifactorial analysis of operative risk with points assigned to factors found to have a significant effect on perioperative cardiac morbidity and mortality. Patients studied were then grouped into classes based on point totals with the following mortality and complication rates:

1. *Class I* (0–5 points), with 0.2 per cent cardiac deaths and 0.7 per cent complications.
2. *Class II* (6–12 points), with 2 per cent deaths and 5 per cent complications.
3. *Class III* (13–25 points) with 2 per cent deaths and 11 per cent complications.
4. *Class IV* (26 or more points), with 56 per cent deaths and 22 per cent complications.

Patients with significant coronary artery disease can decrease the risks of noncardiac surgery by first undergoing myocardial revascularization.[47, 96, 101] Hartzer has shown that

TABLE 4. *Preoperative Risk Factors**

Criteria	Points
History	
Age >70 years	5
MI in previous 6 mos.	10
Physical Examination	
S₃ gallop or JVD	11
Important valvular aortic stenosis	3
Electrocardiogram	
Rhythm other than sinus or PAC on last ECG	7
>5 PVC/min. at any time before surgery	7
General Status	
Po₂ <60 or Pco₂> 50 mm. Hg	3
K+ C3.0 or HCO₃ <20 mEq./liter	
BUN >50 or creatinine >3.0 mg./100 ml.	
Signs of chronic liver disease, ↑SGOT	
Bedridden from noncardiac causes	
Operation	
Intraperitoneal, intrathoracic, or aortic operation	3
Emergency operation	4
TOTAL POSSIBLE	53

*Adapted from Goldman L., et al.: N. Engl. J. Med., 297:848, 1977.

Abbreviations: MI = Myocardial infarction; PAC = premature atrial contraction; PVC = premature ventricular contraction; BUN = blood urea nitrogen; SGOT = serum glutamic-oxaloacetic transaminase; JVD = jugular venous distention.

10 to 15 per cent of asymptomatic patients who require peripheral vascular surgery have significant life-threatening coronary artery disease that can be detected preoperatively.[70] For this reason, routine coronary arteriography and myocardial revascularization have been recommended for appropriate candidates prior to peripheral vascular procedures,[70] but such steps are not generally recommended by most authorities. Certain noninvasive means of preoperatively screening all patients at increased risk for coronary artery disease are recommended, however, such as exercise tolerance tests[7] and radionuclide angiography.[82]

Correction of existing congestive heart failure is strongly recommended prior to operation because a 20 per cent cardiac mortality is associated with uncontrolled failure as opposed to a 5 per cent rate if congestive failure is controlled.[59] In general, all patients with cardiac disease should continue their cardiac medications, including antihypertensives, diuretics, digitalis, propranolol, and antiarrhythmic agents until the time of operation.

Preoperative cardiac arrhythmias are associated with an increased risk of perioperative cardiac death. The severity of arrhythmias often corresponds to the degree of myocardial ischemia with dysfunction.[59, 98] It is generally recommended that preoperative prophylaxis for ventricular ectopy, with lidocaine being the agent of choice, be reserved for patients with either an ischemic event within 48 hours preceding surgery or a history of symptomatic ventricular arrhythmias.[98, 116] Supraventricular arrhythmias occur frequently in the elderly and in those patients undergoing major vascular, intra-abdominal, and especially thoracic (up to 30 per cent)[57] operations. Unfortunately, preoperative ECG findings are not accurate predictors of perioperative development of supraventricular arrhythmias. Trials of perioperative prophylactic digitalis have been performed with mixed results,[80, 152] and the drug is currently recommended only for patients at high risk of developing supraventricular arrhythmias.[132]

Patients with valvular heart disease have a lessened ability to compensate hemodynamically for fluctuations in fluid therapy, drug therapy, or anesthesia, indicating a need for more careful perioperative monitoring of hemodynamic parameters. In Goldman's study,[59] all major valvular abnormalities were associated with a significant risk of worsening congestive heart failure. In general, stenotic valvular disease was found to be more difficult to manage than regurgitant disease, and it is not surprising that significant aortic stenosis itself was found to be an independent risk factor in that study.

In patients with significant aortic stenosis, there is a lesser ability to increase blood flow across the stenotic valve and vasodilation is poorly tolerated because the heart cannot adequately increase its output to compensate for decreased vascular resistance. Consequently, spinal anesthesia, which causes vasodilation, is usually contraindicated for patients with aortic stenosis. These patients also tolerate intravascular volume depletion and atrial arrhythmias poorly. Significant aortic stenosis may require surgical correction before other elective procedures are performed.

Other valvular lesions, although not associated with as high an operative mortality as aortic stenosis, require similar careful hemodynamic considerations. In patients with mitral stenosis, volume overload is poorly tolerated and hence mild hypovolemia is preferred to fluid overload. Chronic atrial fibrillation is often present, and anticoagulation to prevent embolic events is indicated in such patients. Patients with mitral stenosis and normal sinus rhythm may benefit from prophylactic digitalis therapy. Aortic and mitral regurgitation can cause hemodynamic problems when left ventricular function is consequently compromised. Therefore, preoperative echocardiographic or radionuclide assessment of left ventricular function is indicated. In general, vasodilation is tolerated much better in these patients than in patients with stenotic valvular disease, and normal or slightly increased intravascular volumes are optimal for management.[76]

Patients with prosthetic heart valves probably have no higher risk of perioperative cardiac complications than do patients with native valvular abnormalities and similar degrees of cardiac compromise. However, anticoagulant therapy and its possible complications are major considerations in these patients. The incidence of hemorrhagic complications from noncardiac operations for patients with prosthetic valves is approximately 13 per cent.[85] Antibiotic prophylaxis is always indicated for patients with prosthetic valves undergoing any surgical procedure in which bacteremia is even a remote possibility. Similarly, patients with significant native valve disease should also undergo perioperative antibiotic prophylaxis in such instances. Current recommendations by the American Heart Association include parenteral administration of aqueous crystalline penicillin G (or ampicillin) plus gentamicin (or streptomycin) given 1 hour prior to surgery and for two postoperative doses (8 to 12 and 16 to 24 hours postoperatively).[84] Vancomycin may be substituted for penicillin in patients allergic to penicillin.

Pulmonary System

Significant pulmonary complications occur in an estimated 5 to 7 per cent of all operations. The incidence is approximately doubled in abdominal operations, tripled in smokers, and quadrupled in patients with chronic obstructive pulmonary disease. Respiratory insufficiency is the direct cause of approximately one fourth of all postoperative mortalities and contributes to the cause of death in another 25 per cent.[100] Accurate identification and preoperative pulmonary treatment can decrease pulmonary complications.

The greatest decrease in pulmonary function is seen following thoracic procedures with upper abdominal, lower abdominal, and extremity or peripheral surgical sites following in that order.[149] Tidal volume decreases, respiratory rate increases, and the absence of periodic hyperinflation of the lungs occurs following operations that result in exacerbation of incisional pain with deep breathing. These alterations promote atelectasis, which in turn may increase pulmonary compliance. Normal ciliary function in the tracheobronchial tree is also decreased after surgery, and this may contribute to atelectasis as well. It is not surprising then that atelectasis is the most commonly recognized pulmonary complication following surgery.[100, 112]

Risk Factors

Cigarette smoking is definitely associated with the development of a variety of respiratory diseases as well as, in the postoperative setting, with the raising of the closing volume (CV) (Fig. 2). Smoking severely affects respiratory tract mucociliary clearance and creates more viscous and copious secretions. Cessation of smoking is recommended preoperatively to lessen the chance of pulmonary complications. The period of preoperative abstinence should begin at least 4 weeks prior to operation to maximally reduce

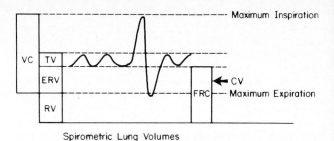

Figure 2. Schematic illustration of normal spirometric lung volumes over time. Maximal levels of inspiration and expiration are shown. Note that the closing volume (CV) is located between maximal expiration and normal exhalation point of tidal volume. TV = Tidal volume; VC = vital capacity; ERC = expiratory reserve volume; RV = residual volume; FRC = functional residual capacity.

postoperative complication rates.[30, 161] Advanced age is associated with expected decreases in static lung volumes, forced expiratory volume (FEV) and flow rates, and pulmonary elasticity. However, age itself is not a risk factor should preoperative pulmonary function studies prove to be normal. Obesity is probably an independent risk factor for postoperative pulmonary complications.[149] The degree of risk is not well defined, however, since the condition of obesity itself is often poorly defined in various studies. Prolonged duration of operation, as well as preoperative dyspnea, bronchitis, cough, or other symptoms of chronic obstructive pulmonary disease, is also associated with greater perioperative pulmonary complications.[147]

Preoperative Screening Tests

Certain laboratory, radiographic, and spirometric evaluations may be indicated preoperatively to quantitate pulmonary pathology and predict postoperative morbidity. The history and physical examination are usually sufficient to identify risk factors and signs of pulmonary dysfunction. However, if sufficient data exist, it is prudent to obtain further diagnostic tests.

The preoperative chest film is an inefficient screening test for detecting pulmonary disease for those under 30.[119, 124] Preoperative chest films are probably indicated in patients from ages 30 to 39 undergoing abdominal procedures and are definitely indicated in patients over age 40, in whom the incidence of bronchogenic carcinoma is increased. Similarly, all patients with significant clinical risk factors previously mentioned should have preoperative chest films made, as should all patients prior to planned thoracic procedures.[27]

Preoperative arterial blood gas determination is an accurate prognostic test for pulmonary problems in the perioperative period.[27] Arterial blood gases are indicated prior to all contemplated pulmonary resections and probably relatively indicated prior to most thoracic procedures. In addition, PO_2 is helpful in further assessing patients with significant clinical risk factors or pulmonary function tests that suggest chronic obstructive or restrictive pulmonary disease.

Pulmonary function tests are helpful in assessing postoperative risks from pulmonary problems. However, there are no reliable studies to indicate which preoperative patients benefit from obtaining such evaluations other than those undergoing pulmonary resection.[19] Obtaining such evaluations should be based on clinical judgment. They are certainly indicated prior to all thoracic procedures and are probably indicated for patients with significant pulmonary risk factors undergoing abdominal surgery and those greater than age 70 with any risk factors.[27]

Various parameters of pulmonary function tests have been associated with increased operative risk.[18] Patients with pulmonary function levels significantly below predicted levels should be assessed for functional improvement following the administration of bronchodilators.[111] Pulmonary function tests can also be used as preoperative predictors of respiratory adequacy following major thoracic or cardiac surgery.[72]

Preoperative spirometric evaluation prior to contemplated pulmonary resection is standard practice. A maximal:minute ventilation of > 50 per cent predicted or an FEV_1 of > 2 liters is considered confirmation of adequate functional reserve.[100] The one-stair flight exercise tolerance test has also been shown to be of value in predicting postoperative death following pneumonectomy.[154] In patients with marginal pulmonary function in whom resection is contemplated, the extent to which the diseased lung is contributing to effective ventilatory function can be accurately estimated by radionuclide ventilation and perfusion lung scanning.[45]

Once the pulmonary operability and operative risk have been established through the various tests just enumerated, a combination of certain measures instituted preoperatively has been shown to be effective in reducing pulmonary risks.[141] These include cessation of smoking, antibiotics, inhalation therapy, segmental postural drainage, chest physiotherapy, and bronchodilators. Patients with chronic obstructive pulmonary disease may benefit from a combination of several of these preoperative measures as well.[64] The relative value of individual measures is far less documented.

In patients with particularly severe chronic obstructive pulmonary disease, bronchitis, or asthma, it may be necessary to postpone operation until pulmonary function is improved. Patients with moderate asthma, as manifested by wheezing and an FEV_1 of 50 to 75 per cent predicted and abnormal arterial blood gases, should be treated with theophylline and hydration and surgery should be postponed.[8] For more severe asthma, steroids may be required. Drugs inducing bronchial irritability (such as cholinergic agents and beta-blockers) should be avoided, as should manipulations that lead to decreased mobilization of pulmonary secretions postoperatively. Preparation should be made preoperatively for adequate intraoperative and postoperative monitoring of respiratory mechanics and blood gases and for postoperative pulmonary toilet.

Endocrine System

Certain specific problems of endocrine dysfunction are either sufficiently common or sufficiently dangerous to warrant special enumeration. In general, for the less common states of endocrine insufficiency, such as hypothyroidism, the preoperative preparation involves simple diagnostic tests to confirm the clinical suspicion of endocrine insufficiency followed by appropriate replacement therapy. Similarly, if the clinical picture is consistent with a state of excess hormone secretion and this is confirmed biochemically, steps should be taken preoperatively to remove or ablate the hormonal excess.

DIABETES MELLITUS

Diabetes mellitus is not a risk factor in surgical procedures if it is well controlled at the time of operation.[54]

The goals of preoperative and perioperative management in these patients are maintenance of a relative state of *mild* hyperglycemia but certainly avoidance of dangerous hypoglycemia. Measurement of serum blood glucose is the single best parameter to monitor insulin requirements.[79] Excess hyperglycemia with an osmotic diuresis and subsequent intravascular volume depletion and creation of a hyperosmolar state are highly undesirable in the immediate postoperative period, when hypovolemia might occur on the basis of other factors. Therefore, blood glucose levels in excess of 250 mg. per ml. are undesirable. During the period of anesthesia, there are no subjective symptoms or levels of consciousness available to indicate hypoglycemia. Therefore, the potentially fatal complication of intraoperative hypoglycemia is one that must always be avoided. Serum glucose levels of 150 to 250 mg. per 100 ml. are not treated with insulin in the immediate perioperative period, and a constant infusion of intravenous fluids containing glucose is maintained throughout the period of anesthesia.

Assessment of the patient's daily insulin requirement should be done prior to operation. The stresses of the procedure precipitate a relative state of hyperglycemia from the physiologic reactions of the body to the stress and trauma of operation. The response to this stress is the release of substances designed to promote catabolism and glucose availability and inhibit insulin release.[104] Type II diabetics may require little if any insulin in the perioperative period, especially if the disease is relatively well controlled by oral hypoglycemic agents. Administration of small doses of regular insulin in the immediate postoperative period may be necessary, however, until oral intake is resumed.

Patients with Type I diabetes, if in uncontrolled ketoacidosis preoperatively, require an intensive period of rehydration and intravascular volume repletion along with continuous infusion of insulin and frequent monitoring of electrolytes and blood glucose levels to obtain a state of adequate control.[128] When control of the diabetic state is obtained, further insulin therapy should be based on maintaining the blood glucose in the range of 150 to 250 mg. per 100 ml.[79] Adjustments of only 20 per cent of daily insulin requirements at a time are recommended for achieving smooth and gradual control of serum glucose levels. A useful guideline to insulin therapy on the morning of operation is to begin an intravenous infusion of 5 per cent dextrose in Ringer's lactate at 75 to 100 ml. per hour prior to insulin administration. This infusion should be kept relatively constant during the operation to ensure adequate glucose administration to prevent hypoglycemia. For Type I diabetics undergoing elective procedures, approximately half the usual morning dose of insulin should be given as regular insulin subcutaneously on call to the operating room. This amount of insulin is usually sufficient to prevent excess hyperglycemia in the immediate perioperative period. If the operation lasts longer than 5 to 6 hours, further insulin can be given based on blood glucose levels.

HYPERTHYROIDISM

Hyperthyroidism results from overproduction of either thyroxine (T_4) or triiodothyronine (T_3) or both. Toxic nodular goiter, Graves' disease, or toxic solitary nodules account for most cases of hyperthyroidism. Preoperative recognition is important to avoid the consequences of intraoperative *thyroid storm*, a syndrome of sudden hyperfunctional changes manifested by a marked sinus tachycardia (atrial arrhythmias may occur) accompanied by hyperthermia, severe agitation, and mental obtundation. This syndrome can be fatal if not properly treated.[106] Propranolol, a beta-blocker, is effective against the cardiovascular collapse seen with thyroid storm and is used as a perioperative prophylactic agent for hyperthyroid patients when its use is not contraindicated.[134] Propylthiouracil (PTU) is an effective inhibitor of T_4 synthesis and is the main agent used to urgently or electively treat hyperthyroidism pharmacologically. Sodium iodide can be used to block the release of thyroxine stored in the thyroid and decrease the vascularity of the gland prior to thyroid resection.

Other measures used in treating hyperthyroid crisis include the administration of glucocorticoids, which inhibit conversion of T_4 to T_3. Acetaminophen should be used to control temperature. Aspirin tends to displace thyroxine from its serum-binding proteins and is contraindicated in hyperthyroidism.[79]

PHEOCHROMOCYTOMA

Pheochromocytomas are rare neoplasms involving the adrenal medulla or, rarely, other catecholamine-secreting tissues in the body. Symptoms may be subtle and few, but include hypertension, diaphoresis, and tachycardia, occasionally occurring in paroxysms. The danger of pheochromocytoma is the associated estimated 10 per cent operative mortality for patients with untreated tumors.[97] Therefore, preoperative recognition and treatment are most important.

Pheochromocytoma is the cause of only 0.5 per cent of all cases of hypertension, but it should be considered in all hypertensive patients, particularly young patients with unexplained hypertension. The tumor may at times be familial and is found as part of the multiple endocrine neoplasia (MEN-II) syndrome.

Pheochromocytoma is treated by surgical excision, and pharmacologic preparation is necessary prior to operation. Phenoxybenzamine is the alpha-adrenergic blocking agent of choice and is given orally twice daily in doses as required to control blood pressure and symptoms of excess circulating catecholamines (usually 60 to 150 mg. per day). Treatment may require from several days to 2 weeks preoperatively before adequate control of hemodynamic instability occurs.[135] At times supplementation with the beta-blocker propranolol is also necessary. Preoperative computed tomography (CT) scanning or angiography is indicated to determine if more than one pheochromocytoma is present (bilateral adrenal involvement occurs in approximately 10 per cent of cases). If the possibility of bilateral adrenalectomy exists, replacement hydrocortisone therapy should begin in the immediate preoperative period.

ADRENAL INSUFFICIENCY

The most common adrenal cortical abnormality present in the perioperative setting is a relative hypoadrenalism referred to as secondary adrenal insufficiency. This is due to glandular suppression in patients taking daily exogenous glucocorticoids. Primary adrenal insufficiency results from primary adrenal failure or Addison's disease. This syndrome is characterized by hyperpigmentation (secondary to elevated levels of adrenocorticotropic hormone, ACTH), hypotension, and hyponatremia (hypoaldosteronism), as well as hyperkalemia (decreased excretion). Systemic symptoms of weakness and anorexia usually accompany these findings. A rise in plasma cortisol following adrenal stimulation with synthetic ACTH confirms the diagnosis.[43]

Replacement steroid therapy for patients with primary or secondary adrenal insufficiency is essential at the time of surgical stress. Otherwise acute adrenal insufficiency as manifested by nausea, vomiting, fever, hypotension, and cardiovascular collapse and death may ensue.[115] Surgical stress results in a rise of plasma cortisol levels to five to ten times normal in 24 hours if stress resolves.[69] Exogenous steroid use can suppress the hypothalamic-pituitary-adrenal axis to the point that the normal postoperative responses to stress fail to occur.

Patients taking supraphysiologic doses of steroids (greater than the equivalent of 7.5 mg. of prednisone per day) for longer than 1 week are susceptible to adrenal suppression for as long as up to a year thereafter.[60] The ACTH stimulation test has been shown to be a good predictor of adrenal adequacy in response to stress.[126] If it is impossible to perform such a test preoperatively, it is recommended that perioperative steroid therapy be given to avoid adrenal crisis. The most commonly used and recommended therapy is intravenous hydrocortisone hemisuccinate or hydrocortisone phosphate. A continuous intravenous drip of 10 mg. per hour or doses of 100 mg. every 8 hours will provide adequate mineralocorticoid and glucocorticoid replacement for patients undergoing major operative procedures. The replacement therapy is continued until stress is no longer present, at which time it is tapered by approximately 20 per cent per day until replacement or preoperative maintenance levels are reached.[60]

Gastrointestinal System

The foremost concern in the preoperative patient with respect to the gastrointestinal system is the functional ability of the alimentary tract and its associated digestive organs to sustain the patient's nutritional requirements. The details of these concerns have already been reviewed. Assessment of hepatic, pancreatic, and intestinal function is also important preoperatively if there is any indication of pathology or functional insufficiency.

LIVER FUNCTION

The liver serves as the major biochemical factory in the body, the site of most intermediary metabolism. Normal liver function should be confirmed prior to elective operations.

A history of alcoholism, particularly a recent episode of excessive ingestion, should prompt investigation for hepatocellular injury. The patient should be questioned regarding jaundice, upper intestinal bleeding, or problems with bleeding during previous surgery. Physical findings of liver disease include the sequelae of chronic alcoholism such as ascites, jaundice, telangiectasias, palmar erythema, hepatomegaly, and gynecomastia. A clinical picture suggesting hepatic insufficiency can be further quantified through laboratory evaluation.

Cholestasis is the failure of the liver to excrete bilirubin, resulting in jaundice if serum bilirubin levels exceed 2 mg. per 100 ml. The causes of cholestasis include an excessive hemoglobin breakdown, hepatocellular injury, and extrahepatic bile duct obstruction. The serum bilirubin is the single best screening test for hepatic excretory function. Extrahepatic biliary obstruction results in a marked elevation of bilirubin and alkaline phosphatase out of proportion to usually only a mild elevation in serum transaminase levels. In contrast, hepatitis, the most common condition associated with hepatocellular injury, is usually characterized by greatly elevated transaminase levels with only mild hyperbilirubinemia. These categorizations, however, are only generalities.[118] Transaminase isoenzymes, fractionation of serum bilirubin into direct and indirect components, and numerous radiologic noninvasive and invasive preoperative studies can now usually characterize the etiology of most causes of hepatic insufficiency.

The liver synthesizes clotting factors II, V, VII, and X, and patients with liver disease require a preoperative check of prothrombin time (PT).[91] Significant hepatocellular damage is usually necessary before inadequate clotting factor synthesis results in a prolongation of PT. Reversible prolongation of PT may result as a consequence of cholestasis present for several weeks or of less severe hepatocellular injury from agents causing hepatitis. In such situations, a 10-mg. dose of intramuscular vitamin K preoperatively will often correct the PT. Failure to respond to such a regimen is an indication of poor hepatic functional reserve and suggests a greater risk for further perioperative hepatic deterioration and failure.[91] Albumin is also synthesized by the liver and hypoalbuminemia of less than 3.5 mg. per 100 ml. suggests either starvation or chronic hepatic insufficiency as seen in chronic liver disease such as cirrhosis.

A classification of patients with cirrhosis-based parameters is depicted in Table 5.[29] Class A patients have adequate hepatic reserve to tolerate anesthesia and elective procedures with minimal additional risk. However, the operative mortality for emergency shunt procedures (for upper gastrointestinal bleeding) for patients in Classes B and C is estimated at 20 to 30 per cent and 40 to 50 per cent, respectively.[88] Operative morbidity and mortality are also excessive in patients with acute alcoholic hepatitis. These patients are usually severely ill, presenting with hepatomegaly, jaundice, fever, right upper quadrant pain, nausea, and vomiting. They have an approximately 50 per cent mortality without operation,[37] and therefore only emergently indicated procedures should be performed. Acute viral hepatitis is also a contraindication to all but emergency operations. Complications of further deterioration of hepatic function, encephalopathy, and operative and postoperative hemorrhagic complications are common in these patients if surgery is performed. It is recommended that resolution of hepatitis as manifested clinically and by return of transaminase levels to normal occur prior to elective operations.

Chronic carriers of hepatitis B have no excessive risk from operations,[88] but the surgeon, anesthesiologist, and operating team must be aware of the danger of hepatitis transmission and take appropriate precautions. Patients in whom chronic persistent hepatitis develops also have no significant excess morbidity from elective procedures, since this is a mild chronic inflammatory condition in which hepatic function usually does not dangerously deteriorate. However, patients with the more aggressive form of chronic active hepatitis and postnecrotic cirrhosis are, as in patients with alcoholic cirrhosis, at increased risk of hepatic failure

from their disease based on the degree of liver damage. The natural history of the disease is a mortality rate of 40 per cent after 5 years.[88] Patients with evidence of marked hepatic functional impairment generally are poor surgical candidates. A course of corticosteroids can at times cause a remission in chronic active hepatitis, and this should be attempted if an elective procedure is indicated.[145]

Patients with obstructive jaundice from extrahepatic biliary duct obstruction can generally be expected to have the best prognosis among patients with preoperative hepatic impairment undergoing operations. Relief of the obstruction usually results in relatively rapid recovery of hepatic function, and the patient's prognosis is usually dependent on the etiology of the obstructing process.

In patients with known symptomatic cholelithiasis preoperatively who are undergoing abdominal operation for other reasons, consideration should be given to incidental cholecystectomy at the time of operation. Such procedures have been safely performed even in as controversial a setting as elective aortic aneurysm repair.[110]

Preoperative evaluation of the biliary tree can now be very effectively performed through the use of various radiologic modalities. Ultrasonography is now the most commonly used rapid noninvasive test for diagnosing cholelithiasis, dilatation of bile ducts, or enlargement of the pancreas. Cholangiography, whether via the percutaneous transhepatic route (PTC) or endoscopic retrograde cholangiopancreatography (ERCP), is frequently used to assess the anatomy of the biliary tree preoperatively in cases of obstructive jaundice.

The remainder of the alimentary tract usually requires only the specific diagnostic tests preoperatively to assess suspected pathology for which surgery is planned. Esophageal problems may require preoperative endoscopy or contrast studies. Reflux is further defined with pH testing. Gastric analysis and serum gastric determination are often helpful in assessing gastric physiologic function in peptic ulcer disease, as are gastroscopy and contrast radiography for defining anatomic problems. Patients with intestinal obstruction may require large amounts of fluid resuscitation prior to operation.[104] Computed tomography, serum amylase, and ERCP may be helpful preoperative tests in assessing pancreatic function and pathology.

Central Nervous System

CEREBROVASCULAR DISEASE

Extracranial cerebrovascular occlusive disease is seen commonly in the elderly population. In these patients, intraoperative hypotension, anoxia, or increased blood viscosity can exacerbate pre-existent compromised cerebral perfusion and result in intraoperative stroke. Therefore, evaluation of findings of cerebrovascular disease preoperatively is important to assess the risk of perioperative stroke.

Coronary artery bypass grafting and major aortic surgery are associated with an approximately 1 to 2 per cent incidence of perioperative stroke.[113, 150] However, patients with preoperative transient ischemic attacks (TIAs) represent a group at an increased risk for developing a stroke following such operations.[26] Preoperative management of patients with cerebrovascular disease initially involves assessment of its severity. Patients who have sustained a frank stroke suffer an instability of cerebral blood flow from 6 to 8 weeks thereafter and elective procedures are contraindicated during this period.[62] Intracerebral hemorrhages require a similar period of time for resolution, and their presence is also a contraindication to operation.

TABLE 5. Classification of Patients with Cirrhosis-Based Parameters*

Class	Serum Albumin (mg./100 ml.)	Ascites	Serum Bilirubin (mg./100 ml.)	Encephalopathy
A	>3.5	No	<2.0	No
B	3.0–3.5	Mild	2.0–3.0	Mild
C	<3.0	Marked	>3.0	Yes

*Adapted from Child, C. G., (Ed.): The Liver and Portal Hypertension, Philadelphia, W. B. Saunders Company, 1964, p. 50.

Studies of the natural history of symptomatic cerebrovascular disease have shown that patients with TIAs have an approximately 37 per cent incidence of developing stroke.[61] Since the morbidity and mortality of uncomplicated carotid endarterectomy is less than this (approximately 1 to 2 per cent),[146] surgical repair of patients with TIAs and angiographically proved significant carotid stenosis or ulceration is indicated. Such repair should be performed prior to other major procedures, except possibly concurrently with coronary bypass.[71]

The role of noninvasive means of estimating carotid occlusive disease is still in the process of being defined. Noninvasive studies are generally good screening procedures, being quite sensitive to abnormalities in carotid flow.[6] Although some surgeons are now advocating performance of carotid artery reconstruction solely on the basis of noninvasive studies,[40] the normal pattern of evaluation has been to perform angiography following noninvasive evidence suspicious for carotid occlusive disease.

Patients with asymptomatic carotid bruits have been the subject of much controversy in the literature regarding whether prophylactic carotid endarterectomy is indicated. Most studies to date support a general conclusion that the asymptomatic carotid bruit that is not associated with significant alteration in hemodynamic flow of the carotid arteries confers no excess risk of neurologic deficit following elective surgery.[9]

Patients with symptoms suggestive of posterior cerebrovascular insufficiency are usually not considered surgical candidates to correct these lesions (with the exception of the subclavian steal syndrome). Instead, treatment with antiplatelet therapy, most commonly aspirin or aspirin and persantine, is indicated. Similarly, patients who cannot or will not undergo carotid endarterectomy for anterior cerebrovascular TIAs should also be treated with aspirin since such therapy has been shown to decrease the incidence of stroke in man.[10]

Seizure Disorders

Patients with seizure disorders must be assessed for the adequacy of control of their disorders on their current medical regimens. If a reliable history of good control is obtained, there is no additional risk for the morbidity that comes from perioperative seizures. If, however, no such documentation is available, measurement of serum levels of anticonvulsants and a period of observation and postponement of elective surgery are advisable.

Administration of anticonvulsants parenterally in the perioperative period, with return to oral intake following resumption of diet postoperatively, is the most common means of perioperative management. Fortunately, the serum half-life of the common anticonvulsants phenobarbital and phenytoin is long, and omission of a few doses is often not critical. Certain metabolic states predispose to seizures. These include uremia, hypernatremia, and hyponatremia (water intoxication). Awareness of these states is essential, since correction of the basic metabolic problem is necessary in addition to administration of anticonvulsants in the patient with seizure disorders. It is recommended that elective operations be postponed when any of these conditions is present.

Alcoholism

Alcoholics are predisposed to many medical problems associated with their disease, such as cirrhosis, poor nutri-

tion, and cardiomyopathy. However, their neurologic problems are also important and are usually preventable as a source of operative morbidity. Delirium tremens is the most serious neurologic complication of chronic alcoholism, resulting from the acute withdrawal from alcohol consumption. The mild symptoms of restlessness and anxiety seen in mild alcohol withdrawal states can progress to hallucination, fever, disorientation, and death. Treatment with sedatives, usually of the benzodiazepine family, is indicated, as is postponement of any contemplated elective operation.[131] Alcoholic withdrawal may also result in grand mal seizures, usually limited in number and occurring several days after cessation of alcohol ingestion. These may be managed by short-term use of anticonvulsants and observation. Neurologic assessment, including electroencephalograms (EEG), is usually normal. Thiamine deficiency in chronic alcoholics may be manifested as Wernicke's syndrome; this can be prevented by the routine preoperative administration of 100 mg. of thiamine intramuscularly to all patients with a history of alcoholism.

Myasthenia Gravis

Myasthenia gravis is an example of the preoperative considerations necessary for the patient with a myopathy. The major considerations include providing adequate ventilatory support in the immediate postoperative period, careful attention to muscle relaxants, anticholinesterase drugs, or other medications particularly affecting muscle strength, and steroid coverage for patients on maintenance prednisone.[44] Patients with myotonic disorders are predisposed to violent muscle contractions after administration of depolarizing neuromuscular blockers, and agents such as succinylcholine should be avoided or used with great caution in these patients.

Renal System

Patients with renal insufficiency or failure pose several special dilemmas in the preoperative period. Diagnostic tests using contrast dye convey a special risk to patients with marginal renal function. Hydration is essential in these patients to prevent or minimize further deterioration in renal function from exposure to the hypertonic dye. Patients requiring chronic dialysis pose the additional associated problems of anemia, usually poor vascular access, often advanced peripheral vascular disease, and usually other end-organ damage as a result of disease processes. The margin for error in fluid balance and medication dosages is also considerably narrower than that in patients with normal renal function. Patients in chronic renal failure receiving continuous abdominal peritoneal dialysis who undergo abdominal operations may require temporary hemodialysis until the peritoneal cavity again becomes useful for dialysis.

The presence of bladder dysfunction postoperatively, specifically difficulty in voiding, is a problem common to even relatively uncomplicated operations such as herniorrhaphy. Rectal procedures may also produce a temporary reflex bladder dysfunction. Use of an indwelling urinary catheter is indicated in all major surgical procedures requiring more than 1 or 2 hours of operating time for dual purposes of both bladder drainage and monitoring urinary output and renal perfusion. Older male patients with significant prostatic hypertrophy as well as younger patients with urethral strictures may be difficult to catheterize. If the disease is associated with any signs of renal compromise

TABLE 6. Preoperative Summary Checklist

Consent obtained
Preoperative orders
  NPO
  Void on call
  Preoperative skin preparation
  Preoperative antibiotics?
  Steroids?
  Cardiac medications?
  Other medications patient usually takes?
  Preoperative sedative?
  IV fluids?

Pertinent x-rays available (including CXR)
Blood (blood products prn) in bank
Preoperative laboratory results
  CBC
  Urinalysis
  Electrolytes, BUN, creatinine
  Coagulation studies?
  Other chemistries/enzymes?
Preoperative ECG?
Special medical problems requiring consultation?
Allergies?

Abbreviations: CXR = Chest x-ray; NPO = nothing by mouth; BUN = blood urea nitrogen; ECG = electrocardiogram; CBC = complete blood count; IV = intravenous; prn = as needed.

such that an obstructive uropathy has been present preoperatively, catheter drainage with correction of the postobstructive diuresis that often ensues is indicated prior to any elective surgery.[73]

CONCLUSION

A useful checklist of common orders that may apply to preoperative preparation in many patients is shown in Table 6. It is a suggestion and is included here with the recognition that it is neither a comprehensive guideline nor one to be used as a substitute for the careful individual attention that must be given each patient.

The maximal benefit of surgical therapy is achieved when an operation appropriate to correct the existing pathologic condition is performed correctly. The events that occur in the operating room are important in determining the patient's prognosis; hence, the surgical team must devote maximal concentration at that time to the performance of the operation. Thorough preoperative preparation of the patient is mandatory to avoid raising concerns for such problems at the critical time of operation. Appropriate consultation with the anesthesiologist and his or her team should be obtained well in advance of operation, particularly with high-risk patients.

The plan of the operation and the expected pathologic findings, as well as any possible alternative findings and subsequent changes in operative treatment they would dictate, should be clear in the surgeon's mind. When the surgical team has both thoroughly prepared the patient for operation with careful attention to detail and is mentally prepared to perform the proposed surgical procedure or its alternatives, the optimal benefits from the operation will follow.

SELECTED REFERENCES

Dudrick, S. J., Wilmore, D. W., Vars, H. M., et al.: Long-term parenteral nutrition with growth, development and positive nitrogen balance. Surgery, 64:134, 1968.
  A landmark article with the first description of the successful use of total parenteral nutrition.

Goldmann, D. R., et al. (Eds.): Medical Care of the Surgical Patient. Philadelphia, J. B. Lippincott, 1982, pp. 31–39.
  A comprehensive text of preoperative and postoperative care, including 38 problem-oriented chapters with a list of contributors.

Goldman, L., Caldera, D. L., Nussbaum, S. R., et al.: Multifactorial index of cardiac risk in noncardiac surgical procedures. N. Engl. J. Med., 297:845, 1977.
  An often quoted study relating preoperative findings to cardiac risk in patients undergoing noncardiac surgery.

Grant, J. P.: Handbook of Total Parenteral Nutrition. Philadelphia, W. B. Saunders Company, 1980, pp. 7–26.
  A brief but comprehensive and well-written text on the important aspects of total parenteral nutrition.

Joint, J. H.: Care of patients with hemophilia and von Willebrand's disease. In Rutman, R. C., and Miller, W. V. (Eds.): Transfusion Therapy: Principles and Procedures, 2nd ed., Rockville, Md., Aspen Systems Corp., 1985, pp. 243–244.
  An excellent summary text of all aspects of transfusion therapy.

Russell, J. C.: Prophylaxis of postoperative deep vein thrombosis and pulmonary embolism. Surg. Gynecol. Obstet., 157:89, 1983.
  An excellent summary article with 203 references on an important and controversial topic.

Souba, W. W., and Wilmore, D. W.: Nutritional considerations. In Vandam, L. D. (Ed.): To Make the Patient Ready for Anesthesia: Medical Care of the Surgical Patient, 2nd ed. Reading, Mass., Addison-Wesley, 1984, pp. 267–295.
  Another useful reference on the proper nutritional preparation for surgical procedures.

Tisi, G. M.: Preoperative evaluation of pulmonary function: Validity, indications and benefits. Am. Rev. Respir. Dis., 119:293, 1979.
  Review article on available data supporting indications for preoperative pulmonary evaluation.

Veterans Administration Ad Hoc Interdisciplinary Advisory Committee on Antimicrobial Drug Usage: Prophylaxis in surgery. J.A.M.A., 237:1003, 1977.
  Recommendations of the VA Ad Hoc Committee for appropriate antibiotic use in the perioperative period.

REFERENCES

1. Adler, M., Quenon, M., Even-Adin, D., et al.: Whole gut lavage for colonoscopy: A comparison between two solutions. Gastrointest. Endosc., 30:65, 1984.
2. Alexander, J. W., Fischer, J. E., Boyajian, M., et al.: The influence of hair-removal methods on wound infections. Arch. Surg., 118:347, 1983.
3. American Heart Association Council on Thrombosis: Prevention of venous thromboembolism in surgical patients by low-dose heparin. Circulation, 55:423A, 1977.
4. American Society of Anesthesiologists: Classification of physical status. Anesthesiology, 24:111, 1963.
5. Antimicrobial prophylaxis for surgery. The Medical Letter, 25:113, 1983.
6. Archie, P. J., Jr., Posey, P. H., and Goodson, D. S.: Improved accuracy of cerebrovascular noninvasive tests using combined methods. Surg. Gynecol. Obstet., 151:791, 1980.
7. Arous, E. J., Baum, P. C., and Cutler, B. S.: The ischemic exercise test in patients with peripheral vascular disease. Arch. Surg., 119:780, 1984.
8. Atkins, P. C.: The risks of surgery in patients with asthma. In Goldmann, D. R., Brown, F. H., Levy, W. K., et al. (Eds.): Medical Care of the Surgical Patient. Philadelphia, J. B. Lippincott, 1982, pp. 422–425.
9. Barnes, R. W., and Marszalek, P. B.: Asymptomatic carotid disease in the cardiovascular surgical patient: Is prophylactic endarterectomy necessary? Stroke, 12:497, 1981.
10. Barnett, H. J. M.: Canadian Cooperative Study Group: A randomized trial of aspirin and sulfinpyrazone in threatened stroke. N. Engl. J. Med., 299:53, 1978.
11. Belding, H. H.: Use of anticoagulants in the prevention of venous thromboembolic disease in postoperative patients. Arch. Surg., 90:566, 1965.
12. Bergentz, S. E.: Dextran prophylaxis of venous thromboembolism. In Bergan, J. J., and Yao, J. S. T. (Eds.): Venous Problems. Chicago, Year Book Publishers, 1978, pp. 529–540.
13. Berger, S. A., and Nagar, H.: Antimicrobial prophylaxis in urology. J. Urol., 120:319, 1978.
14. Beutler, E., and Wood, L.: The in vivo regeneration of red cell 2,3-diphosphoglyceric acid (DPG) after transfusion of stored blood. J. Lab. Clin. Med., 74:300, 1969.

15. Bjornsson, S., Yates, J. W., Mittleman, A., et al.: Major surgery in acute leukemia. Cancer, *34*:1272, 1974.

16. Bodey, G. P., Buckley, M., Sathe, Y. S., et al.: Quantitative relationship between circulating leukocytes and infection in patients with acute leukemia. Ann. Intern. Med., 64:328, 1966.

17. Borow, M., and Goldson, H.: Postoperative venous thrombosis: Evaluation of five methods of treatment. Am. J. Surg., *141*:122, 1981.

18. Boushy, S. F., Belley, D. M., North, C. B., et al.: Clinical course related to preoperative and postoperative pulmonary function in patients with bronchogenic carcinoma. Chest, *59*:383, 1971.

19. Boysen, P. G., Block, A. J., and Moulder, P. V.: Relationship between perioperative pulmonary function tests and complications after thoracotomy. Surg. Gynecol. Obstet., *152*:813, 1981.

20. Browse, N. L., Jackson, B. T., Mayo, M. E., and Negus, D.: The value of mechanical methods of preventing postoperative calf vein thrombosis. Br. J. Surg., *61*:219, 1974.

21. Burdon, D. W.: Principles of antimicrobial prophylaxis. World J. Surg., *6*:262, 1982.

22. Burke, J. F., Quinby, W. C., Bondoc, C. C., et al.: Immunosuppression and temporary skin transplantation in the treatment of massive third degree burns. Ann. Surg., *182*:183, 1975.

23. Butson, A. R. C.: Intermittent pneumatic calf compression for prevention of deep venous thrombosis in general abdominal surgery. Am. J. Surg., *142*:525, 1981.

24. Butterworth, C. E., Jr.: Malnutrition in the hospital. J.A.M.A., *230*:879, 1974.

25. Buzby, G. P., Mullen, J. L., Matthews, D. C., et al.: Prognostic nutritional index in gastrointestinal surgery. Am. J. Surg., *139*:160, 1980.

26. Carney, W. I., Stewart, W. B., DePinto, D. J., et al.: Carotid bruit as a risk factor in aortoiliac reconstruction. Surgery, *81*:567, 1977.

27. Cebul, R. D., and Kussmaul, W. G.: Preoperative pulmonary evaluation and preparation. In Goldmann, D. R., Brown, F. H., Levy, W. K., et al. (Eds.): Medical Care of the Surgical Patient. Philadelphia, J. B. Lippincott, 1982, pp. 367–368.

28. Chetlin, S. H., and Elliott, D. W.: Biliary bacteremia. Arch. Surg., *107*:319, 1973.

29. Child, C. G., and Turcotte, J. G.: Surgery and portal hypertension. In Child, C. G. (Ed.): The Liver and Portal Hypertension. Philadelphia, W. B. Saunders Company, 1964, pp. 1–85.

30. Chodoff, P., Margand, P. M. S., and Knowles, C. L.: Short term abstinence from smoking: Its place in preoperative preparation. Crit. Care Med., *3*:131, 1975.

31. Clagett, G. P., Brier, D. F., Rosoff, C. B., et al.: Effect of aspirin on postoperative platelet kinetics and venous thrombosis. Surg. Forum, *25*:473, 1974.

32. Clarke, J. S., Condon, R. E., Bartlett, J. G., et al.: Preoperative oral antibiotics reduce septic complications of colorectal operations: Results of a prospective, randomized, double-blind clinical study. Ann. Surg., *186*:251, 1977.

33. Coe, N. P., Collings, R. E. C., Klein, L. A., et al.: Prevention of deep venous thrombosis in urological patients; a controlled, randomized trial of low-dose heparin and external pneumatic compression boots. Surgery, *83*:230, 1978.

34. Committee on Control of Surgical Infections of the American College of Surgeons: Control of Infections in Surgical Patients. Philadelphia, J. B. Lippincott, 1976.

35. Committee on Infectious Diseases, Committee on Drugs, and Section on Surgery: Antimicrobial prophylaxis in pediatric surgical patients. Pediatrics, *74*:437, 1984.

36. Condon, R. E., Bartlett, J. G., Nichols, R. L., et al.: Preoperative prophylactic cephalothin fails to control septic complications of colorectal operations: Results of Veterans Administration Cooperative Study. Am. J. Surg., *137*:68, 1979.

37. Conn, H. O.: Steroid treatment of alcoholic hepatitis. Gastroenterology, *74*:319, 1978.

38. Coon, W. W.: Risk factors in pulmonary embolism. Surg. Gynecol. Obstet., *143*:385, 1976.

39. Cranley, J. J., Canos, A. J., and Mahalinjam, K.: Non-invasive diagnosis and prophylaxis of deep venous thrombosis of the lower extremities. In Madden, J. L., and Hume, M. (Eds.): Venous Thromboembolism; Prevention and Treatment. New York, Appleton-Century-Crofts, 1976, pp. 131–153.

40. Crew, J. R., Dean, M., and Johnson, J. M.: Carotid surgery without angiography. Surg. Rounds, Sept. 1985, pp. 18–23.

41. Cruse, P. J. E., and Foord, R.: A 10-year prospective study of 62,939 wounds. Surg. Clin. North Am., *60*:27, 1980.

42. Daly, J. M., Massar, E., Giacco, G., et al.: Parenteral nutrition in esophageal cancer patients. Ann. Surg., *196*:203, 1982.

43. Danowski, T. S.: Outline of Endocrine Gland Syndromes, 3rd ed. Baltimore, Williams & Wilkins, 1976, pp. 293–302.

44. Dawson, D. M.: Neurologic disease. In Vandam, L. D. (Ed.): To Make the Patient Ready for Anesthesia: Medical Care of the

Surgical Patient, 2nd ed. Reading, Mass., Addison-Wesley, 1984, pp. 188–193.

45. DeMeester, T. R., Van Heertum, R. L., Kavas, J. R., et al.: Preoperative evaluation with differential pulmonary function. Ann. Thorac. Surg., *18*:61, 1974.

46. Dudrick, S. J., Wilmore, D. W., Vars, H. M., et al.: Long term parenteral nutrition with growth, development, and positive nitrogen balance. Surgery, *64*:134, 1968.

47. Edwards, W. H., Mulheria, J. G., Jr., and Walker, W. E.: Vascular reconstructive surgery following myocardial revascularization. Ann. Surg., *187*:653, 1978.

48. Eisenberg, D., Silberman, H., Maryniuk, J., et al.: Inapplicability of the prognostic nutritional index in critically ill patients. Surg. Forum, *32*:109, 1981.

49. Eisenberg, J. M., and Goldfarb, S.: Clinical usefulness of measuring prothrombin time as a routine admission test. Clin. Chem., *22*:1644, 1976.

50. Ellison, N., and Ominsky, A. J.: Clinical considerations for the anesthesiologist whose patient is on anticoagulant therapy. Anesthesiology, *39*:328, 1973.

51. Estes, J. E., Jr.: Abdominal aortic aneurysms: A study of 102 cases. Circulation, *2*:258, 1960.

52. Fairfull-Smith, R. J., and Freeman, J. B.: Immediate postoperative enteral nutrition with a nonelemental diet. J. Surg. Res., *29*:236, 1980.

53. Field, R., Jr.: Preoperative hair removal: An unnecessary surgical tradition. Surg. Rounds, March 1983, pp. 66–67.

54. Galloway, J. A., and Shuman, C. R.: Diabetes and surgery: A study of 667 cases. Am. J. Med., *34*:177, 1963.

55. Gehov, M. A., and Cox, M.: Disorders of volume, tonicity, and potassium in the surgical patient. In Goldmann, D. R., et al. (Eds.): Medical Care of the Surgical Patient. Philadelphia, J. B. Lippincott, 1982, pp. 247–249.

56. Genton, E., Gent, M., Hirsh, J., and Harker, L. A.: Platelet-inhibiting drugs in the prevention of clinical thrombotic disease. N. Engl. J. Med., *293*:1174–1178, 1236–1240, 1296–1300, 1975.

57. Ghosh, P., and Pakrash, B. C.: Cardiac dysrhythmias after thoracotomy. Br. Heart J., *34*:374, 1972.

58. Goldman, L.: Cardiac risks and complications of noncardiac surgery. Ann. Surg., *198*:780, 1983.

59. Goldman, L., Caldera, D. L., Nussbaum, S. R., et al.: Multifactorial index of cardiac risk in noncardiac surgical procedures. N. Engl. J. Med., *297*:845, 1977.

60. Goldmann, D. R.: The surgical patient on steroids. In Goldmann, D. R., et al. (Eds.): Medical Care of the Surgical Patient. Philadelphia, J. B. Lippincott, 1982, pp. 113–125.

61. Goldner, J. C., Whisnant, J. P., and Taylor, W. F.: Long-term prognosis of TIA. Stroke, *2*:160, 1971.

62. Gonzulez-Scarano, F., and Hurtig, H.: Management of the surgical patient with cerebrovascular disease. In Goldmann, D. R., et al. (Eds.): Medical Care of the Surgical Patient. Philadelphia, J. B. Lippincott, 1982, p. 519.

63. Gordon-Smith, I. C., Grundy, D. J., LeQuesne, L. P., et al.: Controlled trial of two regimens of subcutaneous heparin in prevention of postoperative deep-vein thrombosis. Lancet, *1*:1133, 1972.

64. Gracey, D. R., Divertie, M. B., and Didier, E. P.: Preoperative pulmonary preparation of patients with chronic obstructive pulmonary disease: A prospective study. Chest, *76*:123, 1979.

65. Grant, J. P.: Handbook of Total Parenteral Nutrition. Philadelphia, W. B. Saunders Company, 1980, pp. 7–26.

66. Greenberg, A., and Goldfarb, S.: Acid-base disturbances in the surgical patient. In Goldmann, D. R., et al. (Eds.): Medical Care of the Surgical Patient. Philadelphia, J. B. Lippincott, 1982, pp. 290–291.

67. Greenfield, L. J.: Pulmonary embolism: Diagnosis and management. Curr. Probl. Surg., *13*:1, 1976.

68. Hallen, B.: Computerized anesthetic record-keeping. Acta Anesthesiol. Scand. (Suppl.), *52*:38, 1973.

69. Haugen, H. N., and Brinck-Johnsen, T.: The adrenal response to surgical trauma. Acta Chir. Scand. (Suppl.), *357*:100, 1966.

70. Hertzer, N. R., et al.: Coronary artery disease in peripheral vascular patients: A classification of 1,000 coronary angiograms and results of surgical management. Ann. Surg., *199*:223, 1984.

71. Hertzer, N. R., Coop, F. D., Taylor, P. C., et al.: Staged and combined surgical approach to simultaneous carotid and coronary vascular disease. Surgery, *84*:803, 1978.

72. Hilberman, M., Kamm, B., Lamy, M., et al.: An analysis of potential physiological predictors of respiratory adequacy following cardiac surgery. J. Thorac. Cardiovasc. Surg., *71*:711, 1976.

73. Hinman, F., Jr.: The pathophysiology of urinary obstruction. In Campbell, M. F., and Harrison, J. H. (Eds.): Urology, Vol. 1, 3rd ed. Philadelphia, W. B. Saunders Company, 1970, pp. 330–332.

74. Hirschmann, J. V., and Invi, T. S.: Antimicrobial prophylaxis: A critique of recent trials. Rev. Infect. Dis., 2:1, 1980.

75. Hirsh, R. A.: An approach to assessing perioperative risk. In Goldmann, D. R., et al. (Eds.): Medical Care of the Surgical Patient, Philadelphia, J. B. Lippincott, 1982, pp. 31–39.

76. Hirschfeld, J. W., Jr.: Surgery in the patient with valvular heart disease. In Goldmann, D. R., et al. (Eds.): Medical Care of the Surgical Patient. Philadelphia, J. B. Lippincott, 1982, pp. 99–112.

77. Homi, J., Reynolds, J., Skinner, A., et al.: General anesthesia in sickle cell disease. Br. Med. J., 1:1599, 1979.

78. Immelman, E. J., Jeffery, P., Benatar, S. R., et al.: Failure of low-dose heparin to prevent significant thromboembolic complications in high-risk surgical patients: Interim report of prospective trial, Groote Schuur Hospital Thrombembolus Study Group. Br. Med. J. 1:1447, 1979.

79. Izenstein, B. Z., Dluhy, R. G., and Williams, G. H.: Endocrinology. In Vandam, L. D. (Ed.): To Make the Patient Ready for Anesthesia: Medical Care of the Surgical Patient. Reading, Mass, Addison-Wesley, 1980, pp. 116–119.

80. Johnson, L. W., Dickestein, R. A., Fruchan, C. T., et al.: Prophylactic digitalization for coronary artery bypass surgery. Circulation, 53:819, 1976.

81. Joist, J. H., Care of patients with hemophilia and von Willebrand's disease. In Rutman, R. C., and Miller, W. V. (Eds.): Transfusion Therapy. Principles and Procedures, 2nd ed. Rockville, Md., Aspen Systems Corp., 1985, pp. 243–244.

82. Jones, R. H., Douglas, J. M., Jr., et al.: Noninvasive radionuclide assessment of cardiac function in patients with peripheral vascular disease. Surgery, 85:59, 1979.

83. Kakkar, V. V., Corrigan, T. P., Fossard, D. P., et al.: Prevention of fatal postoperative pulmonary embolism by low doses of heparin: An international multicentive trial. Lancet, 2:45, 1975.

84. Kaplan, E. L., Anthony, B. F., Bisno, A., et al.: Prevention of bacterial endocarditis. Circulation, 56:139A, 1977.

85. Katholi, R. E., Nolan, S. P., and McGuire, L. B.: The management of anticoagulation during noncardiac operations in patients with prosthetic heart valves: A prospective study. Am. Heart J., 96:163, 1978.

86. Keighley, M. R. B., Baddeley, R. M., Burdon, D. W., et al.: A controlled trial of parenteral prophylactic gentamicin therapy in biliary surgery. Br. J. Surg., 62:275, 1975.

87. Keighley, M. R. B., Burdon, D. W., and Gatehouse, D.: Rate of wound sepsis with selective short-term antibiotic prophylaxis in gastric surgery. World J. Surg., 6:445, 1982.

88. La Mont, J. T.: Anesthesia and surgery in the patient with liver disease. In Vandam, L. D. (Ed.): To Make Ready for Anesthesia: Medical Care of the Surgical Patient. Reading, Mass., Addison-Wesley, 1980, pp. 44–63.

89. Law, D. K., Dudrick, S. J., and Abdou, N. I.: Immune competence of patients with protein-calorie malnutrition. Ann. Intern. Med., 79:545, 1973.

90. Lewin, I., Lerner, A. G., Green, S. H., et al.: Physical class and physiologic status in the prediction of operative mortality in the aged sick. Ann. Surg., 174:217, 1971.

91. Losowsky, M., Simmons, A. V., and Mitoszewski, K.: Coagulation abnormalities in liver disease. Postgrad. Med., 53:147, 1973.

92. Luft, H. S., Bunker, J. P., and Enthoven, A. C.: Should operations be regionalized? The empirical relation between surgical volume and mortality. N. Engl. J. Med., 301:1364, 1979.

93. Lumb, P. D.: Fluids and electrolytes. In Kortz, W. J., and Lumb, P. D. (Eds.): Surgical Intensive Care: A Practical Guide. Chicago, Year Book Medical Publishers, 1984, p. 330.

94. Lumn, J. N., and Elwood, P. C.: Anaemia and surgery. Br. Med. J., 3:71, 1970.

95. MacLean, L. D.: Host resistance in surgical patients. J. Trauma, 19:297, 1979.

96. Mahar, L. J., Steen, P. A., Tinker, J. H., et al.: Perioperative myocardial infarction in patients with coronary artery disease with and without aorta-coronary artery bypass grafts. J. Thorac. Cardiovas. Surg., 76:533, 1978.

97. Manger, W. M., and Gifford, R. W., Jr.: Pheochromocytoma. New York, Springer-Verlag, 1977, p. 5.

98. Marchlinski, F. E.: Arrhythmias and conduction disturbances in surgical patients. In Goldmann, D. R., et al.: (Eds.): Medical Care of the Surgical Patient. Philadelphia, J. B. Lippincott, 1982, pp. 59–77.

99. Marx, G. F., Mateo, C. V., and Orken, L. R.: Computer analysis of post-anesthetic deaths. Anesthesiology, 39:54, 1973.

100. McClelland, R. N. (Ed.): Selected Readings in General Surgery, 9:1, 1982.

101. McCollum, C. H., et al.: Myocardial revascularization prior to subsequent major surgery in patients with coronary artery disease. Surgery, 81:302, 1977.

102. McKenna, R., Galante, J., Bachmann, F., et al.: Prevention of venous thromboembolism after total knee placement by high-dose aspirin or intermittent calf and thigh compression. Br. Med. J., 1:514, 1980.

103. Menkins, J. L., Pietsch, J. B., Cristou, N. V., and MacLean, L. D.: Predicting surgical infection before the operation. World J. Surg., 4:439, 1980.

104. Moore, F. D.: Metabolic Care of the Surgical Patient. Philadelphia, W. B. Saunders Company, 1959, pp. 73–88.

105. Muller, J. M., Brenner, V., Dienst, C., and Pichlmaier, H.: Preoperative parenteral feedings in patients with gastrointestinal carcinoma. Lancet, 1:68, 1982.

106. Nelson, N. C., and Becker, W. F.: Thyroid crisis: Diagnosis and treatment. Ann. Surg., 170:263, 1969.

107. Nichols, R. L.: Use of prophylactic antibiotics in surgical practice. Am. J. Med., 70:686, 1981.

108. Nichols, R. L., and Condon, R. E.: Preoperative preparation of the colon. Surg. Gynecol. Obstet., 132:323, 1971.

109. Nicolaides, A. N.: The current status of small-dose subcutaneous heparin in the prevention of venous thromboembolism. In Bergan, J. J., and Yao, J. S. T. (Eds.): Venous Problems. Chicago, Year Book Medical Publishers, 1978, pp. 517–528.

110. Ouriel, K., Ricotta, J. J., Adams, J. T., and DeWeese, J. A.: Management of cholelithiasis in patients with abdominal aortic aneurysm. Ann. Surg., 198:717, 1983.

111. Pennock, B. E., Rogers, R. M., and McCaffree, D. R.: Changes in measured spirometric indices: What is significant? Chest, 80:183, 1973.

112. Presley, A. P., and Alexander-Williams, J.: Postoperative chest infection. Br. J. Surg., 61:448, 1974.

113. Reul, G. J., Morris, G. C., Howell, J. F., et al.: Current concepts in coronary artery surgery: A critical analysis of 1287 patients. Ann. Thorac. Surg., 14:243, 1972.

114. Rhodes, E. R., Dixon, R. H., and Silver, D.: Heparin induced thrombocytopenia with thrombotic and hemorrhagic manifestations. Surg. Gynecol. Obstet., 136:409, 1973.

115. Roberts, J. G.: Operative collapse after corticosteroid therapy: A survey. Surg. Clin. North Am., 50:363, 1970.

116. Rodstein, M., Wolloch, L., and Gubner, R. S.: Mortality study of the significance of extrasystole in an insured population. Chest, 64:564, 1973.

117. Rombeau, J. L.: Preoperative total parenteral nutrition and surgical outcome in patients with inflammatory bowel disease. Ann. Surg., 196:203, 1982.

118. Rosoff, J., Jr., and Rosoff, L.: Biochemical tests for hepatobiliary disease. Surg. Clin. North Am., 57:257, 1977.

119. Royal College of Radiologists National Study: Preoperative chest radiology. Lancet, 2:83, 1979.

120. Russell, J. C.: Prophylaxis of postoperative deep vein thrombosis and pulmonary embolism. Surg. Gynecol. Obstet., 157:89, 1983.

121. Ryan, J. A., Jr., and Taft, D. A.: Preoperative nutritional assessment does not predict morbidity and mortality in abdominal operations. Surg. Forum, 31:96, 1980.

122. Sagar, S., Massey, J., and Sanderson, J. M.: Low-dose heparin prophylaxis against fatal pulmonary embolism. Br. Med. J., 4:257, 1975.

123. Sagar, S., Nairn, D., Stamatakis, J. D., et al.: Efficacy of low-dose heparin in prevention of extensive deep-vein thrombosis in patients undergoing total hip replacement. Lancet, 1:1151, 1976.

124. Sagel, S. S., Evens, R. G., Forrest, J. V., et al.: Efficacy of routine screening and lateral chest radiographs in a hospital-based population. N. Engl. J. Med., 291:1001, 1974.

125. Salzman, E. W.: Physical methods of prevention of venous thromboembolism. Surgery, 81:123, 1977.

126. Sampson, P. A., Brooke, B. N., and Winstone, N. E.: Biochemical confirmation of collapse due to adrenal failure. Lancet, 1:1377, 1961.

127. Sanders, R. A., and Sheldon, G. F.: Septic complications of total parenteral nutrition: A five year experience. Am. J. Surg., 132:214, 1976.

128. Schade, D. S., Eaton, R. P., Alberti, K. G., and Johnston, D. G.: Diabetic Coma, Ketoacidotic and Hyperosmolar. Albuquerque, University of New Mexico Press, 1981, pp. 127–139.

129. Scholz, P. M., Jones, R. H., Wolfe, W. G., and Sabiston, D. C.: Prophylaxis of pulmonary embolism. Major Probl. Clin. Surg., 25:96, 1980.

130. Schulze, R. A., Jr., Strauss, H. W., and Pitt, B.: Sudden death in the year following myocardial infarction. Relation to ventricular premature contractions in the late hospital phase and left ventricular ejection fraction. Am. J. Med., 62:192, 1977.

131. Sellers, E. M., and Kalant, H.: Alcohol intoxication and withdrawal. N. Engl. J. Med., 294:757, 1976.

132. Selzer, A., and Walter, R. M.: Adequacy of preoperative digitalis therapy in controlling ventricular rate in postoperative atrial fibrillation. Circulation, 34:119, 1966.

133. Seropian, R., and Reynolds, B. M.: Wound infections after preoperative depilatory versus razor preparation. Am. J. Surg., *121*:251, 1971.

134. Shanks, R. G., Hadden, D. R., Lowe, D. C., et al.: Controlled trial of propranolol in thyrotoxicosis. Lancet, *1*:993, 1969.

135. Sjoerdsma, A., Engelmark, K., Waldmann, T. A., et al.: Pheochromocytoma: Current concepts of diagnosis and treatment. Ann. Intern. Med., *65*:1302, 1966.

136. Skillman, J. J., Collins, R. E. C., Coe, N. P., et al.: Prevention of deep vein thrombosis in neurosurgical patients: A controlled, randomized trial of external preventive compression boots. Surgery, *83*:354, 1978.

137. Sohmer, P. R.: Transfusion therapy. *In* Pittiglio, D. H., Baldwin, A. J., and Sohmer, P. R. (Eds.): Modern Blood Banking and Transfusion Practices. Philadelphia, F. A. Davis, 1983, p. 328.

138. Souba, W. W., and Wilmore, D. W.: Nutritional considerations. *In* Vandam, L. D. (Ed.): To Make the Patient Ready for Anesthesia: Medical Care of the Surgical Patient, 2nd ed. Reading, Mass., Addison-Wesley, 1984, pp. 267–295.

139. Spanier, A. H., Pietsch, J. B., Meakins, J. L., et al.: The relationship between immune competence and nutrition. Surg. Forum, *27*:332, 1976.

140. Steen, P. A., Tinker, J. H., and Tarhan, S.: Myocardial reinfarction after anesthesia and surgery. J.A.M.A., *239*:2566, 1978.

141. Stein, M., and Cassara, E. L.: Preoperative pulmonary evaluation and therapy for surgical patients. J.A.M.A., *211*:787, 1970.

142. Stevens, R. H., Cox, M., Feig, P. V., et al.: Internal potassium balance and the control of plasma potassium concentration. Medicine, *60*:339, 1981.

143. Stone, H. H., Haney, B. B., Kolb, L. D., et al.: Prophylactic and preventative antibiotic therapy: Timing, duration, economics. Ann. Surg., *189*:691, 1979.

144. Stone, H. H., Hooper, C. A., Kolb, L. D., et al.: Antibiotic prophylaxis in gastric, biliary, and colonic surgery. Ann. Surg., *184*:443, 1976.

145. Summerskill, W. H.: Chronic active liver disease reexamined: Prognosis hopeful. Gastroenterology, *66*:450, 1974.

146. Sundt, T. M., Sandok, B. A., and Whisnant, J. P.: Carotid endarterectomy: Complications and preoperative assessment of risk. Mayo Clin. Proc., *50*:301, 1975.

147. Tarhan, S., Moffitt, E. A., Sessler, A. D., et al.: Risk of anesthesia and surgery in patients with chronic bronchitis and chronic obstructive pulmonary disease. Surgery, *74*:720, 1973.

148. Tarhan, S., Muffitt, E. A., Taylor, W. F., and Guiliani, E. R.: Myocardial infarction after general anesthesia. J.A.M.A., *220*:1451, 1972.

149. Tisi, G. M.: Preoperative evaluation of pulmonary function: Validity, indications, and benefits. Am. Rev. Respir. Dis., *119*:293, 1979.

150. Treiman, R. C., Foran, R. F., Cohen, J. L., et al.: Carotid bruit: A follow-up report on its significance in patients undergoing an abdominal aortic operation. Arch. Surg., *114*:1138, 1979.

151. Turner, W. W., Landreneau, R. J., Toler, G. F., et al.: How accurate is nutritional risk classification? Surg. Forum, *33*:107, 1982.

152. Tyras, D. H., Stothert, J. C., Kaiser, G. C., et al.: Supraventricular tachyarrhythmias after myocardial revascularization: A randomized trial of prophylactic digitalization. J. Thorac. Cardiovasc. Surg., *77*:310, 1979.

153. Vacanti, C. J., Van Houten, R. J., and Hill, R. C.: A statistical analysis of the relationship of physical status to postoperative mortality in 68,388 cases. Anesth. Analg., *49*:564, 1970.

154. Van Nostrand, D., Kjelsbery, M. O., and Humphrey, E. W.: Preresectional evaluation of risk from pneumonectomy. Surg. Gynecol. Obstet., *127*:306, 1968.

155. Vargish, T., Crawford, L. C., Stallings, R. A., et al.: A randomized prospective evaluation of orally administered antibiotics in operations on the colon. Surg. Gynecol. Obstet., *146*:193, 1978.

156. Veterans Administration Ad Hoc Interdisciplinary Advisory Committee on Antimicrobial Drug Usage: Prophylaxis in surgery. J.A.M.A., *237*:1003, 1977.

157. Wagner, C. W., Nesbit, R. R., and Mansberger, A. R.: The use of intravenous hydrochloric acid in the treatment of 34 patients with metabolic acidosis. Ann. Surg., *46*:140, 1980.

158. Wapnick, S., Guinto, R., Reizis, I., et al.: Reduction of postoperative infection in elective colon surgery with preoperative administration of kanamycin and erythromycin. Surgery, *85*:316, 1979.

159. Warnold, I., and Lundholm, K.: Clinical significance of preoperative nutritional status in 215 noncancer patients. Ann. Surg., *199*:229, 1984.

160. Wasserman, L. R.: The treatment of polycythemia vera. Semin. Hematol., *13*:57, 1976.

161. Wightman, J. A. K.: A prospective survey of the incidence of postoperative pulmonary complications. Br. J. Surg., *55*:85, 1968.

HEMOSTASIS: PATHOPHYSIOLOGY AND MANAGEMENT OF CLINICAL DISORDERS

CHARLES S. GREENBERG, M.D.

5

The hemostatic system functions to initiate blood co-agulation and arrest bleeding. Coagulation is the process that transforms blood from a liquid state into a gel-like clot. The hemostatic system also prevents unwanted clotting and thrombosis from occurring. A complex series of reactions involving plasma proteins, platelets, and the blood vessel have evolved to regulate blood coagulation. Pathologic defects in the hemostatic system may result in either bleeding or thrombosis. Thrombosis is the process in which unwanted blood coagulation produces tissue injury. The pathophysiology of blood coagulation, the laboratory tests, the transfusion products, and the drugs used in treating hemostatic and thrombotic disorders will be described in this chapter.

OVERVIEW OF THE ANATOMIC AND BIOCHEMICAL EVENTS IN HEMOSTASIS

The anatomic and biochemical events involved in he-mostasis are summarized in Table 1. These reactions are listed sequentially to emphasize the multiple steps involved in blood coagulation. Considering these reactions separately is useful for defining the level at which a pathologic defect exists in hemostasis, especially in discussions of clinical disorders (Table 2).

Hemostasis is initiated by tissue injury, which causes endothelial cell disruption and exposure of subendothelial tissues (Table 1). Vasoconstriction is the initial response to injury and occurs through the contraction of smooth muscle cells within the vessel wall. Vasoconstriction functions to reduce blood flow through the damaged vessel. Locally injured neurons and adherent platelets provide the stimulus for vasoconstriction.[18]

Platelets bind to the subendothelium through collagen and other adhesive molecules in the subendothelium. Adherent platelets release both thromboxane A_2 and sero-tonin, which further stimulate vasoconstriction. When platelets release substances from their dense granules and *alpha granules*, additional platelet-platelet interactions oc-cur in a process called *platelet aggregation*. Platelet aggre-

gation is also enhanced by thromboxane A_2, which is synthesized by platelets, and thrombin, which is formed at the platelet surface.[10]

Platelet aggregates form the initial hemostatic plug. In addition, platelets function biochemically to enhance thrombin formation.[17] Thrombin, the enzyme responsible for transforming blood into a fibrin gel, is formed through the plasma proteins in the coagulation system.[14]

Coagulation proteins circulate as inactive molecules until they are activated by a sequence of proteolytic reactions that terminate with the production of thrombin. Thrombin converts soluble fibrinogen into an insoluble fibrin gel that surrounds and strengthens the initial platelet aggregate.[12]

The platelet-fibrin plug is then stabilized to resist the clot-disrupting forces. Blood coagulation factor XIII is converted by thrombin to factor XIIIa, the fibrin-stabilizing enzyme. Factor XIIIa functions to strengthen the fibrin clot and to make it resistant to plasmin, the fibrin-degrading enzyme. This concludes the formation and stabilization of the hemostatic plug.[16]

Blood coagulation reactions are regulated to prevent unwanted and potentially life-threatening thrombosis in uninjured vessels.[22] In a large vessel that supplies blood to many tissues, clotting must be restricted to the surface of the vessel. Otherwise, blood flow to vital tissues supplied by the blood vessel would be impaired. The hemostatic system utilizes several regulatory proteins to localize throm-bin formation and digest fibrin.[22]

After coagulation has been initiated, the fibrinolytic system is activated to dissolve fibrin and preserve vessel patency. The fibrinolytic system utilizes plasmin to degrade fibrin enzymatically. Plasmin is formed from plasminogen by the action of plasminogen activators. The plasminogen activators are released from the vessel wall at the sites of blood clotting.[3]

Once the blood clot has formed and bleeding has stopped, the vascular tissue must be repaired. Platelets release growth factors that aid the repair of injured tissue by stimulating the proliferation of vascular cells and fibro-blasts.[8]

TABLE 1. *Anatomic and Biochemical Events in Hemostasis*

Injury and Vasoconstriction
   Vascular injury disrupts endothelial cells, exposes subendothelial connective tissue, and causes vasoconstriction
Platelet Adhesion
   Platelets adhere to the subendothelium through binding to collagen and factor VIII:vWF
Platelet Release Reaction
   Adherent platelets release ADP, serotonin, and thromboxane A_2
Platelet Aggregation
   ADP and thromboxane A_2 cause platelets to expose membrane receptors for fibrinogen; fibrinogen bound to stimulated platelets induces platelet aggregation
Thrombin Generation
   Tissue injury initiates the blood coagulation system and leads to thrombin formation; thrombin formation is accelerated by the platelets
Fibrin Formation
   Thrombin converts soluble fibrinogen into a network of fibrin strands that reinforces the platelet aggregate
Clot Stabilization
   The platelet and fibrin mass are made resistant to clot-degrading forces through factor XIIIa-catalyzed cross-linking reactions
Fibrin Digestion
   Plasmin, the major clot-dissolving enzyme, proteolytically degrades fibrin; plasmin is formed from plasminogen by plasminogen activators released by vascular tissues
Regulation of Thrombin Formation
   Plasma proteins regulate the formation and function of thrombin in the circulation
Repair of the Injured Blood Vessel
   Platelets release growth factors that facilitate the proliferation of vascular endothelial and smooth muscle cells, which restore the structure of the injured blood vessel

Abbreviations: vWF = von Willebrand's factor; ADP = adenosine diphosphate.

Serious bleeding and thrombotic complications may develop whenever defects exist in the hemostatic system. Clinical disorders of hemostasis are listed in Table 2 and will be described later in the chapter.

ANATOMIC BASIS OF HEMOSTASIS

The Vascular Wall and Endothelial Cells

Endothelial cells line the surface of all blood vessels and are in direct contact with the blood. Under the light

TABLE 2. *Clinical Disorders of Hemostasis and Their Effect on Blood Coagulation Reactions*

Coagulation Reaction	Clinical Disorders
Platelet adhesion	von Willebrand's syndrome
	Bernard-Soulier disease
Platelet release reaction	Storage pool disease
Platelet aggregation	Aspirin ingestion
	Glanzmann's thrombasthenia
Thrombin generation	Hemophilia A and B
	Liver disease
	Vitamin K deficiency
Fibrin formation	DIC syndrome
Clot stabilization	Factor XIII deficiency
Fibrin digestion	α_2-Plasmin inhibitor deficiency
Regulation of thrombin formation	Antithrombin III deficiency
	Protein C deficiency

Abbreviation: DIC = Disseminated intravascular coagulation.

microscope, they appear as a "cobblestone" array of cells lining the vessel wall. Endothelial cells have unique structural features that vary, depending upon the location and size of the blood vessel. Capillaries are the smallest vessel of the microcirculation and are composed solely of endothelial cells and basement membrane.[18]

Capillaries in the brain are composed of endothelial cells with tight continuous, intercellular connections, whereas those in the liver have openings that allow the passage of macromolecules. Plasma components are exchanged by endothelium through vesicles, intracellular channels, or intercellular openings.

The larger blood vessels in the circulation have subendothelium that contains collagen, adhesive glycoproteins, and glycosaminoglycans forming the intima. Beneath the intima, there is a collection of smooth muscle cells, fibroblasts, and collagen called the *media.* The outermost layer is known as the *adventitia* and consists of fibroblasts and collagen.

Endothelial cells are metabolically active and function at several steps in blood coagulation. Endothelial cells synthesize and release the prostaglandin, PGI_2, also called *prostacyclin,* a potent vasodilator and inhibitor of platelet adhesion and platelet aggregation.[20]

Prostacyclin inhibits platelet aggregation by triggering adenylate cyclase in the platelet membrane to produce cyclic adenosine monophosphate (cAMP).[20] The increase in platelet cAMP levels inhibits the expression of the fibrinogen and factor VIII:vWF (von Willebrand factor) receptors on the platelet membrane. The fibrinogen receptor mediates platelet aggregation, whereas the factor VIII:vWF receptor regulates platelet adhesion.[10] Prostacyclin also opposes the vasoconstriction caused by thromboxane A_2 and makes vasoconstriction a transient event.

The synthesis and release of prostacyclin from endothelial cells prevent unwanted accumulation of platelets. Endothelial cells release prostacyclin and increase prostacyclin synthesis when stimulated by thrombin and other substances produced at sites of tissue injury.

In the first step of prostacyclin synthesis, the membrane enzyme phospholipase A releases arachidonic acid from membrane phospholipids[2] (Fig. 1). In the next step, the cyclooxygenase converts arachidonic acid into labile intermediates that are converted by prostacyclin synthetase within endothelial cells to PGI_2.[18]

Platelets can also synthesize arachidonic acid, but they fail to make prostacyclin because they do not contain the prostacyclin synthetase. However, platelets convert arachidonic acid into thromboxane A_2, a potent vasoconstrictor and platelet-aggregating agent (Fig. 1).

Intact endothelium is responsible for maintaining blood in a fluid state. This is illustrated by the failure of blood to clot when a segment of a blood vessel is occluded. If the endothelial cells in the occluded segment are injured, clotting occurs in the injured vessel. The nonthrombogenic property of the endothelium enables surgeons to apply tourniquets to extremities for prolonged periods during orthopedic and vascular procedures.

Blood coagulation is prevented by the endothelium because blood does not contact *tissue factor.* Also known as tissue *thromboplastin,* tissue factor is an important protein for the initiation of blood clotting. Tissue factor can be found intracellularly and is associated with the surface of many cells in the body.[14]

Tissue factor initiates clotting by binding blood coagulation factor VII and converting it to factor VIIa. Factor VIIa leads to thrombin formation through the cascade of reactions in the coagulation pathway. Endothelial cells

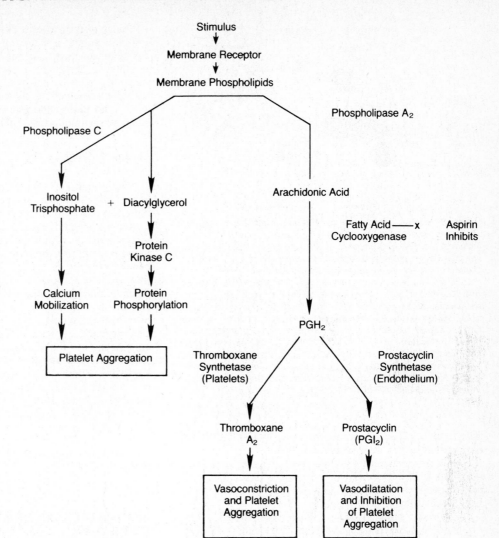

Figure 1. Metabolism of membrane phospholipids in platelets and endothelial cells—role in regulation of platelet and endothelial function.

synthesize tissue factor, but do not express it on their cell surface. This helps to ensure that the endothelium does not initiate blood coagulation. However, once the endothelium has been injured, tissue factor is released or exposed and coagulation reactions are initiated.

The endothelium functions to limit coagulation reactions once they have been initiated by two mechanisms. Endothelial cells have surface receptors for converting the anticoagulant protein, called *protein C*, to its active form. Protein C is a vitamin K–dependent plasma protein that is converted to protein C_a, an anticoagulant, by the combined actions of thrombin and an endothelial surface protein called *thrombomodulin*.[9] Once activated, protein C_a degrades blood coagulation factors Va and VIIIa, important cofactors involved in regulating the rate of thrombin formation. With these cofactors proteolytically degraded, thrombin formation is inhibited. Intact endothelial cells adjacent to sites of tissue injury will therefore limit coagulation reactions. Tissues with endothelial cell injury will not have this protective mechanism, and protein C_a will not be formed.

Heparin-like anticoagulant molecules are also present on endothelial cells. These molecules act as cofactors for converting antithrombin III to a potent inhibitor of the enzymes in the blood coagulation pathways, including factors XIIa, XIa, IXa, Xa, and thrombin.[22]

The endothelium also functions to enhance the degradation of blood clots by activating the fibrinolytic pathway. Endothelial cells synthesize and release proteins known as *plasminogen activators* that activate the fibrinolytic system.[3] The plasminogen activators bind to the fibrin clot and convert plasminogen to plasmin, the major clot-lysing enzyme. Drugs that stimulate the release of endothelial cell plasminogen activators are being developed and tested to reduce the incidence of postoperative thrombosis.[3] Tissue plasminogen activator has been synthesized by modern molecular biology techniques and will soon be available to attempt the selective lysis of pathologic clots within coronary arteries and other vessels.

Platelet Anatomy and Formation of the Hemostatic Plug

Normal hemostasis requires that platelets function properly and circulate in sufficient numbers to form a primary hemostatic plug and arrest bleeding. Platelets are disc-shaped fragments, 2 to 3 microns, that are released from megakaryocytes in the bone marrow. Resting platelets retain their discoid shape by a circumferential band of cytoskeletal microtubules and microfilaments (Fig. 2).

The platelet surface has multiple invaginations that connect with internal membranes, giving them a sponge-like ultrastructure (Fig. 2). Membrane channels inside platelets not connected to the cell surface bind calcium in a manner similar to that in the endoplasmic reticulum of

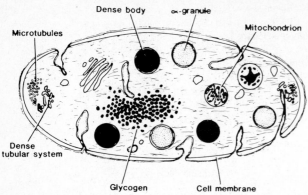

Figure 2. Platelet structure. This diagram summarizes platelet structures seen by electron microscopy. The most external portion includes the cell membrane and submembrane area, including specialized filaments. This forms the wall of the platelet and line channels of the surface-connected canalicular system. The platelet cytoplasm contains microfilaments and a circumferential band of microtubles and glycogen. Embedded in the cytoplasm are mitochondria, alpha granules, and dense bodies. The platelet membrane system includes the surface-connected canalicular system and the dense tubular system, which serve as the platelet sarcoplasmic reticulum and regulator of cellular calcium content. (Modified from White, J. G., and Gerrard, J. M.: Anatomy and structural organization of the platelet. In Colman, R. W., Hirsh, J., Marder, V. J., and Salzman, E. W. (Eds.): Hemostasis and Thrombosis: Basic Principles and Clinical Practice. Philadelphia, J. B. Lippincott Company, 1982.)

muscle cells. The membrane channels allow platelets to have extensive contact with plasma proteins.

Platelets remain in the circulation for an average of 8 days unless they encounter injured tissue and participate in coagulation reactions, bind to the clot, or are removed from circulation by the spleen.

Normally, platelets do not adhere to endothelial cells or to other platelets. However, once the endothelium is injured, platelets will attach, lose their discoid shape, and spread upon subendothelial connective tissues. Adherent platelets release serotonin, adenosine diphosphate (ADP), and adenosine triphosphate (ATP) from dense granules and synthesize and release thromboxane A_2 molecules that further enhance platelet-platelet interaction, increasing the size of the hemostatic plug.[10]

Platelets also contain alpha granules, which contain several coagulation proteins, including factor V; fibrinogen; factor VIII: vWf and fibronectin; and alpha granule–specific proteins, including platelet factor IV, β-thromboglobulin, and platelet-derived growth factor.[10]

The platelet cytoplasm has substantial amounts of contractile proteins, including actin, actin-binding protein, and myosin, which initiate contractile reactions. The glycogen stores and mitochondria in the platelet cytoplasm provide the energy for anaerobic and aerobic metabolism, respectively (Fig. 2).

The contents of the alpha granules, dense granules, and lysosomal granules are released into the surface-connected canalicular system in association with contraction of the actomyosin microfilaments.[10] The intracellular membranes not connected to the cell surface form a dense tubular membrane system (DTS) that has the capacity to bind and release calcium ions. Many of the intracellular responses of platelets to membrane signals are mediated by the increase in cytoplasmic calcium concentration.

Platelet aggregation results in the local accumulation of closely adhering platelets that reduce blood loss through openings in the vessel wall. Platelet aggregates also accelerate thrombin formation by providing specific binding sites for blood coagulation factor Xa and factor V. These binding sites make the platelet surface an efficient site for the assembly of the enzyme system, known as the *prothrombinase complex*, that converts prothrombin to thrombin.[18] The final hemostatic plug is composed of platelets that are surrounded by a network of fibrin strands.

Venous and Arterial Thrombi

Anatomically, venous thrombosis starts in the area immediately behind a venous valve. This is an area in which there is turbulent blood flow. At these sites, platelets adhere to damaged endothelium and fibrin accumulates. Venous thrombi are usually directly attached to the vessel wall and propagate in the direction of blood flow. Erythrocytes become trapped in the mass of platelet and fibrin strands that forms the characteristic red thrombus seen in venous thrombosis. When the vessel lumen is totally occluded, the clot will extend in both directions until it reaches another branch of the blood vessel. Propagating thrombi are especially prone to breaking off from the vessel wall and embolizing into the pulmonary circulation.[13]

Arterial thrombi also tend to occur in areas of turbulent blood flow within the high-pressure, rapidly moving arterial circulation. However, the rapid flow rate in the arterial circulation forces arterial thrombi to remain localized and erythrocytes do not become trapped. The arterial thrombi appear white rather than red because they contain only platelets and fibrin. If arterial thrombi are dislodged, they embolize into the circulation and cause organ injury by blocking the arterial blood supply to the organ(s).[13]

BIOCHEMISTRY AND PHYSIOLOGY OF HEMOSTASIS

Platelet Adhesion

The process by which platelets adhere is an essential event for normal hemostasis. The factor VIII:vWF molecule plays a major physiologic role in regulating platelet adhesion. The smallest subunit of the factor VIII:vWF is synthesized by endothelial cells as a 230,000-dalton polypeptide that circulates as a disulfide bonded aggregate with molecular weights greater than one million daltons.[10] Subendothelial tissues contain factor VIII:vWF, which either has been released from endothelial cells or has been bound from the plasma.

Platelets adhere to the subendothelium by attaching to collagen, factor VIII:vWF, or fibronectin molecules. Adherent platelets change from their usual disc shape to thin, flat, elongated forms that spread over the entire segment of the damaged vessel. Specific binding sites exist on platelets for collagen, factor VIII:vWF, and fibronectin.[10]

Platelets do not adhere readily to damaged vessels if VIII:vWF is absent from plasma or if it is qualitatively abnormal. The clinical disorder resulting from quantitative or qualitative abnormalities in the factor VIII:vWF molecule is known as *von Willebrand's disease*. In recent years, several specific defects have been defined in patients with von Willebrand's disease.[10] These specific types of von Willebrand's disease are described in other texts and are beyond the scope of this chapter.[10]

Platelets bind factor VIII:vWF by a specific glycoprotein receptor on their plasma membrane, known as glycoprotein Ib. In Bernard-Soulier disease, the platelet membrane is missing glycoprotein I and the deficient platelets are unable to adhere to the subendothelial connective tissue.[10] Surgical procedures performed on individuals with von Willebrand's disease or Bernard-Soulier disease result in serious bleeding unless the factor VIII:vWF defect and platelet defect are corrected by the transfusion of either cryoprecipitate or platelets, respectively.[10]

Platelet Aggregation

After platelets adhere to injured vessels, stable platelet-platelet interactions form in the platelet aggregation process. In the absence of platelet aggregation, formation of the primary hemostatic plug fails. Platelet aggregation is a complex reaction involving the platelet release reaction, phospholipases A_2 and C cleavage of membrane phospholipids, alterations in intracellular cAMP levels, mobilization of intracellular calcium, and expression of fibrinogen receptors on the cell surface.

The platelet release reaction is a process analogous to the secretory processes of other cells. During the release reaction, granules fuse with the cell membrane and release their stored contents. Thrombin, subendothelial collagen fibers, epinephrine, and ADP are physiologic stimulators of the release reaction. Alpha granules are stimulated to release before the dense granules. Specific membrane receptors for ADP, epinephrine, collagen, and thrombin have been characterized.[10]

Intracellular cAMP levels have been shown to play a role in regulating platelet aggregation. Substances that increase cAMP levels inhibit platelet aggregation (prostacyclin, dipyridamole) whereas those that stimulate platelet aggregation lower cAMP levels (ADP, epinephrine).[20] Platelet membrane receptors are coupled to membrane adenylate cyclase, the enzyme that synthesizes cAMP. In recent years, second messengers other than cAMP have been discovered which link membrane receptors to secretory processes. A similar system may exist within the platelet. Several platelet agonists stimulate the membrane phospholipase A_2, which releases arachidonate from the membrane phospholipid and a precursor for prostaglandin synthesis. The product of prostaglandin synthesis, thromboxane A_2, enhances the release reaction and platelet aggregation.[20]

More recently, the cleavage of inositol-containing phospholipids by phospholipase C has been shown to serve as a second messenger for platelet agonists.[15] Thrombin-mediated platelet release reaction and aggregation have been associated with phospholipase C cleavage of inositol lipids to produce diacylglycerol and inositol trisphosphate.[1] Diacylglycerol functions within the cell membrane to activate protein kinase C.[1] Protein kinase C phosphosylates molecules necessary for platelet secretion.[15] Inositol trisphosphate acts as a second messenger to mobilize intracellular calcium. Mobilized calcium appears to be essential for platelet secretion and aggregation (see Fig. 1).

The final common pathway for platelet aggregation involves fibrinogen binding to the platelet membrane to enhance platelet-platelet interactions. Platelets do not aggregate when fibrinogen or the fibrinogen receptor is absent.[10]

The fibrinogen binding site on platelets is composed of platelet membrane glycoproteins IIb and III. In a disorder called *Glanzmann's thrombasthenia*, the platelet membrane is deficient in glycoproteins IIb and III; these platelets do not aggregate, although they adhere normally.[10] [People] with Glanzmann's thrombasthenia have a serious [bleeding] bleeding disorder. This further demonstrates that platelet aggregation is required for normal hemostasis.

Blood Coagulation Factors, the Coagulation Cascade, and Thrombin Generation

The coagulation factors that regulate thrombin formation are protein molecules synthesized by the liver. Hepatocytes synthesize most coagulation proteins, including fibrinogen, prothrombin, factors V, VII, VIII:C, IX, X, XI, XII, and XIII, and the coagulation protein inhibitors, antithrombin III, α_2-plasmin inhibitor, and protein C. The major exception to the hepatocyte synthesis of coagulation proteins is the endothelial cell synthesis of factor VIII:vWF. Although factor VIII:C and factor VIII:vWF proteins are synthesized at different sites, they circulate in plasma as a complex.[14] In addition to the synthetic function of hepatocytes, Kupffer cells in the liver function catabolically to remove activated coagulation proteins.

Normal coagulation processes are dependent upon vitamin K. The vitamin K–dependent coagulation factors are protein C and factors II (prothrombin), VII, IX, and X. All of these proteins contain carboxylated glutamic acid residues. The carboxylation reaction is catalyzed by a vitamin K–dependent enzyme system within hepatocytes. The carboxylated forms bind to platelet phospholipids in the presence of calcium and dramatically accelerate coagulation reactions that lead to thrombin formation.[24]

In the absence of vitamin K, coagulation factors are synthesized, secreted, and circulate in a form that fails to accelerate thrombin formation. Warfarin, an oral anticoagulant, inhibits vitamin K–dependent carboxyiation reactions, and the vitamin K–dependent proteins are secreted as nonfunctional forms. This explains the anticoagulant properties of the vitamin K antagonists. Vitamin K deficiency also causes the production of nonfunctional coagulation proteins that may inadvertently result in an anticoagulate state and increase the risk of bleeding.[24]

The initial mass of platelets that covers an injured vessel does not provide an adequate hemostatic barrier unless it has been reinforced by fibrin. The phospholipids on the platelet surface enhance thrombin formation. Thrombin initiates fibrin formation and fibrin stabilization, which strengthens the initial platelet aggregate. Through the combined action of the plasma coagulation proteins and the platelet surface, thrombin is formed. Thrombin leaves the platelet surface, enters the plasma, and converts soluble fibrinogen into insoluble fibrin strands. Disorders in thrombin formation secondary to deficiencies in functional plasma coagulation proteins produce serious bleeding problems. Hemophilia A and B disorders in factor VIII:C and factor IX, respectively, produce serious lifelong bleeding problems. The clinical and laboratory manifestation of hemophilia A and B and other rare coagulation protein deficiencies are beyond the scope of this discussion (see the References listed at the end of the chapter).

The plasma proteins responsible for generating thrombin have been assigned Roman numerals based on the order of their discovery and an internationally accepted nomenclature (Table 3). When the proteins are converted to serine proteases, their active form, they are designated by an "a" after the Roman numeral. The activated serine protease functions in a cascade of reactions that leads to thrombin formation. Factors V and VIII function as cofactors in the *coagulation cascade* and do not directly convert

TABLE 3. Coagulation Proteins

Protein	Plasma Level (mg./100 ml.)	Effective* Hemostatic Level	Replacement Product	Half-Life (Days or Hours)	Function
Fibrinogen	180–360	100 mg./100 ml.	Cryoprecipitate	4 days	Forms the fibrin clot
Prothrombin (Factor II)	10.0	20–40%	Plasma	2–3 days	Produces thrombin and activates fibrinogen; factors V, VIII, and XIII; platelets; and protein C
Factor V	2.0	25%	Plasma	1 day	Cofactor for factor Xa activation of prothrombin
Factor VII	0.1	10–20%	Plasma	6 hours	Activates factors IX and X
Factor VIII:C (Antihemophilic factor)	0.1	25%	Purified factor VIII or cryoprecipitate	8–12 hours	Cofactor for factor IXa activation of factor X
Factor VIII:vWF (von Willebrand's factor)	2.0	25%	Cryoprecipitate	1 day	Mediates platelet adhesion
Factor IX	1.0	20%	Plasma Purified factor IX	1 day	Activates factor X
Factor X	1.0	25%	Plasma	1–2 days	Activates prothrombin
Factor XI	0.5	15–25%	Plasma	2–3 days	Activates factor IX
Factor XII	2.0	< 10%	Not necessary	—	Activates factor XII and prekallikrein
Factor XIII (Fibrin-stabilizing factor)	1.0	5%	Cryoprecipitate	4 days	Covalently cross-links fibrin monomers to each other and α_2-plasmin inhibitor to fibrin

*Values expressed as percent of the normal coagulant activity.

an inactive coagulation protein into a serine protease (Fig. 3).

Two different pathways (*intrinsic* and *extrinsic*) exist for initiating thrombin formation. The proteins in these pathways (known as the coagulation cascade) are responsible for initiating and amplifying thrombin formation (Fig. 3). A small stimulus at the first step of the cascade is catalytically amplified at each step in such a way that large amounts of thrombin are rapidly formed.[14]

The intrinsic system is initiated by contact of plasma proteins (factor XII, prekallikrein, and high-molecular-weight kininogen) with a negatively charged surface, such as glass. The extrinsic pathway initiates thrombin formation through the interaction of factor VII with a substance derived from tissues, tissue factor. Tissue factor is a phospholipoprotein present in most tissues. The division of coagulation reactions into two different pathways is very useful for interpreting laboratory tests of coagulation. However, the sharp distinction between the two pathways fails to explain many aspects of clinical hemostasis. In recent years, there has been evidence that the two pathways function together in forming thrombin.[19]

The physiologic importance of the intrinsic pathway for initiating clotting appears limited, since persons with congenital factor XII, high-molecular-weight kininogen, and prekallikrein deficiency do not bleed either spontaneously or if surgery is performed. In contrast to these individuals, those born with factor XI, factor VIII, and factor IX deficiencies may bleed spontaneously or may have serious bleeding complications following surgery. This suggests that the intrinsic pathway is important for amplifying thrombin formation, although it may not initiate thrombin formation.

Recently, investigators have shown that there are important interconnections between both pathways. After factor VII is activated by tissue factor to form factor VIIa, factor VIIa converts factor IX to factor IXa in the intrinsic

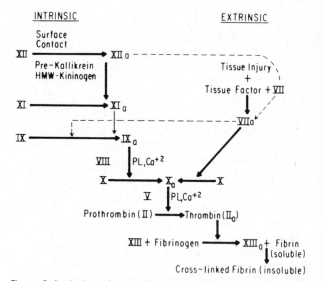

Figure 3. Intrinsic and extrinsic systems of blood coagulation and their interactions. The extrinsic pathway initiates thrombin formation through tissue injury and the exposure of tissue factor. Factor XI binds tissue factor and directly activates factor X to factor Xa. Factors V, factor Xa, the phospholipid surface of platelets (PL), and calcium (Ca⁺²) function as the prothrombinase complex to form thrombin (factor IIa). The intrinsic pathway initiates thrombin formation through surface contact. Factor XIa then activates factor IX to form factor IXa. Factor IXa converts factor X to factor Xa by the combined action of factor VIII:C (factor VIII:C; anti-hemophilia factor), the phospholipid surface and calcium. Factor Xa converts prothrombin to thrombin as described above. Soluble fibrin is formed by thrombin and stabilized by factor XIIIa to form insoluble fibrin. The extrinsic and intrinsic pathways interact through factor XIIa, activating factor VII to factor VIIa and factor VIIa activating factor IX. Furthermore, thrombin feeds back to activate factors VII, XII, IX, VIII, V, and X. These reactions further amplify the formation of thrombin.

pathway.[14] In addition, factor XIIa can convert factor VII to factor VIIa. Furthermore, thrombin, the product of both pathways, can feed back and amplify its own formation by activating protein cofactors utilized in both pathways, i.e., factor V and factor VIII[14]. Factor Xa can also feed back and activate factor VII.[14]

A major pathway for initiating thrombin formation is through the release or exposure of tissue factor. Tissue factor initiates thrombin formation by binding to factor VII in the presence of calcium and phospholipid and then converting factor X to factor Xa. Factor Xa binds to the platelet surface and forms the prothrombinase complex that proteolytically converts prothrombin to thrombin (Fig. 3). The prothrombinase complex plays a central role in generating thrombin. The essential elements for assembling the prothrombinase complex on the platelet surface are factor V, calcium, platelet phospholipid, and factor Xa. In the absence of any of these factors, the rate of thrombin formation and clotting is reduced.[17]

Factor VII can also initiate thrombin formation through activation of factor IX in the presence of tissue factor, calcium, and phospholipid. Then factor IXa can lead to Xa formation, assembly of the prothrombinase complex, prothrombin conversion, and fibrin formation through the intrinsic pathway (Fig. 4).[14]

The intrinsic coagulation pathway functions to activate factor X through the contact factors. The contact factors include factor XII, high-molecular-weight kininogen and prekallikrein. When plasma contacts a negatively charged surface, all three contact factors together activate factor XI. Factor XIa then activates factor IX. In the following reaction, which takes place on a phospholipid surface, factor VIII:C accelerates factor IXa activation of factor X. Factor Xa is assembled into the prothrombinase complex, and thrombin is formed (Fig. 4).

Factor IX and factor XI deficiencies may produce serious lifelong bleeding problems, further illustrating the importance of the intrinsic pathway in amplifying thrombin formation. Clinically, the initiation and amplification of thrombin formation may occur through both the intrinsic and extrinsic pathways. The interactions between the two pathways may be more relevant than attempting to separate the pathways.[19]

Kallikrein, a product of the contact pathway of coagulation, causes *bradykinin* to be released from high-molecular-weight kininogen. Bradykinin, a vasodilator, can cause hypotension. The contact pathway of coagulation is thought to be activated during septicemia, allergic reactions, and transfusion reactions. This may account for the development of hypotension associated with these clinical situations. These findings demonstrate that under certain clinical conditions the intrinsic pathway is activated and has an important role to play in the host response to immunologic stimuli.[5]

Factors Regulating Thrombin Formation

Thrombin formation must be regulated, otherwise fibrin would be formed at sites remote from tissue injury and produce widespread organ injury. Clinically, the continuous and unregulated formation of thrombin in the circulation is known as the *disseminated intravascular coagulation (DIC) syndrome*. Activated antithrombin III is the major physiologic inhibitor of thrombin. Antithrombin III is activated by heparin or heparin-like molecules on endothelial surfaces.[22] Heparin binds to antithrombin III and forms a heparin–antithrombin III complex. The heparin–antithrombin III complex leads to the formation of a covalent complex with one of several serine proteases in the coagulation system, factors Xa, IXa, XIa, or thrombin (Fig. 5).[22] The antithrombin III–protease complex is then cleared by the liver. After formation of the antithrombin III–protease complex, the heparin is released and catalyzes the formation of additional heparin–antithrombin III complexes (Fig. 5).

Thrombin formation is restricted further by thrombin catalyzed activation of protein C at the endothelial cell surface. Activated protein C (protein C_a) degrades factor VIIIa and factor Va and reduces the rate of thrombin formation.[9]

Prostacyclin—as mentioned, a potent vasodilator—is released by endothelium at sites of clotting and facilitates the restoration of blood flow. Restoring blood flow over the site of vascular injury dilutes the concentration of activated coagulation factors, which reduces the rate of thrombin formation. The rate of the enzymatic reactions in the coagulation cascade are dependent upon the local concentration of activated clotting factors.

Fibrin Formation and Stabilization

Converting fibrinogen into a network of stable fibrin strands occurs through the action of thrombin. Thrombin proteolytically releases fibrinopeptides A and B from the fibrinogen molecule-producing fibrin monomer (Fig. 6). The fibrin monomers acquire the ability to associate either with fibrinogen or with other fibrin monomers. When the fibrin monomers associate with each other, they assemble in a staggered overlapping configuration called a *protofibril*. The protofibrils grow in size by forming long rows of molecules that produce fibrin strands. The strands then associate with each other and form a branching network of fibers, producing a gel (Fig. 6).[12]

Blood coagulation factor XIII binds to fibrin and is converted by thrombin to factor XIIIa. Factor XIIIa covalently cross-links adjacent fibrin monomers to each other. Factor XIIIa also cross-links α_2-plasmin inhibitor, the major

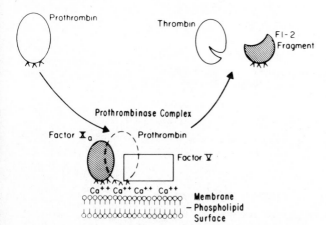

Figure 4. Formation of thrombin by the prothrombinase complex. The phospholipid surface of platelets contains the prothrombinase complex containing factor Xa, calcium, and the cofactor factor V. Soluble prothrombin is cleaved by the prothrombinase complex to form thrombin. The phospholipid binding sites on prothrombin contain the γ-carboxyglutamic acid residues, which are released after thrombin is formed and called the F1-2 fragment. (From Mosher, D. F.: In MacKinney, A. A. (Ed.): Pathophysiology of Blood. New York, John Wiley & Sons, 1984.)

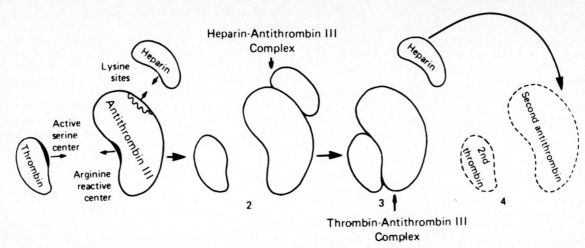

Figure 5. The mechanism of action of heparin and antithrombin III. Heparin binds to antithrombin III through a lysine residue on antithrombin III, forming the heparin–antithrombin III complex (Panel 2). This exposes an arginine group on antithrombin III that covalently binds thrombin and other serine proteases in the coagulation cascade (factors XI, IXa, and Xa) (Panel 3). The antithrombin III–thrombin complex forms, and the heparin is released. The heparin can then catalyze a similar reaction between another antithrombin III molecule and thrombin (Panel 4). The heparin–antithrombin III complex can inhibit most of the serine proteases (factors XIIa, IXa, Xa, and thrombin) in the coagulation system, thereby inhibiting both thrombin formation and thrombin. (Modified with permission from Rosenberg, R. D.: Heparin-antithrombin system. In Colman, R. W., Hirsh, J., Marder, V. J., and Salzman, E. W. (Eds.): Hemostasis and Thrombosis: Basic Principles and Clinical Practice. Philadelphia, J. B. Lippincott Company, 1982.)

inhibitor of plasmin, to the clot. Factor XIIIa cross-linked fibrin is mechanically stronger and resistant to lysis by plasmin.[16] Factor XIII may also facilitate wound healing, since some factor XIII–deficient patients suffer from wound dehiscence and abnormal scar formation.[16]

Digestion of Fibrin by the Fibrinolytic System

When the hemostatic process begins, fibrinolysis is initiated. This close regulation of thrombosis and fibrinolysis serves as an effective mechanism for dissolving fibrin.

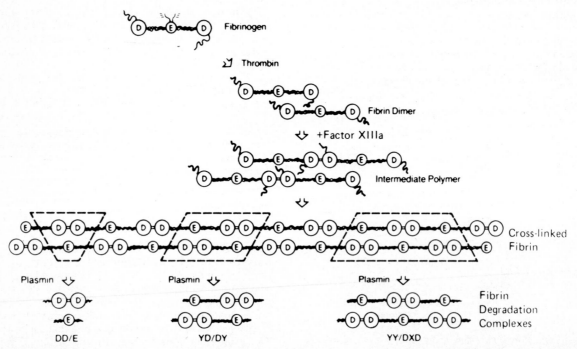

Figure 6. Fibrin formation and plasmin-catalyzed fibrin—degradation of factor XIIIa cross-linked fibrin. Fibrinogen is cleaved by thrombin to produce fibrin monomers that associate and form fibrin dimers. Additional fibrin monomers are then added, and Factor XIIIa catalyzes covalent cross-linking between the D domains in adjacent fibrin monomers. The intermediate fibrin polymer grows to form a two-stranded protofibril. Plasmin degrades cross-linked fibrin fibers by proteolytically cleaving between the D and E domains. The soluble degradation products that are released are high-molecular-weight complexes of cross-linked fibrin non-covalently associated (these are shown in the enclosed boxes). (Modified with permission from Marder, V. J., Francis, C. W., and Doolittle, R. F.: Fibrinogen structure and physiology. In Colman, R. W., Hirsh, J., Marder, V. J., and Salzman, E. W. (Eds.): Hemostasis and Thrombosis: Basic Principles and Clinical Practice. Philadelphia, J. B. Lippincott Company, 1982.)

During fibrin formation, plasminogen binds to fibrin and is therefore situated in the ideal location to initiate clot lysis. Plasminogen remains inactive until a protease known as *tissue plasminogen activator* binds to fibrin and converts plasminogen to plasmin. Tissue plasminogen activator is released from the vessel wall at sites of thrombin formation. Tissue plasminogen activator fails to convert plasminogen to plasmin in the circulation because it must bind to the fibrin surface to function efficiently. When tissue plasminogen activator binds to fibrin, it enhances the proteolytic cleavage of plasminogen to plasmin.[3]

The other important physiologic plasminogen activator, urokinase, is produced in the kidney and is secreted into the urine. Urokinase, unlike the tissue plasminogen activator molecule, can directly convert plasminogen to plasmin in the absence of fibrin.[3]

Streptokinase, a bacterial protein, is used clinically as a plasminogen activator to treat deep venous thrombosis, pulmonary emboli, and myocardial infarction. Streptokinase binds to plasminogen and forms a plasminogen-streptokinase complex that converts plasminogen to plasmin. Both streptokinase and urokinase are capable of converting plasminogen to plasmin within the circulation. The formation of plasmin in plasma causes the degradation of fibrinogen as well as fibrin.[3]

Plasmin functions only briefly in plasma because of a fast-acting plasmin inhibitor (α_2-*plasmin inhibitor*), which rapidly forms a covalent bond with plasmin that inactivates the enzyme. Within the fibrin clot, plasmin functions longer because the concentration of α_2-plasmin inhibitor is lower. Plasmin is eventually inactivated within the clot by α_2-plasmin inhibitor bound to fibrin. Plasma also contains another slower-acting system to inhibit plasmin. Plasma α_2-macroglobulin slowly inhibits plasmin by binding plasmin and prevents it from degrading fibrinogen or fibrin.[3]

Plasmin degrades fibrinogen, which has a trinodular structure by a sequence of proteolytic reactions to form fragments X, Y, D, and E. These reactions are diagrammed in Figure 7. Plasmin digests fibrin strands in a sequence of reactions similar to those diagrammed in Figure 6. Fibrin, which has been stabilized by factor XIIIa, has covalent bonds formed between adjacent D domains on separate fibrin monomer molecules. Soluble fibrin degradation products are released by plasmin cleaving at sites between the D and E domains. Fibrin degradation products are high-molecular-weight complexes of cross-linked fibrin associated noncovalently. The final product of plasmin degradation of cross-linked fibrin is a molecule called D-D dimer and fragment E. D-D dimer is the terminal plasmin digestion product from fibrin that contains the D domains from two adjacent fibrin monomers that have been cross-linked by factor XIIIa. Plasmin-digested fibrinogen degradation products are cleared from the circulation by the liver.

Laboratory Evaluation of the Surgical Patient with a Hemostasis Problem

The physician caring for a patient with a problem in hemostasis must integrate clinical and laboratory information for effective management. This requires correct interpretation of coagulation tests and an appreciation of their limitations. Clinical data obtained from examining the patient and reviewing the history are very important in establishing the correct diagnosis. The clinician must recognize that coagulation tests do not measure the platelet and endothelial cell surface reactions that play a major role during coagulation *in vivo*. This remains a major limitation of coagulation laboratory tests. Most coagulation laboratory

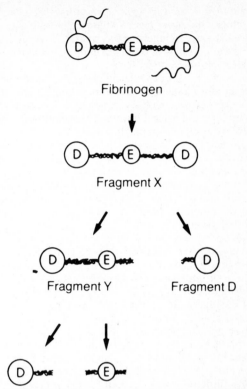

Figure 7. Fibrinogen degradation by plasmin and the fibrinogen degradation products. Fibrinogen is composed of three separate polypeptide chains designated as α, β, and γ chains. The chains have many inter- and intrachain disulfide bonds and are arranged three dimensionally as three nodules. Two identical D nodules are located on either side of the central fragment E. Fragment E contains the region in which fibrinopeptides A and B are cleaved from the α and β chains, respectively. The trinodular structure of fibrinogen is shown at the top of the diagram. The two D domains have extensions that represent portions of the chains. Plasmin degrades the fibrinogen by first releasing these α-chain appendages from the D domains, forming fragment X. Fragment X is then degraded by a specific cleavage between the D and E domains, producing fragments Y and D. Fragment Y is further degraded by another cleavage between the fragment D and E domains to produce fragments D and E. (Reproduced with permission from Marder, V. J., Francis, C. W., and Doolittle, R. F.: Fibrinogen structure and physiology. In Colman, R. W., Hirsh, J., Marder, V. J., and Salzman, E. W. (Eds.): Hemostasis and Thrombosis: Basic Principles and Clinical Practice. Philadelphia, J. B. Lippincott Company, 1982.)

tests are performed with platelet-poor plasma, and artificial phospholipids are substituted for the platelet surface.

Despite these limitations, coagulation laboratory tests do provide accurate information on several specific phases of blood coagulation (Table 4) and on the functional and

TABLE 4. *Common Coagulation Laboratory Tests and Their Relationship to Coagulation Reactions*

Laboratory Test	Coagulation Reaction
Bleeding time	Platelet adhesion and aggregation
Platelet aggregometry	Platelet release and aggregation
Prothrombin time (PT)	Thrombin generation via extrinsic pathway
Activated partial thromboplastin time (aPTT)	Thrombin generation via intrinsic pathway
Thrombin clotting time	Fibrin formation
Reptilase time	Fibrin formation
Fibrin(ogen) split products	Fibrin and fibrinogen degradation

immunologic level of coagulation factors. The coagulation laboratory, therefore, has an important role in the preoperative diagnosis of inherited coagulation disorders, guiding replacement therapy of coagulation protein and monitoring anticoagulation therapy.

The clinical history remains the single most important piece of information available to the clinician. Despite this fact, coagulation laboratory screening tests are used as a substitute for the clinical history. The extent of coagulation laboratory testing required to ensure that the hemostatic system can effectively limit blood loss during minor surgery remains controversial.[21] A complete laboratory evaluation should be obtained prior to major surgery (e.g., thoracic, abdominal, or central nervous system) for any patient who gives a positive response to any of the following questions. Is there a family history of bleeding? Has there been excessive bleeding following either previous surgery or dental work? Have frequent nosebleeds occurred or has nasal packing been required? Has bleeding occurred without trauma into any joint or muscle? Is there bleeding from the gums or skin? Does excessive bleeding or bruising occur following aspirin ingestion?

Coagulation laboratory tests have the capability to measure platelet adhesion and aggregation, the generation of thrombin, and fibrin formation. The bleeding time measures platelet adhesion, release, and aggregation. Platelet aggregometry measures the platelet release reaction and aggregation. The extrinsic and intrinsic pathways for generating thrombin are evaluated by the *prothrombin time* (PT) and *activated partial thromboplastin time* (aPTT), respectively. Fibrin formation is measured by the thrombin time and/or by quantitating the level of clottable fibrinogen (Table 4).

Platelets must be able to adhere and aggregate normally prior to major surgery. The bleeding time measures both platelet adhesion and platelet aggregation. Determination of bleeding time is performed by inflating a blood pressure cuff to 40 mm. Hg and making a standardized 1-mm. cut on the forearm with the aid of a disposable device. After the incision is made, the time required to stop bleeding from the skin incision is recorded. The normal bleeding time is less than 10 minutes. The bleeding time becomes prolonged when the platelet count is below 100,000 per mm.[3] or when there is a defect in either platelet adhesion or aggregation. Aspirin will prolong the bleeding time several minutes over the value obtained before aspirin ingestion. However, any patient with a bleeding time over 12 minutes while receiving aspirin should be evaluated for a platelet adhesion or aggregation abnormality.

Platelet aggregometry has been used to examine platelet aggregation in the laboratory. Platelet-rich plasma is incubated with a platelet agonist (ADP, epinephrine, collagen). The suspension is stirred and changes in light transmission through the platelet suspension are recorded (Fig. 8). Several different responses can be observed, depending upon the type and concentration of the agonist. Low concentrations of ADP may induce only a change in platelet shape, which produces a sudden decrease in light transmission (Fig. 8 [A]). This is followed by the primary wave of aggregation, which is a reversible platelet-platelet interaction (Fig. 8 [B]). The secondary wave of aggregation occurs at higher concentrations of agonist and represents irreversible platelet aggregation (Fig. 8 [C]). The secondary wave of aggregation is mediated by the release reaction and thromboxane A_2 synthesis. In the presence of aspirin, the secondary wave of platelet aggregation is absent (Fig. 8 [C]). A similar defect is found in patients with an inherited

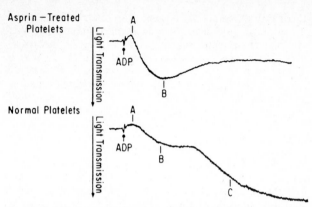

Figure 8. Platelet aggregometry. Platelet aggregation in vitro is assayed by recording the light transmission through stirred, platelet-rich plasma at 37°C. Light transmission increases as platelet aggregates form. The first response is platelet shape change (A); this is followed by a primary wave of aggregation (B), then a secondary wave of aggregation occurs in association with the release reaction. Platelets from a patient who has ingested aspirin are shown. Aspirin-treated platelets display absence of the secondary wave of aggregation, although shape change and primary wave of aggregation have occurred.

storage pool defect, congenital deficiency in thromboxane A_2 synthetases, or cyclooxygenase deficiency.[10]

A recently developed modification of the platelet aggregometer monitors platelet aggregation in whole blood. The instrument has the advantage of measuring platelet aggregation and release in a more physiologic environment containing other blood cells.

Clinically significant bleeding can occur in patients with mild factor deficiencies even though preoperative coagulation tests may be normal. The PT and aPTT will remain normal until the coagulation factor levels are less than 30 per cent. Therefore, patients with mild hemophilia A or B may not be detected unless a careful history suggests a hemorrhagic tendency.[21]

Several inherited disorders of coagulation can produce serious bleeding problems and will not be detected by the PT, aPTT, fibrinogen, or thrombin time. These include von Willebrand's syndrome, factor XIII deficiency, and α_2-plasmin inhibitor deficiency. These disorders can be detected prior to surgery with more specialized and specific laboratory tests.[21]

In the coagulation laboratory, the time required to clot platelet-poor plasma after the addition of tissue factor, calcium, and phospholipid is known as the prothrombin time. Thrombin generation via the intrinsic pathway is measured in the laboratory by the aPTT. The aPTT is performed by incubating platelet-poor plasma with a negatively charged substance (ellagic acid, or celite) in the absence of calcium to form factor XIIa. The time required to form a clot is measured after calcium and phospholipid are added.

A common clinical and coagulation laboratory problem may occur during the preoperative period: the patient with abnormal aPTT who does not report a history of bleeding. The appropriate management of this problem has been detailed. The abnormal test must be confirmed, and a mixing study should be performed. After one part of normal plasma is mixed with one part of the patient's plasma, the 1:1 mixture should produce a normal aPTT. Normal platelet-poor plasma has at least 50 per cent of all the coagulation factors. Even if the patient plasma was totally deficient in an intrinsic pathway coagulation protein, there would be

50 per cent levels in the 1:1 mixture and the aPTT would be normalized. When the 1:1 mixture corrects, one may assume that the patient's plasma is deficient in an intrinsic pathway coagulation factor. When there is no bleeding history, the most common cause for a prolonged aPTT that corrects with a 1:1 mixture is a deficiency in either factor XII, prekallikrein, or high-molecular-weight kininogen. If there is no correction of the aPTT, an inhibitor is present that alters either thrombin or fibrin formation.

The most common inhibitor to be detected with the aPTT is the *lupus* anticoagulant, an immunoglobulin molecule that prolongs the aPTT because it binds the artificial phospholipids used in the aPTT assay. When the lupus anticoagulant binds to phospholipids, it delays clotting *in vitro* because it inhibits the assembly of the prothrombinase complex on phospholipid surfaces used in the assay. Lupus anticoagulants alone do not cause a bleeding problem because the antibody does not inhibit assembly for the prothrombinase complex on the platelet surface *in vivo*.[25] The other causes of an abnormal mixing study are abnormal fibrinogen molecules *(dysfibrinogenemia)* and heparin. They can be identified as a cause for an abnormal mixing study by a prolongation of the thrombin time.

The thrombin time is a sensitive measure of fibrin formation. The test is performed by adding thrombin to platelet-poor plasma and measuring the time required for fibrinogen to be cleaved by thrombin and polymerize, forming a fibrin gel. The normal thrombin clotting time values vary, depending on the thrombin concentration used in the assay. In most laboratories, this is between 10 and 20 seconds. Thrombin clotting times are prolonged when an inhibitor of thrombin cleavage of fibrinogen is present (i.e., heparin, fibrin degradation products, dysfibrinogenemia) or an inhibitor of fibrin monomer polymerization (monocolonal immunoglobulins, fibrin degradation products, or dysfibrinogenemia). The thrombin time is also prolonged when fibrinogen levels are below 80 mg. per 100 ml. or greater than 400 mg. per 100 ml.

Fibrinogen is assayed by a technique similar to the one used for measuring thrombin clotting time, except that more thrombin is added in the assay. At the higher thrombin concentration, the test is made insensitive to therapeutic heparin levels (0.2 to 0.4 units per ml.). Since the assay measures clottable fibrinogen, the nonclottable forms of fibrinogen (called *dysfibrinogens*) will be detected as a reduced level of clottable fibrinogen.

Determination of immunologic fibrinogen levels can enable detection of clottable and nonclottable forms of fibrinogen. Determination of these levels is performed by measuring the size of immunoprecipitate rings that form using agar plates containing anti-fibrinogen antibodies. Normal levels range from between 185 to 360 mg. per 100 ml.

The *reptilase time* is an important test in the evaluation of a patient with an abnormal thrombin clotting time. Although thrombin is inhibited by antithrombin III complexed to heparin, reptilase is not inhibited. Therefore heparin prolongs the thrombin clotting time and has no effect on the reptilase time. Reptilase proteolytically releases fibrinopeptide A and does not release fibrinopeptide B from fibrinogen. The reptilase-derived fibrin monomers polymerize, forming long strands and a fibrin gel. The reptilase time is prolonged as a result of inhibitors of fibrinopeptide A release (dysfibrinogenemia), fibrin degradation products, and inhibitors of fibrin polymerization.

The fibrinolytic system is usually activated whenever thrombin enters the circulation. Laboratory evidence that plasminogen has been converted to plasmin is obtained indirectly through measurements of plasmin-derived fibrin

and fibrinogen degradation products. The fibrin(ogen) degradation products are indirect measures of the presence of plasmin in the circulation. Plasmin formation is physiologically localized to the fibrin clot. However, under pathologic conditions, it may enter the circulation and degrade fibrinogen, factor V, or factor VIII.

Fibrinogen is degraded in a stepwise sequence by plasmin to form fragments X, Y, D, and E (see Fig. 7). These degradation products are indirectly measured by their ability to act as antithrombins and fibrin polymerization inhibitors using the thrombin time. They are also measured directly in serum using a latex agglutination assay. The assay consists of latex particles coated with antibodies to fibrinogen or fragments D and E. If plasma is allowed to clot, there should be less than 10 μg. per ml. of fibrinogen antigen in the serum. If the serum has more than 40 μg. per ml., excessive fibrinolysis is strongly suggested.

Recently, a latex agglutination assay has been developed to quantitate the fibrin-derived D-D dimer produced by plasmin degradation of cross-linked fibrin. This assay has the capability of measuring fibrin-specific degradation products. Currently available fibrin degradation assays do not specifically measure fibrinogen degradation products or detect fibrinogen degradation products.

Management of Hemostatic Disorders in Surgical Patients

Hemostatic disorders in surgical patients can be categorized as a defect in one of the several steps in hemostasis. These will be discussed as (1) disorders of platelets, (2) disorders of thrombin formation, (3) disorders of fibrin formation, (4) disorders of fibrinolysis, and (5) thrombotic disorders.

DISORDERS OF PLATELETS

The most common disorder of platelets in surgical patients is *thrombocytopenia*. Spontaneous bleeding occurs when the concentration of platelets in the circulation is reduced. From clinical experience, spontaneous bleeding occurs when platelet counts are less than 20,000 per mm.[3] The platelet concentration that allows surgery to be safely performed has not been firmly established, although most surgeons and anesthesiologists prefer to have platelet counts higher than 100,000 per mm.[3] The ability of platelets to adhere, aggregate, and limit bleeding declines as the platelet count falls to below 100,000 per mm.[3] However, there are exceptions to this rule. Patients with immune destruction of platelets, called *immune thrombocytopenia purpura* (ITP), may have normal hemostasis when platelet counts are less than 50,000 per mm.[3] because they rapidly produce young hemostatically competent platelets. There are also patients with platelet counts over 100,000 per mm.[3] who bleed because their platelet function is abnormal as a result of drugs, uremia, or an intrinsic platelet disorder, i.e., *storage pool disease*.

The first question that needs to be addressed in evaluating the thrombocytopenic patient is whether the bone marrow is adequately producing platelets. If the platelet count has dropped more than 25 per cent in 24 hours in the absence of blood loss, then platelet destruction, and not decreased marrow production, is the most likely explanation for the thrombocytopenia. The bone marrow aspirate plus biopsy is the most direct method for measuring platelet production. The number of megakaryocytes in the bone marrow is decreased when the marrow has been injured by drugs (e.g., ethanol or cancer chemotherapeutic agents).

Thrombocytopenia in surgical patients is commonly due to enhanced platelet destruction caused by a drug. Surgery alone rarely causes thrombocytopenia, although platelets are utilized at an increased rate to restrict blood loss. During surgery or in the postoperative period, drug-induced thrombocytopenia may result. Heparin and cimetidine are two of the most common agents associated with drug-induced thrombocytopenia. Antibodies directed against the drug or a drug-platelet complex may coat platelets and cause them to be recognized by the reticuloendothelial system and removed from the circulation.

On rare occasions, heparin induces platelets to aggregate in the circulation, producing life-threatening arterial emboli. However, in most situations, heparin-associated thrombocytopenia either reverses spontaneously or soon after the heparin has been discontinued. Surgical patients in whom postoperative septicemia develops frequently become thrombocytopenic. Septicemia causes thrombocytopenia through immunoglobulin binding to platelets, which enhances their clearance from the circulation.

The treatment of thrombocytopenia that is due to increased platelet destruction is dependent upon the etiology. In most cases of drug-induced thrombocytopenia, discontinuing the drug is adequate treatment. When bleeding develops in a thrombocytopenic patient, a platelet transfusion is needed. Platelets are given to patients prophylactically when the platelet count is less than 20,000 per mm.[3] in an effort to prevent spontaneous life-threatening bleeding of the central nervous system. Patients who are receiving heparin and in whom thrombocytopenia develops should be observed carefully for signs of arterial thrombosis. If there has been arterial thrombosis, heparin should be stopped and the anticoagulation should be switched to another form, such as warfarin. When the heparinized patient has mild thrombocytopenia, the clinician has the option of either switching to another type of heparin (i.e., from beef to pork) or of observing the patient closely. If the platelet count drops to less than 50,000 per mm.[3] or if a bleeding problem develops, the heparin should be immediately discontinued.

Abnormal platelet adhesion can occur under any of these circumstances:

1. The platelet membrane receptor for factor VIII:vWF is absent (Bernard-Soulier syndrome).
2. The concentration of factor VIII:vWF is reduced (Type I—von Willebrand's disease).
3. The high-molecular-weight forms of factor VIII:vWF that bind to platelets are reduced (Type II von Willebrand's disease).
4. There is an antibody to the factor VIII:vWF (acquired von Willebrand's disease).[10]

Patients with von Willebrand's disease are at times difficult to diagnose preoperatively unless a careful history has been obtained.

Clinically, these patients may have either a severe or a minor bleeding problem. Laboratory tests to measure factor VIII:vWF are available to define whether patients have (1) a reduced amount of the factor VIII:vWF antigen, (2) factor VIII:vWF antigen that does not facilitate platelet adhesion, or (3) abnormal size of the factor VIII:vWF complex. In patients with a bleeding history and a normal PT and aPTT, these tests should be performed prior to major surgery. The bleeding time is not always abnormal in these patients, although post-aspirin bleeding times are usually prolonged.

Abnormal platelet aggregation occurs in several rare congenital disorders, including (1) storage pool disease (dense granules are deficient in their ADP content); (2) congenital deficiency of cyclooxygenase or thromboxane A_2 synthetase; (3) deficiency in the fibrinogen receptor (Glanzmann's thrombasthenia); (4) deficiency of alpha granules (Gray platelet syndrome); and (5) defective calcium mobilization. Although these are rare clinical disorders, the importance of normal platelet structure-function relationships in hemostasis is evident.[10]

A very common cause of abnormal platelet aggregation is aspirin ingestion. A single dose of aspirin irreversibly inhibits the platelet membrane cyclooxygenase for the entire life span of the platelet. Therefore, platelet aggregation will be abnormal for up to one week after a single dose of aspirin (650 mg.). Aspirin inhibits platelet aggregation, but does not modify platelet adhesion.

Acquired deficiency of the storage pool granules and alpha granules may occur during the DIC syndrome and cardiac bypass surgery.

DISORDERS OF THROMBIN GENERATION

Disorders of thrombin generation are usually diagnosed preoperatively if a careful history has been obtained. On rare occasions, congenital disorders of thrombin formation are diagnosed postoperatively. For example, in a patient with mild factor XI deficiency, bleeding may not occur until after surgery. In contrast, patients with severe hemophilia A (factor VIII deficiency) or hemophilia B (factor IX deficiency) typically have a well-defined history of spontaneous hemorrhage into joints and muscles. With the plasma concentration of the deficient factor increased to an effective hemostatic level (see Table 3), patients with severe hemophilia A or other factor deficiencies may safely undergo surgery.

Vitamin K deficiency frequently develops in surgical patients. Factors II, VII, IX, and X are synthesized without the normal amount of carboxylation of glutamic acid residues in vitamin K deficiency. These molecules fail to generate thrombin normally. Deficiency occurs because of poor dietary intake of foods containing the vitamin, suppression of vitamin K synthesis by antibiotic therapy, malabsorption of fats, or abnormal hepatocyte utilization of vitamin K. In addition, when there is biliary tract obstruction, the vitamin is not absorbed because the bile salts required for normal vitamin K absorption are not entering the gastrointestinal tract.

There are several vitamin K preparations available for treating this deficiency. Surgical patients requiring the parenteral form of vitamin K are advised to receive it subcutaneously to guarantee absorption. If bleeding is occurring, vitamin K and fresh frozen plasma should be given together, since it may take 1 to 2 days for the liver to resynthesize functional vitamin K–dependent factors. Fresh frozen plasma contains sufficient amounts of these factors to aid hemostasis immediately when there is not enough time to wait for the liver to resynthesize the factors.

DISORDERS OF FIBRIN FORMATION

The disseminated intravascular coagulation syndrome presents a serious threat to surgical patients. The pathologic factors that initiate this syndrome in surgical patients are hypotension, septicemia, abscesses, tissue necrosis, and transfusion reactions. Whatever the pathologic event, coagulation reactions are initiated that activate platelets, utilize coagulation factors, deposit fibrin in the microcirculation, and convert plasminogen to plasmin. The laboratory manifestation of this persistent stimulus for coagulation is a combination of abnormal test results, including thrombocytopenia, prolonged PT or aPTT, hypofibrinogenemia, and an elevated level of fibrin(ogen) degradation product. The clinical and laboratory features of this syndrome are a direct result of excessive thrombin and plasmin formation (Fig. 9).[6]

The treatment of the DIC syndrome should be directed at the stimulus that has started the coagulation reactions. This means treating the underlying disease as well as treating the clinical manifestations of bleeding and/or thrombosis. Typically, the stimulus initiating coagulation has been present for several hours by the time the DIC syndrome is clinically recognized.

Once treatment has been directed to the underlying cause, if bleeding continues, replacement therapy for a low platelet count, a low fibrinogen concentration, or a deficiency of coagulation factors should be considered. When arterial or venous thrombosis occurs, heparin therapy is indicated to prevent further embolization and thrombosis. If fibrinolysis is producing serious bleeding, heparin therapy should be started before giving epsilon-aminocaproic acid (Amicar) to inhibit the fibrinolytic system.

In patients with liver disease the level of clottable fibrinogen is frequently reduced (acquired dysfibrinogenemia). The fibrinogen molecule produced by the liver in these patients has an increase in carbohydrate content (sialic acid) which intereferes with fibrin polymer formation. Immunologic levels of fibrinogen are normal in these patients. Clinically, the abnormal fibrinogen molecule produced in liver disease will not cause any bleeding problems when there are no additional coagulation factor deficiencies.

Patients born with abnormal fibrinogen molecules (congenital dysfibrinogenemia) can have either a bleeding or a thrombotic tendency. The dysfibrinogenemic patients with a bleeding tendency may need replacement therapy with cryoprecipitate to correct the defect in fibrin formation prior to surgery. Rarely, individuals are born with normal fibrinogen molecules but with low or absent fibrinogen levels in their circulation (hypodysfibrinogenemia or afibrinogenemia). These patients may also need replacement therapy with cryoprecipitate.

Disorders of the Fibrinolytic System

Clinically, failure to regulate the fibrinolytic system can produce bleeding. During prostate surgery, urokinase bathes tissues and rapidly lyses fibrin. Epsilon-aminocaproic acid inhibits clot lysis by inhibiting plasminogen binding to fibrin. This drug has been used to reduce fibrinolytic activity and bleeding complications in patients undergoing prostate surgery and in hemophiliacs who are undergoing dental procedures. Epsilon-aminocaproic acid should never be given to patients who have a continuous intravascular stimulus for clotting because they need a functional fibrinolytic system to prevent fibrin deposition. Renal failure and other thrombotic complications can occur when patients with intravascular coagulation are treated with epsilon-aminocaproic acid.[11]

Clinically, it is rare to have a primary disorder of fibrinolysis without an underlying stimulus for thrombosis. Patients with malignancy occasionally have tumors that produce large amounts of a plasminogen activator. The plasminogen activator may cause a fibrinolytic state alone, although it is more common for there to be an underlying stimulus for thrombosis (i.e., DIC syndrome) present.

Thrombotic Disorders in Surgical Patients

Surgical patients may experience a disorder of the hemostatic system that produces thrombosis. To prevent thrombosis, the hemostatic system contains three important plasma proteins: (1) antithrombin III, (2) protein C, and (3) protein S.

Recurrent deep venous thrombosis may occur in patients with congenital deficiencies of antithrombin III. This fact emphasizes the clinical importance of antithrombin III in preventing thrombosis on the venous side of the circulation. Acquired antithrombin III deficiency occurs secondary to massive thrombosis, the DIC syndrome, heparin therapy, liver disease, and protein-losing disorders of the kidney and gastrointestinal tract. The acquired antithrombin III deficiency may account for the thrombotic problems that occur in these clinical situations.

During heparin therapy, there is a reduction in the level of antithrombin III. Furthermore, the DIC syndrome may reduce antithrombin III levels by increasing the utili-

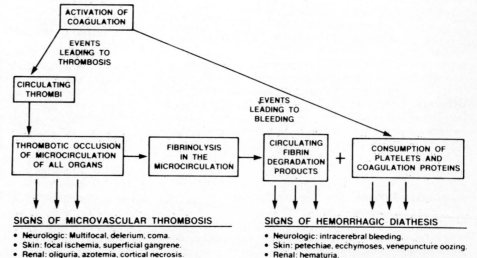

Figure 9. Clinical and laboratory consequences of the disseminated intravascular coagulation syndrome. When there is a strong stimulus for activation of coagulation, a series of events is initiated that leads to either thrombosis or hemorrhage. (Reproduced with permission from Marder, V. J.: Microvascular thrombosis. In Lichtman, M. A. (Ed.): The Science and Practice of Clinical Medicine, vol. 6. New York, Grune & Stratton, 1980.)

zation of antithrombin III to limit thrombin formation. The antithrombin and anti–factor Xa effects of antithrombin III play major roles in the antithrombotic action of antithrombin III.[22] Heparin assays have been recently developed, and they measure heparin levels in clinical samples by quantitating the ability of the heparin–antithrombin III complex in the plasma to inhibit factor Xa or thrombin activity.

Protein C is another plasma protein that functions to limit thrombin formation.[9] An inherited disorder of protein C has been discovered and reported to be associated with recurrent superficial and deep venous thrombosis. Surgical patients have not been reported to acquire a deficiency in protein C unless they develop the DIC syndrome. Protein C is activated at the endothelial cell surface; if autoimmune diseases injure the endothelium or if local trauma modifies the endothelial cell surface, protein C may not be activated. This could produce a vessel segment that would be prone to thrombosis. Research is currently being done in this area.

Protein S is the vitamin K–dependent protein that functions to localize protein C to phospholipid surfaces. In the absence of protein S, protein C activation is impaired and its function is reduced. Congenital deficiency of protein S has been reported to cause a thrombotic disorder similar to that of protein C.[7]

Postoperative deep venous thrombosis is a complication of surgery and bed rest. In patients undergoing intraabdominal surgery for a gynecologic malignancy or in those who undergo reconstructive hip surgery, postoperative deep venous thrombosis is especially prone to develop. Most venous thromboses occur in the veins of the lower extremity because this is an area where blood flow is reduced. Clinically, deep venous thrombosis produces obstruction to blood flow, which initiates an inflammatory response in the veins. A potential complication of a clot in the deep venous system is embolization into the pulmonary circulation.

Pulmonary embolization is the process whereby a clot in the deep venous system breaks off from the vessel wall and enters the pulmonary circulation. Most pulmonary emboli originate from the deep venous system or the pelvic veins and may interfere with pulmonary oxygenation or cardiac function if the embolus obstructs a large segment (usually greater than 60 per cent) of the pulmonary circulation. Arterial emboli from areas of thrombosis in atherosclerotic arteries may produce serious tissue injury and organ dysfunction, depending upon the size and location of the embolus.[13]

The post-phlebitic syndrome is a serious complication of deep venous thrombosis. The syndrome is the direct result of the destruction of the venous valves by thrombi. This produces an increase in hydrostatic pressure in the perforating veins of the calf, which normally directs blood flow from the superficial veins into the deep venous system. When the perforating valves are damaged, the blood flow is forced into the superficial system during muscle contraction of the lower limbs. The increased blood flow induces edema and impairs the function of the subcutaneous tissues. This will ultimately lead to serious discoloration and ulceration of the skin.[13]

Transfusion Therapy in the Surgical Patient

Blood banks can provide the blood and plasma products necessary for effective tissue oxygenation and hemostasis. Surgical patients may require transfusion of red cells, platelets, or plasma components during hospitalization. The effects of blood loss in man will be reviewed briefly, since the pathophysiologic consequences of blood loss must be distinguished from the effects of massive transfusion when severe hemorrhage occurs.

PATHOPHYSIOLOGY OF BLOOD LOSS IN MAN

The pathophysiologic consequences of blood loss in man are dependent upon the extent and rate of blood loss. Furthermore, the physical state of the patient will also determine how well blood loss is tolerated. When 10 to 15 per cent of the circulating blood volume is rapidly lost (within 30 minutes), the great vessels will contract and symptoms are mild. Once 30 per cent of the blood volume has been lost (1.5 to 2.0 liters), most patients have signs and symptoms of shock with apprehension, dyspnea, hypotension, cool skin, tachycardia, and decreased urinary output. Cardiac output drops, and the body redirects blood flow by arteriolar vasoconstriction to the heart and brain at the expense of other vital organs. Tissue oxygen delivery is seriously impaired in the peripheral tissues, producing alterations in metabolism that lead to lactic acidosis. If tissue oxygen delivery is not improved, permanent organ dysfunction may result. In the case of the heart, when the blood pressure drops below a critical value, the coronary arteries become underperfused and this worsens cardiac function and will ultimately lead to death. Once more than 50 per cent of the blood volume has been lost, the vicious circle of decreased tissue perfusion and worsening cardiac output develops that cannot be tolerated. The cause of death in patients who die from shock is organ injury that has resulted from decreased perfusion of peripheral tissues.[4]

Patients with coronary artery disease are unable to tolerate a large loss of blood volume because their coronary arteries cannot vasodilate sufficiently to increase cardiac blood flow when there is a drop in blood pressure. This fact must be considered when deciding when and how vigorously transfusion should be performed.

The factors that regulate tissue oxygen delivery are complex and include pulmonary gas-exchange mechanisms, hematocrit, cardiac output, and hemoglobin oxygen affinity. The hematocrit is the percentage of whole blood volume that is composed of erythrocytes. The normal hematocrit is 35 to 45 per cent. With rapid blood loss, the hematocrit may remain constant because the vascular space contracts to an amount similar to that of the red cell mass. As a rule of thumb, the hematocrit changes 2 to 3 per cent for each unit (500 cc.) of blood lost.

MANAGEMENT OF MASSIVE BLEEDING

Many surgical patients experience shock and massive bleeding. Any delay in obtaining blood for these patients may adversely influence their chances of survival. In this situation, there may be insufficient time to perform a complete cross-match. Under these circumstances, type O-negative blood should be given. In emergencies where the blood type of the patient is known, the blood bank may rapidly provide type-specific blood.

In cases of massive bleeding, every attempt should be made to reduce blood loss. In certain instances, this may mean initiating surgery in a patient who is still bleeding. The next concern should be to restore perfusion to vital tissues. Perfusion is a major priority, since there is a significant reserve in the oxygen-carrying capacity of blood. For these reasons, fluids are immediately infused in bleeding patients to enhance perfusion.

The hemostatic system may fail during massive transfusion therapy of a bleeding patient. This frequently causes confusion regarding the need for blood and whether the transfused blood has caused the hemostatic problem. Once the patient has lost one blood volume (equivalent to the body weight in kg. × 70 cc. per kg. or 5 liters of blood), only 25 to 35 per cent of the patient's original blood remains in the circulation. Therefore, the platelet count of a patient who has received 5 units of blood without receiving platelets will be reduced to a level of 60,000 to 90,000 per cu. mm., assuming the initial platelet count was 250,000 per cu. mm. Therefore, platelet counts less than 60,000 per cu. mm. in a massively transfused patient are due to consumption of platelets by the coagulation process.

There is little evidence to support the concept that blood transfusions lead to hemostatic failure without another cause being present. Most authorities maintain that the hemostatic defects of massive transfusion are a combination of transfusing blood containing the calcium-binding agent citrate, infusion of plasma deficient in functional factors V and VIII, and intravascular coagulation. In conclusion, the hemostatic defect in the massively transfused patient is in part due to increased consumption of platelet and coagulation factors and not simply due to a transfusion and dilution effect.

Sodium citrate chelates calcium ions and prevents blood from clotting during storage. When blood products containing citrate are transfused, the citrate may reduce ionized calcium. Clinically, the magnitude of this effect usually does not produce any adverse problems. The level of ionized calcium that is sufficient for coagulation reactions and for normal cardiac function is normally maintained during massive transfusions. Rarely, a serious depression in ionized calcium levels may develop that requires therapy with intravenous calcium-containing solutions.

Hypothermia regularly occurs in the massively transfused patient because blood is stored refrigerated. Hypothermia may contribute to some of the hemodynamic problems in the massively transfused patient.

TRANSFUSION OF ERYTHROCYTES

There are several major issues that must be considered when initiating transfusion therapy. First, approximately how much blood has the patient lost? Can the patient tolerate further losses? Has bleeding stopped? Is the patient capable of replenishing the lost cellular and plasma factors on his own? Once these questions have been considered and the decision to transfuse erythrocytes has been made, a choice has to be made regarding the type of erythrocyte-containing blood product to transfuse. Erythrocytes are indicated when the red cell mass has been depleted through any one of several pathologic events (blood loss, hemolysis, decreased marrow production) and when there is an urgent need for improvement in tissue oxygen delivery.

Blood for transfusion is collected into a citrate-containing anticoagulant solution that contains glucose (citrate-phosphate-dextrose, CPD). When blood is collected and stored in the refrigerator at 4°C. for more than 6 hours, cellular and plasma components begin to lose their function. The white blood cells and platelets are not functional after 24 hours, factor VIII coagulant activity is reduced after 48 hours, factor V is unstable after 5 days, and red cells are not useful after 3 weeks.[23]

Fresh blood is anticoagulated blood that is less than 6 hours old. Fresh blood is difficult to obtain because of the logistical problem of having a ready supply of donors available. Therefore, its clinical use has been very limited. When available, fresh blood is an excellent choice for the massively bleeding patient. In practice, a unit of packed red blood cells, one unit of fresh frozen plasma, and a unit of platelets will provide the same components as one unit of fresh blood.

Whole blood is anticoagulated blood that has been stored for more than 6 hours and probably has undergone some loss of platelet and factors V and VIII function. Packed red blood cells are obtained by centrifuging whole blood and removing plasma. The red cells that remain have a hematocrit of approximately 75 per cent. Packed red blood cells fulfill the need for increasing the circulating red cell mass without significantly contributing to the plasma volume. Each unit of packed red blood cells transfused raises the hematocrit 2 to 3 per cent. Packed red cells are the most commonly used and most readily available erythrocyte component in blood banks.

Patients may develop severe fever and chills following transfusions of compatible packed red cells. These patients require white cell–poor blood components. This is provided as a washed red cell preparation and must be used within 24 hours. Frozen red cells are the best source of white cell–poor blood and are available for storing extremely rare blood types.

PLATELET TRANSFUSIONS

Platelets can be very useful in the management of the thrombocytopenic patient or in the patient who acquires a platelet defect following surgery. Random single donor platelets are harvested from a single unit of fresh blood that has been centrifuged to remove erythrocytes. One unit of random single-donor platelets contains enough platelets to raise the platelet count 10,000 per mm.[3] when measured 1 hour after transfusion of an adult patient. Transfused platelets survive in the circulation with a half-life of about 6 days. Random donor platelets should be given only to bleeding patients with documented thrombocytopenia (< 100,000 platelets per mm.[3]) or to any patient with a platelet count that is less than 20,000 per mm.[3] Antibodies may develop to the HLA antigens on random donor platelets. In these immunized patients, there is a failure to obtain any increment in the platelet count following a transfusion of random donor platelets. HLA-identical platelets are indicated in patients sensitized to the HLA-antigens. HLA-identical platelets are obtained by separating the blood of a sibling identified as HLA-identical with a plateletpheresis machine. Granulocyte transfusions have recently become technically possible through the use of leukopheresis machines. However, in surgical patients they have no practical use. Lymphocytes, which are metabolically active, are present in platelets and in whole blood and have the capability of initiating a graft-versus-host reaction in the severely immunosuppressed recipient.

PLASMA COMPONENTS AND REPLACEMENT THERAPY

Fresh frozen plasma is prepared by centrifugation to remove the platelets from the plasma remaining after preparation of packed red blood cells. The platelet-poor plasma is stored at −20°C. because activity of factors V and VIII is more stable at −20° than when stored at 4°C. Fresh frozen plasma is indicated for the rapid treatment of the bleeding patient who has a coagulation defect caused by liver disease, warfarin therapy, DIC, or massive red cell transfusions. Fresh frozen plasma is also used in the management of patients who have congenital deficiencies of factors II, V, X, IX, or XI.

Cryoprecipitate is prepared by freezing plasma to −90°C. and allowing it to slowly warm up to 4°C. After rewarming, a gelatinous precipitate remains; the precipitate is enriched in fibrinogen, factor VIII:vWF, and the factor VIII:coagulant protein, compared with the original plasma. A single unit of cryoprecipitate is supplied, 15 to 25 cc. Despite its small volume, cryoprecipitate has a very high protein concentration and will significantly expand the plasma volume. Cryoprecipitate is indicated for the bleeding surgical patient who has a fibrinogen level of less than 100 mg. per 100 ml. Cryoprecipitate is also indicated in the treatment of patients with hemophilia A (factor VIII deficiency) and von Willebrand's syndrome. Each unit of cryoprecipitate contains approximately 200 mg. of fibrinogen, 150 units of factor VIII:vWF, and 100 units of factor VIII:coagulant.

COMPLICATIONS OF TRANSFUSION THERAPY

Blood transfusions carry a risk of inducing hepatitis and other adverse reactions. *Post-transfusion hepatitis* occurs in 8 to 10 per cent of patients receiving a transfusion and is most often due to type non-A, non-B virus (70 per cent) or to cytomegalovirus and hepatitis B virus. More recent epidemiologic data suggest that the *acquired immune deficiency syndrome* (AIDS) is caused by an infectious agent, most likely a virus, which is transmitted through blood products. The infectious agent has been designated HTLV-III (human T cell lymphotropic retrovirus-III).[2] The long-term implications of receiving blood products from a person exposed to the HTLV-III virus remain poorly defined. Clinically, blood products should not be indiscriminately utilized since bioactive substances may have adverse consequences.

Another adverse result is the *hemolytic transfusion reaction*. This reaction usually occurs immediately following the institution of a transfusion and results in severe chest pain, flank pain, fever, chills, and hypotension. Hemolysis occurs intravascularly and produces hemoglobinemia and hemoglobinuria. Intravascular coagulation and acute renal failure are common results of the hemolytic transfusion reaction. These reactions are very rare and are usually due to mistakes in patient or blood identification rather than to a problem in the ability of the cross-match procedure to identify compatible blood.

The *leukoagglutinin reaction* occurs more commonly than the hemolytic transfusion reaction, with a frequency of one per 40 transfusions. It usually occurs late in a transfusion. These reactions are accompanied by only fever and chills.

Since most transfusion reactions are due to leukoagglutinins and since surgical patients are in need of blood, the transfusion may continue if there has been no change in blood pressure, if symptoms are mild and occurred at the end of the transfusion, if plasma and urine show no evidence of hemolysis, or if the patient has undergone transfusion previously and is known to have fever and chills following the administration of blood. In contrast to these mild reactions, severe hemolytic transfusion reactions must be vigorously treated by stopping the transfusion and supporting the blood pressure with fluids and vasopressors.

Clinically, when a patient has received a blood transfusion and fever and chills develop, a decision must be made concerning whether a severe hemolytic transfusion reaction is taking place. The blood transfusion should be stopped, and both patient and blood identification must be re-checked. Urine and plasma should be checked for a brown or red color, which would indicate hemolysis. The unit should be returned to the blood bank and a post-transfusion cross-match plasma specimen obtained.

Post-transfusion purpura is an unusual cause of thrombocytopenia in recently transfused surgical patients. Patients with platelets deficient in the Pl^{A1} antigen and anti-Pl^{A1} antibodies (1 per cent of the population) may develop severe thrombocytopenia following transfusion of blood products containing the Pl^{A1} antigen. These patients may require plasmapheresis and transfusion with Pl^{A1}-negative platelets if life-threatening bleeding develops.[23]

Another unusual but severe transfusion reaction that produces respiratory distress and shock can occur in transfused patients with an IgA deficiency who have anti-IgA antibodies. These patients may require washed red cells to prevent a recurrence of this reaction.[23]

SELECTED REFERENCES

Colman, R. W., Hirsh, J., Marder, V. J., and Saleman, E. W.: Hemostasis and Thrombosis Education: Basic Principles and Clinical Practice. Philadelphia, J. B. Lippincott Company, 1982.
    A comprehensive reference source to be used to answer specific questions in the basic science and clinical areas of hemostasis. Individual chapters are authored by basic scientists and clinical experts in hemostasis. The text will provide the student with an in-depth discussion and extensive bibliography. This is one of the most up-to-date and comprehensive textbooks ever assembled for those interested in blood coagulation.

Hirsch, J., and Brain, E. A.: Hemostasis and Thrombosis: A Conceptual Approach. New York, Churchill Livingstone, 1983.
    This book outlines normal and abnormal hemostatic processes that produce bleeding and thrombotic disorders. There is a diagram for each paragraph that effectively reinforces the written presentation. This book is recommended as the first text to be read by students who are interested in comprehending the hemostatic system. Questions at the end of each chapter emphasize important points.

Hirsh, J., Genton, E., Hirsh, E., and Hull, R.: Venous Thromboembolism. New York, Grune & Stratton, 1981.
    An up-to-date and informative textbook devoted to the pathogenesis, diagnosis, treatment, and complications of venous thromboembolism. The authors have made many significant contributions to this field and have extensive clinical experience.

Koepke, J. A. (Ed.): Laboratory Hematology, vols. 1 and 2. New York, 1984.
    An authoritative textbook that focuses upon the laboratory aspects of hematology. In addition, there are chapters in both volumes that discuss clinical and laboratory aspects of disorders in blood coagulation. The chapters on transfusion therapy and the adverse reactions to transfusion provide a comprehensive review of an important topic. The methods involved in coagulation laboratory testing are reviewed and emphasize the need for quality control in this area.

Mosher, D. F.: *In* MacKinney, A. A., Jr. (Ed.): Pathophysiology of Blood. New York, John Wiley and Sons, 1984.
    This book concisely reviews the basic science and clinical aspects of hemostasis. Case development problems followed by answers serves to emphasize the clinical significance of the hemostatic system.

Petz, L. D., and Swisher, S. N. (Ed.): Clinical Practice of Blood Transfusion. New York, Churchill Livingstone, 1981.
    Edited by two authorities in the areas of immunohematology and transfusion, this textbook reviews immunology, cross-match procedures, methods of blood preservation, and clinical transfusion practices. Chapters 21 and 22 are written by Dr. J.A. Collins, an expert on the pathophysiology of hemorrhagic shock and the problems of transfusion therapy. These chapters emphasize the pathophysiologic consequence of blood loss and outline how different transfusion therapies may influence patient survival.

Thompson, A. R., and Harker, L. A.: Manual of Hemostasis and Thrombosis, 3rd ed. Philadelphia, F. A. Davis Company, 1983.
    This book presents a concise review of hemostasis and thrombosis and is written for medical students. The manual describes a pathophysiologic approach to hemostatic and thrombotic disorders. Its up-to-date citations from the literature make this a valuable book for all health professionals interested in a single-volume text that reviews blood coagulation.

REFERENCES

1. Berridge, M. J., and Irvine, R. F.: Inositol trisphosphate, a novel second messenger in cellular signal transduction. Nature, *312*:315, 1984.
2. Centers for Disease Control Task Force on Kaposi's Sarcoma and Opportunistic Infections: Epidemiologic aspects of the current outbreak of Kaposi's sarcoma and opportunistic infections. N. Engl. J. Med., 306:248, 1982.
3. Collen, D.: On the regulation and control of fibrinolysis. Thromb. Haemost., *43*:77, 1980.
4. Collins, J. A.: Hemorrhage, shock, and burns: Pathophysiology and treatment. *In* Petz, L. D., and Swisher, S. N. (Eds.): Clinical Practice of Blood Transfusion. New York, Churchill Livingstone, 1981, pp. 425–453.
5. Colman, R. W.: Surface-mediated defense reactions: The plasma contact activation system. J. Clin. Invest., *73*:1249, 1984.
6. Colman, R. W., Robboy, S. J., and Minna, I. D.: Disseminated intravascular coagulation: A reappraisal. Ann. Rev. Med., *30*:359, 1979.
7. Comp, P. C., and Esmon, C. T.: Recurrent venous thromboembolism in patients with a partial deficiency of protein S. N. Engl. J. Med., *311*:1525, 1985.
8. Deuel, T. F., and Huang, J. S.: Platelet-derived growth factor: Structure, function, and roles in normal and transformed cells. J. Clin. Invest., *74*:669, 1984.
9. Esmon, C. T.: Protein C: Biochemistry, physiology and clinical implications. Blood, *62*:1155, 1983.
10. George, J. N., Nurden, A. T., and Phillips, D. R.: Molecular defects in interactions of platelets with the vessel wall. N. Engl. J. Med., *311*:1084, 1984.
11. Griffin, J. D., and Ellman, L.: Epsilon-aminocaproic acid (EACA). Semin. Thromb. Hemostasis, *5*:27, 1978.
12. Hermans, J., and McDonagh, J.: Fibrin: Structure and interaction. Semin. Thromb. Hemos., *8*:11, 1982.
13. Hirsh, J., Genton, E., and Hull, R.: Venous Thromboembolism. New York, Grune & Stratton, 1978.
14. Jackson, C. M., Nemerson, Y.: Blood coagulation. Ann. Rev. Biochem., *49*:745, 1980.
15. Lapetina, E. G., Watson, S. P., and Cuatrecasas, P.: Myo-inositol 1,4,5-trisphosphate stimulates protein phosphorylation in saponin-permeabilized human platelets. Proc. Natl. Acad. Sci. U.S.A. *81*:7431, 1984.
16. Lorand, L., Losowsky, M. S., and Miloszewski, K.J.M.: Human factor XIII: Fibrin-stabilizing factor. Prog. Hemost. Thromb., *5*:245, 1980.
17. Majerus, P., et al.: The formation of thrombin on platelet surface. *In* Mann, K. G., and Taylor, F. B. (Eds.): The Regulation of Coagulation. New York, Elsevier, 1980, p. 215.
18. Majno, G., and Joris, I.: Endothelium: A review. Adv. Exp. Med. Biol., *104*:169, 1978.
19. Marlar, R. A., Kleiss, A. J., and Griffin, H.: An alternative extrinsic pathway of human blood coagulation. Blood, *60*:1353, 1982.
20. Moncada, S., and Vane, J. R.: Arachidonic acid metabolites and the interaction between platelets and blood vessel walls. N. Engl. J. Med., *300*:1142, 1979.
21. Rappaport, S. I.: Preoperative hemostatic evaluation: Which tests, if any? Blood, *61*:229, 1983.
22. Rosenberg, R. D., and Rosenberg, J. S.: Natural anticoagulant mechanisms. J. Clin. Invest., *74*:1, 1984.
23. Simpson, M. B., Jr.: Adverse reactions to transfusion therapy: Clinical and laboratory aspects. *In* Koepke, J. A. (Ed.): Laboratory Hematology. New York, Churchill Livingstone, 1984, pp. 1175–1228.
24. Stenflo, J.: Vitamin K, prothrombin, and γ-carboxyglutamin K acid. Adv. Enzymol., *46*:1, 1978.
25. Thiagarjan, P., and Shapiro, S. S.: Lupus anticoagulants. Prog. Hemost. Thromb., *5*:198, 1982.

NUTRITION AND METABOLISM IN SURGICAL PATIENTS

MURRAY F. BRENNAN, M.D. • JAMES H. F. SHAW, M. B., CH.B.

6

THE METABOLIC RESPONSE TO STRESS

Stress and injury are commonly observed phenomena in surgical patients. To evaluate the response of these patients, the degree of stress must be carefully assessed. Numerous rating systems have been applied to differentiate the degree of stress induced by simple elective operations, such as a cholecystectomy, from the major trauma seen as a consequence of a motor vehicle accident, complicated by infection, and multiple organ system failure.

Under normal circumstances, the metabolic response to injury is an adaptive and beneficial reaction on the part of the host. If the injury or insult is short-lived, the response is beneficial. However, if the injury is prolonged or if a secondary event such as infection supersedes, the metabolic response becomes destructive, with massive loss of host-tissue and functional impairment of organ systems.

Neuroendocrine Response

The neuroendocrine response is a neurophysiologic reflex induced by the injury process. The effector arm of this response involves the peripheral and central nervous pathways, in particular the spinothalamic pathways and the reticular formation, with final processing occurring mainly in the medulla, thalamus, and hypothalamus. A simplistic outline of this response is seen in Figure 1.

The efferent response is then initiated in the hypothalamus, the pituitary gland, and the autonomic nervous system to produce the effector arm of the neuroendocrine response (Fig. 2). Activation of the autonomic nervous system induces a marked increase in sympathetic activity. Plasma catecholamine levels are elevated, and the magnitude and duration of this elevation closely parallels the severity of the injury or stress (Table 1).

In physiologic terms, this response can be viewed simplistically as the "fight or flight" response described by Walter B. Cannon in 1936. There are two fundamental physiologic components: hemodynamic and metabolic. The cardiovascular response includes the development of tachycardia, increased cardiac output, mobilization of blood from

peripheral storage areas, and peripheral vasoconstriction (i.e., skin and viscera). The metabolic response includes increases in plasma glucose and free fatty acid (FFA) levels and the stimulation of release of cortisol, catecholamines, and glucagon. These latter three hormones combine to increase gluconeogenesis and lipolysis, thereby mobilizing energy stores.

The alterations in pituitary function result in part from the enhanced secretion of releasing factors from the hypothalamus, which stimulates the release of hormones from the anterior pituitary. Alternatively, the activation of the posterior pituitary promotes the release of antidiuretic hormone (ADH). The anterior pituitary hormonal response results in the release of adrenocorticotropic hormone (ACTH), growth hormone, follicle-stimulating hormone (FSH), thyroid-stimulating hormone (TSH), prolactin, and luteinizing hormone (LH). As a result of increased ACTH activity, plasma cortisol levels increase. This hypercortisolemia of injury has been implicated in the pathogenesis of the increased nitrogen losses that occur during stress; however, recent evidence suggests that this continued cortisol excretion plays a permissive rather than an initiating role in protein catabolism. Elevation in plasma growth hormone levels has been noted in postoperative patients and during physical exertion; however, this response is usually short-lived and the exact significance of the growth hormone release in response to stress is not fully understood. Thyroid hormone activity results in decreased levels of triiodothyronine (T_3) with elevation of reverse T_3. Thyroxine (T_4) levels are usually in the normal range, as are TSH levels. These alterations in thyroid activity have been postulated to be of significance in modulating the changes in metabolic rate. It should be emphasized, however, that the roles played by thyroid hormone, luteinizing hormone, follicle-stimulating hormone, prolactin, and testosterone are probably of minor significance in the metabolic response to stress.

Increased posterior pituitary activity results in the release of ADH, a major feature of the metabolic response to stress. Factors known to promote the release of ADH include the neural pathways just mentioned, and the poorly understood "nonspecific response" to injury. Hypoglycemia is also a strong stimulus to ADH release. The net effect of

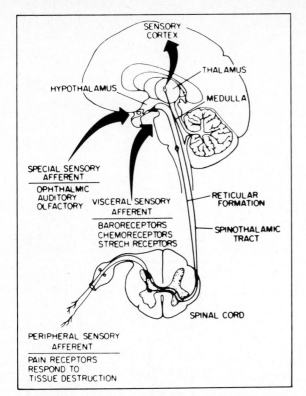

Figure 1. Afferent neurologic pathways transmit sensory perception to higher central nervous system centers. (From Popp, M. B., and Brennan, M. F.: Metabolic response to trauma and infection. In Fisher, J. E. (Ed.): Surgical Nutrition. Boston, Little, Brown and Co., 1983, pp. 479–514.)

increased ADH availability is volume conservation, designed to maintain vascular volume, and tissue perfusion.

The renin angiotensin-aldosterone system is also activated during stress. In severe injury, plasma renin levels increase up to tenfold. As a consequence of the increased secretion of aldosterone, the renal tubules retain sodium and water at the expense of potassium (Fig. 3).

Effect of Metabolic Response on Body Composition

Body composition and calorie equivalence of normal man are illustrated in Figure 4. In response to injury, profound changes in body composition occur. An example of the response of fluid content to sepsis and starvation is shown in Figure 5. The increase in total body water content is a consequence of the increase in extracellular water, with the intracellular water volume actually decreasing.

The metabolic and nutritional consequences of starvation and injury are contrasted in Table 2.

TABLE 1. Increase in Catecholamine Secretion in Response to Injury (% Increase over Control Values)*

Condition	Epinephrine (%)	Norepinephrine (%)
Elective surgical operation	136	289
Burn injury	386	248
Severe sepsis	950	868

*Adapted from Popp, M. B., and Brennan, M. F.: Metabolic response to trauma and infection. In Fischer, J. E. (Ed.): Surgical Nutrition. Boston, Little, Brown and Co., 1983, pp. 479–514.[6]

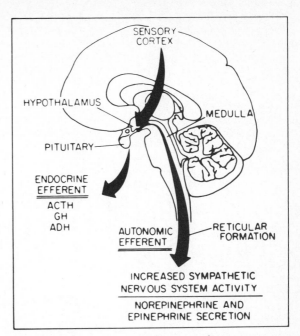

Figure 2. Efferent neurologic pathways mediate automatic and endocrine components of the central nervous system response. (From Popp, M. B., and Brennan, M. F.: Metabolic response to trauma and infection. In Fisher, J. E. (Ed.): Surgical Nutrition. Boston, Little, Brown and Co., 1983, pp. 479–514.)

Changes in Energy Balance

In contrast to what is seen during starvation, energy requirements are generally increased during stress. The changes in energy balance that occur with various types of stress are summarized in Table 3.

Changes in Protein Metabolism

In response to major injury, lean body mass, mainly in the form of muscle, is mobilized, protein is broken down, and amino acids are released. Amino acids may be burned directly for energy by muscle, by liver, and by kidney for gluconeogenesis or may be reutilized for synthesis. Urea synthesis and urinary nitrogen losses are increased, and a state of negative nitrogen balance ensues that persists for the duration of the injury. The use of stable and radioactive isotopes allows us to examine the differential effects of a variety of stresses and injuries on the balance between whole-body synthesis and catabolism. These changes are illustrated in Table 4.

In general, following major trauma or injury, catabolism increases. This increase usually exceeds the increase seen in synthesis and places the patient at risk of lean tissue dissolution. In mild injury, the rate of protein synthesis decreases, whereas catabolism is only mildly altered (Table 4). The mechanisms of nitrogen loss are shown in Table 5.

Changes in Glucose Metabolism

Hyperglycemia is a common accompaniment to injury. This has been variously labeled as "stress diabetes" or hyperglycemia of injury. Although it has been observed often, the mechanism has been elucidated only recently. Gluconeogenic rates can double and even triple in serious injury, and this is reflected by an increase in the rate of

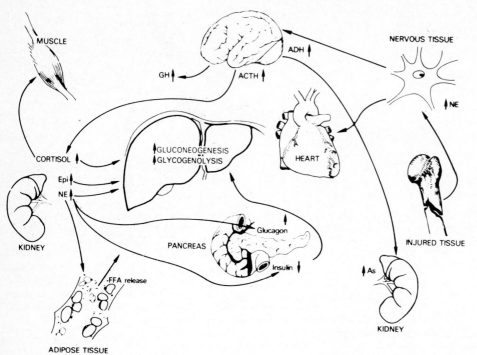

Figure 3. Effect of the neuroendocrine response to trauma on body composition and fluid electrolyte balance.

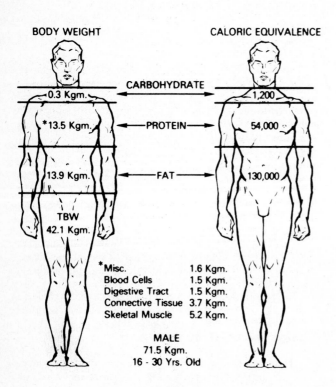

Figure 4. Body composition and caloric equivalents of normal man. (From Brennan, M. F.: Cancer, 43:2053, 1979.)

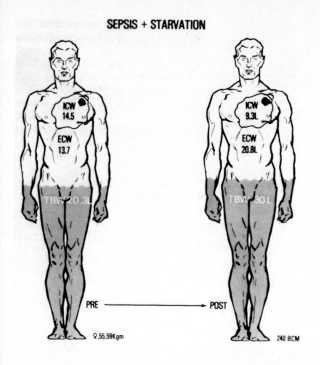

SEPSIS + STARVATION

Figure 5. Body water changes in sepsis and starvation. Drawn from tabular data in the body cell mass.

glucose production. Amino acids and lactate are the main precursors, with a contribution from fat in the form of glycerol.

Although glucose turnover is elevated in patients with severe injury, the amount of this increased glucose production that is directly oxidized is still not clear (Tables 6 and 7). In septic animal models, glucose oxidation may be increased, decreased, or unaltered in response to infection. Most isotopic determinations of glucose oxidation in septic man have demonstrated an enhanced rate of glucose oxidation.

The metabolic substrates utilized to facilitate this enhanced rate of glucose production in stressed individuals have been studied extensively. In severely injured patients, the major substrates are lactate and amino acids released from muscle, in particular alanine and glutamine. This mechanism, whereby peripheral nitrogen can be shunted to the liver for conversion to glucose, is termed the *alanine*

cycle. It is clear, however, that if only nitrogen is contributed to the pyruvate to make alanine or to the glutamate to make glutamine, this would be a nonproductive energy-wasting cycle. The assumption is thus: Not only is the nitrogen contributed to pyruvate; intrinsic muscle carbon fragments are utilized to make new carbon skeletons contained within the alanine. An example of one of these cycles—the *glucose-alanine cycle*— is shown in Figure 6.

Alterations in Fat Metabolism in Trauma and Sepsis

Fat metabolism has been studied much less extensively than has glucose and protein metabolism. Whereas free fatty acids are generally elevated in the plasma of patients following injury or sepsis, there is no clear consensus as to the quantitation of lipolysis and fatty acid oxidation in septic or traumatized man. An increase in glycerol turnover does occur in severely stressed patients in comparison with nonstressed controls. The oxidation of ^{14}C-labeled triglyceride in postoperative patients has been suggested to be elevated. It also appears that the obligatory fatty acid mobilization and oxidation that occur during sepsis and injury are only minimally influenced by the addition of other exogenous substrate. In non-injured man, the addition of lipid infusion does not appear to give any beneficial effect in protein sparing over and above the contained glycerol. This, however, may well not be so in the chronically starvation-adapted patient.

Kinetic studies addressing triglyceride and fatty acid turnover have not been performed in septic patients. Septic animals, however, have been used to study rates of FFA and triglyceride kinetics and oxidation. These data suggest that the rate of appearance of FFA and triglyceride following sepsis is markedly elevated. Furthermore, fat oxidation (in particular, the fatty acids contained in very low density lipoprotein—VLDL) is markedly increased in septic animals (Table 8).

No clear picture emerges concerning fat metabolism in trauma. Several studies have indicated that fat metabolism

TABLE 2. Nutritional and Metabolic Consequences of Starvation and Injury*

Category	Starvation	Injury
Anorexia	+	+
Weight	↓	↓
Basal metabolic rate	↓	↑
Blood glucose	↓	↑
Serum insulin	↓	↑ ↓
Plasma glucagon	↑	↑ ↑
Total plasma amino acids	↓	↑
Urinary nitrogen excretion	↓	↑
Whole-body glucose turnover rate	↓	↑
Whole-body glucose recycling (%)	±	↑
Whole-body protein turnover	↓	↑
Whole-body protein synthesis	↓	↑ ↓
Whole-body protein catabolism	↑	↑
Gluconeogenesis from alanine	↑	↑

*Modified from Brennan, M. F.: N. Engl. J. Med. *305*:375, 1981.[2]

Key: ↑ = a significant increase; ↓ = a significant decrease; ± = either no change or a nonsignificant trend. For anorexia, + denotes its presence.

TABLE 3. Metabolic Consequences of Stress

	Vo_2	N_2 Losses	Equivalent Protein Loss (gm./day)	Equivalent Lean Tissue Loss (gm./day)	Fluid and Electrolyte Losses
Starvation	40%	3–10	19–36	84–280	↓
Surgical operation	+5%	10–12	63–75	280–350	↑
Trauma	+20%	10–15	75–94	350–420	↑ +
Burns	+50%	15+	94+	420+	↑ + +
Sepsis	+50%	20+	125+	560+	↑ + +

Abbreviations: Vo_2 = Oxygen consumption (values indicate per cent increase above basal); N_2 = nitrogen.

TABLE 4. Whole-Body Protein Synthesis and Catabolism Measured by Isotopic Tracer Methodology*

Published Reports	Surgical Problem	Nutritional Intake of Subjects Relative to Controls	Percent Normal Protein Synthesis	Percent Normal Protein Catabolism
1	Severe burn	Variable	↑	↑ +
2	Mild burn	Variable	203	203
3	Trauma	Same	150	179
4	Severe sepsis	Variable	–	200+
5	Sepsis	Same	121	121
6	Elective surgery	Same	77	94
7	Elective surgery	Decreased	88	101

*Modified from Popp, M. B., and Brennan, M. F.: Metabolic response to trauma and infection. *In* Fischer, J. E. (Ed.): Surgical Nutrition. Boston, Little, Brown and Co., 1983, pp. 479–514.[6]

TABLE 5. Nitrogen Losses before, during, and after Various Surgical Procedures*

Surgical Problem	Average Preoperative Loss (gm./day)	Average Duration (Days)	Average Operative N_2 Loss (gm./day)	Average Preoperative N_2 Loss (gm./day)	Average Duration (Days)
Small bowel obstruction	11.0	1	12	75	10
Major burn	630	20	—	—	—
Gastrectomy for bleeding ulcer	91	5	18	75	15
Multiple fracture	190	18	—	150	15
Thyroidectomy	—	—	12	15	5
Pneumonectomy	—	—	57	—	—
Mastectomy	—	—	24	15	10
Cholecystectomy	—	—	12	114	10
Perforated appendicitis	15	1	12	49	10

*Adapted from Dudrick, S. J., and Rhoads, J. E.: Metabolism in surgical patients: Protein, carbohydrate, and fat utilization by oral and parenteral routes. *In* Sabiston, D. C., Jr. (Ed.): Textbook of Surgery. 12th ed. Philadelphia, W. B. Saunders Company, 1981.

TABLE 6. *Glucose Production Rates in Stressed and Nonstressed Post-absorptive Man**

Clinical Situation	Rate of Glucose Production (mg./kg./min.)†
Post-absorptive, normal man	2.5 ± 0.2
Elective operation	2.5 ± 0.3
Severe sepsis	5.1 ± 1.5
Severe burns	3.2 ± 1.6

*Adapted from Shaw, J. H. F., Klein, S., and Wolfe, R. R.: *Surgery, 97:*557, 1985.[7]
†All data obtained via primed constant infusions of either 6-³H-glucose or 6-6d₂-glucose.

may be enhanced, especially in burn patients; however, kinetic studies have not been performed. Kinetic studies in burned animals, however, do indicate an enhanced turnover and utilization of fatty acids and glycerol (Table 9).

Response of Surgical Patients to Substrate Infusion

Provision of exogenous substrate in the form of glucose results in decreased endogenous glucose production and inhibition of body nitrogen loss as the exogenous glucose makes up for that contributed by gluconeogenesis. In normal man, glucose infusion markedly reduces both urinary nitrogen levels and the rate of production of urea (Table 10). In severely injured patients, isotopic tracer studies indicate that glucose infusion will suppress endogenous glucose production but the response is more variable than in normal volunteers. During glucose infusion in injured patients, the rate of glucose oxidation increases, but this increase is less than that seen in normal man (see Table 7). The actual fate of the infused glucose has recently been examined in elective postoperative patients. As the rate of glucose infusion increases, the percentage of the infused glucose that is *directly* oxidized to carbon dioxide (CO_2) decreases. At very high rates of glucose infusion (over 7 or 8 mg. per kg. per min.), the respiratory quotient (RQ) usually exceeds 1.0, indicating net fat synthesis. This suggests that although a moderate amount of glucose is useful in terms of both protein sparing and direct oxidation for energy, a large quantity of glucose is not necessarily better and may actually be harmful in terms of liver fat

TABLE 7. *Glucose Production and Oxidation in Normal Volunteers and Burn Patients in the Basal State and during Glucose Infusion*†*

	Normal Volunteers	Burn Patients
Basal rate of glucose production (mg./kg./min.)	2.5 ± 0.2	3.1–6.6
Basal rate of glucose oxidation (mg./kg./min.)	1.0 ± 0.1	0.7–2.0
Suppression of glucose production during glucose infusion	78 ± 5%	47–100%
Change in glucose oxidation during glucose infusion (mg./kg./min.)	0.2–0.6	0–0.25

*Adapted from Wolfe, R. R., et al.: *Metabolism, 28:*1031, 1979.[9]
†Glucose infusion rate: 2.0–2.6 mg./kg./min.

TABLE 8. *Fat Metabolism in Gram-Negative Septicemia**

	Control	Septic Patients†
Plasma FFA concentration (μmol./kg./min.)	0.45 ± 0.05	0.76 ± 0.21
FFA production (μmol./kg./min.)	11.0 ± 2.1	36.1 ± 4.4
FFA oxidation (μmol./kg./min.)	3.0 ± 0.2	4.7 ± 1.5
Plasma triglyceride concentration (μmol./kg./min.)	0.5 ± 0.05	1.35 ± 0.71
VLDL production (μmol./kg./min.)	0.5 ± 0.1	2.5 ± 0.8
VLDL-FA oxidation (μmol./kg./min.)	0.5 ± 0.2	4.8 ± 1.0

*Adapted from Wolfe, R. R., et al.: *Metabolism, 28:*1031, 1979.[9]
†All septic values are significantly different from control value.
Abbreviations: FFA = Free fatty acid; VLDL = very low density lipoprotein; VLDL-FA = fatty acid contained in VLDL.

deposition and excessive CO_2 production. The excess in CO_2 production in a severely stressed individual with impaired pulmonary function may be deleterious.

These responses are completely consistent with the previous results obtained from observing changes in nitrogen excretion in the urine following high-dose glucose infusion. There is a limit to which this can be suppressed, and further benefit in sparing nitrogen is thus no longer able to be demonstrated.

In patients with severe infection, the response to glucose infusion can differ from that seen in uncomplicated trauma, but it appears to be one of degree only. The ability to suppress gluconeogenesis in mild injury, compared with severe injury and stress, appears to be a factor of quantity alone; and when high-dose glucose is infused, suppression of gluconeogenesis can almost always be obtained.

NUTRITIONAL ASSESSMENT

Malnutrition as a prognostic indicator of outcome in surgical patients has only recently been emphasized. In 1936, Studley recognized that patients with peptic ulcer disease undergoing operations had a much higher mortality

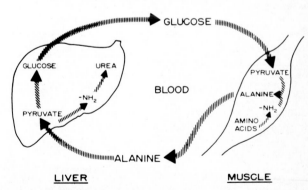

Figure 6. The glucose-alanine cycle. (From Moore, F. D., and Brennan, M. F.: Surgical injury: Body composition, protein metabolism neuroendocrinology. In American College of Surgeons (Ed.): Surgical Nutrition. Philadelphia, W. B. Saunders Company, 1975, pp. 169–222.[5])

TABLE 9. Effect of Thermal Injury on Fat Metabolism*

	Control	Burn Patients
Free fatty acid production (μmol./kg./min.)	11.3 ± 1.0	17.6 ± 2.6†
Glycerol production (μmol./kg./min.)	2.46 ± 0.54	4.2 ± 0.7†
Total fat oxidation (μmol./kg./min.)	11.1	13.8

*Adapted from Wolfe, R. R., et al.: Circ. Shock, 9:383, 1982.[10]
†Significantly higher than control values.

if they had antecedent weight loss. More recently, nutritional assessment of patients has received greater emphasis as a consequence of nutritional surveys done in hospitals. Surgical stress is associated with an increased turnover rate of energy substrates and with associated increases in metabolic rate and loss of whole-body nitrogen. The ability to define indicators of malnutrition in surgical patients has been hampered by the lack of a simple and easily recognizable parameter that is, of itself, responsive to nutritional support. Weight loss has been the factor most commonly used to describe the degree of inanition. Malnutrition, as defined by weight loss alone, is a prognostic factor in most disease states. An acute loss of body weight of 10 to 15 per cent over 2 to 3 weeks has a much more dramatic effect on body function than does a more gradual loss. A total loss of greater than 30 per cent is associated with decreased visceral function, marked morbidity, and a significant incidence of mortality. A decrease of 50 per cent of body weight is usually incompatible with survival.

Signs of malnutrition that may indicate specific deficits are widely recognized, e.g., dry atrophic skin and crusting lesions or trace metal or essential fatty acid deficiency. Other physical signs and observations used to assess malnutrition are illustrated in Table 11.

The assessment of nutritional requirements can be done by the determination of nitrogen balance and oxygen consumption, although the two are not totally interdependent. Facilities for the determination of oxygen consumption of all stressed patients are limited. Accurate determinations, however, can be predicted using various formulas such as the Harris-Benedict equation. This formula has

TABLE 10. Basal Rates of Glucose and Urea Production in Normal Volunteers and Septic Patients and Effect of Glucose Infusion*

	Normal Volunteers	Septic Patients
Glucose		
Basal rate of production (μmol./kg./min.)	2.5 ± 0.1	5.1 ± 1.5
Percent of suppression of endogenous production during glucose infusion (4 mg./kg./min.)	88%	39%
Urea		
Basal rate of production	11.0 ± 1.4	38.3 ± 13.4
Percent suppression during glucose infusion	13%	21%

*Adapted from Shaw, J. H. F., Klein, S., and Wolfe, R. R.: Surgery, 97:557, 1985.[7]

been validated in severely ill and septic postoperative patients and is given below:

Basal energy expenditure (BEE):

For males = 660 + 13.7 W + 5H + 6.8 A
For females = 655 + 9.6 W + 1.7H − 4.7A

with W = Weight in kg., H = height in inches, and A = age in years.

Visceral Protein Assessment

Serum albumin measurement had been used as a classic index of the state of malnutrition. Albumin is the major protein produced by the liver during health, and one third of the total exchangeable albumin is contained within the intravascular space. Two thirds is contained in extravascular tissues, especially skin, muscle, and viscera. The plasma albumin concentration is highly influenced by the degree of hydration, and maldistribution of fluid between intra- and extravascular spaces considerably distorts the serum albumin concentration. The long half-life of albumin (12 to 17 days) does not reflect acute changes in the synthesis and catabolism of the more short-term proteins, which are greatly influenced by acute stress. It is clear, however, that plasma albumin levels, less than 3 gm. per 100 ml., indicate a poor prognosis.

Plasma transferrin, because of its shorter half-life, has been suggested to be a more accurate and sensitive indicator of protein-calorie malnutrition. Transferrin, however, is also dependent on the presence or absence of iron deficiency; thus, interpretation may be difficult.

More important, however, may not be the ability of albumin or transferrin to define malnutrition and to predict outcome, but the failure of such entities to be adequately reflected when nutritional status is improved by nutritional support.

Immunologic Parameters of Malnutrition

Delayed hypersensitivity, total lymphocyte count, serum complement levels, and cellular immune function have all been used to assess the state of immunity in response to malnutrition. It is clear that patients with protein-calorie malnutrition display decreased opsonin activity, and this is associated with depressed complement availability. In addition, any activity that can interfere with protein synthesis will alter the function of T and B lymphocytes, macrophages, lymphokines, and the complement system.

Delayed cutaneous hypersensitivity as an indicator of anergy has been assessed by the intradermal injection of various antigens. The most commonly employed have been *Candida*, purified protein derivative (PPD), and dinitrochlorobenzene (DNCB). The problem, again, is lack of specificity: In patients who are malnourished or ill for whatever reason, anergy may be present, not as a consequence of the nutritional status but, rather, as a result of the underlying disease process. Anergy testing, therefore, is another way in which one can define "whether the patient is sick." The ability of nutritional support to reverse these changes in anergy has been poorly studied. It does not seem clear that in limited patient populations in whom the primary or underlying disease has been controlled, improvement in nutrition alone can reverse residual anergy. When the underlying disease process has not been reversed,

TABLE 11. Merits and Shortcomings of Methods for Documenting Malnutrition

	Merits	Shortcomings	Overall Usefulness
1. Weight loss	Simple to perform	Nonspecific as to tissue type loss, i.e., does not discriminate between loss of muscle, fat, water, etc.	Useful baseline clinical assessment
2. Anthropometric measurements	Useful for surveillance of chronic malnutrition	Limited role in assessment of acute malnutrition	Does not correlate well with measurement of total body nitrogen
3. Creatinine-weight index	Useful for surveillance of chronic malnutrition	Limited role in assessment of acute malnutrition	Not very useful as a single test in surgical patients
4. Serum albumin levels	Useful in chronic malnutrition. Low levels (3 gm./100 ml.) correlate well with increased morbidity and mortality	Nonspecific (not a useful index of host-response to nutritional support)	Useful marker of increased risk of morbidity and/or mortality
5. Serum transferrin levels	More sensitive indicator of chronic malnutrition than plasma albumin (because of shorter half-life)	Nonspecific; misleading in presence of iron deficiency anemia	Same as for albumin
6. Immune profile	Useful marker of chronic malnutrition, decreased protein synthesis; readily performed	Nonspecific, e.g., may be due to underlying disease process and malnutrition; total lymphocyte count does not correlate well with outcome	Useful in conjunction with other clinical tests
7. Prognostic nutritional assessment	Easily performed; uses multiple tests to avoid shortcomings of single tests		Useful; correlates well with outcome
8. Nitrogen balance	Provides a dynamic assessment of protein and energy balance; simple to perform	Underestimates losses (important in trauma and burned patients)	Probably the best single method for dynamically assessing nutritional status and response to nutritional support
9. 3-Methylhistidine excretion	Specific marker of catabolism	Time-consuming assay that provides little information over N_2 balance	Useful research tool; not a clinically practical test
10. Oxygen consumption	Easily performed; provides accurate information regarding energy requirements	Expensive specialized equipment required	Very useful method of assessing energy requirements in surgical patients
11. Isotope dilutional techniques and neutron activation	Highly accurate means of determining total body supplies of protein, fat, water; accurate means for determining rates of muscle catabolism and synthesis and energy metabolism.	Expensive; difficult to perform	Technology research tools; impractical clinically

nutritional support appears unable to have an impact on the reversal of anergy to a significant degree.

Prognostic Nutritional Assessment

Various entities have been combined using multiple indicators of nutritional insufficiency to provide a nutritional index that will indicate outcome. These indices are then used to predict those patients who are at greatest risk for morbidity and mortality from malnutrition and who therefore could be expected to best respond to nutritional support.

The system that has been evaluated most favorably is the *Prognostic Nutritional Index* (PNI), developed by Mullen and colleagues. Plasma albumin, triceps skinfold, plasma transferrin, and delayed hypersensitivity are combined to form an index that predicts outcome. These studies were performed using multivariant analysis of many nutritional parameters that were examined for their ability to predict outcome:

$$PNI \% = 158 - 16.6 \text{ albumin}$$
$$- 0.78 \text{ triceps skinfold thickness}$$
$$- 0.2 \text{ plasma transferrin level}$$
$$- 5.8 \text{ delayed hypersensitivity score}$$

(Delayed cutaneous hypersensitivity is expressed on a scale of 0 to 2, with 0 being nonreactive to antigen and 2 being a response greater than 5 mm. reactivity to a single antigen.)

Experimental Methods

A number of more sophisticated techniques are available for nutritional assessment. Unfortunately, they are not readily applicable to all patients at the bedside and currently can be used only in institutions with applied clinical research facilities. These techniques employ either isotopic infusion techniques or various methods to gain detectable radioactivity following neutron activation of body components.

Whole-body potassium (^{40}K) has long been used as an indicator of potassium content, which in turn reflects lean tissue composition. Isotopic infusion techniques have been based on the use of either stable or radioactive isotopes to determine whole-body protein turnover and, by the knowledge of intake and output, whole-body protein synthesis and catabolism. The most widely used has been the stable isotope ^{15}N glycine, whose enrichment can be measured in an excretory end product (urea or ammonia). With the use of this isotope, estimates of whole body protein turnover, net protein catabolism, and synthesis can be performed. Alternatively, net protein catabolism may be estimated by measuring the rate of oxidation of an essential amino acid, e.g. leucine. These methods are summarized by Waterlow and Stephen.[8]

Gamma ray neutron activation has been employed to analyze absolute levels of calcium, phosphorus, chloride, nitrogen, and sodium by delayed neutron activation analysis. Body composition analysis of protein and fat may be then determined from these data.

Nutritional Support for the Surgical Patient

Nutritional support for the stressed and injured patient can be provided either *parenterally* or *enterally*. Conventionally, the parenteral route is considered either *central* (the nutrient is placed into a large or high-flow vein and therefore can be hypertonic and provide all requirements) or *peripheral* (peripheral veins are used, with less concentrated solutions providing less than complete formulations delivered). However, the majority of surgical patients can be supported by use of the gastrointestinal tract (enteral route), with parenteral nutrition being reserved for those patients in whom the gastrointestinal tract is for one reason or another not available.

PARENTERAL NUTRITION

Vascular Access

The use of parenteral nutrition requires adequate vascular access. This can be obtained by the percutaneous insertion of a central venous catheter in the vast majority of cases. In the short-term hospitalized patient, the percutaneous subclavicular subclavian vein line placement is the preferred method of access. For long-term venous access, the use of the cuffed Silastic (Hickman or Broviac) catheter has considerable advantages. These catheters have recently been manufactured with a double lumen so that in many patients one lumen can be used for infusion of parenteral nutrient mixtures and the other for venous sampling. In the cancer patient, this optimizes both patient comfort and physician monitoring.

Requirements

Nitrogen. Amino acids are usually provided in their synthetic form. Earlier attempts using casein hydrolysates have been superseded by the use of defined amino acid solutions containing both essential and non-essential amino acids in a balanced solution. Special solutions for specific indications are addressed later.

Energy Source. The majority of patients are well served by glucose as an energy substrate. The provision of 150 nonprotein calories to each gram of nitrogen seems adequate for growth and maintenance and will usually prevent the administered nitrogen being burnt for energy. Fat is used as an energy source more commonly in Europe than in the United States, where fat is used largely to prevent essential fatty acid deficiency that may occur during chronic parenteral feeding. It is expected that in the future increasing quantities of fat will be used as an energy source, particularly in those patients in whom high rates of glucose infusion have been shown to be associated with excessive CO_2 production, increased ventilatory demand, and increased catecholamine release.

The basic requirements for vitamins and trace elements are outlined in Tables 12 and 13.

TABLE 12. *Daily Requirements of Trace Elements**

Element	Requirement
Zinc	5.0 mg.
Copper	1.5 mg.
Manganese	0.5 mg.
Iodine	0.5 mg.
Chromium	0.02 mg.†
Selenium	100 μgm.†

*Adapted from Brennan, M. F., and Horowitz, G.: *In* Surgery Annual. Chicago, Year Book Medical Publishers, 1983, pp. 1–35.[3]
†Not established as essential to life in man.

TABLE 13. Daily Vitamin Requirements*

Vitamin	Dosage†
A	3300 I.U.
D	200 I.U.
E	10 I.U.
K	100 mg.
B_1 (Thiamine)	3 mg.
B_2 (Riboflavin)	3.6 mg.
B_3 (Dexpanthenol)	15 mg.
B_5 (Niacin)	40 mg.
B_6 (Pyridoxine)	4 mg.
B_7 (Biotin)	60 mg.
B_9 (Folate)	0.4 mg.
B_{12}	5 μg.

*Adapted from Brennan, M. F., and Horowitz, G.: *In* Surgery Annual. Chicago, Year Book Medical Publishers, 1983, pp. 1–35.[3]
†Provided by one ampule of MVI-12 daily (available from United States Vitamin Corp., Division of Revlon, Tuckahoe, N.Y.)

Indications

Indications for parenteral feeding include gastrointestinal fistula, short bowel syndrome, organ system failure, major burns, severe trauma and sepsis, as an adjunct to cancer chemotherapy, prior to major surgery, acute pancreatitis, and other situations of increased metabolic demand. Any clinical situation that precludes the use of the gastrointestinal tract for nutritional purposes can be evaluated for the need for parenteral nutritional support.

Special Situations

Total parenteral nutrition (TPN) is recommended in the following situations.

Respiratory Insufficiency. In patients with severe injury, high rates of glucose infusion have been shown to be associated with an increase in respiratory quotient and an excessive rate of CO_2 production. When glucose is administered at high rates (in excess of 6 to 8 mg. per kg. per min.), only a small percentage of the infused glucose is directly oxidized and a substantial portion of the remainder is directed to fat synthesis. The respiratory quotient for this lipogenesis is approximately 8.6, and CO_2 production by the host increases markedly. In the patient with a compromised respiratory system, this excessive CO_2 load provides an added stress that is best avoided by providing energy requirements in the form of 30 to 50 per cent fat and the remainder as glucose.

Renal Failure. Patients with established renal failure can be maintained in positive nitrogen balance with decreased plasma urea levels by the provision of essential amino acids or essential amino acid precursors, such as the keto-analogues of essential amino acids. Commercial solu-

TABLE 14. Acute Renal Failure: Comparison of Nutritional Support with Glucose Alone Versus Glucose Plus Amino Acids*

	n	Recovered from ARF and Survived	Discharged from Hospital
Essential amino acids plus glucose	28	21/28 (75%)	61%
Glucose alone	25	11/25 (44%)†	40%

*Adapted from Abel, R. M., et al.: N. Engl. Med. J., *288*:695, 1973.[1]
†Significant difference between groups (p <.05).
Abbreviation: ARF = Acute renal failure.

tions are now available for the patient requiring nutritional support who is in established renal failure. Furthermore, the provision of essential amino acids and glucose has been shown to improve recovery and decrease mortality in patients suffering from renal failure (Table 14).

Hepatic Failure. Recent studies indicate that the encephalopathy that is seen in patients with liver failure is associated with defective peripheral metabolism of amino acids. Increased loads of aromatic amino acids (phenylalanine, tyrosine, and methionine) and an associated decrease in plasma levels of the branched chain amino acids (leucine, isoleucine, and valine) are commonly observed in patients with hepatic failure. There is some evidence that the presence of these abnormal amino acids results in the increased production of false or abnormal central nervous system neurotransmitters. Clinical improvement in patients and animals with liver failure can be shown following treatment with nutrient solutions enriched with branched chain amino acids and deficient in the aromatic amino acids. These formulas are currently being evaluated clinically.

Sepsis. Despite marked advance in clinical nutrition, the support of the septic patient remains a dilemma. Several investigators have proposed that an energy fuel deficit exists in septic man and that this is associated with "insulin resistance" and glucose intolerance. They propose that there is an impaired ability to utilize glucose while the elevations of plasma insulin result in an impairment of lipolysis—which of itself may be contributed to by a lack of available carnitine, resulting in defective utilization of fat. On this basis, some suggestion has been made that a branched chain amino acid solution may improve the support of the septic patient.

Despite the appealing nature of the "energy-fuel deficit" hypothesis, direct isotopic assessment of glucose and fat oxidation in sepsis does not provide substantiation. Although many questions remain unanswered, the data available indicate that the oxidation of glucose, FFA, and the fatty acids contained in VLDL triglyceride are all elevated in sepsis, in contradiction to what is proposed by the energy-fuel deficit hypothesis.

Because of the lack of consensus regarding energy metabolism in sepsis, it is difficult to establish guidelines for nutritional support in septic patients. At present, the same guidelines that apply to surgical patients in general should be used.

Preoperative Parenteral Nutritional Support. In general terms, studies by Smale[7a] and Müller[5] et al. indicate that patients with malnutrition have a lower incidence of mortality and morbidity if they receive parenteral feeding preoperatively.

Complications

The technical and metabolic complications of TPN are summarized in Table 15. Septic complications are also of considerable practical importance. Catheter sepsis in patients receiving TPN is a frequently diagnosed problem. Most commonly, the patient develops clinical signs of sepsis in the absence of any obvious focus. A diagnosis of catheter sepsis is strengthened by the presence of positive blood cultures and confirmed by a positive culture from the catheter tip. Skin bacteria are the usual organisms cultured, the most common being *Staphylococcus aureus*. Fungemia is a less frequent complication, with *Candida albicans* being the most common organism involved. Removal of the catheter is the fundamental management for suspected

TABLE 15. Metabolic Complications of Total Parenteral Nutrition*

Complication	Cause
Glucose metabolism	
Hyperglycemia and nonketotic coma or ketoacidosis	Excessive glucose dose; inadequate insulin or steroid administration; sepsis
Rebound hypoglycemia	Sudden cessation of TPN (persistent insulin secretion due to prolonged islet stimulation by TPN rare)
Amino acid metabolism	
Hyperchloremic acidosis	Excessive chloride content of amino acid solutions
Hyperammonemia	Excessive ammonia in protein hydrolysate solutions or primary hepatic disorders
Prerenal azotemia	Excessive infusion of protein hydrolysate and amino acid solution
Calcium and phosphorus metabolism	
Hypophosphatemia (decreased red cell 2,3-DPG)	Inadequate provision of phosphorus
Hypocalcemia	Inadequate calcium administration or hypoalbuminemia
Hypercalcemia	Excessive calcium, vitamin D, or albumin administration
Vitamin D deficiency or hypervitaminosis-D	Inadequate or excessive vitamin D administration
Essential fatty acid deficiency	
Decreased levels of phospholipids, linoleic, and arachidonic acids	Inadequate provision of essential fatty acids, inadequate administration of vitamin E
Elevation of eicostrienoic acid	
Miscellaneous	
Hypokalemia	Inadequate provision of potassium; diuresis
Hyperkalemia	Excessive potassium administration; renal impairment
Hypomagnesemia	Inadequate provision of magnesium; diabetes
Anemia	Inadequate supply of one or more of the following: iron, folate, B_{12}, copper
Bleeding tendency	Vitamin K deficiency
Elevations of plasma enzymes ALT, AST, alkaline phosphatase	Excessive glucose administration or fat depletion in liver

*Adapted from Dudrick, S. J., and Rhoads, J. E.: Metabolism in surgical patients. *In* Sabiston, D. C., Jr. (Ed.): Davis-Christopher Textbook of Surgery, 12th ed. Philadelphia, W. B. Saunders Co., 1981.

catheter sepsis, although changing the catheter over a guideline is at present being investigated as an alternative procedure. Antibiotic treatment is often unnecessary once the catheter is removed; however, fungemia may necessitate the use of antifungal therapy, especially in the immunocompromised host. The most important aspect in the management of catheter sepsis is prevention. Of particular importance is the meticulous care of the catheter site and tubing. Ideally, the TPN catheter should be used solely for the administration of TPN because this selective use of the catheter has been shown to minimize septic complications.

Results of Parenteral Feeding

The metabolic responses to TPN during starvation and injury are summarized in Table 16. The impact of TPN on

the morbidity and mortality of gastrointestinal fistulas and acute pancreatitis is summarized in Tables 17 and 18, respectively. Data addressing the use of TPN as an adjuvant to cancer chemotherapy are summarized by Brennan.[2]

In patients with short bowel syndrome, TPN has clearly increased survival. Parenteral nutrition is undoubtedly a useful adjunct in the therapy of patients with inflammatory bowel disease, although it is not clear whether TPN is superior to enteral nutrition in these patients. As demonstrated in the previous section, the use of TPN in patients with acute renal failure is an important means of decreasing mortality and morbidity. There is no clear role, however, for TPN in the patient with chronic renal failure, despite positive results from keto-analogue–enriched dietary supplements. Encouraging results have been obtained from studies using intravenous branched chain amino

TABLE 16. Metabolic Response to Total Parenteral Nutrition in Patients with Starvation or Injury*

Response	Starvation	Injury
Weight	↓	↓
Blood glucose	↑	↑
Serum insulin	↓	↓
Plasma glucagon	↑	↑
Plasma amino acids	↓	↑
Urinary nitrogen excretion	↓	↑
Whole-body glucose turnover	↓	↑
Whole-body glucose recycling rate	↓	↑
Whole-body protein turnover	↓	↑
Whole-body protein synthesis	↓	↑
Whole-body protein catabolism	±	↑
Gluconeogenesis from amino acids	↑	↑

*Adapted from Brennan, M. F., and Horowitz, G.: *In* Surgery Annual. Chicago, Year Book Medical Publishers, 1983, pp. 1–35.[3]
Key: ↑ = an increase; ↓ = a decrease; ± = no change.

TABLE 17. Influence of Total Parenteral Nutrition (TPN) on Mortality and Closure Rate for Patients with Gastrointestinal Fistulas*

Author	n	TPN	% Closure	% Mortality
Bury	80	No	79	17
Voitk, et al.	29	No	75	28
Sheldon, et al.	51	Yes	82	16
MacFadyen, et al.	62	Yes	92	6
Agnirre, et al.	38	Yes	79	21
Reber, et al.	114	Yes 71% No 29%	83	22
Soeters, et al.	128	Yes 57% No 43%	61	21

*Adapted from Goodgame, J. T.: *In* Fischer, J. E. (Ed.): Surgical Nutrition. Boston, Little, Brown and Co., 1983, pp. 779–793.[4]

TABLE 18. Effect of Total Parenteral Nutrition (TPN) on Morbidity and Mortality of Acute Pancreatitis*

Author	n	TPN	Renal Failure	Respiratory Failure	Overall Mortality
Goodgame	46	Yes	15%	28%	20%
Gordon	41	No	15%	—	15%
Interiano	50	No	—	18%	10%
Gleidman	26	No	—	—	35%
Fetter	85	Yes	—	22%	14%
Frey	306	No	—	—	25%
Lawson	15	No	—	—	26%

*Adapted from Goodgame, J. T.: In Fischer, J. E. (Ed.): Surgical Nutrition. Boston, Little, Brown and Co., 1983, pp. 779–793.[4]

acid–enriched solutions in patients with acute hepatic decompensation; however, the role of branched chain amino acid–enriched solutions in liver failure is still under investigation. In contrast to the acute situation, there is general agreement that branched chain amino acid–enriched solutions are of little value in chronic liver failure.

Although there is general agreement that in severely burned patients and in individuals with life-threatening sepsis, those who are malnourished generally do worse than those who are well nourished, the role of branched chain amino acid–enriched solutions in severely stressed individuals still requires clarification.

Peripheral Parenteral Nutrition

In patients who are moderately stressed, provision of amino acids with small amounts of either glucose or fat via a peripheral vein improves nitrogen balance and probably facilitates protein synthesis. However, patients who are markedly hypercatabolic, requiring over 3000 calories and 15 gm. of nitrogen per day, clearly are not candidates for this type of regimen and are generally better managed with conventional TPN.

Peripheral parenteral nutrition (PPN) has been shown to be superior in terms of nitrogen balance to the use of 5 per cent dextrose, and in selected patients this constitutes a useful means of providing short-term protein sparing for periods of 1 to 2 weeks while the patient either recovers or is commenced on either TPN or enteral feeding. A standard approach to PPN would be to use a 5 per cent amino acid stock solution as the nitrogen source combined with both glucose and fat as the energy source; e.g., 1500 ml. of 5 per cent amino acid solution mixed with 75 gm. of glucose provides 12 gm. of nitrogen and 300 calories. The addition of 1500 ml. of 10 per cent lipid emulsion added by a Y connector results in a total caloric intake of 1950 calories and 12 gm. of nitrogen.

In PPN, the use of a central venous catheter is avoided and a lower incidence of septic complications is demonstrated. In addition, catheter care is simpler and metabolic complications are less frequent. Alternatively, TPN can result in the provision of more calories and more nitrogen in a smaller total volume, and in many chronically ill patients, peripheral venous access is difficult.

ENTERAL ALIMENTATION

If the gastrointestinal tract is functional, it is the preferred route for nutritional support. Although with use of the gastrointestinal tract the problems of vascular access seen with both TPN and PPN are avoided, this technique is not without risk. In addition, it has been only comparatively recently that suitable formulas have become available for severely ill patients. Furthermore, the development of fine-bore nasogastric tubes has greatly enhanced patient tolerance of enteral alimentation (EA).

As in TPN, the fundamental issue is the provision of amino acids, calories, vitamins, and trace elements in adequate amounts to achieve or approach positive nitrogen balance.

The same basic principles concerning the simultaneous provision of calories and nitrogen apply in EA as in other forms of alimentation (Table 19). A vast array of nutritional formulas exist, and these may be broadly classified into four groups:

1. Blenderized formulas (food reduced to liquid form).
2. Milk-based formulas.
3. Alimental or defined formula diets (space diets).
4. Modular enteral feeding regimens.

A complete account of the composition of the various preparations available is beyond the scope of this text.

Indications for Enteral Feeding

In general terms, patients with an intact gastrointestinal tract who cannot or will not take food by mouth are candidates for enteral feeding. Specific indications include:

1. Gastrointestinal fistulas.
2. Short bowel syndrome.
3. Inflammatory bowel disease.
4. Pancreatitis.
5. Chronic partial bowel obstruction.
6. Renal failure (specific formulas of essential amino acids are available).
7. Hepatic disease (special formulas, enriched branched chain amino acids are available).
8. Severe burns or other trauma.
9. Sepsis.
10. Cancer patients receiving chemotherapy.
11. Head and neck cancer patients with severe dysphagia.
12. Preoperative bowel preparation.

TABLE 19. Guidelines for Enteral Feeding

1. Use fine-bore (1-mm internal diameter) Dubhoff tube (high patient tolerance)
2. Check x-ray after tube placement to ensure correct position
3. Accurately label food container contents
4. Use continuous flow feeding, not bolus technique
5. Initiate feeding with 20% strength feeds, and increase to full strength over 5 days
6. Administer protein and energy source together with Cal:N_2 ratio 150:1
7. Simultaneously administer doses of vitamins and trace elements
8. Monitor as for total parenteral nutrition

Contraindications

Enteral alimentation should not be given if an adequate oral intake can be maintained; if there is ileus, or bowel obstruction; if there is severe vomiting; or if there are high enterocutaneous fistulas.

SELECTED REFERENCES

Annotated References

Blackburn, G. L., and Thornton, P. A.: Nutritional assessment of the hospitalized patient. Med. Clin. North Am., 63:1103, 1979.
This article provides an in-depth review of the methods for assessing nutritional status in surgical patients. Statistics of malnutrition, plus the indications and the efficacy of nutritional support, are also reviewed.

Fischer, J. E. (Ed.): Surgical Nutrition. Boston, Little, Brown, and Co., 1983.
A complete in-depth coverage of metabolism and nutrition in the surgical patient. The account is presented by 46 authors. Specific topics covered include intermediary metabolism, patient evaluation, physiologic alterations in disease, and specific modes of therapy.

Moore, F. D.: Homeostasis: Bodily changes in trauma and surgery: The responses to injury in man as the basis for clinical management. In Sabiston, D. C., Jr. (Ed.): Davis-Christopher Textbook of Surgery, 12th ed. Philadelphia, W. B. Saunders Company, 1981.
This chapter provides a masterly account of the metabolic alterations seen in surgical patients. The author integrates a considerable amount of personal data with pertinent findings from other investigators.

Popp, M. B., and Brennan, M. F.: Metabolic response to trauma and infection. In Fischer, J. E. (Ed.): Surgical Nutrition. Boston, Little, Brown, and Co., 1983, pp. 479–514.
This chapter presents a comprehensive overview of the metabolic and nutritional responses to injury.

Waterlow, J. C., and Stephen, J. M.: Nitrogen Metabolism in Man. London, Applied Science of England (Elsevier), 1982.
This comprehensive text provides explanations of many of the methods of evaluation used in human protein metabolism.

General References

Brennan, M. F.: Uncomplicated starvation versus cancer cachexia. Cancer Res., 37:2359, 1977.

Burke, J. F., Wolfe, R. R., Mullany, C. J., Mathews, D. W., and Brier, D. M.: Glucose requirements following burn injury. Ann. Surg., 190:274, 1979.
Cahill, G. F.: Starvation in man. N. Engl. J. Med., 282:668, 1970.

REFERENCES

1. Abel, R. M., Beck, C. H., and Abbot, W. M.: Improved survival in acute renal failure after treatment with I.V. amino acids and glucose. N. Engl. J. Med., 288:695, 1973.
2. Brennan, M. F.: Total parenteral nutrition in the cancer patient. N. Engl. J. Med., 305:375, 1981.
3. Brennan, M. F., and Horowitz, G.: Total parenteral nutrition in surgical patients. In Surgery Annual. Chicago, Year Book Medical Publishers, 1983, pp. 1–35.
4. Goodgame, J. T.: A critical evaluation of the results of total parenteral nutrition in various disease states. In Fischer, J.E. (Ed.): Surgical Nutrition. Boston, Little, Brown and Co., 1983, pp. 779–793.
5. Moore, F. D., and Brennan, M. F.: Surgical injury: Body composition, protein metabolism and neuroendocrinology. In Ballinger, W. F. II, et al. (Eds.): American College of Surgeons: Manual of Surgical Nutrition. Philadelphia, W. B. Saunders Company, 1975, pp. 169–222.
5a. Müller, J. M., Keller, H. W., Brenner, U., Walter, M., and Holzmüller, W.: Indications and effects of preoperative parenteral nutrition. World J. Surg., 10:53, 1986.
6. Popp, M. B., and Brennan, M. F.: Metabolic response to trauma and infection. In Fischer, J. E. (Ed.): Surgical Nutrition. Little, Brown and Co., 1983, pp. 479–514.
7. Shaw, J. H. F., Klein, S., and Wolfe, R. R.: Assessment of alanine, urea, and glucose interrelationships in normal subjects and in patients with stable isotopic tracers. Surgery, 97:557, 1985.
7a. Smale, B. F., Mullen, J. L., Buzby, G. P., and Rosato, E. F.: The efficacy of nutritional assessment and support in cancer surgery. Cancer, 47:2375, 1981.
8. Waterlow, J. C., and Stephen, J. M.: Nitrogen Metabolism in Man. London, Elsevier, 1982.
9. Wolfe, R. R., Durkot, M. J., Allsop, J. R., and Burke, J. F.: Glucose metabolism in severely burned patients. Metabolism, 28:1031, 1979.
10. Wolfe, R. R., Durkot, M. J., and Wolfe, M. H.: Effect of thermal injury on energy metabolism, substrate kinetics, and hormonal concentration. Circ. Shock 9:383, 1982.
11. Wolfe, R. R., O'Donnell, T. F., Stone, M. D., Richmond, D. A., and Burke, J. F.: Investigation of factors determining the optimal glucose infusion rate in TPN. Metabolism, 29:892, 1980.

ANESTHESIA

LENNART FAGRAEUS, M.D., PH.D.

7

In the middle of the 19th century, two medical discoveries of particular importance to all surgeons were introduced; namely, anesthesia and antisepsis. Together, these discoveries reduced surgical mortality significantly and allowed surgery to expand its horizon in ways previously unimagined. General anesthesia was first introduced by the demonstration of ether anesthesia at the Massachusetts General Hospital in October 1846. This led to a very rapid acceptance of anesthesiology as a separate clinical discipline.

Today, clinical anesthesiologists participate in the preoperative preparation of the surgical patient, providing intraoperative physiologic life-support and immediate and long-term postoperative care. In addition, care of the critically ill patient, respiratory therapy, diagnostic procedures, and treatment modalities of pain are all examples of services expected to be performed by a modern anesthesia department. As a member of a comprehensive patient care team, the anesthesiologist now has the ability to provide safe anesthesia for a number of new and sophisticated surgical procedures, ranging from radical cancer operations and organ transplantations to complicated cardiac operations in patients of all ages.

This chapter provides only a concise and general overview of clinical anesthesia and the various anesthetic procedures available to the patient. It is hoped, however, that the information, which is admittedly personal and only briefly referenced, may become useful in discussions of the indications for a particular surgical procedure, while at the same time provide a basis for consideration of the hazards of the anesthetic procedure.

PREOPERATIVE PREPARATION

In order for the anesthesiologist to make a rational choice of the procedure for a particular patient undergoing surgery, a careful and thorough preoperative evaluation is essential. The purpose of the preoperative clinical workup and subsequent assessment by the anesthesiologist is to derive pertinent information from the patient's medical history, clinical status, physical examination, and laboratory results. This information helps to classify the patient according to the severity of systemic disease. The American Society of Anesthesiology has adopted a uniform system that has five classes as follows:

1. A normal, healthy patient.
2. A patient with mild systemic disease.
3. A patient with severe systemic disease that limits activity but is not incapacitating.
4. A patient with an incapacitating systemic disease that is a threat to life.
5. A moribund patient not expected to survive over 24 hours with or without surgery.

There is a close, but no direct, correlation of physical status on the one hand and anesthesia and surgical mortality and morbidity on the other, but overall morbidity is at least 4 to 5 times greater in Class 3 and 4 patients than in Class 1 patients.

In addition to the above data, other major factors should be considered preoperatively. The *site and type of surgical procedure* to be performed will have a significant impact on the anesthetic requirements, since the anesthesiologist will tailor the anesthetic technique to the type of operation, the patient's condition, and the physiologic effects of the anesthetic agent. The *physiologic and pharmacologic effects* of the various anesthetic agents play important roles and will be discussed subsequently in this chapter. The *experience of the anesthesiologist* is also important. Not all individuals who can administer an anesthetic are necessarily equally experienced in administering all types of anesthetic procedures. In these times of increasing subspecialization, the experience, background, and training of the anesthesiologist become important factors. As a general rule, it is advisable for an anesthesiologist to administer the type of anesthesia with which he has had the most experience. Finally, the *experience, skill, and training of the surgeon* will become important factors for the anesthesiologist. Anesthetic requirements for inguinal herniorrhaphy are obviously different from those for aortic reconstructive surgery, but so are the anesthetic requirements for an appendectomy by an experienced surgeon who takes 20 minutes for the entire operation different from those of a surgeon who is less experienced and who may require 1½ hours of anesthesia.

PREMEDICATION

Traditionally, the aim of premedication has been to render the patient comfortably sedated and free of apprehension. No medication, however, can take the place of an informative, reassuring preoperative visit by the anesthesiologist, who should take enough time to explain to the patient and relatives the anesthetic procedure and its inherent risks. Also included in this discussion should be diet restrictions, preoperative preparations, monitoring of bodily functions, postoperative emergence from anesthesia, and the postoperative location, e.g., recovery room or intensive care unit. This latter information is especially important if prolonged mechanical ventilation with endotracheal intubation may be necessary. Subsequent to presentation of this information, the patient or, when applicable, the relatives should be asked to give informed consent to the chosen anesthetic procedure.

In addition to sedation before surgery, some measure of analgesia should be considered and provided, especially for those preoperative procedures that may be painful, e.g., invasive monitoring or regional anesthesia. A number of sedative agents, including *barbiturates*, *phenothiazines*, and *benzodiazepines*, therefore, are often combined with an analgesic, usually a *narcotic*. The end result should lead to the average healthy adult arriving in the operating suite calm and cooperative. The pediatric patient, however, who is less likely to respond to the anesthetic induction in a cooperative manner, ideally should be sleeping.

ANESTHETIC TECHNIQUES

Techniques may be broadly divided into the categories of *general* and *regional anesthesia*. Since each of these classifications can be subdivided into several others, with techniques being applied singly or in combination and with the use of a multitude of different pharmacologic agents, it follows that the modern anesthesiologist has the ability to be quite flexible in tailoring procedures to the particular needs of the patient. Although a precise technique is not of particular consequence in a healthy young patient scheduled for elective surgery, it may become critically important in an elderly patient scheduled for a major emergency procedure and who has significant concurrent problems, e.g., ischemic heart disease, increased intracranial pressure, or renal failure.

General Anesthesia

The *anesthesia state*, commonly referred to as *general anesthesia*, is characterized by an induced state of unconsciousness during which surgical stimulation elicits only autonomic reflex responses. Thus, the patient should not exhibit any voluntary movements, but changes in respiratory rate and cardiovascular parameters may be observed. The anesthetic state differs from the *analgesic state*, which may be defined as absence of sensibility to pain. This state can be produced by narcotic agents that are able to relieve pain long before unconsciousness occurs. Conversely, barbiturates and tranquilizers do not relieve pain until complete unconsciousness has occurred. A good anesthetic agent should induce a state of unconsciousness together with a state of analgesia sufficient to prevent critical responses to pain while allowing some basic autonomic reflex activity.

General anesthesia can be induced either by administration of *intravenous anesthetic agents* or by *inhalational (gaseous) anesthetics*, which are absorbed into the pulmonary circulation from the alveoli. Although it is obvious that these two principal techniques differ significantly in many aspects, they share one important common factor. In order to provide optimal conditions for surgery, the patient has to be brought to an adequate depth or level of anesthesia. Since the individual response to a general anesthetic varies greatly and there is no reliable dose-response relationship, the dose of anesthetic agent used must be exactly right. As a guideline, anesthesiologists have used the clinical signs of anesthesia (pupillary size, eye motion, and respiratory rate and volume) of which there are four well-defined stages, each of which can be subdivided into different planes.

During the *first stage*, the patient is still conscious but in an analgesic and amnesic state. In the *second stage*, the patient is unconscious but prone to react unpredictably and usually shows an irregular breathing pattern. The *third stage* provides optimal surgical conditions with adequate respirations and stable hemodynamics. However, at its deeper planes, both respiration and circulation show increasing signs of insufficiency until eventually at the *fourth stage* cardiovascular collapse and respiratory arrest develop.

These clinical signs were adopted during the era of ether anesthesia and are now difficult to use, since present-day anesthetic agents affect pupillary size differently and are much more potent respiratory depressants. Therefore, in order to administer adequate anesthetic dosages, more emphasis is today placed on continuous monitoring of heart rate, electrocardiogram (ECG), respiratory rate, and frequent measurements of blood pressure.

INTRAVENOUS ANESTHESIA

Advantages of intravenous anesthesia include better patient compliance, a lack of claustrophobic feeling (as when a mask is applied to the face), rapid onset of unconsciousness, and general convenience for the anesthesiologist. Intravenous agents, therefore, lend themselves to induction of anesthesia except in the very young pediatric patients, in whom the insertion of an intravenous cannula is too much of a stress.

Among the disadvantages, the most prominent ones are the very rapid (sometimes too rapid) induction and the significant cerebral depression achieved, as seen by respiratory arrest necessitating assisted ventilation, and hemodynamic instability. However, this is not to say that the analgesic level may be adequate for surgical stimulation, especially since after a few minutes redistribution of the anesthetic agent into various tissue compartments, together with hepatic and renal biotransformation, may rapidly decrease blood levels to a point where the patient may regain awareness. For this reason, intravenous induction agents are usually used together with *nitrous oxide* or other inhalational anesthetics to achieve sufficient analgesia and with *muscle relaxants* to provide optimal surgical conditions. Besides complex pharmacokinetics, other disadvantages of intravenous anesthesia lie in the fact that it cannot be reversed as easily as can inhalational anesthesia and that there is a potential for drug interaction, especially in the elderly, chronically sick patient who often presents a pharmaceutical challenge.

In spite of these disadvantages, however, intravenous anesthesia is becoming increasingly popular and is today, outside of the young pediatric patient groups, the preferred way to induce and partially maintain anesthesia. An additional reason for the popularity of intravenous anesthesia is that it eliminates the risk of pollution in the operating rooms posed by the inhalational agents, and thereby the exposure by anesthesia personnel to these agents, and reduces the risk of some very special toxic reactions that have been reported in patients under general inhalational anesthesia.

The ultra–short-acting barbiturates, e.g., *sodium thiopental* or *methohexital*, or *etomidate*, a carboxylated imidazole, and a number of tranquilizers, e.g., the *benzodiazepines* and *droperidol*, are the agents most frequently used for induction of general anesthesia or sedation for regional anesthesia. In addition, in recent years, potent analgesics have also been used for general anesthesia, but they are associated with important side effects. For instance, *ketamine* has a sympathetic stimulating effect and is, therefore, contraindicated in patients with hypertension or increased intracranial pressure.

Narcotic agents, e.g., *morphine*, *meperidine*, and *fentanyl*, are well known for causing respiratory depression, which may be particularly dangerous in the postoperative period. However, recent developments in ultra–short-acting narcotics, e.g., the new phenylpiperidine derivatives *alfentanil*, *sufentanil*, and *carfentanil*, are promising, in that they allow patients to regain respiratory function much faster while at the same time provide cardiovascular stability. This latter ability, which is characteristic of most narcotics, is an increasingly important factor today, since more and more surgical patients are elderly and are considered poor anesthetic risks because of cardiovascular system disease. The technique utilizing potent analgesic agents (narcotics), together with a sedative drug of the butyrophenone derivatives (haloperidol or droperidol), has been called *neuroleptanalgesia*. It produces strong analgesia, marked tranquility, and apparent somnolence without loss of consciousness. When nitrous oxide, other inhalational agents, and muscle relaxants are added to produce complete general anesthesia for a major surgery procedure, the technique is referred to as *neuroleptanesthesia*, or balanced anesthesia. It usually provides stable hemodynamics, reduced reflex activity, strong analgesia, and excellent amnesia as well as good antiemetic effects postoperatively and has been used with good results in poor-risk patients.

INHALATION ANESTHESIA

A variety of inhaled agents can produce general anesthesia; these range from inert gases (e.g., argon and xenon), which are not metabolized, to halogenated hydrocarbons (e.g., halothane, enflurane), which undergo partial metabolization by the liver. Nitrous oxide, without question the most widely used inhalational agent today, exhibits minimal biotransformation.

Inhalational anesthetics, while ranging widely in potency, have one important advantage compared with intravenous agents. They can all be administered and reversed in a controlled and rapid fashion, since they are absorbed, as well as excreted, via the lungs (alveoli). Because their potency varies widely, attempts have been made to establish a standard dose or an index of equipotency for each agent by which comparison of the pharmacologic and physiologic properties of various inhalational agents is made possible. The minimal alveolar concentration (MAC) of a given agent, defined as the concentration at which 50 per cent of the patients move in response to a painful stimulation, has been used as such an index since the early 1960s. Although attractively simple and easy to understand, only 1.0 MAC values of different inhaled anesthetics represent equianesthetic levels of general anesthesia. A limitation of the MAC concept is found in the facts that dose-response curves for the various agents vary widely and that multiples of MAC do not represent equianesthetic levels. Another limitation is that the MAC concept compares anesthesia levels only

and is unable to predict physiologic effects on important organ systems, e.g., cardiovascular and renal functions, especially in the chronically ill patient.

Currently, a functional index of anesthetic agents is lacking; in fact it may be impossible to establish since the individual responses to a given concentration of an agent vary widely between patients. Nevertheless, the concept of MAC represents an important step both clinically and in understanding the mechanism of action of inhalation anesthesia.

Nitrous Oxide

Nitrous oxide (N_2O) is undoubtedly the most widely used inhalation anesthetic agent today. It is a non-explosive, inorganic gas, which because of its low blood/gas partition coefficient, allows rapid equilibration between alveoli and pulmonary circulation. Therapeutic concentrations in the arterial blood going to the brain, therefore, are obtained very rapidly. Nitrous oxide is, however, mainly an analgesic, and its major disadvantage is that it cannot induce true anesthesia at normal atmospheric pressure without decreasing the oxygen concentration in the inhaled gas mixture to hypoxic levels. The MAC for nitrous oxide is 105 per cent; i.e., it would require hyperbaric conditions to use nitrous oxide as the sole anesthetic agent. Since that is impractical, it is instead employed together with other more potent anesthetic agents, either intravenous or inhalational. In addition, in order to provide optimal working conditions for major surgery, a neuromuscular blocking agent is frequently added to constitute what is commonly referred to as a *balanced anesthetic technique*.

By use of a balanced technique in which a combination of drugs is used, each at low concentrations or doses, it is possible to reduce the depressant cardiovascular effects of many of the halogenated inhalational agents or the respiratory depressant effects of the narcotics while still providing adequate anesthesia and analgesia and skeletal muscle relaxation.

The use of nitrous oxide, however, is not without risks. One hazard is the potential for nitrous oxide to induce arterial hypoxemia and insufficient oxygen delivery when used in high concentrations, especially in patients with significant pulmonary or cardiac disease. In particular, during thoracic or upper abdominal surgery, intraoperative gas distribution in the lungs will significantly affect ventilation-perfusion ratios, which when added to the patient's preexisting cardiopulmonary disease will further decrease oxygen saturation and delivery.

Two other clinical situations exist in which the physical properties of nitrous oxide have undesirable effects. Both hazards relate to the fact that nitrous oxide is much more (34 times) soluble in blood than in nitrogen. As a result, caution must be exercised when nitrous oxide is administered to patients with inadvertent air in closed-off cavities, e.g., bowel, pleura, and middle ear. When used in concentrations above 50 per cent, nitrous oxide will diffuse rapidly into the nitrogen-containing space, leading to an increase in trapped volume, or, in a nonelastic space such as the middle ear, to an increase in pressure. In such instances, nitrous oxide is best avoided or, if used, should be administered only in low concentrations, i.e., below 40 per cent.

The other physical hazard occurs immediately following surgery and during emergence from anesthesia. If room air is used when the anesthetic agents are turned off, the influx of large quantities of nitrous oxide from the blood into the alveoli could dilute the 20.9 per cent oxygen in room air to unsafe levels, eventually producing diffusion hypoxia. In order to avoid this problem, it is important that the patient is administered oxygen-enriched gas mixtures in the immediate postoperative period.

Halothane

Halothane ($CF_3CHBrCl$) has been the second most widely used inhalational anesthetic over the last 30 years. It is a very potent, non-explosive, halogenated hydrocarbon with an MAC of 0.77 per cent and is, unlike nitrous oxide, a total anesthetic; i.e., it can be used to attain all levels of surgical anesthesia. Halothane also has good patient acceptance, and emergence is associated with a low incidence of nausea and vomiting.

There are some major disadvantages to the use of halothane. Respiration is depressed and respiratory acidosis develops if ventilation is not supported or controlled. Myocardial function is also depressed and cardiac output reduced. In addition, significant vasodilation occurs and can lead to a pooling of blood in the peripheral circulation. Together with the weakened cardiac function, this leads to arterial hypotension, which may become significant and dangerous in the patient who is hypovolemic, secondary to hemorrhage or depletion of extracellular fluid volume as in trauma, intestinal obstruction, or dehydration. However, when used in low concentrations, as in the balanced anesthesia technique, the cardiovascular effects of halothane can be put to good use in deliberately lowering arterial pressure. This technique is commonly referred to as *controlled hypotension* and is often useful because blood and fluid losses can be significantly reduced during extensive surgical procedures or when blood transfusions cannot be administered. It must be emphasized, however, that controlled hypotension can also be induced by other anesthetic agents with vasodilatory effects, e.g., enflurane and isoflurane, or with potent intravenous vasodilators, e.g., nitroprusside and nitroglycerin.

In addition, halothane sensitizes the myocardium to both endogenously produced and extrinsically administered catecholamines. This may lead to cardiac arrhythmias that could be life-threatening. Thus, catecholamine-containing agents are best avoided in patients under halothane anesthesia, and the level of anesthesia should be kept at a deep enough level to avoid significant stress response, i.e., catecholamine release.

Finally, a rare but sometimes disastrous complication is the development of "halothane hepatitis" or even hepatic necrosis. This clinical syndrome has been ascribed to an allergic or hypersensitivity reaction to either halothane or its metabolites and usually consists of the development of a diffuse hepatitis 2 to 5 days following anesthesia. It must be emphasized, however, that many other conditions seen in surgical patients are associated with a hepatitis-like clinical picture. Therefore, the very existence of "halothane hepatitis" is still debated, and the risk involved in the judicious use of halothane has not been proven great enough to ban its use. It must be concluded that halothane still remains a safe and effective inhalation anesthetic when used appropriately.

Enflurane

Enflurane (CHF_2OCF_2CHFCl) is another halogenated hydrocarbon of great potency (MAC of enflurane is 1.68 per cent in oxygen). It represents a group of more recently synthesized compounds tailor-made to combine a stable ether link (for anesthetic effect) with halogen molecules (F for nonflammability and Cl for anesthetic effect). Induction is rapid, and depression of respiratory and cardiovascular systems occurs largely to the same extent as with halothane. Enflurane differs from halothane, however, in several important ways. It has no myocardial sensitizing effects to catecholamines and tends to potentiate the response to neuromuscular blocking drugs. Few, if any, convincing cases of halothane-like hepatotoxicity have been reported. This is possibly due to the fact that the percentage of enflurane that undergoes biotransformation is only a fraction of that observed with halothane. Instead, enflurane appears to have a potential for causing renal dysfunction that is probably associated with increased plasma levels of inorganic fluoride. Although there are no strong data to prove that a given plasma level of inorganic fluoride is nephrotoxic, it would seem appropriate to avoid or limit the use of enflurane in patients with significant preexisting renal disease or those undergoing renal transplantation. Finally, in a small percentage of normal patients the use of enflurane is associated with the development of electroencephalographic (EEG) patterns characteristic of epilepsy. The clinical significance of these abnormal EEG changes, however, seem dubious, especially since they do not appear more frequently in patients with epilepsy. Nevertheless, until the neurophysiologic events leading to these changes have been elucidated, it seems prudent to avoid the use of enflurane in epileptics.

Isoflurane

Isoflurane ($CHF_2OCHClCF_3$) is the most recent addition to the group of potent halogenated hydrocarbons (introduced on the market in 1980). Its MAC is 1.15 per cent in oxygen. Isoflurane is an isomer of enflurane; however, although it can be employed in much the same way, it differs from enflurane in some important aspects. Isoflurane undergoes no or only minimal biotransformation; i.e., it is excreted unchanged via the lungs, and, as such, it comes close to the long-sought concept of the "ideal" anesthetic agent. It depresses the myocardium less than other halogenated agents do, it is a more potent vasodilator, and it potentiates the effects of both major types of muscle relaxants. Although more extensive human studies on the clinical safety features of isoflurane are needed, it may well be the last halogenated agent to be introduced.

Other Inhalational Agents

Many other inhalational anesthetic agents have been used in the past but with mixed success rates. A brief list of previously used inhalational agents include the historically well known *ether* and its related compounds, *chloroform*, *cyclopropane*, *ethylene*, *trichloroethylene*, *fluroxene*, and *methoxyflurane*. Although many of these agents are quite potent and a few of them do not depress respiration and circulation, all share the disadvantage of either being explosive, chemically unstable, or toxic to the liver and kidneys.

NEUROMUSCULAR BLOCKING AGENTS (MUSCLE RELAXANTS)

Commonly, the intravenous neuromuscular blocking agents, also called muscle relaxants, are classified into two groups, i.e., *nondepolarizing* agents, e.g., curare, and *depolarizing* agents, e.g., succinylcholine. It must be emphasized, however, that muscle relaxation can be produced also by other means, e.g., centrally by attaining deep levels of general anesthesia or peripherally by the use of regional anesthesia (local nerve block).

Nondepolarizing agents prevent access of acetylcholine to the receptor site of the myoneural junction. In doing so, they prevent depolarization of the motor end-plate, and no contraction can take place (paralysis). No muscular fasciculation is seen after intravenous administration, in contrast to the case with the depolarizing agents, which work by depolarizing the motor end-plate in a fashion similar to that of acetylcholine. The depolarization then spreads to the muscle fibers, initially causing fasciculation, but eventually making them electrically unresponsive to subsequent stimulation. The result is a flaccid paralysis of the muscles.

Muscle relaxants provide profound muscle relaxation and optimal surgical conditions without the need for deep levels of anesthesia. However, the use of relaxants carries with it significant risks. The most obvious one is the patient's inability to breathe spontaneously, since all muscles, including the respiratory muscles, are paralyzed. This inability to breathe must be compensated by artificial ventilation either manually or by a respirator. Great care must be exercised in delivering an adequate minute volume so that respiratory acidosis or hypoxia does not develop. Duration of action is dose-dependent, but is also influenced by other factors, e.g., electrolyte abnormalities, levels of plasma cholinesterase and administration of antibiotics. If the effect of a muscle relaxant is not reversed, it may extend beyond the duration of the surgical procedure. This would lead to the patient's becoming apneic or too weak to breathe spontaneously after completion of surgery and after emergence from the anesthetic procedure. In the case of a nondepolarizing relaxant, its effect can be reversed by the intravenous administration of anticholinesterase, e.g., neostigmine. Since anticholinesterases usually induce muscarinic stimulation leading to significant bradycardia, atropine or other vagolytic agents must be administered simultaneously. In order for the proper dose for the reversal drugs to be calculated, the magnitude of neuromuscular blockade should be measured. This could be performed by determination of the patient's muscle function, e.g., by the ability to lift the head from the support or the strength of the hand grip. More objective and reliable is an assessment of the patient's respiratory ability by use of a simple respirometer. The combined measurements of tidal volume, vital capacity, and maximal negative pressure that the patient can generate often provide sufficient information of respiratory capacity. This approach, however, suffers from a significant limitation in that it requires a level of cooperation and motivation that may well be lacking in a patient who is tested immediately after the surgical procedure or who has been given narcotics or other long-acting anesthetic agents.

The most reliable way of determining the magnitude of neuromuscular blockade, regardless of anesthetic agents used, is a standardized electrical stimulation of a peripheral motor nerve. This technique also allows frequent assessments of the degree of paralysis during the anesthetic procedure, thereby avoiding overdosage, while at the same time providing a relatively constant degree of muscle relaxation, which will facilitate the surgical procedure. A potential limitation lies in the fact that neuromuscular function, as measured in a peripheral nerve and muscle group, may not be the same as for the respiratory muscles. Different muscle groups have been found to be dissimilar in both sensitivity to various muscle relaxants and in rate of recovery. Final proof of adequacy of ventilation is obtained through repeated arterial blood gas analysis.

Succinylcholine. Succinylcholine is the most widely used depolarizing muscle relaxant. It has a very quick onset, a short duration (3 to 5 minutes), and a rapid recovery phase. Succinylcholine was introduced clinically in 1952 and has since then been mostly used immediately after induction of anesthesia to facilitate intubation of the trachea or to provide muscle relaxation for short surgical procedures. As such, it is given either as a bolus injection or by continuous intravenous infusion. Prolonged paralysis is seen after overdose when the depolarizing block is transformed to a nondepolarizing neuromuscular blockade. Delayed recovery is also seen in patients with low or atypical plasma cholinesterase levels. Side effects include muscle pains (after fasciculation), significant release of potassium from muscle tissue after burns, severe trauma, spinal cord injuries, and the development of malignant hyperthermia and rigidity (incidence approximately 1 per 100,000).

Curare. Among the nondepolarizing muscle relaxants, curare (d-tubocurarine) has been used for centuries by natives of South America as a poison applied to the heads of their arrows. Curare was introduced into clinical practice in 1942. It is a relatively long-acting agent; after a clinical dose of 0.3 to 0.5 mg. per kg., the approximate duration of action is 30 to 40 minutes. When curare or other nondepolarizing agents are used, caution must be exercised with patients suffering from myasthenia gravis, since they are extremely sensitive to these compounds. Other undesirable effects of curare include the risk for histamine release and ganglionic blocking action.

Pancuronium. Pancuronium is not associated with these side effects. It is a relatively new (1972) and a more potent long-acting, nondepolarizing agent than curare. One undesirable effect of this drug is tachycardia secondary to sympathetic stimulation. This may cause problems for patients with ischemic heart disease because of the associated increase in myocardial oxygen requirements.

Gallamine. Gallamine has a shorter duration than do curare and pancuronium. It is an undesirable drug for patients with renal insufficiency or failure, since it is entirely excreted by the kidney.

Metocurine. Metocurine is a more recent nondepolarizing agent that produces less tachycardia than pancuronium and gallamine and less hypotension from histamine release and ganglion blocking action than does curare.

Atracurium. Very recently, atracurium was introduced as a nondepolarizing agent with minimal cardiovascular effects. It is metabolized by means of the Hoffmann elimination, which is a nonenzymatic spontaneous degradation in body tissue that takes place at normal body temperature and pH. It is also hydrolyzed by nonspecific esterases in the plasma. It can, therefore, be used in patients with renal or hepatic failure, and also in patients with low or atypical plasma cholinesterase levels.

Vecuronium. A recent derivative of pancuronium, vecuronium has shown shorter duration than has pancuronium and minimal cardiovascular effects. It is excreted by the liver into the bile and thus can be used in patients with renal disease; however, there may be prolonged effects in patients with hepatic insufficiency.

Regional Anesthesia (Nerve Block)

LIMITATIONS

Regional anesthesia refers to all anesthetic techniques utilizing nerve blocks to obtain complete pain relief. With the afferent nerve impulse flow interrupted (deafferentiated), regional anesthesia comes close to the "ideal" or stress free anesthesia concept; however, it is used less frequently than might be expected because of several limitations:

1. A nerve block takes time to induce, and turnover time between surgical cases may be unnecessarily extended.

2. There is always the risk that the nerve block might not be fully effective, in which case the patient may need a repeat injection (if within safe dose limits of the particular local anesthetic) or may be given a general anesthetic. Either of these steps will further extend the time before surgery, in addition to which the patient is also caused further inconvenience.

3. There is always a possibility that the nerve block either will lead to neurologic complications or, if it affects a significant part of the vascular bed, may cause hemodynamic instability that may be dangerous in the elderly, atherosclerotic patient, the trauma victim, or the hypovolemic patient.

4. Poor patient compliance is always a problem because many patients are afraid of being "awake" and do not wish to listen to the various sounds in the operating room.

Although it may be thought that regional anesthesia is safer than general anesthesia because there is less physiologic disturbance associated with a nerve block, there have been no earlier studies to support this concept. However, recent data from the literature indicate that in selected cases, especially in elderly patients, complications of surgery, e.g., deep venous thrombosis and pulmonary embolism, may be significantly reduced by the use of regional anesthesia. Today, a well-conducted and skillfully applied regional anesthetic will give just as satisfactory results as a good general anesthetic.

CLASSIFICATION

Local anesthetic agents can be classified into two categories: *amino-esters* (procaine, chloroprocaine, and tetracaine), and *amino-amides* (lidocaine, bupivacaine, etidocaine, and mepivacaine). Ester-linked drugs are metabolized through hydrolysis and amides by oxidative dealkylation in the liver. Anaphylactoid reactions are well documented in the case of ester-linked agents, but are very rare after administration of amides.

EFFECTS

Regional anesthesia techniques today range from topical application of a local anesthetic to neural blockade of large parts of the body during spinal or epidural anesthesia. There is a direct relationship between concentration of local anesthetics used and size of nerve affected. Thus, one may go from sympathetic, to somatosensory, and finally motor nerve block by simply increasing the concentration of the local anesthetic used. The duration of a nerve block is directly related to what local anesthetic agent is being used, but for any given agent, higher concentrations will have longer effects. In addition, the duration of a nerve block can be extended by adding a vasoconstrictor, e.g., epinephrine or neosynephrine, to the local anesthetic solution, thereby delaying reabsorption and prolonging the effect.

An important disadvantage of regional anesthesia might be seen with the sympathetic blockade obtained during spinal or epidural anesthesia. During these procedures, large areas of the peripheral vascular bed become dilated and hypotension may develop, secondary to pooling of blood primarily in the venous or capacitance vessels of the circulation. It is, therefore, important to monitor the patient's blood pressure carefully during regional anesthesia. Ideally, before administration of a nerve block that may lead to a sympathetic block of a significant part of the vascular bed, one should consider "preloading" the patient with an appropriate volume of intravenous fluids to prevent a sudden significant hypotensive response. Such a response is exaggerated in patients who already have blood volume deficits, e.g., peritonitis, and hemorrhagic or septic shock.

A promising new field of regional anesthesia relates to the excellent pain control achieved by small amounts of narcotics into the subarachnoid or epidural space. It is known that opioid receptors in the dorsal horn of the spinal cord react with the injected narcotic agent to produce significant spinal analgesia. A major advantage with the use of spinal or epidural narcotics is the long duration after each injection (several times that of any local anesthetic) and the absence of sympathetic block. A disadvantage is that the pain relief is not enough for surgical stimulation, and among the undesirable effects are itching, urine retention, and the risk for late respiratory depression. However, these can be reversed by the administration of a narcotic antagonist, and the technique has found widespread use, particularly for postoperative pain relief.

OTHER ANESTHETIC TECHNIQUES

Acupuncture

Acupuncture is an old technique for pain relief that has been used in the Far East and Asia for some four thousand years. Renewed interest in acupuncture after World War II led to its introduction as a clinical anesthesia modality in the early 1970s in the United States. The theory is that vital forces flow in "meridians" in the body and that these flows are disturbed in disease. A disturbed meridian can be treated by inserting a needle at a specific point in the body, which has over 1000 such acupuncture points. This corrects the disturbance and induces analgesia. Unfortunately, opinions differ widely about the right positions for needle insertion. Naloxone (a narcotic antagonist) inhibits the analgesia effects of acupuncture, thus suggesting that endorphins are involved in creating the analgesic state. Recent controlled studies have shown that acupuncture has an effect similar to that of a placebo. Therefore, enthusiasm for acupuncture for pain relief during surgical procedures has declined. However, it may in selected cases be of value in patients with chronic pain not amenable to more conventional forms of therapy. Complications include infection, serum hepatitis, hematomas, nerve damage, and pneumothorax.

Hypnosis

The use of hypnosis for pain relief was first reported at the end of the 18th century and remained relatively popular for minor surgery until the introduction of inhalation anesthesia in 1846, at which time hypnosis was largely abandoned from surgical practice. The mechanism of hypnosis is not well understood, but it is thought that after the patient has been brought into a trance-like state, a painful sensation is modified by symptom suppression and then interpreted by the patient as an innocuous or comfortable sensation. There is a possibility that hypnosis may occasionally release underlying psychiatric disorders. Although hypnosis was officially approved in the United States in 1958 as a therapeutic tool, it has been of limited clinical value, except in selected cases. Within the field of somatic medicine, the most common use of hypnosis has been for the relief of various painful states, especially during childbirth and in dentistry.

Electrical Anesthesia

By direct application of high-frequency, low-voltage, and low-amperage currents, electrical anesthesia was introduced in the late 19th century, but never received widespread popularity. The various suggested mechanisms potentially leading to a state of anesthesia include interruption of sympathetic transmission by electric current, interference with intracellular ion exchange, and blocking of neuronal circuits. Among the disadvantages are the difficulty in obtaining an adequate anesthetic level and an increase in blood pressure. Therefore, the technique is contraindicated in patients with moderate to severe hypertension. Another disadvantage is the muscle rigidity seen in many patients, a side effect that sometimes requires large doses of muscle relaxants. This technique has little to offer in the modern anesthesiology service.

Regional Hypothermia

It has long been known that cold can produce a local or regional nerve block. Over the past one hundred years, regional hypothermia, or *refrigeration analgesia*, has been used to control pain ranging from infection to cancer. With a lowering of the local temperature, the metabolism is reduced and the nerve conduction impulses are slowed down and finally blocked, as if a local anesthetic had been injected. In some carefully selected poor-risk and malnourished patients, this technique may have some advantage over other more involved anesthetic techniques, especially under field conditions in primitive environments. In the modern clinical setting, however, there is no significant advantage over standard clinical techniques. The application of more intense cold, *cryotherapy*, utilizes the destructive properties of subzero temperatures for minor surgery (e.g., hemorrhoidectomy) or selected nerve blocks for pain relief (e.g., ilio-inguinal, intercostal) or control of arrhythmias by interrupting intracardiac aberrant conduction pathways.

INTRAOPERATIVE MONITORING

It is important that vital signs be adequately monitored during the anesthetic procedure, since this period may well be the most dangerous one in the patient's life. While modern electronic devices offer sophisticated monitoring of a variety of variables, the old "finger-on-the-pulse technique" still maintains its central role for monitoring cardiovascular status, highlighting the fact that the most important feature is the patient-anesthesiologist interface. Repeated clinical examinations are of primary importance. More specifically, the hands, eyes, and ears of the attending anesthesiologist remain the basic tools for measurement and monitoring, supplemented by the stethoscope and blood pressure cuff.

Minimal requirements for monitoring during a standard anesthetic procedure in an otherwise healthy patient include heart rate, ECG, arterial blood pressure, respiratory rate, and body temperature. In addition, a precordial or an esophageal stethoscope allows for continuous evaluation of both heart and breath sounds, whereas for longer cases, urinary output is a useful index of renal function and an indirect measure of cardiovascular function. Except for urinary output, these variables are obtained by noninvasive techniques.

For high-risk patients (e.g., open-heart cases, trauma, severe burns) in whom major shifts in blood volume can be anticipated, intraarterial pressure monitoring is recommended using an arterial catheter. This also allows for frequent blood sampling for blood gas analysis. These patients may also require central venous pressure monitoring by means of a venous catheter positioned in an intrathoracic vein. Usually, about half of the total blood volume is accommodated in the systemic venous system, and only approximately 15 per cent is found in the arterial system; thus, small changes in venous tone and volume capacity can make significant changes in the regulation of the hemodynamics of the circulatory system. In the normal patient, changes in the central venous pressure (right atrial filling pressures) may give some indication of changes in left atrial filling pressures. However, when cardiac function is abnormal, as in the patient with ischemic or valvular heart disease, right and left arterial pressures may not be closely related. In these cases, it becomes necessary to estimate left atrial filling pressures by inserting a pulmonary artery catheter, usually referred to as a *Swan-Ganz catheter*. This is a balloon-tipped, flow-directed flexible catheter that can be floated into one of the major branches of the pulmonary artery. When the balloon is inflated, the pressure measured at the tip of the catheter is an approximation of the filling pressure of the left atrium. The catheter can also be used for measuring the cardiac output by the thermodilution technique. Recently, fiberoptic versions of pulmonary catheters have been introduced that allow continuous measurement of mixed venous oxygen saturation. This variable may serve as an early warning of insufficient oxygen delivery to the body, secondary to low cardiac output, respiratory failure, or increased metabolic demands.

The EEG as a measure of the circulation to the brain is a more sensitive index of the failing heart than the ECG, and it is a valuable monitor during operations involving carotid artery surgery or extracorporeal circulation. The integrated and simplified version of the EEG is used as a cerebral function monitor. The sum of cortical activity has, in recent years, been used to estimate depth of anesthesia. However, a more specific and sensitive method for monitoring selective central nervous system function is the evoked potential technique, e.g., utilizing somatosensory, visual, or auditory stimulation. Peripheral nerve stimulators are frequently used to assess the amount of depression of neuromuscular transmission by muscle relaxants or anesthetic agents.

Finally, the most modern anesthesia machines are equipped with instruments by which continuous analysis of the inspired and expired gas mixtures (oxygen, carbon dioxide, and halogenated hydrocarbons) can be obtained. In addition, simple spirometry (tidal volume and minute ventilation) can be performed with an in-line respirometer connected to the expiratory limb of the breathing circuit. Gas flows can be measured by a pneumotachograph, which is also placed in the breathing circuit. In addition, repeated samples for blood gas determination and acid-base analysis can now be performed either inside or in proximity to the operating room.

In summary, it is obvious that the anesthesiologist, in performing an anesthetic procedure, has at his disposal the equivalent of an acute care laboratory. However, to reiterate, the *hands, eyes* and *ears* of the anesthesiologist remain the basic and most important tools for intraoperative patient monitoring.

THE POSTOPERATIVE VISIT

The close patient-physician relationship that was established during the preoperative visit should be continued and maintained during the postoperative period. A follow-up visit, therefore, is made to all patients within the first 24–hour period postoperatively. The only exceptions would be surgical outpatients who are released from the hospital the same day. The visit provides the patient with an opportunity to relate his experiences to the anesthesiologist, who simultaneously can evaluate the patient for possible complications attributable to the anesthetic procedure. Any complications should be noted and discussed with the patient, especially such adverse reactions that may be important to report to another anethesiologist, should anesthesia and surgery be necessary in the future. Examples of such adverse reactions may include malignant hyperthermia, prolonged effect of muscle relaxants, and allergic reactions, but also unusual upper airway anatomy that may make it difficult to maintain an unobstructed airway or to intubate the patient, and the development of cardiac pathology, e.g., a myocardial infarction. The well-informed patient who is able to warn the anesthesiologist of potential adverse reactions can play a role in significantly reducing the risks during a subsequent anesthetic procedure.

COMPLICATIONS AND SEQUELAE OF ANESTHESIA

Mishaps in connection with anesthesia are infrequent, but the destabilizing effect of the surgical procedure on a particular organ system, together with anesthesia-related depressions in vital bodily functions could, if not identified, quickly turn a minor aberration into a major complication. Anesthesia-related deaths constitute approximately 2 per cent of the overall surgical mortality and can be broken down into four very broad categories:

1. Hypovolemia from inadequate fluid and blood management.

2. Respiratory failure following the use of narcotics and/or muscle relaxants.

3. Inability to maintain an adequate airway, including complications of intubation.

4. Insufficient supervision and care in the immediate postoperative period.

Obviously, the ideal way to manage complications is to prevent their occurrence. Hence, the experienced anesthesiologist is familiar with the surgical procedure and has appropriate knowledge of the physiologic and pharmacologic effects of the anesthesia technique chosen for the particular surgical procedure. Some disease states dictate avoidance of certain drugs or anesthetic techniques, and the following conditions exemplify just a few of many situations in which the skilled anesthesiologist can prevent the occurrence of a major complication.

In order to prevent profound hypotension, a hypovolemic patient should not receive anesthetic agents that produce uncontrollable vasodilatation or significant myocardial depresssion, nor should the patient with increased intracranial pressure be given drugs that will further increase intracranial pressure. Barbiturates are contraindicated for patients with porphyria, and succinylcholine should not be given to patients with atypical pseudocholinesterase or plasmocholinesterase deficiency. If a patient is known to be susceptible to malignant hyperthermia, halogenated hydrocarbons, succinylcholine, and local anesthetic agents of the amide type must be avoided, as should nitrous oxide in those cases where the patient has air in a closed-off body space, e.g., pneumothorax and bowel obstruction.

Finally, major regional anesthesia, e.g., spinal or epidural blockade, should be avoided in the patient with a bleeding disorder or in one who is heparinized because of the risk of uncontrolled bleeding in the epidural space, which could result in spinal cord compression. Although the anesthetic risk can never be eliminated, it can be reduced significantly by appropriate preparation of the patient, choice of anesthetic technique, frequent checking of the anesthesia equipment, and vigilant monitoring of the patient during and after the surgical procedure.

SUMMARY

This general overview of basic anesthesia has been kept very concise and is not intended to provide the reader with skills needed to anesthetize a patient. Nevertheless, it is hoped that this brief introduction to anesthesia will cause the reader to reflect on the overall anesthetic management of the patient and on the essential role of the anesthesiologist as a key member of the surgical care team. For further information, the interested reader is referred to standard comprehensive textbooks listed among the references.

SELECTED REFERENCES

Atkinson, R. S., Rushman, G. B., and Lee, J. A.: A Synopsis of Anaesthesia. Bristol, Great Britain, John Wright & Sons Ltd., 1982.

Bromage, P. R.: Epidural Analgesia. Philadelphia, W. B. Saunders Company, 1978.
This is an excellent text concerning epidural analgesia and includes pharmacologic aspects of local anesthetics.

Churchill-Davidson, H. D. (Ed.): Wylie and Churchill-Davidson's A Practice of Anaesthesia. Chicago, Year Book Medical Publishers, Inc., 1984.

Cousins, M. J., and Bridenbaugh, P. O. (Eds.): Neural blockade. *In* Clinical Anesthesia and Management of Pain. Philadelphia, J. B. Lippincott Company, 1980.

Dripps, R. D., Eckenhoff, J. E., and Vandam, L. D.: Introduction to Anesthesia: The Principles of Safe Practice. Philadelphia, W. B. Saunders Company, 1982.
A highly recommended introductory text. It has been an excellent resource through numerous editions and contains much important data.

Greene, N. M.: Physiology of Spinal Anesthesia. Baltimore, The Williams and Wilkins Company, 1981.

Gregory, G. A.: Pediatric Anesthesia. New York, Churchill Livingstone, 1983.

Krechel, S. W. (Ed.): Anesthesia and the Geriatric Patient. Orlando, Fla., Grune & Stratton, Inc., 1984.

Levine, R. D.: Anesthesiology: A Manual for Medical Students. Philadelphia, J. B. Lippincott Company, 1984.

Miller, R. D. (Ed.): Anesthesia. New York, Churchill Livingstone, 1986.
A current, updated textbook that provides considerable detail of all aspects of anesthesia both theoretical and practical. It is an unusually valuable reference source.

Shnider, S., and Levinson, G.: Anesthesia for Obstetrics. Baltimore, The Williams and Wilkins Company, 1979.

WOUND HEALING AND MANAGEMENT

PETER J. E. CRUSE, M.B., CH.B. • N. TAIT McPHEDRAN, M.D.

8

Wounds heal by an inflammatory reaction, the ultimate purpose of which is to produce a firm scar to unite the injured part and restore function.

HISTORICAL ASPECTS

From the time of the Sumerian Tablet, which made recommendations for treatment of wounds in the dynasty of Ur in Mesopotamia in 2000 B.C., to the present, many have studied the process of wound healing and have designated treatments to enhance this process. Throughout recorded history, treatment of wounds has reflected society's attitude toward illness and disease. The Egyptians applied unguents and dressings, but relied heavily on religious invocations. The Greeks, at the time of Hippocrates, made a step forward by separating the management of illness from religion. For wounds they favored cleanliness and minimal intervention. The Romans disdained fallen gladiators, but using Greek methods, they treated soldiers in well-designed hospitals. In the Middle Ages, the advent of gunpowder changed the methods of warfare. There were more devastating injuries, and boiling oil was poured into wounds in the mistaken belief that toxic products of gunpowder explosion needed to be removed from the wound by heat. Ambroise Paré established a permanent place in medical history when he recognized, and then taught, that gunshot wounds healed more quickly, with improved patient survival, if cauterization was not done. John Hunter, in the late 18th century, first proposed the definition given in the opening paragraph and was the first to advocate leaving war wounds open to heal by second intention (see below).

In modern times, much has been learned about the process of wound healing and some of the factors that impair the process but little or nothing about how it can be accelerated—the quest of the ancients! The process of wound healing is essentially the same for skin, muscle, tendon, bone, and all other body tissues. It is most easily described in relation to a clean, incised wound of normal skin that heals ideally in a sterile environment.

NORMAL SKIN

Normal skin has three layers: epidermis, dermis, and subcutaneous tissues. The *epidermis* has a basal layer of cells that continually multiply to maintain the stratified epithelial layer. This layer is the primary barrier between the exterior and the internal environment of the body. It prevents invasion by bacteria or toxic substances and, together with the underlying dermis, protects the deeper structures from trauma. The skin also prevents loss of body fluid and electrolytes to the external environment. The *dermis* is a layer of dense collagen, and the *subcutaneous tissue* consists of connective tissue surrounding fat globules.

Connective tissue is a continuous fabric of fibrous tissue extending throughout the body. It comprises about 30 per cent of the body weight and consists of collagen, reticulin, and elastin surrounded by ground substance (mucopolysaccharides and mucoproteins). Among the fibers are fibroblasts, fat cells, histiocytes, mast cells, and plasma cells.

Collagen is of particular interest because it is the basic protein from which the framework for all tissues and organs is elaborated. Condensed, it forms ligaments and tendons. Although five distinct types of collagen have been found in various body tissues, all collagen molecules exhibit the following characteristics:

1. Molecules are made up of three peptide chains twisted in a right-handed helix.
2. The amino acid glycine occurs in every third position.
3. Hydroxyproline and hydroxylysine are amino acids unique to collagen.

Collagen is formed in the rough endoplasmic reticulum of fibroblasts. During this process, ascorbic acid is required to hydroxylate proline to hydroxyproline. Thus, in ascorbic acid deficiency (scurvy), collagen production is greatly reduced and wounds heal poorly if at all.

The strength of collagen fibers depends on cross-linking within and between molecules. The most common bond is between an aldehyde group of hydroxylysine and an amino group of another hydroxylysine—called a Schiff base. This cross-linking is inhibited in *lathyrism*, a condition occurring in animals that eat sweet pea seeds (*Lathyrus odoratus*). These animals develop skeletal deformities and aneurysms as a result of loss of tissue tensile strength. *Penicillamine* also reacts with aldehyde groups and blocks cross-linking, but the process is less devastating than in lathyrism. *Ehlers-Danlos syndrome* and *Marfan's syndrome* are rare diseases caused by defects in collagen synthesis and maturation.

THE CLEAN INCISED WOUND

A clean incision through the epidermis, dermis, and subcutaneous tissue will heal by a series of events that proceed concurrently over a period of time. Immediately after injury, the wound fills with blood, which clots. Very soon, acute inflammation develops and epithelium covers the wound. More slowly, scar tissue develops and is remodeled to firmly appose the sides of the wound. Although these tissue processes are discussed separately, it is important to recognize that they are dynamic and all begin to develop within minutes of injury.

Inflammation

Immediately after injury, local vasoconstriction occurs, which stops bleeding, and the blood in the wound clots. Within 5 to 10 minutes, local vasodilatation follows and plasma leaks from small venules into the surrounding tissues. Polymorphonuclear leukocytes and monocytes become viscid and adhere to the endothelium of capillaries. Shortly thereafter, they actively emigrate from the capillary and begin the débridement of damaged cells and blood clots by the process of phagocytosis. Polymorphonuclear leukocytes are most prominent during the early phases of this reaction, but mononuclear cells are more prominent if the inflammatory reaction is prolonged. These mononuclear cells are collectors of debris not readily digested by the polymorphonuclear leukocytes. In chronic inflammation, they are the prominent phagocytes and may become conjoined to form giant cells (e.g., hypersensitivity reaction of tuberculosis).

The inflammatory reaction is localized initially by fibrin obstruction of the lymphatics. Within 2 days, fibronectin, a glycoprotein, accumulates and produces adhesion of fibroblasts, fibrin, and collagen, thus ensuring permanent localization of the reaction.

Injured cells release intracellular enzymes into the extracellular space. Early vasodilatation and permeability are secondary to histamine from mast cells and last about 30 minutes. The prolonged vascular response is due to prostaglandin E_1 and E_2 (and therefore inhibited by acetylsalicylic acid and indomethacin).

Of particular interest is *platelet-derived growth factor* (PDGF). This substance, found in all species, is probably the primary stimulant that attracts cells to the area of injury and triggers their replication to effect repair. The cells of the acute reaction (polymorphonuclear leukocytes, mononuclear cells, mast cells) and the fibroblasts of the latter response all seem to respond to PDGF.

Epithelialization

During the period of intense vascular and cellular reaction, epithelium rapidly regenerates to resume its barrier function. Within 48 hours, a thin layer of epithelium

completely covers a sutured, clean wound. This begins with mitosis of the basal cells of the epidermis and is followed by migration of the epithelium down the wound edges and across the incision. The epithelium migrates as a sheet until it comes into contact with other epithelial cells, at which time all motion ceases. The mechanism of this *contact inhibition* is not well understood, although it has been the subject of much investigation. As the wound matures, the epithelium thickens but never develops rete pegs or the other structures of normal epithelium.

Scar Formation

Within 24 hours, probably stimulated by PDGF, fibroblasts in the subcutaneous tissue migrate from the wound edges along fibrin strands in the wound. Soon collagen is secreted, cross-linking begins, and the process toward firm union between the wound edges is under way. In the healing wound, measurement of hydroxyproline is an index of collagen production. Levels are high from day 4 to 12, and then they diminish quickly. Nonetheless, the tensile strength of the wound continues to increase as the collagen matures. Two main processes are at work during this maturation: (1) cross-linking within collagen molecules and between collagen fibers, and (2) remodeling of the direction of the collagen bundles.

To effect remodeling, existing collagen bundles are dissolved by tissue collagenase; new bundles are formed and aligned to resist lines of tension across the wound. Interweaving and cross-linking between bundles and with the wound edges lead to firm healing. In uncomplicated healing, the strength of collagen and the rate at which it reaches maturity vary with the load placed on the wound. Thus, a skin incision will heal solidly within 2 to 3 weeks; wounds of the abdominal fascia will be reasonably secure within 6 weeks, but will continue to gain strength for at least 6 months; tendons or ligaments require a minimum of 3 months for early healing and continue to gain strength for over a year. The increase in wound breakage strength with time is depicted in Figure 1.

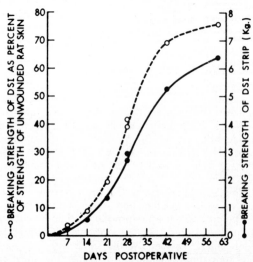

Figure 1. Increase in breaking strength of a healing rat skin wound shown in absolute terms and as a percentage of comparable unwounded skin. Note the prolonged gain in strength of unwounded skin. DSI = Dermal skin incision. (From Levenson, S. M., et al.: Ann. Surg., 161:293, 1965.)

Thus far, healing of a clean, incised wound has been discussed. This is called *healing by first intention*. In a wound in which tissue is lost, healing occurs by *second intention*.

Healing by Second Intention

With tissue loss, wound edges are not apposed and the healing process is modified. The internal milieu of the body must be protected from external bacteria or toxins, and the wound edges must be brought together as well as possible. These objectives are achieved by the simultaneous development of granulation tissue and wound contraction.

Granulation Tissue

An open wound is not at risk to serious infection, an observation originally made by John Hunter. This is because there is free drainage of necrotic cells and because of the development of granulation tissue—a modification of the inflammatory process that resists bacterial invasion and provides a healthy base for epithelial growth from the wound edges.

Initially, blood clot fills the wound and a fibrin network is formed. Phagocytic granulocytes and monocytes begin the process of débridement. Capillary buds and fibroblasts rapidly proliferate into the clot. The capillary buds secrete lytic enzymes to break up the fibrin and permit rapid development of a network. The buds then undergo canalization, forming vascular arcades that provide a rich blood supply of nutrients, oxygen, granulocytes, and monocytes needed to remove dead tissue and clot. Abundant polymorphonuclear cells in the interstitial tissues provide the primary defense against infection and also account for the purulent discharge from granulation tissue as dead cells are extruded. Proliferating fibroblasts accompany these vessels and begin to deposit collagen.

Within 4 to 6 days, healthy pink granulation tissue forms an excellent base to support and nourish advancing epithelium (or a skin graft is applied). As time passes, fibroplasia continues and cross-linking occurs. Many blood vessels atrophy. With final healing, there is a white scar covered with thin epithelium.

Wound Contraction

Wound contraction is a process by which there is diminution in the size of a wound in which there is tissue loss. *Contraction* occurs *early* and must not be confused with *contracture*, or *cicatrization*, which causes diminution in the size of the scar and therefore is a *delayed* event. In wound contraction, there is centripetal movement of the whole thickness of the skin. This can be accomplished only if the skin is mobile. It is therefore more effective in areas where the skin is freely mobile (e.g., the perineum and abdominal wall).

The mechanism of wound contraction is still not clear. It could be brought about by contraction of collagen fibers or by the action of contractile cells in the granulation tissue. Collagen contraction is unlikely because it has never been recorded in a living animal. Furthermore, wound contraction occurs before there is much collagen in the wound, and also contraction occurs normally in scorbutic animals. The most likely mechanism is contraction of contractile fibroblasts (myofibroblasts). These cells are found throughout the body, particularly concentrated around open wounds. There are two theories of how these myofibroblasts pull the wound edges to reduce the size of the wound 80 per cent within a week to 10 days. One theory (the "picture frame" theory) postulates that the myofibrils act beneath the wound edges and draw them forward toward the center. The other theory postulates that the myofibrils in the center of the wound draw the edges toward them. Present evidence favors the picture frame theory, although it is quite possible that both mechanisms occur.

Factors That Impair Wound Healing

LOCAL FACTORS

Oxygenation. Oxygenation is perhaps the most important factor that affects the rate of healing. This is apparent clinically: In well-vascularized areas, such as the face and tongue, wounds heal rapidly; in poorly vascularized tissue, such as tendons and cartilage, wounds heal very slowly. Healing is impaired when sutures or dressings are too tight, in diabetics, or in the elderly in whom small vessel disease is extensive. Following radiation, fibrosis impairs vascularity and healing.

Hematoma. Hematoma or *seroma* impairs healing by increasing the separation of wound edges and the amount of débridement necessary before fibrosis can occur. Blood products are fertile media for bacterial growth and wound infection. A hematoma is the most common impairment of the local resistance of the tissues to infection and, as a consequence, the prevention of hematoma formation is the *sine qua non* of good operative technique.

Surgical Technique. Normal wound healing is a delicate balance between collagen lysis and collagen formation. The enzyme collagenase mobilizes mature collagen as part of the remodeling process. In abdominal wounds, collagenase weakens the fascia up to 5 mm. from the cut edge. Sutures must be placed well beyond this weakened area if they are to hold until healing restores full strength to the repair. Collagen lysis increases if there is infection and by the action of steroids. This explains wound breakdown in patients with infected wounds, especially if steroids are being given.

GENERAL FACTORS

Nutrition. Vitamin C deficiency impairs hydroxylation of proline and lysine so that collagen is not secreted by fibroblasts.

Zinc. Zinc is required in the healing process of patients with severe burns, trauma, or sepsis, but its action is not clear.

Steroids. Steroids impair healing by suppressing the inflammatory response and increasing collagen lysis. Their effect is most marked during the first 4 days after injury. After this, they have little effect except to inhibit the normal resistance to infection.

Sepsis. Systemic sepsis slows healing. The mechanism is not yet established, but it is probably related to the requirement for amino acids to form collagen molecules. This is probably why parenteral feeding improves wound healing in patients with malnutrition or sepsis.

Cytotoxic Drugs. 5–Fluorouracil, methotrexate, cyclophosphamide, and nitrogen mustard *impair* wound healing by suppressing fibroblast replication and collagen synthesis.

COMPLICATIONS OF WOUNDS

Hematoma

Hematoma occurring *early* is the result of failure to control bleeding vessels, and it may occur *late* in patients with hypertension or coagulation defects. Ordinarily, a hematoma may be left to resolve spontaneously, but an expanding hematoma requires reoperation and control of the bleeding.

Infection

Wound infection is still one of the most common complications of surgical procedures and frequently follows a wound hematoma. In 1867, Lister, in his landmark work on antisepsis, noted that hospital gangrene accounted for a mortality between 20 and 100 per cent. Today, wound infection is not often fatal, but it accounts for considerable morbidity. Two primary factors are significant in the pathogenesis of these infections: (1) the dose of bacterial contamination, and (2) the resistance of the patient.

CONTAMINATION OF THE PATIENT

Endogenous Contamination. Contamination from within the patient usually arises from the gastrointestinal, genitourinary, or respiratory tract. It is surprising that at least 500,000 bacteria per gram are required to produce infection in a traumatic wound. This number of bacteria is found normally in the bowel. Bowel preparation with laxatives and enemas, plus antibacterial treatment with antibiotics before operations on the colon, has lowered the incidence of wound infections from this potent source of endogenous contamination.

Exogenous Contamination. Contamination from the environment has proved to be much less important than endogenous contamination in the genesis of wound infection. The operating room ritual of scrubbing, gowning, and field preparation is designed to control this exogenous contamination.

LOCAL RESISTANCE OF THE WOUND

Since the time of Paré, surgeons have recognized the importance of hemostasis, adequate blood supply, débridement of necrotic tissue, and obliteration of dead space in the prevention of wound infections. Closed suction drains reduce infection in operations with a potential dead space, such as hip arthroplasties and mastectomies.

RESISTANCE OF THE PATIENT

Prophylactic Antibiotics. Antibiotics, if present in the wound at the time of injury, enhance the ability of a wound to withstand bacterial contamination. To be effective, they must be present in the wound within, at most, 3 hours after contamination and should be present beforehand in patients undergoing operation. Prophylactic antibiotics are particularly useful for operations on the stomach and duodenum, the biliary tract, and the large intestine. They also are used for operations in which infection would be catastrophic, e.g., vascular or orthopedic prosthetic implantations. They are relatively indicated in patients with diabetes, obesity, malnutrition, or immunosuppression or in those of the geriatric age group who have impaired system resistance.

Delayed Primary Closure. The grossly contaminated wound, after débridement and irrigation, may be left widely open. The open wound is not at risk to infection because there is free drainage of exudate and because granulation tissue forms early. After 4 to 6 days, when healthy granulation tissue is abundant, the wound may be closed with little fear of infection. Billroth, the father of gastrointestinal surgery, used this technique for all abdominal operations in the late 19th century.

Established Wound Infection. Wide drainage is the only effective treatment for established wound infection. Antibiotics are not usually required except in the presence of spreading infection (cellulitis or septicemia). The classic signs of pain, swelling, redness, and fluctuation indicate the need for wide local drainage and delayed primary closure, as discussed previously.

Wound Dehiscence. The incidence of abdominal wound dehiscence is approximately one in every 500 abdominal operations. It is most common after upper abdominal wounds. The longer after operation that dehiscence occurs, the greater likelihood that poor healing is the cause. Abdominal distention, chronic cough, obesity, and old age predispose to wound dehiscence. Wound infection is involved in many patients. Technical factors also predispose wounds to dehiscence and account for the majority of cases. Too-tight suturing, sutures too near the fascial edge, and poor suture material are the important factors in technical errors. The rate of absorption of catgut is variable, and the suture may be absorbed before wound strength has been established.

Discharge of serosanguineous peritoneal fluid is the usual first sign of wound dehiscence. The absence of a palpable healing ridge confirms the impending disaster. If the skin is intact, one can reinforce the wound with adhesive strips or a binder, knowing full well that an incisional hernia will develop and can be repaired later. If evisceration occurs, reoperation is mandatory.

Sinus Tracts. If a wound infection heals, leaving a sinus tract, there is usually a multifilament suture at the base of the sinus acting as a *foreign body*. Silk is the most common offender, and the sinus is maintained by bacterial colonization of the interstices of the multifilament sutures. When the suture is removed, the sinus closes. If the sinus should persist, it is likely that multiple sutures are involved and the wound is apt to require exploration with removal of the sutures.

Keloids. Keloids are exuberant scars caused by a hyperactive repair process. Both collagen deposition and collagen lysis are increased. Keloids are particularly common in dark-skinned races and there is often a history of previous keloids. Hypertrophic scars can be improved by relieving tension, e.g., Z-plasty, if the scar crosses a flexion crease. Elastic compression helps diminish this exuberant response, especially after burns, but its permanent value is not known at this time. Cortisone injection may be useful for small keloids. Lathyrogenic agents such as beta-aminopropionitrile (BAPN) have been used experimentally.

SUMMARY

Wound healing is a dynamic process involving blood elements, blood vessels, fibroblasts, and epithelial cells. Initially, blood in the wound clots, which is followed by an inflammatory response, which débrides dead cells and bacteria. Fibroblasts and blood vessels advance on the fibrin in the clot, collagen is deposited, and, with time, the collagen gains strength by cross-linking and remodeling in the direction of the major stresses. Epithelialization occurs very early to protect the wound from external contamination.

SELECTED REFERENCES

International Review of Connective Tissue Research. New York, Academic Press, 1963 to current.
A continuing series of volumes that present considerable detailed information about the entire subject of wound healing.

Madden, J. W., and Arem, A. J.: Wound healing: Biologic and clinical features. *In* Sabiston, D. C., Jr. (Ed.): Textbook of Surgery: The Biological Basis of Modern Surgical Practice, 13th ed. Philadelphia, W.B. Saunders Company, 1986.
This is an excellent resource for a complete reference of all aspects of wound healing.

Trinkaus, J. P.: Cells into Organs, 2nd ed. Englewood Cliffs, N.J., Prentice-Hall, Inc., 1984.
This monograph presents detailed information concerning cellular aspects of inflammation and wound healing. It provides fascinating reading for the student interested in basic cellular principles.

BURNS

GREGORY S. GEORGIADE, M.D. • W. CHRISTOPHER PEDERSON, M.D.

9

HISTORY

Although burns have occurred since man first encountered fire, the rational treatment of burns and the first studies of their pathophysiology began in the 1900s. Application of scientific principles by observation in large numbers of burn patients came in 1921, when Underhill of Yale studied 20 victims of a fire at the Rialto Theater in New Haven, Connecticut. Noting changes in hemoglobin, hematocrit, and serum chloride levels, he analyzed the content of blisters and provided evidence for protein losses. Another disaster, the Coconut Grove fire of 1942 in Boston, Massachusetts, enabled Cope and Moore to study fluid and protein losses in a large number of patients. These and other studies led to Evans' development of the first surface area–weight formula for computing fluid replacement in burn patients. Later studies at Brooke Army Hospital led to the development of the formulas most widely used today.[3]

With appropriate fluid therapy, increasing numbers of burn patients survived to develop burn wound sepsis. This led to the search for a topical agent to control bacterial growth in the burn wound. Moyer proposed the use of 0.5 per cent silver nitrate applied topically, which was found to protect against bacterial growth on the surface and beneath the burn eschar. Moncrief and Lindberg later described the use of mafenide acetate (Sulfamylon) as an agent effective against gram-positive and gram-negative organisms that penetrated the burn eschar. Because of electrolyte problems encountered with the use of silver nitrate and pain on application of mafenide acetate, Fox developed and popularized silver sulfadiazine (Silvadene) cream.

A major advance in the care of burned patients was the development of the burn unit. With a specialized unit designed for the burn victims, the concept of "team" care of these patients has evolved. This involves personnel with a special interest and training in the care of burn patients, including physicians, nurses, physical and occupational therapists, and technicians.

EPIDEMIOLOGY

Approximately 2 million people suffer burns in the United States each year, with 100,000 being hospitalized and 20,000 requiring burn center care.[16] Deaths from burns have decreased since 1920, and today patients with burns of greater than 50 per cent of the body surface area have a reasonable chance for survival if treated appropriately.[8]

The peak incidence for burns is seen in young adults in the age range of 20 to 29 years, followed by children aged 9 or younger. Burns are infrequent in those aged 80 or more.

About 80 per cent of burns occur in the home. In children under 3 years of age, the most common cause of burns is scald injury. From age 3 to 14, the most frequent cause is flame burns from ignited clothing. From this age group to about age 60, most burns are due to industrial accidents. After this age, burns usually occur in house fires caused by smoking in bed or in association with mental lapses.

Mortality rates for burn injuries have decreased greatly with advances in burn care. Although burns in the very young and elderly patient still carry an increased risk of mortality, figures for the 14- to 44-year-old populations have shown considerable improvement. Estimates of burn mortality are made according to the "LA50," or that percentage of body surface area of second- and third-degree burn that will result in the death of 50 per cent of those patients suffering this injury. Large series of burn patients treated in the 1940s and 1950s reflected LA50 figures of around 45 per cent.[5] Curreri's group recently reported their experience over 16 years, and the LA50 in the 15- to 44-year-old age group was 63 per cent.[7] This improvement is related to advancements in the treatment of burn shock, infection, inhalation injury, surgical nutrition, and wound coverage.

PATHOPHYSIOLOGY OF BURN INJURY

Thermal injury to the body occurs either by direct conduction of heat or by electromagnetic radiation. The degree of burn injury is related to a number of factors, including the conductance of the particular tissue involved, the time in contact with the source of heat energy, and surface pigmentation. Nerves and blood vessels are the structures least resistant to heat conductance, whereas bone is the most resistant. Other tissues are intermediate conductors. Sources of electromagnetic radiation include x-rays, microwaves, infrared waves, ultraviolet rays, and visible light. These can injure tissues either thermally (microwaves) or by ionization (x-rays).

Cells can tolerate temperatures up to 44° C. without significant damage. Between 44° C. and 51° C., the rate of tissue destruction doubles for each degree rise in the temperature and only limited amounts of exposure time can be tolerated. Above 51° C., proteins are denatured and the rate of tissue destruction is very rapid. Temperatures above 70° C. cause extremely rapid cellular destruction, and only extremely brief periods of exposure can be tolerated. At lower heat ranges, the body can effectively dissipate the thermal energy by circulatory changes; however, at higher ranges this is ineffective.

A burn wound is made up of several zones, beginning with a zone of tissue coagulation at the point of maximal injury. Bordering the zone of coagulation is a zone of stasis, which is characterized by sluggish blood flow and is composed of potentially salvageable cells. Surrounding the zone of stasis is a zone of hyperemia in which the cells are minimally involved and should recover fully. With drying or infection, cells in the zone of stasis can be lost and a partial-thickness injury converted to a full-thickness one. One aim of burn treatment is to avoid loss of these two outer zones.

Burns have classically been referred to as first, second, or third degree. A first-degree injury involves only the superficial epidermis and appears as an area of hyperemia and erythema. A second-degree injury involves the deeper layers of the epidermis and parts of the dermis and presents with blistering and/or edema and weeping. A third-degree injury involves all layers of the epidermis and dermis and usually appears as a dry wound, often with coagulated veins visible through the skin surface (Fig. 1).

Although this classification of burn injury has utility and is much in present use, burns are better classified simply as "partial thickness" or "full thickness." Partial-thickness injury includes first- and second-degree burns; full-thickness injury includes third-degree burns. Use of this system of burn depth classification gives a clinical impression as to whether a burn will heal spontaneously or whether it will require grafting. On initial evaluation, however, it is often difficult to assess the depth of injury, particularly in deep dermal (second-degree) burns.

Burn depth is dependent not only on the type of burning agent and time of exposure but also on the thickness of the area of injured skin and its blood supply. Areas with thicker skin require a longer exposure to the heat source to produce a full-thickness burn than do thinner areas of skin. The skin in elderly patients and infants is thinner in all areas than it is in other age groups, and this is an important consideration in estimating burn depth in these patients.

METABOLIC RESPONSE TO BURN INJURY

Burn wounds affect not only the skin and subcutaneous tissue but also have primary or secondary effects on nearly every system of the body. These effects are related directly to the depth and extent of the burn wound. Some of the effects are transient and clinically insignificant; others are long-lasting and profound.

There is a marked increase in capillary permeability in the area of a burn related to factors that are not entirely clear. It is well known, however, that this loss of capillary integrity extends to the whole body in burns greater than 25 to 30 per cent of the body surface area. These larger burns, therefore, result in a massive transudation of isotonic fluid and protein into the extravascular space, with a resulting decrease in the circulating plasma volume. The net effect is one of edema formation, with a lowering of cardiac output and increase in peripheral vascular resistance. At a variable time period after injury, the integrity of the capillaries returns, generally starting at 12 hours and accelerating at 18 to 24 hours after injury. Some increase in capillary permeability can be demonstrated up to 3 weeks after injury, however.[4]

Immediate hemolysis of red cells occurs in the area of the burn; this varies, depending on depth and extent of the injury. This generally involves only a small percentage of the circulating red cell mass; however, scald burns with prolonged immersion can result in significant lowering of the hematocrit. A more significant effect in most patients is a lowering of the life span of the red cells, which may be decreased to 30 per cent of normal.

Besides the marked changes in intravascular volume, there are major alterations in cardiac function. Cardiac output can decrease to 30 per cent of normal values in burns involving 50 per cent or more of the body surface. With fluid resuscitation, this value will rapidly return toward normal; however, in the untreated patient, restoration of normal cardiac output can take up to 36 hours. After this period of time, cardiac function increases to supranormal ranges and may remain there for prolonged periods. The precise cause of the decrease in myocardial function is not clear, but appears to be due to a plasma factor present in significant amounts in burns of greater than 40 per cent total body surface area (TBSA).[2]

Renal function abnormalities are noted in burn patients, primarily related to changes in circulating plasma volume and cardiac output. Although a prolonged decrease in renal plasma flow can result in either high-output or oliguric renal failure in the burn patient, timely and adequate fluid resuscitation obviates these problems.

In addition to fluid losses secondary to loss of capillary integrity, the burn patient experiences increased evaporative water loss. During the first 48 hours, these losses are primarily due to exudate on the surface of partial-thickness wounds. Areas of full-thickness skin loss are initially dry and suffer minimal evaporative losses; however, with softening of the eschar, water losses increase greatly. With extensive full-thickness burns, evaporative losses may reach 6 to 8 liters per day. This loss may be estimated by the formula:

(25 + per cent TBSA burn) × total body surface area in square meters = ml. water lost per hour.

The changes in pulmonary function seen in burn patients are generally the same as those seen in any patient

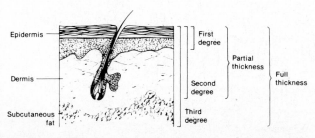

Figure 1. Skin anatomy and relationship to depth of burn.

with trauma. These changes are proportional to the size of the burn wound. The patient with a pulmonary burn injury will have marked changes in pulmonary function, but these are related to local factors and are not due to systemic changes from cutaneous wounds.

Many abnormalities are noted in the plasma and cellular elements of the blood in patients with burns. Changes seen in the plasma include a rise in liver enzymes, a decrease in serum proteins and albumin, and alterations in lipid products. These are directly related to severity of the burn and, with the important exception of the drop in albumin, are generally clinically unimportant. Decreases in the serum albumin are marked in large burns and persist until the wounds are closed. The white blood cell count rises promptly in the burn patient and may stay elevated for long periods of time. A sudden decrease in the white blood cell count in the face of a previous elevation may mark the onset of sepsis. Leukotaxis and phagocytosis have been shown to be defective in patients with wounds as well.[19]

EARLY CARE OF THE BURN PATIENT

First Aid and Emergency Room Care

Initial care of a patient with burns follows the general precepts of care of any trauma patient. Specifically, the patient should be removed from the source of thermal energy, whether it is burning clothing or a high-tension electrical wire. After adequate ventilation and cardiac function are ensured, a rapid general assessment of the injuries should be made as to severity and extent of burn. Some type of clean cover should be placed over the burn wounds and the patient readied for transport. Patients with small burns (less than 20 per cent TBSA) can be transported to the hospital by any reasonable means; however, patients with large burns require placement of an intravenous line and transport by the most expeditious means. Small partial-thickness burns may be treated at the scene by application of cold water to reduce pain; however, this is unwise in large injuries. Prolonged treatment with cold solutions in such patients can lead to hypothermia.

When first seen in the emergency room, the burn patient is again approached as any patient with potentially multiple trauma. If the burn is large and no intravenous line has been placed, a large-bore catheter should be inserted, preferably in an unburned upper extremity. If no such site exists, a line can be placed in the leg or in a central vein if necessary. Venous cutdowns should be avoided in the burn patient because of the high potential for septic complications. An indwelling urinary catheter should also be placed to monitor urinary output during resuscitation. Blood should be drawn for cell counts, serum electrolytes, and creatinine. In patients burned in a closed space or with potential pulmonary injury, arterial blood gases with carboxyhemoglobin levels should be obtained as well. In patients with large burns, blood should be typed and screened for later cross-matching if transfusion becomes necessary.

While the lines are being placed and blood drawn, a systematic history and physical examination of the patient should be undertaken. Important in the history are drug allergies, status of tetanus immunization, and systemic disease processes, all of which can affect or alter treatment. Special attention should be taken in examination of the face and eyes, the pulmonary and cardiac systems, and the abdomen. Patients suffering burns often have other major

injuries, and these can be the cause of lethal complications if initially overlooked. In large burns, a chest x-ray should be obtained in the emergency room when the patient is stabilized. Other appropriate radiologic studies may be done at the same time, depending on the extent of injuries.

Estimating Depth and Extent of Burns

As alluded to earlier, deciding whether a burn is partial- or full-thickness is important before making further decisions as to treatment. First- and third-degree injuries are usually easily identified, but the healing potential of intermediate-depth burns is often difficult to predict with certainty. Indeed, any partial-thickness wound should heal in a period of 3 weeks. Any burn that has not epithelialized during this time period was either underestimated initially or was allowed to desiccate or become infected in the treatment period.

First-degree burns appear red and somewhat raised from the surrounding normal skin. They are painful and often associated with a "stinging" sensation. An example of a first-degree burn is the typical sunburn. *Superficial second-degree burns* present with blistering of the skin and surrounding erythema and are exquisitely tender to touch. If the blisters have burst, the wound will appear wet and weep serum. *Deeper second-degree burns* may have blisters, but after the blisters have burst, the wound will appear blanched and dry. The patient with a deep dermal burn will have somewhat decreased sensation to touch or pinprick in the area of burn; close attention is required so that conversion to full thickness is avoided. A *third-degree burn* will have a parchment appearance to the coagulated skin, often with thrombosed veins visible through the skin. Full-thickness burns are insensate to touch or pinprick.

When the patient is seen in the emergency room, an estimation of the percentage of total body surface area (per cent TBSA) burned is made. This is less important in the small burn (less than 20 per cent); however, initial estimates in larger burns dictate amounts of fluid given for resuscitation. A gross estimate of the area burned can be obtained by the Rule of Nines. In this formula, each anatomic area is given a percentage of TBSA, which is a multiple of nine.

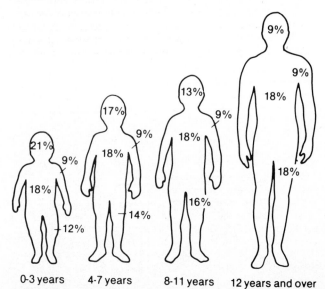

0-3 years   4-7 years   8-11 years   12 years and over

Figure 2. Changes in percentage of body surface area with growth.

Each upper limb represents 9 per cent, each lower limb 18 per cent, the anterior and posterior trunk 18 per cent each, the head and neck 9 per cent, and the perineum and genitalia 1 per cent. This gives an approximate estimate of burn area, but the clinician needs to be aware that the relative percentage of surface area of different anatomic parts of the body will differ in the adult and in the young child. In a child, the head and neck represent a much larger surface area than in the adult and the lower limbs less. To avoid these problems, such charts as the Lund-Browder exist for accurate delineation of TBSA burned in any age patient (Fig. 2). In rapid assessment of small burns, one surface of the patient's hand can be used as an estimate of 1 per cent of body surface area.

Care of the Small Burn Wound

The great majority of burns are small and can be treated on an outpatient basis. These are generally superficial burns less than 15 to 20 per cent TBSA not involving the hands, face, or perineum. Otherwise, burns may be treated safely and effectively at home with close follow-up by the physician.

Care of the small burn wound is directed to maximizing patient comfort and wound healing without complications. The burn wound should be cleansed to remove foreign material and débrided if necessary. Intact blistered skin need not be removed; however, loose nonviable skin in second-degree burns should probably be débrided. After judicious débridement, the wound is gently washed with either a povidone-iodine or similar antibacterial solution.

An occlusive bulky dressing placed over the burn will decrease pain and act to absorb drainage. The choice of topical antimicrobial wound therapy is made by the individual clinician. Partial-thickness burns less than 2 per cent TBSA should probably not be treated with topical chemotherapeutic agents. Burn creams are expensive and not necessary for small superficial wounds. A good choice of wound coverage in small burns is the prepared gauze dressing, which contains a grease base that will adhere less and prevent wound desiccation. Among these are Vaseline, Adaptic, and Xeroform gauzes. Full-thickness wounds or those greater than 2 to 3 per cent TBSA should receive some type of antibacterial treatment. In addition to the creams specifically designed for use in burns, silver sulfadiazine, mafenide acetate, gentamicin cream, or povidone-iodine ointment is equally effective in smaller burns. Several new dressings that obviate the use of bulky dressings and creams have been developed. These may be used very effectively in the clean burn wound seen shortly after injury. Among these products are Op-Site, Biobrane, and Epi-Lock. They are applied directly to the burn after cleansing and débridement of blisters and act to control pain by occlusion and allow re-epithelialization in a moist environment. An excellent option, if available, is the use of human amniotic membrane as a biologic dressing in small clean burns. This requires a system of harvesting and storage, however, and may not be available in all hospitals.[18]

All patients should be given tetanus prophylaxis as with any other wound. Patients who have not had a tetanus toxoid booster within 5 years should receive one routinely. In those patients without prior immunization, tetanus immune globulin as well as the first in the standard series of tetanus toxoid immunizations should be administered.

While advocated by some, routine systemic antibiotic prophylaxis in patients with small burns is rarely indicated.

With close outpatient observation, oral antibiotics may be administered if the wounds show evidence of infection. This is primarily due to *Streptococcus* and will present with increasing erythema around the burn. Penicillin or other anti-streptococcal antibiotics are usually effective treatment. Immunocompromised patients, or those presenting with an already infected wound, should receive some type of broad-spectrum antibiotic coverage as well as topical antibacterial treatment to the wound.

Certain areas require special consideration in outpatient treatment. Patients with burns of the face should have careful examination of the eyes, including fluorescein staining, to exclude a corneal burn. In the case of a suspected ocular burn, an ophthalmologist should be consulted. Burns of the ear should be carefully treated to avoid the complication of chrondritis. This involves the avoidance of pressure to the ear and topical treatment with a burn cream to prevent infection. Facial burns should be treated carefully with silver sulfadiazine, which causes conjunctivitis if it gets in the eye. A better choice of topical treatment for the face is a gentamicin or another polymicrobial ointment. The burned hand should be splinted in the position of function and elevated for the first 24 to 48 hours to minimize edema. Motion should be encouraged after this to avoid joint stiffness. The lower extremity with a small burn should also be elevated initially, especially one involving the feet and ankles.

Follow-up is generally at 2- to 3-day intervals initially. The dressings are carefully removed to avoid damage to regenerating skin and gently cleansed of exudate and loose skin particles. The patient may be instructed in daily cleansing and redressing of the wound. Re-epithelialization should be complete in 2 to 3 weeks, at which time dressings may be discontinued. A light protective dressing may be worn for another week or two, depending on the circumstances and location of the wound. Healing of a burn wound is often accompanied by itching, and this may be relieved somewhat by diphenhydramine hydrochloride (Benadryl) given orally. After complete healing, the new epithelium will be more sensitive than the surrounding skin to sunlight or heat. The patient should be instructed to avoid exposure of the area to intense sunlight or heat for a period of up to 6 months. Likewise, the new skin tends to be relatively dry and scaly from loss of some of the sweat and sebaceous glands secondary to the burn injury. This may be treated with any number of lotions or skin creams while the surface characteristics of the skin slowly improve.

Resuscitation of the Burn Patient

The primary treatment of the patient suffering a large burn is avoidance of complications related to fluid and electrolyte deficits in the immediate postburn period. Estimation of the percentage of TBSA of the burn is the initial step in calculating fluid requirements. Likewise, the patient should be weighed early in the course of treatment for a baseline level to guide later therapy. An indwelling urinary catheter is used as an index of renal perfusion and to evaluate the effectiveness of fluid resuscitation. In the patient with a combination cutaneous burn and pulmonary injury, or in the patient with prior cardiovascular or pulmonary disease, monitoring of central pressures with a Swan-Ganz catheter should be considered.

Several formulas have been developed by different centers for calculation of fluid requirements in burn patients. Among these are the Brooke, Modified Brooke,

Evans, and Parkland formulas. The two systems most in use today are the Modified Brooke and Parkland. These two formulas calculate fluid requirements, based on the total burned area times the patient's weight in kilograms times a volume of lactated Ringer's solution to be given over the first 24 hours post-injury. In both calculations, half of the total fluid is given over the first 8 hours of resuscitation, with a fourth of the total given in each of the succeeding 8-hour periods. While the older Brooke formulation gave free water as 5 per cent dextrose in water, in both formulations the total initial fluid is now administered as lactated Ringer's solution. The volumes of Ringer's solution advocated in the Parkland and Modified Brooke formulas are 4 cc. per kg. per cent burn and 2 cc. per kg. per cent burn, respectively. Either of these gives appropriate levels of fluid for initial calculations of resuscitation requirements as shown by successful use in large numbers of patients. It is important for the clinician involved in resuscitation of burn patients to be aware, however, that any formula should be used only as a guide for estimation of fluid requirements (Fig. 3). Close and careful monitoring of sensorium, urinary output, and central vascular pressures (when appropriate) with subsequent appropriate alterations in fluid therapy dictated by the individual patient's response is the proper method of resuscitation. Altered mental status in the early postburn patient with normal arterial blood gases should alert the physician to a possible decrease in cerebrovascular flow. Urinary output should be in the 30 to 50 cc. per hour range in the adequately hydrated burn patient with otherwise normal renal function. With low urinary output or cardiovascular instability in the face of apparently adequate volumes of intravenous fluid administration, insertion of a thermodilution Swan-Ganz catheter to monitor left and right heart pressures and cardiac output is appropriate. Although these catheters have the potential for vascular and septic complications, their benefits often outweigh the risks for short-term use during initial resuscitation.

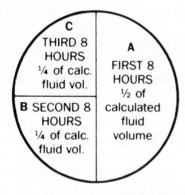

3 ml/kg body wt./% burn

Example: weight = 70 kg.
                                          % burn = 65%

3 cc x 70 kg. wt. x 65% TBS = 13,650 ml

A. First 8 Hours
1/2 x 13,650 = 6825 ml
1/8 x 6825 = 853 ml/hr.

B. Second 8 Hours
1/4 x 13,650 = 3412 ml
1/8 x 3412 = 427 ml/hr.

C. Third 8 Hours
427 ml/hr.

Figure 3. Calculation of minimal fluid resuscitation requirements in the first 24 hours after burn injury.

Resuscitation in children requires alterations of the preceding parameters. A similar formula is used based on the weight in kilograms times the percentage of TBSA burn from a chart such as the Lund-Browder. Total fluid requirements for the first 24 hours are then calculated as 3 ml. per kg. per cent TBSA burn and administered one half in the first 8 hours and one fourth in each of the next 8-hour periods. Sodium bicarbonate is added to each liter of Ringer's lactate. The adequacy of fluid resuscitation is assessed by monitoring of vital signs and urinary output. In children weighing 30 kg. or less, the urinary output should be maintained at 1 ml. per kg. per hour.

From the preceding discussion, it is obvious that no formula is absolutely correct for all patients. A reasonable way to ascertain initial fluid requirements in the burn patient is to use 2 to 4 ml. per kg. per cent TBSA burn. This range can then be used as parameters for fluid administration based on indices of perfusion.

Resuscitation needs after the first 24 hours are determined by ensuring appropriate cardiovascular function and urinary output. In addition, the fluid administered the second day should include replacement of protein losses with albumin or fresh frozen plasma. Because of the large volumes of salt administered in the initial phase of resuscitation, the Parkland and Modified Brooke formulas avoid the use of salt in non–protein-containing fluids in the second 24 hours. In the Parkland formula, colloid is administered in the 700 to 2000 ml. range with D5W as required to maintain adequate urinary output. In the Modified Brooke formula, colloid requirements are calculated as 0.3 to 0.5 ml. per kg. per cent TBSA burn given with D5W. In both calculations, this volume is given during the 25- to 48-hour course.

In the early post-resuscitation period, urinary output is not an appropriate guide by which to assess adequacy of fluid replacement. This is due to the fact that fluid gained during initial resuscitation and sequestered as third space losses is lost between the third and tenth postburn days. To compensate for this fluid mobilization, the burn patient should be allowed a 2 to 3 per cent daily weight loss until the preburn weight is reached. Fluid requirements are calculated on the basis of evaporative losses from the burn wound. The formula for this determination was noted earlier; however, this formula estimates water losses at the lower end of the range of actual loss. In order to determine fluid requirements accurately, daily determinations of serum sodium, osmolality, and body weight are necessary. Generally the fluids administered are either non–sodium-containing or low in salt, again as a result of the large amount of salt administered in the initial phase of resuscitation. The serum sodium and urinary excretion of sodium are monitored closely to determine salt requirements in the intermediate postburn period.

Other Considerations in the Immediate Postburn Period

The patient suffering a burn of greater than 20 to 25 per cent TBSA will frequently have a paralytic ileus. This precludes the use of oral fluids in resuscitation and requires the use of nasogastric intubation and suction to avoid abdominal distention and secondary emeses and aspiration. Likewise, the burn patient is at risk to develop stress ulceration (Curling's ulcer) of the gastroduodenal mucosa. This is best treated by prevention with the use of antacids via the nasogastric tube and/or intravenous H₂ antagonists (such as Zantac). Patients who develop massive gastroin-

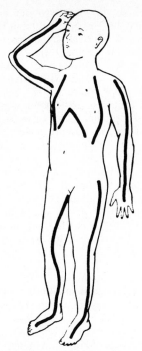

Figure 4. Lines for incision for escharotomy in burn patients.

testinal bleeding or perforation despite prophylaxis may require operative intervention.[15]

The patient requiring analgesia in the early postburn period should be treated with titrated small doses of intravenous narcotics. Full-thickness burns are suprisingly pain-free, and little medication usually is required. Partial-thickness burns, on the contrary, may be exquisitely painful, and large doses of intravenous narcotics may be necessary for control of pain. Inadvertent overdosage with resultant respiratory depression should be treated with the appropriate antagonist.

In the patient with circumferential burns of the chest or extremities, escharotomy may be necessary. A stiff, full-thickness burn may act as a barrier to normal chest excursion, with resultant decreases in pulmonary function. Likewise, in the circumferentially burned extremity, edema in the postburn period may cause cessation of arterial flow as a result of increasing pressure within the surrounding inelastic eschar. Peripheral pulses should be monitored hourly in the patient with extremity burns, particularly if they are circumferential. Palpation of pulses is often unreliable, especially in the face of an overlying burn; therefore, a Doppler flowmeter should be used to determine adequacy of flow. With decreasing chest excursion or evidence of decreasing peripheral pulses, escharotomy should be performed without delay. This can be done in the burn unit without anesthesia, as the eschar is insensitive. Incisions are made on the chest in the anterior axillary lines bilaterally and in the midlateral and midmedial lines of the extremities (Fig. 4). The incision is simply carried deep enough to allow separation of the edges of the eschar. Ventilatory function and/or pulses will return rapidly to normal when an adequate escharotomy is performed.

Initial Care of the Burn Wound

Along with treatment to avoid complications of fluid shifts, care should be directed to maintenance of the burn wound in optimal condition. This ideally prepares the wound for definitive closure and avoids burn wound sepsis.

Systemic antibiotics are not effective in full-thickness burns because of the avascularity of the eschar; thus, topical antimicrobial therapy is the treatment of choice. Early topical treatment attempts resulted in emergence of *Pseudomonas aeruginosa* organisms as significant pathogens responsible for invasive burn wound sepsis. This stimulated the formulation of topical agents with activity against these organisms. Several types of topical antimicrobial therapy exist to avoid bacterial overgrowth in the burn wound. In present widespread use are silver nitrate, mafenide acetate cream, and silver sulfadiazine. Each of these agents has specific advantages and disadvantages when applied topically to the burn wound, and awareness of these is important for appropriate treatment.[6]

Silver nitrate is applied as a 0.5 per cent solution incorporated into gauze dressings placed on the burn. These are then kept moist and wrapped to avoid evaporation of water from the solution, which may cause a potentially toxic rise in the concentration. Silver nitrate has a broad spectrum of antibacterial activity, is painless to the patient, and has no allergenicity. The solution does not penetrate the eschar, however, and thus should be used only in initially clean wounds. The silver nitrate soaks also act to leech cations from the wound. This action, coupled with the fact that free water is absorbed from the solution, may cause electrolyte imbalances. Another disadvantage is the necessity for occlusive dressings, which limits early motion of joints and can lead to later problems in rehabilitation. A relative limitation to the use of this solution is that it discolors normal skin and anything else on contact. It is inexpensive, however, and may be used in patients who have complications associated with use of the other agents.

Silver sulfadiazine is supplied as a 1 per cent suspension in a water-soluble cream. The active compound, however, is only minimally water soluble and thus has little penetration of the eschar of full-thickness wounds. Its application is thus limited somewhat, as with silver nitrate, in that it is best applied to the noncontaminated burn wound. It is painless on application and causes no problems with electrolyte imbalance. There have been rare reports of hypersensitivity, and the agent lacks effectiveness against certain strains of *Pseudomonas*. A unique complication of silver sulfadiazine therapy is the development of an idiosyncratic neutropenia, which may require discontinuation of the agent.[17] In large burns it may be applied without dressings, which allows for close observation of the wound and full motion of involved joints. Silver sulfadiazine is the agent of choice in the treatment of relatively small burns (5 to 20 per cent) seen in the early postburn period to avoid complications of bacterial overgrowth in the wound.

Mafenide acetate is an 11.1 per cent suspension supplied in a water-soluble base. It diffuses across the eschar to provide adequate antimicrobial activity within and beneath the nonviable tissue. It has a broad spectrum of gram-negative activity, but lacks effectiveness against staphylococci. Mafenide acetate is the best agent for use in the already contaminated burn wound and in those with questionable subeschar growth. Its use is complicated by pain and burning on application, which may last 30 minutes. Allergic reactions are seen in about 7 per cent of patients and present as a rash on normal surrounding skin. As a result of its effect as a carbonic anhydrase inhibitor, hyperventilation is seen, particularly in children. Renal compensation from this phenomenon usually occurs; however, systemic alkalosis and pulmonary problems may require decrease in the frequency of application or discontinuation.

The rational use of any agent in the topical treatment of a large burn wound requires daily observation of the wound. It should be understood that topical agents do not sterilize the wound, but act only to control levels of bacteria present. Although overt infection is uncommon in wounds of less than 20 to 30 per cent, larger wounds are more susceptible to overgrowth of bacteria, even with appropriate topical therapy. If signs of conversion of partial-thickness wounds to full-thickness appear (drying, discoloration) or new areas of brownish discoloration appear, a full-thickness biopsy of the wound should be performed. This is done to evaluate the level of bacteria in the wound by quantitative culture techniques. Surface cultures are unreliable as a result of both the presence of the topical antibacterial agents on the wound surface and the potential presence of intra- and subeschar infection. If quantitative cultures reveal bacteria at the level of 100,000 organisms per gram of tissue or greater, invasive burn wound infection is likely. This diagnosis dictates prompt alteration in therapy. Systemic antibiotic therapy appropriate for the offending organism should be initiated, and the care of the wound should be altered. If a nonabsorbable topical agent is being used, it should be changed to mafenide acetate, with its ability to achieve penetration of the eschar. In localized areas of invasion, consideration of subeschar infusion of appropriate antibiotics may be given. If the entire wound is involved, surgical excision and wound coverage with biologic dressings are often necessary for control. Subeschar infection with fungi requires wide local excision of the involved area with appropriate wound coverage. In the face of established burn wound invasion and generalized sepsis, all methods of treatment are poor and mortality is high.[10]

ELECTRICAL BURNS

The passage of high-voltage electrical energy through tissues results in its conversion to thermal energy.[9] This results in a burn that involves not only the skin and subcutaneous tissues but also all tissue in the path of the electrical current. Electrical resistance of tissue is variable, with bone, tendon, and skin being of high resistance and blood and nervous tissue being of low resistance. This results in passage of electrical current preferentially through tissue fluids and along neurovascular bundles. This may result in vascular or nervous injury at some distance from the site of cutaneous burn.

An electrical burn is usually caused by contact with a source of high-voltage energy such as that incurred by a lineman working close to an electrical power source. The limbs are the most common sites of contact, with the arms and hands more frequently injured than the legs and feet. Contact often results in cardiac and/or respiratory arrest, and cardiopulmonary resuscitation is frequently required at the scene of the injury. The wound at the area of entry of the electrical current is usually charred and has a depressed appearance. It may be surrounded by areas of typical thermal burn or normal-appearing tissue. Exit wounds similar to the explosive wounds of exit caused by high-velocity missiles may appear. Arcing of electricity across joints may cause cutaneous thermal burns in areas not involved with entry or exit of the current. The size of the cutaneous wounds is usually misleading and may result in underestimation of the underlying damage to muscle, nerves, and vessel. Extremities with electrical burns are subject to the complication of compartment syndromes as a result of deep muscular or vascular injury. With damage to the underlying muscles, release of myoglobin into the bloodstream and resultant myoglobinuria is frequently seen with electrical injury. Subsequent sequestration of fluid and decreased renal blood flow increase the likelihood of renal damage from myoglobin precipitating in the renal tubules.

The treatment of electrical burns is directed at the cutaneous portion of thermal injury as well as the deeper injury. The area involved in surface burns is calculated in the same way as for a standard thermal injury. Fluids are administered as appropriate for the surface area burned with additional volume to account for damage to underlying muscle. This is approached as in the patient with a crush injury, which is similar in many respects to a high-voltage electrical injury. In the true major electrical injury, massive fluid replacement is necessary to avoid complications. This amount (above and beyond requirements for cutaneous burns) cannot be determined by any formula. Patients with large amounts of myoglobin in the urine will present with port wine–colored urine, and resuscitation of these patients requires urinary outputs in the range of 75 to 100 ml. per hour. Likewise, the urine should be alkalinized with intravenous sodium bicarbonate, which prevents the precipitation of the myoglobin. If the urine does not clear promptly or urinary output remains low despite administration of large volumes of fluid, a forced diuresis should be instituted with mannitol. In the patient with massive muscle injury, doses of mannitol (12.5 gm. per dose) may be required over 12 to 24 hours. Patients who fail to respond to the above measures may require emergency limb amputation or débridement of nonviable muscle. When there is doubt, tissue involved in high-voltage electrical injury should be explored early to assess viability of the underlying muscle. At the time of exploration, débridement of nonviable tissue as well as fasciotomy can be performed.[12]

One potential delayed complication of electrical injury is the development of cataracts. These can be unilateral or bilateral and are usually seen after electrical contact in or around the head. Cataracts caused by electrical injury will become evident from a few days to months after the injury. Ophthalmologic examination is important early in the evaluation of the patient with electrical injury to document pre-existing cataracts or visual disturbances.

The cardiac muscle, likewise, is susceptible to injury from electrical current. An electrocardiogram should be obtained to exclude potential cardiac injury, and continuous cardiac monitoring is important to diagnose and treat arrhythmias. Neurologic injuries also occur, particularly to the spinal cord, but may be difficult to characterize until electrophysiologic testing can be performed. Close attention to the abdomen is important in the immediate post-injury phase because the passage of current through the peritoneal cavity can result in damage to the intestinal tract.

Definitive care of electrical burns follows the general precepts of care for any burn or large wound. With massive tissue loss or amputation, reconstruction with muscle or myocutaneous flaps may be necessary.

CHEMICAL BURNS

Cutaneous injuries from chemicals differ from thermal injuries in that the degree of injury is related directly to length of exposure. In this respect, the physician can directly alter the depth of injury by expeditious treatment. All affected clothing should be quickly removed and the skin examined for areas of injury. Since burn depth is also determined by the concentration of the agent present on the skin, dilution with copious lavage is the next step in patient management. Various specific neutralizing agents have been proposed for various chemicals; however, none offers much advantage over immediate, high-volume irrigation of the wound with water. Some of these may even cause an increase in the severity of injury by releasing heat with neutralization of the offending chemical. Burns with alkali are often little affected by irrigation if the wound is over 1 hour old. An increase in the depth of the burn may be seen with irrigation because of facilitation of passage of hydroxyl ions into the deeper layers of the skin. History is important in determining the exact composition of the chemical because this may dictate therapy after dilution with water lavage.

Burns with phenol, hydrofluoric acid, and phophorus deserve special attention. Phenol is poorly soluble in water, and lavage should be followed with application of a solvent such as polyethylene glycol, propylene glycol, glycerol, vegetable oil, or simple soap and water. High concentrations of absorbed phenol can cause cardiac, renal, and central nervous system effects, and the patient needs close monitoring of these functions. Hydrofluoric acid penetrates the skin rapidly and may cause liquefaction of soft tissues and erosion to underlying bone. Pain is severe with burns of this type, and careful intralesional injection of calcium gluconate is used to neutralize the fluoride ion and alleviate pain. Phosphorus burns require immediate attention to remove all identifiable particles of phosphorus in the wound. This substance ignites when exposed to air-drying and should be placed under water after removal. Application of dilute copper sulfate solution to the wound surface may be necessary to identify small embedded particles of phosphorus.[1]

After removal of the offending chemical, these burns are treated in the standard manner of any cutaneous burn. Small burns are often amenable to outpatient treatment, but larger injuries require standard resuscitation protocols and monitoring for potential systemic effects because of absorption.

INHALATION INJURY

Purely thermal injuries to the pulmonary system are rare in the burn patient, since the only documented way to truly "burn" the tracheobronchial tree is by inhalation of live steam. A victim of a fire is exposed to smoke, which contains many noxious chemicals, including sulfur dioxide, nitrogen dioxide, hydrochloric acid, hydrocyanide, carbon monoxide, and carbon dioxide. Inhalation of agents of this type causes severe pulmonary injuries and accounts for the single most lethal component of burns. Many patients who die at the scene of a fire do so from inhalation injury. Of patients reaching the hospital with burns, inhalation injury is seen in up to 30 per cent. The majority of patients with inhalation injury suffer burns about the head and neck and are often burned in an enclosed space. It is important to note, however, that most patients with head and neck burns do not suffer pulmonary injury.

First aid for the victim with possible inhalation injury consists of removing the patient from the source of noxious gases and of administering oxygen. When first seen in the hospital, all patients with burns sustained in an enclosed space and those with facial burns should be evaluated for inhalation injury. The index of suspicion is higher in patients with singed nasal hairs, oral or pharyngeal edema, hoarseness, or carbonaceous sputum. While the chest film in the immediate postburn period is usually normal, one should be obtained as a baseline and to exclude pre-existing pulmonary disease. Blood gas determination is done to evaluate the presence of carboxyhemoglobin in the blood because carbon monoxide has a 200-fold greater affinity for hemoglobin than does oxygen.

Once a patent upper airway is secured and the patient is hemodynamically stable, flexible fiberoptic bronchoscopy should be performed. If marked pharyngeal edema is present, an endotracheal tube may be passed. Signs of inhalation injury on bronchoscopy include mucosal edema and erythema, erosions, and deposition of carbonaceous material in the airways. [133]Xenon scanning of the lungs can be helpful in diagnosing inhalation injury. A peripheral injection of [133]xenon should be cleared by normal lungs within 90 seconds. Scanning with a gamma camera reveals retention of xenon in injured areas; however, false-positive results may be seen in patients with underlying pulmonary disease.[11]

Patients with inhalation injury are treated symptomatically. Those with evidence of carbon monoxide poisoning are given 100 per cent oxygen by endotracheal tube and followed with serial blood gases until they return to normal levels. Hyperbaric oxygen may be required in the most severe cases. Patients with minimal pulmonary injury may be treated with humidified oxygen by mask along with bronchodilators and mucolytics. In the case of more severe injury, intubation is often necessary. Tracheostomy is to be avoided in the burn patient because of septic complications at the operative site. The airway may be managed very well by a soft cuffed tube placed nasotracheally. Respiratory decompensation may be rapid in the patient with pulmonary injury, and thus close monitoring is essential. All patients with stridor or dyspnea should be intubated. Other relative indications include severe infiltrates on chest x-ray, increased respiratory rate (greater than 35 per minute), decreased lung compliance, increased shunt fraction, and low Po_2. Placing the patient on a T-piece to humidified oxygen may be adequate treatment until edema subsides; however, patients with decreasing Po_2 or worsening ventilatory patterns should be placed on a volume ventilator and positive end-expiratory pressure may be required. In such patients, invasive monitoring should be strongly considered to obviate problems with fluid shifts with further aggravation of pulmonary compromise.

Although steroids have been advocated in the past by some authors, their use in burn patients with inhalation injury is not indicated. No efficacy has been shown, and indeed steroids may be harmful. Antibiotics should be reserved for the patient with established pulmonary infection, since their use for prophylaxis does not prevent infection and may promote the growth of resistant organisms.

DEFINITIVE TREATMENT OF THE BURN WOUND

Healing of burn wounds results from epithelial proliferation along the edges of the wound and in the skin appendages. Epithelial cells from hair follicles and sweat glands grow out onto the surface of the wound and eventually coalesce to provide skin coverage. The deeper the burn, the more of these organelles are destroyed and thus fewer remain to effect coverage of the wound. For this reason, superficial wounds heal more rapidly than deeper wounds. Total healing time for even deep dermal burns should not exceed 4 weeks. Burns healing spontaneously over a protracted time period have a much greater propensity to form hypertrophic scar, and this should be a factor in consideration of other forms of treatment in deep dermal burns.

After the patient is stabilized and has recovered from the major systemic alterations secondary to the burn injury, attention is given to wound coverage. Early coverage of the burn equates with decreased fluid and protein losses and return of function of the burned part. Obtaining closure of the wound may require excision of the burned area or may be done after spontaneous separation of the burn wound eschar.

Two types of excision are employed for burn wounds: One is called tangential excision, and the other involves excision to muscle fascia. In tangential excision, the burned skin is removed in thin layers with a dermatome until the underlying viable tissue is reached. Once the entire wound has been excised down to a normal bed, the wound may be covered with freshly harvested split-thickness skin grafts or biologic dressings with delayed grafting. With small deep dermal or full-thickness burns, early tangential excision and immediate grafting offer an option to prolonged local treatment and delayed healing. When done before bacteria are established in the wound, this technique can result in a closed wound long before healing per primum. In the patient with burns of an entire extremity or surface of the torso, excision to muscular fascia is a reasonable option. Non-infected fascia offers an excellent bed for graft take, and when rapid closure of large wounds is required, this method is an excellent alternative. Burn eschar and underlying subcutaneous fat are removed sharply down to, but not including, the fascia. Split-thickness skin grafts are then placed directly on the fascia.

Split-thickness skin grafts may be taken from virtually any part of the body surface with intact skin. When small areas of burns are being covered, grafts should be taken from areas that will avoid further cosmetic deformity, such as the upper thighs and buttocks. Skin tone varies in different parts of the body, with the head and neck skin being pinker than other areas because of the concentration of underlying capillaries. Small burn wounds of the face should be covered with small grafts taken from the post-auricular or supraclavicular areas to avoid problems with color match.

Several dermatomes exist for obtaining split skin, including the manual Blair-Brown knife, the Padgett dermatome, and the powered Brown and Padgett dermatomes. Harvesting skin with one of the manual techniques requires some experience to obtain usable skin; therefore, the powered dermatomes are more in general use, particularly the Brown. Split-thickness skin is generally taken in the range of 1/12,000 to 1/16,000 of an inch thick by means of setting the dermatome to the appropriate depth. Thinner grafts have a better chance of being accepted than thick grafts; however, they are more prone to contraction as they heal. In the patient with extensive donor site requirements, skin may be reharvested from the same site after allowing re-epithelialization. In these patients, skin is usually harvested in the thin range to increase the rapidity of donor site healing. Before skin on the burn wound is placed, it is usually expanded with a meshing device. This can increase expansion of the skin in ratios from 1.5:1 to 9:1 and allows for escape of serum through the skin and coverage of large recipient areas with limited donor areas. The open interstices in a meshed skin graft placed on a wound epithelialize from the intact surrounding skin graft. Although meshed skin grafts can be utilized successfully on any part of the body, they are generally avoided on the face for cosmetic

reasons. When placed on hand burns, meshed skin should not be expanded to avoid hypertrophic scarring and contraction in areas of graft interstices.[14]

The periphery of skin grafts is held in place with either sutures or staples until healing occurs. Staples have the advantages of ease of application and of decreased bleeding from the skin edges. Wounds covered with skin grafts may be left open or may be covered with an occlusive dressing. The open technique has the advantages of ease of visualization of the wound and motion of the affected part. This is particularly useful in burns of the hand.

In potentially infected wounds, the dressings are removed at 3 days so that the grafts can be inspected. Exudate may be gently cleansed from the wound, and areas of poor contact of the graft to bed may be corrected. If no suspicion of possible wound contamination exists, the dressing may be left intact for 5 to 7 days. At this point in time, the graft should adhere reasonably well to the bed and should show early signs of revascularization. In the case of meshed grafts, it is often prudent to leave some type of dressing over the grafted areas until re-epithelialization of the interstices is complete. This will avoid drying of the areas not covered by skin until they are covered with epithelium.

LONG-TERM CARE AND RECONSTRUCTION

Care of the burn patient does not end with healing of the burn wounds. For healed burn wounds as well as donor sites and skin-grafted areas, special attention is required so that undesirable sequelae and complications may be avoided. After closure of the burn wounds is achieved, the patient will often be subjected to a long series of reconstructive procedures prior to returning as a productive member of society.

As mentioned previously, patients with grafted areas need to be cautioned about problems with exposure. Treatment is aimed to avoid heat and sun exposure as well as local trauma.

A major problem with healing burn wounds is the formation of hypertrophic scarring, particularly in areas such as the anterior neck and across joints. This occurs over a period of weeks to months following healing of the wounds and can proceed to loss of function of the affected parts, even to the point of dislocation of joints as a result of the inexorable pull of scar tissue. Splinting of joints and pressure applied over the area of burn wound have been shown to decrease contracture and hypertrophic scarring.[13] Pressure over areas of burn scars is applied with the use of controlled-pressure garments, which are custom-fitted to the particular patient and the area involved. These must be worn until the scar matures, a period extending from 6 months to a year from the time of healing.

Even with the use of these modes of therapy, operative procedures will be required for certain areas to reconstruct acceptable appearance and function. The face and hands are two such areas in particular. Functionally, the eyelids, nose, and mouth are areas often requiring scar release with Z-plasties or further skin grafting. Severe burns to the face often merit consideration for reconstructive procedures simply to restore a more normal appearance. Recent attention has focused on the use of full-face skin grafting and the use of full-face flaps to replace unacceptable burn scars. Likewise, grafts may be required to replace hair of the scalp and eyebrows.

Release of scarring in the upper extremity is often

necessary to restore a functional limb. This may involve all joints from the axilla to the fingers. Release may often be accomplished with a simple Z-plasty of the involved area; however, severe contractures may need further grafting or flap coverage to restore adequate range of motion. Consideration of scar contracture release should be given early prior to ankylosis of the involved joint, which can lead to further permanent loss of function.

CONCLUSION

The care of burn patients presents many potential challenges to the clinician. With the application of good general principles of care of the traumatized patient and knowledge of the pathophysiology of burn injuries, treatment can be given in a rational way. Uniformly good results can be expected in smaller burns, but larger injuries require close attention to more specific parameters of care.

SELECTED READINGS

Artz, C. P., Moncrief, J. A., and Pruitt, B. A., Jr.: Burns: A Team Approach. Philadelphia, W. B. Saunders Company, 1979.
This comprehensive book written by a number of workers in the field of burn therapy includes chapters concerning basic fundamentals of burn therapy, e.g., early care, local care of the burn wound, anesthesia of the body, types of burns (electrical, flame, chemical), and the general management and rehabilitation of the burned patient.

Davies, J. W. L.: Physiological Responses to Burning Injury. London, Academic Press, 1982.
This excellent book discusses the numerous physiologic responses of the body to the burn injury, e.g., changes in capillary permeability, occurrence and therapy of oligemia, electrolyte changes, renal function, respiratory problems, protein changes and plasma and tissue fluids, hematologic changes, and metabolic, endocrine, and immunologic responses to the burn.

DiGregorio, V. R.: Rehabilitation of the Burn Patient. New York, Churchill Livingstone, 1984.
The rehabilitation of the burned patient is addressed, e.g., occupational therapy, including splinting, positioning, and exercise; management of

pain; psychological stress; treatment of burns of specific areas; burns in children; and post-hospitalization care.

REFERENCES

1. Agee, R. N., Long, J. M., Hunt, J. L., Petroff, P. A., Lull, R. J., Mason, A. D., and Pruitt, B. A.: Use of ^{133}xenon in early diagnosis of inhalation injury. J. Trauma, *16*:218, 1976.
2. Alexander, J. W., Ogle, C. K., Stinnett, J.D., and Macmillan, B. G.: A sequential prospective analysis of immunologic abnormalities and infection following severe thermal injury. Ann. Surg., *188*:809, 1978.
3. Artz, C. P.: History of burns. *In* Artz, C. P., Moncrief, J. A., and Pruitt, B. A. (Eds.): Burns: A Team Approach. Philadelphia, W. B. Saunders Company, 1979.
4. Baxter, C. R.: Fluid volume and electrolyte changes of the early postburn period. Clin. Plast. Surg., *1*:693, 1974.
5. Bull, J. P., and Fisher, A. J.: A study of mortality in a burn unit: A revised estimate. Ann. Surg., *139*:269, 1954.
6. Chen, C. K., Jarrett, F., and Moylan, J. A.: Acute leukopenia as an allergic reaction to silver sulfadiazine in burn patients. J. Trauma, *16*:395, 1976.
7. Curreri, P. W., Luterman, A., Braun, D. W., and Sutures, G.: Burn injury. Ann. Surg., *192*:472, 1980.
8. Demling, R. H.: Improved survival after massive burns. J. Trauma, *23*:179, 1983.
9. Holliman, C. J., Saffle, J. R., Kravitz, M., and Warden, G. D.: Early surgical decompression in the management of electrical injuries. Am. J. Surg., *144*:733, 1982.
10. Hunt, J. L., Mason, A. D., Masterson, T. S., and Pruitt, B. A.: The pathophysiology of acute electrical injuries. J. Trauma, *16*:335, 1976.
11. Janzekovic, Z.: A new concept in the early excision and immediate grafting of burns. J. Trauma, *10*:1103, 1970.
12. Jelenko, C.: Chemicals that "burn." J. Trauma, *14*:65, 1974.
13. Larson, D. L., Abston, S., Evans, E. B., Dobrkovsky, M., and Linares, H. A.: Techniques for decreasing scar formation and contractures in the burn patient. J. Trauma, *11*:807, 1971.
14. MacMillan, B. G.: The use of mesh grafting in treating burns. Surg. Clin. North Am., *50*:1347, 1970.
15. Monafo, W. W., and Ayvazian, V. H.: Topical Therapy. Surg. Clin. North Am., *58*:1157, 1978.
16. Pruitt, B. A.: The burn patient: I. Initial care. Curr. Probl. Surg., *16*:4, 1979.
17. Pruitt, B. A.: The burn patient: II. Later care and complications of thermal injury. Curr. Probl. Surg., *16*:10, 1979.
18. Pruitt, B. A., and Goodwin, C. W.: Stress ulcer disease in the burned patient. World J. Surg., *5*:209, 1981.
19. Thompson, P. D., and Parks, D. H.: Monitoring, banking, and clinical use of amnion as a burn wound dressing. Ann. Plast. Surg., *7*:354, 1981.

PRINCIPLES OF OPERATIVE SURGERY: ANTISEPSIS, ASEPSIS, TECHNIQUE, SUTURES, AND DRAINS

BENJAMIN F. RUSH, JR., M.D.

10

Scientific evaluation of the principles of surgery began barely a hundred years ago but has rapidly progressed. Today, most surgical procedures have been assessed by rigorous scientific methods. It is by these means that such procedures become reproducible and predictable.

Lister's concept that surgical infection is due to the introduction of bacteria into the wound has prevailed. Nevertheless, it is impossible to sterilize skin. In a hospital environment, transient bacteria on the skin surface are more likely to be pathogenic and are present in hair follicles and in the sebaceous and sweat glands of the patient and the surgeon. For many years, skin was cleansed by a scrub with green soap (10 to 15 minutes) followed by a 70 per cent ethyl alcohol rinse. During the course of an operation, bacteria can emerge from the pores of the patient or surgeon to contaminate the skin. In the recent past, hexachlorophene was introduced as an antiseptic that was very bactericidal, leaving a thin film on the skin that was active for many hours. It was also ideal for the surgical hand scrub, since the film lasted for a substantial period and repeated scrubbing built an antiseptic layer that persisted on the hands of the operating team from day to day. Unfortunately, it became apparent that this material could be absorbed through the skin, and significant blood levels were demonstrated in operating room personnel. This, together with the discovery that the compound is teratogenic, led to its disfavor.

One of the oldest compounds for skin antisepsis is tincture of iodine. This was the most effective of all the antiseptics, capable of killing bacteria, yeast, and most spores on contact. Unfortunately, it is irritating to the skin, and a rather high incidence of subjects were allergic to iodine compounds.

The use of iodine has returned in the last decade, with the discovery that it can be linked to polyvinyl compounds and combined with detergents to make an excellent germicidal solution. The antibacterial action depends on the slow release of free iodine from the iodine-containing organic compound. "Iodophors" are effective against both gram-positive and gram-negative bacteria but not spores. The frequency of allergic reactions noted with tincture of iodine is much reduced with these compounds. If a layer of iodophor is left on the skin, the slow release of iodine continues for several hours, protecting the patient through-out the operation from the great majority of skin contaminants (Fig. 1).

The most commonly accepted technique in cleansing the patient's skin is to begin with the area where the incision is to be made and to consider this as the cleanest portion of the area of operation. The skin is cleansed in ever-widening circles from this point. The surgeon never returns the cleansing sponge to the incision site from the periphery. Two or three cleansings of the skin, often with a detergent solution containing an iodophor, may then be followed by an aqueous solution or tincture of the iodophor as a final preparation.

Cleansing of the surgeon's hands and arms is done with a scrub brush, with considerable attention being given to cleansing under the nails and between the fingers. With detergent solutions containing an idophor, an initial scrub of the hands for about 5 minutes is considered adequate.[5]

ASEPSIS

The Operating Team

The apparel and conduct of the operating team are of enormous importance in the aseptic treatment of the surgical patient. Members of the surgical team change from street clothes to clean "scrub suits" before entering the operating room. These suits, formerly white, are now green, gray, or blue in order to reduce glare from the operating lights. In addition to the scrub suit, the hair is covered with an appropriate cap, and, in cases of beards or whiskers, the face will be covered as well with a special hood. Shoes are covered also with surgical "booties." Hoods, caps, booties, and, in many cases, the scrub suit itself are often made of disposable paper and are discarded at the end of the operative procedure.

The mouth and nose are covered by a mask, which is an important barrier to contamination, since the mouth and nose are important sources of bacteria, particularly when the operator talks. Some of the old gauze masks that were popular fewer than 10 to 20 years ago were shown to be highly ineffective, filtering out no more than 10 to 20 per cent of particulate matter. The masks containing fiber glass

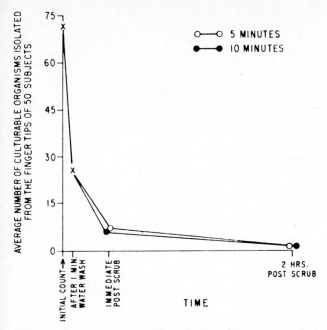

Figure 1. Comparison of the effect of a 5- or 10-minute surgical scrub on skin bacterial counts obtained from 50 subjects using povidone-iodine and a brush. (From Dineen, P.: Surg. Gynecol. Obstet., 129:1181, 1969.)

used today are capable of screening 95 to almost 100 per cent of particulate matter from the nose and mouth.

In a well-prepared operating room, the most important source of contamination, with the possible exception of the patient himself, is the operating team. The cornified layer of skin is constantly shedding, and each flake of skin has many bacteria.[12] It has been demonstrated that contamination is directly related to the number of people in the room, to motion in the room, and to the amount of conversation. Any operating team member with an infection should make this known to the surgeon and should be excluded from the operating suite. Occasionally, members of the operating team are carriers of diseases, with an increased incidence of pathogens on their skin or elsewhere. The presence of such a carrier may lead to a sudden outbreak of infection in the operating suite, and the pathogen should be identified by appropriate cultures.[17]

Preparing the Patient

The removal of hair at the site of the incision is another surgical tradition that is being reassessed. It was customary to shave all hair from the incision site, and patients undergoing an abdominal operation had the hair removed from the nipple lines to the genitalia. Several studies have now confirmed that shaving hair in the area of the incision can increase the incidence of infection in the surgical wound.[4,6,15] This is most severe if shaving is done the night prior to operation; however, even if the area is shaved in the operating room immediately prior to operation, there can be a increase in the incidence of infection. The best technique is either to remove hair with a depilatory or, interestingly enough, not to shave the patient at all. Infection rates with these last two methods are about equal. The mechanism of infection induced by shaving the skin appears to be the multiple small cuts, most being microscopic, that harbor and encourage infection adjacent to the incision.

After hair is removed and the wound site has been cleansed with an antiseptic, the patient is draped in such a

way that all areas uninvolved by the operation are excluded from the surgical field. Usually two, or even four, layers of cloth are used to cover the patient. Cloth drapes, unfortunately, are subject to contamination when wet, and bacteria from the patient's skin can penetrate the interstices of a wet cloth drape. Recently, it has been shown that the safest technique is the use of disposable paper drapes, which are impervious to bacterial transmission, and these drapes are now standard in most operating rooms.

Preparing the Instruments

Instruments and equipment to be used at the operating table can be sterilized by steam heat, chemical solutions, dry heat, or gas methods. The method chosen is usually dependent on the characteristics of the material being sterilized.

STEAM HEAT

The autoclave is a device designed to expose equipment to steam heat under pressure and is applicable to most surgical instruments and supplies. At a pressure of 15 pounds per square inch, the temperature in an autoclave reaches 121°C. The time required to sterilize most surgical packs is 20 minutes.

Another system for steam sterilization, "flash" sterilization, is dependent on the attachment of a vacuum pump to the sterilizer, which removes most of the air and exposes the instruments to pure steam much more rapidly than in an ordinary autoclave in which air is gradually displaced over a period of time by the influxing steam. During the period in which there is a mixture of air and steam in the autoclave, the heat of the mixture, and thus the effectiveness of sterilization, is reduced. A flash autoclave is capable of sterilizing instruments in 3 minutes, and these autoclaves are often used in the operating suite to sterilize instruments that have become contaminated and are needed again quickly.

CHEMICAL STERILIZATION

Another technique for disinfecting equipment, which is not suitable for exposure to steam heat but which can tolerate moisture, is chemical sterilization. Currently, the most popular solutions are 2 per cent aqueous solutions of glutaraldehye. These solutions are highly effective against bacteria spores and viruses. They are often used for disinfection of urologic equipment, such as catheters, and can be used with almost any form of rubber or plastic equipment.

DRY HEAT

Items that can tolerate heat but not moisture or that are not penetrated well by steam can be sterilized with dry heat. A hot air oven at 170°C. will sterilize items in about 1 hour. These ovens are sometimes used for glassware, petroleum jelly–soaked sponges that are not well penetrated by steam, or substances (such as talc) that tend to cake in the presence of moisture.

Other Sources of Contamination

Every attempt is made to render the entire operating suite as free of bacteria as possible. Room air is a potential source of bacteria, although with modern filtration in air-conditioned operating suites and frequent exchange of room air, the concentration of bacteria in the air is minimal. Laminar flow has been used in some operating rooms. This is a system of unimodal air flow in which air enters either at the ceiling and exits through the floor or enters from one wall and exits from the opposite wall, so that there is a one-way flow of air. Nevertheless, this technique has not appeared to improve infection rates significantly over the standard air conditioning system in which room air is exchanged frequently through large filters.[12]

The most dangerous sources of bacteria and other microorganisms in an operating room are the operating team and the patient. If an unprepared bowel is opened during an operation and a small amount of feces spills into the peritoneal cavity, the patient has suddenly been exposed to a concentration of bacteria as great as a billion organisms per gram of feces, probably at a time when the maximal number of organisms in the filtered air can be numbered in the tens or hundreds.

The patient plays another role in the bacterial versus-host relationship, and that is the intrinsic resistance to withstand contamination. Contamination of the patient's tissues from extrinsic sources in a properly conducted operating room environment has been reduced by modern techniques to a very low level, and the vast majority of patients should be able to tolerate this degree of contamination without the development of infection. Should the patient, however, have *suppression* of intrinsic resistance through malnutrition, disease, genetic predisposition, or other causes, it may be impossible to reduce the level of bacterial contamination below a point that will lead to infection.[8, 14] Hunt has emphasized that the remaining strides in reducing the incidence of wound infection probably relate to an increasing knowledge of the complexities of the immune system and to the ability to adjust and enhance them.[7]

OPERATIVE TECHNIQUE

Halsted was an early proponent of the gentle handling of tissues, careful hemostasis, and appropriate irrigation of wounds to enhance healing and prevent infection with surgical procedures. He said:

I believe that the tendency will always be in the direction of exercising greater care and refinement in operating and that the surgeon will develop increasingly a respect for tissue, a sense which recoils from inflicting unnecessary insult to structures concerned in the process of repair.

As his teachings spread, this model of the careful, deliberate, gentle surgeon became widely accepted. It should also be remembered that the longer an operation, the greater the stress to the patient and the risk of wound infection.[4]

Incisions

The incision permits the surgeon to gain access to the operative field. Many incisions have been described in the literature for various indications, and there are a host of eponyms attached to them. However, the principles of selecting an incision are simple and include ensurance of good exposure, allowance of good healing, and an acceptable scar.

In general, incisions are made along the normal skin lines, which are followed by a much finer scar than those

made at angles to the skin lines. There are exceptions, as in an exploratory laparotomy; in this case, a midline (or, occasionally, a paramedian) incision is elected, even though it crosses normal skin lines, because it gives the best access to the abdominal cavity. In children, with their almost circular abdominal cavities, the abdomen can be explored as easily through a transverse incision, and this is usually selected because of its better cosmetic result and increased resistance to disruption. In reoperations, every attempt should be made to use the original approach. The stainless steel surgical scalpel still appears to be the best for skin incisions. High-frequency current, as used in *electrocautery*, produces a skin wound that is four times as susceptible to infection as wounds made by the scalpel (Fig. 2). In prospective trials, it has been shown that electrosurgery almost doubled the infection rate of surgical wounds.[4] Moreover, if a *carbon dioxide laser* is used to make a skin incision, the resulting wound has been shown experimentally to be ten times as susceptible to infection as an electrosurgical incision (Fig. 3).

Dissection during an operation may be sharp or blunt. Sharp dissection is accomplished either with the knife or with scissors. Blunt dissection is used to divide tissue planes

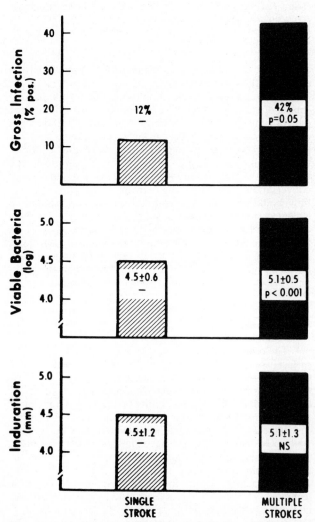

Figure 2. A clean stroke of the knife dividing the skin leads to much less susceptibility to infection than do multiple strokes, as demonstrated in this experimental model. (From Edlich, R., Rodenhaven, G., Thacker, J., and Edgerton, M.: South Plainfield, N. J., Chirurgecon, Inc., 1977.)

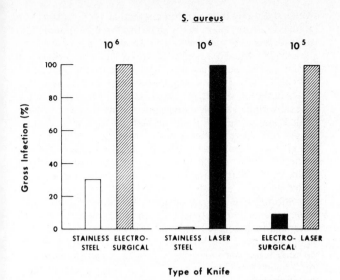

Figure 3. The use of a knife to divide tissues produces a wound much less susceptible to infection than the use of either electrosurgical or laser incisions. Laser-made incisions appear even more likely to induce infection than do electrosurgical incisions. (From Edlich, R., Rodenhaven, G., Thacker, J., and Edgerton, M.: South Plainfield, N. J., Chirurgecon, Inc., 1977.)

and can be done with the tip of the fine dissecting scissors or gently with a finger or the hand holding a surgical sponge. Although the technique of dissection is part of the training of an experienced surgeon and requires personal experience to develop fully, certain principles can be emphasized. One should take advantage of the routes and planes that nature has created. Countertraction is probably one of the most important features of dextrous and smooth surgical dissection, and tension on tissue planes usually develops a line at the point where the planes normally divide. Dissection here leads to a more bloodless division of the structures. The least amount of trauma will be accomplished in dissecting natural tissue planes.

Hemostasis

The most important hemostatic device is the body's own systemic and local mechanisms for controlling hemorrhage. Should these mechanisms fail, the patient will likely exsanguinate, regardless of the attempts made to control bleeding. Thousands of tiny vessels are divided when a scalpel divides the patient's tissues. The majority of these tiny arterioles, capillaries, and venules seal themselves by constriction and by small fibrin clot. The bleeding seen by the surgeon is from larger vessels, some of which are small and bleed minimally and then seal themselves. Even larger vessels require deliberate hemostasis, such as *ligatures* or use of the *electrocautery*. Pressure is sometimes used to obtain hemostasis, at least until (1) the bleeding is reduced, (2) the site can be better visualized, and (3) the vessel is controlled.

Sutures

Sutures are used either for hemostasis or to join divided anatomic structures. There are many techniques for suturing different organs and tissues of the body. However, the principle in selecting sutures is that the suture with the smallest diameter and strength for the specific use is the appropriate one. The strength required is equivalent to the

strength of the tissues being sutured. A suture can be extracted from fat with the application of only 2 pounds of pressure, so that a suture with a tensile strength of 20 pounds is useless in this location and very fine sutures should be used. Application of this principle also yields the minimal residue of foreign body in the patient at the end of the procedure. A ligature provokes an increased risk of infection in being a foreign body. Very rarely, sutures larger than the strength of the tissues required are used in order to provide a larger surface area that will prevent the suture from cutting through soft tissue, such as in closing lacerations of the spleen and liver. Tight sutures may cause necrosis of the enclosed tissues and can also induce an increased susceptibility to infection.

When suturing structures together, the surgeon has the choice of using an *interrupted* or *continuous suture*. The former implies multiple sutures, each one tied individually; the latter indicates a suture tied at one end of a row and then passed through the tissues repeatedly and finished with a tie at the end of the row. Indications for selection of one of these techniques depend on a combination of science, tradition, myth, custom, prior training, and instinct. In general, interrupted sutures are regarded as a safer technique, since failure of one suture does not affect others in the row, while failure of the tie at either end of a continuous suture disrupts the entire row. On the other hand, continuous sutures probably leave less foreign body in the wound (compared with multiple knots) and distribute the stress more uniformly along the row. These traditional and theoretical considerations are gradually yielding to the ubiquitous randomized prospective clinical trial. Richards and colleagues have reported in such a trial that continuous and interrupted sutures in abdominal closure are equally effective.[13]

Cautery

Bovie discovered that high-frequency alternating current in the range of 250,000 to 2,000,000 Hz could be used to incise or coagulate tissue to obtain hemostasis. This technique was first popularized by Cushing in neurosurgery and was subsequently used in other types of surgery.

If the current is undamped, the active electrode (i.e., the small tip of the electrosurgical instrument) acts as a bloodless knife. The cells at the edge of the line of incision disintegrate, although the heat creates mild thermal injury, which may increase susceptibility to infection.[4, 6] If the current is delivered as a damped oscillation, there is a rapid dehydration of living cells that fuse into a hyaline-like structure and the vessels within the mass are coagulated. This type of hemostasis is useful in controlling large numbers of small bleeding vessels, although it is limited to vessels of 2 mm. or less in diameter and is more effective with venous than arterial vessels. The object of the technique is to coagulate only the vessel itself and as little of the surrounding tissue as possible. To achieve this, a fine-tipped clamp is used to occlude the bleeding site and grasp as small an amount of tissue as possible. It is useful to place slight traction on the clamp to isolate the tissue from the remainder of the field. The field should be kept as dry as possible in the vicinity of the clamp in order to avoid dispersing the electric energy away from the point of application. Care must be taken so that the clamp is not touching retractors or other objects in contact with the patient, since areas of tissue that were not intended for coagulation will be injured. Touching the clamp with the monopolar electrode results in a high density of electrical energy at the tip of the clamp, which rapidly flows through the body and exits through the grounding plate, which is placed at some appropriate point under the patient. The grounding plate must be kept as large as possible to disperse the energy at this point so that it will have no effect on the tissues on exit. If the ground plate becomes detached, energy will leave the patient through any available portal, such as electrocardiograph (ECG) leads. Since these are much smaller points of exit, burns of the skin may occur with serious consequences to the patient.

Laser beams are another method of delivering high energy into the patient's tissues and can be used both as a scalpel and for hemostasis. These devices are still rather bulky and awkward for general use and may not have much advantage except for very special applications such as the coagulation or evaporation of tissues through fiberoptic instruments.

Cold also serves to produce hemostasis, and application of dry ice has been used to coagulate small hemangiomas, but it is not ordinarily used for the control of surgical bleeding.

Chemical cautery is most familiar to males who cut themselves shaving and then apply a "styptic pencil." The use of chemical coagulation is an old technique and various styptic formulas are described in early Egyptian, Roman, and Greek writings. Control of these substances is difficult, and if used in a large wound, they may diffuse into and injure considerable amounts of surrounding tissues. Styptics are very effective in controlling bleeding from small cuts such as the defects left by a biopsy forceps in the oral cavity or cervix or those in the skin. Silver nitrate sticks represent a good example of a useful styptic.

PRESSURE PACKS AND COAGULANTS

At times, situations arise in an operation where a wide field of many small bleeding points defeats attempts at specific control of each bleeding vessel. This may require the use of a surgical pack, a long strip of loosely woven bandage 1 to 6 inches in width. Packs bring about control of bleeding by pressure and by providing a lattice of material, which encourages clotting. They may be as small as a few inches of material packed in a deep oozing crevice in a wound or as large as several yards of material used to treat the entire pelvis. Packs are often used in combination with a pressure dressing, providing additional pressure on the exterior of the wound. These are inferior techniques to control bleeding and are often a "last resort" when all other techniques have failed. Packs provoke a high susceptibility to infection and should be removed in 24 to 72 hours.

Certain substances such as collagen or fibrin promote coagulation and are sometimes applied in areas such as the liver or spleen when repair of lacerations is attempted and the pulp of the structures contains a large number and variety of low-pressure vascular spaces. They may be applied as a powder or as a woven fabric or sponge and have the advantage of being slowly absorbed by the tissues.

Sutures

Suture materials are used to join the tissues of the body in the course of a surgical operation. A *suture* usually implies use of the material together with a needle, whereas the same material used to tie a vessel without the use of an associated needle is a *ligature*. Many materials have been used as sutures in the past, including linen, cotton, various plastics, silver, and stainless steel. Sutures are

swedged directly to the end of disposable needles, since the swedged needle is less bulky than the threaded needle and causes less trauma when drawn through tissue.

An *ideal* suture should be strong enough so that only a thin strand is required to draw the tissues together, thereby reducing the amount of foreign body left in the body. It should be easily manipulated and tied and should be reabsorbed and disappear as soon as the tissues have healed and achieved their normal strength. The suture should also have a coefficient of friction high enough to produce a secure closure with the least number of knots, yet low enough so that it will slip through tissues without injury to the surrounding tissues. The totally ideal suture remains to be found.

Sutures can be classified as (1) *naturally occurring materials*, such as catgut, silk, or wire; or (2) *synthetic materials*, including (a) the synthetic collagens (polyglycolic acid, polyglactin), which are absorbable sutures or (b) various non-absorbable plastics, such as polyamides (nylon), polyesters (Dacron), and polyolefines (polyethylene, polypropylene).

NATURAL SUTURES

Of all the many forms of natural sutures used in the past, only catgut, stainless steel wire, and silk are still used.

Catgut. Catgut is made from the submucosa of sheep or porcine intestine. Untreated plain catgut creates a markedly inflammatory action in tissues, with a large cuff of inflammatory cells surrounding the suture on microscopic examination. It is absorbed quite rapidly in approximately 10 days. If catgut is treated with chromic acid, the inflammatory response is reduced, although it remains appreciable. The sutures retain their strength for approximately 21 days and somewhat longer when a large sized suture is used.[10] Since there is a tendency for the catgut knot to slip, the ends of the sutures should be cut approximately a quarter of an inch from the knot.

Stainless Steel Wire. This can be obtained, either as a monofilament or a multifilament suture, and was once the suture of choice in a contaminated wound because of its resistance to infection. Stainless steel has a deservedly poor reputation for its handling qualities because it is stiff and may cut through tissues if too tight. Although this material stimulates less inflammatory response in tissues than does catgut or silk, it has recently been shown to predispose to infection to a greater degree than many of the available plastic suture materials.[6] If stainless steel wire is used, the wire should not be kinked at any point, since the breaking strength at that site is reduced. The knot formed by stainless steel has excellent retention power and rarely slips, but it has the disadvantage, if placed subcutaneously, of being easily palpable by the patient through a thin abdominal wall. Likewise, the ends of stainless steel wire must be carefully inverted away from the skin to avoid irritation or perforation of the skin. For these reasons, stainless steel wire is used less often than the newer plastic sutures.

Silk. Silk has been used for many years. Because it is non-absorbable, it forms a persisting foreign body in the tissues. For this reason, it is now less popular than previously, especially in closure of incisions, and is gradually yielding to substitution of the newer synthetic materials.

SYNTHETIC SUTURES

The *absorbable synthetic sutures*, such as polyglycolic acid and polyglactin, stimulate a minimal inflammatory response in tissues, especially in comparison to catgut.

Unlike catgut, the knots with synthetics are much less likely to slip. The products of degradation of polyglycolic acid have an antibacterial effect, and this may also contribute to the reduction in inflammatory tissue response. These features of the synthetic absorbable sutures have led to their rapid substitution for catgut in many instances.

Non-absorbable sutures have the advantage of retaining their strength in an infected wound to a much greater extent than absorbable sutures and of being the most inert in tissues, compared with even the new synthetic absorbable sutures. Not all non-absorbable sutures are truly non-absorbable. Nylon and silk begin to lose strength after approximately 2 months and by the end of 6 months have little or no remaining tensile strength. Polyesters and poly-olefines, however, maintain their original tensile strength almost indefinitely. In certain situations, such as in suturing prosthetic heart valves, this long-term strength is necessary, since the prosthetic valves may never become thoroughly integrated into the surrounding tissues and need the additional support of the original sutures.

Multifilament polyesters (Dacron) were one of the early synthetics used, but they had the disadvantage of a rather high coefficient of friction, so that there was some resistance to their passage through tissues and the tendency for the knot to snag and not snub up securely to the structures being tied. This has been partially alleviated by coating the sutures with Teflon, facilitating their passage through the tissues and encouraging a better ability for the knot to slide into place.

Monofilament polyamide (nylon) and *polypropylene* seem to produce the least reaction of all currently available material. However, they have such a low coefficient of friction that a minimum of six knots must be placed in order to prevent slippage. This increases the amount of foreign body in the wound, and, in addition, the interstices of the multiple ties have the theoretical disadvantage of creating small protected sites in which bacteria may flourish.

It is obvious that there are a number of considerations in selecting suture material. Natural materials are gradually being replaced by synthetic sutures. In experimental work, *carbon fibers* and *ceramics* are being evaluated for intra-operative implanted materials and have found use as a replacement for tendons. Carbon encourages an in-growth of fiberblasts, which tend to line the carbon fibers.

Adhesives

Closure of the skin with sutures renders the skin closure especially susceptible to infection. Each suture is a small wick that is capable of inducing infection from the contaminated skin surface into the subcutaneous tissues. Silk sutures, with greater capillarity, are more likely to cause this problem, but nylon or polypropylene skin sutures also increase the susceptibility to infection. The skin closure that has proved least likely to cause susceptibility to infection is the use of microporous adhesive tape (Fig. 4). In a controlled series, the infection rate in wounds closed with tape is half that of wounds closed with percutaneous sutures.[2] Unfortunately, these tapes are not applicable in every site. In areas that are moist, such as the axilla and groin, the tape may not adhere effectively. In very active areas also, such as the extremities, tape closures are less secure. However, closure of lacerations or incisions in the trunk and face can be made quite secure with microporous tapes when properly used.

There has been considerable interest in the use of adhesives to replace sutures in repairing structures within

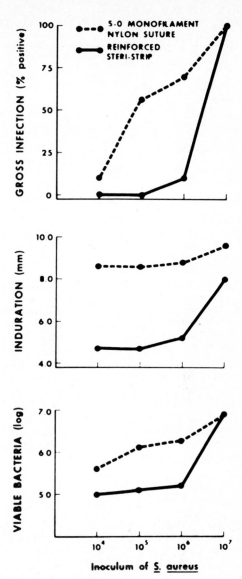

Figure 4. Even fine monofilament percutaneous sutures potentiate infection in a wound, compared with closure with adhesive strips. (From Edlich, R., Rodenhaven, G., Thacker, J., and Edgerton, M.: South Plainfield, N. J., Chirurgecon, Inc., 1977.)

the body. Most of this work is experimental at present, and many adhesives have proved too toxic to tissues to be effective. One area in which adhesives have proved useful is in the fixation of the articulating surface of artificial joints of the hip and other areas with acrylic plastic. Considerable success is reported, but some problems still exist, especially loosening of the adhesive over a period of time. Research is continuing to improve these adhesives and the techniques for applying them.

Staples

The use of staples for joining tissues in the abdomen and chest and for the achievement of hemostasis appears to have found widespread acceptance in this decade. Ravitch published some of his early experiences with a stapler in 1959.[11] Although the early instruments developed in Russia showed great ingenuity, they were somewhat awkward and difficult to load, since each of the tiny tantalum staples had to be loaded individually by hand into the

TABLE 1. Skin Staples in Potentially Contaminated Wounds (Percent of Wounds with Abscess Formation: Ten Mice in Each Category*†)

Inoculum	Percutaneous Sutures			Subcuticular Polyglycolic Acid Sutures	Skin Staples	Unwounded Controls
	Nylon	Silk	Polyglycolic Acid			
10^8	60	90	80	50	40	40
10^7	50	50	70	70	20	20
10^6	40	20	20	30	0	10
Average	50	53	56	50	30	23

*Modified from Stillman, R., Marino, C., and Seligman, S.: Arch Surg., *119*:821, 1984.

†Statistically significant differences by the Fisher exact test are as follows: nylon versus skin staples, P = .029; silk versus skin staples, P = .015; percutaneous polyglycolic acid versus skin staples, P = .007; subcuticular polyglycolic acid versus skin staples, P = .029; and unwounded controls versus skin staples, P not significant.

machine. Subsequently, another instrument maker developed these devices and by the 1970s had introduced a series of improved staplers. The convenience and safety of these instruments gradually became recognized, together with a gradual accumulation of detailed studies in the literature, and demonstrated that reconstruction of organs with these instruments was as effective as the use of hand suturing.[3] Moreover, in certain instances, such as in the esophagus, staple closure was superior to standard sutures.

Staples have a preferred role in many pelvic, abdominal, and thoracic procedures, and their development continues as new concepts are introduced. A row of staples that totally compresses the tissues can be used when hemostasis is the main object of the procedure, such as the transection of a major vessel.[16] Like microporous tape, staple closure of skin incisions has proved more likely to increase resistance to infection than percutaneous closure with silk or nylon (Table 1).

Drains

Drains are used for two primary purposes, the first being the prevention of the accumulation of blood, plasma, or other fluids within the body by allowing them to drain to the exterior. Examples include bile from liver tissue,

blood from an area of extensive oozing within the body where many small bleeding points defy the ability of the operator to control them, and lymph from a site in which lymphatics have been transected and cannot be otherwise controlled. For the benefit of wound drainage, the surgeon must consider the risk of contaminating the wound and increasing susceptibility to infection (Fig. 5). As soon as drainage from the area has diminished to small amounts, the drain should be removed.

A somewhat different situation occurs when an abscess cavity is encountered in the abdomen or other region. In this instance, the abscess is often surrounded by a thick wall that does not collapse when the contained pus is removed. In this situation, pus will continue to accumulate in the cavity and perpetuate the abscess. The final resolution occurs when the cavity gradually fills with granulation tissue, and drainage may be required in this situation for many days or even weeks. In this instance, gross infection is already present and the decision to use a drain is not difficult.

A second and somewhat more controversial use of drains is to establish a path of least resistance adjacent to a healing anastomosis in the abdomen from closure of a viscus. If the closure is doubtful and leakage from the anastomosis is likely, a drain can be placed adjacent to the area. Abdominal drains, however, are quickly surrounded

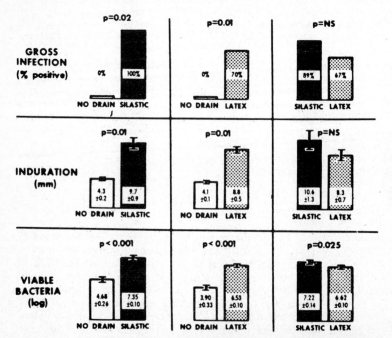

Figure 5. The potentiation of infection in experimental wounds by latex and silicone drains. When drains are used, wounds will almost always be contaminated. (From Edlich, R., Rodenhaven, G., Thacker, J., and Edgerton, M.: South Plainfield, N. J., Chirurgecon, Inc., 1977.)

by the omentum and by fibrinated loops of bowel, which soon form a tract around the drain so that the peritoneal cavity is not drained. This characteristic of abdominal drains must be recognized.[1,9] If the purpose is to provide a sinus tract adjacent to an anastomosis, it must be left for much longer periods. Should the anastomosis leak and form a perianastomotic abscess, the abscess is most likely to break into the sinus tract and find its way to the surface, since this is the route of least resistance. However, this is not guaranteed, and in the presence of a firm, well-formed sinus tract, the abscess may perforate into an adjacent viscus or into the general peritoneal cavity. Finally, there is substantial experimental evidence that a drain adjacent to an anastomosis may encourage anastomotic leaks. Thus, the decision to drain a doubtful anastomosis is fraught with hazards and should be done on rare occasions.

Drains are not prophylactic; they do not prevent anastomotic leaks, nor do they prevent anastomotic abscesses. There was a time, a few decades ago, when surgeons encountering a patient with diffuse soiling of the peritoneal cavity would place drains in all the sites in which abscess formation was most likely, such as the pelvis, pericolic gutters, subphrenic space, and subhepatic space. Patients emerged from the operating room with a porcupine-like collection of abdominal drains extending in all directions. It is now understood that this practice succeeds in creating multiple intra-abdominal sinuses and the drains are draining only their own sinus tracts after a very short time. The so-called prophylactic use of drains for peritoneal contamination has been abandoned.

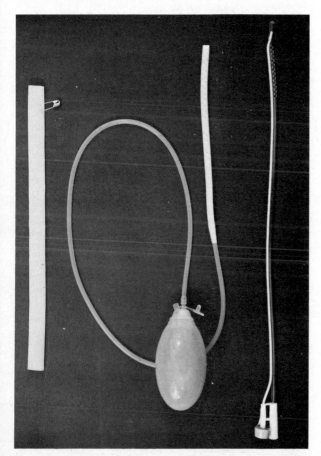

Figure 6. The three commonly used drains. Left, *Penrose.* Center, *Suction. Note attached portable suction device.* Right, *Sump. Note bacterial filter over air vent.*

Three types of drains are used primarily: (1) the Penrose drain (latex rubber), (2) the closed or open suction drain, and (3) the sump drain (Fig. 6). Each of these has its own particular application and indications.

PENROSE DRAIN

Penrose drains are thin, flat, latex rubber tubes of various diameters. They are soft and flexible and do not damage adjacent organs in the abdominal cavity. The drainage action is effected through gravity and capillarity. They are somewhat irritating to the surrounding tissues and will form a firm sinus tract fairly promptly, a useful property if the formation of a well-defined sinus tract is the purpose for the drain. They have the disadvantage of freely draining in either direction; i.e., bacteria growing on the skin or accumulating in the damp environment of an overlying dressing can migrate down the drain just as freely as fluid is drawn up the drain into the dressing. Culture of the tips of these tubes often shows contamination with various organisms within hours after they are inserted. Fortunately, the formation of a firm sinus tract around the tube protects most of the abdomen from this contamination, but the sinus tract is infected.

If these tubes are left in place for more than 48 hours, they should be removed slowly (2 inches a day is recommended) to allow the sinus tract to close from below upward toward the skin. Sudden removal of the entire tube may result in the skin closing first, with the formation of an abscess in the drain tract. If these drains are used to drain an infected wound, such as a breast abscess, a well-defined periappendiceal abscess, or a perirectal abscess, the problem of reverse contamination is probably of little concern. The drain does not usually form a sinus tract as in the peritoneal cavity, but it keeps the skin overlying the abscess open to permit drainage until the abscess cavity has begun to close by granulation.

SUCTION DRAIN

Suction drains are usually firm-walled, multiholed tubes that are inserted into the area to be drained through a rather tightly fitting exit wound through the skin, permitting suction to be applied. They are connected to various types of suction devices, either through a connection to wall suction or frequently to various portable devices that are spring-driven, or otherwise actuated and that can be attached to the patient's pajamas, avoiding restrictions of the patient's movements. Their greatest usefulness is in the removal of accumulated fluids and secretions. They are especially effective under large skin flaps, such as those encountered following radical neck dissection or radical or modified breast dissections. In these areas, they serve to draw the skin down to the underlying tissues rapidly and seem to promote a more rapid coaptation of the overlying skin and the underlying surfaces.

Removal of these tubes is determined by the amount of fluid removed. When the volume of suction has decreased to 50 ml. or less per day, depending somewhat on the size of the space being drained, the tube is usually removed. Ideally, removal within 24 to 72 hours is preferable. In draining of the abdomen, some of these tubes have the disadvantage of eroding into loops of adjacent bowel if left in place for too long a period. Firm-walled tubes of this type should not be left in place in the abdominal cavity for more than a few days, although newer tubes that are much softer and more flexible have been fabricated, especially those made of silicone rubber. Soft tubes of this type can be left in place for much longer periods without as much danger of eroding adjacent bowel. Silicone tubing has the property of minimal irritation to adjacent tissues. If the intention of drainage is to establish a sinus tract, latex Penrose drains or other rubber tubings are superior, since it takes much longer to develop a firm tract around silicone tubing.

Because suction tubes are inserted with a tight fit at the skin, contamination of the tube from the skin surface occurs somewhat more slowly. When these tubes are used in the abdomen, the surrounding sinus tract can be disrupted by irrigating the tube at regular intervals.[1] In fact, it is this principle that permits successful peritoneal dialysis. The disadvantage of irrigating such tubes is the contamination of the peritoneal cavity with bacteria contained within the sinus formed around the tube.

The question of propriety and usefulness of irrigating abdominal drainage tubes is somewhat controversial. In areas outside the abdomen, irrigation of the tubes is less hazardous and can be advantageous if the tube becomes obstructed early while fluids are still accumulating under tissue flaps.

SUMP DRAIN

A number of different configurations are included under the heading of sump drains, but the basic principle is that a multiholed tube is inserted into the wound and formed into a U, so that the distal end of the U is above the surface of the skin. As suction is applied to one end, air is drawn through the other. By this device, pressure in the tube is maintained at atmospheric levels and tissue around the drain is less likely to be drawn into the holes of the tubing.

The sump drain is most useful in the drainage of established *fistulas*, in which relatively large amounts of material must be removed, as in the intestine, pancreatic ducts, or hepatic ducts. In addition to retrograde contamination of the drain from the skin, the sump drain adds contamination from room air drawn into the drainage tract. This does not seem to occur if the suction is kept below 10 pounds per square inch or if contamination can be prevented by the use of a bacterial filter over the air vent.

SELECTED REFERENCES

Edlich, R., Rodenhaven, G., Thacker, J., and Edgerton, M.: Fundamentals of Wound Management in Surgery. South Plainfield, N.J., Chirurgecon, Inc., 1977.
One of the best reviews of the scientific basis of surgical techniques. Experimental data relating to the effects of local anesthesia, hair removal, antisepsis, surgical débridement, mechanical cleansing, dead space, drainage, dressings, and a host of other factors in the creation and care of the operative wound are presented.

Simmons, R. (Guest Editor): Surgical infection. World J. Surg., *4*:367, 1980.

A symposium on surgical infection including nine articles, each with commentaries from distinguished authorities. The last two articles are most applicable to the contents of this chapter, but all are useful. The bibliography is extensive.

Steichen, F., and Ravitch, M.: Stapling in Surgery. Chicago, Year Book Medical Publishers, 1983.
This text reviews the history, experimental background, and instrumentation of suturing with the use of staples. It is written by two of the major pioneers in the field and is superbly illustrated.

Van Way, C. III, and Bverk, C.: Surgical Skills in Patient Care. St. Louis, The C.V. Mosby Company, 1978.
Chapters 1 through 6 cover much of the material in this chapter in somewhat greater detail. Multiple line drawings are used in each chapter. Chapters 7 through 14 deal with the performance of many ward procedures.

Wind, G., and Rich, N.: Principles of Surgical Technique: The Art of Surgery. Baltimore, Urban and Schwarzenberg, 1983.
Profusely and well-illustrated text demonstrating many of the kinesthetic acts of the surgeon. Surgical "ties" are especially well shown, including two-handed, one-handed, and instrument ties.

REFERENCES

1. Agrama, H. M., Blackwood, J., Brown, C., Machiedo, G., and Rush, B.: Functional longevity of intraperitoneal drains. Am. J. Surg., *132*:418, 1976.
2. Carpendale, M., and Sereda, W.: The role of percutaneous suture in surgical wound infection. Surgery, *58*:672, 1965.
3. Chassin, J., Rifkind, K., Sussman, B., Kassel, B., Fingaret, A., Draget, S., and Chassin, P.: The stapled gastrointestinal tract anastomosis: Incidence of postoperative complications compared with suture anastomosis. Ann. Surg., *188*:689, 1978.
4. Cruse, P. J., and Foord, R.: A five-year prospective study of 23,649 surgical wounds. Arch. Surg., *107*:206, 1973.
5. Dineen, P.: An evaluation of the duration of the surgical scrub. Surg. Gynecol. Obstet., *129*:1181, 1969.
6. Edlich, R., Rodenhaven, G., Thacker, J., and Edgerton, M.: Fundamentals of Wound Management in Surgery: Technical Factors in Wound Management. South Plainfield, N.J., Chirurgecon, Inc., 1977.
7. Hunt, T.: Surgical wound infections: An overview. Am. J. Med., *76*:717, 1981.
8. Morris, P., Barnes, B., and Burke, J.: The nature of the irreducible minimum rate of incisional sepsis. Arch. Surg., *92*:367, 1966.
9. Moss, J. P.: Historical and current perspectives on surgical drainage. Surg. Gynecol. Obstet., *152*:517, 1981.
10. Postlethwait, R. W.: Principles of operative surgery: Antisepsis, technique, sutures, and drains. *In* Sabiston, D. C., Jr. (Ed.): Davis-Christopher Textbook of Surgery, 12th ed. Philadelphia, W. B. Saunders Company, 1981.
11. Ravitch, M., Brown, I., and Daviglus, G.: Experimental and clinical use of the Soviet bronchus stapling instrument. Surgery, *46*:97, 1959.
12. Ravitch, M., and McAuley, C.: Airborne contamination of the operative wound. Surg. Gynecol. Obstet., *159*:177, 1984.
13. Richards, P., Balch, C., and Aldrete, J.: Abdominal wound closure: A randomized prospective study of 571 patients comparing continuous vs. interrupted suture techniques. Ann. Surg., *197*:238, 1983.
14. Scrimshaw, N.: Synergism of malnutrition and infection. J.A.M.A., *212*:1685, 1970.
15. Seropian, R., and Reynolds, B.: Wound infections after preoperative depilatory vs. razor preparation. Am. J. Surg., *121*:251, 1971.
16. Stillman, R., Marino, C., and Seligman, S.: Skin staples in potentially contaminated wounds. Arch. Surg., *119*:821, 1984.
17. Walter, C. W.: The surgeon's responsibility for asepsis. Med. Instrumentation, *12*:140, 1978.

SURGICAL INFECTIONS AND CHOICE OF ANTIBIOTICS

RONALD LEE NICHOLS, M.D.

11

The development of a *nosocomial* (hospital-acquired) infection is a prime cause of increased morbidity and mortality in the hospitalized patient. Therefore, any break in infection control can result in septic complications that could potentially cause a greater risk to the patient's well-being than the original disease state or operative procedure. Approximately 20 to 30 per cent of hospitalized surgical patients will become infected, either prior to admission or during hospitalization. A *hospital-acquired* infection is defined as one that manifests itself after 72 hours of admission or after a surgical procedure. Medicine services tend to have higher rates of *community-acquired* infection, whereas surgical wards have increased hospital-acquired infections. Approximately 70 per cent of all hospital-acquired infections occur in patients who have undergone a surgical procedure. The urinary tract, surgical wound, and respiratory tract are the prime sites of infection. These infections, when present, have been estimated to increase the length of hospital stay by an average of one week. The additional cost of hospitalization varies depending on the site of the infection, but it is estimated to average about $7000 per patient.[8] Wound infections increase hospitalization costs the most, urinary tract infections the least, probably less than $1000 per episode. In the United States the annual cost of hospital-acquired infections is $1 billion as a low estimate and up to $10 billion as a high estimate. These economic factors express only a small part of the story, for each hospital-acquired infection has its own tale of sorrow, disappointment, and tragedy.

It is imperative to be aware of the often complex nature surrounding the development of infection in the hospitalized patient. The microbiology of the various infections seen on each of the clinical services, the techniques of diagnosis, the factors that reduce the incidence of the infections, and the strategies of treatment must be offered and stressed at all levels of the educational program. It is hoped that this chapter will serve as a link between the basic science microbiologic curriculum and the development of clinical infection.

HISTORICAL ASPECTS

The idea that living organisms can originate from nonliving matter (*spontaneous generation*) was expressed as early as 384 B.C. by Aristotle. Many others supported this view over the centuries. The *microbic theory of disease* was also expressed by many in writings over the generations, but was first described by Fracastorius in 1545. Ambroise Pare (1510–1590), a military surgeon, was the first to challenge the use of scalding hot oil in wounds. This cruel practice was generally utilized in an attempt to destroy the exudate of suppurating wounds, which was thought to be itself poisonous.

Over a generation later, in the 1670s, Antony van Leeuwenhoek developed the first simple microscope, which he used to discover bacteria and protozoa. In the 1800s, great advances were made by Koch, Pasteur, Lister, Semmelweiss, and many others. Semmelweiss, observing a high death rate in mothers delivering their children in certain clinics in Vienna (child-bed fever), felt that an etiologic agent was carried to the mother by doctors and students. He therefore stressed, in 1847, hand washing before delivery with a solution of chlorine. This technique resulted in a dramatic drop of maternal mortality that had resulted from puerperal fever. His observations resulted in a fierce storm of opposition from the medical community that continued to his death. His tragic death from the very condition to which he had devoted his life, and his inability to convince the medical profession of the truth of his perception, together made him one of our great medical heroes.

Lister, guided and stimulated by the work of Pasteur on the nature of fermentation and putrefaction, was to become the "father of antiseptic surgery." He was the first to stress cleanliness in the operating room and developed a machine to spray carbolic acid into the air of the operating room in an attempt to prevent exogenous contamination during surgery. Many other basic scientists and clinicians throughout the world contributed greatly to the germ theory of disease; however, it is beyond the scope of this chapter to mention them all.

The observation by Fleming in 1928 that penicillin inhibited bacterial growth appeared to offer the breakthrough for the eventual elimination of surgical infections. Despite the subsequent development of hundreds of other antimicrobial agents, infection in the surgical patient continues and attests to the importance of the development of other techniques in addition to the use of antimicrobials for its prevention.

HOST-DEFENSE MECHANISMS

Clinical infection does not necessarily follow bacterial contamination. Since microorganisms are ubiquitous in the environment and endogenous to many of our body systems, the microbiologic isolation of bacteria alone cannot be assumed to be equated with infection. The development of clinical infection following bacterial contamination is the result of a complex interaction between the offending microbe and the patient, as elaborated by host-defense mechanisms. These factors are as follows.

1. Bacterial factors
   a. Amount and type of bacteria present
   b. Bacterial growth requirements (aerobic, anaerobic or facultative) or redox potential
   c. Virulence factors (capsules, surface components, exotoxins, endotoxins, and enzymes)
2. Local tissue factors
   a. Blood supply
   b. Foreign bodies
   c. Necrosis
   d. Hematoma
3. Systemic host-defense factors
   a. Delivery of phagocytes
   b. Neutrophil chemotaxis
   c. Serum factors (opsonins)
   d. Phagocytic activity

Bacterial Factors

The growth and multiplication of bacteria within tissues after the initial contamination depend upon several bacterial factors. Most bacteria require initial concentrations of greater than 10^5 organisms in order to produce a clinical infection. The growth requirements of each microorganism are also critical. Strict *aerobic* organisms are those that grow and multiply only in an environment that has oxygen, whereas strict *anaerobes* flourish only in an oxygen-free environment. However, most enteric bacteria are *facultative*, allowing them to grow and multiply in either setting.

As soon as the bacteria invade the tissues, different substances or enzymes elaborated by the bacteria act to determine the nature of the infection. The presence of streptococci, which frequently produce streptokinase (which initiates the fibrinolytic dissolution of fibrin clots), and hyaluronidase (which depolymerizes the ground substance of tissues) can result in a rapidly spreading infection. In contrast, staphylococci are usually less invasive and normally result in localized abscess formation. Gram-negative enteric bacilli, such as *Escherichia coli*, possess endotoxin in their cell wall; endotoxin is released following bacterial death and may result in clinical septic shock.

Local Tissue Factors

Tissues with good blood supply are more resistant to infection following bacterial contamination, e.g., scalp wounds, in which there is ample blood supply, versus back or buttock wounds, in which there is a more limited blood flow. The importance of this has been proved experimentally by the addition of epinephrine to local anesthetic instilled into a wound, which reduces the number of bacteria needed to produce an infection by decreasing the local blood supply. The presence of necrotic tissue or hematoma within wounds further increases the risk of subsequent

infection. A foreign body within a wound has been shown experimentally to decrease the bacterial inocula necessary for infection from 10^5 staphylococci to as few as only one hundred. Similar results have been demonstrated for clostridial infection when foreign bodies and devitalized muscle are left in the wound. As a result of these findings, it is recommended that in heavily contaminated wounds or in wounds in which foreign bodies or all devitalized tissues cannot be satisfactorily removed, delayed closure will, in most instances, decrease the incidence of serious local infection.

Systemic Host-Defense Factors

Understanding the normal systemic host-defense mechanisms is a complex and critically important issue to the prevention of surgical infections. Infection results from either an intrinsic abnormality or interference in the host-defense process or as a result of an overload of its normal capabilities.

Normally, humans live in an environment of a host of potentially pathogenic bacteria, viruses, and fungi. The intact epithelial surface of the body and mucous membrane barrier allow for the peaceful coexistence between man and the microorganisms. However, when the skin or mucous membrane barrier is broken by trauma, disease states, or surgery, microorganisms may enter sterile tissues. Their entrance excites the normal systemic host-defense mechanisms into action. The scheme of events that subsequently occur is very complex and will be offered in a basic simplified form in this chapter.

Bacteria entering tissues actuate an inflammatory response that attempts to localize the bacteria to the site of invasion. Chemical mediators that cause local vascular constriction are released from serum and bacteria. This is followed by a humoral and cellular response, both of which are important to the containment of the infection and host survival. Antibodies against the invading bacteria will combine with their specific surface antigens to form a complex that enhances phagocytotic activity. Complement is a protein found in serum that nonspecifically also renders the bacteria more susceptible to phagocytosis. This enhancement of phagocytosis by humoral factors is usually referred to as *opsonization*. Neutrophils and mononuclear phagocytes appear at the site of invasion, and a chemotactic response directs these cells to the offending bacteria and phagocytosis begins. The *neutrophil* is the dominant circulating phagocytic cell that protects man from invading bacteria. After phagocytosis of the offending bacteria, intracellular killing occurs. Defects in this schema can lead to a failure of the system and can be seen in patients who are immunosuppressed by either malnutrition disease states or medications. The main steps in this schema are listed as follows.

DEFECTS IN PHAGOCYTE DELIVERY

The migration of the neutrophils and mononuclear cells to areas of bacterial invasion can be reduced in the following situations:

1. Decreased systemic blood flow (as in shock states).
2. Decreased local blood flow (as associated with vascular occlusive states).
3. Presence of devitalized or necrotic tissue or hematoma in the local area of injury.
4. Disease states such as uremia or chronic steroid intake, which reduce vascular reactivity.

5. Decreased production of phagocytes as seen in granulocytopenic states in patients on various chemotherapy regimens or in those receiving large body area irradiation.

ABNORMAL NEUTROPHIL CHEMOTAXIS

Once the neutrophils are in the extravascular tissue, they exhibit random movement until they come within a relatively short distance of an attractive particle (bacterium). At this time they stop their random motion and directly approach the particle because of chemotactic forces. Surgical patients with severe trauma, burns, cancer, and malnutrition are immunosuppressed at the time of bacterial challenge and frequently exhibit anergy (failure to respond to cutaneously injected antigens). This failure has been associated more with defects in neutrophil chemotaxis than with any other immune mechanism.

ABNORMAL SERUM FACTORS (OPSONINS)

At the site of any injury, plasma proteins that include specific antibodies and complement appear. They act as strong opsonizing agents that allow for phagocytosis of the contaminating bacteria. If no prior exposure to the offending bacteria has occurred, little or no specific antibody will be present and phagocytosis will be minimal initially. Rarely, patients with agammaglobulinemia or dysgammaglobulinemia have a further problem because they cannot synthesize a specific antibody. Complement levels and activity can be significantly reduced in chronically malnourished patients or in those affected with acute starvation.

ABNORMAL PHAGOCYTOSIS

Defects in bacterial ingestion by the neutrophil have been reported in various disease states, including (1) uremia, (2) ketosis, (3) several immunologic deficiency states, (4) leukemia, and (5) hyperglycemia.

ABNORMAL INTRACELLULAR KILLING

A decreased rate of intracellular bacterial killing was first reported in congenital chronic granulomatous diseases of childhood. Other disease states occasionally associated with this defect include (1) patients with severe thermal and traumatic injury, (2) malnourished patients and (3) those receiving immunosuppressive therapy.

Host-defense problems are often identified in critically ill surgical patients, including those with (1) leukemia, (2) diabetes mellitus, (3) uremia, (4) burns, (5) trauma, (6) certain solid malignancies, (7) malnutrition, (8) obesity, and (9) inherited immunodeficiency states. The prevention of infection in these patients is difficult and especially requires attention to details of surgical technique, judgment, and the appropriate use of efficacious antibiotics when indicated.

MICROBIOLOGY OF SURGICAL INFECTIONS

During the past two decades, there has been emphasis placed upon the primary role played by the human polymicrobial endogenous microflora in the development of sepsis in the surgical patient.[23] Numerous studies have defined the qualitative and quantitative character of each organ's microflora in both health and disease in order to allow one to better anticipate the microorganisms usually causing infection in each clinical setting. Although each major organ system has different microflora, there are only slight differences when comparisons are made from person to person. With the exception of the use of antibiotic agents, no other factors have been shown to alter these microfloras significantly, a finding that attests to their profound stability.

Human Endogenous Gastrointestinal Microflora

The gastrointestinal tract is the primary reservoir for endogenous bacteria within the human body. The numbers and types of microorganisms increase progressively downward in the gastrointestinal tract (Table 1). In the normal human, the stomach and proximal small intestine support a rather sparse bacterial flora of both aerobes and anaerobes ($<10^4$ per ml.).[3] Acidity and motility appear to be the major factors that inhibit the growth of bacteria within the stomach. Diseases of the stomach and duodenum may compromise these factors. Thus, in cases of bleeding or obstructing duodenal ulcer, gastric ulcer, or carcinoma, the microflora of the stomach usually increases, being composed principally of anaerobes from the oral cavity and aerobic coliforms.

The microflora of the distal small bowel represents a transitional zone between the microflora of the upper and lower gastrointestinal tracts; modest numbers of aerobic and anaerobic microorganisms (up to 10^8 per ml.) are usually present. The largest concentrations of microorganisms are located in the colon, where up to 10^{11} anaerobes per gm. of stool or ml. of intestinal aspirate can be identified. Coliforms also are present in the colon in concentrations of 10^8 per gm. The solid intra-abdominal organs, such as the liver and spleen, rarely harbor a resident microflora in health, whereas the human vagina harbors a microflora that is similar in character but lower in number than in the colon.

This geographical arrangement of microorganisms within the gastrointestinal tract, in part, accounts for the differences in septic complications associated with injuries to the upper and lower intestine. Sepsis that occurs after upper intestinal leaks is generally less severe, with reduced morbidity and mortality, in comparison with sepsis that occurs after leaks that follow colonic injuries.

Microorganisms Causing Infection in Surgical Patients

The Gram stain morphology of the aerobic and anaerobic microorganisms isolated from the various infections observed in surgical patients is listed in Table 2. Most of the causative microorganisms are endogenous to the human body. Certain bacteria such as *Staphylococcus* or *Pseudomonas*, although occasionally part of the human endogenous microflora, usually cause infection by *exogenous* (airborne) contamination. These exogenous bacteria are, therefore, very important causes of wound infection following clean operative procedures (where no endogenous contamination occurs during surgery) and also in the development of respiratory or urinary tract infections in the patients with prolonged periods of hospitalization. The most commonly isolated microorganisms from septic sites on the various surgical services are listed in Table 3.

TABLE 1. Endogenous Gastrointestinal Microflora

Region	Predominant Microflora	Concentration (per gm. or ml. of Aspirate)		Predominant Organisms	
		Aerobes	Anaerobes	Aerobes	Anaerobes
Oropharynx	Slight predominance of anaerobic organisms	10^4 to 10^5	10^5 to 10^7	*Streptococcus* *Haemophilus* *Neisseria* Diphtheroids	*Peptostreptococcus* *Fusobacterium* *Bacteroides melaninogenicus* *Bacteroides oralis*
Esophagus	Slight anaerobic predominance	10^4 to 10^5	10^5 to 10^7	*Streptococcus* *Hemophilus* *Neisseria*	*Peptostreptococcus* *Fusobacterium* *B. melaninogenicus* *B. oralis*
Stomach	Both aerobic and anaerobic (when present)	Microflora absent or minimal if normal gastric acidity and motility present		*Streptococcus* *Escherichia coli* *Klebsiella* *Enterobacter*	*Peptostreptococcus* *B. oralis* *B. melaninogenicus*
Biliary tract	Great aerobic predominance (when present)	No concentrations in healthy person		*E. coli* *Klebsiella* *Enterobacter* Enterococcus	*Clostridium* *Bacteroides fragilis*
Proximal small intestine	Slight predominance of aerobic organisms	10^2	10^1 to 10^2	*Streptococcus* *E. coli* *Klebsiella* *Enterobacter*	*Peptostreptococcus* *B. oralis* *B. melaninogenicus*
Distal ileum	Slight predominance of anaerobic organisms	10^4 to 10^6	10^5 to 10^7	*E. coli* *Klebsiella* *Enterobacter*	*B. fragilis* *Peptostreptococcus* *Clostridium*
Colon	Great predominance of anaerobic organisms	10^6 to 10^8	10^9 to 10^{11}	*E. coli* *Klebsiella* *Enterobacter*	*B. fragilis* *Peptostreptococcus* *Clostridium*

TABLE 2. Source and Clinical Setting of Bacteria Commonly Isolated from Surgical Infections

Bacteria	Usual Origin		Clinical Setting of Infection								Comments
	Endogenous	Exogenous	Septicemia	Endocarditis	Urinary Tract	Biliary	Soft Tissue	Respiratory	Intra-Abdominal	Enterocolitis	
AEROBIC											
Gram-negative bacilli											
Acinetobacter	X				X						Formerly Bethesda-Ballerup group; closely related to *Klebsiella*
Citrobacter	X		X				X				
Enterobacter	X		X		X	X	X		X		Most common cause of
Escherichia coli	X		X		X	X	X		X		urinary tract infections
Haemophilus		X	X					X			
Klebsiella	X		X		X	X	X	X	X		
Legionella		X						X			
Morganella	X		X		X		X				Formerly *Proteus morganii*
Proteus mirabilis	X				X		X				
Proteus vulgaris			X		X		X		X		Formerly paracolon bacillus; may
Providencia		X			X		X	X			produce blue-green pus in
Pseudomonas aeruginosa		X	X		X		X	X	X		wounds
Salmonella		X	X							X	Formerly thought to be
Serratia	X		X		X			X			nonpathogenic; most isolates are hospital-acquired
Shigella		X	X							X	Can mimic Crohn's disease or
Yersinia	X						X			X	appendicitis
Gram-positive bacilli											
Corynebacterium	X						X				
Gram-positive cocci											
Staphylococcus aureus		X	X	X	X		X		X	X	Clusters
Staphylococcus epidermidis		X	X	X			X				Clusters
Hemolytic *Streptococcus*	X		X	X			X	X			Chains
Streptococcus faecalis (enterococcus)	X		X		X	X	X		X		Not usually found as sole pathogen
Streptococcus pneumoniae (pneumococcus)		X	X					X			
ANAEROBIC											
Gram-negative bacilli											
Bacteroides fragilis	X		X			X	X		X		Most common isolate
Bacteroides (other)	X		X				X		X		
Fusobacterium	X						X	X			Tapered, pointed ends
Gram-positive bacilli											
Actinomyces		X					X	X			Branching filamentous forms, found in chronic draining infections of face and abdomen
Clostridium	X	X	X				X	X	X	X	Most species have spores
Gram-positive cocci											
Peptostreptococcus		X	X				X	X	X		Chains

TABLE 3. *Microorganisms Most Commonly Isolated from Postoperative Infection*

Location	Aerobes	Anaerobes
Head and neck	Streptococci	*Bacteroides* (other than *B. fragilis*), peptostreptococci, fusobacteria
Gastrointestinal		
Esophagus	Streptococci	As for mouth
Stomach	Streptococci and coliforms	As for mouth
Biliary	*E. coli*, enterococci	Clostridia
Distal ileum	*E. coli*, *Klebsiella*	*B. fragilis*, peptostreptococci, clostridia
Colon	*E. coli*, *Klebsiella*	As for distal ileum
Gynecologic	*E. coli*, *Klebsiella*	As above
Orthopedic	Staphylococci, streptococci	—
Thoracic	Streptococci, pneumococci	*Bacteroides* (other than *B. fragilis*), peptostreptococci
Cardiovascular	Staphylococci, streptococci	—
Urologic	*E. coli* or *Proteus*	—

Microbiologic Techniques

The techniques for aerobic bacterial culturing and identification have been fairly well standardized throughout the United States. However, great strides have been made in anaerobic microbiology since 1970. Each of the following represents a major advance.

ANAEROBIC CULTURE TECHNIQUES

Anaerobic Jars. These jars are used to incubate solid media in Petri dishes that have been inoculated with the clinical specimens. The jars are made anaerobic either by using disposable hydrogen–carbon dioxide generating envelopes or by repeated vacuum evacuation and replacement by anaerobic gas (10 per cent hydrogen, 5 or 10 per cent carbon dioxide, balance nitrogen). The limited exposure to oxygen during specimen handling and plating has not been shown to affect the majority of important anaerobic bacteria that are isolated from clinical specimens. The jars are incubated in normal laboratory incubators, offer the advantage of using conventional plated media, and are relatively easy to use.

Anaerobic Chamber. The development of the *anaerobic glovebox* or chamber has been a major step forward in the culturing of anaerobic microorganisms. In these chambers, the anaerobic environment is constantly maintained by an air lock and catalyst pellets. An apparent advantage of the glovebox over the anaerobic jar is that, through the gloves, plating and other bacteriologic manipulations can be performed within the anaerobic chamber. This eliminates all danger of oxygen exposure. Furthermore, the glovebox allows for the daily examination of individual Petri dishes and the selection of colonies for identification while it prevents the exposure to oxygen of the remaining Petri dishes. This is an extremely important feature when fast-growing anaerobes are cultured on the same plates as slow-growing, fastidious organisms.

Bio-Bag. The newest method to be developed for growing anaerobes is the use of a disposable gas-imperme-able plastic bag. This bag is large enough for two Petri plates, a small anaerobic gas generator, and an anaerobic indicator. This system is fairly inexpensive and easy to use. It has been shown to keep the plates anaerobic for up to one week.

ANAEROBIC IDENTIFICATION METHODS

There are two types of identification kits currently available. The first relies upon growth of the organism on selected sugars and other substrates. The presence of growth is determined by color changes in chemical indicators added to the media. An incubation time of 24 to 48 hours is required for growth before identification can be made. The second type of kit tests for the presence of preformed enzymes in the bacteria. Only 4 hours of incubation are necessary, since growth of the organism is not required.

All these methods require a Gram stain and the test kit results to identify the organism. Most employ computer-assisted data bases that give bacterial names and probabilities of being correct. Some of the identifications require supplemental tests or *gas chromatography* to yield an acceptable identification.

The use of gas chromatography in the identification of anaerobic organisms is based on the observation that during metabolism these organisms release various acid end products into their surrounding environment. Chromatography may be performed within 2 to 4 days of receiving the initial specimen in the laboratory.

SPECIMEN COLLECTION

Proper collection and transportation of clinical specimens are critical factors in the recovery of the clinically significant bacteria. The sample of discharge or exudate should be collected from the deep, active region of infection to prevent surface contamination and aeration of the specimen. Whenever possible, tissue samples or fluid aspirates rather than swabbed specimens are collected. As with aerobic specimens, the material on the swabs should be processed rapidly to prevent drying and to preserve viability. It is also important to thoroughly saturate the swab with exudate when this collection method is utilized.

Several different transport devices have been developed for the preservation of clinical specimens during the time between collection and bacterial culturing. Anaerobic transport systems may contain an agar with both oxygen-reducing capabilities and indicators of oxygenation. Either the specimen is injected into a vial containing this transport agar, or a swab with the specimen is pushed into a tube full of the agar. An alternative method involves the use of a swab that is placed into an anaerobic environment immediately.

Not all clinical specimens should be routinely cultured for anaerobes because of the difficulty and expense of the anaerobic techniques. Nasal swabs, throat swabs, sputum, feces, voided or catheterized urine, and vaginal swabs routinely show the growth of endogenous microflora, which often complicates the search for the actual infecting microorganisms. For the following types of clinical specimens, the suspicion of *anaerobic sepsis* requires special recommendations for collection.

Cystitis and Urinary Tract Infections. When cystitis and urinary tract infections are highly suspect, urine should be collected by percutaneous suprapubic puncture of the bladder. Voided urine commonly contains anaerobes from the normal urethral flora. Because anaerobes are involved in less than 5 per cent of urinary tract infections, bladder puncture is necessary only when clinical symptoms point to anaerobic sepsis.

Pneumonia, Lung Abscess, and Other Pulmonary Infections. Percutaneous transtracheal needle aspiration provides a reliable sample for culture, since it bypasses areas that are normally colonized with anaerobic flora. Sputum specimens must not be used for anaerobic culture because of the great variety and number of anaerobes normally present in the mouth.

Blood Specimens. Blood specimens should be taken by the usual technique of venipuncture and injected into both aerobic and anaerobic blood culture broths. Specimens other than blood should not initially be put into enrichment broths, since this allows the overgrowth of aerobic organisms and distorts the relative proportion of isolated organisms.

DIAGNOSIS OF SURGICAL INFECTION

A carefully obtained history combined with a thorough physical examination is the most important single step in the diagnosis of surgical infection. When physical findings are initially nondiagnostic, repetitive examinations frequently detect changes that lead to an accurate clinical diagnosis. Failure to repeatedly examine the infected patient is the most common reason for delayed diagnosis and late initiation of appropriate treatment. Nevertheless, the occurrence of deep-seated intra-abdominal infections may tax the ingenuity of the most astute clinician.

Fever is most frequently the first finding observed in patients with surgical infection. When the postoperative patient becomes febrile, it is important to consider the many causes of fever at the different time periods in the postoperative course (Table 4). Strong chills along with the fever indicate bloodstream invasion (septicemia).

Leukocytosis (>15,000 per mm.³) usually accompanies acute bacterial infection. In general, the greater the increase in the total leukocyte count, the more severe the infection. There is also frequently a shift to increased mature and immature forms of neutrophils. In undiagnosed overwhelming infections of long duration, it is not unusual to observe leukopenia (<6,000 per mm.³). This phenomenon appears to be due to the exhaustion of the supply of peripheral leukocytes, which follows bone marrow suppression. The finding of increased numbers of lymphocytes or mononuclear cells tends to favor the diagnosis of a viral rather than a bacterial infection.

When infections involve the skin and soft tissues, the cardinal signs of inflammation are usually present. These include warmth, erythema, swelling, pain, and loss of function. The earliest finding in postoperative wound infection, in addition to fever, is the return of incisional pain, which usually occurs around the fourth to fifth postoperative day.

Infections that are due to predominantly anaerobic microorganisms are often more difficult to diagnose and, in this case, clinical clues are helpful. They include:

1. Infections associated with sites that normally harbor an anaerobic flora. Since anaerobes constitute the predominant flora of the oropharynx, colon, and female genital tract, infections related to these areas are more likely to involve these organisms.

2. A foul-smelling discharge. This is normally diagnostic of anaerobic infection, since most aerobic bacteria are not capable of producing this characteristic odor.

3. Tissue necrosis with abscess formation or gangrene.

4. Infection associated with gas production (tissue crepitance).

5. Gram stain of exudate showing characteristic forms. Many anaerobes have a unique morphology, which permits a presumptive bacteriologic diagnosis.

6. Failure to recover common pathogens with aerobic culture suggests infection involving fastidious organisms such as anaerobes.

7. Failure to respond to antibiotics that are not active against anaerobic bacteria (e.g., aminoglycosides).

The work-up of the infected postoperative patient also includes chest x-ray, urinalysis, and, if indicated, urine culture and antibiotic susceptibility studies. Appropriately obtained cultures and specimens for Gram staining should be sent to the laboratory as soon as possible. Blood cultures obtained shortly after an episode of chills and fever may not be positive because of the ability of the peripheral phagocytes to promptly remove the bacteria entering the bloodstream. Thus, blood cultures, when indicated, should be taken at frequent intervals in the septic surgical patient starting at the first sign of fever.

TABLE 4. *Causes of Fever During Operation and Postoperative Course*

Time	Cause
During operation	Pre-existing infection (lung, kidney, soft tissue, or intra-abdominal)
	Transfusion reaction
	Endocrine crisis (hyperthyroid, pheochromocytoma)
Less than 48 hours postoperatively	Atelectasis
	Early soft tissue infections (streptococci, clostridia)
Postoperative day 3–4	Pneumonia
	Intravascular catheter sepsis
	Urinary tract infection
	Thrombophlebitis
Postoperative day 5–8	Wound sepsis (*Staphylococcus aureus* or polymicrobial enterics)
Postoperative day 9–14	Intra-abdominal abscesses
	Late wound infections due to low virulence bacteria (*Staphylococcus epidermidis*, diphtheroids)

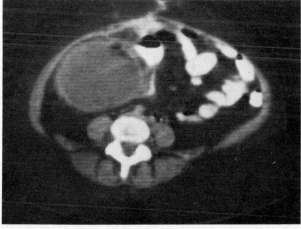

Figure 1. CT scan of abdomen with contrast showing peripheral enhancement and air within the abscess cavity located in the right lower quadrant.

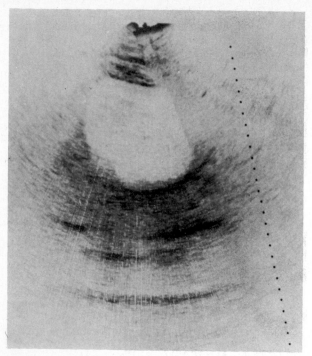

Figure 2. Sonogram of abdomen showing large sonolucent area, which proved to be abscess cavity at operative exploration.

The diagnosis of deep-seated pelvic or intra-abdominal infections frequently requires specialized radiologic examinations in order to identify the area of infection. The choice of which tests are indicated depends largely on the expertise and equipment of the radiology department. The most commonly employed non-invasive tests include radioactive scanning, computed tomography (CT), and ultrasonography (Figs. 1 and 2). Rarely, selective arteriography is indicated in order to localize deep-seated infections.

SURGICAL WOUND INFECTIONS

The overall incidence of postoperative wound infection was reported at 7.5 per cent in a much quoted national study reported two decades ago.[1] This incidence varied by surgeon, hospital, and the surgical procedure performed. The economic, physical, and psychological impact of post-operative wound sepsis mandates the use of preventive methods, the most critical of which are proper operative technique and sound clinical judgment.

Classification

Surgical wounds are generally classified as clean (Class I), clean-contaminated (Class II), contaminated (Class III), or dirty (Class IV).

Clean Wounds. Class I wounds are those in which the gastrointestinal or respiratory tracts have not been entered during the course of operation. The usual causes for post-operative infections in these cases are the aerobic exogenous bacteria, such as staphylococci, which enter the wound during the course of operation. The overall infection rate in clean surgical procedures should be less than 2 per cent.

Clean-Contaminated Wounds. Class II wounds are associated with elective operations in which the gastrointestinal or respiratory tract has been entered during elective surgery. The risk of infection in these cases is higher than in clean surgical procedures and generally is reported to be between 5 and 10 per cent. The primary cause of infection in these patients is the endogenous microflora of the organ that has been surgically resected.

Contaminated Wounds. Class III wounds include those in which acute inflammation (without pus formation) or gross spillage of gastrointestinal contents is encountered at the time of operation. Infections in these cases again are primarily due to the endogenous bacteria, and the infection rate is around 20 per cent.

Dirty Wounds. Class IV wounds include those in which gross pus is encountered at operation usually as a result of organ perforation, and the infections are primarily related to the involved organ's endogenous microflora. Infection rates are most often reported at about 40 per cent.

It can therefore be stated that the primary risk of wound infection in elective clean operations is *airborne* or *exogenous*; in the other categories, postoperative infection is usually due to *endogenous bacteria*, which escape from diseased, traumatized, or surgically resected viscera. Nosocomial infection rates (1980–1983) and surgical wound infection rates (1983) from the Tulane Medical Center Hospital are shown in Figures 3 and 4. By use of the concepts of infection control, the higher hospital nosocomial infection rate found in the 1980–1981 period was reduced in 1982–1983, and the surgical infection rates for Class I (clean) and Class II (clean-contaminated) were in the desired range.

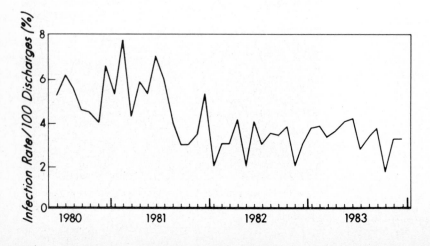

Figure 3. Nosocomial infection rates at Tulane Medical Center Hospital, 1980–1983. The higher rates found from 1980–1981 were significantly decreased from 1982 to 1983 by strict adherence to infection control procedures.

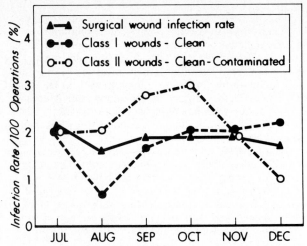

Figure 4. Infection rates for surgical procedures at Tulane Medical Center Hospital, July–December 1983. Although the rates for Class I and Class II operative wounds vary slightly, all rates remain fairly constant and at a low level.

Types of Clinical Wound Sepsis

The majority of postoperative wound infections are uncomplicated, involving only the skin and subcutaneous tissues. Infrequently, they progress to become necrotizing infections, which may involve the fascia and muscle. The usual clinical presentation of uncomplicated wound infection includes local incisional pain and tenderness, swelling, redness, and increased warmth and elevated body temperature, which most often begin between the 4th and 8th postoperative day. The cardinal features of treatment of an uncomplicated wound infection are operative drainage and local wound care. When infection occurs during the first 48 hours after operation, it is characteristically caused by either clostridia or beta-hemolytic streptococci. In such cases, the dramatic clinical presentation may include profound systemic toxicity and rapid local advance of the infection, often involving all layers of the body wall. A high mortality rate (60 to 80 per cent) can be expected unless a rapid diagnosis is made on the basis of clinical presentation as well as results of Gram's stain. Treatment includes parenteral administration of penicillin and aggressive, prompt surgical débridement of all infected tissue.

Non-antibiotic Factors That Influence Wound Infection Rates

This section reviews the factors that have been implicated in influencing the postoperative infection rates in clean operations, in which the exposure to endogenous bacterial contamination is absent or minimal.[14] Many other factors, without convincing evidence, are postulated to influence postoperative wound infection. These include preoperative scrub technique, surgical glove damage, barrier materials, and "laminar flow" air systems in the operating room. Anecdotal experience and commercial interests rather than scientific studies usually account for these associations (Table 5).

DURATION OF PREOPERATIVE HOSPITALIZATION

The longer the preoperative period of hospitalization, the greater the infection rate. Cruse and Foord have

TABLE 5. Factors Influencing the Development of Postoperative Infections in Clean Surgical Procedures: Degree of Importance

Very Important (Infection Rate Doubled)
Period of preoperative hospitalization prolonged
Shaving the operative site on the day prior to surgery
Increased duration of operation
Use of prophylactic abdominal drains
Operation done in the presence of a remote active infection

Important (Infection Rate Significantly Increased but Less Than Doubled)
Failure to shower with antiseptic prior to operation

Unproven Importance (No Significant Increase in Infection Rate)
Surgeon's hand scrub—iodophor versus hexachlorophene
Patient skin preparation—iodophor versus hexachlorophene
Use of plastic skin drapes
Use of "laminar" flow air systems

reported an overall 1.1 per cent infection rate in a large group of patients whose preoperative stay was one day. This infection rate doubled each week that the patient remained in the hospital prior to surgery. Studies have shown that colonization occurs in virtually every patient with nosocomial bacteria within 2 weeks of admission to an intensive care unit. These colonizations usually occur with hospital-acquired antibiotic-resistant organisms.

PREOPERATIVE SHOWERING

Preoperative showering with hexachlorophene-containing antiseptics on the evening prior to surgery is associated with a significantly decreased postoperative infection rate. This decrease in infection rate has not been observed if regular soap is used in the preoperative shower, thus attesting to the value of antiseptics in decreasing the populations of skin bacteria.

PREOPERATIVE HAIR REMOVAL

Razor shaving of the operative site the day before surgery has been demonstrated to increase the postoperative infection rate significantly. This increase is due to the growth and multiplication of skin microorganisms in the damaged epithelium following the razor shave. For this reason, when razor shaving is employed, it should be confined to the immediate preoperative period. However, studies have shown a lower postoperative infection rate if no shaving, use of electric clippers, or a depilatory cream is used prior to surgery.

DURATION OF OPERATION

Generally speaking, each added hour of operation will result in a doubling of the infection rate. Shapiro and coauthors have reported a prospective study of risk factors for infection following hysterectomy.[22] They observed that an increasing duration of operation was associated with a decreasing effect of antibiotic prophylaxis in the prevention of infection at the operative site. The statistically significant benefit of antibiotic prophylaxis in operations lasting 1 hour was lost in operations lasting over 3.3 hours. This finding is undoubtedly related to the pharmacokinetics of antibiotic prophylaxis as well as to increased bacterial wound colonization, which is found in lengthy and complicated operative procedures.

USE OF SURGICAL DRAINS

Clinical and experimental studies have mentioned the dangers of using prophylactic drains in abdominal surgery. Based on the frequent findings of skin bacteria at the interior of the abdominal drains, the "two-way street" concept has been proposed.[21] Increased infection rates have been reported following splenectomy in which drains were employed.[4] The presence of either silicone substances (Silastic) or latex Penrose drains in experimental wounds dramatically enhanced the wound infection rate even in the face of subinfective doses of bacteria. Based on these experimental and clinical studies, it appears safe to conclude that the prophylactic use of abdominal drains is unwarranted and may indeed be a dangerous practice. When drains are required to empty localized collections, they should be placed through sites other than the primary surgical incision.

OPERATION PERFORMED IN THE PRESENCE OF
AN ACTIVE REMOTE INFECTION

Significant increases in postoperative wound infection occur when an elective procedure is done in the presence of an active remote infection.[1] It is therefore prudent to initiate treatment for urinary, pulmonary, or skin infections prior to attempting elective operative procedures.

ANTIBIOTIC PROPHYLAXIS IN THE SURGICAL PATIENT

Great progress has been made in the last decade concerning the appropriate use of antibiotic prophylaxis in the patient undergoing surgery. Well-controlled, prospective, blinded studies have outlined many of the areas in which antibiotic prophylaxis is of benefit as well as those clinical settings in which the risks of antibiotic prophylaxis outweigh the expected value.[6,16]

Historically, the most common errors included the widespread use of antibiotic prophylaxis in clean surgical procedures as well as the faulty timing of their initial administration. Currently, the most common error is the practice of continuation of the antibiotic agents beyond the time necessary for maximal benefit (>72 hours).

In order to administer prophylactic antibiotics appropriately in the various clinical settings on the surgical service where this practice has been of proven value, one must be cognizant of the following nuances, including:

1. The choice of the antibiotic agent should be based on the type of organisms usually known to cause infection.

2. The route of administration must be appropriate.

3. The dosage necessary to attain efficacious tissue or serum levels must be appropriate.

4. The timing of administration should offer the maximal benefits without creating risk of adverse effects.

Basic Principles of Surgical Prophylaxis

In surgery, antibiotic prophylaxis refers to the administration of antibiotic agents to patients without evidence of established infection, with the objective of reducing subsequent postoperative septic complications. Prophylaxis should be limited to patients in whom the development of an infection is likely or in those in whom infection may be associated with a catastrophic end result.[13,25]

TIMING

The effective use of prophylactic antibiotics depends to a great extent on the appropriate timing of their administration. Parenteral antibiotics in effective doses generally should first be given within 1 hour prior to the operation. This timing results in therapeutic drug levels in the wound and related tissues during the operation, but it does not allow for the development of bacterial resistance. Administration of the drugs should be continued for less than 24 hours, a period during which the concentration of bacteria in the wound and dissected tissues may exceed the capacity of the unaided tissues to destroy them and to heal. Continuation of prophylactic drug therapy beyond 24 hours increases the risk of drug toxicity or bacterial superinfection and does not reduce the incidence of subsequent infection. Most believe that two or three doses of antimicrobials beginning just before the operation are sufficient for prophylaxis.

When prophylaxis is accomplished with orally administered antibiotics, as is frequently practiced in elective colon resection, the agents should be given only during the 24 hours prior to operation. Longer periods of preoperative preparation are not necessary and have been associated with the isolation of resistant organisms within the colonic lumen at the time of resection.

ROUTE OF ADMINISTRATION

Among the various routes by which prophylactic antibiotics can be administered, systemic administration by intravenous (IV) infusion (parenteral) is preferred in most surgical patients. Administering antibiotics intravenously in a relatively small volume of diluent over a short period of time (IV bolus) results in high serum levels that are reflected in more rapid entry and higher early concentrations of antibiotics in wound fluid. Administration of equivalent doses of antibiotics either by continuous intravenous infusion or by intermittent intramuscular injection produces lower blood levels and retarded entry of the antibiotics into wound fluid. Oral administration of relatively poorly absorbed antibiotics plays a major role only in elective preparation of patients prior to colon operations.

CHOICE OF ANTIBIOTICS

No one antibiotic agent or combination can be relied on for effective prophylaxis in all the clinical settings found on the surgical services. The agent or agents employed should be chosen primarily on the basis of their efficacy against the microorganisms that usually cause the infectious complications in the clinical setting. For example, in uncomplicated cardiovascular or orthopedic operations, the usual cause of postoperative infections is aerobic streptococci or staphylococci; the organisms responsible for infection following gastrointestinal or gynecologic surgery are more complex, and an appropriate choice of prophylactic antibiotics requires an understanding of the polymicrobial nature of the endogenous microflora at each site. The microorganisms usually responsible for postoperative infections in each surgical discipline have been previously listed in Table 3.

Clean Surgical Procedures

The use of prophylactic antibiotics in "clean" surgical cases should be limited to those in which a prosthetic foreign body has been implanted. Operations in which prophylactic antibiotics are not generally indicated are listed in Table 6. The benefit of the use of antibiotic prophylaxis in these "clean" surgical cases is outweighed by the potential harmful effects of the antibiotic; these include toxic or allergic drug reactions and bacterial or fungal superinfections. Low infection rates in clean cases are best obtained by strict adherence to the principles of good surgical technique. Other factors that help keep the infection rate at a

TABLE 6. Operations in Which Prophylactic Antibiotics Are Not Generally Required

Operative Procedure	Exceptions
General surgery	
Breast biopsy	
Cholecystectomy	Clinical risk factors are present
	Positive intraoperative Gram's stain of bile
Gastrectomy	Gastric ulcer or complications of duodenal disease (bleeding, obstruction, etc.) or gastric malignancy
Head and neck	Anticipate cutting across contaminated area (oropharynx, hypopharynx, nasopharynx)
	Enter dura during such procedures as ethmoidectomy
Inguinal hernia or incisional hernia repair	
Mastectomy (modified or radical)	
Parathyroidectomy	
Soft tissue surgery	Human bite
	Major soft tissue injury
Stripping of varicose veins	
Splenectomy	
Thyroidectomy	
Vagotomy-gastrectomy	Gastric ulcer or complications of duodenal ulcer
Vagotomy-pyloroplasty	Same as above
Gynecology	
Cesarean section	Membranes have been ruptured
Oophorectomy	
Tubal ligation	
Neurosurgery	
All procedures	Large area of dead space or presence of devitalized bone
	Insertion of ventricular shunt or other foreign body
Orthopedic surgery	
All procedures	Open fracture
	Foreign body implanted
	Amputation in presence of gangrene
Thoracic surgery	
All procedures	Penetrating wounds with extensive damage to soft tissue
	Perforation or transection of esophagus
	Transection of bronchial tree
Urology	
All procedures	Patients with positive urine cultures
	Obstructive uropathy
Cardiovascular	
All procedures	Foreign body
	Cardiac bypass employed

minimum have been discussed previously. However, the presence of any foreign body in a clean wound disables wound healing. Early experimental studies have suggested that a foreign body in a wound can result in suppuration with a bacterial inoculum, which of itself does not result in infection.

The risk of development of infections in patients undergoing clean surgical procedures with prosthetic devices, such as total hip replacement, implantation of cardiac valves, or vascular grafts, is low. However, when infection does occur in these clinical settings, the result most often is catastrophic. Prophylactic, systemically administered anti-staphylococcal drugs may reduce the incidence of postoperative infection in these procedures and is therefore recommended. Traditionally, penicillinase-resistant penicillins, such as methicillin, oxacillin, or nafcillin, have been employed for prophylaxis in this clinical setting. Recently, increased numbers of these infections have been reported from *Staphylococcus epidermidis*, an organism that has a significant degree of resistance to this group of semisynthetic penicillins. It is for this reason that first-generation cephalosporins, such as cephalothin or cefazolin, that exhibit good activity against all the organisms commonly causing postoperative sepsis in these cases now appear to be the drugs of choice.

Gastric Surgery

The most common indication for gastroduodenal operation prior to 1975 was chronic non-obstructing duodenal ulcer. Patients undergoing gastric resection for this indication rarely experienced postoperative infection, a finding that led to the general belief that the stomach contents were most often sterile, and antibiotic prophylaxis was not indicated. With the advent of modern medical treatment for chronic duodenal ulcer, the surgeon was called on less frequently to operate for this indication. Gastroduodenal operations are now performed primarily for complications of duodenal ulcer or for gastric ulcer or malignancy, and postoperative infections are common. These findings have resulted in an increased interest in the gastric microflora and the role of antibiotic prophylaxis in the patient undergoing gastroduodenal surgery.

GASTRODUODENAL MICROFLORA

The association of the intragastric acid status and the bacterial flora of the stomach, duodenum, and jejunum has been emphasized since the 1920s. The bacteriostatic action of gastric acid is now well established.

In 1975, we reported the results of a prospective clinical study on the influence of endogenous gastric microflora on the subsequent development of postoperative surgical infections.[19] Two groups of patients were identified as far as subsequent risk of infection:

1. *High risk (>20 per cent postoperative infection rate).* These patients had preoperative compromise of gastric acid or gastric motility and therefore had a gastric microflora present at the time of surgery that was responsible for subsequent postoperative infections. Clinically, these patients were undergoing operation for bleeding or obstructing duodenal ulcer or for gastric ulcer or malignancy.

2. *Low risk (<5 per cent postoperative infection rate).* These patients had normal preoperative gastric acid and motility and had few, if any, bacteria in the stomach at the time of operation. All of these patients had undergone operation for chronic non-obstructing duodenal ulcer.

RECOMMENDATIONS

Antibiotic prophylaxis has proved to be of benefit in patients who fall into the high-risk group.[13,20] Systemically administered cephalosporin agents appear to be the drugs of choice.

Biliary Tract Surgery for Chronic Calculous Cholecystitis

The healthy biliary tract rarely, if ever, harbors bacteria in any significant concentration. In the presence of chronic calculous cholecystitis, bacteria have been isolated in 15 to 30 per cent of the cases.

The bacteria isolated from bile in all disease states of the biliary tract are primarily gram-negative enteric coliforms. *Escherichia coli*, alone or mixed with another organism, is present in 50 per cent of the positive cultures. Other coliforms, e.g., *Klebsiella*, *Enterobacter*, and *Proteus* are less commonly isolated. *Streptococcus faecalis (Enterococcus)* is an aerobic gram-positive coccus that is also frequently isolated. Anaerobic microorganisms are isolated in fewer than 20 per cent of the cases, *Clostridium perfringens* in most studies being the most common.

CLINICAL RISK FACTORS

Positive cultures of bile collected at the time of biliary surgery are associated with an increased risk of postoperative infection. The clinical factors that favor the isolation of bacteria in bile at the time of operation and a corresponding increased risk of postoperative sepsis have been elicited.[5,11] These clinical risk factors include:
1. Age over 70.
2. Previous biliary tract operation.
3. Jaundice.
4. Chills or fever within 1 week of operation.
5. Operation performed within 1 month of an acute attack of cholecystitis.
Prophylactic antibiotics are indicated when one or more of these clinical risk factors are identified preoperatively.

IMMEDIATE GRAM STAINING OF BILE

Certain patients undergoing elective cholecystectomy with no clinical risk factors identified will nevertheless have bacteria in bile. The technique of immediate Gram's staining of bile at the time of operation has been useful in identifying these patients.[12] The bile sample, usually taken from the gallbladder, is sent to the microbiology laboratory for immediate Gram's staining and, if positive, for culture and susceptibility studies at the time of the cholecystectomy. The overall correlation rate of Gram's stain, compared with subsequent bile cultures, is greater than 75 per cent. The use of this technique allows the surgeon to administer appropriate antibiotics during the operation in those patients who did not receive them previously. It also allows for the addition or changes in antibiotics when organisms are seen that were not anticipated.

RECOMMENDATION

Well-controlled studies have shown the benefits of prophylactic antibiotic therapy in patients who had clinical risk factors or a positive intraoperative Gram's stain showing the presence of bacteria in bile.

The initial antibiotic agent chosen should be highly effective against the usual infecting organisms, the facultative gram-negative coliforms. The cephalosporins appear to be the drugs of choice. If a gram-positive rod is seen on Gram's stain, penicillin should be added to the regimen. Equal benefit can be expected from antibiotic agents that give either high serum levels or high bile levels.

Colon Surgery

The human colonic microflora comprises a greater variety of microorganisms, with counts higher than any of the other body's normal flora. As stated previously, anaerobes outnumber aerobes by at least 1000:1.

Employment of effective antimicrobials for oral bowel preparation before elective colon resection requires knowledge of the normal bowel flora, the capacity of various fecal bacteria to produce infections, the frequency with which each species of microorganism is involved in infection, and the patterns of antimicrobial sensitivity of these pathogens. At the risk of oversimplification, the clinically important information can be reduced to a few statements:
1. The predominant organisms of the normal bowel flora contain more than 20 species of resident and transient aerobes and more than 40 species of anaerobes. Most of these microorganisms are not pathogens.
2. *E. coli* and *Bacteroides fragilis* are the most commonly isolated organisms for septic wounds following colon operation. Other pathogenic organisms are found less frequently, so that, for practical purposes, effective antibiotic therapy directed against *E. coli* and *B. fragilis* will control the majority of infectious wound problems.
3. *E. coli* in the colonic flora is sensitive to either oral neomycin or kanamycin; *B. fragilis* is sensitive to oral erythromycin base, metronidazole, or tetracycline.

Based on this knowledge, the combination of neomycin-erythromycin base was chosen for clinical trials because these drugs were likely to be effective in controlling both aerobic and anaerobic fecal pathogens and were not generally used for treatment of infection.[17-18] This bowel preparation, as generally used, is as follows:

(*At home, if possible*)
Day 1: Low-residue diet
    Bisacodyl, one capsule orally at 6:00 P.M.

Day 2: Continue low-residue diet
    Magnesium sulfate, 30 ml. 50 per cent solution (15 gm.) orally at 10:00 A.M., 2:00 P.M., and 6:00 P.M.
    Saline enemas in evening until return clear

(*In hospital*)
Day 3: Clear liquid diet; supplemental intravenous fluids as needed
    Magnesium sulfate, as above, at 10:00 A.M. and 2:00 P.M..
    No enemas
    Neomycin (1 gm.) and erythromycin base (1 gm.) orally at 1:00 P.M., 2:00 P.M., and 11:00 P.M.
Day 4: Operation scheduled at 8:00 A.M.

This preoperative preparation has been shown to be effective in preventing infection following elective colon resection. It appears unclear at this point whether the common practice of adding short-term systemic antibiotics to the oral antibiotic regimen has any additive effects.[7]

TREATMENT OF SURGICAL INFECTION

The proper treatment of deep-seated infections in the surgical patient most frequently requires both surgical and antimicrobial therapy. Prevention of infection, as discussed in previous sections, is most important in decreasing the incidence of these untoward events. General principles of the surgical and medical management of surgical infection will be offered in this section, and the treatment of specific surgical infections will be addressed in later sections of this chapter.

Surgical Intervention

Antibiotic therapy alone will not result in a cure of most surgical infections. Surgical intervention, therefore, is the most critical step in the treatment of these infections. Spreading infections involving the skin, subcutaneous, fascial, and muscular layers are best treated by exploration to determine the extent of involvement. During this exploration, nonviable, necrotic tissue must be widely excised. Tissue death can be assumed when foul-smelling, gangrenous areas are identified. Areas adjacent to this tissue may be incised in order to determine the presence of an active blood supply. Often only one tissue layer (e.g., skin and subcutaneous tissue) will be involved. Rarely, as in clostridial myonecrosis, all layers including skin, subcutaneous fascia, and muscle will be necrotic, necessitating amputation (if the infection is on an extremity) or full-thickness excision (when the infection is located on the body).

The surgical treatment of abscesses requires incision and drainage of these localized collections of pus. Following drainage of the purulent abscess material, which includes bacteria, leukocytes, and debris, frequent antiseptic packing of the space will result in its closing with normal tissues. When abscesses are deep-seated, parenteral antibiotics are also required to prevent the invasion into adjacent tissue planes or the bloodstream during operative drainage. During drainage, manual exploration may detect tissue planes between loculations of pus, which must be broken down in order to release all localized infection. Closed mechanical drainage is necessary for these deep-seated infections in order to provide complete decompression to help prevent recurrence of the infection.

Antimicrobial Therapy

Antimicrobial therapy is a necessary part in the treatment of deep-seated surgical infections or in superficial spreading infections. The chosen therapy should be given parenterally in appropriate doses at regular time intervals. Knowledge of the pharmacokinetics of each agent utilized will help determine the dosage schedule. Frequently, the decision as to which antimicrobial agents to prescribe has to be made empirically before culture and sensitivity results are available.[15] In these cases, a Gram-stained specimen will provide important information that, when combined with the clinical setting, will allow for an efficacious choice. Subsequent changes in the empiric antimicrobial therapy will depend on (1) clinical response, (2) results of culture and susceptibility reports, and (3) presence of drug toxicity or side effects. It is frequently possible to discontinue one or more antimicrobial agents when empiric combination therapy has been chosen, once the culture and susceptibility studies are available. It should be stressed, however, that clinical response rather than laboratory data is most important in decisions regarding any change of the antimicrobial therapy.

The selection of an antimicrobial agent is simplified when a specific pathogen and its susceptibility pattern are known. Such a listing for microorganisms frequently isolated from sites of surgical sepsis, drug of choice, usual parenteral dosage, and alternative agents is cited in Table 7. Although many individual antimicrobial agents are equally effective against each of the specific microorganisms, the choices offered have been made after consideration of efficacy, toxicity, and cost. The dosages listed are those that would be prescribed for a patient of average weight (70 kg.) without any evidence of pre-existing renal or hepatic toxicity. Dose modifications or alternative choices for the antimicrobial agents might be indicated in the presence of renal or hepatic dysfunction with the antibiotics listed in Table 8.

In the critically ill surgical patient, empiric selection of antimicrobial agents is often necessary before culture and sensitivity data are available. These choices are best made on the basis of the most likely pathogen associated with a specific clinical setting (Table 9). This table is simply a guide to the initial therapy of specific infections in which the causative agents have not yet been determined. The limitations of this empirical format for therapy must be emphasized. Gram's stain results and clinical response in addition to subsequent culture and susceptibility results will predicate changes in the initially chosen regimen.

The necessary duration of drug therapy remains one of the true mysteries in the treatment of surgical sepsis. Each infected patient must be observed daily for clinical response and laboratory evidence of decreasing sepsis. Generally, parenteral treatment is required for 5 to 7 days. It is rarely necessary to utilize oral antibiotics after the completion of a parenteral course of efficacious antimicrobials. The duration of treatment is most critical when one has utilized aminoglycoside antibiotics. Evidence suggests that ototoxicity and nephrotoxicity associated with the use of these agents are most influenced by a therapeutic course extending beyond 10 days or by pre-existing organ dysfunction.

Each antimicrobial agent has known side effects and drug toxicity. It is important that one be aware of the adverse effects of each agent utilized. The most commonly reported adverse effects of each group of antimicrobial agents are listed in Table 10. A carefully obtained historical review of previous exposures to antimicrobials will frequently reveal episodes of drug toxicity, an occurrence that should greatly influence the current antimicrobial selection.

Finally, the cost of each antimicrobial agent should be considered. The cost-effective agent should be employed when there is no clear-cut evidence of increased efficacy or decreased toxicity of a more expensive agent. The differences in cost per gram are especially striking when the different generations of cephalosporins are considered (Table 11). The choice of which of these agents or generations should be employed strongly depends on the culture and susceptibility reports in each clinical infection. The attitude of some concerning surgical antibiotic prophylaxis—that the agent with the greatest overall spectrum is desirable—has not been proven by scientific studies and therefore results in unnecessarily high costs.

SPECIFIC INFECTIONS IN THE SURGICAL PATIENT

Intra-abdominal Sepsis

Penetrating abdominal trauma and perforated appendicitis and diverticulitis are among the most common clinical conditions that precede the development of intra-abdominal sepsis.[2] Other predisposing causes include perforation of

TABLE 7. Antimicrobials Useful Against Common Microorganisms Causing Surgical Infection

Microorganism	Drug of Choice	Parenteral Dose	Alternative Agents
Gram-positive cocci			
Peptostreptococci	PEN	1×10^6 units q 6 hr.	CLIN, MET
Streptococcus pneumoniae (pneumococcus)	PEN	1×10^6 units q 6 hr.	CEPH*, ERY
Staphylococcus aureus	PEN-R†	1–2 gm. q 4–6 hr.	CLIND, ERY
Staphylococcus epidermidis	CEPH*	1 gm. q 4–6 hr.	Vancomycin
Streptococcus (beta-hemolytic)	PEN	1×10^6 units q 6 hr.	CEPH* ERY
Streptococcus faecalis	AMP + GENT¶	1 gm. q 4–6 hr. 80–120 mg. q 8 hr.‡	PEN + AMINO§
Gram-positive bacilli			
Actinomyces	PEN	$1–2 \times 10^6$ units q 6 hr.	TET, CEPH*
Clostridium	PEN	$2–4 \times 10^6$ units q 4–6 hr.	TET, CEPH*
Corynebacterium	PEN	1×10^6 units q 6 hr.	ERY, CEPH*
Gram-negative bacilli			
Acinetobacter	GENT	80–120 mg. q 8 hr.‡	Other AMINO§
Bacteroides (except B. fragilis)	PEN	1×10^6 units q 6 hr.	CLIND, MET
B. fragilis	MET	0.5–1 gm. q 6 hr.	CLIND, CEFOX
Citrobacter	GENT	80–120 mg. q 8 hr.‡	Other AMINO§
Enterobacter	GENT	80–120 mg. q 8 hr.‡	Other AMINO§
Escherichia	GENT	80–120 mg. q 8 hr.‡	Other AMINO§
Fusobacterium	PEN	1×10^6 units q 6 hr.	CLIND, MET
Haemophilus	CHLOR	1 gm. q 6 hr.	
Klebsiella	GENT	80–120 mg. q 8 hr.‡	Other AMINO§
Legionella pneumophilia	ERY	1 gm. q 6 hr.	Rifampin
Morganella	GENT	80–120 mg. q 8 hr.‡	Other AMINO§
Proteus mirabilis	AMP	1–2 gm. q 6 hr.	CEPH,* AMINO§
P. vulgaris	GENT	80–120 mg. q 8 hr.‡	Other AMINO§ or TIC
Providencia	CEFOX	1–2 gm. q 6 hr.	GENT, TIC
Pseudomonas aeruginosa	TOB + CARB¶	80–120 mg. q 8 hr.‡ 2–4 gm. q 4–6 hr.	Other AMINO§ and TIC
Serratia	GENT	80–120 mg. q 8 hr.‡	Other AMINO§
Shigella	AMP	1–2 gm. q 6 hr.	CHLOR
Salmonella	CHLOR	1 gm. q 6 hr.	AMP

*First-generation cephalosporin—cefazolin, cephapirin or cephalothin.
†Nafcillin, oxacillin, methicillin—if a methicillin-resistant strain, use vancomycin.
‡Usual dosage in patient without renal impairment; dose should be monitored with serum peak and trough levels.
§Tobramycin, amikacin, or netimycin—determined by sensitivity studies.
¶Combination therapy indicated.
Abbreviations: AMINO = Aminoglycosides; AMP = ampicillin; CARB = carbenicillin; CEFOX = cefoxitin; CEPH = cephalosporin; CHLOR = chloramphenicol; CLIN = clindamycin; ERY = erythromycin; GENT = gentamicin; MET = metronidazole; PEN = penicillin; PEN-R = penicillinase-resistant penicillins; TET = tetracycline; TIC = ticarcillin; TOB = tobramycin.

the stomach or duodenum, spontaneous leak from a gastrointestinal carcinoma, pancreatitis, cholangitis, and intestinal infarction. Intra-abdominal sepsis following elective surgery occurs most often after gastric or colon resection.

Peritonitis occurs initially after the leakage of microorganisms from a diseased or traumatized organ. The dissemination of infection within the peritoneal cavity is

TABLE 8. Antimicrobial Recommendations for Renal and Hepatic Infection

Renal	
Aminoglycosides	Mezlocillin
Amphotericin B	Piperacillin
Azlocillin	Ticarcillin
Carbenicillin	Trimethoprim/Sulfa
Cephalosporins	Vancomycin
Methicillin	
Hepatic	
Clindamycin	Rifampin
Metronidazole	
Either	
Tetracycline	Chloramphenicol

dependent on many factors, including the location and size of the primary leak, the nature of the underlying injury or disease, the presence of adhesions from previous operations, the duration of present illness, and the efficiency of the defense mechanisms of the host. Generalized peritonitis is the most frequently reported type of intra-abdominal infection.

Localization of infection results in intraperitoneal, retroperitoneal, or visceral abscesses. Most often, intraperitoneal abscesses appear in the right lower quadrant in association with appendicitis or perforated duodenal ulcer.[2] Abscesses also appear in the left lower quadrant or in the pelvic, subphrenic, or subhepatic spaces, but they are rarely found in the lesser sac or between the loops of the intestine.

Visceral abscesses are found most commonly in the liver and are seen infrequently in the pancreas, spleen, and kidney. More than 50 per cent of liver abscesses are associated with either cholangitis or appendicitis.

Surgical drainage is the most important step in the proper treatment of intra-abdominal sepsis. When possible, drainage should be accomplished in a dependent fashion. The area of damaged or diseased viscera should be repaired or exteriorized, thereby decreasing the chance of continued

TABLE 9. *Antimicrobial Recommendations for Empiric Therapy of Commonly Seen Bacterial Infections**

Type of Infection	Most Likely Organisms	Systemic Antimicrobial Therapy†
Intra-abdominal		
Peritonitis, intra-abdominal or visceral abscess	Coliforms and *Bacteroids fragilis*	Cefoxitin alone or clindamycin or metronidazole } + aminoglycoside
Biliary tract infection	*Escherichia coli*	Cephalosporin alone or ampicillin plus aminoglycoside
Genitourinary (cystitis, pyelonephritis)		
First episode	*E. coli*	Ampicillin or cephalosporin
Recurrent	Coliforms or enterococci	Ampicillin plus aminoglycoside
Female genital tract		
Postoperative infection	Coliforms, *B. fragilis*	Cefoxitin alone or clindamycin or metronidazole } + aminoglycoside
Pneumonia		
Adult—uncomplicated	*Pneumococcus*	Penicillin G
Following aspiration	Mixed aerobes/anaerobes	Clindamycin ± aminoglycoside
Respiratory-induced (hospital acquired)	*Pseudomonas*	Carbenicillin or ticarcillin or pipericillin or imipenem alone } + aminoglycoside
Skin or soft tissue		
Cellulitis, lymphangitis or erysipelas	Beta-hemolytic streptococci	Penicillin G or cephalosporin
Pyoderma furunculosis (abscess)	*Staphylococcus aureus*	Penicillinase-resistant penicillin or cephalosporin
Decubitus ulcer (if septic)	Mixed aerobes/anaerobes	Clindamycin or metronidazole } + aminoglycoside
Gangrene (crepitant myositis)	Clostridia	Penicillin
Diabetic gangrene	Mixed aerobes/anaerobes	Clindamycin or metronidazole } + aminoglycoside
Human bite	Mixed aerobes/anaerobes	Penicillin G and tetracycline

*Specimens for culture and susceptibility should be sent as soon as possible.
†Changes in therapy are dictated by clinical response and culture results.

TABLE 10. Toxicity of Antimicrobial Agents

Drug	Side Effects of Toxicity	Drug	Side Effects of Toxicity

Penicillins
Primary penicillins
  Penicillin G (benzyl)
  Penicillin
	Hypersensitivity reactions
	  (immediate or delayed)
	Hemolytic anemia
	Central nervous system toxicity
	  (doses > 30–40 million units
	  per day)
		Erythromycins	Nausea
			Vomiting
			Epigastric distress
			Cholestatic jaundice
			  (erythromycin estolate)
			Thrombophlebitis

Penicillinase-resistant
  Methicillin
  Nafcillin
  Oxacillin
	Hypersensitivity reactions (all)
	Interstitial nephritis (meth)
	Drug-induced hepatitis (oxal)
		Clindamycin	Antibiotic-related colitis
			Nausea
			Vomiting
			Epigastric distress
			Abnormal liver functions
			Hypersensitivity reactions
			Thrombophlebitis

Broad-spectrum
  penicillin
  Carbenicillin
  Ticarcillin
  Mezlocillin
  Piperacillin
  Azlocillin
	Hypersensitivity reactions (all)
	Sodium loading (carb)
		Chloramphenicol	Dose-related anemia and
			  leukopenia
			Non–dose-related idiosyncratic
			  aplastic anemia
			Nausea
			Vomiting

Ampicillin	Hypersensitivity reactions High-incidence skin rash Antibiotic-associated colitis	Vancomycin	Ototoxicity Nephrotoxicity Thrombophlebitis Hypersensitivity reactions

Cephalosporins
All generations
	Hypersensitivity reactions
	Cross-over reactions in the
	  penicillin-allergic patient
	Positive direct Coomb's test
	Phlebitis
	Nephrotoxicity (cephaloridine)
	Antibiotic associated colitis
	Liver function abnormalities
	Bleeding diathesis (cefamandole,
	  moxalactam)
	Antabuse-like reaction
	  (cefamandole, moxalactam)
		Sulfonamides	Hypersensitivity reactions
			Anorexia
			Nausea
			Vomiting
			Acute hemolytic anemia
			Hepatitis
			Nephropathy

Aminoglycosides
  Gentamicin
  Tobramycin
  Amikacin
  Netilmicin
	Ototoxic
	Nephrotoxic
	Hypersensitivity reaction (rare)
	Neuromuscular blockade (rare)
		Metronidazole	Nausea
			Vomiting
			Anorexia
			Metallic taste
			Central nervous system—vertigo,
			  ataxia, seizures, peripheral
			  neuropathy
			Neutropenia
			Disulfiram (Antabuse)-like
			  reaction

Other antibiotics Tetracyclines	Nausea Vomiting Epigastric distress Candida overgrowth Antibiotic-related colitis Thrombophlebitis Tooth discoloration Hepatotoxicity Photosensitivity Vertigo	Amphotericin B	Chills Fever Nausea Vomiting Nephrotoxicity Thrombophlebitis Anemia Hypersensitivity

TABLE 11. *Average Daily Dose, Cost and Activity of Parenteral Cephalosporins*

Agent	Equivalent Dosing (gm.)*	Price per Gram†	Daily Cost	Microbiologic Activity‡
First-generation				
Cephapirin	1 q 6 hr.	$ 3.55	$14.20	Gram-positive aerobes + +
Cephalothin	1 q 6 hr.	2.88	11.52	Gram-negative aerobes +
Cefazolin	0.5 q 6 hr.	6.55	13.10	Gram-negative anaerobes −
				Gram-positive anaerobes +
Second-generation				
Cefamandole	1 q 6 hr.	7.15	28.60	Gram-positive aerobes +
Cefonicid	2 q 24 hr.	15.20	30.40	Gram-negative aerobes + +§
Cefoxitin	1 q 6 hr.	8.52	34.08	Gram-negative anaerobes + +¶
Cefuroxime	1.5 q 8 hr.	7.80	35.10	Gram-positive anaerobes +
Third-generation				
Cefoperazone	1 q 8 hr.	11.28	33.84	Gram-positive aerobes +
Cefotaxime	1 q 6 hr.	11.40	45.60	Gram-negative aerobes + +
Ceftizoxime	1 q 8 hr.	11.18	44.72	Gram-negative anaerobes + +#
Moxalactam	1 q 8 hr.	12.20	36.60	Gram-positive anaerobes +

*Dosage recommendation for serious infection.
†Average wholesale prices from Medi-Span Hospital Formulary Pricing Guide, July 1984.
‡+ + = good activity; + = activity; − = no activity.
§No activity against *Pseudomonas*.
¶Only cefoxitin has good *Bacteroides fragilis* activity.
#Moxalactam has best *Bacteroides fragilis* activity.

peritoneal contamination. Unlike patients with superficial wound abscesses in whom drainage alone usually suffices, those with intra-abdominal sepsis are best managed by a combination of surgical drainage and appropriate antibiotic therapy. The *antibiotic agents* chosen should be given parenterally before, during, and after operative drainage to guarantee adequate tissue levels. This factor helps decrease further local invasion, secondary septicemia, and metastatic abscess formation.

Most authors agree that antibiotics effective against both the aerobes and anaerobes of the colonic flora are desirable in the treatment of intra-abdominal infections.[9] Clindamycin and metronidazole are favored for anaerobic coverage while an aminoglycoside is usually chosen for the aerobic coverage. The addition of penicillin or ampicillin to cover the enterococci appears unnecessary unless this organism has been cultured from the infected sites. Single-drug therapy with cefoxitin has been shown to be comparable with combination therapy in recently reported studies.[24] Antibiotic agents advocated for treatment of intra-abdominal sepsis are listed in Table 12. The rational choice of which agent to employ depends largely on efficacy, toxicity, and cost.

Mechanical techniques utilized in the treatment of suppurative peritonitis include saline irrigation and careful débridement of peritoneal debris.[10] Many surgeons recommend irrigation of the peritoneal cavity with antibiotics such as cephalothin or kanamycin or with povidone-iodine solutions. It appears to the author that these approaches are most often unnecessary, unrewarding, and possibly dangerous.

Clostridial Infections

Many species of *Clostridium* are found in the normal human colon. Their isolation on culture in the absence of clinical findings causes great alarm, but is rarely of clinical significance. The worst of the clostridial infections—"gas gangrene" (clostridial myonecrosis) and tetanus—although uncommon, are truly catastrophic events. More frequently, clostridia participate in infections in a less dramatic fashion, either as part of the infecting flora in necrotizing soft tissue infections or as the sole pathogen in antibiotic-related enterocolitis.

GAS GANGRENE

Gas gangrene is a destructive process of the muscle associated with local crepitance and extreme systemic signs of toxemia. A predisposing event such as trauma, gunshot wound, frostbite, or intestinal surgery exposes muscle and subcutaneous tissues to these ubiquitous organisms. In the proper environment of tissue necrosis, low oxygen tension, and adequate concentrations of nutrients, the clostridial spores introduced from the external environment or the gastrointestinal tract are allowed to germinate, with the concomitant production of toxins.

Bacteriology

Clostridia are gram-positive, spore-forming, obligate anaerobes that are widely present in soil. In humans, they can be found in the gastrointestinal and the female genital tract, although they can be isolated occasionally from the surface of the skin and from the mouth.

TABLE 12. *Parenterally Administered Agents Advocated for Coverage of Aerobic and Anaerobic Components of Human Colonic Microflora*

Aerobic Activity	Anaerobic Activity	Aerobic and Anaerobic Activity
Amikacin	Carbenicillin	Cefoperazone
Aztreonam	Chloramphenicol	Cefotaxime
Cefamandole	Clindamycin	Cefotetan
Cefonicid	Metronidazole	Cefoxitin
Cefuroxime	Mezlocillin	Ceftizoxime
Gentamicin	Piperacillin	Imipenem
Netilmicin	Ticarcillin	Moxalactam
Tobramycin		

The most important of the histotoxic species involved in gas gangrene is *C. perfringens*, which is relatively aerotolerant and quite fast-growing. It produces alpha toxin, which is a phospholipase C that splits lecithin. Its activity can be inhibited by specific antitoxin. The alpha toxin has been associated with gas gangrene; it is known to be hemolytic, to destroy platelets, and to cause widespread capillary damage.

Myonecrosis is caused by *C. perfringens* in 80 per cent of patients, and the remaining causative agents are *C. novyi*, *C. septicum*, and *C. bifermentans*. The wounds themselves are also frequently contaminated with other aerobic and anaerobic bacteria, especially when the abdominal wall is primarily involved.

Pathogenesis

The pathophysiology setting of gas gangrene is necrosis of the muscle caused by a compromised blood supply, either through direct injury or underlying vascular disease, in association with contamination by potential pathogens. The conditions for elaboration of the toxin are a low tissue oxidation-reduction potential, anoxia, and local necrosis. These conditions are fulfilled in traumatic wounds associated with sepsis.

The current experience in metropolitan centers is that 60 per cent of cases are related to trauma, one half by automobile accidents, with the remainder being crush injuries, industrial accidents, or gunshot wounds. Other cases of gas gangrene occur postoperatively following colon resections, ruptured appendix, perirectal infection, perforated bowel, and biliary tract or gastroduodenal surgery. A small number of cases of gas gangrene can be traced to vascular insufficiency, usually in diabetics who develop disease in the stump following amputation. Overall, the experience is that two thirds of gas gangrene cases occur in the extremities and one third in the abdominal wall.

Clinical Features

The *incubation period* of gas gangrene is usually 8 hours to 2 days, with an average of 36 hours. There is a sudden onset of *pain* in the wound, increasing in severity and extending somewhat beyond the original borders over the next several hours. The skin initially becomes edematous and tense. It changes color from an initial pale appearance to a magenta hue, often accompanied by large, hemorrhagic bullae. A thin, watery discharge appears early in the course. It may have an unpleasant foul-sweet odor, and on microscopic examination there are abundant gram-positive rods with a remarkable *paucity of inflammatory cells*. The patient initially has a tachycardia that cannot be explained by the height of fever or circulatory changes. Subsequently, a high fever (38 to 40°C.), shock, and renal failure ensue.

The *appearance of the involved muscle* is characteristic, being quite unlike any other soft tissue infection. It must be viewed by direct surgical exposure, since many of the changes are not apparent when inspected through the edges of a traumatic wound. Initially, the muscle is pale and edematous, appearing as a piece of steak that has been seared over a charcoal fire. The muscle, however, does not contract when cut with a scalpel, and further dissection usually reveals beefy, red, nonviable muscle tissue. As the disease progresses, the muscle becomes frankly gangrenous, black, and extremely friable, and the patient is near death. It is important to establish the diagnosis of myonecrosis as early as possible in order to resect all devitalized, necrotic tissue.

The *mental status* of a patient with gas gangrene is an extraordinary feature of the disease process. Despite profound hypotension, renal failure, and advancing crepitance, these patients may be remarkably alert and show extreme sensitivity to their surroundings.

Diagnosis

The *sine qua non* for diagnosis of gas gangrene is *direct visualization of the muscle* to determine the characteristic appearance of the disease. When the infection is limited to the skin and subcutaneous tissue at operation (clostridial cellulitis), the débridement is easier and prognosis much improved (Table 13). The clinical features, as described above, should arouse suspicion early in the course, so that the disease can be recognized and surgically managed with haste. Gas in the wound and surrounding tissue is a relatively late finding, and by the time crepitance is appreciated the patient may be beyond hope of survival. X-ray examination of the affected site reveals gas in the tissues with dissection along the fascial planes; again, however, this tends to be a late finding (Fig. 5). A great help in diagnosis is examination of the wound discharge by Gram's stain. Needle aspiration of the active margin of the skin infection is helpful when wound discharge is not present.

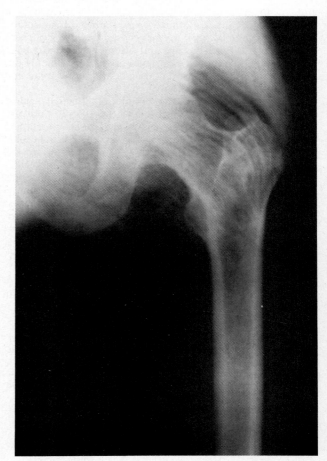

Figure 5. X-ray film of left hip in a patient with clostridial myonecrosis showing gas dissecting through soft tissue and muscle around the joint. Such gas patterns are characteristic of clostridial infections.

TABLE 13. Differential Diagnosis of Necrotizing Soft Tissue Infections

Characteristic	Clostridial Myonecrosis (Gas Gangrene)	Clostridial Cellulitis	Anaerobic Streptococcal Myositis	Synergistic Necrotizing Cellulitis	Necrotizing Fasciitis
Systemic toxicity	Extreme	Absent, mild	Moderate	Moderate to severe	Moderate to severe
Wound pain	Severe	Mild	Occurs late	Moderate to severe	Mild
Tissue induration	Absent	Absent	Absent	Absent	Present, hard
Gas	Present-late	Present	Present	Variable	Variable
Appearance of skin	Tense, white or gangrenous with bullae	Variable	Red, swollen	Swollen; red or gangrenous	Brawny; pale red or gangrenous
Muscle death	Always, extensive	None	Rare, localized	Rare, focal	Rare, localized
Gross characteristic of exudate	Thin, serous; may be sweetish or putrid	Putrid, brown	Seropurulent, sour	Purulent, putrid	Variable
Gram's stain of exudate	Few PMNs, gram-positive rods	Abundant PMNs, gram-positive rods	Many PMNs, gram-positive rods	Variable PMNs, mixed organisms	Many PMNs, variable, sometimes mixed organisms
Etiology	Clostridia	Clostridia	Anaerobic streptococci (± aerobic streptococci, staphylococci)	Mixed-aerobic, anaerobic streptococci, *Bacteroides*, and coliforms	Aerobic and anaerobic streptococci and staphylococci; occasionally *Bacteroides*
Surgical therapy	Extensive removal of all infected muscle and overlying tissue	Excision of involved superficial tissue	Débridement of involved necrotic tissue	Débridement of involved necrotic tissue	Excision of involved fascia and other necrotic tissue
Antibiotic therapy	Penicillin	Penicillin	Penicillin	Aerobic-anaerobic coverage	Aerobic-anaerobic coverage

Abbreviation: PMN = Polymorphonuclear neutrophils.

Complications

The mortality of gas gangrene is 40 to 60 per cent. It is highest in cases involving the abdominal wall and lowest in those affecting a single extremity. Among the signs that prognosticate a poor outcome are *leukopenia*, *low platelet count*, *intravascular hemolysis*, and severe *liver* or *renal* impairment.

Hypotension is an early sign of gas gangrene and can lead to *renal failure* and *irreversible shock*. Release of alpha toxin into the bloodstream can cause severe *hemolysis*, with hemoglobinemia, hemoglobinuria, and renal cortical necrosis.

Treatment

Surgical management is the most important modality of the therapy. As a general principle, all involved muscle should be resected in order to ensure survival. Clearly nonviable muscle, as demonstrated by lack of response to stimulus with the scalpel, should be removed. The major attention should be paid to *adequate excision*; *reconstruction* should be planned at a later stage. Such decisions require fine surgical judgment based on the extent of myonecrosis. The most common error of judgment in this disease is delaying the incision that is required to visualize the involved muscle; even a few hours' delay can be disastrous.

Antibiotic treatment is directed against clostridia in gangrene of the extremities and at a mixed microflora in those cases involving the abdominal wall. Penicillin G has excellent activity against nearly all strains of *C. perfringens*. The normal dose is 3 million units intravenously every four hours (reduce dosage with renal failure).

Antitoxin

The use of clostridial antitoxin is still *controversial*, despite the rather convincing claims from wartime experiences. Furthermore, available supplies are limited now because the manufacturers have generally discontinued production. The antitoxin is believed to neutralize toxin circulating in the bloodstream. The disease in its classic form, however, is characterized by compromised circulation and rapid fixation of toxin to tissue. It should be recalled that antitoxin is available only as a *horse serum* preparation; the large doses recommended for therapy carry a significant risk of immediate anaphylactic reactions as well as delayed reactions such as serum sickness. For these reasons, the use of antitoxin in treating gas gangrene is not recommended, especially when optimal surgical management is available at an early stage.

Hyperbaric Oxygen

The therapeutic use of hyperbaric oxygen (100 per cent) under pressure of 3 atmospheres has been strongly debated. In laboratory conditions, hyperbaric oxygen has generally resulted in killing of bacteria in addition to inhibiting toxin production. It is very difficult to judge the efficacy of this therapy from reading the literature, but this author can avow from personal experience that the effect of hyperbaric oxygen therapy in gas gangrene can be very dramatic. There are certain problems with such a therapeutic modality, not the least of which is the logistics of moving a desperately ill patient to appropriately equipped centers. In addition, hyperbaric oxygen has been shown to have certain untoward effects. Oxygen toxicity produces complications in the central nervous system and lung that can be serious and even life-threatening. It would be reasonable to conclude that patients with gas gangrene should be treated with hyperbaric oxygen if a facility is readily available.

TETANUS

Tetanus is a tragic disease, not only for its severity but because it can be completely prevented by appropriate immunizations. At the present time in the United States,

***TABLE 14.** Diseases to Be Considered with Tetanus Syndrome*

Generalized Tetanus	Trismus	Opisthotonos
Phenothiazine reaction	Dental abscess	Strychnine poisoning
Bacterial meningitis	Mandibular fracture	Rabies
Hypocalcemic tetany	Tonsillitis	Perforated peptic ulcer
Retroperitoneal hemorrhage	Diphtheria	Vertebral osteomyelitis
Epilepsy	Mumps	
Decerebrate posturing	Trichinosis	
Narcotic withdrawal	Retropharyngeal abscess	
	Mandibular osteomyelitis	

tetanus occurs primarily in rural areas or when childhood immunizations have not been performed routinely. The responsible organism, *Clostridium tetani*, is a gram-positive, anaerobic, spore-forming rod that has an ubiquitous distribution in the environment.

Pathogenesis

Most cases of tetanus occur after puncture wounds, lacerations, and crush injuries. The organism finds a receptive environment in the presence of tissue necrosis, anoxia, and other bacterial contaminants. As it germinates, the organisms release the toxin responsible for the clinical syndrome, which interrupts neuromuscular transmission by inhibiting the release of acetylcholine.

Clinical Features

The *incubation period* is variable, from a few days to several weeks. In general, a long latency is associated with more distal injuries and has a better prognosis. Three clinical forms of tetanus are recognized:

1. *Generalized tetanus*, responsible for about 80 per cent of cases. The disease is descending in clinical presentation, often beginning with trismus and progressing to neck stiffness, abdominal rigidity, and tetanic spasms of the extremities. Trismus can produce facial spasm known as *risus sardonicus*. As the spasm progresses, the back muscles are involved with arching of the back (*opisthotonos*). The two most prominent signs of incipient generalized tetanus are trismus and rigid abdominal musculature.

2. *Cephalic tetanus*, occurring with otitis media or traumatic injuries to the head. There is usually isolated cranial nerve involvement, especially the seventh nerve.

3. *Local tetanus*, involving the muscles in an area of injury. This is the mildest form of this disease.

Many diseases are confused with tetanus. Before making this diagnosis, one should consider the conditions listed in Table 14.

Diagnosis

Tetanus is a *clinical diagnosis* based on the physical findings. The organism can be seen in Gram's stains of infected material, but it is often confused with other gram-positive rods and may be difficult to identify in the mixed flora of a grossly contaminated wound. Culturing the organism also is very difficult.

Complications

The muscle spasms and seizures can lead to *fractures* of the spine and long bones. *Pulmonary embolism* has a high associated incidence, and *autonomic dysfunction* can occur, leading to hypertension and cardiac arrhythmias. Also a frequent complication is aspiration pneumonia, which frequently is the cause of death.

Prevention

A "tetanus-prone" wound is characterized by tissue necrosis associated with gross contamination from the environment. Additionally, a delay in treatment may place a wound in this category. Such wounds are at greatest risk to produce tetanus, but it must be emphasized that even minor puncture wounds or needle sticks have been the precursor to severe disease. Although it is a matter of judgment as to who should receive preventive measures, it is best to err on the side of conservatism, especially in non-immunized individuals. The current recommendations for immunization in the presence of a wound appear in Table 15.

A most important feature of tetanus prevention is appropriate wound care, with débridement and cleansing in order to remove any pockets of necrotic tissue and anaerobic dead spaces. With regard to the use of toxoid and *tetanus immune globulin* (TIG), as noted previously, the following points should be made:

1. The *TIG* is human globulin; the older preparations of horse serum should not be employed unless the TIG is unavailable. The *toxoid* should be the combined tetanus-

***TABLE 15.** Recommendations for Tetanus Immunization*

Tetanus Immunization Record	Wound	Recommendation
None or incomplete	Low risk	Toxoid—complete immunization*
Unknown	High risk	Toxoid—complete immunization + TIG†
No booster (within 10 years)	Low risk	Toxoid
	High risk	Toxoid ± TIG
Booster (within 10 years)	Low risk	None
	High risk	Toxoid

*Toxoid = Tetanus and diphtheria toxoids (adult type), 0.5 ml. intramuscularly.
†TIG = Tetanus immune globulin (human), 250 units intramuscularly.

diphtheria (TD) toxoid (adult type) in the form of adsorbed toxoid (with aluminum adjuvant). In this manner, the patient can be immunized against diphtheria as well as tetanus.

2. The usual dose of TIG is 250 units unless there is a severe injury, in which case 500 units can be employed. The TIG should be given with a different syringe and at a different site from the toxoid. In the event that this dose of TD constitutes a primary immunization, the patient should be instructed to return 28 days later to receive the second dose.

3. In general, booster injection of adsorbed toxoid, following an adequate primary vaccination series, should provide protective antibody for 10 years, during which time booster doses are not required. This interval should be shortened to 5 years in the setting of a severe injury. Multiple injections of toxoid, prompted by each injury, can lead paradoxically to lower levels of circulating antibody, so this practice is discouraged.

4. Antibiotic treatment and surgical débridement do not give adequate protection against tetanus. Thus, the immunization status of all patients with contaminated wounds must be ascertained and appropriate treatment should be initiated.

Treatment

The treatment of tetanus is mainly a physiologic exercise in preventing complications. Any toxin that has been elaborated and already fixed to tissues is in an irreversible state, so the disease cannot be interrupted once it has started. Indeed, the spasms and increased muscular contractions can continue for several weeks after the organism has been eradicated.

The initial phases of treatment involve eliminating the organism by surgical débridement and antibiotics, and administration of antitoxin for circulating toxin that has not yet been fixed. The other modalities are directed at physiologic stabilization and nutrition.

1. *Surgical débridement* of any obvious wound should be undertaken in order to remove necrotic tissue.

2. *Antibiotic therapy* should be directed at the organism, and penicillin G is the treatment of choice (3 million units intravenously every 6 hours).

3. *Antitoxin* should be administered for the possibility of binding any circulating toxin. TIG, in a dose of 500 units, is given. During the course of the illness, a full immunizing schedule of toxoid should be provided in order to prevent a second attack.

4. *Prevention of muscle contractions and spasm* is achieved by short-acting barbiturates and muscle relaxants such as chlorpromazine. Diazepam may be used to control seizures. In severe cases, curare-like drugs are required.

5. *Environmental stimuli* should be reduced to a minimum by placing the patient in a quiet, darkened room.

6. *Tracheostomy* should be considered in patients who have had a series of tetanic seizures. It is obviously necessary when curare-like drugs are employed.

7. *Total parenteral alimentation* is an important part of the management of patients with tetanus who may be unable to swallow because of trismus.

CLOSTRIDIAL INTESTINAL DISORDERS

Clostridium is known to cause three types of intestinal illness: (1) food-borne disease, (2) enteritis necroticans, and (3) pseudomembranous colitis. These illnesses are caused by different clostridial strains and their toxins, and each has its own epidemiology and pathogenesis.

Food Poisoning

Food poisoning associated with clostridia is common in the United States. The responsible vehicle is usually a meat product that has been cooked one day, allowed to cool, then is reheated and served the following day.

The most prominent clinical finding is moderate to severe mid-epigastric pain, which is crampy in nature and is usually associated with watery diarrhea. Fever and vomiting are uncommon, although nausea is frequent. The incubation period is 8 to 24 hours, with the usual onset 8 to 12 hours after contact with contaminated food. Fortunately, the disease is rather mild, not lasting more than 24 hours. Surgical intervention or medical therapy is not indicated in this condition.

Enteritis Necroticans

Enteritis necroticans is a severe, necrotizing disease of the small intestine with a high mortality rate. The implicated organism is C. *perfringens* (type C), and the beta toxin appears to be the major cause. Associated with this syndrome is the ingestion of undercooked pork.

Clinical features that appear within 24 hours include acute abdominal pain, bloody diarrhea, vomiting, shock, and, in approximately 40 per cent patients, peritonitis and death. The pathology is an acute ulcerative process of the bowel, usually restricted to the small intestine. The mucosa is lifted off the submucosa, forming large denuded areas. Pseudomembranes composed of the sloughed epithelium are commonly seen, and gas may dissect into the submucosa. There is very little experience with surgical management of this condition. Since vast areas of small bowel are involved in the severe cases, it is unlikely that survival would be improved by aggressive intervention.

Pseudomembranous Colitis

Pseudomembranous colitis is a severe, necrotizing process involving the large intestine that occurs as a complication of antibiotic therapy. Although clindamycin was the antibiotic associated initially with the disease, most cases are now ascribed to ampicillin and cephalosporins. It is now clear that nearly all antimicrobial drugs can cause this condition.

Bacteriology. The responsible pathogen is *Clostridium difficile*, a constituent of the normal flora in approximately 10 per cent of people, which apparently overgrows to large populations in the presence of antibiotics. Many strains of this organism are resistant to antimicrobial agents, although the pattern of resistance is highly variable. However, all strains are sensitive to vancomycin. C. *difficile* elaborates a potent necrotizing toxin that is responsible for the syndrome.

Clinical Features. These can vary from mild diarrhea to necrotizing colitis that leads to perforation. The most common presentation, by far, is mild diarrhea, lasting days to weeks. In some patients, the progression from mild diarrhea to severe disease (pseudomembranous colitis) can be observed, but this course can be interrupted by stopping the offending antibiotic or by instituting appropriate therapy.

Pathologic Features. The pathologic features of pseudomembranous colitis are quite distinctive: Initial events are limited to the superficial mucosa with necrosis and formation of a pseudomembrane that is composed of fibrin with a paucity of inflammatory cells. The underlying submucosa is denuded and hemorrhagic, but lacks the inflammatory reaction that is seen with ulcerative colitis or bacillary dysentery. Severe cases of pseudomembranous colitis display sloughing of the pseudomembrane, transmural extension of the necrosis, and perforation through the serosa into the peritoneal cavity.

Diagnosis. Diagnosis is initially based on the clinical setting of diarrhea, which is related temporally to antibiotic therapy. About half the cases occur during therapy, with the remainder beginning after stopping the antibiotic, usually within the first week, but occasionally up to 4 weeks later. *Sigmoidoscopy* reveals the characteristic appearance of an inflamed, friable mucosa. In more advanced cases, there is a myriad of yellowish plaques or pseudopolyps and a grayish membrane covers the mucosa in a patchy distribution. The late stages show a diffusely ulcerated mucosa. Barium studies of the colon show "fingerprinting" of the bowel wall with fine ulcerations. There is a test for identification of the toxin in the feces by demonstration of a histotoxic effect in tissue cultures.

Therapy. The therapy of antibiotic-associated diarrhea and pseudomembranous colitis is divided into several stages, depending on the severity of the disease.

1. *Mild diarrhea* is treated by removing the offending antibiotic. Intravenous fluid and electrolytes should be administered to dehydrated patients. *Narcotic anti-diarrheals and their analogues must be avoided.*

2. More *severe* forms of *chronic diarrhea* can be treated with vancomycin (250 mg. by mouth four times a day for 7 days). Metronidazole has been used effectively in some cases (500 mg. by mouth three times a day), although it should be recognized that this drug has also been a cause of pseudomembranous colitis in other cases.

3. Pseudomembranous colitis can progress to *toxic megacolon*, a condition that frequently requires emergency surgical intervention.

4. *Corticosteroids* have been unimpressive in treating this condition. However, the authors have had some encouraging results in the therapy of toxic megacolon using large doses of prednisone (60 mg. per day in four divided doses), thereby avoiding total colectomy. Short of this drastic situation, steroids are not recommended because most patients would respond to vancomycin therapy.

5. Cholestyramine has been recommended in patients with pseudomembranous colitis, but the results are variable.

6. Severely ill patients with pseudomembranous colitis may be unable to tolerate oral vancomycin; intravenous metronidazole should be used instead.

Other Necrotizing or Soft Tissue Infections

Several other spreading infections in addition to clostridial myositis and cellulitis involve the soft tissues. Again, the keystone to successful treatment is rapid early diagnosis.

ANAEROBIC STREPTOCOCCAL MYOSITIS

Anaerobic streptococcal myositis is a more indolent process than are other aerobic streptococcal infections. It is caused by various species of anaerobic streptococci (peptostreptococci). Involvement of the muscle and fascial planes usually follows trauma or a surgical procedure. There may be *severe* local pain. The overlying skin appears as a gangrenous wound that emits a foul, watery, brown discharge. Bleb formation is common, and crepitus may be apparent in the surrounding tissue. The gas formation can be extensive, with tracking into the adjacent healthy tissues. On inspection of the muscle, there is redness and edema

with some local destruction. However, there is no myonecrosis, and the muscle contracts when cut with the scalpel. Although there usually is generalized toxicity and fever, the patient is not as ill as those with gas gangrene.

The initial approach to a crepitant skin infection is to obtain a sample of exudate for Gram's stain and open the wound for inspection of muscle and soft tissue. The major distinctions between the diseases caused by anaerobic streptococci and clostridia are listed in Table 13.

SYNERGISTIC NECROTIZING CELLULITIS

Synergistic necrotizing cellulitis is a highly lethal polymicrobial infection that produces extensive necrosis of the skin and soft tissues with progressive undermining along fascial planes. The process may be rather indolent at first, presenting after 7 to 10 days of mild symptoms. Patients are often afebrile or have only low-grade fever, lacking systemic toxicity in the early stages of the infection. The initial skin lesion is a small area of necrotic or reddish-brown bleb with extreme local tenderness. However, the superficial appearance belies the widespread destruction of the deeper tissues. By direct inspection through skin incisions, there is extensive gangrene of the superficial tissues with some local necrosis of fascia and muscle. The discharge is brown, rather thin and watery, with a foul odor; such exudate has been labeled "dishwater pus." Gram stain reveals a *mixed flora* with abundant polymorphonuclear leukocytes. Gas can be palpated in the tissues in 25 per cent of the patients.

The most common site of involvement is the *perineum*, seen in half of patients. The major predisposing causes are *perirectal abscess* and *ischiorectal abscess*; these conditions track to the deeper structures of the pelvis, leading to a severe form of disease.

In approximately 40 per cent of patients, there is involvement of the thigh and leg. Some infections arise in the adductor compartment of the thigh, often extending from an infected amputation stump or diabetic gangrene. Lesions in the lower leg usually are associated with vascular disease or diabetic foot ulcers. The remaining 10 per cent of cases occur in the upper extremities or in the neck, most frequently in patients with vascular disease or diabetes.

Predisposing conditions include diabetes mellitus, which is present in more than 50 per cent of patients, and cardiovascular disease, renal disease, and obesity. This is a *mixed aerobic-anaerobic infection*, consisting of organisms from the intestinal tract. The surgical and medical treatment recommendations are found in Table 13.

NECROTIZING FASCIITIS

A relatively rare infection, necrotizing fasciitis involves subcutaneous tissues with extensive undermining and tracking along fascial planes. Although originally associated with beta-hemolytic streptococci (Group A), it is apparent that the disease can be caused by other microorganisms, including anaerobic streptococci, *Staphylococcus aureus*, *Bacteroides*, and a mixed aerobic-anaerobic flora.

Clinical Features

Clinical features include extension from a skin lesion in about 80 per cent of cases. Often the lesion is initially trivial, such as a minor abrasion, insect bite, injection site, or abscess (the perirectal type being the most frequent).

The initial presentation is that of cellulitis, which advances rather slowly. Over the next 2 to 4 days, however, there is systemic toxicity with high body temperatures. The patient is disoriented and lethargic. The local site of infection shows edema, skin discoloration, and occasionally anesthesia of the skin.

The most distinguishing clinical feature is the "woodenhard" feel of the subcutaneous tissues. In cellulitis or erysipelas, the subcutaneous tissues can be palpated and are yielding, but in fasciitis the underlying tissues are firm and the fascial planes and muscle groups cannot be discerned by palpation. It is often possible to observe a broad erythematous track in the skin, along the route of the fascial plane as the infection advances in an extremity. If there is an open wound, probing the edges with a blunt instrument permits ready dissection of the superficial fascial planes well beyond the wound margins. There is characteristically little pain associated with this procedure.

Bacteriology

Monomicrobial Form. Pathogens in this group are Group A beta-hemolytic streptococci, *Staphylococcus aureus*, and anaerobic streptococci. Staphylococci and hemolytic streptococci occur in about equal frequency, and approximately one third of patients will have both pathogens. In most cases, infection is acquired outside the hospital, and the majority of these infections present in the extremities, approximately two thirds in the lower extremity. There is often an underlying cause, such as *diabetes*, *arteriosclerotic vascular disease*, or *venous insufficiency with edema*. In some instances, a chronic vascular ulcer changes into a more acute process. The mortality in this group is high, approaching 50 per cent in patients with severe vascular disease.

Polymicrobial Form. An array of anaerobic and aerobic colonic organisms can be cultured from the involved fascial plane, from one to 15 bacteria, with an average of five pathogens in each wound.

Diagnosis

It may not be possible to diagnose fasciitis upon initial examination. Overlying cellulitis is a frequent accompaniment. The involvement of the deeper fascial planes is suggested by the following features:

1. Failure to respond to initial antibiotic therapy. Cellulitis usually improves, with lowering of fever and reduction in local signs, within 24 to 48 hours. Fasciitis is a more stubborn infection that shows little improvement in the initial few days.

2. Hard "wooden feel" of the subcutaneous tissue, extending beyond the area of apparent skin involvement.

3. Systemic toxicity, often with altered mental status. Treatment considerations are offered in Table 12.

BETA-STREPTOCOCCAL GANGRENE

Although most spreading infections caused by streptococci are not necrotizing and are easily treated with local care and parenteral penicillin, occasionally these organisms can bring about gangrenous infections similar to the clostridial infections. No predisposing clinical factors have been identified, and these infections may occur following minimal trauma, such as elective surgical incision. Diagnosis is made by Gram's stain and culture results. Gangrenous changes are most often confined to the skin and soft tissues. Appropriate treatment includes penicillin and rapid surgical débridement of all involved tissues.

ECTHYMA GANGRENOSUM

Rarely, during gram-negative septicemia, embolic spread of the causative organisms may produce characteristic skin lesions (ecthyma gangrenosum). These lesions start as pustules that ulcerate and progress to necrotic patches frequently covered with eschar. They are usually multiple and occur in equal distribution on the body surface. These infections usually occur in immunosuppressed, critically ill hospitalized patients. *Pseudomonas aeruginosa* is the usual causative microorganism. Treatment includes surgical débridement of the necrotic lesions and specific anti-pseudomonal antibiotic therapy. Despite adequate therapy, the mortality rate remains high (>60 per cent) in the postoperative patient.

Nosocomial Infections in the Surgical Patient

Pneumonia, urinary tract infections, and intravascular catheter sepsis also occur all too frequently during the postoperative course. The following section details the microorganisms usually implicated as well as the preventive and treatment techniques that should be utilized.

HOSPITAL-ACQUIRED PNEUMONIA

Nosocomial pneumonia occurs in 0.5 to 5 per cent of hospitalized patients. It is second only to urinary tract infection as a cause of hospital-acquired infections. The mortality rate can be as high as 50 per cent if the invading pathogen is a resistant, gram-negative bacillus. The areas within the hospital at greatest risk are intensive care units and burn units, because of the type of illness found there and because of the intrahospital spread of potential pathogens within these areas.

Pathophysiology

The pathogens of pneumonia associated with hospitalization come from three major sources:

1. Contamination of the oropharynx from the hospital environment with subsequent aspiration.

2. Contamination of inhalation therapy equipment.

3. Direct introduction through tracheostomy or endotracheal tubes.

Colonization of the oropharynx with gram-negative bacilli occurs in about 20 per cent of the patients by the end of the first day of hospitalization and in about 45 per cent after 4 days. Patients with pre-existing pulmonary disease are at greatest risk. After colonization, the offending microorganisms are aspirated into the bronchioles and alveoli. Pre-existing broad-spectrum antibiotic therapy also aids in the selection of antibiotic-resistant organisms.

In the mechanisms of entry via the use of contaminated inhalation therapy equipment, hospital-associated bacteria colonize in the breathing circuits, including the tubing, nebulizers, humidifiers, and valves. The organisms may grow to heavy concentrations at these sites, and when this occurs, they may be delivered to the lower respiratory tract by aerosol. Droplet size determines the localization within the lung of such contaminated aerosols. The most dangerous droplets are 1 to 2 microns in diameter and can be delivered directly to the smaller bronchioles and alveoli, thereby bypassing the normal pulmonary defense mechanisms. Therefore, any piece of respiratory equipment that creates such small particles (such as an ultrasonic nebulizer) carries a higher risk of causing pneumonia. Small-volume nebulizers, often used for delivering medication in an intermittent positive-pressure breathing (IPPB) machine, have an intermediate risk of causing pneumonia because of the small reservoir system and the relatively large droplets that are produced. The greatest risk of infection is associated with large-reservoir nebulizers, especially the "mainstream nebulizers," which are attached directly to compressed air or oxygen valves. This equipment produces droplets of varying diameters, including those of 1 to 2 microns. In addition, there is an opportunity to contaminate the nebulizing jet and the large volume of fluid within the reservoir.

Bacteriology

The pathogens responsible for nosocomial pneumonia vary from hospital to hospital, depending on the specific bacterial flora associated with each institution. The gram-negative organisms are the main culprits, many of which are resistant to several antibiotic agents and are well adapted for survival on moist surfaces and even in some decontamination solutions. Common pathogens associated with nosocomial pneumonia include *Pseudomonas aeruginosa*, *Klebsiella*, *E. coli*, *Serratia*, and *Enterobacter*. *Staphylococcus aureus* still on occasion may cause hospital epidemics of pneumonia.

Prevention and Treatment

The use of preventive techniques will not eliminate, but will decrease, the incidence of postoperative pneumonia. These are as follows:

1. Prevent postoperative atelectasis by utilizing established techniques of deep breathing and coughing, blow bottle, incentive spirometry, and so on.

2. Limit or avoid stays in intensive care units.

3. Carefully limit the use of broad-spectrum antibiotics.

4. Remove endotracheal tubes early. Nearly all patients become contaminated with gram-negative bacilli within 2 to 3 days of intubation.

5. When prolonged intubation is necessary, meticulous care in the suctioning and handling of the endotracheal tube is critical. Use sterile gloves and disposable suction catheters.

6. Avoid nebulization with antimicrobial drugs or disinfectants.

7. Every 48 hours, change tubing, nebulizing equipment, and reservoirs in inhalation therapy devices.

8. Completely empty and refill reservoirs every 8 to 12 hours, thus avoiding the buildup of bacterial growth.

9. Use sterile water (not tap water) in reservoirs.

10. Clean the breathing circuits, including tubing, valves and nebulizers, initially to remove particulate material; then disinfect or sterilize.

Once pneumonia is diagnosed, selective systemic antimicrobial therapy given in appropriate doses, in addition to adequate pulmonary support, is indicated.

URINARY TRACT INFECTION

Urinary tract infection is generally the most common type of sepsis in the surgical patient. It is caused by postoperative urinary retention and the use of urethral catheters. Bacteriuria, defined as greater than 10^5 bacteria per ml. of urine is indicative and diagnostic of these infections.

Cystitis versus Acute Pyelonephritis

Most urinary tract infections, in the postoperative patient, are limited to the urinary bladder. If treated promptly and appropriately very few patients will experience upper tract infections. High fever, chills, and leukocytosis are generally indicative of acute pyelonephritis. Single catheterization done appropriately for urinary retention will result in only about a 2 per cent incidence of urinary tract infections in elective surgical patients. In debilitated patients, this incidence may increase to 10 to 20 per cent. Urinary tract infection is most common in patients requiring indwelling urinary catheters. If open drainage is used, virtually all patients will be infected within 2 days; when a closed drainage system is employed, about 5 to 10 per cent per day will become infected.

Bacteriology

Bacteria can reach the bladder or renal parenchyma by retrograde contamination, hematogenous dissemination, inoculation from contiguous infection, or lymphatic spread. The retrograde route is the usual source of infection in the postsurgical patient.

Over 90 per cent of initial urinary tract infections are caused by *E. coli*, the majority of which are highly susceptible to most antimicrobial agents. Antibiotic-resistant strains of *E. coli*, *Klebsiella*, *Enterobacter*, *Proteus*, *Pseudomonas*, *Serratia*, and enterococci are found usually in urinary tract infections associated with multiple courses of antibiotic treatment or repeated instrumentations or catheterization in the face of underlying structural defects.

Prevention and Treatment

The prevention of urinary tract sepsis during the postoperative period depends primarily on adequate hydration and the limited use of urethral catheterization. When catheterization is necessary for urinary retention, a single in-and-out passage should be done with sterile technique. When an indwelling Foley catheter is used, it should be attached to a closed drainage system. In this clinical setting, it is important to follow the patient with urine cultures every 3 to 5 days and after removal of the catheter. The use of preventive bladder irrigation with antiseptics or chronic use of antibiotics should be discouraged in the postoperative patient.

The decision to treat with antibiotics is based on symptomatology and the finding of bacteriuria on culture. The goal of therapy is eradication of bacteria from the urinary tract in order to prevent progressive renal insufficiency. Although the antimicrobial agent chosen should be based on the culture and sensitivity results, it should be remembered that most infections are due to antibiotic-sensitive strains of *E. coli*. Therefore, the treatment chosen should be inexpensive, safe, and well tolerated. Oral ampicillin, tetracycline, or sulfisoxazole are among the agents that fulfill these goals. Parenteral treatment should be employed in the patient with restricted oral intake or in those with upper tract infections.

INTRAVASCULAR CATHETER-RELATED SEPTICEMIA

Like so many mechanical adjuncts to modern surgical practice, intravenous and intra-arterial lines, although necessary, are somewhat risky invasions of the normal skin barrier. The major risk of these intravascular infusion devices is local infection or dissemination to the bloodstream. Organisms can be isolated from the local colonizations in only about 10 per cent of patients with an indwelling catheter.

Risk Factors

The major risk factors that increase the likelihood of intravascular catheter-associated sepsis are as follows:

1. *Phlebitis* is strongly associated with subsequent infection. The development of the local thrombus is usually due to chemical or physical irritation. This sterile thrombus later becomes infected and is the usual source of catheter-related septicemia.

2. The length of time during which the indwelling catheter remains in place is critical. The risk increases after 48 hours and is particularly high after 72 hours.

3. External manipulation of the catheter augments the risk by introducing exogenous microorganisms.

4. The skin flora surrounding the catheter site represents the most common source of pathogens. For this reason, catheters should be inserted with strict aseptic technique and the surrounding area should be kept clean with antiseptic solutions.

5. Remote infections occasionally result in contamination of the catheter tip.

6. The type of infusion fluid may influence the development of contamination and subsequent infection. Fluids that require the addition of other substances (e.g., vitamins, electrolytes) increase the risk of external contamination. Hypertonic solutions, such as used in hyperalimentation, often result in chemical phlebitis, which predisposes the patient to infection.

7. The type of catheter used relates to the risk of infection, *metal* needles having the lowest risk and long *plastic* indwelling catheters having the highest.

8. The location of insertion also is important. Infusions done through cut-downs in the lower extremities are associated with the highest septic complication rate. Subclavian veins become infected more frequently than do peripheral veins in the arm.

The use of a special hospital intravenous team may lower the risk of infection, although this point, to date, has not been verified.

Microbiology

A great variety of bacteria and fungi have been recovered from venous catheters. *Staphylococcus epidermidis* is the most common organism found on the catheter tip and surrounding skin, reflecting its major source from the normal microflora of the skin. It is rarely isolated in the blood culture of patients in whom catheter-related septicemia develops. The most common blood isolates are *S. aureus* and the gram-negative bacilli. *Klebsiella-Enterobacter* group, *Pseudomonas*, and *Serratia* are the most commonly isolated of the gram-negative bacilli.

Treatment

Any febrile spike in the postoperative period should suggest catheter-related sepsis in patients with indwelling plastic intravascular catheters. After other causes of postoperative fever have been investigated and excluded, blood cultures should be drawn and all central lines removed and cultured. The wide majority of cases of catheter-associated septicemia are self-limiting, if so treated. Febrile episodes will cease on catheter removal, and systemic antibiotics are rarely necessary for successful treatment. However, if the catheter is left in place, metastatic infections may result from the continued cyclic septicemia. There is no evidence that systemic antibiotics reduce or in any way alter the incidence of catheter-associated infections. Surgical exploration and excision of the involved segment of vein are indicated if *suppurative phlebitis* occurs.

Hepatitis B

Hepatitis B, formerly called *serum hepatitis*, is caused by a virus that has been termed the "Dane" particle. In contrast to *hepatitis A*, illness frequently is insidious in onset and is associated with extrahepatic manifestations, such as arthritis and skin rashes.

The disease is transmitted primarily by percutaneous inoculation, such as through blood transfusion or needle stick. Recent evidence suggests that the disease can be transmitted through contaminated saliva, semen, or blood introduced onto mucosal surfaces.

The incubation period for hepatitis B is 40 to 180 days (mean 90 days). The virus can be demonstrated in the blood from 1 to 2 months before until 1 to 2 months after the onset of jaundice. Other body secretions, including urine and bile, have been shown to contain the virus.

There is a chronic blood carrier state that can affect up to 10 per cent of normal patients. Several groups of patients are at higher risk of becoming chronic carriers, especially those undergoing chronic hemodialysis, those receiving multiple transfusions (sickle cell anemia, hemophilia), and those with Down's syndrome. The course of the chronic carrier state is quite variable and can range from total lack of symptoms to chronic active hepatitis with or without postnecrotic cirrhosis. Morbidity and mortality are variable, but in general are more severe in this illness than in hepatitis A.

DIAGNOSIS

Several antigen-antibody systems have been described in hepatitis B. The hepatitis B surface antigen (HBsAg) is found on the surface of the virus, and it is the clinical marker for hepatitis B infection. In addition, there are antibody markers to this surface antigen, *anti-HBs*. Immunity to hepatitis B is usually specific and life-long. In order to make a diagnosis of acute hepatitis B, one needs to obtain a positive HBsAg determination.

PREVENTION OF SPREAD OF INFECTION

General Measures

Several general measures are applicable to prevent the spread of hepatitis in surgical units. Surgeons should be aware of several groups of patients who are at high risk of harboring hepatitis B, namely, those maintained on chronic hemodialysis, those from institutions for the mentally retarded, those receiving multiple blood transfusions, those who are homosexuals, or those who are intravenous drug abusers. Many of these patients are asymptomatic carriers and therefore should be screened for HBsAg upon admission.

Procedures in General Medical, Obstetric, and Surgical Units

Patients with acute hepatitis B or with HbsAg-positive blood should be cared for in rooms separate from other patients without hepatitis. Should this not be possible, semiprivate rooms or wards in which blood and instrument precautions are observed should be used. Staff should wear gowns and gloves when handling blood or blood-contaminated objects from HBsAg-positive patients and when doing venipunctures and anytime a potential contact with blood exists. Careful handwashing should be observed both by staff and the hepatitis patient. Masks or other facial coverings should be worn during procedures that might result in splashing of infectious material into the face.

Hepatitis B Immune Globulin

Hepatitis B immune globulin (HBIG) has recently undergone clinical trials in the United States. It is efficacious in certain circumstances, such as needle stick exposure or mucosal exposure to blood containing HbsAg. Current recommendations are a dose of 0.05 to 0.07 ml. per kg. of body weight within a 7–day period of exposure, with a second dose administered 25 to 30 days after the first.

Hepatitis B Vaccine

A vaccine for hepatitis B has been recently licensed and is currently available. The vaccine is a purified inactivated preparation of HBsAg that induces a protective antibody response when given in three successive doses at 0, 1, and 6 months. The vaccine is recommended for health care workers (especially surgeons), homosexual males, hemophiliacs, dialysis patients, and infants born to HBsAg-positive mothers. Side effects have been low and limited to fever and local arm pain.

THERAPY

No specific treatment is available for any of the forms of viral hepatitis. Patients with severe derangement of liver function need to be hospitalized. Severe liver dysfunction is most often reflected in a prolongation of the prothrombin time. No specific diet need be employed. If anorexia is severe, however, intravenous fluids may be necessary. Parenteral vitamin K should be given to hypoprothrombinemic patients, but patients with severe hepatocellular disease usually do not respond. Bed rest need not be strictly enforced, especially in patients who are young and who have previously been healthy. There are no indications for corticosteroids in early uncomplicated hepatitis. Indeed, the use of steroids has not been shown to be beneficial in acute fulminant hepatitis.

Pseudomycotic and Mycotic Infections

PSEUDOMYCOTIC INFECTIONS

Slowly progressive and chronic pseudomycotic infections frequently result in the formation of granulomas and abscesses that spontaneously drain through sinus and fistula tracts. Both *Actinomyces* and *Nocardia* produce these lesions, which resemble those produced by fungi, but are actually bacterial.

Actinomycosis

Actinomyces israelii is a gram-positive, filamentous, anaerobic microorganism often found as part of the normal microflora of the oropharynx. Clinically, these microorganisms cause pulmonary, soft tissue, and intra-abdominal infections. The resultant draining sinuses, most commonly seen in the jaw or lower abdomen, will discharge purulent material containing "sulfur granules" seen on low-power microscopic examination. Mandibular involvement most often precedes the development of the facial form of this disease. In the abdominal forms, the cecum and appendix appear to be the initial sites of infection. Secondary infection of the involved tissue is common. All forms of actinomycosis are treated with penicillin G (5 to 20 units $\times$ 10^6 units daily) given for 4 to 6 weeks. Surgical débridement and excision are frequently necessary in addition to the antibiotic therapy.

Nocardiosis

Nocardia is an aerobic, gram-positive, branching, filamentous microorganism often endogenous to the normal respiratory tract. It can produce clinical syndromes similar to actinomycosis or may produce a specific entity, *madura foot* (mycetoma), which results in extensive bone destruction with little systemic toxicity. Surgical débridement plus long-term sulfonamide therapy (6 to 8 gm. daily) appears to be the treatment of choice.

MYCOTIC INFECTIONS

The majority of fungi of clinical importance grow as either molds or yeasts. Some are biphasic, existing in both forms. Spores produced are easily aerosolized and therefore can result in primary pulmonary infections.

Histoplasmosis

Histoplasma capsulatum induces a primary pulmonary infection following inhalation. Fungemia, which frequently follows, is usually self-limiting. Endemic areas include the eastern-central United States bordering the Mississippi and Ohio Rivers. Over 90 per cent of people living in some of these areas have had primary pulmonary histoplasma infection before age 20.

Clinical syndromes include primary and chronic cavitary pulmonary infection and disseminated histoplasmosis. Disseminated histoplasmosis denotes progressive extrapulmonary involvement, including that of the central nervous system and gastrointestinal tract. Diagnosis is made from specialized stains and cultures as well as from skin and serologic testing.

Thoracotomy frequently is necessary when histoplasmosis presents as a solitary, noncalcified pulmonary lesion. If such a nodule is excised, it is usually not necessary to treat with amphotericin B. Amphotericin B therapy is indicated in prolonged or progressive pulmonary disease or in disseminated disease.

Blastomycosis

Blastomyces dermatitidis is the causative agent of this primary pulmonary infection, which results following inhalation of the organism. It is also referred to as North American blastomycosis and can closely mimic carcinoma.

The causative microorganism is endemic to southeastern and southern central regions in the United States. Diagnosis is made by specialized stains and culture and by skin and serologic testing. Clinical syndromes include primary and chronic pulmonary infection with or without distal site involvement and isolated distal involvement. Distal involvement occurs most frequently in skin, bone, or genitourinary tract.

Primary pulmonary involvement most commonly results in alveolar consolidation with hilar adenopathy. Progressive infection may result in necrosis or in cavitation and empyema. Chronic involvement reveals fibronodular infiltrates with small cavities on chest roentgenogram. Distal involvement of the skin may result in raised, warty, crusted lesions that mimic basal cell carcinoma; bony lesions may appear either as osteolytic or osteoblastic processes.

Treatment with amphotericin B is usually not required in primary acute pulmonary infestation; however, it is required in chronic involvement with or without operative resection and when there is skin, bone, or genitourinary involvement.

Coccidioidomycosis

Coccidioides immitis, the causative microorganism, is endemic to the southwestern United States, especially in the San Joaquin Valley of California and in southern Arizona and New Mexico. The offending microorganism produces primary pulmonary and disseminated disease. Diagnosis is made by specialized stains and cultures and with skin and serologic testing. Primary pulmonary involvement resolves without sequelae in 95 per cent of the patients, whereas in the rest of cases thin-walled solitary nodules develop. Manifestations of cell-mediated immunity, such as erythema nodosum, erythema multiforme, and frank arthritis occur in up to 20 per cent of all patients with pulmonary disease, a much higher incidence than in other fungal infections. Disseminated disease may show rapid progression with involvement of meninges, bone, and skin. Amphotericin B is less effective against *C. immitis* than the other pathogenic fungi, but still remains the drug of choice. Antimicrobial therapy is rarely indicated in primary pulmonary disease; however, it is indicated when operative resection is undertaken or in the disseminated form.

Cryptococcosis

Cryptococcus neoformans, the causative organism, is distributed worldwide and most often associated with pigeon guano. Disease usually involves the pulmonary and central nervous systems; it may also involve the skin or bone or may be generally disseminated. Diagnosis is made primarily on histologic staining, which shows the characteristic yeast form with its thick, unstained capsule. No skin test is presently available, but cultures and serology are helpful in making the diagnosis. Pulmonary or bone involvement may mimic neoplasm. Cryptococcal meningitis is an important opportunistic infection in renal transplant recipients and in other immunosuppressed patients. The development of headaches in these patients should indicate prompt spinal tap examination. Patients with extrapulmonary involvement require combination therapy with amphotericin B and 5–fluorocytosine (flucytosine).

Aspergillosis

Aspergillosis is one of the opportunistic fungal diseases caused by common fungi that are normally nonpathogenic.

The numerous members of the genus *Aspergillus* commonly colonize on mucosal surfaces, but in general invade tissues only in immunosuppressed patients. When organisms are inhaled by the susceptible host, they may cause pulmonary infections that result in an aspergilloma (fungus ball). This condition, although not highly invasive, frequently causes hemoptysis, which may lead to aspiration that can be life-threatening in severe conditions. Invasive pulmonary aspergillosis has become common in patients undergoing cancer chemotherapy or taking steroids and may lead to a rapidly infiltrating lesion with possible dissemination to the central nervous system, heart, liver, or skin. Another form of invasive disease can involve the sino-orbital region. Aspergillomas seldom require operative resection or medical treatment, however, whereas invasive disease may require both amphotericin B and surgical resection.

Candidiasis

Candidiasis is an infection by species of the genus *Candida*, which is frequently isolated as part of the normal flora of the oropharynx and colon. Clinical candidiasis is most frequently caused by *C. albicans*. These opportunistic fungi can invade tissues of those critically ill patients with altered local or systemic immunity. Localized disease usually involves the moist intertriginous skin areas, mouth, vagina, esophagus, or nail beds. Invasive candidiasis is the most important clinical form of the disease. Predisposing factors include patients who are malnourished, multiple abdominal operations, long courses of broad-spectrum antibiotics, use of systemic steroids, hyperalimentation through indwelling catheters, and immunosuppression. Invasion of the bloodstream can be self-limiting, or it can result in widespread metastatic seeding of many organ systems, including the liver, lung, damaged heart valves, and central nervous system. Diagnosis is based primarily on culture results. Positive blood cultures most often indicate invasive disease, except when fungemia is associated with an intravenous catheter, and removal of the catheter may result in clearance of the organism from the bloodstream.

Topical nystatin is useful in treating local candidiasis; high doses of oral nystatin are useful in reducing the numbers of organisms in the intestine, thereby reducing the incidence of fungemia in the critically ill immunodepressed patient. Invasive candidiasis requires parenteral amphotericin B treatment. Combination therapy with flucytosine in this setting is sometimes advocated.

SELECTED REFERENCES

Alexander, J. W., and Meakins, J. L.: A physiological basis for the development of opportunistic infections. Ann. Surg., *176*:273, 1972.
The importance of defects in host resistance in the pathogenesis of surgical infection is emphasized in this article, which focuses on neutrophil function.

Altemeier, W. A., Hummel, R. P., and Hill, E. O.: Changing patterns in surgical infections. Ann. Surg., *178*:436, 1973.
This is a recommended article describing a series of interesting changes that have occurred during the past 28 years. Included have been a marked increase in the incidence of gram-negative infections superimposed on or secondary to antibiotic therapy and an increasing incidence of infections by bacteria formerly considered to have little or no virulence.

Cruse, P. J. E., and Foord, R. A.: A five-year prospective study of 23,649 surgical wounds. Arch. Surg., *107*:206, 1973.
This excellent prospective study of surgical wound infection details the factors that are significant in their occurrence.

Gorbach, S. L., Bartlett, J. G., and Nichols, R. L. (Eds.): Management of Surgical Infections. Boston, Little, Brown and Company, 1984.
This book reviews in-depth current approaches to the diagnosis, prophylaxis, and treatment of most infections found in the surgical patient. The manual format is most appropriate at the medical student level.

REFERENCES

1. Ad Hoc Committee of the Committee on Trauma, National Research Council Division of Medical Sciences: Factors influencing the incidence of wound infection. Ann. Surg. (Suppl.), *160*:32, 1954.
2. Altemeier, W. A., Culbertson, W. R., Fullen, W. D., and Shook, C. D.: Intra-abdominal abscesses. Am. J. Surg., *125*:70, 1973.
3. Bornside, G. H., and Cohn, I., Jr.: The normal microbial flora: Comparative bacterial flora of animals and man. Am. J. Dig. Dis., *10*:844, 1965.
4. Cerise, E. J., Pierce, W. A., and Diamond, D. L.: Abdominal drains: Their role as a source of infection following splenectomy. Ann. Surg., *171*:764, 1970.
5. Chetlin, S. H., and Elliott, D.: Preoperative antibiotics in biliary surgery. Arch. Surg., *107*:319, 1973.
6. Condon, R. E.: Rational use of prophylactic antibiotics in gastrointestinal surgery. Surg. Clin. North Am., *55*:1309, 1975.
7. Condon, R. E., Bartlett, J. G., and Nichols, R. L., et al.: Preoperative prophylactic cephalothin fails to control septic complications of colorectal operations: Results of controlled clinical trial. Am. J. Surg., *137*:68, 1974.
8. Green, J. W., and Wenzel, R. P.: Postoperative wound infection: A controlled study of the increased duration of hospital stay and direct cost of hospitalization. Ann. Surg., *185*:264, 1977.
9. Harding, G. K. M., Buckwold, F. J., Ronald, A. R., Marrie, T. J., Brunton, S., Koss, J. C., Gurwith, M. J., and Albritton, W. L.: Prospective, randomized comparative study of clindamycin, chloramphenicol, and ticarcillin, each in combination with gentamicin, in therapy for intra-abdominal and female genital tract sepsis. J. Infec. Dis., *142*:384, 1980.
10. Hudspeth, A. S.: Radical surgical débridement in the treatment of advanced generalized bacterial peritonitis. Arch. Surg., *110*:1233, 1975.
11. Keighley, M. R. B., Flinn, R., and Alexander-Williams, J.: Multivariate analysis of clinical and operative finding associated with biliary sepsis. Br. J. Surg., *63*:528, 1976.
12. Keighley, M. R. B., McLeish, A. R., Bishop, H. M.: Identification of the presence and type of biliary microflora by immediate Gram stains. Surgery, *81*:469, 1977.
13. The Medical Letter: Antimicrobial prophylaxis for surgery. *23*:77, 1981.
14. Nichols, R. L.: Techniques known to prevent postoperative wound infection. Infect. Control, 3:34, 1982.
15. Nichols, R. L.: Empiric antibiotic therapy for intra-abdominal infections. Rev. Infect. Dis., 5:s90–s97, 1983.
16. Nichols, R. L.: Prevention of infection in high-risk gastrointestinal surgery. Am. J. Med., *76*:111, 1984.
17. Nichols, R. L., Broido, P., Condon, R. E., Gorbach, S. L., and Nyhus, L. M.: Effect of preoperative neomycin-erythromycin intestinal preparation of the incidence of infectious complications following colon surgery. Ann. Surg., *178*:453, 1973.
18. Nichols, R. L., Condon, R. E., Gorbach, S. L., and Nyhus, L. M.: Efficacy of preoperative antimicrobial preparation of the bowel. Ann. Surg., *176*:227, 1972.
19. Nichols, R. L., and Smith, J. W.: Intragastric microbial colonization in common disease states of the stomach and duodenum. Ann. Surg., *182*:557, 1975.
20. Nichols, R. L., Webb, W. R., Jones, J. W., Smith, J. W., and LoCicero, J.: Efficacy of antibiotic prophylaxis in high-risk gastroduodenal operations Am. J. Surg., *143*:94, 1982.
21. Nora, P. F., Vanecko, R. M., and Bransfield, J. J.: Prophylactic abdominal drains. Arch. Surg., *105*:173, 1972.
22. Shapiro, M., Munoz, A., Tager, I. B., Schoenbaum, S. C., and Polk, B. F.: Risk factors for infection at the operative site after abdominal or vaginal hysterectomy. N. Engl. J. Med., *307*:1661, 1982.
23. Swenson, R. M., Lorber, B., Michaelson, T. C., and Spaulding, E. H.: The bacteriology of intra-abdominal infections. Arch. Surg. *109*:398, 1974.
24. Tally, F. P., McGowan, K., Kellum, J. M., Gorbach, S. L., and O'Donnell, T. F.: A randomized comparison of cefoxitin with or without amikacin in surgical sepsis. Ann. Surg., *193*:318, 1981.
25. Veterans Administration Ad Hoc Interdisciplinary Advisory Committee on Antimicrobial Drug Usage: Prophylaxis in surgery. J.A.M.A., *237*:1003, 1977.

SURGICAL ASPECTS OF VIRAL HEPATITIS AND THE ACQUIRED IMMUNE DEFICIENCY SYNDROME (AIDS)

H. KIM LYERLY, M.D. • *KENT J. WEINHOLD, PH.D.* • *DANI P. BOLOGNESI, PH.D.*

12

Surgeons are often involved in performing diagnostic and therapeutic procedures on patients with potentially communicable diseases and in transfusing blood and blood products. Therefore, an awareness and understanding of infectious blood-borne diseases is of considerable importance. *Viral hepatitis* has been recognized as being transmitted by percutaneous inoculation and blood transfusion, and recent advances have led to a greater understanding of the etiology, epidemiology, and pathogenesis of this disease. Another infectious disorder recognized since 1981, the *acquired immune deficiency syndrome (AIDS)*, has been conclusively shown to be caused by a human retrovirus. It has emerged as an increasingly significant clinical entity that can be transmitted sexually, perinatally, and parenterally.

VIRAL HEPATITIS

Viral hepatitis is an infection of the liver by one of four groups of viruses, and the disease may present with a broad range of syndromes ranging from subclinical to lethal. Although infection with any one of the viral agents may lead to clinically similar disease, the viral agents and their characteristics are quite distinct (Table 1). In the majority of patients, viral hepatitis is self-limited, but extrahepatic manifestations or progression to chronic liver disease may occur, depending upon the viral agent.

Type A hepatitis virus (HAV, formerly known as infectious hepatitis) and *Type B hepatitis virus* (HBV, formerly known as serum hepatitis) have long been recognized as being epidemiologically and clinically distinct, and there are specific serologic tests to aid in their diagnoses.[60] *Type non-A, non-B hepatitis* (NANB) is probably caused by at least two different agents and is not diagnosed by a specific serologic test; therefore, it is a diagnosis of exclusion. It is the major cause of post-transfusion hepatitis today. A recently described epidemic type of non-A, non-B hepatitis, spread by water or close personal contact, is a cause of outbreaks of hepatitis in Southeast Asia and North Africa.[65] The fourth type, *delta hepatitis*, is a defective virus that requires the presence of HBV for replication and may occur as a co-infection with acute HBV or as a superinfection of a HBV carrier. Other viral agents may also affect the liver, but usually as part of a more general systemic disease. The nomenclature describing the hepatitis viruses and their associated antigens and antibodies is quite complex and is listed in Table 2. Familiarity with these terms is essential to the understanding of this group of diseases.

Epidemiology

In 1983, approximately 21,500 cases of hepatitis A, 24,300 cases of hepatitis B, 3500 cases of hepatitis non-A, non-B, and 7100 cases of hepatitis, type unspecified, were reported in the United States.[18] Since reporting is incomplete, the actual number of cases is thought to be several times larger.

The incidence of hepatitis A has decreased over the last 15 years, but it is still common in older children and young adults. HAV is primarily transmitted by person-to-person contact, generally through fecal contamination. Hepatitis A virus is present in the feces about 2 weeks preceding and 1 week following the onset of clinical disease, and there is no chronic fecal carrier state.[6] Fecal oral transmission is facilitated by poor personal hygiene, poor sanitation, and intimate contact.[29] Transmission of HAV by blood transfusion has occurred, but this is rare, as a chronic carrier state of HAV in blood has not been demonstrated.

Although hepatitis B is a disease of low endemicity in the United States—with only 0.1 to 0.5 per cent of the population being virus carriers, an estimated 200,000 persons are infected each year. Six to 10 per cent of those infected will become chronic carriers of HBV.[65]

Transmission of HBV occurs via percutaneous or perimucosal routes and includes blood or blood product transfusion, percutaneous inoculation with HBV contaminated material, and perinatal and sexual transmission.[38, 58, 64, 78, 79] HBV is present in high concentrations in blood and virtually all body fluids; however, HBV is not transmitted via the

TABLE 1. Hepatitis Virus Characteristics

	Hepatitis A	Hepatitis B	Hepatitis Non-A, Non-B	Delta Hepatitis
Causative agent	27 nm. RNA virus	42 nm. DNA virus	Two or more agents	35–37 nm. RNA defective virus
Transmission	Fecal-oral, water-borne, food-borne	Parenteral inoculation, direct contact	Same as HBV, also fecal-oral, water-borne	Same as HBV
Incubation period	2–6 weeks	1–6 months	2–20 weeks	Unknown
Infectious period	2–3 weeks in late incubation and early clinical phase	During HBsAg positivity	Unknown	Unknown
Massive hepatic necrosis	Rare	Uncommon	Uncommon	More common
Carrier state	No	Yes	Yes	Yes
Chronic hepatitis	No	Yes	Yes	Yes

Abbreviations: HBV = Hepatitis B virus; HBsAg = hepatitis B surface antigen.

fecal oral route or by food or water contamination. Populations at high risk for infection include homosexual men, intravenous drug abusers, prison inmates, hemodialysis patients, household contacts of HBV carriers, and clients in institutes for the mentally retarded.

Non-A, non-B hepatitis occurs in the United States, with epidemiologic characteristics similar to HBV and appearing most commonly following blood transfusion and parenteral drug use. Multiple episodes of non-A, non-B hepatitis have occurred in the same individuals and may be due to different agents.[51] A carrier state has been confirmed in experimental animal studies, and a carrier state may exist in up to 8 per cent of the population.[18, 81] The recently described epidemic form of non-A, non-B hepatitis occurring in Asia and Africa has been transmitted to experimental animals, and candidate viruses have been identified.[55]

Delta hepatitis is caused by a defective virus that may cause infection only in the presence of active HBV infection. Delta hepatitis may be diagnosed by the detection of delta antigen early in infection or delta antibody late in infection.[73] Routes of transmission appear similar to those of HBV, occurring most frequently in intravenous drug addicts and hemophiliacs in the United States.[74] Of the HBV-positive patients, 3 to 12 per cent are thought to have antibodies to delta antigen.[67]

One major concern to users of blood and blood products is the risk of acquiring hepatitis following blood transfusion. Most whole blood has a relative low risk of inducing infection with HBV because of the relatively low frequency of HBV carriers in the population, the exclusion of potentially infectious donors, and the routine testing of donor blood for hepatitis B surface antigen (HBsAg). Washing and freezing of red cells are thought to reduce the risk of infection, but these procedures do not make them reliably virus-free.[2] The risk of acquiring HBV following transfusion of a single unit of blood is less than 1 per cent; however, the risk may vary for different blood products.[1] High-risk blood and blood products include those derived from commercial (as opposed to volunteer) donors, which may increase the risk of infection by a factor of 10, and those from pooled sources, which include plasma and clotting factors.[43] Serum albumin, thrombin, profibrinolysin, fibrinolysin, immune globulin, and hyperimmune globulins are all considered low-risk preparations.[8, 30, 50, 68] Although the

TABLE 2. Hepatitis Nomenclature

Virus	Antigen		Antibody	
	Name	*Interpretation*	*Name*	*Interpretation*
Hepatitis A (HAV)	HA Ag*	Major antigen, acute infection	Anti-HA	
			IgG	Immune to HAV, detectable at onset, lifetime persistence
			IgM	Indicates recent infection with HAV, positive 4–6 months after infection
Hepatitis B (HBV)	HBsAg	Surface antigen(s), prior exposure to HBV	Anti-HBs	Immune to HBV, passive antibody from HBIG, or immune response to HBV vaccine
	HBcAg*	Core antigen, acute or chronic	Anti-HBc	
			IgG	Early or late convalescence, chronic hepatitis
			IgM	Acute infection, positive 4–6 months after infection
	HBeAg	Core-related antigen, acute or chronic infectivity	Anti-HBe	Late convalescence
Hepatitis non-A, non-B (NANB)	–	–	–	–
Delta hepatitis (HD)	Delta antigen*	Acute delta hepatitis	Anti-HD*	Immune to delta, past exposure

*No commercial test available.

Abbreviations: HBV = Hepatitis B virus; HAV = hepatitis A virus; HBIG = hepatitis B immune globulin; HBsAG = hepatitis B surface antigen; HBcAG = hepatitis B core antigen; HBeAG = hepatitis B e antigen; HA Ag = hepatitis A antigen; HD = delta hepatitis.

incidence of post-transfusion hepatitis arising from HBV has been reduced by these measures, there are no specific tests available to detect the presence of non-A, non-B hepatitis; therefore, most transfusion hepatitis that occurs is most often due to non-A, non-B hepatitis, which occurs in five to ten cases per 1000 transfusions.

Health care workers are also concerned with the risk of acquiring hepatitis following percutaneous inoculation of contaminated material, such as that following needle stick injury. HBV, non-A, non-B, and delta hepatitis may all be acquired via this route. The risk of an unvaccinated person's acquiring HBV following needle stick injury is about 15 per cent without intervention; however, the use of immune globulin and hyperimmune globulin as post-exposure prophylaxis reduces this risk.[18]

The possibility of becoming a *carrier* is also of concern to surgeons and health care workers.[34] Carriers of HBsAg are defined as persons who are HBsAg-positive on at least two occasions 6 months apart. Although all carriers are not infectious, there is no currently available test that makes this distinction. Infectivity correlates best with HBeAg positivity, but a higher degree of infectivity is also seen the closer the HBsAg-positive individual is to acute infection, the higher the titer of anti-HBc and the more immunocompromised the host. In contrast, the presence of antibodies to HBsAg or HBeAg makes the individual less likely to be infectious. The overall incidence of infectious carriers is approximately 16 per cent, but for practical purposes all carriers should be considered infectious and treated as such. Although the risk to patients has not been defined, disease transmission from a physician HBV carrier to patients is considered a rare event that is usually minimized by common hygienic measures and proper surgical technique.[46, 57] Routine determination of HBsAg in asymptomatic physicians is not currently recommended.

Pathogenesis

After a variable incubation period, depending upon the agent, viral replication in the liver cells increases, followed by the appearance of viral components and liver cell necrosis with an associated inflammatory response. In typical cases of viral hepatitis, the pathologic hepatic changes consist of combinations of portal, periportal, and lobular hepatitis with an accumulation of inflammatory cells and parenchymal cell necrosis throughout the liver.[52] Differences in the histopathology generally correlate with the clinical severity and resolve completely with recovery from the acute illness. More severe variants of acute necrosis include bridging, confluent, and massive necrosis. Submassive and massive necrosis is reflected in a more severe clinical course.

Two theories have been proposed for the mechanism of the illness. One suggests direct cytopathogenicity of liver cells by the virus, and the other proposes humoral and cell-mediated immunopathogenic mechanisms for all types of viral hepatitis. Although the immunologic response of the host plays an important role in the pathogenesis of viral hepatitis, it remains ill defined.

Clinical Manifestations

All of the hepatitis viruses may cause a wide spectrum of clinical disease, and the resultant clinical syndrome of each virus is often not distinguishable. Inapparent subclin-

ical disease may occur several times more frequently than symptomatic clinical disease, but the clinical syndrome typically found in about 90 per cent of patients includes jaundice, lassitude, anorexia, weakness, nausea, and dark urine, with fever, vomiting, headache, chills, and abdominal discomfort occurring less frequently.

Abnormalities in the aminotransferases (AST, ALT) and elevations of the alkaline phosphatase and serum bilirubin are laboratory abnormalities that reflect hepatocyte necrosis. Specific serologic tests for viral antigen and antibodies are also abnormal, as demonstrated in Figure 1. In the majority of patients, the illness is self-limited, with 85 to 90 per cent of patients recovering completely 2 to 6 weeks following onset.

In patients with hepatitis A infection, this clinical picture usually develops with no further complications from the virus. Although hepatitis B, non-A, non-B and delta hepatitis usually follow this same pattern of disease, in 10 to 12 per cent of those with clinically apparent disease, extrahepatic manifestations or complications will develop. Extrahepatic manifestations frequently occur in the form of arthralgia, arthritis, and urticaria. HBV infection may result in unique extrahepatic manifestations, including vasculitis and nephritis, which are thought to be due to localization of antigen antibody complexes in affected tissues.[6, 33]

Complications of viral hepatitis include acute *fulminant hepatitis*, which occurs in less than 1 per cent, and is characterized by progressive jaundice, hepatic encephalopathy, coagulation defects, renal failure, and death, which may occur within weeks. No specific therapy—including steroids, hyperimmune globulin, and exchange transfusion—has been found to be useful. *Chronic active hepatitis* (CAH) is a more common complication and may progress to cirrhosis. A prior episode of typical HBV disease may or may not have occurred. Steroids may be beneficial for this condition. Viral hepatitis may also present with a cholestatic picture of liver function abnormalities with profound jaundice but with no anatomic obstruction of the biliary tree. The prognosis is favorable; however, other disorders such as biliary stones, strictures, or tumors must be excluded. Finally, there is a close association between HBV infection and *hepatoma* (hepatocellular carcinoma), suggesting the oncogenic potential of the virus.[5]

Non-A, non-B hepatitis appears to result in chronic hepatitis in approximately 25 per cent of patients. Although chronic hepatitis caused by non-A, non-B hepatitis was once considered to be less fulminant than that associated with HBV, in as many as 30 per cent of patients, non-A, non-B chronic aggressive hepatitis may progress to cirrhosis.[82]

Available evidence suggests that delta hepatitis infection worsens the microscopic appearance of and accelerates the liver disease associated with HBV infection and is more likely to be associated with fulminant hepatitis.[45, 73, 82]

Prevention

General measures, including case finding and attention to standard principles of hygiene, and specific measures directed against the recognized modes of transmission are the principal features of disease prevention in all four types of viral hepatitis.[37] These methods are only partially successful, and need for passive immunity is common. Immune globulins are sterile solutions of antibodies from human plasma. Immunoglobulin (Ig) contains antibodies against

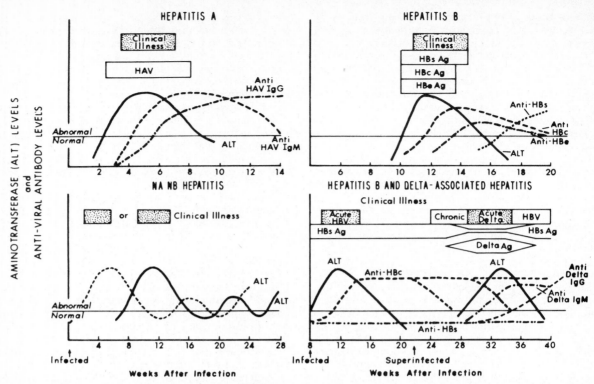

Figure 1. Tests for viral antigen and antibodies. (From Hamilton, J. D.: Viral hepatitis and the surgeon. In Sabiston, D. C., Jr. (Ed.): Textbook of Surgery, 13th ed. Philadelphia, W. B. Saunders Company, 1986, p. 1124.)

hepatitis A virus and HBsAg. Hepatitis B immune globulin (HBIG) is immune globulin prepared from plasma containing high titers of anti-HBsAg. The current recommendations for the use of serum immunoglobulin or HBIG for prophylaxis are summarized in Tables 3 and 4.[18]

Active immunization is now commercially available for HBV. A vaccine prepared from a plasma of chronic carriers of HBsAg has been widely tested, and normal recipients of the vaccine acquire high titers of antibody to HBsAg and are protected against naturally acquired disease. One early concern had been the risk of transmitting the AIDS virus (HTLV-III/LAV), because a portion of the population of HBV carriers used to manufacture the vaccine were in high-risk groups for AIDS. These fears have proved un-

TABLE 3. Hepatitis B Virus Prophylaxis

Source	Exposure	Exposed Person Unvaccinated	Exposed Person Vaccinated
HBsAg-positive	Perinatal	1. HBIG within 12 hours* 2. HBV vaccine within 12 hours; repeat at 1 and 6 months†	
	Sexual	1. HBIG within 14 days	Nothing required
	Percutaneous	1. HBIG immediately‡ 2. Initiate HBV vaccine§	1. Test exposed person for anti-HBs¶ 2. If inadequate antibody, HBIG plus HBV vaccine booster dose
Known source High-risk HBsAg-positive	Percutaneous	1. Initiate HBV vaccine 2. Test source for HBsAG; if positive, HBIG.	Test source for HBsAg only if exposed is vaccine nonresponder; if source is HBsAg-positive, give HBIG immediately plus HBV vaccine booster dose
Low-risk HBsAg-positive	Percutaneous	Initiate HBV vaccine	Nothing required
Unknown source	Percutaneous	Initiate HBV vaccine	Nothing required

*HBIG dose 0.5 ml. IM.
†HBV vaccine dose 0.5 ml. (10 μg.) IM for infants or children younger than 10 years of age.
‡HBIG dose 0.06 ml./kg. IM
§HBV vaccine dose 20 μg. IM for adults. First dose within 1 week; second and third doses, 1 and 6 months later.
¶Exposed persons should be tested for anti-HBs unless they have been tested within the last 12 months, adequate antibody is 10 sample ratio units (SRU) or more by radioimmunoassay or positive by enzyme immunoassay.

TABLE 4. Hepatitis A, Hepatitis Non-A, Non-B, and Delta Hepatitis Prophylaxis

Virus Exposure	Time of Evaluation	Type of Exposure	Immunoglobulin
Hepatitis A	Pre-exposure	Travel to endemic area	Yes
	Post-exposure	Household/sexual	Yes
		School/work	No
		Institution	Yes
		Day care center	Yes
		Medical personnel	Yes
Hepatitis non-A, non-B	Post-exposure	Percutaneous	Yes
Delta hepatitis	Post-exposure	Percutaneous	Recommendations for hepatitis B prophylaxis

founded to date.[12] Serologic and immune profile studies in patients receiving the vaccine have demonstrated no increased incidence of AIDS or antibodies to HTLV-III/LAV, and viral inactivation steps used in processing the vaccine have been shown to inactivate the virus responsible for AIDS.[15, 54] The current recommendations for HBV vaccination are listed in Table 5.[18]

Treatment

There are currently no accepted modes of specific therapy for any of the types of viral hepatitis. Therapy consists of supportive management, with adequate rest, proper nutrition, and the avoidance of hepatotoxins.

ACQUIRED IMMUNE DEFICIENCY SYNDROME

The acquired immune deficiency syndrome is a profound defect in cellular immunity leading to opportunistic infections and unusual neoplasms that was first recognized in homosexual men in 1981.[9, 10] It was subsequently de-

TABLE 5. Hepatitis B Virus Pre-exposure Vaccination Recommendations*

Health care workers

Highest risk: Medical technologists, operating room staff, phlebotomists and intravenous therapy nurses, surgeons and pathologists, and oncology and dialysis unit staff

Increased risk: Dental professionals, laboratory and blood bank technicians, dialysis center staff, emergency medical technicians, and morticians

Clients and staff of institutions for the mentally retarded
Hemodialysis patients
Homosexually active men
Users of illicit injectable drugs
Recipients of clotting factor concentrates
Household and sexual contacts of hepatitis B virus carriers
Inmates of long-term correctional facilities
Heterosexually active persons
Travelers to areas with high levels of endemic disease

Special high-risk populations: Alaskan Eskimos, native Pacific islanders, and immigrants from highly endemic areas

*Prevaccination serologic screening for susceptibility is dependent on (1) cost vaccination, (2) cost of screening for susceptibility, and (3) expected prevalence of immune individuals in the group. Screening is cost-effective in groups with the highest risk of hepatitis B virus infection unless testing costs are extremely high.

scribed in intravenous drug abusers, Haitian immigrants, recipients of factor VIII concentrates, blood transfusion recipients, and children and sexual partners of AIDS patients.[11, 13, 31] AIDS is characterized by a progressive lymphopenia predominantly of helper/inducer T cells that is clinically manifested by susceptibility to life-threatening opportunistic infections and malignancies. AIDS is now known to be due to infection with a human retrovirus named the *human T lymphotropic virus type III* (HTLV-III) by researchers at the National Institutes of Health (NIH) and *lymphadenopathy-associated virus* (LAV) by French workers at the Pasteur Institute.[4, 40, 61] With the emergence of effective laboratory testing for viral antigens and viral antibodies has come the realization that although AIDS represents the most severe manifestation of HTLV-III/LAV infection, there exists a broad spectrum of clinical syndromes.[72] *AIDS-related complex (ARC)* is a syndrome characterized by minor conditions clinically associated with immunosuppression and laboratory evidence of immunosuppression. Other syndromes include *progressive generalized lymphadenopathy (PGL)*, defined as unexplained lymph node enlargement for more than 3 months in two or more non–inguinal node groups, and *lymphadenopathy syndrome (LAS)*, defined as PGL with wasting. Immune thrombocytopenia is associated with HTLV-III/LAV infection as well as non–life–threatening fungal, bacterial, and viral infections.[80] Central nervous system syndromes are also being recognized as manifestations of HTLV-III/LAV infection. Finally, HTLV-III/LAV infection exists in patients who are clinically well but who have laboratory abnormalities of T cell function. The Centers for Disease Control (CDC) definition for AIDS, pediatric AIDS, and the AIDS-related complex is shown in Table 6.[19]

HTLV-III/LAV belongs to a family of human retroviruses characterized by the enzyme *reverse transcriptase*, viral envelope proteins, and a tropism for the helper/inducer (T4) subset of T cells. The T4 cell is centrally responsible for the regulation of immune responses to viral, fungal, and tumor-related antigens. Infection of T4 cells *in vitro* with HTLV-III/LAV causes cell death, which suggests a mechanism for the resultant profound effect on nearly all aspects of cellular immunity *in vivo*, leading to the clinical manifestations of opportunistic infections and neoplasms. Screening for antibodies to HTLV-III/LAV is done by an enzyme-linked immunosorbent assay (ELISA), which is highly sensitive and specific. However, to exclude false-positive results, the diagnosis is usually confirmed by Western blot analysis. Viral antigen can be detected by viral culture, radioimmune precipitation, and immunofluorescence. Currently, viremia is usually confirmed by a culture of peripheral blood lymphocytes and detection of reverse

TABLE 6. *Definition of Acquired Immune Deficiency Syndrome (AIDS) and Related Conditions*

AIDS-Surveillance Definition of the Centers for Disease Control

The occurrence of a disease that is at least moderately predictive of a defect in cell-mediated immunity, occurring in a person with no known cause for diminished resistance to that disease. These diseases include:

- Kaposi's sarcoma (in patients less than 60 years of age)
- Primary lymphoma of the central nervous system
- *Pneumocystitis carinii* pneumonia
- Unusually extensive mucocutaneous herpes simplex of more than 5 weeks' duration
- *Cryptosporidium* enterocolitis of more than 4 weeks' duration
- Esophagitis due to *Candida albicans*, cytomegalovirus, or herpes simplex virus
- Progressive multifocal leukoencephalopathy
- Pneumonia, meningitis, or encephalitis due to one or more of the following:
  - *Aspergillus, C. albicans, Cryptococcus neoformans*, cytomegalovirus
  - *Nocardia, Strongyloides, Toxoplasma gondii, Zygomycosis*, or atypical
  - *Mycobacterium* species (not tuberculosis or lepra)

In the absence of the above opportunistic infections, any of the following diseases if the patient has a positive serologic or virologic test for HTLV-III/LAV:

- Disseminated histoplasmosis
- Isoporiasis, causing diarrhea for over 1 month
- Bronchial or pulmonary candidiasis
- Non-Hodgkin's lymphoma of high grade pathologic type and of B cell or unknown phenotype
- Kaposi's sarcoma (in patients over 60 years of age)

Patients who have a lymphoreticular malignancy diagnosed over 3 months after the diagnosis of an opportunistic disease used as a marker for AIDS will not be excluded. Patients will be excluded if they have a negative result on testing for serum antibody to HTLV-III/LAV, have no other type of HTLV-III/LAV test with a positive result, and do not have a low number of T helper cells or a low T-helper/T-suppressor ratio.

Pediatric AIDS-Provisional Surveillance Definition of the Centers for Disease Control

Same as AIDS in adults, with the following provisions:

A. Congenital infections that must be excluded are:
1. *T. gondii* in patients less than 1 month of age
2. Herpes simplex virus in patients less than 1 month of age
3. Cytomegalovirus in patients less than 6 months of age

B. Specific conditions that must be excluded in children are:
1. Primary immunodeficiency diseases, severe combined immunodeficiency, Di George syndrome, Wiskott-Aldrich syndrome, ataxia-telangiectasis, graft-versus-host disease, neutropenia, neutrophia function abnormality, agammaglobulinemia, or hypoglobulinemia with raised IgM
2. Secondary immunodeficiency associated with immunosuppressive therapy, lymphoreticular malignancy, or starvation

C. Histologically confirmed diagnosis of chronic lymphoid interstitial pneumonitis in a child, unless tests for HTLV-III/LAV are negative

AIDS-Related Complex (ARC)		
Any Two Clinical Features	*Plus*	*Any Two Laboratory Abnormalities*
Fever over 100°F. (37.8°C.) for 3 months or longer		Helper T cells less than 400/mm.^{3}
Weight loss over 10% or 15 pounds		Helper: suppressor ratio less than 1.0
Lymphadenopathy over 3 months		Leukothrombocytopenia, anemia
Diarrhea		Elevated serum globulins
Fatigue		Depressed blastogenesis
Night sweats		Anergy to skin test

transcriptase activity or viral antigens by radioimmunoassay. Current diagnostic testing nomenclature is listed in Tables 7 and 8.[39]

Epidemiology

Since the first patients were reported in 1981, over 20,000 patients with AIDS had been reported by 1986, including over 165 children, and the number of reported cases continues to double every 12 months. The prognosis of these patients is poor, and about one half of adults and two thirds of affected children have died.[32]

In the affected adults, 73 per cent of the cases have been in homosexual or bisexual men, 17 per cent in intravenous drug abusers, 1 per cent in hemophiliacs, 1 per cent in heterosexual contacts of AIDS patients, 2 per cent in recipients of blood transfusions, and 6 per cent in patients with no known risk factors. In the pediatric group, 71 per cent of the cases were in children of AIDS patients, 5 per

cent in hemophiliacs, 16 per cent in recipients of blood transfusions, and 8 per cent in patients with no known risk factors. Forty-seven states have reported cases of AIDS, with the highest numbers in New York, California, Florida, New Jersey, and Texas.[32] There have been over 1200 cases reported in Europe to date.[23] In Africa the epidemiology of AIDS appears much different with male:female ratio close to 1:1.

Transmission of the virus is primarily via sexual contact and secondarily via blood or blood products. AIDS can be transmitted by percutaneous inoculation with contaminated material from AIDS patients or from those at risk of AIDS and perinatally from infected mother to infant. Although HTLV-III/LAV has been isolated from saliva, tears, urine, pleural effusions, and ascites, the epidemiology of HTLV-III/LAV is similar to that of hepatitis B infection and AIDS has not been shown to be transmitted by contaminated food or water or by the fecal oral route.

The extent of HTLV-III/LAV exposure in the general population is unknown. Screening of high-risk groups has

TABLE 7. Clinical Tests for HTLV-III/LAV Virus or Viral Antigen

Test	Comment
Measure of infectious virus	
Culture of peripheral blood mononuclear cells; assay for reverse transcriptase and/or cell free viral antigens	Nonquantitative, repeated samples needed, labor-intensive; may involve transmission to indicator cell lines; main value in confirming positive serology, examining suspected seronegative, viremic patients, or assessing efficacy of antiviral therapy
Test for viral antigens	
ELISA or radioimmunoassay antigenemia assays for measurement of antigens present in serum, plasma, or lymphocytes	Qualitative, independent of infectious virus status; questionable sensitivity; employ competitive radioimmunoassay or "antigen capture" technologies
Test for viral nucleic acid	
"Southern" blot	Detects proviral sequences in DNA, good if no expression of RNA or antigen occurs, but requires cloned virus probes and adequate cells; not routinely available
In situ *hybridization*	Cumbersome due to low frequency of virus-infected peripheral cells

Abbreviations: ELISA = Enzyme-linked immunosorbent assay; HTLV-III/LAV = human T lymphotropic virus type III/lymphadenopathy-associated virus.

demonstrated a significant proportion to have antibodies to HTLV-III/LAV. The presence of antibodies to HTLV-III/LAV is interpreted to mean that there has been prior exposure to the virus and the patient has mounted an immunologic response. In one series, 1 per cent of asymptomatic homosexual men were noted to have antibodies to HTLV-III/LAV in 1978; 73.1 per cent were seropositive in 1985.[22] Eighty-seven per cent of intravenous drug abusers in some series were seropositive.[14, 26, 27, 53, 75, 77, 84] Currently, over 90 per cent of factor VIII hemophiliacs and 39 per cent of factor IX hemophiliacs in the United States are seropositive, but only 4 per cent of those hemophiliacs who have received only frozen red cells have antibodies to HTLV-III/LAV.[17, 35, 36, 66] Less than 5 per cent of Haitian immigrants are seropositive, indicating that Haitian extraction in and of itself is not a risk factor. Screening of potential recruits to the U.S. military has shown a seropositivity rate of up to 200 per 10,000 with a male:female ratio of 2.5:1. It has been estimated that there are 500,000 to 1,000,000 seropositive patients in the United States.[32]

A major concern is the risk of iatrogenic or nosocomial infection with HTLV-III/LAV, although transfusion-associated AIDS represents only 2 per cent of all cases of the syndrome. Blood components implicated in transmission include red cells, platelets, plasma, whole blood, and clotting factors.[11, 13, 17, 31, 35, 36, 66, 69] The risk of acquiring AIDS following transfusion of a single unit of blood appears to be low. The initial screening of blood demonstrated one in 1200 units to represent potentially infectious blood; however, antibody screening now required for all donated blood will eliminate these potentially infectious units.[20] Furthermore, patients with AIDS and those at risk for AIDS are advised not to donate blood or blood products. Heat treatment of certain blood products may eliminate some infectious products from seronegative donors.

The risk of infection from exposure to material contaminated with infectious material is thought to be small.[85] Major prospective evaluations of health care workers who were thought to be inoculated have demonstrated only rare cases of documented seroconversion following needle stick injury, in contrast to the 15 per cent incidence of transmission associated with HBV carrier–associated needle stick injury.[3, 41, 48, 49, 82] HBV and *Cryptococcus* transmission from AIDS patients to health care workers without HTLV-III seroconversion occurring in the health care worker has been reported.[22, 23] The risk to patients of surgeons or health

TABLE 8. Tests for Human Antibody to HTLV-III/LAV That Measure Past Exposure

Test	Comment
Western blot	100% positive in AIDS patients. Virus proteins are separated by electrophoresis, transferred to a membrane, then incubated with human sera. The antigen-antibody complex is identified by a radioactively labeled protein with a high affinity of binding to such complexes (Staph A protein). This test identifies different sets of antibodies to individual viral proteins. Largely qualitative, valuable in following disease progression.
Enzyme-linked immunoabsorbent assay (ELISA)	Detergent-disrupted virion or its parts are absorbed to wells in plastic dishes. These are reacted with an unknown human serum. Antihuman globulin with attached enzyme is added. A colorimetric reagent is the final step. If the human serum bound to virus, subsequent reagents bind and the color develops in a positive test. Largely qualitative.
Radioimmune assay (RIA)	This measures the response only to a single virus protein. Uses purified radiolabeled viral protein, antibody is made in an animal species. The labeled reaction can be competed for by human antibody.
Immune fluorescence	This test is good for antigens on the cell membranes of live cells. A human target cell infected with virus, live or fixed, is reacted with a human serum. Binding is recognized by a fluorescein-labeled antihuman globulin.

care workers who are seropositive is unknown. There is no evidence that health care workers infected with HTLV-III/LAV have transmitted infections to patients.

Clinical Features

No long-term studies regarding the natural history of HTLV-III/LAV infection exist at present. It has been demonstrated that, following inoculation, seroconversion may take place as early as 2 weeks to longer than 6 months from the time of exposure. In a 5-year follow-up of 31 seropositive patients, two developed AIDS and eight developed AIDS-related symptoms, while two thirds remained symptom-free. The long, variable latency period makes interpretation of early data difficult.[7, 48, 59, 63, 83] In some series, seroconversion is followed by AIDS in 6 to 19 per cent of patients. The latency period from seroconversion to AIDS has averaged over 3 years in homosexuals in whom AIDS develops. In transfusion-associated AIDS, the latency period has averaged 29 months, but cases have been reported with latency periods as long as 7 years. The subclinical sequelae of HTLV-III/LAV are currently unknown.

Although a spectrum of syndromes probably represents HTLV-III/LAV infection, the end stage manifestations are the result of depletion of T4 cells with a resultant cellular immune defect leading to opportunistic infections and unusual neoplasms.

Opportunistic Infections

The majority of the morbidity and mortality seen in AIDS patients is related to overwhelming infection. Clinical syndromes that occur frequently include diffuse pneumonia, fever, diarrhea, central nervous system disorders, generalized lymphadenopathy, and esophagitis. Table 9 lists the opportunistic infections recognized most frequently in AIDS patients. These include infections usually seen in hosts, such as renal transplant recipients on immunosuppressive drugs.

Pneumocystis carinii pneumonia is the most common type in AIDS patients. It frequently presents with patchy interstitial and alveolar infiltrates. Diagnosis is most often made on transbronchial or open lung biopsy. Therapy is accomplished with trimethoprim-sulfamethoxazole combinations or with pentamidine; however, rash and drug-related toxicity are frequently seen in AIDS patients. *Cryptosporidium* is a small bowel pathogen that causes persistent debilitating diarrhea. Therapy has been largely unsuccessful.

Cytomegalovirus (CMV) is a major pathogen in AIDS patients with many patients having persistent CMV viremia. Pneumonitis can be caused by CMV and is frequently isolated from open lung biopsy and transbronchial biopsies. Several cases of CMV bowel ulcerations and perforations have been reported, and chorioretinitis and blindness are not infrequently noted in end stage AIDS patients. *Hepatitis B virus* often presents in patients with AIDS as well as the at risk population. Precautions in preventing transmission of HBV in AIDS patients must be followed as well. *Herpes simplex* may cause extensive mucosal cutaneous ulcers in the oral and perineal areas and may be disseminated or demonstrate visceral involvement. *Herpes zoster* may be localized to dermatomal distribution or may be disseminated. Disseminated herpes zoster can best be treated with

TABLE 9. *Opportunistic Infections in Acquired Immune Deficiency Syndrome*

Organisms	Clinical Syndrome
PROTOZOA	
Pneumocystitis carinii	Pneumonia
Toxoplasma gondii	Encephalitis
	Chorioretinitis
	Lymphadenopathy
Cryptosporidium	Enterocolitis
FUNGI	
Candida species	Stomatitis
	Esophagitis
	Enterocolitis
	Gastrointestinal bleeding
Cryptococcus neoformans	Meningitis
	Peritonitis
	Dissemination
Histoplasma capsulatum	Hepatosplenomegaly
MYCOBACTERIUM	
Avium-intracellulare	Hepatosplenomegaly
	Lymphadenopathy
	Enterocolitis
	Pneumonitis
	Debilitation
Tuberculosis	Pneumonia
	Draining lesions
BACTERIA	
Salmonella	Proctocolitis
Shigella	
Campylobacter	
Entamoeba histolytica	
Giardia lambia	
Chlamydia	
Neisseria gonorrhea	
Treponema pallidum	
VIRUSES	
Cytomegalovirus (CMV)	Gastrointestinal bleeding and perforation
	Diarrhea, proctitis, enteritis
	Chorioretinitis
	Hepatitis
	Lymphadenopathy
Epstein-Barr virus	Lymphadenopathy
Hepatitis B and non-A, non-B	Hepatitis
Herpes simplex	Localized skin lesions
Herpes zoster	Disseminated skin lesion

local care and intravenous antiviral therapy; however, the lesions usually recur. *Epstein-Barr* virus may be associated with CNS lymphomas.

Candida infections can be demonstrated in patients presenting with stomatitis, esophagitis, or gastrointestinal bleeding. Candidal esophagitis may be an initial manifestation of AIDS or may appear after opportunistic infection or Kaposi's sarcoma (KS) has occurred. Response to antifungal therapy is usually good; however, frequent recurrences require maintenance therapy on antifungal agents. *Cryptococcus neoformans* is a common cause of meningitis; however, disseminated cases are found also. One patient underwent laparotomy for acute abdominal pain and was found to have disseminated intraperitoneal cryptococcus.[70] Hepatosplenomegaly and retroperitoneal lymphadenopathy may be caused by *histoplasmosis*.

Bacterial infections are primarily associated with proctocolitis with extensive diarrhea and local bleeding termed the "gay bowel syndrome." Venereal diseases, including *Neisseria* gonorrhea or syphilis gonorrhea, present as urethritis, anorectal ulcerations, arthritis, or penile lesions.

Mycobacterial infections are usually associated with atypical mycobacterium, most frequently *Mycobacterium avium-intracellulare*, and are associated with hepatomegaly, lymphadenopathy, diarrhea along with fever, weight loss, and progressive debilitation. *M. avium-intracellulare* is usually resistant to most conventional therapy, but ansamycin plus clofazimine may be tried in combination with other drugs. *Mycobacterium tuberculosis* causes both pulmonary and extrapulmonary disease and is usually controlled with chemotherapy.

The primary role of the surgeon is in distinguishing treatable infectious lesions from neoplasia by biopsy. It is important that specimens be sent for viral, mycobacterial, and fungal cultures and stains as well as pathologic review in all cases.

Malignant Neoplasms

Patients with AIDS are known to have a high incidence of progressive KS, but there has also been an increased incidence of malignant lymphomas. Kaposi's sarcoma was described in 1872 by Moritz Kaposi,[56] and in the classic form of the disease the lesions occur in the lower extremities of older individuals of European or Jewish heritage. This less virulent cutaneous form has a benign course over a decade or more compared with the more virulent African form of KS, which frequently involves the viscera. AIDS patients have an epidemic form of KS that frequently involves the viscera as well as produces skin lesions. The cutaneous lesions of epidemic KS can vary from barely detectable macules or plaques on virtually any cutaneous area to large confluent lesions around the face, torso, and extremities. HTLV-III/LAV is not isolated from the lesions of epidemic KS, but it may trigger the appearance by immunodeficiency or some other stimulus.

Kaposi's sarcoma is the initial manifestation in approximately 30 per cent of patients with AIDS, but it occurs in a larger percentage of homosexuals with AIDS.[76] Cutaneous disease has been treated with irradiation therapy as well as with alpha interferon, and combination chemotherapy has been effective. Visceral involvement may be manifested as gastrointestinal bleeding, perforation, or obstruction or as hemoptysis. Treatment is directed to the individual clinical problem; however, evidence that any therapy is associated with major improvements in survival has not been demonstrated.

Malignant lymphomas of both the Hodgkin's and non-Hodgkin's types have been demonstrated in AIDS patients and in those at risk for AIDS. In a study of 90 patients with non-Hodgkin's lymphoma, 89 per cent presented with extranodal involvement, including 42 per cent in the central nervous system and one third in the bone marrow.[24] Seventeen per cent had primary gastrointestinal involvement, and patients have presented with intestinal perforation.

Squamous cell carcinoma of the tongue and anus as well as cloacogenic carcinoma of the anus-rectum has been described in homosexual men. These tumors have been previously reported in homosexual patients who did not have AIDS and are not thought to be specifically related to HTLV-III/LAV infection. Although hepatoma is frequently associated with HBV infection, which is very common in AIDS patients and the at-risk population, hepatoma has not been reported to date. Moreover, other solid tumors have not occurred in higher frequency in AIDS patients.

However, the shorter life span of these patients may preclude the appearance of neoplasms with slower growth rates. The surgeon is often involved in biopsy of these lesions to distinguish between infection and neoplasm.

Prevention

Prevention of AIDS currently centers around public health measures and education designed to decrease transmission via the currently recognized modes. There has been a decrease in certain sexual practices reported by homosexual men, and the incidence of other sexually transmitted diseases in this population has decreased.[16] However, heterosexual transmission, which has been prevalent in the spread of AIDS in Africa, is being recognized with increasing frequency in the United States.[21, 71]

Screening of blood has resulted in the elimination of some potentially infectious blood; however, there exists the possibility of antibody-negative patients who are viremic. Therefore, it is recommended that AIDS patients or those at risk for AIDS refrain from donating blood or blood products. To diminish the risk in patients receiving coagulation factors, virus inactivation steps are now incorporated in the processing steps of pooled clotting factors.[16] Effective virus inactivation steps are also taken in preparation of hepatitis B vaccine, and no increased risk of AIDS is noted in patients who received this vaccine.

Prevention of infection to health care workers is heavily dependent on isolation measures and education. Current recommendations are listed in Table 10.[25, 28, 62] Development of a vaccine is currently under investigation, although none is available currently.

Treatment

Currently, there are no specific therapies available for the treatment of AIDS. Investigational trials of antiviral drugs and immune system restorative factors, including bone marrow transplantation, are under evaluation. Current therapy is directed toward supportive management of the sequelae of severe cellular immunodeficiency.[86]

TABLE 10. *Precautions for Health Care Workers in the Prevention of Acquired Immune Deficiency Syndrome*

1. Place AIDS patients on blood/body fluid precautions with appropriate identification of the disease on the patient, room, and chart.

2. Sharp items (needles, scalpel blades, and other sharp instruments) should be considered potentially infectious and handled and disposed of with extraordinary care.

3. Protective clothing and coverings should be used to prevent exposure to blood, body fluids contaminated with blood, semen, and aerosols or droplets during patient care or procedures. Hands should be washed thoroughly and immediately if they become contaminated.

4. Clearly label, double bag in impermeable bags, and use gown and gloves when handling AIDS specimens.

5. Notify operating room and laboratory personnel prior to planned procedures on AIDS patients.

6. All nondisposable items and work surfaces should be decontaminated with freshly prepared 1:5 dilution of 5.25% sodium hypochlorite (household bleach).

Among the promising experimental drugs under investigation in Phase I and II clinical trials are the antiviral agents suramin, HPA-23, ribavirin, and azidothymidine (AZT) as well as immunorestorative compounds, including interleukin 2 (IL-2) and gamma interferon. A recently completed trial with AZT revealed increases in circulating helper-inducer T lymphocytes in 15 of 19 patients during the course of therapy as well as a loss of cutaneous anergy in six of the subjects.[86]

SELECTED REFERENCES

1. Centers for Disease Control: Recommendtions for protection against viral hepatitis. Morbid. Mortal. Weekly Rep., *34*:373, 1985.
   A concise reference of recommendations for prophylaxis against viral hepatitis including immune serum globulin (ISG), hepatitis B immune globulin (HBIG), and hepatitis B vaccine.

2. DeVita, V, T., Jr., Hellman, S., and Rosenberg, S. A. (Eds.): AIDS Etiology, Diagnosis, Treatment and Prevention. Philadelphia: J. B. Lippincott Company, 1985.
   A comprehensive monograph of AIDS written by many of the leading investigators.

3. Institute of Medicine: Mobilizing Against AIDS. National Academy of Sciences, 1986.
   A timely summary of facts and ongoing research concerning AIDS.

4. Kulstad, R. (Ed.): AIDS: Papers from Science 1982–1985. American Association for the Advancement of Science, 1986.
   A selection of original papers from Science describing much of the basic research relating to HTLV-III/LAV and AIDS.

5. Vyans, G. H. (Ed.): Viral Heapatitis—1984. Fourth International Symposium on Viral Hepatitis. San Francisco, March 1984.
   Authoritative discussions of a number of topics relating to viral hepatitis are presented in great detail in this volume.

REFERENCES

1. Aach, R. D., and Kahn, R. A.: Post-transfusion hepatitis: Current perspectives. Ann. Intern. Med., *92*:539, 1980.
2. Alter, H. J., Tabor, E., Meryman, H. T., Hoofnagle, J. H., Kahn, R. A., Holland, P. V., Gerety, R. J., and Barker, L. F.: Transmission of hepatitis B virus infection by transfusion of frozen deglycerolized red blood cells. N. Engl. J. Med., *298*:637, 1978.
3. Anonymous: Needlestick transmission of HTLV-III from a patient infected in Africa. Lancet, *2*:1376, 1984.
4. Barre-Sinoussi, F., Chermann, J. C., Rey, F., Nugeyre, M. T., Chamaret, S., Gruest, J., Dauguet, C., Axler-Blin, C., Vezinet-Brun, F., Rouzioux, C., Rozenbaum, W., and Montagnier, L.: Isolation of a T-lymphotropic retrovirus from a patient at risk for acquired immune deficiency syndrome (AIDS). Science, *220*:868, 1983.
5. Beasley, R. P., Hwang, L. Y., Lin, C. C., and Chien, C. S.: Hepatocellular carcinoma and hepatitis B virus. A prospective study of 22,707 men in Taiwan. Lancet, *2*:1129, 1981.
6. Bernstein, L. H., Koff, R. S., Seigel, E. R., Merritt, A. D., Goldstein, C. M., and an Expert Panel: The hepatitis knowledge base—a prototype information transfer system. Ann. Intern. Med., *93*:165, 1980.
7. Blattner, W. A., Biggar, R. J., Weiss, S. H., et al.: Perspective on AIDS from epidemiologic studies of HTLV-III. Ann. Intern. Med. (in press).
8. Boeve, N. R., Winterschied, L. S., and Merendino, K. A.: Fibrinogen-transmitted hepatitis in the surgical patient. Ann. Surg., *170*:833, 1969.
9. Centers for Disease Control: Morbid. Mortal. Weekly Rep., *30*:250, 1981.
10. Centers for Disease Control: Morbid. Mortal. Weekly Rep., *30*:305, 1981.
11. Centers for Disease Control: *Pneumocystis carinii* pneumonia among persons with hemophilia A. Morbid. Mortal. Weekly Rep., *31*:365, 1982.
12. Centers for Disease Control: Hepatitis B virus vaccine safety: Report of an inter-agency group. Morbid. Mortal. Weekly Rep., *31*:465, 1982.
13. Centers for Disease Control: Possible transfusion-associated acquired immune deficiency syndrome (AIDS)—California. Morbid. Mortal. Weekly Rep., *31*:652, 1982.
14. Centers for Disease Control: Antibodies to a retrovirus etiologically associated with acquired immunodeficiency syndrome (AIDS) in populations with increased incidences of the syndrome. Morbid. Mortal. Weekly Rep., *33*:377, 1984.
15. Centers for Disease Control: Hepatitis B vaccine: Evidence confirming lack of AIDS transmission. Morbid. Mortal. Weekly Rep., *33*:685, 1984.
16. Centers for Disease Control: Provisional public health service interagency recommendations for screening donated blood and plasma for antibody to the virus causing acquired immunodeficiency syndrome. Morbid. Mortal. Weekly Rep., *34*:1, 1985.
17. Centers for Disease Control: Changing patterns of acquired immunodeficiency syndrome in hemophilia patients—United States. Morbid. Mortal. Weekly Rep., *34*:241, 1985.
18. Centers for Disease Control: Recommendations for protection against viral hepatitis. Morbid. Mortal. Weekly Rep., *34*:313, 1985.
19. Centers for Disease Control: Revision of the case definition of acquired immunodeficiency syndrome for national reporting—United States. Morbid. Mortal. Weekly Rep., *34*:373, 1985.
20. Centers for Disease Control: Update: Public Health Service Workshop on human T-lymphotropic virus type III antibody testing—United States. Morbid. Mortal. Weekly Rep., *34*:477, 1985.
21. Centers for Disease Control: Heterosexual transmission of human T-lymphotropic virus type III/lymphadenopathy-associated virus. Morbid. Mortal. Weekly Rep., *34*:561, 1985.
22. Centers for Disease Control: Update: Acquired immunodeficiency syndrome in the San Francisco cohort study, 1978–1985. Morbid. Mortal. Weekly Rep., *34*:573, 1985.
23. Centers for Disease Control: Update: Acquired immunodeficiency syndrome—Europe. Morbid. Mortal. Weekly Rep., *34*:583, 1985.
24. Centers for Disease Control: Self-reported behavioral change among gay and bisexual men—San Francisco. Morbid. Mortal. Weekly Rep., *34*:613, 1985.
25. Centers for Disease Control: Summary: Recommendations for preventing transmission of infection with human T-lymphotropic virus type III/lymphadenopathy-associated virus in the workplace. Morbid. Mortal. Weekly Rep., *34*:681, 1985.
26. Cheingsong-Popov, R., Weiss, R. A., Dalgleish, A., Tedder, R. S., Jeffries, D. J., Shannon, D. C., Ferns, R. B., Briggs, E. M., Weller, I. V. D., Mitton, S., Adler, M. W., Farthing, C., Lawrence, A. G., Gazzard, B. G., Weber, J., Harris, J. R. W., Pinching, A. J., Craske, J., and Barbara, J. A. J.: Prevalence of antibody to human T-lymphotropic virus type III in AIDS and AIDS-risk patients in Britain. Lancet, *2*:477, 1984.
27. Cohen, H., et al: International Conference on AIDS. Atlanta, Ga., April 1985.
28. Conte, J. E., Jr., Hadley, W. K., Sande, M., and University of California, San Francisco, Task Force on the Acquired Immunodeficiency Syndrome: Infection-control guidelines for patients with the acquired immunodeficiency syndrome (AIDS). N. Engl. J. Med., *309*:740, 1983.
29. Corey, L., and Holmes, K. K.: Sexual transmission of hepatitis A in homosexual men. N. Engl. J. Med., *302*:435, 1980.
30. Craske, J., Dilling, N., and Stern, D.: An outbreak of hepatitis associated with the intravenous injection of factor VIII concentration. Lancet, *1*:221, 1975.
31. Curran, J. W., Lawrence, D. N., Jaffe, H., Kaplan, J. E., Zyla, I. D., Chamberland, M., Weinstein, R., Lui, K-J., Schonberger, L. B., Spira, T. J., Alexander, W. J., Swinger, G., Ammann, A., Solomon, S., Auerbach, D., Mildvan, D., Stoneburner, R., Jason, J. M., Haverkos, H. W., and Evatt, B. L.: Acquired immunodeficiency syndrome (AIDS) associated with transfusions. N. Engl. J. Med., *30*:69, 1984.
32. Curran, J. W., Morgan, W. M., Hardy, A. M., Jaffe, H. W., Darrow, W. W., and Dowdle, W. R.: The epidemiology of AIDS: Current status and future prospects. Science, *229*:1352, 1985.
33. Dienstag, J. L.: Immunopathogenesis of the extrahepatic manifestations of hepatitis B virus infection. Springer Seminol. Immunopathol., *3*:461, 1981.
34. Dienstag, J. L., and Ryan, D. M.: Occupational exposure to hepatitis B virus in hospital personnel: Infection or immunization. Am. J. Epidemiol., *115*:26, 1982.
35. Evatt, B. L., Gomperts, E. D., McDougal, J. S., and Ramsey, R. B.: Coincidental appearance of LAV/HTLV-III antibodies in hemophiliacs and the onset of the AIDS epidemic. N. Engl. J. Med., *312*:483, 1985.
36. Eyster, M. E., Goedert, J. J., Sarngadharan, M. G., Weiss, S. H., Gallo, R. C., and Blattner, W. A.: Development and early natural history of HTLV-III antibodies in persons with hemophilia. J.A.M.A., *253*:2219, 1985.
37. Favero, M. S., Maynard, J. E., Leger, R. T., Graham, D. R., and Dixon, R. E.: Guidelines for the care of patients hospitalized for viral hepatitis. Ann. Intern. Med., *91*:872, 1979.
38. Feinstone, S. M., and Purcell, R. H.: Non-A, non-B hepatitis. Ann. Rev. Med., *29*:359, 1978.

39. Fischinger, P. J., and Bolognesi, D. P.: Prospects for diagnostic tests, intervention, and vaccine development in AIDS. *In* DeVita, V. T., Jr., Hellman, S., and Rosenberg, S. A. (Eds.): AIDS. Etiology, Diagnosis, Treatment, and Prevention. Philadelphia, J. B. Lippincott Company, 1985.

40. Gallo, R. C., Salahuddin, S. Z., Popovic, M., Shearer, G. M., Kaplan, M., Haynes, B. F., Palker, T. J., Redfield, R., Oleske, J., Safai, B., White, G., Foster, P., and Markham, P. D.: Frequent detection and isolation of cytopathic retroviruses (HTLV-III) from patients with AIDS and at risk for AIDS. Science, *224*:500, 1984.

41. Gerberding, J. L., Moss, A. R., Bryant, C. E., et al.: Risk of acquired immune deficiency syndrome (AIDS) virus transmission to health care workers. Abstracts of the 25th Interscience Conference on Antimicrobial Agents and Chemotherapy. Washington, D.C., American Society of Microbiology, *25*:131, 1985.

42. Goedert, J. L., and Blattner, W. A.: The epidemiology of AIDS and related conditions. *In* DeVita, V. T., Jr., Hellman, S., and Rosenberg, S. A. (Eds.): AIDS. Etiology, Diagnosis, Treatment, and Prevention. Philadelphia, J. B. Lippincott Company, 1985.

43. Goldfield, M., Bill, J., and Colosimo, F.: The control of transfusion associated hepatitis. *In* Vyas, G., Cohen, S. M., and Schmid, R. (Eds.): Viral Hepatitis. Philadelphia, Franklin Institute Press, 1978.

44. Gottlieb, M. S., Schroff, R., Schanker, H. M., Weisman, J. D., Fan, P. T., Wolf, R. A., and Saxon, A.: *Pneumocystitis carinii* pneumonia and mucosal candidiasis in previously healthy homosexual men: Evidence of a new acquired cellular immunodeficiency. N. Engl. J. Med., *305*:1425, 1981.

45. Govindarajan, S., Chin, K. P., Redeker, A. G., and Peters, R. L.: Fulminant B viral hepatitis: Role of delta agent. Gastroenterology, *86*:1417, 1984.

46. Grady, G. F.: Hepatitis B from the medical professions—How rare? How preventable? N. Engl. J. Med., *296*:995, 1977.

47. Hamilton, J. D.: Viral hepatitis and the surgeon. *In* Sabiston, D. C., Jr. (Ed.): Textbook of Surgery, 13th ed. Philadelphia, W. B. Saunders Company, 1986.

48. Henderson, D. K., Saah, A. J., Zak, B. J., et al: Seroepidemiology of HTLV-III among health care professionals. Federation for Clinical Research Meeting, Washington, D. C., May 1985.

49. Hirsch, M. S., Wormser, G. P., Schooley, R. T., Ho, D. D., Felenstein, D., Hopkins, C. C., Joline, C., Duncanson, F., Sarngadharan, M. G., Saxinger, C., and Gallo, R. C.: Risk of nosocomial infection with human T-cell lymphotropic virus III (HTLV-III). N. Engl. J. Med. *312*:1, 1985.

50. Holland, P. V., Alter, H. J., Purcell, R. H., Lander, J. J., Sgouris, J. T., and Schmidt, P. J.: Hepatitis B antigen and antibody in cold ethanol fractions of human plasma. Transfusions, *12*:363, 1972.

51. Hollinger, F. B., Mosley, J. W., Szmuness, W., et al.: Transfusion-transmitted viruses study: Experimental evidence for two non-A, non-B hepatitis agents. J. Infect. Dis., *142*:400, 1980.

52. Ishak, K. G.: Light microscopic morphology of viral hepatitis. Am. J. Clin. Pathol., *65*:787, 1976.

53. Jaffe, W. H., et al. The acquired immunodeficiency syndrome in gay men. Ann. Intern. Med., *103*:662, 1985.

54. Jacobson, I. M., Dienstag, J. L., Zochoval, R., Hanrahan, B. A., Watkins, E., and Rubin, R. H.: Lack of effect of hepatitis B vaccine on T-cell phenotypes. N. Engl. J. Med., *311*:1030, 1984.

55. Kane, M. A., Bradley, D. W., Shrestha, S. M., et al.: Epidemic non-A, non-B hepatitis in Nepal: Recovery of a possible etiologic agent and transmission studies in marmosets. J.A.M.A., *252*:3140, 1984.

56. Kaposi, M.: Idiopatisches multiples Pigmentsarkom der haut. Arch. f. Derm. u Syph., *4*:365, 1872.

57. Kiernan, T. W., and Powers, R. J.: Hepatitis B virus. Inappropriate reactions to transmission risks. J.A.M.A., *241*:585, 1979.

58. Krugman, S., Overby, L. R., Mushahwar, I. K., Ling, C. M., Frosner, G. G., and Deinhardt, F.: Viral hepatitis type B: Studies on natural history and prevention re-examined. N. Engl. J. Med., *300*:101, 1979.

59. Lawrence, D. N., Lui, K-J., Bregman, D. J., et al.: A model-based estimate of the average incubation and latency period for transfusion-associated AIDS. International Conference on AIDS, Atlanta, Ga., April 1985.

60. Lemon, S. M.: Type A viral hepatitis: New developments in an old disease. N. Engl. J. Med., *313*:1059, 1985.

61. Levy, J. A., Hoffman, A. D., Kramer, S. M., Landis, J. A., and Shimabukuro, J. M.: Isolation of lymphocytopathic retroviruses from San Francisco patients with AIDS. Science, *225*:840, 1984.

62. Lotze, M. T.: AIDS: A surgeon's responsibility. ACS Bull., *70*:6, 1985.

63. Maloney, M. J., Cox, F., Wray, B. B., Guill, M. F., and Hagler, J.: AIDS in a child 5½ years after a transfusion. N. Engl. J. Med., *312*:1256, 1985.

64. Mathiesen, L. R., Shinhoj, P., Hardt, F., Nielsen, J. O., Sloth, K., Zoffman, H., Moller, A. M., Wong, D., and Purcell, R. H.: Epidemiology and clinical characteristics of acute hepatitis types A, B, and non-A, non-B. Scand. J. Gastroenterol., *14*:849, 1979.

65. Maynard, J. E.: Epidemic non-A, non-B hepatitis. Semin. Liver Dis., *4*:336, 1984.

66. McGrady, G., et al.: International Conference on AIDS. Atlanta, Ga., April 1985.

67. Nath, N., Fang, C. T., and Berberian, H.: Antibodies to delta antigen in asymptomatic HBsAg reactive blood donors in the United States and its association with other markers of hepatitis B virus. Am. J. Epidemiol., *122*:218, 1985.

68. Oken, M. M., Hootkin, L., and DeJager, R. L.: Hepatitis after Konye administration. Am. J. Dig. Dis., *17*:271, 1972.

69. Peterman, T. A., et al.: International Conference on AIDS. Atlanta, Ga., April 1985.

70. Potter, D. A., Danforth, D. N., Jr., Macher, A. M., Longo, D. L., Stewart, L., and Masur, H.: Evaluation of abdominal pain in the AIDS patient. Ann. Surg., *199*:332, 1984.

71. Redfield, R. R., Markham, P. D., Salahuddin, S. Z., Wright, D. C., Sarngadharan, M. G., and Gallo, R. C.: Heterosexually acquired HTLV-III/LAV disease (AIDS-related complex and AIDS): Epidemiologic evidence for female-to-male transmission. J.A.M.A., *254*:2094, 1985.

72. Redfield, R. R., Wright, D. C., and Tramont, E. C.: The Walter Reed staging classification for HTLV-III/LAV infection. N. Engl. J. Med., *314*:131, 1986.

73. Rizzetto, M.: The delta agent. Hepatology, *3*:729, 1983.

74. Rosina, F., Saracco, G., and Rizzetto, M.: Risk of post-transfusion infection with the hepatitis delta virus: A multicenter study. N. Engl. J. Med., *312*:1488, 1985.

75. Safai, B., Groopman, J. E., Popovic, M., Schupbach, J., Sarngadharan, M. G., Arnett, K., Sliski, A., and Gallo, R. C.: Seroepidemiological studies of human T-lymphotropic retrovirus type III in acquired immunodeficiency syndrome. Lancet, *1*:1438, 1984.

76. Safai, B., Johnson, K. G., Myskowski, P. L., Koziner, B., Yang, S. Y., Cunningham-Rundles, S., Godbold, J. H., and Dupont, B.: The natural history of Kaposi's sarcoma in the acquired immunodeficiency syndrome. Ann. Intern. Med., *103*:744, 1985.

77. Schupbach, J., Haller, O., Vogt, M., Luthy, R., Joller, H., Oelz, O., Popovic, M., Sarngadharan, M. G., and Gallo, R. C.: Antibodies to HTLV-III in Swiss patients with AIDS and pre-AIDS and in groups at risk for AIDS. N. Engl. J. Med., *312*:265, 1985.

78. Snydman, D. R.: Hepatitis in pregnancy. N. Engl. J. Med., *313*:1398, 1985.

79. Szmuness, W., Much, M. I., Prince, A. M., et al.: On the role of sexual behavior on the spread of hepatitis B infection. Ann. Intern. Med., *83*:498, 1975.

80. Stricker, R. B., Abrams, D. I., Corash, L., and Shuman, M. A.: Target platelet antigen in homosexual men with immune thrombocytopenia. N. Engl. J. Med., *313*:1375, 1985.

81. Tabor, E., Seeff, L. B., and Gerety, R. J.: Chronic non-A, non-B hepatitis carrier state: Transmissible agent documented in one patient over a six-year period. N. Engl. J. Med., *303*:140, 1980.

82. Vyas, G. H. (Ed.): Viral Hepatitis—1984. Fourth International Symposium on Viral Hepatitis. San Francisco, Calif., March 1984.

83. Weiss, S. H., Goedert, J. J., Biggar, R. J., et al.: Natural history of HTLV-III seropositive persons from AIDS risk groups. Proc. Am. Soc. Clin. Oncol., *4*:2, 1985.

84. Weiss, S. H., et al.: International Conference on AIDS. Atlanta, Ga., April 1985.

85. Weiss, S. H., Saxinger, W. C., Rechtman, D., Grieco, M. H., Nadler, J., Holman, S., Ginzburg, H. M., Groopman, J. E., Goedert, J. L., Markham, P. D., Gallo, R. C., Blattner, W. A., and Landesman, S.: HTLV-III infection among health care workers. Association with needle-stick injuries. J.A.M.A., *254*:2089, 1985.

86. Yarchoan, R., Weinhold, K. J., Lyerly, H. K., Gelmann, E., et al.: Treatment of AIDS or AIDS-related complex with 3'-azido-3'-deoxythymidine, an inhibitor of HTLV-III/LAV replication. Lancet, *1*:575, 1986.

MANAGEMENT OF THE ACUTELY INJURED PERSON

P. WILLIAM CURRERI, M.D.

13

The most frequent cause of death during the first 3 decades of life among civilians in the United States is traumatic injury. In fact, when one analyzes the cause of death for all age groups, only cancer and cardiovascular disease fatalities outnumber death secondary to traumatic injury. Twelve per cent of all hospital beds within the United States are occupied by traumatized patients. Each year, in excess of 50,000,000 injuries occur in the United States of which 20 per cent prove to be disabling and 0.2 per cent are ultimately fatal. Thus, over 100,000 deaths occur each year as a result of accidental injury. Unfortunately, it is a disease of the young in whom disability has the potential of producing economic disaster, since they make up the largest proportion of the working force.

Although the number of patients dying from severe injury is increasing each year in the United States, the incidence of death and disability has been declining as a result of improved medical and paramedical efforts. Many of the principles utilized in the field and emergency room treatment of injured patients were gained during experience of the military during World War II, the Korean War, and the Vietnam conflict. In each succeeding war, the incidence of mortality and disabling complications was diminished. As an example, the incidence of post-traumatic acute renal failure was reduced to one of 1867 total casualties and one of 600 seriously wounded casualties in the Vietnam conflict, compared with an incidence of one of 1319 casualties and one in every 200 seriously wounded individuals during the Korean War. Primary reasons cited for the increased survival and dramatic decrease in the incidence of renal failure in Vietnam included (1) rapid transport of casualties to definitive treatment centers by helicopter; (2) availability of fresh blood transfusion with type-specific or Type O-negative blood, as well as other electrolyte and plasma expander solutions; and (3) the relative rarity of prolonged hypotension. The average transportation time to definitive treatment centers in Vietnam was only 32 minutes, compared with greater than 4 hours in Korea. It should also be noted that the rapid development of vascular surgical principles during the Korean War led to a significant decrease in the necessity for performing post-traumatic amputations in comparison with similar injuries incurred during World War II.

In civilian populations, improved survival rates are also associated with an organized approach to delivery of care to traumatized individuals. The development of specialized transportation vehicles (ambulances and helicopters) equipped with appropriate monitoring devices and supplies for treatment during transport has promoted the organization of community-wide dispatching systems that allow rapid triage in delivery of patients to a definitive medical center for further diagnostic evaluation and definitive treatment. Extensive training programs for emergency medical technicians and paramedics are now mandated in many communities, and radio-controlled direction to these individuals by physicians in trauma centers allows rapid diagnostic evaluation and early therapeutic intervention even before the patient arrives at the emergency room. Improved diagnostic and therapeutic modalities for the treatment of hypotension, respiratory distress, and cervical spine injury, the control of hemorrhage, the management of head injury, and the management of post-traumatic hypermetabolism have all resulted in improved in-hospital care of the severely injured patient. In addition, emergency medical personnel in major metropolitan areas are now trained in accomplishing safe extraction of individuals trapped following vehicular or industrial accidents. It is the purpose of this chapter to specifically review the priorities required to ensure appropriate immediate care of the trauma victim from the time he is first evaluated until he leaves the emergency room. In addition, principles of diagnosis and treatment with regard to specific organ injury will be summarized.

IMMEDIATE CARE

Of utmost importance during the immediate evaluation of the traumatized patient is the establishment of treatment priorities. In essence, patient management includes (1) a rapid primary evaluation, (2) resuscitation of vital functions, (3) secondary assessment in more detail, and, finally, (4) the initiation of definitive care. The primary survey is designed to identify significant life-threatening or limb-threatening problems. During the resuscitation phase, these life-threatening conditions are treated prior to performing a secondary survey, at which time the patient is examined from head to toe and appropriate diagnostic laboratory studies and radiologic examinations are obtained. It is only then that definitive care directed toward less life-threatening injuries can be begun.

Primary Survey

The primary survey may be accomplished in a few minutes and is designed to identify life-threatening injuries, which must be treated immediately so as to prevent rapid deterioration or further injury secondary to iatrogenic manipulation.

AIRWAY AND CERVICAL SPINE

The physician should first direct attention to the airway and the cervical spine. Airway patency, down to and including the larynx, should be confirmed, and any foreign debris within the airway must be removed. At the same time, specific attention should be directed toward the potential existence of cervical spine fractures, since excessive movement of the cervical spine might convert a simple fracture without neurologic damage into a fracture dislocation with irreversible neurologic injury. Thus, hyperextension of the patient's head and neck in order to establish or maintain an airway or to introduce an endotracheal tube must be avoided until the cervical spine has been assessed by obtaining a cross-table lateral cervical spine x-ray in which all seven cervical vertebrae are visualized.

When upper airway obstruction is identified, a series of simple maneuvers must be undertaken to immediately relieve the obstruction. Most commonly, upper airway obstruction in the unconscious patient occurs as a result of prolapse of the tongue backward toward the posterior pharyngeal wall, which mechanically blocks the entrance to the larynx. Since the tongue has muscular attachments to the mandible, movement of the mandible anteriorly will also bring the tongue forward and relieve the obstruction. One method of accomplishing this is the *chin lift*. The fingers of one hand are placed under the mandible, and the mandible is gently lifted upward while the thumb of the same hand lightly depresses the lower lip to open the mouth. Another technique, the *jaw thrust*, is accomplished by placing the fingers behind the angle of the jaw to move the mandible forward. The palms of each hand are left open along the side of the face, and the thumbs rest on the chin as the jaw is thrust forward. Since these maneuvers do not hyperextend the neck, there is relatively little risk of displacing an unrecognized cervical spine fracture.

Should these actions fail to relieve the obstruction, the physician must proceed to mechanical methods that allow maintenance of the upper airway. These include insertion of an oropharyngeal airway, a nasopharyngeal airway, an esophageal airway, or an endotracheal tube. If a cervical spine fracture has not been precluded by a lateral cervical spine injury, the endotracheal tube should be inserted through the nose in order to avoid hyperextension of the neck, which is required for the insertion of an oral tracheal tube.

Should nasal tracheal intubation be unsuccessful, *surgical cricothyroidotomy* is indicated. This is performed by making a vertical or transverse skin incision that extends through the cricothyroid membrane with subsequent insertion of a small tracheostomy tube. Surgical cricothyroidotomy is preferred to tracheostomy during emergency therapy, since it can be performed rapidly and relatively bloodlessly under less than ideal conditions. In children younger than the age of 12, in whom the cricoid cartilage provides circumferential support to the upper trachea, the insertion of a No. 14-gauge needle through the cricoid cartilage with delivery of intermittent high flows of oxygen may be a preferable method of relieving upper airway obstruction until definitive tracheostomy is performed.

AIR EXCHANGE

The physician must next direct attention to the adequacy of air exchange. Twenty-five per cent of trauma deaths result from chest injuries; many of these may be prevented by prompt diagnosis and correct management once the patient arrives at the hospital. Air exchange can be quickly assessed by listening at the patient's nose and mouth for the movement of air. The patient's chest should be exposed so that intercostal or supraclavicular muscle retractions may be noted and respiratory movement can be assessed by observation, palpation, and auscultation of the chest.

The physician should search for the presence of three life-threatening complications of chest trauma that can be rapidly treated. These include (1) tension pneumothorax, (2) open pneumothorax, and (3) flail chest.

Tension Pneumothorax

A tension pneumothorax results when air leaks into the pleural space either from the lung or through the chest wall through a one-way valve. As air accumulates under pressure within the pleural cavity, the lung is collapsed and the mediastinum and trachea are displaced toward the opposite side. This may interfere with venous return to the heart. This condition is identified by the presence of tachypnea, the absence of breath sounds, the development of cyanosis, and tracheal deviation to the side opposite the tension pneumothorax. It should be managed by rapid insertion of a large-bore needle into the second intercostal space in the midclavicular line of the affected hemithorax. This allows the tension pneumothorax to be converted into a simple pneumothorax until a chest tube can be inserted to re-expand the lung. A glass syringe is traditionally used for this maneuver. If tension exists in the pleural cavity, the barrel will be "blown out" of the syringe. If no tension is present, the syringe prevents air entry into the pleural cavity. Plastic syringes are unsatisfactory for this purpose, since the pressure required to move the barrel is high, making it relatively insensitive.

Open Pneumothorax

An open pneumothorax occurs when the injury has resulted in loss of chest wall integrity as well as when there is injury to the lung. Such wounds may result in continued contamination of the pleural cavity with subsequent development of empyema if not closed. Treatment consists of prompt closure of the chest wall defect with a sterile occlusive dressing, which is taped on three sides to provide a flutter-type valve. During inhalation, the dressing is occlusively sucked over the wound, preventing air from entering. When the patient exhales, the open end of the dressing allows air to escape. Subsequently, a chest tube is inserted in order to maintain expansion of the lung.

Flail Chest

Flail chest is usually seen after a patient has incurred multiple rib fractures, resulting in a segment of chest wall that no longer has bony continuity with the thoracic cage. This segment of the chest wall exhibits paradoxical movement, which results in a marked decrease in effective ventilation and retention of carbon dioxide. The patient should receive humidified oxygen, and the flail segment should be stabilized by direct compression until endotracheal intubation can be accomplished and volume ventilation with a mechanical respirator instituted. Some patients with small flail segments may not require mechanical ventilation if adequate analgesics to control pain allow adequate chest wall expansion. However, if respiratory failure develops, as indicated by the development of tachypnea and hypoxia, prompt internal stabilization of the fractures should be accomplished via endotracheal intubation and mechanical ventilation.

CIRCULATION

The physician next directs attention to evaluation of the circulation. Pulses should be palpated and assessed for quality, rate, rhythm, and anatomic site. If a radial pulse can be palpated, systolic pressure will usually be greater than 80 mm. Hg. Femoral pulses may be palpated at systolic pressures over 70 mm. Hg and carotid pulses at a pressure over 60 mm. Hg. In addition, capillary refill may be evaluated by blanching a finger or toenail. Color will return to the nail bed within 2 seconds in a patient who is normovolemic. In addition, exsanguinating hemorrhage to the outside should be identified and controlled by direct pressure on the wound.

NEUROLOGIC AND PHYSICAL STATUS

Next, a brief neurologic evaluation should be performed to establish level of consciousness and pupillary size and reaction. The level of consciousness can be briefly assessed and classified by determining whether the patient is alert, whether he responds only to vocal stimuli, whether he responds only to painful stimuli, or whether he is unresponsive.

The patient must then be exposed in order to evaluate the presence of external injuries. All clothing must be removed, and the patient must be examined on both the anterior and posterior aspects of the body's surface.

PRESSURE EVALUATION

Finally, a blood pressure should be obtained and the pulse pressure evaluated. A decrease in pulse pressure along with elevated venous pressure and decreased heart tones should suggest the potential of cardiac tamponade. Such patients may exhibit pulsus paradoxus and decreased voltage of the QRS segment on the electrocardiogram (ECG). This condition is initially managed in the emergency room by performing pericardiocentesis utilizing the subxiphoid route. Subsequent exploratory thoracotomy with repair of the injuries to the heart is usually required once cardiac output has been restored following the removal of blood from the pericardial sac by pericardiocentesis.

Resuscitation

After the primary survey is completed, resuscitative measures are instituted in all patients with major injuries. These include the administration of supplemental oxygen and insertion of at least two large-bore intravenous lines. At the same time, a small sample of blood should be withdrawn so that it may be typed and cross-matched and basic diagnostic chemical studies performed. If hypotension has been identified, hypovolemic shock should be anticipated and a balanced salt solution administered at rapid rates. Electrocardiographic monitoring is instituted to detect the development of arrhythmias, and both urinary and gastric catheters should be inserted if not contraindicated.

When hypovolemia results in diminished cardiac output and inadequate peripheral perfusion, aerobic metabolism at the cellular level is markedly impeded. Lactic acidosis as a result of cellular anaerobic metabolism rapidly ensues. In addition, extracellular fluid is lost to the intracellular space as the Na^+–K^+ adenosine triphosphate (ATP) pump fails and extracellular sodium and water cross the cellular membrane in exchange for potassium. Subsequent hyperkalemia and cellular death frequently lead to organ failure. The presence of severe metabolic acidosis is associated with decreased myocardial contractility and therefore further exaggerates the consequences of diminished organ blood flow.

Since hemorrhage is defined as an acute loss of the normal circulating blood volume, it is essential for the physician to possess a means to estimate normal blood volume. Blood volume in the normal male represents approximately 7.2 per cent of ideal body weight and in the adult female approximately 7.0 per cent of ideal body weight. In the pediatric age group, a total blood volume may be calculated at approximately 80 to 90 ml. per kg. of body weight.

Hemorrhage has been classified according to the amount of acute blood loss experienced by the patient. Class I hemorrhage is defined as a loss of up to 15 per cent of the total circulating blood volume; Class II, an acute loss of 20 to 25 per cent of blood volume; Class III, an acute loss of 30 to 35 per cent of blood volume; and Class IV, an acute loss of 40 to 50 per cent of the circulating blood volume.

The severity of hemorrhage may be estimated by presenting clinical symptoms. Class I hemorrhage is manifested usually by a very minimal increase in pulse rate. In Class II hemorrhage, the pulse rate will exceed 100 and the patient begins to display tachypnea. In addition, one might note a rise in diastolic pressure secondary to the elaboration of circulating catecholamines with a resulting decrease in pulse pressure. A patient with Class III hemorrhage will exhibit a pulse rate of greater than 120, marked tachypnea, and a decrease in systolic blood pressure and pulse pressure. Class IV hemorrhage is accompanied by marked tachycardia of greater than 140 with a systolic blood pressure of less than 50 to 60 mm. Hg. Pallor and a decrease in surface temperature may be appreciated.

Hemorrhage in both Class I and Class II may be treated by the administration of a balanced salt solution. Such solutions are administered so as to infuse approximately 3 units of crystalloid solution for every unit of lost blood. Both Class III and Class IV hemorrhage require the administration of both balanced salt solution and whole blood in order to restore hemodynamic stability.

Restoration of circulating blood volume may be assessed by serial evaluation of clinical signs and symptoms, including pulse rate, respiratory rate and blood pressure; restoration of adequate urinary output; reversal of metabolic acidosis; and restoration of normal central venous pressure. If adequate restoration of volume is not accomplished immediately, a persistent state of hypovolemia should be suspected. A fluid challenge test dose consisting of 200 ml. of lactated Ringer's solution administered over a period of 10 minutes frequently improves vital signs and suggests the persistence of hypovolemia. In the pediatric patient, such a fluid challenge consists of 20 to 40 ml. per kg. per hour of lactated Ringer's solution.

HYPOTENSION

Profound hypotension is often initially managed in the field by application of a *pneumatic antishock garment*. This garment is applied to the lower extremities and abdomen and effectively decreases the volume of tissue being perfused. The application of this garment is contraindicated in patients with pulmonary edema, i.e., cardiogenic shock, and in patients with major intrathoracic hemorrhage. When the pneumatic antishock garment has been utilized, it is important that it not be deflated until blood volume and cardiac output have been restored. Gradual deflation of the garment while monitoring arterial pressure is then permissible and should not be unduly delayed, since areas under the garment may be underperfused, resulting in the development of compartment syndromes.

Secondary Examination

Following initial evaluation for life-threatening injury and the initiation of resuscitative measures, the physician begins a definitive examination to detect non–life-threatening, but potentially disabling, trauma. Examination begins with evaluation of pupillary size, a search for hemorrhage within the conjunctiva and fundus, the identification of dislocation of the lens, and a search for evidence of a penetrating injury of the globe. A quick visual test is performed to rule out optic nerve injury. The physician should carefully palpate the bony structure of the face to detect maxillofacial trauma and should carefully evaluate the neck for the presence of distended veins.

After completion of a visual evaluation of the chest, each of the bones of the chest wall should be palpated carefully to detect fractures. The chest is then auscultated and the presence of decreased breath sounds is further evaluated by percussion to detect the presence of a hemothorax or pneumothorax.

The abdomen is then carefully palpated to detect involuntary guarding, which might suggest the presence of a perforated viscus or the rapid accumulation of intra-abdominal blood. Rectal examination is performed in order to identify intraluminal blood, to evaluate the integrity of the rectal wall, to detect a change in anal sphincter tone, and to evaluate the integrity of the urethra.

The extremities and pelvis are then carefully palpated to detect fractures and the presence or absence of peripheral pulses. Finally, an in-depth neurologic examination is performed in order to identify motor and sensory deficits, the presence of skull fractures, or the presence of a closed head injury. In particular, the tympanic membrane should be carefully visualized for the presence of blood and the nose should be evaluated for the presence of cerebral spinal fluid (CSF) discharge. If a potential injury to the spinal column exists, the patient must be adequately immobilized on a spinal board and a semi-rigid cervical collar should be applied.

At this time, a brief past history should be obtained. Information is required with regard to known allergies, current medications, past illnesses, the time of the patient's last meal, and any specific events that preceded the injury. A small proportion of patients will be traumatized as a result of an acute medical illness that may have precipitated the accident.

LABORATORY AND RADIOLOGIC EVALUATION

Further diagnostic laboratory and radiologic evaluation is usually required at this juncture. An anteroposterior chest film, arterial blood gases, and ECG should be obtained to evaluate the potential for previously undetected intrathoracic injury. If intra-abdominal injury is suspected, but not yet confirmed, peritoneal lavage may be considered in certain patients. This particular diagnostic maneuver is most valuable in the patient with altered mental status or neurologic injury in whom the physical examination may be falsely negative. In particular, patients with alcohol or drug overdose, suspected head injury, or demonstrated spinal cord injury should undergo peritoneal lavage. Likewise, it is helpful in identifying the absence of intra-abdominal injury in patients with falsely positive physical examinations. This would include patients with fractures of the lower ribs, pelvis, or lumbar spine. Some patients will have a negative abdominal physical examination but will be unavailable for prolonged monitoring because of the necessity of performing prolonged neurosurgical or orthopedic operative procedures. A negative peritoneal lavage in these patients is helpful in determining the safety of proceeding with operative intervention. Finally, there is a group of patients who show equivocal physical findings on abdominal examination. Peritoneal lavage in such patients will frequently identify a significant intra-abdominal injury.

Peritoneal lavage is contraindicated in the patient who has had multiple previous abdominal operations. Such patients frequently have adhesions of the small bowel to the anterior abdominal wall that prevent the safe insertion of the lavage catheter into the abdominal cavity. In addition, it is clear that lavage should not be performed when there are obvious signs on physical examination indicating the need for exploratory laparotomy.

Prior to performing peritoneal lavage, it is necessary to decompress the urinary bladder by inserting a catheter. After preparation of the abdomen, a small amount of local anesthetic is placed in the midline of the abdomen one third of the distance from the umbilicus to the symphysis pubis. The overlying skin and subcutaneous tissues are then incised through the fascia, and the peritoneum is then carefully incised while upper tension is placed on the anterior abdominal wall with hemostats applied to the fascia. A peritoneal dialysis catheter is then inserted into the peritoneal cavity, and the catheter is aspirated to detect the presence of free blood. If greater than 20 ml. of nonclotting free blood is obtained, the peritoneal lavage is terminated. If no gross blood is obtained, 10 ml. per kg. of Ringer's lactate is allowed to flow into the peritoneal cavity and the patient is then gently rocked. After 5 to 10 minutes, the fluid is siphoned off and sent to the laboratory for examination. A positive test consists of greater than 100,000 red blood cells per cu. mm., greater than 500 white blood cells per cu. mm., or the presence of bile, bacteria, or fecal material within the solution. A positive test implies a 97 per cent chance that significant intra-abdominal injury (necessitating laparotomy) has occurred. A negative lavage implies a 99 per cent chance that no significant intra-abdominal injury is present.

If renal damage is suspected or significant microscopic hematuria is detected, a one-shot infusion intravenous pyelogram (IVP) should be obtained prior to exploratory laparotomy in order to confirm the bilateral presence of kidneys and to prove bilateral renal function. In addition, extravasation of urine can frequently be identified.

Definitive Care

Specific definitive care of major injury is begun as soon as life-threatening problems have been managed and the specific injuries identified by diagnostic means. If immediate operation is not required, continuous monitoring of the patient's physiologic response to treatment is mandatory. Following resuscitation, vital signs should be restored and an hourly urinary output of at least 50 ml. should be obtained in the adult patient. In the pediatric patient, an output of approximately 1 ml. of urine per kg. of body weight per hour usually indicates adequate resuscitation.

HEAD AND SPINAL CORD TRAUMA

Head Injury

Death following severe multisystem trauma most commonly results from closed head injury. The presence of brain injury should be highly suspected in any patient with an alteration of consciousness. Alterations of consciousness may result from injury to the cerebral cortices bilaterally or the brain stem reticular activating system just above the level of the mid-pons. In addition, depression of consciousness may result from decreased cerebral blood flow or increased intracranial pressure.

Closed head injury often manifests itself as progressive neurologic deterioration. Thus, the state of the patient's consciousness at the scene of the accident should be ascertained from prehospital emergency personnel and the patient must be reassessed by neurologic examination at relatively frequent intervals.

On physical examination, a rise in intracranial pressure often is reflected by changes in vital signs. The respiratory rate decreases initially as intracranial pressure rises, but later it may become rapid and respiratory efforts may become noisy or agonal. Systolic blood pressure also rises following an increase in intracranial pressure with a widening of the pulse pressure. Pulse rate usually slows with a rise in intracranial pressure producing initial bradycardia. Preterminally a bradycardia may convert to a tachycardia with very high intracranial pressures. Some patients with significant closed head injury will exhibit hyperthermia, which may need to be controlled in order to prevent seizure activity.

Initial neurologic examination should be confined to assessment of immediate life-threatening injury requiring neurosurgical intervention. Brain function may be evaluated by establishing neurologic response as estimated by the Glasgow Coma Scale. This examination consists of evaluating the patient's ability to open his eyes, respond verbally, and move his limbs. In addition, pupillary responses in both eyes are evaluated. Eye-opening responses may be spontaneous with normal blinking, responsive to verbal stimulation, or responsive only to pain. Most seriously brain injured patients will have no eye-opening response. Verbal responses may be absent in the most seriously brain-injured patient. Intermediate stages of verbal response include the production of incomprehensible sounds, the utilization of inappropriate words, and the presence of confused conversation in response to specific questions. The patient with little brain injury will be oriented with respect to name, age, and place. Motor response in the limbs is evaluated by response to verbal command, response to pain, the presence of abnormal flexion with decorticate posturing, the presence of extensor responses indicating decerebrate posturing, and the absence of any motor response at all. It is important to emphasize that initial evaluation of brain function must be repeated at frequent intervals in order to determine whether such function is improving or deteriorating.

SKULL FRACTURE

Careful examination of the skull by visual inspection and palpation is mandated in the patient with suspected closed head trauma. Palpation should be performed only with a sterile glove in the presence of scalp lacerations, since such lacerations may be in direct communication with the cerebral substance through an open-skull depressed fracture. Frequently, depressed skull fractures may be detected in this manner alone. When closed head trauma is suspected, confirmation by skull x-ray is usually worthwhile to assess the degree of depression.

Skull x-rays may detect linear, non-depressed fractures—which in themselves require no definitive therapy. When linear fractures cross suture lines or arteriole grooves, the potential possibility of delayed epidural hemorrhage should be considered.

Depressed skull fractures require neurosurgical intervention when the fragment is depressed for a distance greater than the thickness of the skull. Failure to intervene operatively may lead to long-term seizure disorders.

Basilar skull fractures are most frequently diagnosed on physical examination. Cerebral spinal fluid (CSF) may be noted to emerge from the ear or the nose. In addition, ecchymosis in the mastoid region, known as *Battle's sign*, also suggests a basilar skull fracture. Frequently, such patients will exhibit blood behind the tympanic membrane.

COMPUTED TOMOGRAPHY AND NUCLEAR MAGNETIC RESONANCE

The utilization of skull x-rays as a diagnostic technique to confirm closed head injury has been supplanted largely by the use of computed tomography (CT) examination of the head. Not only can bony lesions be detected by CT; the presence of intracerebral hematomas, extracerebral hematomas, pneumocephalus, and cerebral edema can also be demonstrated. It has been noted by Quind and Smathers[17] that the presence of sphenoid sinus effusion on the skull radiograph of a traumatized patient represents a very sensitive sign of intracranial damage and thus represents an indication for emergent head CT.

Initial CT may not be sufficient to provide high diagnostic accuracy in patients with confirmed closed head injury. Serial studies have frequently depicted new lesions appearing following admission to the hospital. In general, these include intracerebral hematoma, intraventricular hemorrhage, extracerebral hematoma, progressive cerebral edema, and infarction. Patients displaying such new lesions on serial CT scans have a relatively poor outcome in 80 per cent of cases. In contrast, patients who demonstrate no new lesions on serial examination exhibit only a 20 per cent poor outcome.[11]

Computed tomography has also been used to estimate intracranial pressure following closed head trauma. The presence of intraventricular clot or significant ventricular compression correlates reasonably well with the level of intracranial pressure.[21]

Recently, a technique employing nuclear magnetic resonance (NMR) has been introduced as a new diagnostic tool for the evaluation of brain injury. Initial studies suggest that NMR may be superior to CT for demonstrating extracerebral as well as intracerebral traumatic lesions. In particular, isolated subdural hematomas are more clearly seen on NMR and epidural hematomas may be more easily detected as a result of better visualization of the dura mater.[9]

Several reports have now suggested that CT can be

used for prognostic purposes in evaluation of patients with head injury.[4, 23] The presence of completely or partially obliterated basal cisterns is a particularly poor prognostic sign and is associated with a mortality rate in excess of 65 per cent. Compression of the ventricles, together with the presence of multiple lesions of the brain parenchyma, is also associated with a poor prognosis.

OTHER USES OF COMPUTED TOMOGRAPHY FOLLOWING HEAD TRAUMA

Although an in-depth discussion of facial and orbital injury is beyond the scope of this chapter, it is worthwhile to re-emphasize that greater detail of complex facial fractures can be appreciated from CT than from conventional radiographs. Frequently, this information can be utilized to plan definitive reduction and internal fixation of such fractures prior to operative intervention. Computed tomography has proved superior in the diagnosis of orbital apex and orbital medial wall fractures and in detection of intraocular foreign bodies compared with routine facial radiographs and polytomography. In addition, CT imaging more accurately assesses the degree of comminution and soft tissue injury when utilized to evaluate patients with complex facial fractures involving the middle or upper third of the facial skeleton.[3]

THERAPY OF HEAD TRAUMA

Emergency treatment of the patient with suspected closed head injury includes maintenance of an open airway to ensure brain oxygenation, hyperventilation (particularly when increased intracerebral pressure is suspected), and adequate fluid resuscitation to preserve cerebral blood flow. When shock has been successfully treated, fluid should be restricted to maintenance levels in order to reduce inadvertent iatrogenic intracerebral pressure rise as a result of cerebral edema.

The mainstay of treatment should be careful re-evaluation via monitoring and repeat CT scanning if clinical conditions should deteriorate. Most patients who have been unconscious for 5 or more minutes should be observed in the hospital for a minimum of 24 hours. Many such patients will have suffered simple concussion, which implies no significant anatomic brain injury. Such patients may complain of temporary headache, dizziness, nausea, or amnesia, but they will reveal no localizing signs on neurologic examination. Patients with contusions of the brain usually exhibit more serious alterations in the state of consciousness with or without the presence of focal neurologic signs. They frequently have a history of a prolonged episode of unconsciousness but rarely require surgical intervention.

Patients with intracranial hemorrhage frequently require operative intervention. Computed tomography has allowed rapid diagnosis of intracranial hemorrhage and precise localization. In general, intracranial hemorrhage may be *meningeal* or *intracerebral*. Meningeal hemorrhage may be subdivided into three types, depending on anatomical location: (1) acute epidural hemorrhage, (2) acute subdural hematoma, and (3) subarachnoid hemorrhage.

The most common site of *acute epidural bleeding* is from the middle meningeal artery and is usually associated with linear skull fractures over the parietal or temporal areas that cross the grooves of the middle meningeal artery. Epidural hemorrhage is usually signaled by immediate loss of consciousness, followed by an intervening lucid interval and then a secondary depression of consciousness. During the secondary depression of consciousness, hemiparesis on the opposite side is frequently noted. In addition, a dilated or fixed pupil on the same side as the impact area is almost always noted. Rapid surgical intervention is necessary in order to control the bleeding, thus preventing secondary brain injury.

Subdural hematomas usually result secondary to venous bleeding. These usually present with a slower onset of symptoms and often indicate underlying primary brain injury. When the subdural hemorrhage is identified by a CT scan, its prompt evacuation is usually indicated.

Subarachnoid hemorrhage is associated with blood in the CSF and signs and symptoms of meningeal irritation. Symptoms frequently include headache and photophobia. No emergency therapy is usually required.

Intracerebral and *intraventricular* hemorrhages are associated with a relatively high mortality rate. Neurosurgical intervention is frequently required, particularly if the injury follows penetrating trauma to the skull.

Cervical Spine Injury

When patients exhibit significant trauma of soft tissues or bony structures above the clavicle, a high suspicion of potential cervical spine injury is required. On physical examination, a physician must particularly note the presence of flaccid areflexia, loss of rectal sphincter tone, the presence of diaphragmatic breathing, inability to extend the forearms, responsiveness to pain above the clavicle but not below, the presence of hypotension without other evidence of hypovolemia, and the presence of priapism. In such patients, a lateral cross-table x-ray of the cervical spine should be obtained as an emergency prior to manipulation of the neck. If not employed by prehospital medical personnel during transportation, a semirigid cervical collar should be utilized until it can be verified by x-ray that no significant dislocation or fracture is evident in any of the seven cervical vertebrae. X-rays must be carefully examined to ensure proper contour and alignment of the vertebral bodies and must be carefully scrutinized to detect displacement of bone fragments into the spinal canal or fractures of the vertebrae themselves. Fracture of C1 (atlas) is known as a *Jefferson fracture* and is often associated with a fracture of C2. Such fractures are frequently unstable and must be treated initially with cervical traction tongs or a spine board and semirigid cervical collar. Fractures of C2 (axis) are also often unstable and may require either surgical intervention or halo immobilization.

Fractures of C3 through C7 may be either stable or unstable, depending on the mechanism of injury. Patients with unstable vertebral injuries should be immobilized with a properly applied spine board and a semirigid cervical collar or with the application of cervical traction tongs until they can be transported to a definitive treatment center. Unstable fractures should be suspected when the anterior and posterior elements of the cervical spine are disrupted and when there is greater than 3.5 mm. overriding of a superior vertebra on the adjoining inferior vertebra. In addition, when angulation between two adjoining vertebrae exceeds 11 degrees, an unstable fracture has been identified.

Similar principles should be followed in evaluation of potential spinal trauma in the thoracic or lumbar vertebrae. In addition, on physical examination the physician should palpate the vertebra to detect localized pain, tenderness, or a posterior "step-off" deformity. The presence of pronounced muscle spasm should suggest the potential for fracture of the vertebra or transverse process. Careful neurologic assessment is required, including both sensory and motor function. Such examination will frequently suggest a level of spinal cord injury and may be used as a guide to detect progressive deterioration in spinal cord function.

Many radiologists now recommend computed tomography for evaluation of patients with suspected spinal trauma. Computed tomography often provides more detailed information regarding the extent of fracture displacement and the presence of soft tissue abnormalities within the spinal canal. Intramedullary hematomas, intrinsic cord swelling, and extrinsic cord pressure frequently can be differentiated by CT, which allows better discrimination in selection of patients for specific surgical or medical therapy.[19]

TRAUMA TO THE EXTREMITIES

Physical examination of the potentially injured extremity should await the control of immediate life-threatening injuries. The patient should be completely undressed to provide for adequate examination of the extremities. The physician should inspect each of the four extremities to detect edema, muscle spasm, physical deformity, open wounds, and color. Each extremity is then palpated to detect the presence of tenderness, crepitation, and sensation. Distal pulses should be palpated and, when necessary, a Doppler flowmeter utilized to confirm the presence of arterial and venous blood flow. Gentle pressure on the nail beds will allow examination of capillary refill, which should occur within 1 to 2 seconds.

At this juncture, the patient should be carefully examined for the presence of fractures. Fractures are classified as either *closed* or *open*, depending upon whether or not the fracture communicates with a defect in the skin. The physician should be aware of specific injuries that are frequently associated with fractures or dislocation. For instance, wrist injuries are commonly associated with injury of the elbow and/or shoulder. Calcaneal fractures are often accompanied by fractures of the lumbar spine (L1–L2). Additionally, knee injuries may be associated with fractures or dislocations of the hip, and a fractured femur may be accompanied by a dislocation of the ipsilateral hip.

It should be emphasized that fractures are frequently associated with considerable blood loss into the soft tissue around the fracture. A blood loss of 1 to 1½ units may be expected with a fractured tibia, and 2 or more units of blood may be lost in association with a fractured femur. Pelvic fractures may be associated with retroperitoneal bleeding of 6 or more units of blood.

Immobilization constitutes initial therapy of patients with fractures. Immobilization must be accomplished prior to patient transfer, and, when possible, splints should extend at least one joint above and below the fracture site. Severely angulated fractures may be aligned prior to application of the splint, although it is necessary to recheck distal pulses, skin color, and skin temperature prior to and after aligning angulated fractures. In addition, the physician should remove gross contamination from the wound of open fractures and when possible, prevent contaminated bone ends from re-entering the wound during the application of splints.

Whenever serious extremity injury has occurred, the patient must be constantly monitored for the potential development of a compartment syndrome. Such a syndrome results from muscle edema, bleeding, and reactive vasodilatation following re-establishment of arterial continuity

within enveloping fascial sheets. The resulting compression frequently results in ischemia to the muscle, as well as to the distal structures, secondary to constriction of axial vessels. Symptoms and signs associated with increased compartmental pressures include pain, loss of sensation, and paralysis. If untreated, a distal extremity may exhibit pallor and pulselessness. When necessary, a fasciotomy should be performed promptly to relieve the underlying pressure and to preserve local blood flow.

INJURY TO THE RESPIRATORY TRACT

Trauma to the respiratory tract represents a particularly dangerous injury. Not only may the airway be acutely obstructed; severe acute and chronic sequelae may also result from a delay in diagnosis. Early complications are related to cervical mediastinal infection as well as to interference with pulmonary mechanics secondary to persistent air leaks with inadequate expansion of the lung. Late morbidity is associated with compromised phonation and the development of tracheobronchial stenosis if immediate operative repair of major injuries is not performed.

The Larynx

Laryngeal fractures should be suspected when a patient presents with hemoptysis and subcutaneous emphysema following blunt injury to the neck. The diagnosis is best confirmed by CT of the laryngeal skeleton.[20] Lesions caused by direct trauma include supraglottic fractures, lateral glottic fractures, and cricotracheal separation.

When severe laryngeal injury is suspected, a secure airway should be immediately obtained by a tracheotomy and the patient evaluated for the presence of cervical vertebral injuries. Preoperatively, the patient should also be evaluated for the presence of recurrent laryngeal paralysis.

Supraglottic fractures will result in displacement of the supraglottic structure superiorly and posteriorly. Open reduction of the fractured dislocation may be accomplished through a cervical approach, at which time lacerations of the mucous membrane should be repaired and the fractured dislocation internally splinted around an individually molded stent for a period of 6 weeks.

Lateral glottic fracture occurs when there is a fracture of the thyroid alae in the vertical plane and the ipsilateral vocal cord and arytenoid are torn and denuded. These injuries are managed by excision of the damaged or scarred components of the glottis and mucosal repair.

Laryngotracheal separation may occur at the level of the first tracheal ring. In such cases, the cricoid ring is usually fractured inferiorly and the mucosa of the subglottis is torn and displaced with the trachea into the superior mediastinum. Emergency treatment requires the establishment of a tracheotomy into the open distal trachea. After control of infection (requiring up to 2 weeks) primary surgical repair may be accomplished. The distal trachea is sutured to the cricoid plate and an internal stent is inserted to support the anastomosis for a period of 4 weeks.

Although most injuries to the larynx are caused by blunt injury to the neck, severe injury of the larynx may occur secondary to high-velocity bullet wounds of the neck. These injuries to the larynx are particularly hazardous because of associated dyspnea or asphyxia. Thus, early tracheostomy is frequently required prior to operative exploration. Efforts should be made to accomplish conservative reconstruction of the larynx. However, if such attempts are unsuccessful, total laryngectomy may be required.

The Trachea

The diagnosis of tracheal injury following stab or gunshot wounds of the neck or thorax should be suspected when the patient manifests hemoptysis, subcutaneous emphysema, or the presence of air escaping from a cutaneous wound. If the patient is relatively stable from a hemodynamic and respiratory standpoint, tracheal injury can be confirmed by emergency bronchoscopy.

The management of tracheal injuries is dependent upon the magnitude of the tracheal wound. When it can be established by tracheal bronchoscopy that the injury involves less than one third of the circumference of the trachea or bronchus, and when the wound edges are well opposed without evidence of loss of tracheal tissue, the injury may be managed by temporary oral tracheal intubation in which the cuff is inflated below the tracheal injury to prevent the escape of air and bronchial secretions into the mediastinum. After 24 to 48 hours, the cuff is deflated; it is removed after another 24 hours if there is no progression of pneumomediastinum or subcutaneous emphysema.

In more extensive injuries of the trachea, the patient should be initially intubated with a long endotracheal tube and the cuff inflated distal to the tracheal injury. In the majority of cases, primary repair may be accomplished after débridement of nonviable tissue from the edges of the tracheal wound. Following primary repair, the patient must be carefully monitored for at least 3 months in order to detect the development of tracheostenosis at the site of the anastomosis. The primary symptom of tracheostenosis is the gradual development of dyspnea on exertion.

The Bronchi

Severe blunt trauma to the thorax may result in tracheobronchial disruption. It is believed that tracheobronchial disruption occurs as a result of at least three mechanisms:

1. Sudden, forceful compression of the thoracic cage results in a decrease in the anterior posterior diameter of the thorax and an increase in the transverse diameter. As a result, the lungs are displaced laterally, producing traction on the trachea at the carina where a rupture may occur.

2. In addition, it has been observed that when the trachea and major bronchi are crushed between the sternum and the vertebral column at the same time that the glottis is closed during the moment of impact, intrabronchial pressure may be suddenly increased, resulting in rupture of larger bronchi.

3. Finally, rapid deceleration may result in shearing forces at the point where the respiratory tree is relatively fixed, i.e., the cricoid and carina. Disruption of the right bronchus is more frequently observed than isolated disruption of the left bronchus.

On physical examination, the patient with tracheobronchial disruption may exhibit subcutaneous emphysema, respiratory distress, and hemoptysis. The presence of dyspnea and pneumothorax are less commonly observed. A chest roentgenogram may confirm the presence of a pneumomediastinum, pneumothorax, peribronchial air, obstruction of an air-filled bronchus, or pulmonary infiltrate as a result of aspirated blood. A radiolucent shadow along the anterior aspect of the spine, as a result of air beneath the deep cervical fascia, may be noted on a lateral cervical spine x-ray. In addition, the position of the hyoid bone should be noted on a lateral radiograph of the neck. When the hyoid is located above the level of the third cervical body, tracheal transection should be suspected. The diagnosis is confirmed by tracheobronchoscopy, which remains the definitive method of diagnosis of tracheobronchial disruption. When the patient is clinically unstable, emergency surgical exploration may be required. Repeated bronchoscopic examination is indicated when a patient exhibits unexplained persistent pleural air leaks, lumbar atelectasis, or persistent pneumothorax despite tube thoracostomy.

When the diagnosis of major tracheobronchial disruption has been confirmed, prompt surgical exploration is warranted with primary repair. Delay in operative reconstruction may result in bronchial stricture, empyema, or development of a bronchopleural cutaneous fistula.

ESOPHAGEAL INJURIES

Although the esophagus may be damaged by both penetrating and blunt injury, most esophageal perforations result from gunshot or knife wounds of the neck or thorax. The esophagus represents a highly contaminated gastrointestinal conduit with a bacterial flow that often contains harmful forms of anaerobic bacteria. Furthermore, the esophagus lacks serosa, thus making suture repair of lacerations more tenuous.

Symptoms and Signs

The most common symptoms associated with esophageal injury include cervical or thoracic pain, neck tenderness, dyspnea, and dysphagia. On physical examination, the presence of fever and subcutaneous emphysema may be appreciated. A patient will rapidly display leukocytosis, and chest roentgenograms will often reveal a pneumomediastinum, cervical soft tissue gas, hydrothorax, and pneumothorax.

Diagnosis

The level of the perforation may be confirmed by esophagram and/or esophagoscopy. It should be emphasized that both of these modalities may occasionally give false-negative results in patients with suspected esophageal injury.

Treatment

Injuries in the *cervical esophagus* are effectively treated by prompt cervical exploration, closure of the defect, and soft tissue drainage of the neck. When the injury is confined to the cervical portion of the esophagus, late complications are extraordinarily rare. Injuries to the *thoracic esophagus* must be treated by prompt thoracotomy. The mediastinum is opened widely and the perforation identified. A primary, two-layered repair should be attempted when there is sufficient tissue remaining to accomplish this without narrowing of the esophagus. In most cases, these repairs require reinforcement with some type of soft tissue flap. When the injury is in the *distal esophagus*, a gastric fundic patch may be utilized. Injuries to the *proximal two thirds of the esophagus* may be reinforced utilizing a pleural flap or a rhomboid muscle flap.

It should be recognized that in the presence of extensive tissue involvement following penetrating wounds of the esophagus, primary repair of thoracic esophageal perforations may be associated with a high incidence of failure. In such cases, less morbidity has been observed after defunctionalization of the esophagus is done. The distal esophagus is approached through a thoracotomy and ligated with absorbable sutures below the level of the injury. A cervical esophagostomy is performed to defunctionalize the entire esophagus above and below the point of intrathoracic injury. The patient is then placed on total parenteral intravenous nutrition for a period of about 2 weeks, at which time the esophageal perforation is frequently healed. If a barium swallow confirms healing of the esophageal injury and patency of the distal esophagus (following dissolution of the distal absorbable ligatures on the esophagus), the cervical esophagostomy may be closed.[18]

CHEST TRAUMA

Penetrating Wounds

Although stab wounds and gunshot wounds of the thoracic cavity are not uncommon in modern society, unlike penetrating abdominal trauma, about 80 per cent of penetrating chest injuries are managed conservatively utilizing tube thoracostomy alone. After an adequate airway and intravenous resuscitation of shock have been established, pneumothorax or hemothorax should be treated by placement of a tube thoracostomy through an incision in the fifth or sixth intercostal space at the mid-axillary line. Evacuation of less than 1500 ml. of blood from the pleural cavity should suggest conservative therapy, since most minor bleeding will cease once expansion of the lung is accomplished. When more than one liter of blood is collected from the pleural cavity, consideration should be given to autotransfusing this blood, providing there is no indication of concomitant gastrointestinal injury with communication between the abdomen and the pleural cavity through the diaphragm. When continued bleeding exceeds 250 ml. per hour, exploratory thoracotomy must be considered in order to operatively control a major bleeding vessel, often an intercostal or bronchial artery.

The most frequent sign of intrapericardial injury following penetrating wounds is *cardiac tamponade*, which is demonstrable in 65 to 80 per cent of patients with penetrating myocardial trauma. Since the pericardium is nondistensible, intrapericardial pressure gradually increases, resulting in increased resistance to diastolic filling of both ventricles and a subsequent drop in cardiac output.

The most reliable and specific indicator of tamponade is an elevation of the central venous pressure. It should be noted, however, that increased central venous pressure may be attenuated when pronounced hypovolemia exists. Classic signs of cardiac tamponade include distant heart sounds, pulsus paradoxus, and decreased voltage in the QRS segment on the ECG.

The diagnosis of cardiac tamponade should be strongly suspected in the patient with hypotension, despite the initiation of adequate intravenous fluid resuscitation. When the diagnosis is suspected, immediate pericardiocentesis should be performed in order to evacuate nonclotting blood from the pericardium. The procedure requires the insertion of a 16-gauge polytetrafluoroethylene (Teflon) intravenous catheter into the pericardial sac via the subxiphoid root. The needle is inserted at an angle of approximately 45 degrees to the sternum and 45 degrees to the right of the midline and is advanced toward the left shoulder. If an ECG electrode is placed on the needle, it is possible to appreciate contact of the needle with the myocardium. Removal of as little as 10 ml. of nonclotted blood frequently results in a significant increase in cardiac output. It is important to note that approximately a fourth of these patients will develop recurrent tamponade following initial evacuation of blood. Therefore, emergency thoracotomy should follow as soon as feasible to evacuate clot from the pericardium and to secure hemostasis when cardiac injury is detected. It is important to ensure that tamponade has been relieved prior to the induction of general anesthesia since inhalational gases frequently cause peripheral vascular dilatation and decreased myocardial function, resulting in profound hypotension. A surgical team should be scrubbed and ready for immediate thoracotomy prior to the delivery of anesthesia, and in some instances the performance of a subxiphoid pericardial window under local or light inhalational anesthesia is recommended prior to endotracheal intubation and full anesthetic induction.

In most cases, an anterolateral left thoracotomy in the fifth intercostal space is the preferred incision for exploratory thoracotomy following penetrating injury of the chest. When necessary, the sternum can be subsequently divided transversely and the incision extended into the corresponding intercostal space on the right side. This incision provides the surgeon with exposure to all chambers of the heart and the posterior mediastinal structures. Penetrating wounds of the heart most frequently involve the right ventricle. Injuries of the left ventricle and the right and left atrium are less common. Likewise, transection of the coronary arteries is uncommon and occurs in only approximately 4 to 5 per cent of patients with penetrating injury. Occasionally, patients will arrive in the emergency room without spontaneous respiratory effort or palpable pulses, despite the presence of signs of life at the scene of the accident. Such individuals will frequently benefit from emergency endotracheal intubation, ventilator assistance, and emergency room thoracotomy to obtain temporary control of major intrathoracic hemorrhage. If the patient can be resuscitated in the emergency room, he is immediately transported to the operating room for definitive repair of cardiac or great vessel injury.

Injuries of the heart often may be repaired without the necessity of cardiopulmonary bypass. However, this capability must be available to the operating team in the event that valvular injury, major coronary artery injury, or multiple wounds resulting in torrential hemorrhage is encountered.

Blunt Chest Injury

Blunt chest injuries result from vehicular accidents as a result of abrupt contact between the chest wall and the vehicular steering column. These are typically deceleration injuries, which may result in significant myocardial or pulmonary contusion. There may be little evidence of external injury upon examination of the chest wall. The physician must carefully inspect the chest wall and should be specifically alert to detect the presence of rib or sternal fractures, costochondral separation, and flail chest. Fractures of the first or second rib usually indicate that significant force has been applied to the chest wall, and such fractures are associated with a 14 per cent incidence of significant vascular injury.[13]

A chest x-ray will detect not only rib fractures but also the presence of a widened mediastinum, which suggests vascular injury, and pulmonary infiltrates, suggesting lung contusion. Many radiographic criteria have been utilized to detect the presence of significant vessel injury in the mediastinum. The most frequent injury is a transection of the thoracic aorta, usually just distal to the ligamentum teres. The eight radiographic signs of this injury are a widened mediastinum, the presence of hemothorax, fracture of the first or second rib, fractured clavicle, pulmonary contusion or pneumothorax, an apical cap, depression of the left main stem bronchus, and loss of the normal aortic contour. In practice, superior mediastinal widening and loss of the aortic contour are the most reliable signs of great vessel injury and mandate emergency aortography.[8] Traumatic disruption of the descending aorta is diagnosed by arteriography, and emergency surgical exploration is indicated in order to accomplish primary repair of the aorta. Failure to diagnose and repair such lesions results in a high likelihood of delayed rupture or development of a large false aneurysm.

Pulmonary contusions may be treated conservatively with the delivery of supplementary oxygen and ventilatory support. Such lesions are usually self-limited, and if oxygenation can be maintained, spontaneous recovery may be expected in 5 to 10 days. On the other hand, myocardial contusions may be much more serious in that the patient may exhibit arrhythmias and diminished cardiac output. Complications of myocardial contusion include cardiac rupture and ventricular aneurysm. Myocardial contusion should be suspected following blunt injury to the chest whenever arrhythmias are detected on the ECG. Frequently, there will be signs of severe myocardial muscle damage with elevation of the creatine phosphokinase (CPK) isoenzymes and elevated ST segments on the electrocardiogram. The most frequent cause of death is the sudden appearance of a ventricular arrhythmia accompanied by conduction blocks. Two-dimensional echocardiography has proven to be of help in the confirmation of significant myocardial contusion. This technique can identify right ventricular dilatation, localized myocardial thinning, and segmental wall motion abnormalities.[15]

Patients with myocardial contusion require hospitalization in a coronary care or intensive care unit with continuous cardiac monitoring. Oxygenation must be maintained and ventricular arrhythmias treated promptly. Since most arrhythmias are ventricular in origin, they may be initially managed with the bolus infusion of 50 to 100 mg. of lidocaine.

ABDOMINAL TRAUMA

Diagnosis

The diagnosis of abdominal trauma is difficult if based on history and physical examination alone. This is particularly true in the case of blunt abdominal trauma or penetrating trauma secondary to stab wounds. Approximately 12 per cent of patients admitted to an emergency room with blunt trauma to the abdomen will present with refractory shock and obviously require urgent abdominal exploration. Between 40 and 70 per cent of patients will exhibit signs of peritonitis, including localized tenderness, abdominal guarding, abdominal distension, and mild hypotension.

These patients require exploration of the abdomen following hemodynamic stabilization.

Of patients with significant intra-abdominal injury, however, 20 to 40 per cent will exhibit equivocal signs, or accurate physical examination is impossible because of neurologic injury or mental obtundation. These patients require further diagnostic investigation to exclude injury to solid organs or hollow viscus if late complications are to be avoided.

Peritoneal Lavage

The most widely used diagnostic technique is peritoneal lavage (described earlier in this chapter). However, recently newer types of radiologic techniques that are highly specific for detecting organ injury have been developed. Some of these should be considered in addition to, or in lieu of, peritoneal lavage in selected patients.

Lavage has proved to be a highly sensitive test for detecting intra-abdominal injury after blunt trauma or stab wounds to the anterior abdomen. The accuracy rate of this diagnostic procedure is approximately 97 per cent, but the test is invasive, nonspecific, and relatively inaccurate in evaluating retroperitoneal or diaphragmatic injury. Moreover, the test is so sensitive that it is estimated that between 6 and 20 per cent of patients with positive results of lavage have, in fact, trivial injuries that would not have required abdominal laparotomy. It seems reasonable to continue a search for an equally accurate, but more specific, method with which to detect significant intra-abdominal organ injury.

Surgical Exploration

At the present time, controversy exists with regard to the necessity for mandatory abdominal exploration in the case of penetrating wounds of the abdomen. Currently, most surgeons believe that penetrating wounds secondary to gunshot injuries should be explored operatively, since it is frequently impossible to detect blast injury imparted by the high-velocity missiles utilizing acute diagnostic studies. Not infrequently, small arteriovenous fistulas, ischemic necrosis of hollow viscus walls secondary to tangential injury, or fragmented defects are overlooked even when other radiologic techniques are utilized in addition to peritoneal lavage. Stab wounds to the anterior abdomen do not necessarily require laparotomy. The stab wound is initially investigated under local anesthesia by local exploration with direct visualization. Following routine preparation of the skin, the surgeon incises the overlying skin beginning at the area of the entrance wound and moving in a direction parallel to the suspected route of the stabbing instrument. If the stab wound does not penetrate the anterior rectus fascia, the wound may be irrigated and closed over a small subcutaneous drain. The patient can then be safely discharged from the emergency room. When penetration of the anterior rectus fascia has occurred, the patient may undergo peritoneal lavage. If the examination of return fluid proves negative, the patient may be admitted to the hospital for observation over the next 12 to 24 hours and subsequently discharged. When peritoneal lavage proves to be positive, the patient should be prepared for emergent surgical exploration. Stab wounds superior to the costal margin, but inferior to the nipples, or stab wounds posterior to the posterior axillary line are best managed by local exploration and immediate laparotomy if the investing fascia has been violated.

RADIOLOGY

With blunt abdominal trauma, other diagnostic modalities may be helpful. However, when additional radiologic studies are ordered, the physician must accompany the patient to the radiologic suite and be prepared to abort further diagnostic testing should the patient exhibit signs of clinical deterioration, necessitating immediate operative intervention.

Most patients with extensive abdominal trauma will require routine roentgenography of the pelvis to rule out the presence of extensive pelvic fractures. Pelvic fractures are often associated with significant retroperitoneal venous bleeding that is best treated by nonoperative means. In general, plain roentgenograms of the abdomen are not indicated, since they are of relatively low sensitivity and lack specificity with regard to diagnosis of abdominal injury. Occasionally, roentgenograms supplemented by contrast may be indicated when diaphragmatic rupture is suspected or the physician is highly suspicious of duodenal or genitourinary injury.

ULTRASOUND

Some physicians have advocated utilizing ultrasonography to survey the abdomen for abdominal injury. However, experience with ultrasonography following blunt abdominal trauma is quite limited and requires the presence of an experienced technician and interpreter. This is a totally noninvasive examination requiring only 10 to 15 minutes to accomplish an entire abdominal screen, but the overall sensitivity of the method is not known at the present time. A further disadvantage to the utilization of ultrasonography is the frequent presence of excessive intestinal gas following abdominal injury that interferes with sonographic investigation.

RADIONUCLIDE SCAN

Radionuclide scanning has also been used for specific diagnostic screening following blunt abdominal trauma. Technetium 99m–labeled colloids are utilized to perform swift, noninvasive isotopic studies of the spleen, liver, or kidney. Such an examination requires approximately 20 minutes and is particularly useful for following patients with previously diagnosed insignificant injury of the liver, spleen, or kidneys.

The drawbacks of radionuclide scanning include the fact that the defects are somewhat nonspecific, and organ infarction, abscess, neoplasm, and pseudocysts frequently appear similar to lesions that could have been caused by the trauma. Furthermore, the method does not detect injuries of nonsolid organs, such as a perforation of the small intestine. Therefore, one cannot accomplish a complete screen of the abdomen for traumatic injury as may be obtained by peritoneal lavage or CT scanning.

COMPUTED TOMOGRAPHY

For the past half decade, CT findings have been more extensively utilized in screening the abdomen following blunt trauma. Computed tomography is highly specific for injuries of the spleen, liver, kidneys, pancreas, duodenum, diaphragm, and retroperitoneum. Many experts at trauma centers in the United States have now suggested that CT should largely replace peritoneal lavage as the method of choice for evaluating blunt trauma to the abdomen. False-negative results can be produced by motion artifacts and,

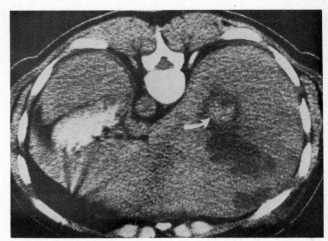

Figure 1. Intrahepatic hematoma resulting from gunshot wound. Irregular plane of low density representing damaged parenchyma and lysed hematoma. High-density focus (arrow) is freshly clotted blood. At laparotomy that preceded the CT scan, a small "nick" was seen on the surface of the liver and the extent of intrahepatic damage was not appreciated. (From Federle, M. P.: CRC Crit. Rev. Diagn. Imaging, 19:257, 1983.)

therefore, the technique is less useful in the inebriated or anxious patient. It should be stressed that if CT scanning is used, peritoneal lavage must not be performed prior to the scanning procedure, since retained lavage fluid may be mistaken for intraperitoneal blood. Likewise, contrast enhancement may be necessary to differentiate hematomas from parenchymal organs, which are relatively isodense. The procedure requires about 20 to 30 minutes and has a 99 per cent accuracy rate when experienced interpreters are available.

The advantages of CT include the ability to visualize the retroperitoneum and to assess the extent of renal damage prior to operative exploration. The technique is not limited by intestinal gas, and it is noninvasive. Its major advantage over peritoneal lavage lies in the fact that it is not only sensitive but is specific for the type and extent of underlying visceral injury (Fig. 1).

Another major advantage is that the amount of intra-abdominal bleeding can be quantitatively assessed and patients with minor solid organ lacerations but with little or no hemoperitoneum may be managed nonoperatively. Abdominal bleeding may be classified as mild or moderate, and these findings may be correlated with clinical assessments. Small hematomas tend to accumulate near the site of origin, whereas free intraperitoneal bleeding is frequently indicated by the accumulation of blood in the pericolic gutters and the pelvis.

The major drawback of CT scanning for detection of intra-abdominal injury is related to institutional facilities and capabilities. A body scanner is required in the immediate vicinity of the emergency room, and expert interpretation of the CT images is required on a 24-hour-a-day basis.

ANGIOGRAPHY

Flush aortography or selective celiac, mesenteric, and renal arteriograms have also been advocated to diagnose specific intra-abdominal organ injury. This methodology reliably detects significant renal, splenic, and hepatic injury and has the additional advantage of estimating tissue viability, since it assesses perfusion of damaged parenchyma. In addition, it is the only diagnostic method that identifies traumatic arteriovenous fistula, arteriobiliary fistula, or pseudoaneurysm. In the case of arteriobiliary fistula, therapeutic embolization may be often accomplished. In addition, angiography will frequently identify arterial pelvic bleeding secondary to severe pelvic fractures. Approximately 18 per cent of patients with pelvic fractures will have identifiable bleeding vessels, usually as a result of laceration of branches of the internal iliac. Approximately 85 per cent of patients with major pelvic bleeding may be successfully controlled with embolization via the arteriographic catheter.[6]

There are contraindications to obtaining abdominal aortograms, including anuria, local infection, allergy to contrast medium, bleeding diathesis, clinical shock, and absence of distal pulses. It must be remembered that angiography is an invasive procedure and therefore has an associated mortality rate of approximately 0.06 per cent and a serious complication rate of 0.4 per cent.[10] Therefore, angiography for blunt abdominal injury is recommended only when it is incidental to needed thoracic aortography and incidental to needed pelvic angiography and when suspected intra-abdominal injury is not diagnosed by the utilization of clinical examination, peritoneal lavage, or computed tomography. In addition, aortography is often diagnostic when intravenous pyelography indicates unilateral nonvisualization of a kidney, since the arteriogram will often differentiate between major renal vascular injury and parenchymal injury.

OTHER TECHNIQUES

None of the diagnostic techniques just described is very helpful in detecting injuries of the genitourinary system. Urethral and bladder injuries are best diagnosed by retrograde urethrography and cystography. A cystogram, as well as an intravenous pyelogram, is indicated when examination of the urine reveals either gross hematuria or significant microscopic hematuria.

Specific Abdominal Organ Injuries

TRAUMATIC RUPTURE OF THE DIAPHRAGM

Traumatic rupture of the diaphragm may be seen after either blunt or penetrating abdominal trauma. It occurs after blunt injury when great force has been applied momentarily to the abdominal cavity. Following blunt injury, the left diaphragm is most frequently ruptured with potential herniation of the stomach, spleen, or colon into the left hemithorax. Loss of integrity of either the left or the right diaphragm should be suspected following penetrating trauma of the upper abdomen or lower chest. When a diaphragmatic rupture is confirmed, associated intra-abdominal injuries should be expected. In a large series of patients with both penetrating and blunt diaphragmatic injury reviewed at the University of Texas Health Science Center in San Antonio, only 8.8 per cent had an isolated diaphragmatic injury.[16]

It is estimated that 3 to 4 per cent of patients surviving serious accidents will exhibit a diaphragmatic rupture. The resulting tear in the diaphragm creates a significant pleuroperitoneal transdiaphragmatic pressure gradient that promotes visceral herniation. Clinical diagnosis by physical examination is seldom possible. Most diaphragmatic ruptures are suspected by examination of a chest film on which the left diaphragmatic leaf cannot be clearly visualized. If gastric herniation has occurred, a large air-filled sac may be present in the left hemithorax, which is devoid of the usual lung markings. If a nasogastric tube is passed into the stomach, it characteristically follows a course through the esophagus into the infradiaphragmatic stomach and then passes back through the diaphragm into the body of the stomach. On occasion, it may be necessary to introduce contrast material into the stomach to demonstrate herniation of the stomach through the diaphragmatic rent. When a patient is seen several days following injury, traumatic rupture of the diaphragm can frequently be confirmed by either real-time sonographic examination or by thoracoscopy. Treatment of the diaphragmatic rupture is usually accomplished by primary repair utilizing non-absorbable sutures. Repair of the defect in the diaphragm may be easily accomplished through either a thoracotomy incision or an abdominal incision. The latter is usually utilized following blunt or penetrating trauma because there is such a high incidence of associated intra-abdominal injury that requires repair.

INJURIES TO THE STOMACH AND SMALL INTESTINE

Penetrating and blunt injuries to the stomach, jejunum, and ileum are relatively easily corrected at surgical exploration. Penetrating injuries require only débridement of the wound edges and simple closure. Occasionally, a number of wounds will be found in the small intestine over a relatively short segment, in which case it may be more efficacious to resect the involved segment and perform a primary anastomosis.

Blunt injuries to the stomach and small bowel are usually secondary to vehicular accidents. Postulated factors for injury include sudden increase in local intraluminal pressure, compression of the small bowel against the vertebral column, and deceleration at or near a point of fixation. The use of lap seat belts has occasionally been responsible for both stomach and small bowel avulsion injuries. The small bowel may occasionally show segments of devascularization secondary to avulsion of the mesentery from the bowel following rapid deceleration. Surgical repair requires the resection of nonviable segments of small bowel and anastomosis of the remaining viable proximal and distal segments. Avulsion injuries of the stomach usually occur near the pylorus at a point where the stomach is anchored by the retroperitoneal duodenum. Such patients may require resection of the distal segment of stomach and re-establishment of bowel continuity via a gastrojejunostomy.

The diagnosis and management of injury to the duodenum are more difficult because of its retroperitoneal position. Duodenal injury occurs in only 3 to 5 per cent of patients undergoing abdominal laparotomy for trauma. Usually, the physical signs and symptoms are unimpressive because of the retroperitoneal location of the organ. Physical examination may reveal slight tenderness with pressure in the right upper abdomen, flank, or back. Frequently, bowel sounds are absent. Peritoneal lavage may not be diagnostic during the first 24 hours following the traumatic incident because of the retroperitoneal location of the duodenum. Plain roentgenograms of the abdomen may show a retroperitoneal accumulation of air along the iliopsoas muscle or the diaphragmatic cura or adjacent to the right kidney. Approximately 15 per cent of patients will exhibit hematemesis or gross blood obtained after passage of a nasogastric tube. The most frequent site of duodenal injury is in the second portion.

At operative exploration, the entire duodenum must be carefully inspected if evidence of retroperitoneal air or hemorrhage is evident. This is accomplished by performing a Kocher maneuver to expose both the anterior and posterior surfaces of the first, second, and third portion of the duodenum. The fourth portion of the duodenum may be inspected by dividing the ligament of Treitz. Operative treatment of duodenal wounds largely depends on the extent of injury to the bowel wall and whether or not there is concomitant injury to the pancreas or the common bile duct.

Perhaps the least significant duodenal injury is the intramural duodenal hematoma leading to intestinal obstruction. This injury is more frequently seen in children and should be suspected when bilious vomiting follows 24 to 48 hours after an episode of blunt abdominal trauma. The diagnosis is confirmed by upper gastrointestinal contrast studies, which reveal a classical "coiled-spring" appearance in the duodenum. Sonography may exhibit echolucencies in the duodenal wall secondary to the hematoma. If coexisting pancreatic injury can be excluded by ultrasound, CT scan, and the absence of amylasemia, most children may be treated conservatively without operative intervention. Nasogastric decompression is accomplished by an indwelling nasogastric tube and the children are begun on total parenteral nutrition. At 5 to 7 days ultrasonography and upper gastrointestinal contrast studies are repeated to confirm improvement in gastric emptying and duodenal transit of gastric contents. If total obstruction still exists or there is subsequent evidence of pancreatic injury, such patients should undergo explorative surgery promptly, at which time the hematoma may be evacuated from the duodenum.

When injuries to the duodenum involve the entire thickness of the bowel wall, a number of operative procedures have been described to accomplish safe repair. The most devastating complication of duodenal repair is breakdown of the suture lines, which results in a lateral duodenal fistula. A complete, isolated tear of the duodenum diagnosed within 24 hours of injury may often be managed by simple primary closure with two layers of sutures. However, if simple closure were to result in significant compromise of the duodenal lumen, alternative means of operative management must be employed. A single-layer closure of the duodenum may be acceptable if it is supported with a serosal patch utilizing a loop of jejunum over the suture line.

Severe duodenal injuries may be treated with pyloric exclusion with simultaneous gastrojejunostomy. In such cases, the duodenal injury is repaired and the duodenum is excluded from the gastrointestinal tract by closure of the pylorus through an anterior gastrotomy. The pylorus is occluded by a running suture of non-absorbable suture or by staples. The gastrotomy through which this procedure is done is then converted to a gastrojejunostomy by anastomosing the stomach to the proximal jejunum (Fig. 2). This procedure allows the duodenum to heal without the passage of gastric acid into the duodenum stimulating pancreatic secretion of enzymes. Even if a fistula results from the duodenal repair, it is now an end fistula rather than a lateral fistula and has a better chance of spontaneously healing following appropriate drainage and conservative therapy with enteral nutrition delivered through a jejunostomy feeding tube.

One might expect a high incidence of marginal ulceration after this procedure, but marginal ulcers have occurred in only approximately 10 per cent of patients undergoing pyloric exclusion and gastrojejunostomy. Such patients may be treated either medically or surgically in the event that marginal ulceration becomes a problem. Because

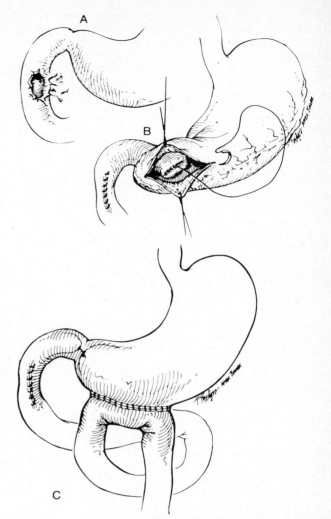

Figure 2. Severe duodenal injury (A) treated by primary repair, gastrotomy, and pyloric exclusion (B). Pylorus is oversewn with running suture. C, Gastrojejunostomy performed at gastrotomy site. (From Martin, T. D., Feliciano, D. V., Mattox, K. L., and Jordan, G. L.: Arch. Surg., 118:632, 1983.)

this procedure is reserved for those with the most extensive isolated injuries to the duodenum, there is a relatively high mortality rate associated with this operation, which ranges from 4 to 22 per cent in various clinical reports.

If significant injury occurs to the duodenum as well as to the head of the pancreas, pancreaticoduodenectomy may be required in order to excise devitalized tissue. Such injuries are relatively rare and are associated with a high incidence of operative mortality (in the range of 35 per cent).

INJURIES TO THE COLON AND RECTUM

Injuries to the colon and rectum most frequently follow penetrating injury of the abdominal cavity. Although blunt abdominal injuries involving the colon and rectum do occur, the liver, spleen, and small bowel are more frequently traumatized in the absence of a penetrating missile. Injuries of the colon and rectum comprise about 5 per cent of blunt intra-abdominal injuries.

Injuries following penetrating injury may be overlooked. It must be remembered that a portion of the ascending and descending colon is retroperitoneal and injuries may therefore not be immediately apparent. Likewise, injuries to the rectum are frequently below the peritoneal reflection and will be missed by intra-abdominal operative exploration if not diagnosed by preoperative endoscopy. All patients with potential rectal injuries should undergo digital examination of the rectum as well as endoscopic inspection to a distance of at least 10 cm. Likewise, the bare areas of the ascending and descending colon must be inspected by reflection of this portion of the colon whenever only one intraperitoneal defect is found on abdominal exploration or whenever the penetrating wound is located in the flank or back. Frequently, these bare areas of the colon will exhibit tangential injuries following stab wounds or gunshot wounds that traverse the retroperitoneum.

There is probably no greater controversy with regard to operative treatment than in the treatment of colon injuries. Management of colon injuries requires considerable clinical judgment and is largely determined by the degree of injury, the presence of other life-threatening associated intra-abdominal injuries, the amount of fecal contamination of the abdomen, and the time lapse between injury and the operative repair. Because these patients have not had preoperative mechanical cleansing of the bowel, most surgeons believe that therapy should be conservative unless the colon injury is minor and there has been little fecal contamination of the abdominal cavity.

Serosal, superficial, or seromuscular tears of the colon that result in no intraperitoneal contamination may be treated by simple suture repair. Isolated injuries of the right colon, without extensive fecal contamination, may be treated by primary resection of the right colon with ileotransverse colostomy. However, when the injury is extensive, when it is associated with other intra-abdominal injuries, or when there exists extensive fecal contamination of the abdomen, more conservative therapy is mandatory. This includes primary repair with exteriorization of the injured colonic segment or excision of the injured colonic segment with the construction of a colostomy or ileostomy with a distal mucous fistula. Injuries of the left colon should be treated by repair and exteriorization, resection with creation of a proximal colostomy and distal mucous fistula, or resection and repair with a completely diverting proximal colostomy. Repair of the colon with exteriorization may allow primary healing with the possibility of returning the colon to the abdominal cavity between 5 and 10 days postoperatively. This technique requires adequate débridement, wide mobilization of the colon so that it can be brought onto the anterior abdominal wall, careful local therapy to the exposed colon in order to keep it moist, and prompt conversion of the exteriorized segment to a colostomy should the wound fail to heal. It should be noted that significant serositis develops in most patients following externalization and the long-term late development of isolated colonic stricture remains a potential risk. If resection of the injured segment with creation of a proximal colostomy and distal fistula is elected, reanastomosis of the colon can usually be accomplished in 4 to 8 weeks.

Injuries of the extraperitoneal rectum require intra-abdominal exploration and creation of a completely diverting colostomy. The distal segment of the sigmoid colon and rectum are then evacuated by lavage with 2 to 3 liters of dilute povidone-iodine solution in order to rid the rectal segment of all particulate fecal matter. The anal sphincter is then dilated and the defect in the rectal mucosa primarily repaired, if possible. Retrorectal suction drains are then inserted through a small incision between the coccyx and the posterior anal wall. Such drains prevent the development of perirectal soft tissue infection and necrotizing fasciitis. Re-establishment of the continuity of the gastrointestinal tract may usually be accomplished at 6 to 8 weeks following the initial injury.[24]

HEPATIC INJURIES

Significant hepatic injury may occur after either penetrating or blunt trauma of the abdomen. In a large series of 443 cases of liver trauma from the San Francisco General Hospital, 42 per cent of the injuries were due to blunt trauma, 32 per cent to stab wounds and 26 per cent to gunshot wounds.[2] Significant injury to the liver usually presents with few localizing signs on physical examination. Hypovolemic shock is not uncommon and may be accompanied by increased abdominal distention as a result of intraperitoneal bleeding from the injured liver. The diagnosis can be confirmed either by abdominal CT scan or peritoneal lavage. Multiple intravenous catheters should be placed in the upper extremity, since large amounts of crystalloid and blood may be required during operation for replacement of exsanguinating hemorrhage from the liver injury.

On entering the abdominal cavity, the surgeon may note brisk bleeding from the right upper quadrant. In such cases, the liver should be encased with large abdominal lap pads and an assistant assigned to compress the liver against the right hemidiaphragm. A brief intra-abdominal exploration is then performed in order to assess associated injuries, which will be present in 80 to 85 per cent of patients. When attention can again be focused on the liver injury, the liver should be carefully inspected to ascertain the degree of parenchymal damage. The liver injury may consist of a simple superficial laceration that is not bleeding, deep lacerations with extensive bleeding, large stellate fractures that involve several segments of the liver, significant arterial disruption with devitalization of one or more segments of the right or left lobe, or avulsion injuries of a lateral segment of the liver parenchyma. If hemorrhage is no longer evident, primary repair of the parenchyma is unnecessary and the abdominal cavity may be closed with drainage of the hepatic defect (in select cases, drainage may not be required). Most surgeons still prefer to drain superficial nonbleeding liver lacerations for 24 to 48 hours to prevent the accumulation of bile, which may temporarily leak from injuries to small biliary ducts. When active bleeding is still present, the hepatic laceration must be explored and hemostasis obtained by individual ligature or the application of stainless steel hemoclips. In a small proportion of cases, bleeding will be so brisk as to interfere with careful exploration of the hepatic laceration. In such cases, temporary hemostasis may be obtained by the Pringle maneuver, in which the hepatoduodenal ligament, including the portal vein, hepatic artery, and common bile duct, is compressed between the thumb and first finger of the operating surgeon. If bleeding is controlled by this maneuver, the surgeon can temporarily place a noncrushing clamp across the hepatoduodenal ligament, thus gaining temporary control of hemorrhage and allowing individual ligation of vessels within the liver parenchyma. If this maneuver is not completely successful in controlling bleeding from the liver injury, a number of alternatives may be considered. The right and left hepatic arteries may be isolated and individually cross-clamped with noncrushing instruments. If this succeeds in gaining hemostasis, the clamps should be serially removed in order to determine the hepatic artery distribution, which is feeding the injured vessels. Either the right or left hepatic artery can be ligated without serious consequences in the human. If continued slow oozing from the hepatic surfaces is still noted, hemostasis may sometimes be accomplished by insertion of a pedicle flap of the greater omentum into a deep liver laceration. If the patient is rapidly deteriorating secondary to hemorrhage, hemostasis may require emergent packing of the injured liver, utilizing intra-abdominal lap pads. The lap pads are brought out through the abdominal wound and gradually removed over the ensuing 48 to 72 hours.

Some patients will exhibit extensive parenchymal damage, excessive bleeding into the liver substance with devitalization of an entire segment or lobe, or injury to the hepatic veins or retrohepatic caval veins with widespread parenchymal liver damage. Such patients frequently require major hepatic resection in order to gain control of hemorrhage. Injury to the hepatic veins is usually associated with brisk hemorrhage from behind the liver when the liver is elevated from the retroperitoneal vena cava. In such cases, the surgeon should consider extending the incision onto the chest by performing median sternotomy. The pericardium is rapidly opened, and a large chest tube may be inserted through the auricle of the right atrium into the inferior vena cava. A side hole is made in the tube at a point that will be positioned just inside the right atrium. Occluding venous tourniquets are then placed around the chest tube just above the entrance of the renal veins into the inferior vena cava and at the intrapericardial portion of the inferior vena cava. A Pringle maneuver is simultaneously performed, thus completing vascular isolation of the liver. The atrial cava shunt allows isolation of the retrohepatic vena cava while at the same time maintaining return of venous blood from the lower portion of the body to the heart. The involved hepatic lobe can then be resected and the injury to the hepatic vein overlying the liver repaired directly.

Mortality following hepatic injury ranges from 3 to 9 per cent, of which approximately 60 per cent is secondary to exsanguination at the time of operation. Most patients can be treated by simple repair and fewer than 10 per cent will require major hepatic resection. Postoperative morbidity, secondary to pulmonary complications and multiple organ failure, is common and requires intensive postoperative critical care.

Late complications of hepatic injury are not uncommon and must be considered when postoperative recovery is prolonged. Intrahepatic abscesses, sterile intrahepatic hematomas, and hematobilia have all been described. In addition, occasional reports of late traumatic, hepatic arteriovenous fistulas with the development of portal hypertension and visceral bleeding have been described. Intrahepatic abscess will require reoperation and drainage. Hepatic arteriovenous fistulas and hemobilia can frequently be detected by selective hepatic angiography, at which time treatment options include selective embolization or operative repair.

Injury to the Pancreas

Because of its retroperitoneal position, injury affecting the pancreas after either blunt or penetrating injury often remains unsuspected. Delay in recognition following blunt abdominal injury often allows the development of local inflammation or systemic sepsis prior to the presentation of acute abdominal signs. Unfortunately, delay in diagnosis is an important factor for the increased morbidity and mortality observed in patients with pancreatic injury. Overall, mortality of such patients is approximately 20 per cent and is often related to the presence of associated injuries of major blood vessels, duodenum, or colon.

Patients with significant injuries of the pancreas may exhibit hyperamylasemia, but most believe there is relatively little correlation between an elevated serum amylase level and pancreatic injury. Diagnosis by peritoneal lavage is often misleading, since hyperamylasemia in the recovered fluid is often not present for 24 to 48 hours because of the retroperitoneal position of the pancreas. Thus, a positive diagnostic peritoneal lavage is helpful, but the absence of red blood cells or increased amylase levels is unreliable in excluding a retroperitoneal injury. Perhaps the best diagnostic test to detect unsuspected pancreatic injury is the abdominal CT scan. Frequently, pancreatic transections or hematomas of the injured pancreas can be detected long before clinical signs are apparent when using this technique.

Treatment

The operative treatment of pancreatic injury is dependent upon the extent of pancreatic trauma discovered at the time of operation. Careful inspection of both the anterior and posterior surfaces of the pancreas is necessary. Patients with simple pancreatic contusion without capsular or ductal disruption and without persistent hemorrhage may be treated by simple drainage using closed-sump suction drains. When major lacerations, fractures, or intraparenchymal hematomas of the body and tail are present, distal pancreatectomy should be performed with salvage of the spleen if technically feasible. The distal pancreatic stump of the remaining pancreas is then oversewn and the transected proximal pancreas closed with interrupted interlocking mattress sutures of non-absorbable suture. Occasionally, the distal stump should be drained into a Roux-en-Y pancreaticojejunostomy if there is severe contusion and edema of the remaining pancreatic head. This procedure is also indicated when patients require a secondary operation after pancreatic injury because of a persistent major pancreatic fistula. Patients with severe hemorrhage or contusion of the head of the pancreas, when it is due to deep lacerations or transections of the proximal pancreas, may be treated by duodenal diverticulization or duodenal diversion as described for duodenal injuries, provided that the main pancreatic duct is uninvolved. In order to determine pancreatic duct injury, a duodenotomy is performed and retrograde cannulation of the ampulla of Vater accomplished. Radiopaque dye may then be injected into the pancreatic duct and examined by intraoperative radiographic examination. Alternatively, intraoperative endoscopic retrograde pancreatography may be performed by an assistant if duodenotomy is contraindicated. If the proximal pancreatic duct or ampulla is injured at a location that precludes reconstruction or if there is combined devascularization injury of both the pancreas and duodenum, pancreatoduodenectomy is indicated. All pancreatic injuries should be drained, and drains should be removed only after feeding has been resumed and the volume of drainage is minimal.

Complications

Postoperative complications of pancreatic injury usually result from inadequate control of leaking exocrine secretion. The patient may develop evidence of pancreatic cutaneous fistulae along drain tracts, pseudocysts, or intra-abdominal abscess formation. Usually, fistulae are relatively minor and transient and persist for less than 4 weeks, provided adequate drainage has been effected.

Pancreatic pseudocysts occur in less than 10 per cent of patients with pancreatic injury and again are often related to inadequate drainage. A persistent pseudocyst may be operatively treated by cystgastrostomy, cystduodenostomy, or cyst Roux-en-Y jejunostomy.

The development of intra-abdominal abscess after pancreatic injury is much less frequent and occurs in approximately 1 per cent of patients with significant pancreatic trauma. Abscess formation usually requires external drainage at a secondary operative exploration following localization by ultrasound or CT scanning.[12]

INJURY TO THE SPLEEN

Splenic injury is most commonly seen after blunt abdominal injury. Patients with major splenic injury may present with mild left upper abdominal tenderness and early signs of hypovolemia. However, it is important to note that, more often than not, such patients do not exhibit frank signs of shock. The injury should be suspected in the patient who exhibits postural tachycardia or hypotension. Fractures of the ribs in the left lower thorax may be present when significant force has been applied to the left upper quadrant. In such patients, diagnosis of left upper quadrant pathology on physical examination is difficult because of pain associated with rib fracture palpation.

Either diagnostic peritoneal lavage or CT scan will reliably detect perisplenic hematomas. At abdominal exploration, the spleen is carefully inspected after division of the lienophrenic, lienorenal, and the lienocolic ligaments. If no other life-threatening complications are encountered on careful abdominal exploration, primary repair of the splenic injury should be attempted. If hemorrhage persists, splenic repair may be accomplished by the placement of interrupted mattress sutures over pledgets, the application of crystalline microcollagen or other hemostatic agents, or a partial splenectomy. Though splenectomy is associated with an increased incidence of post-splenectomy sepsis, splenectomy should be performed promptly if hemorrhage cannot be controlled by more conservative means or if there are other urgent life-threatening injuries that require operative attention. The incidence of post-splenectomy sepsis in splenectomized patients is less than 1 per cent, and such patients can be protected postoperatively by the prophylactic administration of penicillin and immunization with pneumococcal vaccine.

Several pediatric centers have advocated the nonoperative treatment of children with splenic injury whenever possible. Such children are hospitalized and carefully monitored for 10 to 12 days following injury. Fluids and blood components are delivered intravenously to prevent the development of hypovolemia. Spontaneous control of hemorrhage may be documented by performing serial radioactive splenic scans and/or serial CT examination. Upon discharge it is necessary for these children to avoid activities that involve physical contact for a period of 2 to 3 months. This approach to splenic trauma is less enthusiastically endorsed by many pediatric surgeons, since primary splenic repair is usually successful in patients who were previously treated by careful in-hospital observation. Immediate abdominal exploration also avoids the potential of overlooking a serious associated injury.

INJURY TO THE GALLBLADDER AND COMMON BILE DUCT

Perforation of the gallbladder may occur secondary to either penetrating or blunt abdominal trauma. A most important factor predisposing to perforation of the gallbladder following blunt abdominal trauma is the presence of a distended gallbladder. The organ may be distended because of either fasting or alcohol ingestion in normal patients or secondary to obstruction of the cystic duct in patients with cholelithiasis. Usually, the diagnosis may be suspected in patients with signs of peritoneal irritation on physical examination and hypotension that cannot be explained by blood loss. The peritoneal lavage fluid will contain bile. Injuries to the gallbladder, whether due to penetrating or blunt trauma, are best treated by cholecystectomy.

Injuries to the extrahepatic biliary tree are far more difficult to diagnose. Such patients frequently exhibit delayed symptoms of peritonitis. Tangential injuries of the extrahepatic biliary tract are not uncommon following penetrating trauma. Such injuries may be managed by surgical débridement and primary suture closure with T tube drainage of the common duct. Over 90 per cent of patients suffering significant injury to the common bile duct following blunt abdominal trauma will exhibit complete transection of the common duct at a point where the common duct enters the pancreas. An attempt at primary anastomosis of such ducts usually results in postoperative ductal stenosis, since the ducts have not been dilated as a result of distal obstruction. The performance of a biliary enteric anastomosis, i.e., between the proximal common duct and a Roux-en-Y loop of jejunum, is more successful in the treatment of such complete transections.

GENITOURINARY TRAUMA

Urologic injury should be suggested by the presence of either gross or microscopic hematuria, blood appearing at the urinary meatus, anuria or dysuria, fractures of the pubic arch, and the presence of a high-riding prostate on rectal examination. Inability to pass a Foley catheter into the bladder with ease should suggest the possibility of posterior urethral disruption.

The presence of microscopic or gross hematuria requires that the patient be further evaluated by limited intravenous pyelogram in order to diagnose significant genitourinary tract injury. Intravenous pyelography is particularly valuable in the individual who exhibits flank pain, pelvic fractures, or low rib fractures.[7] If it is impossible to easily catheterize the urinary bladder through the urethra or if there is blood at the meatus of the penis, a retrograde urethrogram and cystogram should be obtained following the completion of the IVP. Intravenous pyelography should be performed in patients with penetrating trauma and significant microscopic hematuria, even though abdominal exploration is anticipated. The objective in performing an IVP is to demonstrate that there are bilateral functioning renal units. When one or the other kidney does not appear to function, aggressive further diagnostic evaluation with CT and renal artery angiography is indicated. Computed tomography is a noninvasive method that clearly separates minor injuries from major injuries and provides valuable information for proper management in the operating room.[14] Renal artery angiography will differentiate between the presence of damage to the renal pedicle and renal agenesis. Furthermore, the angiogram may diagnose the development of arterial venous malformations or fistulas and significantly outlines the anatomy of the vascular tree to each kidney.

Therapeutic Management

Management of penetrating injuries to the kidney is usually relatively straightforward. Minor parenchymal injuries may be easily treated with débridement, suture hemostasis, and simple drainage. When significant parenchyma has been devitalized, partial nephrectomy may be necessary. In less than 10 per cent of cases nephrectomy is necessary. When approaching the retroperitoneal space following penetrating injury, it is important to control the renal pedicle along the aorta in order to gain proximal control of the renal artery and vein prior to opening Gerota's fascia. If proximal control is gained prior to inspection of the kidney, temporary occlusion will frequently allow primary repair of a badly injured kidney (Fig. 3).

After blunt abdominal injury, IVP, CT scan, and renal angiography may confirm only minor renal injury without associated intra-abdominal injury. Such patients may frequently be managed nonoperatively and a nephrectomy performed later only if secondary hypertension or other significant complications develop. However, if diagnostic studies confirm the presence of a shattered kidney, a renal pedicle injury, or cortical laceration with disrupted fragments, early surgical intervention may allow salvation of part of the functioning renal parenchyma. Postoperatively, patients need to be regularly monitored in order to diagnose the late development of hypertension, which has been documented as late as 10 years after injury.

Renal Vascular Injury

Vascular pedicle injuries are particularly difficult to manage. Most patients with renal pedicle injuries will eventually develop hypertension and require a nephrectomy even if primary repair is successful. Retrospective analysis of a large series of patients with renal vascular injuries at the Parkland Memorial Hospital suggested that revascularization of an acute renal artery thrombosis is almost always unsuccessful.[22] However, isolated renal vein injuries can frequently be repaired. Renal salvage was accomplished in only 10 per cent of patients with renal artery injury. Therefore, it is now felt that revascularization of traumatic occluded renal arteries should be attempted only when

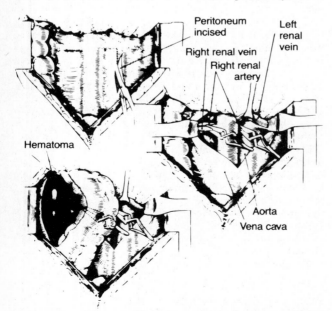

Figure 3. The midline approach to the renal pedicle is illustrated. (From Guerriero, W.: Symposium on genitourinary trauma. Urol. Clin. North Am., 4(1):7, 1977.)

there are bilateral renal injuries. The success rate of repair of the renal vascular pedicle is almost zero at 12 to 18 hours after the injury. Thus, if vascular repair is to be attempted, the diagnosis must be promptly confirmed and the patient should undergo urgent exploration.

Ureteral, Bladder, and Urethral Injury

Ureteral injuries usually result from penetrating wounds. Successful repair depends on prompt recognition of this injury, since fistulas and stricture formation are the inevitable sequelae of a misdiagnosis. If the ureter is not actually severed, it may be drained with or without the presence of an internal stent. When laceration of the ureter is present, primary repair should be done after resection of the damaged segment. An oblique primary anastomosis can frequently be accomplished over an indwelling silastic catheter stent. When the injury is found near the bladder, ureteroneocystostomy may be performed utilizing a nonrefluxing anastomosis tunneled under a bladder flap. It is rare that the damage to the ureter is so severe that primary anastomosis cannot be accomplished, and consideration must then be given to performing a ureteroureterostomy utilizing the opposite intact ureter.

Trauma to the bladder most often accompanies pelvic fractures. The diagnosis is confirmed by retrograde cystogram. Extravasation can usually be seen following maximal distention of the bladder by instillation of contrast material. Whether the injury is extraperitoneal or intraperitoneal, it can usually be treated with wound débridement and closure in two layers. The bladder is then decompressed for 5 to 6 days with either a Foley catheter or suprapubic cystostomy.

Posterior uretheral disruption should be treated initially by percutaneous cystostomy. This allows drainage of the bladder. Secondary repair of the posterior urethral disruption is performed later. The patient is re-evaluated at 6 weeks following the injury, and if urinary continuity is demonstrated with the presence of stricture, a urethrotomy can be performed with a high success rate. If complete disruption remains and there is no urinary continuity, surgical correction of the defect can be performed 3 months following the injury. Anterior urethral injuries are more uncommon, but may result from penetrating missiles or following a straddle injury. Clinically, it is relatively easy to diagnose because there is marked swelling and discoloration of the penis and perineum. These patients may have extensive damage to the spongiosum of the urethra. Early surgical exploration is indicated with mobilization of the urethra and excision of the injured segment with reanastomosis.

VASCULAR TRAUMA

Arterial or venous injury following penetrating or blunt trauma is not uncommon and frequently demands priority with regard to diagnosis and operative treatment. Failure to appreciate even minor arterial injury may lead to the late development of false aneurysm formation or arteriovenous fistula. The diagnosis of vascular injury is dependent upon a high degree of suspicion when external injury occurs in the vicinity of major blood vessels. Although the presence of continued external hemorrhage or the development of a large hematoma may accompany major arterial or venous injury, such classic findings are often absent despite transection of a large vessel.

Physical signs of ischemia of a distal extremity should indicate a high probability of major arterial injury. Absent or weak distal pulses, loss of sensation, and inhibited motor function all may be appreciated in the severely ischemic extremity. However, it should be emphasized that the presence of palpable pulses does not exclude proximal arterial trauma. The vessel may not be circumferentially injured, and pulsations may be transmitted through totally occluded distal vessels. Some series have shown that palpable distal pulses may be appreciated in 25 per cent of cases with proven vascular trauma. The utilization of Doppler ultrasound may be of assistance in detecting the presence or absence of a pulse wave in the swollen extremity. However, the presence of a *pulse wave* does not, in itself, ensure adequate blood flow, although the measurement of systolic *pressure* in distal arteries, utilizing the Doppler ultrasound, may be helpful in estimating the adequacy of distal extremity perfusion. Careful auscultation over an injured extremity is essential in order to detect bruits, which are often indicative of arteriovenous fistula or false aneurysm.

Radiologic Diagnosis

Arteriography remains the single best method for diagnosing arterial injury. Any abnormality of the intima is suggestive of arterial injury and mandates operative exploration of the vessel, providing proximal and distal control of the vessel can be accomplished. However, angiography is an invasive procedure requiring radiologic expertise. Therefore, it is not required when there are clear indications for operative exploration of the vessel or when the patient is hemodynamically unstable. In such cases, arteriography may be performed in the operating room at the time of surgery, if necessary, to delineate obscure injury.

Operative Therapy

The operative approach to most injuries of major vessels encompasses a number of management principles. Preliminary hemostasis should always be accomplished by simple compression. The use of arterial tourniquets or blind application of vascular clamps should be avoided in order to prevent occlusion of blood flow through collateral vessels and inadvertent iatrogenic injury to the ends of transected vessels. Operative exploration should be prompt to avoid irreversible injury to distal muscle and nerves, both of which are particularly susceptible to acute ischemia. Irreversible soft tissue damage is frequently observed after 4 to 6 hours of severe ischemia and, thus, operative repair should be accomplished as soon as possible following diagnosis.

In the operating room, large areas of the external surface of the patient should be prepared with a standard surgical antimicrobial soap solution. It may be necessary to extend initial incisions a significant distance in order to gain proximal and distal control of the injured vessel. In addition, the surgical team must be cognizant of the potential necessity for harvesting vein grafts to repair arterial injury. Thus, appropriate skin preparation of a non-injured extremity should be performed so that such vein grafts may be easily harvested. Preoperative prophylaxis with antibiotics is required in order to decrease the potential for wound infection or infection of synthetic material utilized to repair major arteries. Intraoperative systemic anticoagulation is usually contraindicated unless the patient is known to have isolated vascular trauma. Patients with multisystem trauma often exhibit a consumptive coagulopathy that may be exaggerated by systemic anticoagulation. Following proximal and distal control of the injured vessel, some surgeons may infuse the distal arterial tree with a heparin-saline solution in order to prevent distal intravascular coagulation if a prolonged delay in arterial repair is contemplated.

The initial incision should be generous so that non-injured proximal and distal portions of the vessel can be identified and controlled prior to entering the hematoma around the site of injury. If distal control cannot be easily attained because of the anatomic location of the injury, control of back bleeding may be accomplished by insertion of a Foley catheter intraluminally with inflation of the balloon of the catheter when the catheter has been positioned distal to the injury.

After ensuring proximal and distal control, the hematoma surrounding the vessel must be carefully removed from the injured portion of the vessel and the artery or vein carefully inspected. Even though the artery may remain intact, the presence of a contusion of the arterial wall usually indicates underlying intimal damage and the subsequent development of an intimal flap with late arterial occlusion. All devitalized tissue must be removed, even if this débridement results in a significant gap between the proximal and distal ends of the vessel that will not permit end-to-end anastomosis.

Several alternatives are available to accomplish arterial or venous reconstruction. Lacerations of major arteries or veins may frequently be repaired by simple closure with a continuous vascular suture. If this technique would result in significant stenosis of the lumen, a small patch may be sewn to the lacerated edges of the vessel utilizing either autologous vein or synthetic material. If complete transection of the vessel has occurred, the vessel may be repaired by direct end-to-end anastomosis, providing the suture line is not under excessive tension. Should a significant portion of the artery require resection, either a synthetic interposition graft must be inserted or a venous graft may be fashioned utilizing the greater saphenous vein from the lower extremity or the cephalic vein from the upper extremity. In general, such grafts should be taken from a non-injured extremity because concomitant venous trauma with subsequent phlebothrombosis of deep veins may occur, in which case the saphenous vein may be required for venous return during the postoperative period. When major intra-abdominal vascular injury has occurred in combination with injuries to the gastrointestinal tract, great care must be taken to prevent infection of the vascular reconstruction. The insertion of synthetic materials should be avoided in such patients, and if end-to-end anastomosis cannot be accomplished, serious consideration should be given to interruption of the aorta or iliac arteries with the simultaneous performance of an extra-anatomic reconstruction. Extra-anatomic reconstruction with synthetic material may be accomplished by anastomosing the axillary artery to the femoral artery via a subcutaneous route or by performing a femorofemoral cross-over graft at the level of the symphysis pubis.

Arterial and venous injuries are commonly associated with major fractures when the vessels are proximal to the bone. For instance, fractures of the distal femur may be associated with injuries to the popliteal artery. If rapid reduction and fixation can be accomplished, it is particularly helpful in protecting the integrity of the vascular repair. When the vascular repair must be accomplished prior to fixation of the fracture, it is necessary for the surgeon to protect this anastomosis during manipulation of the fracture segments.

At the conclusion of the procedure, an operative arteriogram should be obtained prior to closure of the incision. In this way, distal embolization or thrombosis may be appreciated and embolectomy with a Fogarty catheter may be accomplished. Distal run-off is particularly important to guarantee flow through the repaired vessel over a prolonged period of time following arterial reconstruction.

Whenever distal ischemia of soft tissue is suspected, serious consideration should be given to the performance of fasciotomies at the conclusion of the procedure in order to avoid compartment syndrome. Fasciotomy should be considered in patients with evidence of sensory or motor dysfunction and in patients exhibiting severe crush injury. The necessity for postoperative decompression of muscular compartments should also be considered when there has been a preoperative delay of more than 4 to 6 hours, intraoperative severe hypotension or shock, or a concomitant injury to a major vein.

Penetrating Neck Trauma

Penetrating wounds of the neck are particularly worrisome because so many major vascular structures pass through the neck to supply the intracerebral circulation. Previously, it had been customary to explore all wounds of the neck that penetrated the platysma muscle in order to exclude injury to the carotid vessels and the jugular veins. However, mandatory exploration of the patient with no clinical signs of injury results in a very high negative exploration rate approaching 90 per cent. During the past decade, many groups have advocated selective management of patients with penetrating wounds to the neck in order to decrease the frequency of an entirely negative neck exploration.

To accomplish this, the neck is divided into three anatomic zones. Zone 1 is considered that level below the cricoid cartilage; Zone 2, the level of the neck between the cricoid cartilage and the angle of mandible; and Zone 3, that area of the neck above the angle of mandible. Symptomatic patients with clinical signs of hemorrhage or expanding hematoma, dysphagia, hematemesis, dysphonia, hoarseness, hemoptysis, subcutaneous emphysema, or neurologic deficit require immediate operative exploration. Injury to a major structure of the neck is usually present in over 90 per cent of such patients. Ancillary studies in this group of patients are utilized only to help plan an operative approach, particularly when the injuries occur in Zone 1 or Zone 3. However, when the patient remains asymptomatic, diagnostic ancillary procedures may allow observation alone and obviate the necessity for operative intervention. Injuries in Zone 1 may be evaluated by chest roentgenogram, arteriography (aortic arch and four-vessel angiography), and fluoroesophagography. Since injuries in Zone 2 are rarely occult, an *asymptomatic* patient with penetrating trauma in this area may be serially observed. Should there be clinical suspicion of an injury in the neck involving the pharynx, esophagus, or trachea, a lateral neck film may reveal air in the soft tissues. Injuries in Zone 3 require arteriography to identify internal carotid artery lesions that occur very high in the neck near the entrance of the carotid artery into the skull. Arteriography helps to identify those patients in this group who are best managed by arterial ligation, extracranial-intracranial bypass or simple anticoagulation.

Injury to the Brachiocephalic Vessels

Injuries of the subclavian artery most frequently are associated with penetrating trauma. Since the artery lies behind the clavicle, there are often associated injuries of the ribs, clavicle, brachial plexus, and lung.[1] The presence of a bruit over the artery, together with hematoma formation and a pulse deficit in the distal artery, is highly suggestive of subclavian artery injury, although the extensive collateral arterial network of the shoulder may allow enough blood flow to the extremity to prevent signs of distal ischemia.

Exposure of the brachiocephalic vessels may be difficult. The right subclavian, innominate, and proximal right carotid arteries are best exposed through a median sternotomy with extension of the incision into the right part of the neck. If adequate exposure of the distal subclavian vessel cannot be obtained by this approach, the medial portion of the clavicle may be resected. Additional exposure can be obtained by adding an incision in the third interspace anteriorly, allowing rotation of a flap (including the sternum and ribs) that is reflected laterally to expose the vessel.

The left subclavian and left proximal common carotid arteries may be exposed through a left anterior third interspace thoracotomy. The second and third portions of the subclavian artery can frequently be visualized following resection of the medial portion of the clavicle.

Isolated Venous Injury of the Lower Extremity

If both major arterial and venous injuries of the lower extremity are present, the arterial repair should be given the highest priority. When possible, major veins should be repaired also, providing that the patient is hemodynamically stable and that there is no significant additional life-threatening injury. If an isolated venous injury is present in the lower extremity, every effort should be made to repair the injury utilizing lateral suture repair, end-to-end anastomosis, venous patch graft, or nonreversed saphenous vein graft. The management of injured major veins by simple ligation frequently results in severe venous stasis, intractable edema, and potential tissue nonviability. Although postoperative phlebothrombosis is not uncommon following major venous repair, long-term disability from venous stasis is less frequent compared with patients who undergo venous ligation. Increased venous patency may be improved by temporarily increasing venous flow through the injured portion of the vein by performing a distal (temporary) arteriovenous shunt.

Arterial Injuries Associated with Lower Extremity Fracture

Since the arterial and venous conduits of the lower extremity are intimately associated (from an anatomic standpoint) with the posterior aspect of the distal femur and tibia, fractures of the distal femur, as well as dislocations of the knee, frequently result in significant vascular injury. After institution of resuscitative measures to correct volume deficits and provide adequate oxygenation, the fracture should be splinted and reduced if possible. Immediately following stablization of the fracture, the pulses should be examined by palpation and Doppler pressure. When vascular injury is suspected, angiography should be performed immediately. Femoral artery injuries usually may be repaired by resection of nonviable vessels with subsequent end-to-end anastomosis or insertion of a reversed saphenous vein graft. Injury to the popliteal vessel usually requires the insertion of a saphenous vein graft because a considerable distance of the artery is frequently injured. If injury has occurred to the arteries distal to the popliteal trifurcation, patients may be managed selectively. In most patients distal viability will be maintained if at least one of the three major arteries remains patent and the ankle:brachial artery pressure ratio exceeds 0.5. Fasciotomy may be required if early signs of a compartment syndrome are recognized.

If recognized, femoral artery injuries are easily repaired with excellent results and few amputations. Because there is frequently a diagnostic delay following popliteal artery disruption, subsequent amputation has been required in approximately 18 to 25 per cent of patients.[5] Since injuries to vessels distal to the popliteal trifurcation are frequently associated with severe comminuted fractures, extensive soft tissue defects, and heavy contamination, revascularization attempts are associated with only a 25 per cent success rate. Such patients frequently require the utilization of musculocutaneous flaps or transfer of free flaps from remote areas in order to obtain soft tissue coverage of the vascular repair.

Orthopedic stabilization of the fracture may be accomplished by external skeletal fixation, although immediate internal fixation has been advocated in selected cases when there is no serious associated injury and when contamination is minimal. Unfortunately, the presence of associated nerve deficits, as well as significant soft tissue injury, often prevents normal postoperative function, even when vascular reconstruction efforts have been successful.

SNAKE ENVENOMATION

Snake envenomation accounts for significant morbidity and mortality in the United States annually. The treatment of patients suffering snakebite consists primarily in the timely administration of antivenom. Wound débridement as primary therapy, without the administration of antivenom, is associated with a 16 per cent incidence of significant wound complication.

The symptoms and signs of progressive envenomation include nausea, emesis, hypesthesia, fasciculation, hypotension, oliguria, and hemorrhage. Hemorrhage frequently follows the development of a consumption coagulopathy and the development of disseminated intravascular coagulation (DIC). The degree of envenomation may be semiquantitatively graded from 0 to 4, as described by Parrish. An initial dose of intravenously administered antivenom may be predicted utilizing this grading system, and the dosage may be supplemented with additional antivenom when persistent abnormal symptoms or signs are noted or when the coagulation profile remains abnormal. Usually, antivenom administration may be completed within 24 hours following the injury, although as many as 100 vials of antivenom may be necessary in the most severely injured patient. The most frequent complication is the later development of serum sickness.

ANTITETANUS PROPHYLAXIS

All injured patients should be evaluated for the adequacy of protection against tetanus. It should be recalled that men over the age of 60 and women over the age of 40 are often not protected against tetanus, since they may never have been fully immunized or they may not have received necessary booster doses of tetanus toxoid. Antitetanus prophylaxis is extraordinarily important, since the case fatality rate of tetanus remains at approximately 50 per cent.

Protective levels of antibody are frequently found in fully immunized individuals for 10 or more years after their last booster dose. Thus, patients should not receive unnecessary tetanus prophylaxis, since this not only leads to unnecessary expense, but may result in allergic responses. Patients with a risk of tetanus may be treated either actively or passively utilizing tetanus toxoid or human tetanus immunoglobulin. The evaluating physician must estimate the risk of the subsequent development of tetanus based on contamination of the wound and the presence of ischemic or nonviable tissue. In general, patients who have been fully immunized and who have received a tetanus toxoid booster within the past 5 years do not require further antitetanus treatment, regardless of the extent of injury. Likewise, no treatment is required in the fully immunized patient who has received a tetanus toxoid booster 5 to 10 years previously if the wound is not tetanus prone. If such a patient has any risk of tetanus, as determined by wound examination, tetanus toxoid should be administered. Tetanus toxoid should also be administered to all patients who have previously been fully immunized and who have not received a tetanus toxoid booster during the past 10 years. If the patient gives a history of incomplete immunization or gives an uncertain history, human tetanus immunoglobulin should also be administered when the physician believes that the wound is at moderate risk for harboring anaerobic organisms, including those responsible for the subsequent development of tetanus.

SUMMARY

The treatment of traumatized individuals has markedly improved over the past several decades as a result of better prehospital care and additional efforts to establish in-hospital protocol to ensure efficient triage, diagnosis, and treatment of life-threatening injuries. A thorough knowledge of the principles elucidated in this chapter will allow the physician, regardless of level of specialization, to provide emergency care, utilizing a set of priorities to ensure maximal survival, as well as optimal restoration of function.

SELECTED REFERENCES

Federle, M. P.: CT of abdominal trauma. CRC Crit. Rev. Diagn. Imaging, 19:257, 1983.
This monograph is edited by an authority well known for his pioneering efforts in utilizing the CT scan as a diagnostic aid in the study of trauma at the San Francisco General Hospital. The author utilizes excellent artist drawings to define the anatomy viewed on subsequent CT scans, allowing the nonradiologist to easily recognize intra-abdominal injury. Characteristic trauma, as seen by CT, of the liver, spleen, pancreas, duodenum, colon, and kidney is illustrated.

Hryshko, F. G. and Deeb, Z. L.: Computed tomography in acute head injuries. J. Computed Tomog. 7:331, 1983.
These authors have summarized the characteristic alterations of CT scans after a variety of head injuries. The review is beautifully illustrated and emphasizes important diagnostic points in assessing the patient with closed head injury by CT. All types of cranial fractures and intracranial hemorrhage are examined.

Robbs, J. V. and Baker, L. W.: Cardiovascular trauma. Curr. Prob. Surg. 21:1, 1984.
This monograph by two senior cardiovascular surgeons reviews diagnos-

tic and therapeutic considerations for a variety of cardiovascular injuries. Both intrapericardial wounds and peripheral vascular injuries are examined. The authors have outlined the pathophysiologic alterations that follow vascular trauma and concisely outline a diagnostic and management plan for each injury. They document the success of their therapeutic protocols by presentation of clinical outcome from their own experience, which is obviously extensive.

REFERENCES

1. Busuttil, R. W. and Acker, B.: Management of injuries to the brachiocephalic vessels. Surg. Gynecol. Obstet., *154*:737, 1982.
2. Carmona, R. H., Lim, R. C., Jr., and Clark, G. C.: Morbidity and mortality in hepatic trauma: A 5–year study. Am. J. Surg., *144*:88, 1982.
3. Daffner, R. H., Gehweiler, J. A., Jr., Osborne, D. R., and Roberts, L., Jr.: Computed tomography in the evaluation of severe facial trauma. Comput. Radiol., 7:91, 1983.
4. Espersen, J. O., and Petersen, O. F.: Computerized tomography in patients with head injuries: Assessment of outcome based upon initial clinical findings and initial CT scans. Acta Neurochir., *65*:81, 1982.
5. Flint, L. M., and Richardson, J. D.: Arterial injuries with lower extremity fracture. Surgery, *93*:5, 1983.
6. Gilliland, M. G., Ward, R. E., Flynn, T. C., Miller, P. W., Ben-Menachem, Y., and Duke, J. H., Jr.: Peritoneal lavage and angiography in the management of patients with pelvic fractures. Am. J. Surg., *144*:744, 1982.
7. Guice, K., Oldham, K., Eide, B., and Johansen, K.: Hematuria after blunt trauma: When is pyelography useful? J. Trauma, *23*:305, 1983.
8. Gundry, S. R., Williams, S., Burney, R. E., Cho, K. J., and MacKenzie, J. R.: Indications for aortography in blunt thoracic trauma: A reassessment. J. Trauma, *22*:664, 1982.
9. Han, W. S., Kaufman, B., Alfidi, R. J., Yeung, H. N., Benson, J. E., Haaga, J. R., El Yousef, S. J., Clampitt, M. E., Bonstelle, C. T., and Huss, R.: Head trauma evaluated by magnetic resonance and computed tomography: A comparison. Radiology, *150*:71, 1984.
10. Jones, T. K., and Walsh, J. W.: Diagnostic imaging in blunt trauma of the abdomen. Surg. Gynecol. Obstet., *157*:389, 1983.
11. Kobayashi, S., Nakazawa, S., and Otsuka, T.: Clinical value of serial computed tomography with severe head injury. Surg. Neurol., *20*:25, 1983.
12. Linos, D. A., King, R. M., Mucha, P., Jr., and Farnell, M. B.: Blunt pancreatic trauma. Minn. Med., March 1983. p. 153.
13. Livoni, J. P., and Barcia, T. C.: Fracture of the first and second rib: Incidence of vascular injury relative to type of fracture. Radiology, *145*:31, 1982.
14. McAninch, J. W., and Federle, M. P.: Evaluation of renal injuries with computerized tomography. J. Urol., *128*:456, 1982.
15. Miller, F. A., Jr., Seward, J. B., Gersh, B. J., Tajik, A. J., and Mucha, P., Jr.: Two-dimensional echocardiographic findings in cardiac trauma. Am. J. Cardiol., *50*:1022, 1982.
16. Miller, L., Bennett, E. V., Jr., Root, H. D., Trinkle, J. K., and Grover, F. L.: Management of penetrating and blunt diaphragmatic injury. J. Trauma, *24*:403, 1984.
17. Quinn, S. F., and Smathers, R. L.: The diagnostic significance of posttraumatic sphenoid sinus effusions: Correlation with head computed tomography. J. Comput. Tomogr., *8*:61, 1984.
18. Popovsky, J.: Perforations of the esophagus from gunshot wounds. J. Trauma, *24*:4, 1984.
19. Post, M. J. D., Green, B. A., Quencer, R. M., Stokes, N. A., Callahan, R. A., and Eismont, F. J.: The value of computed tomography in spinal trauma. Spine, 7:417, 1982.
20. Stanley, R. B., Jr.: Value of computed tomography in management of acute laryngeal injury. J. Trauma, *24*:359, 1984.
21. Tabaddor, K., Danziger, A., and Wisoff, H. S.: Estimation of intracranial pressure by CT scan in closed head trauma. Surg. Neurol., *18*:212, 1982.
22. Turner, W. W., Jr., Snyder, W. H., III, and Fry, W. J.: Mortality and renal salvage after renovascular trauma; A review of 94 patients treated in a 20–year period. Am. J. Surg., *146*:848, 1983.
23. Van Dongen, K. J., Braakman, R., and Gelpke, G. J.: The prognostic value of computerized tomography in comatose head-injured patients. J. Neurosurg., *59*:951, 1983.
24. Vitale, G. C., Richardson, J. D., and Flint, L. M.: Successful management of injuries to the extraperitoneal rectum. Am. Surg., *49*:159, 1983.

SURGICAL COMPLICATIONS

JAMES A. SCHULAK, M.D. • ROBERT J. CORRY, M.D.

14

The goal of all surgical procedures is to either cure the patient of disease or palliate him. However, complications may follow even a successful procedure and, when severe, may cause serious disability or even death. In the vast majority, surgical complications are transient problems and, while causing temporary concern, can be successfully managed. This is especially true if the complication is recognized early and appropriate measures to resolve it are expedited. Moreover, many complications can be predicted prior to their occurrence because of circumstances of either the patient's illness or the operation.

The aim of this chapter is to review a variety of complications encountered following operations. Emphasis will be placed on both recognition of the signs and symptoms of surgical misadventure and an understanding of the resultant pathophysiologic abnormalities so that appropriate remedial measures can be taken.

After completion of a surgical procedure it is essential to *monitor* the patient for signs indicative of a complication, including fever, tachycardia, dyspnea, hypotension, oliguria, jaundice, abdominal distention, and excessive pain. Mental status changes, such as anxiety, confusion, somnolence, stupor, and coma, are also very important. Since most surgical complications are manifested by one or more of these signs, it is imperative that the clinician not only understand the pathophysiology of these responses but be equally familiar with the more common complications specifically associated with the changes that occur. A brief summary of these signs and their causes is shown in Table 1.

POSTOPERATIVE FEVER

An elevation in temperature is frequently observed following operation. However, it is not necessarily indicative of a serious complication. For example, fever may be due to atelectasis, mild transfusion reaction, dehydration, drug therapy (especially penicillin and cephalosporin antibiotics), or phlebitis at the site of an intravenous line. In all of these situations, however, the patient's temperature rarely exceeds 38 to 38.5°C., and fever of a greater degree often signals the presence of a more serious condition. Although infections such as pneumonia, cystitis, intraperitoneal abscess, central venous nutrition (CVN) line contamination, and wound sepsis are the most common causes of fevers greater than 38°C., other equally significant postoperative complications should be considered. These include

hyperthermia induced by anesthesia, deep vein thrombophlebitis, pulmonary embolism, myocardial infarction, acalculous cholecystitis, and pancreatitis. Finally, it should be remembered that fever may be a component of the patient's underlying disease and as such is not indicative of a postoperative complication. Common examples include metastatic or lymphoproliferative malignancies and hyperthyroidism.

Etiology

Since the etiology of postoperative fever is quite variable, an organized approach is necessary in establishing a diagnosis. The type of operation performed as well as the time course of fever appearance may be helpful in reducing the list of possible causes. For example, atelectasis more commonly occurs in the early postoperative period, whereas wound infections usually become manifest 4 to 5 days later. There are exceptions, making preconceived concepts misleading. As an illustration, casual attribution of early post-

TABLE 1. *Physical Signs and Symptoms of Surgical Complications with Common Associated Conditions*

Sign	Associated Conditions
Fever	Atelectasis, transfusion reactions, drug therapy, infections, thrombophlebitis, pulmonary embolism
Tachycardia	Anxiety, hypovolemia, hypoxemia, fever, cardiac arrhythmia, sepsis, pain
Tachypnea and dyspnea	Anxiety, atelectasis, pneumonitis, pulmonary edema, pulmonary embolus
Hypotension	Hypovolemia, sepsis, cardiac failure, anaphylaxis
Oliguria	Hypovolemia, renal failure, urinary tract obstruction
Jaundice	Hemolysis, hepatitis, sepsis, central venous nutrition, biliary tract obstruction, biliary fistula
Abdominal distention	Paralytic ileus, intra-abdominal hemorrhage, bowel obstruction, constipation
Wound pain	Infection, dehiscence
Change in mental status	Hypoxemia, sepsis, drug therapy, alcohol withdrawal, stroke, fever, postoperative psychosis

operative fever to atelectasis without careful inspection of the wound may lead to a consequential delay in the diagnosis of a streptococcal or clostridial wound infection that may occur within the first 24 hours after operation. It is necessary, therefore, to evaluate each patient thoroughly with a complete physical examination and review of the clinical situation.

Evaluation

The most common postoperative fever is of pulmonary origin from either atelectasis or pneumonitis. Accordingly, inspection of the patient's breathing pattern and auscultation of the lungs are essential components of the initial fever workup. Routine chest films, however, are not advocated unless physical signs of pneumonia are present or the fever persists despite institution of measures designed to re-expand the lungs following atelectasis.[9] Blood cultures should be obtained as part of the initial evaluation in all patients with a fever above 38.5°C. Positive cultures may be the first indication of an intra-abdominal abscess, generalized sepsis, or central venous line infection. Since urinary tract infection is the most frequently encountered nosocomial infection, removal of a urinary catheter alone can arrest the fever.

Additional laboratory tests are indicated in immunosuppressed patients, such as those receiving cancer chemotherapy and organ transplant recipients on immunosuppressive therapy, since the variety of possible infections in these patients is great. Fungal, parasitic, and viral infections are common in this group, thus warranting inclusion of the appropriate culture and serologic analyses in their work-up. In addition, fever may be the first sign of allograft rejection in transplant patients, as is discussed in Chapter 15.

Wound Infection

Wound infection remains an important cause of postoperative fever and patient morbidity; therefore, examination of the wound is also a mandatory component of a postoperative work-up for fever. As suggested earlier, wound sepsis can be present within 24 hours following operation if the causative organisms are streptococci or clostridia. Infections that are due to the latter are extremely serious, e.g., clostridial myonecrosis (gas gangrene) can develop rapidly with grave consequences. More commonly, however, fever resulting from wound infection usually occurs after the fourth postoperative day, as a somewhat longer incubation period is necessary for the frequently causative endogenous enteric gram-negative or exogenous staphylococcal contaminants to reach significant levels. Early in the postoperative course, the fever may be of low grade, being associated with simple cellulitis. As the septic process progresses with development of a subcutaneous abscess, the fever pattern may change to one of high-degree daily spikes, such as would be seen with an intra-abdominal abscess. Tenderness, erythema, edema, crepitation, and purulent discharge are hallmarks of this latter stage of wound infection and, with few exceptions, indicate the need for immediate surgical drainage. Although antibiotic therapy may be useful in treating wound cellulitis, unless systemic sepsis is present, such therapy is generally of little value after adequate débridement and drainage have been accomplished. A more extensive consideration of wound infection, prevention, and antibiotic prophylaxis is presented in Chapters 8 and 11.

MENTAL STATUS ABNORMALITIES

Changes in mental status following operation are of particular concern to the patient, the family, and the surgeon. Variable presentations include failure to awaken following operation, somnolence, confusion, disorientation, agitation, convulsions, and coma. These may follow physiologic abnormalities that affect the brain, such as hypoxia, hypoglycemia, uremia, elevated blood ammonia, and the like. Similarly, mental status may be altered by various "overdoses" of drugs, such as narcotic analgesics, tranquilizers, and cimetidine in the elderly. Specific intracranial lesions can also cause disorders of consciousness and orientation. Those more commonly observed in the postoperative period include strokes, septic emboli, and brain abscesses as well as unrecognized injuries in victims with multiple trauma.

Failure to Awaken Following Operation

Failure to awaken after anesthesia is most often due to transient failure to recover rapidly from the anesthetic agents administered during the operation and is usually self-limited. A cerebrovascular accident, however, must be considered in all patients with preoperative carotid bruits, those undergoing operations in whom the carotid artery was occluded, and in those with significant hypotensive periods either before or during the operation. Computed tomographic (CT) scans have become most useful in making an early diagnosis of this complication. More commonly, agitation and anxiety are encountered in the immediate postoperative period. Fortunately, simple explanations and solutions, such as pain, discomfort from indwelling endotracheal and nasogastric tubes, or inability to empty a full bladder, are often readily apparent. Agitation and anxiety may also be due to either arterial hypoxemia or intra-abdominal hemorrhage, both of which require expedient evaluation and appropriate intervention. Pharmacologically induced somnolence may occur in narcotized elderly patients, especially those with renal failure. Fortunately, this complication is easily reversed with naloxone. Some patients may develop hallucinations after administration of either meperidine or, more commonly, pentazocine and will improve after being changed to a different parenteral analgesic agent.

Disorientation

Agitation or disorientation that occurs several days after operation is more likely to be due to metabolic disorders. Diabetic patients frequently develop either hyperglycemia, which when severe enough can blunt cognition, or insulin-induced hypoglycemia, with its subsequent somnolence or coma. Because untreated hypoglycemia is more injurious to the brain than hyperglycemia, rapid intravenous infusion of dextrose is indicated in all diabetic patients who suddenly become unconscious. Diagnosis is confirmed by their reawakening within minutes of the infusion and by an abnormally low (less than 50 mg. per 100 ml.) blood glucose value from a sample drawn just prior to dextrose administration.

Similarly, sudden cessation of hypertonic intravenous nutrition may lead to hypoglycemic coma owing to the persistent pancreatic release of insulin. The latter can be obviated by use of a tapering regimen when CVN is no longer necessary or by the peripheral infusion of 10 per cent dextrose when central venous lines suddenly fail. Patients receiving CVN for prolonged periods may also develop tremulousness and agitation due to hypocalcemia and hypomagnesemia. Hypocalcemia is also a common complication of parathyroidectomy and thyroidectomy, especially in patients who have undergone a subtotal parathyroid resection for renal osteodystrophy. Severe "bone hunger" may result in difficult to manage calcium homeostasis abnormalities for several days to weeks after operation. Conversely, hypercalcemia may induce a state of somnolence or coma and is more commonly encountered in patients with metastatic neoplasia. Intravenous hydration with saline and induction of diuresis with furosemide or ethacrynic acid are the first lines of therapy in such patients, whereas use of corticosteroids, mithramycin, and ethylenediaminetetraacetic acid (EDTA) should be reserved for those in deep coma or with life-threatening cardiac arrhythmias.

Delirium Tremens

Alcoholic patients may manifest a withdrawal syndrome as a result of the sudden cessation of alcohol. The symptoms range from mild agitation and tremors to complete disorientation with hallucinations and convulsions. This syndrome, known as *delirium tremens,* may be accompanied by hyperpyrexia, dehydration, and even adrenal insufficiency and requires immediate medical attention. Intravenous hydration as well as measures to reduce fever should be instituted. Sedation should be induced with agents such as chlordiazepoxide, thorazine, paraldehyde, or chloral hydrate. Mechanical restraints should be used if necessary. Rarely, intravenous alcohol may be used in patients who are difficult to control. Deficiencies in vitamin B and magnesium are involved in the pharmacology of this syndrome; therefore, these nutrients should be added to the therapeutic regimen. Convulsions are treated with anticonvulsant agents such as barbiturates, magnesium sulfate, and diphenylhydantoin. Prophylaxis of delirium tremens may be the best treatment and continuance of alcoholic beverages in moderation postoperatively may be appropriate in selected patients.

Psychiatric Disturbances

Psychiatric disturbances after operation are frequently seen in elderly patients, patients undergoing cardiac operation, those experiencing prolonged stays in an intensive care unit (ICU), and in patients with cancer. In regard to the latter, this complication presents primarily as apathy and depression, especially in those who have experienced a major alteration in anatomy, such as mastectomy, colostomy, and limb amputation. Frequently, elderly patients lose orientation at night and become confused or even combative with medical personnel. This syndrome, commonly referred to as "sundowning," may be explained by the loss of familiar surroundings and supportive family.

Treatment consists of reassurance from both the surgeon and nursing staff. Attempts at reorienting such patients with frequent nursing visits and exposure to radio and television are often helpful. In addition, family should be encouraged to spend as much time as possible with the disoriented elderly patient, as this may help to allay their temporary paranoia. Occasionally, use of restraints is necessary to prevent the patient from hindering his care by the disruption of intravenous lines, drains, and monitoring devices. Tranquilizing agents, however, should be used cautiously in the elderly, as they may not only be the cause of some forms of "postoperative psychosis" but have the potential to precipitate respiratory and hemodynamic failure.

"ICU-itis"

Hallucinations, disorientation, and delirium are also frequently encountered in patients who are in an ICU-type setting. Although metabolic factors (e.g., hypoxia and electrolyte disturbances) are sometimes implicated in the development of this "ICU-itis," environmental factors, such as complete loss of chronologic orientation, as well as complete dependence upon nursing personnel also play major roles in its etiology. As with the elderly, constant reassurance, physiologic recovery, and transfer from an ICU with continuous activity usually suffice to correct the disorder. It should be remembered that patients with a history of psychiatric disturbances prior to operation, although often temporarily improved during the immediate postoperative period, are prone to exacerbations during convalescence.

Somnolence

Finally, sudden disorientation or somnolence may be the first sign of occult sepsis. Often the patient has undergone an intestinal resection and anastomosis without apparent sequelae. Five to seven days later, the first sign of trouble may be a mental status change that precedes development of the usual signs of peritonitis because of anastomotic disruption or abscess. In such patients, failure to readily find a metabolic cause for the problem warrants a thorough search for occult infection.

INFECTION

Infection following operation on either the thoracic or abdominal cavity may range in severity from simple wound cellulitis to life-threatening abscess and septicemia. Wound cellulitis and infection have been discussed earlier in this chapter and in more detail in Chapters 8 and 11. Although wound sepsis certainly adds to patient morbidity, it rarely is a cause of death. Conversely, major postoperative intraabdominal and intrathoracic infections greatly increase patient morbidity, cost of care, and mortality. These types of infections present as either well-localized abscesses or generalized peritonitis or mediastinitis. If not recognized early and dealt with definitively, they are frequently the cause of systemic sepsis and its most dreaded sequela, *multiple organ failure.* Therefore, expeditious diagnosis and appropriate intervention are mandatory. However, diagnosis needs to be accurate, as an unnecessary operation in search of occult sepsis may be just as detrimental to the patient's recovery as is delayed necessary surgery.

General Considerations

PHYSICAL FINDINGS

The diagnosis of major postoperative infections is determined by numerous factors, including physical findings, particularly fever and pain, as well as laboratory data, especially the leukocyte count and differential analysis. In addition, a high index of suspicion relating to the operation performed is important. Fever, especially of low grade, is common postoperatively and is usually attributed to atelectasis. However, a temperature elevation above 38.5°C. that occurs 4 to 5 days or later after operation should be considered to be caused by infection until proven otherwise. Leukocytosis is usually present for several days following operation owing to demargination of the intravascular white cell pool, but this value should return to normal within several days. In contrast, leukocytosis occurring later, especially with fever and a predominance of immature cellular forms (a left shift), is very likely indicative of an infection and requires investigation.

FEATURES OF THE OPERATION

Another major consideration in making the diagnosis of postoperative infection is the personal knowledge of the surgeon relative to the features of the operation. For example, patients who have undergone extirpation of a perforated viscus with widespread peritoneal soilage or those who have a less than perfect bowel anastomosis are at greater risk for an intraperitoneal abscess than those with a clean peritoneal cavity and a flawless surgical procedure. Radiologic evaluation using ultrasonography, CT, and isotopically tagged leukocyte scintigraphy is often very successful in demonstrating even the smallest of abscesses and, as such, is extremely beneficial as an adjunct to expert clinical acumen. Moreover, ultrasonography and CT may provide such accurate localization of the abscess as to allow relatively safe direct percutaneous catheter drainage, thus obviating the need for reoperation in selected cases.[10]

Intra-abdominal Infection

Intra-abdominal infections may present as either an abscess or generalized peritonitis. The morbidity varies immensely, depending upon both the type and the extent of infection and ranges from spontaneous rectal drainage of a pelvic abscess after appendectomy to generalized multimicrobial fecal peritonitis following complete disruption of a bowel anastomosis. Nevertheless, therapeutic principles are constant irrespective of the type of infection. An accurate diagnosis must be made, and expedient evacuation of pus with adequate dependent drainage must be achieved. The causative factors should be corrected, such as with resection or exteriorization of a perforated viscus. Finally, judicious use of systemic antibiotics is indicated in the treatment of an abscess when accompanied by systemic sepsis and in all patients with generalized peritonitis. Antibiotic therapy (discussed in Chapter 11) should be as specific as possible, thus emphasizing the importance of cultures of the evacuated pus. Until such data are available, however, the antibiotic regimen chosen should be of broad spectrum, including coverage for aerobic gram-negative enteric bacteria as well as anaerobic bacteroides species.

ABSCESS

Intraperitoneal abscesses occur most commonly in both lower quadrants and the pelvis. However, they may occur at any site in the peritoneal cavity[2] (Fig. 1). Common procedures leading to this complication are appendectomy and colon resections, especially with low colonic anastomoses. Pelvic abscess is even more probable if sepsis was present at operation, as with perforation of the appendix or a sigmoid colon diverticulum. The patient may have a complete recovery in the immediate postoperative period,

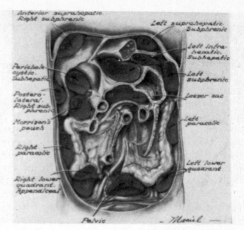

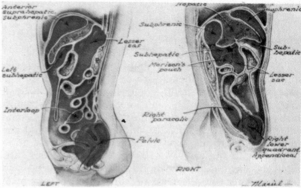

Figure 1. Locations of intra-abdominal abscesses. (From Welch, C. E., and Hardy, J. D.: Advances in Surgery, Vol. 5. Chicago, Year Book Medical Publishers Inc., 1971, p. 305.)

without typical signs such as intermittent spiking fevers, chills, leukocytosis, or pelvic pain until a week or more after operation. Malaise that lingers and is without apparent explanation is often associated with a later diagnosis of an abscess. Simple digital rectal and vaginal examination suffices to establish the diagnosis by the presence of a tender mass either on the side of the operative procedure or in the pelvis. Confirmatory evidence may be gained by demonstration of a fluid-filled mass on an ultrasonogram or CT scan. If low, the abscess may be drained through the rectum or, in females, through the vagina. Alternatively, a small lower abdominal incision may be necessary to completely evacuate larger pelvic collections.

Subphrenic and Subhepatic Abscesses

Subphrenic and subhepatic abscesses are more common following operations on upper abdominal organs. Systemic signs and systems include those described earlier as well as upper abdominal fullness and flank, pleuritic, or shoulder pain. The diagnosis may be suggested on plain upright chest x-ray films by a pleural effusion on the side of the abscess, an elevated hemidiaphragm, the presence of air bubbles or an air-fluid level beneath the diaphragm, or an anterior displacement of the gastric air shadow. Subphrenic abscesses are usually demonstrated best by CT. When CT is not available, these abscesses can also be demonstrated, on combined lung and liver-spleen scintigraphy, by a widened space between the visceral images being revealed. Drainage of subphrenic abscesses may be accomplished through either an extraperitoneal or intraperitoneal approach, with extraperitoneal drainage being attempted most frequently either posteriorly through the bed of the twelfth rib (Fig. 2) or, especially with suprahepatic abscesses, anteriorly using a subcostal but extraserosal incision. When multiple abscesses or persistent visceral leakage is suspected (or in the obese), an intraperitoneal approach is often indicated.

Subhepatic abscesses may be encountered after operations on the biliary tract or the duodenum. Caution should be taken in interpreting ultrasonograms of this region, since many patients develop a benign uninfected subhepatic fluid collection following right upper quadrant operation that does not require drainage. Although surgical drainage of subphrenic and subhepatic abscesses is widely practiced, the CT scan or ultrasonographic approach to percutaneous catheter aspiration is often successful and may obviate the need for reoperation.

Other Intraperitoneal Abscesses

Other intraperitoneal abscesses include those loculated by the omentum and/or visceral surfaces as well as those in the solid organs. These may be multiple and difficult to image owing to their small size, requiring laparotomy for definitive diagnosis. The recent development of leukocyte scintigraphy provides a helpful technique in the diagnosis of intra-abdominal abscess of the interloop type. Patients with an interloop abscess may present with localized signs of pain and tenderness as well as partial bowel obstruction in addition to the usual systemic findings. When such abscesses are single and near the fascial surface, direct percutaneous aspiration may be possible. Laparotomy, however, with wide exploration and débridement of the

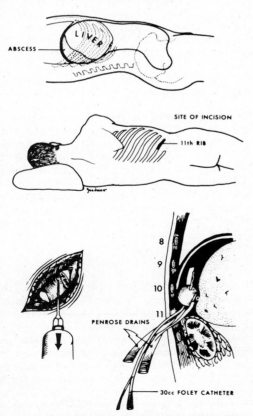

Figure 2. Posterior drainage of subphrenic abscess. (From Sabiston, D. C., Jr. (Ed.): Davis-Christopher Textbook of Surgery, 12th ed. Philadelphia, W. B. Saunders Company, 1981, p. 427.)

peritoneal cavity, is often necessary to achieve complete resolution. Visceral abscesses most commonly occur in the liver, but may also be present in the spleen, pancreas, kidney, and female adnexae. They should be suspected when the development of specific organ dysfunction, such as jaundice (liver), thrombocytosis (spleen), or hyperglycemia (pancreas), presents in conjunction with systemic signs of sepsis. Visceral abscesses are usually best demonstrated by CT scanning.

PERITONITIS

Generalized peritonitis in the postoperative period usually follows peritoneal sepsis at the original operation or following anastomotic breakdown. The latter is classically encountered 5 to 7 days after operation and should be considered in any patient with unexplained tachycardia, fever, change in mental status, and abdominal pain. The diagnosis is often based on clinical findings but may be confirmed by demonstration of extravasation using water-soluble contrast (Gastrografin) radiography in patients with upper gastrointestinal or colonic anastomosis. The diagnosis of small intestinal perforation by use of contrast roentgenography is difficult unless controlled infusion enteroclysis is employed. Conversely, careful use of paracentesis may be helpful in demonstrating the presence of bile, leukocytes, amylase, food particles, or bacteria in the aspirated fluid, as such findings strongly suggest the diagnosis of perforation.

Anastomotic Breakdown

With anastomotic breakdown, reoperation is urgently necessary. The anastomosis can be revised in some patients when the disruption involves either the small bowel or stomach. However, in the presence of widespread contamination, especially with colonic leaks, exteriorization of the bowel with fecal diversion is preferred. In addition, all quadrants of the peritoneal cavity should be thoroughly cleansed with copious saline irrigation. Some also recommend the use of antibiotic irrigation and extensive débridement of purulent layers on the peritoneum surfaces; however, the latter practices are controversial.

Perforation

Postoperative spontaneous perforation of the bowel is a rare event with a clinical picture similar to that seen with an anastomotic leak. This complication, which generally is secondary to an occult intraoperative injury such as a serosal tear or electrocautery burn, also requires immediate operative repair. Some bowel injuries and anastomotic leaks, however, may develop an enterocutaneous fistula without generalized peritonitis or abscess formation. Although operative intervention may ultimately be necessary in some patients, these fistulas can at times be managed successfully without operation. The bowel may be placed at rest by instituting CVN and allowing the fistulas to heal spontaneously. Fistulas that develop in ischemic or irradiated bowel, that are associated with the presence of a foreign body, or that occur in a loop of bowel that is either obstructed distally or involved with malignancy, are unlikely to close without a surgical procedure.

Intrathoracic Infections

Postoperative infection in the thorax can occur in the lung itself (such as pneumonia and pulmonary abscesses) or in the pleural space or mediastinum.[18] Incomplete or inappropriate therapy of pulmonary infections, especially those caused by *Staphylococcus* or *Klebsiella,* may lead to parenchymal necrosis and development of a lung abscess. Cavitation and abscess formation often follow tuberculous or fungal infection as well as pneumonias secondary to aspiration. The diagnosis of lung abscess is primarily made by roentgenographic examination in conjunction with clinical manifestations of infection. Therapy consists of long-term administration of antibiotics, with accurate identification of the causative organisms and their sensitivity to the various antibiotics. When aspiration is the causative factor, antibiotic coverage for *anaerobic* organisms is mandatory. Whereas chest physiotherapy and postural drainage may be sufficient to effect spontaneous drainage in many patients, bronchoscopic evacuation of the abscess may ultimately be necessary in others. Occasionally, operation is indicated for lung abscess when symptoms persist, when thick-walled abscesses do not resolve, when the lesion cannot be distinguished from malignancy, or with development of severe hemoptysis. In these situations, lobectomy is the procedure of choice.

Empyema

Empyema is a collection of pus in the pleural space and may occur following any thoracic operation, especially potentially contaminated procedures such as lobectomy for abscess, esophageal resection and anastomosis, or exploration for penetrating chest trauma. Postpneumonectomy pleural space infections are encountered occasionally. When empyema follows pulmonary resection, the presence of a bronchopleural fistula must also be considered. Diagnosis of empyema is made by aspiration of pleural fluid or pus. Therapy usually consists of prolonged drainage by a chest tube, often requiring placement of more than one tube to ensure adequate drainage. Simple aspiration, however, may be effective if the effusion is due to transdiaphragmatic contamination of an established intra-abdominal infection, providing the latter is also being drained. In addition, systemic administration of antibiotic therapy is indicated in all patients with pleural space infections, whereas intrapleural instillation may be necessary for postpneumonectomy empyema. Operative intervention for empyema is reserved for those with multiple loculations that cannot be adequately drained by tube thoracostomy and those who develop a thickened pleural peel that inhibits reexpansion of the lung. In such instances, débridement and decortication are performed as well as limited pulmonary resection of any destroyed lung.

Mediastinitis

Mediastinitis is one of the most dreaded postoperative complications, as it frequently leads to death. It is most commonly observed following esophageal operations in which intraoperative contamination results from spillage of enteral contents or in which an anastomotic leak develops. Esophageal perforation following endoscopy or dilatation procedures is also a common cause of this infection. Rarely, mediastinitis may occur following "clean" cardiac procedures and is almost always due to intraoperative contamination. As with other closed space infections, the clinical course may be one of rapid deterioration with progression to shock and respiratory insufficiency, emphasizing the need for prompt recognition and therapy.

Early signs of mediastinitis include fever, tachycardia, leukocytosis, and chest pain. Subcutaneous emphysema may also be evident if proximal esophageal perforation or anastomotic disruption has occurred. The diagnosis is strongly suggested by the presence of hydropneumothorax or air-fluid levels in the mediastinum on chest film. Confirmatory evidence for esophageal injury can be obtained by extravasation of contrast media on Gastrografin swallow. Broad-spectrum antibiotic therapy and nasogastric aspiration may suffice for treatment of small esophageal perforations due to an endoscopic accident. However, prompt operative intervention with drainage and repair of the esophageal defect is usually indicated for other cases of mediastinitis as well as those initially treated nonoperatively if resolution does not occur promptly.

PULMONARY INSUFFICIENCY

Pulmonary insufficiency is probably the most common physiologic complication observed in the postoperative period. Its incidence is dependent not only on patient characteristics, including age, personal habits, and intrinsic disease, but on the clinical course during and after operation. Predisposing factors clearly associated with development of postoperative pulmonary compromise include old age, poor nutritional status, a history of smoking, existence of either obstructive or restrictive pulmonary disease, operations of long duration, especially those employing thoracoabdominal incisions, sepsis, a stay in the ICU, and failure of other major organ systems. The morbidity resulting from pulmonary complications is varied and ranges from the transient asymptomatic fever of mild atelectasis to the adult respiratory distress syndrome (ARDS). Fortunately, the signs and symptoms of pulmonary complications are not subtle, and early diagnosis, based on the presence of tachypnea, dyspnea, fever, cough, anxiety, auscultatory abnormalities, blood gas alterations, and chest film findings, is readily made.

General Considerations

The primary role of the lung is to provide gas exchange with the uptake of oxygen, its transfer to the red blood cell, and the subsequent elimination of carbon dioxide. Although clinical criteria are helpful in assessing the quality of this process, laboratory evaluations are essential if accurate diagnosis and treatment of pulmonary insufficiency are to be effective. Arterial gases are more representative of the actual state of respiration and are more easily interpreted; therefore they should be used when possible in preference to venous samples.

Intrapulmonary Factors

Three important values are the partial pressures of oxygen (P_{O_2}) and carbon dioxide (P_{CO_2}) as well as blood pH. Several major factors often influence P_{O_2} levels, including the concentration of inspired oxygen (FI_{O_2}), ventilatory mechanics, including respiratory rate, tidal volume, and dead space, and imbalance in ventilation and perfusion. The latter, commonly referred to as intrapulmonary shunting, is of critical importance in the management pathogenesis of ARDS.

The normal P_{O_2} ranges from 80 to 100 torr, and values greater than 100 torr indicate inspiration of oxygen in a concentration greater than that of room air. It is not necessary to achieve such high values therapeutically, how-

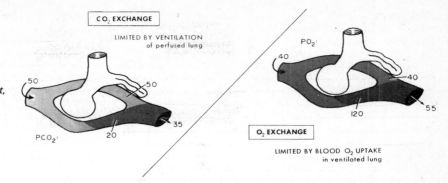

Figure 3. Intrapulmonary shunt. (From Bartlett, R. H.: Surg. Clin. North Am., 60:1325, 1980.)

ever, because with values above 95 torr hemoglobin is already fully saturated with oxygen. Interpretation of low Po_2 values, on the other hand, requires knowledge of the Pco_2 as an index of the ventilatory state and of the FIO_2. For example, a low Po_2 with a high Pco_2 and adequate FIO_2 suggests inadequate ventilation. In this situation, improving ventilation by increasing either the tidal volume or rate of breathing may both decrease the hypercarbia and improve oxygenation.

Conversely, a low or normal Pco_2 (40 torr or less) and a high FIO_2 (greater than 40 per cent) indicates a significant problem with gas exchange at the alveolar-capillary level. This usually follows poor ventilation (either due to atelectasis or pulmonary edema) of perfused alveoli with the subsequent development of an intrapulmonary shunt (Fig. 3). Appropriate therapy would initially include increasing the amount of oxygen available for exchange by raising the FIO_2.

DECREASED CARDIAC OUTPUT

In addition to intrapulmonary factors, decreased cardiac output can also contribute to a fall in arterial Po_2 by further decreasing oxygen saturation of venous blood. In patients with an intrapulmonary shunt, the significant contribution to arterial Po_2 made by the residual oxygen concentration of venous blood is thus eliminated.

VENTILATION

Interpretation of Pco_2 values is less complicated in that it is primarily influenced by *ventilation*. A normal Pco_2 concentration is approximately 40 torr, and significantly greater values suggest the presence of inadequate ventilation. Hypoventilation might be observed normally in nonintubated patients with obstructive pulmonary disease or in those who are intubated with mechanical ventilation with either an inappropriately slow breathing rate, low tidal volume, or excessive dead space. Values for Pco_2 are best interpreted in concert with those for pH, since not only does carbon dioxide concentration affect pH, but its value may also indicate whether appropriate respiratory compensatory mechanisms are functioning in the presence of metabolic disorders. For example, the normal physiologic pH ranges from 7.38 to 7.41. Lower values indicate acidosis, which, if accompanied by a high Pco_2 (greater than 40 torr), suggests hypoventilation as the cause. Similarly, an alkalotic pH in conjunction with low Pco_2 is also indicative of a respiratory cause, in this case overventilation. Discordance from these relationships, especially in the case of a low pH and normal to low Pco_2, suggests either inability of the respiratory mechanism to compensate for a metabolic disorder, as is observed with early ARDS, or, more ominously, a metabolic acidosis too severe for correction by alterations in respiratory mechanisms.

SPIROMETRY

To preoperatively evaluate a patient's ventilatory status and better understand the use of mechanical ventilation in the postoperative period, familiarity with the basic principles of spirometry is essential. A schematic spirogram showing the subdivisions of lung volumes is depicted in Figure 4. These volumes can be either measured directly or extrapolated through use of routine pulmonary function studies. In addition, functional parameters, such as determining the fraction of forcibly expelled air in 1 second (forced expiratory volume, or FEV_1), can be measured and, in conjunction with blood gas analysis data, used to complete the preoperative pulmonary assessment. Restrictive lung disease caused by obesity, pulmonary fibrosis of any etiology, or thoracic cavity immobility due to a chest wall deformity will be manifested by a reduced vital capacity. Obstructive pulmonary disease is predicted by an FEV_1 that is less than 80 per cent and an elevated Pco_2. Knowledge of these parameters in addition to the patient's preoperative baseline blood gas analysis data is essential before embarking on thoracic procedures, especially those that include pulmonary resection. Moreover, with such data predictions can be made regarding the patient's potential for developing postoperative respiratory difficulties following any type of surgical procedure.

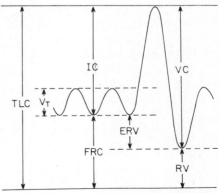

Figure 4. Lung volume subdivisions. TLC = Total lung capacity; V_T = tidal volume; IC = inspiratory capacity; FRC = functional residual capacity, i.e., lung volume at end-expiration; ERV = expiratory reserve volume; RV = residual volume, i.e., lung volume after forced expiration from FRC; VC = vital capacity, i.e., the maximal volume of gas inspired from RV. (From Sabiston, D. C., Jr. (Ed.): Davis-Christopher Textbook of Surgery, 12th ed. Philadelphia, W. B. Saunders Company, 1981, p. 2036.)

Atelectasis

ETIOLOGY

Atelectasis, defined as either incomplete expansion of or collapse of all or part of the lung, occurs to some degree in all patients who undergo operation. The etiology of atelectasis is variable but includes bronchial mucous plugs, extrinsic compression from hemopneumothorax, and simple alveolar hypoventilation, of which the latter is by far the most common. This occurs because of the decreased tidal volume or "shallow" breathing that is often precipitated by incisional pain during the first several days after operation. The resultant reduction in functional residual volume of the lung predisposes to closure of the lower bronchi, thereby creating the typical pattern of basilar atelectasis. Atelectasis of this type occurs more frequently in elderly patients and smokers as well as those who are obese and those who have a reduced functional residual capacity (FRC).

Three additional factors that predispose to the development of atelectasis in the postoperative patient include a supine position for prolonged periods (this also reduces FRC), ventilation with gas high in oxygen concentration (oxygen is more readily absorbed from obstructed alveoli, thus allowing alveolar collapse to occur sooner), and a reduction in pulmonary surfactant following an operation (this substance normally lines the alveolar membranes and is essential for reduction of the surface tension necessary to maintain normal lung volume). Patients with atelectasis may present with tachypnea and anxiety due to mild hypoxia, but infrequently do they have dyspnea. More commonly, the primary manifestation of atelectasis is a low-grade fever.

TREATMENT

The treatment of atelectasis is directed toward re-expansion of the lungs, which usually results in rapid resolution of the symptoms. This can be accomplished by early postoperative ambulation. Walking not only allows fuller diaphragmatic excursion and, therefore, better lung expansion than can be achieved in a reclining position; it also increases FRC, which in itself reduces atelectasis. Of particular importance in patients who are not ambulatory, pulmonary re-expansion can also be induced by use of breathing and coughing exercises. Expensive bedside devices, such as incentive spirometers and blow bottles, have been used, but many question their real value, and better results can be achieved by repeated encouragement from the medical and nursing staff for the patient to simply breathe deeply and cough at hourly intervals. Conversely, use of intermittent positive pressure breathing (IPPB) devices for the treatment of atelectasis is not advised, as their efficacy is not proven.

Of equal therapeutic importance with improving breathing mechanics in the treatment of atelectasis is the provision of adequate analgesia. It should be remembered that patients do not become addicted to narcotics by using these agents for several days, but they can develop significant morbidity if adequate pulmonary toilet is not maintained, especially when coughing is avoided because of postoperative pain. Atelectasis that is progressive and accompanied by dyspnea or increasing fever may be due to a major mucous plug. The diagnosis is confirmed by demonstration of lobar collapse on chest x-ray, as illustrated in Figure 5.

Treatment may be initiated with aggressive chest physiotherapy but may require bronchoscopy for extrication of

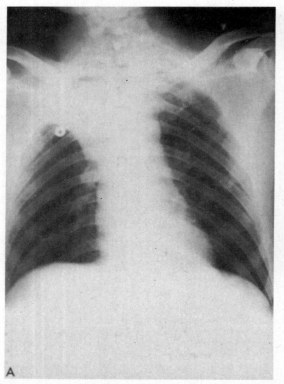
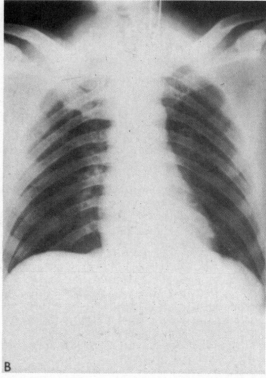

Figure 5. Pulmonary atelectasis. A, Before bronchoscopy. B, After bronchoscopy. (From Sabiston, D. C., Jr., and Spencer, F. C. (Eds.): Gibbon's Surgery of the Chest, 3rd ed. Philadelphia, W. B. Saunders Company, 1976, p. 181.)

the plug and re-expansion of the collapsed segment of lung. Fever of greater than 38.5°C that does not readily resolve with the previously mentioned measures in a tachypneic or dyspneic patient should never be attributed to simple atelectasis. Radiologic evaluation is immediately warranted in such patients, as either a pneumonia or complete lobar collapse may be present. Blood gas analysis is also indicated, since the presence of severe arterial hypoxia suggests the development of either ARDS or a pulmonary embolus (diagnosis and treatment of this major pulmonary complication is considered in detail in Chapter 42).

Pneumonia

Postoperative pneumonia, although not causing pulmonary insufficiency as defined by ventilator dependency or even development of major oxygenation deficiency, nevertheless represents a common form of postsurgical pulmonary complication. Pneumonia developing in a postoperative patient is by definition a nosocomial infection and has a greater potential for morbidity and mortality.[20] Nosocomial pneumonias rank only behind urinary tract infection and intravenous cannula site phlebitis in frequency of occurrence and are especially common in surgical patients. The incidence of this complication has been estimated at between 2 and 17 per cent in surgical patients, depending upon the presence of various risk factors. These include old age, presence of underlying pulmonary or cardiovascular disease, previous pneumonia, a smoking history, long preoperative hospitalization, thoracic or upper abdominal incisions, immunosuppressive therapy (either prophylactic for transplantation or antineoplastic chemotherapy), and, most important, the necessity for ventilatory support, especially with prolonged intubation. Although increased patient morbidity and hospital stay are almost certain consequences of this complication, the risk of death also has a high probability (28 to 57 per cent in one study).[20]

PATHOGENESIS

The pathogenesis of postoperative pneumonia includes contamination of the lungs through aspiration, inhalation, or lymphohematogenous spread of the causative organism from other infected sites in the patient. Of these potential pathways, aspiration is the most common mechanism. Nasogastric and endotrachial intubation, frequently required after operation, enhance the possibility of aspiration by interfering with the normal defense mechanisms of swallowing, coughing, and gagging. Owing to stringent policies regarding the maintenance of ventilatory equipment, direct contamination of the airspace from inhalation of bacteria in the ventilator itself is rare. Nevertheless, this possibility needs to be considered in all ventilated patients with pneumonia, especially those in an ICU where other pneumonias have been diagnosed. Finally and of less likelihood is the lymphohematogenous spread of organisms from other sites of infections, such as the bladder, wound, or abscess. Irrespective of the portal of entry for contaminating bacteria in the postoperative patient, a situation favorable for the development of pneumonia exists owing to a temporarily altered immune response in many surgical patients.

DIAGNOSIS

The diagnosis of postoperative pneumonia is generally straightforward and is based upon the presence of specific signs and symptoms of fever, tachypnea, cough, rales, or consolidation on pulmonary auscultation and sputum production. Chest roentgenography is mandatory in initial evaluation of all patients with suspected pneumonia, as it may not only confirm the presence of pneumonitis but also may aid in the determination of etiology. For example, demonstration of lobar consolidation suggests a bacterial cause, interstitial infiltrates suggest a viral cause, and other patterns, such as patchy consolidation, are indicative of pneumonia due to *Legionella pneumophila.* Radiologic evaluation, however, may be of little value in diagnosing pneumonia in the patient with concomitant ARDS, as the bilateral "white lungs" in this situation often obscure further delineation of pulmonary disease.

Confirmatory evidence is obtained through isolation of a culture-proven pathogen, which requires the collection of adequate sputum samples that contain leukocytes and minimal epithelial cells. This can be achieved by endotracheal lavage and aspiration in the intubated patient but may be very difficult to accomplish in nonventilated patients. If a nonintubated patient cannot produce a satisfactory specimen through coughing, either nasotracheal or transtracheal aspiration may be necessary. In immunosuppressed patients, in whom early and specific antibacterial therapy is of even greater importance, diagnosis is often aggressively made by use of transpleural needle aspiration, bronchoscopy, or even open lung biopsy. All specimens should be evaluated by Gram's stain, as this may be helpful in selecting appropriate antibacterial therapy. If infection with *L. pneumophila* is suspected, the aspirate or biopsied material should also be evaluated with direct fluorescent antibody techniques, as it may be difficult to obtain culture results that indicate that this organism is the pathogen.

TREATMENT

Treatment of postoperative bacterial pneumonia is based upon selection of an appropriate antibiotic as well as adequate pulmonary toilet. Consideration of the clinical setting as well as Gram's stain results is helpful in choosing such an agent prior to obtaining culture and sensitivity reports, as the latter may not be available for several days. Gram-negative rods on sputum smear usually indicate choice of an antipseudomonal agent as well as one that also covers the other common pathogens. For example, combination therapy in such a patient might include an aminoglycoside and a third-generation cephalosporin. When gram-positive cocci are found, an antibiotic covering both staphylococci and streptococci is appropriate and might include either a first-generation cephalosporin or a penicillinase-resistant penicillin. In patients in whom aspiration is suspected, it is important to include an agent that provides anaerobic coverage. In addition, if *Legionella* is a possibility, inclusion of erythromycin in the therapeutic regimen is indicated. In any case, it should be emphasized that such broad-spectrum therapy needs to be specifically tailored to the causative organism once the culture data are available to decrease the possibility of both superinfection with other organisms and development of resistant strains.

Acute Respiratory Insufficiency

CLINICAL PRESENTATION

Acute respiratory insufficiency, especially in its most severe form (ARDS), is one of the most serious of all postoperative complications. Postoperative respiratory failure may present as two distinctly different syndromes and in two different contexts. The first and most common is one of prolonged ventilator dependency following endotracheal anesthesia. This may be encountered as either failure of the patient to meet acceptable criteria for extubation following operation (see hereafter) or the urgent necessity for reintubation and resumption of ventilator support after an apparently successful extubation. As might be expected, this complication is most frequently experienced by elderly patients with pre-existing pulmonary disease, by patients who have prolonged operations, and by those who are nutritionally depleted and therefore lack adequate energy for the muscular work of respiration. In addition, pulmonary edema, which can develop unexpectedly during an operation, may also significantly alter pulmonary gas exchange and thereby impede successful extubation in the early postoperative period.

Pharmacology

Pharmacologic factors also must be considered in patients with this complication. Anesthetic agents such as methoxyflurane can accumulate in the adipose tissue of the obese and be released in a rebound fashion, causing respiratory depression after the patient has been extubated. Similarly, muscle relaxants administered during the operation may also accumulate and interfere with resumption of spontaneous ventilation. This may occur more readily in patients in renal failure, since curare is excreted by the kidney, but is also occasionally seen in patients who have received continuous infusion of the shorter-acting depolarizing agents, such as succinylcholine. In addition, intraperitoneal irrigations with neomycin can also impede the return of spontaneous ventilation, as it is readily absorbed by the peritoneum and may potentiate the action of the longer-acting nondepolarizing neuromuscular blocking agents, such as curare and pancuronium. In either situation, the muscles of respiration may become or remain paralyzed for prolonged periods unless the situation is reversed with neostigmine. Postoperative suppression of ventilatory drive, especially in elderly patients with chronic obstructive disease, is most common secondary to overdosage of narcotic analgesics. Pharmacologic reversal with the narcotic antagonist naloxone may be helpful in this situation.

Extubation

Successful extubation can be predicted in the majority of patients if the following criteria are met and include evidence that neuromuscular blockade is reversed by adequate inspiratory excursions as well as movement of other muscle groups: a P_{CO_2} that is appropriate for the pH (usually 40 torr or lower), a breathing rate of 15 to 25 breaths per minute, and a tidal volume of 5 to 7 ml. per kg. Absolute criteria for P_{O_2} are difficult to determine, again because of the many factors that influence this parameter. Nevertheless, a general rule is that the P_{O_2} should be at least 65 to 70 torr with the patient breathing room air. Similarly, indications for reintubation also include both clinical and laboratory criteria. Respiratory distress with an increasing rate of greater than 30 to 40 breaths per minute usually cannot be maintained for long periods before muscular exhaustion ensues. In addition, a low tidal volume of less than 300 ml. per breath will not permit adequate gas exchange. The resultant physiologic manifestation of such a breathing pattern is carbon dioxide retention with P_{CO_2} in the 45- to 50-torr range and arterial blood hypoxia with a P_{O_2} of less than 65 torr.

Adult Respiratory Distress Syndrome

Adult respiratory distress syndrome is the second major type of acute postoperative pulmonary insufficiency and may be simply defined as the inability of the patient to satisfactorily ventilate himself without mechanical intervention. This syndrome is distinctly different from the previously described syndrome of prolonged ventilator dependence in that pathologic changes occur in the lungs that are responsible for the physiologic aberrations that accompany this complication. The term ARDS is a misnomer, since acute respiratory failure of this type has been observed in the pediatric age group as well. Moreover, throughout the years this syndrome has had many names, depending upon what currently was thought to be its etiology. Some of these terms include shock lung, wet lung, posttraumatic respiratory insufficiency syndrome, and pulmonary fat embolism syndrome. As indicated by this variable nomenclature, ARDS may occur in the setting of massive trauma, shock from any cause, intracranial injury, burns, sepsis, pancreatitis, long bone fractures, and multiple transfusions.

The clinical manifestations of ARDS are usually those of tachypnea, anxiety, ventilatory fatigue due to the decreased compliance of "stiff lungs," increased arteriovenous shunting with hypoxemia, and, frequently, a lower than expected P_{CO_2}. The chest film may be normal in the early course. However, progressive bilateral pulmonary infiltration invariably develops and pulmonary function studies reveal a decrease in both compliance and functional residual capacity.

Pathophysiology

As suggested by the multiple names given this syndrome, the pathophysiology of ARDS may include multiple factors. The final outcome, however, is the same because the lung has only one way to morphologically respond to injury. The early phase of ARDS is characterized by both endothelial and alveolar membrane injury. This results initially in the development of interstitial edema and inflammation. As alveolar membrane permeability increases, fluid and protein accumulates in the alveolar airspace as well, producing severe pulmonary edema and the development of hyaline membranes. Concomitant with this is a loss of alveolar Type II cells and a decrease in their production of surfactant. This process reduces compliance, further decreases the FRC, and favors progressive atelectasis. As the number of nonventilated but perfused alveoli increases owing to edema and atelectasis, intrapulmonary shunting also increases, with a resultant decrease in P_{O_2}. Normally, the shunt fraction is approximately 5 per cent, but with ARDS it may reach values as high as 35 to 40 per cent.[6]

Neither reducing the amount of intravenous fluid resuscitation nor increasing the amount of inspired oxygen will be adequate to overcome this situation in the majority of patients. Multiple clinical trials have been performed comparing the role of intravenous crystalloid and colloid solution administration in the etiology of this complication, with the consensus being that the increased hydrostatic pressure of the former is not implicated in its development. Moreover, administration of oxygen is effective only if the alveoli are open, thus suggesting the need for institution of other measures in the therapy of this syndrome.

Treatment

Mechanical Ventilation

The treatment of ARDS is primarily one of support utilizing mechanical ventilation and is most effective when initiated early in the syndrome. Although in some instances simple ventilation with a slightly increased tidal volume and FIO₂ is all that is necessary, the best results are obtained with addition of positive end-expiratory pressure (PEEP). Prior to institution of PEEP, however, a brief trial of diuretics may be indicated to exclude the possibility that the insufficiency is due to simple pulmonary edema. Moreover, patients with renal failure may benefit from urgent dialysis in this situation. When these measures fail, the use of PEEP or, in intubated patients breathing spontaneously, continuous positive airway pressure (CPAP) is clearly indicated and has produced a marked increase in salvage of patients with this devastating complication.[4] PEEP acts by both preventing further alveolar collapse and promoting reinflation of alveoli already collapsed. The end result is an increase in functional residual capacity, a decrease in the extent of arteriovenous shunting, and better oxygenation. Moreover, the use of PEEP permits reduction in the FIO₂ necessary to prevent hypoxemia, which is also important in preventing the development of oxygen toxicity and pulmonary fibrosis.

Positive pressure ventilation is not without complications, however, as alveolar rupture with subsequent development of pneumothorax, tension pneumothorax, pneumomediastinum, and, rarely, pneumoperitoneum have been observed in patients treated with PEEP. More commonly, a decrease in cardiac output ensues owing to multiple hemodynamic factors but predominantly reduced venous return with subsequent decreased left ventricular stroke volume.[15, 19] The potential for these complications warrants routine examination with serial chest films and careful monitoring of the cardiovascular system with a Swan-Ganz catheter.

When the diagnosis of ARDS is made, the patient is intubated and ventilated with a volume-regulated respirator. PEEP is added in increments of 3 to 5 cm. of H₂O until an adequate Po₂ (greater than 60 torr) is achieved using the lowest possible FIO₂. Generally, an attempt is made to maintain the FIO₂ at 50 per cent or less (the level at which pulmonary damage from oxygen toxicity could occur) while not exceeding a PEEP of 15 cm. of H₂O. Nevertheless, the goal of therapy is satisfactory oxygenation, and, therefore, increases in both PEEP and FIO₂ above these guidelines are at times necessary. In this situation, consensus currently dictates careful increases in PEEP with cardiovascular support through intravascular volume supplementation and judicious use of inotropic agents if cardiac output falls rather than prolonged ventilation with FIO₂ levels of 80 to 100 per cent.[24]

In addition to PEEP, the use of intermittent mandatory ventilation (IMV) has also been instrumental in improving the outcome of patients with ARDS. This technique allows the patient to breathe spontaneously while providing supplementary ventilator-driven breaths at a predetermined rate as necessary. IMV thereby reduces the need for both sedation and paralysis while preserving somewhat the tone of respiratory muscles. Moreover, it has been postulated that use of IMV may produce improved pulmonary and cardiovascular function and simultaneously make weaning from ventilator dependency an easier task.[4] Finally, as ARDS resolves and ventilator support is no longer necessary, many patients benefit from a period of CPAP breathing prior to extubation.

Treatment of Underlying Disorders

A comprehensive approach to ARDS includes not only ventilator support but also treatment of the underlying disorders. Nutrition must be maintained through either enteral or intravenous alimentation. Foci of sepsis require eradication by expeditious drainage of abscesses, débridement of necrotic tissues, and administration of appropriate antibiotics. The probability of ventilated patients developing a pneumonia is enhanced, thereby mandating constant surveillance. Pulmonary edema may respond to the administration of diuretics, although care must be taken not to decrease the vascular volume too greatly lest a fall in cardiac output ensue that requires inappropriate decreases in PEEP.

Overall, the understanding and management of ARDS have improved to the point where young patients, who experience resolution of their underlying disease, are expected to survive. Nevertheless, persistence of the inciting cause or, more ominously, development of multiple organ failure usually suggests a poor prognosis.

RENAL FAILURE

Renal insufficiency is a serious complication whether it occurs in the surgical or nonsurgical patient; however, it has added significance in the former, as it is associated with mortality rates of 50 per cent or higher.[22] A urinary output of less than 500 ml. per day or less than 0.5 ml. per kg. per hr. is defined as oliguria and is a hallmark of impending acute renal failure (ARF). Complete anuria is rare and is seen primarily in patients with a postrenal obstruction or irreversible cortical necrosis. Renal insufficiency may also be manifested by nonoliguric or even high-volume urinary output and as such may not be appreciated early in its course. In addition to classifying renal insufficiency according to the quantity of urine production, this complication has been classically subdivided into three categories depending upon the site of abnormal physiology: (1) prerenal azotemia (hypovolemia), (2) renal azotemia (renal injury), and (3) postrenal azotemia (obstructive uropathy).

The development of renal insufficiency is more common in elderly patients, especially those undergoing cardiovascular procedures with either cardiopulmonary bypass or cross-clamping of the aorta. This complication may occur in any age group if the appropriate predisposing factors are present. Patients with a mild pre-existing renal impairment, those who have undergone angiography immediately prior to operation, those who have experienced periods of hypotension during the operation, or those who have received potentially nephrotoxic drugs after operation are the most likely candidates for development of renal insufficiency. In addition, any condition that causes hemodynamic instability in the postoperative period, such as cardiac failure or sepsis, also places the patient at significant risk to develop ARF.

Prerenal Azotemia

ETIOLOGY

Renal hypoperfusion is the most common cause of prerenal azotemia in surgical patients. Because prerenal azotemia is readily reversible if promptly recognized and treated, it must be suspected in any patient who develops oliguria or biochemical renal dysfunction. Renal perfusion and subsequent function are dependent upon multiple factors, including cardiac output, blood pressure, intravascular volume, and the neuroendocrine forces that affect both glomerular filtration rate (GFR) and salt and water excretion. Thus, initial evaluation of the oliguric patient is directed toward determining whether abnormalities in any of these factors exist. For example, cardiac tachyarrhythmias may be accompanied by incomplete left ventricular filling and subsequent decreased cardiac output. More commonly, however, a decreased vascular volume is the primary cause of reduced renal blood flow and decreased GFR. This can be recognized by both clinical findings and laboratory testing.

Hypovolemia should be suspected in patients who have sustained serious trauma or who have experienced excessive blood loss from hemorrhage during or after operation. In addition, patients with high-volume fluid losses, either measurable ones, such as nasogastric tube aspiration and ileostomy drainage, or unmeasurable ones, such as ascites and third space sequestration, are also at increased risk. Clinical findings such as tachycardia, hypotension, decreased skin turgor, and anxiety are suggestive of decreased vascular volume.

With prerenal azotemia the kidney is still uninjured; therefore its response to hypoperfusion is predictable. Urine concentration will be increased as the kidney attempts to conserve water and sodium. This produces an increased specific gravity (usually greater than 1.020), urinary osmolality of greater than 500 mOsm. (may be greater than 1000 mOsm.), and urinary sodium concentration of less than 20 mEq. per liter. Moreover, the urine to plasma urea concentration and plasma urea to creatinine concentration ratios are both greater than 10. Finally, the urine sediment in prerenal azotemia is normal.

TREATMENT

Because the vast majority of surgical patients with signs of prerenal azotemia are fluid depleted, treatment is directed toward adequate rapid replacement in those without obvious congestive heart failure. This can be accomplished by administering an intravenous fluid bolus of between 500 and 1000 ml. of either normal saline or Ringer's lactate over a short period (30 to 60 minutes). Usually, this expands the vascular volume sufficiently to increase urinary output to a satisfactory level. If not, a second bolus should be administered, and, if possible, either central venous pressure (CVP) or pulmonary wedge pressure (PWP) should be measured. Values of less than 12 mm. Hg in either case are indicative of a persistently decreased vascular volume and warrant continued fluid resuscitation until either urinary output improves or the vascular compartment is replenished.

Once an adequate output (30 to 50 ml. per kg.) has been re-established, one should ensure that the underlying cause is also treated. Significant hemorrhage should be treated by blood transfusion, whereas infusion rates for maintenance intravenous solutions should be readjusted to more accurately approximate the ongoing fluid losses. Diuretics are not indicated in the treatment of hypovolemia-induced prerenal azotemia, as pharmacologically induced diuresis in the absence of adequate fluid resuscitation may only compound the situation by causing further dehydration.

Other causes of prerenal azotemia, including congestive heart failure (CHF), gastrointestinal bleeding with intraluminal stasis, and intravenous administration of high concentrations of amino acids in the patient with marginal renal function, require a somewhat different therapeutic approach. This is especially true in oliguric patients with CHF, in whom the problem is decreased cardiac output compounded by an excessive intravascular volume. Here, reduction of the CVP or preload is desired, and therefore

institution of fluid restriction and administration of diuretics are usually necessary, as may be the cautious use of inotropic agents. Increases in blood urea nitrogen (BUN) that are disproportionate to both the serum creatinine level and urinary output may indicate the presence of blood in the gut or may simply be a manifestation of intravenous alimentation. In either situation, renal dysfunction *per se* is not the cause, and thus urgent measures to improve renal function are not indicated. Rather, control of the hemorrhage or reduction in the CVN rate may be all that is necessary.

Renal Azotemia

Renal azotemia, or acute renal failure, is primarily seen in the setting of persistent and severe renal hypoperfusion and therefore should be suspected in the same types of patients who are at risk for developing prerenal azotemia. Most commonly ARF is of the oliguric variety; however, it may present with normal- to high-volume urine output as well. Although the etiologies of oliguric and non-oliguric renal failure overlap, it has been suggested that high-output ARF may be more frequently due to nephrotoxic agents than oliguric ARF.[3] In addition, it is felt that nonoliguric ARF patients experience a less morbid hospital course, require less dialysis, and have a greater overall survival than those with oliguria. However, oliguric ARF alone, as suggested earlier, is associated with a mortality of 50 per cent or more in surgical patients. When ARF is accompanied by failure of other organs, such as jaundice and liver dysfunction, gastrointestinal hemorrhage, or respiratory failure, the probability of death is even greater.

Renal ischemia is the prominent factor in the pathophysiology of ARF and produces injury to both the glomeruli and the renal tubules. Acute tubular necrosis (ATN), once thought to be the predominant element in ARF, is manifested morphologically by dilated distal tubules that are composed of flattened epithelium and that contain leukocyte casts and necrotic cells.[5] In addition, interstitial edema, a mild cellular infiltrate, and focal areas of necrosis and regeneration are seen in the proximal tubules. Whether or not these morphologic changes actually result in tubular dysfunction, however, is somewhat controversial. Conversely, experimental evidence suggests that glomerular blood flow and subsequent filtration are markedly decreased following either ischemic or nephrotoxic insult and, therefore, may also contribute significantly to the cause of oliguria.[7] In contrast to what is observed in the renal tubules, the glomeruli appear normal microscopically except for the presence of fibrin deposition, and thus an anatomic explanation for decreased glomerular filtration is not available. Nevertheless, in ARF a shunting of blood away from the renal cortex does occur. Whether this is due to neuroendocrine forces, such as the sympathetic nerve stimulation and catecholamine release that accompany shock, the activation of the renin-angiotensin system, or simple intraglomerular vascular obstruction is not clear.

DIAGNOSIS

The diagnosis of ARF is based on the presence of renal dysfunction in predominantly oliguric patients in whom both prerenal and postrenal causes of azotemia have been eliminated. Unlike prerenal azotemia, the kidney in ARF is injured, and therefore its response to renal hypoperfusion is inappropriate. Despite oliguria, salt conservation does not occur and urine sodium is usually elevated (greater than 40 mEq. per liter). Concentrating ability is lost, which results in the production of isosthenuria with urine osmolality less than 400 mOsm. and, in the absence of glycosuria and proteinuria, a specific gravity of approximately 1.010. The urine/plasma urea concentration ratio is usually less than 4, and the plasma urea to plasma creatinine concentration ratio is less than 10. Examination of the urine sediment may reveal tubular cells and casts as evidence of the parenchymal injury. Renal scintigraphy demonstrates reduced blood flow in comparison to the aorta and non-clearance of the tracer on the parenchymal phase. A comparison of laboratory values and clinical criteria commonly used to differentiate prerenal and renal azotemia are presented in Table 2.

TREATMENT

Most patients with incipient ARF should be treated with a trial of fluid resuscitation as outlined previously for those with prerenal azotemia, as it is sometimes difficult to distinguish between the two at onset. Renal blood flow may be increased in some instances by the administration of dopamine, since this agent enhances both renal and splanchnic flow when used in low, nonvasopressive doses (2 to 5 μg per kg. per min.). Furosemide, administered intravenously in large doses (100 to 1000 mg.), may be helpful in establishing the diagnosis, since the prerenal kidney responds with a diuresis whereas the kidney in ARF does not. In addition, both furosemide and mannitol are reported to have a vasodilatory effect on the renal vasculature and therefore may be of some therapeutic benefit early in the course. Recent experimental evidence suggests that there may eventually be a clinical role for the use of oxygen radical scavengers such as superoxide dismutase or calcium channel blockers such as verapamil in the early post-injury stage of ARF. Clinical trials have not yet been performed for either of these agents.

After the diagnosis of ARF is established, therapy primarily consists of fluid restriction if intravascular volume is adequate. For most patients, intake is restricted to between 500 and 700 ml. per day. This is a total maintenance fluid requirement and must include all supplemental intravenous administrations, such as "piggy-backed" drugs. However, it is appropriate to replace large, ongoing losses, such as nasogastric tube and ileostomy drainage, in addition to the maintenance regimen.

All potentially toxic, renal-excreted substances should be either withdrawn from therapy or their dosage adjusted appropriately. The most important of these are potassium and aminoglycoside antibiotics. Supplemental potassium should be eliminated from intravenous solutions, and antibiotics containing potassium salts should be matched to their sodium equivalents. Conversely, patients with high-output ARF may actually excrete potassium in addition to their extensive water losses. Urine electrolyte analysis is therefore helpful so that potassium supplementation rather than restriction can be provided if necessary. Nutrition may also play an important role in reversing the parenchymal injury in ARF. Both clinical and experimental evidence demonstrates the efficacy of administration of essential amino acids and hypertonic glucose (renal failure CVN) in shortening the recovery.[1]

RECOVERY

For survivors of ARF, the usual duration of renal dysfunction is 7 to 21 days, with some dysfunction persisting for several weeks longer. Complete resolution of the renal injury that lasts longer than 4 weeks, although occasionally observed, is rare. During this period of renal impairment, serum creatinine values generally rise at a steady rate of approximately 2.0 mg. per 100 ml. per day, whereas the extent of BUN elevation is less predictable. Recovery from ARF is manifested by a return of normal urine output and may be accompanied by a rapid decrease in the solutes. Some patients, especially those suffering from the oliguric variety of ARF, may actually experience a short polyuric phase during early recovery. Because the period of oliguria may be of short duration, dialysis therapy in addition to the previously described measures is not always necessary. Dialysis should be withheld until complications of uremia develop, such as pruritus, coagulopathy with gastrointestinal bleeding, somnolence, and coma. These symptoms are usually associated with BUN values of greater than 150 mg. per 100 ml., but their occurrence is variable and it is difficult to use BUN concentration as a sole guide to the need for therapy. However, development of fluid overload with subsequent congestive heart failure and pulmonary edema, uncontrollable acidosis or hyperkalemia, and the presence in the blood of toxic, renally excreted substances all necessitate urgent dialysis.

DIALYSIS

Hemodialysis

Dialysis therapy can be accomplished by hemodialysis or peritoneal dialysis. Hemodialysis allows for a more expeditious correction of hyperkalemia and acidosis and the removal of toxic substances than does peritoneal dialysis, although excess intravascular fluid can be removed efficiently by either method. Hemodialysis requires vascular access, and this can be achieved readily by percutaneous cannulation of either the subclavian or femoral vein with a large-bore catheter. If this is not possible, an arteriovenous shunt can be constructed using Teflon cannulas and Silastic tubing as described by Quinton and Scribner. The two most frequently used sites for shunt placement are the wrist through the radial artery and cephalic vein (Fig. 6) and the ankle through the posterior tibial artery and saphenous vein. Common complications of hemodialysis for ARF include cardiovascular instability with hypotension due to massive fluid fluxes; convulsions due to the dialysis disequilibrium syndrome that results from too rapid correction of uremia; and contamination of the access cannula and subsequent bacteremias and possible sepsis.

TABLE 2. Laboratory and Clinical Criteria for Differentiation of Prerenal and Renal Azotemia

Criterion	Prerenal Failure	Renal Failure
Urinary specific gravity	>1.020	1.010
Urinary sodium	<20 mEq./L.	>40 mEq./L.
Urinary osmolality	>500 mOsm.	<400 mOsm.
Urine/plasma urea concentration	>10	<4
Plasma urine/plasma creatinine	>10	<10
Urinary sediment	Normal	Epithelial cells and casts
Response to fluid resuscitation	Diuresis	No diuresis
Response to furosemide administration	Diuresis	No diuresis

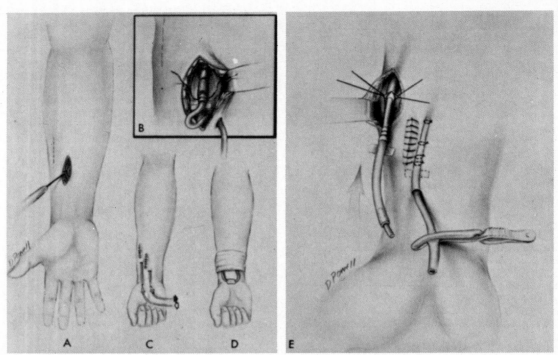

Figure 6. *Arteriovenous shunt for hemodialysis. A, Exposure of artery and vein. B, Cannulation of radial artery. C, Shunt in use during dialysis. D, Shunt incorporated in dressing between dialyses. E, Cannulation of vein. (From Sabiston, D. C., Jr. (Ed.): Davis-Christopher Textbook of Surgery, 12th ed. Philadelphia, W. B. Saunders Company, 1981, p. 478.)*

Peritoneal Dialysis

Short-term (1 to 3 days) peritoneal dialysis is achieved by percutaneous catheter placement using the type of catheter and technique commonly employed in diagnostic peritoneal lavage for abdominal trauma. This is not feasible in patients with multiple abdominal scars (because of the possibility of inadvertently injuring intestine that may be adherent to the abdominal wall) or in patients requiring long-term therapy. In the latter cases, a "mini-laparotomy" is performed to place the catheter. Peritoneal dialysis can be safely performed in the early postoperative period, providing the patient has a securely closed wound that will not leak the dialysate. Because anticoagulation is not necessary, this type of dialysis may be particularly advantageous in patients with a bleeding diathesis. In addition, the presence of early generalized peritoneal sepsis is not an absolute contraindication to this type of dialysis, since the frequent dialysate exchanges may aid in eliminating the bacterial contaminant by mechanical lavage.

Similarly, peritoneal dialysis may be the dialysis therapy of choice for patients with the ARF that accompanies severe pancreatitis, again because of the added benefit of removal of the intra-abdominal toxins released by the injured pancreas. Conversely, the presence of established peritonitis with extensive coverage of the intestine with fibrin, multiple intestinal adhesions, or extensive intraperitoneal hematomas is not conducive to achieving efficient peritoneal dialysis because of a reduced peritoneal surface area. Complications of percutaneously placed peritoneal dialysis catheters primarily involve injury to underlying viscera with hemorrhage and sepsis. Contamination of the catheter and/or dialysate with subsequent peritonitis remains the most common complication in both the acute and chronic forms of therapy.

Postrenal Azotemia

ETIOLOGY

Postrenal azotemia refers to the development of renal failure secondary to obstruction of urinary outflow. This complication most commonly occurs in elderly males with bladder outlet obstruction and benign prostatic hypertrophy or bladder atony and dysfunction secondary to acute bladder dilatation. This problem can be averted by preoperative bladder catheterization in patients who are predisposed to its development. Anuria in a patient with an indwelling catheter may be due to catheter kinking or blockage with blood clots. If catheter patency is established, complete anuria implies bilateral ureteral obstruction, which is very rare. Nevertheless, unrecognized bilateral ureteral injury does occasionally occur during pelvic operations, owing to either misplaced sutures or inadvertent laceration. In addition, extrinsic obstruction due to neoplasia or retroperitoneal fibrosis has also been associated with the development of postrenal azotemia, and therefore these possibilities need to be excluded.

DIAGNOSIS

The diagnosis of postrenal azotemia depends on a high index of suspicion, elimination of prerenal and renal causes of failure, and demonstration of the obstruction either by resolution of the problem with bladder catheterization or demonstration of obstruction with retrograde ureteral contrast roentgenography. Relief of obstruction to urinary flow may be temporarily achieved by the retrograde passage of ureteral catheters or by percutaneous pyelostomy. This often results in massive postobstructive diuresis with attendant fluid and electrolyte losses. Prompt intervention prevents development of permanent renal parenchymal damage and should be the primary therapeutic goal.

Special Circumstances

Several conditions in postoperative patients are associated with renal failure or oliguria not due to hypovolemia-induced decreased GFR *per se* and therefore warrant separate consideration. Transfusion reactions caused by the administration of mismatched blood may include as part of their sequelae massive hemolysis, hemoglobinemia, hemoglobinuria, and possible renal shutdown. Similarly, and somewhat more common, is the renal failure that may develop as a consequence of severe *myoglobinuria,* as might be observed in crush injuries and other conditions in which extensive muscle ischemia and necrosis occur. The etiology of ARF in both cases is the same, i.e., a result of obstruction of the renal microcirculation with hemoglobin or myoglobin precipitates and casts. Besides elimination of the causative factors, such as the immediate cessation of the blood transfusion, therapy of this particular form of ARF consists of hydration, administration of furosemide and mannitol to encourage diuresis, and alkalinization of the urine with systemic administration of sodium bicarbonate to retard cast formation.

INCREASED INTRA-ABDOMINAL PRESSURE

Patients who develop massive abdominal distention and increased intra-abdominal pressure secondary to hemoperitoneum may develop oliguric ARF even in the face of adequate intravascular volume and normal blood pressure. The exact etiology of this phenomenon is uncertain although it does not appear to be due to either decreased cardiac output or ureteral obstruction. Rather, it may be secondary to renal vein compression and is associated with intra-abdominal pressures of greater than 25 mm. Hg as estimated by measuring the intrabladder pressure through an indwelling Foley catheter as described by Kron and associates.[14] Urgent reoperation with abdominal decompression often produces prompt diuresis with resolution of the renal failure.

INAPPROPRIATE SECRETION OF ADH

Oliguria may be due to inappropriate secretion of antidiuretic hormone (ADH), which promotes increased water resorption from the urine by enhancing distal tubular permeability. The syndrome consists of decreased urine output, edema, water toxicity with severe hyponatremia, nausea, vomiting, and eventual mental status and neurologic changes. The inappropriate ADH syndrome is encountered most frequently in patients who have either sustained head trauma or undergone neurosurgical procedures. In addition, some patients with small cell carcinoma of the lung may also develop the syndrome through ectopic production of ADH. The diagnosis is confirmed by demonstration of high urinary sodium values in the presence of hyponatremia. Attempts to correct the low serum sodium level by intravenous sodium administration are contraindicated, as this results in further water retention with worsening of the hyponatremia. Rather, treatment simply consists of water restriction, as the condition is usually self-limited.

POSTOPERATIVE JAUNDICE

Jaundice is a frequently encountered complication following operations of any type and may have many different causes (Table 3). Hyperbilirubinemia may be due to the overproduction of bile pigments, which may occur with massive hemolysis; decreased ability of the liver to process the pigment load, as is the case with hepatic parenchymal disorders such as hepatitis; or obstruction of the biliary ductal system. The initial step in evaluating the newly jaundiced patient is to determine to which of these broad categories the problem is attributed. Helpful in this regard are the details of the patient's operation and clinical course. For example, an alcoholic patient may be prone to develop hepatitis, whereas massive intraoperative transfusion often leads to hemolysis, and biliary tract procedures are more apt to result in ductal obstruction than are other types of operations. Also of importance in making an accurate diagnosis is the qualitative and quantitative analysis of the type of hyperbilirubinemia.

Bilirubin is measured as either a conjugated (direct) or as unconjugated (indirect) pigment, the combination of the two giving a value of total bilirubin. Because the biotransformation of bilirubin occurs in the liver, determination of its predominant type is often very helpful in localizing the source of jaundice. In addition, analysis of the urine for bilirubin adds confirmatory evidence. Unconjugated bilirubin is not water soluble and is not present in the urine even when present in high concentration in the serum, whereas direct hyperbilirubinemia is manifest by dark urine.

Urinary bilirubin, however, should not be confused with the presence of *urobilinogen*. Urobilinogen is a renal-cleared, enteric-formed, colorless metabolite of unconjugated bilirubin. The urinary concentration of urobilinogen is partially dependent upon the presence of bilirubin in the gut. Thus, by using this type of information, one can predict, for example, that a patient with hemolysis-induced jaundice will have an elevated urine urobilinogen and low urine bilirubin, whereas a patient with an obstructed common bile duct presents with the exact opposite picture.

TABLE 3. *Common Causes of Postoperative Jaundice*

Hemolysis
    Extravasated blood, hematomas, etc.
    Transfusion reactions
    Drug reactions
    Sepsis
Hepatic parenchymal disease
    Exacerbation of pre-existing liver disease
    Viral hepatitis
    Shock-induced injury
    Intrahepatic abscess
Cholestasis
    Drug induced
    Sepsis
    Central venous nutrition
Biliary tract disease
    Choledocholithiasis
    Inadvertent bile duct ligature
    Bile fistula or leak
    Cholecystitis
    Pancreatitis with bile duct obstruction
    Bile duct stricture due to injury

Hemolysis

Hemolysis of transfused blood and reabsorption of extravasated blood are the most common sources of increased pigment in the postoperative period. Therefore, as an initial step in the evaluation of indirect hyperbilirubinemia, it should be determined whether conditions that lead to either exist. Intra-abdominal, retroperitoneal, and pelvic hematomas are frequently the source of extravasated blood. The presence of these lesions is usually readily recognized or suspected because of the circumstances of either the patient's operation or trauma.

ETIOLOGY

The cause of intravascular hemolysis, however, is sometimes more difficult to identify. Intraoperative or early postoperative hemolysis, when due to transfusion of mismatched blood, may be manifest by fever, chills, a bleeding diathesis, and possibly renal failure and therefore should be recognized immediately so that appropriate therapeutic measures can be taken. Transfusion of banked rather than fresh blood with its decreased red blood cell life span is a frequent cause of postoperative hemolysis, the extent of which is dependent upon the quantity of blood administered. Hemolysis may also be precipitated by administration of various drugs because of intrinsic red cell defects, hemoglobinopathies, or autoimmunity. The latter can be verified by development of a Coomb's-positive reaction and readily responds to discontinuation of the causative drug. Many patients with Coomb's-positive autoimmune hemolytic anemia do not have an obvious cause. Hemolysis, especially in children, may be associated with sepsis, although the specific pathophysiology of this variant is not understood.

DIAGNOSIS

The extent of clinical jaundice associated with hemolysis is usually mild unless either parenchymal liver disease is coexistent or the patient has an underlying hemoglobinopathy, such as sickle cell anemia or thalassemia. Diagnosis of hemolysis is confirmed by an elevated unconjugated serum bilirubin fraction, reduced serum haptoglobin concentration, and normal liver enzyme profile. Therapy of hemolytic jaundice is directed toward correction of the underlying cause. There is also the need for patience, since it is a self-limited process. Although mild cases are not harmful, massive hemolysis may precipitate renal failure owing to hemoglobinuria.

Hepatic Parenchymal Dysfunction

Hepatic parenchymal disorders are responsible for the development of jaundice in many patients. Hepatocellular injury may predate the operation in patients with active hepatitis, cirrhosis, or alcoholism in whom "recurrent" jaundice may represent an exacerbation of their underlying disease. However, the injury may be either drug-induced or associated with peri- and postoperative shock. The latter variant of liver dysfunction is often a component of the multiple organ failure syndrome.

DRUG-INDUCED HEPATITIS

Anesthesia-induced hepatitis is an often implicated but rarely proven event that has been associated with administration of either halothane or methoxyflurane to patients who presumably have a hypersensitivity to these agents.[23] Initial exposure to these anesthetics may result in only a mild, nonicteric hepatitis that is commonly never diagnosed. With subsequent exposure, however, jaundice may be severe and accompanied by extensive hepatic necrosis, as manifest by marked elevation of liver enzyme concentrations, an enlarged tender liver, and encephalopathy.

SEVERE TRAUMA

Hypotension and hypoxia are frequently encountered both in patients with severe trauma and in the course of many major operations and, although more commonly thought of in the context of postoperative renal failure, may be responsible for liver cell anoxic injury as well.[17] In addition, septic shock is also a frequent precipitating event for the development of liver injury. The resultant hepatic abnormality is one of decreased cellular excretion of bilirubin and intrahepatic cholestasis.

The magnitude and duration of jaundice in this setting are dependent upon the extent of the liver injury. Generally, jaundice develops within several days of either operation or the occurrence of septic shock and may persist for weeks. As with anesthesia-induced jaundice, elevations in alkaline phosphatase and transaminase concentration are also observed. Diagnosis of this type of liver failure is based on demonstration of the appropriate clinical setting as well as exclusion of other causes of hepatic injury. Again, therapy is supportive with adequate supplemental nutrition to foster parenchymal repair and regeneration. Of importance in this regard, especially in patients with encephalopathy, is the use of branched-chain amino acids in the hyperalimentation regimen.[8]

OTHER CAUSES

In addition to shock, cholestatic jaundice may also be due to many other causes, such as drug therapy (e.g., chlorpromazine, cyclosporine), sepsis, and use of CVN. The etiology of sepsis-related hyperbilirubinemia is not fully understood but is probably due to a combination of factors, including liver hypoperfusion and hemolysis. CVN-related cholestasis, however, is associated with liver enlargement that occurs secondary to excessive hepatic storage of carbohydrates and fat. Bilirubin concentration is only mildly elevated and is usually accompanied by liver enzyme abnormalities as well. Therapy for CVN-associated jaundice includes either a reduction in carbohydrate administration, temporary cessation of therapy, or, paradoxically, an increase in the proportion of calories administered as intravenous fat. Central venous nutrition may also precipitate the development of acalculous cholecystitis and its accompanying mild hyperbilirubinemia. Lastly, hepatic congestion and cholestasis due to right heart failure are not uncommon findings in elderly patients or patients following cardiac operations.

VIRAL HEPATITIS

Viral hepatitis, although a common cause of postoperative jaundice and liver dysfunction, more frequently is not observed until several weeks or more after operation owing to the necessary incubation periods of the various pathogens. Because of diligent screening protocols for hepatitis-associated antigen (HAA), hepatitis B is somewhat less prevalent than in the past, as are cytomegalovirus (CMV) and Epstein-Barr virus–associated infections. Non-

A, non-B viral hepatitis is currently the most commonly diagnosed postoperative liver disease, presumably transmitted by blood products. Nevertheless, as part of the early jaundice evaluations, serologic evidence should be sought for the presence of either CMV or HAA, as this may aid in diagnosis but may also have long-term prognostic importance, especially in regard to the latter pathogen.

Biliary Tract Obstruction and Injury

Biliary tract obstruction is a rare cause of postoperative jaundice that is most commonly observed in patients with biliary tract procedures. Hyperbilirubinemia is of the conjugated variety, associated with an absence of urinary urobilinogen and accompanied by a marked rise in serum alkaline phosphatase. A noticeable lack of bilious material in the nasogastric tube aspirate provides early, suggestive evidence that ductal obstruction has occurred. Initially the patient is often asymptomatic; however, severe pruritus may eventually ensue owing to increased serum bile salt concentration. In addition, the presence of fever and chills suggests the development of cholangitis and its attendant sepsis. Early recognition of this complication is essential so that appropriate antibiotic therapy can be instituted and expedient surgical or endoscopic drainage accomplished.

DIAGNOSIS

Diagnosis of biliary obstruction is confirmed using radiologic techniques; however, hyperbilirubinemia associated with a sudden increase in the volume of T-tube bile drainage as well as serum hyperamylasemia is suggestive of distal ductal obstruction. If the patient has a T-tube in place, the first step is to obtain a cholangiogram. This may demonstrate ductal obstruction caused by the tube itself owing to either partial dislodgment or faulty placement as illustrated in Figure 7 or to the less common and more catastrophic complication of a mistakenly ligated bile duct. In addition, this study may also reveal the presence of a missed or "retained" common bile duct stone that has subsequently impacted in the distal bile duct.

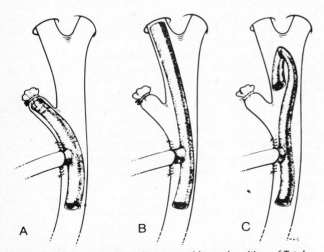

Figure 7. Postoperative jaundice caused by malposition of T-tube. A, Common hepatic duct obstruction by inadvertent placement of proximal limb in cystic duct stump. B, Drainage of right hepatic duct with left hepatic duct obstruction. C, Obstruction of common hepatic duct by a too long and kinked proximal limb. (From Greenfield, L. J. (Ed.): Complications in Surgery and Trauma. Philadelphia, J. B. Lippincott Company, 1984, p. 520.)

Alternatively, the cholangiogram may suggest the presence of ampullary edema and pancreatitis secondary to either the instrumentation or cholangiography of the original procedure. Cholescintigraphy with ^{99m}technetium-labeled iminodiacetic acid (IDA) derivatives may be useful in diagnosing the presence of obstructive jaundice in patients without a common bile duct drain in place. Although these agents permit visualization of the biliary tract in the presence of bilirubin levels as high as 30 mg. per 100 ml., they do not provide sufficient resolution to determine anatomic detail, such as the differentiation between a bile duct stone and a stricture. Nevertheless, the ultimate absence of tracer in the duodenum is strong evidence for obstruction as the cause of jaundice in such patients. Ultrasonography of the bile ducts may also be helpful by demonstrating choledochal calculi and ductal dilation. The latter findings, however, may require several days, and thus this test is not one of first choice. Lastly, percutaneous transhepatic cholangiography (PTC) and endoscopic retrograde cholangiopancreatography (ERCP) provide the most definitive imaging of the biliary ductal system in patients unable to undergo T-tube cholangiography and therefore may be necessary in some cases to document the complication.

TREATMENT

The appropriate therapeutic measures and surgical options for the patient with postoperative obstructive jaundice are considered in Chapter 27. Briefly, urgent reoperation is indicated in all patients with a ligated duct or T-tube dislodgment occurring in the first five postoperative days. In regard to the latter, sufficient time has not yet elapsed to ensure formation of an adequate peritubal tract. With the former, a short segment resection of the ligated portion of duct with either end-to-end anastomosis or enteric diversion to a Roux-en-Y limb may be necessary. Malpositioned biliary tract drains simply need to be operatively repositioned and secured in place. T-tube dislodgment recognized after a week should be treated by tube removal, as the peritubal fibroblastic tract is usually sufficiently developed by then to prevent generalized peritoneal bile spillage. Ampullary edema, if the causative factor, usually resolves spontaneously so that as long as bile can drain externally through the T-tube therapy is expectant. Small bile duct stones may pass spontaneously with time; however, larger ones usually require definitive management. Although reoperation is sometimes necessary, more often the use of various nonoperative techniques in the rapidly advancing field of interventional radiology is preferable.[21] Basket retrieval under fluoroscopic guidance through a well-developed (6-week) T-tube tract is the most commonly performed and successful method for removing bile duct calculi. Newer techniques include endoscopic papillotomy and stone extraction via the duodenum as well as attempts to dissolve stones with solvents such as cholic acid or monooctanoin. As with the basket retrieval of stones, the latter approach also requires the presence of an indwelling bile duct drain.

BILE LEAK

Besides biliary tract obstruction, jaundice due to a surgical mishap may be secondary to a bile leak or fistula. Fortunately this is not a frequently encountered problem, as the morbidity in some patients may be significant. Bile leakage is most commonly encountered following operations on the biliary tract. Persistent bile drainage from the hepatic bed of the gallbladder may occur following chole-cystectomy. In addition, the cystic duct may drain either because the ligature has slipped or because its placement was neglected.

Bile duct suture lines, whether part of a choledochal enteric anastomosis or a simple choledochotomy closure, may also disrupt and result in development of a biliary leak. Less common, but even more devastating, are missed occult injuries of the biliary tract that may occur after any operation in the upper abdomen. This occurs because ductal injury is an anticipated complication of procedures on the biliary tract and therefore easy diagnosis is the rule, whereas its potential presence is often denied by the responsible surgeon after nonbiliary tract operations. Two additional iatrogenic causes of bile extravasation being encountered with increasing frequency are bile duct perforation due to ERCP and pericatheter bile leakage from PTC procedures. Lastly, bile may collect intraperitoneally as a result of liver trauma.

Intraperitoneal bile leaks cause jaundice either because of the concomitant obstruction of the distal bile duct or because the bilirubin is subsequently reabsorbed directly into the blood via the visceral peritoneal surfaces. If a drain was placed at the original operation and remains functional, no other intervention may be necessary, providing complete bile diversion has not ensued (e.g., gallbladder bed and cystic duct leaks, partial anastomotic disruptions and small perforations), as many of these injuries heal spontaneously. Conversely, when drainage persists for more than 5 days, when the bile fistula is complete, and when bile collections occur in undrained patients, reoperation is required for drainage and repair. Failure to do so expeditiously places the patient at risk for the development of bile peritonitis, bile ascites, and septic shock. Prior to operation, however, radiologic evaluation using ERCP or PTC may be helpful in some cases to delineate the nature of the injury (Fig. 8).

Much rarer causes of postoperative jaundice include extrinsic obstruction of the distal bile duct as a result of hematoma or pseudocyst; pyogenic liver abscess following liver trauma or resection; ligation of the hepatic artery; and intrinsic metabolic disorders such as Gilbert's disease and Dubin-Johnson syndrome.

ALIMENTARY TRACT DYSFUNCTION

Dysfunction of the gastrointestinal tract following most major operations, especially those upon the abdomen, is an expected complication. The severity of dysfunction may range from simple loss of appetite or hiccoughs to a paralytic ileus that precludes resumption of oral alimentation, usually for 3 to 4 days. Fortunately, these complications are functional and usually self-limited. Problems such as early postoperative small bowel obstruction and stress ulceration of the gastric mucosa require prompt recognition and intervention and may also lead to major morbidity and reoperation. Therefore, it is important that the surgical team be aware so that preventive measures can be employed when appropriate and the patient can be adequately counseled preoperatively to help allay postoperative anxiety.

Anorexia, Nausea, and Vomiting

Anorexia is very common postoperatively. Although loss of appetite invariably accompanies intra-abdominal procedures, it may also occur after any operation. This is mediated by the hypothalamus and is generally associated

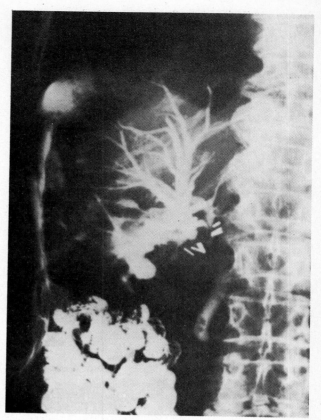

Figure 8. Percutaneous transhepatic cholangiogram demonstrating biliary tract leak. (From Greenfield, L. J. (Ed.): Complications in Surgery and Trauma. Philadelphia, J. B. Lippincott Company, 1984, p. 518.)

with decreases in gastrointestinal motility, as with paralytic ileus (see further). In addition, anorexia is often associated with the presence of intra-abdominal inflammation, carcinoma, intestinal obstruction, hepatitis, congestive heart failure, and adrenal insufficiency. The symptom itself is nonspecific and therefore of little value in making precise diagnoses of postoperative disorders. Nevertheless, regaining of an appetite is generally a sign that the patient is recovering from illness, whereas persistent anorexia suggests that occult disease persists.

Nausea and vomiting are also frequently encountered postoperatively and may be secondary to paralytic ileus, mechanical small bowel obstruction, intra-abdominal abscess and inflammation (especially if in the epigastrium), and the administration of various drugs commonly given surgical patients. General anesthetics and opiate analgesics are most often implicated in this regard. Treatment consists of limiting the patient's oral intake to liquids and use of antiemetic agents. Nausea and vomiting caused by paralytic ileus and bowel obstruction require a more aggressive therapeutic approach. In addition to the psychological debilitation that accompanies prolonged periods of vomiting, well-known physiological consequences also occur. Hypovolemia, hypokalemia, and alkalosis are the predominant early metabolic aberrations that may ultimately require correction if vomiting persists. Aspiration pneumonia is also an important complication of vomiting.

Diarrhea

Diarrhea is a common manifestation of gastrointestinal disease prior to operation but is rarer after operation. For example, diarrhea may be part of the symptomatology in patients with inflammatory bowel disease, Zollinger-Ellison syndrome, chronic pancreatitis, villous adenoma, and thyrotoxicosis and therefore may be encountered frequently in patients awaiting operation. Diarrhea occurring after operation is more likely to be due to mechanical, infectious, or physiologic consequences of the procedure. Diarrhea is often the first sign of various inflammatory conditions, such as pelvic abscess and enterocolic or gastrocolic fistulas. Moreover, in regard to the latter, the resultant diarrhea is a direct result of the distal colon being rapidly filled with liquid from the upper gastrointestinal tract. It may also be the presenting sign of a fecal impaction, and all patients with this complication need a rectal examination and proctoscopy. A barium enema may be helpful in making a diagnosis, but it also may be therapeutic by facilitating the dislodgment of impacted feces. Lastly, in patients being treated with large amounts of magnesium-containing antacids, diarrhea may also develop.

Colitis

Colitis resulting from infections should always be entertained as a possible diagnosis for diarrhea after operation. Although *Salmonella, Shigella* (colitis), and staphylococci (enteritis) predominate as causative organisms, parasitic and protozoan infections are also occasionally seen. More ominously, however, is the development of pseudomembranous enterocolitis, which, if unrecognized or misdiagnosed, can lead to prolonged morbidity and death. This complication is frequently due to administration of various antibiotics, of which clindamycin, lincomycin, and ampicillin are most often involved. The disease presents early (3 to 5 days after operation) with cramping abdominal pain that may be difficult to distinguish from that normally expected after abdominal operations. Fever and chills follow with development of diarrhea. Proctoscopic examination usually reveals an edematous and friable colonic mucosa covered with the thin yellow plaques or pseudomembranes. Diagnosis is confirmed by demonstration of the organism *Clostridium difficile,* which causes the illness by release of a toxin. The disease may be mild with self-limited diarrhea, or progressive, with the development of intractable diarrhea, toxic colonic dilatation, and perforation. Therapy is supportive with immediate cessation of the causative agents, fluid and electrolyte resuscitation, and administration of the antibiotic vancomycin (to which most strains of *C. difficile* are sensitive). In the rare event of toxic megacolon or perforation, urgent total abdominal colectomy is indicated.[13]

Constipation

Constipation has many causes. In the immediate postoperative period it may be due to paralytic ileus and self-limited. Constipation is often seen in elderly patients, many of whom are laxative abusers. These patients have essentially lost the normal colonic muscular tone and have difficulty in spontaneously initiating a bowel movement. Diabetic patients with gastrointestinal neuropathy are similarly affected. In both situations, early intervention with stool-softening agents and cathartics may be indicated. When oral intake is satisfactory, a diet high in bulk fiber may also be helpful in establishing a regular pattern of defecation. Rectal examination should be performed periodically to evaluate the possibility of stool impaction. Low

impactions can be manually removed; however, extrication of fecal masses higher in the rectosigmoid usually require the use of multiple enemas. Lubricating agents, such as mineral oil, given by the oral route may be helpful, and caution should be taken in prescribing osmotically active preparations if total or near total obstruction is present, since they may cause the patient to become markedly distended and further increase discomfort. Fecal impaction not successfully resolved may rarely lead to development of a stercoral ulcer and subsequent colonic perforation and fecal peritonitis. In constipated patients, that is, those who have not passed flatus or feces, the possibility of a postoperative bowel obstruction should also be considered. As with diarrhea, pharmacologic intervention may also cause constipation, and the most common agents are the aluminum-containing antacids and the analgesic codeine.

Paralytic Ileus

ETIOLOGY

Paralytic ileus is defined as either a lack of peristaltic activity or disorganized contraction of the intestine that results in the inability of enteral contents to be propelled normally. The etiology is believed to be splanchnic sympathetic nerve stimulation, which produces a reflex loss of peristalsis. Although most commonly associated with intraperitoneal operations or inflammatory-type processes (abscess, hematoma, peritonitis), retroperitoneal injuries and operations may also cause ileus.

CLINICAL PRESENTATION

Regardless of the cause, absence of progressive peristalsis results in the accumulation and stasis of both swallowed air and intraluminal fluid in the stomach and small bowel. This process causes the usual symptoms of nausea and bloating, abdominal distention, and vomiting. Gaseous distention may be severe enough to cause the patient extreme discomfort, especially if it results in an acute gastric or colonic dilatation. The abdomen is commonly distended and even tympanitic to percussion in severe ileus. Peristaltic bowel sounds are either absent or infrequent, helping to distinguish this entity from postoperative mechanical bowel obstruction, in which bowel sounds consist of hyperactive "tinkles," and peristalsis may even be visible through the abdominal wall. The roentgenographic picture of paralytic ileus (Fig. 9) is one of gas-filled loops of bowel throughout the abdomen, including both large and small intestines, whereas mechanical small bowel obstruction is suggested by the presence of air-fluid levels and no colonic gas.

TREATMENT

Treatment of paralytic ileus consists of aspiration of the stomach with a nasogastric tube and provision of adequate intravenous fluids, as a significant third space loss may ensue if the condition persists for more than several days. Resolution normally progresses from the gastric antrum (2 to 3 hours), to the small bowel (6 to 8 hours), to the right colon (24 to 48 hours), and eventually to the sigmoid colon (48 to 72 hours). Therefore, retention of nasogastric intubation for longer than 2 to 3 days is generally unnecessary, as the small intestine has regained both its absorptive and propulsive capabilities. Passage of flatus is an indication that resumption of oral alimentation is safe.

Paralytic ileus persisting for greater than 4 days suggests that other factors need to be considered. Peritonitis,

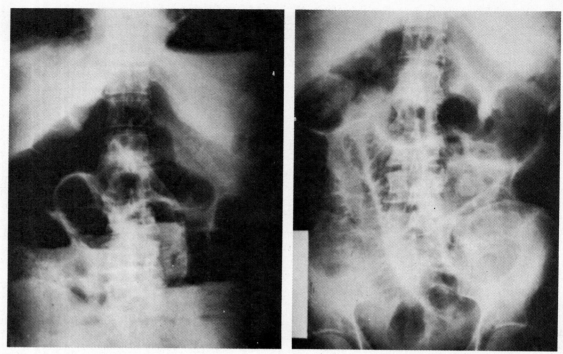

Figure 9. Roentgenographic demonstration of paralytic ileus. (From Sabiston, D. C., Jr. (Ed.): Davis-Christopher Textbook of Surgery, 12th ed. Philadelphia, W. B. Saunders Company, 1981, p. 1001.)

either incompletely treated from the initial operation or newly developed due to anastomotic leak, intraperitoneal abscess, or hematoma as well as metabolic disorders such as severe hypokalemia, are possible explanations.

Postoperative Bowel Obstruction

DIAGNOSIS

Bowel obstruction in the early postoperative period may be difficult to distinguish from prolonged paralytic ileus, as both can be present in the first week after operation. The diagnosis should be suspected in patients who do not regain bowel function in the expected time course and who, in addition, demonstrate the clinical and roentgenographic criteria outlined previously. When there is doubt, the diagnosis can be confirmed by use of barium contrast enteroclysis (Fig. 10). Because early mechanical bowel obstruction is often due to either anastomotic edema or filmy adhesions, both of which may be self-limited, the use of such x-rays should be reserved for perplexing cases. A slightly prolonged period of nasogastric intubation and patience may be all that are necessary. Although long intestinal tubes (Cantor, Miller-Abbott) have been advocated for use in these situations, their use requires accurate placement in the duodenum and frequent nursing care to ensure proper advancement.

OPERATIVE INTERVENTION

Operative intervention for postoperative bowel obstruction should be elected when the patient has evidence of a complete or closed loop obstruction or for suspected volvulus with intestinal gangrene. These more severe variants of postoperative bowel obstruction may be due to

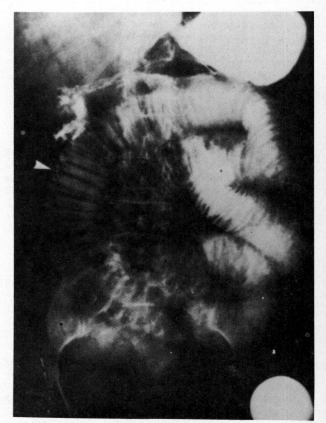

Figure 10. Barium contrast study of patient with small bowel obstruction. (From Cheung, L. Y., and Ballinger, W. F.: Hardy's Textbook of Surgery. Philadelphia, J. B. Lippincott Company, 1983, p. 461.)

internal herniation through a mesenteric defect or to a dense adhesion, both situations in which spontaneous resolution is unlikely. In such patients, signs of peritonitis with fever, rebound tenderness, and leukocytosis are often present, indicating the urgent necessity for exploration. In addition, failure of spontaneous resolution of a partial obstruction within a week of onset, even with the absence of peritonitis, often indicates re-exploration, as the morbidity of such an operation may actually be less than that of prolonged intubation and intravenous alimentation. Frequently these latter operations are of short duration, as either a single band adhesion or adherence of the bowel to a fascial suture is all that is found.

Acute Gastric Mucosal Hemorrhage

Hemorrhage from diffuse gastric mucosal ulceration is the most life-threatening variant of postoperative gastrointestinal tract dysfunction. This entity, commonly termed *acute stress ulceration,* is the gut componer* of the multiorgan failure syndrome, although it may frequently present as an isolated complication. The clinical picture is one of brisk upper GI bleeding that occurs in a severely ill patient, often in shock and on a ventilator, who has had either a major operation or extensive trauma. Endoscopically, diffuse shallow mucosal ulcers and hemorrhagic oozing are seen throughout the stomach, whereas only rarely are specific bleeding points demonstrated.

The etiology of this disorder is believed to be an increased back diffusion of hydrogen ions across the gastric mucosa with subsequent acid-induced injury. Localized ischemia may also be an essential component.

If the hemorrhage is not due to a duodenal ulcer, therapy consists of the usual resuscitative maneuvers, treatment of the underlying condition, and neutralization of the gastric pH. Before the therapeutic importance of achieving gastric neutrality was appreciated, many patients were subjected to near total gastrectomy as the only means of stopping the often lethal hemorrhage. This approach, although occasionally still necessary, has fortunately been replaced by medical management with administration of antacids and histamine receptor–blocking agents such as cimetidine.[11] Because of the extreme morbidity associated with this complication, all patients who are at risk for developing it should be treated prophylactically with these agents immediately following operation.

Other Forms of Gastrointestinal Dysfunction

Many other variants of gastrointestinal dysfunction may occur following operations on the gastrointestinal tract. For example, diarrhea may be encountered after resection of the terminal ileum owing to decreased bile salt absorption and subsequent irritation of the colon. Vagotomy and drainage procedures for peptic ulcer may also be accompanied by diarrhea as well as the classical "dumping" syndrome with symptoms of palpitation, nervousness, and abdominal bloating. Major resection of the small intestine (greater than 75 per cent) often leads to the development of the short bowel syndrome, and adequate nutrition cannot be maintained by the usual diet. Gastric resection with either Billroth I or II reconstruction may result in a variety of postgastrectomy symptoms, including the development of pain, esophagitis, and frequent bilious vomiting or an inability to empty the gastric pouch. Similarly, delayed gastric emptying may also accompany parietal cell vagot-

omy. Total abdominal colectomy with ileoproctostomy produces frequent defecation early after operation. However, with time the rectosigmoid colon adapts, with a reduction in bowel movements to three to five daily. Patients with small intestinal stomata are prone to fluid and electrolyte depletion, whereas both ileostomies and colostomies occasionally require early revision because of ischemia and frequently develop late peristomal hernias or stenosis.

MULTIPLE ORGAN FAILURE

Failures of individual organ systems are severe insults to the postoperative patient but when isolated are usually not lethal. When multiple organs fail, either in combination or in sequence, a chain of events follows that may end in death. The syndrome of multiorgan failure is one created by the advances in medical therapy that currently permit prolonged survival of the severely injured or septic patient. The major organs affected are the heart (cardiovascular shock), lungs (ARDS), kidneys (ARF), gastric mucosa (stress ulceration), and liver (jaundice), and these complications may occur in any sequence (Fig. 11).

Coagulopathy

In addition to failure of the solid organs, other systems may become inadequate in such patients. Coagulopathy is frequently encountered in septic and multiply transfused patients and may be due to a combination of thrombocytopenia and dilution of clotting factors in patients whose blood volume has been replaced during a short period. Treatment consists of transfusion of platelets, fresh frozen plasma, and fresh whole blood. Septic patients may develop disseminated intravascular coagulation (DIC), in which the clotting factors, platelets, fibrinogen, prothrombin, and factors V and VIII are consumed throughout the microcirculation. The diagnosis of DIC is based on demonstration of reduced circulating levels of these labile clotting factors, thrombocytopenia, and elevated prothrombin and partial thromboplastic times. Treatment is directed toward correction of the underlying disorder, such as with drainage of an abscess, removal of the gangrenous organ, and administration of broad spectrum antibiotics. Unlike dilutional coagulopathies, replacement therapy is less helpful if the consumption continues. Extensive fibrinolysis may accompany DIC, in which case the judicious use of ϵ-aminocaproic acid (EACA) may also be indicated.

Immunodysfunction

Severe injuries, including extensive burns, general anesthesia, and surgical procedures are immunosuppressive and therefore enhance development of infection and sepsis.[12] In addition, elderly patients, malnourished patients, diabetics, and patients with neoplastic diseases, especially of lymphoproliferative type, may also develop immunodysfunction. Almost all parameters of immune function have been demonstrated to be abnormal in such patients. These include leukocyte chemotaxis, phagocytosis, and intracellular killing. Abnormalities in both T and B lymphocyte function have also been demonstrated. Cell-mediated immunity (T cell) is impaired, as is the ability to make antibody (B cell) in severely burned patients. Similar

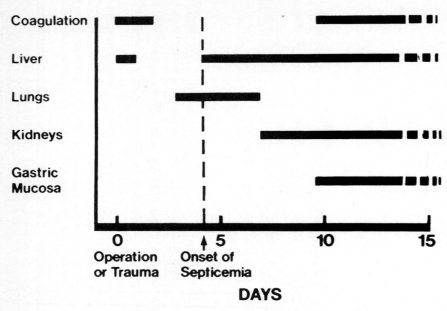

Figure 11. Sequence of organ failure in the multiple organ failure syndrome. (From Borzotta, A. P., and Polk, H. C., Jr.: Surg. Clin. North Am., 63:332, 1983.)

observations have been made in malnourished patients with the demonstration of reversible skin test anergy.

Although it is increasingly clear that many patients with multiple organ failure have immunodeficiency, there is unfortunately no satisfactorily proven therapeutic approach to management of this problem other than providing adequate nutritional support and being aware of the possibility of early sepsis. Ultimately, assessment of immune status in the critically ill by determination of circulating lymphocyte subsets (currently accomplished with monoclonal antibody techniques) may allow for early identification of the severely immunocompromised. Administration of broad spectrum hyperimmune globulin, interferon, or various immunostimulatory agents may allow for a less morbid postoperative recovery.[16]

Asplenic patients are also immunocompromised with or without multiorgan failure. The role of the spleen is important in the production of antibodies and in the opsonization of particulate antigens. Without a spleen, patients are more susceptible to development of sepsis owing to encapsulated bacteria such as pneumococci, and administration of specific antipneumococcal vaccines is therefore appropriate.

Nutritional Support

An important aspect of the care of patients with multiple organ failure is the provision of adequate nutritional support. Although this may be achieved by enteral feedings through a gastrostomy or jejunostomy, the use of CVN is more appropriate during critical illness. Not only does CVN ensure total absorption of the caloric load, but it bypasses the need for the gastrointestinal tract, which may have dysfunction due to periods of ischemia. Critically ill patients are highly catabolic, and this should be considered in planning the daily caloric requirements. Infusion of as much as 5000 calories daily may be necessary to reach an anabolic state.

Sepsis

Finally, the sudden development of individual or multiple organ failure in a postoperative patient apparently

recovering from operation may be due to occult sepsis. When obvious sources such as pneumonia, urinary tract infection, and CVN line contamination have been eliminated, attention should be directed toward the abdomen. Physical signs and symptoms may not always be present, and a CT scan of the abdomen is frequently helpful in establishing the source. Approximately half of patients re-explored for sepsis with multiple organ failure have showed abdominal findings not obvious prior to operation.[6] Intraperitoneal abscess is the most common finding, and whereas diagnosis preoperatively is often desirable, general abdominal re-exploration may be the best option. This approach permits expeditious diagnosis and treatment, often before irreversibile organ failure ensues.

SELECTED REFERENCES

Altemeier, W. A., Culbertson, W. R., Fullen, W. D., and Shook, C. D.: Intra-abdominal abscesses. Am. J. Surg., 125:70, 1973.
This is a review of a large series of patients who developed postoperative intra-abdominal abscesses. Superb illustrations of the anatomy of intra-abdominal abscesses are presented together with detailed tables that index pertinent clinical bacteriologic and epidemiologic data. In addition, this study considers the polymicrobial nature of most intra-abdominal abscesses and emphasizes the significant patient mortality and morbidity of this complication.

Baue, A. E.: Multiple systems failure. *In* Dudrick, S. J., Baue, A. E., Eiseman, B., MacLeen, L. D., Rowe, M. I., and Sheldon, G. F. (Eds.): Manual of Preoperative and Postoperative Care. Philadelphia, W. B. Saunders Company, 1983.
This is an overview of the predisposing factors as well as operative and postoperative conditions that contribute to the development of multiorgan failure. A practical therapeutic approach is reviewed.

Greenfield, L. J. (Ed.): Complications in Surgery and Trauma. Philadelphia, J. B. Lippincott Company, 1984.
This is a comprehensive text that covers the broad topic of surgical complications in depth. Included are chapters on anesthesia, shock, renal failure, respiratory failure, and wound healing. In addition, complications that may follow operations on all major organs are presented. The mortality, morbidity, and percentage of incidence of various complications of commonly performed operations are reviewed.

REFERENCES

1. Abel, R. M., Beck, C. H., Jr., and Abbott, W. M.: Improved survival from acute renal failure after treatment with intravenous essential

L-amino acids and glucose. Results of a prospective double blind study. N. Engl. J. Med., *288*:695, 1973.

2. Altemeier, W. A., Culbertson, W. R., Fullen, W. D., and Shook, C. D.: Intra-abdominal abscesses. Am. J. Surg., *125*:70, 1973.

3. Anderson, R. J., Linas, S. L., Berns, A. S., Henrich, W. L., Muller, T. R., Gabow, P. A., and Schrier, R. W.: Non-oliguric renal failure. N. Engl. J. Med., *296*:1134, 1977.

4. Civetta, J. M., and Augenstein, J. S.: Acute respiratory failure following surgery and trauma. *In* Greenfield, L. J. (Ed.): Complications in Surgery and Trauma. Philadelphia, J. B. Lippincott Company, 1984.

5. Danielson, R. A.: Differential diagnosis and treatment of oliguria in post-traumatic and postoperative patients. Surg. Clin. North Am., *55*:697, 1975.

6. Ferraris, V. A.: Exploratory laparotomy for potential abdominal sepsis in patients with multiple organ failure. Arch. Surg., *118*:1130, 1983.

7. Finn, W. F., Arendshorst, W. J., and Gottschalk, C. W.: Pathogenesis of oliguria in acute renal failure. Circ. Res., *36*:675, 1975.

8. Fischer, J. E.: The effect of normalization of plasma amino acids on hepatic encephalopathy in man. Surgery, *80*:77, 1976.

9. Freischlag, J., and Busuttil, R. W.: The value of postoperative fever evaluation. Surgery, *94*:358, 1983.

10. Glick, P. L., Pellegrini, C. A., Stein, S., and Way, L. W.: Abdominal abscess. A surgical strategy. Arch. Surg., *118*:646, 1983.

11. Hastings, P. R., Skillman, J. J., Bushnell, L. S., and Silen, W.: Antacid titration in the prevention of acute gastrointestinal bleeding. A controlled, randomized trial of 100 critically ill patients. N. Engl. J. Med., *298*:1041, 1978.

12. Howard, R. J.: Effect of burn injury, mechanical trauma, and operation on immune defenses. Surg. Clin. North Am., *59*:199, 1979.

13. Keighley, M. R. B.: Antibiotic-associated pseudomembranous colitis—pathogenesis and management. Drugs, *20*:49, 1980.

14. Kron, I. R., Harmon, K., and Nolan, S. P.: The measures of intra-abdominal pressure as a criterion for abdominal reexploration. Ann. Surg., *199*:28, 1984.

15. Luce, J. M.: The cardiovascular effects of mechanical ventilation and positive end-expiratory pressure. J. A. M. A., *252*:807, 1984.

16. McIrvine, A. J., and Mannick, J. A.: Lymphocyte function in the critically ill surgical patient. Surg. Clin. North Am., *63*:245, 1983.

17. Nunes, G., Blaisdell, F. W., and Margaretten, W.: Mechanism of hepatic dysfunction following shock and trauma. Arch. Surg., *100*:546, 1970.

18. Skinner, D. B., and Myerowitz, P. D.: Recent advances in the management of thoracic surgical infections. Ann. Thorac. Surg., *31*:191, 1980.

19. Smith, P. K., Tyson, G. S., Jr., Hammon, J. W., Jr., Olsen, C. O., Hopkins, R. A., Maier, G. W., Sabiston, D. C., Jr., and Rankin, J. S.: Cardiovascular effects of ventilation with positive expiratory airway pressure. Ann. Surg., *195*:121, 1982.

20. Talbot, G. H.: Nosocomial pneumonia in the surgical patient. Infect. Surg., *3*:557, 1984.

21. Teplick, S. K., Haskin, P. H., Matsumoto, T., Wolferth, C. C., Jr., Pavlides, C. A., and Gain, T.: Interventional radiology of the biliary system and pancreas. Surg. Clin. North Am., *64*:87, 1984.

22. Tilney, N. J., Morgan, A. D., and Lazarus, J. M.: Acute renal failure in surgical patients. *In* Tilney, N. J., and Lazarus, J. M. (Eds.): Surgical Care of the Patient with Renal Failure. Philadelphia, W. B. Saunders Company, 1982.

23. VanThiel, D. H., and Lester, R.: Postoperative jaundice. Mechanisms, diagnosis and treatment. Surg. Clin. North Am., *55*:409, 1975.

24. Weisman, I. M., Rinaldo, J. E., and Rogers, R. M.: Positive end-expiratory pressure in adult respiratory failure. N. Engl. J. Med., *307*:1381, 1982.

TRANSPLANTATION

JEREMIAH G. TURCOTTE, M.D. • DARRELL A. CAMPBELL, JR., M.D.
DONALD C. DAFOE, M.D. • DOUGLAS M. BEHRENDT, M.D.
MARVIN M. KIRSH, M.D. • WILLIAM H. MARKS, M.D.

15

Organ transplantation is now an established clinical science that provides effective therapy for end-stage disease of several major organs. With the introduction of the new immunosuppressant cyclosporine, there has been a resurgence of interest in heart, heart-lung, liver, and pancreatic transplantation and an enhancement of interest in renal transplantation. This chapter discusses the immunobiology of transplantation, multiorgan donation, organ preservation, and the current status and technique of transplantation of individual major organs. A brief description of transplantation of islet cells and the small intestine and autotransplantation of tissues is also included.

IMMUNOBIOLOGY OF ORGAN TRANSPLANTATION

A successful transplant will reverse the symptoms and many of the complications of end stage organ failure, improve chances for long-term survival of individual patients, and, in many instances, be cost-beneficial to society. Unfortunately, in some patients an irreversible immune response may intervene and cause rejection of the allograft. Since rejection is a war waged at the cellular level, the ability to care for transplant patients successfully requires an understanding of transplantation immunobiology. This section discusses the role of cell surface antigens, immunocompetent cells, and antibody in the pathogenesis of rejection and reviews the strategies for successful transplantation of allogeneic tissues.

Cell Surface Antigens

The emergence of the acquired immune deficiency syndrome (AIDS) as a distinct and fatal disease entity has highlighted the degree to which we depend on a functioning immune system for protection against exogenous pathogens. Alloantigens, or "non-self" antigens, are also considered by the immune system to be exogenous even if they are not pathogens. A healthy immune system in the absence of immunosuppression will quickly recognize and "reject" alloantigen-bearing tissue.

Rejection of a transplanted organ depends upon recognition by the host lymphocytes that the transplanted organ is foreign or "non-self." The ability of host lympho-cytes to make this distinction depends upon the presence on donor cells of distinctive cell surface proteins called *histocompatibility antigens*. These antigens are distinct from the differentiation antigens discussed later (e.g., T4, T8) in that the differentiation antigens are identical from one individual to another. The "distinctiveness" of histocompatibility antigens is an inherited trait determined by a specific chromosomal area called the major histocompatibility complex (MHC). In man the MHC is designated the human lymphocyte antigen HLA locus. The HLA locus is on human chromosome 6. In the mouse the analogous chromosomal area is termed H-2 and is on chromosome 17.

The HLA complex contains genes that code for the development of two general types of cell surface antigens named Class I and Class II antigens. Class I and II antigens differ in function, structure, and distribution. Class I antigens generally serve as distinctive "targets" for immune responses, whereas Class II antigens play an important role in the initiation of the immune response. Class I antigens contain a 44,000-molecular-weight (M.W.) glycoprotein and a 12,000-M.W. subunit called a beta-2-microglobulin. Class II antigens are made up of a 34,000-M.W. glycoprotein called the alpha chain and a 28,000-M.W. glycoprotein called the beta chain but no beta-2 microglobulin (Fig. 1). Class I antigens are found on the cell surface of all nucleated cells; Class II antigens have a much more limited distribution and are found only on B cells, some macrophages, sperm, and epidermal cells. Class II antigens are not found on resting T cells, but may appear on such cells after activation.

Within HLA, three separate loci (called the A, B, and C loci) code for the synthesis of Class I type antigens, and a fourth (called the D locus) codes for the synthesis of Class II antigens. Inherited information at each locus codes for the synthesis of slightly different versions of the same type of molecule; these different versions are called *alleles*, and they account for the distinctiveness of one individual's cells. There are not, however, an infinite number of alleles (Table 1). At present the A locus is thought to code for any one of only 20 different alleles, the B locus codes for one of 32 possible alleles, the C locus codes for one of six alleles, and the D locus codes for one of ten possible alleles. Because we are diploid organisms, we have two "sixth" chromosomes, one chromosome being inherited from the mother and one from the father. Because HLA alleles are

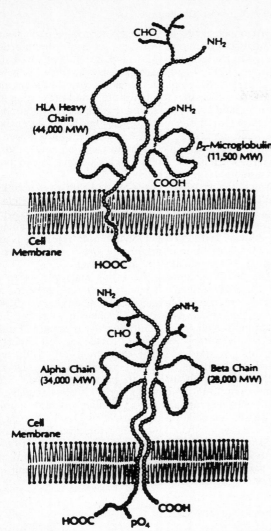

Figure 1. Class I and Class II histocompatibility antigens. Top, a Class I type histocompatibility antigen is depicted. This type of antigen is composed of a 44,000 molecular-weight (M.W.) heavy chain and 11,500-M.W. beta₂-microglobulin subunit. Bottom, a Class II type histocompatibility antigen is shown. This type of antigen is composed of two different glycoprotein chains but no beta₂-microglobulin subunit. (From Najarian, J. S.: Hosp. Pract. 131:61, 1982.)

codominant, there are actually two different A locus alleles expressed on the cell surface, two different B locus alleles, two different C locus alleles, and on B cells and macrophages two different D locus alleles.

Differentiated Cells Participating in the Rejection of Foreign Tissue

The process of rejection invokes several interrelated immune mechanisms. The rejection response is mediated through the action of lymphocytes, macrophages, antibody molecules, and soluble mediators.

T LYMPHOCYTES

The central importance of the T (thymus-derived) lymphocyte in the process of allograft rejection is confirmed from the repeated observation that animals depleted of T

cells, but not other cell types, are incapable of rejecting a transplant. Most current antirejection therapy is designed to eliminate T cells temporarily or to alter their function substantially.

T cells are lymphocytes derived from hematopoietic stem cells, which further differentiate in the thymus. The process of differentiation involves accumulation of immature cells in the cortex of the thymus, with subsequent migration to the medulla and release into the peripheral blood as mature T cells. A particularly important trait acquired by T cells during thymic differentiation is the requirement that they recognize foreign antigen only in conjunction with specific types of autologous protein, i.e., Class II or, in some cases, Class I antigen. This "corecognition" of foreign antigen and autologous protein is often referred to as antigen recognition with "histocompatibility restriction." T lymphocytes can be distinguished from B lymphocytes by the absence of immunoglobulin on the T cell surface membrane. T cells also bear certain distinctive antigens. One particularly important T cell antigen is designated T3. Because it appears on all T cells regardless of their specialized function, it is called a "pan T cell" antigen. Another antigen, T11, is also a "pan T cell" antigen, but this antigenic marker also defines immature T cell forms.

Specialized subtypes of mature T cells emerge from the thymus. These specialized T cell subsets can be divided into two broad categories.

TABLE 1. HLA Antigens*

HLA Class I			HLA-Class II	
HLA-A	HLA-B	HLA-C	HLA-D	HLA-DR
A1	B5	CW1	DW1	DR-1
A2	B7	CW2	DW2	DR-2
	B8			
A3	B12	CW3	DW3	DR-3
	B13			
9	B14	CW4	DW4	DR-4
	B15			
10	B17	CW5	DW5	DR-5
	B18			
11	B27	CW6	DW6	DRW6
	B37			
25	B40		DW7	DR-7
	BW4			
26	BW6		DW8	DRW8
	BW16			DRW9
28	BW21		DW9	DRW10
	BW22			
29	BW35		DW10	
	BW38			
AW19	BW39			
	BW41			
AW23	BW42			
	BW44			
AW24	BW45			
	BW46			
AW30	BW47			
	BW48			
AW31	BW49			
	BW50			
AW32	BW51			
	BW52			
AW33	BW53			
AW34				
AW36				
AW43				

*The recognized HLA antigens are listed by sublocus, that is, HLA-A, HLA-B, HLA-C, and HLA-D. The locus for HLA-DR antigens is either within the HLA-D sublocus or tightly linked to it on chromosome 6.

Helper/Inducer T Cells

The preponderance of lymphocytes circulating in the peripheral blood at any given time are T cells, and the majority of the T cells present belong to the "helper" or "inducer" subset. The "helper" designation refers to the role that these cells play in assisting B cells to differentiate into plasma cells with subsequent production of specific antibody. T cells have many other important functions as well. The B cell response to most protein antigens is completely dependent upon T cell help. T cell help in some cases requires direct T cell–B cell contact. This is termed "cognate help." In other instances T cells provide assistance by secreting soluble mediators called lymphokines. This is termed "factor dependent help." The role that the helper T cell subset plays in allograft rejection clearly involves cooperation with B cells in the production of antibody to the foreign alloantigen. The term "inducer" refers to the role that this subset of T cells plays in the recognition of antigen and subsequent amplification of specific immune responses. This subject is described in more detail in a later section. Helper/inducer T cells can be identified using monoclonal antibodies, which recognize an antigen specific for this subset. A common designation for this specific antigen in humans is T4.

Suppressor/Cytotoxic T Cells

Another major T cell subset includes cells that have suppressor or cytotoxic activity. Currently, cells with either one or the other function are considered to be in the same subset. "Suppressor" T cells function to regulate the immune response. They may, for example, limit the amount of T cell help available to participate in the previously mentioned T helper cell–B cell interaction, which would effectively "turn off" a given antibody response. The mechanism by which suppression occurs is poorly understood but usually involves the production of soluble suppressor molecules, which transmit the "turn-off" signal. Suppressor T cells are identified by a differentiation antigen called T8. This subset of T cells has attracted the interest of transplant biologists because it seems logical that long-term acceptance of an allograft would involve establishment of a suppressor subset programmed to suppress host response to specific foreign antigens. Such a phenomenon has in fact been documented in several human transplant patients.

T cells capable of killing another cell on direct cell-cell contact are called cytotoxic T cells, and these cells also bear the T8 differentiation antigen. It seems likely that this type of cell participates in the rejection of allogeneic tissue. The helper T4 cell subset recognizes foreign antigen in conjunction with an antigen-presenting cell and then secretes a soluble mediator, interleukin-2, which causes clonal expansion of the cytotoxic T8 cell line. Evidence that these cells play an important role in the process of rejection comes from the observation that cells bearing T8 antigen can be readily eluted from rejecting transplants.

B Cells

B lymphocytes are precursors of antibody-producing plasma cells and are derived originally from hematopoietic stem cells. These cells are distinguished by the presence of immunoglobulin on their cell surface. B cells bind antigen to their cell surface and then interact with helper T cells or soluble mediators before differentiation and antibody production.

Macrophages and Dendritic Cells

Mononuclear phagocytic cells are not lymphocytes but are equally important in protecting the host from infection. These cells are referred to as monocytes when circulating in peripheral blood and macrophages when fixed in parenchymal organs. Macrophages function early in the immune response by processing foreign protein and presenting it to other lymphoid cells in an immunogenic form. Macrophage presentation of antigen to T cells has been extensively studied and appears to involve internalization followed by antigen re-expression in conjunction with an autologous or "self" Class II antigen. Helper T4 cells then "corecognize" antigen and autologous protein.

Macrophages also produce a soluble lymphokine termed *interleukin 1* (IL-1), which allows helper T cells to produce another lymphokine, interleukin-2 (IL-2), which in turn initiates T cell clonal expansion. The relevancy of this pathway to the subject of allograft rejection is that many types of immunosuppressive drugs act in part by inhibiting IL-1 production by macrophages.

The ability of antigen-presenting macrophages to express Class II antigen also has much relevancy for the subject of organ transplantation. The macrophages present within donor organs are routinely shed into the recipient circulation following transplantation. By presenting foreign Class II antigen, these shed cells provide the first important information to the recipient that "non-self" cells have invaded the "self" milieu. Immunogenic donor cells shed into the recipient circulation are called "passenger" cells. The most important type of "passenger" cell is actually not a traditional macrophage but a peculiar-looking mononuclear sessile cell called a dendritic cell. Dendritic cells, so called because of their long thin cytoplasmic projections, express an extremely high concentration of Class II determinants on their cell surface and are potent immunogens. Most parenchymal organs, including liver, heart, and kidney, contain dendritic cells.

Natural Killer (NK) Cells

Natural killer (NK) cells are probably lymphoid in origin but do not bear the distinctive cell surface markers associated with T or B cells. These cells display cytocidal activity, as does the subset of cytotoxic T8 cells, but, in contrast to the latter, NK cells display very little specificity for antigen. NK cells were originally recognized by their ability to lyse a wide variety of different tumor cell lines. It is now appreciated that NK cells also participate in the process of allograft rejection and can be eluted easily from a rejecting organ.

Advances in molecular biology now permit the precise identification and quantification of various specialized groups of cells. These advances have been made possible by the use of monoclonal antibodies. These antibodies are made by chemically fusing an antibody-producing plasma B cell with a cultured mouse myeloma cell line. Clones of such fused cells are selected that are producing an antibody of a single specificity (monoclonal) to the desired antigen. Monoclonal antibodies have been developed that recognize the differentiation antigens just described, and it is common practice in clinical transplantation to periodically assess the composition of the peripheral blood in the hope that changes in T cell subsets will herald the onset of transplant rejection. Although it is somewhat controversial, some clinicians feel that the T4:T8 ratio rises during an acute rejection episode. The T4:T8 ratio falls dramatically during

TABLE 2. *Flow Cytometric Analysis* of Cell Populations in the Peripheral Blood*

Marker Description†	Per Cent in Peripheral Blood (Normal Individual)
T11 Pan T cell	80
T3 Mature cell	70
T4 Helper/inducer	46
	Normal ratio 1.9
T8 Suppressor/cytotoxic	24
B1 Mature B cell	10

*Flow cytometry refers to an automated technique used to analyze cell populations. In the application described here, peripheral blood lymphoid cells are combined with various mouse monoclonal antibodies and subsequently stained with a fluoresced goat anti-mouse antibody. This technique is referred to as indirect immunofluorescence or the "sandwich" technique. Flow cytometric analysis is used to quantitate the number or percentage of fluoresced cells present for each specific monoclonal antibody.

†Marker description here refers to a group of antibodies described by Schlossman et al. and made available by Coulter immunology. Other similar antibodies with different designations are marketed by the Ortho Company and Becton Dickerson Company.

and after a viral infection. A profile of lymphoid cell phenotypes found in the blood of a normal individual is shown in Table 2.

Initiation of the Immune Response to Foreign Antigens

The mere presence of alloantigen on foreign tissue is not sufficient to elicit an immune response. Killed allogeneic cells, which express alloantigen, will not "turn on" the process; likewise, certain nonlymphoid parenchymal cells express alloantigen but will not induce immunity. These observations have led to the "two-signal" model of immune induction whereby transplantation antigen and a "second signal" of costimulator are required before the cascade of immune events begins. Such a "second signal" is produced only by metabolically active lymphoid cells. In the case of an organ transplant, one could imagine two general means by which the host would become sensitized. In the first, the donor "passenger cell," i.e., the dendritic cell, would provide large amounts of Class II transplantation antigen on its cell surface while also providing a ready source of costimulator (Fig. 2). In the second, pathway donor parenchymal or endothelial cells, which cannot provide costimulator because they are not lymphoid cells, would at least shed alloantigen into the recipient circulation, which, in turn, would be scavenged by host macrophages. Host macrophages would process and present foreign antigen in the usual way and provide a "host derived" costimulator (Fig. 3). Evidence exists that the former mechanism of induction is the more important of the two. If this is correct, then removal of donor passenger cells from transplanted organs prior to transplantation would have favorable effects on subsequent immunologic events.

Regardless of whether donor dendritic cells or host macrophages present the "two-signal" message, it seems clear that the recipient of this information is the helper subset of T cells (Th). After antigen recognition, helper T cells produce a large amount of lymphokine, interleukin-2 (see Fig. 2). IL-2 causes rapid clonal expansion of other T cells, particularly the T8 cytotoxic subset. As mentioned earlier, although it is donor Class II antigen on passenger cells that initiates antidonor immunity, the expanded cytotoxic clone (Tcy subset) focuses primarily on the foreign Class I antigens, which are distributed widely throughout the offending transplant. All cells bearing the Class I antigenic target are potential victims. Some proportion of Th subset cells subsequently become "memory" cells with the capability of responding rapidly on re-exposure to antigen. The suppressor subset of T cells also enters into this process. Such cells are activated by antigen exposure, clonally expand, and, via the production of soluble mediators, act to regulate the tempo of the rejection response.

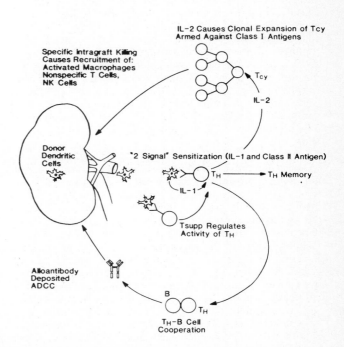

Figure 2. Response of the immune system to an allograft. In this schematic view of the development of immunity to an allografted kidney donor dendritic cells are shed into the recipient's circulation. Dendritic cells provide a rich source of foreign alloantigen and also a source of interleukin-1 (IL-1). The helper subset of T cells is the primary recipient of the "2 signal" message; the cells then may produce the interleukin-2 necessary to drive clonal expansion of cytotoxic T cells (Tcy). The helper subset of T cells also interacts with B cells to result in production of alloantibody directed at the transplant. A subpopulation of T helper cells also presumably become "memory" cells with the capability to rapidly respond to antigen rechallenge. T suppressors are also activated by antigen exposure, and these cells are thought to regulate the activity of T helper cells and thus control the tempo of the immune response.

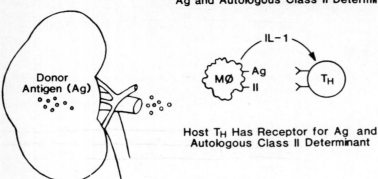

**Hosts Macrophage (MØ) Presents
Ag and Autologous Class II Determinant**

Host T$_H$ Has Receptor for Ag and
Autologous Class II Determinant

Figure 3. Alternate mechanism for sensitization to alloantigen from a renal transplant. By an alternate mechanism, the host macrophage processes soluble antigen shed from the transplant. Antigen is then presented to the T helper population of cells in conjunction with an autologous Class II determinant and macrophage-derived IL-1. This is antigen presentation with a "histocompatibility restriction," i.e., T helpers must have a receptor for antigen and also a receptor for autologous Class II determinants for antigen recognition to occur.

Rejection

CELLULAR MECHANISMS ACCOUNTING FOR REJECTION

Most of the information available about effector mechanisms responsible for allograft rejection has been derived using a "smoking gun" approach; if a particular cell type is present in the rejecting allograft, its guilt is assumed. Using this concept and particularly by identifying the T cell subsets with immunofluorescent antibody, a picture of rejection emerges that implicates many specific and nonspecific immune mechanisms.

A large proportion of cells invading allografted tissue are T cells. Most of the T cells present bear the T8 marker, indicating that they belong to the suppressor/cytotoxic subset. The T4 helper/inducer subset usually comprises a smaller percentage of infiltrating cells. Mononuclear phagocytic cells are quite prominent during a rejection episode, accounting for 30 to 50 per cent of cells. In many cases the percentage of infiltrating cells that are macrophages increases over time. In contrast to cytotoxic T cells, which attack cells very specifically, macrophages never display antigen specificity and are instead recruited to act nonspecifically, presumably as the result of earlier antigen-specific events. The ability of the macrophage to kill allogeneic cells is, however, substantial and probably relates to macrophage release of reactive oxygen intermediates. T cells are usually seen in close association with blood vessels, and macrophages are most often adjacent to parenchymal cells. B cells usually comprise 10 to 15 per cent of infiltrating cells, and it is tempting to imagine that these cells produce antidonor antibody *in situ*. Granulocytes usually comprise only a small (2 per cent) percentage of cells infiltrating an allograft.

In addition to specific Tcy-mediated killing and nonspecific macrophage-mediated killing, several other mechanisms are important during the process of allograft destruction. First, large numbers of NK (natural killer) cells with cytotoxic activity against donor cells are often detected during the early phase of the rejection process. Second, the deposition of antidonor antibody in the transplanted organ facilitates specific killing of allogeneic cells by uncommitted T cells. This process, called *antibody-dependent cell-mediated cytotoxicity* (ADCC), can be detected throughout the course of the rejection process. Finally, deposition of antidonor antibody in the transplanted organ is associated with complement fixation, cell death, and recruitment of inflammatory cells. The end result is a graft whose vascular endothelial cells are damaged and swollen and whose interstitium is invaded by hordes of host cells. A typical histologic picture of acute rejection is shown in Figure 4.

The signs and symptoms that occur as the result of the rejection process depend upon the immune mechanism by which rejection takes place, the intensity of the process, and the type of organ being transplanted.

HYPERACUTE REJECTION

Hyperacute rejection is a form of rejection that occurs dramatically in renal transplantation but rarely, if ever, in cases of heart or liver transplantation. In this type of rejection pre-existing antigraft antibodies in the recipient serum recognize foreign graft antigens immediately after blood perfuses the newly implanted kidney. Such antibody may be present as the result of (1) exposure to the foreign HLA antigens in previous blood transfusions, (2) exposure to paternal HLA antigens of a fetus during pregnancy, (3) previous kidney transplants, or (4) exposure to cross-reacting viral or bacterial antigens. When antibody recognizes foreign antigen, complement is fixed and graft destruction begins immediately. On a clinical level, the downhill sequence of events occurs promptly and becomes obvious in either the operating room or the recovery room. Urine production becomes bloody and then ceases entirely. The patient is often febrile and hypertensive and looks quite ill. This type of rapid antibody-mediated rejection is usually irreversible and often requires prompt transplant removal.

ACCELERATED REJECTION

Accelerated rejection is a variant of hyperacute rejection. This occurs when the recipient has been previously exposed to donor foreign antigen, but the serum antibody level to these antigens is low or absent. In this circumstance the donor-recipient crossmatch will be negative. The new graft acts as a "booster," and a rapid and more intensive anamnestic response begins sooner than would classic acute rejection. The patient may become febrile with rapid decline in renal function on the second to sixth post-transplant day. Sometimes this process reverses, but it is difficult to control with antirejection therapy.

ACUTE REJECTION

Acute rejection is a process mediated primarily by cells rather than antibody. In contrast to hyperacute rejection, which occurs very rarely, acute rejection is a rather constant feature of transplantation. The clinical onset of rejection is quite variable and depends upon the degree of antigen disparity between donor and recipient and also the type and dose of immunosuppressive drugs being used.

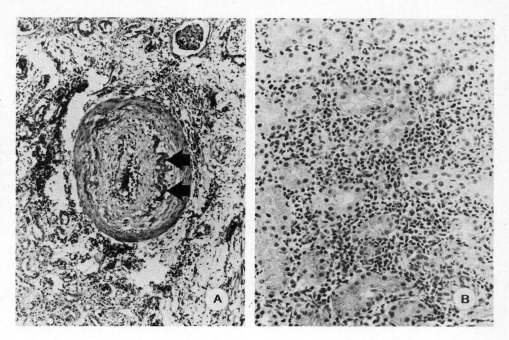

Figure 4. Acute rejection of a renal allograft. A, Vascular alteration in severe acute rejection. There is a necrotizing vasculitis present with fibrinoid necrosis (arrows) and neutrophilic infiltration of the vessel wall (H & E × 330). B, Acute cellular rejection with an intense mononuclear cell infiltrate in the interstitium with edema and active tubular breakdown (H & E × 208).

The clinical signs and symptoms associated with this process are well documented with kidney transplantation. After an initial 7 to 10 day period of relative calm, the patient becomes lethargic and febrile. The febrile response is probably the result of either host release of interleukin-1 (formerly termed endogenous pyrogen) by macrophages or the damaged allogeneic cells releasing their contents (pyrogens) in the host circulation. As donor vascular endothelium becomes edematous, the kidney becomes relatively ischemic, the patient becomes hypertensive, and renal function deteriorates. The allograft usually swells. Although there are no intact nervous connections to the recipient, the enlarging inflamed organ presses against parietal peritoneum, and the patient often experiences pain at the operative site. If the swelling is pronounced, the transplant may partially occlude the iliac veins, producing scrotal or labial edema and ipsilateral leg edema. In contrast to hyperacute rejection, which is not treatable, a high percentage of acute rejection episodes (85 to 95 per cent) are reversible. Usually high doses of intravenous or oral steroids are administered. Sometimes antithymocyte globulin is given when rejection fails to respond to steroid pulse therapy. Recent monoclonal antibodies specifically directed at T3 and T12 lymphocyte subsets have been used clinically to reverse rejection.

The clinical events associated with the rejection of other organs are considerably less obvious than those seen when kidneys are transplanted. Acute rejection following heart transplantation, for example, may be manifest clinically only by a falling cardiac output and blood pressure. Because these findings occur late in the process, the diagnosis of cardiac allograft rejection depends upon routine endomyocardial biopsy rather than clinical signs or laboratory tests. The diagnosis and management of rejection are discussed in more detail in the sections on individual organs.

CHRONIC REJECTION

Chronic rejection is an indolent form of rejection with few clinical signs. In the case of renal transplantation, the syndrome is characterized by salt retention, weight gain, progressive proteinuria, and a gradual and inexorable rise in the serum creatinine. The immune mechanisms responsible for this process are not well understood, but clearly both cell-mediated and humoral mechanisms are involved. Histologically, chronic rejection is characterized primarily by occlusion of vessels and tubular atrophy (Fig. 5). Immunofluorescent studies demonstrate the presence of immunoglobulin, complement components, and fibrinogen throughout the graft. Chronic rejection may occur as early as 7 to 10 days following transplantation but ordinarily is not seen until after the first postoperative month. In contrast to acute rejection, chronic rejection responds poorly to treatment with steroids.

Strategies for Successful Transplantation of Allogeneic Tissue

AVOIDING HYPERACUTE REJECTION

Determining that the prospective recipient does not possess circulating antigraft antibody is of great importance, particularly in the field of renal transplantation. Because solid organ transplants generally express blood group antigens as well as histocompatibility antigens, such antibody could be in the form of naturally occurring antibodies to blood group antigens (isoantibodies) or antibody directed at cell surface HLA determinants (lymphocytotoxic antibodies). Accordingly, two straightforward tests are done prior to transplantation. First, ABO cross-matching is done so that donor and recipient are compatible for red blood cell group antigens. The same rules of blood transfusion apply to organ donation; blood groups are matched if possible, but an "O" type donor is a "universal donor" and an AB type recipient is a "universal recipient." When ABO compatibility exists, a "lymphocytotoxic cross-match" is done to test for the presence of antigraft antibody in recipient serum. As stated previously, this is much more important for renal transplantation than for liver or heart transplantation.

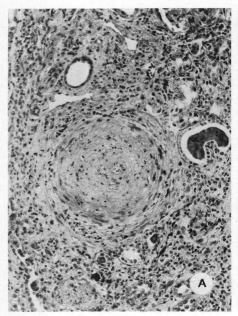
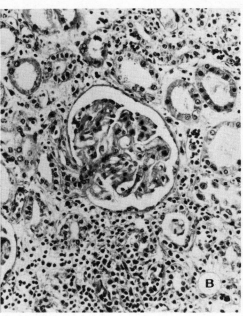

Figure 5. Chronic rejection of a renal allograft. A, Vascular alterations in chronic rejection. Note the marked thickening of the vessel wall with obliteration of the vessel lumen (H & E × 330). B, Glomerular and tubulointerstitial alterations in chronic rejection. The glomerulus has an increased amount of mesangial matrix plus irregularly thickened glomerular capillary loops. The tubulointerstitial component of the biopsy reveals marked tubular atrophy with increased interstitial fibrosis and mononuclear cell infiltration (H & E × 330).

The lymphocytotoxic cross-match is as simple as the ABO cross-match. Recipient serum is incubated with donor lymphocytes in the presence of rabbit complement for 4 hours. Killing of more than 20 per cent of donor lymphocytes during incubation is evidence that antigraft antibodies are present. A more sophisticated analysis is sometimes done in which peripheral blood T and B cells are separated prior to cross-match testing. Although the issue is somewhat controversial, antibodies directed at B cells but not T cells do not generally cause hyperacute rejection, and transplantation is often done if the recipient possesses only anti–B cell antibodies to the donor. Under no circumstances is transplantation done if antibody to donor T cells is detected. Antibody levels wax and wane, and an older serum sample from a recipient is often found to contain antidonor antibody while the most recent specimen does not. In this circumstance, transplantation is usually not done because of the fear that low levels of antibody are present but for some reason not detectable and that a hyperacute or anamnestic accelerated rejection would occur.

MINIMIZING ANTIGENIC DISPARITY

An organ transplanted between identical twins never undergoes rejection. Conversely, an organ transplanted between completely unrelated individuals usually undergoes severe rejection, and potent immunosuppressive drugs are required to reverse the process. Attempts to match donor 1503and recipient antigens as much as possible would seem logical to minimize the intensity of the rejection process. This general principle is clearly true in the case of related renal transplantation and bone marrow transplantation and somewhat less obvious in the case of cadaveric renal transplantation and may not be true at all in the case of liver and heart transplantation.

HLA TYPING IN RELATED RENAL TRANSPLANTATION

Humans have two kidneys, but each one is capable of sustaining life individually. For this reason it is possible for a healthy individual to donate one kidney to a relative.

Such a transplant is called a related renal transplant. The other type of kidney transplant, called a cadaveric renal transplant, means that the donor organ has been removed from an unrelated individual who has experienced "brain death." There are many advantages of voluntary related donation, including the fact that the donor may be preselected on the basis of close antigenic similarity to the recipient. In the absence of an identical twin, the best results are obtained if donor and recipient are HLA identical, indicating that they have inherited the same parental sixth chromosomes, somewhat less promising if donor and recipient are HLA semi-identical (share one chromosome 6), and even less promising if donor and recipient are HLA nonidentical (do not share either chromosome 6).

The inheritance of HLA antigens follows straightforward rules of Mendelian genetics. The haplotype status of family members is easily determined using serologic techniques in which various alleles of the A, B, C, and D locus are defined. Usually only the HLA-A and HLA-B alleles are typed. HLA alleles are codominant. The allele on both the maternal and paternal chromosome 6 is expressed. Usually four HLA alleles, that is, two HLA-A and two HLA-B, are identified in an individual. Identity of the four allele products in the donor and the four products in the recipient would indicate HLA identity. Two of the alleles identical with HLA semi-identical individuals and none of the typed alleles would be expected to be shared in the HLA nonidentical case. Parent-child transplants are always one-haplotype matches. The probability that siblings will be HLA identical is 25 per cent, HLA semi-identical 50 per cent, and HLA nonidentical 25 per cent.

MIXED LYMPHOCYTE CULTURE

The mixed lymphocyte culture (MLC) is an assay used to gain information about antigenic disparity at the HLA-D locus. This assay takes advantage of the observation that lymphocytes cocultivated in vitro between donor and recipient will proliferate rapidly if one cell population expresses HLA-D locus products that are different from HLA-D locus products expressed in the other cell population. The rate of cellular proliferation is measured and is taken as a rough index of HLA-D disparity. We are most interested in the response of recipient lymphocytes to donor lymphocyte antigens. The donor cells are usually inactivated with radiation or mitomycin-C so that only the rate of proliferation of recipient cells will be measured. A very high percentage (98 per cent) of HLA identical donor-recipient pairs shows low reactivity in MLC, whereas only 20 per cent of HLA semi-identical pairs demonstrate low reactivity in MLC. Given a choice of HLA semi-identical donors, the potential donor whose cells stimulate the least proliferation in MLC is preferable. Because this is a functional *in vitro* assay, the MLC has been called a "transplant in a test tube." One disadvantage of the MLC is that the *in vitro* incubation requires 5 to 6 days. Thus, MLC cannot be used in the selection of cadaveric donors because these organs may be reliably preserved for only 1 to 2 days.

DONOR-RECIPIENT MATCHING USING CADAVERIC DONORS

With cadaveric transplantation identical chromosomes are not shared between donor and recipient, and one can only hope that some individual HLA-coded alleles are identical by random chance. For many years only A and B locus products were typed because it was determined early that matching for C locus products did not correlate with the success of transplants and because matching for D locus products was technically difficult. After many years of matching for A and B locus products in cadaveric renal transplantation, investigators have learned that there is a small but consistent benefit to antigen matching. An unrelated donor recipient pair with all four HLA-A and HLA-B locus products matched will have a 10 per cent greater chance of success at 1 year and possibly an even greater improved success rate at 5 years. Unfortunately, given the diversity of allelic products at the A and B loci, the chance of "four antigen match" between two unrelated individuals is small (0.015 per cent). A major logistic program would be required to match a significant number of cadaveric donor recipient pairs, and the overall influence on results would be minimal. Further, the extreme potency of modern immunosuppressive drugs has tended to supersede small benefits to be gained from A and B locus matching. Many programs no longer select donor and recipient on the basis of this information.

Matching the D locus products has more potential for improving transplantation results. First, the locus is less polymorphic, i.e., there are far fewer allelic products coded for by this locus so that the chances for matching between unrelated individuals is greater (see Table 1). Second, because HLA-D codes for Class II type antigens, which are involved in the inductive phase of the immune response, one would hope that matching for this type of antigen would tend to limit the perception of "foreignness" by recipient cells. As mentioned earlier, the MLC assay used to define HLA-D locus products is not applicable to cadaveric transplantation because it requires 5 to 6 days to perform. Only recently has it been possible to type D locus type products serologically, a process requiring only a few hours. The typed alleles are probably not exactly the same antigens as those measured in MLC, but they are very similar and the responsible locus is known to be very close or tightly "linked" to the true HLA-D locus. For this reason, the serologically defined antigens are referred to as HLA-DR (D-"related") antigens. DR matching has an important influence on results in renal transplantation. Substantial benefit is obtained only when both HLA-DR alleles are identical between donor and recipient. The DR locus is less polymorphic than other loci, and donor and recipient can be matched for both DR products in many cases.

For reasons that are unclear but that may be related to differential expression of antigen on different types of organs, matching for any kind of antigen does not appear helpful in liver or heart transplantation.

Immunosuppression

All transplants, except those utilizing identical twins, require immunosuppression to prevent rejection. Traditional immunosuppression has involved a combination of glucocorticoid drugs and azathioprine (Imuran) with large intravenous doses of steroids administered to reverse acute rejection episodes. This regimen, called "conventional immunosuppression," has been effective but suffers from a lack of specificity, with general depression of the immune system resulting commonly in infectious complication. The following paragraphs describe immunosuppressive drugs currently in use in most programs. Some centers are developing a "triple drug" maintenance regimen of prednisone-cyclosporine-azathioprine, all in low doses in the hope of improving effectiveness but lowering infectious complications. A general trend is toward reduced steroid dosages and development of drugs capable of more specifically depressing antiallograft immunity.

CORTICOSTEROIDS

Corticosteroid drugs were first used to reverse a clinical rejection episode in 1960. Since that time, steroids have been incorporated as a basic component of all types of immunosuppressive regimens. Over the years many dose-related side effects and complications have been recognized. The current approach to immunosuppressive therapy utilizes much smaller doses of drug than were used previously.

Steroids are administered from the time of transplantation at a daily maintenance dose. Initially large doses are given, but over the course of a few weeks the dose is tapered to the lowest tolerated maintenance dose. When acute rejection intervenes, three or four "pulses" consisting of large doses of intravenous or oral steroids are given daily or every other day. The precise mechanism by which a beneficial effect is obtained from steroids is not clearly understood. Probably the most important effect, elucidated only recently, relates to the observation that the *in vitro* generation of cytotoxic T cells is impeded in the presence of steroids. More specifically, steroids are known to block the production of interleukin-1 by the macrophage and interleukin-2 by helper T cells (Fig. 6). Other mechanisms are also important and may relate to anti-inflammatory properties rather than immunosuppressive effects *per se*. Steroids stabilize lysosomal membranes, an attribute that may be particularly important when considering the important cytocidal effect of activated macrophages.

AZATHIOPRINE

Schwartz and Damashek demonstrated in 1959 that the purine analogue 6-mercaptopurine produces specific tolerance in rabbits. Later azathioprine, a less toxic derivative of 6-MP, was introduced into clinical practice. This drug is metabolized in the liver into 6-thioinosinic acid, which in turn inhibits the synthesis of both DNA and RNA (see Fig. 6). As a consequence of its effects on nucleic acid synthesis, the widespread cellular activation characteristic of the re-

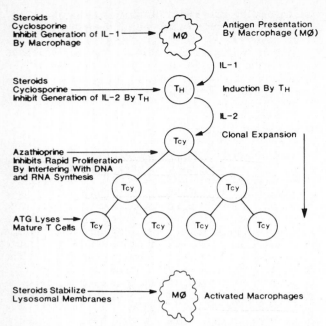

Figure 6. Sites of action of immunosuppressive drugs. Many of these drugs have other important actions and side effects throughout the body. For instance, azathioprine is a general purine antimetabolite that interferes with purine synthesis throughout the body.

jection phenomenon is partially inhibited. Azathioprine by itself is not sufficiently immunosuppressive in the great majority of circumstances to allow for the successful transplantation of an allograft, and steroids are always administered concomitantly. Because of its effects on actively dividing cells, azathioprine also has a substantial bone marrow toxicity, and hematologic parameters must be evaluated regularly in patients receiving this drug. Azathioprine is catabolized by xanthine oxidase; therefore, the dosage of azathioprine is greatly reduced in patients also receiving allopurinol, a xanthine oxidase inhibitor.

Cyclosporine

Cyclosporine is a drug isolated from the mycelia of *Tolypocladium inflatum* Gams, a fungus found in the soil of southern Norway. Borel first described the immunosuppressive effects of cyclosporine in 1976. In succeeding years, this class of drugs has been investigated extensively. The consensus is that cyclosporine is the most potent immunosuppressive substance yet discovered. In most centers the percentage of patients with successful cadaveric renal transplants 1 year following transplantation has increased by 20 per cent following institution of a cyclosporine-prednisone immunosuppressive regimen. Furthermore, cyclosporine is not associated with the broad depression of recipient immunity usually seen with other immunosuppressive drugs. Cyclosporine appears to act principally at the level of the T cell with little effect on B cells and antibody production. The primary immunosuppressive effect involves the relatively specific inhibition of interleukin-2 generation by helper T cells, with resultant inhibition of clonal expansion (see Fig. 6). However, cyclosporine administration also causes inhibition of the production of interleukin-1 by monocytes. Many observers have noted an alteration in the balance of T cell subsets in cyclosporine-treatment patients

such that the T4 "helper" subset is depressed in relation to the T8 suppressor/cytotoxic group. Cyclosporine may have a suppressor "sparing" effect, and a preponderance of suppressor T cells may provide an immunologic advantage to the transplant recipient.

Substantial nephrotoxicity occurs with the administration of cyclosporine. This side effect requires careful monitoring of drug dosage and serum levels. Usually a drug dose can eventually be found that is immunosuppressive but not nephrotoxic. An early concern about development of lymphomas in cyclosporine-treated patients has not been borne out on subsequent analysis. In a large series the incidence of malignancy was 0.5 per cent, a figure even lower than that for patients treated conventionally with a prednisone-azathioprine regimen. Other side effects, such as tremor, gum hypertrophy, hirsutism, hypertension, and hyperkalemia, have also been observed.

Heterologous Antiserum Directed Against Human T Cells

Because T cells bear distinctive antigens not found on other cells, it is possible to produce heterologous antibodies that will specifically lyse human T cells. Commonly such antibody is generated by injecting human thymocytes into horses or rabbits; the resultant preparation is called antithymocyte globulin (ATG). A similar preparation may be made against a human lymphoblastoid line (ALG for antilymphoblast globulin). Regardless of the details of antibody production, heterologous anti–T cell serum is very effective in reversing acute rejection episodes. Unfortunately, because the immunogen (thymocytes or lymphoblastoid lines) is often not completely pure, antibodies to other antigens are also formed and may cause serious problems, such as thrombocytopenia. Because T cells are actually lysed after administration of this reagent, patients often temporarily suffer significant symptoms such as rigors and high fever.

Monoclonal Antibody

Kohler and Milstein first described the technology for making monoclonal antibodies. Such relatively "pure" antibodies can also be made against specific T cell differentiation antigens and used for immunosuppressive purposes. Currently, ongoing investigations are evaluating a monoclonal anti-T3 and anti-T12, both "pan" T cell antigens. In the future monoclonal antibodies to subset antigens such as T4, T8, and IL-2 will undoubtedly be developed. Side effects, such as thrombocytopenia, have not been seen using these preparations. Despite the inherent attractiveness associated with the use of mouse monoclonal antibodies for the treatment of rejection, a limiting feature is that the recipient will recognize the mouse antibody as foreign and may rapidly make antibody against the injected monoclonal antibody combining site. This anti-"idiotypic" antibody would preclude further use of the monoclonal antibody. Presumably such a phenomenon would not limit the effectiveness of the cruder horse preparations because they contain hundreds of anti–T cell specificities, not all of which could be blocked by the host immune response.

Immunologic Tolerance

Tolerance is defined as a specific unresponsiveness to antigen induced by previous exposure to that antigen. A distinction is made whether tolerance is developed to autologous tissue (self-tolerance) or is the result of manipulation of the immune system (acquired tolerance). The subject of acquired tolerance is of great interest to transplant biologists. Induction of specific tolerance to an allograft would presumably spare the function of the rest of the immune system, and the significant incidence of infection associated with nonspecific immunosuppression would be avoided. Before reviewing the attempts to induce specific tolerance in clinical transplantation, it is helpful to review some of the more well-understood mechanisms accounting for tolerance in experimental animals.

CLONAL DELETION

In 1949, Burnet and Feiner proposed a theory to explain why an individual's immune system does not attack its own tissues. According to Burnet's hypothesis, the clone of lymphoid cells capable of recognizing "self" antigens is deleted at some point in early embryologic development. Deletion of this clone results in lifelong unresponsiveness to "self" antigens.

Experimentally, injection of antigen into an animal at birth often results in long lasting tolerance to that antigen, and in some instances the clonal deletion theory has been implicated. Particularly good evidence for this mechanism comes from the observation that transfer of syngeneic (same strain) lymphoid cells from a nontolerant animal reverses the tolerance, i.e., no additional mechanism prevents the transferred normal cells from reacting to the involved antigen. However, in some well-described cases, transfer of normal syngeneic cells does not reverse neonatal tolerance, suggesting that the phenomenon may be the result of other mechanisms as well.

TOLERANCE INDUCED BY PREADMINISTRATION OF ANTIGEN

The optimal immune response to antigen depends upon a number of factors, including the dose of antigen used, molecular weight, solubility, and other physical characteristics of the antigen in question and the route and timing of the administered substance. The optimal response will depend upon the genetic background and capabilities of the injected animal and, in the case of response to an allograft, the type of histocompatibility barrier to be overcome. If conditions of immunization are not optimal a suboptimal or weak immune response may occur, and in some cases a specific long-lasting tolerance results. Many experimental models have been used to investigate conditions under which antigen-induced tolerance to allografts occurs.

Usually the antigen used has been whole blood, blood products, or more purified lymphoid cells from thymus, lymph node, or spleen. The intravenous route of administration of antigen is clearly more tolerogenic than other routes, and in the case of adult animals it is helpful if the recipient is partially immunosuppressed in some way. Soluble antigen is usually more tolerogenic than cell-bound antigen. Depending upon the system studied, both Class I and Class II antigens are capable of inducing tolerance. The strain combination tested is of primary importance. Often a tolerogenic protocol in one strain combination is completely ineffective in another combination. This observation relates to the recent recognition that the immune response to MHC antigens is controlled by specific inherited immune response genes. In interpreting rodent experiments, it is important to note that tolerance induction is particularly easy in rats but not necessarily easy in other species, including man. A particular risk of antigen pretreatment protocols is that the recipient becomes sensitized rather than tolerant to the administered antigen. If this occurred in a human setting, hyperacute rejection might result. Rats generally do not develop hyperacute rejection because of substantial differences in mechanisms for complement fixation.

TOLERANCE INDUCED BY ADMINISTRATION OF ANTIDONOR ANTIBODY

Passive administration of antidonor antibody at the time of transplantation may result in tolerance to the involved antigen. This phenomenon, known as immunologic enhancement, was originally thought to be the result of "masking" or covering up of the involved antigen by antibody so that immune recognition was inhibited. The weight of evidence currently suggests that it is the ability of the administered antibody to promote opsonization of antigen reactive cells that is of critical importance. In this latter model, the enhancing antibody or antigen antibody complexes bind to host T cell receptors and the complexed antigen reactive T cell is quickly eliminated (opsonized) by the host reticuloendothelial system. Antibodies to both Class I and Class II antigens are effective in certain models. Noncytotoxic antibody is also often effective in causing enhancement, an observation of interest to clinicians since with this type of antibody the dangers of causing hyperacute rejection would be reduced. Unfortunately, noncytotoxic antibody fragments (Fab-2 fragments), which have specificity for antigen but do not fix complement, are not effective in producing enhancement.

TOLERANCE INDUCED BY THE GENERATION OF ANTI-IDIOTYPIC ANTIBODY

Administered antigen generates the production of anti-antigen antibody. The antigen-specific combining site on the antibody molecule is called the *idiotype*. Idiotypes are also found on the cell surface of certain lymphoid cells, predominantly the T cells. Because the idiotype is very specific for the foreign antigen, it is in some ways "foreign" itself and the host develops "anti-idiotypic" antibody. Such an anti-idiotypic antibody functions to limit the immune response to antigen since it blocks the receptor for antigen on cells or antibody molecules. One might theoretically limit the immune response to an allograft by stimulating the generation of anti-idiotypic antibody. This has been accomplished in a rat cardiac allograft model, but whether such a technique could be used in humans is unknown.

TOLERANCE MEDIATED BY SUPPRESSOR CELLS

Any of the foregoing circumstances under which tolerance occurs may be mediated by subpopulations of cells capable of suppressing the immune response. The most studied examples involve suppressor T cells, which release soluble mediators called *suppressor factors*. These factors act to limit the participation of helper T cells in generating an immune response. Interestingly, the suppressor factors often demonstrate a histocompatibility restriction, so that suppressor factor elicited in one animal would not necessarily be effective on transfer to another animal. Although there are many examples of nonspecific suppression, the most thoroughly studied instances of suppression involving organ transplants describe a suppressor population that is antigen specific. For example, the recipients of long-lasting related renal transplants have been found to have in their blood suppressor T cells capable of suppressing *in vitro* immune responses to donor cells but not unrelated cells.

ATTEMPTS TO INDUCE TOLERANCE IN TRANSPLANT PATIENTS

Based on the experimental work previously described, a number of innovations have been added recently to the more traditional strategies of immunosuppression. Attempts have been made to actively deplete donor organs of "passenger cells" prior to transplantation in the hope of decreasing the immunogenicity of the organ. Cadaveric donors have been pretreated with high doses of cytotoxic drugs prior to organ removal in the hope that these high doses would result in lysis of lymphoid or macrophage passenger cells in the transplanted organ. These trials have met with limited success. Sensitization may have occurred by an alternative mechanism whereby donor endothelium sheds antigen alone and this antigen is then processed by host macrophages.

In other trials, recipients have been given solubilized HLA antigens or buffy coat extracts of donor cells prior to transplantation, but no clear beneficial effect has been noted. Enhancement by the administration of antidonor antibody has also been attempted. Intact antidonor antibody was not given for fear of eliciting hyperacute rejection. Instead, antidonor antibody was first treated with papain, an enzyme that cleaves off the antibody receptor for complement (Fc receptor). This treatment produces Fab fragments, which have specific combining sites for donor antigen but do not fix complement. Using this strategy, hyperacute rejection would not result. Unfortunately, Fab fragments are known to be relatively ineffective in producing enhancement experimentally. Clinical trials with Fab fragments have also been disappointing.

PRETRANSPLANT BLOOD TRANSFUSIONS

Pretransplant blood transfusions have been demonstrated by many groups to improve results. Antigen is administered in the form of allogeneic white blood cells and platelets from the blood donor. An attractive hypothesis to explain these observations is that after exposure to such antigen both helper and suppressor T cell subsets are activated, but the kinetics of activation differ so that helper T cells are active early, followed by a slower onset of activation of suppressor T cells. If an organ transplant is then performed subsequent to transfusion, when the T suppressor subset is predominant, rejection would be suppressed.

Whether this is the correct mechanism, most transplant centers require that cadaveric transplant recipients be "preconditioned" with three to five preoperative blood transfusions. Such a hypothesis requires that the suppressor generated be relatively nonspecific since it is unlikely that donor blood and donor organ from different individuals would share substantial amounts of antigen. A more specific type of preconditioning can be utilized in related renal transplantation. Donor-specific transfusions involve preoperative administration of 200 ml. of blood obtained from the prospective donor every 2 weeks on three occasions prior to transplantation. If sensitization does not occur, the transplant is then performed. The results with such protocols have been very successful even though the mechanism is not fully understood. The use of donor-specific transfusions is discussed more fully in the section on renal transplantation.

Today transplant surgeons primarily depend upon nonspecific immunosuppressive drugs to prevent or reverse rejection. Clearly the direction for the future is to induce tolerance or selectively interdict an immune response with the use of purified antigen, monoclonal antibody, or immunocompetent cells directed toward a specific target receptor.

MULTIORGAN PROCUREMENT AND PRESERVATION

The need for donor organs is directly related to the success of the transplant procedure. With improved patient and organ graft survival, age limitations and other indications tend to be liberalized. The history of kidney transplantation exemplifies this trend. In contrast to the initial strict guidelines, kidney transplants are now performed in infants, in adults up to age 60 or 65, in patients with diabetes mellitus, and in patients with other chronic diseases that previously would have precluded their receiving a transplant. The availability of cadaver organs has not kept pace with the expanding need. As a result, the list of patients awaiting a kidney transplant continues to lengthen despite the fact that increased numbers of kidney transplants are performed each year. In 1984, the American Council on Transplantation published estimates of the number of patients awaiting transplant and the need for transplantation of major organs (Table 3).

Availability of Donors

The potential number of cadaveric donors in the United States has been estimated to be approximately 20,000 annually. At present, only about 4000 cadaver donors are being utilized despite the great need for more organs. The age limit for heart donation is 35 years, a restriction that further limits the availability of this organ. The Battelle Institute has estimated that the potential for cardiac donors is 16,000 per year and the total number of potential recipients is 14,111. Heart, heart-lung, lung, and liver donor organs must be of a size appropriate for the individual recipient. As a result, it is especially difficult to find a suitable donor of these organs for children.

The reasons why only a small proportion of potential cadaveric donors are actually utilized are complex. The most correctable cause is the failure of physicians and nurses to identify appropriate donors and inquire about donations with family members. Recently, the states of New York, Oregon, and Michigan passed "mandatory request" laws. These laws require that hospitals establish a system that assures that a qualified individual will approach families when it is obvious that their relative is about to expire. In fact, bereaved families often obtain much solace from the knowledge that someone else might benefit from what otherwise is the tragic loss of a family member.

TABLE 3. *Status of Organ Transplantation in 1984**

	Performed	**Waiting List**
Bone marrow	865	N/A
Cornea	23,500	3,500
Heart	400	100
Heart/lung	17	50
Kidney	6,730	11,000
Liver	308	300
Pancreas	87	50

*These estimates were provided by The American Council of Transplantation. The true need is larger than the "waiting list." For instance, the need for kidney transplants is estimated at 20,000 per year and for heart transplants at 16,000 per year.

Organ Sharing and Organ Procurement Agencies

Transplantation is by its very nature a cooperative effort between donor and recipient, between donor hospital and recipient hospital, and between the multiple physicians necessarily involved with the procurement and transplantation of an organ. In the early years of kidney transplantation it was recognized that regional organizations were necessary to coordinate these efforts. There are now 110 hospital-related and 51 independent organ procurement agencies in the United States. These agencies in turn cooperate with each other, thus providing an informal network that spans the entire United States and interacts with agencies in other countries. These organizations provide a 24-hour telephone communication system, lists of patients awaiting cadaveric transplantation, histocompatibility typing, organ procurement and preservation teams, systems for billing hospital and physician costs, educational programs, and follow-up data. In 1984, the federal government established the Task Force on Organ Transplantation, which is expected to make recommendations for a more formal national network, including a national listing of patients awaiting organ transplantation.

Brain Death

In the United States the concept of "brain death" is now generally accepted. Previously an individual was declared dead when a physician judged that his heart had stopped. Now a person can be legally declared dead if a physician judges that his brain function has been so severely and irreversibly damaged that life cannot be sustained without artificial support. Such patients always require support with a respirator. Organs can be removed before cardiac activity ceases, thus avoiding injury from anoxia and ischemia.

Presently 30 states have brain death laws. These laws state that the declaration of "brain death" by a physician constitutes legal death. Most of the established guidelines for confirming the presence of "brain death" are based on the Harvard criteria published in 1968. Many hospitals have now established their own criteria for "brain death" and organized committees to evaluate individual potential organ donors. To avoid any possible conflict of interest, the patient's personal physician and members of the transplant team are not included as members of these committees. With experience, most institutions have made the criteria for "brain death" less rigid. For example, the required interval between isoelectroencephalograms has been eliminated or reduced from 24 to 12 hours. The criteria currently utilized at the University of Michigan are outlined in Table 4. The great majority of cadaveric organ donors have expired from head injuries, cerebrovascular accidents, brain tumors, or brain ischemia secondary to such events as cardiac arrest and drug overdose.

Criteria for Organ Donation

The general and organ-specific criteria for donation are listed in Tables 5 and 6. Because potential organ donors are near death and frequently have abnormalities such as pulmonary infiltrates and bacteriuria, there is a tendency to preclude patients inappropriately as possible organ donors. Usually it is best to have the patient evaluated by a physician experienced in organ transplantation before deciding that there is a contraindication to donation.

TABLE 4. *Guidelines for the Establishment of Brain Death at the University of Michigan Medical Center**

Clinical Examination
1. Absent cerebral function. No response to external stimuli. Absent decerebrate or decorticate responses.
2. Absent brainstem function. The following reflexes are absent:
   a. Pupillary light and reflex
   b. Corneal reflex
   c. Oculocephalic reflex
   d. Oculovestibular reflex
   e. Respiratory reflex, i.e., apnea off respirator, no respiratory reflex when P_{CO_2} is 60 torr or greater.

Confirming Studies
1. Electrocerebral silence by electroencephalogram (EEG) at normothermia and in the presence of a negative drug screen. This examination is strongly recommended unless not feasible.
2. Four-vessel cerebral angiography demonstrating no intracranial flow. This test may be used if EEG not feasible.
3. Brainstem auditory evoked potentials (BAEPS) are used to confirm the loss of brainstem functions in drug-induced coma. Brainstem reflexes may be suppressed by certain drugs but BAEPS are resistant to CNS suppressant drugs. Not necessary on a routine basis.

*Note that only one EEG is required.

Related donors are utilized routinely only for kidney transplantation. The University of Minnesota is the only institution using related donors for pancreas transplantation at the present time. Living volunteers must have normal function of the donor organ and no risk factors that would increase operative mortality or morbidity.

Management of the Cadaver Donor

Once a patient has been declared dead, every effort should be made to avoid injury to the transplantable organs. The cadaver donor is monitored and provided the same physiologic support in an intensive care unit as a living patient. Frequently cadaver donors are dehydrated because fluids have been restricted to avoid cerebral edema. Intravascular volume is restored and balanced electrolyte solutions, blood transfusions, and adrenergic drugs, such as dopamine or dobutamine, are administered as needed to maintain a normal blood pressure and a urinary output of 50 to 100 ml./hr. Vasoconstrictive doses of dopamine are discouraged because of potential injury to the organs and to avoid depletion of catecholamines if heart transplantation is contemplated. Injury to the hypothalamus may induce diabetes insipidus. This is treated with pitressin or oxytocin. At times a central venous catheter or a Swan-Ganz catheter is placed to assist in monitoring. The administration of

TABLE 5. *General Criteria for Organ Donors*

Appropriate age and size
Brain death
Reasonably stable cardiovascular system
No systemic sepsis
No contamination of abdomen for kidney, liver, or pancreas transplants
No malignancy except primary brain cancer or skin cancer
No chronic hypertension
No hepatitis antigenemia
No diabetes mellitus*

*Diabetes mellitus is only a relative contraindication. Some groups will use kidneys or livers in patients with diabetes if renal or liver function is normal.

TABLE 6. *Specific Cadaveric Donor Criteria for Individual Organs*

Kidney
  1 to 55 years of age
  Admitting creatinine less than 1.5 mg./100 ml.
  No history of chronic renal disease

Liver
  Few months to 50 years of age
  Normal liver function tests
  No history of hepatitis or chronic liver disease
  Compatible liver size (donor weight within + 10 per cent to
    − 20% of recipient weight)

Heart
  Less than 35 years of age
  No cardiac disease
  No cardiac arrest
  No traumatic chest injury
  Normal chest x-ray
  Normal electrocardiogram
  Compatible heart size

Pancreas
  1 to 50 years of age
  No history of diabetes in immediate family
  No history of pancreatitis
  Near normal serum amylase
  Glucose level does *not* have to be normal

mannitol has been demonstrated to be of benefit for kidney preservation. Some groups also administer steroids to the donor as an adjunct to organ preservation.

As much history as possible is obtained from family members, especially concerning such chronic diseases as hypertension, diabetes mellitus, chronic heart, liver, or kidney disease, cancer, and substance abuse. Blood, urine, and tracheal cultures are routinely obtained. Blood studies usually include hematocrit, white blood cell count, electrolytes, glucose, liver and renal function studies, hepatitis antigen and antibody studies, CMV antibody titers, and, most recently, HTVL-III antibody studies, especially in patients at risk for acquired immune deficiency disease. Fever, leukocytosis, positive cultures from endotracheal tubes or urinary catheters, and mild abnormalities on chest x-ray are not in themselves contraindications to donation.

Organ Preservation

Much of the morbidity and mortality associated with transplantation can be directly attributed to less than optimal organ preservation. Excellent function of the transplanted organ in the early postoperative period avoids many problems later. Good organ preservation begins with proper preoperative and intraoperative management of the cadaver donor. Hypotension and anoxia must be avoided, the organs and tissues must be handled gently, and the length of warm ischemia during removal of the organ from the donor must be kept to a minimum. Careful *ex vivo* preservation techniques are essential. The length of rewarming time during revascularization of the organ should also be kept to a minimum. The kidney will usually tolerate 30 minutes of warm ischemia well. There will be an increasing incidence of postoperative acute renal failure with 30 to 60 minutes of warm ischemia. After 2 hours of warm ischemia most kidneys are nonviable. The duration of warm ischemia that the heart, liver, and pancreas will tolerate is significantly less.

COLD STORAGE

Hypothermia at 2 to 4°C. is the most effective modality available to preserve organs. By slowing the rate of chemical reactions and decreasing energy utilization, the damaging effects of hypoxia and ischemia are minimized. Organs may be cooled *in situ* in the donor by quickly perfusing the organ through a previously placed aortic cannula with cold electrolyte solution just after clamping the aorta below the diaphragm. Normothermic ischemia is thus kept to a minimum. The extirpated organs are then flushed free of blood with a 2 to 4°C. preservation solution. Most transplant groups use a solution that has a high potassium and low sodium concentration and large concentrations of relatively impermeable solute such as glucose, phosphate citrate, and mannitol. The most widely used solutions are those developed by Collins, Sacks, and Ross. The flushed organ is then immersed in cold electrolyte solution, placed in a sterile plastic bag or container, and stored at approximately 4°C., usually by surrounding the container with ice.

Cold storage is the least expensive and simplest form of preservation. It is the only method currently available for the storage of the heart, liver and pancreas. Safe limits for the length of preservation using cold storage are 4 hours for heart, 6 hours for pancreas, 8 hours for liver, and up to 30 hours for kidney.

HYPOTHERMIC PULSATILE PERFUSION

The technique of hypothermic pulsatile perfusion was developed to extend the safe duration of preservation beyond that achievable with simple hypothermia. This technique requires an organ preservation machine and combines hypothermia at 6 to 10°C. with pulsatile or continuous roller pump type perfusion and a special oxygenated perfusate. Pulsatile perfusion at a relatively low pressure of 40 to 60 torr systolic and 20 to 40 torr diastolic is thought to open microcirculation and deliver substrate to parenchymal cells. Usually a protein-rich solution, such as cryoprecipitated plasma, plasma protein fraction, silica gel–treated plasma, or a mannitol solution with electrolyte composition similar to extracellular fluid, is utilized. Belzer, of the University of Wisconsin, a pioneer in the development of pulsatile perfusion, has recently obtained excellent results with a new perfusate containing adenosine and gluconate.

At the present time pulsatile perfusion is utilized only for cadaveric kidney preservation. Successful transplantation of kidneys with prompt function has been reported with preservation times up to 72 hours. There is some evidence that this technique is preferable to simple hypothermia if there has already been damage to the kidney in the donor or if preservation times of greater than 24 to 30 hours are anticipated. High perfusion pressures and low flow of perfusates through the graft suggest injury to the kidney and allow a selective discarding of kidneys. However, pulsatile perfusion is expensive and has a greater risk of microbial contamination, embolization, and endothelial damage than simple hypothermia. Currently, there is considerable investigation into the potential of pulsatile perfusion to increase the safe preservation times for heart, liver, pancreas, and heart-lung donor organs.

The Multiorgan Donor Operation

An increasing number of families are consenting to donation of more than one organ from a deceased relative.

Both corneas, both kidneys, the heart, and either the liver or the pancreas can be utilized from a single donor. The celiac axis and the portal vein are used to reconstruct the blood supply to either a pancreas or a liver transplant. For this reason, it is not anatomically feasible to utilize the pancreas and liver from the same donor.

The removal of organs for transplantation is conducted as for any major operation. The procedure is performed in an operating room with the assistance of an anesthesiologist. As with any major procedure, blood transfusions and other supportive measures may be necessary. If the donor's cardiovascular status is stable, the operative procedure is performed in a careful, unhurried fashion.

A long sternal splitting midline incision extending from the sternal notch to the pubis is made (Fig. 7). The blood vessels and other vital structures of each major organ are then dissected free of surrounding tissue. The exact order in which each of the organs are mobilized or removed varies with the preference of the surgical team and the condition of the donor. Protection of the heart from any warm ischemia is the first priority, since obviously this organ must immediately function well in the recipient. A common operative sequence is to isolate the major structures to the heart first, then the liver or pancreas, and finally the kidneys. Cannulas are then inserted into the distal aorta and the vena cava, and the superior mesenteric artery is occluded. The aorta and the vena cava are clamped at the level of the diaphragm. The intra-abdominal organs are then quickly cooled by *in situ* perfusion of 4°C. electrolyte solution. The heart is then promptly removed. Both kidneys are removed en bloc with the attached aorta and vena cava. The liver or the pancreas is then removed with a patch of aorta attached to the celiac axis. If the donor becomes unstable at any point during the intra-abdominal

dissection the procedure can be interrupted, the intra-abdominal organs cooled *in situ*, and the heart promptly removed. Auxiliary procedures include removal of the spleen and mesenteric lymph nodes for histocompatibility testing.

Portions of the iliac artery and vein are removed and used as vascular extensions for reconstruction of the blood supply to the graft in the recipient when necessary. Details of the donor operation are included in the sections on each individual organ. The operation is concluded with closure of the wound. Frequently several surgical teams, one from each of the centers planning to use a donor organ, participate in the operation. To reduce the cold preservation time these teams usually use air transport if the recipient hospital is distant from the donor hospital.

RENAL TRANSPLANTATION

Historic and Experimental Basis

Renal transplantation is now universally accepted as a highly successful treatment for end-stage renal disease (ESRD). Since its introduction, morbidity and mortality have been greatly reduced. The procedure has been demonstrated to be both cost-effective and cost-beneficial. For most patients renal transplantation is the treatment of choice for ESRD. In 1984, 6730 renal transplant operations were performed in the United States.

EARLY EXPERIENCE

Renal transplantation was an experimental and controversial method of treatment when it was first introduced over 30 years ago. In the early 1950s, Hume, of the Peter Bent Brigham Hospital, achieved short-term success with cadaveric grafts in which no immunosuppression was used. The first identical twin transplant was performed at the same hospital by Murray in 1954. This early experience with renal isografts was useful in developing and establishing the standard surgical technique. Encouraged by their success with isografts, additional attempts were made to transplant allografts using relatively crude forms of immunosuppression. In 1959, total body radiation was successfully used by Hamburger in Paris and Murray in Boston with nonidentical twin transplants. Total body radiation was associated with a high morbidity and mortality. In the early 1960s, experiments using the antimetabolite 6-mercaptopurine as an immunosuppressant led to a major improvement in the success of clinical allografting. Subsequently, the use of azathioprine, an analogue of 6-mercaptopurine, and steroids resulted in an effective combination that could be used clinically. Episodes of acute rejection were successfully reversed with supplemental high doses of steroids. Azathioprine and steroids became the mainstays of maintenance immunosuppressive therapy for the next 20 years.

CROSS-MATCHING

In the mid 1960s, transplant centers began to utilize cross-matches prior to transplantation. As discussed in the section on immunobiology, a transplant cross-match detects preformed antibody directed against donor antigens during incubation of the potential donor's white blood cells with the recipient's serum. During the 1960s, antilymphocyte globulin (ALG) was also introduced. This biologic agent is

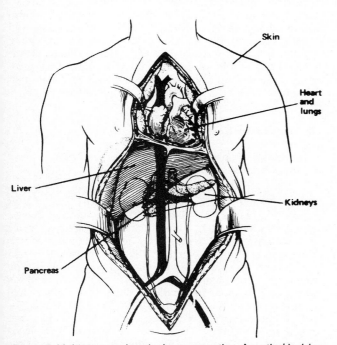

Figure 7. Multiorgan cadaveric donor operation. A vertical incision from sternal notch to pubis is made. The blood vessels and other vital structures to the donor organs are isolated. Organs are removed in sequence as described in the text. Every effort is made to minimize warm ischemia time using such techniques as in situ perfusion with cold electrolyte solution or precooling with infused cold electrolyte solution before excising the organ.

Labels in figure: Skin, Heart and lungs, Liver, Kidneys, Pancreas a heterologous antiserum to human lymphocytes that is raised in another animal species. Graft survival was increased by 10 to 15 per cent when ALG was used for 1 or 2 weeks after transplantation in combination with maintenance azathioprine and steroid treatment.

HLA HISTOCOMPATIBILITY TYPING

Another advance during this decade was the development of HLA histocompatibility typing. It seemed reasonable to anticipate better graft survival if the recipient received a kidney that was well matched with respect to histocompatibiliy antigens. Furthermore, the introduction of pulsatile hypothermic perfusion of cadaver kidneys provided at least 24 hours of satisfactory kidney preservation, allowing transport of organs between transplant centers to optimize the histocompatibility match. With living related donor kidney transplants, attention to matching the HLA antigens was found to be of great benefit. On the other hand, in cadaveric renal transplantation there was a 5 to 15 per cent improvement in long-term results at best when well-matched transplants were compared with poorly matched transplants. There continues to be debate over the merits of "matching" when unrelated or cadaveric donors are utilized.

By the 1970s, transplantation of living related donor kidneys had met with substantial success. Approximately 75 per cent of living related donor kidney recipients were dialysis independent 1 year after transplantation. One-year cadaver graft survival during this era was about 50 per cent. Patient mortality was 15 to 25 per cent at 1 year following cadaveric renal transplantation, and 5 to 10 per cent following related renal transplantation.

BLOOD TRANSFUSIONS

An interesting chapter in the history of renal transplantation is the change in policy regarding the use of blood transfusions in transplant recipients that occurred during the late 1970s. During those years the puzzling observation of a higher graft survival in the range of 15 to 20 per cent in patients who had received multiple random donor blood transfusions was corroborated by many centers. For many years blood transfusions had been given sparingly to patients awaiting renal transplantation to avoid sensitization to foreign antigens. Sensitization would make it difficult to find a suitable kidney to which the recipient had no preformed antibody. By the early 1980s a complete reversal in philosophy regarding blood transfusions had occurred. Many centers now required that a minimal number of random blood transfusions be given to potential cadaver allograft recipients to take advantage of this poorly understood phenomenon.

DONOR-SPECIFIC TRANSFUSIONS

Although living related donor renal transplantation had yielded satisfactory results and a 1-year mortality rate of less than 5 per cent at many centers, there remained a need for improvement. When the donor and recipients shared one haplotype only and the mixed leukocyte culture (MLC) studies showed a lack of a D locus match, the 1-year graft survival rate was only 65 to 70 per cent. In this circumstance the use of donor-specific transfusions (DST) was undertaken. DSTs are an innovative approach whereby the host is purposely exposed to donor antigen. Recipients receive three 200-ml. blood transfusions obtained from the potential related donor. If a positive cross-match does not develop, the subsequent transplant from the blood donor may have a survival of over 90 per cent at the end of 1 year. Significant titers of donor-specific antibody developed in about 30 per cent of potential recipients; the transplant cross-match became positive and transplantation using this particular donor was then contraindicated. Sensitization could be reduced to 10 per cent if the DSTs were given while the recipient was maintained on low-dose azathioprine.

MONOCLONAL ANTIBODIES

Another event of importance in the early 1980s was the use of hybridoma technology to raise monoclonal antibodies against cell surface markers. Monoclonal antibodies directed at lymphocytes, for example, were investigated as treatment for acute rejection of renal allografts and found to be of some benefit. The use of monoclonal antibodies in transplantation science remains in its embryonic stage, but this technology could lead to the development of potent, highly specific immunosuppression. Recently, a monoclonal antibody directed at the T3 subset of lymphocytes has been reported to temporarily reverse over 95 per cent of rejection episodes.

CYCLOSPORINE

The most recent advance in transplantation is the introduction of the immunosuppressive agent cyclosporine. This drug was first used in human renal transplantation in England in 1978 and was released for use in clinical transplantation in the United States in 1983. Soon thereafter the 1-year graft survival of cadaveric renal transplant at many transplant centers increased to 75 to 85 per cent. Use of the new agent was associated with fewer infectious complications, less frequent and milder rejection episodes, and shorter hospitalizations. A host of side effects, including troublesome nephrotoxicity, also became evident. Nevertheless, cyclosporine is the most effective immunosuppressant available. Analogues of the parent compound that have fewer side effects are currently under investigation.

The Transplant Recipient

SELECTION AND EVALUATION OF CANDIDATES FOR RENAL TRANSPLANTATION

The general and specific criteria for renal transplantation are listed in Tables 5 and 6. Patients are almost always on dialysis before transplantation, but in some instances, especially when a related donor is available, patients receive a transplant before complications of renal failure, such as bone disease, ensue. Whether a kidney transplant is recommended for patients who meet the general criteria frequently depends upon the physician's judgment and the wishes of the individual patient. Physiologic rather than chronologic age must be considered. The 32-year-old diabetic with coronary artery disease may well be at greater risk than a "healthy" 60-year-old nonsmoker with newly diagnosed renal failure. The primary disease responsible for ESRD in the renal transplant candidate must be considered, since certain diseases tend to recur in the renal allograft (Table 7).

Successful renal transplantation yields a higher rate of rehabilitation and is more cost-effective than chronic dialysis. Mortality rates for those selected patients who re-

TABLE 7. *Diseases That May Occur in the Allograft**

Membranoproliferative glomerulonephritis
IgA nephropathy
Focal glomerulosclerosis
Lupus nephritis
Antiglomerular basement membrane disease
Diabetic glomerulosclerosis (Kimmelstiel-Wilson syndrome)
Oxalosis
Cystinosis
Obstructive nephropathy

*The presence of disease in the recipient is not a contraindication to transplantation, since frequently the disease either does not recur or recurs in a mild form. Oxalosis was previously considered an absolute contraindication, but with appropriate management successful transplants have been performed in these patients.

ceive renal transplants are low and similar to the best dialysis center mortality rates. Despite these compelling arguments for renal transplantation, only about 10 per cent of ESRD patients in the United States are referred for renal transplantation. The reasons for the apparent underutilization of this modality are multifactorial. The risk of immunosuppression and surgery, the shortage of cadaver donor kidneys, and satisfaction with dialysis are some valid reasons why ESRD patients do not seek a kidney transplant. Under ESRD federal regulations, a multidisciplinary committee must be organized at each transplant or dialysis center to determine the best course of treatment for each ESRD patient.

HISTORY AND PHYSICAL EVALUATION

The evaluation of the renal transplant candidate begins with a careful history and physical examination. The prospective renal transplant recipient and his family are apprised fully of the risks and benefits of renal transplantation. The possibility of living related donor kidney transplantation is investigated. ABO blood group and histocompatibility testing of the patient and family members who wish to be considered for donation is completed. If living related donation is not an option, the patient is placed on a waiting list for a cadaver kidney transplant.

PREPARATION FOR TRANSPLANTATION

Most patients require access to the bloodstream for chronic hemodialysis in preparation for transplantation. Either a radiocephalic arteriovenous fistula or a prosthetic vascular conduit between an artery and vein is used to establish a high-flow access for hemodialysis. Another dialysis mode, continuous ambulatory peritoneal dialysis (CAPD), requires the placement of a "permanent" peritoneal dialysis catheter for multiple daily dialysate exchanges.

Occasionally other operations are necessary to prepare a patient for transplantation. The objective is to correct any conditions that might jeopardize the recipient after he has been placed on immunosuppression. Bilateral recipient nephrectomy is performed if the kidneys harbor infection or are the cause of intractable hypertension. Some polycystic kidneys that cause symptoms of recurrent infection, cyst rupture, or hemorrhage or are large enough to encroach upon the site of the transplant are also removed before transplantation. The native kidneys are of value to the ESRD patient because of their role in erythropoietin production, vitamin D metabolism, and, in some cases, fluid

balance through continued urine production. Thus, they should not be removed routinely.

Correction of obstruction of the urinary collecting system or the establishment of a satisfactory urinary reservoir with bladder augmentation or an ileal loop may be required. Splenectomy is sometimes warranted for pancytopenia due to hypersplenism, since a low white blood cell count or low platelet count may limit the dose of azathioprine or ALG that can be administered. Splenectomy as an adjuvant to immunosuppression is no longer indicated. Subtotal parathyroidectomy for symptomatic secondary hyperparathyroidism may be advisable before transplantation, especially if the patient is hypercalcemic or has already developed significant complications of hyperparathyroidism. If a renal transplant candidate has uremic pericarditis and pericardial effusion unresponsive to vigorous dialysis, a pericardectomy may be necessary. Ulcer surgery in the patient with a history of ulcer disease has been advocated to avoid related complications in the peritransplant period. However, the appropriate use of histamine H2 receptor antagonists has replaced the use of prophylactic ulcer surgery. Most patients need only establishment of vascular access for dialysis prior to transplantation.

Related Donor Selection

Approximately 70 per cent of renal transplants performed currently use cadaver donor kidneys. The remaining kidney transplants are from living related donors. Living related donation has several advantages: (1) a prolonged waiting period is avoided; (2) suboptimal function after transplantation due to acute tubular necrosis is seldom experienced, whereas dialysis is temporarily needed in up to 50 per cent of cadaveric transplants; and (3) most important, there is a definite patient survival advantage when using a donor related kidney. The donor operation carries a mortality rate of 0.1 per cent or less. After a brief period of adaptation and hypertrophy, the single kidney provides 75 to 80 per cent of the renal function present before donation. The longevity of the donor is not significantly decreased as compared with the normal population. Some have questioned the appropriateness of volunteer donation since the results with cadaveric transplantation have improved. Psychological testing has documented an improvement in donor self-esteem. Nevertheless, the prospective donor must be carefully counseled and made aware of the risks involved. Loss of time from work caused by 5 to 7 days of hospitalization and 4 to 6 weeks of convalescence should be discussed. The motivation of the donor to donate must be unequivocal and free of coercion from family or other sources.

COMPATIBILITY TESTING

The first steps in evaluation are testing for ABO blood group compatibility, performing a transplant cross-match between donor and recipient, and HLA and DR histocompatibility testing. As discussed previously, ABO compatibility must exist and the cross-match must be negative. Donors are not usually accepted if there is no match for either HLA haplotype. With a one haplotype match, a mixed lymphocyte culture is frequently performed to determine the best donor if more than one is available or to decide if preoperative blood transfusions or other modifications in the immunosuppressive program would be indicated. The type of renal disease in the ESRD patient must also be considered. Certain familial renal diseases, such as

Alport's syndrome or polycystic kidney disease, which also might have been inherited by the prospective donor, must be excluded. Donor renal function should be normal as assessed by creatinine clearance. The presence of significant proteinuria or microscopic hematuria on urinalysis precludes donation and warrants careful follow-up. Systemic illnesses that may affect renal function, such as hypertension or glucose intolerance, are contraindications to donation. Infectious disease in the donor and a history of malignancy, except for skin cancer and hepatitis antigenemia, are other contraindications.

INVASIVE DIAGNOSTIC STUDIES

If the donor is medically suitable, more invasive diagnostic studies are obtained. An intravenous pyelogram is obtained to investigate structural abnormalities. An arteriogram is also obtained to delineate the renal vasculature; the presence of multiple renal arteries may determine which kidney is used and occasionally may preclude donation.

Cadaver Donor Selection and Kidney Preservation

The criteria for selection of suitable cadaveric donors are described in the previous section and in Tables 5 and 6. The number of patients awaiting a kidney transplant continues to increase more rapidly than the number of transplants performed primarily because of a shortage of cadaveric kidney donors (see Table 3). Kidneys can be preserved either by simple hypothermia for 24 hours or by hypothermic pulsatile perfusion for up to 72 hours as described in the previous section. At the present time, there is no consensus concerning the preferred method of preservation. It is obvious that the current preservation techniques are imperfect, since 30 to 50 per cent of recipients of cadaveric kidneys require dialysis temporarily after the operation while the kidney that has been injured as a result of ischemia is recovering. The incidence of primary nonfunction, that is, failure of the transplanted kidney to function, is about 1 per cent.

Surgical Technique

VOLUNTEER DONOR NEPHRECTOMY

Donor nephrectomy is a major operation. The kidney may be approached transperitoneally or retroperitoneally via a flank incision. The latter approach is preferred by most centers (Fig. 8). A rib may be resected to expedite the dissection. With minimal manipulation of the kidney, an adequate length of the artery and vein is obtained. The ureter is transected at the pelvic brim. The periureteral tissue is preserved to ensure that the blood supply to the ureter is preserved. When the kidney is mobilized fully, the patient is temporarily heparinized, the vessels divided, and the kidney removed promptly to minimize warm ischemia time. The metabolic rate of the kidney is reduced rapidly by flushing with a cold perfusate, and the kidney is then immediately transplanted. Major postoperative complications are uncommon, but can include hemorrhage, pneumothorax, and wound infection. Operative mortality is less than 0.1 per cent.

CADAVER DONOR NEPHRECTOMY

A bilateral donor nephrectomy is performed on the heart-beating, brain-dead cadaver in the careful manner of

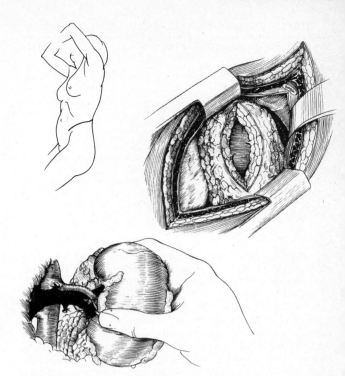

Figure 8. Volunteer nephrectomy through a flank incision. When necessary, a rib may be removed to improve exposure. After transecting the skin, subcutaneous tissue, and flank muscles, the kidney is approached retroperitoneally through Gerota's fascia. The renal vessels are skeletonized to their junction with the aorta and vena cava. The renal vessels are skeletonized and divided at their junction with the aorta and vena cava. The aorta is divided at the pelvic brim.

a routine elective operation. The principles described in the section on multiorgan preservation also apply when only the kidneys are to be removed. Although the kidneys may be removed individually, the preferred technique is en bloc removal of both kidneys together with a segment of aorta and vena cava to avoid injury to renal vessels (Fig. 9). The kidneys and major vessels are skeletonized except for the perihilar fat and periureteral tissue, which are left undisturbed to protect the blood supply to the collecting system. The donor is then heparinized. The aorta and vena cava are clamped above the renal vessels if only the kidneys are to be donated, and the kidneys are flushed with cold electrolyte solution through a catheter placed in the distal aorta. The aorta and vena cava are divided and the kidneys submerged in an iced solution. The kidneys are flushed with preservation fluid through the aorta. Many surgeons do not employ in situ perfusion and simply rapidly remove the kidneys individually or en bloc with the aorta and vena cava. Lymph nodes and the spleen are also removed to provide cells for tissue typing. The abdomen is closed in the routine manner. With increasing frequency, cadaveric donor nephrectomy is part of a multiorgan donor operation as described previously.

THE RENAL TRANSPLANT OPERATION

On admission of the recipient, a history and physical examination are repeated to establish that no contraindications to transplantation have arisen recently. Common interim complications are viral rhinitis, bacterial peritonitis associated with a peritoneal dialysis catheter, and sepsis

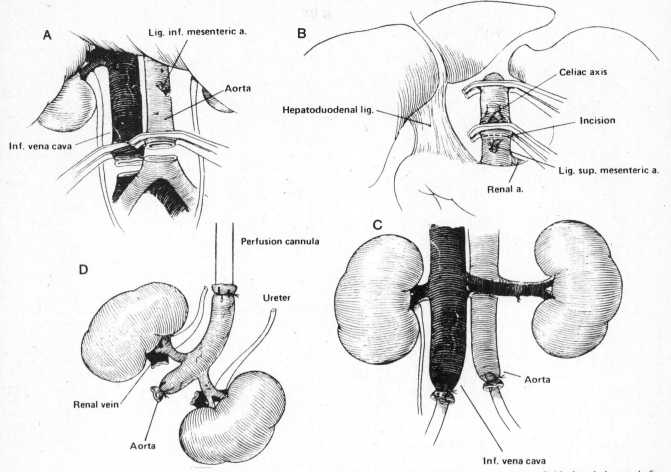

Figure 9. En bloc removal of cadaveric kidneys for transplanation. A, The distal aorta and inferior vena cava are divided and clamped after both kidneys and ureters have been mobilized. B, The proximal aorta is clamped either above or below the celiac axis, depending on the proximity of the renal arteries. C, Kidneys are then cooled in situ by perfusing cold electrolyte solution through a cannula in the distal aorta. Kidneys are then removed en bloc. D, Both kidneys can be perfused conveniently on an organ preservation machine through a single cannula.

associated with an angioaccess prosthesis. Preoperative dialysis is indicated if hypervolemia or hyperkalemia is present. In some centers a central venous catheter is routinely placed prior to operation to monitor fluid replacement. Several studies have documented that the incidence of postoperative acute renal failure can be greatly reduced by optimization of volume status just prior to transplantation.

Renal transplants are implanted retroperitoneally in the pelvis through a lower abdominal curvilinear incision (Fig. 10). The heterotopic position is used because of the ready accessibility of iliac vessels and because the ureter, which is necessarily shortened during the donor operation, can then easily reach the bladder. The end of the renal vein is anastomosed to the side of the recipient external iliac vein, and the renal artery is anastomosed either end-to-end to the internal iliac artery or end-to-side to the external iliac or common iliac artery (see Fig. 10). Re-establishment of vascular continuity usually requires 30 to 45 minutes. Anastomosis times of longer duration increase the incidence of acute tubular necrosis postoperatively. The ureter is then reimplanted into the anterior dome of the bladder, or an internal ureteroneocystostomy (Leadbetter-

Politano) to the posterior wall of the bladder near the trigone is fashioned. In either procedure a short submucosal tunnel is constructed to reduce ureteral reflux.

Postoperative Care

In the immediate postoperative period attention is again directed at optimizing volume status. Generally, a crystalloid solution, such as 5 per cent dextrose in half-strength saline, is used to replace urinary output, with additional replacement as needed to maintain central venous pressure. The urethral catheter is irrigated every 30 to 60 minutes to remove any blood clots that may have formed in the bladder and that could cause obstruction of the catheter. Serum potassium must be monitored frequently, since hyperkalemia often results from intraoperative administration of muscle relaxants and blood products. Most transplant surgeons administer prophylactic antibiotics, especially with cadaveric transplants. Oliguria, excessive diuresis, hypertension, and hyperglycemia are frequently encountered and should be treated appropriately.

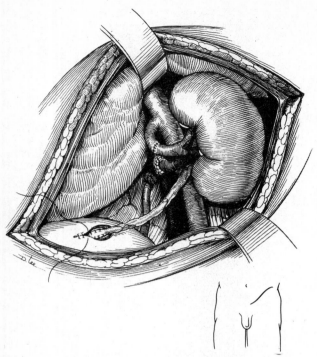

Figure 10. Implantation of a kidney transplant into the iliac fossa. The end of the renal vein is anastomosed to the side of the external iliac vein and the end of the renal artery to the divided end of the internal iliac artery. An external ureteral neocystostomy is being fashioned by implanting the ureter into the anterior dome of the bladder.

Diagnosis and Treatment of Acute Renal Allograft Rejection

An abrupt decline in renal function usually heralds the onset of acute renal allograft rejection. An elevation of serum creatinine of 0.3 mg. per 100 ml. or more in a 24-hour period is considered evidence of rejection unless some other cause for the elevated creatinine is apparent. Compatible clinical symptoms and signs, such as fever, malaise, hypertension, ipsilateral leg edema, or abdominal pain at the site of transplantation, help confirm the diagnosis. Progressive oliguria is often noted during acute rejection. A number of clinical entities that mimic rejection should be excluded either before or concurrently with the initiation of antirejection treatment. These include acute tubular necrosis, vascular thrombosis, hyperacute rejection, ureteral obstruction, peritransplant lymphocele, and cyclosporine toxicity. Technetium sulfur colloid radionuclide scans, ultrasonograms, percutaneous renal biopsies, and, occasionally, renal arteriograms are used to clarify the diagnosis. Elevation of serum creatinine also occurs with cyclosporine nephrotoxicity. This diagnosis is difficult to verify and is often a diagnosis of exclusion. A percutaneous renal transplant biopsy is often helpful to distinguish acute rejection from cyclosporine nephrotoxicity. Cyclosporine nephrotoxicity is not associated with systemic complaints or oliguria. The serum creatinine may also be artifactually elevated in diabetic patients with high blood glucose levels.

Acute rejection is treated with high doses of intravenous or oral steroids. Intravenous steroids are usually administered at intervals varying from every 8 to 48 hours for 3 to 6 days. Increased doses of oral steroids are usually tapered over a 1- to 2-week period. When steroid pulse therapy fails, some groups add antithymocyte globulin or

anti-T3 monoclonal antibody as a "rescue protocol." About 95 per cent of acute rejection episodes can be reversed.

Complications

IMMUNOSUPPRESSION

Renal transplant patients are subject to the same spectrum of postoperative complications as other patients undergoing major operations but are also at risk for complications related to chronic immunosuppression. Technical problems, such as arterial or ureteral stenosis, ureteral leaks, and postoperative hemorrhage, are seen occasionally. The most common complication encountered following transplantation is infection. In the early postoperative period, urinary tract infections, infections of indwelling intravenous lines, wound infections, pneumonia, or deep peritransplant abscesses may be encountered. An arterial anastomosis rarely becomes infected. When this occurs a pseudoaneurysm forms and the transplant must be removed promptly so that fatal exsanguination from the suture line does not occur.

In the late postoperative course, the chronically immunosuppressed patient is subject to systemic viral, bacterial, and fungal infections. The most common virus encountered is cytomegalovirus (CMV), a herpes virus that is either transmitted via the transplanted kidney or reactivated in the host. This infection typically occurs 5 to 6 weeks following transplantation and is characterized by the onset of fever, malaise, and leukopenia. The severity of the illness varies greatly, but fatalities may occur, particularly in patients with no detectable levels of pre-existing antibody to CMV prior to transplantation. Systemic *Candida* infections and *Candida* esophagitis may occur. Interestingly, *Candida* and cytomegalovirus infections often occur simultaneously. Systemic herpes simplex and zoster viral infections are also seen. Uncommon pneumonias, such as fungal pneumonias and *Pneumocystis carinii* pneumonia, are occasionally seen in the transplant population. A diagnosis of *P. carinii* pneumonia is usually made either empirically or by open lung biopsy, since the organism cannot be cultured from sputum. Treatment is with intravenous trimethoprim-sulfamethoxazole (Bactrim) initially, but pentamidine is used later if the patient does not respond.

LYMPHOCELES

Lymphoceles are peritransplant collections of lymphatic fluid that result from either operative transection of lymphatics coursing along the iliac vessels or lymphatic leak from the allografted kidney. Lymphoceles can be large and obstruct the ureter, resulting in hydronephrosis, oliguria, and edema of the ipsilateral leg. Most lymphatic fluid accumulations gradually resolve without operative intervention. When operation is required, the preferred procedure is to drain lymphatic fluid into the peritoneal cavity via a surgically established peritoneal "window."

URINOMA

A urinoma is a peritransplant collection of extravasated urine that has leaked from the ureteroneocystostomy or an area of infarction of the renal parenchyma or calyceal collecting system. When a urinoma is encountered, the source of urine leak must be quickly identified so that it can be repaired and drained. Often an external nephrostomy tube is used in this situation to divert the urinary stream while healing occurs.

COMPLICATIONS RELATED TO STEROID ADMINISTRATION

Some complications are directly related to chronic steroid administration. The long list of steroid complications include a cushingoid appearance, alopecia, buffalo hump, hypertension, centripetal obesity, striae, pancreatitis, ulcer disease, and osteomalacia. The incidence and severity of these complications can be reduced dramatically by reducing the steroid dose. If the dose can be reduced to 10 mg. of prednisone per day, most of these complications will either not occur or be minimal.

NEOPLASMS

There is a small but consistent increase in the incidence of neoplasms in patients on long-term immunosuppression whether it be prednisone and azathioprine or prednisone and cyclosporine. Most of the neoplasms encountered are of lymphoreticular origin. Patients receiving cyclosporine may develop a peculiar B cell lymphoproliferative disorder that initially appears to be a lymphoma but that disappears on discontinuance of the medication.

Results

The success of renal transplantation is typically expressed in terms of the percentage of transplants functioning and the percentage of patients surviving at 1 and 5 years following transplantation. Much work has been done to identify some of the factors that correlate with success or failure (Table 8). A subset of patients has been defined who do particularly poorly with a conventional prednisone-azathioprine regimen. These patients are termed "high responders" because of *in vitro* results indicating a high level of lymphocyte responsiveness to allogeneic cells and nonspecific stimulators. Many of the positive and negative correlations described with conventional immunosuppression are lost when cyclosporine is used. With cyclosporine, preoperative blood transfusions and antigen matching may not provide any additional benefit. The risk of failure with a "high responder" patient is also dramatically lowered with a cyclosporine-prednisone regimen.

RELATED RENAL TRANSPLANTATION

Related renal transplantation results in the best patient survival and graft function. Typically 1-year patient survival with HLA identical transplantation is 98 per cent, whereas 1-year graft function is greater than 90 per cent. These results are so good and so consistent that most transplant surgeons use conventional immunosuppression in this category, reserving cyclosporine for the more difficult HLA semi-identical and cadaveric donor transplant. HLA semi-identical transplants are divided into groups with "high" or "low" reactivity in MLC. High responders are often treated with preoperative transfusions. In a recent report describing 131 patients using preoperative donor specific transfusions, there was no patient mortality and a 1-year graft function rate of 93 per cent. Low responders are usually transplanted with conventional immunosuppression. Some controversy now exists with regard to the use of cyclosporine in related renal transplantation, since it appears that excellent results can also be obtained with this drug in the absence of donor-specific transfusions. HLA nonidentical donors have seldom been used because most data suggest that these transplants fare no better than those from cadaveric donors.

CADAVERIC RENAL TRANSPLANTATION

Cyclosporine-prednisone immunosuppression is used with cadaveric transplantation. Three randomized and three large concurrent trials have recently compared cyclosporine with conventional azathioprine-prednisone. One-year patient survival ranged from 88 to 97 per cent with the cyclosporine groups, which was similar to the survival of the azathioprine groups. Four of the six trials, however, demonstrated a significant improvement in 1-year graft survival with cyclosporine (72 to 83 per cent) as opposed to azathioprine (52 to 76 per cent).

LONG-TERM RESULTS

Cyclosporine has been used clinically for only a few years. Published data on long-term function reflect the use of conventional immunosuppression with prednisone and azathioprine. The actuarial graft survival of large series of kidney transplants collected by Terasaki at the University of California at Los Angeles is depicted in Figure 11. Most of these patients were treated with a conventional azathioprine-prednisone protocol. Since the introduction of preoperative blood transfusions, cyclosporine, and monoclonal antibody has substantially improved 1-year results, there is good reason to be confident that the long-term results will also be substantially improved utilizing these more modern immunosuppressive agents.

TABLE 8. *Factors Associated with Improved Results in Renal Transplantation* Using Prednisone and Azathioprine*

Good HLA or DR match, especially with related donors
Preoperative blood transfusions
Splenectomy (controversial)
Bilateral recipient native nephrectomy (controversial)
Length of time on dialysis more than 1 year
Good function of first allograft
Loss of first allograft from technical complications or slow chronic rejection rather than acute rejection
Nonresponder, i.e., failure to develop antilymphocyte antibodies despite many blood transfusions

*With the introduction of improved immunosuppression, especially the drug cyclosporine, these factors may no longer be important. Early results with cyclosporine indicate that most kidney recipients do well regardless of whether these factors are present.

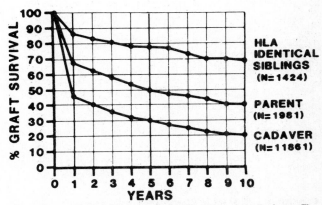

Figure 11. Actuarial survival rates of first kidney transplants. The transplants were performed between 1969 and 1979. No failures were excluded on the basis of technical error. (From Terasaki, P. I., et al.: Cell. Immunol., 62:277, 1981.)

LIVER TRANSPLANTATION

Historic and Experimental Background

In 1956, Cannon of Los Angeles reported the first experimental orthotopic liver transplant. Initial clinical trials were undertaken in 1963 and 1964 in Denver by Starzl, in Boston by Moore, and in Paris by Demirleau. Clinical success as measured by extended survival was not achieved until July 23, 1967, when Starzl implanted a liver into an 18-month-old girl with hepatocellular carcinoma. The infant lived for 13 months before dying of metastatic cancer. Routine success awaited the introduction of a new immunosuppressant, cyclosporine A; Calne, of Cambridge, England, reported the first clinical trials evaluating this drug in 1978 and 1979.

Several circumstances peculiar to liver transplantation account for the delay in this operation becoming a practical therapeutic procedure. Much experimental work and many lessons from clinical trials had to accumulate before a therapeutic threshold was attained.

COMPLEXITY OF OPERATION

The first problem is the sheer magnitude of the procedure. Three major operations are required: donor hepatectomy, recipient hepatectomy and implantation of the hepatic allograft. The combined duration, complexity, and technical requirements of these procedures represent a quantum jump in magnitude of operative intervention compared with most other surgical procedures. Attempts to reduce the complexity of the operation, such as placing the graft in a heterotopic position, thus avoiding recipient hepatectomy, have met with success in only a few patients. Many grafts were compromised by attempting to simplify the biliary anastomosis by constructing the more convenient cholecystojejunostomy or cholecystoduodenostomy rather than the more demanding choledochocholedochostomy or choledochojejunostomy.

IMMUNOLOGIC REQUIREMENTS

The immunologic requirements for transplanting a liver also differ from those of other organs. In the pig, rejection is often very mild, and porcine recipients have survived for many months without any immunosuppression. Dogs with liver transplants have also survived for many months following discontinuation of immunosuppression. However, two attempts at transplantation in humans without immunosuppression resulted in prompt rejection of the graft. Hyperacute rejection has not been observed in human liver transplants even when the presence of antidonor T warm antibodies have been demonstrated in the donor-recipient cross-match. Liver allografts also seem to be resistant to AB blood isoantibody incompatibilities. Until these phenomena are better understood and until more clinical experience has been gained, most transplant surgeons require or prefer a negative donor recipient cross-match and ABO compatibility, and all groups use potent immunosuppressive protocols. Whether results will correlate with HLA or DR histocompatibility also remains to be defined.

PERFUSION WITH PORTAL BLOOD

For normal function the liver requires perfusion with portal blood. Experimental observations have confirmed that when either a normal liver or a transplanted liver is deprived of portal blood the liver will atrophy and hepatic insufficiency will ensue. Much of this information was gleaned from work related to development of portosystemic shunts for the treatment of patients with portal hypertension and bleeding varices. Starzl believes that the important hepatotrophic factors are the high concentration of insulin and glucagon present in the portal blood draining from the pancreas. The need for perfusion with portal blood limits the choice of sites for implanting a liver graft and is a major reason why the orthotopic position is preferred.

Associated Conditions

Most patients who are candidates for liver transplantation are suffering from advanced stages of hepatic insufficiency with associated coagulopathies and portal hypertension. The management of these conditions, especially intraoperatively, needed to be learned largely through trial and error before hepatic transplantation could be successful routinely. Portal hypertension and coagulation defects are the major reasons that continuous hemorrhage occasionally requires the replacement of as many as 200 units of blood during the recipient operation. The liberal use of plasma, platelets, factor VIII cryoprecipitate, and protamine during the operation is mandatory to control coagulation. The objective of treatment is to prevent a severe coagulation defect rather than correct it after it appears. The coagulation defects, especially during the anhepatic and early post-reimplantation phases, are not fully understood, and the appearance of heparin-like activity has been observed.

During the anhepatic phase, when both the vena cava and the portal vein are cross-clamped, there is limited return of blood from the lower body to the heart. Portal hypertension is intensified in this interval. Children tolerate this interruption of flow reasonably well, but cardiovascular instability and kidney damage may result in adults. Recently, a venovenous bypass system for temporarily shunting blood from the portal system and infradiaphragmatic systemic venous system to the axillary vein has been developed. This reduces blood loss, stabilizes blood pressure and cardiac output, and reduces kidney injury and the need for postoperative hemodialysis. Shaw and colleagues from the University of Pittsburgh reported that in 36 patients in whom the bypass was employed, the mean number of transfusions required was 18.9 units and no patient required hemodialysis during the first postoperative week. This bypass system does not require systemic heparinization, and this development will undoubtedly reduce the morbidity and mortality associated with liver transplantation.

SUMMARY

Many individuals have contributed to the field of liver transplantation, and hundreds of articles have appeared in the literature. There is no doubt, however, that, without the leadership of Starzl and Calne, liver transplantation would still be largely confined to the experimental laboratory. Through innovation, hard work, and perseverance for more than 25 years, these two surgeons are responsible for most of the advances that have made liver transplantation a clinical reality. Both patients and health professionals are greatly indebted to them.

Donors, Recipients, and Liver Preservation

The general and specific criteria for organ donation listed in the previous section also apply to cadaveric donors

TABLE 9. General Criteria for Liver Transplantation*

Absolute

1. Irreversible chronic liver disease without effective medical or surgical therapeutic alternatives other than transplantation. The liver disease is progressive to the point of significant interference with the patient's quality of life or ability to work.
2. A thorough understanding by the patient and family of the magnitude of the operation and its sequelae including lifetime follow-up.
3. A strong motivation to undergo the procedure.
4. A reasonable expectation that the quality of life will be improved.
5. A reasonable risk for operation and tolerance of immunosuppressive therapy.
6. Sufficient social stability to provide assurance that patient will cooperate with the follow-up and the immunosuppressive program.

Relative

50 years of age or younger.

*These criteria represent the consensus of a Michigan State Medical Society committee of physicians and others with expertise in transplantation.

TABLE 11. Inborn Errors of Metabolism for Which Hepatic Transplantation Has Been Performed*

Alpha-1-antitrypsin deficiency
Byler's disease
Crigler-Najjar syndrome, Type I
Galactosemia
Glycogen storage disease, Types I and IV
Hemachromatosis
Protoporphyria
Sea-blue histiocyte syndrome
Tyrosinemia
Wilson's disease

*With increasing experience not all of these diseases may be appropriate indications for liver transplantation, since the patients may have nonhepatic manifestations of their disease that will not improve or the disease may recur promptly in the transplant.

of livers (see Tables 5 and 6). Obviously, there should be no history of chronic liver disease. Liver function studies should be normal unless there is an adequate explanation for slight abnormalities associated with terminal illness of the patient. The donor liver must be approximately the same size as the recipient liver. One guideline is to utilize donors whose weight is no more than 10 per cent greater or 20 per cent less than that of the potential recipient. If major discrepancies in size exist, it is difficult to do the suprahepatic vena caval anastomosis, the liver may not fit well into the right upper quadrant, the recipient and donor vessels may kink or be difficult to approximate, and it may be very difficult to close the abdomen, especially if the bowel also becomes edematous during the procedure.

The general criteria for liver transplantation are listed in Table 9. The specific diseases for which a liver transplant is indicated are listed in Table 10. Most groups will not recommend a liver transplant for patients who are addicted to alcohol or drugs. A considerable number of transplants

TABLE 10. Specific Diseases for Which Liver Transplantation is Indicated

Cirrhosis
Alcoholic
Cryptogenic
Primary biliary
Secondary biliary
Posthepatic
Bleeding varices with end-stage liver disease*
Budd-Chiari syndrome
Biliary atresia
Neonatal hepatitis
Chronic active hepatitis
Sclerosing cholangitis
Caroli's disease
Subacute hepatic necrosis
Congenital hepatic fibrosis
Hepatic adenomatosis
Fibrolamellar hepatocellular carcinoma
Inborn errors of metabolism

*Most end-stage liver diseases can be treated with liver transplantation. Contraindications include portal vein thrombosis, hepatitis antigenemia, alcoholism, substance abuse, and primary or metastatic hepatic cancer with the possible exception of fibrolamellar hepatocellular carcinoma.

have been performed in patients with hepatocellular carcinoma. Unfortunately, the cancer recurs quite promptly in most patients so that enthusiasm for transplantation in this group of individuals has waned. As indicated by results with a small group of patients, fibrolamellar hepatocellular carcinoma may be an exception. This cancer has a better prognosis than other types of primary liver tumors, and there has been less recurrence following liver transplantation compared with other histologic types of liver cancer. The inborn errors of metabolism for which hepatic transplantation has been performed are listed in Table 11. In some of these diseases, such as alpha-1-antitrypsin deficiency, the results of liver transplantation have been very good. With others, such as sea-blue histiocyte syndrome, more experience will be needed to determine if significant palliation or a cure can be obtained. At least two patients with hemophilia-A have received liver transplants because they have developed posthepatitic cirrhosis. In both instances the hemophilia was also essentially cured since the liver proved to be a major source of factor VIII. Liver transplantation is not only therapeutic but can be regarded as a clinical experimental model that will provide significant information about inborn errors of metabolism and other diseases.

In general, all patients with irreversible end-stage liver disease who meet the general criteria are potential candidates for a liver transplant. The major exceptions are patients with hepatocellular carcinoma and active substance abusers.

Serious liver disease often progresses very slowly in many patients. Other patients may go from a state of relative well-being and normal activity to a preterminal state within a matter of days, especially if a serious infection or gastrointestinal hemorrhage occurs. Because of this unpredictability, it is especially difficult to decide when a patient has reached the stage at which a liver transplant should be considered. The natural history of the patient's specific disease must be known to make this judgment. Candidates should be in relatively good physiologic condition. Sherlock, a distinguished British gastroenterologist, emphasized at the NIH Consensus Conference on Liver Transplantation in 1983 that the prognosis is poor for most patients with cirrhosis or chronic hepatitis when they have experienced a serious complication of liver disease (Table 12). When one of these complications is present the patient should be evaluated and either promptly transplanted or followed at least monthly to observe signs of progression. In addition, it is known that patients who are so ill as to require care in an intensive care unit do not fare nearly as

TABLE 12. *Prognostic Indicators of Cirrhosis and Chronic Hepatitis**

Steadily increasing jaundice—2-mg. increase every 6 months
Presence of ascites—40 per cent 2-year survival
Refractory ascites—6-month average survival
Encephalopathy without a precipitant—6-month average survival
Increasing prothrombin time despite vitamin K—6-month average survival
Spontaneous peritonitis or septicemia—6-month average survival
Recurrent variceal hemorrhage—6-month average survival

*These guidelines are modified from those presented by Sherlock at the 1983 NIH Consensus Conference on Liver Transplantation.

well as those who are admitted from home or who are hospitalized in a general hospital setting immediately prior to the transplant.

Surgical Technique

ANATOMY

The attachments of the liver within the abdominal cavity are the right and left coronary and triangular ligaments and their reflections to the diaphragm superiorly, the falciform ligament and round ligament anteriorly, the vena cava and its peritoneal reflections posteriorly, and the lesser omentum and hepatoduodenal ligament containing the hepatic trinity medially. These structures must be divided to remove the liver from the donor.

The liver has a dual afferent blood supply through the portal vein and through the hepatic artery. Venous drainage is via the right and left hepatic veins and small hepatic veins from the caudate lobe, which drain directly into the vena cava. The arterial supply to the distal common bile duct is from small branches of gastroduodenal artery, a branch of the common hepatic artery. The gastroduodenal artery should be preserved if the distal common duct is used to re-establish bile duct continuity.

Standard hepatic artery anatomy is present in only about 55 per cent of patients. Total or partial replacement of the right hepatic artery to the superior mesenteric artery (18 per cent) and of the left hepatic artery to the left gastric artery (25 per cent) are common variations. Awareness of these variations is essential for adaptation of the appropriate arterial reconstruction. Variations in portal vein anatomy are much less common. Variations in cystic duct anatomy that alter the surgical procedure, such as a distal insertion of the duct into the common duct, are sometimes encountered.

The nerve supply to the liver follows the hepatic arteries. Parasympathetic innervation is through the vagus nerves and sympathetic innervation through the celiac plexus. The consequences of completely denervating the liver are unknown, with the possible exception that gallbladder emptying is impaired with division of the vagus nerve. This may predispose to the development of cholelithiasis, and many surgeons remove the donor gallbladder during the transplant operation.

DONOR HEPATECTOMY

The donor operation is usually a part of a multiorgan donor procedure as described previously. A long midline vertical incision, including a midline sternotomy, from sternal notch to pubis, is made (see Fig. 7). The major initial maneuvers in donor hepatectomy are to first divide the ligamentous attachments and then isolate the hepatic artery–celiac axis complex and adjacent aorta, portal vein, common bile duct, and the vena cava above and below the liver. To isolate the hepatic artery and celiac axis, the gastroduodenal, right gastric, and splenic arteries are divided. Often a cannula is placed in the divided splenic vein as a conduit to precool the liver with cold lactated Ringer's solution prior to interrupting the blood supply to the liver. The gallbladder is vented and irrigated free of bile. This prevents autodigestion during preservation. Many surgeons remove the gallbladder. The common bile duct is divided during the course of dissection of the trinity.

While the kidney is isolated for donor nephrectomy, cannulas are placed in the distal aorta and vena cava. The sequential order of maneuvers to remove the liver is to divide the common bile duct adjacent to the pancreas, begin precooling the liver through the splenic vein catheter, divide the superior mesenteric artery and vein, cross-clamp the aorta just below the diaphragm, cool the liver and kidneys by infusing cold electrolyte solution through the distal aortic catheter, excise the celiac axis with a button of aorta, and divide the suprahepatic vena cava above the diaphragm along with a cuff of diaphragm. The liver and vena cava are freed from their posterior attachments from above downward, and finally the infrahepatic cava is divided to release the liver (Fig. 12).

The liver is then flushed with a preservation solution, such as EuroCollins' solution, and then immersed in 4°C. balanced electrolyte solution. With simple hypothermia the liver can be preserved safely for a maximum of 8 hours.

RECIPIENT HEPATECTOMY AND IMPLANTATION OF THE LIVER

The recipient operation is usually begun as soon as the abdomen of the donor is explored and a suitable graft is identified. Overlapping the donor and recipient operations reduces the preservation time and thus the ischemic injury to the liver. The two operations are coordinated via telephone. A Swan-Ganz pulmonary artery catheter, a central venous catheter, and an arterial line are inserted for monitoring cardiovascular hemodynamics. Several larger-bore intravenous lines are required for administration of blood and fluids. Coagulation panels are obtained every 30 to 60 minutes to guide replacement of coagulation products. All blood and fluids are prewarmed to help maintain body temperature. Some teams use a special pump system for rapid infusion of blood when needed. A thromboelastograph, a machine that rapidly provides a qualitative estimate of coagulation defects based on the shape of the blood clot, is used by some teams to assist in replacing coagulation factors. A specialized and highly skilled anesthesiology team is essential for a successful outcome.

The right or left axillary vein and saphenofemoral junction are first isolated for later placement of the venovenous bypass catheters. Blood is returned to the heart from the portal vein and the femoral vein and distal vena cava with a special vortex pump via the axillary and subclavian veins. Venovenous bypass is not necessary in pediatric transplant patients. The liver is exposed through a generous bilateral subcostal transverse incision with a vertical midline extension to the xiphoid process. The superior wound edge and rib cage are elevated with a strong retractor fixed to the operating table. The ligamentous attachments of the liver are divided, and the proper hepatic artery, portal vein, common bile duct, and inferior vena cava above and below the liver are isolated and encircled with tapes. These vital structures are not divided until the

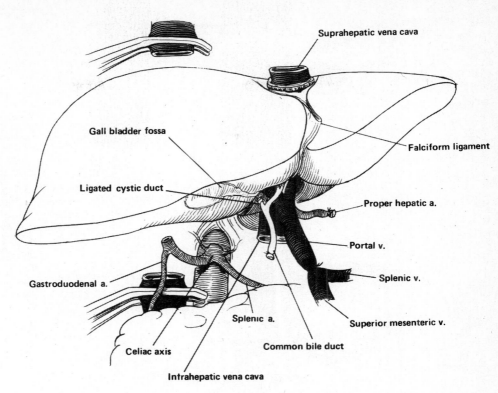

Figure 12. Donor hepatectomy. Note that the vena cava is usually divided above the diaphragm in order to give a more adequate length of cava for reanastomosis. Usually, a cannula is inserted into the splenic vein for precooling and intraoperative cooling of the liver. Rather than divide the proper hepatic artery, we now usually include the entire hepatic artery and celiac axis with a surrounding button of aorta with the donor graft.

Labels on figure: Suprahepatic vena cava · Gall bladder fossa · Falciform ligament · Ligated cystic duct · Proper hepatic a. · Portal v. · Splenic v. · Gastroduodenal a. · Splenic a. · Superior mesenteric v. · Celiac axis · Common bile duct · Infrahepatic vena cava

donor liver actually arrives in the operating room. The bile duct is then divided and the systemic portion of the venovenous bypass system activated after placing catheters in the saphenofemoral junction and axillary vein. The portal vein is divided and a cannula placed in the end of the portal vein for decompression of the portal venous system into the venovenous bypass. The vena cava is transected above the renal veins and the proper hepatic artery divided distal to the gastroduodenal artery. Finally, the suprahepatic cava is divided as it disappears into the liver. The liver is then excised from above downward. Recipient hepatectomy is frequently the most difficult portion of the operation. The presence of portal hypertension increases blood loss. The diseased liver may be enlarged and adherent to adjacent structures. Adhesions from previous operations may complicate the dissection.

The donor liver is reimplanted by reanastomosing the vena cava above the liver, the portal vein, the donor celiac or hepatic artery to the recipient proper hepatic artery, and, lastly, the infrahepatic vena cava (Fig. 13). In children the celiac axis of the donor is sometimes anastomosed to the side of the aorta. The exact sequence and type of anastomoses performed vary with surgical preference and the anatomy encountered. During the procedure it is helpful to continue flushing the liver with cold electrolyte solution through the previously placed cannula in the donor splenic vein. This cools the liver, removes potential air emboli, and, most important, flushes potassium and other harmful metabolic products that accumulate in the liver during the preservation period. Some surgeons use a final warm flush. Cardiac arrest may occur soon after the liver is revascularized if flushing is not thorough.

The final step in the procedure is to re-establish biliary tract continuity. Most surgeons now employ an end-to-end choledochocholedochostomy and insert a T-tube into the recipient portion of the common bile duct to stent the anastomosis. When the common duct is diminutive or diseased, as is frequently the case in children with biliary atresia, a Roux-en-Y choledochojejunostomy is constructed. Considerable time is then spent in obtaining hemostasis. Drains are placed about the liver and the wound closed. The recipient operation usually requires about 12 hours but may vary from 6 to 18 hours or more.

Postoperative Care

RESUSCITATION

Recipients are returned to the surgical intensive care unit. Postoperative stabilization may require all the skills of the intensive care team. The postoperative course of the patient will vary substantially depending upon the preoperative status of the patient, blood loss during the operation, continuing hemorrhage, and, most important, whether the liver functions well promptly. Respiratory function, cardiovascular hemodynamics, liver function, coagulation status, renal function, blood sugar, and fluid and electrolyte balance are monitored closely and supported appropriately. Most transplant teams utilize prophylactic antibiotics. Hemodialysis is sometimes required to treat acute renal failure.

IMMUNOSUPPRESSION

The immunosuppressive regimen consists of a combination of cyclosporine and steroids. Protocols vary with each transplant team but generally are similar to those used in kidney transplantation. Typically in adults 17 mg./kg. of oral cyclosporine is administered preoperatively. Postoperatively, 2.5 mg. per kg. of cyclosporine is administered

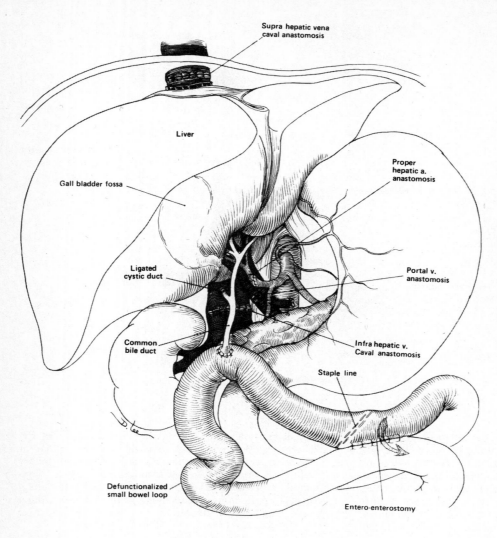

Supra hepatic vena
caval anastomosis

Liver

Gall bladder fossa

Ligated
cystic duct

Common
bile duct

Defunctionalized
small bowel loop

Proper
hepatic a.
anastomosis

Portal v.
anastomosis

Infra hepatic v.
Caval anastomosis

Staple line

Entero-enterostomy

Figure 13. Orthotopic liver transplant. The inferior vena cava is anastomosed above the liver. Then the portal vein or hepatic artery is rejoined. Usually, after either of these vessels has been rejoined, the clamps are removed and liver perfusion begun. Finally, the vena cava below the liver is reanastomosed. In this illustration an end-to-side modified loop choledochojejunostomy is depicted. This procedure is used when the common duct of the recipient is diseased or very small such as in children. In most adults, an end-to-end choledochocholedochostomy is performed.

intravenously every 8 hours until oral intake is resumed. A tapering oral schedule beginning with 17 mg. per kg. in two divided doses is then begun. Serum levels of cyclosporine are monitored daily and doses adjusted to maintain a therapeutic level of about 200 mg. per ml. Cyclosporine may be lost in the bile drained externally through the T-tube. Pediatric patients may require higher doses of cyclosporine to achieve therapeutic levels.

Methylprednisolone, 50 mg. intravenously every 6 hours, is begun preoperatively or immediately after the operation. The dose is tapered during the first week to 20 or 30 mg. per day. Oral prednisone is begun when feeding resumes. Doses are adjusted in proportion to weight for pediatric patients.

REJECTION

Acute rejection is difficult to diagnose in the liver transplant recipient. Declining liver function may be due to rejection, preservation injury to the liver, vascular thrombosis, biliary obstruction, ascending cholangitis, hepatic abscess or necrosis, or perihepatic sepsis. The details of the clinical course of the patient are important in making the differential diagnosis. Rejection is often manifested by a rise in serum bilirubin and liver enzymes and a decrease in T-tube drainage. The character of the bile may change

and become more clear in color. Hepatic nuclear scans, T-tube cholangiograms, arteriograms, computed tomograms, and percutaneous liver biopsy are used to confirm the diagnosis. The histologic picture of acute rejection consists of an infiltration of lymphocytes in the hepatic trinities and around central veins with destruction of bile ducts and venous endothelium. Cholestasis and hepatocyte necrosis may be present.

Rejection is usually treated with three to four large intravenous pulses of methylprednisolone, 10 to 30 mg. per kg., given daily or every other day. Rejection unresponsive to steroid pulses is sometimes treated with a course of antithymocyte globulin. Prompt retransplantation is feasible for irreversible rejection and other causes of liver loss. In 1984, 25 per cent of the approximately 150 liver transplants performed at the University of Pittsburgh were second transplants.

Complications

As with other transplant patients, bacterial, fungal, and viral infections of all types are the most common complications. Intrahepatic or perihepatic sepsis is a special problem in the liver transplant patient. This can result from leaks or stenosis of the biliary anastomosis, ascending cholangitis, or necrosis of liver tissue. Preservation injury, vascular complications, and rejection can lead to ischemia or necrosis of hepatic parenchyma. This compromised tissue is an ideal locus for development of a hepatic abscess. Percutaneous or operative drainage may be required. Cholestatic jaundice with serum bilirubin up to 35 to 40 mg. per 100 ml. may occur secondary to ischemic injury during preservation. If not too severe, this cholestatic condition resolves in 1 to 4 weeks. Other complications peculiar to the liver transplant patient are leaks or stenoses of the biliary anastomosis, thrombosis of the hepatic artery, portal vein, or vena cava, abscesses secondary to intra-abdominal hematomas, and renal failure. Renal failure can result from intraoperative hypotension, sepsis, or injury to the kidney while the vena cava is clamped or as a complication of cyclosporine therapy. Use of the venovenous bypass system has reduced the need for early postoperative hemodialysis.

Results

There are several variables that are known to influence the success of liver transplantation. Children tend to do better than adults. Patients whose general physiologic status is stable do better than patients who are in hepatic coma and require support in an intensive care unit. The outcome may also vary with the primary recipient disease. For instance, the results in patients with primary biliary cirrhosis have usually been superior to those seen in patients with alcoholic cirrhosis. The high recurrence rate of hepatocellular carcinoma has made results in patients with this disease very poor.

At this relatively early stage in the evolution of liver transplantation, most groups tend to report their entire experience as a single cohort. Patients with different primary diseases and varying operative risks are often grouped together. This tends to confuse the interpretation of reported results and makes it difficult to put the results of one group in perspective with those of another group. The situation is analogous to the early days of the development of portosystemic shunt surgery during which reports tended to group together patients with varying degrees of hepatic reserve and different etiologies for their portal hypertension.

The most important variable influencing the results of liver transplantation is the introduction of cyclosporine. Prior to the introduction of this immunosuppressant, the groups with the largest experience in the world reported one-year survival rates of 25 to 50 per cent. In addition, only recently has it been appreciated that patients will do well after a second or, occasionally, even a third liver transplant, thus improving overall patient survival. With the use of cyclosporine, three experienced groups, Starzl at the University of Pittsburgh, Calne at Cambridge University, and Pichlmayr of Hanover, West Germany, have reported 1-year actuarial survivals of approximately 70 to 80 per cent. Results of other groups with less experience have not been as successful, but often patients treated with the older azathioprine steroid regimen are included in these reports. There is no doubt that liver transplantation is a very worthwhile endeavor for many patients with end-stage liver disease. Opportunities for improvement include simplification and standardization of the operation, clarification of appropriate indications and contraindications for operation, prompt retransplantation when necessary, and improvements in our ability to diagnose as well as treat rejection.

PANCREATIC TRANSPLANTATION

Historic and Experimental Basis

In 1966 at the University of Minnesota, Lillihei performed the first human pancreas transplant. The procedure consisted of a segmental or tail-of-pancreas graft with the pancreatic duct ligated. The splenic artery and vein from the pancreatic graft were anastomosed to the iliac vessels. The patient was insulin independent for only 6 days, and the graft was removed at 6 weeks. This pioneering effort began the era of clinical investigation into pancreatic transplantation.

Clinical trials of transplantation of the entire pancreas with a segment of duodenum soon followed. These efforts met with little success. There was a fairly high rate of leakage of various types of anastomoses of the pancreatic duct or duodenum. Techniques of ductal drainage into the ureter (Gliedman), the jejunum (Toledo-Pereyra), and a retroperitoneal jejunal limb (Dickerman and Turcotte) and free drainage of the peritoneal cavity (Sutherland, Goetz, and Najarian) were investigated in animals. None of these techniques when applied to humans in the early 1970s was clearly superior.

In 1978, Dubernard introduced a safer technique of segmental pancreas transplantation with occlusion of the pancreatic duct by intraductal injection of a synthetic polymer. This method avoided the problem of providing drainage of the exocrine secretion of the pancreas. The disadvantage of this procedure is that the obstruction of the pancreatic duct induces fibrosis of the gland, which eventually compromises insulin secretion. Currently there has been a resurgence of interest in transplantation of the entire pancreas along with the short segment of duodenum or periampullary button of duodenum. The duodenum is anastomosed either to the small intestine or into the urinary bladder.

Pancreas transplantation is still under development. The precise indications, best surgical technique, and preferred immunosuppressive regimen are unknown and vary from one group to another. As of 1984, more than 350 pancreas transplants have been recorded in the pancreas registry kept by Sutherland at the University of Minnesota. There is a growing body of experimental evidence that suggests that, with careful maintenance of normoglycemia, the complications of diabetes will be prevented or delayed in onset. Unfortunately, even with the most careful medical program or insulin pump therapy, a reasonable pattern of normoglycemia cannot be maintained in many patients. Pancreatic transplantation has the potential of being the most sensitive and effective means of maintaining normoglycemia. In addition, glucagon and other hormones may be provided that will stabilize blood sugar levels and prevent the development of complications.

Recipients

Pancreatic transplantation is indicated for patients with Type I diabetes mellitus, formerly known as juvenile onset diabetes. Exogenous insulin therapy prevents diabetic ketoacidosis and prolongs the lives of these patients. However, over time most patients develop complications because of the diabetes and have a shortened life span. The disease affects young, lean individuals and is associated with the development of severe complications, such as retinopathy, peripheral neuropathy, Kimmelstiel-Wilson syndrome of the kidney, and gastroenteropathy.

Type I diabetics are insulin deficient owing to destruction of the insulin-producing islets of Langerhans in the pancreas. Current theory suggests that islet destruction is the result of viral or other environmental insult superimposed upon a susceptible genetic background. Approximately 10,000 individuals in the United States develop insulin-dependent diabetes each year. In its 1974 report, the National Commission on Diabetes estimated that each year in the United States 300,000 people die owing to the vascular complications of all forms of diabetes. The approximate total cost of this disease in 1979 was estimated to be eight billion dollars.

There is no consensus or uniform practice concerning the exact indications for pancreatic transplantation. The general criteria as listed in the previous section usually include an age limit of 50 years. All groups restrict transplantation to Type I juvenile diabetics. However, pancreatic transplants have been performed simultaneously with kidney transplants, sequentially after a kidney transplant, or in diabetic patients who have good kidney function and do not require a kidney transplant. The procedure has been used most commonly after the onset of one or more of the complications of diabetes, but many transplants have been performed in patients who desire it before the onset of complications. A positive transplant cross-match is a contraindication to transplantation. There is not enough experience to determine whether a good HLA or DR histocompatibility match improves results. Experience at the University of Minnesota has demonstrated that related grafts have a better actuarial survival at 1 year than cadaver grafts.

Donors

Most groups use only cadaver donors as a source of pancreatic allografts. The general criteria and specific criteria for pancreatic donors have been listed previously (see Tables 5 and 6). Many cadaver donors are hyperglycemic because of the administration of steroids and dextrose and the endogenous discharge of catecholamines. Hyperglycemia *per se* is not a contraindication to pancreas donation. Mild hyperamylasemia is also not a contraindication but must be evaluated in the context of the overall picture. The pancreas is usually removed as part of a multiorgan donor operation. A choice is made between using either the liver or the pancreas. Both grafts are based on the same vascular supply, that is, the portal or splenic veins and the celiac axis. Most transplant surgeons do not wish to risk the liver or the pancreas or prolong ischemia times by attempting to remove both organs from the same donor. Living related donors are utilized at the University of Minnesota. The body and tail of the pancreas are removed, leaving the spleen and sufficient pancreatic tissue to avoid diabetes in the donor. Because of the magnitude of the operation, the potential morbidity, and the potential for diabetes to develop later in life, most transplant groups are reluctant to use volunteer donors.

The pancreas is preserved by simple hypothermia. After removal from the donor, the pancreas is flushed with a special cold perfusate. Usually a EuroCollins' type solution or a silica gel–filtered plasma solution is used. Maximum safe storage time is 6 hours. Hypothermic pulsatile perfusion has been investigated in animals and has extended the preservation of canine pancreatic grafts to 24 hours.

Poor preservation of the pancreas is one of the factors that may lead to early vascular thrombosis of the graft.

Surgical Technique

SEGMENTAL GRAFT

The body and tail of the pancreas to the left of the portal vein are excised from the donor. The segmental graft is placed in the iliac fossa or within the abdomen. Usually the donor splenic artery and vein are anastomosed to the recipient's iliac vessels (Fig. 14). This technique is used with both cadaver and volunteer donor grafts. The duct in the transplanted segment may be ligated, occluded with polymers such as neoprene, or drained into the bladder or intestine.

PANCREATICODUODENAL GRAFTS

The entire pancreas and a portion of the duodenum are removed from the donor. The donor operation is similar to standard pancreaticoduodenectomy but with a more extensive dissection of the major vessels. The entire portal vein to its bifurcation and the celiac access, together with intact splenic, hepatic, and gastroduodenal arteries, are preserved with the graft. The common bile duct and superior mesenteric artery and vein are divided and ligated. Either a short segment of duodenum or a button of duodenum about the ampulla of Vater is preserved. The celiac axis and the portal vein are then anastomosed to the iliac vessels. Some groups also anastomose the superior mesenteric artery. The segment of duodenum or a periampullary button is then anastomosed directly to the side of a loop of small bowel, a Roux-en-Y limb of small bowel, or into the urinary bladder (Fig. 15; see Fig. l4).

Sollinger and Belzer at the University of Wisconsin have pioneered the use of the urinary bladder as a conduit for the exocrine secretions. The bladder is conveniently located for this anastomosis and is usually sterile. Surprisingly, the loss of protein and electrolytes in the pancreatic secretion does not seem harmful to the recipient and the urine does not activate the pancreatic enzymes. Some transplant groups perform this procedure intra-abdominally, whereas others prefer to perform the procedure and place the graft entirely retroperitoneally.

The spleen has been transplanted as part of a composite graft with the entire pancreas and a portion of the duodenum in a few patients (see Fig. 14). Early vascular thrombosis is one of the common complications of pancreatic transplantation. Inclusion of the spleen with the graft was thought to provide a physiologic arteriovenous fistula that might reduce the incidence of vascular thrombosis. In addition, there is some evidence to suggest that an immunologic advantage might be conferred. However, some patients developed graft versus host disease when the spleen was included, necessitating removal of the spleen. In addition, there is no clear-cut evidence that vascular thrombosis has been reduced as compared with other techniques.

Postoperative Care

IMMUNOSUPPRESSION AND REJECTION

At most pancreatic transplant centers, the same immunosuppressive program is used for pancreatic transplants

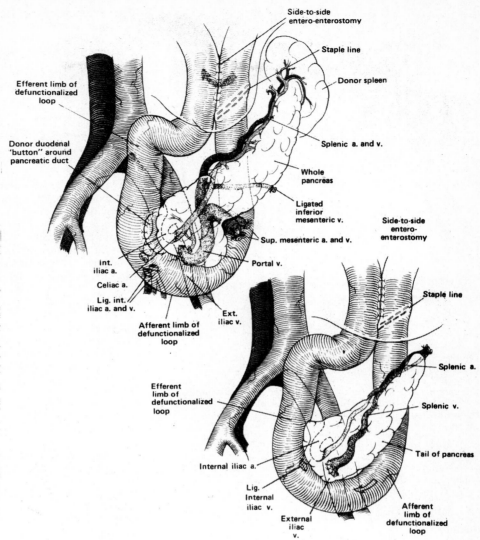

Figure 14. Pancreaticoduodenal graft with spleen and segmental pancreatic graft.

Top illustration, *The entire pancreas and spleen have been transplanted into the iliac fossa. The portal vein is anastomosed to the side of the iliac vein and the celiac axis anastomosed to the end of the divided internal iliac artery. A periampullary button of duodenum is implanted into the side of a modified Roux-en-Y loop of jejunum. The insertion of a staple line distal to the enteroenterostomy prevents any intestinal contents from passing by the duodenal-jejunal anastomosis and effectively converts this loop into a functional Roux-en-Y. Most groups have abandoned transplanting the spleen along with the pancreas, as discussed in the text.*

Bottom illustration, *A segment of pancreas is implanted into the retroperitoneal iliac fossa. The splenic vein is anastomosed to the side of the external iliac vein, and the splenic artery or celiac axis is anastomosed to the end of the divided internal iliac artery. We prefer to use the internal iliac artery rather than the side of the external iliac artery because the vascular supply to the leg is less at risk if there is any complication with this anastomosis or if the graft needs to be removed. The cut edge of the pancreas is inverted into the lumen of the jejunum with a two-layer anastomosis.*

as for kidney transplantation. The use of cyclosporine has improved results. Rejection seems more difficult to prevent or control in the pancreas transplant patient than in patients with other types of organ transplants. Many groups now utilize triple therapy, that is, cyclosporine, steroids, and azathioprine. Usually a low dose of azathioprine, that is, approximately 1.5 mg./kg., is used to supplement the other drugs. Early results with triple drug therapy in both pancreatic and heart transplantation are promising.

The diagnosis of rejection is made when there is a persistent elevation in blood glucose and/or hyperamylasemia. Unfortunately, these laboratory abnormalities are rather late signs of rejection. Experimental studies have demonstrated that the rejection process is well advanced, with necrosis of both acinar and islet tissue by the time hyperglycemia occurs. Other markers of rejection, such as decreased serum insulin and 24-hour urinary glucose C-peptide ratio, are useful to confirm the presence of rejection but are either too cumbersome or too time-consuming to be of use clinically. The treatment of pancreas transplantation rejection is similar to that used for kidney transplants and consists mainly of high doses of steroids and/or the use of antilymphocyte globulin. When the kidney and the pancreas are transplanted simultaneously, rejection of the kidney is usually apparent before changes in blood glucose or amylase occur. In this sense, the kidney can be used as a more sensitive indicator for initiating antirejection therapy.

COMPLICATIONS

The complications associated with pancreatic transplantation are those specific to the operation plus the usual complications associated with immunosuppression. The pancreatic graft is particularly susceptible to vascular thrombosis during the first few postoperative days. About 25 per cent of grafts are lost from this complication. With more careful attention to preservation and careful placement of the graft, the incidence of this complication seems to be decreasing. Aspirin and dipyridamole, heparin, or low-molecular-weight dextran is often administered during the early postoperative period to help prevent thrombosis. Leaks from the duodenal or pancreatic ductal anastomosis and acute pancreatitis also occur and frequently result in graft loss. Bacterial and fungal infections are common problems, since these patients are both diabetic and im-

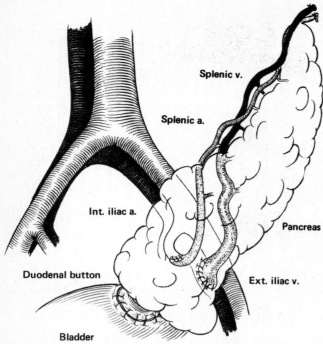

Figure 15. Pancreaticoduodenal allograft utilizing the urinary bladder. The operation may be done retroperitoneally or intra-abdominally. The end of the portal vein is anastomosed to the side of the external iliac vein. The end of the celiac axis is anastomosed to the end of the divided internal iliac artery. The periampullary button of duodenum has been implanted into the dome of the bladder.

munosuppressed. Some groups routinely administer ketoconazole prophylactically to prevent *Candida* and other fungal infections.

Results

The postoperative mortality for patients undergoing pancreatic transplantation is approximately 10 per cent, and actuarial survival at 1 year is approximately 80 per cent. Until recently, the overall probability of a cadaveric transplant recipient remaining independent of exogenous insulin at the end of 1 year was only 20 to 30 per cent. Rejection has been the most common cause of graft loss. Results with related grafts are better, and over 50 per cent of these grafts are functioning at 1 year. The University of Minnesota has reported that, with HLA identity between the related donor and the recipient, the success rate has been 100 per cent when technical failures are excluded. The longest duration of functional pancreatic allograft of a transplant is over 5 years.

More current results with cadaveric pancreatic transplants are encouraging. With greater experience and as more groups contribute to the development of pancreatic transplantation, many of the technical details of the operation have been improved. The use of cyclosporine, triple-drug therapy, and antithymocyte globulin or monoclonal antibody for treatment of rejection has also improved results. For instance, Corry, of the University of Iowa, recently reported a 57 per cent 1-year actuarial graft function rate and an 82 per cent 1-year patient survival rate with 20 consecutive cadaveric pancreatic transplants. In this technique, the entire pancreas and a small segment of

duodenum are transplanted retroperitoneally. The duodenum is anastomosed to the side of a loop of small bowel that is brought into the retroperitoneum. A kidney from the same donor is transplanted during the same operation. At the University of Michigan the pancreas and a similar small segment of duodenum are transplanted intraperitoneally and anastomosed to the bladder.

ISLET CELL TRANSPLANTATION

History

In 1973, amelioration of chemically induced diabetes in rats by transplantation of isolated pancreatic islets into the peritoneal cavity was reported. Since these exciting initial reports, several investigators have accomplished successful islet transplants in large animals. Islet transplantation into humans was performed in the mid-1970s, but no long-term islet graft survivals occurred in over 70 attempts. Recent work in rodents has rekindled interest in islet transplantation by demonstrating prolonged acceptance of islet grafts, even with major antigenic disparity without immunosuppression. In these experiments, islet graft immunogenicity is altered by tissue culture, exposure to hyperbaric oxygen, specific antibody pretreatment, or ultraviolet irradiation. This body of experimental work suggests that islet transplantation without recipient immunosuppression could become a clinical reality in the foreseeable future.

Advantages

Islet transplantation is appealing for several reasons. Isolated islets can be transplanted without the necessity of a major recipient operation. Islets can be stored in tissue culture or cryopreserved for long periods of time, allowing pooling of islets and optimal matching of donor and recipient. Islets can be transplanted in "physiological" sites, such as the spleen or liver, allowing insulin delivery into the portal venous system. In theory, one donor could provide islets for several recipients. Only 10 per cent of the islet mass from one pancreas is necessary to establish normoglycemia in a diabetic host. With present techniques, however, the isolation of islets is laborious and inefficient, with a yield of less than 5 per cent of islets from a single human pancreas. Exocrine cell contamination of the islet preparation is a source of several complications.

Results

Unfortunately, there has been no long-term success with transplantation of allogeneic islets. Most often, the islets have been infused into the portal vein and engrafted into the liver. Even with successful initial engraftment, the function of the islets is lost after several months for reasons that are not completely understood. If too many islets or clusters of cells are infused into the portal system, portal hypertension and bleeding varices can result. Recently there have been attempts to infuse islets into the spleen or place them under the capsule of the kidney, but unfortunately there is still no long-term success. Because of the relative simplicity of the procedure and the success achieved in altering the immunogenicity of islets, there is still great interest and active investigation related to islet cell transplantation.

HEART AND HEART-LUNG TRANSPLANTATION

Historic and Experimental Basis

Carrel and Guthrie, during the course of their Nobel Prize–winning experiments in vascular surgery, removed hearts from puppies and sutured them into the necks of adult dogs. Some of these transplanted hearts were able to beat for a number of hours. Surprisingly, this work was not resumed until the 1930s, when Mann and associates at the Mayo Clinic performed heterotopic heart transplants in puppies and recognized for the first time that the grafts were lost not because of surgical technique but rather because of a poorly understood rejection process. In 1960 and 1961, Lower and Shumway reported the first successful orthotopic heart and heart-lung transplants in animals utilizing local cooling for periods up to 7 hours. Their initial contributions related to surgical techniques and to the demonstration that myocardial viability could be preserved by means of topical cooling. Subsequent work at Stanford under Shumway's leadership has been chiefly responsible for establishing the scientific basis for the methods currently utilized. His group demonstrated that the heart undergoes rejection like any other organ beginning at about 1 week after transplantation. This process could be inhibited with the immunosuppressive agents utilized for renal transplantation. During the course of these studies and later ones in humans, it was also demonstrated that orthotopic heart grafts, although totally denervated, are capable of supporting the entire cardiac output, maintaining normal sinus rhythm, and responding appropriately to exercise. Other crucial contributions were the endocardial biopsy technique developed by Caves for monitoring cardiac rejection and the studies of rejection histology by Billingham.

In December 1967, Barnard, in Capetown, South Africa, successfully performed the first human orthotopic heart transplant. During the subsequent year there was such widespread enthusiasm for heart transplantation that over 100 were performed. Unfortunately, survival was very low, and it became apparent that much remained to be learned about the management of infection and rejection. During the next decade, only Shumway, Lower, Barnard, and their associates persisted, and the clinical results slowly improved so that by 1980 over half of the patients were surviving more than 1 year. With the introduction of cyclosporine A in 1980, results improved dramatically, rekindling interest to the point that, in 1983, 172 transplants were accomplished in 13 centers in the United States.

COMBINED HEART AND LUNG TRANSPLANTATION

The earliest experimental work in combined heart and lung transplantation was performed by the Russian surgeon Demekov in the 1940s. Without the use of hypothermia or cardiopulmonary bypass, he was able to successfully transplant the heart and lungs in 2 of 67 dogs. The longest survival was 5 days. Even in the modern era the longest survival that could be achieved in dogs after orthotopic heart-lung transplantation was only 10 days. The majority of dogs died of respiratory insufficiency caused by denervation of the lung. In a landmark study, Nakae demonstrated that only in the primate is normal respiratory control possible after cardiac and pulmonary denervation. Reitz and associates performed the first long-term successful combined heart and lung transplants in primates in 1980. Buoyed by these successful experiments and the increasing success with human cardiac transplants, the Stanford group began a clinical program of heart-lung transplantation in 1981.

HETEROTOPIC HEART TRANSPLANTATION

Barnard's group had long been interested in heterotopic heart transplantation, that is, implanting the donor heart parallel with the native heart as an assist pump for one or both of the diseased ventricles. The original purpose of this technique was to permit heart transplantation in patients with elevated pulmonary vascular resistance in whom an orthotopic heart transplant ordinarily would lead to right heart failure and death. Two other advantages of this technique are that the recipient's own heart is preserved, allowing the possibility that it might recover, and that survival of the recipient is not dependent solely upon the "new" heart should it be rejected. Barnard performed the first clinical heterotopic implant in 1974, and subsequently he and others have reported a number of patients undergoing heterotopic transplantation in association with corrective procedures to the recipient's heart. The 1-year survival approximates 76 per cent, with graft survival being 66 per cent.

Recipients

HEART TRANSPLANTATION

To be considered an appropriate candidate for cardiac transplantation, a patient must have terminal, otherwise untreatable heart disease with less than a 10 per cent likelihood of surviving 6 months. In the Stanford series, 46 per cent of such patients have suffered from advanced ischemic heart disease and 45 per cent from idiopathic cardiomyopathy. Normally, only patients 55 years of age or younger are selected. Only a few children have undergone cardiac transplantation, but they need not be excluded, as evidenced by the recent successful transplant performed in a 2-year-old child. There must be normal function or reversible dysfunction of the liver and kidneys and no evidence of active infection, recent pulmonary infarction, insulin-requiring diabetes, pulmonary vascular resistance greater than 8 Wood units, or any other systemic illness that would limit recovery or long-term survival. Of particular importance is psychological and social evaluation of potential recipients to ensure that they possess the personal and family resources to undergo the extreme stress of the operation and the prolonged and intensive follow-up required.

HEART-LUNG TRANSPLANTATION

In many patients with terminal acquired heart disease, secondary pulmonary hypertension develops either because of pulmonary edema and stasis or as a result of multiple pulmonary emboli. These patients cannot be treated by isolated orthotopic heart transplantation because the normal donor right ventricle cannot handle the increased work load imposed upon it acutely by the pulmonary hypertension. For these patients, joint heart-lung transplantation and heterotopic heart transplantation are the only alternatives. Children with congenital heart disease with either irreversible vascular disease from prolonged left to right shunting or marked hypoplasia of pulmonary arteries that makes correction impossible can also be better treated by combined heart and lung or heterotopic heart transplantation. Finally, combined heart-lung transplantation rather than isolated lung transplantation may well be the best treatment for patients with certain primary lung diseases.

The combined replacement of the heart and lung has several advantages over isolated lung transplantation:

1. All the diseased tissues are replaced and removed.

2. There is immediate blood supply to the tracheal anastomosis, since the coronary-bronchial vascular beds are undisturbed.

3. Assessment of rejection of both the heart and lung grafts may be made by endomyocardial biopsy, whereas there is presently no good technique for assessing rejection of the lung alone.

Patients usually considered for this procedure are young adults with primary pulmonary hypertension of unknown etiology. Patients with end-stage chronic obstructive lung disease, interstitial fibrosis, and cystic fibrosis also might be candidates. However, uncertainty about recurrence of the disease, the fact that the tracheobronchial tree is rarely sterile, and the possibility of other organ involvement make these latter groups of patients less than ideal candidates. In patients with severe emphysema and secondary changes in thoracic volume, transplantation with donor organs of normal volumes may be impractical, and these patients should not be considered candidates for heart and lung transplantation at the present time.

Donors

No accurate estimate exists of the number of organ donors potentially available. The acceptable donor must be younger than 35 years of age and free of any evidence of cardiac disease or cardiac trauma and diabetes (see Tables 5 and 6). Donors for combined heart and lung transplantation are especially difficult to obtain because of the tendency for those with brain death to develop pulmonary edema and for the intubated patient to develop tracheobronchial infection and pneumonia. An additional important requirement is that there be a close size match. The donor's lung must fit within the fixed capacity of the recipient's thoracic cage to avoid compression of the transplanted lung, which could lead to atelectasis and shunting.

The heart-lung donor should be intubated with a high-compliance, high-volume, low-pressure endotracheal tube connected to a volume-cycled respirator and ventilated with an inspired oxygen fraction (FIO_2) of 40 per cent or less. It is useful to use a size 8 or 9 tube so that the endoscopic bronchoscopy can be performed if necessary. The addition of 3 to 5 cm. H_2O of positive end-expiratory pressure (PEEP) and intermittent "sighing" helps to prevent alveolar collapse. The arterial oxygen tension on an FIO_2 of 40 per cent should be greater than 90 torr. The central venous pressure should be maintained as low as possible (below 10 cm. H_2O) by means of fluid to prevent alveolar collapse. The arterial oxygen tension on an FIO_2 of 40 per cent should be greater than 90 torr. The central venous pressure should be maintained as low as possible (below 10 cm. H_2O) by means of fluid restriction and diuresis to help prevent neurogenic pulmonary edema, especially if the lungs are to be used as well as the heart.

Surgical Technique

DONOR OPERATION

Procurement of the donor heart is often accomplished in conjunction with surgical teams obtaining other organs.

The superior and inferior venae cavae are clamped to allow the heart to empty. An incision is then made in the right pulmonary veins for cardiac decompression. One liter of 4°C. physiologic solution is infused via the aortic root. This arrests cardiac metabolism and preserves the heart up to 4 hours. The superior vena cava is then suture ligated, the aorta is clamped and sutured or stapled at the level of the innominate artery, and the four pulmonary veins, inferior vena cava, and pulmonary artery bifurcation are divided. The heart is then immersed in 4°C. physiologic solution within sterile containers and transported to the recipient operating room.

Experience has shown that ischemic periods of up to 4 hours are safe utilizing these simple preservation methods. Since less than 1 hour of ischemic time is utilized in implanting the heart, up to 3 hours after available for procurement and transportation, allowing for distant heart procurement. In 1977, Stanford initiated a program for distant heart procurement and found only slight ultrastructural differences and no functional differences from hearts obtained on site. Thus, with attention to careful coordination of transportation and operating rooms, donor hearts are now transported for distances of up to 1000 miles, greatly expanding the available donor pool.

A limiting factor in heart-lung transplantation is preservation of the donor lung. The preferred method of heart-lung procurement at present is to utilize partial cardiopulmonary bypass with perfusate at a temperature of 4 to 6°C. The advantages of donor hypothermic cardiopulmonary bypass are that this technique (1) ensures cardiovascular stability during heart-lung mobilization, (2) permits meticulous hemostasis of the donor mediastinum, thus avoiding postimplantation hemorrhage from donor collateral vessels, and (3) provides satisfactory lung preservation and maintenance of lung function. Preservation of the lung for periods greater than 2 hours has not proved safe. Therefore, only on-site donors should be used.

RECIPIENT OPERATION

The heart transplant recipient is prepared as for any open heart procedure with appropriate monitoring lines. There is close coordination between the donor and recipient operating rooms so that the donor heart may be implanted into the recipient as soon as available. At the appropriate time, a median sternotomy incision is made, cardiopulmonary bypass is initiated, and the diseased heart is excised at the atrioventricular junction, leaving generous cuffs of right and left atria, ascending aorta, and main pulmonary artery.

The donor heart is then sutured to the recipient bed (Fig. 16). The donor and recipient atria are anastomosed with a continuous suture, and then the pulmonary artery and ascending aorta are sutured. During this time, donor heart hypothermia is maintained by administration of another 500 ml. of cardioplegic solution, continuous external irrigation with cold physiologic solution, and irrigation of the interior of the heart through a left atrial cannula. The latter serves also as a means of removing air from the donor cardiac chambers.

After completion of the aortic suture line, the aortic clamp is removed, allowing the donor heart to be perfused with the recipient's blood. At this point, the heart is defibrillated if necessary and allowed to beat and recover from its anoxic period while the pulmonary artery anastomosis is completed.

In heart-lung transplants, it is essential to remove the heart and lungs without injury to the vagus, phrenic, or

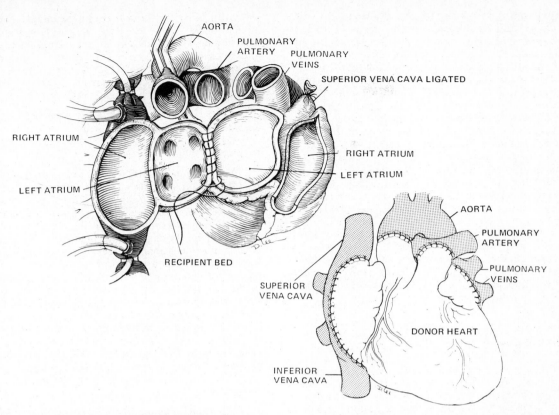

Figure 16. Transplantation of the heart into the recipient. The right and left atria of the donor heart are anastomosed to the recipient atria with a continuous suture. Then the pulmonary artery and aorta are sutured. Finally, the cardiopulmonary bypass is discontinued.

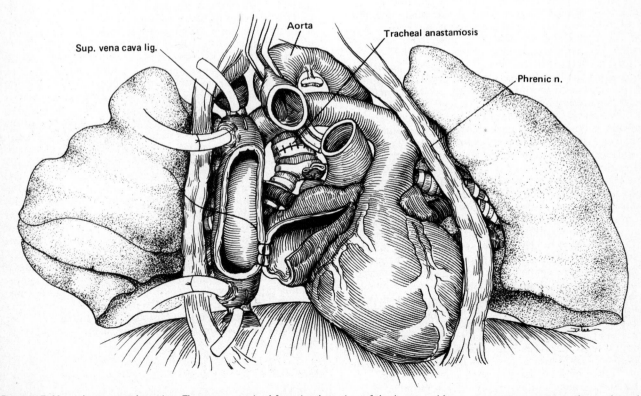

Figure 17. Heart-lung transplantation. The steps required for reimplantation of the heart and lungs are to reanastomose the trachea, then the right atrium of the donor heart to the right atrium of the recipient, and finally rejoin the donor and recipient ascending aorta. The cardiopulmonary bypass is then discontinued.

recurrent laryngeal nerves and to carefully ligate the bronchial arteries. After a complete anterior pericardiectomy is performed, the patient is placed on cardiopulmonary bypass. The recipient's heart is removed, leaving a posterior cuff of right atrium in place for reimplantation. The left lung is then excised, and the left bronchus is stapled proximally before it is divided to minimize the risk of contamination of the surgical field. The right lung is then removed followed by the remnants of the pulmonary artery. A small segment is left in place in the region of the ductus ligamentum to preserve recurrent laryngeal nerve function. Finally, the trachea is divided just above its bifurcation and the remnants of the major bronchi are removed.

Implantation of the donor organs begins with the tracheal anastomosis (Fig. 17). The trachea is sutured with a continuous suture of 3-0 polypropylene, adjusting for size discrepancy at the membranous portion of the trachea. The atrial anastomosis is performed, followed by the aortic anastomosis, both with a continuous suture of 3-0 polypropylene. After removal of the aortic cross-clamp, the heart and lungs are resuscitated as for isolated heart transplantation. Ventilation is begun, and, when the heart is fully resuscitated, bypass is discontinued.

Postoperative Care

Postoperatively, the patients are hemodynamically monitored and supported in the same manner as any patients having open heart surgery. They are extremely dependent upon catecholamine supplementation for 3 or 4 days, and a dopamine or isoproterenol infusion is started before bypass is discontinued. Isoproterenol is particularly beneficial in supporting the heart rate, which tends to be slow owing to denervation. Antibiotics are discontinued after 2 days. Because of the hazard of pulmonary infection, the patient is weaned from the ventilator and extubated as soon as possible. Monitoring lines and chest tubes are removed promptly. A program of physiotherapy is begun the first postoperative day, with great stress placed on pulmonary hygiene. Hypertension complicates administration of both cyclosporine and steroids. These patients usually require antihypertension medications such as prazosin, hydralazine, and captopril. They tend to retain salt and water and normally require substantial doses of diuretics such as furosemide and hydrochlorothiazide.

One unique problem of the heart-lung transplant patient is the development of a "reimplantation response" characterized by interstitial pulmonary edema with attendant pulmonary congestion and decreased lung compliance. This usually occurs within 48 hours postoperatively and lasts from 1 to 3 weeks. The likely causes are (1) disruption of the pulmonary lymphatic system, (2) surgical trauma to the donor lung, (3) changes in the pulmonary oncotic pressure, and (4) denervation. Optimal pulmonary function during this time is achieved with vigorous diuretic therapy and fluid restriction and, at times, prolonged ventilatory support. The radiologic appearance of the reimplantation response is similar to that seen with rejection or infection; therefore, care must be taken to exclude the presence of these conditions. A second major problem is decreased pulmonary gas exchange due to both the reimplantation response described previously and rejection. After extubation, these patients require supplemental oxygen and careful and frequent monitoring of arterial blood gases.

During the first week, daily serum cyclosporine trough levels should be obtained. Electrolytes, serum creatinine, liver function tests, and a complete blood count are obtained daily. These patients, although having normally functioning hearts, as a rule have chronically weakened musculoskeletal systems. A program of nutritional and physical rehabilitation extending over several months is often required. The patient may be discharged after several negative endocardial biopsies.

Immunosuppression

PREDNISONE AND AZATHIOPRINE

The immunosuppressive regimen originally found to be effective in animals and then in humans consisted of loading doses of azathioprine and methyl prednisolone followed by maintenance doses of prednisone and azathioprine. Dosage was regulated on the basis of the white cell count, which may be profoundly depressed by azathioprine. Antithymocytic globulin (ATG) was added to this regimen following the demonstration of its efficacy in 1973. Rejection in patients treated with these drugs could be detected in the early stages by a reduction in R-wave voltage on serial electrocardiograms. Although management of these patients is frequently complicated by severe infection because of depression of the immune system and by rejection episodes necessitating courses of steroids and ATG, results have generally been good in experienced hands and this method continues to be used in some centers.

CYCLOSPORINE

The fungal metabolite cyclosporine A was first applied to cardiac transplantation in 1980. With this agent there has been a dramatic decrease in lethal infections and rejection episodes in the early postoperative period. Although it is possible that long-term survival rates will not be greatly different with cyclosporine A than with conventional immunosuppression, most believe that patient morbidity and hospital stay have been dramatically reduced.

The protocol we employ is derived from that used at Stanford and our own experience with kidney recipients. Twelve hours preoperatively the patient is given an oral loading dose of 17 mg. per kg. of cyclosporine. This is followed by an additional 2 mg. per kg. administered intravenously 1 hour preoperatively to assure that the newly grafted heart is exposed to maximum immunosuppression when first contacting the recipient. Postoperatively cyclosporine A is given in a dose of 2 mg. per kg. every 12 hours intravenously until the patient is tolerating oral feedings, at which time oral administration of 5 mg. per kg. is begun every 12 hours. Serum trough levels are determined daily, and the amount of cyclosporine is adjusted to maintain a level of 200 to 400 mg. per 100 ml. During reperfusion of the donor heart in the operating room, the patient receives 1 gm. of methylprednisolone intravenously. Prednisone is administered in doses of 50 mg. every 12 hours for three doses and then orally b.i.d. The prednisone dosage is rapidly tapered over the next 2 weeks until a maintenance level of 10 to 20 mg. daily is reached. Antithymocyte globulin is no longer utilized as part of the initial treatment program but is reserved for reversing acute rejection episodes.

PROTOCOL FOR CARDIOPULMONARY TRANSPLANTATION

The immunosuppressive protocols generally used for cardiopulmonary transplantation differ significantly from those used for isolated heart transplants because of fear that the early high doses of steroids might inhibit tracheal healing. Oral cyclosporine, 18 mg. per kg., is given as soon as the donor is found to be acceptable. Postoperatively, cyclosporine, 3 to 18 mg. per kg. per day, is given in divided doses by nasogastric tube or orally and adjusted according to blood levels. Methylprednisolone, 500 mg., is administered intravenously for three doses, but no further steroids are given for 2 weeks. Jamieson and colleagues also use rabbit antithrombocyte globulin, 2.5 mg. per kg. intramuscularly, on the day of the operation and for 2 days thereafter or until circulating T cells fall below 5 per cent. Additional immunosuppression is achieved during the first 2 weeks with oral azathioprine. It is given immediately postoperatively and maintained at 1.5 mg. per kg. After 14 days, oral azathioprine is discontinued and low-dose oral prednisone, 0.2 to 0.3 mg. per kg. in divided doses, is begun. Long-term maintenance therapy after 2 weeks is with cyclosporine and prednisone.

Unfortunately, with cyclosporine immunosuppression no noninvasive diagnostic test for rejection has been found reliable, so that routine endocardial biopsy is necessary. The bioptome designed at Stanford by Caves is introduced into the internal jugular vein by percutaneous technique and guided under fluoroscopic control to the right ventricular septum, where several 3-mm. tissue samples are obtained for microscopic examination. The procedure is performed weekly for the first 3 months and then less often when rejection episodes have been controlled.

Complications

REJECTION

In the first 2 months after transplantation many patients undergo one or more rejection episodes (Fig. 18). Thereafter the frequency declines. With azathioprine immunosuppression, rejection could be predicted by a decrease in R-wave voltage on electrocardiogram and by the development of a gallop rhythm, arrhythmias, or congestive failure on clinical examination. In contrast, rejection is usually clinically silent in patients treated with cyclosporine and can be detected only by means of routine endocardial biopsy. Low-grade fever, leukocytosis, a diminished requirement for antihypertensive medications, and an in-

crease in the ratio of T4/T8 lymphocytes may provide clues that rejection is occurring. These findings are suggestive but not diagnostic of rejection. Rejection of the lungs, fortunately, does not occur without concomitant cardiac rejection; therefore, endocardial biopsies can be utilized to monitor rejection in heart-lung recipients. Reitz and associates have found that the frequency and severity of rejection episodes following cardiopulmonary transplantation are not greater than with isolated cardiac transplantation and that rejection of the lung does not occur without histologic changes in the heart biopsies. They also found that lung rejection does not seriously affect pulmonary function during the course of cardiac rejection except in the early post-transplantation period when diffuse interstitial edema may be present.

Biopsies are graded in three categories: (1) *mild*—lymphocyte infiltration only; (2) *moderate*—lymphocyte infiltration with scattered myocyte necrosis; and (3) *severe*—widespread myocyte necrosis and lymphocyte infiltration. Mild rejection need not be treated. However, patients with moderate or severe rejection episodes are given a 3-day "pulse" of methylprednisolone, 10 mg. per kg. intravenously, with the maintenance prednisone and cyclosporine doses held constant. If steroid pulse therapy fails to reverse the histologic findings or if myocyte necrosis is very severe or there is clinical deterioration, a course of ATG is administered. Some programs utilize a 3-day course of intramuscular rabbit ATG and others use a 14-day course of intravenous equine ATG, 17 mg. per kg. Steroid pulses may be accompanied by hypertension and therefore are administered with caution and careful monitoring.

INFECTION

A major advantage of cyclosporine immunosuppression over azathioprine is a major reduction in the incidence of serious problems from postoperative infections due to chronic immunosuppression. In one study, these occurred in 70 per cent of azathioprine-treated patients but only in 47 per cent of cyclosporine-treated patients in the first 3 postoperative months. More recent experience has revealed that, although the incidence of infection has been only slightly less with cyclosporine, the morbidity and mortality have been much reduced (Fig. 19). Most of these infections are pulmonary, and many are caused by unusual organisms

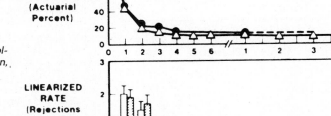

Figure 18. Incidence of rejection episodes following cardiac transplantation. (From Jamieson, S. W., et al.: Heart Transplant., 3:225, 1984.)

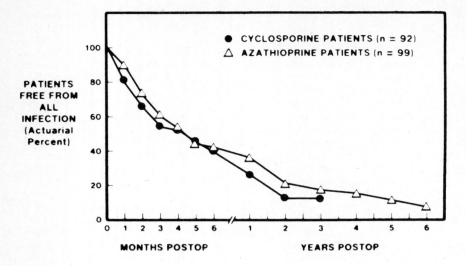

Figure 19. Actuarial probability of being free from infection following cardiac transplantation. The patients treated with cyclosporine are compared with patients treated with azathioprine. The two groups are not randomized. (From Jamieson, S. W., et al.: Heart Transplant., 3:225, 1984.)

such as *Legionella,* herpes virus, and fungi. Vigorous diagnostic efforts are required if there is any new pulmonary infiltrate suggesting pneumonia, any change in mental function suggesting meningitis, or any other unexplained signs or symptoms. Patients on steroids are normally hypothermic; any slight fever is cause for concern.

GRAFT ATHEROSCLEROSIS

Occasional patients experience early, silent occlusive atherosclerosis of the graft coronary arteries leading to infarction, sudden death, or congestive failure. Angina does not occur because the heart is denervated. For this reason, all transplant patients should have routine postoperative coronary angiography. Risk factors appear to be donors over 35 years of age, frequent rejection episodes, persistent hypertriglyceridemia, and HLA-A$_2$ incompatibility. This last complication is probably related to immunologic injury to the epithelium, since it is not unique to cardiac grafts. In an effort to reduce this risk, patients are maintained on aspirin and dipyridamole after transplantation, and their blood lipids and cholesterol are carefully controlled. Because of its diffuse distribution and rapid progression, graft coronary atherosclerosis is not amenable to bypass grafting, leaving retransplantation as the only option. At last report, 15 patients have undergone retransplantation at Stanford for this problem with nine short-term survivors (Table 13).

TABLE 13. Survival Following First and Second Cardiac Transplants*

	Patients	Survival at 3 Months (%)
First retransplant		
Immediate graft failure	3	0
Acute rejection	5	3 (60)
Graft atherosclerosis	14	9 (64)
Constrictive disease	1	1 (100)
Second retransplant		
Immediate graft failure	1	1 (100)
Graft atherosclerosis	1	0

*From Jamieson, S. W., et al.: Heart Transplant., 3:225, 1984.

OTHER COMPLICATIONS

Patients receiving cyclosporine develop a fine interstitial myocardial fibrosis, which does not appear to lead to cardiac dysfunction. They may also experience renal toxicity, hirsutism, a fine tremor, hypertension, and other less common side effects. These latter complications usually improve or disappear when the dose of cyclosporine is decreased. Some patients have been switched from cyclosporine to azathioprine late postoperatively to reverse their renal impairment. Side effects of chronic steroid administration also occur. Patients who have had combined heart-lung transplants tend to have problems raising secretions. Some have developed a pattern of restrictive lung disease. Therefore, prolonged pulmonary physiotherapy and careful follow-up are required.

Results

One-year survival rates following cardiac transplantation have steadily improved from approximately 20 per cent in the 1960s to over 80 per cent currently, with an improvement in the projected actuarial 5-year survival to approximately 50 per cent (Fig. 20). The major causes of death continue to be rejection and infection. The quality of life among the survivors has been excellent, especially in contrast to their marked preoperative disability. Ninety-seven per cent have been asymptomatic, and 82 per cent have been rehabilitated sufficiently to return to employment, homemaking, or school (Table 14). This high rate of rehabilitation is no doubt in part due to the careful selection of transplant recipients. Patients usually carry on relatively normal lives while adhering to the rigorous postoperative follow-up required.

To date, approximately 38 patients have undergone combined heart-lung transplantation. Seventy per cent of the patients are alive and well 1 year following the operation. The two longest-surviving patients are living 24 and 36 months postoperatively. Although the number of patients undergoing heart-lung transplantation is not large, the operation holds great promise for those patients with end-stage cardiopulmonary disease who cannot be treated by conventional methods or isolated heart transplantation.

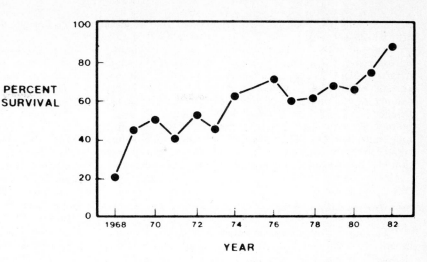

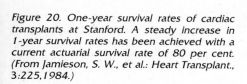

Figure 20. One-year survival rates of cardiac transplants at Stanford. A steady increase in 1-year survival rates has been achieved with a current actuarial survival rate of 80 per cent. (From Jamieson, S. W., et al.: Heart Transplant., 3:225,1984.)

Conclusions

In the past 15 years, cardiac transplantation has progressed rapidly from an experimental procedure to an acceptable therapeutic modality for the patient with terminal heart disease. No doubt, even greater advances will be made with the development of newer immunosuppressive agents, improvement in the logistics of bringing donors and recipients together, and development of techniques to store donor hearts for a prolonged period of time.

The costs are substantial. At Stanford, where long experience and high volume should have allowed maximal efficiency, the last reported average hospital stay is 45 days at an average cost of $57,000 in hospital charges. The ongoing costs of outpatient visits, follow-up hospitalization, and medication add $10,000 to $20,000 a year to this. Funding for these considerable costs is variable. Clearly, for cardiac transplantation to be widely utilized, reliable sources of funding need to be found. Rather than absolute costs, more consideration should be given to cost-benefit ratios, since many of these patients return to work, pay taxes, and become contributing members of society.

LUNG TRANSPLANTATION

Historic and Experimental Basis

In 1947, Demikhov performed the first recorded orthotopic experimental pulmonary transplant in modern times; no immunosuppression was used. Ten days was the longest survival achieved. Numerous investigators then attempted pulmonary transplantation in the laboratory. Several technical advances led to success, including utilization of a transected cuff of left atrium from the donor that included the orifices of the pulmonary veins to help prevent pulmonary venous thrombosis; construction of a distensible pulmonary artery anastomosis by spatulating both the donor and recipient pulmonary arteries; and reinforcement of the bronchial suture line with a pedicle omental graft or by telescoping the transplanted bronchus within the recipient bronchus. Investigators learned that a single lung transplant can provide total respiratory function while accommodating the entire pulmonary blood flow at acceptable pulmonary artery pressures.

Ideal preservation of the donor lung is of paramount importance. Procurement of lungs from donors in distant hospitals is not feasible today because it prolongs preservation time beyond our present capabilities. Lungs can be preserved reliably for only about 2 hours. Techniques that extend the ischemic tolerance of lung grafts include constant inflation and ventilation as well as hypothermic perfusion and storage. The best solutions for lung preservation are of the intracellular type with a low sodium and a high potassium concentration and a large amount of phosphate base, e.g., Collins' and Sacks' solutions.

Recipient and Donor Criteria

The current criteria for a single lung transplant are compatible ABO blood type between donor and recipient, absence of recipient antibodies to donor lymphocytes, and comparable size of the donor and recipient hilar structures. Cadaveric donors must have at least one normal lung on chest roentgenogram, a nonpurulent and relatively organ-

TABLE 14. Rehabilitation following Cardiac Transplantation: One-Year Survivors (N = 106)*

	No.	Per Cent
New York Heart Association functional status		
Class I	103	97
Class II	2	
Class III	1	
Class IV	0	
Rehabilitated		
Yes	87	82
No	19	
Work activity		
Employed full time	45	
Employed part time	14	
Homemaker	8	
Student	10	
	77	73
Retired by choice		
Medical disability	19	
	10	

*From Pennock, J. I., et al.: J. Thorac. Cardiovasc. Surg., 83:168, 1982.

ism-free lung by fiberoptic bronchoscopy, and a donor arterial oxygen tension over 250 torr with an FIO_2 of 1.0.

Patients with a variety of terminal pulmonary diseases unresponsive to all medical therapy are candidates for single lung transplant. These diseases include pulmonary fibrosis, chronic emphysema, cystic fibrosis, bronchiectasis, posttraumatic pulmonary insufficiency, alpha-1 antitrypsin deficiency, and silicosis. Patients with moderate to severe pulmonary hypertension are treated by combined heart-lung transplantation. The contraindications for isolated lung transplantation are the same as for heart-lung transplantation except that older individuals are suitable candidates.

Surgical Technique

The surgical techniques developed in the experimental laboratory form the basis for those used in patients. A standard thoracic posterolateral incision provides good exposure in both the donor and the recipient. In the recipient the inferior pulmonary ligament is divided, the pericardium opened, and the appropriate pulmonary artery circumferentially mobilized. Similarly, the junction of the pulmonary veins and left atrium is freed. The mainstem bronchus is dissected free of adventitia to its bifurcation at the carina. A similar dissection is performed in a donor of comparable size or slightly larger size than the recipient. After application of vascular clamps, the pulmonary artery, main bronchus, and left atrium are divided, leaving a generous cuff of the latter. The atrial anastomosis is constructed in two layers with a continuous cardiovascular suture. The bronchial anastomosis is re-established with interrupted absorbable suture, and the pulmonary artery anastomosis is accomplished with a one-layer continuous arterial suture (Fig. 21). The bronchial anastomosis is usually reinforced with an omental pedicle graft.

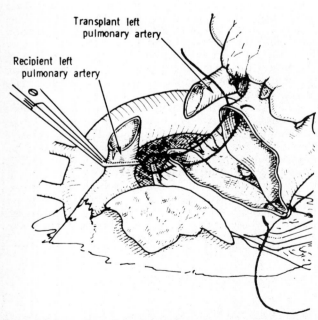

Transplant left
pulmonary artery

Recipient left
pulmonary artery

Figure 21. Lung allograft implantation, anterior view. Implantation is begun by placing two horizontal mattress sutures at each end of the left atrial cuff. Note spatulation of donor and recipient pulmonary arteries by transecting them diagonally. (From Veith, F. J., and Richards, K.: Ann. Surg., 171:555, 1970.)

Postoperative Care

The postoperative management of recipients with isolated lung transplants is very similar to that employed for patients undergoing combined heart-lung transplantation. The cornerstone of immunosuppression is cyclosporine. Maintenance prednisone treatment is omitted for the first 2 weeks after the operation because of the risk of impaired healing of the tracheal anastomosis. After 2 weeks prednisone therapy is initiated. The patients are then maintained on low-dose steroid and cyclosporine therapy. A potential complication peculiar to transplantation of pulmonary tissue, whether unilateral or combined with a cardiac graft, is the phenomenon known as "reimplantation response." This has been discussed in the section on heart-lung transplantation.

Lung allograft rejection may manifest itself clinically by shortness of breath and/or nonproductive cough. Radiographically, there is opacification of the transplanted lung, and physiologically there is evidence of ventilation/perfusion abnormalities. Superimposed infection may complicate the rejection episode. Early accurate diagnosis is important for proper treatment of rejection. Transthoracic needle biopsy has proved to be of value in establishing the diagnosis. Rejection episodes have been treated with a 3-day course of "pulse" therapy with methylprednisolone and a 10- to 14-day course of antithymocyte globulin.

Results

The success of clinical lung transplantation has lagged behind that achieved with other organ transplants. Since the first human lung transplant by Hardy in 1963, only 37 additional attempts have been recorded in the intervening years. Until recently the long-term results were disappointing. The longest survivor lived only 10 months after the operation. Recently, Cooper, at the University of Toronto, successfully transplanted a right lung in a 58-year-old man with terminal pulmonary fibrosis. The patient is alive and well 18 months following operation and is working full time with minimal symptoms. Cooper also successfully transplanted a left lung in a 35-year-old woman with pulmonary fibrosis. She is alive and well 6 months following operation. Both patients experienced several episodes of rejection, which were successfully treated.

With Cooper's encouraging results, interest in isolated lung transplantation has been rekindled. The development of cyclosporine as an effective immunosuppressive agent offers promise that allograft rejection can be controlled in humans and increases the prospects for long-term clinical success with this procedure. Unfortunately, even with the development of more effective preservation techniques, the scarcity of adequate donor lungs will be a major limiting factor in clinical lung transplantation.

SMALL BOWEL TRANSPLANTATION

Small bowel transplantation has the potential to rehabilitate the intestinal cripple. The number of patients in need of small bowel replacement is not known. However, there are sufficiently large numbers of patients with the short bowel syndrome to support a home hyperalimentation industry, and many other patients expire owing to poor nutrition or other complications. The adult population of patients is derived from persons suffering mesenteric vascular thrombosis or embolus, iatrogenic injuries, trauma, volvulus, strangulated bowel obstruction, mesenteric involvement with resectable tumors, and resection of more than 75 per cent of the small bowel for any reason, such as recurrent bowel obstruction. Short bowel problems in children result largely from necrotizing enterocolitis, volvulus, trauma, and complications of malrotation and intussusception.

Historic and Experimental Basis

Lillehei and others at the University of Minnesota reported the first successful canine model of small bowel transplantation in 1959. The major contribution of early experimental work was to demonstrate the technical feasibility of the procedure and adequate nutritional function of the autograft after complete division of blood vessels, lymphatics, and nerves. Without immunosuppression, animals with allografts survived about 7 to 14 days. Death apparently resulted from what is now recognized as graft versus host disease (GVHD). When immunosuppression with azathioprine and prednisone was added, survival to 38 days was recorded. Most noteworthy was the demonstration that immunosuppressed animals developed a picture of classic rejection rather than GVHD. Radiation of the allograft prior to transplantation (150 rads) has also prevented the development of GVHD in the dog. More recently it appears that cyclosporine immunosuppression is even more effective in avoiding GVHD. GVHD has been prevented by cyclosporine in the rat and dog, and preliminary trials in the pig indicate similar results. With the use of cyclosporine, dogs and pigs have survived with total small bowel allografts for more than 550 days. These animals survive without signs of rejection or GVHD but with variable function of the graft. Most successful long-term survivors have received cyclosporine by the intravenous or intraperitoneal route. Both routes of administration avoid the problem of variable absorption of cyclosporine through the transplanted small intestine.

Surgical Technique

The best technique for transplantation of the small bowel has not been defined. Vascular thrombosis is common and has occurred in up to 60 per cent of animals in some experimental series. Most clinical attempts have ended in early thrombosis of the graft for reasons that are not obvious. When the entire small bowel is transplanted, usually the superior mesenteric artery and vein are anastomosed to the aorta and vena cava. Venous drainage through the splanchnic venous system may have some physiologic advantage, but it is technically more difficult to isolate or identify a suitable open branch of the portal vein in patients who have already lost most of their small intestine. It is also possible to transplant smaller segments of small bowel, and there is one report of transplantation of the distal small bowel and right colon in humans.

Results

Deterling performed the first two human small bowel transplants in 1964 at Boston Floating Hospital. Both were implanted in children; one patient died after 12 hours and a second within several weeks. In five of the seven reported cases of small bowel transplantation either the graft or the patient was lost in the early postoperative period. In the sixth patient the transplant survived a longer period of time, and histologic sections demonstrated that it had undergone acute rejection. Fortner reported the seventh case in 1972. The bowel functioned for 2 months, but the patient died on the 176th postoperative day from sepsis. With the use of cyclosporine there is increasing success in experimental small bowel transplantation, and this may lead to additional clinical attempts in the near future.

AUTOTRANSPLANTATION OF TISSUES AND ORGANS

Historic and Experimental Basis

Over the centuries virtually every tissue and organ in the body has been transferred from one location to another. The skulls of prehistoric man contain trephination defects repaired with bone flaps. The first recorded use of autotransplantation techniques is contained in the Sushruta Samhita, a Sanskrit text from India that was written over 2000 years ago. This text has remarkably detailed descriptions of pedicle grafts for reconstruction of the nose, ear, and lip. The technique of a staged tubular pedicle graft was described by Tagliacozzi in 1587. In modern times autografts of various tissues and organs have become important techniques in every surgical discipline.

The terms "autotransplantation" and "autografting" describe the transfer of an organ, tissue, or cells from one area of the body to another ectopic position. A free graft, such as a split-thickness skin graft, implies that the tissue is transferred without an attempt to preserve or reanastomose the vascular supply of the graft. When pedicle grafts are used, the blood supply is maintained through the base of the pedicle until the graft is revascularized from ingrowth of capillaries and small vessels in its new location (Fig. 22). With the development of microvascular techniques, it is now possible to transfer entire organs or large composite grafts to distant sites on the body by anastomosing the main artery and vein without having to depend upon a pedicle for an interim blood supply (Fig. 23). This type of graft is sometimes referred to as a free pedicle graft or flap or an autotransplant when an entire organ is transferred to an ectopic location.

Oxygen and essential nutrients can be provided to dispersed cells or thin grafts via serum or interstitial fluid from surrounding tissues until the ingrowth of capillaries can occur. Capillary ingrowth occurs as quickly as 4 or 5 days in split-thickness grafts. Thick grafts or whole organ grafts require reanastomosis of their arterial and venous blood supply. Some autografts simply serve as a framework for ingrowth of cells from adjacent tissue and thus do not require preservation of their nutrient supply. Many bone grafts are not truly living but simply provide a lattice that is slowly resorbed or into which living cells migrate. Likewise, interposition nerve grafts serve as conduits for wallerian regeneration of axons. Preservation of nerve supply to grafts is a problem that has been only partially solved. Free transfer of muscles often does not result in a good functional result because of a lack of a nerve supply, and reinnervation of extremity or digit reimplants may take many months. In the remainder of this section, we will list the more important types of autografts and discuss those that are commonly used in surgical practice.

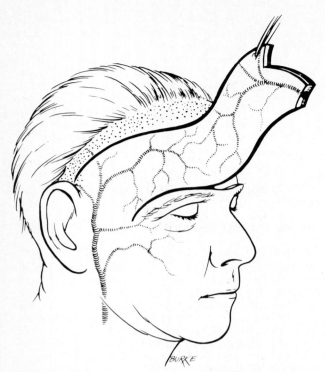

Figure 22. Pedicle skin graft. The graft circulation is through vessels entering at the base of the pedicle. The pedicle can be used for reconstruction of the nose, jaw, or other parts of the face and scalp. After the graft has healed into its new position, the base of the flap can be divided. The graft will survive as a result of the ingrowth of small vessels and capilliaries.

Skin Grafts

Skin grafts are the oldest and most widely utilized form of autografting. In 1804, Baronio demonstrated that it was possible to transplant skin from one site to another in sheep. Split-thickness skin grafts were originally obtained with the use of a long, thin knife, such as the Goulian knife. Today most grafts are obtained with a motor-driven dermatome utilizing a vibrating blade. With modern dermatomes the thickness and dimensions of the graft can be more precisely controlled. The major indications for the use of various types of skin grafts are to cover cutaneous

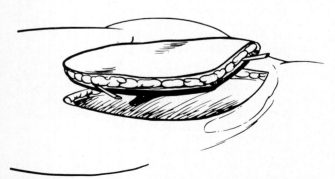

Figure 23. Tensor fasciae latae graft. This is a myocutaneous flap. The major artery and vein are preserved. The major artery and vein can be reanastomosed using microsurgical technique. The graft can be transferred to virtually any part of the body.

TABLE 15. *Commonly Employed Types of Skin Grafts*

Split-thickness free grafts
Full-thickness free grafts
Pedicle grafts of full thickness skin
Free full-thickness grafts with vascular anastomoses
Myocutaneous pedicle and free grafts
Hair transplant punch grafts
Cultured epidermal cells
Composite grafts of skin and cartilage
Cadaver allografts and xenografts

defects, reconstruct body parts such as the nose or lips, and reline cavities such as the mouth and vagina (Table 15).

SPLIT-THICKNESS GRAFTS

Split-thickness grafts usually vary in thickness from 12/1000 to 18/1000 of an inch. If the rete pegs of the dermis or the epithelium of the skin appendages remains, the skin of the donor site will re-epithelialize. Split-thickness grafts require a well-vascularized, relatively clean graft site, since their survival depends upon the exchange of serum and interstitial fluid for the first 4 or 5 days and the rapid ingrowth of capillaries within that time. All open wounds are contaminated with bacteria, but split-thickness skin grafts will usually survive if there are fewer than 10^5 organisms per gram of tissue in the graft bed.

PEDICLE GRAFTS

The length of a pedicle graft is limited by the breadth of its base. The usual guideline is that the pedicle or flap should not be more than two times longer than the width of the base, but there are many exceptions to this rule. These grafts depend upon the capillaries and small vessels in the dermis and subcutaneous tissue for their blood supply. The development of myocutaneous grafts permits the length of these pedicles or flaps to be much longer. These flaps are planned so that the blood supply is based upon a major regional vessel, such as the thoracoacromial artery for a pectoralis major flap (Fig. 24). Muscle is fed by this larger vessel, and the viability of the skin is maintained through small feeder vessels throughout the length of the muscle. Myocutaneous flaps can also be used in much more contaminated areas, probably because their blood supply is so much more abundant than pedicle flaps.

EXTENSIVE GRAFTING

The patient with an extensive burn may require up to 90 per cent of his body to be resurfaced with skin grafts. Special techniques have been developed to meet this requirement. Split-thickness autografts may be expanded into a mesh that will cover a larger area. The epidermal cells will migrate to cover a bare area of 2 to 3 cm. in diameter. Recently, epidermal cells have been grown in tissue culture. They greatly increase in number while in culture and can then be used to cover a much greater area of exposed surface. Burn patients are also partially immunosuppressed by virtue of the large physiologic insult that has occurred. For this reason, it is feasible to use human cadaver allografts or even pig xenografts to temporarily cover the wound. Surprisingly, many of these grafts do not reject promptly and instead survive for many weeks.

Skin may be expanded with the use of a subcutaneous prosthesis that is slowly inflated over a period of days or

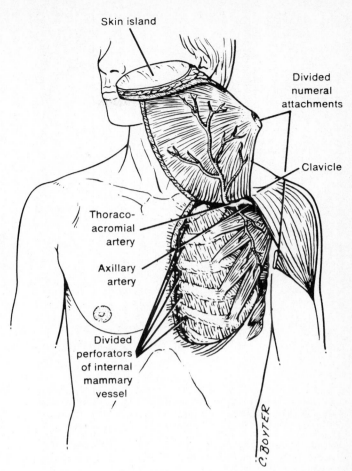

Figure 24. Pectoralis major myocutaneous flap. This flap is based on the thoracoacromial artery. The island of skin can be moved long distances to repair defects on the head, neck, or chest wall. In this illustration, the thoracoacromial artery remains intact. However, the vessels could be divided and anastomosed to distant sites using microvascular techniques.

weeks (Fig. 25). The expanded area of skin may be used as a flap or as a source of split-thickness grafts.

PUNCH GRAFTS

Hair transplants are now performed routinely. Usually a "punch" technique is used. A small cylinder or "punch" of hair-bearing skin is excised and transferred to the scalp.

Vascular Autografts

Vascular grafts have been used since the early 1900s following the experimental work of Carrel in 1905. The grafts derive their nutrition either by direct absorption from the vascular lumen or through small vessels that connect to the lumen of the graft. Vein grafts are among the most commonly employed autografts. The greater and lesser saphenous veins and occasionally the internal jugular vein or a forearm vein are most commonly employed. These veins generally have sufficient strength to withstand arterial pressure, but sometimes dilatation or aneurysm formation occurs. When valves are present in the vein, the graft may be "reversed," so that the one-way valves are oriented to permit passage of arterial blood. Arterial autografts are used less often because there are only a few medium- or large-sized arteries in the body of any length that can be

removed without causing distal ischemia. The internal iliac and internal mammary arteries can be excised without harm and are used occasionally for vascular reconstruction.

INDICATIONS

Table 16 lists some common indications and procedures in which vascular grafts are used. The coronary artery bypass has become one of the most common operations in the United States. Usually saphenous veins and occasionally internal mammary arteries are used for this procedure. The

TABLE 16. *Some Common Indications for the Use of Vascular Autografts*

Vein autografts
   Segmental replacement of arteries—renal artery stenosis
   Bypass of occluded vessels—coronary artery bypass
   Patch angioplasty of stenosed vessels
   Vascular shunts—mesocaval shunt, angioaccess shunts
   Replacement of large veins and vein valves—femoral vein
     reconstruction for chronic venous insufficiency

Arterial autografts
   Segmental replacement of arteries—renal artery stenosis,
     coronary artery bypass
   Endothelial cell seeding of prosthetic grafts

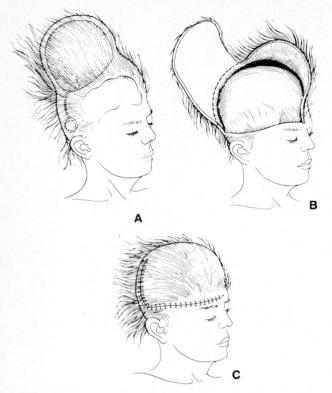

Figure 25. *Skin expansion. A Silastic balloon is placed beneath the subcutaneous tissue. The balloon is slowly expanded over time. The skin can be greatly expanded by this technique. In this illustration the scalp is being greatly expanded (A). Flaps are then fashioned from the expanded skin (B). The flaps are sewn into place to repair a scalp defect (C). The expanded skin grows hair like the normal scalp from which it was derived.*

greater saphenous vein is frequently employed for bypass operations in peripheral vascular surgery such as the femoral-popliteal artery bypass. The internal jugular vein is occasionally used for interposition mesocaval or portacaval shunts for treatment of portal hypertension. Small patches of vein are commonly employed for patch reconstruction of stenosed segments of vessels such as following carotid endarterectomy. Vein autografts are less prone to thrombosis than plastic prostheses and for this reason are preferred for reconstruction or bypass of smaller vessels. Vein grafts also resist infection and can be successfully employed in contaminated fields such as following traumatic wounds.

Vein grafts have been used to reconstruct an incompetent femorosaphenous venous system and thereby alleviate chronic venous insufficiency in the lower extremity. The usual procedure has been to replace a segment of femoral vein with an autograft containing a competent valve. Unfortunately, most of these attempts have failed because of the high incidence of thrombosis.

ENDOTHELIAL SEEDING

Another interesting experimental use of autogenous tissue is the endothelial seeding of prosthetic materials. Endothelial cells are procured from autologous vessels, cultured *in vitro*, and then used to coat the surface of a prosthetic material such as Dacron. The objective is to provide a prosthesis with an endothelial surface to prevent clotting. This method has the potential for avoiding thrombosis in grafts of very small diameter and avoiding problems with thrombosis in artificial implants, such as the artificial heart.

Musculoskeletal Grafts

Successful *muscle grafts* require an intact neurovascular supply. This can be accomplished by swinging the graft on a pedicle or with microvascular techniques. This requirement significantly limits the usefulness of muscle autografts. Muscle grafts with intact blood supplies have been reported to be partially reinnervated within 5 months. Muscle grafts are used in the treatment of facial paralysis and to restore function in the hand. Free muscle grafts with microvascular anastomosis have also been utilized to restore function of the anal sphincter. The muscular component of the myocutaneous graft serves primarily as a conduit for blood supply.

Bone grafts of various types are commonly employed in several surgical specialties. In most cases the bone does not survive and serves mainly as a skeletal framework for the ingrowth of new bone and bone cells. With cortical grafts only the most superficial cells survive; with cancellous bone more cells survive. Bone grafts are used to stabilize fractures, especially with delayed healing, to supplement the arthrodesis of joints, and to reconstruct skeletal and skull defects. Cancellous bone is usually obtained from the iliac crest. Cortical grafts come from the ribs, wing of the ilium, the fibula, and the diaphysis of long bones. Since, in most cases, the bone simply serves as a skeletal matrix, cryopreserved or radiation-preserved bone allografts are utilized commonly.

Cartilage is a privileged tissue in that it does not undergo rejection. The mucoprotein matrix surrounding the chondrocytes protects these cells from rejection. Fresh autografts of cartilage and preserved allografts are used commonly for reconstructing the nose, the ear, and the orbit. Table 17 lists some common types of muscle, bone, cartilage, joint, and fascial grafts.

Nerve Autografts

Nerve autografts are employed to bridge defects in motor nerves caused by trauma or as a result of the excision of neoplasms. The greatest success is obtained in a reconstruction of pure motor nerves. Common indications are repair of the ulnar, medial, and radial nerves of the arm and forearm and of the facial nerve. Sensory nerves, such as the sural, superficial radial, lateral femoral cutaneous, and auricular nerve, may be used as donor segments. Before axons can enter the grafted segment, wallerian degeneration takes place in both the distal damaged nerve and the graft. Axon regeneration progresses at a rate of approximately 1 mm. per day. Thin nerves are usually employed because thick nerves will undergo necrosis centrally. When repairing

TABLE 17. *Musculoskeletal Autografts*

Muscle
Pedicle muscle grafts with intact neurovascular supply
Free grafts with microvascular anastomosis

Bone and cartilage
Reconstruction of facial bones, nose, and ear
Cancellous bone chips to facilitate healing of fractures, arthrodesis of joints, and bone cavities
Inlay and onlay grafts of bone segments to stabilize fractures and bone reconstructions
Preserve allografts of bone or cartilage
Extremity and digit reimplantation
Joint transplantation

Fascia
Abdominal and chest wall hernia repairs

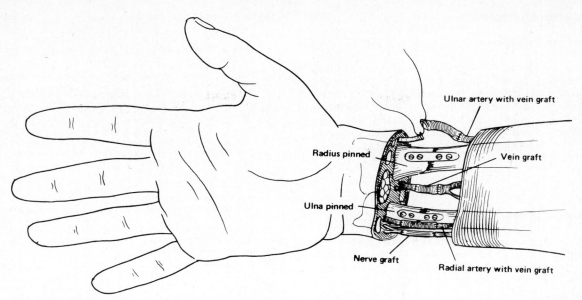

Figure 26. Reimplantation of the hand. The fractures are stabilized with metal plates. The ulnar and radial arteries and the major vein have been reconstituted with interposition vein grafts. An interposition nerve graft has also been used. The tendons will also be repaired.

a large nerve, several thin grafts may be bundled parallel to each other to form a so-called cable graft. Use of microsurgical techniques to obtain more accurate interposition of the grafts has improved results. However, the delay in nerve fibers crossing the suture line and intermixing of fibers at each suture line are unresolved problems that diminish success.

Composite and Other Autografts

Various complex composite grafts have been transplanted with increasing success through the use of microsurgical techniques. These include transplantation of digits, arms, forearms and hands, entire joints, and epithelial growth plates (Fig. 26).

Endocrine Autografts

Transplantation of endocrine tissue holds great appeal. Theoretically, small quantities of tissue may be sufficient to correct a deficiency of a particular hormone. However, many hormones, such as thyroid and corticosteroids, can be replaced with synthetic hormones, so that there is a limited application for endocrine autotransplantation.

PARATHYROID

Parathyroid autotransplantation is the most commonly employed endocrine autograft. Wells of Duke and Washington Universities has clarified the indications and techniques. Small fragments or slices of parathyroid are placed into muscle pockets. These fragments survive by absorption of nutrients until blood supply is re-established. They respond to the usual stimuli and may grow by hypertrophy or hyperplasia if necessary. When it is suspected that insufficient parathyroid tissue remains after a thyroidectomy, small fragments can be implanted into the sternocleidomastoid muscle. Fragments are sometimes implanted into the forearm when most of the parathyroid tissue has

been removed for treatment of severe secondary hyperparathyroidism or generalized parathyroid hyperplasia. Parathyroid tissue can also be cryopreserved and implanted into the forearm muscle at a later date if necessary.

ISLET CELLS

Occasionally it is necessary to remove all or most of the pancreas for benign disease. The most common circumstance in which this occurs is the surgical therapy of chronic pancreatitis. The islet cells of the resected tissue have been isolated in a fashion identical to that used for autografts of islet cells. Cells are then injected into the portal system or the spleen. Unfortunately, these cells have functioned effectively for only a few months.

PANCREAS

Attempts have also been made to autotransplant the tail or a segment of pancreas to a heterotopic location, such as femoral vessels in the groin. This technique has been attempted in patients who require removal of most of their pancreas for benign disease such as chronic pancreatitis. The technique has met with limited success because of the problem of draining the exocrine secretion and the fact that the function of the islets is frequently already compromised from the underlying pancreatic disease.

OTHER ENDOCRINE TRANSPLANTS

Experimental attempts to transplant virtually every other endocrine organ have been reported. Fragments or slices of the thyroid, pituitary, ovary, and testes have been successfully transplanted in man. Woodruff has recommended that slices of ovary be transplanted into the rectus muscle at the time of oophorectomy. However, synthetic hormone replacement is the treatment of choice in most instances.

Gastrointestinal Autografts

There are few indications for the utilization of gastrointestinal autografts. The mesentery of the bowel is usually of sufficient length that a vascular pedicle can be maintained and the segment of bowel merely transposed to the desired location. Free autografts have been used for the replacement of the hypopharynx and cervical esophagus. Usually a segment of jejunum is excised with preservation of its main arterial and venous blood supply. Vascular continuity is re-established using microsurgical techniques by anastomosing the artery to a branch of the carotid artery and jugular vein.

Bone Marrow Grafts

Both allografts and autografts of bone marrow are being employed with increasing frequency. The usual indication is the treatment of various leukemias, lymphomas, and aplastic anemias. A special problem of bone marrow allografting is the occurrence of graft versus host disease. Rejection or graft versus host disease does not occur with autografts or bone marrow grafts between identical twins.

Bone marrow is usually obtained by aspirating the marrow cavity of the sternum, iliac crest, or ribs. The patient with leukemia or other malignancy is then treated with high-dose irradiation or intensive chemotherapy. Hematopoiesis is restored by injecting the stored and cryopreserved marrow. This procedure has been helpful in the treatment of non-Hodgkin's and Burkitt's lymphoma and has been used experimentally in various solid cancers, such as melanoma and ovarian cancer. The marrow can be altered while out of the body by treatment with radiation, or selected populations of cells can be deleted from the marrow with the use of monoclonal antibodies.

Bench Surgery

Bench surgery is a form of autotransplantation. An organ is removed from the body and is protected by simple hypothermia. A partial resection or repair is then performed and the organ reimplanted into the body. This technique is most commonly used with kidneys for such procedures as heminephrectomy, resection of distal renal artery aneurysms, or repair of a traumatic injury.

SELECTED REFERENCES

Annotated References

Calne, R. Y.: Liver Transplantation. New York, Grune & Stratton, Inc., 1983.
This book is a comprehensive review of both experimental and clinical transplantation. The details of pre- and postoperative care, operative technique, diagnosis of rejection, histology of rejection, and the results of the Cambridge group are included.

Cooper, E. L.: General Immunology. Elmsford, N.Y., Pergamon Press, 1982.
This textbook is more general and less detailed than Fundamental Immunology. *The book is clearly written and a pleasure to read.*

Kahan, B. D.: Cyclosporine Biological Activity and Clinical Applications. New York, Grune & Stratton, Inc., 1984.
A thorough review of the mechanisms of actions, immunosuppressive properties, and pharmacokinetics of cyclosporine is included. The last portion of the book summarizes clinical trials with cyclosporine in kidney, heart, lung, liver, pancreas and bone marrow transplantation. There is an extensive discussion of cyclosporine toxicity.

Morris, P. J. (Ed.): Kidney Transplantation: Principles and Practice. 2nd ed. London, Grune & Stratton, Ltd., 1984.
Dr. Morris has put together an informative, up-to-date text covering all aspects of renal transplantation. Both practical and theoretical issues are well addressed by the selected expert authors.

Morris, P. J.: Tissue Transplantation. New York, Churchill Livingstone, 1982.
This concise volume summarizes the general field of transplantation. Specific chapters summarize advances in each organ category.

Paul, W. E.: Fundamental Immunology. New York, Raven Press, 1984.
William Paul is an internationally respected immunologist. He has assembled a comprehensive and very detailed review of current thinking in immunology. The topics are well chosen and invariably written by authorities in the field.

Simmons, R. L., Finch, M. E., Ascher, N. L., and Najarian, J. S. (Eds.): Manual of Vascular Access, Organ Donation and Transplantation. New York, Springer-Verlag, 1984.
This atlas contains many handsome illustrations that clearly demonstrate the surgical techniques used in multiorgan transplantation. The accompanying text complements the illustrations. The authors are from the University of Minnesota, an institution with a history of innovation and achievement in transplantation.

Tilney, N. L., and Lazars, J. M. (Eds.): Surgical Care of the Patient with Renal Failure. Philadelphia, W. B. Saunders Company, 1982.
This text provides a thorough background on patients with renal failure. The multisystem effects of acute and chronic renal failure are emphasized. The discussions on dialysis and transplantation are balanced and non-polemical.

Toledo-Pereyra, L. H. (Ed.): Basic Concepts in Organ Procurement, Perfusion and Preservation for Transplantation. New York, Academic Press, Inc., 1982.
The editor of this volume has compiled an excellent, very readable text. The text includes chapters on historic development in organ preservation, diagnostic criteria, and legal status of brain death, kidney donation, and reviews of preservation of specific organs. Along with basic concepts in organ preservation science, the book deals with the socioeconomic issues of transplantation.

Immunobiology

Kahan, B. D.: Individualization of cyclosporine therapy using pharmacokinetic and pharmacodynamic parameters. Transplantation, *40*:457, 1985.
Krensky, A. M., and Clayberger, C.: Diagnostic and therapeutic implications of T cell surface antigens. Transplantation, *39*:339, 1985.
Steinmiller, D.: Which T cells mediate allograft rejection? Transplantation, *40*:229, 1985.

Multiorgan Donation

Bart, K. J., Macon E. J., Whittier, F. C., Baldwin, R. J., and Blount, J. H.: Cadaver kidneys for transplantation. A paradox of shortage in the face of plenty. Transplantation, *31*:379, 1981.
Beecher, H. K. (Chairman, Ad Hoc Committee of the Harvard Medical School to Examine the Definition of Brain Death): Special communication. A definition of irreversible coma. J.A.M.A., *205*:337, 1968.
Starzl, T. E., Hakala, T. R., Shaw, B. W., Jr., Hardesty, R. L., Rosenthal, T. J., Griffith, B. P., Iwatsuki, S., and Bahnson, H. T.: A flexible procedure for multiple cadaveric organ procurement. Surg. Gynecol. Obstet., *158*:223, 1984.

Organ Preservation

Belzer, F. O., and Southard, J. H.: The future of kidney preservation. Transplantation, *30*:161, 1980.
Toledo-Pereyra, L. H.: Organ preservation. J. Surg. Res., *30*:165, 1981.

Renal Transplantation

Dupont, E., Wybran, J., and Toussaint, C.: Glucocorticoids, steroids and organ transplantation. Transplantation, *37*:331, 1984.
Salvatierra, O., Vincenti, F., Amerd, W. J. C., Garavoy, M. R., Potter, D., and Feduska, N. J.: The role of blood transfusions in renal transplantation. Urol. Clin. North Am., *10*:243, 1983.
Terasaki, P., Toyotome, A., Mickey, M. R., Cicciarelli, J., Iwaki, Y., Cecka, M., and Tiwari, J.: Patient, graft and functional survival rates: An overview. *In* Terasaki, P. (Ed.) Clinical Kidney Transplants. Los Angeles, UCLA Tissue Typing Laboratory, 1985.

Liver

Pichlmayr, R., Brolsch, C., Wonigeit, K., Neuhaus, P., Siegismund, S., Schmidt, F. W., and Burdelski, M.: Experiences with liver transplantation in Hannover. Hepatology, *4*(Suppl.):565, 1984.

Shaw, B. W., Jr., Gordon, R. D., Iwatsuki, S., and Starzl, T. E.: Hepatic retransplantation. Trans. Proc., 7:264, 1985.

Starzl, T. E., Iwatsuki, S., Van Thiel, D. H., Gartner, J. C., Zitelli, B. J., Malatack, J. J., Schadel, R. R., Shaw, B. W., Jr., Hakala, T. R., Rosenthal, J. T., and Porter, K. A.: Evolution of liver transplantation. Hepatology, 2:614, 1982.

Williams, R., Calne, R. Y., Roles, K., and Polson, R. J.: Current results with orthotopic liver grafting in Cambridge/King's College Hospital series. Br. Med. J., 290:49, 1985.

Pancreas

Corry, R. J., Naghiem, D. D., Schulak, J. A., Beutel, W. D., and Gonwa, T. A.: Surgical treatment of diabetic nephropathy with simultaneous pancreatic duodenal and renal transplantation. Surg. Gynecol. Obstet., 162:547, 1986.

Scharp, D. W. (Ed.): Progress Symposium. Transplantation of pancreatic islet cells. World J. Surg., 8:1, 1984.

Sutherland, D. E. R., Goetz, F. C., and Najarian, J. S.: One hundred pancreas transplants at a single institution. Ann. Surg., 200:414, 1984.

Heart, Heart-Lung

Copeland, J. G., Griepp, R. B., Bieber, C. P., et al.: Successful retransplantation of the human heart. J. Thorac. Cardiovasc. Surg., 73:242, 1977.

Jamieson, S. W., Oyer, P., Baldwin, J., et al.: Heart transplantation for end-stage ischemic heart disease: The Stanford experience. Heart Transplant., 3:224, 1984.

Jamieson, S., Reitz, B., Aye, P., et al.: Combined heart-lung transplantation. Lancet, 1:1130, 1983.

Lung

Veith, F., Kamholz, S., Mollenkopf, F., and Montefusco, C.: Lung transplantation in 1983. Transplantation, 35:271, 1983.

Small Bowel

Kirkman, R. L.: Small bowel transplantation. Transplantation, 37:429, 1984.

PRINCIPLES OF SURGICAL ONCOLOGY

E. CARMACK HOLMES, M.D. • BARRY D. MANN, M.D.

16

PRINCIPLES OF CANCER SURGERY

The surgeon's role in the total management of the cancer patient can be presented in the following categories: (1) prevention, (2) diagnosis, (3) treatment, (4) palliation, (5) reconstruction, and (6) follow-up.

Prevention

The development of cancer can often be prevented by the recognition and prophylactic treatment of conditions associated with a high incidence of malignant disease. Ulcerative colitis and familial polyposis, for example, are associated with the subsequent development of carcinoma of the colon. Prophylactic total colectomy is frequently indicated for these high-risk patients. Barrett's esophagus, a columnar epithelium-lined esophagus, usually the consequence of prolonged reflux esophagitis, is associated with a 10 per cent incidence of adenocarcinoma of the esophagus. Although prophylactic surgery is usually not indicated, these patients must be followed closely. Testicular carcinoma develops with greater frequency in patients with undescended testicles than in other patients. Correction of cryptorchidism can eliminate this risk.

Surgeons must understand the pathology and natural history of premalignant lesions. Proper treatment and careful follow-up of patients with conditions such as leukoplakia, cervical dysplasia, and atypical nevi can prevent the development of malignancy.

Malignancy cannot always be anticipated. Frequently, however, it can be recognized early, and early recognition is associated with the best prognosis. The armamentarium for the detection of subclinical, asymptomatic cancer is increasing. Examples of detection methods include *mammography*, useful for screening for breast cancer in women over 50 as well as women over 35 at high risk due to family or previous personal history; the *Papanicolaou (Pap) test*, an effective screening technique for carcinoma of the cervix; *stool examination for occult blood*, a simple and important part of any complete physical examination; and *sigmoidoscopy*, occasionally recommended as a screening test for colon cancer in patients over 50.

Diagnosis

Diagnosis in patients presenting with malignant disease involves general diagnostic skills, which are beyond the scope of our discussion. However, several pertinent points specific to oncologic diagnosis warrant mention.

The patient with cancer can present initially with metastases to lymph node groups or other organs. Intelligent management demands an understanding of the differential diagnosis. Abnormal lymph nodes in the *cervical* region, for example, require a search for a primary tumor in the oropharynx, nasopharynx, hypopharynx, or larynx. Thyroid carcinomas and lymphomas also may metastasize to cervical lymph nodes. *Supraclavicular* adenopathy is seen frequently from metastatic breast cancer or carcinoma of the lung or esophagus. A supraclavicular metastasis also may represent a malignant primary tumor below the diaphragm, such as carcinoma of the stomach, pancreas, colon, or cervix. An abnormal *axillary* lymph node in a female should initiate a careful breast examination and a mammogram, if examination is unrevealing. Inguinal adenopathy is commonly seen with tumors of the anal or genital area. Melanomas and lymphomas can metastasize to any of the aforementioned lymph node groups.

The most common target organs for metastatic disease are lung, liver, bone, and brain. The clinical setting and evidence of multiple lesions generally discriminate between a primary tumor arising in the organ and metastases. Knowledge of the metastatic pattern of the various tumor types is the key to expeditious work-up and institution of proper treatment.

The surgeon is frequently called upon to perform a diagnostic biopsy. Biopsy considerations must take into account the plan for definitive surgery. Excisional biopsy refers to the complete excision of a tumor mass with little or no margin of normal tissue. The tumor itself is not violated. Excisional biopsy is appropriate for most tumors. In certain instances, however, incisional biopsy is preferable. For example, the treatment of soft tissue sarcoma requires wide margins around the primary site. An incisional biopsy facilitates the recognition of clean surgical planes by leaving the tumor *in situ* until the definitive operation is performed.[8]

Because tumors have a tendency to seed and contaminate incisions, the biopsy incision should be placed so that it can be included in a subsequent definitive surgical resection. A biopsy site that is far removed from the potential operative incision can jeopardize plans for definitive treatment. New attitudes toward breast biopsy illustrate this point. Formerly, the circumareolar incision was popular for breast biopsy because it avoided unnecessary scars if a lesion proved benign. However, since the advent of breast-preserving procedures, the circumareolar incision is no longer universally appropriate. If a cancer is biopsied around the areola, the areola must be sacrificed in the subsequent resection, thus negating the cosmetic advantage of a breast-preserving procedure.

The diagnosis of a cancer frequently can be obtained by needle biopsy. Fine-needle biopsy is a technique of cell aspiration. It is relatively simple and yields single cells or clumps from which an accurate diagnosis can be made by an experienced pathologist. However, negative needle aspirations do not exclude malignancy due to potential sampling errors.

Biopsy needles have slightly larger bores than other needles and are designed to extract a core of tissue with recognizable architecture. The Tru-Cut needle is an example.[18] Although there is theoretical concern about spreading cancer cells by introducing needles into tumors, this has not been a problem. As a general caveat, a biopsy should be performed only by a surgeon who is well acquainted with the differential diagnosis and the options for definitive surgical treatment. Finally, when handling tissue of any kind, specific coordination with the pathologist is essential to be sure that specimens are handled properly. Improper handling may preclude essential tissue examinations such as electron microscopy.

Treatment

The ultimate surgical goal is the safe conduct of surgery and the prevention of local recurrence. Tumors should be resected *en bloc* with adequate normal tissue margins; the line of resection should never contain visible or palpable tumor. Obtaining an "adequate" surgical margin is an important but somewhat arbitrary concept. Acceptable margins may vary according to histologic types, anatomic location, and plans for further therapy. For example, previously it was generally accepted that a margin of 5 cm. including the muscular fascia was required for adequate resection of a primary melanoma. Over the past decade, however, stratification by Clark's level (see "Malignant Melanoma" later in this chapter) has shown that acceptably low recurrence rates can be obtained with narrower surgical margins for shallow melanomas. Modifications are also made for anatomic location. Wide margins of skin can be obtained easily on the trunk, but margins on the face require modification to be cosmetically acceptable.

The magnitude of surgical resection can be modified for the treatment of certain tumor types by the use of adjuvant therapeutic modalities. Segmental breast resections, for example, when combined with radiation therapy, are thought to be as effective as radical mastectomy for prevention of local recurrence. Similarly, when adjuvant radiation therapy and chemotherapy are added to surgery for soft tissue sarcoma, very low local recurrence rates can be obtained with less radical excisions.[8]

Concern for the potential inadvertent dissemination of tumor cells during surgery has led to the development of a variety of surgical practices. For example, for surgery of the colon, some surgeons perfuse the bowel lumen with tumoricidal solutions and the tumor is not handled ("no-touch technique") until the venous supply of the bowel has been ligated. Although these techniques have gained acceptance because of their theoretical value, their actual contribution to the prevention of local recurrence is controversial.[11]

When a tumor cannot be removed completely, should it be removed at all? A popular hypothesis is that "debulking" or "cytoreductive" surgery may benefit the cancer patient by reducing tumor bulk, thereby creating circumstances more favorable for radiation or chemotherapy. Debulking has proved effective for management of ovarian cancer, a fact that may relate to the unique surface-spread pattern of this malignancy. However, in general, debulking of tumors results in increased blood loss, increased risk of tumor cell dissemination to new areas, and increased overall risk to the patient.

Tumors that metastasize to regional lymph nodes are best handled by en bloc resection of the tumor and the tissues containing the primary nodal drainage area. This applies particularly to visceral lesions of the stomach and colon, where the regional nodes are in close anatomic proximity. When the lymph node drainage areas are far from the primary site (as in melanoma), the surgeon must decide whether the potential for metastases and therapeutic benefit warrants regional node removal.[5]

Surgical excision has an important role in the treatment of metastatic disease. There are indications for the surgical removal of solitary cerebral, hepatic, and pulmonary metastases. New developments in perfusion and infusion chemotherapy have given surgery a new role in the treatment of hepatic metastases and in-transit metastases of the extremity. The surgical treatment of metastatic disease is covered in greater detail hereafter.

Palliation

Even if disseminated metastatic disease is present, surgery can often provide relief from pain and other symptoms. Gastrointestinal bypasses, for example, can restore the alimentary tract obstructed with unresectable tumor. Palliative colon resection may be justified, even when disseminated disease is present, to prevent the development of obstruction and bleeding. An abdominoperineal resection for rectal cancer should be performed even in the face of hepatic metastases if it can be easily accomplished. Removal of the rectum prevents bleeding and pain that may occur if the rectum is left in place.

Reconstruction

Reconstructive surgical techniques aid in the rehabilitation of cancer patients following definitive surgical therapy. For years reconstruction has played an important part in the rehabilitation of patients who have undergone surgical resections of the head and neck. Continued developments in this area have made radical surgery functionally and cosmetically more acceptable. Similarly, breast reconstruction has significantly enhanced the quality of life for women who have undergone mastectomy.

Follow-up

Surgical responsibility for the cancer patient does not end when the incision has healed. Careful clinical follow-

TABLE 1. Cancer Follow-Up*

Primary Cancer Site	Common Sites of Recurrence	Tests†
Head and neck cancers	Local, cervical nodes	Chest x-ray every 6 to 12 mos.
Breast	Axillary and supraclavicular	Chest x-ray every 6 mos.
	Chest wall, liver, bone	Mammogram every 1 to 2 yrs.
		Bone scan every 2 yrs. if warranted‡
Lung	Lung, liver, bone, brain	Chest x-ray every 6 mos.
Colon	Liver, lung, peritoneum	Barium enema every 1 to 2 yrs.
		Colonoscopy or sigmoidoscopy every yr.
		Digital and guaiac tests every 3 mos.

*Modified from Rubin, P.: Clinical Oncology for Medical Students and Physicians, 6th ed. Philadelphia, American Cancer Society, 1983.

†All follow-up visits should include careful physical examination.

‡Probably unnecessary as routine in patients with Stage I disease.

up of the cancer patient is mandatory. Physical examination, as well as radiographic, endoscopic, and serological testing (where indicated), should be performed at appropriate intervals. In general, early recognition of cancer recurrence is associated with a more favorable outcome. It should also be remembered that patients with certain types of malignancies have a higher incidence of second primary tumors. An example of appropriate follow-up for some common malignancies is shown in Table 1.

ETIOLOGY OF CANCER

It is difficult to identify a single causative agent for most human tumors. Although there are many known environmental carcinogens associated with the development of cancer, other factors such as genetic predisposition, inherent genetic instability, age, sex, the immune response, and oncogenic viruses are related to the development of human neoplasms.

As early as 1775, Sir Percivall Pott suggested that carcinoma of the scrotum was an occupational hazard of 18th century English chimney sweeps. Subsequently, in Germany, carcinoma of the bladder was found frequently in workers in the aniline dye industry. The high incidence of carcinoma of the lung in German miners was noted in the late 19th century and was subsequently found to be caused by exposure to radioactive materials inhaled by the miners. More recently, uranium miners in the western United States have been noted to have a high risk of developing lung cancer from exposure to radioactive uranium. Other agents related to the development of cancer are benzpyrene, asbestos, tobacco smoke, and vinyl chloride. Even agents that are used to treat cancer, such as ionizing radiation and several chemotherapeutic agents, are known to be carcinogenic.

Viruses cause cancer in a number of animal models. In the early 1900s, Rous demonstrated that cancer could be induced in chickens by a virus. Subsequently, many viruses were shown to induce a variety of different cancers in a wide spectrum of animals. Although both DNA and RNA viruses have been implicated, the RNA viruses have received the most attention. These viruses contain the enzyme reverse transcriptase, which allows the RNA virus to replicate DNA genetic material. For this reason, these viruses are referred to as retroviruses.

One DNA virus that is closely associated with human cancer is the EB (Epstein-Barr) virus. First isolated in Africans with Burkitt's lymphoma, it is also associated with nasopharyngeal carcinomas. This virus is known to be the causative agent of infectious mononucleosis, and its close association with the previously mentioned tumors makes it a likely candidate as an etiologic agent in human malignant disease. More recently, the human T cell leukemia viruses (HTLV) were described. This family of viruses is capable of suppressing T-cell lymphocytes and transforming these lymphocytes into malignant T cell leukemias. The evidence that this virus is the causative agent in human T cell leukemia is quite convincing. In addition, this same family of viruses may cause acquired immune deficiency syndrome (AIDS). In this syndrome, it is postulated that the virus alters T cell regulation to give rise to severe immunologic deficiency. In this immune deficiency state, the patient is susceptible to a variety of fatal infections. A virulent form of cancer, Kaposi's sarcoma, is frequently associated with this immune deficiency state. Interferon, with its antiviral and immunoregulatory effects, has been effective in treating this tumor.

Thus, the evidence is rapidly mounting that viruses play an important role in the induction of human cancer. The mechanism of viral oncogenesis relates to the ability of the virus to insert DNA genetic material (oncogene) into the genetic apparatus of the infected cell. This viral DNA, or oncogene, then codes for the unrestricted proliferation necessary for cancer formation.

Immune deficiency states also predispose to the development of malignant disease. It is well known that transplant recipients who are treated with immunosuppressive agents, such as steroids, have a high incidence of cancers, particularly those of the lymphatic system and Kaposi's sarcoma. Withdrawal of the immunosuppressants frequently results in tumor regression. Children who are born with congenital defects in their immune responses, such as agammaglobulinemia, ataxia telangiectasia, and the Wiscott-Aldrich syndrome, have a high degree of fatal malignant disease during the first 5 to 10 years of life. Indeed, most cancer patients have immunologic defects, such as impairment of delayed cutaneous hypersensitivity reactions. Thus, alterations in the immune response can be related to the development of neoplasia.

There are many hereditary cancers. Retinoblastoma is one example. Although nonhereditary cases of retinoblastoma do occur, it has been calculated that 40 to 50 per cent are inherited. Gardner's syndrome is another example of a familial carcinoma in which family members frequently have multiple polyps of the colon that become malignant. Several other conditions are associated with an abnormally high familial incidence of leukemias or carcinomas.

In recent years, nutrition has been recognized as an important factor in the development of a variety of diseases, including cancer. Animal studies have shown that mice maintained on a low-fat diet have a decreased incidence of breast cancer. Epidemiologic studies have shown that populations that subsist on low-fat diets have a lower incidence of breast and colorectal cancer. Whereas carcinoma of the breast is uncommon in Japan, it is relatively common in Japanese women who move to the United States and adopt the customary high-fat diet currently consumed in this country. Diet may also predispose to colorectal cancer. It is hypothesized that high-fat diets facilitate absorption of carcinogens and slow the transport time through the intestine; thus low-fat, high-roughage diets may protect against colon cancer. In summary, carcinogenesis may require exposure to environmental carcinogens superimposed on genetic predisposition, the presence of latent oncogenic viruses, or special aspects of dietary intake.

PATHOLOGIC STAGING IN ONCOLOGY

Certain aspects of tumors are important as prognostic indicators. The tissue of origin and the degree of histologic differentiation are important considerations in this regard. Tumor "grade" is a histologic parameter. Tumors are frequently graded according to their degree of differentiation and the number of mitotic figures per high power field under the microscope. Tumors are usually graded as Grade I, II, III, or IV, with Grade I being the most highly differentiated and Grade IV being the most poorly differentiated.

In addition to these histologic considerations, tumor "stage" describes the anatomic distribution of the tumor. The American Joint Committee for Cancer Staging and End Results Reporting has developed a staging system called the TNM System (Table 2), which characterizes the anatomic extent of the malignancy at the time of diagnosis. Having a unified staging system assists in more accurate prediction of the prognosis and provides for more meaningful comparison of results reported from different institutions. The letter "T" represents the primary tumor with the appropriate numbers describing the size of the tumor and the functional impairment caused by direct extension of the tumor. The letter "N" represents the regional lymph node involvement or the presence of lymph node involvement in different anatomic locations. The letter "M" represents distant metastases, and the absence of metastases is designated by "MO" (see Table 2). The TNM classification may be a clinical classification or a postsurgical pathologic classification. As a clinical classification, the TNM is determined by clinical assessment prior to surgical intervention. As a postsurgical classification, the TNM classification is based on the examination of the specimen removed at the time of surgery. Thus, with the TNM classification and the knowledge of the site of origin and the degree of differentiation, one can, with considerable accuracy, predict the clinical course.

A variety of techniques have been developed to more accurately stage solid tumors. Since treatment frequently depends on the stage of the disease, in some instances major surgery is performed solely to obtain more accurate staging information. For example, in lung cancer the presence or absence of mediastinal nodal involvement is an important determinant of clinical management. The mediastinum can be evaluated through a small cervical incision, and lymph nodes in the paratracheal area can be sampled for staging purposes. In addition, the right and left hilar areas can be explored through limited parasternal incisions to assess the nodes in these areas. Surgical staging procedures are particularly useful in patients with Hodgkin's disease. The presence of tumor in the spleen, liver, or retroperitoneal lymph nodes significantly alters the medical management of these patients, and, therefore, a staging laparotomy is frequently indicated. In addition, axillary lymph node dissections are indicated in patients with breast cancer to determine whether the patient needs postoperative adjuvant chemotherapy.

Other factors that are important in determining survival and response to surgery are age and sex. Frequently, younger patients have more rapidly progressive tumors and older patients may have more indolent tumors. In some instances, sex is important in determining prognosis. Females with melanoma have a better prognosis than do males. Knowledge of the tissue of origin is helpful. A diagnosis of small carcinoma of the lung indicates disseminated disease regardless of the clinical stage. On the other hand, patients with basal cell and squamous cell carcinoma of the skin almost never develop metastatic disease. The interval to recurrence also varies depending on the tissue of origin. Squamous carcinomas of the lung and head and neck almost always recur within 3 years of surgical treatment; papillary carcinomas of the thyroid can recur after an interval of 20 years. However, many tumors are totally unpredictable. Malignant melanoma, for example, may spread and destroy the host very rapidly or may remain dormant for 10 years or more before recurring.

It is extremely important to conscientiously attempt to stage patients based on the TNM classification, the grade of the tumor, and site of origin so that treatment can be appropriately designed.

TABLE 2. TNM Staging System

Tumor	
TX	Tumor cannot be assessed
T0	No evidence of primary tumor
TIS	Carcinoma *in situ*
T1, T2, T3, T4	Progressive increase in tumor size and regional involvement
Nodes	
NX	Regional lymph nodes cannot be assessed clinically
N0	Regional lymph nodes not demonstrably abnormal
N1, N2, N3, N4	Increasing degrees of regional lymph node involvement
Metastases	
MX	Not assessed
M0	None known
MI	Distant metastases present

Abbreviations: T = Primary tumor; N = regional lymph nodes; M = distant metastases.

PRINCIPLES OF RADIATION BIOLOGY AND THERAPY

Principles and Methods of Delivery

Radiotherapy involves the treatment of malignant disease with ionizing radiation. It can be used alone with curative intent or in combination with surgery and/or chemotherapy. It is also an important palliative tool. The basic mechanism of action of all forms of radiation therapy is the production of ionization within tissues, causing the formation of free radicals and resulting in lethal chemical changes within the cell.

Ionizing radiation can be electromagnetic or particulate. X-rays and gamma rays are electromagnetic radiations without mass or charge. Whereas the mechanism of action of both is similar, x-rays are produced by the interaction of moving electrons with matter, whereas gamma rays are the emission products of radioactive isotopes (e.g., iridium 192 and cobalt 60). X-rays and gamma rays create charged ions by causing "secondary" electrons to be ejected from the atoms within the target tissue.

Examples of particulate radiation are electrons, protons, alpha particles, neutrons, negative pi mesons, and heavy ions. At present, electron beams and beta rays (electrons produced during nuclear decay) are the most useful clinically. The other forms of particulate radiation are being actively investigated.

The interaction of radiation with matter is quantified as the amount of energy absorbed per unit mass. This is known as the *absorbed dose*. The commonly used unit is the rad, which represents 100 ergs of energy absorbed per gram of tissue. One hundred rads is equivalent to 1 gray (Gy) and represents the absorption of 1 joule per kilogram.

The energies of the various forms of radiation are measured in electron volts. An x-ray beam of 1000 electron volts is designated 1 keV. All photon or x-ray beams above one million (1,000,000) electron volts (1 meV) are known as megavoltage beams. The ranges of electromagnetic radiations used in clinical practice are as follows:

1. *Superficial radiation*—x-rays from 10 to 125 keV.
2. *Orthovoltage radiation*—x-rays from 125 to 400 keV.
3. *Megavoltage radiation*—generally several million volts.
4. *Gamma ray sources*—radioactive cobalt 60 produces gamma rays having average energies in the 1.25 megavoltage range (1.17 to 1.33 meV).

The important difference among these various radiations is that as the energy increases, the penetration of the x-rays into the tissue increases (Table 3). Superficial radiation, therefore, is appropriate only for superficial tumors. Megavoltage radiation has replaced orthovoltage radiation in the treatment of deep tumors. Compared with orthovoltage, megavoltage is "skin-sparing." The maximal dose is not reached in the skin but occurs at some depth below the surface, and 50 per cent of the maximal dose can achieve considerable penetration. In addition, the more homogeneous delivery and better focusing possible with present-day megavoltage equipment minimizes injury to adjacent organs, permits reduction in the amount of radiation given to normal tissues, and is better tolerated by the patient.

TABLE 3. *Skin Sparing and Depth at 50% Dose for Commonly Used External X-Ray Therapy Beams**

Maximal Beam Energy	Depth at Which Max. Dose Is Delivered (cm.)	Depth at Which 50% Dose Is Delivered (cm.)
250 keV (x-ray unit)	Surface	7
1.25 meV (cobalt 60)	0.5	11
Linear Accelerators		
4 meV	1.0	14
6 meV	1.5	16
10 meV	2.0	18
15 meV	3.0	20
Betatrons		
25 meV	4.0	23
35 meV	5.0	26

*After Coia, L. R., and Moylan, D. J.: Therapeutic Radiology for the House Officer. Baltimore, Williams & Wilkins, 1984.

Two general types of application technique are used in radiation therapy: *teletherapy*, which uses an external beam, and *brachytherapy*, in which the radioactive source is implanted in the patient. The goal of the radiation therapist is to maximize the dose absorbed by the tumor and minimize absorption by normal tissue. In teletherapy, the size of the treatment field, the number of the treatment beams, and the beam direction can be modified to achieve the desired distribution of absorbed energy (Fig. 1).

Brachytherapy, or short-distance radiation therapy, takes advantage of the principle that a rapid decrease in energy absorption occurs with increasing distance from a radiation source. Radioactive isotopes are implanted directly into a target site to deliver high-intensity radiation over a very limited area. Brachytherapy is most frequently employed in gynecologic and head and neck tumors, usually in combination with external beam radiation.

Radiobiology

Irradiation causes an immediate transfer of energy to tissue. The resulting ionization causes a loss of cellular

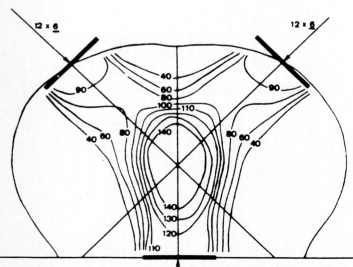

Figure 1. Treatment plan in which three external beams of 12 × 6 cm. are used. Central axes are at 120-degree angles to each other. Beam arrangement maximizes dose at center of target.

reproductive capability and eventual cell death. The percentage of cells killed and the time to cell death depend on cellular kinetics. Different types of tissues vary in their susceptibility.[9]

The survival curves for normal and malignant tissue are similar (Fig. 2). The "shoulder" of the curve is evidence that the cell can accumulate radiation damage before death occurs. When the lethal dose has been accumulated, the curve becomes a constant slope, indicating a direct logarithmic dose-response relationship.

Several factors determine cellular radiosensitivity. In general, normal and malignant cells are most sensitive during mitosis. Therefore, rapidly dividing cells, such as lymphoid tissue, bone marrow, intestinal villi, testes, and ovaries, are the most sensitive. In contrast, mature neurons, bone, cartilage, and muscle are relatively radioresistant. Radiosensitivity of malignant cells is also related to the degree of tissue oxygenation. Fully oxygenated cells are approximately two-and-one-half times more radiosensitive than hypoxic tumor cells.

Since the earliest use of ionizing radiation, it was discovered empirically that fractionation of the dose induced a greater anti-tumor effect and minimized normal tissue reactions. This empiric fact may relate to differences in the repair capabilities of normal and malignant tissue. With each dose of radiation, some cells are damaged but not killed. Cells can repair sublethal damage within 2 to 6 hours of radiation. The repair mechanisms of normal tissue seem to be more efficient than those of malignant tissues. Therefore, fractionated dosages remain in the sublethal range for a larger population of the normal cells, thus sparing normal tissues. Smaller dose fractions require a larger total dose to achieve the same degree of killing, and larger fractions require a smaller total dose.

It is thought that fractionation of radiation doses may improve overall therapeutic effectiveness. Theoretically, each radiation exposure kills the well-oxygenated cells preferentially. This permits the hypoxic cells to "reoxygenate" by gaining greater access to capillaries. In addition, cells that have been in a relatively resistant phase of the cell cycle during one fraction may "redistribute" to a more vulnerable phase. Thus, in theory, fractionation both lessens the toxicity to normal tissue and increases the total number of tumor cells that can be killed by permitting "reoxygenation" and "redistribution."

Tissue Response to Radiation Therapy

Rapidly dividing tissues are injured easily by radiation but renew themselves with relative rapidity. When turnover is rapid, clinical injury may be apparent within days, but healing occurs rapidly if the total delivered dose has not been excessive.

The stroma and the microvasculature in all tissues, including tissues with a static population such as nerve or muscle tissue, are affected by radiation. Acute damage is characterized by vascular dilatation, local edema, and inflammation. Endarteritis may occur, obliterating the capillary lumen. Radiation enteritis and pneumonitis are clinical manifestations of this process. Later, atrophy, ulceration, and fibrosis occur. In addition, late effects of radiation on static populations become apparent. Such consequences, fortunately uncommon, include focal brain necrosis, radiation myelitis, spinal cord transection, and osteoradionecrosis.

Tumor Response to Radiation Therapy

The interdependent elements of fraction size, total dose, interval between fractions, and total duration of treatment comprise the dose-response relationship. These parameters can be varied according to the clinical situation. In general, the required lethal dose for different human tumors ranges from 2000 rads in 2 weeks to 8000 rads in 8 weeks, with the usual range from 4500 to 7000 rads. Daily fractions are in the range of 200 rads, with 3 to 5 fractions delivered weekly. Doses and fractionation are further modified according to tumor type, stage of disease, and whether the intent of radiation is curative or palliative.

The common denominator of clinical radiosensitivity is tumor shrinkage. Radiosensitivity is determined by numerous factors, including histologic type, tissue of origin, mitotic rate, cellular death, absorption, tissue oxygenation, tumor vascularity, and anatomic location. Though radiosensitivity is determined by a complex interplay of factors, it can be predicted with some accuracy on the basis of histologic type alone. Tumor types have been categorized into the following:

1. *Markedly sensitive* types include germ cell tumors (seminoma, dysgerminoma); lymphoproliferative tumors (Hodgkin's disease, lymphoma, leukemia); myelomas; and embryonal tumors (neuroblastoma, Wilm's tumor, and retinoblastoma).

2. *Moderately sensitive* types include squamous cell carcinomas (originating in the skin, alimentary tract, and respiratory tract) and adenocarcinomas from a variety of organ systems.

3. *Relatively radioresistant* types are melanomas, mesenchymal tumors, (sarcomas), and tumors of neural origin (glioma, astrocytomas).

Radiosensitivity and radioresistance do not imply curability or incurability. Radiocurability depends upon the tumor's anatomic location, its natural history, and the tolerance of adjacent normal tissues. For example, although

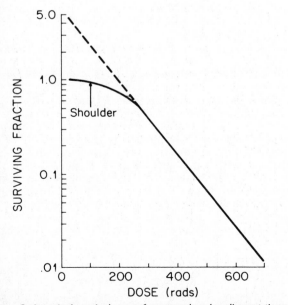

Figure 2. A typical survival curve for normal and malignant tissues. The "shoulder" represents range of sublethal dose; when exceeded, the relationship becomes logarithmic.

malignant lymphomas are highly radiosensitive, they are cured by radiation alone only in their earliest stages because of their tendency to disseminate. Squamous cell carcinoma and adenocarcinoma, on the other hand, are histologic types that are only "moderately radiosensitive," yet local control and cure frequently have been achieved by radiation therapy. Early stage squamous cell carcinomas of the oral cavity, larynx, oropharynx, nasopharynx, skin, and lip can be treated successfully by radiation therapy. Radiation therapy can be curative for localized adenocarcinoma of the breast and prostate.

Relative radioresistance does not imply that radiation therapy has no place in the treatment of patients with tumors. Soft tissue sarcomas are relatively radioresistant, but, when combined with surgery, radiation therapy improves local control. Similarly, following surgical resection, radiation can be a helpful adjunct to regional control of bulky lymph node metastases of melanoma, despite the fact that it is a relatively "radioresistant" tumor.

Clinical Uses

Radiation therapy plays three major roles in cancer treatment: (1) it can be used singly as the primary curative method; (2) it can be used as an "adjuvant" to either surgery (preoperatively or postoperatively) or chemotherapy; and (3) it can be used as a means of palliating symptoms.[17] The following paragraphs introduce its range for treatment of various types of tumors. For a more detailed review, the reader should consult the radiation therapy texts referenced at the end of this chapter.

Head and Neck Cancer. Both radiation therapy and surgery offer excellent local control for early squamous cell carcinomas of the head and neck. In general, radiation therapy carries a lower risk of morbidity and offers better functional and cosmetic results. When used postoperatively, radiotherapy decreases local-regional recurrences. Lymph node metastases from primary squamous cell carcinomas can be managed successfully with radiotherapy. When nodal metastases are bulky or multiple, a combination of surgery and radiation therapy offers the best chance for local control.[9]

Breast Cancer. Radiation therapy plays an important role in the management of primary and metastatic breast cancer. Studies have shown that radiation and conservative tumor resection (lumpectomy, segmental resection, or quadrantectomy) produce results similar to those seen following radical mastectomy in patients with small primary tumors. For the T1 and T2 lesions, radiation can be offered as primary therapy. Cosmetic results following excision and radiation are generally quite satisfactory.

When given postoperatively, radiation therapy decreases the incidence of local recurrence. Radiotherapy is the treatment of choice for locally recurrent breast cancer and plays a major role in the management of inflammatory breast cancer. It provides very effective palliation for metastases to bone.

Lung Cancer. Surgical excision is the treatment of choice for operable lung cancers. Radiation therapy is the treatment of choice for locally advanced, unresectable disease. An occasional cure is obtained (5 to 10 per cent), and many benefit from relief of local symptoms. Small cell carcinoma of the lung, usually metastatic by the time of discovery, is best treated by a combination of chemotherapy and radiation.

Gastrointestinal Tract Tumors. Radiation therapy is useful for the treatment of esophageal carcinoma. Some esophageal tumors are squamous cell in origin. Tumor cells spread longitudinally through the rich lymphatics of the esophagus, which frequently makes the results of the surgical treatment disappointing. For lesions of the proximal third of the esophagus, radiation and surgery have produced equivalent results.

Radiation therapy is very useful for the treatment of gastric lymphomas following surgical resection.

Radiation is effective as a preoperative adjuvant to surgery for rectal cancer. Studies have shown improved survival and fewer local recurrences in patients receiving preoperative radiation prior to abdominoperineal resection. Radiation therapy also has been shown to decrease the risk of local recurrence when administered postoperatively. Radiation therapy is an alternative to surgery for the primary treatment of rectal cancer in patients with small, well-differentiated, low-lying cancers and in patients considered to be at high risk for major surgery.

Female Genital Tract. Radiation therapy plays an important role in the primary treatment of cervical and vaginal malignancies. The normal tissues of the cervical and vaginal mucosa have great tolerance for radiation, and the vaginal and uterine cavities are accessible to brachytherapy (intracavitary implants).

Well-differentiated, Stage I adenocarcinoma of the uterus is treated by surgery alone. For stages of uterine cancer that are more advanced and for lesions that are not well-differentiated, preoperative intracavitary radiation combined with external beam therapy decreases pelvic and vaginal tumor recurrences.

Radiation therapy has been shown to be of value in improving local control of ovarian tumors when the disease is confined to the pelvis. Because of the distinctive pattern in which ovarian carcinoma spreads beyond the pelvis, radiation can be delivered to the entire peritoneal cavity, including the undersurfaces of the diaphragm.[17]

Male Genital Tract. Seminoma is highly radiosensitive and can be cured even when it is widely disseminated. Following orchiectomy, treatment consists of radiation therapy to the ipsilateral pelvic, renal hilar, and para-aortic lymphatics. When nodal metastases have been below the diaphragm, the mediastinal and supraclavicular nodal areas are irradiated as well.

Radiation therapy is highly effective for local control of prostatic carcinoma. For Stage A lesions, therapy is confined to the prostatic bed; in Stages B and C, the entire pelvis is in the radiation field.

Hodgkin's and non-Hodgkin's Lymphoma. Radiation therapy in conjunction with combination chemotherapy has made a significant impact of the treatment of Hodgkin's disease. Because of the predictable pattern of spread in Hodgkin's disease, a nearly 90 per cent 5-year survival has been achieved for the early stages (I, II, and IIIA) of the disease. For more advanced stages, chemotherapy is the mainstay of treatment. For those patients achieving remission with chemotherapy, radiation is directed to sites of regressed lymph nodes because of the high probability of residual microscopic disease. Increased survival rates have been noted.

Whereas non-Hodgkin's lymphomas are extremely sensitive to radiotherapy, their radiocurability is more difficult owing to the less orderly progression of the non-Hodgkin's lymphomas and because these patients frequently present with widespread disease. Chemotherapy is the main treatment, although radiation should be administered to areas of identifiable involvement.

Clinic ects on Normal Tissue

When a tumor in any area of the body is being treated, the immediate side effects and long-term complications must be considered. These must be weighed against the potential benefits of radiotherapy. The following generalizations serve as a guide to anticipated clinical effects.

General Systemic Effects. General fatigue, loss of appetite, nausea, and vomiting can be present. These symptoms are especially prominent when the liver and epigastrium are in the radiated field and when the dose fraction is high.

Skin. Radiation dermatitis can be minimized by megavoltage therapy, but it is inevitable when intensive radiotherapy directed toward skin, as in breast cancer with skin involvement.

Head and Neck. Mucositis may occur, particularly when the oropharynx is treated. Deterioration of dentition can occur and dysphagia may interfere with nutrition. Good dental prophylaxis can prevent most dental complications. Dry mouth and loss of taste can occur with higher doses. Osteoradionecrosis of the mandible occurs occasionally with high doses.

Gastrointestinal Tract. Esophagitis is common when the esophagus is in the radiated field. Decreased appetite is the most common symptom of abdominal irradiation, and diarrhea can occur. Cicatrix formation and stenosis may be complications but are fortunately uncommon. When the pelvis is irradiated, proctitis and tenesmus can occur.

Soft Tissues. Growing cartilage is very radiosensitive and can result in epiphyseal changes in children. Muscular atrophy may occur in children, and fibrosis may occur in adults.

Bone Marrow. Suppression of blood elements, aplasia, and pancytopenia can occur.

Lung. Acute and chronic pneumonitis are proportional to the volume of lung irradiated and a function of the time course of treatment.

Emergent Uses of Radiotherapy

There are three common oncologic situations in which radiation should be considered part of emergency treatment.[4]

Spinal Cord Compression. Ninety five per cent of spinal cord compressions are due to extramedullary malignant disease. Most often this syndrome is caused by metastatic cancer originating in the lung, breast, prostate, or kidney. Radiation therapy is the treatment of choice in most cases of spinal cord compression. For acute paraplegia or rapidly progressing symptoms, neurosurgical intervention should be considered.

Superior Vena Cava Syndrome. Obstruction of the superior vena cava is usually caused by lung cancer or lymphoma involving the mediastinum. The syndrome presents as facial edema, conjunctival edema, and distention of the neck veins. Initial treatment usually consists of high-dose fractions (300 to 400 rads daily) for the first 3 days, diuretics, and occasionally steroids. The response is usually rapid and gratifying.

Airway Compression. Compression of the trachea or carina results most frequently from carcinoma of the lung, trachea, and esophagus. Radiation therapy is often indicated for lesions not amenable to surgery and for incompletely resected lesions.

Palliative Uses

Radiotherapy can effectively palliate some symptoms of bone, brain, and hepatic metastases. As with all types of palliative therapy, performance status, life expectancy, extent of disease, and anticipated benefit must be considered carefully in the design of therapy.

Bone Metastases. These occur frequently from cancers of the breast, prostate, lung, thyroid, and kidney. Radiotherapy will provide significant pain relief in 80 per cent of patients. When more than 50 per cent of the cortex of a weight-bearing bone has been destroyed by tumor, initial surgical management should be considered to prevent pathologic fracture.

Brain Metastases. These are common from carcinoma of the lung, breast, kidney, and melanoma and gastrointestinal malignancies. Most are multiple. The median survival of patients with brain metastases without treatment is 1 month. With whole brain radiation (usually 2000 to 4000 rads in 1 to 3 weeks), median survival can be extended to 4 to 6 months. Most patients experience some degree of short-lived symptomatic improvement. Corticosteroids for control of increased intracranial pressure are an important adjunct to treatment.

Hepatic Metastases. These occasionally respond to radiation with pain relief and improvement of hepatic function. Symptomatic improvement is noted in 50 to 75 per cent of patients.[4]

Combined Modality Therapy

RADIATION AND SURGERY

Improved local-regional control has been demonstrated by combining surgery and radiotherapy for a variety of tumors. The intent of preoperative radiation is to diminish the viability of cancer cells, thereby making their spread through lymphatic or vascular channels less likely. A theoretical advantage of preoperative administration is that the tumor vasculature has not been disturbed by surgery and therefore the cells are less hypoxic and more radiosensitive. In some instances, a reduction in tumor size induced by preoperative radiation may make an unresectable tumor resectable. Often, the magnitude of the required operation will be diminished. Preoperative radiotherapy has been useful for the management of head and neck tumors, soft tissue sarcomas, superior sulcus tumors of the lung, and rectal cancer.

Postoperative radiation therapy has several theoretical advantages over preoperative therapy: (1) there is no delay in operation; (2) there is no impairment of wound healing; and (3) if the lesion proves to be less extensive than initially thought, the patient is spared unnecessary irradiation. Postoperative radiotherapy has been shown to enhance local control in the treatment of brain tumors, head and neck cancers, gastrointestinal lymphomas, soft tissue sarcomas, gynecologic tumors, and carcinoma of the breast, lung, and rectum. When postoperative radiotherapy is planned, the surgeon's operative notes should be carefully detailed. Anatomic extent, fixation, invasion, and suspicious regions of nodal metastases should be described. *If a mass is unresectable, it should be outlined with clips to serve as guides for the radiotherapist.*

RADIATION AND CHEMOTHERAPY

The combination of radiotherapy and chemotherapy has the appeal of combined local and systemic treatment.

Chemotherapy has been administered before, during, and after delivery of radiotherapy. In each case, the rationale for its employment is somewhat different.

Chemotherapy has been administered before radiation in order to "debulk" massive primary tumors. This technique has occasionally proved valuable for cancer of the head and neck; however, no increase in ultimate survival has been shown. In carcinoma of the breast and in sarcoma, tumor reduction can make a tumor more easily managed by one of the "local therapies," i.e., surgery or radiation. Pretreatment with chemotherapy provides an invaluable *in vivo* assay of the tumor's sensitivity to the drugs administered.

Chemotherapeutic drugs have been used concomitantly with radiotherapy as "radiosensitizing agents" with the hope of obtaining a synergistic effect upon the tumor. Some drugs that appear to have radiosensitizing properties include doxorubicin hydrochloride (Adriamycin), 5-fluorouracil (FU), bleomycin, hydroxyurea, methotrexate, *cis*-platinum (Cisplatin), and actinomycin D. A dramatic example has been the improvement in local control of Ewing's sarcoma from 67 to 95 per cent by the simultaneous administration of vincristine and cyclophosphamide during the course of radiotherapy.

When chemotherapy is delivered after primary radiation or surgery, the rationale for its use is treatment of any micrometastases that may be present. This type of adjuvant therapy has been successful for breast cancer, testicular tumors, soft tissue sarcomas, and several solid tumors in children.[11]

PRINCIPLES OF CANCER CHEMOTHERAPY

Recognition of the fact that cancer was rarely localized led to a search for systemic treatment. Knowing that synthetic chemicals and natural products were effective for erradication of bacterial and parasitic infections spurred hopes that drug therapy could be helpful for the treatment of cancer. It was for an antiparasitic agent, in fact, that Ehrlich first used the term "chemotherapy" in the early 20th century.

Successful anticancer drug therapy was achieved in the early 1940s when Huggins and Hodges used estrogens to induce regression of prostatic cancer. Shortly thereafter, as an outgrowth of research in gas warfare, the anticancer potential of the alkylating agents was realized. When an explosion in Naples Harbor was associated with significant lymphoid hypoplasia in those exposed, nitrogen mustard became the treatment for lymphoid malignancies. Nitrogen mustard was first used to treat Hodgkin's disease and lymphosarcoma in 1943.[11]

Many new anticancer agents have been introduced in the last several decades. The potential of the corticosteroids and the antifolates was recognized in the early 1950s, and the antimetabolite analogues of the purines and pyrimidines were introduced shortly thereafter. The vinca alkaloids and the nitrosoureas were developed for clinical use in the early 1960s and doxorubicin was released for use in 1968. Some of today's most useful agents, such as the antiestrogens, are recent developments of the 1970s.

The early days of "chemotherapy" established strong images for the lay public as well as many physicians, because treatment with anticancer drugs appeared to be a futile exercise associated with severe toxicity. The discipline of medical oncology has done much to dispel these unwarranted notions. At present, chemotherapy is used successfully for a variety of malignant diseases, including Hodgkins' disease and the non-Hodgkins lymphoma, Burkitt's lymphoma, testicular tumors, trophoblastic tumors, Wilms' tumor, sarcoma of childhood, and carcinoma of breast. Although severe toxicities have by no means been eliminated, progress has been made in minimizing excessive morbidity.

Biologic Basis of Cancer Chemotherapy

Three decades of empiricism have shown that many cancer drugs are most effective when delivered intermittently, for repeated courses, and as multidrug combinations. These empiric clinical findings have their basic basis in the kinetics of cellular killing, the mechanism of drug action, the heterogeneity of tumor cell populations, and the cellular development of drug resistance.

A clinically detectable tumor has 10^9 cells. Only a percentage of these cells, known as the "growth fraction," is actively dividing at any time. Growth fraction can range from less than 10 per cent for a typical adenocarcinoma to nearly 90 per cent for some rapidly growing lymphomas. When a tumor is in its early stage most of its cells are in the proliferative phase. As the tumor mass increases, the growth fraction decreases. Therefore, tumor growth slows as the tumor becomes larger.

The killing of tumor cells by anticancer agents is described as "first-order kinetics." This means that a constant percentage of tumor cells rather than constant number of cells is killed by each exposure to the drug. Even though a clinically detectable tumor may become undetectable after treatment, microscopic residual disease is still present. For instance, if a tumor burden of 10^9 cells is reduced by a drug capable of killing 99.999 per cent of the cells, 10^4 cells will remain. A single exposure to one drug cannot produce 100 per cent killing. Administration of chemotherapy in repeated cycles and in the maximal dose tolerated is an attempt to reduce the absolute number of remaining tumor cells to zero by the multiplicative effect of fractional cell kill. "First-order kinetics," therefore, provides the necessity and rationale for the administration of repeated, intermittent cycles of chemotherapy.

Every replicating cell passes through relatively well-defined "phases." The cycling of the phases is termed the cell cycle. A cycle for a "typical" cell is described in Fig. 3. Synthesis (S) and mitosis (M) are easily identified for replicating cells. They are punctuated by "gaps" referred to as G_1 and G_2. Gaps are not dormant periods. They are simply phases during which the major expenditures of cellular metabolism are not directly related to DNA synthesis or replication.

Chemotherapeutic agents are generally labeled "cell cycle specific" or "cell cycle nonspecific" according to whether or not their mechanism of action is related to a specific phase(s) of the cell cycle.

Although isoenzyme typing of tumor cells suggests that tumors arise from single clones of malignant cells, recent studies show that solid tumors are particularly heterogeneous. Newly developed techniques for *in vitro* cloning of solid tumors have shown that tumors are composed of cells with differing biochemical, morphologic, and drug-response characteristics. This heterogeneity provides the rationale for the use of drug combinations, as not all cells within a tumor will be sensitive to any one drug. In addition, cell populations that were sensitive initially may subsequently develop resistance. Cellular mechanisms for the development of resistance include (1) changes in cell permeability

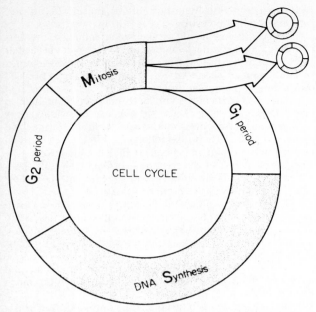

Figure 3. Typical cell cycle featuring phases of DNA synthesis (S) and mitosis (M) with "gaps" (G_1 and G_2).

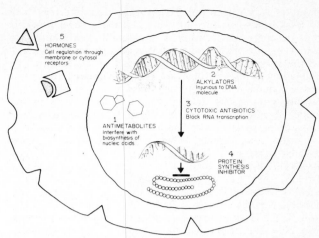

Figure 4. Mechanisms of action of anti-neoplastic agents. 1, Antimetabolites *interfere with synthesis of nucleic acids.* 2, Alkylating agents *injure the DNA molecule directly.* 3, Antibiotic derivatives *inhibit DNA-directed RNA synthesis.* 4, Protein synthesis inhibitors *interfere with synthesis of macromolecules.* 5, Hormones and anti-hormones *affect cellular metabolism via cell-surface or cytosol receptors.*

to drug, (2) changes in activating or deactivating enzymes, (3) alterations within target enzymes for drug, (4) more effective DNA repair, and (5) changes in metabolism that circumvent blocks imposed by chemotherapeutic drugs.[2] Overcoming the problem of drug resistance is a major justification for combination regimens.

Mechanisms of Action of Antineoplastic Agents

The rational and safe use of antineoplastic drugs requires a fundamental understanding of their mechanisms of action, means of administration, metabolism, and potential toxicity. Design of effective drug combinations depends upon an understanding of their pharmacodynamics. Theoretically, more effective and less toxic chemotherapeutic regimens can be produced by combining drugs that have different mechanisms of action and different side effects.[7]

The major categories of antineoplastic agents exert their influence on cells by interfering with cellular processes at four points: (1) biosynthesis of the nucleic acids, (2) incorporation of the nucleic acids into strands of DNA and DNA self-replication, (3) translation from DNA to RNA, and (4) synthesis of proteins necessary for cell survival. A fifth category of anticancer drug regulates cellular behavior by (5) combining with cytoplasmic or cell-surface receptors (Fig. 4). The major categories of antineoplastic agents, their mechanisms of action, and common clinical examples are listed in Table 4.

Antimetabolites. The biosynthesis of the nucleic acids can be inhibited at the level of their production or at the

TABLE 4. *Antineoplastic Agents: Mechanisms of Action*

General Category	Mechanism	Examples
Antimetabolites	Interference with biosynthesis of nucleic acids	5-Fluorouracil (5-FU)
		Methotrexate
		6-Mercaptopurine (6-MP)
Alkylators	Injurious to DNA molecule	Mechlorethamine (Mustargen)
		Cyclophosphamide (Cytoxan)
		Phenylalanine mustard (Melphalan)
		Chlorambucil (Leukeran)
Cytotoxic antibiotics	Block RNA transcription	Doxorubicin (Adriamycin)
		Mithramycin (Mithracin)
		Mitomycin-C (Mutamycin)
		Bleomycin (Blenoxane)
Enzyme and synthesis inhibitors	Interference with synthesis of macromolecules	Vincristine (Oncovin)
		Vinblastine (Velban)
		Asparaginase (L-asparaginase)
Hormones and hormone blockers	Cell regulation through membrane or cytosol receptor	Estrogens*
		Progestogens*
		Glucocorticoids*
		Antiestrogens*
Others	See text	Dacarbazine (DTIC)
		Cis-platinum (Platinol)
		VP-16 (Vindesine)

*Indicates general class of compounds, not specific drugs.

point of DNA incorporation. Drugs that interfere with DNA synthesis at this level are cell cycle–specific agents and are appropriately called antimetabolites. Methotrexate and 5–FU are examples. Methotrexate competitively inhibits the enzyme dihydrofolate reductase, which catalyzes the reduction of dihydrofolate to tetrahydrofolate. This enzymatic reduction is required for nucleic acid synthesis, and its inhibition blocks production of both purines and pyrimidines. 5–Fluorouracil inhibits thymidylate synthetase and in so doing blocks thymidine incorporation into DNA.

Alkylating Agents. Whereas antimetabolites function as false substrates, alkylating agents injure the DNA molecule directly. These drugs are termed alkylating agents because they are able to substitute alkyl groups ($R-CH_2-CH_2^+$) for the hydrogen atoms of some organic compounds. Although many cellular substances are "alkylated" in this way, DNA is the primary target for these anticancer agents. The alkylating agents interfere with the proper incorporation of base pairs by cross-linking abnormal base pairs. In addition, alkylation produces breaks in the linkage of the twin strands of DNA so that replication cannot occur. There are five chemical classes of alkylating agents: (1) the nitrogen mustard derivatives, (2) ethylenimine derivatives, (3) alkyl sulfonates, (4) triazene derivatives, and (5) the nitrosoureas.

Antibiotics. Several anticancer agents are derived from strains of the soil fungus *Streptomyces*. These "antibiotic" derivatives exert their tumoricidal effect by binding to the DNA in a fashion that blocks DNA-directed RNA synthesis. Doxorubicin, actinomycin D, mithramycin, and mitomycin C are useful clinical examples.

Enzymatic and Protein Inhibitors. Following successful manufacture of RNA from DNA, the cell produces both structural and functional proteins for continued cell survival. Several antineoplastic agents interfere with protein synthesis at this point. For example, the naturally occurring vinca alkaloids (vinblastine and vincristine) are alkaloid extracts from the periwinkle plant. These drugs interfere with protein synthesis. Specifically, synthesis of the protein tuberin is blocked, spindle activity is destroyed, and mitotic arrest results.

The enzyme L-asparaginase is used in the treatment of acute lymphoblastic leukemia. It exploits a difference in enzyme content between normal and malignant cells. By depriving cells that have little or no asparagine synthetase of asparagine, this enzyme blocks synthesis of proteins that are vital to cell survival.

Receptor Blockers. Tumor cells can be influenced by the binding of a variety of hormones and antihormones to membrane or cytoplasmic receptors. The result of this influence is regulation of cell activity, not reproductive death as with the other classes of antineoplastic agents mentioned previously. Nonetheless, tumor activity is suppressed and clinical regression occurs. Estrogens are clinically useful for treatment of prostate cancer and postmenopausal breast cancer. Both estrogens and antiestrogens are important for treatment of metastatic breast cancer. The recent recognition of and ability to quantitate estrogen receptor proteins in the cellular cytoplasm has provided a method for predicting clinical response to hormonal manipulation. When high levels of estrogen receptors can be identified on breast cancer tissue, the patient has a 60 to 80 per cent chance of responding to hormonal manipulation. In the absence of estrogen receptors, less than 10 per cent of patients will respond to these agents. Tamoxifen, a nonsteroidal estrogen antagonist, is capable of competitive ... to cytoplasmic estrogen receptors and is considered ... rmonal treatment for postmeno-

pausal patients with metastatic breast cancer. Its efficacy can be predicted by estrogen receptor analysis.

Progestational agents are known to influence the normal epithelium of the female genital tract and the acinar epithelium of the breast. These agents have been useful for the treatment of carcinoma of the uterus and can be used for hormonal manipulation of metastatic breast cancer.

The glucocorticoids exert their influence by binding to intracellular receptors. These steroids cause a wide variety of biochemical and metabolic changes within normal and malignant cells. Their "lympholytic" effect makes them useful for treatment of malignant hematopoietic diseases. They also are useful for treatment of hypercalcemia associated with malignant disease and treatment of tumor-associated edema of the brain or spinal cord.

There are several useful anticancer drugs whose mechanisms of action cannot be classified in the categories listed. Most have "alklylator-like" activity, although their cytotoxic mechanism is not by strict alkylation. Several agents warrant mention:

1. *Dacarbazine* (DTIC) is a triazene derivative that has some effectiveness against melanoma. It functions much like an alkylator.

2. Cis-*platinum* is a heavy metal compound. It forms a positively charged complex in aqueous solution and interacts with nucleophilic sites to form covalent links with DNA, RNA, or proteins. *Cis*-platinum is highly effective for treatment of ovarian carcinoma, testicular carcinoma, and squamous cell carcinoma of the head and neck.

3. *VP-16* is a new synthetic derivative of podophyllotoxin, an extract of the mandrake plant. It inhibits nucleoside transport in tissue culture, although its mechanism of action *in vivo* has not been elucidated. The drug is useful for treatment of the lymphomas, small cell cancer of the lung, and testicular tumors.

Guidelines for Clinical Use

Before treatment with chemotherapy can begin, histologic diagnosis of malignant disease must be obtained. The extent and stage of the disease must be determined; this requires a complete physical examination with appropriate radiographic and radioisotopic tests. At times, as in

---

TABLE 5. *Means of Assessing Response**

Definitions
Complete response (CR): disappearance of all signs and symptoms of malignancy
Partial response (PR): At least 50% reduction in tumor volume†

Clinical Determinations
Size by physical examination or radiologic or radioisotopic measurement
Regression of malignant effusion or ascites
Improvement in organ function, e.g., improved renal function after obstructive uropathy

Laboratory Determinations
Peripheral white blood count (leukemia)
Serum markers: paraproteins (myeloma), CEA, hCG, alpha-fetoprotein

---

*Modified from Haskell, C. M.: Cancer Treatment, 2nd ed. Philadelphia, W. B. Saunders Company, 1985.

†Estimated by the sum of the products of the greater and lesser diameters of all lesions; assumes the appearance of no new lesions.

Abbreviations: CEA = Carcinoembryonic antigen; hCG = human chorionic gonadotropin.

TABLE 6. Karnofsky Performance Scale

Condition	Percentage	Comments
Able to work and carry on normal activity. No special care needed.	100	Normal, no complaints, no evidence of disease.
	90	Able to carry on normal activity.
	80	Normal activity with effort, some signs or symptoms of disease.
Unable to work. Able to live at home, care for most personal needs. Varying degrees of assistance are needed.	70	Cares for self. Unable to carry on normal activity or to do active work.
	60	Requires occasional assistance but is able to care for most personal needs.
	50	Requires considerable assistance and frequent medical care.
Unable to care for self. Requires equivalent of institutional or hospital care. Disease may be progressing rapidly.	40	Disabled, requires special care and assistance.
	30	Severely disabled, hospitalization is indicated although death not imminent.
	20	Hospitalization very necessary.
	10	Moribund, fatal processes progressing rapidly.
	0	Dead.

Hodgkin's disease, exploratory laparotomy may be required for accurate staging. Finally, a determination must be made as to whether the objective is curative or palliative. The anticipated benefits of the treatment must be weighed against the potential toxicity. A means for assessing objective response to treatment (Table 5) and a technique for monitoring drug toxicity should be available. The patient's subjective and functional status must be considered as well as the structure of his social support system. The Karnofsky performance index (Table 6) is frequently used to assign a numerical value to patient performance status. This value can be helpful in communication between physicians and for evaluating results of clinical trials.

In Table 7, the common malignancies are grouped according to the effectiveness of chemotherapy in their management. In Group I diseases, complete remissions occur in 50 to 60 per cent of patients. In the diseases listed in Group II, chemotherapy induces regression and prolonged survival, but actual cures are rare. For the neoplasms in Group III, chemotherapy has been less effective.[11]

Drug Toxicity

The ideal anticancer drug exhibits *selective* toxicity, i.e., it kills tumor cells but has no effect on normal tissues. Unfortunately, there is no such drug. Drugs operate through metabolic processes, and, to date, there are no known significant qualitative differences in the metabolic properties of malignant and normal tissues. The degree of selective toxicity, therefore, depends upon quantitative differences, often minimal, between normal and malignant cells.

Clinically useful drugs are those that exhibit greater toxicity to malignant cells than to normal cells. The margin between therapeutic benefit and toxicity, however, is frequently narrow.

Over the past two decades, progress in drug administration and sequencing has improved antitumor effects while minimizing drug toxicity. However, all drugs affect normal cells. The most evident effects are upon the cells that divide most rapidly, i.e., the bone marrow, the epithelial cells of the gastrointestinal tract, and the hair follicles. The major toxicities of the common chemotherapeutic agents are now described.

Bone Marrow. This most critical toxicity for many of the drugs can result in leukopenia, with risk of infection, and in thrombocytopenia, with risk of bleeding. Certain alkylating agents (mitomycin C) cause cumulative myelosuppression. Severe toxicity, manifested by WBC <1000, granulocyte count <250, and platelet count <25,000, may warrant hospitalization and treatment.

Gastrointestinal Tract. Anorexia, nausea, and vomiting are common with many agents; symptoms can be suppressed by antiemetics, although their effectiveness is variable.

Immunosuppression. Most of the commonly used drugs suppress both humoral and cellular immunity. Patients can become targets for opportunistic infections. The immunosuppressive effects are usually self-limited when drugs are withdrawn.

Cardiorespiratory System. Myocardial damage can occur with doxorubicin and cyclophosphamide (Cytoxan). Cardiac toxicity is the dose-limiting factor of doxorubicin, and pulmonary fibrosis can occur with large doses of bleomycin, cyclophosphamide, or mitomycin-C.

TABLE 7. Solid Tumor Sensitivity to Chemotherapy

Group I—high rates of complete remission (60 to 90%) potentially curative (50 to 60%)
Hodgkin's disease
Testicular tumors
Ewing's sarcoma
Embryonal rhabdomyosarcomas } + radiation
Wilm's tumor

Group II—major responses (60 to 70%), but not curative
Myeloma
Ovarian
Breast
Small cell of lung

Group III—chemotherapy less effective
Colon
Stomach
Pancreas
Lung
Head and neck
Melanoma
Brain tumors
Renal cell

Hepatic System. An uncommon system for toxicity, but drugs that can cause hepatotoxicity (e.g., mithramycin and methotrexate) should be avoided in patients with decompensated liver disease.

Genitourinary System. Hemorrhagic cystitis occurs with cyclophosphamide. Kidney damage occurs with high doses of *cis*-platinum, and uric acid nephropathy can be induced by release of purines in response to several tumoricidal agents. Proper hydration and allopurinol will prevent nephropathy.

Central Nervous System. Mild to moderate neurologic manifestations are seen with several agents. Peripheral neurotoxicity is common with large doses of vincristine.

Sterility. The alkylating agents cause sterility, a particular concern in the treatment of young adults. Sperm storage before the initiation of chemotherapy should be considered for young males.

Teratogenicity. Congenital malformations occur when chemotherapeutic drugs are administered to pregnant women, particularly if these drugs are administered during the first trimester.

Mutagenicity. Most anticancer agents are mutagenic, i.e., they can induce new malignant tumors. Second malignancies occur with increased frequency in patients who have been treated for Hodgkin's disease, multiple myeloma, and other solid tumors.

Combination Chemotherapy

As discussed previously, the inherent heterogeneity of tumors, the nature of cellular kill by "first-order kinetics," and the ability of tumors to develop resistance to drugs require the use of drug combinations for effective therapy. Most successful chemotherapeutic combinations have been derived, for the most part, by empiric trials. Drugs with different mechanisms of action and different predominant toxicities are chosen for most combination regimens. Because myelosuppression is generally the most profound toxicity and is common to almost all anticancer agents, the drugs of a regimen must not have the same points of maximal myelosuppression (measured as the nadir of the granulocyte count). These principles are illustrated well by some of the common drug regimens. "MOPP," for example, (mechlorethamine, Oncovin, procarbazine, and prednisone) is a standard drug regimen for treatment of Hodgkin's disease and other lymphomas. Each agent has a different mechanism of action: mechlorethamine (nitrogen mustard) is an alkylating agent; procarbazine depolymerizes DNA; vincristine (Oncovin) destroys spindle protein; and prednisone is a "lympholytic" steroid. The former three drugs cause myelosuppression, and the nadir of their granulocyte counts is staggered: mechlorethamine (7 to 15 days); vincristine (4 to 5 days); procarbazine (25 to 36 days).

PVB, called the "Einhorn regimen," is a combination of *cis*-platinum, vinblastine, and bleomycin and is very effective for treatment of testicular neoplasms. The drugs have different mechanisms of action and their major toxicities are directed against different organ systems. Vincristine poisons the mitotic spindle and is primarily neurotoxic; bleomycin causes scission of the DNA and its primary toxicity is pulmonary fibrosis; *cis*-platinum is akin to the alkylators and exerts its major toxicity on the kidney.

To introduce the "vocabulary" of combination chemotherapy, some of the common regimens and their primary uses are listed in Table 8.

Adjuvant Therapy

Many solid tumors have already metastasized at the time of initial surgery. Experimental data suggest that micrometastases are more susceptible to chemotherapy than clinically detectable tumors. Therefore, chemotherapy should be more effective when administered in the postoperative period when gross clinical disease is absent.[19] The use of surgical adjuvant therapy in breast cancer illustrates this concept.

The National Surgical Adjuvant Breast Project began trials in 1957 in which women with potentially curable breast cancer were given thiotepa for 2 days following surgery. After 5 years there was no significant difference in disease recurrence between the treated patients and the controls; however, there was a distinct subset of women who had a prolonged disease-free interval. This group of premenopausal women had more than four positive axillary lymph nodes. Subsequently, L-phenylalanine mustard was used with similar results. Again, premenopausal patients with greater than four positive nodes had prolonged disease-free intervals. More recent adjuvant studies have employed drug combinations, such as CMF (cyclophosphamide, 5–FU, and methotrexate), which has become a "standard" breast adjuvant. In controlled trials, this combination has been shown to prolong the disease-free interval in premenopausal women with positive lymph nodes. There is also some evidence, although not conclusive, that when given in adequate doses, this regimen will prolong disease-free survival in postmenopausal women as well.

The availability of beneficial adjuvant therapy demands that patients undergoing surgery be carefully staged. In patients with breast cancer, this requires pathologic assessment of the axillary lymph nodes. In general, patients with Stage I solid tumors (pathologically negative lymph nodes) do not require adjuvant therapy. However, because patients with positive lymph nodes may benefit from adjuvant therapy, accurate staging is a critical part of any cancer operation.

Adjuvant chemotherapy has been shown to be bene-

TABLE 8. *Common Drug Regimens*

Regimen	Drug	Use
MOPP	(**m**echlorethamine, **O**ncovin, **p**rocarbazine, **p**rednisone)	Hodgkin's and non-Hodgkin's lymphomas
ABVD	(**A**driamycin, **b**leomycin, **v**incristine, **D**TIC)	Hodgkin's and non-Hodgkin's lymphomas
PVB	(*cis*-**p**latinum, **v**inblastine, **b**leomycin)	Testicular tumors
CMF	(**c**yclophosphamide, **m**ethotrexate, 5-**F**U)	Popular breast adjuvant
FAC	(5-**F**U, **A**driamycin, **c**yclophosphamide)	Breast cancer
MOCA	(**m**echlorethamine, **O**ncovin, **c**yclophosphamide, **A**driamycin)	Small cell, lung cancers
CAP	(**c**yclophosphamide, **A**driamycin, *cis*-**p**latinum)	Lung, ovarian cancers
FAM	(5-**F**U, **A**driamycin, **m**itomycin-C)	Gastric tumor

ficial for patients with carcinoma of the breast, neuroblastoma, testicular tumors, or sarcoma. It also may be beneficial for carcinoma of the lung, squamous cell carcinoma of the head and neck, and cancer of the esophagus.

Although it is appealing on a biologic basis to assume that chemotherapy should always be beneficial in a setting of micrometastatic disease, antineoplastic agents are not without significant potential toxicity. Therefore, adjuvant therapy should be administered only when known to be of benefit or within the framework of a carefully performed prospective randomized trial.

Predictive Assays

The ultimate in rational design of chemotherapy would be to have an *in vitro* test to predict the chemosensitivities of each tumor. The clonogenic assay, or stem cell assay, has been developed for this purpose. Single cell suspensions of tumor cells are exposed *in vitro* to chemotherapeutic agents. When these cells are plated in agar, viable stem cells form tumor colonies. The subsequent development of colony units on the plates exposed to drugs is then compared with control plates, and a percentage of tumor cell inhibition is determined. Several investigators have shown that there is a degree of correlation between these *in vitro* tests and clinical responses. Particularly, these tests predict quite accurately those agents that are ineffective. To date, however, these tests have been of limited clinical use. Thus, the assay remains largely experimental and, at present, holds greatest promise for screening of new anticancer agents.

TUMOR IMMUNOLOGY AND IMMUNOTHERAPY

For many years immunologists suspected that the immune response plays an important role in the tumor-host relationship. However, it was not until the early 1950s that tumor antigens were conclusively demonstrated. In these studies, immunization with tumor cells protected animals from future tumor inoculations. These antigens were, therefore, called *tumor-specific transplantation antigens*. It was subsequently demonstrated that passive or adoptive protection could be transferred to non-immunized animals with lymphocytes from animals immunized against the tumor. It is, therefore, well established that animal tumors contain tumor antigens that are capable of eliciting immune responses that produce protection against tumor growth.

Tumor antigens have been demonstrated in a variety of human tumors. Melanoma patients have antibodies that react with melanoma cells. Generally, a patient's antibodies will react to autologous melanoma cells as well as melanoma cells from other patients.[16] In the case of Burkitt's lymphoma, Epstein-Barr (EB) viral antigens can be detected in the tumor cells and patients with Burkitt's lymphoma have antibodies that react to these viral antigens. In addition to melanoma and Burkitt's lymphoma, tumor antigens have been demonstrated in neuroblastomas, colon cancer, and sarcomas. These antigens have been detected by a variety of immunologic techniques, including immunofluorescence, delayed cutaneous hypersensitivity reactions, complement fixation, and lymphocyte- as well as antibody-mediated cytotoxicity.

Despite these observations, only occasionally does the presence of antibody to these antigens correlate with prognosis. In some instances, the antibody titer correlates with the tumor burden. Sarcoma patients with high tumor volumes have low antibody titers, and those who are clinically free of disease have high titers. These correlations are not consistent with stage of disease and are not sufficiently reliable to use clinically.

Another group of antigens that are found in human neoplasms are not specific for the individual tumor and are referred to as *tumor-associated antigens*. The first of these described was the carcinoembryonic antigen (CEA), which occurs in fetal tissue as well as malignant tissue. Although this antigen was originally thought to be specific for adenocarcinomas arising in the gastrointestinal tract, it has subsequently been described in a variety of carcinomas, including breast cancer, pancreatic cancer, lung cancer, and lymphomas and in the sera of patients with hepatitis, cirrhosis, pancreatitis, and inflammatory disease of the colon. CEA does correlate with the extent of colon cancer. Thus, patients with Duke's C and D lesions have high levels of CEA, and those with early lesions may have a normal or slightly elevated CEA level. CEA has been useful for following patients after surgical resection of colon cancer. Persistent elevation of CEA following surgery suggests a recurrence.

Another tumor-associated antigen is the *alpha-fetoprotein* (AFP), which is elevated in patients with hepatomas. This substance is clinically useful for the diagnosis of hepatoma. It is frequently associated with nonseminomatous testicular tumors and is occasionally present in the sera of patients with gastric and prostatic cancer. Approximately 85 per cent of patients with hepatoma will have an elevated AFP, and, as with CEA, this marker is quite useful for following the clinical course of patients. Because CEA and AFP do occur in other disease states, both benign and inflammatory, they are not definitive screening tests; however, they are quite useful as markers of response in those patients who are undergoing or have undergone therapy.

Another group of antigens are the *oncofetal antigens* (OFA). In contrast to AFP and CEA, the OFA is capable of inducing antibody production in patients. These oncofetal antigens have been found in a variety of human neoplasms, including carcinomas, sarcomas, and melanomas. They are also found in fetal brain tissue. OFA can be found in the urine of patients with tumors, and some investigators have correlated urinary antigen levels with the tumor burden. In theory, OFA could be used to monitor tumor burden during and after therapy.

Although it has been difficult to demonstrate that immune responses to human tumors increase resistance to cancer, there are a number of observations that indicate that cancer immunity exists in humans. Over 100 cases of spontaneous regression of malignant tumors have been documented. In addition, in patients who have been disease-free for 10 to 15 years after treatment of the primary tumor, a recurrence may develop. This indicates that some host mechanism was suppressing the growth of the tumor. The high incidence of neoplasia in patients with AIDS, congenital immune deficiency syndromes, and transplant recipients also suggests the importance of the immune response in cancer control. In addition, it has been noted that the presence of tumor cells in the peripheral blood and in the drainage of operative wounds following surgery does not correlate with recurrence. Finally, it is well known that patients with cancer have depressed immunocompetence. Patients with depressed cellular immunity, as demonstrated by the absence of delayed cutaneous hypersensitivity reactions or abnormal *in vitro* lymphocyte proliferative responses, have a much poorer prognosis than patients who have intact cell-mediated immunity. An intact cellular immune mechanism does not correlate closely with survival, but, in almost all instances, depression of cell-mediated immune responses is indicative of a poor clinical course.

Therefore, there is considerable evidence that the immune response is important in the host-tumor relationship. However, the precise mechanisms are quite complex and manipulation of the immune response for therapy remains experimental.

A major contribution to the study of the immunology of cancer is the development of the hybridoma technique for producing monoclonal antibodies. These antibodies have greatly facilitated our ability to study tumor biology. The great advantage of monoclonal antibody over conventional antisera is that conventional antisera raised in animals have antibodies that react with many different antigens. Monoclonal antibodies are antibody clones with specificity for a single antigenic determinant. Monoclonal antibodies are derived by the fusion of immunized murine lymphocytes with murine myeloma cells. The fusion process allows the resulting hybridized lymphocyte to grow continuously in tissue culture. By a process of serial dilution and selection, a single clone of lymphocytes (hybridoma) producing the desired antibody can be isolated, and the resulting supernate will contain the one antibody produced by that single clone.

These antibodies have many applications. Monoclonal antibodies can be used to classify neoplasms, which classification would be difficult using other histologic techniques. For instance, monoclonal antibodies to lymphocyte cell surface markers can be used to characterize human lymphomas. Many other monoclonal antibodies are available to the pathologists for classification of a variety of tumors. Monoclonal antibodies to many human tumor antigens have been produced, including alpha-fetoprotein, CEA, a variety of lymphocyte antigens, including T cell–and B cell–specific antigens, bone marrow cells, melanoma, lung, kidney, prostate, and pancreatic tumors. In theory, monoclonal antibodies can identify tumor-related antigens in the sera of patients and can be used to monitor response to therapy. Monoclonal antibodies can be conjugated with radioisotopes and diagnostic imaging can be performed. Finally, monoclonal antibodies can be conjugated with radioactive substances, chemotherapy agents, and cellular toxins such as diphtheria toxin and ricin for use in direct therapy against cancer. The use of monoclonal antibodies for therapy is experimental, and the clinical trials that have been performed to date have produced equivocal results. However, a monoclonal antibody has been used to successfully treat a B cell lymphoma patient who was refractory to standard antineoplastic regimens.

IMMUNOTHERAPY

The specificity of the immune response makes immunotherapy an attractive anticancer modality. However, for a variety of reasons immunotherapy has not realized its expected potential. For instance, animal studies have indicated that immunotherapy is effective against only a limited amount of tumor and, therefore, is potentially only effective against microscopic disease or in conjunction with other more potent modalities such as surgery, radiation therapy, and chemotherapy. A variety of agents have been used as immunotherapeutic drugs. The most popular of these agents is BCG, or Calmette-Guérin bacillus. This agent is an attenuated strain of *Mycobacterium bovis* that augments the immune response in animal systems. In order for BCG to be effective, the host must be immunocompetent, the tumor burden must be relatively small, and the agent should come into close contact with the tumor cells. BCG has been evaluated in many human cancers. The results have been equivocal. However, the use of BCG by direct intratumor injection is effective for several cutaneous cancers.

Another bacterial agent, *Corynebacterium parvum*, has been evaluated as an immunotherapeutic agent. Whereas BCG is a live attenuated bacillus, *C. parvum* is a nonviable agent. *C. parvum* is similar to BCG in its immunologic characteristics, and intralesional injection can also induce regression. *C. parvum* has been used in a variety of clinical studies both alone and in combination with chemotherapy, surgery, and radiation therapy, but none of these studies has produced consistent results.

Levamisole is a low-molecular-weight chemical and is an effective anthelmintic drug. It was subsequently discovered to augment delayed hypersensitivity reactions in cancer patients. Because of its ability to stimulate the immune response, levamisole was initially used to treat immunosuppressed cancer patients. It has been tested extensively, and there have been no consistent findings that demonstrate its efficacy in patients with cancer. It has, however, been used effectively in other nonmalignant conditions such as rheumatoid arthritis and herpes infection.

Other forms of immunotherapy employ allogeneic tumor cells or autologous tumor cells to stimulate the immune response. Frequently these tumor cell vaccines are used in combination with agents such as BCG or Freund's adjuvant. The immunogenicity of these tumor cells can be augmented by treating them with a variety of enzymes such as neuraminidase. However, many trials to evaluate this form of active specific immunotherapy have shown no consistent beneficial effect.

Immunotherapy remains most effective when used for various skin tumors. Skin carcinomas can be made to regress after the induction of local delayed cutaneous hypersensitivity with certain chemicals that are applied topically to the tumor. In addition, BCG causes regression of cutaneous metastases of malignant melanoma following direct intralesional injection. This form of treatment is quite effective and has become a standard therapeutic maneuver for the treatment of in-transit metastatic melanoma. In addition, local cutaneous recurrences of breast cancer also respond to intralesional injection of BCG. Finally, superficial carcinoma of the bladder responds to intralesional BCG injection.

Epidermoid carcinoma of the skin is also sensitive to immunotherapy. Patients can be sensitized to *dinitrochlorobenzene* (DNCB), and subsequent application of this chemical will give rise to local delayed cutaneous hypersensitivity reactions that result in regression of basal cell or squamous cell carcinoma of the skin.

Immunotherapy has also been evaluated in combination with other treatments such as surgery, chemotherapy, and radiation therapy. When used in combination with these other cytoreductive modalities, this treatment is referred to as "adjuvant immunotherapy." There have been many studies evaluating adjuvant immunotherapy; however, most have been ineffective or, at best, equivocal.[20]

The role of immunotherapy as an adjunct to surgery remains quite limited and experimental. Since most of the immunotherapeutic treatments have limited toxicity, the combination of chemotherapeutic agents and nonspecific and specific immunotherapy is theoretically attractive.

However, in spite of many clinical trials to date, no consistent chemoimmunotherapy regimens have been shown to be effective in patients with solid tumors.

Thus, the great expectations for dramatic effects of immunotherapy for malignant disease have not been realized. A considerable amount of research continues with a variety of biologic response modifiers. Research continues into the potential application of interferon, T cell growth factor (interleukin-2), monoclonal antibodies, and other immunotherapeutic agents in cancer therapy. Among these new agents, IL-2 in combination with lymphokine-activated killer cells has the greatest promise, especially in melanoma and hypernephroma.

Adoptive immunotherapy is an approach to cancer in which immune cells with antitumor reactivity are systematically administered to a tumor-bearing host and can either directly or indirectly mediate the regression of established tumor. If immune cells with antitumor reactivity can be developed, their specificity and sensitivity can result in cells capable of attacking tumor but not normal tissues, and thus a low morbidity of treatment would be expected. The major obstacle to the development of this therapy as a practical option has been the inability to produce immune cells with antitumor reactivity. No general methods have yet been developed for the generation of immune cells reactive with tumor antigens.

A new approach to raising immune lymphoid cells with antitumor reactivity was described in 1980.[10a] Peripheral blood lymphocytes of normal individuals and cancer patients can be activated in culture with IL-2 leading to expression of cytotoxic activity toward a wide spectrum of histologically distinct fresh autologous tumor cells. These lymphokine-activated killer (LAK) cells represent a lytic system distinct from natural killer (NK) or cytotoxic T-lymphocytes (CTL). Although the biologic role of these LAK cells is presently not known, their attributes point toward an important function in immune surveillance and in host defense against cancer.

A variety of animal models have been developed utilizing the adoptive transfer of immune cells that can mediate the regression of established tumors; however, LAK cells and IL-2 must be infused concurrently for optimal benefit. Preliminary clinical studies have demonstrated the feasibility of infusing large amounts of IL-2 and large numbers of activated lymphoid cells into patients, and tumor regression has been demonstrated.[17a] Significant fluid retention has emerged as a complication of this therapy, but further clinical trials are planned.

SOFT TISSUE SARCOMA

The term "soft tissue sarcoma" refers to malignancies that arise in mesodermal structures. These tumors of connective tissue are generally characterized by a common morphologic appearance and similar clinical patterns. Soft tissue sarcomas represent less than 1 per cent of all newly diagnosed malignant tumors, although approximately 4500 new cases occur in the United States each year; of these, 1600 patients will die of their disease.[5]

The etiology of soft tissue sarcoma is unknown. Most soft tissue sarcomas arise *de novo*, although malignant degeneration of benign tumors is known to occur. Of all patients with von Recklinghausen's disease (multiple benign neurofibromata), approximately 10 per cent will develop neurofibrosarcoma. Chronic lymphedema has been associated with the development of lymphangiosarcoma, most commonly in postmastectomy patients who received post-operative radiotherapy in addition to radical mastectomy (Stewart-Treves syndrome). Fibrosarcomas and rhabdomyosarcomas have been reported to occur years after significant radiation exposure.[8]

Soft tissue sarcomas can occur anywhere in the connective tissues of the body. Approximately 40 per cent occur in the lower extremity, and 75 per cent of lower extremity sarcomas occur above the knee. Fifteen per cent of sarcomas occur in the upper extremity, 30 per cent occur on the trunk, and smaller percentages occur in the retroperitoneum and about the head and neck. Soft tissue sarcomas are the sixth most frequent tumor in children and are usually rhabdomyosarcomas of the head and neck area.

There are at least 35 different malignant variants of soft tissue sarcoma.[8] The most frequently encountered histologic types (which comprise 80 per cent of these neoplasms), include liposarcoma, malignant fibrous histiocytoma, synovial cell, rhabdomyosarcoma, fibrosarcoma, and undifferentiated sarcomas. Histologic type does not strongly influence prognosis or type of treatment. The most important prognostic factors for soft tissue sarcoma are the histologic grade and the size of the tumor. Initially, these tumors were classified according to their suspected cell of origin. However, in a study by the American Joint Committee on Staging and End Results Reporting, it was found that even expert pathologists could not agree on the histogenesis of nearly 30 per cent of these tumors. When a large series was reviewed, however, it became clear that by segregating the tumors into Grades I, II, and III, as determined by the number of mitoses per high-powered field, a significant correlation with survival could be obtained. A clinicopathologic staging system was then devised that integrated histologic grade into the TNM system. This classification correlates well with metastatic potential and prognosis. Stage I tumors have a 80 to 90 per cent 10-year survival, Stage II 60 per cent, Stage III 25 per cent, and Stage IV, "disseminated metastatic disease," 3 per cent.

Soft tissue sarcomas expand radially, respecting fascial plane barriers, and spread along the path of least resistance, generally within fascial compartments. As they increase in size, encroaching upon surrounding normal tissues, a so-called pseudocapsule develops from the pressure against the surrounding tissues. The pseudocapsule contains tumor cells, and "shelling out" of any such tumor will result in local tumor recurrence. Regional lymph node involvement is less than 5 per cent (somewhat higher in rhabdomyosarcoma and in synovial cell sarcoma). Hematogenous spread occurs early, and pulmonary metastases are usually the first, and frequently the only, site of disseminated disease. Local recurrence can indicate disseminated metastases in about one third of patients.

Patients with sarcomas usually present with an asymptomatic soft tissue mass that may have been present from weeks or months. Although history of trauma often calls attention to the "bump," it is not etiologically related. Physical examination cannot distinguish between benign and malignant soft tissue lesions. Therefore, all soft tissue lesions must be biopsied unless it is clear that the lesions have been present for a period of years without change. Preoperative assessment of the patient with a sarcoma should include a chest x-ray and either whole lung tomography or a computed tomography (CT) scan of the chest to exclude metastatic disease to the lung. A CT scan of the primary site often aids in the assessment of the involved muscular compartments. Arteriograms are sometimes helpful for defining vascular displacement or venous invasion.

Because definitive treatment ultimately requires removal of wide margins around the primary anatomic site, excisional biopsy should be avoided for any soft tissue sarcoma greater than 3 cm. in diameter. Excisional biopsy obscures the tumor's proper anatomic position and obfuscates definitive management. For lesions greater than 3 cm., incisional biopsy is the diagnostic procedure of choice. The incision should be placed longitudinally in an area that can be excised readily when the definitive operation is performed. Although needle aspiration biopsy or Tru-Cut biopsy can establish the diagnosis of sarcoma, a larger sample is frequently needed to establish the precise histologic grade of the lesion.

Surgical Treatment

Because soft tissue sarcomas extend along fascial plains, all types of surgical excision have been associated with high incidences of local recurrence. Simple excisions, or enucleations, around the pseudocapsule were associated with a 90 to 95 per cent rate of local recurrence. Consequently, it was recommended that involved muscle groups be excised from origin to insertion. This improved local control; however, recurrence rates of 30 to 35 per cent were unacceptably high. Extremity amputations reduced local recurrences to 20 per cent but included such radical procedures as forequarter amputation and hemipelvectomy for proximal upper and lower extremity lesions. Thus, it became clear that surgery alone was probably inadequate treatment for soft tissue sarcoma.

Early efforts to treat soft tissue sarcomas with radiotherapy suggested that they were radioresistant. Response rates of less than 20 per cent were probably due to the fact that the treated tumors were frequently large and hypoxic. More recent studies, however, have shown that radiation therapy after surgical excision of all gross tumor (without a particularly wide margin of resection) can reduce local recurrence to 20 per cent. Studies have also suggested that preoperative radiation therapy is effective for decreasing local recurrence rates. Protocols in which 5000 to 6000 rads precede gross excision of tumor have significantly decreased rates of local recurrence to 15 per cent. However, such high doses of radiation to an extremity can result in significant morbidity.

The advent of Adriamycin in 1968 provided the first effective chemotherapy for soft tissue sarcoma. When response rates in adults with metastatic disease were reported to be 30 to 40 per cent, the drug subsequently was used as an adjunct to surgical treatment. Recent studies using Adriamycin alone and in combination with other agents as adjuvant treatment have demonstrated reduced incidences of systemic metastases.[6] Several groups have shown that high doses of Adriamycin could be delivered to soft tissue sarcoma of the extremity by intra-arterial infusion. By exploiting the ease of access to the major vessels of the extremities, it was shown that high concentrations of drug could be delivered and that some cell necrosis would occur. Improved rates of local recurrence were obtained with intra-arterial perfusion of the tumor followed by surgical excision.

Present trends in the treatment of soft tissue sarcoma now include an integration of pre- or postoperative radiation and/or chemotherapy. In several centers, these multimodality treatment protocols have shown local control rates and ultimate survival comparable to or better than those of amputation. Such multimodality protocols, the basis of which is the preservation of the extremity, have become known as "limb salvage procedures." One such protocol employs preoperative intra-arterial doxorubicin combined

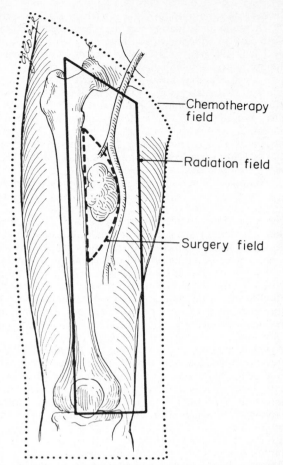

Chemotherapy field

Radiation field

Surgery field

Figure 5. Multimodality therapy for soft-tissue sarcoma. The "shrinking field" concept permits limitation of the surgical field while minimizing local recurrence.

with preoperative radiation therapy in high-dose fractions.[8] The theoretical concept is one of a "shrinking field" of treatment. Chemotherapy treats the whole extremity; radiation therapy treats the whole compartment; and excision of the tumor is a relatively localized phenomenon (Fig. 5). This combined modality protocol has reduced local recurrence rates to 3 per cent.

MALIGNANT MELANOMA

Melanoma is a malignant cancer of the pigmented cells of the skin. It is increasing on the North American continent, particularly in the southeastern and southwestern United States, and is now more common than Hodgkin's disease. Melanoma is particularly common in fair-skinned individuals of northern European extraction who settled in Australia and other areas close to the equator. It is unusual in blacks but can occur in the subungual areas and in the less pigmented areas such as the soles of the feet. Sun exposure has been implicated but not proved as a causative factor, whereas genetic factors may be important because relatives of patients with melanoma have a fourfold increase in risk of the disease. There are families whose members have multiple primary melanomas. Melanoma is uncommon before puberty and is rare in patients under 12 years of age.

Melanomas generally arise in pre-existing nevi but can occur *de novo*. Certain clinical features may suggest malignant degeneration in a nevus, e.g., changes in color, in particular darkening or deepening to a purple or a blue-black hue; changes in size or shape; nodularity; and associated ulceration, bleeding, or pruritus. Any of these changes is an indication for biopsy. In some instances, primary malignant melanomas may regress partially or completely. When this regression occurs, there is a paradoxical lack of pigmentation associated with a whitish "halo" area. Thus, it is possible for an individual to present with metastatic melanoma to the regional lymph nodes without evidence of a primary tumor.

Melanomas usually undergo two growth phases: (1) a *radial* growth phase, which may be brief or may last for several years, in which the melanoma spreads peripherally at the level of the basement membrane of the epidermis; and (2) a *vertical* growth phase, in which the metastatic potential of the melanoma increases dramatically and is associated with penetration into the dermis and, eventually, the subcutaneous tissue.[3]

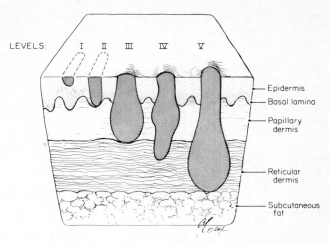

Figure 6. Diagram of Clark's microstaging indicating levels of invasion.

Classification

Melanoma is generally classified into three types:

1. *Lentigo maligna melanomas* usually occur in the elderly on areas exposed to the sun, such as the face and neck. These lesions tend to be large with a flat surface. Lentigo maligna rarely has a significant vertical growth phase but enlarges by radial growth and has a low metastatic potential.

2. *Superficial spreading melanoma* is the most common of the three types. These melanomas occur in a younger age group than lentigo maligna, do not have a predisposition to areas exposed to the sun, and tend to have long periods of radial growth before vertical invasion.

3. *Nodular melanoma* represents 20 per cent of all melanomas. These lesions are typically nodular and deeply pigmented. Generally, there is no evidence of radial or intraepidermal growth, and they usually have an extensive vertical growth component.

Melanomas can also occur in the mucous membranes of the lip and anus as well as in the subungual areas. However, these lesions are quite rare and represent less than 2 per cent of all melanomas.

Microstaging

Suspicious nevi should be totally excised along with a small amount of adjacent normal skin. For larger lesions, an incisional biopsy should be performed through the portion of the lesion that appears to be most nodular, irregular, or deeply pigmented. This biopsy should also include a portion of adjacent skin. Cauterization and shave biopsies are not appropriate for melanoma. The shave biopsy precludes accurate microstaging. The development of microstaging systems by Clark and Breslow has added considerably to our understanding of the pathogenesis and prognosis of patients with melanoma (Fig. 6). A Clark's Level I melanoma is completely contained within the epidermis. It is frequently referred to as melanoma *in situ* since the basal lamina is intact. It is also referred to as atypical melanocytic hyperplasia, which emphasizes its benignity. Clark's Level II melanoma invades to the papillary dermis but not beyond. Clark's Level III melanoma invades down to the interface between the papillary and reticular dermis. Clark's Level IV melanoma penetrates into the

reticular dermis, and Clark's Level V melanoma penetrates into the subcutaneous tissues. Survival and likelihood of regional lymph node metastases correlate very closely with Clark's levels of penetration. The more deeply penetrating lesions have a greater likelihood of regional lymph node metastases and a poorer prognosis.

With Breslow's classification system, the thickness of the melanoma is directly measured on the histologic slide by an oculomicrometer. The depth of penetration correlates well with the overall survival. Patients with melanomas less than 0.75 mm. thick have an excellent prognosis, whereas melanomas penetrating between 0.76 and 1.5 mm. have significant metastatic potential. Patients with melanomas greater than 1.5 mm. thick have the highest incidence of regional lymph node metastases and the poorest overall survival. Clark's levels also correlate with survival. The 5-year survival of patients with Clark's Level II melanoma is in excess of 90 per cent. Five-year survival for all patients with a Clark's Level III melanoma is approximately 70 per cent, Level IV 55 per cent, and Level V about 20 per cent. Knowledge of the pathologic status of the regional lymph nodes allows more accurate prognostication. Patients without regional lymph node metastases have a 75 per cent 5-year survival, and those with four or more nodes involved have a 25 per cent or less 5-year survival.

Management

The initial work-up must include a careful examination for evidence of regional lymph node involvement. Melanomas of the head and neck metastasize to the parotid and cervical lymph nodes. Melanomas of the upper extremity metastasize to the axillary lymph nodes and those of the lower extremity to the inguinal lymph nodes. Melanomas on the trunk may metastasize to either the axillary or inguinal lymph node area or both. When lymphatic drainage is ambiguous, injection of radiolabelled colloid into the area of the truncal melanoma will demonstrate the pattern of lymphatic drainage. These scans assist the surgeon in selecting the appropriate nodal group when regional lymph node dissection is considered. Careful observation for a second primary lesion is important.

All biopsies should be carefully evaluated by a competent pathologist to determine the type of melanoma and its depth of penetration. For patients who have no evidence on physical examination of regional lymph node metastases, the work-up should include a chest X-ray, complete blood count, and liver chemistries. For patients who have clinical evidence of regional lymph node involvement, liver and brain scans are also indicated. Extensive work-up for metastatic disease in patients with negative regional lymph nodes on physical examination is not necessary.[12]

Following work-up, melanomas should be treated by a wide excision of the primary lesion. For many years it was thought that a 5-cm. margin was necessary. This dogma has been challenged, and it is apparent now that less than 5 cm. may be adequate. Most oncologists feel that a margin of 3 cm. from the edge of the pigmented area is sufficient. For Levels I or II melanoma, a margin less than 3 cm. is usually adequate. For more deeply penetrating lesions, however, a margin of at least 3 cm. is recommended. Lesions that penetrate into the subcutaneous fat (Level V) should be excised along with the underlying fascia.

The role of regional lymph node dissection in patients with melanoma is controversial.[11] When the regional lymph nodes are clinically palpable, most agree that a radical regional lymphadenectomy should be performed. However, in the absence of clinically suspicious nodes, regional lymph node dissection is much more controversial. The morbidity associated with deep inguinal node dissection can be significant. Fortunately, axillary and cervical lymphadenectomies have very little morbidity and almost no cosmetic deformity. Regional lymph node dissections are useful for staging because the presence of nodal involvement significantly affects prognosis. Whether or not regional lymphadenectomy is therapeutic remains to be determined. It is generally agreed that regional lymph node dissection is not indicated in patients with Clark's Level II melanoma or a melanoma with Breslow thickness of less than 0.75 mm. Since patients with Level III melanomas greater than 0.75 mm. thick have a 15 to 20 per cent incidence of positive nodes and patients with Levels IV and V melanomas have a 30 to 35 per cent incidence of positive nodes, many surgeons feel that these patients should undergo regional lymphadenectomy. Although there are no prospective randomized trials to support the therapeutic value of regional lymphadenectomy for clinically negative nodes, most surgical oncologists will perform regional lymph node dissection in patients who have lesions that are greater than 1.5 mm. thick and in all patients with Clark's Levels IV and V melanomas.

Following surgery, a few patients may develop satellitosis or in-transit metastases. Satellitosis refers to the development of recurrent melanoma in the skin within 5 cm. of the surgical scar. In-transit metastases refers to metastatic cutaneous lesions in the dermal lymphatics that occur between the scar and the site of the regional lymph node dissection. In-transit metastases may respond well to BCG injection, and hyperthermic chemotherapeutic regional perfusion of the extremity may be beneficial for controlling locally recurrent or in-transit melanoma.

Historically, melanoma has been quite resistant to chemotherapy. At the present time, DTIC is considered the best single agent. More recently a combination of bleomycin, vincristine, methyl-CCNU, and DTIC has shown considerable promise.

Adjuvant chemotherapy or immunotherapy has not been useful for patients with melanoma. However, recent results with IL-2 and LAK cells have been very encouraging.

SURGICAL MANAGEMENT OF METASTATIC DISEASE

Logic would lead one to assume that once tumor cells have disseminated hematogenously, further surgery is not indicated. However, experience suggests that this is not the case in certain patients. Gradually over the last 20 years surgical intervention has become more and more common in patients with metastatic disease. In some instances surgery is performed strictly for palliation, such as in patients with CNS metastases. However, in others, resection of metastatic disease is associated with a significant prolongation of disease-free survival and, in some instances, cure. Malignancies tend to have an affinity for certain metastatic sites. For instance, soft tissue sarcomas have a predilection for the lung, colorectal cancers for the liver, and breast cancer for the bone. These sites are frequently the first site of metastases and in some instances may be the only clinical site of metastatic disease. Autopsy data have indicated that patients with soft tissue sarcomas may die from pulmonary metastases but have no evidence of disease elsewhere. The most frequent sites of surgical resection for metastases are the lungs, liver, and central nervous system.

Surgical intervention may be indicated in patients who have metastases to the spinal cord to relieve pain or other distressing systems such as motor paralysis. Indeed, on occasion, resection of a solitary brain metastasis is indicated and may be associated with a significant prolongation of survival.

Five-year survival following resection of pulmonary metastases may increase, in selected patients, from 30 to 60 per cent.[13, 14] Even patients with multiple bilateral pulmonary metastases may benefit from resection. In recent years, several criteria have been established to help surgeons select patients for resection of pulmonary metastases. The factors that must be considered include:

1. A primary tumor that is adequately controlled.
2. Metastatic disease confined to the lung and no other evidence of visceral metastases.
3. The number of metastatic nodules.
4. The histologic type of the primary lesion.
5. The tumor growth rate or doubling time.
6. The availability of effective chemotherapy.

As a general rule, no patient should be considered for resection of pulmonary metastases unless the primary tumor is controlled. The histologic type is an important consideration. Patients with testicular tumors respond very well to resection of their pulmonary metastases. Five-year survival rates are increased to 60 per cent following surgical resection. On the other hand, patients with breast cancer, gastrointestinal tumors, and melanoma do not benefit significantly from pulmonary resection. Patients with soft tissue sarcomas and hypernephromas frequently derive considerable benefit from resection of pulmonary metastases. This is especially true if the tumor doubling time or the growth rate of the metastases is slow and the interval from the treatment of the primary and the onset of the metastases is long. In general, the 5-year survival following resection of pulmonary metastases in patients with soft tissue and bone sarcomas is between 25 and 35 per cent.

Patients with hepatic metastases may also respond well to resection.[14] Most hepatic metastases are from a colorectal primary tumor. Unfortunately, most of these metastases involve the liver diffusely or involve other organs as well as the liver. Occasionally, however, patients present with lesions confined to areas of the liver that are anatomically suitable for resection. In these patients, hepatic resection can result in 2-year survival rates as high as 40 to 50 per cent. In general, patients with one solitary metastatic lesion have a more favorable outcome than patients with multiple lesions, and those patients who have a long disease-free interval between the resection of their primary and the onset of hepatic metastases have a better prognosis.

The morbidity and mortality from hepatic resection

have declined markedly in the past 10 years. Currently, in experienced hands, the mortality is between 4 and 7 per cent.[15] Therefore, patients who have a solitary hepatic metastasis, who are free of other metastatic disease, and in whom the primary has been controlled should be considered for hepatic resection.

Because most patients with hepatic metastases are not candidates for hepatic resection, other modalities have been investigated. Systemic chemotherapy has not had a significant impact on hepatic metastases from colon cancer. 5-fluorouracil remains the drug of choice, but the response rate rarely exceeds 15 per cent. Other forms of therapy, therefore, have been explored. Most recently, continuous infusion of the hepatic artery with chemotherapy has been advocated. This technique involves the insertion of a catheter into the hepatic artery and the implantation of a continuous infusion pump in the subcutaneous tissue of the abdomen. Because 5-FU is metabolized by the liver, large doses of this agent can be infused continuously into the liver with very few side effects. Response rates to continuous hepatic artery infusion are quite high when compared with response rates to systemic chemotherapy.[1]

While no prospective randomized and properly controlled trials have been used to evaluate hepatic artery infusion, comparisons to historic controls indicate a significant prolongation of survival. Most oncologists feel that hepatic artery infusion is an effective form of therapy for hepatic metastases in carefully selected patients.

SELECTED REFERENCES

Balch, C. M., Urist, M. M., Soong, S., and McGregor, M.: A prospective Phase II clinical trial of continuous FUDR regional chemotherapy for colorectal metastases to the liver using a totally implantable drug infusion pump. Ann. Surg., 198:567, 1983.
The results of the treatment of 81 patients with liver metastases from colorectal cancer by hepatic artery infusion are reviewed. The results are compared with those of stratified historical controls. The results and toxicity are discussed.

Burk, M. W., and Morton, D. L., (Eds.): Adjuvant treatment of cancer. Surg. Clin. North Am., 61(6), 1981.
This monograph describes the current status of adjuvant therapy such as irradiation, chemotherapy, and immunotherapy following surgical removal of a variety of solid tumors. Melanoma, breast cancer, colon cancer, genitourinary cancer, and lung cancer are among those covered.

DeVita, V. T., and Schein, P. S.: The use of drugs in combination for the treatment of cancer: Rationale and results. N. Engl. J. Med., 288:998, 1973.
More detail on the biologic rationale for combination chemotherapy. The kinetics of cell-kill are discussed. Empirical findings are examined in light of background theory.

Goldie, J. H., and Coleman, A. J.: The genetic origin of drug resistance: Implications for systemic therapy. Cancer Res., 44:3643, 1984.
This paper discusses the various mechanisms for the development of drug resistance by tumor cells. The theory behind the use of non–cross-resistant drugs and other treatment strategies is discussed.

Hill, G. J.: Historic milestones in cancer surgery. Semin. Oncol., 6:409, 1979.
A historical review detailing the evolution of the principles of cancer surgery. Ancient, medieval, and renaissance ideas are discussed. Focus is on developing concepts and techniques of the 20th century. Major individual contributions are identified.

Huth, J. F., Holmes, E. C., Vernon, S. E., Callery, C. D., Ramming, K. P., and Morton, D. L.: Pulmonary resection for metastatic sarcoma. Am. J. Surg., 140:9, 1980.
The principles of the surgical management of pulmonary metastases are discussed. The prognostic variables and the surgical techniques are discussed.

Irie, R. F., Sze, L. L., and Saxton, R. E.: Human antibody to OFA-I, a tumor antigen, produced in vitro by Epstein-Barr virus-transformed human B-lymphoid cell lines. Proc. Natl. Acad. Sci., 79:5666, 1982.
This paper describes the production of antibodies to a tumor antigen by human lymphocytes. These antibodies were specific for tumors of neuroectodermal origin such as melanoma, glioma, and neuroblastoma.

Iwatsuki, S., Shaw, B. W., and Starzl, T. E.: Experience with 150 liver resections. Ann. Surg., 197:247, 1983.
Forty-three patients with liver metastasis underwent hepatic resection. Mortality was less than 5 per cent and the 3-year survival rate was in excess of 50 per cent.

Kern, D. H., and Bertelsen C. A.: Present status of chemosensitivity assays. Intl. Adv. Surg. Oncol., 7:187, 1984.
An updated account of the methods, results, and reproducibility of in vitro chemosensitivity assays. Relevance to clinical practice is examined.

Rosenberg, S., Tepper, J., Glatstein, E., et. al.: The treatment of soft-tissue sarcomas of the extremities: Prospective randomized evaluation of (1) limb-sparing surgery and radiation compared to amputation and (2) the role of adjuvant chemotherapy. Ann. Surg., 196:305, 1982.
An excellent example of a prospective randomized trial designed to compare multimodality therapy and amputation and to test the efficacy of adjuvant chemotherapy.

Terry, W. D., and Rosenberg, S. A. (Eds.): Immunotherapy of Human Cancer. New York, Elsevier Holland Inc., 1982.
This monograph summarizes the experience to date of immunotherapy of human cancer. It is based on a symposium on immunotherapy and reviews the world experience.

REFERENCES

1. Balch, C. M., Urist, M. M., Soong, S., and McGregor, M.: A prospective phase II clinical trial of continuous FUDR regional chemotherapy for colorectal metastases to the liver using a total implantable drug-infusion pump. Ann. Surg., 198(99):567, 1983.
2. Chabner, B.: Pharmacologic Principles of Cancer Treatment. Philadelphia, W. B. Saunders Company, 1982.
3. Clark, W. H.: Tumor progression in primary melanoma. In Clark, W. H. (Ed.): Human Malignant Melanoma. New York, Grune and Stratton, 1979, pp. 15–31.
4. Coia, L. R., and Moylan, D. J.: Therapeutic Radiology for The House Officer. Baltimore, Williams & Wilkins, 1984.
5. Copeland, E. M.: Surgical Oncology. New York, J. Wiley & Sons, 1983.
6. DeVita, V. T., Hellman, S., and Rosenberg, S. A.: Cancer: Principles and Practice of Oncology. Philadelphia, J. B. Lippincott, 1982.
7. DeVita, V. T., and Schein, P. S.: The use of drugs in combination for the treatment of cancer: Rationale and results. N. Engl. J. Med., 288:998, 1973.
8. Eilber, F. R.: Soft tissue sarcoma of the extremity. Curr. Probl. Cancer, 8(9):1, 1984.
9. Fletcher, G. H.: Textbook of Radiotherapy, 3rd ed. Philadelphia, Lea and Febiger, 1980.
10. Gallo, R. C., and Wong-Staal, F.: Certain thoughts on the viral etiology of cancer. Cancer Res., 44:2743, 1984.
10a. Grimm, E. A., and Rosenberg, S. A.: The human lymphokine-activated killer cell phenomenon. Lymphokines, 9:279, 1984.
11. Haskell, C. M.: Cancer Treatment, 2nd ed., Philadelphia, W.B. Saunders Company, 1985.
12. Holmes, E. C., Moseley, H. S., Morton, D. L., Clark, W., Robinson, D., and Urist, M. M.: A rational approach to the surgical management of melanoma. Ann. Surg., 186:481, 1977.
13. Holmes, E. C., and Morton, D. L.: Pulmonary resection for sarcoma metastases. Orthop. Clin. North Am., 2:805, 1977.
14. Huth, J. F., Holmes, E. C., Vernon, S. E., Callery, C. D., Ramming, K. P., and Morton, D. L.: Pulmonary resection for metastatic sarcoma. Am. J. Surg., 140:9, 1980.
15. Iwatsuki, S., Shaw, D. W., and Starzl, T. E.: Experience with 150 liver resections. Ann. Surg., 19:247, 1983.
16. Morton, D. L., Eilber, F. R., Joseph, W. L., Wood, W. C., Trahan, E., and Ketcham, A. S.: Immunological factors in human sarcomas and melanomas: A rational basis for immunotherapy. Ann. Surg., 172:740, 1970.
17. Prosnitz, L. R., Kapp, D. S., and Weissberg, J. B.: Radiotherapy. N. Engl. J. Med., 309:771, 1983.
17a. Rosenberg, S. A., Lotze, M. T., Muul, L. M., et al.: Observations on the systemic administration of autologous lymphokine-activated killer cells and recombinant interleukin-2 to patients with metastatic cancer. N. Engl. J. Med., 313:1485, 1985.
18. Rubin, P.: Clinical Oncology for Medical Students and Physicians, 6th ed. Philadelphia, American Cancer Society, 1983.
19. Schabel, F. M.: Rationale for adjuvant chemotherapy. Cancer 39:2875, 1977.
20. Terry, W. D., and Rosenberg, S. A. (Eds.): Immunotherapy of Human Cancer. New York, Elsevier Holland, Inc., 1982.

THE BREAST

EDWARD M. COPELAND III, M.D. • KIRBY I. BLAND, M.D.

17

The breast is an embryologic structure unique to the class *Mammalia*—thus the designation mammary gland. It is a modified sweat gland, variable in number among subgroups of the mammalian species. Single pairs of mammary glands are observed in man, apes, and monkeys (except for marmosets). The breast remains a dormant, nonfunctional structure in the male, whereas breast development in the female is active and under neuroendocrine control of the anterior pituitary gland and ovary. Remarkable functional and pathological alterations occur in the breast and span the interval from menarche, pregnancy, and lactation to post menopause. The various normal and pathologic conditions that occur as a result of these physiologic alterations demand a comprehensive knowledge of the events that occur in the pre- and postmenopausal female. Such information is necessary for the diagnosis and appropriate therapy of diseases of the breast.

EMBRYOLOGY AND DEVELOPMENTAL ANATOMY

In the human embryo, the breast is first recognized as a "milk streak" in approximately the sixth week of fetal development. An area of ectodermal thickening, known as the *milk bud*, develops in the pectoral portion of the torso of the embryo. This distinct linear elevation extends bilaterally from the axilla to the vulva and is known as the *milk line* or *mammary ridge* (Fig. 1). The pectoral location of the breast in humans is shared only with higher primates of the mammalian species.

By week 9 of intrauterine development, the milk line has atrophied, except in the pectoral region, and the first recognition of a breast primordium, the nipple bud, is apparent. By the 12th week of embryogenesis, the nipple bud is invaded by squamous epithelium of the ectoderm. At month 5, mesenchymal connective tissue infiltrates the breast primordium and differentiates into 15 to 20 solid filaments, which are symmetrically distributed beneath the skin of the nipple bud. Mammary ductules develop as ventral ingrowths from these embryologic remnants, subdivide into primary milk ducts, and terminate in lobular buds. Subsequently these buds proliferate into acini after ovarian estrogenic stimulation begins. During intrauterine growth, primary milk ducts branch and subdivide extensively. By the seventh to eighth intrauterine month, ducts cannulate to form lumina that correspond to the immature lactiferous ducts. At birth, the nipple bud has a central depression corresponding to the area penetrated by the lumina of the primary milk ductules. Shortly after birth, penetration of the nipple bud is complete; it everts and is further invaded by basaloid cells that become deeply pigmented to form the areola.

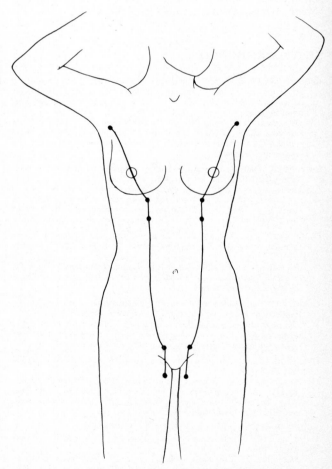

Figure 1. The milk line. Following development of the milk bud in the pectoral area of ectodermal thickening, the "milk streak" extends from the axilla to the groin. By week 9 of intrauterine development, atrophy of the bud occurs except for supranumerary nipples or breasts.

Anatomy

With its musculocutaneous and fatty components, the mammary gland occupies a position between the third and seventh ribs and extends in width from the parasternal to the mid or anterior axillary lines. The mesenchymal portion of the breast resides primarily on the pectoral fascia and the serratus anterior muscle. Commonly, breast tissue will extend into the fold of the axillary space, the so-called axillary tail of Spence. In the male, the glandular and ductule components of the mamma remain rudimentary and undeveloped with short ducts and incompletely developed acini. The flat appearance of the male breast is secondary to a deficiency of nipple-areolar development and parenchymal density and fat.

The virginal breast of the female assumes a typical hemispheric configuration with distinct flattening above the nipple. Unlike the prepubertal breast, the multiparous breast has experienced pituitary and ovarian stimulation, is much larger, and has a denser stroma and ductal component.

The *adult mammary gland* (Fig. 2) represents a modification of the ectodermal vestige of a modified sweat gland and is thus confined to the superficial and deep layers of superficial fascia of the anterior chest wall. The deep layer of superficial fascia crosses the retromammary space to fuse with the pectoral (deep) fascia. A distinct space known as the retromammary bursa exists on the posterior aspect of the breast between the deep layer of superficial fascia and the investing fascia of the pectoralis major muscle. As a result of its loose areolar connections, this distinct bursa contributes to the mobility of the breast on the chest wall. The deep pectoral fascia is intimately related to the sternum and is superolaterally bound to the clavipectoral fascia. These deep fascial envelopes are contiguous inferiorly with the rectus abdominus tendon. Approximately two thirds of

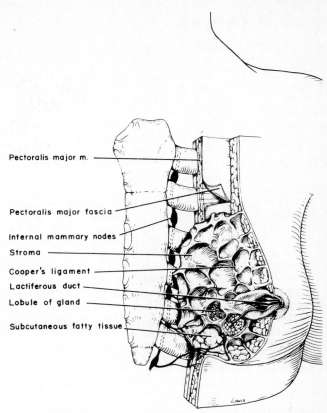

Figure 3. *Tangential view of breast on chest wall. The interposed fibroseptae (Cooper's ligaments) provide stromal support of breast parenchyma. A diffuse lymphatic system is interposed and parallels the extensive ductal network in a periductal or perilobular position and drains the 15 to 20 glandular lobules.*

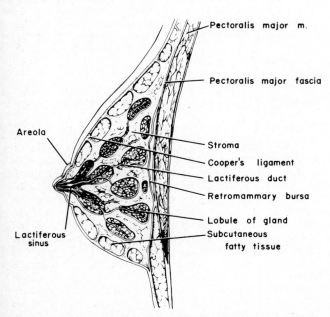

Figure 2. *Cross-sectional (sagittal) view of mammary gland. The breast is invested by superficial and deep fascia. The retromammary bursa contributes to mobility of the gland. The diffuse lactiferous ductal network converges in the subareolar space from glandular lobules to empty into the sinus recess beneath the nipple.*

the breast is intimately related and fascially attached to the pectoralis major muscle. A dense condensation of clavipectoral fascia, known as Halsted's ligament (costoclavicular ligament), extends from the most medial portion of the clavicle to the first rib. Directly beneath this ligament course the subclavian artery and vein through the thoracic inlet. The axillary vessels are surrounded by a dense vascular sheath, which continues as the roof from the axillary space to fuse with the deep fascial contributions of the pectoralis major muscle.

At maturity, the glandular portion of the breast assumes a roughly circular configuration. Fibrous septae interdigitate the mammary parenchyma and extend from the deep pectoral fascia (posterior superficial fascial layer) to the superficial layer of fascia within the dermis. These anterior suspensory ligaments were described by Cooper and insert perpendicular to the delicate superficial fascial layers of the corium (Fig. 3). Together with the retromammary bursa, Cooper's ligaments allow considerable mobility of the posterior aspect of the breast while providing structural support of the lobular and parenchymal components of the organ. Breast size is a correlate of genetic, dietary, and hormonal influences. The postmenopausal breast consistently reveals a disappearance of parenchymal fat and involution of the active, proliferative glandular components, both resulting due to cessation of ovarian stimuli. The nonlactating breast weighs between 150 to 225 grams, whereas the lactating breast may be greater than 500 grams.

Anomalies of Development

For both sexes, developmental anomalies occur as a result of complete or imperfect suppression of the breast anlagen during the multiple phases of embryogenesis. An accessory breast represents the progressive development of the ventral milk line with more than a single pair of the breast primordia. As a result, *supernumerary (accessory) nipples* or *breasts* may persist in unilateral or bilateral positions. This anomaly is estimated to occur in approximtely 1 to 2 per cent of Caucasians and is more common in the female, with a ratio of 2:1. Supernumerary mammary development is considered inheritable with autosomal dominant penetrance. In the majority of presentations, only a diminutive nipple is evident, and the most common clinical presentation is a small nipple and areola bud. These anomalous structures typically occupy a position on the ventral surface of the patient consistent with the embryologic "milk streak" and are thus anatomically restricted to sites between the axilla and inguinal fold. The most common presentation is in the milk line of the inframammary area or the axilla. This embryonic abnormality is more frequent in Orientals than Caucasians.

The rare occurrence of *amastia*, with complete absence of one or both breasts, is a result of developmental arrest of the ventral breast primordium. Unilateral amastia is more common. In the unilateral defect, persistence of a rudimentary breast may be associated with absence and/or underdevelopment of other structures of the anterior and lateral chest wall or arm.

Neurovascular Supply

NERVE SUPPLY

The cutaneous nerve supply of the breast is segmental and originates from T2 to T6 dermatomal segments. The first interspace is supplied primarily by nerves to the subclavius muscle. The dermatomal segments of these areas may be completely or partially denervated after elevation of skin flaps for modified or radical mastectomy. With dissection of skin flaps in the axilla, a major branch of the intercostobrachial nerve may be identified and sacrificed. This nerve is composed primarily of fibers from the lateral cutaneous branches of the second and third intercostal nerves and courses perpendicular and anterior to the latissimus dorsi muscle.

The *intercostobrachial nerve* is not to be confused with either the thoracodorsal or the long thoracic nerve of Bell. The *long thoracic nerve*, or external respiratory nerve of Bell, supplies the serratus anterior muscle and arises from the roots of C5, C6, and C7 to descend posterior to the brachial plexus and the axillary vein and lie on the serratus anterior muscle.

The *thoracodorsal nerve* innervates the latissimus dorsi muscle and arises from the posterior cord of the brachial plexus (C5, C6, and C7). It passes behind the medial cord and axillary vessels to course lateral to the long thoracic nerve and enter the anterior border of the latissimus dorsi muscle. From a functional point of view, it can be sacrificed with relative impunity. Paralysis of part or all of the latissimus dorsi muscle will result in its atrophy, making it of minimal value as musculature for myocutaneous reconstructive efforts. The functional loss is forceful apposition of the upper arm to the lateral chest wall, hindering primarily stevedores and bellmen, who need to carry items clasped between their upper arm and chest wall. Injury to the long thoracic nerve with serratus paralysis results in much greater functional morbidity from shoulder weakness and produces the "winged scapula" deformity.

The lateral pectoral nerve takes origin from the lateral cord of the brachial plexus to supply the pectoralis major and minor muscles. It courses medial to the pectoralis minor muscle and must be preserved when doing a modified radical mastectomy to avoid pectoralis major muscle atrophy. In distinction, the medial pectoral nerve, taking origin from the medial cord of the brachial plexus, courses lateral to the pectoralis minor muscle and supplies both the pectoralis major and minor muscles. This nerve is usually sacrificed when removing the pectoralis minor muscle as part of a modified radical mastectomy. If the lateral pectoral nerve is preserved, the pectoralis major muscle will not atrophy, and, after modified radical mastectomy, chest wall architecture will conform to the pectoralis major muscle and not to the rib cage.

BLOOD SUPPLY

The generous arterial supply to the breast and overlying skin is from branches of the *internal mammary and lateral thoracic arteries* and the *acromiothoracic branch of the axillary artery*.[3] The venous drainage system includes the *intercostal veins*, which traverse the posterior aspect of the breast from the second through the sixth intercostal spaces to enter the vertebral veins posteriorly. Additionally, the intercostal veins may enter the azygos system centrally to terminate in the superior vena cava. The deep venous system of the breast parallels the lateral thoracic and pectoral branches of the acromiothoracic artery (Fig. 4).

The *axillary vein*, into which these tributaries drain, collects all venous supply to the superior and lateral portions of the breast and also drains the pectoral muscles. The perforating veins of the *internal mammary venous system* drain the medial portion of the breast and pectoralis major muscle. This venous plexus traverses the rib interspaces to terminate in the innominate vein and, therefore, represents a direct embolic route to the pulmonary capillary network. All the veins of the breast have multiple anastomotic channels.

Lymphatic Drainage and Routes for Metastases

LYMPHATICS

Lymphatic flow is primarily unidirectional. However, with obstruction, e.g., as a result of developmental, neoplastic, or inflammatory processes, a reversal with bidirectional egress of lymph via rich lymphatic networks may be evident and may account for the observation of neoplastic proliferations in sites remote from the primary neoplasm. Delicate lymph vessels of the corium are valveless, and flow parallels the major venous channels. They also encircle the lobular parenchyma to enter regional lymph nodes in an orderly fashion. The unidirectional flow of lymph is from the periphery toward the right heart. Multiple lymph capillaries anastomose and fuse to form fewer lymph channels that terminate in the large left thoracic duct or the smaller right lymphatic duct (see Fig. 4). Two accessory directions exist for lymph drainage from the breast to nodes of the apex of the axilla via the *transpectoral* and the *retropectoral* routes.[3] Lymphatics of the transpectoral route occupy that position between the pectoralis major and minor muscles and were described by Rotter, a German pathologist. The lymphatics of this chain bear his

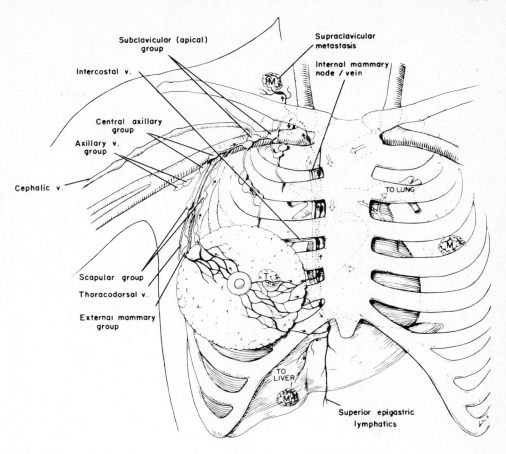

Figure 4. Venous drainage of the mammary gland and relationship to lymphatics, which parallel major venous tributaries. Three principal groups of deep veins serve as vascular routes for metastases: intercostal veins, axillary veins, and internal mammary veins. Visceral metastases to lung or liver are possible via lymphatic or principal vascular drainage routes of the breast that communicate with major venous trunks.

name—Rotter's nodes. The retropectoral lymphatics drain the superior and internal portions of the breast, arborize posterior and lateral to the surface of the pectoralis major muscle, and terminate at the apex of the axilla.

An appreciation of the major nodal groups is essential to thoroughly understand breast lymphatic drainage and to appropriately assess clinical involvement with disease. The principal axillary nodal groups[3] (Fig. 5) include:

1. *External mammary group* (Level I). Parallel the course of the lateral thoracic artery from the sixth rib to the axillary vein and occupy the lateral margin of the pectoralis major muscle and medial axillary space.

2. *Subscapular (scapular) group* (Level I). Contiguous with thoracodorsal branches of the subscapular vessels. They extend from the axillary vein to the lateral thoracic wall.

3. *Axillary vein group* (Level I). The most laterally placed and numerous group of nodes of the axilla. They are ventral and caudal to the axillary vein.

4. *Central nodal group* (Level II). Centrally located between the posterior and anterior axillary folds and occupy a superficial position beneath the skin and fascia of the mid axilla.

5. *Subclavicular (apical group)* (Level III). The highest and most medial of the lymph nodal groups. They are located at the juncture of the axillary vein with the subclavian vein at the level of Halsted's ligament.

These nodal groups are different from the levels of axillary nodes used by pathologists to describe the area of metastatic involvement within the axillae. Level I nodes are in the lateral axilla, lateral to the border of the pectoralis major and minor muscles. Level II nodes are deep to the insertion of the pectoralis minor muscle on the coracoid process, and Level III nodes are medial to the pectoralis minor muscle.

METASTASIS

This rich lymphatic network also has cross-connections within the breast parenchyma and the skin of the contralateral breast and axilla. These communicating dermal lymphatics allow metastatic involvement of the contralateral breast and axilla. Additionally, musculofascial components of the chest wall have extensive lymphatic drainage, which parallels the course of their major intercostal blood supply.

Invasive neoplasms of the lateral breast have preferential lymphatic drainage toward the lateral axilla. In contradistinction, invasive breast neoplasms of the medial quadrants have preferential drainage toward the internal mammary nodal groups. Bidirectional metastases may be observed with central or subareolar lesions. Internal mammary lymphatics terminate in subclavicular nodal groups. The right internal group enters the right lymphatic duct, and the left internal group enters the main thoracic duct. Supraclavicular nodal metastases indicate distant spread of the malignant process. These lymph nodes are at the confluence of the jugular and subclavian veins and are situated beneath the lateral, inferior margin of the sternocleidomastoid muscle. Once these nodes are involved, the disease by definition is no longer regional (Stage IV).

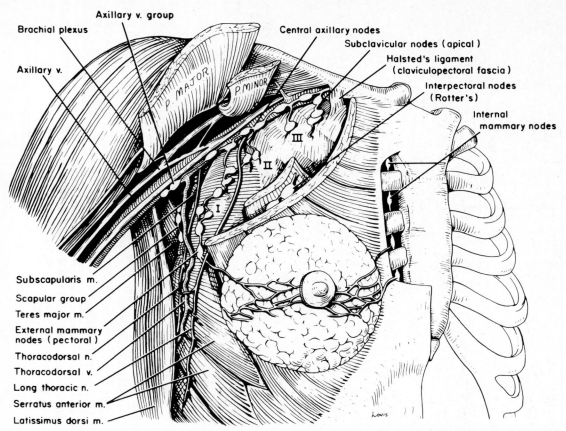

Figure 5. Lymphatic drainage of the breast. Unidirectional flow of lymph toward the axilla or the internal mammary nodes is depicted. The five basic axillary nodal groups include (Level I) external mammary group, subscapular (scapular) group, and axillary vein group; (Level II) central nodal group; (Level III) subclavicular (apical) group. The interpectoral (Rotter's) group is interposed between the pectoralis major and minor. Subareolar and central primary tumors have bidirectional lymphatic flow to the axilla and/or the internal mammary chain.

Physiology

The phases of breast development occur as a result of the mammotropic effects of anterior pituitary and ovarian hormonal secretion. The gonadotropic, luteinizing hormone (LH) and the gonadotropic, follicle-stimulating hormone (FSH) are secreted from basophile cells located in the anterior pituitary gland. The pituitary acidophile cells produce the luteotropic lactogenic hormone prolactin (LTH). Additionally, neurohumoral pathways from the hypothalamus have a biofeedback role for the production and/or release of the gonadotropic hormones.

Following FSH stimulation for development of mature ovarian graafian follicles, estrogen synthesis occurs in the ovary in the presence of minute quantities of LH. Circulating estrogen then initiates the production of LH, which inhibits basophile cell production of FSH. An increased level of LH and a simultaneous decrease in the amount of FSH will initiate ovulation and the formation of a nonfunctional corpus luteum. LTH initiates the release and secretion of progesterone and estrogen from the corpus luteum. Finally, the process is repeated and estrogen production from the ovary is initiated following stimulation of the follicle by FSH in the presence of trace amounts of LH (Fig. 6). Both production and release of LH, and perhaps LTH, from the anterior pituitary are inhibited by estrogens and progestogens circulating in high concentrations.

Activation of FSH release from the basophile cells of the pituitary initiates menarche. Additionally, estrogen production and ovulation cannot occur prior to the synthesis and release of LH from the gonadotropic basophile cell. The synthesis and/or release of LTH can be inhibited by therapeutic doses of estrogens, progestogens, and/or androgens. The evacuation of a gravid uterus and the simultaneous cessation of secretion of placental hormones will initiate increased release and synthesis of LTH from the anterior pituitary.

Under neurohumoral control of the hypothalamus and pituitary, feedback control of the gonadotropins allows the ovarian follicle to produce and release estrogen (estrone, estradiol) with synchronous synthesis and release of progesterone and estrogen from the corpus luteum. In pregnancy, the presence of chorionic gonadotropin (hCG) initiates maintenance and production of progesterone and estrogen from the corpus luteum.

ADOLESCENCE

In the *adolescent breast*, estrogen initiates growth of the epidermal portion of the breast bud with ingrowth of lactiferous ducts, myoepithelial cells, and the alveoli of breast parenchyma (Fig. 7A). The additive effect of progesterone initiates the development of acinar (secretory) tissues of the breast (see Fig. 6). The sudden cessation of

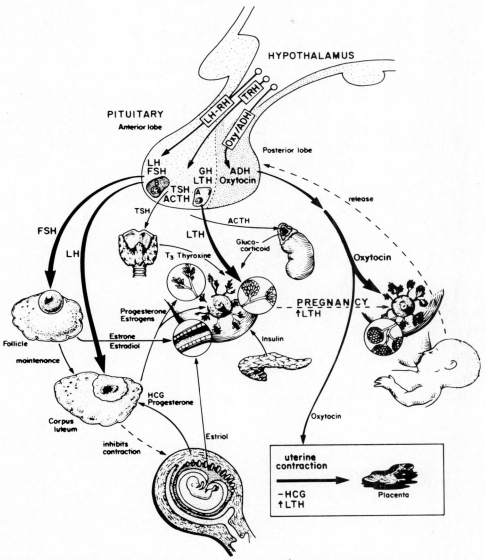

Figure 6. Neuroendocrine control of breast development and function with relationships to gonadotrophic hormones of the anterior pituitary and ovary. Basophile secretion of LH and FSH is responsible for ovarian synthesis and release of progesterone and estrogen, respectively. The mammotropic effects of estrogen and progestin initiate myoepithelial and alveoli development. Acidophile cell secretion of LTH is initiated following evacuation of the gravid uterus and is mammotropic to lobular alveoli. The suckling reflex initiates oxytocin release from the posterior pituitary and is stimulatory to alveoli myoepithelial cells to initiate milk release. Neuroendocrine organs other than the pituitary and ovary provide hormones (glucocorticoid, GH, insulin, thyroxine) that are trophic to ductal and glandular maintenance and growth.

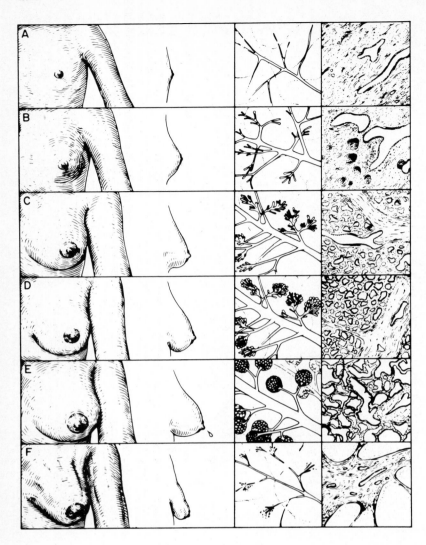

Figure 7. Phases of mammary gland development; anterior and lateral views. Microscopic appearance of ducts and lobules in phases of development, growth, and maintenance. A, Prepubertal (childhood). B, Puberty. C, Mature (reproductive). D, Pregnancy. E, Lactation. F, Postmenopausal (senescent) state.

gonadotropic pituitary hormone or target organ hormone secretion of estradiol or progesterone will, thus, have detrimental effects on breast development, maintenance, and function. With the establishment of cyclic ovarian function in *puberty*, the mammotropic effects of estrogen become evident (Fig. 7B). The ductal and sinus recesses of epithelial development become more evident. Distinct lobules are formed. Concurrent with the mammotropic effects of estrogenic compounds, stromal elements enlarge with parallel growth and replication of duct epithelium. Breast growth is isometric with enlargement and pigmentation of the nipple and areola. The additive effects of estrogen and progesterone contribute to completion of the formation of the lobular and acinar structures of the *mature breast* within 12 to 18 months after the onset of menarche (Fig. 7C). Subsequent enlargement and progressive development of lactiferous ducts and acini occur with hormonal stimuli from each estrogen cycle and with pregnancy. Eventual breast size and contour correlate with body fat content and habitus.

PREGNANCY

In *pregnancy*, milk synthesis and release are initiated around the fifth month (Fig. 7D). Lactation occurs as a result of the intense stimulation from LTH released from the anterior pituitary, acidophile cell. Milk release (letdown) occurs at the time of the suckling reflex from direct stimulation by oxytocin on myoepithelial cells of the breast alveoli (see Fig. 6). Synthesis of oxytocin occurs in the hypothalamus. Neuroendocrine organs (adrenal, thyroid, pancreas) other than the ovary contribute hormones (glucocorticoid, growth hormone [GH], insulin) that are trophic to mammary ductal and glandular growth and maintenance. With established *lactation*, the glandular tissue of the breast parenchyma eventually replaces the fatty components of the interstices of the breast lobules as the latter continue to proliferate (Fig. 7E). Following termination of lactation, stromal and ductal involution is initiated but remains incomplete. Until ovarian hormonal stimulation ceases, the hypertrophic and hyperplastic glandular tissues that develop as a result of the pregnancy are partially maintained.

MENOPAUSE

With *menopause* the estrogenic and progestational effects of ovarian function cease and progressive involution is initiated. Regression to an atrophic or hypoplastic epithelium is apparent within the ducts and lobules, and the stroma is replaced with dense periductal fibrous tissue (Fig.

7*F*). Dilatation of the lactiferous duct network in isolated lobules occurs. Lobular acini are depleted of their columnar epithelium and may enlarge and form macrocysts. On examination, the senile or postmenopausal breast is often asymmetric with irregularities of the lobular component and formation of cysts of varying sizes. As the fat content and supporting periductal fibrostroma are depleted, the senescent breast becomes a pendulous, homogeneous structure with loss of contour and configuration.

ASSESSMENT OF BREAST DISEASE

History and Examination

HISTORY

The dissemination of factual information about the natural history and incidence of breast cancer is often responsible for the patient's awareness of breast disease. A comprehensive history should be obtained before a physical examination is undertaken. Detailed inquiry into associative risk factors, such as age, parity, and menstrual and nursing history, is important. Age of menarche and cyclic alterations with menses are significant correlates of benign and malignant disease. Questions concerning previous surgical procedures, especially oophorectomy, adrenalectomy, or pelvic surgery, are important to ascertain the possible effects of cessation of endogenous estrogen secretion. A history of previous hormonal therapy, including oral contraceptives and exogenous estrogens, is important. The presence and nature of a nipple discharge, as well as its association with cyclic ovulation, may provide important clues about etiology.

Approximately 75 to 85 per cent of breast masses are recognized by the patient prior to seeking medical attention. Growth characteristics, reproducibility of the examination during the menstrual cycle, and nipple discharge are pertinent items of information. Pain (mastodynia) with breast swelling and fullness in the immediate premenstrual or postmenstrual period is suggestive of a benign, hormonally sensitive breast lesion. Inquiry into the family history of breast cancer and into constitutional symptoms, including weight loss, fever, hemoptysis, chest pain, anorexia, and bony skeletal pain, is important when the index of suspicion of malignancy is high.

EXAMINATION

Visual Inspection

Prior to palpation, the physician should sit facing the patient, who should be disrobed to the waist, and observe symmetry and skin changes such as fixation, elevation, retraction, and color. Examination is first conducted with the patient's arms at her sides and then on the hips. Contraction of the pectoral muscles will accentuate breast contour. Recognition of diffuse edema as a result of bacterial cellulitis or from endolymphatic permeation of the dermal lymphatics with tumor emboli is important. Segmental entrapment of Cooper's ligaments may produce skin retraction and dimpling, and may be associated with peau d'orange (Fig. 8). This physical finding usually accompanies a deeply palpable, solid mass, which most commonly represents a malignant neoplasm but occasionally may be fat necrosis.

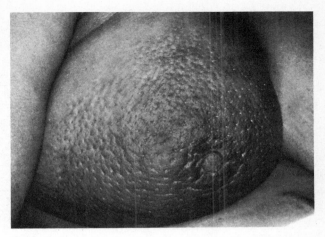

Figure 8. Large, invasive ductal carcinoma with advanced peau d'orange changes.

Palpation of the Breast and Axilla

Systematic palpation of common metastatic sites should be conducted prior to examination of the breast. Examination of the supraclavicular and axillary fossae requires both superficial and deep palpation to identify nodal metastases (Fig. 9*A*). Figure 9*B* depicts the best position for examining the axilla. The patient should be seated with the arm supported by the examiner. Relaxation of the muscles of the shoulder girdle is important, and gentle fingertip pressure best identifies small lymph nodes. Large, bulky extramammary metastases may be obvious to the patient and the physician, and precise documentation of location and size is important during the initial clinical examination. The five nodal groups previously described should be examined, and the palpating fingers should be positioned in the axillary fold so that all infraclavicular structures lateral to Halsted's ligament are evaluated. The examining fingertips compress the axillary contents against the chest wall musculature and the rib cage.

Full extension of the arm with the hand resting on the top of the head flattens the breast against the chest wall and is comfortable for the patient (Fig. 9*C*). Repositioning the patient in the supine position may allow a more thorough examination, particularly with extension and external rotation of the shoulder. A systematic examination of all quadrants of the breast is completed. The object of the evaluation is to detect small lesions that are discrete from the surrounding breast fat and stroma. Lesions that are well circumscribed, painful, and totally separable from adjacent parenchyma usually are not malignant, whereas painless lesions with indistinct borders, classically may be malignant. Distinguishing between benignity and malignancy is impossible on physical examination alone. Clinical judgment and biopsy are required. During the woman's reproductive years the breast has a normal lobular architecture that can be confusing for the patient during breast self-examination. The patient should be instructed how to examine her breasts. The discovery of lesions with three-dimensional characteristics should alert the patient to return to her physician.

The *nipple and areola* should be examined carefully. The presence of nipple inversion should be documented, and, if unilateral, carcinoma should be suspected. The

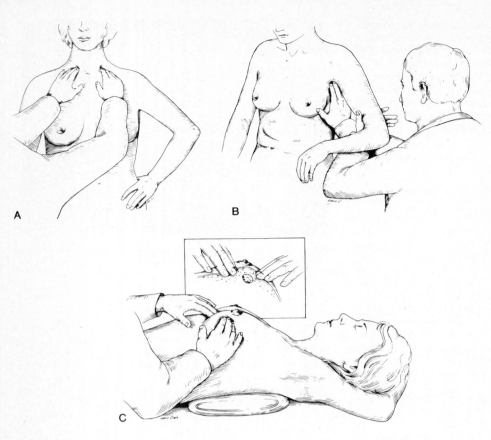

Figure 9. Patient examination. A, examination of supraclavicular and cervical nodes following visual inspection. B, Palpation of axilla. C, Palpation of breast in supine position with digital palpation of focal lesion (inset).

normal, inverted nipple can usually be everted to a correct anatomic position; inability to perform this maneuver warrants biopsy. Benign disease can also involve the nipple-areola complex. Eczema and subareolar inflammatory states are common in the postpartum period during lactation. The presence of an eczematoid, crusty, scaly eruption of the areola is pathognomonic of *Paget's disease* of the nipple. These lesions commonly weep or bleed on contact. Biopsy of Paget's disease confirms a primary ductal carcinoma that has invaded the nipple and skin of the areola to produce the described clinical findings.

Breast Self-Examination

Lay press and media exposure of the epidemiologic frequency and distribution of breast cancer has increased public awareness. The necessity of frequent examination in order to diagnose breast cancer at an early and more favorable stage has been emphasized. The active efforts of the American Cancer Society (ACS) to support public information and education programs have focused on breast self-examination (BSE). A survey by the ACS in 1976 indicated that the percentage of adult women who regularly examine their breasts had increased from 6 to 24 per cent since 1973. Exposure to educational programs also reduces the patient's anxieties about the disease process. Foster and colleagues[16] studied a large group of women with breast carcinoma to determine the relationship between BSE and the clinical and pathologic stage of disease at first diagnosis. Approximately one quarter of patients evaluated performed monthly BSE, whereas half had never performed the examination. A more frequent performance of BSE was associated with the detection of a more favorable clinical stage of breast cancer, fewer axillary lymph node metas-

tases, and a predictably better survival. Other supportive studies suggest that over two thirds of patients who regularly practice BSE will discover neoplasms when the tumor is smaller and will thereby have a more favorable prognosis.

Patients should be carefully instructed to begin a systematic BSE between the ages of 20 and 25. Examination should be done in front of a mirror and in both the sitting and supine positions with the arm hyperextended as described for the physician examination. Ideally, the examination should be conducted 5 to 10 days after the end of menstrual flow when the breasts are least edematous and tender. Also, the examination may be done while the patient is in the shower. A bit of soap and water on the fingertips accentuates tactile sensation. All quadrants of the breast should be examined in an organized and compulsive manner, usually beginning at the periphery and working toward the nipple in a circumferential manner much like the spokes of a wheel.

Roentgenography

XEROMAMMOGRAPHY

In a collaborative effort, the ACS and the National Cancer Institute demonstrated the efficacy of mammography, by low-dose x-ray examination, to detect occult neoplasms otherwise unidentified by experienced examiners. The current application of conventional mammographic techniques and xeromammography (XMM) represents the major modality used to detect such occult, nonpalpable lesions. For purposes of discussion, XMM and the conventional biplane mammogram may be considered to have equivalent diagnostic potential. Both radiographic studies are done in a cephalocaudal and mediolateral projection with reproduction of the XMM pattern on a selenium plate in a positive or negative mode to accentuate tissue density. These radiographic beams consist of electromagnetic energy of very short wavelengths such that matter is variably penetrated as a function of tissue density. The most radiopenetrable substance is fat, whereas the most radiodense (radiopaque) deposits are calcium salts, which are present in approximately 35 to 45 per cent of malignant and premalignant lesions. These deposits occupy the periductal or perilobular position. The extent of calcification is a function of epithelial cell replication and thus accounts for the high frequency of microcalcifications in benign epithelial hyperplasia and noninvasive and invasive neoplasms.

Indications

Routine breast imaging is most useful in detecting breast neoplasms prior to their clinical appearance. The large, fatty breast of the postmenopausal woman and the active dense breast of the young individual are difficult to examine by palpation. Xeromammography is indicated to evaluate a palpable mass and enable one to distinguish between fibrocystic disease and malignancy. The study is of particular value in detecting any unsuspected abnormalities in the contralateral breast of an individual with breast cancer. This technique increases the diagnostic yield approximately twofold over physical examination alone.

Recommendations

At present, recommendations for breast cancer detection suggested by the ACS include: (1) a mammogram every year for asymptomatic women aged 50 years or over; (2) a baseline mammogram for women aged 35 to 39; (3) mammography every 1 to 2 years for women aged 40 to 49, depending on the physical examination and previous mammographic findings as well as additional risk factors; (4) a physical examination by an experienced professional every 3 years for women aged 20 to 40; (5) and an examination every year for those women aged 40 and over.

Radiographic Presentation

Characteristically, xeroradiographic patterns show distortions of the normal breast parenchyma adjacent to malignant tumors. These distortions appear as long or short spicules, or strands of tissue, that radiate from the tumor site. Tissue retraction occurs in the direction of the tumor, and marginal distinction of the malignant tumor from normal parenchyma is lost. The breast cancer may have a stellate appearance on XMM (Fig. 10*A*). Thickening of the skin is apparent on XMM when lymphatic obstruction produces overlying skin edema (peau d'orange). Inflammatory breast cancer represents a lethal, aggressive clinicopathologic variant that is recognizable on XMM. Asymmetric widening of the subcutaneous spaces and prominent subcutaneous lymphatics are seen. Lymphatic vessels appear radiographically engorged by tumor and can be identified in enlarged spaces that radiate as fine streaks perpendicular to the skin (Fig. 10*B*).

Microcalcifications

Soft tissue masses require differentiation between fibronodular or cystic benign lesions of the breast and cancer. The borders of benign lesions are often smooth, and the spiculated or stellate appearance is absent. Microcalcifications may be apparent in both benign and malignant lesions or may be absent from both. Nevertheless, microcalcifications are often the identifying features of an occult, early breast cancer. Microcalcifications scattered in a random fashion throughout the breast, linearly arranged in the configuration of blood vessels, or large (1 to 2 mm.) and single usually represent a benign process. Clustered microcalcifications, often arranged in patterns such as the "spokes of a wheel," are suspicious of malignancy. These calcifications may represent fibrocystic disease, fat necrosis, lobular or intraductal carcinoma *in situ*, or invasive breast cancer (Fig. 10*C*). The identification of an occult area of microcalcification will often necessitate histologic confirmation using radiographically assisted biopsy techniques. Needle localization with XMM documentation of needle position in both craniocaudal and lateral projections allows accurate removal of that portion of the breast containing the suspicious specimen (Fig. 10*D*). The specimen should then be filmed to definitely confirm that the microcalcifications are within it (Fig. 10*E*).

Reliability

The possibility of a carcinoma being present clinically and the XMM failing to reveal it (false-negative) exceeds 10 per cent in many clinics. The false-positive diagnosis of carcinoma is much less (< 5 per cent), and diagnostic accuracy increases as a correlate of the quality of XMM imaging technique and the experience of the radiologist. The incidence of false-negative XMM is too great to utilize this radiographic technique to exclude the diagnosis of carcinoma in a suspicious, solitary breast mass. Additionally, dense, multinodular breasts of advanced fibrocystic disease and small breasts that are difficult to film commonly invalidate the interpretation of xeromammographic images and may obscure the diagnosis of occult malignancies.[6] *Radiographic imaging should not, therefore, be considered a uniformly reliable method to exclude the diagnosis of cancer.* Histologic confirmation of clinically suspicious (radiographically negative) lesions by biopsy is appropriate to avoid such interpretive errors.

THERMOGRAPHY

Electromagnetic heat patterns emitted from malignant lesions may be measured by special thermographic plates. This noninvasive diagnostic modality has no irradiation risk. Nonetheless, this modality is still considered to be investigative, and the accuracy for diagnosis of malignant lesions is less than 70 per cent. False-positive results are more common than with conventional mammography or xeromammography, thereby sharply restricting the usefulness of the study.

SONOGRAPHY

Ultrasound mammography is a noninvasive method for reproducing high-resolution tomographic sections through the breast. The development of a gray scale unit has greatly improved the quality of ultrasonographic images. This modality has the advantage of differentiating a solid breast mass from a cystic breast mass. This adjunctive parameter may complement the XMM without any additional risk of irradiation. The newer gray scale diagnostic accuracy of ultrasound approaches 80 to 85 per cent with low false-negative (7.6 per cent) and false-positive (18 to 20 per cent) rates.[11]

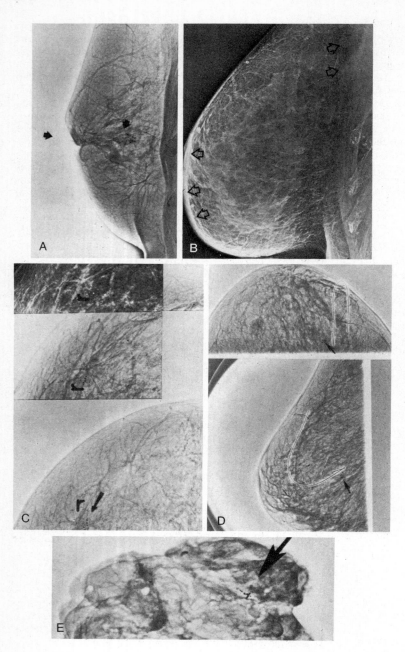

Figure 10. A, *Xeromammographic (XMM) appearance of scirrhous carcinoma with distortions of normal parenchyma (arrow) adjacent to the dense tumor mass. (Courtesy Dr. J. E. Tiestra.)* B, *Inflammatory breast carcinoma. Lymphatic vessels replaced with tumor emboli are identified as fine streaks that radiate perpendicular (arrow) to the skin surface. Enlarged axillary lymph nodes are evident. (Courtesy Dr. J. B. Buchanan, Louisville, Ky.)* C, *Stippled microcalcifications (arrow) in breast carcinoma with magnification views, positive and negative modes. Calcifications are irregular in size and shape and occur in small clusters or in linear configurations.* D, *XMM-guided needle localization for microcalcifications (arrow) of occult cancer.* E, *Specimen radiogram documenting excision of microcalcifications (arrow).*

Techniques for Breast Biopsy

A histopathologic diagnosis should be established for solid, benign, and malignant lesions of the breast. Varying techniques can be utilized to establish the diagnosis after procurement of fluid or tissue.

CYTOLOGIC EXAMINATION

Cystic fluid obtained from needle aspiration of macrocysts of the breast parenchyma can be centrifuged and the sediment examined cytologically. This technique is also useful for histologic examination of nipple discharges. Slide preparation and fixation is similar to that for the Papanicolaou smear. The infrequent diagnosis of neoplastic cells obtained from macrocysts of the breast reflects the rarity

of cystic cancers. All guaiac- or Hemoccult-positive nipple discharge and cystic fluid should be examined cytologically. Clear, turbid, green, or brown fluid, however, is typical of fibrocystic disease, and the yield of malignant cells from cytologic examination of such fluid is so low as to call into question the cost-effectiveness of the procedure.

NEEDLE ASPIRATION CYTOLOGY

A small-bore needle is inserted into a solid mass and suction is applied so that typical cells can be retrieved into the needle, aspirated onto a slide, and examined cytologically. The specimen may be immediately air-dried or fixed in alcohol with subsequent staining with hematoxylin and eosin. Although over half of the cases can be diagnosed utilizing this technique, reproducibility and confirmation are directly correlated with the experience of the cytologist and the slide preparation technique. A negative report does not exclude the diagnosis of carcinoma; however, false-positive reports are extremely rare. A positive diagnosis directly correlates with the size of the neoplasm, the number of aspiration attempts, and the experience of the examiner.

NEEDLE BIOPSY

A solid, definable breast mass may be amenable to needle biopsy. Various needle biopsy devices (Vim-Silverman, Menghini, Trucut) are available to obtain representative core sections of the breast neoplasm. This simple procedure is done under local anesthesia for superficial tumors that are well circumscribed but central or deep in breast parenchyma. A false-positive diagnosis is extraordinarily rare, and the diagnosis can be established in approximately 80 per cent of cases. Adequate tissue sampling is related to the size and consistency of the neoplasm and the experience of the individual obtaining the biopsy specimen. The procedure should be limited to lesions greater than 1 cm. in size. Care must be exercised to avoid penetration through the tumor into the pectoralis major or serratus anterior muscles. Implantation of tumor cells into these structures may be a source of locoregional recurrence. Biopsy tract implantation may occur between the skin and the tumor, and planned excision of the biopsy tract with the primary neoplasm should be an integral part of definitive therapy at mastectomy.

Needle biopsy can be done in an outpatient setting under local anesthesia at minimal cost and with negligible patient morbidity. Inferential data suggest that needle biopsy has less potential to disseminate tumor cells within the breast than does an open biopsy, during which time the primary neoplasm is transected. This technique has a higher yield and lower false-negative rate than needle aspiration cytology. The false-negative results still remain too high to use needle biopsy to exclude the diagnosis of cancer; thus, adequate tissue sampling with open techniques is advised when the diagnosis is inconclusive.

OPEN BIOPSY TECHNIQUES

Open biopsy remains the definitive method for diagnosing carcinoma of the breast. The decision between an *excisional* or *incisional biopsy* is dependent upon the size of the primary neoplasm and the ability to extirpate the lesion intact via an appropriate incision. Open techniques rarely yield false-positive or false-negative reports. Figure 11A depicts classic nonradial incisions. They may be circumareolar (Fig. 11B) or within the superior or inferior halves of the breast in directions that parallel Langer's lines. Excisional biopsy (Fig. 11C) is the best treatment of benign tumors of the breast (e.g., fibroadenoma, fat necrosis, intraductal papilloma, fibrocystic disease) and may be both diagnostic and therapeutic. The ability to totally extirpate a solitary lesion that exceeds 3 cm. in diameter is dependent on the location of the tumor and the size of the breast. Removal of large portions of breast tissue for benign conditions is to be avoided to minimize the cosmetic deformity. Attempts at total extirpation of suspicious neoplasms greater than 3 cm. in size often result in, at least, partial transection of the neoplasm, particularly if the surgeon is using local anesthesia in the outpatient setting. Breast cancer cells may be released into the wound and may disseminate through the breast as easily as do red cells if there is a delay of several days before definitive mastectomy. Suspicious neoplasms that exceed 3 cm. are best biopsied via needle or incisional techniques immediately

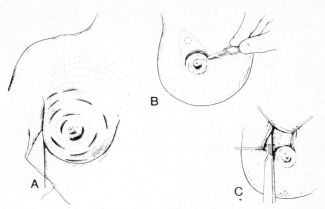

Figure 11. Open biopsy techniques. A, *Sites for nonradial incisions placed parallel to Langer's lines.* B, *Circumareolar incision for access to lesion in 11 o'clock axis.* C, *Development of skin flaps for excisional biopsy.*

prior to planned mastectomy. The mastectomy incision can easily encompass the biopsy wound without entry into it, and no time will elapse to allow any "free" tumor cells to permeate the breast or future skin flaps.

The application of mammography to detect *occult lesions* and sites of *microcalcification* often requires special techniques to facilitate biopsy. An identified nonpalpable tumor or sites of suspicious microcalcification may be localized by XMM-directed needle placement. The patient is then transferred from the radiology suite to the operating room, where the area of needle localization is explored through a counterincision (Fig. 12). Specimen radiography

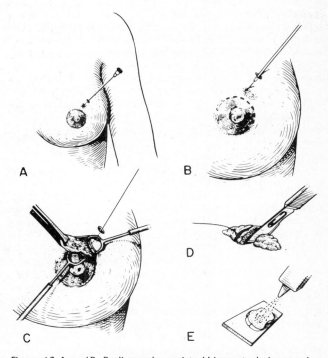

Figure 12. A and B, *Radiography-assisted biopsy techniques using the Kopan needle for xeromammographic localization.* C, *Circumareolar counter incision with retrieval of hook of Kopan needle in radiographically imaged microcalcifications.* D, *and* E, *Bread loafing of biopsy specimen to identify tumor with microcalcifications employing specimen radiography.* (From Bland, K. I., and Buchanan, J. B.: Preoperative localization of nonpalpable (occult) lesions of the breast. In O'Leary, J. P., and Woltering, E. A. (Eds.): Techniques for Surgeons. New York, John Wiley & Sons, 1985.)

is done to confirm that the site of suspicious microcalcifications was resected adequately. Also, methylene blue (approximately 0.1 to 0.2 cc.) may be injected through the radiographically placed needle. Identification of the vital stain in the resected specimen is indicative of an adequate excision, assuming that the needle was positioned properly. Permanent histologic sections are usually required to document the presence of minimal breast cancer.

BENIGN BREAST DISEASE

Proliferative and Nonproliferative Breast Disease ("Fibrocystic" Disease, Chronic Cystic Mastitis)

The first description of benign cystic disease of the breast is credited to Sir Astley Cooper, who subsequently classified its various forms as cystic disease, mastodynia, and adenosis. These forms are interrelated, and together they constitute the most common abnormality of female sexual maturity. Subsequent descriptions by Schimmelbusch (1890) of the microscopic features of cystic disease confirmed the process to be a proliferation of epithelial elements with formation of cysts and loss of normal interacinar connective tissue. Although controversy over the variants of proliferative and nonproliferative diseases exists, for purposes of discussion mastopathy of this type should be considered synonymous with chronic cystic mastitis, benign mastopathy, mammary dysplasia, and cystic disease of the breast.

Etiology

Proliferative diseases (PD) and nonproliferative diseases (nonPD) of the breast are the most frequently diagnosed lesions of the breast and are pathologic processes that occur as a consequence of cyclic, ovarian stimulation of the epithelial and lobular components of the mamma. Development of PD and nonPD after menarche and clinical regression following menopause strongly implicate estrogens and progestins in the etiology. Additionally, prolactin and, more recently, methylxanthines (caffeine) have been suggested as causative agents. The absolute prevalence is unknown, yet autopsy specimens from elderly women contain variable pathologic evidence of PD and nonPD of the breast in virtually 100 per cent of cases. Progression to a disease state with macrocysts, fibrosis, and epithelial proliferation invariably occurs as the result of the dynamic influences of ovarian stimulation. Epithelial changes in rodents treated with exogenous estrogen range from duct adenosis to cystic alterations and from ductal epithelial proliferation to atypia and carcinoma.

Etiology of this entity thus appears to be multifactorial, but the essential factor of relative hyperestrinism initiates epithelial hyperplasia. Also, genetic factors, mammotropic pituitary hormones, and other circulating, nongonadal hormones (e.g., thyroxin, growth hormone, insulin) are operative. Estrogen increases stromal ground substance, which has the propensity to fibrous reorganization. The time of active stimulation of the hormonally sensitive components of the breast corresponds to the peak incidence of the disease, i.e., during the reproductive years, and regression of symptoms follows removal of estrogen and progesterone stimuli at the time of menopause or castration.

Cystic Changes

The cystic changes may be microcystic or macrocystic. Examination of the typical patient reveals diffuse breast fullness and fibronodularity. Cysts of nonproliferative disease may be solitary or multiple and are usually well demarcated, mobile, smooth, and nontender. Both small and large cysts may have a characteristic appearance (e.g., blue-dome cyst of Bloodgood) and may be managed by aspiration (Fig. 13). The fluid recovered is usually clear or straw-colored; however, when the cysts are longstanding, the color becomes gray-green and turbid. Bloody cystic fluid warrants cytologic evaluation and biopsy if a residual mass is palpable after aspiration. These solid lesions may suggest a cystic carcinoma or the presence of a primary cancer coexistent with cystic mastitis.

The frequently applied term "fibrocystic disease" is not descriptive; rather, it denotes a wide variety of histopathologic events in which sclerosing adenosis (epithelial proliferation), fibrous dysplasia (stromal proliferation), blunt duct adenosis (proliferation of ducts without acini), or apocrine metaplasia of ductal epithelium may coexist. None of these terms indicates an inflammatory process, although rarely macrocysts may become spontaneously or iatrogenically inflamed. Despite this multitude of associated benign pathologic entities, clinical manifestations relate almost exclusively to ovarian hormonal stimuli.

Histology

It is becoming increasingly evident that histologic variables, such as degree and character of the *hyperplastic epithelial proliferation*, represent a continuum from *hyperplasia* to frank *neoplasia*. Furthermore, the greater the number of histologic subsets, the more probable that these variables are similar and share comon pathologic features. Dupont and Page[12] have more recently separated the aforementioned histologic lesions of benign breast tissue biopsies into three prognostically predictive categories: (1) nonproliferative lesions (nonPD), (2) proliferative disease without atypia (PDWA), and (3) atypical hyperplasia (AH).

The common *nonproliferative lesions* are typified by mild hyperplasia, cysts, epithelial calcification (calcific densities), and fibroadenomata. These lesions made up 70 per cent of this operative series of benign breast masses. In distinction, *proliferative disease without atypia* constituted 26.7 per cent of the breast masses and includes florid and moderate hyperplasia, atypical lobular hyperplasia, papillomata, and sclerosing adenosis. Advanced proliferative

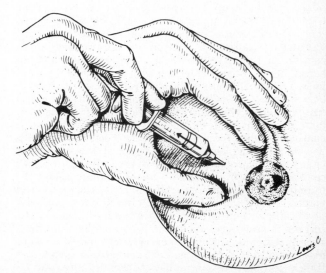

Figure 13. Technique for needle aspiration of cystic lesion of the breast.

lesions, or *atypical hyperplasia*, are composed of both ductal and lobular subtypes and are considered to possess marginal features of *carcinoma in situ*.

CLINICAL PRESENTATION

Patients with PD and nonPD usually complain of pain and fullness in one or both breasts immediately prior to beginning menstrual flow. Over the next 10 to 14 days, the symptoms gradually subside. Pain may radiate down the arm in the distribution of the sensory fibers of the intercostobrachial nerve and is referred to this area from the upper outer quadrant of the breast. Small or large cysts may appear during this time and regress spontaneously. Symptomatic lesions may occur at any time but are most common immediately after menarche and in the perimenopausal period. It is during this latter period that differentiation from a malignant lesion is most difficult.

DIAGNOSIS

Although histologic identification of the coexistence of PDWA and cancer is common, evidence for the relationship of the two entities remains circumstantial. Haagensen reported a fourfold increase in the incidence of cancer in patients previously treated for "fibrocystic" disease without distinction of its proliferative and atypical hyperplastic components. The prevalence of PD and nonPD, however, is so great that the association between the entity and cancer is probably inevitable and coincidental. The diagnosis of cancer by physical examination in an individual with extensive PD or nonPD is difficult. A family history of breast cancer adds additional significance to the risk for carcinoma. Any cystic lesion should be aspirated. If cystic breast disease is the prevailing diagnosis, the patient may be allowed to complete another menstrual cycle and then undergo re-evaluation by physical examination. If the lesion regresses, the diagnosis is confirmed; if it remains, biopsy is considered. Approximately 25 per cent of patients subjected to biopsy should have a malignant neoplasm, or the method of case selection for biopsy has not been appropriately discriminating. The screening of asymptomatic women may yield a much higher cancer-biopsy ratio (approximately 1:6 to 8).[6]

THERAPY

Therapy for physiologic nodularity, other than biopsy to exclude cancer, is directed toward control of pain. Reassurance and mild analgesics usually are all that are required. Androgenic steroids may diminish breast size and pain but are not justified because of their masculinizing side effects. Exogenous cycling of the menstrual period with the oral contraceptives norethynodrel and mestranol (Enovid) has produced good to excellent responses in over half the patients evaluated objectively. The addition of high doses of progesterone may sustain the response. Recently, a synthetic androgen, danazol, has been of therapeutic value. It diminishes secretion of FSH and LH and initiates reduction of ovarian estrogen. Also, it appears to actively compete with estrogen at cellular receptor sites within the breast parenchyma. The side effects of amenorrhea, edema, hot flashes, acne, and muscle cramps are common; the cost of the medication is high, and it must be taken several weeks or months for best results. Its use should be limited to patients with severe symptoms. In patients who respond to danazol, the results are dramatic and objective regres-

sion of palpable disease occurs, Recently, caffeine, cyclic nucleotides, and saturated dietary fats have been implicated as mechanistic agents for benign and malignant disease. The role of foodstuffs and vitamin deficiencies as possible causative agents of breast disease is plausible but unproven to date.[20]

Gynecomastia

Enlargement of the breast in the prepubertal or pubertal male is a consequence of the developmental hormonal milieu. Classically, it occurs between the ages of 13 and 17. The responsible mechanism is poorly understood, but a hyperestrogenic state relative to endogenous androgen secretion is the best explanation. Gynecomastia perhaps occurs secondary to a delay in reversal of the androstenedione-testosterone ratio, normally an event of puberty. Correlation with assays of circulating sex hormones has been disappointing. Enlargement and tenderness of the breast bud may be bilateral or unilateral. Reassurance for the patient and parent is the only therapy required.

Gynecomastia may be the result of a definable etiology. For example, hormonally active tumors may produce gynecomastia, and an examination of the testicles for unsuspected masses should be part of the patient's evaluation. Estrogen is metabolized by the liver; consequently, patients with cirrhosis often develop bilateral gynecomastia. Exogenous injection of estrogen, e.g., for treatment of prostatic carcinoma, and specific drugs, such as digoxin, phenytoin (Dilantin), and marijuana, may produce gynecomastia.

Once the diagnosis is established, the hypertrophic breast tissue may be resected via a circumareolar incision to re-establish a flattened breast contour. Typically, histologic studies confirm the absence of acinar growth and a background of proliferative breast stroma and lactiferous ducts.

Senescent hypertrophy is an event of the male menopause that usually involves both breasts but at different times. The breast tissue is typically enlarged, firm, and tender. This finding usually occurs between the ages of 50 and 70 and spontaneously regresses within 6 to 12 months. Differentiation from carcinoma is essential because cancer of the breast in males accounts for 1 per cent of all breast carcinoma, and peak incidence is in this age group. Should doubt exist, open biopsy should be done.

Galactocele

Obstruction of a lactiferous duct and distention with milk may follow termination of pregnancy and cessation of prolactin stimulation of the breast. The typical location is the subareolar region. The engorged duct is tender, and efforts at manual decompression are usually unsuccessful. The lesion is best managed by excision via a circumareolar incision.

Inflammatory States of the Breast

ACUTE INFLAMMATION

Acute inflammatory conditions of the breast most often are a result of retrograde bacterial infections secondary to disruption of the epithelial interface of the nipple-areola complex. The most common bacteria recovered are of the

Staphylococcus and *Streptococcus* species. These inflammatory states are related to lactation and usually occur within the first weeks of breastfeeding. The inflammatory process may progress to diffuse breast cellulitis with loculated central and subareolar abscesses. Streptococcal infections produce diffuse cellulitis without localization until late in the course of the disease when the patient may present with bacteremia and systemic manifestations. *Staphylococcus aureus* abscesses are typically well circumscribed, fluctuant, and multilocular (Fig. 14). When the abscess is deep in the breast, diagnosis may be difficult.

Periareolar abscesses most often occur in the nonlactating breast. These lesions are frustrating for both patient and physician and may require frequent incision and drainage. On occasion, extensive ablative surgical procedures may be necessary for persistent abscess cavities and sinus tracts.

The presence of an advanced unilocular or multilocular abscess requires immediate surgical intervention and adequate drainage. Cultures for aerobic and anaerobic bacteria, fungi, and atypical tuberculous organisms are imperative. Prior to receiving the culture results, a penicillin derivative is administered. Thorough débridement of the abscess via a circumareolar incision or multiple incisions placed in the direction of Langer's lines is recommended. In the postpartum state, discontinuation of the suckling reflex and the use of a breast suction pump may be advantageous to empty stagnant milk ducts and prevent progressive stasis and bacterial overgrowth in central abscess cavities. Persistent lactation may require intramuscular injections of testosterone enanthate-estradiol valerate (Deladumone) or oral bromocriptine (Parlodel) to induce cessation of lactation and breast involution.

Chronic Inflammation

Chronic inflammatory conditions with abscess formation are relatively uncommon. Although it is less frequently

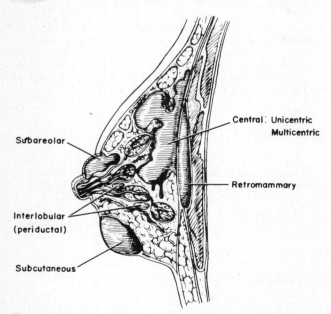

Figure 14. Sagittal section of breast with potential abscess sites. Typical central abscess may be multicentric or focal. Retromammary abscess may be seen in chronic infectious or neoplastic processes (e.g., tuberculosis, carcinoma). Extensive deep abscess may be multilocular and communicate with subcutaneous or subareolar sites. The painful subcutaneous, interlobular, or subareolar abscess may present with diffuse cellulitis.

found than two decades ago, the ubiquitous tuberculous organism still remains the most common cause of chronic bacterial mastitis. The breast tuberculoma is usually nontender and typically has multiple, subcutaneous sinus tracts that extend from deep within the breast to sites of subcutaneous cavitation. Cellulitis may be an associated finding. The demonstration of acid-fast tubercule bacilli in the lesion or at culture is diagnostic. Therapy consists of adequate drainage similar to that for acute or chronic bacterial abscesses and the initiation of antituberculous therapy. Extensive biopsy of the abscess cavity, especially if chronic, is necessary to exclude the possibility of a coexisting invasive cancer.

Mondor's Disease: Thrombophlebitis of the Superficial Thoracoepigastric Vein

The finding of a palpable cordlike thickening of the superficial distribution of the thoracoepigastric vein as it traverses the lateral thorax to the anterior axillary line is diagnostic of Mondor's disease. The patient has acute pain over the superolateral breast or axilla, often related to local trauma. The significance of this process is its differentiation from other benign or malignant diseases of the breast. Symptomatic treatment with heat and analgesics is all that is required.

Nipple Discharge

Nipple discharge occurs in 3 to 9 per cent of patients as a result of alteration in the normal physiologic consequences of duct epithelial secretion. The discharge may be indicative of an inflammatory, proliferative, or neoplastic process. Discharges of pathologic significance usually empty spontaneously from the ductal sinus recesses of the nipple ampullae. Discharges elicited by "milking" segments of the breast parenchyma or the nipple-areola complex are most often benign.

Character of Discharge

The character of the discharge is pathognomonic of the etiology. Four basic discharge types are recognized: bloody, milky, serous, and yellow.

Bloody Discharge. A bloody discharge is the most common type in reported series (50 to 75 per cent) and may vary from bright-red to brown in color. In active breast clinics, however, the most common discharge will be dark-green in color, although the patient may mistake it for blood, since a dark discharge from any orifice is usually interpreted as blood. Dispersing a drop of the discharge on a gauze sponge will usually identify the true color, and a Hemoccult test will confirm blood if doubt exists. The majority of bloody discharges are benign and result from epithelial proliferations that occur as a component of cystic disease or an *intraductal papilloma*. Differentiation from bloody nipple discharge emanating from an *intraductal papillary carcinoma* is important. A solitary mass in a postmenopausal patient who presents with bloody nipple discharge should be considered a malignant process necessitating confirmation by biopsy and/or Papanicolaou smear. In the spectrum of diagnoses, malignancy accounts for 9 to 14 per cent of bloody nipple discharges, whereas intraductal papilloma is the most common diagnosis followed by cystic disease and duct ectasia. Haagensen reported that 11.5 per cent of spontaneous nipple discharges were of malignant origin, of which 55 per cent were bloody.

When a lesion is not identifiable by clinical examination

or mammography, exploration of the subareolar space is indicated. Often the patient will describe a tender, palpable, circumareolar or subareolar mass in a specific breast quadrant that periodically empties with squeezing or on direct compression of the mass. In this instance, precise localization and excision are possible. Radiographic imaging by contrast ductography will occasionally permit preoperative localization of the dilated duct and demonstrate a filling defect.[9]

Milky Discharge. With the consistency and composition of milk, this type of discharge may be evident several months post partum and after cessation of lactation. Milky discharge has no relationship to the development of carcinoma. The production and release of LTH can be inhibited by appropriate doses of estrogen, androgen, and progestins. Infrequently, milky discharge is a symptom of acromegaly and occurs as a result of the mammotropic effect of growth hormone on breast acini.

Serous Discharge. This thin, translucent, and straw-colored discharge may occur spontaneously as a result of normal menses, cyclic oral contraceptives, or early in pregnancy. Intraductal papilloma may be etiologic and can be demonstrated by contrast ductography prior to surgical excision.

Yellow Discharge. This type is indicative of cystic disease or a galactocele. It is associated infrequently with carcinoma. Cytology of the discharge, although desirable, is rarely of diagnostic value.

RARE CAUSES OF DISCHARGE

Rare conditions causing nipple discharge are unrecognized surges in circulating serum prolactin initiated by the acidophilic, lactogenic cells of the anterior pituitary. Elevated levels have been noted in 25 per cent of patients with nipple secretion of various etiologic types and occur most commonly from normal physiologic mechanisms associated with nursing, intercourse, pregnancy, and stress.[27] Additionally, oral contraceptives, antihypertensive agents, and some psychotropic drugs may raise serum prolactin levels.

Approximately one third of patients with secondary amenorrhea and one fourth of patients with galactorrhea have elevated serum prolactin levels. Elevated prolactin values implicate a continuum of pathologic disorders of the neuroendocrine system that produce anovulatory syndromes, hirsutism, sterility, obesity, acne, and loss of libido. Anovulatory syndromes associated with galactorrhea may resolve spontaneously following inhibition of prolactin secretion by bromocriptine or clomiphene. Diligent follow-up is required, however, since a responsible pituitary neoplasm may not be detected until several years later. Multiple determinations of serum prolactin and radiographs of the sella turcica are indicated. Bromocriptine (Parlodel) or clomiphene (Serophene) therapy may be used to control the growth and symptoms of prolactin-producing pituitary microadenomas.[27]

Benign Neoplasms

FIBROADENOMA

Fibroadenoma is a solid, encapsulated, well-circumscribed neoplasm and is the most common breast lesion in women under 25 years of age. The great majority (80 per cent) are solitary. The neoplasm usually presents as a rubbery, firm, nontender, lobulated, mobile breast mass 1 to 4 cm. in size. It is hormonally dependent and may fluctuate as much as 1 cm. in diameter under the estrogenic influences of normal menses, pregnancy, lactation, or the use of oral contraceptives. Rapid growth may be apparent during pregnancy or lactation. Treatment is by excisional biopsy and should be advised because involutional regression is rare. The gross appearance is different from that of any mammary tumor. The edges are sharp, and the cut surface is grayish-white to pink and grossly homogeneous. Histologically, there is a pericanalicular arrangement of lobules that contain dense stroma and proliferative epithelium. A variant may show remarkable epithelial proliferation of mature, irregular, closely packed glands with a secretory epithelium (Fig. 15).

Fibroadenomas removed during lactation are quite cellular and have been mistaken on frozen section for well-differentiated adenocarcinomas. The pathologist examining a fibroadenoma removed during pregnancy should always be informed that the lesion came from a lactating breast.

Giant Fibroadenomas

Giant fibroadenomas or *giant intracanalicular myxomas* are 10 cm. or greater in diameter. In this variant, the connective tissue is more active and proliferative than that in the smaller fibroadenoma. Large polypoid masses appear to project into parenchymal channels and are covered by epithelium that produces a mosaic of distorted variations. These large lesions often result in distortion of the breast, and excision appears to result in an even worse deformity.

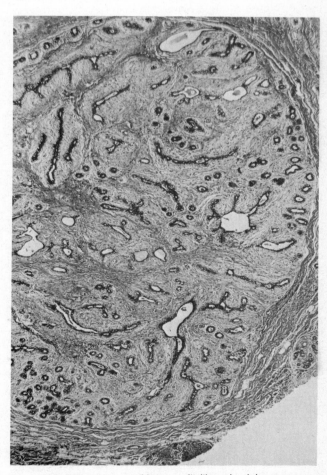

Figure 15. Fibroadenoma. Narrow, slit-like, glandular spaces are surrounded and indented by connective tissue. A sharply demarcated nonencapsulated lobular mass is characteristic (10X). (Courtesy Dr. R. L. Hackett.)

This lesion, however, is a true neoplasm and compresses the surrounding normal breast tissue. Several months after simple excision, this compressed tissue re-expands to return the breast to its original contour.

Cystosarcoma Phyllodes

A rare variant of fibroadenoma, cystosarcoma phyllodes, accounts for less than 1 per cent of all benign and malignant lesions of the breast. Its name is a misnomer, since it is rarely malignant and usually not cystic. Its origin may be from a pre-existing cellular fibroadenoma that now contains one or more components of mesenchymal origin. Differentiation from a fibroadenoma is based on a greater degree of stromal cellularity, cellular pleomorphism, hyperchromatic nuclei, and a significant number of mitotic figures. The characteristic protrusion of polypoid masses of hyperplastic stroma into compressed canaliculi to produce a leaf-like appearance suggested the term phyllodes (Gr. *phyllon*, leaf, and *eidos*, form) to Johannes Müller in 1838. The lesion often attains a large teardrop appearance. The overlying skin is not involved, yet it may be erythematous and warm and may contain multiple dilated veins. Histologically, 25 per cent of these lesions will appear malignant; 10 per cent will metastasize. Malignant transformation occurs in the stromal (mesothelial) component of the tumor, and metastases are almost invariably by the hematogenous route to the lungs rather than to axillary lymph nodes.

These neoplasms are not well encapsulated, and microscopic projections of tumor may penetrate the surrounding breast parenchyma. Simple excision or enucleation commonly leads to local recurrence. These tumors often are difficult to clinically distinguish from an advanced adenocarcinoma; however, they rarely involve skin. Lesions occupying a major portion of the breast are best managed by total mastectomy. Since regional nodes are rarely involved, node dissection is unnecessary. Smaller lesions may be managed by wide local excision with a minimal 1-cm. margin of normal breast parenchyma. More radical procedures appear unjustified, since this neoplasm behaves as a low-grade, soft tissue sarcoma rather than a carcinoma of glandular origin.[10]

Fat Necrosis

A benign lesion of breast parenchyma, fat necrosis may masquerade as a carcinoma. It most often results from trauma to the breast, and a history of recent breast injury can be elicited in greater than 50 per cent of cases. Often an area of ecchymosis surrounds the tender, firm, ill-defined mass that has the clinical characteristics of carcinoma on both physical and XMM examination. Even peau d'orange and skin retraction may exist. Excisional biopsy is indicated for diagnosis and to alleviate the pain and cosmetic deformity that commonly accompany the lesion. Distinction from carcinoma must be verified histologically. Microscopically, a chronic inflammatory response with foreign body giant cells, cyst formations, and angular calcifications containing cholesterol crystals differentiate this lesion from cancer.

Intraductal Papilloma

The presence of a bloody or serous nipple discharge in a premenopausal female without an associated parenchymal breast mass suggests an intraductal papilloma. These lesions typically occur in the major lactiferous channels of the subareolar-nipple complex. They are usually 1 to 2 mm. in diameter and soft and often are not palpable. They appear as raspberry-like projections from the side wall of the ducts and may attain sizes greater than 1 cm. Intraductal papillomas are benign, although intraductal papillary carcinoma has been reported to occur as a transformation from the papillary proliferation of this lesion. Cytologic characteristics and evidence of invasion are the most important differential criteria.

These lesions are treated by wedge resection of the duct mechanism. Should no papilloma be found in the suspected duct, a segmental resection of the subareolar breast should be completed. More radical procedures are not justifiable unless clear documentation of an invasive lesion is confirmed.

Mammary Duct Ectasia (Plasma Cell Mastitis)

Lesions are painful and show an associated mass, dermal fixation, and/or nipple inversion. Breast edema and inflammatory changes may also be present. The lesions are benign but mimic carcinoma by their clinical and radiographic appearance. Microscopically, there is dilatation of atrophic ducts, retention of acellular debris, and an infiltration of plasma cells. Because of the diffuse nature of the lesion and the clinical suspicion of carcinoma, multiple biopsies are necessary to confirm the benignity of this lesion.

Granular Cell Myoblastoma

Granular cell myoblastoma is an uncommon neoplasm of mesodermal origin. The typical lesion is smaller than 2 cm. in diameter and may be confused both clinically and radiographically with an early adenocarcinoma. Local excision is curative.

CANCER OF THE BREAST

Epidemiology

Carcinoma of the breast is the most common site-specific neoplasm in women and is the leading cause of death from cancer in females 40 to 44 years of age. Breast cancer represents 26 per cent of all female cancers and is responsible for 18 per cent of the cancer-related deaths in women (Fig. 16). Approximately 123,000 invasive breast carcinomas were diagnosed in the United States in 1986, from which about 39,900 women will die. Until the past decade, breast cancer was unchallenged as the leading cause of cancer-related mortality. However, in 1985, lung cancer surpassed breast carcinoma as the leading cause of cancer-related death in women (Fig. 17). Mortality from breast cancer has remained stable, whereas the overall incidence of the disease in the United States has increased. This relative decrease in mortality rate reflects the detection of an increased percentage of early breast cancers. Between 1959 and 1964, 5-year survival rates were 63 and 46 per cent for Caucasian and black women, respectively, whereas similar figures for the 1973 to 1980 period were 74 and 62 per cent. Increase in public awareness, mammography, and improved adjuvant therapy are most responsible for this increase in overall survival.

Breast cancer is a common disease. Presently, approximately 1 out of every 14 women (7 per cent) will develop

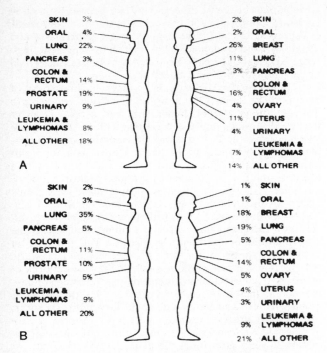

A

SKIN	3%		2%	SKIN
ORAL	4%		2%	ORAL
LUNG	22%		26%	BREAST
PANCREAS	3%		11%	LUNG
			3%	PANCREAS
COLON & RECTUM	14%		16%	COLON & RECTUM
PROSTATE	19%		4%	OVARY
URINARY	9%		11%	UTERUS
			4%	URINARY
LEUKEMIA & LYMPHOMAS	8%		7%	LEUKEMIA & LYMPHOMAS
ALL OTHER	18%		14%	ALL OTHER

B

SKIN	2%		1%	SKIN
ORAL	3%		1%	ORAL
LUNG	35%		18%	BREAST
PANCREAS	5%		19%	LUNG
			5%	PANCREAS
COLON & RECTUM	11%		14%	COLON & RECTUM
PROSTATE	10%		5%	OVARY
URINARY	5%		4%	UTERUS
			3%	URINARY
LEUKEMIA & LYMPHOMAS	9%		9%	LEUKEMIA & LYMPHOMAS
ALL OTHER	20%		21%	ALL OTHER

Figure 16. A, Estimate of the incidence of cancer in 1986 by site and sex. B, Estimate of cancer-related deaths in 1986 by site and sex. (Courtesy E. Silverberg, Department of Epidemiology and Statistics, American Cancer Society.)

breast cancer. Fifty per cent of these women will succumb to this disease. Although women currently report suspicious masses earlier to their physician, the mortality rate remains high and directly relates to the stage of disease at diagnosis.

Mormon, Seventh-Day Adventist, Alaskan Indian and Eskimo, American Indian, Mexican-American, Japanese, and Philippino women living in Hawaii have a lower per capita incidence of breast cancer, whereas nuns and Jewish women have a higher than average incidence of the disease. These variations in incidence are multifactorial and, perhaps, related to genetic, environmental, dietary, ethnic, and hormonal factors.

DIETARY INFLUENCES

Human populations in countries with an increased incidence of breast cancer tend to have a high dietary fat intake. Additional circumstantial evidence for fat as a causative agent comes from an observation made in Japanese women. As their dietary fat intake increases, the incidence of breast cancer increases. Japanese women who migrate to the United States have a low incidence of breast cancer, similar to women in Japan. For second- and third-generation offspring of these migrants, however, incidence rates approach those of Caucasian women born in the United States. These studies strongly implicate environmental rather than genetic factors, and the difference in dietary fat intake between the native Japanese and American-Japanese woman is dramatic. Fat as a causative factor is supported by the low incidence rates among Seventh-Day Adventists, who also have a much lower than average dietary fat consumption. The investigation of the relationship between fat and breast cancer has just begun, and, no doubt, additional variables will be discovered.

MULTIPLE CANCERS

Women with carcinoma of one breast have an increased risk of developing carcinoma of the opposite breast. For women under the age of 50, this risk approaches 0.7 to 1.0 per cent per year over that of the general population. Multiple primary cancers involving the breast, endometrium, and ovary occur more frequently together than is expected by chance alone. Generally, in women with cancer at one of these sites, there is a twofold risk for developing cancer at one of the other sites.

GENETIC FACTORS

Anderson[2] and Lynch and coworkers[24] have demonstrated that the greatest risk of breast cancer is for a woman under the age of 50 whose sister and mother both had breast cancer. The female relatives of a woman with bilateral breast cancer have a risk five and one-half times higher than that of the general population, and if bilateral breast cancers occur before menopause, the risk for relatives increases ninefold. Early onset and/or bilaterality should alert the physician to the possibility of *familial breast cancer*. An improved 5-year age-adjusted relative survival is evident when compared with *sporadic* nonfamilial breast cancer managed in conventional fashion. Interpretation of risk factors, appropriate genetic counseling, and surveillance of family members are important aspects of the physician's management of the patient with breast cancer.[24] The risk for female relatives of a woman who has cancer in only

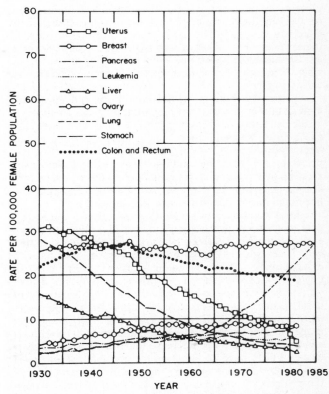

Figure 17. Age-standardized female cancer death rates in the United States by site, 1930 to 1985. A stable mortality rate for breast cancer is evident in U.S. women comparative to declining death rates for liver, gastric, and uterine carcinoma. An increase in death rate has been observed for lung, pancreas, ovary, and leukemia. Lung cancer surpassed breast carcinoma as the leading cancer-related mortality for females in 1985.

one breast is slightly greater than that of the average female population.

HORMONAL INFLUENCES

Childbearing and Fertility. Nulliparous and infertile women have a higher probability (30 to 70 per cent) of developing breast cancer than do parous women. Additionally, with decreasing age at the time of her first pregnancy, the risk will proportionately decrease. Women who have their first full-term pregnancy at 18 years of age or younger have a breast cancer risk that approximates one third that for gravid women 35 years or younger. This increased risk may be related to anovulatory menstrual cycles and may be associated with persistent exposure to endogenous estrogens in the absence of adequate serum concentrations of progesterone. Furthermore, women having their first full-term pregnancy after age 30 have an even higher risk for breast cancer than do nulliparas. A possible explanation for these findings is that early full-term pregnancies prevent cellular dedifferentiation, whereas first full-term pregnancies beyond the age of 30 act as tumor promotors on breast ductal cells, which have already undergone malignant transformation.

Breastfeeding and Menopause. Long-term nursing ($\geq$ 36 months in a lifetime) was once considered to reduce the risk of breast cancer. This observation is no longer considered valid. However, women whose menopause occurs after the age of 55 have twice the risk of developing breast cancer compared with women whose menopause begins before age 45. Artificially induced menopause appears to protect against breast cancer. The protection is lifelong and results, no doubt, from the removal of the endogenous effects of estrogen. The earlier the age of oophorectomy, the lower the risk. Women who have had oophorectomy at age 35 or younger have one third the risk of breast cancer when compared with women whose natural menopause was age 50 or later.

Hormonal Roles. Despite laboratory and epidemiologic data that implicate hormonal mechanisms as etiologic in the causation of breast cancer, considerable uncertainty exists as to which hormones may be operative and their interrelationships. Certainly, a central role for estrogens, prolactin, progesterone, androgens, and other hormones is an attractive hypothesis, yet evaluation of these endogenous hormones is difficult because of the natural variations in hormonal milieu operative within an individual.

Oral Contraceptives and Estrogen Replacement. To date, epidemiologic studies of oral contraceptive and estrogen replacement therapies have not indicated an association with a change in risk for breast cancer. In patients with cystic disease and fibroadenoma, perhaps hormonally related diseases, the use of oral contraceptives for 2 to 4 years has been associated with a decreased incidence of breast cancer. This protective effect has been related specifically to the progesterone content of the pill. Long-term usage of oral contraceptives in patients with no breast abnormality appears to decrease the risk of benign breast disease but to have no effect on the absolute risk of breast cancer. Oral contraceptives, most likely, protect against those forms of nonproliferative disease that are not associated with an increased risk of breast cancer, i.e., those diseases in which atypical hyperplasia of the epithelium is not evident.[20]

PROLIFERATIVE DISEASE AND ATYPICAL HYPERPLASIA

Women with a history of proliferative disease and/or atypical hyperplasia have an identifiable increase in risk for development of breast cancer. This risk persists at least 30 years after diagnosis and correlates best with hyperplastic disorders of ductal epithelium. Atypical hyperplasia and hyperplasia accompanied by calcification represent high risks. No clear-cut relationship between breast cancer and fibroadenoma has been established.

Dupont and Page evaluated women having biopsy of benign breast lesions. Women with biopsies of *proliferative* disease *without* atypical hyperplasia had a risk of cancer that was 1.9 times the risk in women with *nonproliferative* lesions (Table 1). The risk for women with atypical hyperplasia (atypia) was 5.3 times that in women with nonproliferative lesions. A family history of breast cancer had little effect on the risk for women with nonproliferative lesions. However, the risk for women with atypia and a family history of breast cancer was 11-fold that for women who had nonproliferative lesions without a family history. Calcification increased the cancer risk almost fourfold if the biopsy confirmed proliferative disease. The presence of cysts and a family history of breast cancer enhanced the risk 2.7 times. These authors conclude that the majority of women (70 per cent) having breast biopsy for benign disease are not at increased cancer risk since they do not have atypical hyperplasia and/or a family history of breast cancer. The adverse effect of positive family history for the patient with atypical hyperplasia becomes appreciable at approximately 20 years after biopsy (Fig. 18).

IONIZING RADIATION

There is a relationship between exposure to ionizing radiation early in life and breast cancer risk. This risk is linear in a dose-response relationship. Women who have received irradiation as infants for abnormalities such as thymic enlargement or as adolescents for the treatment of acne are considered to be in a high-risk group and deserve

TABLE 1. *Effect of Hyperplasia, Age, Family History, and Calcification on the Risk of Breast Cancer**

Relative Risk	Relative Risk†	P Value
PDWA/non-PD, age 20–45	1.9	0.012
PDWA/non-PD, age 46–55	1.4	0.49
PDWA/non-PD, age > 55	5.6	0.11
PDWA with CAL/non-PD no CAL	2.3	0.008
AH with CAL/non-PD with CAL	8.6	0.0006
AH with CAL/non-PD no CAL	8.3	<0.0001
Cysts, no FH/neither cysts nor FH	1.3	0.19
Cysts with FH/no cysts but FH	2.1	0.14
Cysts with FH/neither cysts nor FH	2.7	0.0004
PDWA/non-PD	1.9	0.003
AH/non-PD	5.3	<0.0001
CAL/no CAL	1.3	0.19
PDWA, no FH/non-PD no FH	1.9	0.007
PDWA with FH/non-PD with FH	2.0	0.25
PDWA with FH/non-PD no FH	2.7	0.004
AH without FH/non-PD no FH	4.3	<0.0001
AH with FH/non-PD with FH	8.4	0.0003
AH with FH/non-PD no FH	11.0	<0.0001

*Modified from Dupont, W. D., and Page, D. L.: N. Engl. J. Med., *312*:146, 1985.

†As compared with the risk in women from Atlanta (Third National Cancer Survey).

Abbreviations: PDWA = Proliferative disease without atypia; AH = atypical hyperplasia; CAL = calcification; FH = family history of breast cancer (mother, sister, or daughter); age = age at time of entry biopsy.

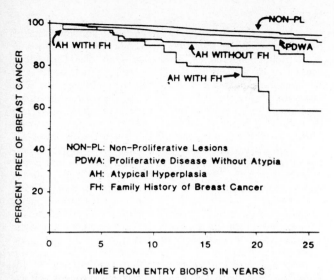

Figure 18. Proportion of patients free of invasive breast cancer as a function of time since the entry biopsy. (From Dupont, W. D., and Page, D. L.: N. Engl. J. Med., 312:150, 1985.)

careful follow-up. Whether young women who receive therapeutic doses of radiation therapy to the mediastinum and neck for treatment of Hodgkin's disease are at greater risk is as yet unknown.

The controversy over routine *mammography* of asymptomatic women between 35 and 50 years of age is an intriguing one. Physicians working in the Breast Cancer Detection Center in Atlanta, Georgia, published a survey of 5810 women in the 35- to 50-year age group who had been examined over a 5-year period.[23] Carcinoma of the breast was detected in 32 women, 43 per cent of the lesions were *in situ*, and the predicted survival rate based on pathologic findings for the 32 women was 87.1 per cent; in other words, 28 women should be cured. The Advisory Committee on the Biological Effects of Ionizing Radiation (BEIR) reports that exposure to an estimated 90 to 100 rads will result in a doubling of the incidence of breast cancer. An extrapolation from these data indicates that 1 rad absorbed by the breast will increase the risk of breast cancer from 7 to 7.07 per cent annually.

Although there is no evidence that the risk increases as the dose of radiation from mammography accumulates over time, Letton and coworkers[23] have assumed that it does, and they have applied this mathematical principle to the cumulative risk of breast cancer to which their asymptomatic patients have been exposed. Using current mammographic techniques, 0.46 rad is absorbed per mammogram; this dose, if cumulative, should change the risk for 5 years from 7 to 7.162 per cent. Therefore, of the 5810 women examined in 5 years, breast cancer should be induced in nine women, of whom at least six should be cured by proper cancer management. Thus, using these theoretical calculations, breast cancer should be detected in 32 asymptomatic women at the risk of inducing breast cancer in nine. If the same mortality rates are used in both groups, three times more women should be saved by mammography than would be killed by it. Also, most early breast cancers are detected with the initial mammogram, and the risk of inducing breast cancer by one examination is extremely small when compared with the clinical value of the information obtained from the study.

Natural History

Patients rarely proceed through the varying stages of breast carcinoma without an attempt at some form of therapeutic intervention. The natural history of breast cancer, however, was reported by Bloom and associates[7] from the records of 250 patients with *untreated* breast cancer housed in the cancer charity wards of Middlesex Hospital in London between 1805 and 1933. The median survival was 2.7 years after initial diagnosis. The 5- and 10-year survival rates for these untreated patients were 18 and 3.6 per cent, respectively. Only 0.8 per cent survived for 15 years. Autopsy data confirmed that 95 per cent of these women died of breast cancer, whereas only 5 per cent died of intercurrent disease. Almost 75 per cent of the patients had ulceration of the breast at the time of their demise. Mean survival of untreated breast cancer patients obtained from the world literature is 38.7 months (range 30.2 to 39.8 months). Breast cancer, therefore, may not be a rapidly lethal disease, although 60 per cent of patients who will develop metastases do so within the first 2 years after mastectomy.

Breast tumors contain a heterogeneous population of cells with differing biologic capabilities for growth, metastases, estrogen receptor activity, and response to chemotherapy. This observation has led many medical oncologists to believe that, once discovered, breast cancer by definition is a systemic disease. Yet appropriate therapy of tumors localized to the breast and regional lymph nodes prolongs survival in over half the patients. Table 2 documents the

TABLE 2. *Observed Survival for Patients with Breast Cancer Relative to Clinical and Histologic Stage**

Clinical Staging (American Joint Committee)	Crude 5-Yr. Survival (%)	Range Survival (%)
Stage I Tumor < 2 cm. in diameter Nodes, if present, not felt to contain metastases Without distant metastases	85	82–94
Stage II Tumors < 5 cm. in diameter Nodes, if palpable, not fixed Without distant metastases	66	47–74
Stage III Tumor >5 cm. OR Tumor any size with invasion of skin or attached to chest wall Nodes in supraclavicular area Without distant metastases	41	7–80
Stage IV With distant metastases	10	—

	Crude Survival (%)		5-Yr. Disease-Free Survival
Histologic Staging (NSABP*)	5-Yr.	10-Yr.	(%)
All patients	63.5	45.9	60.3
Negative axillary lymph nodes	78.1	64.9	82.3
Positive axillary lymph nodes	46.5	24.9	34.9
1–3 positive axillary lymph nodes	62.2	37.5	50.0
> 4 positive axillary lymph nodes	32.0	13.4	21.1

*Reprinted with permission from Henderson, I. C., and Canellos, G. P.: N. Engl. J. Med., 302:17, 1980.

Abbreviation: NSABP = National Surgical Adjuvant Breast and Bowel Project.

direct relationship of survival to advancing clinical and histologic stages of the disease. These data suggest a direct correlation between survival and early pathologic stage. Patients with T1 breast cancers with no nodal involvement have an 82 per cent 5-year survival free of disease, whereas metastatic involvement of axillary lymph nodes may diminish 5-year disease-free survival to 35 per cent.[21, 22]

As noted from the Middlesex Hospital data and from literally hundreds of other clinical reports, 5-year survival in breast cancer does not equate to cure. Breast cancer may recur many years later, even 30 years or more. Thus, results from new treatment programs for breast cancer, and there are many, cannot be evaluated fully until at least 10 years have elapsed. For a breast cancer patient, the most common cause of death between 5 and 10 years after mastectomy is metastatic breast cancer.

METASTASIS

The classic physiologic concept taught by Handley suggested that breast cancer metastasized by centrifugal dissemination into and via the lymphatics to establish first regional and then systemic disease. Primary breast tumors do not contain lymphatic connections; entry into endolymph is initiated by direct invasion. Thereafter, convection currents in the interstitial fluid drain and transport neoplastic cells to regional nodes. Lymph node arrest may be transient, and neoplastic cells that traverse the sinusoids and medullary portions of the lymph nodes retain the capacity for metastasis to remote organs. The regional axillary and internal mammary nodal basins retain a certain "holding capacity" for a specific cell fraction and volume. When this threshold is exceeded, additional emboli pass through the efferent channels and gain access to the systemic venous and lymphatic circulation. This hypothesis does not recognize that neoplastic cells in the breast directly invade venules to establish hematogenous metastases. Viable, circulating neoplastic cells have been detected in effluent venous samples of human blood. No doubt, most of these neoplastic cells are destroyed by immunobiologic mechanisms yet to be described; nonetheless, small fractions of viable cells do survive in the circulation to initiate metastatic growth of selected cell populations at distant sites.

For most breast neoplasms, there is a long preclinical (occult) and prediagnostic interval during which tumor and/or host factors can modulate metastatic formation. For example, if a tumor doubled in size every 100 days, the time required for a single malignant cell to grow into a clinically detectable, 1-cm. mass (10^9 cells) would be slightly more than 8 years. Metastases presumably occur at any time following the first few doublings of the neoplasm. Growth rates of tumors at distant sites also have a wide range; thus, primary breast lesions may be diagnosed many years before metastases are detected. Many human and experimental tumor cells possess tumor-associated antigens that can initiate host reactions that are lethal to the neoplastic cells. A large number of interrelating polypeptides that counteract metastatic growth have been identified, but their exact mechanism of action is yet to be described.

Metastatic involvement of regional lymph nodes represents the most important prognostic variable.[28] Tumor size is an additional prognostic indicator and directly correlates with the probability of lymph node metastases. As noted in Table 2, the number of lymph nodes involved with metastatic disease is inversely proportional to patient survival. Interestingly, patients with occult axillary lymph node metastases may have 5-year survivals that closely parallel those of patients whose lymph nodes are free of tumor.

HISTOLOGY

Histologic differentiation of the cell and the nucleus has an influence on survival. Histologic criteria commonly used include degree of tubule or glandular formation; regularity of nuclear features, including size, shape, and frequency of mitoses; and degree of hyperchromatism. The more anaplastic the cellular features, the worse the prognosis. In the somewhat obsolete nuclear grading system described by Black and Speer[5], there is progression from Grade III through Grade I as the lesion grade increases from well differentiated to highly anaplastic. Some pathologists still use this grading system for the entire cell population; currently, however, nuclear Grade III connotes anaplasia, whereas nuclear Grade I indicates a well-differentiated nucleus.[28] Lymphatic or venous invasion within or surrounding the biopsy specimen portends a bad prognosis. Lesions that are nuclear Grade III and have local lymphatic invasion usually have associated lymph node metastases. Even in the absence of nodal involvement, however, the probability of distant metastases is high. Patients in this population usually have negative estrogen receptor activity and, possibly, are candidates for adjuvant chemotherapy.

Staging

Clinical staging is based on physical examination to determine the extent of involvement of the breast by the neoplastic process (e.g., edema, ulceration, fixation). Additionally, a comprehensive evaluation of ipsilateral axillary and supraclavicular lymph nodes and the contralateral breast and axilla are required.

CLASSIFICATION SYSTEMS

Consistent classifications have evolved over the past four decades and are essential for the comparison of treatment results among institutions and different investigators. Three clinical staging systems have evolved: the Manchester, the Columbia Clinical Classification, and the TNM (tumor, nodes, metastasis) systems. Initially, the Manchester system, developed in 1940 at the Christie Hospital and Holt Radium Institute in Manchester, England, was widely adopted. Subsequently, the more comprehensive Columbia Clinical Classification (Table 3), formulated by Haagensen and Stout, replaced the Manchester classification.

The *TNM system* was developed as a worldwide standard staging system. This international system was reported initially at the meeting of the International Union Against Cancer in São Paulo, Brazil, in 1954. The American Joint Committee on Cancer Staging and End Results Reporting has since modified it slightly (Table 4).

The essentials of the initial examination include:
1. Physical examination
2. Bilateral breast imaging by a validated technique, i.e., xeromammography
3. Usual admission clinical pathology examinations to include a profile of liver enzymes
4. Chest roentgenogram
5. Skeletal roentgenologic survey

Selected examinations include:
1. Radionuclide liver scan or abdominal computed tomography (CT) when there is:
   a. Abnormal liver profile
   b. Hepatomegaly

Table 3. *Columbia Clinical Classification*

Stage A:	No skin edema, ulceration, or solid fixation of the tumor to the chest wall. Axillary nodes not clinically involved.
Stage B:	No skin edema, ulceration, or solid fixation of the tumor to the chest wall. Clinically involved nodes, but less than 2.5 cm. in transverse diameter and not fixed to overlying skin or deeper structures of the axilla.
Stage C:	Any one of the five grave signs of advanced breast carcinoma: 1. Edema of the skin of limited extent (involving less than one third of the skin over the breast) 2. Skin ulceration 3. Solid fixation of the tumor to the chest wall 4. Massive involvement of axillary lymph nodes (measuring 2.5 cm. or more in transverse diameter) 5. Fixation of the axillary nodes to overlying skin or deeper structures of the axilla
Stage D:	All other indications of more advanced breast carcinoma, including: 1. A combination of any two or more of the five grave signs listed under Stage C 2. Extensive edema of the skin (involving more than one third of the skin over the breast) 3. Satellite skin nodules 4. The inflammatory type of carcinoma 5. Clinically involved supraclavicular lymph nodes 6. Internal mammary metastases as evidenced by a parasternal tumor 7. Edema of the arm 8. Distant metastases

2. Radionuclide bone scan for any of the following conditions:
   a. Advanced local disease (T3, T4)
   b. Lymph node metastasis (N1, N2, N3)
   c. Distant metastases (MI)
   d. Bone pain in the absence of any of the above

BONE SCANNING

The role of isotopic bone scans in the staging of breast cancer is somewhat controversial. The incidence of abnormal bone scan findings in patients with operable breast cancer varies widely. From initial studies, it appears that in individuals with abnormal bone scans metastatic disease soon develops. The majority of abnormal findings at preliminary examination, however, occur in patients with extensive regional disease. The prevailing opinion today is that bone scans are too sensitive to be of cost-benefit value in the preoperative staging of patients with relatively early breast cancers (T1, T2, T1N1). In these patients, a skeletal roentgenologic survey often must be correlated with the bone scan to identify such benign conditions as arthritis, bone islands, and healed fractures, which are interpreted to represent potential sites of metastasis on the bone scan. The current value of bone scanning is not so much in the initial examination of patients with early breast cancer but rather in their sequential postoperative follow-up, since bone scanning is one of the more sensitive indicators of evolving metastatic disease. Patients who have suspicious skeletal roentgenologic survey findings or clinically palpable metastatic disease in the axilla or supraclavicular region should receive isotopic bone scans during the preoperative period to provide a baseline for future evaluation. Certainly, any patient who complains of bone pain should have this localized area investigated thoroughly.

COMPUTED TOMOGRAPHY

In some institutions, computed tomography (CT) has replaced radionuclide liver scanning in augmenting diagnostic accuracy. Again, this subject is controversial. Depending on the accuracy of the studies in any one institution, those patients who have elevated hepatic biochemical values deserve liver imaging. Isotopic or CT scanning of the brain is unnecessary unless physical examination or history indicates central nervous system involvement with metastatic disease. Sites of metastatic disease, in order of decreasing frequency, include bone, liver, lung, skin, extra regional lymphatics, and brain. Any organ, however, may be involved with metastatic disease (Table 5).

AXILLA OR CLINICAL STAGING

Since the axillary lymph node basin is the major regional drainage for carcinoma of the breast, approximately 40 to 50 per cent of patients seen today will have pathologic involvement of this site at initial presentation. Detection of axillary involvement on physical examination is fraught with diagnostic hazards. Between 20 and 25 per cent of examinations are inaccurate. In other words, with reasonable frequency, the axillary lymph nodes are thought to contain metastatic disease and pathologically are negative, whereas with equal frequency the axillary nodes are thought to be free of disease when, in fact, pathologically they are involved. Since the status of the axillary lymph nodes correlates significantly with survival, at the very least, a sufficient sample of axillary lymph nodes (approximately 8 to 10 lymph nodes) is required to adequately determine the future status of the patient and indicate the need for adjuvant hormonal therapy, chemotherapy, or radiation therapy. Pathologic staging of the resected specimen is, in effect, more important than clinical staging. Clinical staging initially dictates the type of operative procedure selected, but pathologic staging determines prognosis and the necessity of adjuvant therapy.

Histopathologic Classification

Mammary cancers can be classified according to gross characteristics (scirrhous, colloid, medullary), histogenesis (duct, lobule, acini), histologic characteristics (adenocarcinoma, epidermoid carcinoma, sarcoma, etc.), and invasive criteria (infiltrating, *in situ*). With few exceptions, the majority (85 per cent) take origin from the lactiferous ducts, and the preponderance of mammary cancers are adenocarcinomas. Current terminology commonly denotes histology and is based on the lesion's predominant architecture, yet many patterns may be observed in any one breast cancer. The following classification was originally proposed by Foote and Stewart:

I. Paget's disease of the nipple
II. Carcinoma of duct origin
    A. Noninfiltrating (*in situ*, intraductal)
    B. Infiltrating
        1. Adenocarcinoma with productive fibrosis (scirrhous, simplex)
        2. Medullary
        3. Comedo
        4. Colloid

TABLE 4. TNM Classification

Definitions: TNM Classification

Primary Tumor (T)
[ ] TX   Minimal requirements to assess the primary tumor cannot be met
[ ] T0   No evidence of primary tumor
[ ] Tis Paget's disease of the nipple with no demonstrable tumor
         (*Note*: Paget's disease with a demonstrable tumor is classified according
         to the size of the tumor)
T1* Tumor 2 cm. or less in greatest dimension
[ ] T1a No fixation to underlying pectoral fascia or muscle
[ ] T1b Fixation to underlying pectoral fascia or muscle
         (Check below in addition to T1a or T1b)
         [ ] i Tumor $\leq$ 0.5 cm.
         [ ] ii Tumor > 0.5 $\leq$ 1.0 cm.
         [ ] iii Tumor > 1.0 $\leq$ 2.0 cm.
T2* Tumor more than 2 cm. but not more than 5 cm. in its greatest
    dimension
[ ] T2a No fixation to underlying pectoral fascia or muscle
[ ] T2b Fixation to underlying pectoral fascia or muscle
T3* Tumor more than 5 cm. in its greatest dimension
[ ] T3a No fixation to underlying pectoral fascia or muscle
[ ] T3b Fixation to underlying pectoral fascia or muscle
T4 Tumor of any size with direct extension to chest wall or skin
   (*Note*: Chest wall includes ribs, intercostal muscles, and serratus anterior muscle but not pectoral muscle)
[ ] T4a Fixation to chest wall
[ ] T4b Edema (including peau d'orange), ulceration of the skin of the breast, or satellite skin nodules confined to the same breast
[ ] T4c Both of the above

Lymph Nodes (N)
Definitions for clinical-diagnostic stage

[ ] NX   Minimal requirements to assess the regional nodes cannot be met
[ ] N0   Homolateral axillary lymph nodes not considered to contain growth
[ ] N1   Movable homolateral axillary nodes considered to contain growth
[ ] N2   Homolateral axillary nodes considered to contain growth and fixed to one another or to other structures
[ ] N3   Homolateral supraclavicular or infraclavicular nodes considered to contain growth, or edema of the arm

Lymph Nodes (N)
Definitions for surgical-evaluative and postsurgical resection-pathologic stages
[ ] NX   Minimal requirements to assess the presence of distant metastasis cannot be met
[ ] N0   No evidence of homolateral axillary lymph node metastasis
[ ] N1   Metastasis to movable homolateral axillary nodes not fixed to one another or to other structure
         [ ] N1a Micrometastasis $\leq$ 0.2 cm. in lymph node(s)
         [ ] N1b Gross metastasis in lymph node(s)
                 [ ] i Metastasis more than 0.02 cm. but less than 2.0 cm. in one to three lymph nodes
                 [ ] ii Metastasis more than 0.2 cm. but less than 2.0 cm. in four or more lymph nodes
                 [ ] iii Extension of metastasis beyond the lymph node capsule (less than 2.0 cm. in total dimension)
                 [ ] iv Metastasis in lymph node 2.0 cm. or more in dimension
[ ] N2   Metastases to homolateral axillary lymph nodes that are fixed to one another or to other structures
[ ] N3   Metastasis to homolateral supraclavicular or intraclavicular lymph node(s)

Distant Metastasis (M) All time periods
[ ] MX   Not assessed
[ ] M0   No (known) distant metastasis
[ ] M1   Distant metastasis present
         Specify _____

Indicate on diagram primary tumor and regional nodes involved.
Examination by _____ M.D.
Date _____

Tumor Size _____ x _____ x _____ cm.

Predominant Lesion
Measured on   [ ] Patient [ ] Mammogram
                 [ ] Pathologic specimen
Location   [ ] OUQ   [ ] Nipple/areola
(multiple when   [ ] OLQ   [ ] IUQ   [ ] ILQ
  necessary)

Lymph Nodes   Total number _____
Number with metastasis _____

Table continued on opposite page

TABLE 4. TNM Classification Continued

Stage Grouping

[ ] Clinical-diagnostic (cTNM)
[ ] Surgical-evaluative (sTNM)
[ ] Postsurgical resection-pathologic (pTNM)

[ ] Stage Tis	*in situ*
Stage X	Cannot stage
[ ] Stage I	[ ] T1ai, N0, M0
	[ ] T1aii, N0, M0
	[ ] T1aiii, N0, M0
	[ ] T1bi, N0, M0
	[ ] T1bii, N0, M0
	[ ] T1biii, N0, M0
[ ] Stage II	[ ] T0, N1a or N1b; M0
	[ ] T1a or T1b; N1a or N1b; M0
	[ ] T2a or T2b; N0, M0
	[ ] T2a or T2b; N1a or N1b; M0
[ ] Stage IIIA	[ ] T0, N2, M0
	[ ] T1a or T1b; N2, M0
	[ ] T2a or T2b; N2, M0
	[ ] T3a or T3b; N0, M0
	[ ] T3a or T3b; N1, M0
	[ ] T3a or T3b; N2, M0
[ ] Stage IIIB	[ ] Any T, N3, M0
	[ ] Any T4, any N, M0
[ ] Stage IV	[ ] Any T, any N, M1

*Dimpling of the skin, nipple retraction, or any other skin changes except those in T4b may occur in T1, T2, or T3 without affecting the classification. (*Note*: Cases of inflammatory carcinoma should be reported separately.)

 5. Papillary
 6. Tubular
III. Carcinoma of lobule origin
 A. Noninfiltrating (*in situ*)
 B. Infiltrating

Histologic patterns of rarely encountered epithelial types include squamous call carcinoma, melanoma, adenoid cystic carcinoma, sweat gland carcinoma, and carcinoma with mesenchymal metaplasia of chondromatous or osseous types. Fifty per cent of breast cancers are located in the upper outer quadrant, 25 per cent are in the juxta-areolar area, and the remainder are distributed randomly throughout the medial half of the breast.

PAGET'S DISEASE

A chronic, eczematoid eruption of the nipple was described by Sir James Paget in 1874. The neoplasm constitutes approximately 1 to 3 per cent of all breast carcinomas. At presentation, the surface of the nipple-areola complex is encrusted, scaly, hyperemic, and enlarged. Symptoms are burning, itching, tenderness, and occasional bleeding.

The neoplasm arises as an intraductal adenocarcinoma and involves the epidermis of the nipple and areola by intraepithelial spread. Physical findings commonly precede the identification of a definable, palpable, subareolar mass. Approximately 25 to 35 per cent of patients have axillary nodal metastases at presentation. In general, however, Paget's disease has a better prognosis than most breast cancers because the nipple-areolar changes lead to an early diagnosis.

Biopsy of the nipple and the associated subareolar intraductal carcinoma is diagnostic. The tissues beneath the nipple contain dilated, thick ducts filled with grumous, pasty material (cellular debris). Microscopically, the carcinoma extends up the duct system superficially to produce the characteristic epidermal changes and also extends downward into the duct mechanism to reach and replace lobular epithelium. This intraductal lesion is often multifocal. Ducts throughout the entire breast may be dilated as a result of the obstruction of the central collecting ducts at the ampulla of the nipple. Pathognomonic of this entity is the presence of very large, pale, vacuolated cells (Paget cells) in the rete pegs of the epithelium. These cells show large, hyperchromatic nuclei and mitoses. This lesion may be confused with superficial melanoma; however, the presence of typical pagetoid cells and the associated physical findings are diagnostic of this entity even in the absence of a subareolar

TABLE 5. Sites of Metastases from Breast Cancer in Three Collected Series (%)*

Organ	160 Cases†	43 Cases‡	100 Cases§
Lung	59	65	69
Liver	58	56	65
Bone	44	—	71
Pleura	37	23	51
Adrenals	31	41	49
Kidneys	Not recorded	14	17
Spleen	14	23	17
Pancreas	—	11	17
Ovaries	9	16	20
Brain	—	9	22
Thyroid	—	—	24
Heart	—	—	11
Diaphragm	—	—	11
Pericardium	5	21	19
Intestine	—	—	18
Peritoneum	12	9	13
Uterus	—	—	15
Lymph nodes	72	—	76
Skin	34	7	30

*Modified from Harris, J. R., et al.: Cancer of the breast. *In* DeVita, V.T., Jr., Hellman, S., and Rosenberg, S. A. (eds.): Cancer: Principles and Practice. Philadelphia, J. B. Lippincott Company, 1985, p. 1127.
†Warren and Witman.
‡Saphillo and Parker.
§Haagenson.

TABLE 6. *Relationship Between Morphologic Types of Invasive Breast Cancer, Lymph Node Involvement, and Patient Survival**

Type	Frequency	% With Nodal Involvement	% Survival	
			5 Yrs.	10 Yrs.
Duct with productive fibrosis	78	60	54	38
Lobular	9	60	50	32
Medullary	4	44	63	50
Comedo	5	32	73	58
Colloid	3	32	73	59
Papillary	1	17	83	56

*Modified from McDivitt, R. W., et al.: Tumors of the breast. *In* Atlas of Tumor Pathology, Series 2, Fascicle 2. Washington, D.C., Armed Forces Institute of Pathology, 1968.

mass. The associated ductal malignancy is most usually invasive, but, with some frequency, Paget's disease may be associated entirely with intraductal carcinoma *in situ.*

NONINFILTRATIVE *in situ* CARCINOMA OF DUCTAL ORIGIN

Mammary carcinoma develops biphasically with intraepithelial stages that transform into infiltrating carcinoma after latent periods of varying duration. The common sites for tumor development are in the extralobular terminal ducts. The lactiferous ducts have the highest cell kinetic activity after stimulation by mammotrophic hormones in both the reproductive and senescent breast. There are also the areas of atypical hyperplasia in fibrocystic disease. Cells have the microscopic characteristics of malignancy but do not invade the basement membrane of ductal epithelium. If left untreated, an invasive adenocarcinoma will invariably result, albeit the time for development of that invasive neoplasm may be measured in years or even decades. Intraductal *in situ* carcinoma formerly constituted approximately 1 per cent of all mammary carcinomas. Currently, however, the diagnosis is increasing in frequency because of improved patient education and mammography. It may present as an occult finding on mammography or be associated with a palpable mass. Multicentricity within the ipsilateral breast is common. The incidence of synchronous involvement of the opposite breast is controversial and is variously reported to be from 0 to 35 per cent.

INFILTRATING DUCTAL CARCINOMA WITH PRODUCTIVE FIBROSIS

This neoplasm represents 75 to 78 per cent of invasive mammary carcinomas and is associated with desmoplasia and fibrosis (Table 6). The tumor has been termed *scirrhous carcinoma* or *carcinoma simplex.* As a result of the desmoplastic response, intervening Cooper's ligaments, in route from the deep layer of investing fascia to the superficial fascia surrounding the breast, are involved. As hyalinization occurs, these ligaments are entrapped within the expanding desmoplastic border of the neoplasm. The shortening of Cooper's ligaments by this process produces the characteristic physical finding of dimpling of the skin directly over the neoplasm, particularly when the patient's arm is elevated directly above her head. This form of skin dimpling is not a grave sign since it does not indicate direct skin involvement by the cancer. Diffuse skin infiltration with involvement of Cooper's ligaments may produce *peau d'orange* or extensive edema of the skin.

The tumor offers great resistance when sectioned in the pathology suite, and the divided surfaces may be calcified with yellow, chalky streaks infiltrating like pseudopods into the surrounding normal breast structure. Neoplastic cells are arranged in small clusters or in single rows

to produce "Indian filing," which occupy the irregular cleft spaces between collagen bundles (Fig. 19). A broad spectrum of well-differentiated to highly anaplastic variants may be observed within the same tumor mass, or there may be relative homogeneity of differentiation throughout the specimen.

MEDULLARY CARCINOMA

In approximately 3 to 5 per cent of mammary malignancies, there is a circumscribed appearance termed by Moore and Foote as medullary carcinoma. This neoplasm is thought to originate from large ducts and is characterized by its soft, hemorrhagic gross appearance. It is usually mobile and located deeply within the breast. At diagnosis, the skin is often stretched over a bulky, spherical mass that exceeds 3 cm. in diameter. A history of slow progression in growth may be apparent, although the tumor may rapidly enlarge secondary to hemorrhage or necrosis.

On cut section, the tumor may appear to have a capsule; however, a zone of encircling fibrosis and lymphatic infiltration is apparent on histologic examination. Central liquefaction necrosis is a usual feature and leads to the mistaken diagnosis of carcinoma developing within a previously existing cyst. Microscopically, a highly cellular tumor composed of oval or polygonal large cells with basophilic cytoplasm, vesicular nuclei, and prominent nucleoli is evident. These distinguishing features may be

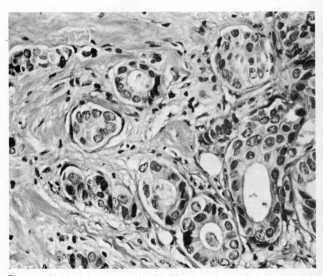

Figure 19. Photomicrograph of infiltrating ductal carcinoma with productive fibrosis (scirrhous carcinoma). Ductal formation is recognized in multiple sites with stromal invasion. An extensive desmoplastic response is evident (62.5×). (Courtesy Dr. R. L. Hackett.)

apparent only in the intact tumor cells that occupy the periphery of the areas of cystic degeneration. A generous infiltration of lymphocytes accompanies the neoplasm and represents an important histologic characteristic. This lesion has a better 5-year survival than invasive ductal or lobular carcinoma. It must be differentiated from cystosarcoma phyllodes, which it mimics clinically. The prognosis for medullary carcinoma is more grave than for cystosarcoma phyllodes, and metastases to axillary lymph nodes are reported in over 40 per cent of patients (see Table 6).

COMEDOCARCINOMA

An invasive ductal carcinoma, comedocarcinoma makes up approximately 5 to 10 per cent of all breast cancers, and like its *in situ* variant it has characteristic plugs of pasty material expressible from the surface of the neoplasm. Its slow growth may extend over several years. McDivitt and associates[25] noted that the average size of the lesion at presentation was 5.0 cm., that one third of the patients had axillary metastases at initial treatment, and that 5- and 10-year survival rates were 73 and 58 per cent, respectively, after appropriate mastectomy. Grossly, the tumor is well circumscribed, firm, and grayish in color. Microscopically, cores of highly cellular, epithelial tissue with focal calcification are seen occluding the ducts (Fig. 20). With invasion, it mimics other histologic patterns with glandular formation, papillary structures, and productive fibrosis.

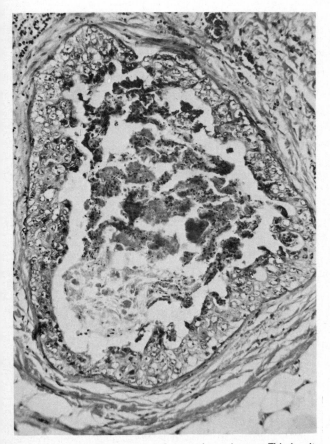

Figure 20. Photomicrograph of comedocarcinoma. This *in situ* carcinoma of ductal origin features irregular cells with variable nuclei. Central necrosis with diffuse microcalcification of cellular debris is characteristic (25×). (Courtesy Dr. R. L. Hackett.)

COLLOID CARCINOMA

An adenocarcinoma of ductal origin, colloid carcinoma is also known as a *mucinous adenocarcinoma* because of the gelatinous material that constitutes a major portion of the neoplasm. It is relatively rare and has a slow growth potential with late metastases. McDivitt and coworkers[25] identified 32 per cent of their patients as having axillary lymph node involvement, and the 5- and 10-year survival rates were 73 per cent and 59 per cent, respectively (see Table 6). This lesion is similar to comedocarcinoma prognostically. Grossly, the tumor is well demarcated but not encapsulated. When cut, strings of mucoid material adhere to the scalpel. Microscopically, there are many small multilocular cysts containing amorphous material that stains blue with hematoxylin-eosin. Between the cyst spaces, parenchyma is infiltrated by columns of malignant cells that often contain a single vacuole producing the classic "signet ring" appearance.

This lesion must be distinguished from *benign granular cell myoblastoma*, and multiple microscopic sections from the tumor often must be processed to identify the malignant features of the neoplasm. Frozen sections are rarely diagnostic.

PAPILLARY CARCINOMA

Of the truly invasive adenocarcinomas of ductal origin investigated by McDivitt and colleagues,[25] papillary carcinoma had the lowest frequency of axillary nodal involvement and the best 5- and 10-year survival rates. These lesions are usually bulky and centrally located and typically appear in a younger age group (35 to 40). Central hemorrhage and necrosis may occur, and nipple discharge is common. Histologically, large sheets of viable cells form a papillary pattern. Characteristically, cells show hyperchromatism, loss of polarity, and numerous mitoses. These histologic criteria are often necessary to distinguish an invasive papillary carcinoma from a benign intraductal papilloma.

TUBULAR CARCINOMA

Tubular carcinoma is a recently described well-differentiated ductal lesion that forms tubules and constitutes approximately 1 per cent of all breast cancers. It frequently mimics sclerosing adenosis of fibrocystic disease and must be differentiated from focal atypical hyperplasia. When the malignant breast lesion is composed of more than 75 per cent tubular components, the prognosis is excellent. Long-term survival approaches 100 per cent if the breast carcinoma contains 90 per cent or more of the tubular components. This pathologic entity constitutes the one circumstance in which only local excision of the tumor may uniformly result in cure.

LOBULAR CARCINOMA

Carcinomas originating in the terminal ductules of the lobules have histologic features that distinguish them from lesions arising in the larger, lactiferous ducts. The noninvasive variety is known as lobular carcinoma *in situ*. The terminal lobules are packed with small, hyperplastic, uniform cells often arranged in rows or beads with a few mitoses but hyperchromatism and nuclear anaplasia (Fig. 21). The gross and microscopic features of invasive lobular carcinoma are often indistinguishable from those of conventional adenocarcinomas, and the prognostic variables and survival, likewise, are similar. Haagensen identified coexisting lobular neoplasia with other forms of invasive breast cancer in 7.2 per cent of operative specimens.

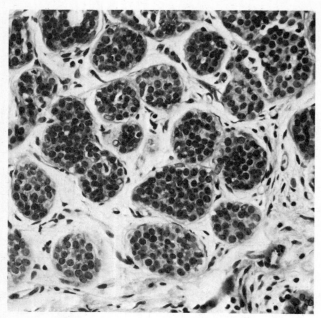

Figure 21. Lobular carcinoma in situ. Lobular acini are distended with tumor cells whose nuclei are uniform and bland in appearance with few or no mitoses. Cells are contained within acinar borders, and evidence for invasion beyond the acini or lobule is absent (62.5×). (Courtesy Dr. R. L. Hackett.)

The true incidence of lobular carcinoma is uncertain. Lobular carcinoma *in situ*, as a single entity, accounts for about 3 per cent of all tumors, whereas infiltrating lobular carcinoma constitutes approximately 10 per cent of all breast cancers.

INFLAMMATORY CARCINOMA

A relatively rare clinicopathologic entity, inflammatory carcinoma constitutes approximately 1.5 to 3 per cent of breast cancers. No specific histologic type predominates. Inflammatory carcinoma denotes the clinically characteristic features of erythema, peau d'orange, and skin ridging with or without the presence of a palpable mass (Fig. 22). The skin over the lesion is often warm, diffusely scaly, and indurated. The breast is commonly hot with the characteristic appearance of cellulitis. A definable tumor mass may be absent, but the breast is diffusely "brawny" and the nipple is often retracted. The diagnosis can be made by a generous biopsy of skin and subcutaneous tissue. The subdermal lymphatics and vascular channels contain microscopic foci of highly undifferentiated tumor emboli. Despite its name, inflammatory cells are not abundant. The disease is rapidly progressive, and 75 per cent of patients have palpable axillary metastases at the time of initial presentation. This carcinoma should be distinguished from contiguous extension of a subdermal, scirrhous carcinoma that invades the skin to produce peau d'orange and inflammation. Inflammatory carcinoma has a distinctly different clinical course and prognosis from those of an adenocarcinoma that has grown to involve the overlying skin. Classically, the average 5-year survival for patients with inflammatory breast cancer is 3 to 5 per cent; whereas, when properly treated, patients with adenocarcinomas that focally invade skin have a 5-year survival rate that approaches 30 per cent.

EPIDERMOID CARCINOMA

Epidermoid carcinoma is encountered infrequently, although foci of squamous metaplasia are not unusual within invasive ductal carcinomas. The pure variant of epidermoid carcinoma arises from metaplasia within the lactiferous ducts. These neoplasms have no distinctive clinical characteristics. Metastases occur almost exclusively via the lymphatic route and are present in approximately 25 per cent of patients treated by mastectomy.

SARCOMA OF THE BREAST

Cancers of nonepithelial origin rarely occur in the mammary gland. Donegan identified sarcomas of the breast in 0.7 per cent of over 2600 patients with breast cancer. Primary lesions include *hemangiosarcoma, fibrosarcoma, liposarcoma, rhabdomyosarcoma, leiomyosarcoma,* and *osteogenic sarcoma. Lymphangiosarcoma* of the arm or shoulder area arises in patients who have extensive and long-standing arm edema after ipsilateral axillary dissection. Often these patients have also received radiation therapy to the axilla. The combination of complete surgical dissection of the axilla and comprehensive radiation therapy to the same area almost ensures that all collateral lymphatic vessels draining lymph from the arm into the systemic circulation will be eradicated. Lymphedema is an unavoidable complication unless the surgical and radiotherapeutic procedures are planned to avoid disruption of the collateral lymphatics supplied from the upper arm. Lymphangiosarcoma is usually unresponsive to radiation therapy or chemotherapy. Radical four-quarter amputation of the extremity has been proposed to manage the ulcerative complications in the arm and palliate the massive and progressive lymphedema. Five-year survivals from this disease are uncommon. The etiology is controversial; the method of prevention, however, is well established—postoperative irradiation of the entire axilla after modified or

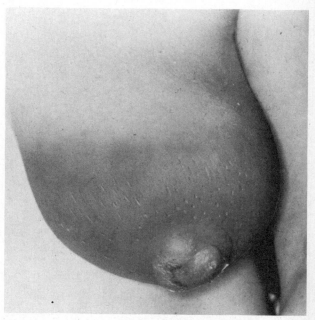

Figure 22. Inflammatory carcinoma. The clinicopathologic features of erythema, hyperemia, peau d'orange, and skin ridging coexist with the findings of a palpable subareolar breast carcinoma.

radical mastectomy should be avoided, if possible, to eliminate the progressive fibrotic obliteration of the lymphatic vessels draining lymph from the upper extremity.

Although *cystosarcoma phyllodes* was presented earlier in the section on benign breast disease, the overall incidence of malignancy in this lesion is debatable. In most series, 10 to 13 per cent of these lesions either metastasize or have the features of a highly anaplastic lesion. Malignant histology appears to correlate with pain, large size of the neoplasm ($\geq$ 7 cm. in diameter), and advancing age (over 52 years). Although lymph node metastases have been reported, this lesion disseminates principally via the bloodstream, and pulmonary metastases are the most common first site of therapeutic failure.

Treatment

Treatment begins with the initial patient interview. The physician should frankly discuss the possibility that a suspicious lesion might be cancer and recommend a remedy. After all, the patient has come to the physician because of a palpable breast mass and she may already fear having breast cancer. Both patient and physician should have a clear understanding of the course of action to be taken in the diagnosis and treatment of a breast lesion, particularly if the biopsy reveals a breast cancer.

Biopsy

The initial step in therapy is biopsy of the suspicious breast mass. Excisional breast biopsy as an ambulatory procedure is acceptable. For the surgeon who is inexperienced with this technique, however, excisional biopsy under local anesthesia can be difficult. The lesion may be deeper in the breast than initially anticipated, and bleeding can be troublesome. The planned mastectomy should be completed following pathologic confirmation of malignancy.

Expeditious mastectomy is advised because hematoma created by the biopsy may dissect throughout tissue planes and produce a large ecchymotic area in the breast. This area of ecchymosis potentially contains viable cancer cells released into the wound during the open or needle biopsy. The indistinct borders of an infiltrating adenocarcinoma make these lesions more likely to be incised during the biopsy procedure, particularly if the operating surgeon is using local anesthesia.

Should malignant cells be released into the biopsy site, they may be contained locally for only a short period of time. When several days elapse between incisional biopsy and mastectomy, the areas beneath the skin of the breast containing ecchymotic areas and, possibly, viable cancer cells may enlarge. These ecchymotic areas represent the migration of red cells from the biopsy site, and, and, hypothetically, cancer cells may migrate an equal distance. These areas of ecchymoses may have resolved clinically when the condition is evaluated by the surgeon for the definitive procedure. Thus, when breast flaps are elevated, areas of skin and subcutaneous tissue that potentially harbor cancer cells may not be removed en bloc with the mastectomy specimen and chest wall cancer may recur. A "disturbed breast" indicates that large ecchymotic areas surround the biopsy site. The chest wall recurrence rate after mastectomy in these patients was as great as 25 per cent until perioperative radiation therapy was utilized to sterilize potentially viable cancer cells remaining in the skin flaps. Currently, local recurrence rates for disturbed breasts approximate 4 per cent.

Baker[4] has published the results of 153 consecutive breast biopsies done under local anesthesia. Nineteen patients proved to have adenocarcinoma, and all patients were admitted to the hospital within 1 to 3 days of biopsy for further diagnostic studies and mastectomy. Under these circumstances, outpatient breast biopsies appear to be safe, particularly if the surgeon is familiar with the technique, has rapid paraffin section diagnostic capability, and can obtain time in the operating room on relatively short notice. If this clinical setting is not available and the lesion cannot be completely excised, outpatient breast biopsy of a suspicious lesion should not be attempted. Only a few women refuse to be anesthetized without knowledge of the histologic diagnosis. When they do refuse, biopsy can be done in the operating room under local anesthesia immediately before mastectomy if the frozen section diagnosis indicates that this procedure is necessary.

Outpatient breast biopsy is indicated for breast lesions that have an increased probability of being benign. Certainly, this procedure is cost-effective and the morbidity from a general anesthetic is eliminated. Those lesions that are suspected of being malignant, however, should be handled very cautiously so that all the specimen is removed, particularly if there is to be a delay of more than 72 hours prior to definitive mastectomy.

Treatment Options

All therapeutic options and the treatment of choice should be discussed with the patient prior to biopsy, particularly if the preoperative evaluation indicates that the lesion is malignant. The physician has the responsibility of discussing all treatment options with the patient preoperatively. Publications in the lay press have made patients aware of breast cancer treatment techniques and reconstructive procedures. Such information can be misinterpreted, and the patient can make diagnostic and therapeutic value judgments based on information published in nonmedical journals. More and more frequently, women are seeking the treatment they think is proper rather than the therapy prescribed by the physician. This conflict may lead to inadequate treatment of the local malignant process in an attempt to preserve the breast from what the patient may interpret as an overzealous surgeon. With few exceptions, a decision regarding the operative procedure should be made *prior to biopsy*. In this regard, fine-needle aspiration for cytologic confirmation of the malignant process can be quite valuable.

Surgery, chemotherapy, and radiotherapy techniques have advanced significantly in the past 3 decades such that the treatment of breast cancer should be integrated among each of these modalities. For example, large breast cancers (greater than 5 cm. in size) with matted, axillary metastases will often shrink in size with the use of preoperative chemotherapy, allowing the surgeon to complete a cytoreductive, planned mastectomy without the use of skin grafts. Following mastectomy, radiation therapy to the chest wall and internal mammary and supraclavicular lymph nodes will eradicate residual microscopic disease in skin flaps or regional lymph nodes outside the operative field. With the use of combination multimodal therapy, local control of the disease to the chest wall is achieved, and any systemic metastases will have been treated initially by the preoperative chemotherapy.

The therapeutic aim of the radiation therapist and the surgeon is control of local disease, whereas the aim of the medical oncologist is control of systemic disease. The medical oncologist has the most difficult job, for although drugs for breast cancer are effective, complete control of documented metastasis, to date, has been achieved infrequently. Proper use of radiotherapy portals to encompass dissected surgical planes provides control of chest wall disease and can be accomplished without increasing the morbidity from either the surgical procedure or the radiation therapy.

LOCAL CONTROL OF CHEST WALL DISEASE (APPROPRIATE COMBINATION OF SURGICAL PROCEDURES AND RADIATION THERAPY)

Adenocarcinomas of the breast that are smaller than 5 cm. in diameter, limited to the lateral aspect of the breast, and without pectoral fascia or skin fixation (T1a, T2a) usually can be treated by surgery alone, provided lymph node metastases are absent in the pathologic specimen. When lymphatic metastases are present or when the adenocarcinoma is centrally or medially located, a combination of surgery and postoperative radiation therapy is often used to ensure local chest wall control of the malignant process.

Stages I and II Breast Cancer

For Stage I and Stage II breast cancer (see Table 2), the type of surgical procedure done and the areas that will receive radiation therapy depend upon the location of the primary lesion in the breast and the presence or absence of axillary lymph node metastases. Neoplasms in the lateral aspect of the breast drain primarily via the axillary lymphatic channels, and disease can be eliminated from the chest wall by *modified radical mastectomy*. The limits of

this dissection include the lateral border of the sternum medially, the latissimus dorsi muscle laterally, the clavicle superiorly, and the superior border of the rectus muscle inferiorly (Fig. 23).

The breast is removed from the chest wall via flaps created within the superficial investing fascia of the dermis. The location of this investing fascia determines the thickness of the skin flaps. The surgeon must remove all breast tissue from these flaps, and with the investing fascia used as a guide, all breast tissue is excised en bloc with the specimen. The breast is resected from the pectoralis major muscle, and the axillary contents are dissected from the axillary vein inferiorly to Halsted's ligament medially. To ensure that Levels I, II, and III lymph nodes are removed, the pectoralis minor muscle should be divided from its insertion on the coracoid process and origin from the ribs. Thus, the specimen includes the breast, the nipple-areola complex with associated overlying skin, the axillary contents, and the pectoralis minor muscle.

Laterally located cancers with multiple axillary lymph node metastases may be associated with internal mammary or supraclavicular lymph node metastases in as many as 25 to 30 per cent of patients; consequently, radiation therapy is advisable to treat these two lymph node basins (i.e., "peripheral lymphatics").

Medially located cancers primarily drain via the lymphatic channels of the internal mammary vessels and may be associated with internal mammary lymph node metastases 10 to 30 per cent of the time. If axillary metastases are present, the incidence of internal mammary node disease may be as great as 50 per cent. If no axillary metastases are noted clinically, medial cancers are treated by modified

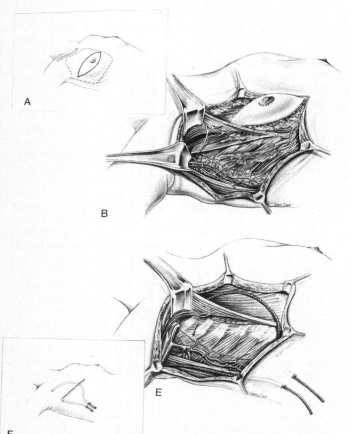

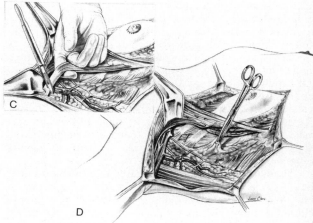

Figure 23. Technique for modified radical mastectomy. A, Transverse incision and area for planned flap elevation. B, Limits of dissection. C, Mobilization and division of pectoralis minor muscle from coracoid process prior to axillary dissection. D, Retraction of pectoralis major muscle with extension of shoulder to provide access to Level I, II, and III nodal groups following excision of pectoralis minor muscle. E, Completed dissection with preservation of neural innervation to pectoralis major. F, Closure with suction catheters in place.

radical mastectomy and postoperative peripheral lymphatic irradiation. If axillary metastases are identified pathologically in more than 20 per cent of the removed axillary lymph nodes, chest wall radiation therapy is added, since in-transit metastatic disease coursing to the axilla via subdermal lymphatics from medially located primary neoplasms may remain in the skin flaps and may be a source of locoregional recurrence.

Centrally located lesions that are attached to the pectoralis major fascia and *medially located lesions* with clinically palpable axillary lymph node metastases that are smaller than 2.5 cm. in size are treated by *radical mastectomy* and peripheral lymphatic and chest wall *radiation therapy*. These cancers are most likely to metastasize through the transpectoral and retropectoral routes (Rotter's nodes) as well as via lymphatics coursing along the neurovascular bundle medial to the pectoralis minor muscle. Preservation of this bundle is necessary to maintain innervation of the pectoralis major muscle and to prevent its atrophy following modified radical mastectomy (see Fig. 23). In the *radical mastectomy*, this neurovascular bundle with associated lymphatic channels and areolar tissue are removed with the specimen to ensure adequate extirpation of regional disease. Radical mastectomy is technically an easier procedure than modified radical mastectomy because the pectoralis major muscle is detached from its insertion into the bicipital groove of the humerus. Once this large muscle is reflected from its humeral and clavicular attachments, the surgeon can directly visualize the axilla and proceed with dissection of the lymphatic and areolar contents of this regional site. Also, the breast remains attached to the pectoralis major muscle and is removed when the pectoralis major muscle is detached from its costal margins. Otherwise, the axillary dissection is similar to that described for modified radical mastectomy, except that both lateral and medial pectoral nerves and associated lymphatic structures are removed with the specimen. An alternative form of treatment is *extended simple mastectomy*, as described hereafter, and radiation therapy to the peripheral lymphatic and apical axillary lymph nodes and the chest wall. Radiation therapy is relied upon to sterilize Rotter's nodes and the pectoralis muscle is left intact.

The responsibilities of the surgeon and the radiation therapist are to provide the patient with the best chance for local control of chest wall disease and ensure minimal morbidity and mortality related to the therapy. Complete surgical dissection of the axilla should not be followed by axillary radiation therapy because the incidence of lymphedema of the ipsilateral arm is increased greatly with combination modalities. Major lymphatic channels are removed surgically, and the remaining lymphatic collateral channels may be destroyed by radiation therapy. Furthermore, the axilla dissected for operable disease should not require radiation therapy after a modified radical or radical mastectomy.

Stage III Breast Cancer

As a rule, moderate doses of radiation therapy (e.g., 5000 rads over 5 weeks) will sterilize lymph nodes 1 cm. in size or less. In the management of Stage III disease for axillary metastases that exceed 2.5 cm. in size and are fixed and matted, the surgical procedure should be directed toward the removal of the primary cancer and lymph nodes *unlikely* to be sterilized by radiation therapy. The probability of control of regional nodal disease is inversely related to the size of the lymph nodes. Metastatic cancer in smaller,

centrally located axillary lymph nodes contiguous with axillary structures and not adequately resected may be sterilized by radiation therapy. The breast and Level I lymph nodes are removed in what has been termed an *extended simple mastectomy*: Level II and III lymph nodes remain on the chest wall to be sterilized by radiation therapy. By such combined treatment, the bulky disease is removed surgically and the microscopic disease is controlled by irradiation. Lymphedema of the arm is uncommon because collateral lymphatic channels entering through the apical axilla are undisturbed. An extended simple mastectomy differs from a modified radical mastectomy in that the pectoralis minor muscle is not detached from the coracoid process and removed and Level II and III nodal basins are not dissected. Both the medial and lateral pectoral nerves are left intact, and the medial border of the dissected specimen is the lateral border of the pectoralis major and minor muscles.

Adenocarcinomas greater than 5 cm. in diameter and associated with minimal clinical axillary disease (Stage IIIA) are often biologically favorable lesions and are best treated by preoperative radiation therapy and either an extended simple, a radical, or modified radical mastectomy. The therapeutic choice is dependent upon the location of the lesion and the dose of radiation therapy delivered to the apex of the axilla.

Stage IV Breast Cancer

Patients with distant metastases (Stage IV), including supraclavicular lymph node metastases, are treated primarily with chemotherapy, but control of local chest wall disease is best obtained by a limited surgical procedure, possibly combined with radiotherapy. The choice of these procedures is individualized for each patient, and the timing of the procedure(s) should be dictated by the medical oncologist since the patient's primary problem is control of distant metastases.

TYLECTOMY, AXILLARY SAMPLING (DISSECTION), AND RADIATION THERAPY

Conservative breast surgery has received much attention lately. These procedures are variously termed *segmental resection, lumpectomy,* or *tylectomy*.

"Lumpectomy" is not a word in the English language, and the preferred term is tylectomy. The breast may be preserved if adequate removal of all primary breast cancer can be accomplished without incision into cancerous tissue. For appropriately selected patients, maintenance of an adequate cosmetic appearance of the breast is the goal of the procedure that achieves control and cure rates equivalent to those of modified radical mastectomy. Frozen section evaluation of the margins of the resected specimen should be performed to ensure that all breast cancer has been removed en bloc with the specimen. A margin that contains breast cancer warrants further excision of breast tissue.

Following reconstruction of the remaining breast tissue, a sampling of the axillary lymph nodes is completed. If *adjuvant chemotherapy* is to be used appropriately, the status of the axillary lymph nodes must be determined. Axillary sampling is done via a curvilinear incision between the lateral border of the pectoralis major and latissimus dorsi muscles 4 to 6 cm. below the apex of the axilla. The lateral axillary contents that would be removed with an extended simple mastectomy (Level I) are taken (usually 10 to 13 lymph nodes). More recently, in some centers complete axillary dissection is being recommended. Indications for tylectomy, axillary sampling, and comprehensive radiation therapy to the breast include (1) a small breast cancer (less than 4 cm. in size), (2) clinically negative axillary lymph nodes, (3) a breast of adequate size to allow a uniform dose of radiation therapy, and (4) a radiation therapist experienced with this modality of treatment. If the therapist is not familiar with this radiotherapy technique, the results of primary radiation therapy for breast cancer can be both therapeutically and cosmetically unsatisfactory. The breast may become painful, fibrotic, edematous, and ulcerated.

Emphasis should be placed on removal of all the primary breast cancer. If viable cancer cells remain within the breast, they will be incorporated into the scar of the healing wound and are uniformly poorly oxygenated. For radiation therapy to be maximally effective, well-oxygenated tissues are necessary. Marginally oxygenated and anoxic cancer cells located within scar tissue may not be eradicated by radiation therapy. A recurrence of breast cancer in the scar would be anticipated. Early in the experience with tylectomy, recurrences were commonly observed within the scar and usually occurred in patients who had undergone biopsy in other institutions prior to referral for primary radiation therapy. Currently, our practice is to re-excise the scar in such patients and complete the axillary sampling procedure. Approximately 50 per cent of patients who have had the scars re-excised were found to have viable cancer cells present in the wound after what was initially deemed an adequate excisional biopsy. In those centers where re-excision of the scar is not advocated, the external beam irradiation dose is usually boosted by the implantation of iridium[192] needles in the area of the scar.

Survival results for these forms of conservative therapy for patients who meet the treatment criteria appear similar at 5 and 10 years to the survival data for patients who are treated by modified radical mastectomy. The long-term effects of irradiating the breast are not yet known, and patients wishing this treatment should be apprised of this future uncertainty. Properly done, tylectomy, axillary sampling, and comprehensive radiation therapy can give a very satisfactory cosmetic result. Breast cancer cannot be considered cured, however, by tylectomy alone, since several

studies have shown the disease to be multifocal within the ipsilateral breast.

If the lymph nodes removed during the axillary sampling procedure contain metastatic cancer, adjuvant chemotherapy should be considered in the postoperative period. In approximately 20 per cent of patients, the axillary lymph nodes are clinically negative yet pathologically positive. The decision as to when these patients should receive adjuvant therapy in relation to the course of comprehensive radiation therapy has not yet been determined.

Radical Mastectomy vs. QU.A.RT.

A randomized, prospective clinical trial reported by Veronesi and associates (Wolmark, Selected References) of Milan, compared radical mastectomy with quadrantectomy, axillary node dissection, and breast irradiation (QU.A.RT.). Between 1973 and 1980, 701 women with lesions 2 cm. or smaller and clinically negative axillae (T1NOMO) were assessed; mean time on study was 8 years. No significant differences between the two groups were apparent in local/regional recurrence, relapse-free survival, or overall survival (Figs. 24 and 25). Two per cent of patients in each group developed a local recurrence, and an additional 2 per cent demonstrated a regional treatment failure. Relapse-free survival at 8 years was 79 per cent in the mastectomy group and 80 per cent for patients managed by the QU.A.RT. protocol; the proportion of patients surviving was 82.5 and 85 per cent, respectively. In node-positive patients, prolonged survival favored the QU.A.RT. group (82 vs. 79 per cent), although this difference was not statistically significant. The study concluded that eligible patients with small breast lesions treated by QU.A.RT. protocol have no demonstrable disadvantage with regard to disease-free survival or overall survival compared with similar patient groups managed by radical mastectomy.

Segmental Mastectomy

In 1976, a randomized prospective trial (B-06) was conducted by Fisher and colleagues,[14] of the National Surgical Adjuvant Breast and Bowel Project (NSABP), to evaluate breast conservation and tumor control by segmen-

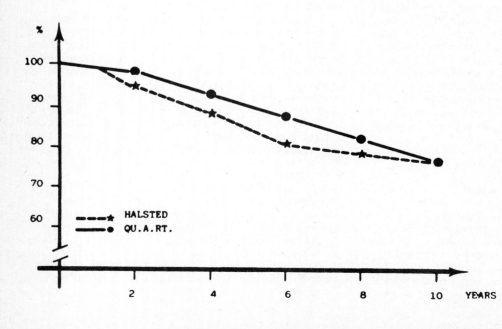

Figure 24. Disease-free survival of patients treated with Halsted mastectomy and with quadrantectomy, axillary dissection, radiotherapy (QU.A.RT.). (From Veronesi, U., et al.: World J. Surg., 9:678, 1985.)

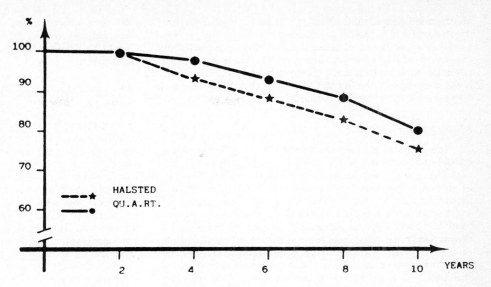

Figure 25. Overall survival of patients treated with Halsted mastectomy and with quadrantectomy, axillary dissection, radiotherapy (QU.A.RT.). (Reproduced with permission from Veronesi, U., et al.: World J. Surg., 9:679, 1985.)

tal mastectomy in the treatment of Stage I and II breast tumors 4 cm. or smaller in size. Women were randomly assigned to total mastectomy, segmental mastectomy alone, or segmental mastectomy followed by breast irradiation. All patients had axillary dissections, and patients with histologically positive nodes received adjuvant chemotherapy (melphalan and 5-fluorouracil).

Estimates based on data from 1843 women accrued in the B-06 study indicate that treatment by segmental mastectomy, with or without breast irradiation, achieves local disease-free, distant disease-free, and actuarial survival rates at 5 years equal to those of patients who had total mastectomy. Mean follow-up at the time of the report was 39 months, and definitive end-results must await 10-year analysis. Nevertheless, results from the study are important. Table 7 shows a comparison of the variable 5-year survival rates for the three treatment groups. Local recurrence in the operated breast was 8 per cent for patients who had segmental mastectomy and breast irradiation, whereas local recurrence was 28 per cent for those women who had segmental mastectomy without radiation therapy. The study, therefore, established the importance of radiation therapy in controlling recurrence of breast cancer in the ipsilateral breast for patients with negative axillary lymph nodes. Also of note was the local recurrence in the breasts of patients with positive lymph nodes, all of whom received adjuvant chemotherapy. ~so had chemo

For node-positive patients with and without treatment with radiation therapy, local breast recurrence rates after segmental mastectomy were 2 and 36 per cent, respectively. The 2 per cent figure is significantly lower than the corre-

sponding 8 per cent recurrence rate in women with negative axillary nodes and thereby indicates that radiation therapy may sensitize breast cancer to the cancericidal effects of chemotherapy (or vice versa).

ADVANCED LOCAL DISEASE

Prior to the advent of current forms of combination chemotherapy, *inflammatory breast cancer* had 5-year survival rates of only 3 to 5 per cent. With the use of any one of the combination chemotherapeutic programs (i.e., cyclophosphamide, doxorubicin [Adriamycin] and 5-fluorouracil) to be discussed later, approximately 60 to 75 per cent of individuals with inflammatory breast cancer will have a dramatic regression of the breast lesion. The breast cancer and any axillary metastases may disappear entirely by clinical examination. Following two to three drug cycles, an extended simple mastectomy may be done to remove the remaining malignant disease from the chest wall. The skin flaps, peripheral lymphatics, and apical axilla are then treated with comprehensive radiation therapy. With this multimodal form of treatment, 5-year survival from inflammatory breast cancer has improved to about 30 per cent.

Combination chemotherapy has also been valuable in the treatment of Stage III disease. Often axillary lymph node metastases may be large and matted. Grave signs (edema, ulceration, peau d'orange, and skin or pectoralis major muscle fixation) may exist; thus, completion of an extended simple mastectomy may not be technically possible. With the use of preoperative chemotherapy, these malignant deposits often regress in size, thereby allowing

TABLE 7. *Comparison of Local Disease-Free Survival, Distant Disease-Free Survival, and Survival After Five Years of Follow-up**

	Disease-Free Survival		Distant Disease-Free Survival		Survival	
	%	P Value	%	P Value	%	P Value
Total mastectomy	66	—	72	—	76	—
Segmental mastectomy	63	0.9†	70	0.7	85	0.06
Segmental mastectomy	72	0.04†	76	0.4	85	0.07
plus radiation		0.02‡		0.2		0.8

*Reprinted with permission from Fisher, B., et al.: World J. Surg., 9:682, 1985.
†Compared with total mastectomy group.
‡Compared with segmental mastectomy group.

an extended simple mastectomy to be done without the use of skin grafts. The use of comprehensive radiation therapy to the chest wall and peripheral lymphatics ensures better control of any disease remaining on the chest wall. As a result of these multimodality approaches, chest wall recurrence rates have been limited to 4 to 6 per cent, and 5- and 10-year survivals have been 45 and 28 per cent, respectively.

BREAST RECONSTRUCTION

Ideally, mastectomy should be done via a transverse or oblique incision. If an oblique incision is used, off-shoulder gowns may be worn without the medial portion of the scar being visible. Laterally, however, the oblique incision should not extend into the apex of the axilla, for scarring could result in limitation of shoulder and arm motion. The ablative operative procedure should be planned with the plastic surgeon in mind, but local control of the neoplasm should not be compromised to preserve cosmetic appearance. The major criticism of breast reconstruction has been the potential for delay in diagnosing recurrent cancer on the chest wall. For Stage I breast cancer, chest wall recurrence as a first sign of failure is unusual; when it occurs, it does not appear until several years after the initial mastectomy. Also, if proper local treatment for breast cancer has been completed initially, local chest wall recurrence rates for Stage I and early Stage II disease should approach 0 to 2 per cent. Additionally, the breast prosthesis is placed most frequently beneath the pectoralis major muscle in a position where it would not obscure a superficial recurrence in the skin and subdermal connective tissues.[19]

Immediate chest wall reconstruction at the time of mastectomy for an invasive breast cancer is not ideal, since the status of the axillary lymph nodes is not known. If radiation therapy or chemotherapy is to be used in an adjuvant setting, breast reconstruction should await completion of these treatment modalities. Certainly, chest wall radiation therapy in a person with an implant is not recommended, and capsular scarring around the breast prosthesis may be stimulated by some forms of chemotherapy, particularly doxorubicin. Therefore, reconstruction may be done at any time the plastic surgeon deems it feasible after the pathologic state of the axillary lymph nodes is known and any adjuvant therapy has been completed.[19]

Immediate breast reconstruction may be done for individuals who have intraductal carcinoma *in situ* or lobular carcinoma *in situ* or for patients who are undergoing a prophylactic mastectomy.

PROPHYLACTIC MASTECTOMY

Patients in a high-risk category with breasts that are difficult to evaluate by both physical examination and mammography are candidates for prophylactic mastectomy. Any type of incision may be used, but the important issue is the removal of all breast tissue from the chest wall. *Subcutaneous mastectomy* done via an inframammary incision often does *not* allow removal of breast tissue from the axillary tail, subareolar sites, or within the nipple. One of two procedures should be done as prophylaxis against breast cancer: (1) *simple mastectomy*, sacrificing the nipple-areola complex, or (2) *total glandular mastectomy*, in which a periareolar incision is extended laterally so that all breast tissue may be removed from the chest wall and axilla by direct vision. The nipple is detached from the areola by a circumferential incision and removed with the specimen.

By such a mechanism, all breast tissue can be removed yet the areola remains intact, the nipple can be reconstructed, and a prosthesis may be inserted during the same operative procedure.

RESULTS OF ATTEMPTS AT LOCAL-REGIONAL CONTROL OF DISEASE

Montague and coworkers[26] reviewed the results of local-regional treatment of breast cancer utilizing surgery and radiation therapy either alone or in combination. In 301 patients treated by radical mastectomy alone, 12 per cent had positive lymph nodes and 5- and 10-year survival rates were 72.6 and 55.0 per cent, respectively. For 368 patients treated with radical mastectomy and postoperative radiation therapy, 63 per cent had positive axillary lymph nodes and 5-and 10-year survival rates were 74.3 and 57.0 per cent, respectively. In the group of patients who received preoperative radiation therapy followed by radical mastectomy, only 29 per cent had histologically positive axillary lymph nodes and 5- and 10-year survival rates were 71.6 and 57.0 per cent, respectively. The number of patients with *clinically* positive axillary lymph nodes before treatment was the same for both groups, i.e., those who received radiation therapy preoperatively and those who received it postoperatively. Thus, it must be assumed that radiation therapy sterilized approximately half of the clinically positive lymph nodes in the *preoperative radiation therapy* group, since the percentage of axillary lymph nodes histologically positive was half that in the group of patients receiving *postoperative radiation therapy*.

Another interesting observation from these results is that the 5- and 10-year survival rates were the same in all three groups, although the percentage of lymph nodes that were histologically positive differed significantly among the groups. None of these patients had chemotherapy prophylactically; therefore, some credit should be given to radiation therapy for equalizing the survival figures. This patient population was selected for presentation in this chapter because no chemotherapy was utilized. Although this patient group was treated by radical mastectomy, predictably the results would have been similar for modified radical mastectomy.

In Montague's series, patients with outer quadrant lesions who had radical mastectomies, histologically normal axillary lymph nodes, and no radiation therapy had 5- and 10-year survival rates of 76 and 58 per cent, respectively. Patients who had medial quadrant lesions with histologically normal axillary lymph nodes and who had received radical mastectomies followed by radiation therapy had 5- and 10-year survival rates of 87 and 76 per cent (P< 0.005), respectively. These differences in survival were also identified in patients with histologically positive axillary lymph nodes. These results suggest that the use of radiation therapy may have improved the long-term survival, particularly in patients with primary breast cancers in the medial portion of the breast. It must be emphasized, however, that this study is one of the few that equates the use of local radiation therapy with an increase in survival. Almost all studies indicate that radiation therapy improves the chance for local control of the disease, but this usually does not equate with an improvement in overall survival rates. Also, these patients were retrospectively evaluated over a 20-year interval at the M. D. Anderson Hospital and Tumor Institute dating back to the 1950s and 1960s. Many of these lesions were large. More recent studies indicate that patients with lesions smaller than 2 cm. in size (T1, NO) have an 85 per cent 5-year survival that diminishes very little at 10 years.

These data also revealed that patients with extended simple mastectomies who were followed by comprehensive radiation therapy for breast cancers that were technically unsuitable for resection, i.e., edematous, large, ulcerated lesions with large matted axillary lymph nodes, had a 23 per cent 10-year survival rate without the addition of chemotherapy. These data indicate that long-term survival can be obtained for select patients by tailoring the surgical procedure and the radiation therapy to the patient's individual needs. The 23 per cent 10-year survival rate for this group implies that not all patients with advanced regional disease necessarily have disseminated breast cancer. This observation should be recalled when evaluating the results of adjuvant chemotherapy trials for advanced local breast cancer. In other words, a 23 per cent 10-year survival rate in patients with advanced Stage III disease treated with chemotherapy cannot necessarily be attributed to the use of chemotherapy in the adjuvant setting.

The more recent analysis of the 10-year results of a randomized clinical trial comparing radical mastectomy and total mastectomy with and without radiation was reported by Fisher and associates[15] of the NSABP. Patients were treated by (1) radical mastectomy, (2) total ("simple") mastectomy without axillary dissection but with regional irradiation, or (3) total mastectomy without irradiation with the proviso that axillary dissection be performed if nodes became clinically positive. Life-table estimates were obtained for 1665 women enrolled in the study (mean 126 months). No significant differences for local disease-free, distant disease-free, or overall survival (approximately 57 per cent) rates were observed at 10 years for the three groups. Additionally, no differences were evident between patients with clinically positive nodes treated by radical mastectomy and those treated by total mastectomy without axillary dissection but with regional radiotherapy (Figs. 26 and 27).

The end results of this study indicate that the *location*

of a breast tumor does not influence prognosis and that irradiation of internal mammary nodes in patients with medial quadrant lesions does not enhance survival. This study also demonstrated that the results obtained at 5 years accurately predict outcome at 10 years. This multi-institutional study concludes that the variations of local and regional treatment utilized in the analysis are not important to determine survival of patients with carcinoma of the breast.

MINIMAL BREAST CANCER

Minimal breast cancer, defined as invasive breast cancer smaller than 0.5 cm. in diameter, *in situ* intraductal, or *in situ* lobular breast cancer is seldom associated with lymph node metastasis. Gallagher and Martin[18] utilized whole organ subserial sections of breast specimens removed for cancer to outline phases in the progression of adenocarcinoma from intraepithelial origin to invasion and local spread. These studies have given credibility to the hypothesis that adenocarcinoma of the breast begins as epithelial atypia, progresses to noninvasive carcinoma, and then proceeds to frank invasion.

Frazier and co-workers[17] reported 176 patients with minimal breast cancer treated during a 20-year interval. Of these patients, 138 had intraductal carcinoma *in situ*, 21 had minimally invasive carcinoma, and 17 had lobular carcinoma *in situ*. Thirty-four patients were asymptomatic and were diagnosed by mammography; 99 patients had breast masses discovered by self-examination; 32 patients had nipple discharge; 6 patients were asymptomatic but had masses discovered during routine physical examination; 3 patients had localized breast pain but no discrete mass; and 2 patients had palpable axillary lymph nodes. Axillary lymph nodes were removed as part of the primary treatment in 114 patients. Four patients had lymph nodes containing metastatic breast cancer. Two of these patients had intraductal carcinoma *in situ*, and two patients had minimally invasive carcinoma.

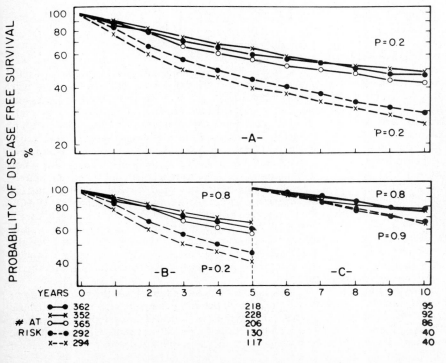

Figure 26. Survival free of disease through 10 years (A), during the first 5 years (B), and during the second 5 years for patients free of disease at the end of the fifth year (C). Patients were treated by radical mastectomy (solid circle), total mastectomy plus radiation (x), or total mastectomy alone (open circle). There were no significant differences among the three groups of patients with clinically negative nodes (solid line) or between the two groups with clinically positive nodes (broken line). (From Fisher, B., et al.: N. Engl. J. Med., 312:675, 1985.)

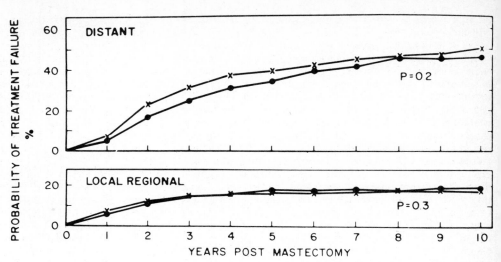

Figure 27. Local or regional and distant treatment failures as the first evidence of disease in patients with clinically positive nodes who were treated by radical mastectomy (solid circle) or total mastectomy and radiation (x). There was no significant difference in distant or local and regional disease between the two groups. (Reproduced with permission from Fisher, B., et al.: N. Engl. J. Med., 312:676, 1985.)

Follow-up of these 176 patients ranges from 1 to 21 years. Eighty-four per cent are living with no evidence of cancer; 4.0 per cent are living with breast cancer; 4.0 per cent have died of breast cancer; and 8.0 per cent have died of diseases other than breast cancer. If patients who had invasive adenocarcinomas in their opposite breast are excluded, eight patients (6.3 per cent) in the minimal cancer group developed metastases, all of whom had intraductal carcinoma *in situ*.

As for patients in whom the opposite breast was at risk, carcinoma developed in 7.7 per cent of those with minimally invasive carcinoma, in 18.3 per cent of those with intraductal carcinoma *in situ*, and in 50.0 per cent of those with lobular carcinoma *in situ*. The median time interval for development of a subsequent *contralateral invasive breast cancer* was 84 months, whereas the median time interval for discovery of a *contralateral noninvasive breast cancer* was only 19 months. Thus, a distinctly longer time interval was involved in the development of an invasive breast cancer. These data support the theory of Gallagher and Martin[18] that breast cancer develops from a stage of intraepithelial atypia and progresses to a stage of frank invasion. The 20-year actuarial survival rate for the 176 patients was 93.2 per cent. If patients who had invasive carcinoma of the contralateral breast were excluded from the survival statistics, no patients with lobular carcinoma *in situ* or minimally invasive carcinoma have died, and the *predicted* 20-year actuarial survival rate for the group is 95.9 per cent.

Intraductal carcinoma in situ appeared to have a slightly more virulent pattern than did lobular carcinoma *in situ*, since axillary metastases were identified in this group. Patients with intraductal carcinoma *in situ* should have at least an extended simple mastectomy, since important information regarding the prognosis and the need for potential adjuvant therapy may be obtained by knowing the status of the Level I axillary lymph nodes.

The proper treatment for *lobular carcinoma in situ* is more controversial. Both breasts are at equal risk for developing invasive breast cancer when this diagnosis is confirmed. This risk, nationwide, may be as high as 30 per cent in either or both breasts over the ensuing 20-year period, and the type of invasive breast cancer may be either ductal or lobular. The histologic study of lobular carcinoma *in situ* documents a frequency of *multicentricity* in the ipsilateral breast of 60 to 90 per cent, and 20 to 45 per cent of women with the disease have synchronous, or develop

metachronous, contralateral breast carcinoma. Thus, the treatment recommended for the *ipsilateral* breast containing lobular carcinoma *in situ* should be recommended for the *contralateral* breast as well. Some women may elect to forego a mastectomy, have careful follow-up, and risk the development of invasive breast cancer in the future. Other women prefer to have bilateral simple mastectomies and immediate breast reconstruction.

Minimal breast cancers that demonstrate invasion should be treated by surgical and radiotherapeutic modalities outlined previously in this chapter. The temptation must be resisted to treat small invasive lesions with limited surgical procedures. Certainly, these small cancers are amenable to tylectomy, axillary sampling, and comprehensive radiation therapy. The excellent actuarial and definitive survival rates for patients with minimal breast cancer indicate the favorable prognosis and the need for continued emphasis on early detection, particularly the necessity for breast self-examination, refinements in mammographic techniques, and an increase in public education on the proper treatment for breast cancer.

Systemic Therapy

Current clinical trials indicate that chemotherapy and, possibly, hormonal therapy, when given to patients with axillary metastasis but no distant metastases (adjuvant therapy), prolong the disease-free interval and may increase survival rates. Similarly, in patients with established distant metastasis, therapy with several drugs that are less effective as single agents has resulted in more than a 50 per cent response rate when used in combination. The most common combinations are (1) cyclophosphamide (Cytoxan), methotrexate, and 5-fluorouracil (CMF) and (2) 5-fluorouracil, doxorubicin (Adriamycin), and cyclophosphamide (FAC). These same combinations are often used in the adjuvant setting as well. Other drugs, such as vincristine and prednisone, have been added to these regimens, but often the slight increase in response rate does not justify the additional toxicity, particularly the neurotoxicity from vincristine.

Although the response rates from these combinations vary from 20 to 70 per cent, complete response rates (those patients in whom all evidence of disease disappears) have consistently been less than 20 per cent. Undoubtedly, the heterogeneity of the cell population within a breast cancer prevents total response. Multiple cell populations have variable response rates to the administered drugs. Also, this heterogeneity may explain why multiple drug combinations with different sites of action within the cell have a better overall response rate than do single agents.

Toxicity associated with cytotoxic drugs for breast cancer is similar to that of chemotherapy for other malignancies, i.e., nausea, vomiting, myelosuppression, thrombocytopenia, alopecia, and increased fatigability. However, these toxic effects are reversible when the drugs are discontinued. Cardiomyopathy is a cumulative, dose-limiting side effect of doxorubicin. Only 550 mg. per square meter may be given to one patient, and cardiomyopathy, when it occurs, usually is not reversible.

HORMONE RECEPTORS

Specific proteins within the cytosol of breast cells bind and transfer appropriate steroid molecules into the cell nucleus to exert a specific hormonal effect. The most widely used receptor proteins are the estrogen and progesterone receptors. These assays usually require approximately 1 gm. of fresh tissue, and the receptors are heat labile. The electric cautery current (Bovie) should not be used when removing tissue on which estrogen or progesterone receptor activity will be measured. The surgeon obtaining the biopsy material should be aware of the heat lability of these receptors. Also, the circulating nurse in the operating room and the pathologist examining the tissue must prepare the tissue for estrogen and progesterone receptor assay as soon as possible, since both of these receptor proteins may decay in activity within 30 minutes of removal from the patient. Tissue cytosol is obtained by homogenation and centrifugation of the prepared specimen, which is incubated with H^3-tritium-labeled estradiol 17^β. Labeled, unbound hormone is removed from the incubation mixture, and the bound estrogen sediment is measured by multipoint titration with Scatchard plot analysis. The binding capacity is expressed in femtomoles of H^3-estradiol bound per mg. of cytosol protein. Values of 10 femtomoles or more per mg. are considered *receptor positive*, whereas values of less than 3 femtomoles per mg. are *receptor negative*. Intermediate values are considered borderline. The degree of positivity is proportional to the differentiation and histologic subtype of the lesion. Ninety per cent or more of well-differentiated ductal and lobular carcinomas are estrogen receptor (ER) positive. Sequential studies of ER activity in the same patient usually reveal no significant change between the primary and metastatic sites, nor is there often any change as metastatic sites evolve in different areas of the body.

Estrogen Receptor Activity

A strong correlation exists between the presence of ER activity and the clinical response to various forms of endocrine therapy. Less than 10 per cent of ER-negative patients respond, whereas greater than 60 per cent of ER-positive patients respond to exogenous estrogens or endocrine ablative procedures.

Prior to the use of ER activity as an indicator of hormonal therapy, the rationale for the use of endocrine treatment in patients with metastatic breast cancer was empirical. A poorly understood, but well-established, paradox was that the patient who responded to the administration of pharmacologic doses of estrogen may subsequently respond to the withdrawal of estrogen. Oophorectomy, adrenalectomy, and hypophysectomy were the endocrine ablative procedures commonly used to treat metastatic disease. *Oophorectomy* was utilized as treatment for premenopausal patients with either skin or bony metastasis with a documented disease-free interval of at least 18 months between treatment of the primary lesion and discovery of the metastasis. Visceral metastases, particularly to the liver and lungs, respond poorly to any form of hormonal manipulation. Pharmacologic doses of exogenous estrogen were reserved for postmenopausal women who had an 18-month disease-free interval and metastases primarily to skin or bone. Response rates in each of these clinical settings was approximately 30 per cent. *Adrenalectomy* and *hypophysectomy* were used for both premenopausal and postmenopausal patients and were often effective in those individuals who had previously responded to either oophorectomy or exogenous estrogens. This response rate also approximated 30 per cent. Those individuals who had rapid onset of metastatic disease or who failed hormonal manipulation were treated with conventional chemotherapy.

Interestingly, now that hormonal receptor assay is available, the correlation between strongly positive receptor activity and the response to hormonal manipulation has become obvious. Receptor activities have allowed the medical oncologist to decide which patients are candidates for either additive hormonal or ablative endocrine procedures. The estrogen receptor has thus become a marker of hormone-dependent breast cancer and has greatly simplified the approach to oncologic treatment protocols for Stages I through IV disease.[1]

Progesterone Receptor Activity

Progesterone receptor (PR) activity in the cytosol should also be measured concomitant with the ER determination of the primary tumor. Premenopausal patients have a lower incidence of ER-positive activity (30 per cent) compared with postmenopausal patients (60 per cent). These data would indicate that premenopausal patients have a much lower response to hormonal manipulation. Indeed, the response rate of pre- and postmenopausal patients is similar, and PR activity may be more indicative of an opportunity for response to hormonal manipulation in the premenopausal patient. Not infrequently, a premenopausal patient will have a tumor that is strongly PR-positive yet may be ER-negative. This biochemical profile indicates a high correlation for response of the malignancy to hormonal therapy.

Antiestrogen Therapy

The antiestrogen tamoxifen (Nolvadex) was originally developed as an antifertility drug; however, it was noted to induce ovulation in infertile women and to cause regression of breast cancer lesions. Approximately one third of the patients initially treated with tamoxifen showed objective evidence of regression of metastatic disease. This regression correlated closely with positive ER and/or PR activity. Antiestrogens block the uptake of estrogen by the target tissue following cytosol binding to the ER. The lack of response at one dose level may be improved by escalating the dose. The most striking advantage of tamoxifen is the almost complete absence of side effects. There may be a "flare" of bone pain and hypercalcemia when tamoxifen therapy is initiated, but this effect is short-lived. Pharmacologic doses of estrogens may also produce this flare of bone pain and may also initiate nausea, vomiting, and fluid retention.

Adrenalectomy

The rationale for adrenalectomy in postmenopausal females, particularly those who responded to exogenous estrogens, was the ablation of all estrogenic stimuli. Following menopause, the adrenal becomes the major production site of endogenous estrogens. Aminoglutethimide, originally introduced as an anticonvulsant, has been found to suppress corticosteroid synthesis. This compound blocks the enzymatic conversion of cholesterol to δ-5-pregnenolone and inhibits conversion of androstenedione to estrogen in peripheral tissues. With therapy, adrenal suppression is evident with an associated fall in cortisol secretion and a biofeedback increase in adrenocorticotropic hormone (ACTH) that can override the aminoglutethimide blockade. Consequently, glucocorticoid therapy is required to suppress ACTH secretion. This "medical adrenalectomy" with aminoglutethimide has been compared prospectively with hypophysectomy and surgical adrenalectomy. In both instances, medical therapy was at least equivalent to surgical ablation and appears to be an acceptable alternative. Neither permanent adrenal insufficiency nor acute crises were observed. Side effects include lethargy, ataxia, and dizziness but are dose-dependent and transient.

ADJUVANT CHEMOTHERAPY

The initial studies by Fisher and associates[13] and Bonnadonna and colleagues[8] suggested that additive chemotherapy given prior to clinically detectable distant metastases may enhance survival for breast cancer patients. The goal of this therapy is the eradication of well-established but unidentified micrometastases. The original recommendations were to use adjuvant chemotherapy of multiple combinations in premenopausal women with three or more positive axillary lymph nodes. More recent data indicate that this therapeutic benefit can also be established in women with one to three abnormal lymph nodes either before or after menopause. The addition of tamoxifen to the chemotherapeutic regimen in ER-positive patients appears to provide even greater protection against the development of distant metastasis.

Obviously, the strategy is to improve the 5- and 10-year disease-free survival rates for patients with regional lymph node metastasis to equal those of patients who have no axillary lymph node involvement. It is too early to determine whether the goal of therapy has been achieved, yet an increase in survival of 10 to 20 per cent over that anticipated for patients with either Stage II or Stage III disease at 5 years is being recognized with regularity in most clinical trials.

Timing and Dosage

As mentioned previously, individuals with advanced Stage III disease may respond to preoperative chemotherapy so that the lesions become surgically operable. The timing and dosages of chemotherapy given to patients with bulky local-regional disease but unidentifiable distant metastases have not been established firmly. For example, preoperative chemotherapy followed by surgery and then radiation therapy appears to be the most ideal method of combination treatment of inflammatory breast carcinoma. Patients who are treated by tylectomy, axillary sampling, and breast irradiation and who have positive axillary lymph nodes also require adjuvant chemotherapy. The questions remain: When should it be administered? Before radiation therapy or after? And if before, how many cycles of chemotherapy should be administered prior to initiating radiation therapy?

Certainly radiation therapy in these clinical circumstances is indicated, since regional lymph node basins and the breast remain intact. Some chemotherapeutic agents increase the desmoplastic response (scarring), particularly when used in combination with radiation therapy. For example, the use of doxorubicin in combination with radiotherapy might produce an unsightly, painful, fibrotic breast. Clearly, those individuals who undergo either modified radical or radical mastectomy and have multiple positive axillary lymph nodes and/or a bulky, anaplastic primary lesion should receive chemotherapy for several cycles (2 to 3 months) prior to initiating radiation therapy to enhance control of chest wall disease after the surgical procedure. It has not been clearly established whether adjuvant chemotherapy will contain local chest wall recurrences as effectively as adjuvant radiotherapy, and until such data are confirmed, radiation therapy should be used as outlined in this chapter to ensure that local-regional disease is controlled.

Summary

There is no clinical evidence that adjuvant chemotherapy is of value for patients with Stage I breast cancer; however, patients whose primary lesions invade blood vessels and lymphatics or are nuclear Grade III (anaplastic) should be considered carefully for adjuvant chemotherapy. The long-term side effects of chemotherapy, however, are not yet identified. Potentially, the drugs may increase the incidence of hematopoietic malignancies later in life. Possibly, tamoxifen may be an ideal adjuvant drug used singularly in high-risk patients with Stage I breast cancer, particularly if ER activity is positive. Answers to these questions await future randomized, prospective trials.

COMBINATION CHEMOTHERAPY FOR METASTATIC DISEASE

Responses to combination chemotherapy (FAC, CMF, or other combinations) have been observed for metastases to bone, liver, soft tissue, lung, and occasionally brain. Randomized, prospective trials comparing cytotoxic chemotherapeutic drugs indicate an increase in response rates from approximately 25 per cent with single agents to between 50 and 60 per cent using combination therapy. Also, median survival for combination therapy in those individuals who do respond is longer than that obtained with single drugs. Relationships between the responsiveness to chemotherapy and ER status have been controversial. Several studies have noted a direct correlation, whereas others have found exactly the opposite. Again, the heterogeneity of the cell population within the breast cancer probably dictates response dynamics. No reproducible parameters to evaluate the heterogeneity of the cell population are yet available. Most trials do identify a significantly longer chemotherapy-induced response in those patients who previously were responders to hormone therapy and who have ER-positive reactivity.

Age, menstrual status, family history of breast cancer, extent of axillary nodal involvement, size of primary, and type of surgery appear to have little influence as predictors for responses to chemotherapy. A prolonged disease-free interval usually does indicate a response advantage. The median duration of response to combination chemotherapy ranges between 12 and 18 months. Once failure has occurred, the use of another combination of cytotoxic agents may result in a remission (partial or complete). Patients who achieve a complete remission have a median survival of 32 months. Patients who experience a relapse from combination chemotherapy are still eligible for hormonal manipulation, particularly if they are ER-positive and have not previously been treated by hormonal manipulation. Patients who have rapidly progressive disease and a short disease-free interval should be treated with cytotoxic chemotherapy in lieu of hormonal therapy. For hormonal therapy to be of objective value, approximately 2 to 3 months are required before an objective response can be realized. This may be too great an interval to observe individuals who have rapidly progressive disease. Whether the addition of tamoxifen to combination cytotoxic regimens can enhance the response advantage awaits the completion of concurrent, randomized, prospective trials.

Breast Cancer in Pregnancy and Lactation

From 0.4 to 3.8 per cent of reported breast cancers occur in pregnant and/or lactating females. The average age of a pregnant patient with concomitant breast cancer is 34 years. This association of pregnancy and breast cancer, in the past, had been thought to be a poor prognostic circumstance. The profound estrogen and progesterone stimulation of breast cancer cells reportedly increased the risk of distant metastasis. More recent studies have indicated that, stage for stage, carcinoma of the breast in a pregnant female is associated with a prognosis similar to that for the nonpregnant woman. There are, however, more patients with Stage II and III breast cancer diagnosed during pregnancy compared with the general population of women with this disease. Whether this later stage at diagnosis is secondary to the hormonal milieu of the pregnancy or to a delay in diagnosis because of the physiologic changes in the breast coincident with pregnancy are unknown. Certainly, women may ignore a mass in the breast or may not identify it because of the increased density of the lactating breast.

DIAGNOSIS

Emphasis should be placed on the prompt histologic diagnosis of any mass in the breast of a pregnant or lactating woman. Mammography is usually less effective because of breast engorgement. The use of needle aspiration may distinguish a solid from a cystic mass and creates no risk for the fetus. Risk of spontaneous abortion during mastectomy is approximately 1 per cent and correlates with the duration of gestation.

THERAPY

Therapy for the pregnant patient is identical to that for the nonpregnant patient. Patients who have advanced breast cancer require the appropriate use of chemotherapy and radiation therapy. If the diagnosis is made in the first or second trimester of pregnancy, termination of the pregnancy is recommended. In the third trimester, treatment may be delayed until a term delivery or labor may be induced prematurely in order to preserve a healthy, viable child as well as provide appropriate treatment for the mother. No delay, however, should exceed 4 weeks. Lactation should be suppressed promptly in the postpartum patient even if biopsy identifies a benign lesion, as milk from transected lactiferous ducts will drain through the biopsy site.

THERAPEUTIC ABORTION

A patient who becomes pregnant during a postoperative course of irradiation therapy or chemotherapy to control an aggressive primary lesion should consider therapeutic abortion. Both radiation therapy and chemotherapy are potentially teratogenic, particularly in the first 12 weeks of gestation. Current recommendations suggest that no more than 500 millirads should be administered or intrauterine development may be impaired.

RECURRENCE

Childbearing in a woman who has had breast cancer may not increase the overall recurrence rate; however, the disease-free interval in patients who have recurrence, theoretically, may be shortened, particularly in ER-positive patients. Consequently, childbearing or estrogen-containing compounds should be considered cautiously before either is recommended to a woman who is at risk for recurrent disease. In patients who are at reasonable risk for recurrent disease and in whom estrogens might be useful as an antineoplastic agent, oral contraceptives or other estrogen-containing compounds should not be prescribed.

Carcinoma of the Male Breast

The incidence of breast carcinoma in men represents less than 1 per cent of all breast cancer. The incidence is reported to be highest among Britons and North Americans, where it constitutes 0.4 to 1.5 per cent of all cancers in men. Gynecomastia may be a presenting feature in nearly 20 per cent of individuals, and male breast cancer has been associated with estrogen therapy, high endogenous estrogen levels, Klinefelter's syndrome, irradiation, and trauma. Clinical features of male breast carcinoma are similar to those seen in women: breast mass, nipple retraction and discharge, skin fixation and ulceration, and pain. The neoplasm is rare in young males but escalates sharply in incidence in older populations. The greatest number of patients affected are between 60 and 69 years of age. This carcinoma appears to be more hormonally dependent (ER-positive) than the typical adenocarcinoma of females. Stage for stage, males with breast cancer appear to have the same survival advantages as do females. The overall prognosis in most series, however, is poor because of an advanced stage of disease at diagnosis. Often, at least one grave sign, usually skin fixation, is present.

The local tumor is best managed by modified radical mastectomy and comprehensive postoperative irradiation in select cases. Orchiectomy and administration of estrogenic steroids may induce remission of metastatic disease. The use of hormone manipulation in the adjuvant setting is uncertain, as so few cases are available for study, yet response rates should be equal to those in women, as should response to adjuvant or therapeutic combination cytotoxic chemotherapy.

SELECTED REFERENCES

Beahrs, O. H., and Meyers, M. H.: American Joint Committee on Cancer. Manual for Staging of Cancer. Philadelphia, J. B. Lippincott Company, 1983.
  This manual was developed by the American Joint Committee on Cancer (AJCC) to provide comprehensive state-of-the-art staging for cancers at various anatomic sites. The student of breast disease is provided a succinct

classification with TNM staging to allow reporting of cancer survival and end results.

Copeland, E. M. III: Surgical Oncology. New York, John Wiley & Sons, 1983.
This book provides a review of cancer of multiple organs with an in-depth review of the principles of diagnosis and treatment of malignant neoplasms of the breast. Details of the techniques for various forms of surgical treatment of breast cancer are described.

Donegan, W. L., and Spratt, J. S.: Cancer of the Breast, 2nd ed. Philadelphia, W. B. Saunders Company, 1979.
This book reflects the extensive experience of the authors with breast carcinoma at a state cancer hospital. This comprehensive volume provides an excellent basis for the epidemiology, diagnosis, clinical assessment, therapeutic modalities, and statistical considerations applied in the management of breast cancer.

Haagensen, C. D.: Disease of the Breast, 3rd ed. Philadelphia, W. B. Saunders Company, 1985.
This classic volume is recommended as a standard text for the student of disease of the breast. This volume reflects the personal experience of a single surgeon in the management of benign and malignant processes of the breast. His meticulous concern for evaluation, pathologic assessment, and therapeutic approaches support the biologic basis on which these decisions are formulated.

Harris, J. R., Hellman, S., Canellos, G. P., and Fisher, B.: Cancer of the breast. *In* DeVita, V. T., Jr., Hellman, S., and Rosenberg, S. A. (Eds.): Cancer: Principles and Practice of Oncology, 2nd ed. Philadelphia, J. B. Lippincott Company, 1985.
This chapter on breast cancer offers the student an excellent treatise on the management of carcinoma of the breast. Therapeutic considerations in the selection of multimodal approaches are analyzed, and objective data are provided that support these various treatment options. The chapter is well supported with concise tables and figures and has an excellent bibliography. Additional sections objectively document contemporary radiotherapeutic approaches for locally advanced and early breast cancer. The section on therapy of systemic disease reviews the rationale for application of steroid receptors for hormonal and cytotoxic chemotherapy. A detailed review of chemotherapy for breast cancer analyzes the historic applications of single and combination agents effective in the management of this neoplasm.

Margolese, R. G.: Breast Cancer. New York, Churchill Livingstone, 1983.
This recent publication comprises the overviews of select authorities on breast cancer. Chapters are organized to provide a comprehensive review of controversial and/or difficult management problems for this neoplasm. The sections on etiology of breast carcinoma and hereditary breast carcinoma are exceptional. The chapter on chemotherapy and the application of steriod hormone receptors is meritorious.

McDivitt, R. W., Stewart, F. W., and Berg, J. W.: Tumors of the breast. *In* Atlas of Tumor Pathology, Series 2, Fasicle 2. Washington, D. C., Armed Forces Institute of Pathology, 1968.
This atlas of the histology of benign and malignant breast neoplasms is a recognized classic treatise of the subject. Detailed gross and microscopic descriptions of the pathology are well supported with illustrations and objective data necessary to the student of this disease.

Pilch, Y. H.: Surgical Oncology. New York, McGraw-Hill, 1984.
This book chapter on breast cancer is well organized and presents an authoritative approach to screening and xeromammographic evaluation of breast disease. The author emphasizes the rationale for the various forms of surgical therapy for operable disease. The results of the NSABP trials conducted within the past decade are reviewed. Illustrations, tables, and bibliography are comprehensive and well supportive of the text.

Wilson, R. E.: The breast. *In* Sabiston, D. C., Jr. (Ed.): Textbook of Surgery: The Biological Basis of Modern Surgical Practice, 13th ed. Philadelphia, W. B. Saunders Company, 1986.
This chapter on breast diseases is an authoritative perspective of various benign and malignant processes. The text provides an excellent overview to the principles applicable in the management of primary breast diseases. The text is well supported with tables, illustrations, an extensive bibliography, and selected bibliographic review of contemporary articles and historic monographs. The succinct summaries of the histopathologic types of breast carcinoma and the logic of therapeutic approaches are meritorious.

Wolmark, N.: Progress symposium—progress in carcinoma of the breast. World J. Surg. *5*:653, 1985.
This volume of World Progress in Surgery provides a thorough and enlightening review of the contemporary approaches of the National Surgical Adjuvant Breast Project, National Cancer Institutes (U. S. and Italy), and select national and European trials for the therapy of primary breast cancer. This compilation of trials succinctly summarizes the results of breast conservation procedures. The applications of radiotherapy and chemotherapy in various stages of disease are included with end results reported in these large clinical prospective studies.

REFERENCES

1. Allegra, J. C.: The use of steroid hormone receptors in breast cancer. *In* Margolese, R. (Ed.): Contemporary Issues in Clinical Oncology: Breast Cancer. New York, Churchill Livingstone, 1983, p. 187.
2. Anderson, D. E.: Some characteristics of familial breast cancer. Cancer, *28*:1500, 1971.
3. Anson, B. J., and McVay, C. B.: Thoracic walls: Breast or mammary region. *In* Surgical Anatomy. Philadelphia, W. B. Saunders Company, 1971, p. 339.
4. Baker, R. R.: Outpatient biopsies. Ann. Surg. *185*:543, 1977.
5. Black, M. M. and Speer, F. D.: Nuclear structure in cancer tissues. Surg. Gynecol. Obstet. *105*:97, 1957.
6. Bland, K. I., Kuhns, J. G., Buchanan, J. B., Dwyer, P. A., Heuser, L. F., O'Connor, C. A., Gray, L. A., Sr., and Polk, H. C., Jr.: A clinicopathologic correlation of mammographic parenchymal patterns and associated risk factors for human mammary carcinoma. Ann. Surg., *195*:582, 1982.
7. Bloom, H. J. G., Richardson, W. W., and Harres, E. J.: Natural history of untreated breast cancer (1805–1933); Comparison of untreated and treated cases according to histological grade of malignancy. Br. Med. J. *5299*:213, 1962.
8. Bonadonna, G., Brusamolino, E., Valagussa, P., et al.: Combination chemotherapy as an adjuvant treatment in operable breast cancer. N. Engl. J. Med., *294*:405, 1976.
9. Chaudary, M. A., Millis, R. R., Davies, G. C, and Hayward, J. L.: Nipple discharge: The diagnostic value of testing for occult blood. Ann. Surg., *196*:651, 1982.
10. Contarini, O., Urdaneta, L. F., Hagan, W., and Stephenson, S. E., Jr.: Cystosarcoma phylloides of the breast: A new therapeutic proposal. Am. Surg. *48*:157, 1982.
11. Crymes, J. E.: Current status of mammography. CRC Crit. Rev. Diagn. Imaging, *11*:297, 1979.
12. Dupont, W. D., and Page, D. L.: Risk factors for breast cancer in women with proliferative breast disease. N. Engl. J. Med., *312*:146, 1985.
13. Fisher, B., Carbone, P., Economou, S. G., et al.: L-Phenylalanine mustard (L-PAM) in the management of primary breast cancer. N. Engl. J. Med., *292*:117, 1975.
14. Fisher, B., Bauer, M., Margolese, R., et al: Five-year results of a randomized clinical trial comparing total mastectomy and segmental mastectomy with or without radiation in the treatment of breast cancer. N. Engl. J. Med., *312*:665, 1985.
15. Fisher, B., Redmond, C., Fisher, E. R., et al.: Ten-year results of a randomized clinical trial comparing radical mastectomy and total mastectomy with or without radiation. N. Engl. J. Med., *312*:674, 1985.
16. Foster, R. S., Jr., Lang, S. P., Costanza, M. C., Worden, J. K., Haines, C. R., and Yates, J. W.: Breast self-examination practicer and breast cancer stage. N. Engl. J. Med., *299*(6):265, 1978.
17. Frazier, T. G., Copeland, E. M., Gallager, H. S., et al: Prognosis and treatment in minimal breast cancer. Am. J. Surg., *133*:697, 1977.
18. Gallager, H. S., and Martin, J. E.: Early phases in the development of breast cancer, *24*:1170, 1969.
19. Gilliland, M. D., Barton, R. M., and Copeland, E. M. III: The implications of local recurrence of breast cancer as the first site of therapeutic failure. Ann. Surg., *197*:284, 1983.
20. Golinger, R. C.: Collective review: Hormones and the pathophysiology of fibrocystic mastopathy. Surg. Gynecol. Obstet. *146*:273, 1978.
21. Henderson, I. C., and Canellos, G. P.: Cancer of the breast: The past decade. I. N. Engl. J. Med., *302*:17, 1980.
22. Henderson, I. C., and Canellos, G. P. Cancer of the breast: The past decade. II. N. Engl. J. Med., *302*:78, 1980.
23. Letton, A. H., Wilson, J. P., and Mason, E. M.: The value of breast screening in women less than 50 years of age. Cancer, *40*:1, 1977.
24. Lynch, H. T., Albano, W. A., Danes, S., Layton, M. A., Kimberling, W. J., Lynch, J. F., Cheng, S. C., Costello, K. A., Mulcany, G. M., Wagner, C. A., and Tindall, S. L.: Genetic predisposition to breast cancer. Cancer, *53*:612, 1984.
25. McDivitt, R. W., Stewart, F. W., and Berg, J. W.: Tumors of the breast. *In* Atlas of Tumor Pathology, Series 2, Fasicle 2. Washington, D. C., Armed Forces Institute of Pathology, 1968.
26. Montague, E. D., Tapley, N., and Barker, J. L.: Radiotherapy in the management of nondisseminated breast cancer. *In* Fletcher, G. H., (Ed.): Textbook of Radiotherapy, 3rd ed. Philadelphia, Lea & Febiger, 1980, pp. 527.
27. Newman, H. G., Klein, M., Northrup, J. D., Ray, B. F., and Drucker, M.: Nipple discharge: Frequency and pathogenesis in an ambulatory population. N.Y. State J. Med., *83*:928, 1983.
28. Wilkinson, E. J., Hause, L. L., Hoffman, R. G., Kuzma, J. F., Rothwell, D. J., Donegan, W. L., Clowry, L. J., Almagro, U. A., Choi, H., and Rimm, A. A.: Occult axillary lymph node metastases in invasive breast carcinoma: Characteristics of the primary tumor and significance of the metastases. *In* Sommers, S. C., and Rosen, P. P. (Eds.): Pathology Annual II. New York, Appleton-Century-Crofts, 1982, p. 67.

THE THYROID

JOHN R. FARNDON, M.B., B.S.

18

The thyroid gland functions primarily to secrete thyroxine (T_4), a hormone essential for bodily metabolism. The thyroid is the site of a number of congenital, metabolic, immunologic, inflammatory, and neoplastic disorders of considerable surgical interest.

EMBRYOLOGY AND RELATED DEVELOPMENTAL ABNORMALITIES

The thyroid gland is first recognized as a thickening of the endoderm of the floor of the pharynx in early somite embryos. The thickening eventually evaginates to form a diverticulum known as the *tuberculum impar*. This forms a bilobed structure attached to the buccal cavity by a narrow stalk—the *thyroglossal duct*. The connecting cord of cells eventually ruptures as the embryo develops, and the developing thyroid is found as a mass of cells draped across the upper part of the developing trachea. Proximity with the aorta and its branches in the early phase of development explains why lobules of glandular tissue may remain adherent to the aorta and its branches and accounts for the occasional presence of thyroid tissue in the adult thoracic cavity. Rarely, the whole gland descends into the thorax. In normal development the thyroglossal duct is completely reabsorbed but may persist in whole or in part. The caudal end of the duct may persist and gives rise to the pyramidal lobe of the gland. A small lobule of thyroid tissue may persist in the tongue (the *lingual thyroid*). The point of attachment of the thyroglossal duct can be seen as a small depression at the junction of the anterior two thirds and the posterior one third of the tongue—the *foramen cecum*.

The thyroglossal duct usually atrophies by the sixth week of intrauterine life. Follicles are apparent in the thyroid gland of the 50-mm. embryo, and colloid is apparent in the 60-mm. embryo, with evidence of glandular function soon after this stage.

Thyroglossal Duct Cyst

The thyroglossal duct cyst is a midline cyst that arises in a remnant of the thyroglossal duct (Fig. 1). The cyst and its associated duct have a variable relationship with the hyoid bone; it may lie behind or in front of, or may occasionally pass through, the body of the bone, and the cyst itself can occur anywhere from the foramen cecum to the suprasternal notch.

Thyroglossal duct cysts occur at all ages but are most common in childhood at about 5 years. They are usually midline and occur in the region of the hyoid bone. They present as painless cystic swellings that move on swallowing and on protrusion of the tongue—a demonstration of the persistent attachment to the foramen cecum. The cyst might present initially with infection within it. Surgical treatment involves *excision of the cyst and its associated tract, which may extend through the hyoid bone to the base of the tongue.* Inadequate treatment can result in recurrence of the cyst, in repeated infections, or in the development of an external fistula or sinus.

Lingual Thyroid

Failure of descent of the thyroid precursor can lead to the development of the gland totally within the substance of the tongue, and thyroid scans (described later) can confirm the absence of thyroid tissue in sites other than the ectopic lingual position. Thyroid tumors can occur in the ectopic gland. More commonly, patients may present with a swelling of the tongue; this produces difficulty in swallowing, difficulty in breathing, or a change in the quality of speech. Surgical excision is necessary for the symptomatic gland producing obstruction. Autotransplantation of the excised thyroid tissue has been advocated to prevent hypothyroidism.[15]

ANATOMY AND PHYSIOLOGY

The thyroid (from the Greek *thyreos*, a shield) is a brownish-red, highly vascular endocrine gland consisting of right and left lobes connected across the midline by an isthmus (Fig. 2). Each lobe reaches superiorly as far as the oblique line of the thyroid cartilage; the isthmus overlies the second and third tracheal rings, and the lowest level of the lobe is usually about the fourth or fifth tracheal ring. The gland is invested in the pretracheal layer of the deep cervical fascia. It usually weighs about 25 gm. in the adult, is slightly heavier in women, and enlarges physiologically at puberty and during menstruation and pregnancy.

The medial surface of each lobe is molded over the larynx and trachea. Superficially, the gland is covered by the sternothyroid, by the sternohyoid, and below by the anterior border of the sternocleidomastoid muscles. Superiorly, the gland is in relation to the cricothyroid. The

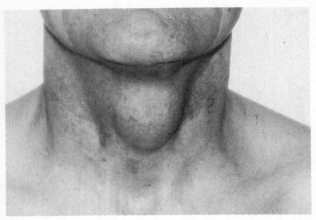

Figure 1. A midline cystic swelling just above the isthmus of the thyroid gland proved to be a thyroglossal duct cyst.

external branch of the superior laryngeal nerve passes deep to this part of the gland on its way to supply this muscle. Posterolaterally, the thyroid is in contact with the carotid sheath, the recurrent laryngeal nerves and the esophagus behind. The parathyroid glands are usually found related to the posterolateral surface of the thyroid. These anatomic points are important in the surgical approach to the thyroid gland, and clearly the recurrent laryngeal nerve and superior laryngeal nerve should not be damaged during operations on the thyroid. Similarly, the parathyroids should be observed in thyroid operations.

The blood supply to the thyroid is very rich and is increased in thyroid overactivity. It is mandatory that the arterial supply be precisely understood and carefully controlled during operations on the gland. The superior thyroid arteries arise from the external carotid artery on each side and pass down the pharynx and larynx to break into branches around the upper pole of the gland, especially on the anterior surface of each lobe. These superior arteries anastomose extensively with the terminal branches of the inferior thyroid artery, which arises from the thyrocervical trunk, a branch of the first part of a subclavian artery. The inferior artery crosses to the posterolateral aspect of each lobe from behind the carotid sheath and divides into branches as it approaches the gland. The recurrent laryngeal nerve usually lies posterior to the branches of the inferior thyroid artery but may lie in front of the artery or, in fact, between its branches, and the surgeon can never assume that the nerve is safe just because the inferior thyroid artery is intact. Increased flow within these arteries, which enlarge in thyrotoxicosis, often leads to an audible murmur (*thyroid bruit*), which is a useful physical sign in thyroid overactivity.

Thyroid veins begin to form on the surface of the gland and can easily be damaged in exploration. The superior thyroid vein courses with the superior thyroid artery and drains directly into the internal jugular vein. It is usually ligated with the artery.

A separate and very definite middle thyroid vein occurs in most instances and drains directly into the internal jugular vein. This vein can be quite short if the thyroid gland is enlarged, and its division can be difficult in some surgical explorations.

The inferior thyroid veins drain blood from the lower poles of each lobe and course to the left brachiocephalic vein.

Because some forms of thyroid cancer (notably medullary and papillary) drain predominantly into the lymphatic vessels, it is important to understand that the lymphatic drainage of the thyroid gland is into nodes lying in the groove between the trachea and esophagus and into nodes in the internal jugular chain.

Applied Surgical Anatomy

Occasionally, the recurrent laryngeal nerves can be involved in a thyroid disease process that affects their function. Malignant disease can infiltrate the nerves and cause malfunction, producing loss of abduction in the affected vocal cords. Sensation beneath the vocal cords is absent on the affected side. Because this lack of function could equally be ascribed to surgical damage, it is therefore an essential component of the preoperative examination of the patient to assess recurrent nerve function by indirect laryngoscopy. If a total lobectomy is to be performed, the recurrent laryngeal nerve on that side becomes very much more at risk and needs to be identified and followed exactly in its course with protection of its integrity. It is often easier to identify the nerve in the tracheoesophageal groove as it courses upward toward the thyroid gland. On the right, the recurrent nerve can more often be direct and not recurrent. This occurs in association with coarctation of the aorta. The nerve courses in proximity to the branches of the inferior thyroid artery and then on the posterior aspect of each lobe at the level of the thyroid cartilage as it passes under the inferior constrictor muscle to gain entry into the larynx. Injury can occur with even the most gentle handling of the nerve. The delicate vessel coursing the length of the nerve needs only to be observed for one to realize how easily intraneural bruising might occur.

During operation the larynx is handled from without and is intubated from within by endotracheal intubation. Hoarseness occurs rather commonly after thyroid surgery and may not be attributable to nerve damage in every instance. In addition to indirect laryngoscopy preoperatively, the examination should be repeated 2 weeks postoperatively. If nerve damage occurs or is inevitable in thyroid malignant disease, the opposite vocal cord eventually compensates for the paralyzed side. Bilateral nerve damage and cord paralysis produce permanent hoarseness, an inadequately protected airway, and total sensory impairment below the vocal cords. Tracheostomy is required in this situation.

The superior laryngeal nerve divides into the internal and external laryngeal branches, the former being sensory to the mucous membrane of the larynx above the vocal folds, and the latter (the smaller of the two branches) descends with the superior thyroid artery, but on a deeper plane to supply the cricothyroid muscle. Damage to the superior laryngeal nerve can occur when the superior thyroid vessels are being ligated. The result is a loss of the tensor function of the cricothyroid with ensuing loss of at least half an octave of the upper voice range and loss of sensation in the larynx above the vocal folds. Clinically, this causes a characteristic voice change; occasionally, the sensory disturbance also causes coughing, especially on drinking liquid.

Inadvertent damage or removal of the parathyroid glands produces hypocalcemic tetany. The position of the parathyroid glands in health and disease is described in Chapter 19, "The Parathyroid Glands."

Physiology and Function Tests

The normal human thyroid gland is able to concentrate iodide from the blood at a rate of about 2 μg. per hour.

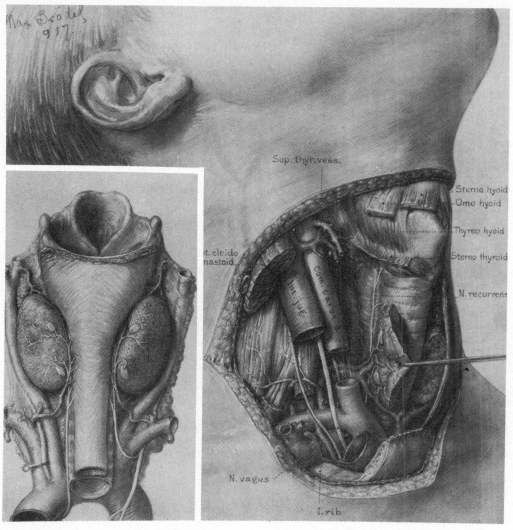

Figure 2. Dissection showing anatomic structures of the neck, especially those in the region of the thyroid gland. The nerve to the left of the vagus is the phrenic. Note location of parathyroid glands and recurrent laryngeal nerve. The amount of thyroid gland on the right side of the trachea is twice the amount that is left after subtotal thyroidectomy. (Drawings from dissections made by Mr. Max Brodel for Professor W. S. Halsted; original art in Brodel Collection, Art As Applied to Medicine. The Johns Hopkins University School of Medicine.)

Although this propensity to maintain iodide is not unique to the gland, the ability to synthesize thyroid hormones occurs only in the thyroid. Once within the thyroid follicular cell, the iodide is oxidized by a peroxidase enzyme system so that any iodine within the gland is found in thyroid hormones or their immediate precursors. The active form of iodine combines with molecules of the amino acid tyrosine, attached to thyroglobulin, to form monoiodotyrosine and diiodotyrosine. Two molecules of diiodotyrosine couple to form thyroxine and one molecule of monoiodotyrosine and one of diiodotyrosine form *triiodothyronine* (T_3) (Fig. 3). Hormone-containing molecules of thyroglobulin are then stored in the colloid until they are required for secretion. Upon secretion, colloid is hydrolyzed to release thyroid hormones with iodotyrosines that have not been coupled; these are rapidly reconverted to iodide and tyrosine by an enzyme within the thyroid gland, preventing their release into the bloodstream and their loss from the body via the urine. Some thyroglobulin molecules are not hydrolyzed and escape directly from the thyroid cell into the bloodstream. Thyroglobulin, therefore, is not totally confined to the thyroid cell and colloid, and this substance,

as with other thyroid hormones, provides a useful marker in thyroid cancer (see later).

Thyroxine and triiodothyronine are *usually* released together from the thyroid, and measurement of one, therefore, is *usually* indicative of the secretory rate of the other. The concentration of T_4 in the circulation is 30 to 50 times greater than that of T_3. With earlier thyroid hormone assays, therefore, T_4 was measured, and this parameter became the major index of thyroid function. A very large proportion of the T_4 in the circulation binds to plasma protein and is inactive. Only the unbound hormone is active, and since changes in the thyroxine-binding proteins occur frequently in clinical situations (although these do not alter greatly the unbound concentration of hormone), the overall concentration may shift in proportion to the protein changes. Any determination of T_4, therefore, should be accompanied by some estimate of free thyroxine.

Triiodothyronine is thought by some to be the only thyroid hormone to have any effect on the tissues. Ten to 20 per cent of T_3 is secreted directly by the thyroid gland, and the remainder is produced by deiodination of T_4 occurring in various tissues. In some cases, the thyroid

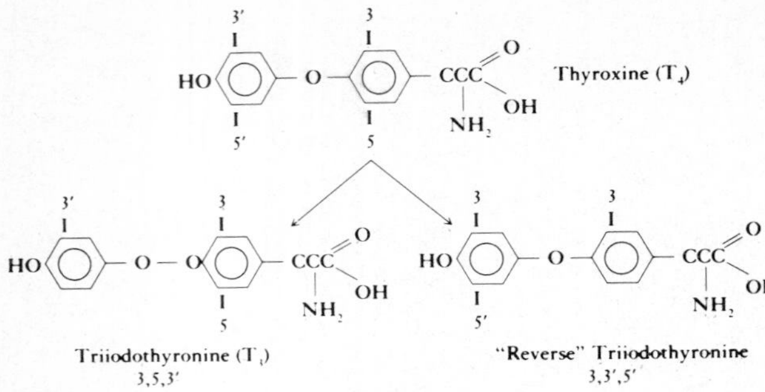

Triiodothyronine (T₃)
3,5,3'

"Reverse" Triiodothyronine
3,3',5'

Figure 3. Formation and structure of thyroxine and triiodothyronine.

gland secretes T_3 as the major hormone and normal or low T_4 levels are found. If T_3 is in excess, this can produce thyrotoxicosis and the phenomenon sometimes called T_3 *thyrotoxicosis.*

Triiodothyronine is also bound to circulating proteins, and again concentrations of total T_3 may vary because of change in protein concentration without metabolic consequences. It is exceedingly difficult to measure free T_3. Further confusion occurs during chronic illnesses and following operation when an inactive or impotent form of T_3 is produced. In this instance, the iodine radicals are placed in different positions within the molecule to produce "reverse" T_3.

Thyroid-stimulating hormone (TSH) is produced by the pituitary gland to regulate the functional activity of the thyroid (Fig. 4). Concentrations of TSH become elevated before there is measurable reduction in serum T_4 or T_3. This hormone is not protein-bound and is not affected by nonthyroidal illnesses. The lower range of normal values cannot be detected by current assays, and therefore a true absence of the hormone is difficult to distinguish from an undetectable level that may be observed in some normal subjects. The elevated levels seen in primary hypothyroidism help confirm this diagnosis. Measurements of TSH are not useful in the diagnosis of hyperthyroidism, but a low thyroxine concentration with a low or undetected TSH level is indicative of pituitary or hypothalamic disease.

Radioisotope Thyroid Scans

Iodine-123 (^{123}I) and iodine-131 (^{131}I) emit gamma rays, and measurement of uptake of these isotopes by the thyroid gland following a standard dose allows a measure of iodine incorporation into the gland. Iodine-131 is the commonly used iodide isotope because it does not have to be freshly made each day. The degree of uptake by iodine in scans can assist in the differential diagnosis of thyrotoxicosis. The use of ^{99m}technetium pertechnetate provides similar information and in addition may allow better diagnosis of malignancy within the thyroid.[2]

Response to Thyrotropin-Releasing Hormone

An injection of thyrotropin-releasing hormone (TRH) into a normal subject causes thyrotrophs in the pituitary to secrete TSH, and the greatest response is seen after about 20 to 30 minutes. In hyperthyroidism caused by excessive thyroid function, pituitary secretion of TSH is suppressed and TRH is ineffective in stimulating TSH release. This classic response is of value in patients with suspected

hyperthyroidism who appear clinically euthyroid and may have normal thyroid hormone levels but in whom hyperthyroidism is suspected because of the presence of Graves' eye signs or a nodular goiter (thyroid enlargement).

In primary hypothyroidism, TSH rises to abnormally high levels after TRH administration. When hypothyroidism exists in the presence of a normal or low TSH level and there is little or no response of TSH to TRH administration, the diagnosis is likely to be of pituitary hypofunction.

Interpretation of Thyroid Function Tests

Measurement of thyroxine and estimations of free thyroxine usually confirm a clinical suspicion of hyperthyroidism or a euthyroid state. When hyperthyroidism is suspected and normal T_4 and binding tests are observed, a T_3 level may demonstrate T_3 thyrotoxicosis. If doubt still remains, a TRH stimulation test will usually confirm or refute the diagnosis of hyperthyroidism.

In the diagnosis of hypothyroidism, determination of a TSH value should provide biochemical confirmation of the diagnosis. When thyroid hypofunction is due to pituitary or hypothalamic disease, observation of thyroid hormones and TSH levels should clarify the situation. Again, a TRH stimulation of TSH will help confirm the site of disease.

DIAGNOSIS AND INVESTIGATION OF THE PATIENT WITH THYROID DISEASE

Physicians and surgeons with an interest in thyroid disease are usually at an advantage regarding the way in which patients present. Occasionally, subtleties of disturbed biochemistry lead to difficulty is diagnosing thyroid disease,

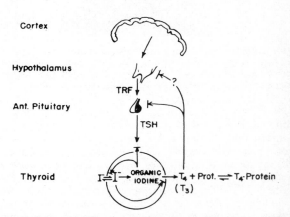

Figure 4. Schema of the homeostatic regulation of thyroid function. Secretion of thyroid-stimulating hormone (TSH) is regulated by a negative feedback mechanism acting directly on the pituitary and is normally inversely related to the concentration of unbound hormone in the blood. Release of TSH is induced by the thyrotropin-releasing factor (TRF), secretion of which appears to set the level of pituitary feedback mechanism. Factors regulating secretion of TRF are uncertain, but may include the free hormone in the blood and stimuli from higher centers. Autoregulatory control of thyroid function is also shown. High concentrations of intrathyroidal iodide decrease the rate of release of thyroidal iodine. In addition, the magnitude of the organic iodine pool inversely influences the iodide transport mechanism and the response to TSH. (From Ingbar, S. H., and Woeber, K. A. In Williams, R. H. (Ed.): Textbook of Endocrinology, 5th ed. Philadelphia, W. B. Saunders Company, 1974.)

but there is no problem in diagnosing clinically obvious thyrotoxicosis or myxedema even in the absence of any thyroid enlargement. The most common presentation of thyroid disease to the physician or surgeon is usually thyroid enlargement—diffuse, multinodular, or apparently single nodular enlargement.

Modest thyroid enlargement (goiter) is common, present in approximately 10 per cent of all females in geographic areas that are not deficient in iodine. Most goiters worldwide result from iodine deficiency, either directly or from the ingestion of goitrogens in items of diet peculiar to that particular area of the world. These clinical situations present no difficulty in diagnosis or management. It is the numerous other forms of thyroid enlargement that present difficulty in diagnosis and management, and clinical algorithms have been constructed to aid investigation and treatment.[27]

In some clinical situations, diagnosis and therapy can be made and instituted almost without investigation. The presence of a hard mass in one or both thyroid lobes with fixation to deeper structures and skin, associated hard lymphadenopathy, pressure effects on the trachea and esophagus, and possible recurrent nerve palsy strongly suggest a diagnosis of invasive thyroid malignancy. Obvious agitation, tremor, a visible goiter, and exophthalmos indicate a diagnosis of hyperthyroidism (Graves' disease). In most clinical situations, however, these helpful clinical diagnostic features are absent and a diagnosis must be achieved by a careful clinical examination and appropriate investigation. Thereafter, appropriate treatment can be determined.

It is helpful to divide these diagnostic problems into three groups based upon the clinical examination of the thyroid with the presence of (1) diffuse enlargement, or goiter, (2) an apparently solitary nodule, or (3) multinodular thyroid enlargement.

Diffuse Goiter

The most frequent cause of a thyroid problem (Fig. 4), when there is no obvious thyrotoxicosis, is a simple *diffuse goiter*, which is especially common in young females. In some cases, this progresses to multinodular goiter over a period of 10 to 20 years.

Some patients have exophthalmic Graves' disease. Although ocular manifestations of the disease may be present, no signs, symptoms, or biochemical features of hyperthyroidism are present. The TRH test is abnormal in a majority of patients, and thyroid antibodies will be present in about 50 per cent. Other patients may have positive clinical signs and symptoms and supportive biochemical changes of thyrotoxicosis, allowing a diagnosis of Graves' disease.

Drug therapy may produce a diffuse goiter, one of the most common agents being lithium carbonate, used in the treatment of manic-depressive illness. Lithium produces an antithyroid action, and sometimes elevated levels of TSH can be detected, with some patients becoming overtly hypothyroid.

Dyshormonogenesis is a rare condition in which genetically determined defects in thyroid hormone synthesis occur. This usually presents in childhood or young adulthood with a goiter and degrees of hypothyroidism.

Thyroiditis

Patients with various forms of thyroiditis may present with diffuse enlargement of the gland. The most common form is *Hashimoto's disease*, which occurs in middle-aged women who often have a family history of thyroiditis, myxedema, and pernicious anemia. Occasionally, the patient presents with signs and symptoms of hyperthyroidism. Thyroid antibodies are almost always present, and the diagnosis can usually be confirmed on *fine-needle aspiration biopsy* (described later). The condition occasionally simulates malignancy, but if the diagnosis is confirmed without doubt, treatment with T_4 replacement allows further confirmation of the diagnosis, in that the gland becomes softer and smaller with the passage of time as the patient is maintained in a euthyroid state.

De Quervain's thyroiditis was first described at the turn of the century and is associated with a fairly sudden onset of pain in the neck, malaise, night sweats, slight enlargement of the thyroid, and complete suppression of iodine or technetium uptake by the gland. Again, needle biopsy usually confirms the diagnosis when disruption and dissolution of the thyroid follicles are seen with an infiltrate of giant cells. The disease is self-limiting.

Riedel's thyroiditis is exceedingly rare and is characterized by a hard, woody fibrosis of the thyroid gland, often producing tracheal compression.

The Solitary Thyroid Nodule

It is important to recognize that approximately half the patients found by clinical examination to have a single nodule are subsequently demonstrated at operation or by thyroid scan to have multinodular disease.

The sudden appearance of a rapidly enlarging nodule within the gland usually indicates hemorrhage into a solitary thyroid cyst. This often resolves spontaneously without further diagnosis or treatment. The majority of patients, however, require further investigation by isotope scanning or ultrasonography of the neck. Isotopic scanning with [99m]technetium, ^{131}I, or ^{123}I allows the nodule to be characterized as "cold," "neutral," or "hot." Little or no isotope concentration in a nodule characterizes the nodules as cold. Since over 10 per cent of these nodules can represent thyroid carcinoma, such patients are candidates for aspiration biopsy or surgical exploration.[19] Ultrasonography should identify solitary cystic lesions, and if they are less than 4 cm. in diameter, these are usually benign. Patients with a neutral or hot nodule who are clinically and biochemically euthyroid can undergo needle biopsy; if benign cells are found, annual examination should follow. In about a fifth of such patients who show negative TRH stimulation, the condition will progress to hyperthyroidism within 5 years. Patients with thyrotoxicosis and a hot nodule require radioiodine or surgical therapy.

Differentiated thyroid tumors can present with a solitary thyroid nodule, and clearly aggressive surgical therapy is usually required if this diagnosis is made. A diagnosis can be confirmed by fine-needle biopsy (see later).

Multinodular Goiter

A diagnosis of multinodular goiter can be made on clinical grounds or unexpectedly by the use of isotope or ultrasound scanning of a supposedly solitary nodule. This usually represents benign disease, but rapid, painless enlargement of a long-standing, multinodular goiter must raise the possibility of malignant change. If there are no compressive symptoms, patients with a multinodular goiter can be observed with periodic examination. If hyperthyroidism is present or develops, treatment is indicated and approximately one quarter of patients who are initially clinically euthyroid with a multinodular goiter will eventually show clinical or biochemical evidence of hyperthyroidism. Overt hyperthyroidism (often of the T₃ variety) is likely to develop in these patients within a few years.[27] Some malignant tumors occur in a multifocal fashion, and a complacent diagnostic attitude cannot be adopted in patients with a multinodular goiter.

FINE-NEEDLE ASPIRATION FOR CYTOLOGIC DIAGNOSIS IN THYROID ENLARGEMENT

The use of fine-needle aspiration biopsy to allow cytologic studies has revolutionized the diagnosis and treatment of thyroid disease. Previous sections in this chapter have described how the clinical diagnosis of thyroid carcinoma can be difficult, and apart from serum calcitonin in medullary thyroid carcinoma there are no specific biochemical markers. The features of ultrasound examination of the neck and the results of isotopic scanning are not sufficiently specific to allow confident diagnosis of benign disease in all solitary or multinodular disease.

The technique of fine-needle aspiration biopsy for cytologic studies must not be confused with *large-needle biopsy*, in which a core of tissue is removed from the thyroid and a diagnosis made on histologic examination. Large-needle biopsy is limited to tumors of at least 2 cm. in diameter, and complications such as hemorrhage and recurrent nerve palsy may occur. There is often local discomfort from the biopsy procedure, and this makes it difficult to obtain the patient's agreement for a second or third biopsy.

Aspiration biopsy has no limitation in regard to the size of tumor, provided that the lesion is palpable. Local anesthetic is not required, and multiple punctures can be performed with very good patient acceptance, even in children. Numerous areas within the lesion can be sampled. Minor intraglandular hematomas occasionally occur, but the technique is not associated with complications or with risk of seeding of malignant cells.[7]

Equipment needed for the biopsy is simple and inexpensive, consisting of a syringe, needle, and syringe holder (Fig. 5). The mechanism of biopsy is shown in Figures 6 and 7. The cytologic characteristics of benign and malignant thyroid tumors are well described.[18] If a trained pathologist and cytologist can be present in the clinical setting, a

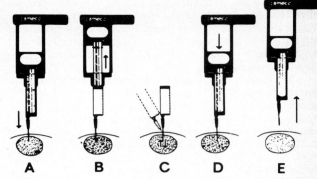

Figure 6. Biopsy procedures. A, The needle attached to its syringe and held in the holder is inserted in the thyroid swelling that will undergo biopsy. B, Suction is pulled on the syringe handle. C, With suction being maintained, the needle is moved in and out of the swelling in different directions. D, Suction is released on the syringe. E, The needle and syringe are then withdrawn from the thyroid swelling.

diagnosis can be made immediately on an outpatient basis and the diagnosis and treatment can be discussed directly with the patient.

Anaplastic and medullary carcinoma can be distinguished readily, and a diagnosis of papillary and Hürthle cell tumors can be made on cytologic smears. It is exceedingly difficult to distinguish between benign and malignant follicular tumors. Most cytologists make a diagnosis of "follicular neoplasm" without specifying its character with the understanding that the lesion should undergo surgical treatment in any event.

Multinodular colloid goiter accounts for 80 per cent of lesions subjected to biopsy and is easily diagnosed. Differ-

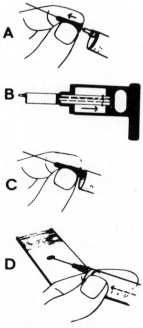

Figure 7. Preparing a cytologic smear suitable for microscopic examination. A, The needle is taken from the syringe. B, Air is pulled into the syringe. C, The syringe and needle are reconnected. D, The syringe plunger is pushed gently down, expressing cellular material onto the microscope slide.

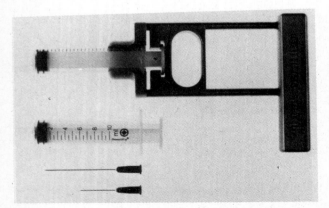

Figure 5. The materials required for fine-needle aspiration biopsy are simple and consist of a syringe, disposable needle, and a syringe holder for better control during biopsy.

ent types of thyroiditis and metastatic disease to the thyroid can also be distinguished, and needle biopsy obviates the need for neck exploration.[7]

In many series, the accuracy of aspiration biopsy for cytologic study compared with eventual histopathology of diagnosed malignant tumors of the thyroid is high. The incidence of false-positive diagnoses is exceedingly rare. False-negative results range from 7 to 30 per cent. It is this latter group that presents the greatest difficulty. How can operation be withheld in a patient with a suspicious thyroid enlargement when cytologic studies have revealed benign disease? If younger (less than 25 years) and older patients (more than 60 years) in whom a risk of malignancy in a solitary thyroid nodule might be as high as 60 per cent are excluded, other patients can be safely treated nonoperatively with thyroxine medication. The patient is carefully followed with further biopsies. Patient acceptance of this technique allows operation to be limited to those at greatest risk of malignancy.

Aspiration biopsy for cytologic study has been performed for over 30 years. The technique has been shown by many centers to have an overall diagnostic accuracy of 94 per cent and a sensitivity for cancer of 89 per cent.[14] Prospective use of the technique in the investigation and diagnosis of thyroid enlargement is beginning to influence the need for operation in patients with asymptomatic thyroid swelling. The frequency of operative intervention can be decreased by 25 per cent, and the proportion of operations for neoplasia can be increased from 30 to 50 per cent. When performed at the first clinic attendance, the approach allows a sound basis for selective operation and leads to economy in the management of thyroid enlargement.[1]

HYPERTHYROIDISM

When a clinical diagnosis of thyrotoxicosis is suspected, two questions need to be answered: (1) Is the patient thyrotoxic? and (2) What is the underlying condition? The answers usually can be obtained by a careful clinical examination and application of the simple investigations detailed earlier.

Presentation

The symptoms and signs of thyrotoxicosis are well known and are depicted in Table 1. The diagnosis is often more difficult in the elderly, and thyrotoxic atrial fibrillation may be difficult to diagnose in this group.[11] In the differential diagnosis, anxiety neurosis, occult neoplasms or

TABLE 1. *Symptoms and Signs of Thyrotoxicosis*

Symptoms	Signs
Irritability, emotional lability	Tremor
Sweating, heat intolerance	Warm, moist skin
Palpitations	Tachycardia, atrial fibrillation
Shortness of breath	Heart failure
Fatigue, muscle weakness	Myopathy
Prominent eyes	Lid retraction, lid lag
Increased appetite	
Weight loss	
Goiter with or without a bruit	
Diarrhea	
Menstrual irregularities	
Hair loss and pruritus	

infections, and chronic pulmonary disease (with the patient on bronchodilator drugs) are common mimics of thyrotoxicosis.

The diagnosis should be confirmed by measurement of circulating T_4 and T_3. Toxicosis from T_3 is more likely to be associated with a nodular goiter. The TRH stimulation test can be used in borderline cases. Newer immunometric assays for TSH, capable of detecting concentrations as low as 0.05 milliunits per liter (mU/L), may discriminate between normal low basal concentrations in euthyroid subjects and abnormally low levels in hyperthyroid patients and may eventually obviate the need for the TRH–releasing test.

The three most common causes of hyperthyroidism are Graves' disease, toxic adenoma, and toxic multinodular goiter. The diagnosis of Graves' disease is strengthened by the identification of a positive family history of thyroid problems, the presence of exophthalmos or other eye signs, pretibial myxedema, and the measurement and detection of antithyroid antibodies. Of patients with Graves' disease, 80 per cent have positive antimicrosomal antibodies.

An isotopic scan confirms the presence of a diffuse active goiter in Graves' disease or a clinical diagnosis of a solitary toxic adenoma, or it may show multiple hot nodules consistent with a diagnosis of toxic multinodular goiter.

Less than 10 per cent of cases of thyrotoxicosis are caused by subacute thyroiditis, thyrotoxicosis factitia (abuse of thyroid medication), struma ovarii, a TSH–dependent disease with or without a pituitary tumor, and a functioning thyroid carcinoma.

Treatment

Three options are available for the patient with thyrotoxicosis: (1) medical therapy, (2) ablative treatment with ^{131}I, and (3) surgical resection.

MEDICAL THERAPY

Beta-adrenergic receptor blocking drugs (e.g., propranolol) and antithyroid drugs (e.g., carbimazole, methimazole, and propylthiouracil) can be used and are most appropriate in the initial treatment of Graves' disease. Remission occurs in about 50 per cent following a period of therapy for 12 to 18 months. Medical therapy is *not* recommended in the treatment of toxic adenoma because the disease recurs once the treatment is stopped. Antithyroid drugs given over a period of 12 or 18 months can produce a long-standing remission. Relapse occurs in up to 50 per cent of patients, and at that point treatment options include a further course of antithyroid drugs or therapy with ^{131}I and operation.

Beta-blocking agents provide symptomatic relief without interfering with thyroid function tests. These are useful in conditions in which the thyrotoxicosis is transient (e.g., in subacute thyroiditis). The drug can be used as the sole preparation for operation, and if proper attention is given, continuation of the therapy after subtotal resection and adjusting the dose, *thyrotoxic storm* need not be a problem.[9]

RADIOIODINE TREATMENT

Debate continues regarding definitive therapy for thyrotoxicosis: radioiodine ablation or surgical resection. Some restrict the use of radioiodine treatment to the elderly, and recommend limiting its use in children or young women of childbearing age. However, two studies have shown that the risk of carcinogenesis, genetic damage, and fetal damage by the use of radioiodine *is not increased* in this form of therapy.[20, 22] Long-term studies have shown therapeutic benefit. Care has to be taken to watch for the development of insidious hypothyroidism if this condition is not induced by the initial dose. Ablative doses of ^{131}I are recommended with T_4 replacement.[23] Some suggest that initial treatment should be based upon patient preference between operation and radioiodine therapy once initial medical control has been gained or once relapse occurs.[12] If radioiodine is chosen, it must be ensured that the female is not pregnant and pregnancy should be avoided for about 12 months following therapy.[26]

For patients with thyrotoxicosis caused by a toxic multinodular goiter, a diffuse toxic goiter (Graves' disease), or a single toxic adenoma (producing pressure symptoms in patients younger than 40 or in older patients), there is generally a preference for surgical treatment. *Subtotal thyroidectomy* provides excellent long-term results.

Prior to operation, control of the thyrotoxic state is essential. Conventional preparation consists of carbimazole with the addition of potassium iodide in the 7 days before operation. This treatment usually results in the lowering of thyroid hormone concentration to the normal range within 6 weeks. If operation cannot be delayed for this length of time, propranolol or another nonselective beta-blocker can be given in combination with potassium iodide for 10 days before operation.[10]

Subtotal resection of the thyroid gland results in long-term euthyroidism in over 90 per cent of patients.[3] Toft and others reported that 80 per cent of patients were euthyroid by the end of the first year, 15 per cent were permanently hypothyroid, and 5 per cent experienced relapse of thyrotoxicosis.[28] The incidence of postoperative hypothyroidism is sometimes overestimated. In about one third of patients undergoing operation, low serum concentrations of total T_4 and elevated concentrations of TSH are demonstrated 3 months after operation without signs or symptoms of hypothyroidism. These biochemical changes usually revert to normal by 6 months, and permanent hypothyroidism therefore must not be diagnosed until 6 months after operation. Patients who have been treated with subtotal thyroidectomy should undergo long-term review for detection and treatment of hypothyroidism. The measurement of serum concentrations of TSH appears to delineate a group in whom there is a greater risk of developing hypothyroidism, and in patients with elevated TSH concentrations hypothyroidism develops at a rate of about 5 per cent each year. This marker, however, is not foolproof, and many patients remain otherwise biochemically euthyroid; indeed, recurrent hyperthyroidism will ensue in some.[12] The incidence of recurrent laryngeal nerve injury and damage to the parathyroid glands with surgical procedures for thyrotoxicosis should be low.[3]

Since thyroid disease is much more common in women, hyperthyroidism occurring during pregnancy is not a particularly rare event; its usual cause is Graves' disease. Patients with the thyrotoxicosis of Graves' disease tend to have remission during pregnancy and exacerbation during the postpartum period. Immunologic mechanisms might account for this pattern in pregnancy. Radioactive iodine therapy is contraindicated during pregnancy, and medical therapy is the mainstay of treatment. Beta-blocking agents can be used safely in this situation, and they may be useful in the rapid control of thyrotoxicosis. Subtotal thyroidectomy should probably be reserved for patients with hypersensitivity to antithyroid drugs and poor compliance and

for the very rare cases in which the drugs are ineffective. Preoperative preparation is as important in the pregnant patient.[4]

SURGICAL MANAGEMENT

The extirpation of the thyroid gland typifies better than any operation the supreme triumph of the surgeon's art.

Halsted, 1920

The indications for surgical exploration of the thyroid gland include:

1. *Therapeutic.* Reduction of *functional mass* in hyperthyroid conditions; subtotal thyroidectomy in Graves' disease or toxic multinodular goiter, or excision of a toxic adenoma.

2. *Therapeutic.* Reduction of *compressive mass;* subtotal thyroidectomy in nontoxic multinodular goiter or lobectomy for thyroid cysts or single nodules (e.g., colloid nodule) that produce compression of trachea or esophagus.

3. *Extirpation of malignant disease.* Usually total thyroidectomy with node dissection; for some tumors, unilateral lobectomy is indicated.

4. *Palliation.* Excision of incurable tumor mass that produces disturbing compressive symptoms: anaplastic, metastatic, or lymphomatous tumors.

Incision and Exposure

A curvilinear skin incision is made (convex downwards) 2 cm. above the suprasternal notch and the clavicles, extending laterally as far as the sternocleidomastoid muscle. The incision is deepened through the platysma muscle, and superior and inferior skin flaps are then developed beneath it. The midline raphe between the strap muscles is divided longitudinally. In some patients with large goiters or lobar swellings, a surgeon may elect to divide the strap muscles horizontally to improve surgical access. A plane of dissection is then developed beneath the strap muscles superficially and the capsule of the thyroid gland more deeply. Care must be taken not to rupture the small branches of the thyroid veins that are present on the surface of the gland.

Subtotal Resection

Subtotal resection will be performed identically for the right and left lobes, with mobilization being the same on each side. Subtotal resection is performed in cases of toxic multinodular goiter, nontoxic multinodular goiter, or Graves' disease. The principle of the resection is to excise the majority of each lobe dividing the superior thyroid vessels, the middle thyroid vein and the inferior thyroid veins, leaving the inferior thyroid artery intact. The portions of the gland excised are the anterolateral aspects of each lobe, the isthmus, and the pyramidal lobe. In some patients with a very marked increase in the blood supply to the gland, the inferior thyroid artery can be ligated in continuity or temporarily occluded with a small clamp until the resection is complete. A common goal is to protect and preserve the recurrent laryngeal nerves and the parathyroid glands. It has been emphasized that in ligation of the superior thyroid vessels care must be taken not to injure the external laryngeal branch of the superior laryngeal nerve because this produces significant voice change.[16] The residual thyroid remnant of the left lobe should be approximately 3 to 4 gm. This can be judged by assessing various sizes of thyroid on a weighing scale. The lobe can be excised completely

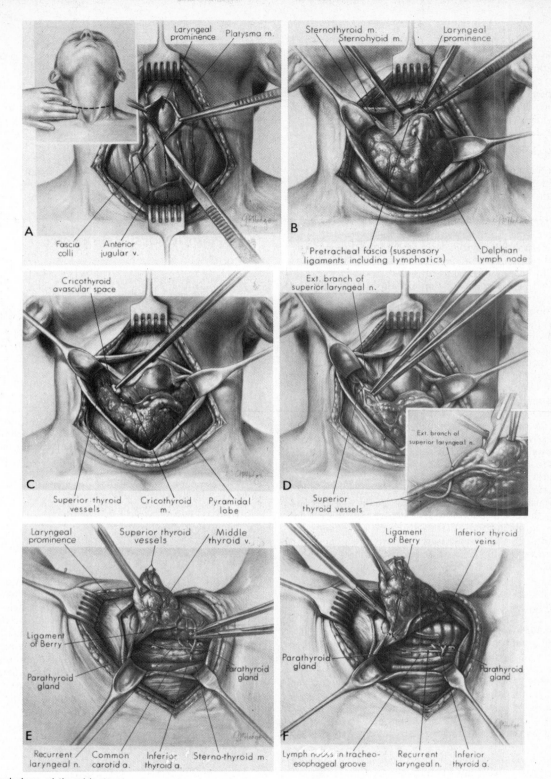

Figure 8. Technique of thyroidectomy.

  A, *With the head extended, a curvilinear transverse incision is made approximately 3 cm. above the clavicular heads. After elevation of superior and inferior flaps, the cervical fascia is divided in the midline.*

  B, *The sternohyoid and sternothyroid muscles are elevated, allowing exposure of the isthmus and lobes. The suspensory ligament is divided at the level of the thyroid cartilage to allow resection of the pyramidal lobe and delphian lymph nodes.*

  C, *The cricothyroid space is opened to allow exposure of the superior pole vessels.*

  D, *The branches of the superior thyroid vessels are dissected free and clamped separately to avoid injury to the external branch of the superior laryngeal nerve.*

  E, *The thyroid gland is rotated anteriorly, exposing branches of the inferior thyroid artery, recurrent laryngeal nerve, and parathyroid glands. The terminal branches of the inferior thyroid artery are divided after the recurrent laryngeal nerve is identified and protected. Blood supply to the parathyroid glands should be preserved if possible.*

  F, *The recurrent laryngeal nerve is carefully protected during division of the ligament of Berry. The lobe and isthmus are then elevated to the midline completing resection of the lobe.*

  (From Thompson, N. W., Olsen, W. R., and Hoffman, G. L.: Surgery, 73:913, 1973.)

by division of the isthmus, or it can be kept in continuity with the isthmus, which is dissected free from the underlying trachea.

Identical excision is then performed on the right side. Throughout the operative procedure, meticulous attention is paid to hemostasis.

Total Lobectomy

Total lobectomy is performed for malignant tumors of the thyroid gland and when the underlying unilobar disease is uncertain. Some surgeons also prefer to perform this procedure on one side for multinodular disease and to leave a slightly larger remnant within the opposite lobe.

When dissection of a lobe is performed, for a malignant tumor, the superior thyroid vessels, middle thyroid vein, and inferior thyroid veins need to be divided. This allows the gland to be mobilized and retracted medially to reveal the final major vascular attachment, the inferior thyroid artery. The parathyroid glands and recurrent laryngeal nerve are identified and protected (Fig. 8). If the parathyroid glands are on the surface of the thyroid, they may have to be initially removed with the thyroid and subsequently transplanted (see Chapter 19). The thyroid lobe is retracted medially, with two parathyroid glands visible in proximity to the terminal branches of the inferior thyroid artery and the recurrent laryngeal nerve covered by a fascial ligament (ligament of Berry). The nerve is identified as a thin, white structure running beneath the ligament and usually beneath the terminal branches of the inferior thyroid artery. The nerve has a tiny vessel running in its substance and must not be damaged. The lobe is slowly and carefully retracted from the ligament of Berry and the recurrent nerve until it is totally separated from the trachea.

In some malignant tumors, such as the follicular and medullary variants, bilateral total lobectomy is recommended with central lymph node compartment dissection. Following completion of the excision of the gland and nodes, hemostasis is assessed and the wound is closed in layers. Drainage is not necessary, provided hemostasis has been secure.

Complications of Thyroidectomy

The complications of thyroidectomy are listed, with a *current* commentary on methods of avoiding these complications.

1. *Hemorrhage.* This risk is minimal, but great care must be taken in securing hemostasis with the judicious use of drains. Hemorrhage is always possible following thyroidectomy. Should this occur, it is usually a surgical emergency in which prompt decompression of the neck and return of the patient to the operating room are required as quickly as possible.

2. *Problem of opening a large vein and causing air embolism.* With current anesthetic procedures, intermittent positive pressure ventilation, and careful surgical technique, this danger should be minimal and is quite rare.

3. *Injury to the recurrent laryngeal nerve.* This produces partial or total (if bilateral) paralysis of the larynx. Adequate surgical anatomic knowledge and care at operation should prevent injury to this nerve or to the superior laryngeal nerve.

4. *Forcing an abnormal amount of a secretion of the gland into the circulation by pressure.* This is a reference to a thyrotoxic storm, now rarely seen because of adequate

patient preparation blocking the overactive thyroid gland in patients operated upon for thyrotoxicosis.

5. *Sepsis extending to the mediastinum.* Again, this complication should not be seen in current surgical clinics. Antibiotics are not required as prophylaxis. Attention to adequate hemostasis at operation performed in a properly ventilated operating room with appropriate instruments and ligatures should be associated with negligible infection.

6. *Postoperative hypothyroidism.* The development of hypothyroidism following surgical resection of the thyroid is rarely observed today. It is guarded against by appropriate clinical and biochemical checks postoperatively.

MALIGNANT TUMORS OF THE THYROID

Thyroid cancer is rare, affecting less than 1 per cent of all patients with malignant disease and accounting for only six deaths per million of the population per year in most areas of the world.[6] Thyroid tumors appear to have a higher incidence in areas of endemic goiter. When iodine intake is high in the population, papillary carcinoma is the form usually seen, although this is also the most common thyroid tumor, especially in young adults. There appears to be a close relationship between *a history of irradiation of head and neck in infancy or childhood* and the subsequent development of thyroid cancer. The dose of irradiation can be as low as 100 rads, and the interval between exposure and tumor can be as long as 30 years. Follicular carcinoma arises in an older group of patients and is usually seen in countries where iodine intake is low. Undifferentiated and anaplastic tumors occur in an even older age group and are more common in women.

The main types of malignant thyroid tumor are characterized in Table 2.

Differentiated Tumors

PAPILLARY CARCINOMA

Papillary carcinoma accounts for the majority of thyroid tumors and occurs in late childhood or early adult life. The tumor grows slowly and spreads primarily to lymph nodes. The lesion often presents as a solitary thyroid nodule, and the diagnosis usually can be made by fine-needle biopsy and cytologic study. Occasionally, the lesion is removed without preceding cytologic diagnosis; if lobectomy or even subtotal lobectomy has been performed, there is little evidence to support an aggressive return to the neck for completion of thyroidectomy, provided that the tumor

TABLE 2. Malignant Thyroid Tumors

Differentiated Tumors
Follicular cell origin
Papillary carcinoma
Follicular carcinoma
Hürthle cell carcinoma, subtype of follicular carcinoma
Parafollicular C cell origin
Medullary thyroid carcinoma
Undifferentiated Tumors
Anaplastic carcinoma
Tumors of Nonthyroid Cells
Lymphoma
Metastatic tumors (hypernephroma, melanoma, bronchial and gastrointestinal neoplasms)

was not transected. If nodes are enlarged, ideally they should be removed by a central dissection along with a total thyroidectomy. The character of metastatic nodes from a papillary tumor usually allows ready dissection of the nodes from surrounding tissues without the requirement for disabling and extensive neck dissection, especially in young patients.

Small amounts of residual thyroid tissue or metastatic nodes can be ablated by radioactive iodine therapy later. This form of therapy is followed by an excellent prognosis, especially in children. Men older than 40 years of age appear to do less well than women. The presence of involved lymph nodes often does not result in a less favorable prognosis. This usually occurs in the younger patient in whom the tumor is rarely aggressive.

FOLLICULAR CARCINOMA

Follicular carcinoma has a peak incidence at around 45 years of age, often presenting as a solitary nodule. Often there is distant spread at presentation, for example, with a secondary deposit in a bone or metastases within the lungs. Diagnosis can be obtained on fine-needle biopsy. A follicular neoplasm that has been diagnosed on fine-needle biopsy should be treated by total lobectomy on the affected side. Frozen section characterization of the tumor is unreliable, and in many cases definitive diagnoses are awaited before further treatment is determined. Histologic evidence of a less differentiated tumor that has infiltrated the capsule or surrounding blood vessel should indicate completion of the thyroidectomy. Ablation of any small residual pads of thyroid by radioactive iodine should be performed in the postoperative period. Secondary tumor may take up significant amounts of isotope, which can be used as a scan to assess tumor burden as well as a therapeutic modality. After isotope therapy, fully suppressive doses of thyroxine are administered. Assessment of TSH levels is done to ensure that the dose has been suppressive. If the tumor is sufficiently well differentiated, the tumor and its metastases may take up iodine; in this situation further treatment with radioiodine can be successful. Additional iodine scans are useful for monitoring recurrence of the tumor.

HÜRTHLE CELL CARCINOMA

Hürthle cell carcinoma is a rare cancer that is histologically related to the well-differentiated malignancies of the thyroid. This form is probably a distinct clinical entity in its own right. The tumor and its metastases do not absorb radioactive iodine, and treatment is primarily surgical, involving total thyroidectomy. With this approach, survival rates approach 60 per cent at 10 years. It is likely that the Hürthle cell carcinoma is a moderate-grade malignancy.[13]

MEDULLARY THYROID CARCINOMA

Medullary thyroid carcinoma is a rare variant, and, like Hürthle cell carcinoma, it accounts for perhaps 3 per cent of all thyroid carcinomas. It occurs sporadically in the population and in various familial settings in which the tumor is inherited as an autosomal dominant character.[8] The tumor has a distinctive histologic appearance with a characteristic solid stroma that usually contains amyloid. The tumor is derived from the parafollicular C cells. Although these cells do not accumulate iodine, they produce *calcitonin*, a hormone that serves as a biochemical marker for the tumor. Measurement of calcitonin in its basal and

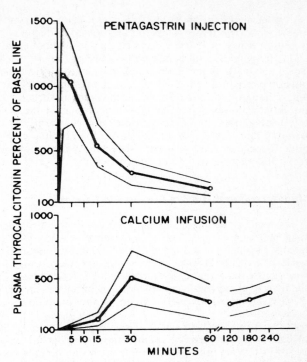

Figure 9. Combined responses of seven patients with elevated baseline levels of plasma CT to pentagastrin injection and calcium infusion. Each patient received both tests on separate days, with pentagastrin injection being the initial test in four of the patients and calcium infusion being the initial test in three of the patients. Open circles and solid lines represent the mean responses, and the shaded area indicates the range of the standard errors. (From Hennessy, J. C., et al.: J. Clin. Endocrinol. Metabol., 39:487, 1974.)

stimulated concentrations in the serum allows a biochemical diagnosis of this tumor before it is clinically apparent. Stimulation of calcitonin is achieved by injection of pentagastrin or calcium (Fig. 9). The responses to therapy are depicted in Table 3. Similarly, the hormone acts as a marker of recurrence or progression of disease. In its familial settings, medullary thyroid carcinoma may be associated

Table 3. Plasma Calcitonin Levels and Prognosis*

Group	Preoperative CT (pg./ml.)	RLNM† (%)	Postop. CT† (%) (>300 pg./ml.)	DM (%)	DTH (%)
1	250–1000 (n = 25)	1(4)	1(4)	0	0
2	1000–5000 (n = 36)	3(8.3)	6(16.7)	0	0
3	5000–10,000 (n = 8)	2(25)	1(12.5)	0	0
4	>10,000 (n = 23)	13(57)	14(61)	4(17)	2(8.7)

*From Wells, S. A., Jr., and Baylin, S. B.: The multiple endocrine neoplasias. *In* Sabiston, D. C., Jr. (Ed.): Textbook of Surgery, 13th ed. Philadelphia, W. B. Saunders Company, 1986.

†Group 1 or Group 2 vs. Group 4, P<0.001.

Abbreviations: Preop CT = Preoperative stimulated plasma CT level; Postop CT = postoperative stimulated plasma CT level; RLNM = regional lymph node metastases; DM = distant metastases; DTH = death.

with hyperparathyroidism and the presence of pheochromocytomas. The tumor is aggressive to varying degrees; it is most benign in its pure familial setting without other endocrinopathies, and its behavior is most aggressive when associated with other endocrinopathies and a particular phenotypic habitus characterized by a marfanoid appearance (the presence of neuromas on the mucosal surfaces of the mouth and eyes) and by ganglioneuromas of the gastrointestinal tract. In the former pure familial variant, death is rarely due to the tumor, whereas in the multiple endocrine associated syndrome with the abnormal phenotype, survival is rare beyond 20 or 30 years of age.[29]

Undifferentiated Tumors (Anaplastic Carcinoma)

Anaplastic carcinoma usually occurs in women older than 60 years of age. The patient often presents with a history of having noted a rapidly enlarging swelling in the neck, often with difficulty in breathing and swallowing and with hoarseness. Examination reveals a hard, fixed mass in the thyroid gland with lymphadenopathy often present. The disease is often widely metastatic to the lungs and bones at presentation.

The results of surgical resection are poor, but some palliation is obtained by radiotherapy. Tracheostomy is occasionally required because of tracheal compression. Generally, chemotherapy is not effective in the management of this tumor.[24]

Tumors of Nonthyroid Cells

LYMPHOMA

Lymphoma is a rare form of thyroid cancer, occurring typically in middle-aged to elderly women who present with a rapidly enlarging, painless, diffuse, firm thyroid mass. Histologically, the lesion is usually of a diffuse large cell type and Hashimoto's disease can be found in the background in over one third of patients.

Treatment consists of thyroidectomy and irradiation. Five-year survival can be greater than 80 per cent when the tumor is confined to the thyroid gland and 40 per cent when the disease is also extrathyroidal.[5]

METASTATIC TUMORS

Probably because of high vascularity, metastases occur in the thyroid, and in most cases they arise from a hypernephroma. Melanoma, pancreatic carcinoma, and bronchial and gastrointestinal tumors occasionally metastasize to the thyroid. The symptoms from these metastases are usually overshadowed by those of the primary tumor and other secondary deposits, and the thyroid disease is usually of little consequence.

Survival and Follow-up of Patients with Differentiated Thyroid Cancer

Because most differentiated thyroid cancers retain the ability to accumulate iodine and produce thyroglobulin, these characteristics are considered in the follow-up of patients with differentiated thyroid carcinoma arising from the follicular cells. The detection of thyroglobulin in the serum following thyroidectomy might predict recurrent disease capable of producing this protein. Similarly, metastases of the tumor outside the neck can be detected by the uptake of ^{131}I in scans. It is suggested that both the iodine scan and measurement of thyroglobulin be used in the long-term follow-up of patients with these tumors.[21] Rising levels of thyroglobulin associated with positive iodine scans can then be followed by therapeutic doses of iodine for ablation of metastases.

It has been difficult to obtain objective data concerning the biologic behavior of these tumors and of the survival characteristics of patients who present with *different forms* of the disease. An early attempt at this analysis was made by the European Organization for Research on the Treatment of Cancer/Thyroid Cancer Cooperative (EORTC). This group derived an index that included age at diagnosis, anaplastic cell type, presence or absence of metastases, sex of the patient, tumor size, and presence or absence of less differentiated medullary or follicular forms. From the derived score, five risk groups were characterized. Results of further studies, however, have now suggested that the sex of the patient is not important. It appears that age at diagnosis, presence of locally advanced disease, distant metastases, histologic features of invasion of the thyroid capsule, and presence of marked cellular atypia remain significant adverse factors. The mortality of patients with differentiated thyroid carcinoma is directly proportional to the age of the patient. Further studies are required to analyze survival for each histologic type and possibly subsets of patients with histologic or epidemiologic variants of each tumor (e.g., the different forms of medullary thyroid carcinoma, familial or sporadic).[25]

SELECTED REFERENCES

Dickinson, P. H.: Colour Atlas of Subtotal Thyroidectomy. Single Surgical Procedures Series, Vol. 5. London, Wolfe Medical Publications Ltd., 1983.
Although this relatively short atlas concerns subtotal thyroidectomy alone, points covering total lobectomy are also discussed. The atlas is richly illustrated and makes clear all the important anatomic features relevant to operative procedures on the thyroid gland. It also provides detail about preoperative patient preparation and postoperative care.

Geelhoed, G. W.: Problem Management in Endocrine Surgery. Chicago, Year Book Medical Publishers Inc., 1983.
This excellent monograph is worthy of thorough reading. Each endocrine disease is discussed relative to management problems, diagnosis, preoperative preparation, anesthetic management, operative technique, postoperative care, pharmacologic management, and follow-up. The text emphasizes the fascination of endocrine disease for the surgeon whether as a student or practicing technician.

Kaplan, E. L. (Ed.): Surgery of the Thyroid and Parathyroid Glands, Vol. 6. *In* Clinical Surgery International. New York, Churchill Livingstone, 1983.
This book is recommended for selected reference reading for diseases of the thyroid and the parathyroid glands. It is a collection of chapters by internationally recognized authors covering the more important aspects of diagnosis and management of patients with thyroid disease. Some of the more difficult and controversial therapies for thyroid cancer, such as external radiation and chemotherapy, are presented. Each chapter is supported by a complete bibliography. This book is highly recommended for the student who wishes to read in depth about thyroid disease.

Thompson, N. W., and Vinik, A. I. (Eds.): Endocrine Surgery Update. New York, Grune & Stratton, 1983.
This is another excellent reference concerning detailed presentation of endocrine disorders by a highly qualified group of contributors.

REFERENCES

1. Al-Sayer, Z. M., Krukowski, Z. H., Williams, V. M. M., and Matheson, N. A.: Fine needle aspiration cytology in isolated thyroid swellings: A prospective two-year evaluation. Br. Med. J., 290:1490, 1985.
2. Beierwaltes, W. H.: Are thyroid scans of value in evaluating most

thyroid nodules? *In* Thompson, N. W., and Vinik, A. I. (Eds.): Endocrine Surgery Update. New York, Grune & Stratton, 1983, p. 18.

3. Bradley, E. L., DiGirolamo, M., and Tarcan, Y.: Modified subtotal thyroidectomy in the management of Graves' disease. Surgery, 87:623, 1980.

4. Burrow, T. N.: The management of thyrotoxicosis in pregnancy. N. Engl. J. Med., 313:562, 1985.

5. Devine, R. M., Edis, A. J., and Banks, P. M.: Primary lymphoma of the thyroid: A review of the Mayo Clinic experience through 1978. World J. Surg., 5:33, 1981.

6. Duncan, W.: Thyroid cancer. *In* Recent Results in Cancer Research. New York, Springer-Verlag, 1980.

7. Engzell, U., Espoti, P. L. and Rubio, C.: Investigation on tumour spread in connection with aspiration biopsy. Acta Radiol. (Stockh.), 10:385, 1971.

8. Farndon, J. R., Leight, G. S., Dilley, W. G., Smallridge, R. C., Harrison, T. S., and Wells, S. A.: Familial medullary thyroid carcinoma without associated endocrinopathies: A distinct entity. Br. J. Surg., 73:278, 1986.

9. Farndon, J. R., Routledge, P. A., Shand, D. G., and Wells, S. A.: Changes in plasma alpha-1-acid glycoprotein concentrations and plasma protein binding on propranolol during operation for thyrotoxicosis. J. Clin. Surg., 1:106, 1982.

10. Feek, C. M., Sawyers, J. S. A., Irvine, W. J., Beckett, G. J., Ratcliffe, W. A., and Toft, A. D.: Combination of potassium iodide and propranolol in preparation of patients with Graves' disease for thyroid surgery. N. Engl. J. Med., 302:883, 1980.

11. Forfar, J. C., and Toft, A. D.: Thyrotoxic atrial fibrillation: An underdiagnosed condition? Br. Med. J., 285:909, 1982.

12. Halnan, K. E.: Risks from radioiodine treatment of thyrotoxicosis. Br. Med. J., 287:1821, 1983.

13. Har-el, G., Hadar, T., Segal, K., Levy, R., and Sidi, J.: Hürthle cell carcinoma of the thyroid gland. Cancer, 57:1617, 1986.

14. Harsoulis, P., Leontsini, M., Economou, A., Gerasimidis, T., and Smbarounis, C.: Fine needle aspiration biopsy cytology in the diagnosis of thyroid cancer: Comparative study of 213 operated patients. Br. J. Surg., 73:461, 1986.

15. Kamat, M. R., Kulkarni, J. N., Desai, P. B., and Jussawalla, D. J.: Lingual thyroid: A review of 12 cases. Br. J. Surg., 66:537, 1979.

16. Kark, A. E., Kissin, M. W., Auerbach, R., and Meikle, M.: Voice changes after thyroidectomy: Role of the external laryngeal nerve. Br. Med. J., 289:1412, 1984.

17. Lennard, T. W. J., Wadhera, V., and Farndon, J. R.: Fine needle aspiration biopsy in diagnosis of metastases to the thyroid gland. J. Roy. Soc. Med., 77:196, 1984.

18. Lowhagen, T., Willems, J. S., Lundell, G., Sundblad, R., and Granberg, P.-O.: Aspiration biopsy cytology in diagnosis of thyroid carcinoma. World J. Surg., 5:61, 1981.

19. Messaris, G., Kyriakou, K., Vasilopoulos, P., and Tountas, C.: The single thyroid nodule and carcinoma. Br. J. Surg., 61:943, 1974.

20. Pochin, E. E.: Leukaemia following radioiodine treatment of thyrotoxicosis. Br. Med. J., ii:1545, 1960.

21. Ramanna, L., Waxman, A. D., Brachman, M. B., Sensel, N., Tanasescu, D. E., Berman, D. S., Catz, B., and Braunstein, G. D.: Correlation of thyroglobulin measurements and radioiodine scans in the follow-up of patients with differentiated thyroid cancer. Cancer, 55:1525, 1985.

22. Saenger, E. L., Thoma, G. E., and Tompkins, E. A.: Incidence of leukaemia following treatment of hyperthyroidism: Preliminary report of the cooperative thyrotoxicosis therapy follow-up study. J.A.M.A., 205:855, 1968.

23. Scott, G. R., Forfar, J. C., and Toft, A. D.: Graves' disease and atrial fibrillation: The case for even higher doses of therapeutic iodine-131. Br. Med. J., 289:399, 1984.

24. Sokal, M., Harmer, C. L.: Chemotherapy for anaplastic carcinoma of the thyroid. Clin. Oncol., 4:3, 1978.

25. Tennvall, J., Biorklund, A., Moller, T., Ranstam, J., and Akerman, M.: Is the EORTC prognostic index of thyroid cancer valid in differentiated thyroid carcinoma. Cancer, 57:1405, 1986.

26. Toft, A. D.: Thyroid surgery for Graves' disease. Br. Med. J., 286:740, 1983.

27. Toft, A. D.: Thyroid enlargement. Br. Med. J., 290:1066, 1985.

28. Toft, A. D., Irvine, W. J., Sinclair, I., McIntosh, D., Seth, J., and Cameron, E. H. D.: Thyroid function after surgical treatment of thyrotoxicosis. N. Engl. J. Med., 298:643, 1978.

29. Wells, S. A., Williams, M. D., Dilley, W. G., Farndon, J. R., Leight, G. S., and Baylin, S. B.: Early diagnosis and treatment of medullary thyroid carcinoma. Arch. Intern. Med., 145:1248, 1985.

THE PARATHYROID GLANDS

NORMAN W. THOMPSON, M.D. • *IAN R. GOUGH, M.B., B.S.*

19

HISTORIC ASPECTS

The parathyroid glands were first discovered in 1849 in a one-horned Indian rhinoceros by Sir Richard Owen, curator of the Hunterian Museum. Owen's brief report was virtually ignored. The first detailed description of the parathyroid glands in man as well as animals was by Ivar Sandström in 1880, then a medical student at the University of Uppsala, Sweden. Sandström's precise gross and microscopic description of the parathyroid glands likewise received little attention. Gley, in 1891, "rediscovered" the parathyroid glands and furthermore made the observation that their excision caused tetany in experimental animals, and this discovery had important surgical implications. The syndrome Gley described was identical to that which had been observed by Billroth following total thyroidectomy.

Von Recklinghausen is credited with describing the characteristic bone changes of severe hyperparathyroidism (osteitis fibrosa cystica) in 1893. However, Askanazy was the first to note a parathyroid tumor in a patient who had died with this disease in 1904. Erdheim, a few years later, noted at autopsy that patients with severe characteristic bone changes had large parathyroid tumors or diffuse hyperplasia. He and other European pathologists believed this was the result of the bone disease rather than its cause. It was not until the independent experiments by Hanson, in 1924, and Collip, in 1925, using parathyroid extract, that the true cause of the bone disease was suspected.

In 1926, the first parathyroidectomy was performed by Mandl in Vienna. His patient had severe bone disease and a pathologic fracture. Mandl initially transplanted normal human parathyroid glands into the neck of his patient with the hope of alleviating the bone disease. Serendipitously, at reoperation 6 weeks later, he removed a large "adenoma" that he discovered while searching for the rejected transplanted glands. When his patient improved, Mandl correctly surmised that the bone disease was caused by the tumor. In America, the first parathyroid exploration was undertaken shortly thereafter, based on experimental evidence that characteristic bone disease was due to parathyroid hypersecretion. This patient's adenoma was not found during his first neck exploration in New York. It was finally found in the mediastinum 5 years later in 1932, after six operations performed in Boston by Cope and Churchill. Unfortunately, renal calcinosis caused the patient's death 6 weeks after operation. Meanwhile, the first successful parathyroidectomy in the United States was reported by Barr in 1929. From 1924 until 1963, the physiology of calcium metabolism and its regulation by the parathyroid glands were gradually elucidated. After the discovery of a radioimmunoassay for parathyroid hormone by Burson and Yalow in 1963 and the widespread availability of serum calcium analysis, the diagnosis and surgical treatment of hyperparathyroidism rapidly became common events. Currently, it is estimated that approximately 1 in 1000 individuals seen in an outpatient clinic has primary hyperparathyroidism, a disease once considered rare.

ANATOMY

Normally, there are two superior and two inferior parathyroid glands. However, some individuals may have five or more glands (5 per cent), and a small percentage have only three glands large enough to be detectable at operation or autopsy.[1, 25] The superior parathyroid glands are derived from the fourth pharyngeal pouch of the embryo and descend a relatively short distance to their usual position posterior to the lateral lobes of the thyroid within 1 to 2 cm. cephalad to the intersection of the inferior thyroid artery and recurrent laryngeal nerve. Most often they are in approximately the same position on each side. However, when enlarged they frequently migrate through the pretracheal fascia into the prevertebral space or descend on a vascular pedicle into the posterior mediastinum. In some individuals, they may be flattened beneath the fascia investing the thyroid or may lie within a superficial cleft of the thyroid. It is very rare for a superior gland to be truly intrathyroidal.

The inferior parathyroid glands are more variable in position. They, like the thymus, are derived from the third pharyngeal pouch of the embryo. Their most common position is anterior to the recurrent laryngeal nerve near the lower pole of the thyroid. However, about 20 per cent descend further caudally and lie within the upper lobes of the thymus. Furthermore, about 2.5 percent of inferior parathyroid glands are truly intrathyroidal, usually within the lower third of the gland. Rarely, an inferior gland may fail to descend properly and can be found within the carotid sheath or upper neck above the level of the thyroid gland. An inferior gland may be situated at any point between the hyoid bone and the anterior mediastinum below the arch of the aorta. The relationship between the position of the inferior glands on each side is less symmetric as compared with the superior glands.

The arterial blood supply to both superior and inferior parathyroid glands is usually by individual end arterial branches of the inferior thyroid artery on each side, although inferior parathyroid glands in the mediastinum are usually supplied by a branch from the internal mammary artery. Venous drainage is via adjacent thyroid veins into the internal jugular or innominate veins.

The number of parathyroids is also variable, although it is rare for fewer than four to be present. In normals or patients with a single parathyroid adenoma, about 5 per cent have more than four glands, usually five and occasionally six. However, when there is diffuse enlargement of all of the glands, such as in secondary hyperparathyroidism or the familial hyperplasia, up to 20 per cent of individuals have detectable supernumerary parathyroids. It therefore seems likely that this latter figure is closer to the true incidence. It is extremely rare to have more than six parathyroid glands.

The combined weight of the parathyroid glands in a normal adult is 160 mg. or less. A normal gland averages 30 to 40 mg., and the upper limit is considered to be 60 mg. The normal parathyroid gland is commonly a flattened ovoid, and the average size is $5 \times 3 \times 1$ mm., but the shape and size of individual glands are quite variable. The usual color is yellow-brown but varies, as does the size and weight, with the fat content and vascularity of the gland. Young or malnourished people have very cellular glands, whereas obese people have large amounts of extracellular fat within the parathyroid capsule.

Parathyroid glands contain three main types of cells, which are recognized by their different staining characteristics on light microscopy.[11] The cell varieties are chief cells (the most numerous), oxyphil cells (which increase in number with increasing age), and water clear cells. All cell types secrete parathyroid hormone. Transitional cell types are common. All of the cells are probably derived from the same stem cell. Hyperplastic glands and adenomas usually demonstrate a predominance of chief cells.

PARATHYROID HORMONE

Parathyroid hormone (PTH) is a single-chain polypeptide of 84 amino acids. It is synthesized in the rough endoplasmic reticulum of the parathyroid cells as pre-pro-PTH, which has 115 amino acids. Proteolytic enzymes cleave 25 amino acids from the amino N-terminal end to produce a 90 amino acid polypeptide, pro-PTH, and further cleavage results in the 84 amino acid chain, which is secreted as "intact" PTH. PTH may be secreted directly, but most is stored in granules awaiting stimuli for secretion.[11] The major controlling influence is ionized calcium concentration, although magnesium is necessary for secretion. Low-ionized calcium concentration stimulates PTH secretion, and high-ionized calcium concentration suppresses PTH secretion. Suppression is incomplete in chronic hypercalcemia of any cause, and a basal rate of PTH secretion persists.

Most PTH is secreted as intact hormone, but some smaller fragments may also be secreted. The biologic activity of PTH is contained in the 34 amino acids at the N-terminal end. PTH is metabolized in the liver, kidneys, and bone. The biologic half-life of the N-terminal portion is only a few minutes. The remainder of the molecule containing amino acids 35 through 84 is referred to as the carboxyl (C)-terminal portion and has a half-life of approximately 1 hour. The half-lives of both fragments are prolonged in patients with renal insufficiency.

Radioimmunoassays are available that are directed toward the N-terminal, mid-portion, and C-terminal portions of PTH. The N-terminal assay may be useful in special circumstances, such as selective venous catheterization studies for localization of parathyroid tumors, or in the assessment of parathyroid autotransplant function, because concentration gradients between the venous effluent of the parathyroid tissue and background systemic PTH are greater for this short half-life fragment. However, the C-terminal assay, which measures both "intact" PTH and the C-terminal fragment, is the most diagnostically useful in patients with primary hyperparathyroidism. It is elevated in the peripheral blood in more than 90 per cent of patients with this disease.

CALCIUM HOMEOSTASIS

PTH and vitamin D are the major factors controlling calcium metabolism. Both have actions that increase serum calcium concentration. The physiologic role of calcitonin, a hypocalcemia-inducing hormone, is not yet fully understood.

PTH binds to receptors in bone and kidney and activates adenylate cyclase, thereby generating cyclic adenosine $3' 5'$ monophosphate (cyclic AMP), which in turn regulates other intracellular enzymes.

PTH acts on bone to accelerate bone resorption and enhance bone remodeling by inducing both osteoclastic and osteoblastic activity. Its action on the renal tubules is to decrease resorption of phosphate and bicarbonate and to increase resorption of calcium. PTH has an indirect role in increasing gastrointestinal absorption of calcium by enhancing the effect of vitamin D. Vitamin D_3 (cholecalciferol) is formed in the skin by the action of ultraviolet light on 7-dihydrocholesterol; it is then hydroxylated in the liver to 25-hydroxycholecalciferol and further activated by 1-alphahydroxylase in the kidney to a potent metabolite, 1,25-dihydroxycholecalciferol. PTH increases the conversion of 25-hydroxycholecalciferol to 1,25-dihydroxycholecalciferol. Vitamin D also favors positive calcium balance, mainly by increasing intestinal absorption. Although one action of vitamin D is to mobilize calcium from bone, it increases calcium and phosphate in the extracellular fluid, and its net effect is to promote mineralization and remodeling of bone.

HYPERCALCEMIA

Hypercalcemia is the characteristic biochemical finding in primary hyperparathyroidism. In normal populations and hospital outpatients, the incidence of hypercalcemia is between 0.1 and 0.5 per cent. Most of these persons will have primary hyperparathyroidism even though about half will be asymptomatic at the time of diagnosis.[14, 21] In contrast to ambulatory populations, the incidence of hypercalcemia in hospitalized patients is about 5 per cent. Nearly two thirds of these patients will prove to have cancer, and only one quarter will have primary hyperparathyroidism.

When hypercalcemia is reported on a biochemical screen, the test should be repeated on blood samples taken without venous stasis and corrected for serum albumin. If hypercalcemia is confirmed, additional laboratory studies should be obtained including BUN, serum creatinine, chloride, phosphate, alkaline phosphatase, and C-terminal PTH assay.

A careful history will be of great assistance in eliciting symptoms of hypercalcemia (Table 1) and obtaining clues

TABLE 1. Clinical Manifestations of Hypercalcemia

1. General: Thirst, polydipsia, weight loss
2. Renal: Polyuria, renal colic (calculi)
3. Gastrointestinal: Constipation, anorexia, nausea, vomiting, abdominal pain
4. Neurologic: Lethargy, proximal muscle weakness, peripheral neuropathy, depression, insomnia, memory loss, confusion, coma
5. Musculoskeletal: Bone pain, arthralgia
6. Cardiovascular: Hypertension, heart block
7. Metastatic calcification: Band keratopathy, chondrocalcinosis, calcification of tendons

regarding the etiology (Table 2). Although the diagnosis of primary hyperparathyroidism can be made with confidence in most patients after appropriate investigation, all the other causes of hypercalcemia must be considered and excluded.

Primary hyperparathyroidism is much more common in persons over the age of 40 and is twice as common in females as in males. Apart from the features of hypercalcemia listed in Table 1, additional clinical findings associated with primary hyperparathyroidism may include osteoporosis, osteitis fibrosa cystica, pathologic fractures, nephrocalcinosis, renal insufficiency, hyperuricemia and/or gout, pseudogout, peptic ulceration, and pancreatitis. It is uncommon for an enlarged parathyroid gland to be palpated in the neck, but this examination should always be done. In most patients with primary hyperparathyroidism in whom a nodule is palpated, the nodule will be in the thyroid rather than a parathyroid gland; however, when the serum calcium is relatively high, the likelihood of detecting a palpable parathyroid adenoma is increased. The classic clinical features of primary hyperparathyroidism may be summarized as the disease of "bones, stones, abdominal groans, and psychic moans."

HYPERPARATHYROIDISM

Pathology

Hyperparathyroidism may be primary, secondary, or tertiary. Primary hyperparathyroidism is the most common cause of hypercalcemia. The parathyroid pathology is a single adenoma in approximately 80 per cent, two adenomas in 2 per cent, hyperplasia of all glands in approximately 15 per cent, and carcinoma in 0.5 to 1 per cent.[2, 5, 13, 19, 25]

TABLE 2. Causes of Hypercalcemia

1. Hyperparathyroidism
2. Malignancy with bone metastases
3. Malignancy without bone metastases (squamous carcinoma of lung or head and neck, renal, ovarian)
4. Hematologic malignancies (multiple myeloma, lymphoma, leukemia)
5. Granulomatous diseases (sarcoidosis, tuberculosis, berylliosis)
6. Excessive vitamin D or vitamin A
7. Milk-alkali syndrome
8. Thiazide diuretics
9. Immobilization of young patients or patients with Paget's disease
10. Benign familial hypocalciuric hypercalcemia
11. Other endocrine disorders (thyrotoxicosis, hypothyroidism, acute adrenal insufficiency)

Hyperplasias and adenomas nearly always involve the chief cells. Rarely, lipoadenomas and functioning parathyroid cysts may occur.

The etiology of hyperparathyroidism is not known in most cases, but a history of head or neck irradiation is found in approximately 10 to 20 per cent of patients with primary hyperparathyroidism in North America and Europe.[15] There is a genetic basis for the diffuse hyperplasia occurring in patients with the multiple endocrine neoplasia (MEN) syndromes. The parathyroids are involved in all patients with the MEN I syndrome and about a third of patients with MEN IIa syndrome. Many other patients with hyperplasia have familial hyperparathyroidism without other endocrinopathies. The remainder have sporadic hyperplasia of all parathyroid glands with no apparent etiologic factors present.

There are three varieties of multiple endocrine neoplasia. As an aid to memory, MEN I can be considered as a syndrome of three "Ps" and the two MEN IIs as syndromes of two "Cs," each of the three syndromes having one additional feature. The three "Ps" of MEN I refer to the endocrine organs involved with primary adenomas or hyperplasia: the pituitary, parathyroids, and pancreas. The additional feature that may occur is adrenal cortical hyperplasia with Cushing's syndrome secondary to excessive adrenocorticotropic hormone (ACTH) from the pituitary adenoma. The two "Cs" of MEN II refer to the hormones produced, calcitonin and catecholamines, from medullary carcinoma of the thyroid and pheochromocytoma, respectively. The additional feature in MEN IIa is parathyroid hyperplasia in about a third of patients, and the additional feature in MEN IIb is the phenotypic expression of Marfanoid body proportions, characteristic facies, and neuromas of lips, tongue, and gastrointestinal tract.

There are no absolute criteria by which pathologists can distinguish an adenoma from hyperplasia in a single parathyroid gland. Careful visual examination of all other glands by the surgeon at operation and biopsy of at least one other gland are necessary before a firm diagnosis can be made. The amount of extracellular parenchymal fat, and in particular the intracellular (intracytoplasmic) fat, can be helpful in distinguishing normal parathyroids from hyperplastic or adenomatous glands. There is a striking decrease or absence of both in most adenomatous and hyperplastic glands.

Chronic hypocalcemic states stimulate the parathyroid glands, and the eventual result is secondary hyperparathyroidism. The causes include dietary deficiency of calcium or vitamin D, intestinal malabsorption, and, most commonly, chronic renal insufficiency.

In renal insufficiency, phosphate retention occurs and phosphate complexes with calcium in extracellular fluid resulting in a relative hypocalcemia. The diseased kidney synthesizes less 1,25-dihydroxycholecalciferol, and this deficiency also tends to produce hypocalcemia because of decreased calcium absorption. Furthermore, in uremia a contributing factor may be end-organ unresponsiveness causing resistance to calcium absorption by the gastrointestinal tract and resistance of bone to the actions of PTH. The parathyroid glands respond by gradually becoming hyperplastic, increasing their PTH secretion. Interpretation of PTH levels in serum must take into account the greatly prolonged half-life of the C-terminal PTH fragment in the presence of diminished renal excretion. The N-terminal PTH assay in secondary hyperparathyroidism is more accurate in determining parathyroid function. Serum calcium levels are low, normal, or high, depending on the stage of the secondary hyperparathyroidism.

Tertiary hyperparathyroidism is a variant of secondary hyperparathyroidism. The term is used by some authors to describe the phase of the disease in which the parathyroid glands have hypertrophied to such a size that they are no longer physiologically responsive to the serum ionized calcium concentration and their relatively autonomous function produces hypercalcemia.

Diagnosis

The diagnosis of primary hyperparathyroidism must be established with certainty prior to operation. The essential biochemical abnormality, present in at least 90 per cent of patients, is an elevated serum calcium level with a simultaneously elevated C-terminal PTH level.[7] It is essential that the calcium and PTH assays be done on the same serum sample and that the tests be repeated if the results are inconclusive.

In the past, before sensitive C-terminal PTH assays were available, the combination of hypercalcemia and "inappropriately normal" intact or N-terminal PTH levels was used to establish the diagnosis of primary hyperparathyroidism. This unsatisfactory criterion was used because of technical difficulties in the radioimmunoassay of various fragments of PTH but is no longer necessary when a reliable C-terminal PTH assay is used.

It has been estimated that up to 20 per cent of patients with malignancy-associated hypercalcemia, without bone metastases, have increased radioimmunoassayable PTH. This situation is sometimes described as ectopic hyperparathyroidism or pseudohyperparathyroidism, although it is thought that the substances detected are polypeptides similar to but different from parathyroid PTH.[12, 23] Osteoclastic activating factor and prostaglandins are two other humoral factors secreted by some malignant tumors that have been implicated in hypercalcemia because of their effects on bone. However, most commonly, the hypercalcemia in malignancy is caused by osteolysis associated with skeletal metastases. Therefore, the hypercalcemia in malignancy is usually not associated with increased PTH levels. In most patients with increased PTH levels, malignancy can be distinguished from primary hyperparathyroidism after a search for the primary tumor and evidence of metastases if the history suggests this possibility. In some cases, when both diseases are present, this may be more difficult. The PTH levels associated with malignancy are invariably lower for a corresponding calcium level than they are with primary hyperparathyroidism. The erythrocyte sedimentation rate (ESR) is more likely to be elevated and the hemoglobin and hematocrit levels lower in malignancy than in primary hyperparathyroidism, although anemia may occur in primary hyperparathyroidism. Serum alkaline phosphatase is an indicator of bone disease in both malignancy and hyperparathyroidism. Occasionally, the hydrocortisone suppression test will be helpful in the differential diagnosis. In this test, 150 mg. of hydrocortisone is given daily for 10 days and is considered positive if the serum calcium falls more than 1 mg. per 100 ml. The hypercalcemia associated with most malignancies and diseases other than primary hyperparathyroidism will show suppression. The test is rarely falsely positive in patients with hyperparathyroidism. Steroids consistently lower the hypercalcemia of sarcoidosis, and this may be useful in both diagnosis and therapy. The serum protein electrophoretic pattern will be abnormal in multiple myeloma and also in many patients with sarcoidosis.

Thiazide diuretics decrease excretion of calcium by the kidney and may increase serum calcium up to 0.5 mg. per 100 ml. above the upper limit of normal range (8.5 to 10.5 mg. per 100 ml.). Levels of serum calcium above 11 mg. per 100 ml. should not be attributed to thiazide diuretics alone.

Parathyroid hormone acts on the proximal kidney tubules to decrease phosphate and bicarbonate resorption with a resultant tendency to acidosis and an increase in serum chloride levels. The serum phosphate is low in most patients with primary hyperparathyroidism but may be normal or even elevated if the disease has impaired renal function. Relatively subtle changes in serum chloride and phosphate levels can be detected by the chloride-phosphate ratio measured in mEq. per liter and mg. per 100 ml. This value will be 33 or greater in 90 per cent of patients with primary hyperparathyroidism and less than 33 in nearly all patients with hypercalcemia from other causes.[18] Any patient initially considered to have primary hyperparathyroidism with a ratio below 33 should be very carefully evaluated for another cause of hypercalcemia.

Measurement of 24-hour urinary calcium excretion usually shows moderately increased levels in primary hyperparathyroidism because the excretion of increased amounts of calcium in the serum overrides the action of PTH on the renal tubules. However, the urinary calcium is also normal or elevated in most patients with other causes of hypercalcemia. Only subnormal levels are really helpful and should lead to consideration of the diagnosis of benign familial hypocalciuric hypercalcemia. The action of PTH on the renal tubule is mediated by cyclic AMP, which is excreted in the urine in increased amounts in about 90 per cent of patients with primary hyperparathyroidism. Although this test is sensitive, it lacks specificity.[12] Roentgenographic changes of osteitis fibrosa cystica are now rarely found in patients with primary hyperparathyroidism, and routine films of the hands and skull are infrequently useful in the diagnosis.

In some patients with relatively mild primary hyperparathyroidism, the serum calcium may fluctuate and may even be within the normal range occasionally. Follow-up and repeat investigations will eventually confirm the diagnosis. In other patients, some additional factor such as reduced intestinal absorption, hypoalbuminemia, or increased renal loss may be acting to reduce serum calcium levels. These situations have been termed *normocalcemic hyperparathyroidism*. Correction of the additional process unmasks hypercalcemia and allows the diagnosis to be established.

A scheme of investigations for the differential diagnosis of hypercalcemia, which includes evaluation of the complications of hyperparathyroidism, is shown in Table 3.

Management of Severe Hypercalcemia

Severe hypercalcemia may be fatal. Hypercalcemic crisis is usually associated with serum calcium levels greater than 14 mg. per 100 ml. but may occur at lower levels. However, not all patients with serum calcium levels above 14 mg. per 100 ml. will have severe symptoms. Patients with severe hypercalcemia typically have a combination of many of the features listed in Table 1. Dehydration and renal insufficiency are particularly important. After urgent measures have been taken to lower the serum calcium level, patients with primary hyperparathyroidism should have a neck exploration as soon as possible.[22] Because PTH testing

TABLE 3. *Investigation of Hypercalcemia*

Serum:
    Calcium, phosphate, albumin (three occasions), creatinine,
       chloride, uric acid
    Alkaline phosphatase
    C-Terminal PTH
Blood
    Complete blood count
    Protein electrophoresis*
    Erythrocyte sedimentation rate*
Urine
    Microscopy and culture
    Calcium
    Cyclic AMP*
X-rays
    Chest and abdomen
    Thoracic and lumbar spine*
    Hands and skull*
    Intravenous urogram*

*Optional.

may cause delay, the diagnosis in these patients may have to be made on the basis of the other clinical findings.

These patients should be treated initially with intravenous saline, and after rehydration and sodium replacement is complete furosemide may be administered. Furosemide inhibits calcium resorption in the ascending limb of the loop of Henle and therefore increases calcium excretion in the urine. Most patients require potassium replacement when renal function has been restored. Some patients require magnesium supplementation as well after this initial therapy.

If the serum calcium level remains high, mithramycin may be used. Mithramycin is a cytotoxic agent that inhibits osteoclast resorption of bone. It is administered intravenously as a single dose and is usually effective for variable periods of time ranging from 24 hours to 1 week.[22] Rebound hypercalcemia occurs rapidly, and repeated doses may cause thrombocytopenia, qualitative defects of platelet function, and renal and hepatic toxicity. Therefore, definitive operation should be performed early and prolonged drug therapy avoided.

Diphosphonates are a recently developed group of compounds with metal-complexing properties that affect the growth and dissolution of poorly soluble calcium salts. The first diphosphonate used in patients caused osteomalacia, but newer agents, including aminohydroxypropylidene diphosphonate (APD) and dichloromethylene disphosphonate (Cl_2MDP), inhibit osteoclastic bone resorption without affecting the mineralization of newly formed osteoid.[8, 24] APD and Cl_2MDP may be given orally or parenterally and appear to be effective in the treatment of malignancy-associated hypercalcemia. Their side effects have not yet been completely documented, and the availability of Cl_2MDP is currently restricted.

Other agents that now have limited roles in the management of severe hypercalcemia are phosphates, steroids, indomethacin, calcitonin, and cimetidine. Although intravenous phosphates are relatively effective in lowering serum calcium, they may worsen the patient's condition by causing metastatic calcification in the heart, lungs, kidneys, and other vital areas. They are contraindicated in hypercalcemic crisis regardless of etiology.[22] Oral phosphates bind calcium in the gut but may also promote some soft tissue calcification. They have been used in the longer-term control of malignancy-associated hypercalcemia. Glucocorticoids, such as prednisone, may be used in malignancy-associated hypercalcemia and are helpful in approximately 50 per cent of patients. Steroids have no role in the management of primary hyperparathyroidism except in the diagnostic suppression test. Indomethacin, like cortisone, inhibits prostaglandin synthesis and has been useful in patients with malignancy-associated hypercalcemia caused by prostaglandin hypersecretion. Calcitonin may be effective in lowering the serum calcium if given in frequently repeated large doses. Despite a few promising reports of a calcium lowering action, cimetidine has subsequently proved to be of no real value in the management of primary hyperparathyroidism.

Management of Primary Hyperparathyroidism

There is no satisfactory nonsurgical treatment of hyperparathyroidism. Although various dietary and drug programs have been tried, none has been effective. Diphosphonates may be feasible in the short term prior to operation, but they have not yet been adequately studied.[8]

Management of the patient with mild hypercalcemia and no symptoms created a dilemma that clinicians had not encountered in the past because the disease was rarely, if ever, diagnosed solely on biochemical findings. Only one long-term study of a large number of patients with asymptomatic hyperparathyroidism has allowed assessment of the natural history of the untreated disease.[21] During a 10-year period, 142 patients were studied; 23 per cent died of apparently unrelated causes, 25 per cent developed complications or progressive hypercalcemia, all but 3 of whom had neck explorations, and 13 per cent were lost to follow-up. It was not possible to predict which patients would develop progressive hypercalcemia and complications. Furthermore, many patients were unwilling to comply with annual clinic visits and repeated investigations.

Often patients with apparently asymptomatic primary hyperparathyroidism do have abnormalities (neuropsychiatric, skeletal, neuromuscular, renal, or cardiovascular) that are detectable by careful investigation and evaluation. For instance, successful parathyroid surgery results in normalization of blood pressure in approximately one third of hypertensive patients with hyperparathyroidism.[6] Some complications of the disease, such as renal impairment, may become irreversible if untreated for long periods of time.

Parathyroid exploration is advocated because it is safe (current mortality of 0 to 0.1 per cent), associated with little morbidity, and offers a definitive cure of the disease in 95 per cent or more of the patients when done by an experienced surgeon.[5, 19, 25] Although some asymptomatic patients with primary hyperparathyroidism with mild or intermittent hypercalcemia (11 mg. per 100 ml. or less) may be managed by close observation, we believe that virtually all patients with biochemically proven disease should undergo neck exploration. A concomitant severe medical problem may be a contraindication to an operation in a small number of patients. The cost of surgical treatment is currently estimated to be approximately equivalent to 5 years of medical follow-up.[14]

OPERATIVE STRATEGY

The diagnosis of primary hyperparathyroidism should be established before a neck exploration is undertaken. The only diagnosis to be established by operation is the type of parathyroid disease present in the individual patient, e.g., adenoma, hyperplasia, and carcinoma. Preoperative investigations to localize hyperfunctioning parathyroid

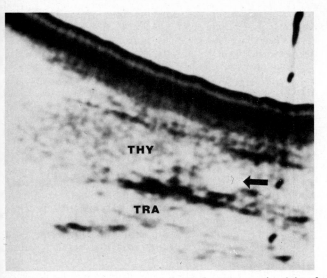

Figure 1. Ultrasound of the neck (sagittal section to the right of the midline) showing a hypoechogenic right inferior parathyroid adenoma 1 cm. in diameter (arrow) adjacent to the inferior pole of the right lobe of the thyroid (THY) and anterior to the trachea (TRA).

tissue are generally unnecessary in a patient initially being explored. An experienced surgeon is far more reliable in determining the location of hyperplastic parathyroid glands than any single test or combination of tests, which may be expensive, invasive, and misleading. Nevertheless, two noninvasive studies currently being widely evaluated because of improving techniques are cervical ultrasonography (Fig. 1) and thallium-technetium scintiscanning. Despite present limitations, continued improvement may make their routine use justified in the future. Selective arteriography and selective venous PTH sampling are specifically unwarranted before an initial neck exploration.

The goals of surgical management are identification and excision of the hyperfunctioning parathyroid gland(s) while preserving the normal glands or the equivalent of one normal-sized (40 mg.) hyperplastic gland. In most cases, these goals can be accomplished during the initial neck exploration. It is imperative that the surgeon not leave the neck without these goals accomplished except in the 1 or 2 per cent of patients in whom the hyperplastic parathyroid gland(s) is within the mediastinum, below a level that cannot be explored from the neck.

The operative strategy is to identify four or more parathyroid glands in all patients so that an accurate assessment of the specific disease process can be made. In patients with adenomas, the enlarged gland is excised while the remaining normal glands are preserved.[9, 25] For confirmation of normal parathyroid tissue, the pathologist may assist the surgeon by performing immediate frozen section examination of small biopsies of one or more of the apparently normal glands. The biopsies are carefully taken from an area of the gland opposite its blood supply. Recently, some pathologists have utilized fat stains because intracellular fat is absent or markedly decreased in 90 per cent of adenomatous and hyperplastic parathyroid glands. However, the pathologist cannot reliably distinguish an adenoma from hyperplasia by examination of a single gland. This fact emphasizes the need for the surgeon to visualize all of the glands and to biopsy at least one that is apparently normal. Because an intravenous infusion of methylene blue stains parathyroid tissue more deeply than other tissues, it

is used intraoperatively by some surgeons to assist in identifying parathyroid glands. Most surgeons, however, rely on the natural appearance of normal glands and use frozen section biopsies only to confirm their macroscopic diagnosis.

In patients with hyperplasia of all glands, the surgeon should be able to make the correct assessment after finding more than two enlarged glands. Although most frequently all of the glands are enlarged in patients with hyperplasia, in some the enlargement may be asymmetric and thus misleading. The majority of surgeons remove all of the hyperplastic glands except the equivalent of one normal-sized, well-vascularized parathyroid (40 mg.). However, some surgeons advocate total parathyroidectomy with immediate autotransplantation of multiple 1-mm. fragments of half of one gland into a forearm muscle in most patients with diffuse hyperplasias. Another alternative is to cryopreserve some parathyroid tissue and transplant only if the patient is shown to be hypoparathyroid after several months. In patients with primary or secondary hyperplasia, the upper thymus should be routinely removed even when four parathyroids have already been found because of the increased incidence of enlarged supernumerary glands (15 to 20 per cent). This is particularly important in the MEN I syndrome.

Carcinoma of the parathyroid is uncommon (0.5 to 1 per cent) but can usually be recognized at operation by its characteristic appearance. Most often there is a thick, pale, irregular capsule around the enlarged parathyroid gland, which is firmer than the characteristically soft adenoma. There may be invasion of adjacent structures as well. En bloc excision of the surrounding tissues and any involved local lymph nodes usually controls the disease for many years providing the tumor has not been ruptured at operation. When the disease is grossly localized, surgical excision is curative in about half of the patients.[2]

OPERATIVE TECHNIQUE OF PARATHYROID EXPLORATION

Exploration of the parathyroid gland is done under general anesthesia with endotracheal intubation. The patient is positioned, as for a thyroid operation, with the neck extended. A slightly curved transverse incision is made approximately 2 cm. above the clavicles, in or parallel to a skin crease, and carried down through the platysma muscle. Superior and inferior flaps are raised deep to the platysma and superficial to the anterior cervical veins, which are enclosed within the investing layer of deep cervical fascia. The strap muscles are separated in the midline from the top of the thyroid cartilage to the sternal notch and retracted laterally. The pretracheal fascia investing the thyroid is opened, and the thyroid gland is exposed and mobilized. The middle thyroid veins are ligated and divided to enable the thyroid lobes to be rotated anteriorly and medially. It is important throughout the procedure to maintain meticulous hemostasis because blood staining of the tissues obscures the parathyroid glands. The normal parathyroid glands must be dissected very carefully to preserve their fragile blood supply. It is important to avoid breaking the capsule of enlarged glands because such hyperplastic tissue can be inadvertently implanted, causing subsequent recurrence.

The fascia between the carotid sheath and upper thyroid lobe is sharply divided posteriorly to the depth of the prevertebral fascia because this allows exploration of the prevertebral space in the neck, including the retropharyngeal area, the upper posterior mediastinum, and the tracheoesophageal groove. Exploration in these locations, as well as the posterior aspect of the upper half of the thyroid lobes, will nearly always reveal the superior parathyroid glands, which are always accessible through a cervical incision (Fig. 2). The inferior parathyroid glands are more variable in position, as noted in the section on anatomy, but can be found via a cervical incision in 98 per cent of patients. Inferior parathyroids that are not found after a careful exploration, including dissection of the upper thymus, may be revealed after deliberate removal of the thymus by carefully teasing it out of the mediastinum through the cervical incision. Fewer than 2 per cent of patients with a hyperfunctioning inferior parathyroid gland will require sternal splitting. Exploration of the deeper mediastinum should probably not be done as part of an initial parathyroid exploration unless the patient has been in hyperparathyroid crisis.

It is usually unnecessary and undesirable to ligate either the superior or inferior thyroid arteries. The recurrent laryngeal nerves will rarely be injured if the surgeon is aware of their close and variable relationship to the parathyroid glands. An inferior gland adenoma is invariably anterior to the recurrent laryngeal nerve, but the nerve may be adherent to its posterior surface, whereas a superior gland adenoma is posterior or lateral to the recurrent laryngeal nerve. The nerve may be adherent to the anterior or medial surface of a large superior gland adenoma. After hemostasis is obtained, the wound is closed by reapproximating the muscle layers in the midline. The details of the operation should be carefully recorded in the patient's chart. It is also very helpful to include an illustration of the positions of the parathyroid glands: "One picture is worth a thousand words." Skin sutures or clips are removed on the second postoperative day and replaced with sterile adhesive strips. The cosmetic result is usually excellent.

RESULTS

An experienced endocrine surgeon will identify four parathyroid glands in more than 95 per cent of patients, and in patients whose disease is caused by a single adenoma 99 per cent or more will be permanently cured. The initial failure and recurrence rates are higher in patients with hyperplasia of all glands.[4, 10, 20] Successful identification of the parathyroid pathology may be more difficult in patients with relatively mild "biochemical" primary hyperparathyroidism.[19, 25] Some patients with persistent hypercalcemia

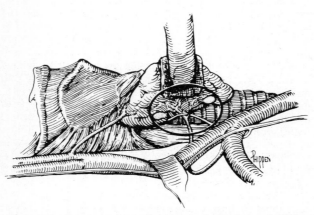

Figure 2. The majority of parathyroid glands are located within a 2-cm. radius of the intersection of the recurrent laryngeal nerve and inferior thyroid artery.

after operation will subsequently be proven to have a diagnosis other than or in addition to primary hyperparathyroidism. The operative mortality is negligible in all but the very elderly or those with severe concomitant disease or hypercalcemic crisis.

Injury to the external branch of the superior laryngeal nerve is extremely rare. Injury to the recurrent laryngeal nerve should also be rare, although temporary unilateral nerve palsy is reported in approximately 1 per cent and permanent nerve palsy in 0.1 per cent. Acute dyspnea immediately postoperatively is uncommon but may be caused by a hematoma compressing the trachea or from bilateral recurrent laryngeal nerve palsy. Hematomas should be evacuated immediately, and bilateral vocal cord palsies require reintubation and sometimes tracheostomy if more than transient. Occasionally, the operation precipitates acute gout or acute pancreatitis.

The most significant postoperative complication after a successful parathyroidectomy is hypocalcemia. Serum calcium levels may drop precipitously, particularly in patients with very high preoperative calcium levels and those with bone disease. Low ionized serum calcium levels increase neuromuscular excitability. Clinical features of acute hypocalcemia include the following:

1. Paresthesia, particularly around the mouth and fingertips.

2. Positive Chvostek's sign (contraction of facial muscles on percussion over the facial nerve).

3. Trousseau's sign (flexion of metacarpophalangeal joints and extension of the interphalangeal joints when a sphygmomanometer cuff is applied above systolic arterial pressure for 3 minutes).

4. Tetany with carpopedal and laryngeal spasm.

These clinical signs, however, are variable, and serum calcium levels should be monitored at least once per day for 3 days postoperatively. Depending on the severity of the hypocalcemia, management consists of oral or intravenous calcium supplements and/or rapidly acting vitamin D preparations. If intravenous calcium is required, it should be given as the gluconate preparation because calcium chloride is locally necrotizing if extravasated. Most hypocalcemia is transient, but permanent hypoparathyroidism requiring long-term vitamin D therapy occurs in about 1 to 2 per cent of patients after parathyroid surgery.

REOPERATION

Recurrence of hypercalcemia after an interval of 6 months or more following a successful operation may be due to hyperplasia of a known parathyroid remnant or overlooked gland, a second adenoma, or another disease.[4] Persistence of hypercalcemia after an initial operation is a different problem, usually due to an inadequate exploration and an overlooked adenoma. The patient should be referred to an expert parathyroid surgeon. In such cases, the diagnosis should be carefully reviewed and confirmed by repetition of serum biochemical studies including C-terminal PTH levels. In most cases, review of the original operative notes and pathologic report will provide clues as to the position of undetected parathyroid glands. If the undetected gland is a superior parathyroid, unilateral neck exploration is all that is required. If the undetected gland(s) are inferior parathyroids, localizing studies may now be indicated. No individual technique is consistently reliable, although a combination of investigations should localize the hyperfunctioning parathyroid tissue in about two thirds of pa-

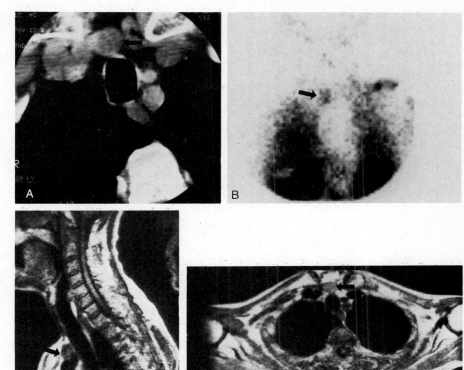

Figure 3. Scans of patient with a 1.5-cm. diameter adenoma of the right inferior parathyroid gland (arrow) in the anterior mediastinum below the manubrium sterni. At the first operation, the other three (normal) parathyroid glands had been identified, but the adenoma was not found.

A, CT scan.

B, Thallium/technetium scintiscan. The computer has subtracted the thyroid image so that it appears white while the image of the parathyroid gland persists.

C, NMR scan (sagittal section to the right of the midline).

D, NMR scan (horizontal section). It is noteworthy that there is no artefact from the shoulder girdle, a problem which often interferes with interpretation of CT scans at this level.

tients.[3] Noninvasive investigations should generally be employed first (Fig. 3). These studies include:

1. Ultrasound.

2. Computerized axial tomography with intravenous contrast.

3. Nuclear magnetic resonance imaging.

4. Isotope scanning combining thallium and technetium.

5. Percutaneous selective venous sampling for PTH assay (N-terminal).

6. Selective arteriography.

Selective arteriography for suspected mediastinal parathyroid adenomas should be limited to catheterization of the internal mammary arteries in order to minimize inadvertent injection of the vertebral arteries and neurologic complications associated with this procedure. Sternal split and full mediastinal exploration is required in fewer than 2 per cent of all patients with primary hyperparathyroidism even though 20 per cent of inferior glands are found in thymic tissue.

Secondary and Tertiary Hyperparathyroidism

The objective of medical management of secondary hyperparathyroidism is normalization of serum calcium and phosphate levels to suppress PTH secretion. In patients with chronic renal failure, the principles of management include (1) administration of oral phosphate binders, such as non-absorbable antacids containing aluminum hydroxide, (2) calcium supplementation with oral preparations and calcium concentrations in dialysis solutions sufficient to promote positive calcium balance, (3) correction of metabolic acidosis by the use of oral sodium bicarbonate and dialysate buffers, and (4) use of vitamin D preparations such as 1,25-dihydroxycholecalciferol to enhance the absorption of dietary calcium. This drug is potent and effective in improving calcium balance, in decreasing PTH production, and in enhancing bone mineralization. However, hyperphosphatemia must first be corrected. The therapy should be initiated and monitored carefully because metastatic calcification occurs when the product of the serum calcium (mg. per 100 ml.) and serum phosphate (mg. per 100 ml.) exceeds 70.

Most patients can be successfully managed for many years on hemodialysis by using these measures, and the potential problem usually resolves after successful renal allotransplantation. However, after several years of dialysis, 10 to 25 per cent of patients develop progressive secondary hyperparathyroidism that can no longer be controlled by medical measures. These long-term hemodialysis patients, along with a few patients despite successful renal transplants, have nonsuppressible parathyroid hyperplasia. This has been termed *tertiary hyperparathyroidism* by some authors, although it probably represents a severe degree of secondary hyperparathyroidism. In this situation, the serum PTH levels rise progressively. These patients typically have high normal or elevated serum calcium levels and renal osteodystrophy. Bone roentgenograms show progressive changes (Fig. 4), and rising serum alkaline phosphatase levels reflect the degree of osteoclastic activity present. Many patients also have neuromuscular weakness, pruritus, and metastatic calcification in blood vessels and viscera. These patients benefit from parathyroidectomy.[16, 17]

Total parathyroidectomy, by eliminating PTH production, exposes the patient to the risk of developing osteomalacia despite therapy with calcium and vitamin D. At present, it is considered advisable to leave a small portion

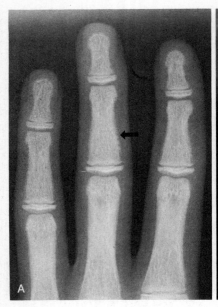
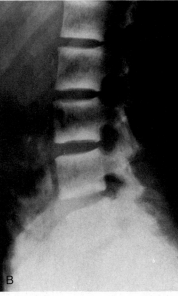

Figure 4. Renal osteodystrophy. A, Subperiosteal resorption of bone on the radial aspect of phalanges (arrow). B, "Rugger-jersey" spine with alternating zones of osteoporosis and osteosclerosis.

of functioning parathyroid tissue, but the method of achieving this is controversial. Some surgeons perform subtotal parathyroidectomy, removing three or more glands while preserving approximately 40 mg. of viable parathyroid tissue with its normal blood supply. Others consider the risk of subsequent cervical recurrence sufficient to justify total parathyroidectomy and immediate autografting of fragments of half of a gland into a forearm muscle.[17] The autotransplantation procedure is successful in 80 to 90 per cent of patients, although it may be many months before the patient can be weaned from calcium and vitamin D. Forearm autograft function can be monitored by comparing PTH assays (N-terminal) in the cubital vein draining the graft site with those of background systemic PTH. If the graft subsequently hyperfunctions and causes hypercalcemia, a portion of the grafted muscle area can be excised under local anesthesia without the risk of a repeat cervical operation.

Profound hypocalcemia frequently follows parathyroidectomy in secondary hyperparathyroidism and requires correction with a rapidly acting vitamin D preparation such as oral 1,25-dihydroxycholecalciferol and intravenous calcium gluconate as well as careful regulation of calcium levels in the dialysis fluid.

Hypocalcemia

The causes of hypocalcemia are listed in Table 4. The management of hypocalcemia related to chronic renal failure has been discussed previously.

The most common cause of hypocalcemia is operative injury or excision of the parathyroids during either a thyroidectomy or parathyroid exploration. With precise technique, the serious complication of permanent hypocalcemia can be avoided in nearly all patients. Total thyroidectomy for primary carcinomas of the thyroid can be consistently done with an incidence of permanent parathyroid deficiency of less than 2 per cent. Great care must be taken to avoid inadvertent excision of normal glands as well as injury to their blood supply. Specifically, the technique of inferior thyroid artery ligation proximal to the end

arteries supplying 90 per cent of parathyroid glands must be avoided. When normal parathyroids, initially attached to the thyroid or actually within the thyroid parenchyma, cannot be left *in situ*, they should be immediately sectioned in 1-mm. fragments and transplanted into a cervical muscle. During parathyroid explorations, every effort should be made to preserve the blood supply to normal glands while locating them and during any subsequent biopsies. Normal-appearing glands should never be excised or even biopsied until all of the parathyroids have been identified or their normal and ectopic locations explored. Formerly, many surgeons excised an enlarged gland (adenoma) and biopsied all of the other normal-sized glands. Most experienced surgeons currently identify the normal glands visually and biopsy only one to exclude hyperplasia. This appears to appreciably decrease the incidence of both transient and permanent hypoparathyroidism.[9]

Reoperative parathyroid surgery is associated with the greatest risk of permanent hypoparathyroidism, particularly when an inexperienced surgeon has either excised or injured normal parathyroids during the initial unsuccessful exploration. A successful reoperation may be complicated by permanent hypoparathyroidism if all of the normal parathyroids have been previously injured. In this setting, forearm transplantation of parathyroid tissue must be considered, even though it is hyperplastic. If there is recorded

TABLE 4. Causes of Hypocalcemia

1. Hypoparathyroidism
   a. Postoperative
   b. Idiopathic
   c. Neonatal (associated with maternal hypercalcemia)
2. Renal insufficiency
3. Intestinal malabsorption of calcium (gut disease or vitamin D deficiency)
4. Pseudohypoparathyroidism
5. Drugs (phosphates, barbiturates)
6. Acute pancreatitis
7. Hypoalbuminemia
8. Hypomagnesemia

evidence of previous excision of two or more glands, parathyroid tissue should be cryopreserved at reoperation. Should the patient prove to be permanently hypocalcemic, a parathyroid transplant can be performed 3 or 4 months later.

A common cause of hypocalcemia following a successful operation for primary hyperparathyroidism even when the normal glands have not been injured is "hungry bones." This is seen most frequently in elderly women with severe osteoporosis. These patients may have normal rather than elevated serum phosphate levels and biochemical evidence of normal parathyroid hormone levels. Nevertheless, their rapidly remineralizing bones contribute to hypocalcemia. Supplementation with large amounts of oral calcium preparations for up to 3 months usually corrects this deficiency.

Long-term management of transient (3 to 6 months) or permanent hypoparathyroidism is accomplished with oral calcium gluconate or carbonate and vitamin D. Cholecalciferol, 1,25-dihydroxycholecalciferol, and the synthetic vitamin D–like compound dehydrotachysterol are all satisfactory but vary in their duration of action and cost. Treatment must be individualized and monitored by serum calcium and phosphate levels at least twice yearly. This is very important because hypercalcemia may develop insidiously. Furthermore, chronic hypocalcemia, even when asymptomatic, can cause avoidable complications. These include osteomalacia, cataracts, cerebral and cerebellar calcification, epilepsy, and dryness of the skin and hair.

SELECTED REFERENCES

Kaplan, E.L. (Ed.): Surgery of the Thyroid and Parathyroid Glands. Clinical Surgery International, Vol. 6. New York, Churchill Livingstone, 1983.
This book contains 9 chapters on the thyroid and 11 chapters on the parathyroids. All chapters are concise and well written by an outstanding group of clinician-scientists. The subjects covered are hyperparathyroidism: incidence, diagnosis, and problems; operative strategy in primary hyperparathyroidism; reoperation for suspected hyperparathyroidism; hyperparathyroidism as part of the MEN I and MEN II syndromes; irradiation to the neck and hyperparathyroidism; clinical and biochemical differentiation of primary hyperparathyroidism from malignancy-associated hypercalcemia; the dilemma of asymptomatic hypercalcemia; secondary hyperparathyroidism; comparison of subtotal parathyroidectomy and total parathyroidectomy and autotransplantation; and postoperative hypoparathyroidism: diagnosis and management.

Thompson, N.W., and Vinik, A.I. (Eds.): Endocrine Surgery Update. New York, Grune & Stratton, 1983.
This book contains 31 chapters by multiple authors: six chapters are devoted to the parathyroid glands. Included is an authoritative review of the value of parathyroid hormone assays in current clinical practice as well as evaluations of the clinical and laboratory features of primary hyperparathyroidism and parathyroid localization studies. Current medical and surgical management of secondary hyperparathyroidism is reviewed, as is primary hyperparathyroidism in children. The techniques of initial parathyroid exploration and reoperative parathyroidectomy are presented in detail. The authors incorporate references to their extensive experience at the University of Michigan Medical Center.

Wells, S.A., Jr.: The parathyroid glands. *In* Sabiston, D.C., Jr. (Ed.): Textbook of Surgery: The Biological Basis of Modern Surgical Practice, 13th ed. Philadelphia, W. B. Saunders Company, 1986, p. 620.
This chapter presents the surgical management of hyperparathyroidism in detail, and the bibliography contains numerous significant historical references.

REFERENCES

1. Akerström, G., Malmaeus, J., and Bergström, R.: Surgical anatomy of human parathyroid glands. Surgery, *95*:14, 1984.
2. Anderson, B. J., Samaan, N. A., Vassilopoulou-Sellin, R., Ordonez, N. G., and Hickey, R. C.: Parathyroid carcinoma: Features and difficulties in diagnosis and management. Surgery, *94*:906, 1983.
3. Brennan, M. F., Doppman, J. L., Kurdy, A. G., Marx, S. J., Spiegel, A. M., and Aurbach, G. D.: Assessment of techniques for preoperative parathyroid gland localization in patients undergoing reoperation for hyperparathyroidism. Surgery, *91*:6, 1982.
4. Clark, O. H., Way, L. W., and Hunt, T. K.: Recurrent hyperparathyroidism. Ann. Surg., *184*:391, 1976.
5. Cowie, A. G. A.: Morbidity in adult parathyroid surgery. J. Roy. Soc. Med., *75*:942, 1982.
6. Daniels, J., and Goodman, A. D.: Hypertension and hyperparathyroidism. Am. J. Med., *75*:17, 1983.
7. DiBella, F. P., and Hawker, C. D.: Parathyrin (parathyroid hormone): Radioimmunoassays for intact and carboxyl-terminal moieties. Clin. Chem., *28*:226, 1982.
8. Douglas, D. L., Kanis, J. A., Paterson, A. D., Beard, D. J., Cameron, E. C., Watson, M. E., Woodhead, S., Williams, J., and Russell, R. G. G.: Drug treatment of primary hyperparathyroidism: Use of clodronate disodium. Br. Med. J., *286*:587, 1983.
9. Edis, A. J., Beahrs, O. H., van Heerden, J. A., and Akwari, O. E.: "Conservative" versus "liberal" approach to parathyroid neck exploration. Surgery, *82*:466, 1977.
10. Edis, A. J., van Heerden, J. A., and Scholz, D. A.: Results of subtotal parathyroidectomy for primary chief cell hyperplasia. Surgery, *86*:462, 1979.
11. Futrell, J. M., Roth, S. I., Su, S. P. C., Habener, J. F., Segre, G. V., and Potts, J. T.: Immunocytochemical localization of parathyroid hormone in bovine parathyroid glands and human parathyroid adenomas. Am. J. Pathol., *94*:615, 1979.
12. Goltzman, D., Stewart, A. F., and Broadhus, A. E.: Malignancy-associated hypercalcemia: Evaluation with a cytochemical bioassay for parathyroid hormone. J. Clin. Endocrinol. Metab., *53*:899, 1981.
13. Harness, J. K., Ramsburg, S. R., Nishiyama, R. H., and Thompson, N. W.: Multiple adenomas of the parathyroids: Do they exist? Arch. Surg., *114*:468, 1979.
14. Heath, H., Hodgson, S. F., and Kennedy, M. A.: Primary hyperparathyroidism: Incidence, morbidity, and potential economic impact in a community. N. Engl. J. Med., *302*:189, 1980.
15. Hedman, I., Hansson, G., Lundberg, L. M., and Tisell, L. E.: A clinical evaluation of radiation-induced hyperparathyroidism based on 148 surgically treated patients. World J. Surg., *8*:96, 1984.
16. Memmos, D. E., Williams, G. B., Eastwood, J. B., Gordon, E. M., Cochrane, C. L., Gower, P. E., Curtis, J. R., Phillips, M. E., Rainford, D. J., and de Wardener, H. E.: The role of parathyroidectomy in the management of hyperparathyroidism in patients on maintenance haemodialysis and after renal transplantation. Nephron, *30*:143, 1982.
17. Rothmund, M., and Wagner, P. K.: Total parathyroidectomy and autotransplantation of parathyroid tissue for renal hyperparathyroidism: A one- to six-year follow-up. Ann. Surg., *197*:7, 1983.
18. Reeves, C. D., Palmer, F., Bacchus, H., and Longerbeam, J. K.: Differential diagnosis of hypercalcemia by the chloride/phosphate ratio. Am. J. Surg., *130*:166, 1975.
19. Russell, C. F., and Edis, A. J.: Surgery for primary hyperparathyroidism: Experience with 500 consecutive cases and evaluation of the role of surgery in the asymptomatic patient. Br. J. Surg., *69*:244, 1982.
20. Russell, C. F., Edis, A. J., and Purnell, D. C.: The reasons for persistent hypercalcemia after cervical exploration for presumed primary hyperparathyroidism. Br. J. Surg., *70*:198, 1983.
21. Scholz, D. A., and Purnell, D. C.: Asymptomatic primary hyperparathyroidism: 10-year prospective study. Mayo Clin. Proc., *56*:473, 1981.
22. Schweitzer, V. G., Thompson, N. W., Harness, J. K., and Nishiyama, R. H.: Management of severe hypercalcemia caused by primary hyperparathyroidism. Arch. Surg., *113*:373, 1978.
23. Simpson, E. L., Mundy, G. R., D'Souza, S. M., Ibbotson, K. J., Bockman, R., and Jacobs, J. W.: Absence of parathyroid hormone messenger RNA in nonparathyroid tumors associated with hypercalcemia. N. Engl. J. Med., *309*:325, 1983.
24. Sleeboom, H. P., Bijvoet, O. L., van Oosterom, A. T., Gleed, J. H., and O'Riordan, J. L. H.: Comparison of intravenous (3-amino-1-hydroxypropylidene)-1,1-biphosphonate and volume repletion in tumour-induced hypercalcemia. Lancet, *2*:239, 1983.
25. Thompson, N. W., Eckhauser, F. E., and Harness, J. K.: The anatomy of primary hyperparathyroidism. Surgery, *92*:814, 1982.

THE PITUITARY AND ADRENAL GLANDS

STEFANIE S. JEFFREY, M.D. • ORLO H. CLARK, M.D.

20

THE PITUITARY AND HYPOTHALAMUS

Normal Anatomy

The pituitary gland normally weighs about 0.5 gm. and measures 13 × 10 × 6 mm. It lies within the bony confines of the sella turcica in the sphenoid bone at the base of the skull. The sella turcica forms the anterior, posterior, and inferior borders of the pituitary. Superiorly, the pituitary is bounded by the diaphragma sellae, which is a fibrous reflection of the dura. Although in 50 per cent of individuals the diaphragma sellae tightly adheres to the pituitary stalk, in 40 per cent there is an opening around the pituitary stalk greater than 5 mm. and in 10 per cent of patients the diaphragma is very thin. The anatomic relationship of the diaphragma sellae to the pituitary stalk is important clinically and may determine the pathways of extension of pituitary tumors (Fig. 1). In patients with an incomplete diaphragma sella, pituitary tumors may preferentially extend superiorly into the region of the optic chiasma and suprasellar cistern. If the diaphragma sellae tightly adheres to the pituitary stalk, pituitary tumors extend inferiorly into the sphenoid sinus. The lateral boundary of the sella turcica is formed by the cavernous sinus, which contains the intracavernous portion of the internal carotid arteries and cranial nerves III, IV, and VI.

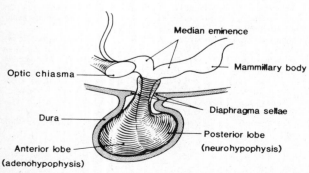

Figure 1. Anatomic relationships of hypothalamus, diaphragma sellae, and pituitary.

Anatomists and physiologists divide the pituitary gland into the *anterior lobe (adenohypophysis)* and the *posterior lobe (neurohypophysis)*. Arterial blood to the anterior lobe comes from two sources: (1) the superior hypophyseal artery, which is a branch of the internal carotid artery, and (2) a rich, physiologically important portal venous system from the median eminence (Fig. 2). This portal system transports neurohumors from the hypothalamus to the adenohypophysis. There may also be retrograde flow in this system. Arterial blood to the posterior lobe arises from the inferior hypophyseal arteries. These systems are largely separate. Venous blood from the pituitary drains into the cavernous sinus.

The neuronal connections between the pituitary and the hypothalamus differ for both the neurohypophysis and the adenohypophysis. The axons that connect the neurohypophysis to the hypothalamus originate from cells in the supraoptic and paraventricular nuclei (Fig. 3). These are referred to as *magnocellular neurons* because of the relatively large size of their cell bodies. It is here within the magnocellular neurons of the supraoptic and paraventricular nuclei that large protein molecules known as *neurophysins* are synthesized. The neurophysins act as carriers for the smaller polypeptides *oxytocin* and *vasopressin*. When linked with the larger neurophysin molecules, they are referred to as *prohormones*. After originating from the magnocellular neurons, these prohormones are carried to the posterior pituitary, where the smaller octapeptides, oxytocin, and vasopressin are separated from the neurophysins and secreted into the blood.

The *parvicellular neurons* in the hypothalamus have small cell bodies and control secretion from the adenohypophysis. Within the parvicellular neurons are specific releasing and inhibiting factors that regulate polypeptide secretion from the anterior pituitary. These factors are synthesized in the hypothalamus and extend down the parvicellular axons to the median eminence of the neurohypophysis. They are then transported to the anterior pituitary via the portal venous system from the median eminence (Fig. 2). The anterior pituitary contains cells with specific receptors for the various hypothalamic releasing or inhibiting factors (Table 1). In general, one specific cell type in the anterior pituitary is thought to secrete one specific polypeptide hormone; however, the gonadotropic cell is known to secrete both luteinizing hormone (LH) and follicle-stimulating hormone (FSH).

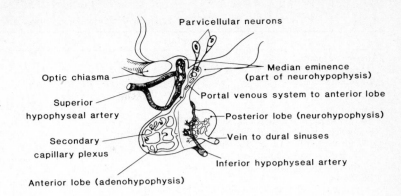

Figure 2. Vascular system of pituitary.

Physiology

THE ANTERIOR PITUITARY

The following hormones are secreted by the anterior pituitary gland: growth hormone (GH), adrenocorticotropic hormone (ACTH), prolactin (PRL), thyroid-stimulating hormone (TSH), FSH, LH, endorphins, and enkephalins.

Growth Hormone

Growth hormone (GH, somatotropin) is a large polypeptide, made up of 191 amino acids (M.W. 21,500), that is secreted by somatotropic cells of the anterior pituitary. The secretion of GH is stimulated by growth hormone–releasing factor (GRF), synthesized in the parvicellular hypothalamic neurons. *Somatostatin,* also known as growth hormone–inhibiting factor (GIH), is another hypothalamic factor. It directly inhibits the secretion of GH. Growth hormone secretion increases during periods of physical exercise, stress, hypoglycemia, or protein depletion, and after the administration of various drugs, such as L-dopa, epinephrine, insulin, glucagon, and morphine derivatives. Hypothalamic secretion of GH occurs periodically throughout the day, with a prominent surge during the early morning hours. The major metabolic effects of GH include stimulation of the growth of the musculoskeletal system and solid viscera. In addition, it directly increases the serum glucose level.

ACTH

Adrenocorticotropic hormone is synthesized by corticotropic cells in the adenohypophysis and is a peptide made up of 39 amino acids (M.W. 4500). The secretion of ACTH is regulated by both feedback from adrenocortical hormones (primarily cortisol) and by corticotropin releasing factor (CRF). The secretion of ACTH follows a diurnal rhythm, with peak secretion during times of sleep in the early morning and the lowest concentration of hormone in the late afternoon and evening. In addition to direct stimulation by the hypothalamus, a variety of other factors may increase ACTH secretion including: stress, trauma, fever, hypoglycemia, and exposure to extreme cold.

ACTH is initially synthesized as part of a larger precursor molecule (prohormone) known as *pro-opiocortin.* This precursor molecule contains a number of active polypeptides, including ACTH, that are later cleaved from this molecule (Fig. 4). The primary metabolic effects of ACTH are to stimulate the growth of the adrenal cortex and the production and secretion of adrenocorticosteroid hormones.

Prolactin

Prolactin is a large, 198-amino acid polypeptide hormone (M.W. 22,000) that is similar to growth hormone and is secreted by the lactotrophic cells of the adenohypophysis. Hypothalamic regulation of prolactin is primarily through the inhibition of its secretions by prolactin-inhibiting factor (PIF). A specific prolactin-releasing factor (PRF) has not yet been identified; however, both thyrotropin-releasing hormone (TRH) and somatostatin increase levels of prolactin. There is a two- to threefold increase in serum prolactin level above baseline level during sleep. Exercise, pregnancy, and lactation are all associated with elevated levels of prolactin. Drugs such as oral contraceptives, reserpine, and chlorpromazine increase prolactin, whereas

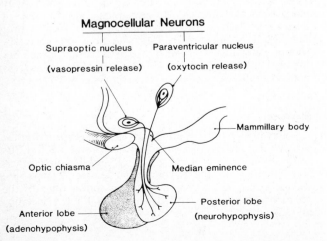

Figure 3. Neuronal connections between the pituitary and hypothalamus.

TABLE 1. Hypothalamic Hormones Affecting the Pituitary

Hormone	Effect
Posterior pituitary	
Arginine vasopressin	
Oxytocin	
Anterior pituitary	
Stimulating	
Growth hormone–releasing hormone (GRH)	Increased GH; decreased TSH response to TRH
Corticotropin–releasing hormone (CRH)	Increased ACTH
Thyrotropin-releasing hormone (TRH)	Increased TSH; increased PRL
Gonadotropin-releasing hormone (GnRH)	Increased LH; increased FSH
Melanocyte-stimulating hormone (MSH)	Increased MSH
Inhibiting	
Prolactin-inhibiting hormone (PIH, dopamine)	Decreased PRL
Somatostatin (growth hormone–inhibiting hormone (GIH)	Decreased GH
Melanocyte-stimulating hormone–release-inhibiting hormone (MRIH)	Decreased MSH

Abbreviations: GH = growth hormone; TSH = thyroid-stimulating hormone; ACTH = adrenocorticotropic hormone; PRL = prolactin; LH = luteinizing hormone; FSH = follicle-stimulating hormone.

L-dopa and dopamine agonists inhibit its release. The major metabolic effects of prolactin are related to lactation in pregnant females, and it has some effects on testosterone synthesis in males.

Thyroid-Stimulating Hormone

Thyroid-stimulating hormone is a glycoprotein (M.W. 28,000) that is synthesized by the thyrotropic cells of the adenohypophysis. Thyrotropin-releasing hormone is a tripeptide secreted by the hypothalamus that increases TSH synthesis and release. In addition to hypothalamic control, circulating thyroid hormones directly inhibit TSH release. The primary function of TSH is to stimulate thyroid growth and the synthesis of thyroid hormones. Peak release of TSH occurs in the early morning.

FSH and LH

Follicle-stimulating hormone and luteinizing hormone are glycoproteins (M.W. 29,000 for each) secreted by cells known as gonadotrophs. Structurally, both FSH and LH have identical alpha subunits with different beta subunits. Hypothalamic regulation of both FSH and LH is under the control of a single factor known as *gonadotropin-releasing hormone* (GnRH), which is secreted in a pulsatile fashion. FSH and LH undergo cyclical secretion in response to a complex interaction of estradiol, progesterone, and gonadotropin pulsations during the follicular and luteal phases of the menstrual cycle. A major surge in LH (and, to a much lesser extent, FSH) occurs just prior to ovulation.

In men, FSH promotes spermatogenesis and stimulates testicular growth. LH stimulates production of testosterone from the Leydig cells of the testes. In women, FSH aids in the development of ovarian follicles and is directly related to steroid production by the ovary. LH has its primary function in the stimulation of the corpus luteum and stimulates estrogen and progesterone production.

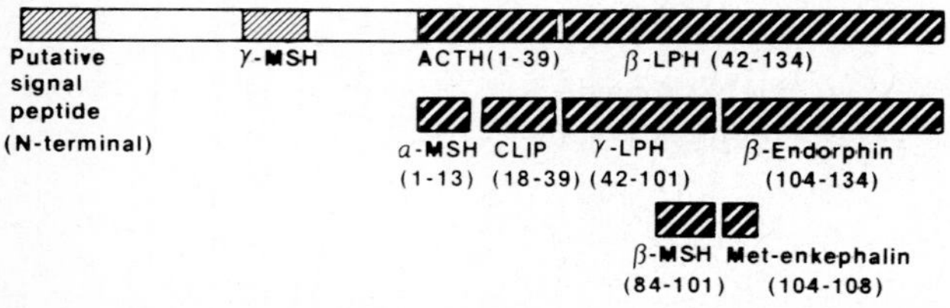

Endorphins and Enkephalins

Endorphins and smaller peptide fragments of endorphins known as enkephalins (Fig. 4) are peptides that bind to opiate receptors in the brain and gut. Their physiologic role is not well understood, but it may be related to pain perception and may possibly influence neural respiratory activity. A "hyperendorphin syndrome" has been suggested with clinical features of prolonged apnea and lethargy. It can be reversed by the narcotic antagonist naloxone.

THE POSTERIOR PITUITARY

Antidiuretic hormone (ADH) and oxytocin are secreted by the posterior pituitary gland.

Antidiuretic Hormone

The magnocellular neurons of the supraoptic and paraventricular nuclei synthesize a large prohormone complex that then migrates to the posterior pituitary. The prohormone complex is then cleaved with separation of antidiuretic hormone (ADH, arginine vasopressin) and its carrier protein neurophysin. The primary factors controlling the regulation of ADH secretion are related to plasma volume and plasma osmolarity. With increasing concentrations of plasma osmolarity above a threshold level of 285 mOsm., there is a direct increase in ADH secretion. This decreases urinary water loss. Conversely, reduced serum osmolarity directly inhibits the secretion of ADH. Significant decreases in the overall plasma volume also stimulate ADH release.

Oxytocin

Oxytocin is also synthesized as a large prohormone within the magnocellular neurons. It is cleaved from its neurophysin in the posterior pituitary. Suckling directly acts as a stimulus for the hypothalamic release of oxytocin. Oxytocin also has a major effect on contractions of the pregnant uterus and in milk secretion by the lactating breast.

Figure 4. Adrenocorticotropic hormone (ACTH) and endorphin precursor molecule (pro-opiomelanocortin). (From Nakanishi, S., et al.: Nature, 278:423, 1979.)

Pituitary Tumors

RADIOLOGIC EVALUATION

Although plain skull films and conventional tomography may provide useful information regarding enlargement of the sella turcica, contrast-enhanced computed tomography (CT) has emerged as the imaging method of choice for diagnosing pituitary tumors. CT has virtually replaced other invasive techniques such as angiography and pneumoencephalography. Following injection of intravenous iodinated contrast, the normal pituitary stalk and body demonstrate significant enhancement. The excellent density discrimination of CT affords ready detection of abnormal pituitary enlargement and extension of pituitary tumors either inferiorly into the sphenoid sinus or superiorly through the diaphragma sellae into the suprasellar cistern and region of the hypothalamus and optic chiasm. Coronal and sagittal reformations of thin axial slices are particularly helpful to fully evaluate the extent of pituitary lesions. Only if there is CT evidence of a possible aneurysm is angiography routinely performed for suspected pituitary lesions. Magnetic resonance imaging (MRI) has recently also proved useful for evaluating the pituitary and eliminates the need for intravenous contrast agents.

CLASSIFICATION

The prior classification of pituitary tumors was based on differentiation of cell types based on light microscopy. Tumors were divided into chromophobic, eosinophilic, and basophilic cell types. With the development of immunohistochemistry, pituitary tumors are now classified according to the type of specific hormone that is secreted by the tumor. Thus, there are both *endocrine-active* and *endocrine-inactive* tumors.

Endocrine-Inactive Tumors

Endocrine-inactive tumors ("chromophobe adenomas" under the old nomenclature) occur with equal frequency in men and women. Clinically, these tumors may present with visual disturbances by compression of the optic chiasma, resulting in bitemporal hemianopsia. Other symptoms are secondary to compression of the adenohypophysis, with loss of hormonal function of GH, gonadotropic secretion, thyrotrophic hormone, and, finally, ACTH. Rarely, diabetes insipidus occurs through decreased secretion of vasopressin.

The differential diagnosis of endocrine-inactive pituitary tumors includes juxtacellular meningiomas, aneurysms, hypothalamic gliomas, chordomas, teratoid tumors, gliomas of the optic chiasma, metastatic tumor, and granulomas. In a small percentage of patients, tumor necrosis occurs with hemorrhage. This may be associated with rapid loss of vision and subarachnoid bleeding. In addition, it may result in panhypopituitarism. This dramatic clinical event has been termed *pituitary apoplexy*. Hyperplastic pituitary glands during pregnancy may also infarct post partum, resulting in Sheehan's syndrome (postpartum hemorrhage with hypopituitarism). Treatment of non–endocrine-secreting adenomas includes either surgical resection or radiation therapy. A transsphenoidal surgical approach is usually used, although large bulky lesions sometimes require craniotomy.

Endocrine-Active Tumors

Acromegaly. This syndrome results from excess secretion of GH by an endocrine-active pituitary tumor. Giant-ism develops in children, acromegaly in adults. The classic coarse features of acromegaly—overgrowth of the hands, feet, and face—may take years to develop. However, newer assays for serum GH now permit much earlier diagnosis. In addition to the skeletal and skin manifestations (increased perspiration and body odor), hypersecretion of GH may result in cardiomegaly and valvular dysfunction as well as hypertension, carpal tunnel syndrome, and accelerated atherosclerosis. If untreated, patients with the full-blown syndrome of acromegaly may die from cardiovascular disease.

Other endocrine-associated problems with acromegaly are primarily related to decreased gonadotrophin secretion and development of diabetes mellitus. Large GH-secreting tumors may also extend above the diaphragma sellae and compress the optic chiasma, resulting in visual field defects.

The therapy of acromegaly is directed to decreasing GH levels below 5 ng. per ml. The therapeutic options include medical therapy with the long-acting dopamine agonist bromocriptine, transsphenoidal adenomectomy, and radiation therapy. Large tumors are almost always treated surgically. Radiation is added if the tumor is incompletely resected or if elevated levels of GH are noted postoperatively. Patients with mild disease may undergo medical therapy, transsphenoidal surgical resection, or primary radiation therapy. If a small microadenoma is present, this can be removed entirely by surgical resection; however, with extremely large lesions, radical hypophysectomy may be required. Patients treated with either supervoltage radiotherapy, proton beam radiotherapy, or radioactive seed implantation respond more slowly than those treated surgically and may develop symptoms of hypopituitarism many years after radiation therapy. Medical therapy with bromocriptine reduces GH levels in 60 to 80 per cent of patients, but in only about 40 per cent do the levels become normal (less than 10 ng. per ml.). Bromocriptine is therefore usually used only in acromegalics in whom adequate reduction of GH levels has not been achieved with surgery or irradiation or for preoperative symptomatic relief.

Cushing's Disease. Excess pituitary secretion of ACTH results in hypercortisolism, known as Cushing's disease. Patients with this disease have a typical body habitus with truncal obesity, thin extremities, buffalo hump, and moon facies. *Cushing's syndrome* refers to the general clinical manifestations in patients with hypersecretion of adrenocortical hormones; *Cushing's disease* refers to the pituitary as the specific cause of this syndrome. In the past, it was felt that a pituitary etiology was evident in only a minority of patients with Cushing's syndrome, but recent evidence has demonstrated that up to 80 per cent of these patients, in fact, have pituitary microadenomas, diffuse hyperplasia, or multiple small adenomas that can be cured by transsphenoidal surgery. The success rate of transsphenoidal surgery in Cushing's disease is about 85 per cent. The results of surgical treatment in patients with macroadenomas and in those with suprasellar extension is much poorer (about 25 per cent success rate). Transsphenoidal microsurgical hypophysectomy has replaced bilateral adrenal resection at many centers as the treatment of choice for Cushing's disease. Total hypophysectomy is necessary to correct the hypercortisolism in about 10 per cent of patients, and postoperative radiation may be required for patients with unresectable tumors and persistent hypercortisolism. Heavy-particle proton beam therapy and the use of local implantation of yttrium, gold, or strontium are therapeutic alternatives. Evaluation of the patient to determine whether there is a pituitary tumor, an adrenal tumor, or an ectopic tumor (such as a bronchial adenoma or oat cell carcinoma that secretes ACTH) is discussed subsequently in this chapter.

Prolactin-Producing Tumors (Prolactinomas). These lesions are the most common endocrine-active pituitary tumors. In females hypersecretion of prolactin may produce the amenorrhea-galactorrhea syndrome. In males hypersecretion of prolactin may produce impotence and decreased libido. Because the metabolic and physiologic disturbances are often more subtle in men, the diagnosis is usually established earlier in women.

In many instances, radiologic imaging with contrast-enhanced CT may not demonstrate small prolactin-secreting microadenomas. Thus, the diagnosis may be established only by documenting elevated levels of prolactin. The normal level of prolactin is less than 20 ng. per ml., and in patients with levels exceeding 150 ng. per ml. a prolactinoma is almost invariably present. However, it is important to point out that mild elevations of prolactin may be produced by renal failure, hypothyroidism, cirrhosis, drugs, stress, nipple stimulation, spinal cord lesions, hypothalamic lesions, or estrogen therapy. The ectopic production of prolactin has also been reported with lung tumors, but is quite rare. These various conditions must be excluded before a confident diagnosis of a prolactinoma can be established.

The treatment of prolactinomas is somewhat controversial at this time because the natural history of this lesion is unknown. Both medical therapy with bromocriptine and transsphenoidal resection are effective in most patients. Surgery is recommended for larger or growing lesions (macroadenomas). Patients with prolactinomas over 2 cm. in diameter or with basal prolactin levels over 200 ng. per ml. may require combined therapy with surgery, radiation, and bromocriptine.

Craniopharyngiomas

Craniopharyngiomas are the most important *nonpituitary tumors* that arise in the vicinity of the sella turcica. They originate from embryologic rest cells of Rathke's pouch and occur most often in children and young adults. These tumors are predominantly cystic and contain calcifications in 75 per cent of cases. This latter finding helps to make this diagnosis. Craniopharyngiomas are usually suprasellar rather than intrasellar in location. A variety of clinical symptoms may be produced by craniopharyngiomas, depending on the size and location of the lesion, including pituitary deficiency with absent or arrested puberty, diabetes insipidus, visual field defects, headache, and, in children, dwarfism. Complete surgical resection is often impossible, so that limited resection with a combination of drainage of the cystic component and subsequent radiation therapy is frequently used.

The Empty Sella Syndrome

The empty sella syndrome is usually the result of asymptomatic expansion of the sella turcica owing to a defect in the diaphragma sellae and herniation of the subarachnoid meninges and cerebrospinal fluid (CSF) into the sella. It occurs most often in middle-aged, obese women and in autopsy studies is found in from 5 to 26 per cent of persons. Other possible causes of the empty sella syndrome include degenerating and necrosing tumors, drained cysts, or a healed stage of a giant cell granuloma, gumma, or

other inflammatory lesion. In the past, pneumoencephalography was required for diagnosis and demonstrated injected air within the sella turcica. Currently, high-resolution CT or MRI is the imaging method of choice. This technique demonstrates CSF within the enlarged sellae.

THE ADRENAL GLAND

Normal Anatomy

The adrenals are pyramid-shaped organs weighing approximately 4 to 6 gm. each. The right adrenal is suprarenal in location; the left adrenal is located along the superior medial aspect of the upper pole of the left kidney (Fig. 5). The adrenals have a rich blood supply with considerable variation in their arterial anatomy. Classically, there are three main adrenal arteries: (1) the superior branch arises from the inferior phrenic artery; (2) the middle branch arises directly from the aorta; and (3) the inferior branch arises from the renal artery.

In contrast to the arterial anatomy, the venous anatomy is rather constant because there usually is a single vein draining the adrenal. On the left, the adrenal vein drains into the left renal vein; on the right, the adrenal vein is short and drains directly into the inferior vena cava.

Histology

The *adrenal cortex* is both physiologically and histologically different from the *adrenal medulla*. The cortex of the adult adrenal is derived from mesoderm and demonstrates three separate functional zones: (1) the zona glomerulosa, (2) the zona fasciculata, and (3) the inner zona reticularis (Fig. 6). Aldosterone is synthesized in the zona glomerulosa. Cortisol and other corticoids are synthesized in the zona fasciculata and zona reticularis. Production of adrenal androgens and small amounts of estrogens occur in both the zona fasciculata and zona reticularis. The adrenal medulla comprises chromaffin cells from ectodermal cells of the neural crest.

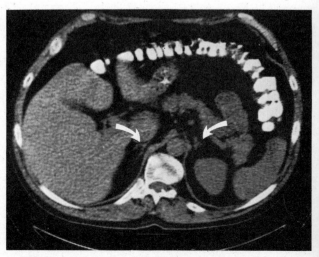

Figure 5. CT scan demonstrating position of normal adrenal glands in relation to kidneys.

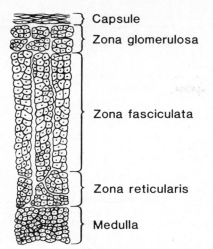

Figure 6. Diagrammatic representation of human adrenal cortex histologic structure.

Physiology

THE ADRENAL CORTEX

The adrenal cortex is the primary site of synthesis of glucocorticoids (cortisol and corticosterone), mineralocorticoids (aldosterone), androgens (adrenostenedione and dihydroepiandrosterone), and estrogens (estradiol). Cortisol is the primary glucocorticoid, and the stimulation for its secretion is initially related to corticotropin-releasing factor (CRF) acting on the anterior pituitary to release ACTH. ACTH then directly stimulates synthesis of cortisol from the zona fasciculata and zona reticularis of the adrenal cortex. A negative feedback system regulates cortisol secretion. Increasing serum levels of cortisol inhibit CRF release from the hypothalamus, which in turn causes decreased production of ACTH and thus lower serum levels of cortisol. During periods of extreme stress, direct stimulation from higher cortical levels in the central nervous system (CNS) may override the feedback mechanism and increased secretion of CRF and ACTH persist despite the increased level of serum cortisol.

Secretion of cortisol follows a well-established and remarkably constant circadian rhythm. Peak periods of cortisol secretion occur early in the morning at approximately 6:00 A.M. The lowest level of cortisol secretion is generally around midnight. In patients with Cushing's syndrome, this pattern of diurnal variation in cortisol levels is lost.

Cortisol is secreted into the systemic circulation in a metabolically inactive state bound to a large binding globulin protein known as *transcortin*. Unbound cortisol becomes metabolically active when it is taken up by cell membranes. A small percentage of plasma cortisol (15 per cent) is also bound to albumin, and approximately 10 per cent is free within the plasma. The free level of plasma cortisol may be increased by decreasing the number of transcortin proteins without increasing secretion of free hormone from the adrenal gland.

Cortisol is metabolized in the liver to inactive metabolites. It is reduced to dihydrocortisol and tetrahydrocortisol and then conjugated with glucuronic acid. Cortisol is also converted to cortisone, which is reduced and conjugated. The conjugated forms are freely water-soluble and are readily excreted in the urine. 17-Hydroxycorticosteroids may be measured in the urine. Although the amount of cortisol excreted into the urine is small, it may be measured directly and reflects the overall synthesis of adrenal cortisol.

The metabolic effects of glucocorticoids are far-reaching. Cortisol and corticosterone promote hepatic gluconeogenesis and may result in clinically apparent diabetes mellitus. There is a direct catabolic effect on fat cells, muscle, lymphatic tissue, and skin fibroblasts, resulting in release of fatty acids, glycerol, and amino acids. The characteristic truncal or centripetal obesity seen in patients with Cushing's syndrome is a direct result of redistribution of fat from a prolonged increase in cortisol secretion. In addition, glucocorticoids affect wound healing and inflammatory response and are both immunosuppressive and anti-inflammatory agents. Increased glucocorticoid levels cause increased urinary calcium levels and result in osteoporosis and kidney stones. Psychiatric disturbances such as depression also are related to increased endogenous secretion or exogenous administration of glucocorticoids.

Androgen secretion is also dependent upon ACTH levels, although there is no direct negative feedback mechanism on either the pituitary or hypothalamus from increased levels of androgens. Androgens undergo hepatic conjugation with glucuronide similar to that of cortisol. Both androgens and estrogens are synthesized in far greater concentrations by the gonads than by the adrenals. Abnormally high levels of androgens are seen in the pathologic conditions of adrenogenital syndrome, congenital adrenal hyperplasia, and some adrenal cortical tumors.

Androgens directly stimulate growth of body hair and development of muscle mass as well as growth of the genitalia. Abnormally high levels of androgens in developing girls result in masculinization with clitoral hypertrophy and labial fusion. In young males this produces mild enlargement of the genitalia.

The primary mineralocorticoid of the adrenal is *aldosterone*, and its major metabolic function is related to sodium metabolism. Stimulation of the adrenal cortex for production of aldosterone is complex and relates to ACTH, the renin-angiotension system, and serum concentrations of both sodium and potassium. In general, the renin-angiotension system is the primary regulatory mechanism governing aldosterone secretion. Renin is secreted from the juxtaglomerular cells of the afferent arterioles of the renal glomerulus. Primary factors inducing renin secretion include a decrease in serum sodium concentration or a decrease in mean renal arterial pressure. In turn, renin secretion stimulates the production of angiotensin I, which is then converted to angiotensin II. Angiotensin II is an extremely potent vasoconstrictor and acts directly upon the glomerulosa cells of the adrenal cortex to stimulate aldosterone secretion. The main metabolic effects of aldosterone result in reduced serum potassium levels, metabolic alkalosis, and hypertension.

THE ADRENAL MEDULLA

The primary secretions of the adrenal medulla include the catecholamines dopamine, norepinephrine, and epinephrine. All three of these biogenic amines are stored within cytoplasmic granules, which are released by exocytosis into the extracellular fluid following cellular excitation.

In addition to its cardiovascular effects, epinephrine has a profound effect on glucose and lipid metabolism. Epinephrine enhances glycogenolysis in both liver and muscles and, along with norepinephrine, can promote release of free fatty acids from the adipose tissue.

End-organ response to epinephrine and norepinephrine can be grouped according to alpha or beta receptors.

The active catecholamines may be rendered inactive by the enzymatic action of catechol-o-methyltransferase (COMT) or monoamine oxidase (MAO). These inactive metabolites (normetanephrine, metanephrine, vanillylmandelic acid [VMA], and methoxy-hydroxy-phenylglycol) can be measured directly in the urine and are clinically useful in diagnosing pheochromocytoma.

Diagnosis of Adrenal Lesions

A variety of methods have been used to diagnose adrenal lesions, ranging from invasive studies (such as adrenal angiography and venography) to noninvasive studies (such as ultrasound and nuclear medicine scans). To date, CT of the adrenals appears to yield the greatest degree of anatomic resolution. With high-resolution equipment, it is possible to diagnose adrenal lesions on the order of 1 cm. The major CT criteria for adrenal disease include alterations in either the density or the configuration of the gland. In most instances, the normal adrenal has a V-shaped or "inverted Y" appearance and is of uniform density. Adrenal tumors are often of lower density than the normal adrenal gland and cause a rounded or convex margin to the adrenal gland (Fig. 7).

It is not uncommon for incidental adrenal masses to be noted by computed tomography that is performed for other clinical indications. Most of these lesions are benign, nonfunctioning adenomas. When smaller than 4 cm. in size and without endocrine activity, these lesions can be followed with a repeat CT scan to quantitate tumor size in 6 months. If there is a known primary malignancy, fine-needle aspiration biopsy of the adrenal tumor under CT guidance is a reliable method for establishing the presence of an adrenal metastasis. If an adrenal mass increases in size or is associated with endocrine activity, surgical removal is recommended. Although CT is a relatively sensitive method for diagnosing adrenal lesions, it is not specific in suggesting the underlying nature of the lesion. In general, however, large lesions (greater than 5 cm.) suggest the diagnosis of adrenal carcinoma. Bilateral adrenal masses are seen with pheochromocytomas, adrenal metastases, and bilateral adrenal hemorrhage. The latter may occur spontaneously and is most common in older patients, in pregnant patients, in patients who are anticoagulated, in those who

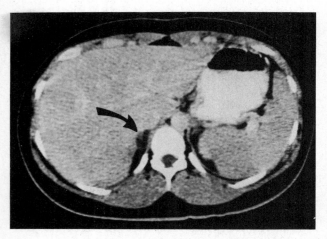

Figure 7. Abdominal CT scan demonstrating a right benign adrenal adenoma in a 30-year-old woman with primary hyperaldosteronism.

TABLE 2. Clinical Manifestations of Cushing's Syndrome*

Manifestation	Incidence (%)
Obesity	95
Hypertension	85
Glucosuria and decreased glucose tolerance	80
Menstrual and sexual dysfunction	76
Hirsutism and acne	72
Striae	67
Weakness	65
Osteoporosis	55
Easy bruisability	55
Psychiatric disturbances	50
Edema	46
Polyuria	16
Ocular changes	8

*From Frohlich, E. D.: Pathophysiology: Altered Regulatory Mechanisms in Diseases. Philadelphia, J. B. Lippincott Co., 1984.

have infection, in those who have hypertension, in those who are malnourished, or in those who are under severe stress.

In patients with primary aldosteronism, very small lesions (less than 1 cm.) may not be detected with CT. Adrenal venous sampling, documenting elevated levels of aldosterone, is still required to lateralize a functioning adrenal adenoma in some patients. A simultaneous serum cortisol level should be obtained to ensure that the sample has been obtained directly from the adrenal vein and has not been diluted.

Cushing's Syndrome

Cushing's syndrome is the clinical syndrome associated with excess cortisol secretion. Instead of the normal circadian rhythm of high corticosteroid secretion in the morning and low corticosteroid level in the evening, there is usually a constant level of secretion without diurnal variation. The *principal reason* for the excess cortisol secretion may be a pituitary source of excess ACTH, such as from a pituitary adenoma or hyperplasia (80 per cent). The excess of pituitary secretion of ACTH causes bilateral adrenal hyperplasia and excess cortisol production. This is known as *Cushing's disease*. A *second reason* for excess corticosteroid secretion is an ectopic source of ACTH production (10 per cent). The most common of these is oat cell carcinoma of the lung. Additional ectopic sources include carcinoid tumors, bronchial adenomas, and tumors of the pancreas, thymus, parotid, liver, thyroid, esophagus, and other organs. Along with ectopic ACTH production, ectopic melanocyte-stimulating hormone (MSH) may also be secreted, causing hyperpigmentation. The *third group of disorders* causing Cushing's syndrome is primary overproduction of cortisol by an adrenal adenoma, carcinoma, or bilateral nodular dysplasia (10 per cent).

CLINICAL FEATURES

The symptoms and signs of Cushing's syndrome are the result of an excess secretion of cortisol. These are listed in Table 2. The most specific of these are muscle wasting, truncal obesity, hirsutism, fungal infections (tinea versicola), purple striae, easy bruisability, and hyperpigmentation. If left untreated, the disease is usually fatal as a result of the effects of muscle wasting, atherosclerosis, hypertension, or infection. Cushing's syndrome is more common in women than men and has a peak incidence between 20 to 30 years of age.

DIAGNOSIS

There are a variety of tests used to diagnose Cushing's syndrome and to differentiate between a pituitary, ectopic ACTH, or an adrenal source for this disorder. In general, in pituitary Cushing's or ectopic Cushing's syndrome, plasma ACTH levels are elevated, whereas in adrenal Cushing's syndrome, ACTH levels are suppressed (Table 3).

Cortisol Levels

In patients suspected of having Cushing's syndrome, if plasma cortisol levels fail to be suppressed with an overnight 1-mg. *dexamethasone suppression test,* urinary free cortisol levels should be measured. Patients with Cushing's syndrome have high levels of free cortisol, 17-hydroxycorticosteroids and 17-ketosteroids in the urine. Plasma cortisol levels may be normal or high, but they remain relatively constant without the normal diurnal variation. This may be detected by measuring plasma cortisol at 8 A.M. and midnight: the morning level should normally be two to three times as high as the midnight level. If it is not, the patient is experiencing abnormal secretion.

Dexamethasone Suppression Test

The first step in diagnosing a person suspected of having Cushing's syndrome is to perform a dexamethasone suppression test. Dexamethasone is a potent synthetic corticosteroid. At low doses (2 mg. per day), it will block pituitary production of ACTH by interfering with the normal feedback mechanism: The hypothalamus detects the circulatory synthetic corticosteroid and "turns off" the pituitary. With a fall in ACTH, there will be a resultant fall in cortisol production by the adrenal gland in normal patients. Thus, in normal patients who receive a midnight dose of 1 mg. of dexamethasone, plasma cortisol levels will be suppressed to almost nil the next morning (overnight dexamethasone suppression test). Patients with Cushing's syndrome, on the other hand, lack a normal feedback mechanism and continue to produce high levels of plasma cortisol, unsuppressed by the low-dose dexamethasone. To determine whether the etiology is pituitary or extrapituitary, higher doses of dexamethasone are given. In most patients with excess pituitary production of ACTH, cortisol secretion will be suppressed to 50 per cent of baseline levels in a challenge with high doses of dexamethasone (8 mg. per day). In patients with high levels of cortisol production from ectopic ACTH secretion or from autonomous function of adrenal tumors, cortisol levels will not be suppressed appreciably with either a low-dose or high-dose dexamethasone suppression test.

Metyrapone Test

Metyrapone (Metoprone) is a compound that interferes with 11-hydroxylation in the adrenal cortex. Instead of producing cortisol, the adrenal gland produces 11-deoxycortisol, which does not negatively feed back on the pituitary. The pituitary, in turn, increases ACTH secretion and more 11-deoxycortisol is produced. This is detected in the urine as increased 17-hydroxycorticosteroid. Patients with normal adrenal function respond to metyrapone, and this test has been used to determine whether a person can respond to stress. In patients with pituitary Cushing's disease, there is a greater than normal increase in urinary 17-hydroxycorticosteroid level to metyrapone. Patients with adrenal tumors and most patients with ectopic ACTH-producing tumors do not respond.

ACTH Measurement

ACTH is measured by radioimmunoassay. In patients with a pituitary cause of Cushing's syndrome, serum ACTH levels should be elevated. The diurnal rhythm of ACTH secretion will be absent. In some centers, ACTH levels are also measured from selective venous catheterization of jugular or more proximal veins (petrosal sinus). An increased level on one side suggests a pituitary tumor. Once a pituitary etiology has been excluded by a high-dose dexamethasone suppression test and/or a metyrapone test, measurement of plasma ACTH will usually differentiate between an ectopic source of ACTH (very high ACTH levels) and autonomous adrenal hypersecretion (suppressed ACTH levels resulting from high cortisol levels and suppression of the normal pituitary).

Radiographic Studies and Scans

Once a pituitary source of excess ACTH production is suspected, a CT scan of the pituitary should be done to determine whether a pituitary lesion can be identified. In the past, posteroanterior (PA) and lateral skull films were used to observe enlargement or erosion of the sella turcica. It is currently known that in as many as 40 to 80 per cent of pituitary adenomas or microadenomas causing Cushing's disease the sella appears normal by conventional radiographs. Pituitary tumors can now be identified directly by CT scanning in most patients, and this is therefore the preferred localization procedure.

If an adrenal etiology is postulated, a CT scan of the abdomen should be obtained to demonstrate an adrenal adenoma, carcinoma or bilateral nodular dysplasia. In patients with adrenal adenomas or carcinoma, the contralateral adrenal is often atrophic or suppressed, whereas in nodular dysplasia both adrenals are enlarged.

TABLE 3. Typical Laboratory Results in Normal Subjects and Patients with Cushing's Syndrome*

	Normal	Adrenal Tumor	Cushing's Disease	Ectopic ACTH Syndrome
Plasma cortisol	10–25 µg.%	High	High	Very High
	Rhythmic	No Rhythm	No Rhythm	No Rhythm
Plasma ACTH	0.1–0.4 mU%	Low	High	High
17-OHCs response to ACTH	3–5 Fold Rise	+,0	+,0	+,0
Response to metyrapone	2–4 Fold Rise	0	+	+,0
Response to dexamethasone	0–3 mg./d	No Fall	Partial Fall	No Fall

*Adapted from Liddle, G. W.: Am. J. Med. *53*:638, 1972.
Abbreviations: 17-OHCs = 17-hydroxycorticosteroid; ACTH = adrenocorticotropic hormone.

Another localization technique is ^{131}I-iodocholesterol scanning. Since cholesterol is the precursor of cortisol, scanning the adrenals will give information about function. Cushing's disease causing bilateral adrenal hyperplasia will show bilateral increased uptake of the isotope. Adrenal adenoma will usually show unilateral uptake of the isotope. Adrenal carcinoma shows either a low-isotope uptake in the malignant adrenal tumor or no uptake on either side.

TREATMENT

Multiple modalities are available for the treatment of Cushing's syndrome. Intelligent use of these modalities requires a certainty as to the diagnosis and etiology behind the excess cortisol production. The different modalities will be discussed first and then will be grouped under the various disorders causing Cushing's syndrome.

Modalities of Treatment

Chemotherapy. Metyrapone will lower cortisol secretion by blocking 11-hydroxylation in the adrenal cortex. It has few side effects, but does not work well in cases of metastatic adrenal carcinoma.

Aminoglutethimide (Elipten) blocks the conversion of cholesterol to prednisolone and thus lowers cortisol levels. Side effects include fever, skin rashes, and lethargy. There is also a concomitant decrease in adrenal secretion of mineralocorticoids and androgens.

Mitotane (O,p'DDD) is an insecticide that causes necrosis of adrenocortical cells and inhibits cortisol synthesis in the zona fasciculata and zona reticularis without affecting aldosterone production. Its side effects can be severe, and they include anorexia, nausea, inability to concentrate, slurring of speech, nystagmus, and elevated serum cholesterol and alkaline phosphatase levels.

Cyproheptadine, a serotonin antagonist, and bromocriptine, a dopaminergic-like drug, have each been used to treat pituitary causes of Cushing's syndrome with varying success. Increased appetite and weight gain have been major side effects in cyproheptadine therapy.

Radiation. Cobalt 60 (^{60}Co) irradiation of the pituitary gland to a total dose of 4000 to 5000 rads will cause remission of Cushing's disease, especially in patients younger than 40 years of age, usually without causing hypopituitarism. In fact, the normal circadian rhythm of cortisol secretion may be restored. The therapeutic response time is slow, however, often taking 6 to 18 months. Other forms of external irradiation, such as heavy-particle (proton) irradiation, are associated with higher rates of remission of Cushing's disease (80 per cent versus 50 per cent for ^{60}Co radiotherapy), but are also associated with a higher incidence of post-irradiation panhypopituitarism. Implants of yttrium-90 and gold-198 have been used with success in small tumors and may be used safely in children.

Surgery. Pituitary surgery can be performed through either a transsphenoidal or a transcranial approach, the former being the less traumatic and the preferred method for small tumors. Resection of a pituitary microadenoma is successful in 50 to 100 per cent of patients. ACTH secretion is often lost for 6 to 12 months after surgery, so that postoperative replacement with cortisone should be given. If no adenoma is found, a total hypophysectomy may be performed. These patients will require permanent endocrine replacement. Total hypophysectomy is usually unacceptable for patients in their reproductive or sexually active years.

Adrenalectomy is the treatment of choice for an adrenal adenoma or adrenal carcinoma. Total adrenalectomy has been used for bilateral adrenal hyperplasia in Cushing's disease and in some patients with ectopic ACTH production. Complications of adrenalectomy include infection and wound dehiscence in those patients with poor wound healing capabilities. Deaths have been reported from pulmonary embolism. The use of preoperative metyrapone, low-dose heparin, prophylactic antibiotics, and preoperative vitamin A (to counteract corticosteroid effects by stabilizing lysosomal membranes) has reduced postoperative morbidity. An important late complication of bilateral total adrenalectomy is *Nelson's syndrome*. This is characterized by the continued growth of a pituitary tumor once cortisol inhibition has been removed. This develops in more than 30 per cent of patients, usually within 2 to 5 years after adrenalectomy, and can result in a locally invasive or incurable pituitary tumor. In some centers, therefore, preoperative pituitary irradiation has been used prior to total adrenalectomy to prevent the occurrence of Nelson's syndrome.

Treatment for Disorders Causing Cushing's Syndrome

Ectopic ACTH Production. Paraendocrine sources of ACTH account for about 10 per cent of patients with Cushing's syndrome. Many of these tumors are highly malignant, the most common being oat cell carcinoma of the lung. The next most frequent tumors are carcinoma of the pancreas, thymoma, bronchial adenomas, and carcinoid tumors. Often the metabolic effects of the tumor are more prominent than the effects of cortisol excess, so that the patient appears cachectic rather than cushingoid.

Metabolic alkalosis is often present. Because of associated MSH secretion, hyperpigmentation may also become apparent. Treatment is directed to resection or therapy of the primary tumor. If this is not successful or if no lesion can be found, bilateral adrenalectomy may be palliative. Metyrapone or mitotane may also be helpful. Hypophysectomy is contraindicated.

Adrenal Adenoma. About 10 per cent of patients with Cushing's syndrome have an adrenal adenoma. It is more common in females than males. Treatment is unilateral adrenalectomy, and patients do very well postoperatively. Supplemental steroid replacement therapy is necessary for at least several months until the suppressed adrenal recovers.

Bilateral Nodular Dysplasia. This rare syndrome is the most common cause of Cushing's syndrome in children, accounting for about 2 per cent of all patients with Cushing's syndrome. Girls are affected more often than boys, and most of these lesions are malignant in patients younger than 15 years old. Surgical treatment includes either total adrenalectomy or total removal of one gland and subtotal removal of the other.

Adrenocortical Carcinoma. Either functioning or nonfunctioning, adrenocortical carcinoma is a rare malignant lesion occurring typically in patients between 30 to 50 years of age. It is a very aggressive malignancy that is rarely cured by current surgical or medical therapy. Delay in diagnosis until the lesion has metastasized and is quite large is a major contributing factor to the poor prognosis. Endocrine functioning tumors are found in approximately half of the patients, and virilization, Cushing's syndrome, feminization, or hyperaldosteronism may occur. In addition to hormonal assay in functioning tumors, diagnosis of an adrenal mass is most often made by computed tomography.

Therapy for adrenocortical carcinoma generally includes both surgical resection, frequently including the kidney, and adjuvant chemotherapy with mitotane. Treatment with mitotane should begin within 2 weeks of the operative procedure. Unfortunately, there are few long-term survivors.

Primary Aldosteronism (Conn's Syndrome)

Conn's syndrome is the clinical syndrome that results from excessive secretion of aldosterone. Hypertension and hypokalemia are the major presenting features. Primary aldosteronism is a curable form of hypertension and accounts for 1 to 2 per cent of all hypertensive patients. It is due to the presence of an adrenal adenoma, bilateral adrenal hyperplasia, or, rarely, adrenal carcinoma. In fewer than 5 per cent of patients, the adenomas are bilateral. The cause of bilateral adrenal hyperplasia is unknown, but may be related to aldosterone stimulation from a pituitary neurotransmitter, possibly serotonin.

Secondary aldosteronism is due to decreased renal artery perfusion pressure, such as in renal artery stenosis. In response, there is increased renin secretion from the renal juxtaglomerular apparatus and increased release of aldosterone from the zona glomerulosa as a result of increased levels of renin and angiotension. Other causes of secondary aldosteronism include cirrhosis, congestive heart failure, and nephrotic syndrome. Bartter's syndrome is a unique cause of hyperaldosteronism, with hyperplasia of the juxtaglomerular cells, increased renin levels, hypokalemic alkalosis, and normotension. These patients frequently present as children with growth failure, polyurea, and weakness. Primary aldosteronism is associated with low renin levels; secondary and other forms of aldosteronism are associated with high renin levels. The size of the adrenal adenoma in patients with primary aldosteronism is usually small (about 1 cm.), and tumor size has little correlation with the amount of aldosterone secreted.

CLINICAL FEATURES

Primary aldosteronism usually occurs in women 30 to 50 years old. Children and young adults are occasionally affected. Although patients with normotensive primary aldosteronism have been described, hypertension and hypokalemia are present in almost all patients and weakness is a common complaint. The hypertension is usually moderate, with diastolic blood pressure in the range of 100 to 130 mm. Hg. The reason for the hypertension is poorly understood. Sodium retention and potassium wasting by the renal tubule is a direct effect of aldosterone. Low potassium levels cause proximal muscle weakness and cramps. Hypokalemia has toxic effects on the kidney, producing a nephrogenic form of diabetes insipidus causing polyuria and polydipsia. Headache, fatigue, and electrocardiographic T-wave and ST segment abnormalities are also prominent symptoms and signs.

Routine laboratory tests show a decreased serum potassium level associated with an increased serum bicarbonate level and a high-normal or increased serum sodium level. The urine potassium level is inappropriately high compared with the serum potassium level.

DIAGNOSIS

The diagnosis of primary hyperaldosteronism is based on finding high aldosterone levels in combination with low plasma renin levels. All antihypertensive medications should be stopped for a period of 3 weeks (methyldopa or clonidine may be used for dangerous rises in blood pressure). Aldosterone levels are measured in the supine position after sodium loading with normal saline infusion or a high-sodium diet. Renin levels are measured under conditions causing increased stimulation (such as the upright position, a low-sodium diet, or following two doses of furosemide).

Scanning methods can be used for tumor localization. CT scans of the adrenals are used to identify adenomas, but bilateral hyperplasia usually cannot be differentiated from normal adrenal glands. ^{131}I-iodocholesterol scanning is done in patients who have stopped taking antihypertensive medication for at least 3 weeks. Dexamethasone suppression of normal adrenal cortical activity helps improve the precision of this procedure. Tumors greater than 1 cm. and hyperplasic adrenal glands are localized with high accuracy.

Selective adrenal vein catheterization for aldosterone sampling is the most sensitive way of detecting excess aldosterone secretion. Ratios of plasma aldosterone to plasma cortisol levels are used to correct any dilutional effect of inaccurate catheter placement. Samples from an adrenal vein draining an adenoma will show an abnormally high aldosterone to cortisol ratio.

THERAPY

The treatment of primary aldosteronism that is due to an adrenal adenoma is unilateral adrenalectomy done via a posterior approach. Preoperatively, spironolactone (200 to 400 mg. daily) is given along with potassium replacement. Postoperatively, aldosterone levels and renin levels normalize and potassium wasting stops. Hypertension improves in most cases and is cured in 60 to 80 per cent of patients. Transient hypoaldosteronism with hypotension and hyperkalemia may be seen rarely and resolves within a few days.

In contrast to the surgical treatment of primary aldosteronism, patients with idiopathic aldosteronism due to bilateral adrenal hyperplasia should be treated medically with spironolactone, an aldosterone antagonist. Side effects of therapy include gynecomastia and impotence in men. Other potassium-sparing antihypertensive medications include amiloride and triamterene. These medications are used for treatment in some patients. Cyproheptadine, a serotonin antagonist, has also been shown to decrease aldosterone levels in patients with bilateral adrenal hyperplasia.

Adrenogenital Syndrome

The majority of infants with adrenogenital syndrome have a partial or complete deficiency of the 21-hydroxylase enzyme necessary for cortisol synthesis. Because of decreased cortisol levels, pituitary secretion of ACTH results in adrenocortical hyperplasia. In patients with partial enzyme deficiency, increased ACTH produces normal levels of cortisol; however, greatly increased levels of adrenostenedione are secreted by the hyperplastic adrenals. This, in turn, is metabolized to testosterone causing virilization in females and hypertrophy of the genitalia in males. If there is complete absence of the 21-hydroxylase enzyme, there is no cortisol production and thus infants born with this entity develop adrenal insufficiency as well as virilization.

In addition to the clinical features of virilization, the adrenogenital syndrome may be diagnosed by demonstrating markedly elevated levels of plasma 17-hydroxyproges-terone. Prenatal diagnosis of the enzyme deficiency is now possible with amniocentesis and HLA typing.

Treatment of adrenogenital syndrome involves administration of cortisol and genital reconstruction in selected females. In infants with complete enzyme deficiency and adrenal insufficiency, both mineralocorticoids (fludrocortisone acetate [Florinef acetate]) and glucocorticoids (cortisol) must be given.

In rare instances, other enzyme deficiencies may impair cortisol synthesis and result in the adrenogenital syndrome. These include 11-β-hydroxylase, 3-β-hydroxydehydrogenase, and 17-hydroxylase. Adults in whom adrenogenital syndrome develops generally harbor a malignant adrenal neoplasm. They therefore differ from infants, who usually have bilateral adrenal hyperplasia.

Adrenocortical Insufficiency (Addison's Disease)

In the past, adrenocortical insufficiency was primarily due to bilateral adrenal tuberculosis. This is a rare occurrence today, and the most common etiology of Addison's disease at present is autoimmune destruction of the adrenal cortex. Another cause of acquired adrenal insufficiency is bilateral adrenal hemorrhage that may occur spontaneously, most often in anticoagulated, hypertensive, and poorly nourished persons. It is also seen in meningococcal septicemia (Waterhouse-Friderichsen syndrome), during pregnancy, in burn patients, and in patients with sepsis or intra-abdominal infection. Rare cases of hereditary and familial Addison's disease have been reported. The combination of autoimmune adrenal insufficiency and hypothyroidism is known as Schmidt's syndrome. This is also frequently associated with diabetes mellitus.

CLINICAL FEATURES

The clinical presentation of adrenal insufficiency is quite variable, ranging from chronic illness lingering for months or years to fulminant Addisonian crisis presenting with shock and coma. Failure to recognize and treat adrenal insufficiency may result in significant mortality. In acute adrenal insufficiency, there may be cardiorespiratory collapse, severe asthma, abdominal pain, or sudden collapse and death. Few laboratory test results are abnormal, although plasma cortisol levels are low and ACTH levels are increased. Treatment must be instituted before the laboratory test results are available.

In patients with chronic adrenal insufficiency, clinical signs and symptoms are secondary to both glucocorticoid and mineralocorticoid deficiency. Major symptoms of chronic glucocorticoid deficiency include lethargy, weakness, weight loss, hyperpigmentation, hypotension, nausea, vomiting, salt-craving, and abdominal pain. Increased MSH typically results in hyperpigmentation of the extensor surfaces, buccal mucosa, and palmar surfaces. Mineralocorticoid deficiency results in significant electrolyte disturbances, including hyponatremia, hypercalcemia, and hyperkalemic acidosis. Hypotension due to decreased plasma volume is often present; this is often seen in conjunction with decreased cardiac size and cardiac output, proximal muscle weakness, and cramps.

Routine laboratory tests may show an increased serum potassium level associated with normal or decreased serum sodium and chloride levels. An increased blood urea nitrogen (BUN) and creatinine and eosinophilia as well as hypoglycemia are often observed. Urinary 17-ketosteroid

excretion is low in the male and virtually absent in the female, and the serum ACTH level is increased. Inability to respond to exogenous ACTH (250 μg. intravenously or intramuscularly of cosyntropin [Cortrosyn]) is a useful confirmatory test.

THERAPY

Treatment of acute Addisonian crisis requires large amounts of intravenous fluids and corticosteroids (hydrocortisone, initially 300 mg. intravenously daily). In patients with more chronic forms of adrenal insufficiency replacement therapy with cortisone acetate is given orally (20 mg. hydrocortisone in the morning and 10 mg. in the evening). Treatment with mineralocorticoid (fludrocortisone acetate, 0.1 mg. daily) is usually not necessary.

Pheochromocytoma

Pheochromocytoma is a chromaffin cell tumor arising from cells of neural crest origin in the adrenal medulla or in extra-adrenal sympathetic nervous tissue. The organ of Zuckerkandl is para-aortic nerve tissue located in the region of the inferior mesenteric artery and aortic bifurcation. It is a common site of extra-adrenal pheochromocytoma. It is also the only extra-adrenal site to produce both epinephrine and norepinephrine. Like the adrenal medulla, the organ of Zuckerkandl contains the enzyme phenylethanolamine-N-methyltransferase (PNMT), which converts norepinephrine to epinephrine. Thus, pheochromocytomas arising in the adrenal medulla or organ of Zuckerkandl may produce both epinephrine and norepinephrine. Other extra-adrenal pheochromocytomas produce only norepinephrine. Most pheochromocytomas (85 to 90 per cent) are located in the adrenal medulla, with right-sided involvement slightly more common than left. About 10 per cent are bilateral, found more frequently in children. About 10 per cent of pheochromocytomas are malignant, found more frequently in females and rarely in children. Thirty to 40 per cent of extra-adrenal pheochromocytomas are malignant and 20 per cent of familial tumors are malignant. About 10 per cent of pheochromocytomas occur in children, usually males. There is an association with the autosomal dominant multiple endocrine neoplasia (MEN) Type IIa (*Sipple's syndrome*): pheochromocytoma, medullary cancer of the thyroid, and parathyroid hyperplasia, as well as an association with the rarer MEN Type IIb: pheochromocytoma, medullary cancer of the thyroid, multiple mucosal neuromas, and ganglioneuromatosis. There is also an association of pheochromocytoma with von Recklinghausen's disease (neurofibromatosis) and von Hippel–Lindau disease (retinal angiomatosis and hemangioblastoma of the cerebellum or spinal cord). Pheochromocytoma sometimes presents during pregnancy.

CLINICAL FEATURES

Signs and symptoms of pheochromocytoma are related to circulating catecholamine levels and amount of epinephrine and norepinephrine release. These include hypertension, tachycardia, sweating, palpitations, tremor, anxiety, abdominal pain, constipation, fever, weight loss, and glucose intolerance. Untreated tumors may cause myocarditis, congestive heart failure, ventricular fibrillation, stroke, and gastrointestinal infarction. Hypertension may be paroxysmal or persistent. Children with pheochromocytomas usually show persistent hypertension, as do patients with malignant pheochromocytomas. Paroxysmal catecholamine release may occur spontaneously, in response to tumor palpation, stress, exercise, or even micturition (especially in the case of pheochromocytomas present in nerve tissue adjacent to the bladder wall). Symptoms may be similar to those of thyrotoxicosis, carcinoid syndrome, or variants of migraine syndrome.

DIAGNOSIS

When pheochromocytoma is suspected, screening tests should be done to measure norepinephrine, epinephrine, and the metabolites normetanephrine, metanephrine, and VMA in the urine. Provocative testing with glucagon, histamine, and tyramine to cause a hypertensive episode is rarely used today because other tests make it unnecessary and because such provocative tests are associated with morbidity. If clinical features and biochemical testing strongly suggest the diagnosis of pheochromocytoma, the patient is placed on alpha-adrenergic blockade for 2 to 3 weeks before tumor localization is attempted. Alpha-adrenergic blockade is done with phenoxybenzamine (Dibenzyline). This relieves some of the vasoconstriction, but it results in hypovolemia. Patients should therefore be vigorously hydrated during this treatment. Side effects of phenoxybenzamine include postural hypotension, nasal congestion, weakness, nausea, and inability to ejaculate. If tachycardia or arrhythmias are present, a beta-adrenergic blocker such as propranolol (Inderal) is added. Propranolol should not be used in patients with asthma, chronic obstructive pulmonary disease, or congestive heart failure. Beta blockade should never be initiated before alpha blockade because cardiac failure or a hypertensive crisis may result from unopposed alpha stimulation and resultant vasoconstriction in a patient with an unresponsive heart.

Localizing techniques include CT scanning, ^{131}I-metaiodobenzylguanidine (^{131}I-MIBG) scanning, selective venous sampling for catecholamines and their metabolites, and selective arteriography. CT scanning is the most accurate technique for localizing pheochromocytomas within the adrenal gland. Adrenal scanning with ^{131}I-MIBG is the most accurate method for localizing ectopically situated pheochromocytomas. MIBG is concentrated in the adrenal medulla and all adrenergic tissue. At usual doses, normal adrenal glands are usually not visualized. ^{131}I-MIBG scanning also determines whether a mass seen by other diagnostic techniques has adrenergic function. Phenoxybenzamine, propranolol, and alpha-methylparatyrosine (AMPT), an alternative drug that decreases catecholamine synthesis, do not appear to inhibit adrenergic uptake by ^{131}I-MIBG.

Selective arteriography is rarely used, but demonstrates the highly vascular nature of most pheochromocytomas. All patients must be prepared with alpha blockers, however, because arteriography may precipitate a hypertensive crisis. Intravenous pyelography identifies 50 per cent of the patients with pheochromocytomas.

TREATMENT

The treatment of patients with pheochromocytoma is by surgical excision. This is done after preoperative adrenergic blockade and vigorous rehydration. Careful monitoring is essential for managing intraoperative hypertension, tachyarrhythmias, and post-removal hypotension. Intraoperative hypertension is most often treated with intravenous sodium nitroprusside (Nipride), a direct smooth muscle relaxant, because of its rapid onset of action. Phentolamine (Regitine), a rapid-acting alpha blocker, is

more physiologic than nitroprusside, but is used less frequently. The patient should receive phenoxybenzamine and should be well hydrated prior to and during the operation, in order to avoid hypotension after removal of the tumor. As little tumor manipulation as is possible should be done during the operative procedure so that a large surge of catecholamines is not released into the circulation. Also, the tumor should not be fractured, to avoid the possibility of seeding tumor cells into the peritoneal cavity. Despite localizing techniques, most authors still recommend an anterior surgical approach in order to examine both adrenals and the para-aortic sympathetic chain. Some surgeons perform bilateral adrenalectomies in patients with familial pheochromocytomas because of the high incidence of another pheochromocytoma (sometimes malignant) developing in the contralateral gland. Operative mortality is less than 2 per cent. About 90 per cent of patients with episodic hypertension become normotensive. The 5-year survival for patients with malignant pheochromocytoma is about 30 to 40 per cent. Metastases are most commonly found in bone, lymph nodes, liver, and lung. Metastatic disease may be treated by surgical debulking procedures, combination chemotherapy, and symptomatic treatment using phenoxybenzamine and AMPT. Radiation may help decrease pain in bony metastases, and high doses of ^{131}I-MIBG have recently been used for palliative or adjunctive treatment.

SELECTED REFERENCES

Annotated References

Ezin, C., et al. (Eds.): Pituitary Diseases. Boca Raton, Fla., CRC Press, Inc., 1980.
This monograph provides a good summary of pituitary structure and function. Chapters cover pathology, clinical disorders, diagnostic radiology, surgery, and radiation therapy of the pituitary gland.

Givens, J. R. (Ed.): Hormone-Secreting Pituitary Tumors. Chicago, Year Book Medical Publishers, Inc., 1981.
This is an excellent text that represents the proceedings of a 1981 symposium on "Functioning Pituitary Tumors: Diagnosis and Treatment." It covers basic pituitary physiology, including recent neuroendocrine peptide physiology as well as chapters on the clinical diagnosis and alternatives of management of Cushing's disease, acromegaly, and prolactinomas. Following each section are panel discussions.

Thompson, N. W., and Vinik, A. I.: Endocrine Surgery Update. New York, Grune & Stratton, 1983.
This reference provides exceptional current information with extensive bibliographies on the following subjects:
1. *"The Diagnosis and Medical Management of Cushing's Syndrome" (D. E. Schteingart).*
2. *"Indications for Surgical Treatment of Cushing's Syndrome" (R. B. Welbourn).*
3. *"Adrenocortical Carcinoma" (N. W. Thompson).*
4. *"Primary Aldosteronism" (R. J. Grehim and M. D. Gross).*
5. *"The Localization and Treatment of Pheochromocytomas with ^{131}I-MIBG" (W. H. Beierwaltes).*
6. *"Adrenal Incidentaloma—Shadow or Substance" (L. P. Sonda and M. D. Gross).*
7. *"Pituitary Surgery for Endocrine Disorders" (W. F. Chandler).*

General References

Aron, D. C., et al.: Cushing's syndrome: Problems in management. Endocr. Rev., *3:*229, 1982.
Burch, W.: A survey of results with transsphenoidal surgery in Cushing's disease. N. Engl. J. Med. *308:*103, 1983.
Chrousos, G. P., et al.: The corticotropin-releasing factor stimulation test: An aid in the evaluation of patients with Cushing's syndrome. N. Engl. J. Med. *310:*622, 1984.
Conn, J. W.: Primary aldosteronism: A new clinical syndrome. J. Lab. Clin. Med., *45:*6, 1955.
Copeland, P. M.: The incidentally discovered adrenal mass. Ann. Intern. Med. *98:*940, 1983.
Cushing, H.: The basophil adenomas of the pituitary body and their clinical manifestations (pituitary basophilism). Bull. Johns Hopkins Hosp., *50:*137, 1932.

Farndon, J. R., Fagrams, L., and Wells, S. A.: Recent developments in the management of phaeochromocytoma. *In* Johnston, I. D. A., Thompson, N. W. (Eds.): Endocrine Surgery. London, Butterworth, 1983.

Javadpour, N., Woltering, E. A., and Brennan, M. F.: Adrenal neoplasms. Curr. Probl. Surg., *17:*1, 1980.

Luton, J. P., et al.: Treatment of Cushing's disease by O,p'-DDD: Survey of 62 cases. N. Engl. J. Med., *300:*459, 1979.

March, C. M., et al.: Longitudinal evaluation of patients with untreated prolactin-secreting pituitary adenomas. Am. J. Obstet. Gynecol. *139:*875, 1981.

Melby, J. C.: Assessment of adrenocortical function. N. Engl. J. Med. *285:*735, 1971.

Nelson, D. H., Meakin, J. W., and Thorn, G. W.: ACTH-producing pituitary tumors following adrenalectomy for Cushing's syndrome. Ann. Intern. Med., *52:*560, 1970.

Odell, W. D., and Nelson, D. H.: Pituitary Tumors. Mount Kisco, N.Y., Futura Publishing Company, 1984.

Streeten, D. H. P., Tomycz, L., and Anderson, G. H.: Reliability of screening methods for the diagnosis of primary aldosteronism. Am. J. Med., *67:*403, 1979.

Tyrell, J. B., et al.: Cushing's disease: Selective transsphenoidal resection of pituitary microadenomas. N. Engl. J. Med. *298:*753, 1978.

Wieland, D. M., et al.: Imaging the primate adrenal medulla with [123I] and [131I] metaiodobenzylguanidine. J. Nucl. Med. *22:*358, 1981.

Zerios, N. T., and Martin, J. B.: Management of hormone-secreting pituitary adenomas. N. Engl. J. Med., *302:*210, 1980.

THE ESOPHAGUS

ANDRÉ DURANCEAU, M.D. • EDWIN LAFONTAINE, M.D.

21

ANATOMY

The esophagus is a muscular tube approximately 25 cm. long, extending from the pharynx to the stomach. It begins in the neck at the level of the cricoid cartilage, opposite the sixth cervical vertebra, where it is in continuity with the pharynx. It is positioned in the midline at the level of the upper esophageal sphincter and deviates slightly to the left as far as the thoracic inlet. As it descends, it gradually crosses to the right at the level of the fourth thoracic vertebra. The esophagus returns to the left of the spine in its distal third and passes through the diaphragmatic hiatus at the level of the tenth thoracic vertebra.

The *cervical esophagus* lies posteriorly between the prevertebral layer of the deep cervical fascia, the longus colli muscle, and the vertebral column. Anteriorly, it is attached by loose connnective tissue to the membranous wall of the trachea. The recurrent laryngeal nerves ascend on each side in the tracheoesophageal groove, where the posterior part of the thyroid gland and the corresponding common carotid artery lies bilaterally. The thoracic duct ascends for a short distance along the left side of the esophagus and flows into the confluence of the subclavian and internal jugular veins.

The *thoracic esophagus* begins at the inlet opposite the body of the first thoracic vertebra between the trachea and the spine. Through its course in the thorax it comes in contact with the tracheal bifurcation and the left mainstem bronchus. It passes behind and to the right of the aortic arch, the left subclavian artery, and the left recurrent laryngeal nerve (Figs. 1 and 2*A*). As it descends, it is covered by the posterior pericardium and the adjacent left atrium (Fig. 2*B*). Posteriorly it lies on the prevertebral fascia and the longus colli muscles. At the level of the fourth thoracic vertebra it overlies the thoracic duct, where it crosses to the left. Posterolaterally are the hemiazygos on the left and the azygos on the right. The arch of the azygos, in close contact with the right lateral esophageal wall at the level of the fourth thoracic vertebra, drains into the superior vena cava. The esophagus lies parallel to the descending aorta in the lower posterior mediastinum (Fig. 2*C*). The vagus nerves form a plexus, which is in close contact with the esophagus, below the hilum of the lungs. At the level of the diaphragmatic hiatus the vagi form two trunks, the right lying behind and the left in front of the esophagus. The mediastinal pleura covers the esophagus in between these major structures on both the right and left.

The *abdominal esophagus* is anchored to the diaphragmatic hiatus by the phrenoesophageal membrane resulting from the investment on the esophageal wall of the transversalis and endothoracic fascia. After emerging between the right crus of the diaphragm, the abdominal esophagus enters the stomach in continuity with the lesser curvature. It is 1.5 cm. in length and lies anterior to the aorta.

The esophagus is constricted at four levels (see Fig. 6): (1) at the upper esophageal sphincter, 15 cm. from the incisor teeth; (2 and 3) where it is in contact with the aortic arch and where it is crossed by the left mainstem bronchus at 22 and 28 cm., respectively, from the incisors; and (4) at the level of the lower esophageal sphincter and diaphragm at 40 cm. from the incisor teeth. These constrictions are of clinical importance, since they may cause difficulties during endoscopic and dilatation procedures. They are also the sites of incarceration for ingested foreign bodies and esophageal injury after caustic ingestion.

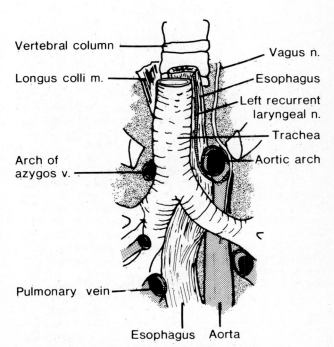

Figure 1. The esophagus and its relationship with intrathoracic structures.

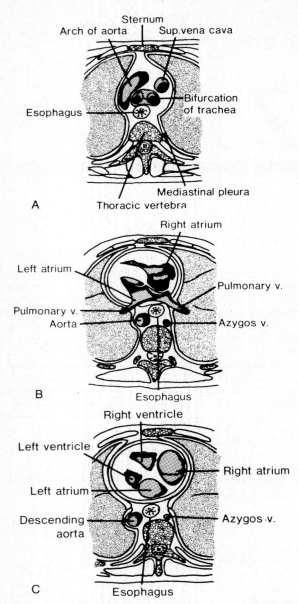

Sternum
Arch of aorta — Sup. vena cava

Esophagus

Bifurcation of trachea

Mediastinal pleura

A   Thoracic vertebra

Right atrium

Left atrium

Pulmonary v.

Pulmonary v.
Aorta

Azygos v.

B   Esophagus

Right ventricle

Left ventricle

Right atrium

Left atrium

Descending aorta

Azygos v.

C   Esophagus

Figure 2. A, Esophageal anatomy at the level of the tracheal bifurcation and aortic arch. B, Thoracic anatomy at the level of the lung hilum. C, The esophagus in the lower posterior mediastinum.

The muscular wall of the esophagus, except for the absence of a serosa, follows the basic pattern of the rest of the alimentary tract. It comprises an external, or fibrous, layer and muscular, submucosal, and mucosal layers. The external layer is an adventitia of irregular connective tissue and nerves. The muscular layer of the esophagus is composed of an outer longitudinal and an inner circular layer. Striated muscle predominates in the upper third, whereas smooth muscle covers the distal third. The longitudinal muscular layer invests most of the esophagus except in its most proximal part. At that level, the outer layer forms two diverging longitudinal bands, which are attached to the cricoid cartilage, thus exposing the circular muscle posteriorly. The inner layer of circular muscle is thinner than the longitudinal layer and is continuous with the inferior

constrictor muscle of the pharynx above and the oblique fibers of the stomach below.

The submucosal layer contains mucosal glands, blood vessels, nerves, and a rich network of lymphatic vessels. Lymphatic drainage tends to run longitudinally in the wall of the esophagus for various lengths before penetrating the muscular layer to reach the regional lymph nodes. Superiorly the drainage is to the deepest cervical nodes near the origin of the inferior thyroid artery behind the carotid sheath. In the thoracic part they drain into the preaortic glands of the posterior mediastinum and to the tracheobronchial lymph nodes. The lower portion may drain along the origin of the left gastric artery to the preaortic glands of the celiac axis. This peculiar nonsegmental lymphatic drainage explains why lymphatic and lymph node metastases are found at a distance from a primary malignant lesion.[21]

The mucosal layer consists of a nonkeratinized stratified squamous epithelium. At the gastroesophageal junction, the stratified epithelium is abruptly succeeded by the simple columnar epithelium of the stomach. The junction is visible to the naked eye as a transverse or crenated line where the pink but pale smooth esophageal lining is replaced by the red and larger folds of the gastric mucosa. The distal 1 or 2 cm. of the esophageal lumen is lined by columnar epithelium.

The arterial supply of the cervical esophagus is from the inferior thyroid branch of the thyrocervical trunk. The thoracic esophagus is supplied by direct branches from the descending thoracic aorta and the bronchial arteries. The lower portion of the esophagus is supplied by branches of the left gastric and left inferior phrenic arteries. The venous drainage of the cervical esophagus is to the inferior thyroid veins. The thoracic esophagus drains into the azygos, hemiazygos, and accessory azygos veins. The abdominal esophagus drains partly into the azygos vein and partly into the left gastric vein, which empties into the portal vein. It is of interest to know that an anastomosis exists in the lower portion of the esophagus between the portal and systemic venous systems. In the case of portal obstruction, varicosities of these veins occur and may result in serious bleeding.

The innervation of the esophagus derives from the vagus nerves and the sympathetic system. The upper esophageal sphincter and the cervical esophagus receive vagal fibers from the recurrent laryngeal nerves and sympathetic fibers from the cervical sympathetic trunks accompanying the inferior thyroid arteries. The thoracic esophagus receives its innervation from the esophageal plexus formed by both vagi. Sympathetic innervation comes from the thoracic sympathetic trunks and the greater splanchnic nerves. The abdominal esophagus is supplied by the anterior and posterior vagal trunks reconstituted from the esophageal plexus and by branches from the greater splanchnic nerves. These nerves form a plexus containing groups of ganglion cells located between the two layers of the muscular coat, Auerbach's plexus and, in the submucosal layer, Meissner's plexus.[8]

PHYSIOLOGY

Esophageal function can be assessed through manometric recordings. These evaluate the finely tuned mechanisms of action that should result in comfortable swallowing.

Pharynx

Voluntary swallowing starts with an upward and posterior thrust of the tongue with closure of the soft palate by contraction of the velopharyngeal muscles. The pharynx then becomes a closed cavity. Upon motor stimulation from the deglutition centers, a peristaltic wave passes down the pharynx resulting in intraluminal pressures of 200 to 600 mm. Hg. The single contraction peak occurs during 0.2 to 0.5 second and progresses aborally through the pharynx at a speed of 9 to 25 cm. per second.[4,10]

Upper Esophageal Sphincter

The body of the esophagus is closed proximally by the upper esophageal sphincter (UES). This is a high-pressure zone created by the sling action of the cricopharyngeus muscle, which is attached to both posterior ends of the cricoid cartilage. Through vagal and glossopharyngeal stimulation, the cricopharyngeus is maintained in a tonic state at rest with a resulting pressure of 20 to 80 mm. Hg.[4] During deglutition, inhibition of the tonic innervation to the sphincter occurs with relaxation of the high-pressure zone to ambient cervical esophageal resting pressure. This relaxation occurs simultaneously with the pharyngeal contraction, a coordination that allows the normal accommodation of the bolus propelled by the pharynx. A postdeglutitive contraction closes the sphincter, generating pressures that are often twice the resting sphincter pressure. The normal resting pressure is then resumed in the UES (Fig. 3).

With the closure of the UES, the peristaltic contraction starts to sweep the cervical esophagus. Both mechanisms prevent the regurgitation of the swallowed bolus from the cervical esophagus back into the pharynx.[4,10]

Esophageal Body

In response to cholinergic stimulation, the esophageal body contraction travels with a velocity of 2 to 5 cm. per second. The striated portion of the esophagus shows a slower activity. The contraction accelerates in the smooth muscle part to slow down again in the distal esophagus, just before the lower sphincter.

The resting pressure in the esophageal body reflects the negative intrathoracic pressure. In the proximal half of the esophagus, contraction pressures may vary between 20 and 70 mm. Hg, whereas the contractions generate pressures of 50 to 100 mm. Hg in the distal half of the esophagus. Contraction duration is from 4 to 6 seconds (Fig. 4A).

Swallowing induces a peristaltic wave that progresses down the esophagus. This is called a *primary contraction*. In the absence of deglutition, esophageal distention or irritation may initiate a normal propulsive wave. This is *secondary peristalsis*, a response to local stimuli of the normal esophageal wall. Tertiary contractions are nonpropulsive and are characterized on the manometric recording by a simultaneous pressure rise at different recording levels. They occur spontaneously or in response to a deglutition. Tertiary contractions are usually considered to be abnormal, but occasionally they can be observed in healthy individuals (Fig. 4B).[4,10]

Lower Esophageal Sphincter

The esophagus is separated from the stomach by a physiologic sphincter that creates a high-pressure zone of 2 to 4 cm. in length. Myogenic and neurogenic mechanisms help maintain the resting tone of the distal sphincter (lower esophageal sphincter, LES) with probable hormonal influences.

The resting tone of the remainder of the esophagus varies with the recording techniques. It usually ranges between 15 and 25 mm. Hg and results in a positive pressure barrier against gastroesophageal reflux. Upon swallowing and while esophageal peristaltic wave progresses in the esophageal body, relaxation to resting intragastric pressure occurs, allowing proper transit of the alimentary bolus from esophagus to stomach. This relaxation is essential for normal sphincter function, and the opening period of the sphincter must accommodate the duration of esophageal body contraction (Fig. 5). As it crosses the sphincter area, the peristaltic wave creates a closing contraction; the LES then goes back to normal resting pressure.

Distal sphincter pressures may vary from moment to moment in any individual. Neurologic, myogenic, and hormonal influences have been mentioned. Mechanical influences are important, and emotions, although poorly quantifiable, may have an effect on LES function as well as on the rest of the esophagus. Theophylline, alcohol, nicotine, nitroglycerin, and diazepam as well as fats and chocolate are known to result in distal sphincter hypotension. Conversely, Urecholine and metoclopramide as well as protein meals increase the LES resting pressure.[4,10]

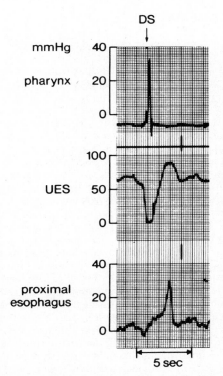

Figure 3. Normal function of the upper esophageal sphincter (UES). (From Hurwitz, A. L., Duranceau, A., and Haddad, J. K.: Disorders of esophageal motility. In Major Problems in Internal Medicine, Vol. 16. Philadelphia, W. B. Saunders Company, 1979.)

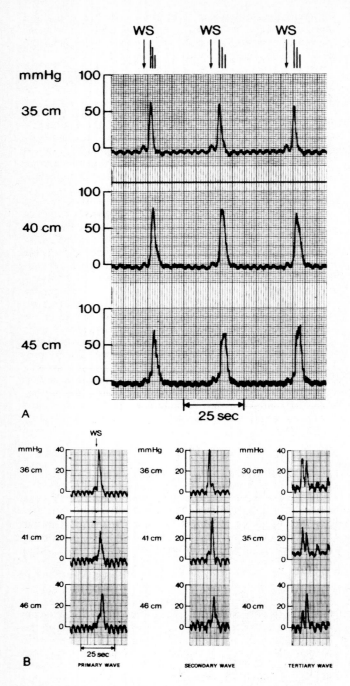

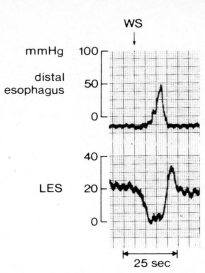

Figure 5. The normal lower esophageal sphincter (LES). (From Hurwitz, A. L., Duranceau, A., and Haddad, J. K.: Disorders of esophageal motility. In Major Problems in Internal Medicine, Vol. 16. Philadelphia, W. B. Saunders Company, 1979.)

on the esophagogram is a prime indication. Even in the presence of a normal barium study of the esophagus, this procedure should be done to evaluate symptoms such as dysphagia, heartburn, hemorrhage, and chest pain. The procedure can also be done for therapeutic purposes; dilatation of strictures, removal of foreign bodies, sclerotherapy of varices, and fiberoptic positioning of endoluminal prosthesis.

Normal Evaluation

The examination is performed on a patient who has fasted overnight. Premedication is variable with the situation and patient. General anesthesia is rarely required. Pharyngeal anesthesia is obtained using a lidocaine spray and intravenous diazepam as a relaxant. Meperidine can be added as an analgesic and atropine sulfate to reduce secretions. Today most studies are done with the flexible instrument. However, the removal of foreign bodies and deeper biopsies for undiagnosed esophageal strictures are better accomplished with the rigid instrument.

It is important to describe the relationship of an abnormal finding to the anatomic landmarks (Fig. 6). The esophageal mucosa is normally glistening, pale pink, sometimes almost white. The walls are usually collapsed. Peristalsis is noted, but endoscopy is not accurate in the diagnosis of motor disorders. The presence of a distended esophagus or retained debris may be caused by achalasia or a distal benign or malignant obstruction. An endoscopic hiatal hernia or spontaneous reflux of gastric juice into the esophagus during the examination suggests, but is not pathognomonic of, gastroesophageal reflux. The gastroesophageal junction may have a linear or serrated appearance. The pale, glistening esophageal mucosa changes to a deeper red color, representing the gastric columnar epithelium. It is important to complete the study with a good examination of the stomach and duodenum.

Figure 4. A, Peristalsis. Normal peristalsis in the esophageal body. (Reprinted with permission from Duranceau, A., Devroede, G., Lafontaine, E., et al. Surg. Clin. North Am. 63:777, 1983.) B, The primary wave is the normal response to voluntary deglutition. The secondary wave is the peristalsis induced by distention or irritation. Tertiary contractions occur either after swallowing or spontaneously and they are nonpropulsive. (From Hurwitz, A. L., Duranceau, A., and Haddad, J. K.: Disorders of esophageal motility. In Major Problems in Internal Medicine, Vol. 16. Philadelphia, W. B. Saunders Company, 1979.)

ENDOSCOPY IN THE ASSESSMENT OF ESOPHAGEAL PATHOLOGY

Esophagoscopy can be performed for either diagnostic or therapeutic purposes. The finding of an esophageal lesion

Esophageal Pathology

The diagnostic yield of esophagoscopy for endoluminal lesions is influenced by the total number of biopsy speci-

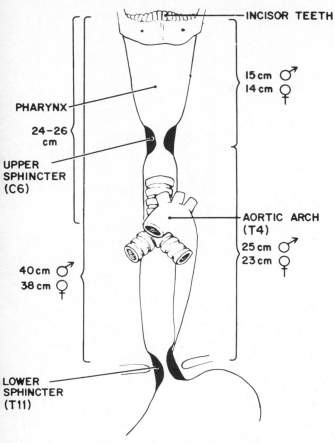

INCISOR TEETH

15 cm ♂
14 cm ♀

PHARYNX

24–26 cm

UPPER SPHINCTER (C6)

AORTIC ARCH (T4)

25 cm ♂
23 cm ♀

40 cm ♂
38 cm ♀

LOWER SPHINCTER (T11)

Figure 6. Anatomic narrowings and landmarks in the esophagus. (From Lafontaine, E., and DeMeester, T. R.: Esophageal carcinoma. In Copeland, E. M. III (Ed.): Surgical Oncology, Vol. 17. New York, John Wiley & Sons, 1983, p. 291.)

mens obtained, the presence of esophageal obstruction, and the growth pattern of the tumor. Ulcerative and exophytic tumors are readily accessible for direct biopsies. An infiltrative tumor is usually covered with normal mucosa at its margins. In the presence of an obstruction it may present as a benign stricture. An adequate biopsy is difficult to obtain, especially when using the flexible endoscope. In this situation, a brush cytology is more effective in establishing the diagnosis, since the brush can be advanced through the stenotic lumen to obtain cells from the center of the tumor. The combination of brush cytology and biopsy gives the best diagnostic yield for tumors of the esophageal body and cardia (Table 1). Biopsy specimens obtained with the rigid endoscope have a slightly higher diagnostic yield than those obtained with the flexible instrument, but when brush cytology is added to the latter the difference is negligible. If the stricture is too tight, it may be necessary to dilate it progressively before obtaining biopsies and brushings. The cervical area of the esophagus must be assessed carefully on withdrawal of the endoscope, since lesions in this area can be easily missed with the flexible instrument during its initial blind insertion.

Esophagoscopy is particularly important in the assessment of gastroesophageal reflux,[7] particularly in detecting the complications of abnormal reflux. Mild or Grade I esophagitis is simple reddening of the mucosa; confluent superficial ulcerations are signs of Grade II esophagitis; ulcerative esophagitis with progressive fibrosis results in Grade III esophagitis; and fibrous stricture means Grade

IV esophagitis. The Barrett esophagus is readily identified when intestinal or gastric metaplasia secondary to reflux has replaced the normal or ulcerated esophageal mucosa. Endoscopically, it presents as a bright red slushy or velvet-appearing mucosa that extends proximally from the esophagogastric junction for varying distances. In the endoscopic assessment of reflux esophagitis, a gastric ulcer or gastritis that easily mimics the symptoms of reflux esophagitis must be excluded. Duodenal ulcer disease with resultant pyloric stenosis and eventual potentialization of reflux must be diagnosed.[11]

Perforation, hemorrhage, cardiopulmonary problems, and sepsis are the primary complications of endoscopy. Perforation occurs in less than 1 per cent of all procedures. The most frequent site is the hypopharynx, but perforation may occur at the other anatomic narrowings along the esophagus. Perforation of the esophagus with the rigid instrument may be the result of full-thickness biopsies of the esophageal wall. It is particularly important to obtain the barium esophagogram before doing an upper digestive endoscopy. Proper radiologic assessment of endoluminal lesions or an abnormal esophageal axis by the endoscopist should minimize the risks of esophageal trauma during the procedure. The contraindications to fiberoptic endoscopy are often relative. The presence of neck deformities or a large Zenker's diverticulum may result in perforation during the blind passage of the instrument. Other abnormalities noted on the esophagogram must be carefully assessed. Thoracic aortic aneurysms, cardiopulmonary instability, and agitation may become contraindications to the performance of the endoscopic examination.

CAUSTIC BURNS OF THE ESOPHAGUS

Chemical injuries to the esophagus can result from the ingestion of caustic substances, either alkaline or acid. They are mostly household cleaning agents. Medication tablets such as potassium chloride, ascorbic acid, and doxycycline are also known to produce esophageal burns. The extent of injury to the esophageal wall depends on the nature and concentration of the substance, time of exposure, and amount ingested.

Pathophysiology

Caustic burns to the esophagus usually result from accidental ingestion in children or suicidal attempts in adults. Depending on the ingested agent, significant esophagitis will appear in up to 50 per cent of the victims.

The alkaline caustic agents sodium and potassium hydroxide cause immediate liquefaction necrosis with diffusion of the agent through the layers of the esophagus. Immediate cell destruction occurs with vascular thrombosis

TABLE 1. Diagnostic Accuracy of Biopsy and Cytology in Esophageal Malignancies*

Carcinoma	Biopsy and Brush Cytology	Tissue Biopsy	Brush Cytology
Esophageal body	37/37 (100%)	30/37 (81%)	37/37 (100%)
Cardia	32/36 (88.8%)	27/37 (75%)	27/35 (77.2%)

*From Proella, J., Reilly, R. W., Kirsner, J., et al.: Acta Cytol., 21:399, 1977.

and secondary bacterial invasion. Sloughing of the necrotic tissue with deposition of granulation tissue results in a fibrotic stricture. Alkaline caustic burns are located at three levels where the esophageal transit is slower: (1) the upper esophageal sphincter area, (2) the mid-esophagus where the aorta and the left mainstem bronchus cause anatomic narrowing, and (3) the distal esophagus just above the LES. By contrast, hydrochloric and sulfuric acids will result in coagulation necrosis on the exposed surface. A bolus of acid in the esophagus will usually cause superficial burns without severe esophageal strictures. However, long exposure on the wall of the stomach will result in severe burns with gastric destruction and fibrotic strictures.

When there is severe damage, a full-thickness injury to the esophageal wall or stomach occurs. Perforation, mediastinitis, peritonitis, abscesses, and fistula formation may develop.[13]

Symptoms and Signs

ACUTE PHASE

Following the ingestion of a caustic substance, local burns in the oropharynx may cause odynophagia. Laryngeal burns result in respiratory difficulties and hoarseness. Neck and chest pain are present with esophageal damage. Destruction of the mucosa with vessel thrombosis causes progressive sloughing. Bacterial invasion occurs, resulting in fever and tachycardia. Esophageal obstruction with dysphagia is secondary to edema in the acute phase, but symptoms will usually lessen when the necrosed tissue sloughs in the esophagus and granulation begins. A life-threatening situation is present with free perforation in the mediastinum and resultant sepsis.

Respiratory symptoms are severe if burns of the airways occur by aspiration. Voluntary clearing of secretions is hampered by pain and edema. Extensive injury to the intra-abdominal esophagus or stomach results in abdominal pain and signs of peritoneal irritation.

CHRONIC PHASE

Proliferation of the granulation and fibrous tissue causes progressive dysphagia in the 5th or 6th week after injury. Continuing sepsis suggests mediastinal infection. Fistula formation with the tracheobronchial tree or the cardiovascular system results in continuous pulmonary infection or massive hemorrhage, respectively.[19]

Evaluation

An evaluation with contrast material is essential to assess the initial damage caused by the caustic agent. Ulcers, narrowing, intramural retention of material, and esophageal air trapping can be observed. Perforation must be excluded. Radiographic control of the esophagus and stomach after 2 weeks and on a periodic basis subsequently will document the development and extent of the injury (Fig. 7). Air in the mediastinum, a blurred esophageal line, or evidence of pulmonary infection is seen on the chest film.

Early endoscopic evaluation is recommended after caustic ingestion if no pharyngeal or laryngeal burns are present. If lesions are observed in the esophagus, the endoscopic procedure should not be pushed distally because

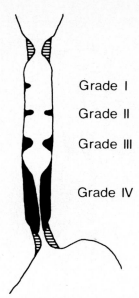

Figure 7. Classification of caustic injuries. Grade I: Short fibrous stricture involving less than the complete circumference. Grade II: String-like anular stricture of the mucosa and submucosa. Grade III: Dumbbell stricture with muscularis damage on less than 0.5 inch. Grade IV: All strictures more than 0.5 inch. (Adapted from Marchand, P.: Caustic strictures of the esophagus. Thorax, 10:171, 1955.)

of the risks of perforation. In the absence of esophageal injury at the initial evaluation, the patient is re-evaluated at one month and after a year.[9]

Treatment

ACUTE PHASE

Full damage to the esophageal wall is present within 30 seconds of exposure to a concentrated alkaline agent. Unless there is uncertainty about the ingested poison, attempts at neutralization or gastric lavage are probably unnecessary when a patient is seen in the emergency room. Dilution of the ingested agent and attempts at neutralization need to be done on site. Respiratory and hemodynamic stability are ensured by ventilatory assistance, if needed, and intravenous fluids. High-dose antibiotics that will cover the oropharyngeal flora should be given to prevent bacterial invasion through the damaged tissues. Steroids combined with the antibiotics may decrease the incidence and severity of stricture formation.

Total esophageal destruction may require emergency esophagectomy with cervical esophagostomy, gastrostomy, or jejunostomy. Subsequent reconstruction using stomach or an isoperistaltic colon interposition will re-establish the digestive continuity.

CHRONIC PHASE

Treatment of the caustic injury in the chronic phase is oriented toward the management of the established stricture. Three weeks after the injury, periodic dilatations of the narrowed esophagus using Maloney bougies, or the more recent Savary bougies that are passed on a guided wire, should ensure proper esophageal diameter for comfortable swallowing. Surgical bypass of the esophagus is indicated when complete stenosis is present. Marked irregularity and pocketing of the esophagus, the development of a fistula, difficulties in maintaining an adequate esophageal lumen, or an uncooperative patient also favor a surgical approach. Subsequent esophagectomy may be considered, since a higher incidence of carcinoma is present in the damaged esophagus.[13, 19]

PERFORATION OF THE ESOPHAGUS

Esophageal perforation can be spontaneous or may result from a variety of causes. Upper gastrointestinal endoscopy and esophageal dilatation are the most frequent reasons for perforation. Operations such as truncal vagotomy, esophageal myotomy, hiatal hernia repair, and pulmonary and mediastinal procedures may also result in iatrogenic perforation. Blunt or penetrating trauma to the chest and abdomen may result in esophageal perforation and rupture. The diseased esophagus is more easily perforated, especially in the presence of a deep esophageal ulcer or a recent caustic burn or during diagnostic or therapeutic manipulation of esophageal carcinoma (Table 2).

Pathophysiology

SPONTANEOUS OR POST-EMETIC RUPTURE

Vomiting creates a marked increase in intra-abdominal pressure with sudden overdistention of the proximal stomach and distal esophagus. This stretching may result in tears of various depth at the esophagogastric junction. Mucosal and submucosal lacerations are called Mallory-Weiss lesions and will result mainly in bleeding. When a full-thickness rupture of the esophageal wall occurs after vomiting, it is commonly called spontaneous or post-emetic perforation or the Boerhaave syndrome.

The location of the rupture may be influenced by the presence or absence of a hiatal hernia. In the presence of a sliding hernia, the maximal pressure is exerted in the herniated stomach and the rent usually occurs at the cardia, involving both stomach and esophagus. In the absence of a hernia, maximal pressure is applied to the distal esophagus, and a 1- to 3-cm. tear usually results on the left posterolateral wall just proximal to the esophagogastric junction.[25]

IATROGENIC RUPTURE

Endoscopic examination is the most frequent cause of esophageal perforation, with an incidence of less than 1 per cent in most reported series. The cervical esophagus at the level of the cricopharyngeus is damaged more often by tearing the posterior wall of the esophagus between the spine and the esophagoscope. Dilatations are the second most frequent cause of iatrogenic rupture of the esophagus and are seen mainly if no guiding wire is used. Hydrostatic dilatation of the distal esophageal sphincter area may result in a 1 to 4 per cent incidence of perforation. Esophageal intubation may result in a through-and-through rupture of the esophageal wall. The Levin tube, the Sengstaken-Blakemore tube when inflated to compress bleeding esophageal varices, and the push-through or pull-through tubes used for esophageal carcinoma palliation have been incriminated in this complication. Posterior or mediastinal surgery may result in esophageal trauma. Endotracheal intubation

TABLE 2. Esophageal Perforation*

Cause	Occurrence (%)
Spontaneous or Post-emetic	12
Iatrogenic	
Endoscopy	
Dilatations	76
Operative	
Foreign body	7
Trauma	
Penetrating	5
Blunt	
Esophageal pathology	
Caustic lesion	
Esophageal ulcer	
Carcinoma	

*Adapted from Postlethwait, R. W.: Surgery of the Esophagus. Norwalk, Conn., Appleton-Century Crofts, 1986.

of the newborn, thyroid or tracheal surgery, and the performance of a tracheostomy have all been reported as causing esophageal rupture (Table 3).

FOREIGN BODIES

When swallowed, a foreign body can be impacted at three levels, which are the natural narrowings of the esophagus: (1) the cricopharyngeal area, (2) the level of the aortic arch and the left mainstem bronchus, and (3) the lower esophageal sphincter area. Erosion through the esophageal wall with free rupture is seen mainly with sharp objects. Periesophageal inflammatory reaction usually prevents free perforations by the foreign body and will wall off the perforation, favoring local abscess or fistula formation in the mediastinum.

Chest pain, dysphagia, and odynophagia are the main symptoms of a patient who is usually conscious of having swallowed a foreign body. Free perforation, when it occurs, has a clinical presentation similar to that of a spontaneous or iatrogenic rupture. Fistula formation within the mediastinum can be seen with the tracheobronchial tree, resulting in free aspiration, or with the cardiovascular system, resulting in massive hemorrhage.

EXTERNAL TRAUMA

Gunshot and stab wounds may result in extensive esophageal damage at any level. Rupture of the esophagus from blunt abdominal trauma is rare, and injury mechanism is similar to that of the post-emetic rupture.

ESOPHAGEAL DISEASE

Total destruction of the esophageal wall can be seen after caustic ingestion. Esophageal ulcers secondary to

TABLE 3. Iatrogenic Perforation*

Cause	Occurrence (%)
Esophagoscopy	51
Dilatation	26
Esophagoscopy and removal of foreign body	7
Esophagoscopy and dilatation	6
Nasogastric intubation	5
Endotracheal intubation	5

*From Janssens, J., and Valembois, P. R.: Traumatic lesions of the esophagus. *In* Vantrappen, G. R., and Hellemans, J.: Diseases of the Esophagus. New York, Springer-Verlag, 1974.

chronic reflux esophagitis and carcinoma of the esophagus may also perforate in the natural evolution of the disease. The clinical presentation of these perforations is dependent on the amount of periesophageal inflammation. When considerable mediastinal reaction is present, pain and odynophagia are the dominant symptoms. If insufficient periesophageal inflammation exists, free perforation will be observed.

Symptoms and Signs

When post-emetic injury to the esophagus occurs, the patient will complain of a low substernal burning or tearing pain. The pain may be extremely intense with neck, back, or left shoulder radiation. Tachypnea, dyspnea, and pleuritic pain usually follow. Abdominal tenderness may be present if the rupture involves the intra-abdominal esophagus. Mediastinal contamination is immediate and virulent. If the pleura is intact, air and the esophageal contents remain in the periesophageal space with progression of the contamination along the cellular planes of the posterior mediastinum (Fig. 8A). On examination, the patient may be in pain with diaphoresis, fever, tachycardia, and hypotension. Subcutaneous emphysema is present in 50 per cent of the patients. Hypoventilation of the left lung with evidence of a pleural effusion is usually present. Hydropneumothorax is found if tearing of the mediastinal pleura has occurred with the emetogenic injury or if necrosis of the pleura has resulted from the mediastinal infection (Fig. 8B). Rarely, the mediastinal infection will progress to involve both pleural cavities, causing bilateral effusions (Fig. 8C).

Iatrogenic injury to the esophagus with perforation results in severe pain, fever, and tachycardia shortly after the procedure. The site of the pain will usually reflect the localization of the injury. Neck pain is common. Substernal pain radiating to the back is present when the esophageal body is perforated within the thorax. Epigastric pain or diffuse abdominal tenderness may result in an exploratory laparotomy when the perforation communicates with the peritoneal cavity. Dysphagia and odynophagia appear most often if the perforation occurred 24 to 48 hours previously. Fever, subcutaneous emphysema, and pain on palpation can be noted. These symptoms, especially if persistent, should lead to full radiologic evaluation of the esophagus.

Pain, dysphagia, and odynophagia are usually present when an impacted foreign body, an esophageal ulcer, or a carcinoma progressively erodes the esophageal wall. A history of foreign body ingestion, chronic reflux symptoms,

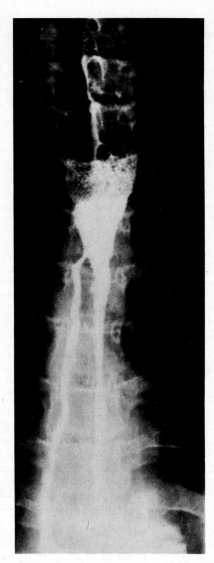

Figure 9. Esophageal perforation resulting from dilatation of a caustic stricture.

or recent progressive obstruction is frequently present. Since the process of perforation in these situations is slow, the resulting inflammation usually prevents free perforation and favors abscess or fistula formation within the mediastinum.

Esophageal rupture is rare following trauma. It must be excluded when there is evidence of mediastinal emphysema, hydropneumothorax, hematemesis, or bloody drainage from a nasogastric tube following blunt or penetrating injury.

Diagnosis

When a clinical picture suggests esophageal perforation, a chest film and an esophagogram should be obtained. (Fig. 9). The chest x-ray will usually show mediastinal emphysema and left pleural effusion with or without pneumothorax. Widening of the mediastinum can be seen, especially with a history of trauma. The esophagogram should be obtained with the patient upright and supine. It

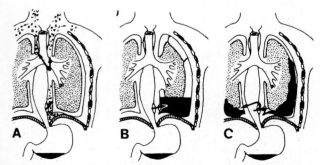

Figure 8. Clinical and radiologic presentation of esophageal perforation. A, Localized mediastinal emphysema. B, Left hydropneumothorax. C, Bilateral hydrothorax. (Adapted from Naclerio, E. A.: Am. J. Surg. 93:291, 1957.)

is essential to locate precisely the site of the perforation. A water-soluble contrast medium should be used initially, followed by liquid barium if no perforation is identified. Cervical spine films may reveal retropharyngeal tissue thickening and air trapping.

Endoscopic evaluation is not indicated because of the possibility of diffusing the mediastinal contamination, increasing the esophageal damage, or introducing acute tension pneumothorax.[16,23]

Management

When an esophageal perforation is diagnosed, the principles of management are as follows: (1) surgical exploration, (2) débridement of all devitalized tissue, (3) appropriate closure of the laceration to prevent continuous soiling, and (4) drainage. Depending on the site of the perforation, the extent of the systemic response, and the time between perforation and diagnosis, the approach may vary, but the management principles remain unchanged.[16] Neck perforations are usually secondary to endoscopic manipulations, and on exploration the rupture site is not easily found. Wide exposure of the posterior pharyngoesophageal junction is mandatory to ensure proper drainage, and secondary healing usually occurs within 15 to 20 days.

Thoracic perforations are managed more aggressively with special attention to the type and duration of the perforation. Lacerations with thoracic contamination result in a mortality of 20 to 30 per cent if the repair is accomplished in the first 24 hours of the rupture. The mortality exceeds 60 per cent when more than 24 hours have passed since the perforation.

An early perforation with a rupture site that can be adequately débrided and repaired with drainage should give satisfactory results. However, perforations treated more than 24 hours after the event, patients with a failed initial repair, and patients with perforation of a diseased esophagus should have the esophagus excised with the establishment of a cervical esophagostomy and a gastrostomy. Control of the sepsis with satisfactory nutrition should permit later reconstruction using a gastric or colon interposition graft.

Intramural or walled-off perforations in a patient with stable vital signs and no evidence of sepsis can be managed by intravenous antibiotics, parenteral nutrition, and inhibition of gastric secretion during alimentary restriction (Fig. 10).

OROPHARYNGEAL DYSPHAGIA

Oropharyngeal dysphagia, also described as cervical or proximal dysphagia, is a symptom complex characterized by difficulty in propelling food or liquid from the oral cavity into the cervical esophagus. There are a large number of disorders that can produce oropharyngeal dysphagia[12,18] (Table 4).

Pathophysiology

NEUROLOGIC DISORDERS

Neurologic disorders are the most common cause of oropharyngeal dysphagia and the most difficult to treat. Cerebrovascular accidents, particularly when involving the

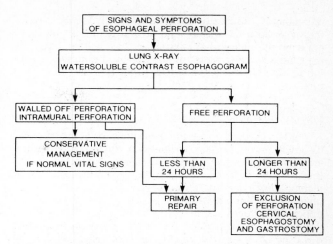

Figure 10. Diagnosis and management of esophageal perforation.

vertebrobasilar arteries or the posteroinferior cerebellar arteries, cause difficulties in bolus formation and propulsion. Patients with Parkinson's disease show hesitancy in bolus preparation with difficulties in initiating swallows. Amyotrophic lateral sclerosis with its loss of lower motor neurons and their regulatory systems may result in dysarthria and dysphagia with repetitive aspiration from absent voluntary deglutition. Peripheral neuropathy may cause oropharyngeal symptoms in the diabetic, the alcoholic, or the patient with poliomyelitis. Recurrent laryngeal nerve paralysis from neoplastic invasion or iatrogenic injury may be responsible for significant oropharyngeal dysphagia.

NEUROMUSCULAR DISEASES

Myasthenia gravis, a disease of the motor end plate, may result in dysphagia, especially if repetitive efforts at swallowing are made. Abnormalities in striated muscle function exist in various forms of muscular dystrophies,

TABLE 4. Etiology of Oropharyngeal Dysphagia

Neurologic	
Central	Cerebrovascular accident
	Parkinson's disease
	Amyotrophic lateral sclerosis, tumors
Peripheral	Peripheral neuropathy
	Recurrent laryngeal nerve palsy
Neuromuscular	
Motor end-plate disease	Myasthenia gravis
Skeletal myopathy	Muscular dystrophy
	Inflammatory disease
	Metabolic myopathy
Structural lesions	
Intrinsic	Abnormal function of upper esophageal sphincter with no evident neurologic or muscular disease
	Pharyngoesophageal diverticulum (Zenker)
Extrinsic	Local lesions with external compression
Iatrogenic	
Cervical surgery	Tracheostomy, thyroidectomy, laryngectomy
Radiation therapy	
Gastroesophageal reflux	

inflammatory disease of the muscle, and metabolic myopathies, as seen in hyper- and hypothyroidism. In these patients, the pharyngeal contractions normally initiated by the pharynx are rendered powerless by the muscular condition. The UES acts as a barrier to the passage of the food bolus instead of being a finely tuned part of deglutition.

STRUCTURAL LESIONS

When there is no specific neurologic or neuromuscular disorder, oropharyngeal dysphagia is considered structural and intrinsic to the upper esophageal sphincter. These intrinsic abnormalities, when observed, will show either incomplete or absent relaxation and/or incoordination of pharyngeal contraction with the relaxation phase of the upper sphincter. Patients with esophageal or Zenker's diverticulum are included in this group, in whom simultaneous contractions of the pharynx and the upper esophageal sphincter occur, generating repetitively high contraction pressures in the pharynx against a prematurely closed sphincter. Outpouching of mucosa and submucosa through the muscularis of the distal pharyngeal wall occurs just proximal to the upper sphincter area. The functional abnormalities are not seen in all patients during the recording of their pharyngoesophageal motility, indicating that the problem may be intermittent with slow progression over the years (Fig. 11).

Local structural lesions, either external or internal to the pharyngoesophageal junction, may result in proximal dysphagia. A high esophageal stricture or a pharyngoesophageal carcinoma may be responsible. Extrinsic compression by osteophytes is rare. A large mediastinal goiter or cervical lymphadenopathies may compress the cervical esophagus and cause dysphagia.

IATROGENIC CAUSES

Any surgical procedure in the neck that causes scarring may be responsible for limitation of the excursion of the larynx during the act of swallowing. Dysphagia and aspiration may result from abnormal bolus propulsion. Ablative surgery such as laryngectomy may cause functional abnormalities of the sphincter. Radiotherapy with its resultant fibrosis causes dense scarring of the tissues. Stricture at the pharyngoesophageal junction following irradiation is particularly difficult to manage.

GASTROESOPHAGEAL REFLUX

When irritant material flows from the gastric cavity into the esophagus, the normal function of the upper esophageal sphincter may be altered. The abnormalities observed are either elevation of the resting pressure or the appearance of premature closure of the sphincter against pharyngeal contraction. Almost 50 per cent of patients with gastroesophageal reflux may present with referred symptoms to the neck. When esophagitis and stricture have resulted from gastroesophageal reflux, the sole manifestation of these complications may be oropharyngeal dysphagia, and only a complete esophageal investigation will establish the proper diagnosis.

Symptoms

The most troublesome symptoms in all these categories of patients are dysphagia and aspiration. The patient with a neurologic condition will frequently present with absent or poor voluntary deglutition more than with dysphagia per se. If voluntary swallowing remains adequate, a blocking sensation or the feeling that the bolus sticks in the cervical region is frequently mentioned. The pooling of food and liquid in the larynx will eventually lead to aspiration and coughing with symptoms of either acute pulmonary infection or chronic lung disease. Dysarthria and sensory and motor deficits can be present.

When muscular disorders are involved, voluntary swallowing is usually normal. It is the poor pharyngeal pump working against a normal-toned sphincter that causes the dysphagia, food incarceration, and oropharyngeal regurgitations. Poor velopharyngeal muscle control leads to the development of a nasal speech and pharyngonasal regurgitations. Increased alimentation time and diet modification progressively occur and may result in weight loss. At the same time, tracheobronchial aspiration occurs regularly with food at mealtime and with saliva during sleep. As long as a good cough reflex is retained, bronchorrhea might be the only resulting symptom. Pulmonary infection, seen in nearly 25 per cent of patients, supervenes when the defense mechanisms fail. Voice alterations, bilateral palpebral ptosis, and voluntary muscle wasting may also be observed.

When the patient with oropharyngeal dysphagia has a pharyngoesophageal diverticulum, the dysphagia and aspiration may be severe. Initially caused by upper esophageal

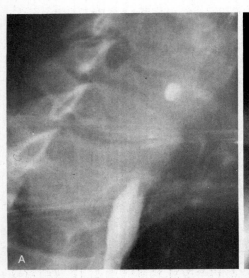
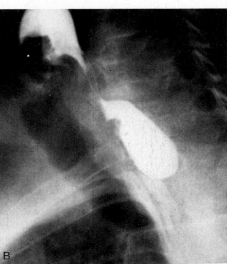

Figure 11. A, *Pharyngoesophageal diverticulum.* B, *Ten years later,* showing the slow progression of the disorder.

sphincter dysfunction, the appearance and development of the diverticulum may produce posterior compression of the proximal esophagus and add a mechanical component to the dysphagia. Freshly eaten food may be regurgitated immediately after eating or while the patient is lying down, occasionally leading to dangerous aspiration and suppurative lung disease. When the pouch contains food and liquid, a bothersome bruit can be heard on swallowing with compression of the neck tissues.

When mechanical obstruction is caused by pharyngeal, laryngeal, or cervical esophageal cancer, dysphagia will progress without remission. Pain on swallowing may be present. The recent appearance of hoarseness suggests recurrent laryngeal nerve palsy.

Evaluation

Following complete subjective and objective evaluation, the patient should be examined using a dynamic cinepharyngoesophagogram. This examination will allow the documentation of the rapidly occurring events with the movements of the tongue and soft palate. Pharyngeal contraction and its symmetry, coordination with upper sphincter opening, and contraction can be assessed. The presence of a cricopharyngeal bar or a pharyngoesophageal pouch can be demonstrated. Complete evaluation of the distal esophagus and stomach is always necessary to exclude other conditions.[10]

Because of the laryngeal excursion, manometric studies when performed with the actual recording techniques will not reveal all the functional abnormalities resulting in oropharyngeal dysphagia. In a certain proportion of swallows for all categories of patients, esophageal motility studies may show incomplete or absent relaxation of the upper sphincter or its incoordination with pharyngeal contraction. Pharyngeal contraction pressures are usually underestimated, and the sphincter resting pressures must be observed with the perspective of its axial asymmetry. One of the major advantages of performing motility studies in the patient with oropharyngeal dysphagia is the actual observation of the patient's swallowing habits for nearly 1 hour.

Endoscopic evaluation of the patient with oropharyngeal dysphagia is important if an endoluminal lesion is suspected. Performance may be more thorough and safer under general anesthesia using initially direct laryngoscopy followed by the introduction of the esophagoscope under direct vision. The use of esophagoscopy may be especially hazardous when performed in the patient with a diverticulum.

Treatment

Treatment of the patient with oropharyngeal dysphagia may be strictly medical when control of the underlying disorder is necessary. Such is the case for the vast majority of the neurologic conditions The specific use of L-dopa in Parkinson's disease or of cholinesterase inhibitors in myasthenia gravis may relieve the swallowing difficulties. Specific conditions such as myotonic dystrophy, skeletal myopathy from hypo- or hyperthyroidism or polymyositis may respond to treatment with appropriate drugs.

Bougienage will improve a stricture resulting from previous surgery or irradiation. The immediate effects of dilatation on functional disorders of the upper sphincter may be improvement of the dysphagia. However, the results are usually of short duration.

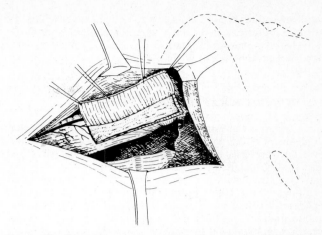

Figure 12. Cricopharyngeal myotomy for oropharyngeal dysphagia. (From Duranceau, A. C., Jamieson, G. G., and Beauchamp, G.: Surg. Clin. North Am., 63:833, 1983.)

Cricopharyngeal myotomy will result in lowering the resistance to bolus transit from pharynx to esophagus in selected patients suffering from oropharyngeal dysphagia. The best surgical results are obtained in patients with intact voluntary deglutition, normal antepulsion and retropulsion of the tongue, and specific abnormalities on the cine studies and/or the motility recordings. Patients with pharyngoesophageal diverticula should always be considered for surgical treatment.

The operation is usually performed through a left neck approach. When there is no diverticulum formation, meticulous sectioning of the distal pharynx, cricropharyngeus muscle, and adjacent cervical esophageal muscle with unwrapping of the pharyngoesophageal junction of its muscular envelope is the operation of choice (Fig. 12). When

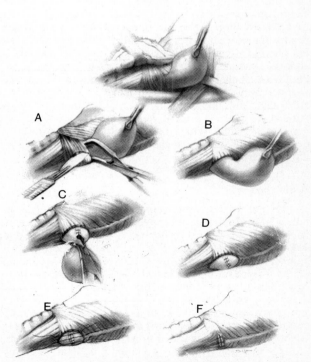

Figure 13. Zenker's diverticulum. A and B, Myotomy and diverticulum suspension. C through E, Diverticulectomy. (From Payne, W. S.: Esophageal diverticula. In Shields, T. W. (Ed.): General Thoracic Surgery, 2nd ed. Philadelphia, Lea & Febiger, 1983.)

a diverticulum is present, a myotomy with diverticulopexy can be preferred. However, if the diverticulum is too large for the retropharyngeal space, a diverticulectomy must then accompany the myotomy (Fig. 13).

MOTOR DISORDERS OF THE ESOPHAGUS

Disorders of esophageal function occur when the usual response to voluntary deglutition results in abnormal contraction patterns in the esophageal body and sphincters. Such abnormalities can be characterized by hypomotility, such as in achalasia and scleroderma. An exaggerated response with high contraction pressures and defective peristalsis is seen in diffuse esophageal spasm. Coordination abnormalities in the upper esophageal sphincter usually cause oropharyngeal dysphagia. When the resting pressure in the lower esophageal sphincter is low or nonexistent, gastroesophageal reflux may occur. If the abnormality is in sphincter relaxation or coordination, dysphagia may appear secondary to the functional obstruction by the sphincter.

Hypomotility Disorders

ACHALASIA

Achalasia is a rare condition (1 per 100,000) that equally affects males and females, generally in the young adult and middle age categories. The symptoms and natural evolution of this condition are caused by the total absence of peristalsis in the esophageal body coupled with imcomplete or failure of relaxation in the lower esophageal sphincter.[6]

Etiology

The etiology of achalasia may be single or multiple. Neurogenic causes are either central or peripheral. Centrally, destruction of the dorsal motor nucleus of the vagus results in motor abnormalities similar to those of achalasia. Peripherally, section or resection of the vagi will cause abnormal esophageal body contractions and dysfunction of the lower esophageal sphincter. Infection with the parasite *Trypanosoma cruzi* is known to result in achalasia of the esophagus and multisystemic disease. Although rare, a familial incidence is present, suggesting the possibility of a hereditary factor. Whatever the cause, the end result is denervation of the esophagus with loss of ganglion cells in the esophageal plexus.[6]

Symptoms

Dysphagia is the most common symptom. Regurgitation will be present in more than 70 per cent of patients. Pain on swallowing or odynophagia will occur in less than 30 per cent of patients, and pulmonary complications will be seen in approximately 10 per cent of all cases. Although ideally divided into three clinical stages, achalasia symptoms may be totally erratic in their development.

The natural evolution of achalasia can be followed with the symptoms of these three stages. During the initial period, substernal dysphagia is the main symptom. Regurgitation of freshly ingested food and odynophagia are present as well. Symptoms are intermittent at this stage and may be increased by stress or cold liquids. Progression of achalasia to Stage II is underlined by milder symptoms with less dysphagia, less odynophagia, and occasional re-

gurgitations. The milder symptoms are explained by a wider esophagus. The resulting increase in pressure of the food column forces passive opening of the distal sphincter. The symptoms of Stage III are those of a decompensated esophagus; dysphagia and regurgitation are present. The baggy esophagus is chronically filled with ingested material that does not progress normally into the gastric cavity. Frequent episodes of nocturnal regurgitation and aspiration result in recurrent pneumonias and pulmonary abscesses. At this stage, compression symptoms by the large esophagus may cause substernal discomfort.

Investigation

Radiology. The chest roentgenogram may reveal a widened mediastinum from a dilated esophagus containing

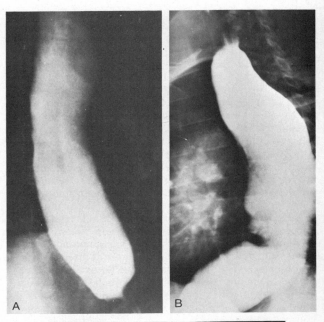

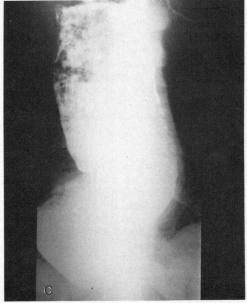

Figure 14. Achalasia. A, *Mild.* B, *Moderate.* C, *With severe dilatation and food retention.*

an air-fluid level. Signs of chronic pulmonary aspiration may be seen. Cinefluoroscopic evaluation of the esophagus will reveal three stages. Stage I, or mild achalasia, shows either no or slight dilatation with minimal retention of contrast material proximal to the lower esophageal sphincter. Vigorous contractions of the esophagus can be seen in this stage and may be difficult to differentiate from diffuse esophageal spasm. Stage II, or moderate achalasia, shows more dilatation with weak nonperistaltic contractions and a tapered esophagogastric junction, suggesting a tightly closed and nonrelaxing distal sphincter. Stage III achalasia shows a very large esophagus with food retention and often a sigmoid-like appearance (Fig. 14).

Manometric Evaluation. The motor abnormalities seen in achalasia are diagnostic.[10] After voluntary swallowing, the UES is the only area that functions normally. In the esophageal body, the resting pressure is elevated from the dilatation and retention of debris. After swallowing, aperistalsis is seen at all levels in the esophagus. The resulting contractions are mirror-like and of poor amplitude. Occasional spontaneous tertiary contractions may be observed (Fig. 15A). The LES shows normal or high resting pressures with imcomplete or absent relaxation on swallowing (Fig. 15B).

In achalasia, a denervation hypersensitivity can be elicited by injecting bethanechol chloride (Urecholine) during the recording of esophageal function. Hyperreaction of esophageal body activity is then seen with higher resting pressure, increased incidence of spontaneous activity, and higher contraction pressures following deglutition. These observations are frequently accompanied by chest pain and regurgitation from esophageal spasm. This positive response to cholinergic stimulation can be abolished by intravenous atropine (Fig. 15C).

Endoscopy. The endoscopic features of achalasia are indirect evidence of a malfunctioning esophagus with stasis. A dilated esophageal body with retained food and liquid, inflammation in the areas of stasis, and a lower esophageal sphincter tonically closed but opening on pressure are the main endoscopic features of achalasia. Endoscopic evaluation is always essential to exclude coexistent esophageal cancer or other causes of stricture.

Treatment

The philosophy of achalasia management is palliation, since the motor abnormalities remain unchanged following all forms of treatment. Efforts are directed toward removal of the functional obstruction of the distal esophageal sphincter.

Two therapeutic approaches can be proposed to the achalasia patient. The esophagogastric junction can be pneumatically or hydrostatically dilated with a bag dilator that is fluoroscopically placed to straddle the lower sphincter area. Inflating the bag to a pressure of 300 to 500 mm. Hg to obtain a maximal bag diameter of 3.0 to 3.5 cm. for

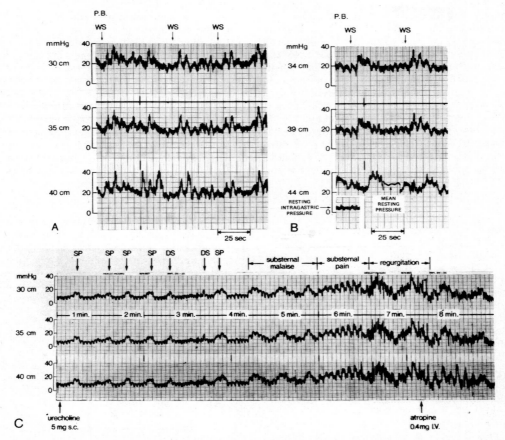

Figure 15. Achalasia. A, Esophageal body function in achalasia. Weak, nonpropulsive waves occur with every swallow. The resting pressure is elevated. B, Lower esophageal sphincter in achalasia. The pressure gradient is either normal or high. Incomplete or absent relaxation is recorded on swallowing. C, Denervation hypersensitivity of achalasia. Hyperactivity appears with cholinergic stimulation and is abolished by intravenous atropine. (From Hurwitz, A. L., Duranceau, A., and Haddad, J. K.: Disorders of esophageal motility. In Major Problems in Internal Medicine, Vol. 16. Philadelphia, W. B. Saunders Company, 1979.)

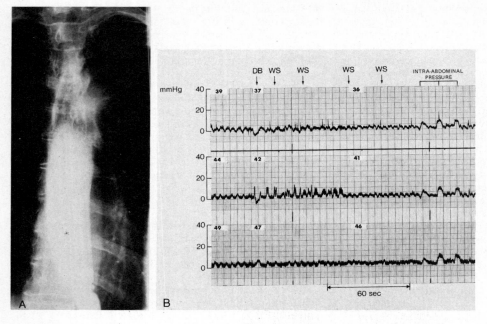

Figure 16. Scleroderma. A, Atonic esophagus of scleroderma with patulous cardia allowing free gastroesophageal reflux. B, Aperistalsis in scleroderma. No gastroesophageal sphincter is identified between the intragastric position at 44 cm. and the intraesophageal position at 41 cm. Esophagus and stomach form a single communicating cavity. (From Hurwitz, A. L., Duranceau, A., and Haddad, J. K.: Disorders of esophageal motility. In Major Problems in Internal Medicine, Vol. 16. Philadelphia, W. B. Saunders Company, 1979.)

a period of 30 to 60 seconds should significantly reduce the LES pressure. Following pneumatic dilatation, the most dreaded complication is perforation, which occurs in up to 4 per cent of patients. Gastroesophageal reflux occurs in 17 per cent of patients following this procedure. Overall good symptomatic results are seen in 60 per cent of patients.

Esophagomyotomy of the esophagogastric junction is the surgical alternative in the treatment of achalasia. A section of the longitudinal and circular muscle layers of the distal 7 to 10 cm. of the esophagus is usually made through a left thoracic approach. The net result of this operation is a significant decrease in the distal sphincter resting pressure without improvement in motor function of the distal esophagus. Good to excellent results are usually obtained in 85 per cent of patients. The incidence of gastroesophageal reflux varies from 3 to 52 per cent. An antireflux procedure may be considered after the surgical treatment of achalasia but must take into account the powerless and aperistaltic esophageal body.[17]

SCLERODERMA

Scleroderma is a collagen disease that causes atrophy of the smooth esophageal muscle and collagen deposition in the submucosa of the esophageal wall. The distal digestive tract is affected as well, and overall hypomotility of the gut results from these pathologic changes.

Patients with scleroderma usually present with reflux symptoms, namely regurgitations and heartburn. These are worsened by the fact that the esophagus is either hypo- or aperistaltic. Because of this lack of defense mechanisms, acid and pepsin will sojourn longer in the esophageal cavity, causing more damage ot the esophageal wall. With increasing reflux esophageal ulcers, bleeding and stricture may develop. Dysphagia is either functional from the motor disorder or mechanical from stenosis. Raynaud's phenomenon is present in up to 90 per cent of patients. This observation correlates with loss of esophageal peristalsis without influencing the contractile strength of the esophageal smooth muscle.

Investigation

Barium studies will show abnormal peristalsis in the majority of patients. With esophageal dilatation, gastro-

esophageal reflux can be seen radiologically but the results are usually an underestimation of the true incidence of reflux, as demonstrated by the 24-hour esophageal pH monitoring. Stricture formation may involve long segments of the distal esophagus.

Esophageal motility studies are the only true indicators of the esophageal abnormalities present. The motor dysfunction can be highly variable and does not depend on the duration of the disease or the symptoms. Both extremes of motor dysfunction can be seen. There is the occasional patient with normal or minimally disturbed peristalsis and contraction pressure. More often, the patient has a totally paralyzed esophagus without distal sphincter. In these patients, the stomach and esophagus form a single cavity, where reflux occurs freely. Various stages of progression of the disease can be seen in between these two extremes. Esophagoscopy shows varying degrees of esophagitis with frequent deep ulcerations and strictures (Fig. 16).

Treatment

The management of the patient with scleroderma is directed toward prevention or treatment of esophageal complications. An aggressive medical treatment must be attempted first with simple mechanical antireflux measures and the use of H^2 blockers. With the presence of muscle cell damage and collagen infiltration, stimulation of esophageal and gastric emptying as well as attempting to increase LES resting pressure with metoclopramide or bethanechol may not bring a significant response.

When severe esophagitis persists and the general condition of the patient is favorable, a modified antireflux procedure, taking into account the absence of propulsive force in the esophageal body, should be performed to limit the esophageal damage from the refluxing material.

Hypermotility Disorders and Diffuse Esophageal Spasm

Symptomatic idiopathic diffuse esophageal spasm (SIDES) is a rare condition, especially if one expects a good correlation between clinical, radiologic, and manometric diagnosis. It is most important to exclude all evidence of previous esophageal or other pathologic conditions that could explain the symptoms. Chronic gastroesophageal reflux, alcoholism, diabetes, or the presbyesophagus of old age can account for significant functional abnormalities. The esophagus damaged by a caustic substance or infiltrated by a tumor, or the patient with central or peripheral neurologic disease can present with markedly deranged esophageal motility. Patients with such previous history should be classified as having secondary diffuse esophageal spasm.[1]

The clinical picture is that of an anxious, "high-strung" individual, male or female, presenting increased symptoms with stressful situations. Esophageal colics causing significant odynophagia is the main symptom. The pain may radiate to the mid-scapular region or may be very similar to angina with neck, left shoulder, and arm radiation. The relationship with food ingestion and the absence of substernal pain on exercise are important subjective points to investigate. Simple dysphagia with food regurgitation may be present, but it is usually accompanied by odynophagia.

Investigation

When reasonable doubt exists in the differential diagnosis between angina and esophageal disease, the patient must be evaluated initially to exclude coronary disease. Cine-esophagography may reveal simultaneous contractions mainly in the distal two thirds of the esophageal body. The esophagus may show dilatation proximal to the functional obstruction of the spastic area. Frequent association with hiatal hernia and epiphrenic diverticulum has been noted (Fig. 17*A*).

Endoscopy must be performed to exclude any endoluminal lesion. Occasionally this procedure may be difficult to perform if too much spasticity is present.

Manometrically normal esophageal function is usually seen in the proximal esophageal sphincter and in the proximal third of the esophagus. Normal esophageal function is then replaced by nonpropulsive high-pressure, repetitive contractions of long duration, which occur in the distal two thirds of the esophagus (Fig. 17*B*). Spontaneous

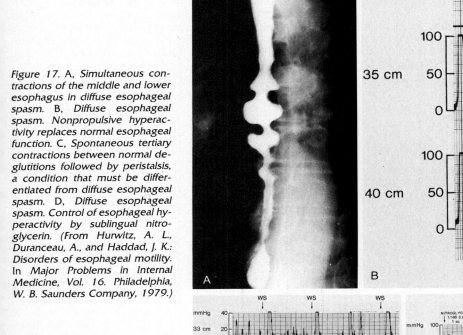

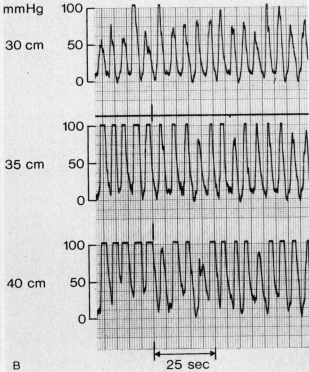

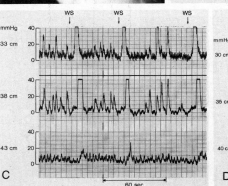

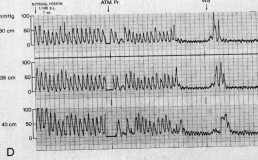

Figure 17. A, *Simultaneous contractions of the middle and lower esophagus in diffuse esophageal spasm.* B, *Diffuse esophageal spasm. Nonpropulsive hyperactivity replaces normal esophageal function.* C, *Spontaneous tertiary contractions between normal deglutitions followed by peristalsis, a condition that must be differentiated from diffuse esophageal spasm.* D, *Diffuse esophageal spasm. Control of esophageal hyperactivity by sublingual nitroglycerin.* (From Hurwitz, A. L., Duranceau, A., and Haddad, J. K.: Disorders of esophageal motility. In Major Problems in Internal Medicine, Vol. 16. Philadelphia, W. B. Saunders Company, 1979.)

tertiary contractions are also seen. The lower esophageal sphincter may show a normal relaxation in 50 per cent of swallows, but frequent incomplete or absent relaxation is observed with premature sphincter closure. One must be very careful in branding a patient with the diagnosis of diffuse esophageal spasm, especially if normal contractions appear after deglutition, but frequent spontaneous tertiary waves between deglutitions form the basis of the esophageal abnormalities (Fig. 17C).

Treatment

Once the diagnosis is established, conservative management is mandatory with periodic re-evaluation at 3 and 6 months and removal of all initiating stimuli. Short- and long-acting nitrites and diazepam will lower the contraction pressures (Fig. 17D). Calcium channel blockers may be used in lowering the vigorous contraction pressures. Pneumatic dilatation of the lower esophagus and sphincter should not be expected to improve the symptoms if the distal sphincter functions normally.

If intractable symptoms persist after this trial period, a long esophagomyotomy over the abnormal motility zone established manometrically should be performed. Careful selection of patients should be made through conservative initial diagnosis and management. An accurate diagnosis will improve the low incidence (67 per cent) of good to excellent results seen in this group.[17]

Coordination Disorders and Esophageal Diverticula

Abnormalities in coordination are observed in association with pharyngoesophageal and epiphrenic diverticula of the esophagus. Pharyngoesophageal diverticula are discussed in the section on oropharyngeal dysphagia.

Mid-esophageal or traction diverticula must be differentiated from these two types of pulsion diverticula. They are usually found at or near the tracheal bifurcation. They show a large opening collar, and the whole wall of the esophagus is usually deformed by an adjacent chronic inflammatory reaction. Usually, no symptoms are present unless a local complication has resulted within or near the diverticulum (bleeding, fistula formation, perforation). Esophageal function in these patients is normal. These diverticula rarely require treatment.

The epiphrenic diverticulum is a condition of unknown etiology, but more frequently it is attributed to a pulsion mechanism from within the esophageal lumen. Its frequent association with primary motor disorders of the esophagus (achalasia, diffuse spasm) suggests that the abnormal contractions with esophageal segmentation may result in outpouching of mucosa and submucosa through the esophageal muscularis. The muscularis mucosa may be hypertrophied from the high esophageal pressures generated by accompanying abnormal contraction.[10] The symptoms are very similar to those of diffuse spasm and include dysphagia, odynophagia, and regurgitation of undigested food.

Investigation

Radiologic evaluation usually shows a diverticulum in the distal third of the esophagus. Projection to the right is common, and abnormal contractions may be seen on the esophageal wall. Endoscopic evaluation must exclude any associated lesion.

Manometric evaluation must be performed to document the presence or absence of a primary motor disorder. Some diverticula are associated with a perfectly normal esophagus. Others may be associated with significant contraction abnormalities and incoordination of the LES (Fig. 18A and B).

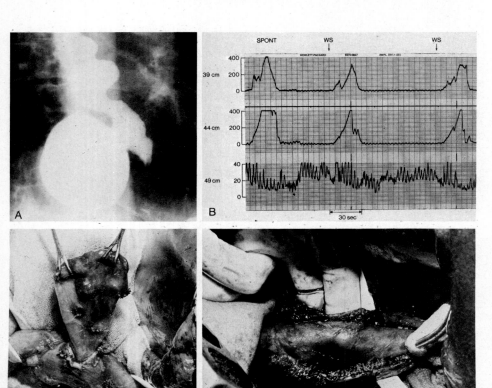

Figure 18. Epiphrenic diverticulum.
A, Abnormal esophageal contractions causing dysphagia and odynophagia.
B, Broad, nonpropulsive, and very high pressure contractions in the esophageal body against a poorly coordinated lower esophageal sphincter.
C, Large epiphrenic diverticulum protruding through the esophageal musculature.
D, Long esophageal myotomy contralateral to the diverticulectomy site. Significant muscle hypertrophy is present.
(A and B from Hurwitz, A. L., Duranceau, A., and Haddad, J. K.: Disorders of esophageal motility. In Major Problems in Internal Medicine, Vol. 16. Philadelphia, W. B. Saunders Company, 1979.)

Treatment

Surgical treatment is indicated only if significant symptoms or complications are present. If the diverticulum is small, an esophageal myotomy that will include the abnormally functioning muscle and the diverticulum-forming area should result in disappearance of symptoms. If the diverticulum is large, a diverticulectomy must be performed with an intraesophageal bougie in place to protect lumen integrity. An esophageal myotomy is then included, covering the abnormal motility area. This is essential to prevent disruption of the suture line in the immediate postoperative period and recurrence of the diverticulum on a long-term basis. A hiatal hernia, if present, should be repaired at the same time (Fig. 18C and D).

GASTROESOPHAGEAL REFLUX AND HIATAL HERNIA

Gastroesophageal Reflux

Gastroesophageal reflux is a normal physiologic event. It occurs more frequently during the waking hours, especially after meals, and only infrequently during sleep. Reflux episodes are related to swallowing when the LES relaxes; in the awake and upright position, it averages 72 episodes per hour and increases to 192 during meals. Recorded incidences of reflux decrease to seven or fewer per hour during sleep, which coincides with a decrease in the frequency of swallowing. At night, i.e., when in the recumbent position, there is a decrease in intra-abdominal pressure and a higher, more stable resting pressure in the sphincter. Physiologic reflux is rapidly cleared from the esophagus, regardless of the position, by swallowing or spontaneous secondary peristalsis.[20]

Symptomatic gastroesophageal reflux may occur in the upright, supine, or mixed position. Patients with supine reflux have fewer episodes, but they are longer lasting, resulting in excessive acid exposure of the mucosa and more severe damage. Biopsy-proven esophagitis is more prevalent in supine than in upright reflux. The duration of reflux episodes is longer in symptomatic patients. Therefore, it is likely that the length of time acid bathes the esophageal mucosa is a critical factor.[2] Heartburn is the primary symptom. This is manifested by substernal burning pain or discomfort with possible radiation to the neck or jaw. Radiation to the arms may simulate pain of cardiac origin.

Regurgitation may or may not be accompanied by heartburn. Both symptoms are exacerbated by meals or postural changes. Some patients present initially with complications of reflux without prior heartburn or regurgitation. Dysphagia and odynophagia may be secondary to a reflux-induced stenosis or to a motility disorder secondary to reflux. Nocturnal episodes of coughing, morning hoarseness, asthma-like syndromes, or recurrent pneumonitis suggest aspiration from gastroesophageal reflux. Anemia may be present but is rarely secondary to massive bleeding. Chest pain of a more severe nature may be caused by spasm of the esophageal muscle triggered by abnormal reflux. Other patients present with symptoms that mimic gastroduodenal, biliary, or pancreatic diseases. During pregnancy, 25 per cent of patients will present daily symptoms of gastroesophageal reflux.

PATHOPHYSIOLOGY

Multiple contributory factors determine whether or not a given individual develops clinical reflux esophagitis. These factors include the tissue resistance of the esophageal mucosa, the efficacy of the antireflux mechanism, the volume and composition of the gastric fluid, and the efficiency of esophageal clearance and gastric emptying.

Anatomic and physiologic factors contribute to the development of reflux. The positive intra-abdominal pressure and negative intrathoracic pressure produce a gradient across the diaphragm that promotes migration of the stomach cephalad with shortening of the intra-abdominal length of the LES. Both pressure and length of the LES exposed to the positive pressure of the abdomen are known to predict the efficiency of the sphincter against reflux. Positive intragastric pressure also places stress on the antireflux barrier, the lower esophageal sphincter. This is accentuated by coughing, straining, pregnancy, and delayed gastric emptying secondary to pyloric stenosis or duodenal pathology. Thus, gastroesophageal reflux would occur continuously were there not some physiologic barrier at the esophagogastric junction.

A consensus exists that the intrinsic LES tone is the major mechanism that prevents gastroesophageal reflux. Numerous studies now provide manometric evidence of a physiologic LES that maintains a high pressure zone during resting conditions and relaxes with swallowing, esophageal distention, vagal stimulation, or other events such as vomiting. Anatomic studies suggest the existence of a thickened elliptical and circular musculature for a length of 3 to 4 cm., corresponding to the physiologic LES. A number of peptides from the gastrointestinal tract have been proposed as possible physiologic regulators of lower esophageal sphincter pressure. These concepts remain controversial. Pharmacologic doses of gastrin will increase LES tone in the normal individual. Progesterone causes a decrease of the LES resting pressure during pregnancy.

The phrenoesophageal membrane anchors the esophagus in the diaphragmatic hiatus and maintains a fixed intra-abdominal segment of LES exposed to the positive pressure of the abdominal cavity. This segment of the esophagus then follows Laplace's law, which states that if equal pressure is applied to dissimilar-sized tubes the smallest one collapses first. This implies a mechanical effect that decreases the likelihood of reflux.

Gastroesophageal reflux occurs by several different mechanisms associated with feeble resting LES pressure or transient LES relaxations. Patients with reflux esophagitis have more frequent episodes of acid reflux and longer exposure to the refluxed material.[3]

The defense mechanisms of the esophagus against reflux are the efficiency of esophageal clearance, esophageal mucosal resistance, and saliva. The intensity of symptoms does not necessarily correlate with the volume of reflux, the presence or absence of an accompanying hiatal hernia, or the severity of endoscopic and histologic esophagitis. However, esophageal damage correlates with the frequency and time of exposure of the irritant material with the esophageal mucosa. Patients with upright reflux have more frequent episodes of reflux but present with less damage than those with supine reflux because of rapid esophageal clearance and the effect of gravity.

In the normal individual, reflux produces instantaneous secondary peristalsis that rapidly empties the lower esophagus of the refluxed material. With the progression of reflux esophagitis, there is development of a dysmotility that prolongs the contact time between the reflux material and the esophageal mucosa. The resultant decrease in esophageal clearance increases esophageal damage. Saliva neutralizes small volumes of acid and the main effect is to induce deglutition. This accounts for the high frequency of swallowing in the awake subject with consequent improvement in esophageal clearance.

The esophageal mucosa is sensitive to acid, pepsin, or bile acids. The effect of these irritants is to alter mucosal permeability, allowing back diffusion of hydrogen ions into the esophageal wall and causing further tissue damage. Individuals show a wide range of mucosal resistance to reflux. Endoscopic findings show little or no correlation with the severity of symptoms.

With failure of the defense mechanisms, there is progression of esophagitis to ulcer formation, fibrosis, and stricture formation. The process of regeneration may lead to the replacement of the esophageal mucosa by a columnar-lined epithelium (Barrett's esophagus). This condition is associated with a higher incidence of esophageal malignancies.[3]

DIAGNOSIS

Clinical Presentations

The single most important diagnostic method is a carefully obtained history. Symptoms of heartburn and regurgitation of sour-tasting material virtually establish the diagnosis of symptomatic gastroesophageal reflux. In these patients, additional information obtained by radiography and endoscopy is sufficient to determine the extent of the problem related to reflux. A more exhaustive investigation is required for patients with atypical symptoms to document the presence of reflux and to exclude other conditions that can have a clinical presentation consistent with gastroesophageal reflux.

Radiology

Radiologic evaluation is the initial step. Evidence of aspiration pneumonia or an irreducible intrathoracic hiatal hernia may be seen on routine chest films. Barium esophagogram is not a sensitive test, but in the presence of free reflux at fluoroscopy the correlation with significant gastroesophageal reflux disease is good with a specificity of 85 per cent. Reflux damage to the esophageal mucosa may be demonstrated by double contrast techniques. Irregularity of the fully distended esophagus, ulcerations, incomplete esophageal distensibility, stricture formation, and the thick mucosal folds of Barrett's esophagus are all signs of esophageal injury. Associated gastric or duodenal pathology must be excluded.

Motility Studies

Esophageal manometry is performed to assess LES tone and motor function of the esophageal body. Overall, a lower esophageal sphincter pressure of less than 10 mm. Hg shows a poor sensitivity but a good specificity of 85 per cent in patients with proven reflux. Preoperative motility studies may also be important in the evaluation of the propulsive force of the esophageal body.

Endoscopy

The endoscopic criteria for esophagitis are hyperemia, erosions, friability, exudations, ulcerations, bleeding, and stricture. With individual differences in mucosal resistance, a number of patients with symptomatic gastroesophageal reflux may show a normal-appearing mucosa. Endoscopy detects an inflamed esophageal mucosa but not reflux. Other conditions, such as foreign body or caustic ingestion, motor disorders with esophageal stasis, or specific infections, can result in abnormalities of the esophageal mucosa.[7]

pH Monitoring and Perfusion Studies

The measurement of esophageal pH is the most sensitive (88 per cent) and specific (98 per cent) method of detecting gastroesophageal reflux. Different techniques of monitoring are available varying from the single measurement to the continuous 24-hour pH monitoring. The acid perfusion test may be useful to relate thoracic symptoms to esophageal disease. Simultaneous recording of esophageal motility may document the dysmotility associated with impaired clearance. A recent addition to the diagnostic armamentarium for the documentation of gastroesophageal reflux is *scintiscanning*. The clinical value of this test remains to be established. Gastric emptying scans, on the other hand, are useful to exclude associated disorders of delayed gastric emptying.[2,22]

THERAPY

Conservative Management

The principles of conservative management are directed toward the relief of symptoms and the prevention of further reflux and its associated complications. Mechanical and pharmacologic methods exist to improve the efficacy of the lower esophageal sphincter. Conservative therapy should also be directed toward correcting abnormalities in esophageal clearance and gastric emptying. Neutralization and inhibition of the reflux material are essential to the control of this condition.

Mechanical means to decrease the frequency and volume of reflux are weight reduction and the avoidance of tight garments. Using gravity by instructing the patient to elevate the head of the bed by 6 inches or to avoid lying down after meals significantly decreases esophageal acid exposure. Certain foods, such as fats, chocolate, and alcohol, have been shown to impair LES function, and their restriction is indicated. Smoking causes a marked reduction in LES pressure. Citrus juices, tomato products, and coffee have been associated with exacerbation of heartburn. Drugs such as calcium-blocking agents, theophylline, valium, and morphine will decrease LES pressure. Antacids are given to neutralize gastric secretion and to increase LES pressure by alkalinization of the antrum. Patients are advised to take small meals to avoid gastric distention. Dietary restriction, weight reduction, and the use of antacids are the mainstays of gastroesophageal reflux treatment.

In those patients who do not respond to this simple therapeutic regimen, more vigorous therapy is indicated. Bethanechol is used to increase the LES tone and improve esophageal clearance. Metoclopramide has similar effects on the LES and improves gastric emptying. Cimetidine decreases gastric acid production without influencing the motility function of the upper digestive tract. Five to 10 per cent of patients with gastroesophageal disease will fail to respond to medical therapy.[20]

Surgical Management

The indications for a surgical approach are established complications of gastroesophageal reflux. Ulcerative esophagitis, stenosis, intestinal metaplasia, bleeding, and aspiration are formal indications. Patients with objective documentation of reflux who remain symptomatic after a year of well-controlled conservative management should also be considered for surgery. Antireflux surgery should restore an adequate pressure in the lower esophageal sphincter while re-establishing an adequate intra-abdominal segment of esophagus. This operation may be performed through a

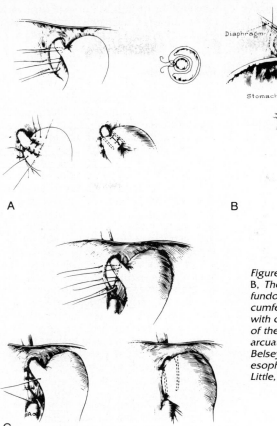

A

B

C

Figure 19. A, *The Nissen total fundoplication.*
B, *The Belsey Mark IV repair creates a partial
fundoplication on 75% of the esophageal circumference. C, The Hill posterior gastropexy
with closure of the posterior hiatus and fixation
of the esophagogastric junction to the median
arcuate ligament. (A–C from* Skinner, D. B.,
Belsey, R. H. R., Hendrix, T. R., et al.: Gastroesophageal Reflux and Hiatal Hernia. Boston,
Little, Brown and Company, 1972.)

thoracic or an abdominal approach. Vagal innervation must
always be protected, and narrowing of the diaphragmatic
hiatus is accomplished to prevent hernia recurrence. A
thoracic or a thoracoabdominal approach is preferred in
patients with strictures that will require intraoperative dilatation or with recurrent disease after previous antireflux
surgery. The abdominal approach is selected in most patients without severe esophagitis and in patients with severely restricted pulmonary function. Surgical management
with an antireflux procedure is an effective form of treatment that prevents reflux, relieves symptoms, and promotes
the healing of the esophagitis lesion.[22]

Different techniques of repairs are available. The Nissen total fundoplication (Fig. 19A) may be performed
through either an abdominal or thoracic approach. After
dissection at the gastroesophageal junction, taking care to
preserve the vagal nerves, the dissected portion of the
fundus is passed posteriorly to wrap the distal esophagus
over a length of 4 cm. A 44-French Mercury bougie is
usually used as an intraesophageal stent to protect the
lumen integrity. The Belsey Mark IV operation (Fig. 19B)
is performed only through a left thoracic approach. It
creates a partial fundoplication over 75 per cent of the
circumference of the distal 4 cm. of the esophagus. The
Hill posterior gastropexy (Fig. 19C) is always performed
via the abdominal route. The cardia is mobilized in a
fashion similar to that used in the other procedures, taking
care to expose the median arcuate ligament overlying the
aorta just proximal to the celiac axis. Posteriorly, sutures
are placed in the crura of the diaphragm to narrow the
orifice at the hiatus. The gastropexy is then performed by
sutures anchoring the gastroesophageal junction as well as
the posterior and anterior smaller curvature of the stomach

to the median arcuate ligament. Intraluminal manometry is
used during the Hill operation to ascertain the calibration
of the cardia.

In the past, results of antireflux operations have been
based on the subjective reporting of symptoms or on the
absence of radiologic recurrence of hiatus hernia or reflux.
A more objective follow-up should include manometric
values of the lower esophageal sphincter as well as 24-hour
pH monitoring. A success rate of about 90 per cent is
claimed for most repairs based on follow-up periods of up
to 7 years. The mortality rate is about 1 per cent.

The morbidity of these procedures is important in
assessing their benefits. Dysphagia may be secondary to
local edema immediately after repair. The inability to belch
or vomit and abdominal distention after meals are present
generally after a total fundoplication. Disruption of these
repairs leads to recurrence of reflux symptoms. Slipping of
the total fundoplication results in symptoms of esophageal
obstruction.

Peptic Stricture

Strictures usually begin just above the squamocolumnar junction. They vary in extent from edema to submucosal
fibrosis to eventual destruction of the esophageal wall. The
principal symptom is dysphagia to solids that progresses to
liquids. Most patients will give a prior history of heartburn
and regurgitation. Other causes of dysphagia, such as
malignancy or motility disorders must be excluded.

Esophageal stricture is a surgical indication. Initial
therapy consists of a progressive dilatation regimen to
obtain an adequate esophageal lumen. This may be the

only treatment for the patient who is a poor surgical candidate, who will then benefit from the addition of the usual conservative management. The dilatable strictures are then treated by a standard antireflux procedure or an elongation procedure, such as the Collis gastroplasty, accompanied by an antireflux technique. This type of repair is constructed from the lesser curvature of the stomach to lengthen the damaged esophagus and should allow a tension-free fundoplication under the diaphragm (Fig. 20).

The undilatable stricture represents an esophagus with marked inflammation and fibrosis. The patients with such a condition or for whom repetitive attempts at stricture correction have failed will require resection. Reconstruction will then be done with colon, jejunum, or stomach.[22]

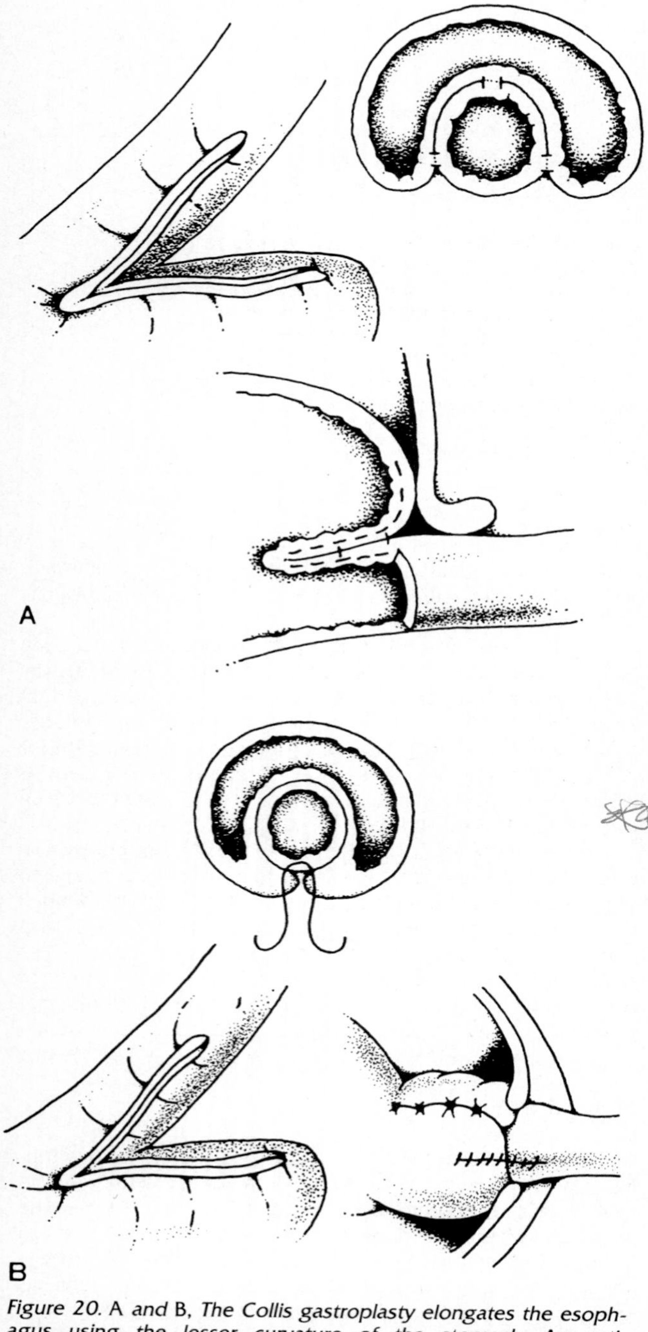

Hiatal Hernia

A hiatal hernia is noted on upper gastrointestinal series in about 10 per cent of the adult population. Of this group it is estimated that only 5 per cent have persistent symptomatic reflux. Hiatal hernias are divided into four types.

The commonly seen Type I sliding hiatal hernia (Fig. 21A) causes no specific symptoms or complications. If asymptomatic, the patient does not require further investigation or treatment. However, an associated hiatal hernia is present in 80 per cent of the population with proven gastroesophageal reflux. In the sliding hiatal hernia, the esophageal hiatus is usually enlarged. The phrenoesophageal membrane is stretched but intact circumferentially. When such a hernia is large and irreducible, complications within the herniated stomach may occur. These complications include occult and massive bleeding from stasis ulcers and represent a surgical indication.

The Type II hiatal hernia is paraesophageal (Fig. 21B). It is caused by a specific defect in the phrenoesophageal membrane. The stomach herniates most often through this defect and the esophageal hiatus. This type of hernia tends to increase progressively secondary to a continuously positive intra-abdominal pressure coupled with the negative intrathoracic pressure. This may progress to acute intrathoracic gastric dilatation and volvulus with the risk of obstruction, strangulation, and perforation. Stasis in the intrathoracic stomach may lead to ulcer formation and bleeding. This type of hernia is lethal and should be repaired surgically when diagnosed.

The Type III hernia is a combination of Types I and II (Fig. 21C). When abdominal organs other than the stomach are contained within the hernial sac, it is classified as Type IV.

Specific symptoms of a Type II, III, or IV hernia are related to the gastric pouch within the sac. Dysphagia results from compression of the distal esophagus by the dilated gastric pouch or from the acute angulation of the esophagogastric junction. Other symptoms are postprandial fullness, early satiety, and vomiting. When gastric volvulus occurs, the classic clinical triad of complete dysphagia, inability to vomit, and inability to introduce a nasogastric tube is diagnostic. In Type IV, symptoms may be related to the presence of the large or the small bowel within the hernia.

Figure 20. A and B, The Collis gastroplasty elongates the esophagus using the lesser curvature of the stomach. An antireflux procedure is added using a partial or a total fundoplication around the gastroplasty.

TUMORS OF THE ESOPHAGUS

The causes of esophageal carcinoma are numerous and complex, with incidence and predisposing factors differing widely in various parts of the world and among diverse ethnic groups. In the United States, the incidence is low (6:100,000 in men and 1.6:100,000 in women). Esophageal cancer constitutes 7 per cent of all gastrointestinal tract cancers and is responsible for about 8000 deaths per year. In the Hunan province of China, the Transkei of South Africa, and the Gonbad region of Iran the incidence is approximately 100:100,000.

Tobacco and excessive alcohol intake, known etiologic factors in carcinoma of the oral and respiratory tracts, are also implicated in carcinoma of the esophagus. Tylosis, a genetic disorder inherited by an autosomal dominant trait

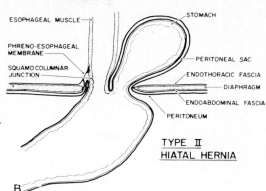

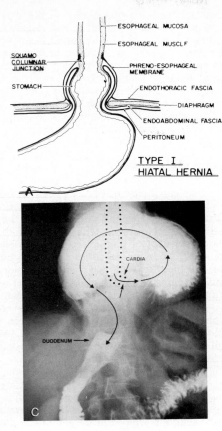

Figure 21. Hiatal hernia. A, Sliding (Type I). B, Paraesophageal (Type II). C, Complete herniation of the stomach above the diaphragm. The duodenum is positioned near the cardia and the stomach is upside down in the mediastinum. Surgical correction is the only treatment when such a hernia is found. (A and B from Skinner, D. B.: Hiatal hernia and gastroesophageal reflux. In Sabiston, D. C., Jr. (Ed.): Davis-Christopher Textbook of Surgery, 12th ed. Philadelphia, W. B. Saunders Company, 1981, p. 823.)

and characterized by marked hyperkeratosis of the palms and soles, has been clearly associated with esophageal cancer. These patients have a 95 per cent probability of succumbing to carcinoma of the esophagus before age 65. Achalasia, Barrett's esophagus, the Plummer-Vinson syndrome, and lye stricture of the esophagus have all been associated with an increased incidence of esophageal cancer.[24]

The American Joint Committee for Cancer Staging and End Results Reporting divided the esophagus into three areas. The cervical esophagus extends from the pharyngoesophageal junction to the level of the thoracic inlet 18 cm. from the incisor teeth, and 15 per cent of carcinomas are located in this area. The upper and middle thoracic esophagus extends from the thoracic inlet to a point 10 cm. above the esophagogastric junction. This is usually located at the level of the 8th thoracic vertebra, 31 cm. from the upper incisor teeth. It is in this area that most esophageal cancers are located (50 per cent). The lower thoracic esophagus, the last 10 cm., contains about 35 per cent of carcinomas.

Pathology

Benign neoplasms of the esophagus are rare. Leiomyomas, polyps, and cysts make up more than 95 per cent of these lesions. The most common are leiomyomas (75 per cent). They occur in the distal esophagus, and half of the affected patients are asymptomatic. Symptomatic patients will present with dysphagia, pain, and nonspecific digestive complaints. The mucosa overlying a leiomyoma is intact. Enucleation is the treatment of choice, but resection may be required for the larger lesions. Other benign tumors of

nonepithelial origin, such as fibromas, lipomas, and neurofibromas, are rare. A histologic classification of esophageal tumors based on the World Health Organization is presented in Table 5.

Benign tumors of epithelial origin such as papillomas, polyps, adenomas, and cysts are also rare. Polyps must be differentiated from carcinomas. Most polyps originate in the cervical esophagus, and a long narrow pedicle may extend into the distal esophagus. Dysphagia is the usual presentation, and regurgitation of the polyp into the mouth has been reported.

TABLE 5. *Histologic Classification of Esophageal Tumors**

Epithelial tumors
Benign
  Squamous papilloma, polyps
Malignant
  Squamous cell carcinoma, adenocarcinoma, adenoid cystic
    carcinoma, mucoepidermoid carcinoma, adenosquamous
    carcinoma, undifferentiated carcinoma

Nonepithelial Tumors
Benign
  Leiomyoma
Malignant
  Leiomyosarcoma

Miscellaneous Tumors
  Carcinosarcoma, malignant melanoma, myoblastoma

Metastatic Tumors to the Esophagus
  Breast, oral cavity, stomach, kidney, prostate, testicle

*Ota, K., and Shin, L. H.: Histological Typing of Gastric and Esophageal Tumors. World Health Organization, 1977.

Squamous cell carcinoma is the most common tumor and accounts for 95 per cent of all malignant lesions in the esophagus. An early lesion usually appears as a flat, grayish, plaque-like thickening of the mucosa. Eventually, this lesion ulcerates with a marked tendency to involve the wall circumferentially and causing luminal narrowing. The esophagus lacks a serosa, and involvement of the surrounding structures is common. The most frequently involved are the trachea, left mainstem bronchus, pericardium, diaphragm, and the large vessels.

Esophageal cancer tends to spread along the submucosal lymphatic plexus, forming satellite nodules under the mucosa at variable distances from the primary tumor. When large, they may also ulcerate into the lumen and masquerade as second primary tumors. Metastasis to lymph nodes distally from the primary lesion stems from the extensive longitudinal and nonsegmental pattern of lymphatic drainage. The most frequent sites of distant metastases are the liver, lung, bone, and kidney.

True adenocarcinomas of the esophagus represent 2 to 4 percent of esophageal malignancies. These lesions usually develop from deep mucous glands or from a columnar-lined esophagus. Malignant non-epithelial tumors of the esophagus are generally leiomyosarcomas. Lymph node and distant metastases are less frequent with this type of tumor. These patients have a better prognosis than do patients with squamous cell carcinoma.

Staging

Carcinoma of the esophagus is staged according to the criteria of the American Joint Committee for Cancer Staging and End Results Reporting (Table 6). Classifications may be determined clinically or at the time of surgical exploration. Accurate staging is obtained only when pathology information is available from the surgical specimen. Stage I disease represents a tumor that involves less than 5 cm. of esophagus without obstruction. There is no circumferential, extraesophageal, nodal, or distant organ involvement. A Stage II lesion involves more than 5 cm. of esophageal length, produces obstruction, or involves the entire circumference of the esophagus without extraesophageal spread. In a cervical lesion, there may be palpable,

movable regional lymph nodes. A Stage III lesion is any esophageal cancer at any level with extraesophageal spread or distant metastases. In the cervical esophagus, metastatic lymph nodes are fixed. Any intrathoracic esophageal cancer with any positive regional lymph node is Stage III. Stage I disease is rarely found in North America. In China, mass cytology screening for this lesion is conducted yearly by scraping the mucosa with an endoesophageal balloon. Seventy per cent of detected cancers are in an early stage, in contrast to 5 per cent in North America.

Clinical Presentation

Early carcinoma of the esophagus is usually asymptomatic. By the time symptoms appear, the lesion is often incurable. Dysphagia and weight loss are the most frequent complaints, occurring in 90 per cent of the patients. At least 60 per cent of the lumen must be obstructed for the patient to experience dysphagia, which occurs late in the course of the disease. Once dysphagia occurs, it progresses rapidly from solids to liquids. The average duration of symptoms is 3 to 4 months and relates poorly to the size, local complications, or survival. In 10 per cent of patients, dysphagia may be absent or minimal even in the presence of an extensive tumor. In these patients, symptoms arise from invasion of the tumor into adjacent structures or from metastases.

Patients over 45 years old complaining of dysphagia should always be carefully observed. Carcinoma as the cause of dysphagia exceeds 70 per cent in this group. Benign esophageal lesions and functional disorders are responsible for the symptomatology in the remaining patients.

Other symptoms and signs result from progression of the disease. These include back pain from spinal involvement, persistent cough from tracheobronchial compression or invasion, cough on swallowing and pneumonia secondary to an esophagotracheal fistula, dysphonia by involvement of the left recurrent laryngeal nerve, Horner's syndrome, and superior vena cava obstruction. Exsanguinating hemorrhage may occur by penetration of the aortic wall. Other ominous findings indicating advanced disease are pleural effusion, ascites, hepatomegaly, palpable cervical or supraclavicular lymph nodes, and bone pain. The oropharynx should be inspected for the presence of a concomitant lesion, which occurs in 10 to 15 per cent of patients.

Investigation

Patients with dysphagia must undergo at least two studies: an esophagogram and an esophagogastroscopy. A small neoplasm can easily be overlooked, especially in the cervical region because the barium transit is rapid at this level. Lesions at the cardia can also be easily missed or can masquerade as achalasia. To exclude the presence of a stricture, both brushings and biopsies must be obtained. When both techniques are done, a pathologic diagnosis can most often be established (see Table 1).

Once a firm diagnosis is obtained, several questions should be answered before deciding on the therapy. Local resectability and the presence or absence of distant metastases must be ascertained by the history, physical examination, and radiologic evaluation. Routine chest films can reveal the presence of a posterior mediastinal tumor with tracheobronchial compression and bony erosion. Metastatic pulmonary nodules or pneumonia secondary to an esophagotracheal fistula may be present. Phrenic nerve involvement can be suspected from diaphragmatic elevation.

TABLE 6. *Staging for Esophageal Carcinomas*

Category	Stage	Extent of Lesion
Primary tumor		
T_1	I	Lesion 5 cm. long, not involving whole circumference and not extending beyond esophagus
T_2	II	Lesion 5 cm. long or involving total circumference
T_3	III	Direct extraesophageal spread
Lymph nodes		
N_0	I	No nodes
N_1	II	Local nodes positive (ipsilateral-cervical)
N_2	II	Bilateral cervical nodes (for cervical lesion only)
N_3	III	Nodes positive and fixed
N_x		Nodes not assessable
Metastases		
M_0	I	No distant metastases
M_1	III	Distant nodes* or metastases

*Thoracic tumor—cervical or celiac; cervical tumor—thoracic or celiac.

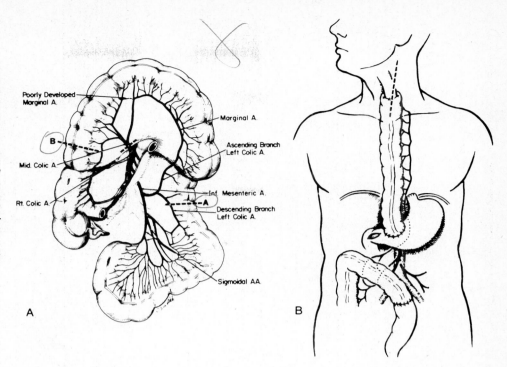

Figure 22. A, Isoperistaltic colon interposition can be pedicled on the left colic artery or the middle colic artery. (From Lafontaine, E. R., and DeMeester, T. R.: Carcinoma of the esophagus. In Copeland, E. M. III (Ed.): Surgical Oncology, Vol. 17. New York, John Wiley & Sons, 1983.) B, The colon is passed behind the stomach and is brought to the neck through the posterior mediastinum or via a substernal tunnel. (From Ellis, F. H., Jr.: Esophagogastrectomy for carcinoma: Technical considerations based on anatomical location of lesion. Surg. Clin. North Am., 60:277, 1980.)

In addition to localization and description of the tumor, the esophagogram is important in the assessment of local resectability. Deformation of the esophageal axis suggests extraesophageal extension and fixation to adjacent mediastinal structures. Advanced local disease is confirmed by demonstration of a tracheoesophageal fistula.

Azygography can provide information as to the patency of the azygos vein overlying the spine. When obstructed, the lesion is usually locally unresectable. *Bronchoscopy* should be done to exclude tracheobronchial involvement. Because of the high frequency of other malignancies in the upper and lower respiratory tract, a careful examination of the oropharynx, larynx, and tracheobronchial tree must be performed. *Mediastinoscopy* can be used to assess the paratracheal lymph nodes. Biopsies should be done for palpable cervical or supraclavicular lymph nodes. Computed tomography (CT) is proving useful to assess local extension to adjacent mediastinal structures and the presence of enlarged lymph nodes.

The presence of metastases to the lungs, liver, and bone should be excluded by appropriate studies. In addition, routine assessment of nutritional status and pulmonary function is essential to determine the operative risk. All these studies attempt to establish a clinical staging and local resectability of the tumor.[15]

Therapy

The main goal of therapy is palliation of dysphagia. Owing to the advanced stage of the disease when diagnosed, most tumors are incurable. With improving preoperative evaluation, the resectability rate should be in the range of 80 to 90 per cent. The main causes of inoperability are the presence of distant metastases, advanced local disease with invasion of the tracheobronchial tree, aorta, or spine, and the general status of the patient.

Preoperative correction of the nutritional deficit is essential, and improvement of pulmonary function is of utmost importance. This is accomplished by cessation of smoking, chest physiotherapy, antibiotics and bronchodi-

lators. Correction of congestive heart failure or other conditions should be completed prior to surgery.

The choice of the optimal surgical therapy remains controversial. When the tumor is resectable, most patients are treated by a standard esophagectomy. The objectives are to achieve a complete excision of the tumor and palliate dysphagia for the remainder of the patient's life.

En bloc esophagectomy and blunt esophagectomy without thoracotomy are variants of the standard operation. When the tumor is locally unresectable, palliation of dysphagia can be obtained by substernal stomach or colon bypass (Fig. 22). Esophageal intubation by endoscopy or laparotomy is an alternative[5] (Table 7).

With the lymphatic anatomy of the esophagus and the majority of carcinomas being in the middle and lower portion, a near-total esophagectomy with anastomosis in the apex of the right chest or in the neck should be favored. The approach is that of Ivor Lewis. The initial stage is a laparotomy for exploration, gastroduodenal mobilization, and pyloromyotomy (Fig. 23A). The lymphatic drainage of the esophagus flows along the lesser curvature of the stomach down to the level of the 4th branch of the left gastric artery. The gastric tube is thus prepared to resect the cardia in continuity with the small curvature of the stomach. A right thoracotomy follows the abdominal operation. Resection of the esophagus and lymphatic drainage

TABLE 7. Esophageal Carcinoma

Possible Treatments

Total esophagectomy (standard, radical, blunt)
Total esophagectomy with laryngectomy and neck dissection
Radiation therapy
Palliative intubation (push-through, pull-through)
Bypass procedure with resection or exclusion
Chemotherapy

Reconstruction Options after Esophageal Resection

Gastric interposition (Fig. 22)
Colon interposition (Fig. 23)
Reverse or isoperistaltic gastric tubes
Jejunal interposition or free transplant

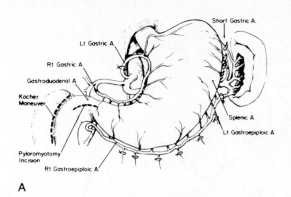

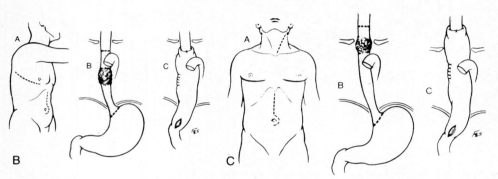

Figure 23. A, *Gastroduodenal mobilization and pyloromyotomy in preparation for gastric replacement of the esophagus. (From Lafontaine, E. R., and DeMeester, T. R.: Carcinoma of the esophagus. In Copeland, E. M. III (Ed.): Surgical Oncology, Vol. 17. New York, John Wiley & Sons, 1983.) B, Ivor Lewis procedure. A right thoracic approach follows the abdominal operation. Reconstruction is completed by a terminolateral esophagogastrostomy in the apex of the chest. C, Reconstruction through a left cervical approach. The stomach can be placed retrosternally or through the posterior mediastinum if the esophagus has been removed. (B and C from Ellis, F. H., Jr.: Esophagogastrectomy for carcinoma: Technical considerations based on anatomical location of lesion. Surg. Clin. North Am., 60:275, 1980.)*

are completed after pulling the stomach into the chest. The continuity is re-established by a terminolateral anastomosis at the apex of the right chest[14] (Fig. 23B). As an alternative to the Lewis procedure, the stomach can be passed retrosternally while the patient is supine and reconstruction is performed through a left cervical incision. This is followed by a right posterolateral thoracotomy to resect the esophagus (Fig. 23C). The location in the anterior mediastinum of the reconstruction is thought preferable to prevent obstruction of the interposed gut by persistent or recurrent tumor. Pulmonary complications and anastomotic failure are the most frequent causes of morbidity and death after surgical treatment. Current mortality is 10 to 15 per cent.

Radiotherapy offered as curative treatment does not control the disease, and 80 per cent of the patients present with recurrent esophageal obstruction within a year. When used as adjuvant preoperative therapy, it may play a role in improving resectability but fails to improve survival. Curative or adjuvant chemotherapy now brings a definite but short response of the tumor without significant benefit in survival.

The average duration of life after the diagnosis is established is less than 3 months for the untreated patient. Survival depends on the extent of the disease at the time of resection. Lymph node involvement and extraesophageal extension carry a poor prognosis with few 5-year survivors. Stage I lesions without nodal involvement carry a 20 per cent 5-year survival.[5]

SELECTED REFERENCES

Dodds, W. J., Hogan, W. J., Helm, J. F., and Dent, J.: Pathogenesis of reflux esophagitis. Gastroenterology, 81:376, 1981.
  Excellent review article on the different mechanisms involved in the production of gastroesophageal reflux. All the contributory factors to the development of reflux are explained in detail.

Hurwitz, A. L., Duranceau, A., and Haddad, J. K.: Disorders of esophageal motility. *In* Major Problems in Internal Medicine; Vol.16. Philadelphia, W.B. Saunders Company, 1979.
  A monograph that is a complete summary on esophageal manometric technique and the approach to the patient with disordered swallowing. Oropharyngeal dysphagia, disorders of motility in the esophageal body, and abnormalities of the lower esophageal sphincter are reviewed. The physiologic effects of surgery on the esophagus are presented.

Mannel, A.: Carcinoma of the esophagus. Curr. Probl. Surg., 14:554, 1982.
  The overall presentation, assessment, and treatment of the patient with carcinoma of the esophagus are reviewed. Precise up-to-date information is presented.

Postlethwait, R. W.: Surgery of the Esophagus. Norwalk, Conn., Appleton-Century-Crofts, 1986.
  The most comprehensive text and review on the whole spectrum of esophageal diseases. An up-to-date book that covers the subject in a complete but concise manner with a first-class bibliography for each individual chapter.

Skinner, D. B., and DeMeester, T. R.: Gastroesophageal reflux. Curr. Probl. Surg. 13:5, 1976.
  Detailed review of the various tests and their accuracy in predicting the presence of reflux. An excellent review of gastroesophageal reflux treatment with descriptions of the most frequently used operative procedures.

REFERENCES

1. Bennett, J. R., and Hendrix, T. R.: Diffuse esophageal spasm: A disorder with more than one cause. Gastroenterology, 59:273, 1970.
2. DeMeester, T. R., Johnson, L. F., Joseph, G. J., Toscano, M. S., Hall, A. W., and Skinner, D. B.: Patterns of gastroesophageal reflux in health and disease. Ann. Surg., 184:459, 1976.
3. Dodds, W. J., Hogan, W. J., Helm, J. F., and Dent, J.: Pathogenesis of reflux esophagitis. Gastroenterology, 81:376, 1981.
4. Duranceau, A. C., Devroede, G., Lafontaine, E., and Jamieson, G. G.: Esophageal motility in asymptomatic volunteers. Surg. Clin. North Am., 63:777, 1983.
5. Earlam, R., and Cunha-Melo, J. R.: Esophageal squamous cell carcinoma: I. A critical review of surgery. Br. J. Surg., 67:381, 1980.
6. Ellis, F. H., and Olsen, A. M.: Achalasia of the esophagus. *In* Major Problems in Clinical Surgery, Vol. 9. Philadelphia, W.B. Saunders Company, 1969.

7. Gibbs, D.: Endoscopy in the assessment of reflux esophagitis. Clin. Gastroenterol., *5*:135, 1976.

8. Gray's Anatomy, 36th Ed. Williams, P., and Warwick, R. (Eds.). New York, Churchill Livingstone, 1980.

9. Haller J. A., Andrews, H. G., White, J. J., Tamer, M. A. and Cleveland, W. W.: Pathophysiology and management of acute corrosive burns of the esophagus: Results of treatment in 285 children., J. Pediatr. Surg., *6*:578, 1971.

10. Hurwitz, A. L., Duranceau, A., and Haddad, J. K.: Disorders of esophageal motility. *In* Major Problems in Internal Medicine, Vol. 16. Philadelphia, W. B. Saunders Company, 1979.

11. Johnson, L. F., DeMeester, T. R., and Haggitt, R. C.: Endoscopic signs for gastroesophageal reflux objectively evaluated. Gastrointest. Endosc. *22*:151, 1976.

12. Kilman, W. J., and Goyal, R. K.: Disorders of pharyngeal and upper esophageal sphincter motor function. Arch. Intern. Med., *136*:592, 1976.

13. Kirsh, M. M., and Ritter, F.: Caustic ingestion and subsequent damage to the oropharyngeal and digestive passages. Ann. Thorac. Surg. *21*:74, 1976.

14. Lewis, I.: The surgical treatment of carcinoma of the esophagus; With special reference to a new operation for growths of the middle third. Br. J. Surg. *34*:18, 1946.

15. Mannel, A.: Carcinoma of the esophagus. Curr. Probl. Surg., *14*:554, 1982.

16. Michel, L., Grillo, H. C., and Malt, R. A.: Esophageal perforation. Ann. Thorac. Surg., *33*:203, 1982.

17. Murray, G. F.: Operation for motor dysfunction of the esophagus. Ann Thorac. Surg. *29*:184, 1980.

18. Palmer, E. D.: Disorders of the cricopharyngeus muscle: A review. Gastroenterology, *71*:510, 1976.

19. Postlethwait, R. W.: Surgery of the Esophagus. Norwalk, Conn., Appleton-Century-Crofts, 1986.

20. Richter, J. E., and Castell, D. O.: Gastroesophageal reflux. Pathogenesis, diagnosis and therapy. Ann Intern. Med., *97*:93, 1982.

21. Rouvière, H.: Anatomie des lymphatiques de l'homme. Paris, Masson & Cie, 1932.

22. Skinner, D. B., and DeMeester, T. R.: Gastroesophageal reflux. Curr. Probl. Surg. *13*:5, 1976.

23. Skinner, D. B., Little, A. G., and DeMeester, T. R.: Management of esophageal perforation. Am. J. Surg. *139*:760, 1980.

24. Warwick, G. P., and Harrington, J. S.: Some aspects of the epidemiology and etiology of esophageal cancer with particular emphasis on the Transkei, South Africa. Adv. Cancer Res. *17*:81, 1973.

25. Watts, H. D.: Lesions brought on by vomiting: The effect of hiatus hernia on the site of injury. Gastroenterology, *71*:683, 1976.

THE ACUTE ABDOMEN

JOHN A. MORRIS, JR., M.D. • JOHN L. SAWYERS, M.D.

22

GENERAL CONSIDERATIONS

Pain, anorexia, nausea, vomiting, and fever are characteristic manifestations of an acute abdominal disorder. Important signs on physical examination include tenderness, guarding, and changes in intestinal peristalsis. The critical distinction, however, is not between the acute and nonacute abdomen but between the *surgical* abdomen and the *nonsurgical* abdomen. The identification of the surgical abdomen depends on the use of three basic diagnostic components: the history, physical examination, and ancillary tests.

History

The history can be divided into several major categories: age, sex, abdominal pain, and systemic symptoms.

AGE AND SEX

The very old and very young each represent approximately 10 per cent of patient presentations with acute abdominal pain. However, patients over the age of 65 have twice the incidence of surgical disease (30 per cent) as a cause for their abdominal pain compared with those patients below the age of 65.[3] In the adult age group, females are more likely to present with abdominal pain than males, but those males who do present with these symptoms have a higher incidence of *surgical* disease. The genitourinary system commonly causes abdominal pain in females. In decreasing order of presentation, common genitourinary causes of abdominal pain in women include pelvic inflammatory disease, urinary tract infection, dysmenorrhea, and ectopic pregnancy.

PAIN

Pain is the hallmark of the acute abdomen. It may be characterized by its mode of onset, character, precipitating factors, or its localization. There are three types of onset of abdominal pain: explosive, rapid, and gradual.

The patient suddenly seized with *explosive,* agonizing pain is most likely to have ruptured a hollow viscus into the free peritoneal cavity or to have sustained a vascular accident. Colic of renal and biliary origin may be sudden in onset but seldom causes pain so severe as to prostrate the patient. The patient with *rapid* onset of pain that quickly becomes worse is likely to have acute pancreatitis, mesenteric thrombosis, or strangulation of the small bowel. The patient with *gradual* onset of pain is likely to have peritoneal inflammation, such as that seen in appendicitis or diverticulitis.

The severity of the pain may be characterized as excruciating, severe, dull, or colicky. *Excruciating* pain unresponsive to narcotics suggests an acute vascular lesion such as rupture of an abdominal aneurysm or infarction of the intestine. Patients with intestinal infarction characteristically have pain out of proportion to both physical and laboratory findings. Pain that is *severe* but readily controlled by medication is characteristic of peritonitis from a ruptured viscus or acute pancreatitis. *Dull,* vague, poorly localized pain suggests an inflammatory process and is a common initial presentation of appendicitis. *Colicky* pain, characterized as cramps and rushes, is suggestive of gastroenteritis. The pain from mechanical small bowel obstruction is also colicky but has a rhythmic pattern with pain-free intervals alternating with severe colic. Peristaltic rushes may be heard during the severe colic. The peristaltic rushes associated with gastroenteritis are not necessarily coordinated with the colicky pain.

A useful clinical feature is the relation of the *location* of pain distribution to organ involvement. The site of abdominal pain is a reflection of the type of nerve stimulation and the organ's embryologic origins. Poorly localized pain sensations from the abdomen are mediated through the autonomic nervous system associated with the intraabdominal viscera. The spinal nerve fibers provide well-localized innervation from the parietal peritoneum, diaphragm, and pelvic walls. Poorly localized pain can usually be ascribed to one of three abdominal areas: the epigastrium, the periumbilical area, and the hypogastrium.

The stomach and duodenum originate from the foregut, and pain from these organs is typically felt in the *epigastrium.* The small intestine and proximal colon nourished by the superior mesenteric artery are derived from the midgut, and pain in this portion of the gastrointestinal tract is *periumbilical.* Pain that originates in the distal two thirds of the colon is embryologically derived from the hindgut and is characteristically referred to the *hypogastrium* (Fig. 1).

Flank pain and pain in the costovertebral angle are associated with renal or ureteral stones or with pyelonephritis. Renal pain may also be associated with pain in the ipsilateral testis. Irritation of the diaphragm may result in pain in the region of the distribution of C4. Thus inflammatory processes of the liver or spleen or a subdiaphrag-

A. FOREGUT DERIVATIVES
B. MIDGUT DERIVATIVES
C. HINDGUT DERIVATIVES

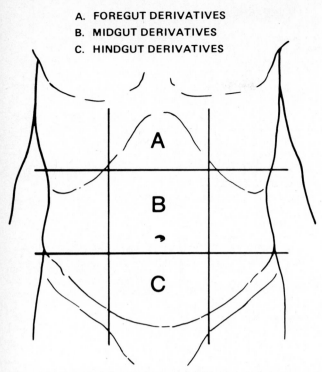

Figure 1. Location of abdominal pain is related to the embryologic development of the involved organs.

matic collection of fluid from a perforated ulcer may refer pain to the shoulder.

Significant information is derived by eliciting the aggravating or alleviating factors associated with pain. For example, heartburn may be experienced only when abdominal pressure is increased. Pain that improves with ingestion of antacids suggests peptic ulcer disease, whereas pain exacerbated by a fatty meal suggests cholecystitis.

Obtaining a careful history for *systemic symptoms* is important in any acute abdominal evaluation. Although some degree of fever is common to most surgical emergencies, it is unusual for a patient with a surgical abdomen to present with fever and *chills*. Surgical conditions that do present with high fever and chills include pylephlebitis and suppurative cholangitis. More commonly, abdominal pain accompanied by high fever and chills is associated with *medical* disease including pelvic inflammatory disease and urinary tract infections. Other systemic symptoms that should alert the physician to the possibility of medical disease include profuse diarrhea, active joint symptoms, skin eruptions appearing at the onset of abdominal pain, and urethral or vaginal discharge. Anorexia, nausea, and vomiting are frequent concomitants of acute abdominal disease. They may help distinguish medical from surgical disease. If nausea and vomiting precede the onset of abdominal pain, surgical disease is less likely.

The assessment of the symptoms of diarrhea, constipation, and obstipation is a critical part of any history for abdominal pain. If it can be ascertained that the patient has passed no gas per rectum and has had no bowel movements for 24 hours, the probability of bowel obstruction is high. Diarrhea is commonly associated with gastroenteritis, but it may be associated with surgical disease such as appendicitis. Bloody, repetitive diarrhea indicates a diagnosis compatible with ulcerative colitis, Crohn's disease, dysentery, or colonic ischemia.

The past medical history should include all previous hospitalizations and operations. In difficult diagnostic problems, questioning should include an extensive family history (Table 1) as well as history of medications, exposure to toxins, and foreign travel.[16]

Physical Examination

When a patient presents with abdominal pain, the history is a data base for review of the diagnostic possibilities, but the decision as to whether or not to operate is made on the basis of *physical examination,* which should be performed in an orderly and systematic manner. The six major features of physical examination include (1) inspection, (2) auscultation, (3) palpation, (4) percussion, (5) rectal/genital examination, and (6) special tests and signs.

INSPECTION

The patient's general appearance may provide a clue to the nature of the disease. Changes in mental status, skin color and turgor, and sunken eyes may all be manifestations of severe hypovolemia and impending cardiovascular collapse. The patient with isolated visceral pain, such as that found in bowel obstruction, may change position frequently, but if the pain is localized or general peritoneal irritation is present, the patient often avoids movement.

The patient's anatomic position in bed is noteworthy. Patients with extensive peritonitis often bring their knees up to relax abdominal tension. Patients with an inflammatory condition in contact with the psoas muscle may flex the corresponding thigh. Patients with severe pancreatitis may sit up in bed with their knees drawn to their chest, rocking back and forth in paroxysms of pain.

The abdomen should be inspected for signs of distention. In thin individuals with long-standing bowel obstruction, rushes may be seen on the anterior abdominal wall. Pulsation in the epigastric area is compatible with aneurysmal disease.

AUSCULTATION

Auscultation is performed prior to palpation because palpation may change the character of bowel sounds. The technique of auscultation requires gentle placement of the bell of the stethoscope on the anterior abdominal wall beginning with the left lower quadrant, then in all four quadrants. An auscultation period of 2 to 3 minutes is necessary to determine that no bowel sounds are present. This time also allows the uninterrupted observation of the patient's face and demeanor. High-pitched bowel sounds occurring in rushes that coincide with pain are indicative of small bowel obstruction.

PALPATION

Of all aspects of the physical examination, *palpation* is probably the most important to the surgeon. Inguinal, femoral, and ventral hernia sites must be carefully examined

TABLE 1. *Familial Conditions Causing Acute Abdomen*

Acute intermittent porphyria
Familial hyperlipoproteinuria
Familial Mediterranean fever
Hemochromatosis
Sickle cell disease

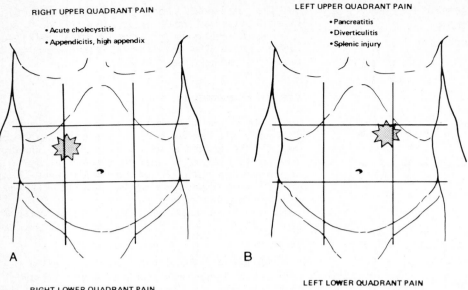

RIGHT UPPER QUADRANT PAIN

- Acute cholecystitis
- Appendicitis, high appendix

LEFT UPPER QUADRANT PAIN

- Pancreatitis
- Diverticulitis
- Splenic injury

A   B

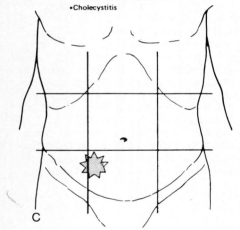

RIGHT LOWER QUADRANT PAIN

- Appendicitis
- Pelvic inflammatory disease
- Cholecystitis

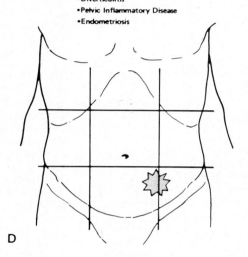

LEFT LOWER QUADRANT PAIN

- Diverticulitis
- Pelvic Inflammatory Disease
- Endometriosis

C   D

Figure 2. A–D, *Location of abdominal pain from various acute abdominal conditions.*

in every patient with abdominal pain. Incarceration of a segment of bowel in a small femoral hernia can easily be overlooked. The only sign of a Richter's hernia may be point tenderness over the hernia site. Coughing often elicits pain in the abdomen, and the patient should be asked to indicate with one finger the point of maximal intensity. This localizes the lesion when generalized peritonitis is not present and provides the clinician with an initial list of working diagnoses (Fig. 2).

Palpation should begin as far away from the pain epicenter as possible, and it should be performed gently with one finger. Gradually, the finger should move toward the area of maximal tenderness. It is then necessary to establish the presence of guarding or "spasm." Place the hand gently over the rectus muscle and depress slightly and request the patient to take a deep breath. If spasm is voluntary, the surgeon will feel the underlying rectus muscle relax. If there is true spasm, however, the surgeon feels a taut, rigid muscle throughout the respiratory cycle. Often this maneuver will establish the presence of peritonitis.

If the lesion is located within the abdominal wall, the tenderness will persist. However, if the lesion is intraperitoneal, the tenderness will decrease as long as the rectus

muscles remain tense.[17] In pelvic inflammatory disease, rigidity is often absent. In elderly feeble patients, muscular rigidity may be absent despite peritonitis. Gastroenteritis is characteristically accompanied by diffuse abdominal tenderness with no muscular rigidity.

PERCUSSION

Percussion of the abdomen should always be performed with great gentleness. It is useful in estimating the amount of distention associated with bowel obstruction and can be used to exclude the presence of a distended urinary bladder as a cause of acute abdominal pain. Perhaps most important, percussion is useful in eliciting costovertebral angle tenderness associated with urinary tract infection or gallbladder disease.

RECTAL AND PELVIC EXAMINATIONS

No examination for surgical causes of abdominal pain is complete without a rectal and/or vaginal examination. In males specific palpation of the contents of the scrotal sac, including testes and epididymis, is essential. Rectal examination in the male is performed with the patient lying on his side with a well-lubricated finger gently introduced into the rectum. By pressing anteriorly, posteriorly, and laterally, the whole lower pelvis can be evaluated.

Anteriorly, one may detect an enlarged prostate, distended bladder, or enlargement of the seminal vesicles. Laterally, tenderness due to an inflamed appendix or an abscess on the lateral wall of the pelvis can be elicited. Posteriorly, palpation may indicate the presence of an inflammatory mass on the pyriformis or in the depression of the sacrum. Following rectal examination, the finger should be examined for the presence of blood or pus, and a small sample of stool should be tested for occult blood by the guaiac test. In patients with a colostomy or ileostomy, digital examination of the stoma is mandatory.

In the female, bimanual examination is essential, and a speculum should be inserted and cultures of the cervix obtained. Bimanual palpation includes a search for cervical tenderness associated with pelvic inflammatory disease as well as palpation of the uterus and both adnexa. A rectal examination, performed simultaneously with vaginal examination, will delineate both inflammatory and neoplastic processes within the cul-de-sac.

SPECIAL TESTS AND SIGNS

Two tests are of primary clinical importance in confirming a diagnosis already made by history and physical examination. The tests include the *iliopsoas* test and the *obturator* test.

The *iliopsoas* test is used to confirm the presence of an inflamed focus in the corresponding psoas muscle (Fig. 3). The patient is placed with the nonpainful side dependent and with one hand stabilizing the pelvis and the other hand placed on the knee; the leg on the painful side is moved in an anteroposterior direction. Pain will be caused by this maneuver if the psoas muscle is rigid from either reflex or direct irritation. This test is not useful if abdominal rigidity is already present.

With the *obturator* test, the patient is placed in the supine position with the knee flexed, and the hip joint is

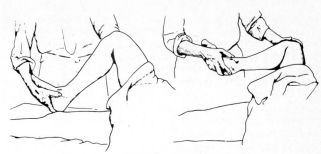

Figure 4. Steps in performing the obturator test.

put in internal and then external rotation (Fig. 4). If the test is positive, external rotation will cause hypogastric pain. A positive sign is associated with a perforated appendix, localized abscess, or the presence of an obturator hernia.

There are three signs commonly associated with examination of the acute abdomen:

1. *Cullen's sign* is periumbilical discoloration, which is present in the patient with extensive hemoperitoneum. Although the sign is dramatic when present, it is frequently not evident despite serious intraperitoneal hemorrhage.

2. *Murphy's sign* is helpful in diagnosing an acutely inflamed gallbladder. The examiner exerts pressure in the right upper quadrant and the patient is asked to inhale deeply. The inspiration causes the liver to descend, causing the inflamed gallbladder to strike the examining fingers. The patient consequently experiences pain and the inspiratory effort stops.

3. *Rovsing's sign* is present when right lower quadrant pain is caused by palpation of the left lower quadrant (Fig. 5). It is often associated with appendicitis.

Confirmatory Tests

In the patient presenting with abdominal pain, the diagnostic possibilities are considered while the history is

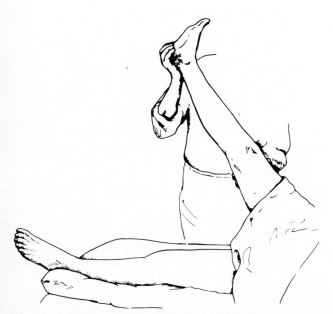

Figure 3. Iliopsoas test may confirm the presence of an inflammatory process near the psoas muscle.

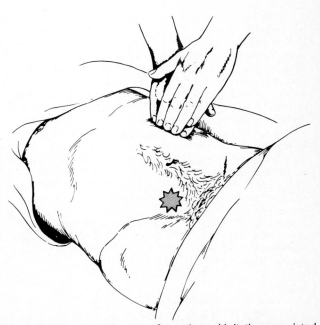

Figure 5. Rovsing's sign, a test for peritoneal irritation associated with appendicitis.

obtained. The physical examination limits the list of possible diagnoses to the most likely diagnosis with several alternatives. Confirmatory tests provide additional information to aid the surgeon in planning therapy. In a majority of patients the decision to operate or not operate is made on the basis of the history and physical examination.

Confirmatory tests are divided into two major categories: x-ray examination and laboratory examination. It is estimated that more than 4 million plain films of the abdomen are obtained each year in the United States at a cost of more than $300 million.[5] It is incumbent on the physician to be selective in patients in whom additional confirmatory tests are ordered.

X-RAY EXAMINATION

The films obtained in an acute abdominal series have traditionally been the most commonly ordered confirmatory test in these patients. This series consists of a flat and upright film of the abdomen and an anteroposterior view of the chest. The upright chest film is the best film for determining free air in the abdomen. It is helpful also in excluding thoracic disease as a cause of nonoperative abdominal pain. Plain abdominal radiographs should be ordered in those patients with moderate to severe abdominal pain and tenderness in whom the diagnosis is uncertain or in patients who have a clinical suspicion of bowel obstruction, renal stones, or ischemia. Abdominal films are not helpful in those patients with convincing evidence of appendicitis, gynecologic disease, mild abdominal pain, or abdominal pain that has persisted longer than 1 week.

Once it has been decided to order an acute abdominal series, one must approach the films in a systematic fashion, looking specifically at the solid viscera, hollow viscera, abdominal lines, calcifications, and extraintestinal air (Fig. 6). The outlines of the liver, spleen, and kidney are clearly definable on plain abdominal films. The presence of cystic masses in any of the viscera must be noted. Displacement of the kidney may indicate a urologic lesion as a cause for the acute abdominal process. Enlargement of the splenic shadow or displacement of the kidney may also suggest a renal origin of the abdominal pain.

Gas patterns within hollow viscera provide important information. These gas patterns are more readily recognized if the stomach has been decompressed by a nasogastric tube. Residual gas within the stomach suggests a high-grade obstruction of the small bowel or perhaps pyloric obstruction secondary to duodenal ulcer disease. Dilated loops of small bowel disease with air fluid levels and no gas in the colon are suggestive of small bowel obstruction. Marked dilatation and rotation of the cecum or sigmoid colon are typical of volvulus. Marked dilatation of the entire colon suggests colonic obstruction, and one should identify the fact that there is no air in the rectal vault. Massive dilatation of the colon with a history of acute colitis indicates toxic megacolon. Free air under the diaphragm or outlining loops of small bowel is highly suggestive of visceral perforation. An encapsulated air shadow outside the contours of the bowel may indicate a localized perforation of the intestine. Air in the biliary tract is diagnostic of a communication between the gastrointestinal tract and the biliary tree and may be seen with gallstone ileus. Air in the portal venous system may be seen in pylephlebitis or with gangrenous bowel.

Two helpful *abdominal lines* are peritoneal fat lines and the psoas shadow. Peritoneal fat lines are obscured when fluid is present in the abdomen. This fluid may be due to ascites, blood, or pus. Obliteration of the psoas

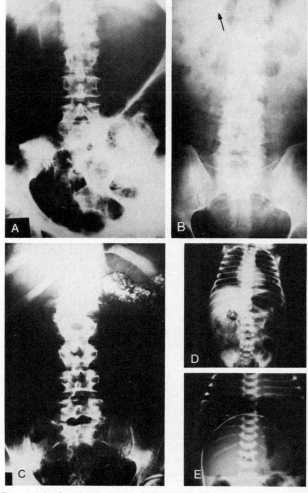

Figure 6. A, *Cecal volvulus.* B, *Gallstone.* C, *Pancreatic calcifications.* D, *Air in the portal vein and obscured peritoneal fat lines.* E, *Free air in abdomen.*

shadow may indicate a retroperitoneal hematoma or abscess.

A thorough search for *calcifications* should always be made. There may be discrete opaque masses such as gallstones, kidney stones, or fecalith, or the calcifications may be subtler, such as is found in lymph nodes, soft tissue masses, the wall of the aorta with associated atherosclerosis, or the pancreas with chronic pancreatitis.

Ultrasound is the test of choice in those patients with suspected gallstone disease as an etiology for abdominal pain. In addition, ultrasound is helpful in the diagnosis of gynecologic disorders leading to abdominal pain including ectopic pregnancy.

For those patients presenting with hematuria and colicky abdominal pain and in whom renal calculi are suspected, a plain film of the abdomen and *intravenous pyelogram* are the procedures of choice. Occasionally, a *barium enema* may be performed in the patient with an acute abdomen. This is usually done after acute abdominal series demonstrate intussusception or in patients in whom the suspected diagnosis is diverticulitis.

LABORATORY TESTS

A complete blood count and serum electrolytes are routinely obtained in patients presenting with abdominal pain. The hematocrit reflects chronic changes in plasma volume, and an elevated hematocrit may reflect dehydration secondary to vomiting or fluid sequestration. A low hematocrit may indicate pre-existing anemia or chronic bleeding.

An elevated white blood count is usually significant. However, it is common for elderly patients to have normal or low white blood counts even in the presence of established peritonitis.[18] A lymphocytosis may suggest a viral infection or gastroenteritis. Marked leukopenia may suggest a primary blood disorder or overwhelming sepsis.

Even more important than the initial blood count is the trend toward a progressively rising leukocyte count, indicating the progression of an inflammatory or septic process. A left shift on the peripheral blood smear is another strong indication of an inflammatory condition, even in the presence of a normal or mildly elevated white count.

The serum amylase should be obtained if pancreatitis is suspected. It may also be elevated in patients with mesenteric thrombosis, intestinal obstruction, or perforated duodenal ulcer. The elevation of the serum amylase is not a reflection of the severity of pancreatitis, and the amylase level may be normal in patients with severe hemorrhagic pancreatitis just prior to cardiovascular collapse. In patients with chronic pancreatitis, serum amylase levels may be only mildly elevated.

Examination of the urine is essential and provides helpful clinical information. In patients presenting with acute onset of abdominal pain, pyuria is indicative of urinary tract infection, hematuria is suggestive of renal calculi, and glycosuria suggests diabetes but may be associated with other catastrophic abdominal conditions. Urine specific gravity reflects the kidney's ability to concentrate and is commonly elevated in patients with acute abdominal pain and dehydration.

In summary, the intelligent approach to the patient with abdominal pain includes a detailed history that takes into account the patient's age, sex, systemic symptoms, and past medical history. These facts provide a framework for more detailed questioning about the pain, its mode of onset, character, precipitating factors, and location. At the completion of the history-taking process, the physician should have in mind a working diagnosis and several alternatives. The physical examination is used to support or reject the working diagnosis; more important, however, physical examination is an essential component of the operative/nonoperative decision. Confirmatory tests are also used to support or reject the working diagnosis. They should be employed judiciously and used only if the results will alter therapy.

SPECIFIC CAUSES OF THE ACUTE ABDOMEN

Common causes of acute abdominal pain can be divided into three major pathologic groups: (1) inflammatory lesions, (2) obstructive lesions, and (3) vascular disorders. Each of these pathologic conditions has a characteristic pain pattern that helps the clinician establish the working diagnosis. Inflammatory lesions present with a gradual onset of dull, poorly localized pain. Obstructive lesions present with a crampy, colicky pain interspersed with pain-free intervals. Vascular lesions present with explosive or rapid onset of excruciating pain that may be unrelieved by narcotics. A series of common causes of abdominal pain listed by pathologic grouping is shown in Table 2.

TABLE 2. *Pathologic Grouping of Common Causes of Acute Abdominal Pain*

Inflammation
Appendicitis
Diverticulitis
Cholecystitis
Perforated peptic ulcer
Acute pancreatitis

Obstruction
Adhesive bands
Hernia
Intussusception
Carcinoma
Diverticular disease
Volvulus

Vascular Disorders
Aortic aneurysm rupture
Acute mesenteric ischemia

Appendicitis

Acute appendicitis is the most common cause of the surgical acute abdomen in patients under the age of 30. One patient out of 15 can expect to develop acute appendicitis during his lifetime. Acute appendicitis is actually more than a single disease entity. In terms of physical signs and symptoms, appendicitis is a prototype disease that proceeds through inflammation, obstruction, and ischemia within a variable time frame. The patient's symptoms reflect the state of the disease process in the time course of the illness.

NATURAL HISTORY

In most patients, and especially in those in younger age groups, appendicitis is due to hyperplasia of submucosal lymphoid follicles, causing obstruction of the appendiceal lumen. Mucosal secretion continues despite the obstructed lumen, and pressure within the appendix builds. As intraluminal pressure increases lymphatics become obstructed, leading to appendiceal edema. This is the stage of acute focal appendicitis characterized by early bacterial extravasation. Because the appendix and the small bowel have the same nerve supply, visceral pain is first perceived as dull, vague pain in the periumbilical area.

The second stage of appendicitis, acute suppurative appendicitis, is characterized by a further rise in intraluminal pressure, venous obstruction, focal ischemia, and serosal irritation. When the inflamed serosa of the appendix is adjacent to the peritoneal peritoneum, the patient experiences migration of the periumbilical pain to the right lower quadrant. This well-localized somatic pain heralds the compromise of arterial blood supply, and the ischemia results in small infarcts along the antimesenteric border of the appendix. This stage of gangrenous appendicitis is associated with increased bacterial extravasation and localized contamination of the peritoneal cavity. Progression leads to perforation and either a localized periappendiceal mass or generalized peritonitis.

Thus, appendicitis progresses through an inflammatory stage, an obstructive stage, an ischemic stage, and a perforative stage, all of which reflect different physical signs and symptoms. Unfortunately, the time frame for the progression of these clinical events is highly variable. Appendicitis is rare in infancy. Approximately 10 per cent of patients with appendicitis are less than 10 years of age or

REFERRED PAIN

The initial pain of appendicitis is usually felt in the epigastrium.

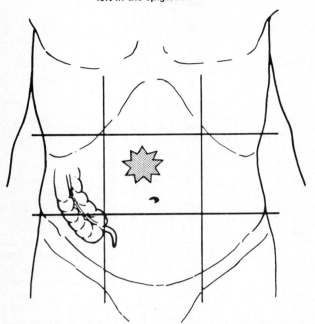

Figure 7. Acute appendicitis initially presents as periumbilical pain.

greater than 50 years of age. The very young and the very old are at higher risk for perforation because atypical presentations are common in these two groups, and infants have few ways to communicate the onset of a problem. Acute appendicitis has a peak incidence in the teens and early 20s with a decline after age 30.

Patients with acute appendicitis present with abdominal pain, and the location of the pain depends on the stage of the disease and the location of the appendix. Typical appendicitis presents with a history of dull, vague, epigastric or periumbilical pain accompanied by anorexia (90 per cent), nausea (80 per cent), and vomiting (65 per cent) (Fig. 7).[13] The incidence of this symptom complex is nearly identical in acute appendicitis, mesenteric adenitis, gastroenteritis, and abdominal pain of unknown cause.

The diagnosis of appendicitis at this stage is difficult. Patients in whom pain has not localized and in whom the duration of symptoms is less than 8 hours can usually be hydrated and observed. As the disease progresses from acute focal appendicitis to acute suppurative appendicitis, typically the pain localizes in the right lower quadrant. If, however, the appendix is retrocecal, the pain localizes in the right flank, mimicking renal colic. If the patient is in the third trimester of pregnancy, the appendix may be displaced cephalad and the pain may be localized to the right upper quadrant.

PHYSICAL EXAMINATION

Patients with appendicitis rarely show signs of systemic toxicity. They may walk in a slightly bent manner. Their attitude in bed tends to be immobile, often with the right leg flexed (Fig. 8). Direct inspection of the abdomen is usually unremarkable, and neither auscultation nor percussion is particularly helpful in the patient with appendicitis. Gentle palpation of the abdomen is critical in making the

decision whether operation is indicated in a patient with suspected appendicitis. Palpation should begin in the left lower quadrant, proceeding to the left upper quadrant, the right upper quadrant, and concluding with an examination of the right lower quadrant. Occasionally, in late appendicitis a mass can be detected. The presence of right lower quadrant tenderness with right lower quadrant muscle spasm is an indication for operation unless there is some other clue that appendicitis may not be the primary diagnosis.

Rectal and pelvic examinations should be performed in all patients with appendicitis. In atypical appendicitis, pain may not localize from the periumbilical region, but right lower quadrant rectal tenderness can be elicited. The presence of cervical tenderness or discharge in a young female with right lower quadrant pain leads one toward the diagnosis of pelvic inflammatory disease. Rovsing's sign may be positive in the presence of suppurative appendicitis. The psoas and obturator signs may also be present in appendicitis, but they are less reliable than Rovsing's sign.

CONFIRMATORY TESTS

Acute abdominal series is not helpful in patients in whom the diagnosis of appendicitis is clear. However, in those patients with atypical presentation in whom the possibility of perforated ulcer, bowel obstruction, or nephrolithiasis is being entertained, x-rays may be helpful. An intravenous pyelogram may uncover a urinary tract disorder such as renal colic. In the past, barium enema has been suggested as a helpful adjunct to the diagnosis of appendicitis in complicated cases. Because this modality is time-consuming and frequently leads to equivocal results, it is now seldom used.

Typically some three quarters of patients with acute appendicitis present with a white count greater than 10,000. The median white count is about 12,000; however, a white count greater than 20,000 is cause to re-evaluate the diagnosis. Less than 4 per cent of patients with acute appendicitis have both a normal differential and a normal total white count. Examination of the urine is useful in excluding other causes of right lower quadrant pain. The presence of bacteria or significant hematuria suggests a general urinary etiology for the pain. However, a significant number of young males with appendicitis will present with occasional white blood cells in the urine.

DIFFERENTIAL DIAGNOSIS

Differential diagnosis of appendicitis is a function of age and sex. Patients may be divided into three age groups: children (defined as age 10 or younger), the elderly (defined as age 50 or older), and teenagers and adults (defined as

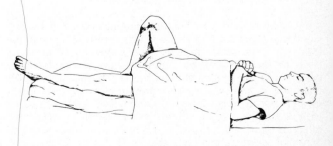

"ATTITUDE" APPENDICITIS

Figure 8. Typical position of patient with acute appendicitis.

age 10 to 50). Because appendicitis is infrequent in the younger age group, it is often considered a more serious disease. Not only is it diagnosed late, but in children the omentum tends to be short and may fail to wall off a perforation of the appendix. Appendicitis is rare below the age of 3 but increases progressively between ages 3 and 10. The differential diagnosis of acute abdominal pain in infancy includes colic, acute gastroenteritis, intussusception, incarcerated hernia, and volvulus. Recurrent bouts of partial intestinal obstruction in infants can be secondary to congenital causes such as intestinal stenosis, anular pancreas, and midgut malrotation.

In the preschool age group (2 to 5 years), appendicitis remains rare. Other causes of acute abdominal pain in this age group include acute gastroenteritis, pyelonephritis, Meckel's diverticulum, and intussusception. School age children (5 to 10 years) show a steady increase in the incidence of appendicitis with age. Gastroenteritis and mesenteric lymphadenitis are the most common inflammatory disorders in this age group. Gastroenteritis typically presents as vomiting that precedes the onset of pain and is often associated with diarrhea. It is rarely associated with localizing signs or muscular spasm. Bowel sounds are usually hyperactive, and rectal examination is rarely positive in gastroenteritis although it is frequently reported to be positive in this age group in patients with appendicitis.

Mesenteric adenitis is often preceded by an upper respiratory tract infection and associated with a vague abdominal discomfort that often begins in the right lower quadrant. Abdominal examination reveals only mild right lower quadrant tenderness that is often not well localized.

Diagnosis of appendicitis in the elderly is often difficult. Frequently these patients present late with equivocal physical findings, and often (30 per cent) the leukocyte count is below 10,000.[18] Chills and fever more frequently accompany appendicitis in older patients. Subnormal temperatures are associated with an abscess or generalized peritonitis. More than 30 per cent of elderly patients have a ruptured appendix at the time of operation. The differential diagnosis in this group of patients includes diverticulitis, perforated ulcer, acute cholecystitis, carcinoma, intestinal obstruction, and mesenteric vascular disease. In teenagers and young adults the differential diagnosis of appendicitis is related to gender. The differential diagnosis in the male with localized right lower quadrant pain includes four genitourinary causes: acute pyelonephritis, renal calculi, torsion of the testicle, and epididymitis. Acute pyelonephritis and renal calculi can be suspected on the basis of urinalysis, and testicular torsion and epididymitis should be suspected on the basis of physical examination. Other confounding diagnoses in the young male include mesenteric adenitis and acute gastroenteritis. These entities are responsible for about a 10 per cent incidence of negative exploration for appendicitis in young males.

Whereas the incidence of appendicitis in females between the ages of 10 and 30 years is approximately half that of males, the incidence of negative exploration is consistently over 20 per cent. This inconsistency is due to the high incidence of genitourinary disease in females. In decreasing order of frequency, diagnostic errors in young females include (1) pelvic inflammatory disease (30 per cent), (2) other gynecologic diagnoses (15 per cent), (3) mesenteric adenitis (13 per cent), (4) gastroenteritis (6 per cent), (5) urinary tract infections (6 per cent), (7) cholelithiasis (3 per cent), and (8) unknown (15 per cent). The incidence of pelvic inflammatory disease in young females with abdominal pain makes the diagnosis of appendicitis more difficult. Lewis and colleagues[13] found that if

the onset of abdominal pain occurred within 7 days of menses the incidence of pelvic inflammatory disease was twice that of appendicitis. If, however, the menstrual period began 8 or more days prior to the onset of abdominal pain, appendicitis was twice as likely as pelvic inflammatory disease. Such a history, together with a proper pelvic examination, can help delineate this difficult subgroup of female patients.

Diverticular Disease

NATURAL HISTORY

Diverticular disease is the term applied to the wide spectrum of clinical conditions associated with the presence of multiple diverticula of the mucosa through the colonic wall. Three quarters of patients with diverticular disease are asymptomatic. The remainder have varying degrees of abdominal pain frequently accompanied by bowel irregularity. Approximately 25 per cent of patients with symptomatic diverticular disease have a course complicated by hemorrhage, inflammation, obstruction, or perforation. Symptomatic diverticulosis is a condition characterized by localized abdominal pain without evidence of peridiverticular inflammation.

Diverticulitis, or acute diverticular inflammation, is the most common complication of diverticulosis. Diverticulitis results from micro- or macroperforations of the diverticulum. The subsequent inflammatory reaction is either localized to the pericolic fat or walled off by adjacent organs, forming a diverticular abscess. At times, the abscess may extend into adjacent organs, forming a fistula. The most common sites of fistula formation include colovesical, colocutaneous, colovaginal, and coloenteric.

The formation of diverticula involves at least two factors: a pressure gradient between the colonic lumen and serosa, and areas of weakness in the colonic wall. The taeniae of the colon constitute three longitudinal muscle coats for the colon, and the serosa is weak between the taeniae. It is weaker still at those sites along the mesenteric border of the colon where perforating blood vessels penetrate the serosa. The herniation of the mucosa occurs alongside these penetrating arteries. As the diverticulum develops, it changes from a small, wide-mouthed structure into a flask-shaped structure prone to fecal entrapment. As fecal material becomes entrapped, the mucosa becomes irritated and diverticulitis ensues. If the fecal pellet erodes into a nutrient artery, hemorrhage may occur. Myochosis, contracting and thickening of the colonic wall evident on barium enema, results from hypertrophy of the colonic muscle layers. However, the degree of myochosis does not seem to be related to the potential for the development of either diverticulitis or other serious complications of diverticular disease.[14]

The frequency of diverticular disease is dramatically correlated with advancing age and the adaptation of Western dietary habits. Patients with diverticular disease have a statistically significant increase in frequency of gallstones, hiatal hernia (Saint's triad), ischemic heart disease, varicose veins, and hemorrhoids.

The major symptom of diverticulitis is abdominal pain. The abdominal pain is crampy and most often localized in the left lower quadrant. During the attacks the patient may experience constipation or diarrhea. Disturbance in bowel habits portends a worse prognosis than if normal bowel function is present. Also, the presence of nausea, vomiting, or persistent urinary symptoms, abdominal distention, and a palpable abdominal mass is associated with a higher complication rate and worse prognosis. Many patients who present with serious complications such as perforations are completely asymptomatic until a few hours prior to admission.

Barium enema in some patients with left-sided abdominal pain shows only myochosis with no evidence of actual diverticular disease. However, some patients have extensive diverticular disease without any symptoms. From a number of observations it is surmised that the natural history of diverticular disease in a majority of patients proceeds from myochosis to the development of diverticula, and in about one third of patients the number of diverticula and the extent of colonic involvement increase with time. Of all patients with colonic diverticula, it is estimated that 20 to 25 per cent develop diverticulitis. Of those patients who do develop diverticulitis, about one third will have *recurring* episodes. Most recurrences take place within the first 5 years, and as the prevalence of attacks increases the morbidity also rises.[14]

Although diverticular disease had in the past been considered a disease of the elderly, it is now recognized as having an increased incidence in young patients.[6] It is no longer uncommon to have patients younger than 40 years of age present with diverticulitis and its complications.

PHYSICAL EXAMINATION

Patients with asymptomatic diverticular disease have a normal physical examination. Consequently, physical findings in diverticular disease depend on the presenting complications. Patients who present with rectal bleeding may have an otherwise normal physical examination. Diverticular disease is the second most common cause of large bowel obstructions, and the physical presentation is described hereafter. Patients with diverticulitis present with tenderness over the involved area of the colon, usually the sigmoid. If the perforation is contained, the tenderness is localized, but generalized peritonitis can be associated with an uncontained perforation. Occasionally, a discrete mass can be felt in the left lower quadrant.

CONFIRMATORY TESTS

Barium enema is the procedure of choice to document diverticula. In addition, the barium enema is useful in excluding other entities in the differential diagnosis, including carcinoma and inflammatory bowel disease. Barium enema is contraindicated in those patients with clear evidence of free perforation. In patients who present with massive lower gastrointestinal bleeding, visceral angiography or radioisotope scanning may be useful in localizing the bleeding point. Pertinent laboratory tests include a complete blood count with differential.

Acute Cholecystitis

NATURAL HISTORY

Acute cholecystitis is characterized by right upper quadrant abdominal pain and tenderness, usually associated with mild fever and leukocytosis. Approximately 95 per cent of patients who have acute cholecystitis are thought to have obstruction of the cystic duct due to an impacted gallstone. Pain is caused by distention and inflammation of the gallbladder. In the experimental animal, however, acute obstruction of the cystic duct does not necessarily lead to acute cholecystitis. Bacteria are thought to play only a minor role in the early stages of acute cholecystitis. Recent evidence from the laboratory indicates that the trauma within the gallbladder from gallstones may release phospholipase within the mucosal cells of the gallbladder. This is followed by conversion of lecithin and bile to lysolecithin, a toxic compound that may increase the inflammatory response. Factors influencing the severity of cholecystitis include age of the patient, diabetes mellitus, and secondary bacterial invasion. In most patients the symptoms subside, but in some the disease progresses with abscess formation and gangrene.

Only 5 per cent of patients develop acute cholecystitis without the presence of gallstones. Acute acalculous cholecystitis is associated with prolonged fasting and is commonly seen in patients on prolonged total parenteral nutrition. Sludge, considered to be a precipitate of calcium bilirubinate, develops in the gallbladder. The role of bile stasis and sludge is not entirely understood but probably is important in patients with acute acalculous cholecystitis.

PHYSICAL EXAMINATION

The initial symptom in most patients with acute cholecystitis is pain in the right upper quadrant, which may radiate to the back. Nausea and vomiting are present in about one half of the patients, and mild icterus has been reported in about 10 per cent. Most patients have temperature in the range of 38 to 39°C., and the gallbladder is palpable in about one third of patients. Muscle guarding and a positive Murphy's sign are usually present.

Leukocytosis with a white count of 12,000 to 15,000 and a serum bilirubin ranging from 2 to 4 mg. per 100 ml. may be seen. This slight elevation of bilirubin is thought to be secondary to inflammation of the common bile duct caused by the contiguous inflamed gallbladder. There may be a slight increase in the alkaline phosphatase and, in some patients, the serum amylase.

CONFIRMATORY TESTS

Plain x-rays of the abdomen will show gallstones in approximately 10 to 15 per cent of patients. Oral cholecystogram is not of value in these patients, and the intravenous cholecystogram is now seldom employed. The imaging study most frequently used is an ultrasound, which may show the presence of gallstones, sludge, or thickening of the gallbladder wall. If there is uncertainty regarding the diagnosis, a radionuclide excretion scan (HIDA scan) may be ordered. Technetium [99]m-labeled derivatives of iminodiacetic acid (IDA) are excreted in high concentration of the bile. Visualization is obtained by a gamma camera. Within 15 to 30 minutes of intravenous injection of the radionuclide, an image of bile ducts and gallbladder should be seen in the normal individual with visualization of the intestine within 1 hour. However, in patients with acute cholecystitis, good images of the bile duct but no image of the gallbladder are characteristic and indicate cystic duct obstruction, substantiating the diagnosis of acute cholecystitis. However, in many patients the clinical history, physical examination, laboratory findings, and ultrasound examination are sufficient to make the diagnosis.

DIFFERENTIAL DIAGNOSIS

The differential diagnosis includes acute peptic ulcer disease, acute pancreatitis, acute appendicitis from a high-lying appendix, the Fitz-Hugh–Curtis syndrome of gonococcal perihepatitis, alcoholic hepatitis, pneumonia in the right lung, and acute myocardial infarction. Most of these can be excluded by appropriate ancillary tests.

TREATMENT

Initial treatment is to correct dehydration and electrolyte balance with appropriate intravenous fluids. A nasogastric tube may be inserted and antibiotics started. Cefazolin (2 to 4 gm. per day) or parenteral ampicillin (4 gm. daily) has been found to be an appropriate antibiotic. The bacteria generally present are *E. coli* and *Klebsiella*.

For several years there has been controversy regarding the timing of operation with recent studies favoring early cholecystectomy. This has been supported by controlled randomized trials that indicate that the death rate is slightly lower with early operation. The duration of the illness and cost of hospitalization are also lower. Concern about the technical aspects of removal of the gallbladder during early operation have not been confirmed in the randomized studies. Advocates of delaying operation thought that most patients' symptoms would subside on nonoperative treatment, and an elective cholecystectomy could be performed 4 to 6 weeks later. However, most surgeons now believe in early cholecystectomy performed within 1 or 2 days of admission to the hospital after confirmation of the diagnosis by the previously mentioned evaluation.

Urgent operation is indicated in patients who are diabetic. The mortality in diabetic patients is increased to approximately 15 per cent.

Cholecystostomy is seldom used now but is indicated in patients whose general condition is very precarious or in whom local complications are present. Cholecystectomy is preferred whenever possible. The overall mortality rate associated with acute cholecystitis has been reported in the range of 5 per cent, but death seldom occurs in good risk patients. Patients dying from acute cholecystitis have generally been elderly and/or have diabetes mellitus.

Whenever technically possible, an operative cholangiogram is obtained at the time of cholecystectomy, since common duct stones are reported to be present in approximately 15 per cent of patients presenting with acute cholecystitis.

Perforated Peptic Ulcer

NATURAL HISTORY

Perforations of the gastrointestinal tract cause sudden severe upper abdominal pain. Patients frequently recall the precise onset of the pain. The most common perforation of the gastrointestinal tract is from a perforated duodenal ulcer, and the second most common is from perforated gastric ulcers. Patients may have had preceding chronic symptoms of peptic ulcer disease, but in other patients acute perforation may be the first manifestation of the disorder. A chemical peritonitis is caused by the leakage of duodenal and/or gastric contents. An outpouring of fluid from the peritoneal surface results. There is generally sufficient acid from the stomach so that a bacterial peritonitis does not develop until late. However, the initial chemical peritonitis causes pain so severe that the patient usually lies quietly with knees flexed.

Perforated duodenal ulcers usually lie anterior, but occasionally a posterior ulcer may also be present. Rarely is acute bleeding an associated finding. The prognosis is related to the time interval between perforation and surgical closure. Mortality rates are reported in the range of 15 per cent and increase with age of the patient.

PHYSICAL EXAMINATION

Patients generally complain of epigastric tenderness and involuntary muscle spasm. Characteristically this has been described as boardlike rigidity. Peristaltic sounds are reduced, and fever is generally low grade. There may be considerable variation in the findings. In about one third of the patients, the onset of pain is not dramatic and may lead to long delays in diagnosis. This is particularly true of patients who are hospitalized for other illnesses. Some perforations may be sealed by the adjacent liver or overlying omentum and present only later as subhepatic or subdiaphragmatic abscesses.

CONFIRMATORY TESTS

The white count is elevated to about 12,000 but after 12 to 24 hours rises to 20,000 or more. Serum amylase shows a slight elevation due to absorption of the enzyme by the peritoneal cavity. Loss of fluid into the peritoneal cavity may cause hemoconcentration and a rise in the hematocrit.

Plain x-rays of the abdomen reveal free air in the peritoneal cavity in approximately 80 per cent of patients. A chest x-ray with the patient in the upright position is more likely to show free air than are x-rays of the abdomen. If the patient is too sick to be upright, a left lateral decubitus film may demonstrate free air. The presence of free air in the peritoneal cavity with a sudden onset of abdominal pain is diagnostic of a perforated peptic ulcer.

In those patients in whom no free air is demonstrated but a perforated ulcer is suspected, an emergency gastrointestinal series may be performed using a water-soluble contrast material. The escape of the contrast material from the intestinal lumen confirms the diagnosis. Some surgeons have advocated passing a nasogastric tube and injecting air into the stomach, with the belief that this will demonstrate free air on the x-ray films.

DIFFERENTIAL DIAGNOSIS

Acute pancreatitis and acute cholecystitis may cause pain similar to that experienced by the patient with a perforated peptic ulcer. Generally, however, the pain is acute in onset and is not accompanied by free air. The serum amylase is considerably higher in most patients with acute pancreatitis. Colonic diverticula and acute appendicitis are possible causes of free perforation. Occasionally, a small duodenal perforation may occur with slow leakage of fluid down the right lateral peritoneal gutter, producing pain and abdominal muscular rigidity in the right lower quadrant, mimicking acute appendicitis. Patients operated on with a diagnosis of acute appendicitis who have a normal appendix or a mild periappendicitis with fluid in the right gutter should be suspected of having a perforated duodenal ulcer, which may necessitate a second incision to close the perforation.

TREATMENT

Patients suspected of having a perforated duodenal ulcer should have intravenous fluids started, blood drawn for appropriate laboratory studies, and a nasogastric tube inserted to empty the stomach. These should be done prior to x-ray studies to determine the presence of free air. Intravenous antibiotics such as cefoxitin or cephazolin should be given preoperatively. As soon as the patient's condition is stabilized by fluid resuscitation, operation is indicated.

The abdomen is explored through an upper midline incision. The perforation is generally found in the anterior wall of the duodenum. Traditional treatment has been to close the perforation with an omental patch, a procedure described by Roscoe Graham. The fluid that has leaked from the gastrointestinal tract is aspirated from the peritoneal cavity, followed by copious irrigation of the abdominal cavity with sterile saline.

Since about two thirds of patients will continue to have ulcer symptoms following patch closure of the perforated duodenal ulcer, there has been increasing interest in performing a definitive procedure to control the ulcer diathesis in addition to closing the perforation. Recently, proximal gastric vagotomy (highly selective vagotomy, parietal cell vagotomy) has been performed following patch closure of the perforation. Proximal gastric vagotomy provides minimal postgastrectomy sequelae so that the patient is not at risk for the dumping syndrome, postgastrectomy diarrhea, or reflux gastritis. Patients who have severe pre-existing disease or extensive contamination of the peritoneal cavity should not have a definitive operative procedure but only patch closure of the perforated duodenal ulcer. Perforated gastric ulcers are best treated by distal gastric resection to include the antrum and the site of the perforated ulcer. With early recognition and prompt surgical intervention, mortality and morbidity rates are low and most patients survive.

Acute Pancreatitis

NATURAL HISTORY

Acute pancreatitis is characterized by the sudden onset of epigastric pain, which frequently radiates to the back and is accompanied by nausea and vomiting. The most common etiology of acute pancreatitis is alcoholism or cholelithiasis. Characteristically, the serum amylase and, later, the urine amylase are elevated. The pathologic process may cause a relatively mild acute attack due to edematous pancreatitis. The disease may worsen with the onset of hemorrhagic pancreatitis, which is accompanied by a high mortality rate and morbidity characterized by pancreatic pseudocyst, abscess, and pancreatic ascites. In the more common edematous pancreatitis, the pancreas and surrounding retroperitoneal tissues are infiltrated with large amounts of interstitial fluid. Fluid losses, if not replaced, may be so massive as to cause hypovolemic shock. The more severe hemorrhagic pancreatitis is accompanied by bleeding into the parenchyma of the pancreas and surrounding retroperitoneal areas. Extensive pancreatic necrosis may occur.

Characteristically, patients suffer severe epigastric pain following a large meal (Fig. 9). Pain radiates through to the back and is constant and associated with nausea and vomiting. Depending on the amount of fluid loss in the pancreas and peripancreatic area, the patient may develop severe dehydration with hypertension and rapid pulse rate. Myocardial function is depressed—probably because of a circulating toxin affecting cardiac performance.

PHYSICAL EXAMINATION

The abdomen is frequently slightly distended with tenderness in the epigastric area with voluntary abdominal wall spasm. Bowel sounds are diminished to absent, and the temperature is slightly elevated. In severe cases of hemorrhagic necrotizing pancreatitis, a bluish discoloration may be present in the flank (the so-called Grey Turner's sign) with similar discoloration in the periumbilical area, a sign described by Thomas Cullen. This occurs in 1 to 2 per cent of patients and is secondary to dissection of blood retroperitoneally into the flank and/or periumbilical area.

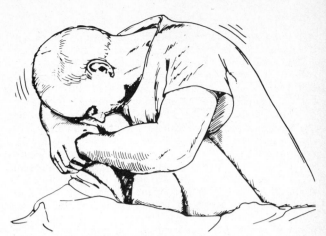

Figure 9. Typical "attitude" of patient with acute pancreatitis.

CONFIRMATORY TESTS

Because of dehydration the hematocrit is elevated, but in hemorrhagic pancreatitis it may be low because of blood loss. The white count is elevated in the range of approximately 12,000. A striking finding is an elevated serum amylase, which rises within 6 hours of the onset of pain with values that may extend above 1000 I.U. per 100 ml. Liver function tests are usually normal except for the serum bilirubin, which may be slightly elevated but seldom above 2 mg. per 100 ml. It is generally thought that the serum amylase concentrations are higher in acute biliary pancreatitis, and lower values are more frequently seen with acute alcoholic pancreatitis.

The urinary clearance of amylase increases during acute pancreatitis because of a decrease in tubular reabsorption of amylase. In very severe pancreatitis, a serum calcium concentration falls because calcium combines with fatty acids. The fatty acids come from the fat in the retroperitoneal area owing to the action of lipase. Serum calcium levels may also fall because of impaired reabsorption from bone owing to the action of calcitonin, which is liberated by high levels of glucagon.

A plain film of the abdomen shows abnormalities in approximately 60 to 70 per cent of patients. The most characteristic finding is the so-called sentinel loop, which is an isolated dilatation of a segment of gut, usually the transverse colon but sometimes a segment of jejunum or duodenum near the pancreas. The colon cut-off sign is another characteristic finding of acute pancreatitis and is due to gas distending the right colon that abruptly stops in the mid-transverse colon owing to colonic spasm adjacent to the pancreatic inflammation. In patients with chronic pancreatitis with intermittent attacks, calcification may be seen in the pancreas. Chest x-rays may show a sympathetic pleural effusion, usually in the left pleural cavity. Upper gastrointestinal series will show a widened duodenal loop, an occasional defect from an edematous ampulla of Vater.

The abdominal CT scan has become quite useful, and changes seen in the pancreas are secondary to inflammation, hemorrhage, or development of pseudocysts and abscesses. Ultrasound may demonstrate a gallstone in patients who have gallstone pancreatitis. Following subsidence of an attack of acute pancreatitis, further evaluation of the pancreatic duct may be done by an endoscopic retrograde cholangiopancreatography.

DIFFERENTIAL DIAGNOSIS

Elevated serum amylase levels may occur with other acute abdominal conditions such as gangrenous cholecystitis, perforated peptic ulcer, mesenteric infarction, and small bowel obstruction. The amylase levels in these conditions seldom rise above 500 I.U. per 100 ml. Since many of these conditions require urgent surgical intervention and acute pancreatitis does not require operative intervention in most cases, it is important to establish the correct diagnosis. However, if the diagnostic dilemma persists, exploratory celiotomy may be indicated on the basis that acute surgical conditions cannot be eliminated in the differential diagnosis. The mortality rate from exploratory laparotomy when the inciting cause proved to be acute edematous pancreatitis has not been excessive.

Treatment

Treatment of acute pancreatitis includes resting the pancreas by reducing stimuli to pancreatic secretion and re-establishing homeostasis. Patients are given intravenous fluid replacement to correct the third space loss of fluid into the retroperitoneum. Impressive amounts of fluid may be necessary to maintain circulating blood volume and adequate blood pressure. Patients with severe hemorrhagic pancreatitis may require blood transfusions as well as fluid therapy.

Patients are placed on nothing by mouth, and a nasogastric tube to aspirate gastric secretions, eliminating vomiting and preventing acids remaining in the duodenum from stimulating pancreatic secretion, is customary. Resumption of oral intake should be delayed until the patient is much improved and amylase levels have returned to normal. Analgesic drugs are indicated, but morphine and other medications causing spasm of the sphincter of Oddi should be avoided. Antibiotics in randomized studies have been found not to be indicated for acute edematous alcoholic pancreatitis but are useful for biliary pancreatitis and severe hemorrhagic pancreatitis. Replacement of calcium and magnesium is indicated, and in those rare occasions when hypocalcemia is refractory, parathyroid extract in doses of 200 units intravenously every 4 hours for six doses has been beneficial. Hypomagnesium is common in alcoholics, and magnesium should be replaced when indicated by low serum levels.

Pulmonary complications with severe pancreatitis are common. Hypoxemia develops in about 30 per cent of patients with acute pancreatitis. Frequent evaluation of blood gases is indicated. A form of adult respiratory distress syndrome may exacerbate the oxygen deficit. Supplementary oxygen therapy is indicated for PaO_2 levels below 70 mm. Hg. Diuretics may be helpful in eliminating excessive fluid. Nutrition should be maintained by total parenteral nutrition (TPN), which avoids stimulation of pancreatic enzymes. Elemental diets given orally or by tube feedings stimulate pancreatic secretions and should be avoided in favor of TPN. Controlled randomized trials of histamine (H_2) blockers, anticholinergic drugs, glucagon, and aprotinin (Trasilol) have shown no therapeutic benefit. Peritoneal lavage has been advocated for severe cases of pancreatitis to remove the toxins in the peritoneal fluid. Although patients seem to improve initially with peritoneal lavage, there has been no improvement in the overall survival rate.

Operative intervention is not indicated, except for the complications of pancreatitis or for diagnostic celiotomy when the diagnosis is in question. For biliary pancreatitis, operation is necessary to remove the gallbladder and any stones that might be present in the extrahepatic biliary system. The timing of operation is controversial. Most surgeons favor operation on these patients during the period

TABLE 3. *Prognostic Signs Used to Identify Risk of Life-Threatening Complications of Acute Pancreatitis**

At Admission or Diagnosis
Age over 55 years
White blood cell count over 16,000/mm.[3]
Blood glucose over 200 mg./100 ml.
Serum lactic dehydrogenase over 350 I.U./liter
Serum glutamic oxaloacetic transaminase over 250 Sigma-Frankel U./100 ml.

During the Initial 48 Hours
Hematocrit fall greater than 10%
Blood urea nitrogen rise more than 5 mg./100 ml.
Serum calcium level below 8 mg./100 ml.
Arterial Po_2 below 60 mm. Hg.
Base deficit greater than 4 mEq./liter
Estimated fluid sequestration more than 6000 ml.

*From Ranson, J.H.C.: Curr. Probl. Surg., *16*:1, 1979.

of hospitalization but prefer to wait until the patient recovers from the initial attack. However, if pancreatitis progresses and the patient's illness becomes worse, then operation may be indicated on an urgent basis. Patients with hemorrhagic necrotizing pancreatitis not responding to medical therapy may benefit by operation to débride necrotic pancreas, insertion of a T tube to drain the common bile duct, and placement of multiple large sump drains in the peripancreatic area. Gastrostomy and tube jejunostomy may be performed at this time. Total pancreatectomy has been advocated in the past, but the mortality rate is excessive in most series.

The mortality rate from acute pancreatitis is approximately 10 per cent. In patients with hemorrhagic necrotizing pancreatitis the mortality rate exceeds 50 per cent. Ranson[15] has pointed out certain factors that are related to morbidity and mortality (Table 3). Although the initial treatment is medical, surgical intervention may benefit patients who do not respond to medical treatment and is certainly indicated for the complications of acute pancreatitis such as abscess, pseudocyst, and pancreatic ascites.

Intestinal Obstruction

There are four major causes of intestinal obstruction: (1) mechanical obstruction of the lumen, (2) lesions of the bowel wall, (3) lesions extrinsic to the bowel, and (4) inadequate motility. Obstruction can occur anywhere along the GI tract, but we will concern ourselves with those obstructions of the large and small bowel. As a general rule, the more proximal the level of the obstruction the more acute the symptoms. High-level obstructions in the small bowel are associated with the acute onset of severe colicky abdominal pain and are often associated with multiple episodes of vomiting. In large bowel obstruction the onset of symptoms is relatively chronic. The symptoms of bowel obstruction are not static. Obstruction can lead to ischemia followed by perforation and systemic vascular collapse.

Natural History

Intestinal obstruction is relatively rare in infancy, with intestinal atresia or stenosis being most common in the neonate and intussusception becoming more common as the infant approaches the preschool age. In the preschool age, intussusception, volvulus, and incarcerated hernia are the most common causes of bowel obstruction.

Small bowel obstruction in the adult is most commonly caused by postoperative adhesive bands. Incarcerated inguinal hernias are now the second most common cause of small bowel obstruction. Frequent causes of large bowel obstruction in the adult include carcinoma, diverticular disease, and fecal impaction.

PATIENT HISTORY

Proper history for intestinal obstruction is based on intelligent questioning of the patient as to the onset and type of pain, the presence of vomiting, changes in bowel habits, and past medical history.

The history of pain should focus on three areas: the onset of the pain, its distribution, and its character.

Typically, the onset of pain in small bowel obstruction is relatively acute, whereas in large bowel obstruction the pain is more insidious in onset. The distribution of pain in small bowel obstruction is epigastric or periumbilical, whereas in large bowel obstruction the pain is most often described in the hypogastrium. Characteristically, obstruction presents with colicky episodic pain, which is often intensified by deep inspiration.

Vomiting is characteristic of bowel obstruction. It is occasionally feculent, and one should always note the relationship of the onset of pain to the onset of vomiting.

The patient should be questioned as to constipation, obstipation, and the recent passage of flatus. A history of either melena or blood-tinged stool suggests carcinoma as a cause of large bowel obstruction.

The patient should be questioned about previous episodes of pain that mimic the current episode. The patient may give a history characteristic of previous diverticular disease suggesting the basis of the current obstruction. In addition, one should obtain a history of previous operations or the use of psychotropic drugs.

PHYSICAL EXAMINATION

Intestinal obstruction presents with episodic pain. The patient is often comfortable between episodes of pain. Persistent pain in the face of a picture of obstruction portends strangulation and imminent perforation and constitutes a surgical emergency.

Patients may show systemic evidence of dehydration as well as abdominal distention. Occasionally, in a thin individual with signs of late intestinal obstruction a peristaltic wave along the abdominal wall can be noted.

When evaluating a patient for intestinal obstruction, auscultation is performed prior to palpation or percussion. One listens for bowel sounds for several minutes. The bell of the stethoscope should be placed on the abdomen with little or no pressure applied. In obstruction one will hear hyperactive bowel sounds with rushes and high-pitched "tinkles."

Adynamic ileus is a major differential diagnosis for intestinal obstruction, and this condition is characterized by hypoactive bowel sounds on physical examination.

Gentle palpation of the acute abdomen in patients with intestinal obstruction reveals varying degrees of distention and tenderness. It is essential that all potential hernia sites be diligently palpated to exclude this common cause of obstruction. Gentle percussion of the abdomen in the obstructed patient may reveal hyperresonance.

Rectal examination is of paramount importance in all patients being evaluated for intestinal obstruction. Often, fecal impaction is the cause of obstruction in elderly or institutionalized patients. Gross blood or guaiac positivity in patients being evaluated for large bowel obstruction is consistent with the presence of carcinoma. It is not unusual to be able to palpate an obstructing rectal carcinoma on rectal examination.

In summary, small bowel obstruction is characterized by acute abdominal pain, which is colicky in nature and usually located in the epigastrium or periumbilical area. Small bowel obstruction is often associated with vomiting, and the most common causes of small bowel obstruction include adhesive bands and external hernias. Obstruction of the large bowel is more insidious in onset and is often associated with nausea rather than vomiting. Obstruction of the large intestine accounts for only 15 to 20 per cent of all bowel obstructions. Of these, colorectal carcinoma is responsible for 60 per cent of patients with large bowel obstruction, and diverticulitis is responsible for 20 per cent.

CONFIRMATORY TESTS

The diagnosis of intestinal obstruction is suspected by history and physical examination and is confirmed by the performance of an acute abdominal series.

The flat x-ray of the abdomen is used to distinguish the level of obstruction and abnormally large quantities of gas in the bowel. One can usually determine whether the small intestine, colon, or both are distended.

Gas in the small bowel outlines the valvulae conniventes. Patients with mechanical small bowel obstruction have minimal amounts of colonic gas. Patients with colonic obstruction, on the other hand, show little small bowel gas if the ileocecal valve is competent. Colonic haustral markings are typically present in large bowel obstruction. Haustral markings are differentiated from valvulae conniventes by the fact that haustral markings occupy only a portion of the transverse diameter of the bowel.

The upright abdominal x-ray film in patients with mechanical small bowel obstruction characteristically shows multiple air fluid levels. Unfortunately, these air fluid levels also occur in patients with adynamic ileus.

The chest x-ray is the best way to identify free air beneath the diaphragm, which is indicative of a perforated viscus. In addition, it identifies pulmonary pathology, which can occasionally cause symptoms similar to those of an acute abdomen.

In summary, the diagnosis of bowel obstruction is made by history and confirmed by physical and x-ray examinations. The treatment of bowel obstruction is surgical, and when the diagnosis is suspected immediate surgical consultation should be obtained.

Acute Mesenteric Ischemia

Ninety-eight per cent of patients with acute mesenteric ischemia present with severe abdominal pain. Other common symptoms include nausea, vomiting, diarrhea, and gastrointestinal bleeding. All too often the diagnosis of acute mesenteric ischemia is made so late that the entire small bowel is infarcted by the time the patient reaches the hospital. With early diagnosis and surgical treatment, it is now possible to salvage ischemic bowel.

NATURAL HISTORY

There are four major causes of acute mesenteric ischemia. These include embolization (45 per cent), nonocclusive disease (35 per cent), arterial thrombosis (15 per cent), and venous thrombosis (5 per cent).

TABLE 4. Acute Mesenteric Ischemia:
Gastrointestinal Symptoms

Symptom	Incidence (%)
Abdominal pain	98
Nausea	60
Vomiting	58
Diarrhea	25
Gastrointestinal bleeding	22

Whereas the incidence of venous thrombosis and non-occlusive mesenteric disease appears to be decreasing, the incidence of embolic disease seems to be increasing. The incidence of acute thrombosis is unchanged, but these patients tend to have a worse prognosis than patients with embolization.

A recent review by Eskin (personal communication) of 40 patients treated with acute mesenteric ischemia reveals that most of these patients were over 60 years of age and had a variety of underlying medical conditions. Cardiac disease, diffuse peripheral vascular disease, chronic obstructive pulmonary disease, diabetes mellitus, and hypertension are the most commonly associated disorders.

Abdominal pain occurred in almost all patients. The duration of symptoms ranged from a few hours to several days. Nausea and vomiting were present in approximately 60 per cent of patients, diarrhea was present in 25 per cent, and 22 per cent of patients had either gross blood per rectum or guaiac positive stool (Table 4).

PHYSICAL EXAMINATION

The hallmark of acute mesenteric ischemia is the sudden onset of pain out of proportion to physical findings. The patients are often writhing in pain but present with nonspecific findings on physical examination. The mucosa of the intestine is more sensitive to ischemia than the serosa, therefore the onset of pain corresponds with the onset of mucosal ischemia. However, physical findings do not become evident until the serosa becomes involved—perhaps several hours after the onset of pain (Table 5).

CONFIRMATORY TESTS

Laboratory data in patients with acute intestinal ischemia often are nonspecific. Leukocytosis, hyperamylasemia, and metabolic acidosis occur, but these abnormal findings occur late in the disease process and often are not present at the time the patient is seen initially (Table 6). Normal laboratory tests may provide the inexperienced physician a false sense of security in these patients.

Plain x-rays of the abdomen frequently are nonspecific or show an ileus pattern. Free air may be present after the gangrenous intestine has ruptured. The key to early diagnosis of acute mesenteric ischemia is mesenteric arteriog-

TABLE 5. Acute Mesenteric Ischemia:
Findings on Initial Physical Examination

Finding	Incidence (%)
Hypotension	48
Tachycardia	68
Fever	56
Hypovolemia	40
Abdominal tenderness	47

TABLE 6. Acute Mesenteric Ischemia:
Laboratory Data on Admission

Laboratory Data	Incidence (%)
Hematocrit	
<35	30
35–45	48
>45	22
White blood cell counts	
<10,000 cells/mm.^{3}	15
10,000–20,000	40
>20,000	45
Acid base balance (ABG)	
Base deficit	70
Normal	5
Base excess	25
Serum amylase	
Hyperamylasemia	73
Normal	27

raphy. If the arteriogram shows a block due to embolus or thrombus, operation is indicated for embolectomy and resection of gangrenous bowel.

After arterial flow is restored to the mesenteric vessels, the bowel is returned to the abdomen, and a waiting period of approximately 35 to 45 minutes ensues. The bowel is then inspected, obviously infarcted bowel is resected, and a conventional anastomosis is constructed. Fluorescein dye and the use of intraoperative Doppler flow monitoring aid in differentiating viable from nonviable bowel.

Seideman has emphasized the importance of a second look procedure approximately 24 hours after resection. The second look procedure is performed after the patient has been stabilized and is reserved for those patients in whom additional resection may be necessary.

In summary, acute mesenteric ischemia is difficult to diagnose. Improved results may be achieved by early recognition of patients at high risk, which include elderly patients with significant underlying atherosclerotic disease. The diagnosis of acute mesenteric ischemia should be considered in all patients with abdominal pain out of proportion to findings on physical examination. Vomiting and diarrhea associated with gastrointestinal bleeding may occur. Laboratory tests typically show metabolic acidosis in conjunction with a leukocytosis and hyperamylasemia. Abdominal x-rays tend to be nonspecific, and the most specific study is mesenteric arteriography.

Abdominal Aortic Aneurysm

Abdominal aortic aneurysms are a relatively infrequent cause of abdominal pain. However, when a patient presents with abdominal pain and a pulsatile supraumbilical abdominal mass, immediate surgical consultation must be obtained.

A majority of abdominal aortic aneurysms are secondary to atherosclerosis. Other less common causes of aortic aneurysms include inflammatory, traumatic, and congenital conditions. Because the vast majority of abdominal aneurysms are atherosclerotic in nature, there is a significant male predominance, as high as 8 to 1 in some series. Ninety-five per cent of aneurysms are infrarenal in origin and occur in patients over the age of 65. Two thirds of patients with abdominal aortic aneurysms have associated iliac artery aneurysm.

NATURAL HISTORY

The natural history of aortic aneurysms is highly variable. However, just like the underlying atherosclerosis, the aneurysmal dilatation is progressive. As a rule of thumb, one can expect an aneurysm to grow at the rate of 4 to 5 millimeters a year. However, this is exceedingly variable from patient to patient.

As the aneurysm grows, the risk of rupture increases. The 5-year risk of aneurysm rupture is a function of size. The sharply increased risk of rupture beyond the diameter of 6 cm. has prompted a 5-cm. figure to be used as an indication of elective repair of asymptomatic abdominal aortic aneurysms. However, 10 per cent of all ruptured abdominal aortic aneurysms are smaller than 5 cm. in diameter.

The pathophysiology of abdominal pain associated with aortic aneurysm is either bleeding into the aneurysm wall or actual perforation of the aneurysm and bleeding into the surrounding retroperitoneal adventitia. In a small number of cases, the abdominal pain is associated with the rapid onset of hypotension and free rupture into the peritoneal cavity. Obviously this constellation of events requires surgical intervention.

As with all patients presenting with abdominal pain of vascular origin, patients with rupture of an abdominal aortic aneurysm have a high incidence of underlying pulmonary and cardiovascular disease.

PHYSICAL EXAMINATION

The principal manifestation of ruptured abdominal aortic aneurysms is back or flank pain, often associated with shock. Ruptured abdominal aortic aneurysm is a relatively common diagnosis in older patients who present with shock and no obvious source of blood loss. Consideration of ruptured abdominal aortic aneurysm should be part of the differential diagnosis of myocardial infarction presenting with hypotension. Both groups of patients present with ischemic ECG changes, and patients with an inferior wall myocardial infarction may complain of back or flank pain. Patients with hypotension secondary to myocardial infarction will present with jugular venous distention, whereas patients with hypovolemia secondary to a ruptured aneurysm will have flat neck veins.

Ruptured aortic aneurysms have two major presentations. One is a free rupture into the peritoneum, which results in rapid exsanguination. Symptoms include the abrupt onset of abdominal pain, rapidly progressive hypovolemic shock, and progressive abdominal distention. These patients require immediate operation.

The second, more common, presentation is a contained rupture. These patients present with the sudden onset of severe abdominal pain or back pain with hypotension that initially responds to fluid resuscitation. The patient often has a history of hypertension. A pulsatile supraumbilical abdominal mass is palpable in 85 per cent of patients.

Another helpful clue to the presence of aneurysmal disease is a careful physical examination for associated occlusive vascular disease. The presence of a bruit over the bifurcation of the carotid arteries is not uncommon in patients with abdominal aortic aneurysm. The hypotensive patient may not have a pulsatile mass unless the blood pressure exceeds 80 mm. Hg.

CONFIRMATORY TESTS

Patients who present with hypotension and a physical examination compatible with a ruptured abdominal aneurysm need urgent operative intervention. Time does not permit confirmatory tests. Routine blood work, electrolytes, and renal function tests are helpful in the postoperative management of the patient but do not contribute to the diagnosis. In the unstable patient the simplest and fastest test to diagnose the presence of abdominal aortic aneurysm is a cross-table lateral film of the abdomen. Eighty-five per cent of abdominal aortic aneurysms are calcified and can be seen on cross-table lateral film. In the stable patient with a contained rupture, ultrasonography, CT scanning, or aortography is the diagnostic procedure of choice, depending on the preference of the surgeon. Both ultrasound and CT scan accurately show the size of the aneurysm and the periaortic hematoma. Aortography, on the other hand, although less accurate in showing the size of the aneurysm, does demonstrate the patient's arterial anatomy.

In summary, patients presenting with abdominal flank or back pain and a pulsatile supraumbilical abdominal mass should be suspected of having a ruptured abdominal aortic aneurysm. The diagnosis can often be confirmed by cross-table lateral abdominal film showing calcification of the abdominal aorta. If the patient presents with abdominal or back pain and refractory hypotension, one must suspect a free intraperitoneal rupture of the abdominal aortic aneurysm; immediate surgical exploration is mandated.

GYNECOLOGIC CAUSES OF ABDOMINAL PAIN

Females have a higher incidence of abdominal pain than do males. The incidence of general surgical disease as a cause for acute abdominal pain is lower than that contributed by gynecologic disease.

Common gynecologic etiologies for abdominal pain include ectopic pregnancy, septic abortion, pelvic inflammatory disease, tubal ovarian abscess, Fitz-Hugh–Curtis syndrome, and mittelschmerz.

Females with abdominal pain should be questioned about possible pregnancy, i.e., recent amenorrhea, intercourse without contraception, and breast tenderness. A history of vaginal bleeding, the relation of menses to the onset of pain, and trauma, including rape and septic abortion, are helpful. Physical examination includes bimanual pelvic examination and rectal as well as an abdominal examination.

Ectopic Pregnancy

Ectopic pregnancy is the most common potentially life-threatening gynecologic disorder presenting with abdominal pain. It should be suspected in any patient with menstrual irregularities, vaginal bleeding, and crampy lower abdominal pain. Classically the bleeding precedes the onset of abdominal pain. The bleeding is often minimal at first but may increase over time.

Ectopic pregnancy is associated with the use of an intrauterine device, a previous history of pelvic inflammatory disease, or previous tubal pregnancy. The principal cause of death in patients with ectopic pregnancy is rupture of the fallopian tube and its adjacent vascular supply. These patients initially present with abdominal pain and peritoneal signs. They may, however, progress to significant bleeding into the abdomen, developing distention and hypotension.

Confirmatory tests include a pregnancy test, but a negative pregnancy test does not necessarily preclude the diagnosis. Other useful laboratory adjuncts include culdocentesis and laparoscopy.

Pelvic Inflammatory Disease

Pelvic inflammatory disease and salpingitis characteristically present in a female with diffuse lower abdominal pain and high fever. Temperature is increased in general surgical disease but may be elevated to 39.5 to 40.0° C. (103 to 104° F.) in patients with pelvic inflammatory disease. The pain and fever of pelvic inflammatory disease classically occur during or just after the menstrual period, a fact that is occasionally helpful in distinguishing pelvic inflammatory disease from appendicitis. In addition, patients with pelvic inflammatory disease may have a previous history of salpingitis or vaginal discharge.

On physical examination, vaginal discharge is often present and purulent. The hallmark of pelvic inflammatory disease is exquisite cervical tenderness elicited on cervical motion. In addition, the cervix is usually warm and hyperemic, and the uterus may be tender. There may be bilateral adnexal tenderness. A unilateral adnexal mass in this setting is highly suggestive of salpingitis with tubal ovarian abscess. Confirmatory tests include marked leukocytosis and culdocentesis, which may reveal purulent fluid.

Endometriosis

Endometriosis is characterized by the development of endometrial glands and stroma in areas outside of the uterus. Such areas may undergo histologic changes during the menstrual cycle. Endometrial implants characteristically occur in the pelvis and uterosacral ligaments but may occur anywhere within the abdomen. Endometriosis of the ovaries generates large "chocolate cysts," or endometriomas. Endometrial implants on the bowel may cause cyclic gastrointestinal tract bleeding.

Patients with endometriosis may be completely asymptomatic; however, they may complain of moderate to severe pain associated with menstrual cycle. Typically, the patient is in her late 20s and has never been pregnant.

Clinically, the diagnosis can be suspected by feeling tender nodules along the uterosacral ligaments or posterior cul-de-sac. The diagnosis can be confirmed at laparoscopy or laparotomy.

Gonorrhea in the Female

Acute uncomplicated gonorrhea in the female often causes dysuria, frequency, increased vaginal discharge, and anal/rectal discomfort. Asymptomatic gonococcal infection in the female involves, in descending order of frequency, the endocervix, the urethra, the anal canal, and the pharynx. Extension of the infection from the endocervix to the fallopian tubes occurs in 10 to 15 per cent of women with gonorrhea, resulting in acute salpingitis. Approximately half of all women with acute salpingitis have gonorrhea. The clinical diagnosis of salpingitis is imprecise, and, at laparoscopy, less than three fourths of clinically suspected cases of salpingitis are confirmed. Fifteen per cent of patients have other findings at laparoscopy, including appendicitis, ectopic pregnancy, diverticulitis, endometriosis, and hemorrhagic ovarian cysts.

The spread of gonococcal infection to the upper abdomen may cause gonococcal perihepatitis (Fitz-Hugh–Curtis syndrome) manifested by right upper quadrant or bilateral upper abdominal pain and tenderness. This syndrome clinically may mimic acute cholecystitis and may even be associated with mild liver function abnormalities.

Mittelschmerz

Mittelschmerz, or midcycle pain, is common in women with regular menstrual periods who are not taking birth control pills. Mittelschmerz is significant in that it is high on the list of differential diagnoses in young women suspected of having appendicitis. Mittelschmerz may present with lower abdominal pain, and there is rarely fever or abdominal uterine bleeding. Physical examination at the time of mittelschmerz may reveal some lower quadrant tenderness with or without rebound. Bimanual examination may show localized tenderness, and a pelvic mass may be present. Lack of fever and a negative pregnancy test in the absence of significant leukocytosis support the diagnosis.

Septic Abortion

Septic abortion commonly occurs following illegal abortion using nonsterile technique. Rarely, it may occur after legal abortion. Incomplete evacuation of the products of conception results in sepsis. The infection is usually rapidly progressive, marching through the myometrium, and may involve the adnexa and pelvic peritoneum. Antibiotic coverage should be designed to include both aerobic and anaerobic bacteria. Septic pelvic thrombophlebitis is a frequent complication.

Clinical findings include fever, leukocytosis, diffuse pelvic tenderness, and a foul-smelling vaginal discharge. Patients may present in frank septic shock, and toxic shock syndrome must be excluded.

GENITOURINARY CONDITIONS ASSOCIATED WITH ABDOMINAL PAIN

Urologic conditions associated with abdominal pain can be divided into our three pathophysiologic divisions of pain: inflammation, obstruction, and ischemia (Fig. 10). Common inflammatory causes of abdominal pain within the genitourinary system include acute pyelonephritis, acute cystitis, and epididymitis. Ischemic causes of abdominal pain include the referred pain of testicular torsion and obstructive causes include nephrolithiasis.

Organisms commonly associated with acute pyelonephritis include *E. coli*, *Proteus mirabilis*, *Klebsiella*, and *Staphylococcus saprophyticus*. Typically, the infection migrates into the upper urinary tract from the bladder. Pyelonephritis is characterized by dysuria, frequency, or urgency in the presence of flank pain or tenderness. Patients may have significant signs of systemic illness including fever, often as high as 39.5 °C. (103° F.). In children, pyelonephritis may be accompanied by nausea and vomiting, and urinary tract symptoms may be minimal.

Uncomplicated bacterial cystitis is a urinary tract infection confined to the bladder and not involving the kidneys. It is more common in women and is associated with the same organisms that commonly present with upper urinary tract infection. Although it is uncommon for these patients to have frank abdominal pain, suprapubic discomfort and tenderness are common. These patients have minimal systemic symptoms and are usually afebrile.

Both upper and lower urinary tract infections are diagnosed by urinalysis and microscopic examination. The "clean" catch urine should be examined within an hour after it is obtained. Both proteinuria and hematuria are commonly found in patients with infection of the urinary

REFERRED PAIN

Flank pain or testicular pain is associated with

- Nephrolithiasis
- Uterolithiasis
- Pyelonephritis

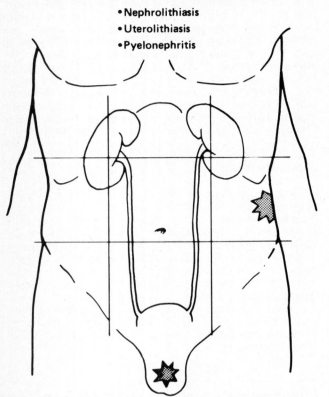

Figure 10. Referral patterns of pain from genitourinary conditions.

and the diagnosis is made if no flow is appreciated. Unfortunately, there are significant false-negative results with this test.

Urolithiasis

Stones within the urinary tract are a common cause of abdominal and flank pain. Stones usually form in the renal pelvis, and symptoms occur either with the passage of the stone into the ureter or as a result of infection. Chronic dehydration is an important cause of stone formation and may be responsible for the high incidence of urolithiasis in tropical climates or in patients with chronic diarrhea. The patient often has a previous history or a family history of stone formation.

The initial symptom of urolithiasis is unilateral flank pain that rapidly becomes excruciating. The crampy pain begins in the side or the back and may radiate to the lower part of the abdomen, genitalia, or the inner thigh. As the stone progresses distally in the urinary tract, the pain may also progress. This characteristic migration of pain is typically for urolithiasis and may help differentiate this pain from other causes of abdominal pain.

Confirmatory tests include microscopic examination of the urine. Less than 5 per cent of patients who present with urolithiasis and abdominal pain lack hematuria. Fifteen per cent of patients with urolithiasis will present with systemic symptoms, including pyuria, fever, and dysuria—all indicative of nephrolithiasis with concomitant infection.

Over 90 per cent of renal calculi are radiopaque; consequently, a plain film of the abdomen should be obtained prior to intravenous pyelography. Intravenous pyelograms may reveal the calculi, the point of obstruction, or delayed visualization of the obstructed side.

SELECTED REFERENCES

Sabiston, D. C., Jr. (Ed.): Textbook of Surgery. Philadelphia, W. B. Saunders Company, 1986.
   This is the classic standard textbook of surgery. Each chapter in the book is written by a noted authority. This comprehensive work covers all aspects of surgery. The student should refer to this textbook for in-depth information regarding surgical disorders of the abdomen.

Silen, W.: Cope's Early Diagnosis of the Acute Abdomen, 16th ed. London, Oxford University Press, 1983.
   Cope's monograph on the acute abdomen has been the introduction to evaluation of surgical patients for generations of medical students. The book is superbly illustrated. The usual abdominal disorders are discussed in detail, but the book is easily read.

Way, L. W. (Ed.): Current Surgical Diagnosis and Treatment, 7th ed. Los Altos, Calif., Lange Medical Publications, 1985.
   This book, originally edited by the late Dr. Bert Dunphy, has been recently revised by his associate, Lawrence Way. The chapter on the acute abdomen details the pathophysiology of surgical abdominal disorders and provides a discussion of diagnosis and treatment.

Welch, C. E., and Malt, R. A.: Abdominal Surgery, Parts I, II, and III. N. Engl. J. Med., *308*:624, 685, 753, 1983.
   Every few years the New England Journal of Medicine *publishes a series of review articles. Drs. Welch and Malt from the Massachusetts General Hospital have reviewed the recent literature regarding surgical abdominal disease. They have reported a survey of this information in a three-part article. This provides a concise summary of recently published articles on acute abdominal disorders. The reference list is extensive.*

tract. Urine cultures should be obtained in all patients suspected of having cystitis or pyelonephritis.

Epididymitis

Epididymitis, or inflammation of the epididymis, tends to occur in sexually active men over the age of 20. There may be a history of previous urinary tract infection or urethritis. On physical examination there is often a unilateral tender epididymis. Microscopic examination of the urine may show leukocytes, suggesting a concomitant urinary tract infection. Prehn's sign is helpful in differentiating epididymitis from torsion of the testicle. Pain relieved by elevating the scrotum is suggestive of epididymitis. In torsion, the pain is exacerbated by moving the scrotum.

Testicular Torsion

Testicular torsion tends to occur in young men and is rare over the age of 25. The onset of pain is abrupt and severe and may be associated with nausea and vomiting. Tenderness is initially noted only in the testicle; however, with persistent ischemia the pain may be described as lower abdominal in nature. Testicular torsion is a urologic emergency that requires operative intervention.

The Doppler has been described as a simple, rapid method for distinguishing torsion of the testicle from epididymitis. The Doppler is placed over the involved testicle,

REFERENCES

1. Almy, T. P., and Howell, D. A.: Diverticular disease of the colon. N. Engl. J. Med., *302*:324, 1980.
2. Beal, J. M., and Raffensperger, J. G.: Diagnosis of Acute Abdominal Disease. Philadelphia, Lea & Febiger, 1979.

3. Brewer, R. J., Golden, G. T., Hitch, D. C., Rudolf, L. E., and Wangensteen, S. L.: Abdominal pain: An analysis of 1,000 consecutive cases in a university hospital emergency room. Am. J. Surg., *131:*219, 1976.

4. Brickman, I. D., and Leon, W.: Acute appendicitis in childhood. Surgery, *60:*1083, 1966.

5. Eisenberg, R. L., Heineken, P., Hedgcock, M. W., Federle, M., and Goldberg, H. I.: Evaluation of plain abdominal radiographs in the diagnosis of abdominal pain. Ann. Intern. Med., *97:*257, 1982.

6. Eusebio, E. B., and Eisenberg, M. M.: Natural history of diverticular disease of the colon in young patients. Am. J. Surg., *25:*308, 1973.

7. Gilmore, O. J. A., Brodribb, A. J. M., Browett, J. P., Cooke, T. J. C., Griffin, P. H., Higgs, M. J., Ross, I. K., and Williamson, R. C. N.: Appendicitis and mimicking conditions: A prospective study. Lancet, *1:*421, 1975.

8. Hill, G. A., Patterson, S. P., Johnson, L. H., White, H. J., Jr., and Ling, F. W.: Unusual cause of acute abdomen in the puerperium. J. Tenn. Med. Assoc., *July:*390, 1984.

9. Hubbell, D. S., Barton, W. K., and Solomon, O. D.: Leukocytosis in appendicitis in older persons. J.A.M.A., *175:*139, 1961.

10. Lee, P. W. R.: The leukocyte count in acute appendicitis. Br. J. Surg., *60:*618, 1973.

11. Lee, P. W. R.: The plain x-ray in the acute abdomen: A surgeon's evaluation. Br. J. Surg., *63:*763, 1976.

12. Lee, R. A., Johnson, C. E., and Symmonds, R. E.: Appendicitis during pregnancy. J.A.M.A., *193:*966, 1965.

13. Lewis, F. R., Holcroft, J. W., Boey, J., and Dunphy, J. E.: Appendicitis: A critical review of diagnosis and treatment in 1,000 cases. Arch. Surg., *110:*677, 1975.

14. Parks, T. G.: Natural history of diverticular disease of the colon. Clin. Gastroenterol., *4:*53, 1975.

15. Ranson, J. H. C.: Acute pancreatitis. Curr. Probl. Surg., *16:*1, 1979.

16. Steinheber, F. U.: Medical conditions mimicking the acute surgical abdomen. Med. Clin. North Am., *57:*1559, 1973.

17. Thomson, H., and Francis, D. M. A.: Abdominal wall tenderness. Lancet, *2:*1053, 1977.

18. Thorbjarnarson, B., and Loehr, W. J.: Acute appendicitis in patients over the age of sixty. Surg. Gynecol. Obstet., *Dec.:*1277, 1967.

23

I

Surgical Anatomy, Physiology, and Pathology

WALLACE P. RITCHIE, JR., M.D., PH.D.
ALICE R. PEREZ, M.D.

The stomach, duodenum, and pancreas act together as an elegantly integrated unit to initiate the digestion of swallowed foodstuffs. Each has a specific role. The stomach secretes a highly caustic acid and a powerful proteolytic enzyme that begins the digestion of protein. It also mixes and grinds ingesta and delivers it as small particles in an orderly fashion into the duodenum. This organ, in turn, acts in association with the pancreas and hepatobiliary tree to adjust intraluminal pH and osmolarity, to promote further hydrolysis of protein and carbohydrate, and to alter dietary fat into an absorbable form. On occasion, the process can go awry, leading to autodigestion of the gastric or duodenal mucosa. The result is a "peptic" ulcer. In addition, a variety of neoplasms may develop in the stomach that may require the attention of the surgeon. In the present chapter, the normal anatomy and physiology of the stomach and duodenum will be reviewed, the operative treatment of peptic ulcers of these organs will be outlined, and the surgical therapy of several other benign and malignant conditions of the stomach and duodenum will be discussed.

SURGICAL ANATOMY OF THE STOMACH AND DUODENUM

The stomach is the first organ of the alimentary canal in the abdominal cavity (Fig. 1). It is pear-shaped and is bounded superiorly by a physiologically competent lower esophageal sphincter and inferiorly by an easily demonstrable pyloric sphincter. Although it is fixed at its upper and lower ends, its midportion is mobile. The wall of the stomach has four layers: an outer serosa, a coat of smooth-muscle fibers (the muscularis propria), the submucosa, and an inner mucous membrane. The external surface of the organ is divided into anatomic regions based approximately on the cell types found in the subjacent mucosa. The proximal stomach (body) contains the vast majority of the stomach's complement of parietal cells, the source of hydrochloric acid (HCl) and intrinsic factor, and of chief cells,

the major source of pepsinogen. Additional cell types include surface epithelial cells, which secrete mucus and bicarbonate into the gastric lumen; mucous neck cells, which also secrete mucus and are precursors of both surface epithelial cells and parietal cells; and mast cells, which contain histamine. The body is bounded superiorly by the cardia (that portion of the stomach immediately below the gastroesophageal junction) and the fundus (the portion of the stomach lying to the left and superior to the gastro-esophageal junction). The cardia and fundus differ from the body only in that the numbers of parietal and chief cells are fewer. The most distal portion of the stomach is the antrum, which contains mucus-secreting glands as well as G cells, the source of the hormone *gastrin*. The stomach has two curvatures, the greater and lesser, and two surfaces, the anterior and the posterior. The anterior stomach is bounded superiorly by the diaphragm, anteriorly by the rectus abdominis muscle, and on the right by the left lobe of the liver. The posterior gastric wall is related to the pancreas, the left adrenal and kidney, the spleen, and the diaphragm. The greater curvature is proximate to the transverse colon; the lesser curvature abuts the liver.

The duodenum curves around the head of the pancreas in a C-shaped fashion, beginning at the pylorus and ending at the ligament of Treitz. It is approximately 10 inches long and is divided, by convention, into four parts: superior (first part), descending (second part), horizontal (third part), and ascending (fourth part). In its course, it receives the common bile duct and both the minor and major pancreatic ducts. Except for the absence of peritoneum on its posterior surface, the layers of the duodenal wall are analogous to those of the stomach. In all but its origin and termination, it is a retroperitoneal organ. Several mucosal cell types can be identified, including absorptive cells lining intestinal villi, goblet cells secreting mucus, a few G cells, and Brunner's gland cells, which secrete a mucoid alkaline fluid.

The stomach and duodenum are extremely well vascularized organs, deriving their blood supply from a rich network of anastomotic interconnections (Fig. 2). Both the

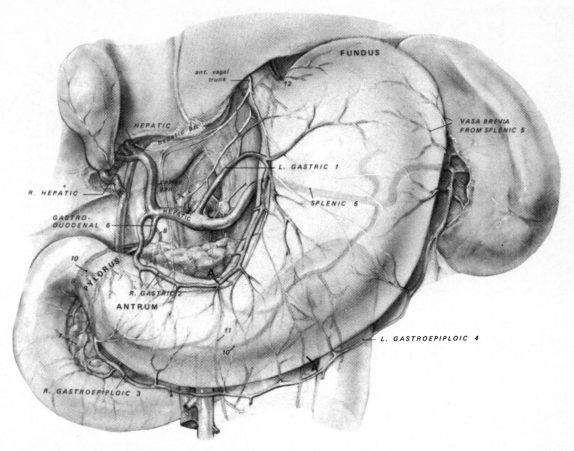

Figure 1. Anatomy of the stomach and duodenum. Grossly, the stomach is divided into fundus (the area superior to the gastroesophageal junction), body, and antrum. The antrum begins proximally at about a line drawn from A *on the lesser curvature to* A' *on the greater curvature and extends distally to the pylorus. There are only two important physiologic divisions, the fundic gland (parietal cell) area and the pyloric gland (antral) area. The junction of these two histologic zones is again roughly at a line between* A *and* A'. *The blood supply to the stomach is carried by six major vessels and by six other vessels of lesser consequence.*

The most important vessels are: 1, left gastric artery; 2, right gastric artery; 3, right gastroepiploic artery; 4, left gastroepiploic artery; 5, splenic artery via the vasa brevia; 6, gastroduodenal artery. The remaining vessels are indicated by a number only in the illustration: 7, superior pancreaticoduodenal artery; 8, supraduodenal artery of Wilkie; 9, retroduodenal artery; 10, transverse pancreatic artery; 11, dorsal pancreatic artery; and 12, left inferior phrenic artery.

The anterior (left) vagus is shown dividing into a gastric and a hepatic branch. Just behind it is also shown the posterior (right) vagus dividing into a gastric and a celiac branch. The duodenal-jejunal flexure is shown here behind the stomach. Its position is variable, and it may often be seen on x-ray protruding above the lesser curvature of the stomach just to the left of the midline.

(From Thompson, J. C.: In Sabiston, D. C., Jr. (Ed.): Textbook of Surgery, 13th ed. Philadelphia, W. B. Saunders Company, 1986, p. 811.)

celiac axis and the superior mesenteric artery are involved. After arising from the superior portion of the abdominal aorta, the celiac axis immediately divides into the left gastric, the hepatic, and the splenic arteries. The left gastric artery supplies the lesser curvature and the lower esophagus. It anastomoses with the right gastric artery, which is one of the branches of the hepatic artery. The greater curvature receives its blood supply from the right gastroepiploic artery, a branch of the gastroduodenal artery (itself a branch of the hepatic), from the left gastroepiploic artery, and from the short gastric arteries, both of which are derived from the splenic artery.

The gastroduodenal artery also supplies the duodenum. Its proximity to the posterior duodenal wall just distal to the pylorus renders it susceptible to acid peptic digestion with consequent massive upper gastrointestinal hemorrhage. The terminal branch of the gastroduodenal artery is the superior pancreaticoduodenal, which anastomoses with the inferior pancreaticoduodenal artery, the first branch of the superior mesenteric artery.

The parasympathetic nerve supply to the stomach and duodenum is also of some importance. The vagus nerves traverse the thoracic cavity as two branches proximate to the esophagus. After forming a plexus in the region of the esophageal hiatus, the anterior and posterior vagus nerves (also known as the nerves of Latarjet) emerge. The left anterior trunk innervates not only the stomach but also the duodenum, pancreas, liver, gallbladder, and bile ducts via its hepatic branch. The right posterior trunk supplies the stomach and, via its celiac branch, joins the celiac plexus to innervate the remainder of the small bowel and the colon up to the level of the splenic flexure. Of clinical importance, both vagus nerves send twigs through the esophageal musculature that provide additional parasym-

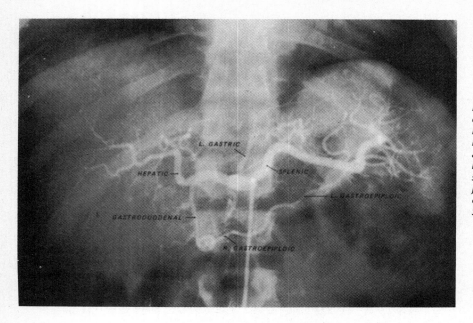

Figure 2. The blood supply of the stomach demonstrated by selective celiac angiography. The angiographic catheter is shown hooked into the orifice of the celiac artery, and injection of radiopaque material outlines the major vessels supplying the stomach (see Fig. 1). (From Thompson, J. C.: In Sabiston, D. C., Jr. (Ed.): Textbook of Surgery, 13th ed. Philadelphia, W. B. Saunders Company, 1986, p. 812.)

pathetic innervation to the proximal acid peptic-secreting portion of the stomach. The antrum, in turn, is innervated by branches of both nerves, where distribution resembles a crow's foot.

SURGICAL PHYSIOLOGY OF THE STOMACH AND DUODENUM

Gastric Acid Secretion

Hydrochloric acid is secreted in the proximal stomach by parietal cells (Fig. 3). Current evidence suggests that these cells contain three distinct receptors on their basolateral membranes: an H_2 receptor, responsive to histamine liberated from mast cells; a gastrin receptor, responsive to the peptide hormone gastrin; and a muscarinic receptor, responsive to acetylcholine released during cholinergic vagal stimulation. A "potentiating interaction" exists between the H_2 receptor and the gastrin and muscarinic receptors so that the acid secretory response to both gastrin and acetylcholine is significantly enhanced if the H_2 receptor locus is saturated. This phenomenon accounts for the demonstrated efficacy of H_2 receptor antagonists in reducing gastric acid production in response to acetycholine or gastrin stimulation alone. Once the gastrin and muscarinic receptor sites are occupied, calcium enters the interior of the cell and membrane-bound adenylate cyclase is activated. These events, in turn, stimulate the production of cyclic adenosine monophosphate (AMP), which acts on an $H^+ - K^+$·ATP-ase located in the apical cell membrane to promote secretion of H^+ in exchange for absorption of luminal K^+. A variety of inhibitors of gastric-acid production interact in this system: H_2 receptor antagonists competitively inhibit at the H_2 receptor locus; atropine blocks the muscarinic receptor; the prostaglandins inhibit activation of adenylate cyclase; omeprazole destroys membrane-bound $H^+ - K^+$ ATP-ase. A schematic illustration of the neurohumoral events occurring in digestion of a meal is shown in Figure 4.

Once secreted, concentrated HCl travels up the gastric pit, where it is only slightly diluted by nonparietal secretion.

Thus it arrives in the gastric lumen at a concentration that far exceeds that of the subjacent tissue. In any other semipermeable membrane of the body, this would promote massive diffusion of H^+ into the mucosa. Under ordinary circumstances, however, this does not occur in the stomach, a capacity of the gastric mucosa that has been termed the "gastric mucosal barrier." The capacity of the stomach to resist autodigestion because of this barrier has been termed "cytoprotection." Factors thought to promote this function include the existence of a viscid mucous gel at the apices of the cells at greatest risk; the surface epithelial cells; the capacity of surface epithelial cells to secrete bicarbonate into the mucus; the ability of the gastric mucosa to increase its nutrient blood flow in response to topical injury; and the ability of the mucosa to restore itself ("restitution") once surface cells are damaged. Endogenous prostaglandins, with which the mucosa is abundantly supplied, may modulate many of these factors.

The physiologic stimulus to gastric acid production is the ingestion of a meal. By convention, three distinct yet interrelated phases of secretion have been described.

The first is properly called the vagal or cephalic phase. The sight, smell, or thought of food excites neural centers in the cortex and hypothalamus. Signals are then transmitted through the vagus nerves to the stomach. Acid production resulting from vagal excitation results primarily from direct vagal stimulation of the parietal cells via muscarinic receptors. The vagus also has the capacity to stimulate release of gastrin from antral G cells. However, the overall contribution of vagally released gastrin to acid production during the cephalic phase is probably small. Vagal excitation also causes the release of mucus from surface epithelial cells and of the pre-enzyme pepsinogen from chief cells. Pepsinogen becomes fully active as the pH of intragastric content falls to 3.0 or lower. Although the magnitude of the acid response seen during the cephalic phase surpasses that produced during the other phases of secretion, its duration is short and therefore accounts for only 20 to 30 per cent of the total volume of gastric acid produced in response to a meal.

The gastric phase of secretion is mediated by the hormone gastrin (Fig. 5). This peptide is released from G

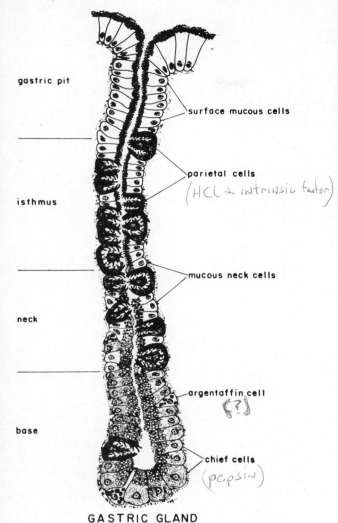

gastric pit

surface mucous cells

parietal cells

(HCL & intrinsic factor)

isthmus

mucous neck cells

neck

argentaffin cell

(?)

base

chief cells

(pepsin)

GASTRIC GLAND

Figure 3. A diagram of a simple tubular gastric gland from the fundus or corpus region of a bat stomach. (From Ito, S., and Winchester, R. J.: J. Cell Biol., 16:541, 1963.)

transient; several important mechanisms capable of inhibiting further acid production are also activated. The first, and most important, relates to intragastric pH. When the pH of intraluminal content in contact with the antrum falls below 2.5, gastrin release is almost completely arrested in normal individuals. Conversely, if antral pH rises to greater than 5, antral gastrin release continues. In addition, it is now clear that the vagus contains inhibitory fibers going to the antrum capable of modulating gastrin release in response to other stimuli. Intramucosal cholinergic reflex arcs may also inhibit both gastrin release and gastric acid production at the parietal cell level. Finally, transfer of an acid chyme into the proximal duodenum also serves to inhibit gastric acid production. Secretin, a hormone released from the proximal duodenum as the pH of duodenal chyme falls, inhibits gastrin release in normal man and, in addition, stimulates pancreatic bicarbonate secretion, leading to neutralization of acid within the duodenum. A second hormone, cholecystokinin (CCK), is released by intraluminal

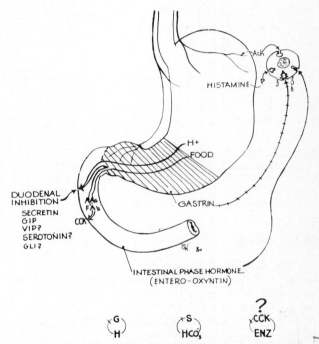

Figure 4. Schematic summary of some of the neurohumoral events that occur when a meal is eaten. Acetylcholine (Ach) is released from vagal nerve endings. Histamine is apparently released from stores within the mucosa. Gastrin is released by food (by a mechanism that is pH-sensitive) from antral mucosa (shaded area). Food in the small bowel stimulates release of the intestinal phase hormone. Each stimulant acts on the parietal cell (perhaps, as shown, each by means of a separate receptor on the cell membrane to stimulate secretion of H+). Delivery of acidified chyme into the duodenum evokes a series of events (some probably reflex, some humoral) that inhibit further gastric secretion. Some of the agents involved are listed. Amino acids and fatty acids (from partially digested food) cause release of cholecystokinin (CCK).

Three feedback mechanisms, which act to halt hormone release, are shown diagrammatically across the bottom as typical endocrine closed-loop relationships: acid (H+) halts release of gastrin (G), and HCO3− halts release of secretin (S). Intraduodenal enzymes (ENZ) may halt release of CCK, but this has not been proved.

(From Thompson, J. C.: In Sabiston, D. C., Jr. (Ed.): Textbook of Surgery, 13th ed. Philadelphia, W. B. Saunders Company, 1986, p. 815.)

cells in response to vagal excitation, antral distention, and the presence of partially digested protein in contact with antral mucosa. Several forms of gastrin have been identified, the most prominent of which is a heptadecapeptide. The active component of the molecule is contained within the C terminal pentapeptide sequence. The gastric phase of secretion persists for the several hours required for gastric emptying; therefore, it accounts for approximately 60 to 70 per cent of the total acid output seen in response to a meal.

The final and least understood phase of gastric acid production is the intestinal phase, which occurs after complete gastric emptying and continues as long as chyme remains in the proximal small intestine. The postulated mediator of this phase (entero-oxyntin) has not been isolated. In any case, it accounts for only 5 to 10 per cent of total acid output seen after eating. It is important to emphasize that each of these phases is interrelated and that the final common pathway for acid production in response to a meal is the parietal cell itself.

Once initiated, gastric acid production does not proceed indefinitely. Not only is the stimulus (the meal)

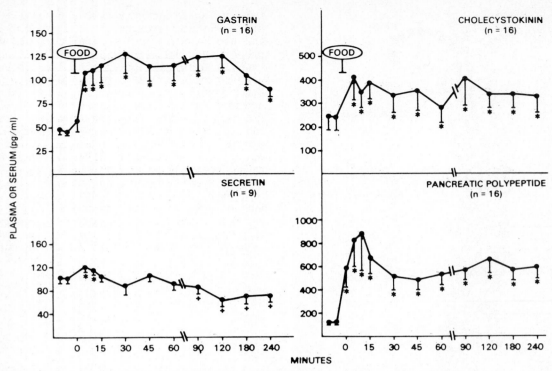

Figure 5. Pattern of release of gastrin, secretin, cholecystokinin, and pancreatic polypeptide. (From Thompson, J. C.: In Sabiston, D. C., Jr. (Ed.): Textbook of Surgery, 13th ed. Philadelphia, W. B. Saunders Company, 1986, p. 816.)

fat and protein and acts as a competitive inhibitor of gastrin at the parietal cell level. It seems likely (although not yet proven) that other intestinal peptides may play an equally important role in the inhibition of gastric acid production under physiologic circumstances.

Gastric Motility

The stomach must serve as a commodious reservoir for large volumes of ingested solids and liquids and, at the same time, must ensure that this material is delivered to the duodenum as small particles in isosmotic solution at physiologic pH. Gastric emptying of liquids is modulated primarily by the proximal stomach. From the resting volume of less than 100 ml., the body of the stomach is capable of increasing its intraluminal volume more than 15 times without an appreciable rise in intragastric pressure. This phenomenon is known as "receptive relaxation" and is partially mediated by the vagus nerve. Thus, following vagal denervation of the proximal stomach, receptive relaxation is absent, the proximal stomach cannot accommodate as well, intragastric pressure rises, and accelerated gastric emptying of liquids results.

Gastric emptying of solids is more complex. As solid food reaches the antrum, antral muscular contractions increase in both frequency and amplitude. This response is also mediated, at least in part, by the vagus. Initially, the pylorus remains closed so that forward propulsion of intestinal foodstuffs is followed by their retropulsion into the proximal stomach, resulting in a mixing and grinding action. Once solid food is an appropriate particle size (approximately 5 mm.), the pylorus opens in response to an integrated peristaltic wave (the antropyloric pump), permitting solid food to empty into the duodenum. Although the precise mechanism(s) of control for this elegantly integrated

motor activity has not been completely elucidated, it is clear that the integrity of the vagus nerve plays a major role. Once food has entered the duodenum, gastric motility is inhibited. Physical factors (temperature, pH, and osmolarity of intraduodenal chyme) and physiologic factors (vagal afferents, cholecystokinin, perhaps other peptides) are involved in this response, which is most profound when the duodenum is exposed to fat.

Physiology of Gastric and Duodenal Digestion

Ingested carbohydrates, fats, and proteins cannot be absorbed in their dietary forms. Therefore, they must be "digested" into absorbable components. The stomach and duodenum are responsible primarily for initiating digestion while absorption takes place in the more distal small intestine. Exceptions include alcohol, certain electrolytes, and ferrous ions, which can be absorbed directly from the stomach.

Dietary proteins consist of long-chain polypeptides, which must be hydrolyzed to component amino acids prior to absorption. This process is initiated in the stomach by the release of pepsinogen, which, in the presence of gastric acid, is converted to pepsin, an exopeptidase. In the duodenum, partially digested protein and fat cause the release of cholecystokinin, which, in turn, acts in concert with vagal stimulation to stimulate secretion of pancreatic trypsin, chymotrypsin, and carboxypeptidase. Each is secreted as an inactive precursor, which is subsequently activated by the duodenal hormone *enterokinase*. In their active forms, these enzymes promote further digestion of proteoses, peptones, and polypeptides, which are ultimately absorbed in the distal small intestine as amino acids.

The principal form of ingested dietary fat is *triglyceride*, three fatty acids linked to glycerol. The pancreatic enzyme that hydrolyzes triglycerides, *lipase*, is insoluble in fat, so that initially the large fat globules entering the duodenum are fragmented into smaller units by a process known as *emulsification*. Bile salts are required for this activity. Once emulsified, triglycerides are then hydrolyzed to fatty acids and monoglycerides. Hydrolysis alone is insufficient to ensure absorption, however, so that these moieties must be rendered water-soluble by bile acids, which form them into "micelles" (hydrophilic bile salts attached to hydrophobic free fatty acid and monoglyceride).

Digestion of carbohydrates is somewhat less complex. The process is initiated by salivary amylase, which hydrolyzes ingested sugars into maltose and isomaltose. The reaction continues in the stomach until sufficient acid is secreted to inactivate the enzyme. The greater part of dietary carbohydrate is hydrolyzed in the duodenum by pancreatic amylase, reducing polysaccharides to the disaccharides lactose and sucrose. These sugars, in turn, are reduced to monosaccharides by enzymes located in the brush borders of the intestinal mucosal cell and are subsequently absorbed as such.

PEPTIC ULCER DISEASE

An *ulcer* is a disruption in the integrity of what is normally a contiguous sheet of cells. A "peptic" ulcer is one that requires for its development the presence of acid and pepsin. In this sense, all ulcerative lesions of the upper gastrointestinal tract are peptic in origin. By convention, an ulcer involves the full thickness of the mucosa, whereas less than full-thickness lesions are termed *erosions*. Two major variants of peptic ulcers are commonly encountered in clinical practice: duodenal ulcers and gastric ulcers.

Duodenal Ulcer

The number of hospitalizations for duodenal ulcer disease has fallen precipitously in the United States over the past 15 years. Some feel that this is a reflection of a decreased incidence of the disease in the population as a whole. Nevertheless, approximately 1 in 15 Americans can expect to suffer from duodenal ulcers during his or her lifetime. The disease occurs more often in middle-aged males than females and is characterized by frequent episodes of exacerbation and remission. In general, duodenal ulcer is a benign condition without excessive mortality or morbidity except in the first year after diagnosis. Thus, 80 to 90 per cent of patients can be treated successfully by nonoperative means.

Anatomically, duodenal ulcers are found in three major locations:

1. Most commonly, distal to the pylorus on the posterior duodenal wall. (As noted previously, the proximity of these ulcers to the gastroduodenal artery can precipitate massive hemorrhage.)

2. Less commonly, distal to the pylorus on the anterior duodenal wall. (Free perforation into the peritoneal cavity can result.)

3. Least commonly, in the pyloric channel. (This location can predispose to obstruction.)

PATHOGENESIS

Over the past decade, much new information has been obtained from patient-related studies that enhance our understanding of the pathogenesis of duodenal ulcer disease in man. It is important to recognize that the disease is heterogeneous and that not all abnormalities are present in every patient. In general, however, patients with duodenal ulcer have approximately twice the number of parietal cells as do normal individuals. This fact is reflected by an increased capacity to secrete acid, both in response to exogenous stimulants (histamine or pentagastrin) and in response to the physiologic stimulus of a meal. Meal-stimulated acid secretion also persists for a longer period of time in patients than in normals. Current evidence also suggests that the individual parietal cells in patients with duodenal ulcer are more sensitive to any given stimulant. Hydrogen ion delivery to the duodenum is greater in patients with duodenal ulcer; in some individuals, this is a consequence of a rapid rate of gastric emptying. The gastrin response to a meal is also significantly exaggerated in duodenal ulcer disease.

Defects in resistance factors have also been identified. Gastrin release in response to a meal is incompletely inhibited at low pH in duodenal ulcer subjects, suggesting a defective acid "brake" on antral gastrin release. In addition, distention of the antrum, which ordinarily inhibits gastric acid production in normal individuals, appears to augment secretion in patients. On the other hand, other inhibitory mechanisms, particularly as they relate to humoral factors (secretin, cholecystokinin) are normal. The study of abnormalities in duodenal resistance factors is in its infancy; as information accumulates, it is likely that additional defects will be identified.

Genetic factors may also play an important role in the pathogenesis of duodenal ulcer. The gene for blood group O is associated with a higher incidence of the disease compared with other blood groups. Similarly, patients who fail to secrete ABO antigens into saliva and gastric juice are at increased risk. It has also been demonstrated that elevated circulating pepsinogen levels are inherited as an autosomal dominant trait. The presence of this trait renders an individual five times as likely to develop duodenal ulcers. Finally, familial duodenal ulcer has been described, suggesting that genetic factors may be important in some patients.

DIAGNOSIS

In the majority of patients, the diagnosis of duodenal ulcer disease is not difficult because the history is quite typical: intermittent episodes of burning epigastric pain aggravated by fasting and temporarily relieved by eating or by the ingestion of antacids. Occasionally, the pain will radiate through to the back, raising the suspicion that the ulcer has penetrated into the pancreas. Definitive diagnosis is established by the finding on upper gastrointestinal barium studies of an active ulcer crater, a deformed duodenal bulb, or edematous duodenal folds (Fig. 6). In the usual case, endoscopic confirmation of the presence of the ulcer and analysis of gastric acid output are not required.

INDICATIONS FOR OPERATION

Longitudinal studies of large numbers of patients with duodenal ulcers indicate that the vast majority (80 to 90 per cent) live in harmony with their disease, often requiring no medication whatsoever. In 10 to 20 per cent of instances, however, surgical intervention will be required. The classic indications for operative therapy include hemorrhage, perforation, obstruction, and failure of nonoperative management ("intractability").

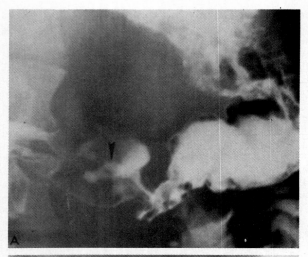

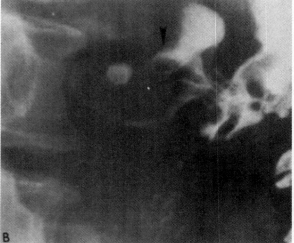

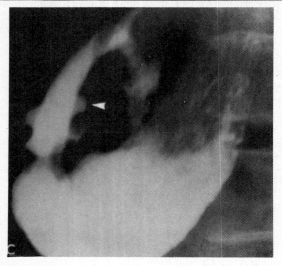

Figure 6. Supine left posterior oblique projections of the duodenal cap showing a duodenal ulcer filled with barium (A and B). A circular collection of barium is also visible (ring sign) (arrow). Supine right posterior projection (C) shows that this is an ulcer in the anterior wall of the duodenum in which only the walls of the crater are coated with barium. A second ulcer in the posterior wall is also visible (arrow). (From Berk, R. N.: In Teplick, J. G., and Haskin, M. E. (Eds.): Surgical Radiology—A Complement in Radiology and Imaging to Sabiston, D. C., Jr. (Ed.): Davis-Christopher Textbook of Surgery, Vol. 1. Philadelphia, W. B. Saunders Company, 1981, p. 439.)

Approximately 10 per cent of patients with duodenal ulcer disease can expect to experience ulcer-related bleeding. In the majority of instances, the magnitude of the hemorrhage is mild, and it will stop spontaneously. In some patients, however, hemorrhage is massive: at least 1000 ml. of replacement volume is required to resuscitate the patient, and at least 500 ml. every 6 to 8 hours is needed to maintain hemodynamic stability. Patients at risk for massive hemorrhage or early rebleeding in the hospital are those with visible vessels in the ulcer crater and those who are actively bleeding at the time of admission. The mortality of hemorrhage from duodenal ulcer is increased as the magnitude of the bleed and the age of the patient increase. In the hands of a skilled endoscopist, a correct diagnosis can be accomplished in 95 to 100 per cent of instances. Whether or not endoscopy should be employed routinely in all patients with upper gastrointestinal bleeding is controversial. It is clear, however, that those patients with massive bleeding should undergo endoscopy. The likelihood that surgical intervention will be required is great, and operative mortality is significantly reduced if a bleeding site has been identified preoperatively.

Ulcers located on the anterior duodenal wall may perforate into the free peritoneal cavity, resulting in the sudden onset of severe generalized abdominal pain associated with a rigid abdomen on examination. In two thirds of instances, patients with perforation will have a long history compatible with chronic duodenal ulcer disease; conversely, perforation may be the index symptom in as many as a third of patients. An erect abdominal film will demonstrate free air under the diaphragm in approximately 85 per cent of instances. In the remaining cases, a lateral decubitus film may reveal air between the liver and the abdominal wall. Occasionally, Rigler's sign will be encountered: the capacity to visualize both the mucosal and serosal surfaces of the small intestine on abdominal roentgenograms. Laboratory studies will usually reveal a leukocytosis with increased immature forms. Occasionally, an elevated serum amylase will be noted as duodenal luminal content spills into the peritoneal cavity and is absorbed systemically.

Gastric outlet obstruction may be a consequence of cicatricial scarring in the region of an ulcer that has undergone repeated cycles of activation and healing. Alternatively, obstruction may be due to edema secondary to ulcer reactivation. Differentiation is important, since the former almost always mandates surgical intervention while the latter may not. Clinical features include nausea, fullness, vomiting, and weight loss. In severe cases, marked dehydration and electrolyte imbalance may ensue. The finding of a dilated stomach that fails to empty on upper gastrointestinal barium studies establishes the diagnosis. Initial treatment should be directed toward decompressing the stomach, correcting electrolyte and volume deficits, and providing maximal nonoperative antiulcer therapy. If the obstruction persists on this regimen, surgical management is warranted.

The final indication for operative therapy is intractability, i.e., the inability of maximal nonoperative treatment to provide symptomatic relief. Simple in concept, the fact remains that there may be as many intractable patients (those who cannot comply with such regimens) as there are intractable ulcers. In the pre-cimetidine era, this was the most common indication for operation. Current evidence suggests that the introduction of H_2 receptor antagonists has reduced the relative numbers of patients coming to operation on this basis by approximately 20 per cent. Conventional surgical wisdom holds that patients operated on for intractability are more prone to the development of disabling *postgastrectomy syndromes* (described later in this

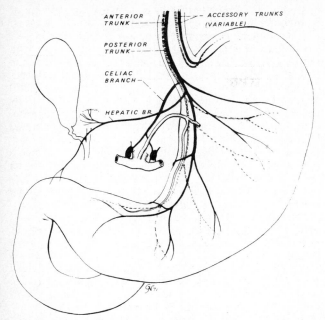

Figure 7. Anatomy of the vagus nerves in relation to the stomach. Both anterior (left) and posterior (right) vagi give off gastric branches. The anterior vagus has a hepatic branch that may send fibers to the region of the pylorus; the posterior vagus has a celiac branch that goes to the celiac ganglia and plexus and from there goes to contribute to the innervation of other abdominal viscera. The remaining fibers descend within the gastrohepatic ligament along the lesser curvature as the anterior and posterior nerves of Latarjet. These give branches to the fundus and cross inferiorly at the incisura angularis onto the antrum, to whose muscle fibers they provide innervation. (From Thompson, J. C.: In Sabiston, D. C., Jr. (Ed.): Textbook of Surgery, 13th ed. Philadelphia, W. B. Saunders Company, 1986, p. 839.)

chapter). This is untrue: The results following operation for intractability are indistinguishable from those seen when the same procedure is employed for one of the other indications.

OPERATIONS FOR DUODENAL ULCER

The aim of operative therapy for duodenal ulcer is to cure the disease (something nonoperative approaches rarely achieve) without producing excessive immediate or long-term morbidity. Based on an understanding of the pathophysiology of duodenal ulcer, several options are available: interruption of the cephalic phase of secretion (vagotomy) (Fig. 7), interruption of the cephalic phase and ablation of the gastric phase (vagotomy and antrectomy), or ablation of the gastric phase in combination with removing a generous portion of the end organ, the parietal cell mass (subtotal gastrectomy). It is unfortunate that those procedures with the highest potential for cure are also those most likely to produce untoward postoperative sequelae.

Subtotal gastrectomy consists of resection of the distal two thirds to three quarters of the stomach with restoration of gastrointestinal continuity either as a gastroduodenostomy (Billroth I) or gastrojejunostomy (Billroth II) (Fig. 8). For many years, this operation was the mainstay of surgical therapy for duodenal ulcer disease. Long-term follow-up, however, indicates that recurrent ulcers can be anticipated in 3 to 5 per cent of patients, that operative morbidity is substantial, and that the incidence of unpleasant postgastrectomy syndromes, particularly early postpran-

dial dumping, is high (approximately 30 per cent). For these reasons, the operation has justifiably been abandoned by most surgeons.

The most popular resective procedure in use today is a distal gastrectomy (antrectomy) combined with section of the truncal vagus nerves at the esophageal hiatus (Fig. 9). This procedure is associated with the lowest recurrence rate of any ulcer operation (less than 2 per cent at 5 years) and is relatively safe in accomplished hands. Unfortunately, the incidence of postoperative diarrhea and dumping remains high (10 to 20 per cent).

Truncal vagotomy associated with a drainage procedure is currently the most popular operation in use in the United States. Its efficacy depends solely on its capacity to interrupt the cephalic phase of secretion. The drainage procedure is necessitated by the fact that denervation of the antrum impairs the capacity of the distal stomach to empty solids. Thus, movement of ingesta into the duodenum must be facilitated. A variety of techniques are available to accomplish this end. The most popular is to perform one of several available types of pyloroplasty (Heineke-Mikulicz, Finney, Jaboulay). All aim to enlarge the gastric outlet. An alternative approach is to create a gastrojejunal anastomosis at the most dependent portion of the stomach. Both types of drainage procedures are equally efficacious in promoting gastric emptying; neither is superior in reducing the risk of recurrent ulcer. Truncal vagotomy and drainage is a safe procedure with a mortality rate of less that 1 per cent. Its main disadvantage is that the risk of recurrent ulcer disease is relatively high (10 per cent recurrence in 10 years, 30 per cent in 15 years). In

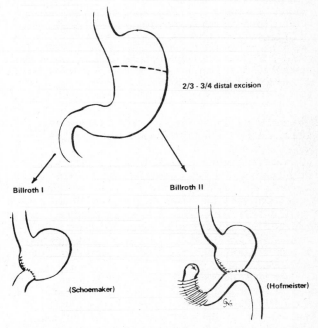

Figure 8. Types of reconstruction after subtotal gastric resection. Resection removes 66 to 75 per cent of the distal stomach, thereby excising the entire antral-gastric mechanism as well as a large portion of the parietal cell mass. Reconstruction of continuity of the gastrointestinal tract may be performed either with a gastroduodenostomy (Billroth I) anastomosis or with a gastrojejunostomy (Billroth II) anastomosis. The Schoemaker modification of the Billroth I anastomosis includes partial closure of the lesser curvature of the stomach, as does the Hofmeister modification of the Billroth II anastomosis. (From Thompson, J. C.: In Sabiston, D. C., Jr. (Ed.): Textbook of Surgery, 13th ed. Philadelphia, W. B. Saunders Company, 1986, p. 838.)

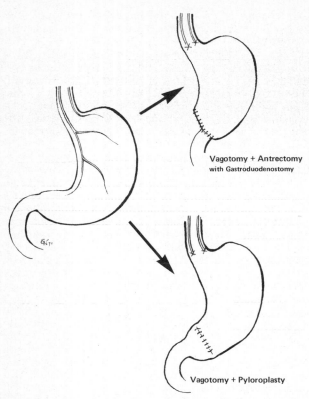

Figure 9. Acceptable operations for duodenal ulcer disease. Because the aim of any surgical procedure for duodenal ulcer is the diminution of acid output, vagotomy should be a part of any such operation if there is no specific contraindication. The choice, therefore, lies between vagotomy plus antrectomy and vagotomy plus drainage. Current information would indicate that gastroenterostomy (with gastric stoma immediately proximal to pylorus) is equally as good a drainage procedure as pyloroplasty. (From Thompson, J. C.: In Sabiston, D. C., Jr. (Ed.): Textbook of Surgery, 13th ed. Philadelphia, W. B. Saunders Company, 1986, p. 841.)

addition, even though gastric reservoir function is preserved, early postprandial dumping occurs in 10 to 15 per cent of instances.

Selective vagotomy is a variant of truncal vagotomy, which enjoyed a brief moment in the sun. In this procedure, the entire stomach is denervated but the vagal branches to the liver and the celiac plexus are preserved. It was thought that an intact visceral vagal innervation would reduce the incidence of postoperative dumping and diarrhea. Unfortunately, this has not been the case in most studies because the presence of the necessary drainage procedure promotes rapid gastric emptying.

The latest innovation in the operative therapy of duodenal ulcer is parietal cell vagotomy, a procedure that attempts to denervate the partietal cell mass only (Fig. 10). Thus, the motor function to the antrum and pylorus is maintained intact, with the result that gastric emptying of solids is normal. For this reason, a drainage procedure is unnecessary. As a result, the incidence of early postprandial dumping is almost completely eliminated. Mortality and morbidity are low, and recurrence rates at 5 years approximate those of truncal vagotomy and drainage. The procedure is a difficult one and should be performed only by surgeons experienced in the technique. In fact, several studies show lower recurrence rates in the hands of those who perform the procedure frequently. Significantly, the

operation is contraindicated in patients with prepyloric or pyloric ulcers because of excessively high recurrence rates.

The operative approach to patients with bleeding or perforation requires special comment. In the patient with massive hemorrhage, it is mandatory to resuscitate the patient adequately prior to operation. As mentioned, endoscopy is a highly useful (perhaps even indispensable) adjunct to confirm the diagnosis. Although it is generally agreed that an acid-reducing procedure is appropriate, controversy exists as to which of the several available should be employed. It is our opinion that truncal vagotomy associated with oversewing of the bleeding ulcer through a pyloroplasty accomplishes adequate control with minimal risk of rebleeding and low operative mortality and morbidity. Similarly, no consensus exists as to the appropriate procedure for the perforated duodenal ulcer. Current evidence suggests, however, that simple closure of the ulcer with an omental patch is appropriate if the patient is unstable, if the degree of peritoneal soiling is great, or if the ulcer is acute. On the other hand, if the patient is stable, if the amount of contamination is minimal, and if the ulcer is clearly chronic, an acid-reducing procedure can be performed safely. Most surgeons prefer a truncal vagotomy with pyloroplasty to include the ulcer.

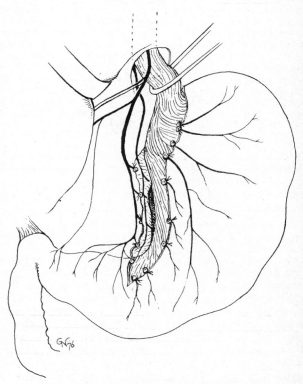

Figure 10. Technique for selective proximal vagotomy. Fundic branches of the gastric divisions of the anterior and posterior vagi are severed and ligated at the attachment of the gastrohepatic ligament to the lesser curvature of the stomach as well as around the circumference of the fundoesophageal junction. The antral branches of the descending nerves of Latarjet are preserved. It is important that the lower esophagus be completely skeletonized so as to divide any vagal fibers that might reach the fundus by way of the distal esophagus. The hepatic branches of the anterior vagus and the celiac branch of the posterior vagus are preserved. (From Thompson, J. C.: In Sabiston, D. C., Jr. (Ed.): Textbook of Surgery, 13th ed. Philadelphia, W. B. Saunders Company, 1986, p. 841.)

Benign Gastric Ulcer

Ulcerations of the mucous membrane of the stomach proper are encountered less commonly than are duodenal ulcers. They occur in older patients, often in association with malnutrition, and are slightly more common in males than in females. The most prevalent type (Type I) heals readily with nonoperative therapy, but has a marked tendency to recur. An additional clinical challenge is to differentiate such ulcers from gastric carcinomas.

PATHOGENESIS

Not all gastric ulcers are etiologically similar. Three types have been distinguished; the Type III benign gastric ulcer (15 per cent of the total) is prepyloric in that it is found within 2 cm. of the pylorus. The etiology of ulcers is probably similar to that of duodenal ulcer; i.e., they are in this location "duodenal ulcers that have gone astray." Therefore, when operative therapy is required, a procedure appropriate to duodenal ulcer should be employed. Type II benign gastric ulcer (20 per cent) are those found in association with a duodenal ulcer that has obstructed the gastric outlet. The "Dragsted hypothesis" suggests that these ulcers result from antral stasis, which produces hypergastrinemia. The subsequent relative hypersecretion of acid leads to ulceration of the stomach at the "point of least resistance," the junction of the acid-peptic secreting and antral mucosae at the level of the incisura on the lesser curvature. As with the Type III ulcers, an operation appropriate for duodenal ulcer gives excellent results.

The most common of the benign gastric ulcers (65 per cent) is Type I. These also occur on the lesser curvature, usually at the incisura but occasionally more proximal. In contrast to Type II ulcers, however, Type I ulcers are always solitary. On occasion, they may be found on the greater curvature, where distinction from gastric carcinoma can be difficult. Considerable clinical and experimental evidence suggests that these ulcerations are a consequence of an incompetent pylorus that permits excessive reflux of upper intestinal content into the stomach. This, in turn, results in the gradual development of an atrophic gastritis that migrates proximally over time. Atrophic gastric mucosa is demonstrably more susceptible to acid-peptic digestion than is normal mucosa, perhaps as a consequence of excessive "back diffusion" of acid. Thus, despite the fact that patients with Type I ulcers are usually normo- or hypochlorhydric on gastric secretory testing, the ulcer is properly classified as peptic. Ulceration usually occurs at the junction of the normal acid-secreting mucosa and the non–acid-secreting gastritic mucosa. Of all peptic ulcers of the upper gastrointestinal tract, this type is most clearly related to defects in mucosal resistance. In fact, excessive ingestion of nonsteroidal anti-inflammatory compounds (NSAIDs) has been clearly implicated in the development of these ulcers in certain subsets of patients.

DIAGNOSIS

The clinical manifestations of gastric ulcer are quite variable. As with duodenal ulcer, pain is the most common presenting complaint. However, the sequence of pain relieved by food is not nearly as clear in gastric ulcer; in fact, food may exacerbate the patient's complaints. Thus, weight loss is a frequent accompaniment of the disease. In addition, it is not uncommon to encounter completely asymptomatic gastric ulcers, particularly in users of NSAIDs. Under these conditions, bleeding or perforation may be the index clue as to their presence.

The definitive diagnosis of gastric ulcer is made radiographically and endoscopically. An upper gastrointestinal barium study will detect the ulcer in more than 95 per cent of instances. Gastroscopy is an important adjunct in this situation because it is frequently difficult to distinguish a benign from a malignant ulcer radiographically. Besides allowing direct visualization of the ulcer, multiple biopsies can be obtained for histologic examination.

When benignity is ensured, a trial of nonoperative therapy is indicated. This approach is usually successful with a benign ulcer. Failure to heal on an adequate regimen suggests malignancy and is an indication for operation. Even in those patients who do heal, relapse may occur in as many as two thirds. In the opinion of most surgeons, this circumstance is also an indication for operation. Finally, 10 to 15 per cent of benign gastric ulcers can either bleed or perforate, necessitating urgent surgical therapy.

OPERATIONS FOR BENIGN GASTRIC ULCER

As indicated previously, patients with Type II and Type III benign gastric ulcers should be subjected to operations appropriate for duodenal ulcer. In Type I benign gastric ulcer, the performance of a distal gastrectomy to include the ulcer without concomitant vagus section is associated with a 95 per cent cure rate. Most surgeons prefer reconstruction as a Billroth II gastroduodenostomy. Some feel that a truncal vagotomy should be added if the ulcer is a consequence of NSAID abuse. Truncal vagotomy with drainage procedure may also be appropriate if the ulcer is concomitantly excised. Early results with parietal cell vagotomy have been salutary, but the long-term recurrence rates have yet to be identified.

The morbidity and mortality associated with bleeding and perforated gastric ulcer are considerably greater than that seen under similar circumstances with duodenal ulcer. This is so because delay in diagnosis of perforation is common and because elderly patients do not tolerate a major upper gastrointestinal hemorrhage as well as do younger patients. The aim of operation under these conditions is to excise the ulcer and to perform an acid-reducing procedure, either distal gastrectomy or truncal vagotomy and drainage. Parietal cell vagotomy is probably inappropriate under these emergent circumstances.

Can lead to colonization of stomach and aspiration pneumonia.

STRESS EROSION AND ACUTE HEMORRHAGIC GASTRITIS

Stress erosions are multiple, punctate, hemorrhagic lesions of the proximal stomach that develop in the setting of severe and unremitting physiologic stress (Fig. 11). In contrast to the more usual chronic ulcerations of the upper gastrointestinal tract, they rarely penetrate deeply into the mucosa and are unassociated with chronic inflammatory cell infiltration. In the absence of effective prophylaxis, stress erosions will progress and coalesce in 20 per cent of instances to form multiple ulcerations resulting in upper gastrointestinal hemorrhage of life-threatening severity. This condition is known as acute hemorrhagic gastritis. Certain populations are predictably at risk: those hospitalized in intensive care units (in 5 per cent bleeding may originate from this source), those sustaining severe trauma

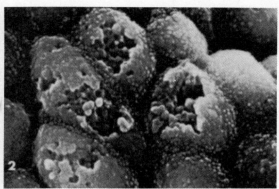

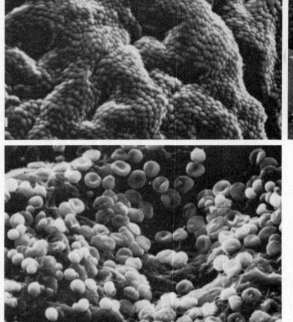

Figure 11. Surface morphology of the stomach in stress ulcer disease. 1, A three-dimensional surface view of stomach mucosa shows many folds, gastric pits, and numerous epithelial cells (× 375). 2, High magnification shows four altered surface epithelial cells, which exhibit membrane disruption and loss of portions of their apical region (× 8000). 3, This region covered by fibrin with enmeshed erythrocytes corresponds to grossly hemorrhagic area (× 2000). (From Lucas, C. E., Sugawa, C., Riddle, J., et al.: Arch. Surg., 102:266, 1971.)

(20 per cent), and those with greater than 35 per cent total body surface area thermal burns (up to 50 per cent). Specific risk factors include large transfusion requirements, the adult respiratory distress syndrome, oliguric renal failure, post-traumatic hepatic dysfunction, and, most important, development of systemic sepsis from any source.

Pathogenesis

Four unique pathophysiologic features characterize the development of stress ulcers. In the first instance, they are acute in onset, suggesting that a sudden rather than chronic or gradual disruption of normal homeostatic mechanisms is responsible. Second, they are multiple in number, suggesting that the condition is a disease of the entire mucous membrane. Third, they are located primarily in the proximal stomach, suggesting that acid and pepsin are important in their evolution. Finally, stress ulcers are not usually associated with hypersecretion of gastric acid, suggesting that resistance factors are more important to its development than are aggressive factors.

When these distinctive features are used to define stress ulcer disease, it is clear that the acute gastric mucosal lesion seen following massive trauma or major burns conforms well to the definition. On the other hand, the acute gastric or duodenal ulcer associated with isolated central nervous system trauma (so-called *Cushing's ulcers*) may well represent a different pathophysiologic entity. This type of injury is associated with high acid output and elevated levels of circulating gastrin. Furthermore, Cushing's ulcers are frequently solitary, often occur in the duodenum, and have a marked tendency to perforate. Conversely, the acute hemorrhagic gastropathies associated with the abuse of drugs and alcohol resemble stress ulcerations in many respects. Indeed, they may have a similar pathophysiology, albeit at the opposite end of the spectrum. Nevertheless, it is inappropriate to consider them as true stress ulcers because the setting in which they develop is unrelated to any massive physiologic insult and their clinical course is substantially more benign.

Stress ulceration and its clinical endpoint, acute hemorrhagic gastritis, are the ultimate expression of failed cytoprotection, the capacity of the gastric mucosa to prevent autodigestion. All of the barriers that normally contribute to cytoprotection could, in theory, be defective in the setting in which stress ulcer disease develops. Perhaps the most important of these is an impaired ability of the gastric mucosa to increase its blood flow in the presence of acid "back diffusion." Considerable experimental and clinical evidence suggests that both excessive luminal acid loss and mucosal ischemia are indispensable to the development of stress ulcer. It is probable that ulcerogenesis is a function of the rate of decline of intramucosal pH, the absolute level of intramucosal pH achieved, and the duration at which intramucosal pH remains outside acceptable physiologic limits.

Diagnosis and Clinical Course

If patients at risk are subjected to endoscopy within 24 to 48 hours following the precipitating insult, more than 60 per cent will demonstrate stress erosions. However, the clinical onset of hemorrhage is often delayed for 5 to 10 days and is usually manifested by painless hematemesis or the appearance of bright red blood in the nasogastric tube. Melena and hematochezia are much less frequently encountered. On occasion, the development of acute hemorrhagic gastritis will be heralded by deteriorating vital signs suggestive of hypovolemia. The diagnosis should be suspected whenever a critically ill patient develops painless upper gastrointestinal tract hemorrhage. Upper endoscopy is the diagnostic modality of choice and will result in a correct identification of the bleeding source in more than 90 per cent of instances. In contrast, barium studies are inaccurate (because of the superficial nature of the lesion) and may even be counterproductive if arteriographic localization of the bleeding site is required.

The aims of therapy in established acute hemorrhagic gastritis are four: (1) resuscitation and stabilization of the patient, (2) control of the hemorrhage, (3) prevention of recurrent bleeding, and (4) patient survival. Unfortunately, it is frequently possible to achieve the first three without accomplishing the fourth because of the setting in which acute hemorrhagic gastritis develops.

TREATMENT

A variety of nonoperative therapies have been advocated for this condition. Regrettably, they are either demonstrably ineffective (antacid titration, systemic H_2 receptor blockade) or effective only temporarily and associated with high morbidity and mortality (selective intra-arterial vasopressin). Operative therapy is only slightly more efficacious. Options include truncal vagotomy and drainage, truncal vagotomy and hemigastrectomy with oversewing of proximal lesions, vagotomy with extensive subtotal gastrectomy (also incorporating oversewing of proximal lesions), and total gastric devascularization. Total gastrectomy has also been advocated, but is inadvisable because of the high associated operative mortality. With the exception of total gastric devascularization, which has been tried in only a few patients, all operative approaches are associated with a relatively poor initial control rate and a high rate of rebleeding. This is especially true following nonresective procedures. Under any circumstance, however, mortality after operation is excessively high (30 to 40 per cent). For these reasons, the best treatment for acute hemorrhagic gastritis is its prevention. Based on what is known of the pathophysiology of the disease, the general methods of accomplishing prophylaxis should include restoration of circulating blood volume, maintenance of a normal cardiac output, correction of acid-base imbalances, and provision of adequate parenteral nutrition. More specific attempts at prevention should include measures to reduce the mass of intraluminal acid and, in the future, could include attempts to strengthen the individual barriers to autodigestion already mentioned.

Two general approaches have been used to control intraluminal pH: intravenous H_2 receptor-blocking agents (primarily cimetidine) and intragastric antacid titration to maintain intraluminal pH above 3.5 or 4. Which form of prophylaxis is most effective has been a matter of some debate. However, several well-designed prospective trials have recently been published that attempt to answer this question. None has demonstrated that cimetidine is in any way superior to antacids; one showed equivalence but only in terms of the endoscopic appearance of the gastric mucosa following thermal injury. Several common themes were apparent in the remaining studies: Intragastric instillation of antacid was invariably more effective in maintaining the pH of gastric aspirate at 3.5 or above than was cimetidine, irrespective of dosage. When cimetidine-resistant patients were crossed over to antacid treatment, prompt control of pH was achieved in virtually every instance. Bleeding was encountered in 2 to 18 per cent of the cimetidine-treated patients compared with 0 to 5 per cent in the antacid-treated groups, differences that were statistically significant. The reasons for the relative "failure" of cimetidine to provide adequate prophylaxis are unclear. In part, they may relate to inadequate drug delivery resulting in inade-

quate control of pH. It has also been suggested that cimetidine fails because, coincident with inhibition of acid secretion, the availability of buffer to the mucosa in the form of the "alkaline tide" is also appreciably reduced.

In the future, better forms of prevention for those few patients in whom current prophylactic regimens are inadequate may be developed. Two classes of compounds may fulfill this need. The first, *sucralfate*, is a basic sulfated aluminum salt of sucrose that forms a viscid and impermeable gel over the lesion because its negative charge binds to positively charged exposed protein. This, in turn, may promote healing of the subjacent gastric erosion. The second class of compounds, the *prostaglandins*, are normally present in abundance in the gastric mucosa. In experimental animals, they are cytoprotective against a variety of noxious insults when given exogenously in both antisecretory and non-antisecretory doses. In man, there is some evidence to suggest that prostaglandins may be efficacious not ony as prophylaxis but also as treatment of established acute hemorrhagic gastritis.

ZOLLINGER-ELLISON SYNDROME

In 1955, Zollinger and Ellison described a triad of findings in a small group of patients with intractable ulcer disease: massive hypersecretion of acid, leading to a virulent duodenal and jejunal ulcer diathesis, associated with a non–beta islet cell tumor of the pancreas. They postulated that an endocrine pancreatic peptide was the offending secretagogue, a postulation that was proved 9 years later by the demonstration of large amounts of gastrin in a resected specimen. It is now clear that Zollinger-Ellison (Z-E) tumors are microscopic in 50 per cent of patients, multiple in two thirds, and clinically malignant in more than 60 per cent. Although malignant gastrinoma may be indolent and compatible with long survival, it usually proves fatal to the patient because of extensive metastatic disease. Approximately 20 per cent are truly solitary (arising either in the pancreas, in the gastric antrum, or in the duodenum) and are therefore amenable to curative resection. Even when cure cannot be effected, it is possible to remove most macroscopic tumor in 60 per cent of instances.

The presence of a Zollinger-Ellison tumor should be suspected in patients who demonstrate multiple ectopically situated ulcers or a rapid recurrence after routine ulcer surgery. Associated radiographic signs include giant rugal folds, an indication of an eightfold increase in parietal cell mass, increased gastric and intestinal secretions, and a rapid transit time. In fact, diarrhea is a frequent presenting complaint (occasionally, the only presenting complaint). The diagnosis is established by the finding of massive hypersecretion of gastric acid (basal acid output greater than 10 mEq. per hour, maximal acid output greater than 50 mEq. per hour) and/or basal hypergastrinemia, which increases, paradoxically, by greater than 400 pg. per ml. when the patient is given purified secretin. The combination of these studies serves to differentiate the syndrome from other causes of elevated serum gastrin, namely, pernicious anemia, antral G cell hyperplasia, postvagotomy states, and retained gastric antrum following gastrectomy.

Occasionally, the Z-E syndrome is found in association with multiple endocrine adenopathies, a variant known as the MEA-1 or *Wermer's syndrome*. MEA-1 consists of hyperfunctioning tumors of the parathyroid, pituitary, and pancreatic islet cells. In the presence of hypercalcemia, parathyroidectomy frequently ameliorates the peptic ulcer diathesis despite persistent hypergastrinemia. The MEA-1 syndrome is inherited as an autosomal dominant trait with variable degrees of penetrance, so that the entire syndrome need not always be present in any given patient.

For many years the standard approach to the treatment of patients with isolated Z-E syndrome was to remove the target organ completely, i.e., to perform a total gastrectomy. This approach evolved from the recognition that direct attack on the primary tumor usually failed to extirpate all the gastrin-producing tissue and that less radical acid-producing procedures did not control ulcer complications. With the demonstration that H_2 receptor blockade markedly decreased acid output (although without affecting serum gastrin levels) and provided symptomatic control in most patients with Z-E syndrome, treatment options have expanded greatly.

In general, three approaches are currently employed. The first continues to rely on total gastrectomy to control the clinical manifestations of the disease. The principal advantage of this approach is that sure control of the ulcer diathesis is achieved and that resection of accessible or solitary tumors can be accomplished. Some also believe that total gastrectomy leads to tumor regression in as many as 10 per cent of instances. The long-term nutritional sequelae of this procedure in patients with Z-E syndrome are few and well tolerated because gastrin is a trophic hormone for small intestinal mucosa. In addition, severe dumping is largely avoided if the patient is reconstructed by a Roux-en-Y esophagojejunostomy. The principal disadvantage of this approach is that a small but definite (5 to 10 per cent) operative mortality exists, even in the hands of the most experienced surgeons.

A second option is "pharmacologic gastrectomy" using H_2 receptor antagonists. The advantage of this approach is that the risks associated with operation are avoided and at the same time control of the hypersecretory state with resolution of symptoms is accomplished, at least initially, in 80 per cent of patients. The disadvantages of the regimen include the fact that (1) the patient must be totally compliant with a lifelong medication schedule; (2) tachyphylaxis develops with time; (3) complications, when they occur, can be catastrophic; and (4) the opportunity to cure the disease is lost.

A third approach subjects each patient to exploratory laparotomy when the diagnosis is made. The aim of operation is to stage the disease in terms of metastatic spread and to remove as much tumor as is technically possible. In addition, resection of solitary gastrinomas can be accomplished if they are present. Some advocate the addition of parietal cell vagotomy at the time of laparotomy because this markedly lowers basal and stimulated acid output and therefore reduces the dosage of cimetidine required. This approach does not preclude the performance of a total gastrectomy at a later date. At the present time, superiority of one approach over another has yet to be demonstrated.

COMPLICATIONS OF GASTRIC SURGERY

All operative procedures designed to ameliorate the peptic ulcer diathesis have a common and rational basis: reduction in the capacity of the stomach to secrete acid. On occasion, this goal may not be achieved, resulting in recurrent ulcer. Even if the goal is realized, the patient may experience untoward sequelae known collectively as the *postgastrectomy syndromes*: a group of conditions, each with unique pathophysiologic features and clinical signs and symptoms that result from loss of gastric reservoir function, from ablation or bypass of the pylorus, or from parasympathetic denervation, either alone or in combination.

Recurrent Ulcer

Failure to accomplish adequate reduction in gastric acid production may result in recurrent ulceration following operation, a circumstance seen more often after operations for duodenal ulcer disease than for gastric ulcer disease. Patients who undergo nonresective procedures are at greater risk than are those in whom a portion of the stomach has been removed. Thus, parietal cell vagotomy for duodenal ulcer is associated with a 5-year recurrence rate of 10 to 15 per cent, compared with approximately 10 per cent with truncal vagotomy and drainage, 4 per cent after subtotal gastrectomy, and 1 to 2 per cent after truncal vagotomy and antrectomy. Most recurrences are evident within the first 2 years after resection, but tend to accumulate with time when nonresective procedures are employed. Recurrent ulcers are located on the enteric side of the anastomosis following resection, but they may occur with equal frequency in the intestine and stomach following nonresective procedures. Diagnosis is not difficult; most patients experience the renewed onset of typical peptic ulcer pain. Confirmation of the diagnosis is made endoscopically. Barium studies are notoriously unreliable because of the distorted postoperative anatomy.

Incomplete vagus section is the most common cause of recurrent ulcer, accounting for more than 80 per cent of cases. A variety of tests are available to measure the completeness of vagotomy postoperatively, the most popular being sham feedings. The classical *Hollander test*, which depends upon the induction of hypoglycemia with insulin, is rarely employed today because it is dangerous, the results being insensitive and nonspecific. Criteria for a "positive" test result, indicating incomplete vagotomy, include a fasting intragastric pH of less than 3.5, a fall of more than 2 pH units during testing, or an increase in acid concentration of greater than 20 mEq. per liter over a 2-hour period. Other causes of recurrent ulcer include the existence of a previously unrecognized gastrinoma, an inadequate resection of the parietal cell mass, retention of antrum at the duodenal stump, and an excessively long afferent limb following gastroenterostomy. Most recurrent ulcers are readily treated using H_2 receptor-blocking agents. Should these fail, re-vagotomy with resection or re-resection is indicated except in the patient with a gastrinoma, as discussed earlier.

Early Postprandial Dumping

Early postprandial dumping is the most common of the postgastrectomy syndromes, occurring in up to 50 per cent of patients after partial gastrectomy, in 30 per cent of patients after truncal vagotomy combined with drainage, and in approximately 5 per cent of patients following parietal cell vagotomy. The syndrome consists of a constellation of gastrointestinal and vasomotor signs and symptoms that occur within the first half hour after the ingestion of a meal. The gastrointestinal components include epigastric fullness, nausea, crampy abdominal pain, vomiting, and explosive diarrhea. Vasomotor components include sweating, weakness, dizziness, pallor followed by flushing, palpitations, and tachycardia. It is fortunate that the complete expression of the syndrome is rarely present in any given patient. In general, gastrointestinal components are more common than vasomotor ones.

The syndrome occurs as a consequence of rapid gastric emptying of hyperosmolar chyme from the residual stomach into the small intestine. This, in turn, causes movement of extracellular fluid into the intestinal lumen in an attempt to achieve isotonicity. The resultant decrease in circulating plasma volume has been postulated as being responsible for the vasomotor components of the syndrome. In addition, however, current evidence suggests that distention of the proximal small intestine liberates a variety of humoral substances (e.g., serotonin, bradykinin, and enteroglucagon) that may account for the facial flushing, the increased small intestinal motility, and the explosive diarrhea encountered in severe cases.

The diagnosis of early postprandial dumping is usually made on clinical grounds alone: characteristic postprandial symptomatology relieved by assuming a supine position. In most instances, sophisticated diagnostic evaluation is unnecessary. On occasion, it may be helpful to determine the rate of gastric emptying of solids and to assess peripheral blood flow using venous occlusive plethysmography and mercury strain gauge manometry. Provocative testing using hypertonic glucose solutions can also be undertaken if the diagnosis is equivocal.

In more than 90 per cent of instances, symptomatic patients can be successfully treated without operative therapy. Specific measures include frequent feeding of small meals rich in protein and fat and low in carbohydrate, and the avoidance of liquids with meals. In some patients, the ingestion with the meal of the gel-forming carbohydrate *pectin* is of added benefit. Posture may also be incorporated into the regimen because the assumption of the recumbent position slows gastric emptying and minimizes plasma volume changes. When operative therapy is required, the interposition of an antiperistaltic 10-cm. loop of jejunum between the gastric remnant and the small intestine has ben reported to be quite successful. Alternatively, creation of a Roux-en-Y limb may also be effective.

Late Postprandial Dumping Syndrome

The late postprandial dumping syndrome, also known as *reactive hypoglycemia*, is less common than its early counterpart, affecting fewer than 2 per cent of postgastrectomy patients. Symptoms occur much later than those of early dumping, usually 1½ to 3 hours following the ingestion of a carbohydrate-rich meal. Typically, patients complain of diaphoresis, tremulousness, tachycardia, and lightheadedness. The symptoms are characteristically relieved by the ingestion of carbohydrate.

The basic defect responsible for late postprandial dumping is the same as that responsible for early dumping: rapid gastric emptying. In this instance, however, the ingestion of a specific foodstuff, carbohydrate, is responsible. When sugars are delivered to the small intestine as a bolus, they are rapidly absorbed, thus producing a marked increase in blood glucose levels. Hyperglycemia triggers the release of large amounts of insulin, which over the course of the next 2 hours not only normalizes blood sugar but also, in symptomatic patients, "overshoots" the end point, resulting in profound hypoglycemia. This, in turn, stimulates the adrenal glands to release catecholamines, the end result being that symptoms indistinguishable from insulin shock are produced.

Nonoperative therapy is aimed toward normalizing the glucose tolerance curve, an aim that can be achieved by adding pectin to the diet. This compound impairs intraluminal digestion of starches and of sucrose and therefore delays carbohydrate absorption. Additional measures include the use of frequent small feedings of carbohydrate-poor meals and the ingestion of carbohydrate when symptoms begin. Should these approaches fail, the interposition of a 10-cm. antiperistaltic loop between the residual gastric pouch and the intestine delays gastric emptying and flattens the glucose tolerance curve with consequent alleviation of symptoms in the majority of patients in whom it has been employed.

Loop Obstruction

AFFERENT LOOP SYNDROME

The afferent loop syndrome is a consequence of obstruction of an afferent limb, i.e., the limb of a gastroenteric anastomosis leading to the stomach. Thus, it can occur only following gastrectomy with reconstruction as a Billroth II gastrojejunostomy. Two forms are distinguished: chronic and acute, the chronic form being more common.

The basic defect in the *chronic* afferent loop syndrome is intermittent obstruction of the limb after eating, most often a consequence of an excessively long afferent loop. Typically, patients complain of epigastric fullness and crampy abdominal pain shortly after the ingestion of the meal. The symptoms are relieved by vomiting. The vomitus is usually projectile and almost invariably contains bile but no food. This clinical picture is a consequence of meal-stimulated hepatobiliary and pancreatic secretion, resulting in the delivery of large volumes of bile and pancreatic juice to the duodenum. In the presence of partial or complete obstruction of the afferent limb, the loop rapidly distends, resulting in epigastric discomfort and cramping. Once the pressure in the loop is sufficiently great to overcome the obstruction, it decompresses itself into the stomach, resulting in projectile vomiting and the immediate relief of symptoms. The vomitus lacks food because the ingested meal has already passed into the efferent limb.

The *acute* form of afferent loop obstruction occurs early after operation. Although less common than the chronic form, it is also more lethal. The syndrome is the consequence of complete blockage of the afferent limb and results in a closed-loop type of obstruction. Patients typically complain of constant abdominal pain and vomiting. The volume of vomitus is small, and it may not contain bile. Delay in diagnosis is a frequent occurrence because the physical examination of the postoperative patient is difficult to interpret. Also, the condition is often incorrectly attributed to postoperative pancreatitis. In fact, hyperamylasemia is commonly seen because the increased hydrostatic pressure of the obstructed loop causes reflux of duodenal content into the pancreatic duct. As the obstruction persists, the afferent loop may strangulate with catastrophic results.

The treatment of both the acute and chronic forms of the syndrome is operative correction. The most expeditious and successful method of correcting the problem is to eliminate the loop. In our opinion, the creation of a long-limb Roux-en-Y with implantation of the afferent limb distal to the gastroenteric anastomosis is usually associated with an excellent outcome. The existence of the acute afferent loop syndrome may present special problems, because if the loop is gangrenous, a pancreaticoduodenectomy is required.

EFFERENT LOOP OBSTRUCTION

Efferent loop obstruction is also an infrequent complication of gastric surgery. It occurs most commonly in the immediate postoperative period, but can manifest itself years following the original procedure. The obstruction is usually a consequence of internal herniation of the efferent limb, usually posterior to the gastroenteric anastomosis. Patients complain of colicky epigastric pain, similar in character to that observed with small bowel obstruction. Radiographic studies may reveal evidence of a high small bowel obstruction. Operative therapy is almost always required. If, as is usually the case, a retroanastomotic hernia is found, it must be reduced and the retroanastomotic space must be obliterated.

Early Satiety

Early satiety, also known as the *small stomach syndrome*, is the consequence of excessive loss of gastric reservoir function. The greater the magnitude of resection, the greater the likelihood the syndrome will develop. Characteristically, patients complain of an extremely unpleasant sensation of fullness after ingesting only small amounts of food. Vomiting usually ensues if the patient attempts to increase oral intake. In severe cases, only small liquid meals are tolerable. Anemia and malnutrition frequently develop in such instances.

A variety of nonoperative measures have been advocated; none has achieved conspicuous success or patient acceptance. In fact, it has been estimated that early satiety is the postgastrectomy syndrome most refractory to nonoperative therapy. When operation is undertaken, the aim of the procedure is to create an adequate substitute gastric reservoir using a variety of surgically created pouches. Unfortunately, no operative procedure can completely ameliorate the symptoms of early satiety. Therefore, the best treatment of the small stomach syndrome is to avoid it in the first place.

Postvagotomy Diarrhea

Increase in stool frequency may be experienced by as many as 30 per cent of patients following transection of the vagus nerves. In most instances, the condition is either self-limiting or easily managed nonoperatively. Although the etiology of postvagotomy diarrhea remains obscure, it is believed that alterations in bile acid excretion or metabolism may play a role. Specifically, it has been suggested that vagal denervation of the hepatobiliary tree results in inadequate mixing of bile acids with intestinal chyme. Therefore, increased amounts of bile acids reach the colon, where they produce a cathartic effect. This postulation is supported by the fact that the bile acid binding resin *cholestyramine* is effective in more than 80 per cent of instances in which it has been tried. Operative therapy is rarely necessary; when required, a 10-cm. reversed jejunal segment placed 70 to 90 cm. from the ligament of Treitz gives excellent results.

Alkaline Reflux Gastritis

Excessive reflux of upper intestinal contents into the stomach following gastrectomy or pylorus ablating procedures has been implicated as a cause of a specific set of postoperative signs and symptoms: burning mid-epigastric pain unrelieved by antacids and frequently aggravated by food, bilious vomiting, hypochlorhydria, endoscopic gastritis (erythema of the entire mucous membrane of the stomach), weight loss, and anemia. In the majority of patients, a gastric resection with gastrojejunostomy reconstruction is the index procedure performed. Less frequently, the syndrome is encountered in association with reconstruction by a gastroduodenostomy or in patients undergoing truncal vagotomy and drainage. The exact incidence is unknown, but is probably less than 3 per cent of all patients undergoing gastric surgery. The factors in upper intestinal content that might be responsible for producing symptoms are unknown, but could include the bile acids, lysolecithin, pancreatic enzymes, or combinations of all three.

Although the diagnosis can be suspected on historical grounds, it is imperative that excessive reflux be established in an objective manner because a poor outcome can be anticipated in up to 50 per cent of patients when remedial operation is based on symptoms alone. Several methods are available to quantitate reflux, including the measurement of intragastric bile acid concentration and the development of reflux indices using gamma-scintigraphy. Normal values for these parameters have also been established.

When the presence of excessive reflux has been documented in typically symptomatic patients, a trial of nonoperative therapy is warranted. This should include H_2 receptor antagonists and the frequent ingestion of aluminum-containing antacids (aluminum binds bile salts). The use of cholestyramine, a bile salt binding resin, and metoclopramide, a promotility agent, has also been advocated; their efficacy, however, is questionable. When an operation is undertaken, conversion of the previous operative procedure to a long-limb (45 cm.) Roux-en-Y has brought salutary results: improvement in histologic gastritis, recovery of the capacity to secrete HCl, and permanent elimination of reflux. Complications have been few (marginal ulceration, significant delays in gastric emptying), bilious vomiting has been completely eliminated, and two thirds of patients are free of epigastric pain for at least 3 years postoperatively.

Gastric Stump Cancer

Carcinoma of the gastric stump occurs in approximately 3 per cent of patients undergoing gastrectomy, a far greater incidence than that observed in comparable but unoperated individuals. A latent period of 7 to 20 years is common. Patients usually present with symptoms that are indistinguishable from those of recurrent ulcer, and the diagnosis can be established only by endoscopy and biopsy. In experimental animals, the incidence of carcinoma is greatest following gastroenterostomy alone, less common following resection with Billroth II gastrojejunostomy, and least common following resection with Billroth I gastroduodenostomy. The pathogenesis of stump cancer, therefore, may be related to excessive reflux of upper intestinal content, which in turn promotes the development of atrophic gastritis, a premalignant lesion. In the face of hypochlorhydria, bacteria, particularly anaerobes, can proliferate in the stomach and can convert ingested nitrates to nitrites, precursors of carcinogenic nitrosamines. The concomitant presence of a susceptible membrane and a potent carcinogen may be the *sine qua non* for the induction of malignancy. Operative therapy is mandatory. Unfortunately, survivorship is poor, almost without exception. For this reason, many recommend lifelong follow-up for patients who have undergone resection in an effort to detect malignancy early.

Miscellaneous Conditions

The excretion of greater than normal amounts of fat in the stool is relatively common following all types of operative procedures on the stomach. In most instances, the absolute magnitude of fecal fat loss is small and of no clinical consequence. In a few cases, however, fat malabsorption may lead to fatty acid–induced diarrhea and to significant deficiencies in fat-soluble vitamin uptake. *Steatorrhea* may be the consequence either of inadequate micellization of ingested fat or of the development of the *blind-loop syndrome*. Steatorrhea, in turn, may predispose to the development of osteomalacia because fat malabsorption results in hypovitaminosis D. In severe cases, spontaneous fractures may develop. Most patients can be adequately treated by increasing vitamin D intake.

A *microcytic hypochromic anemia* can be demonstrated in more than 50 per cent of patients following gastrectomy. The cause is unclear, but it may relate to impaired iron absorption or to subliminal blood loss from the perianastomotic region. On rare occasions, a *megaloblastic anemia* may develop. Both B_{12} malabsorption and folate deficiency may contribute to this condition.

A few patients will be affected by *lactose intolerance* following gastrectomy. It is thought that these individuals have an intrinsic but unrecognized preoperative lactase deficiency that, for reasons that are poorly understood, becomes manifest only in the postoperative period. Treatment consists of avoiding lactose-containing foodstuffs.

OTHER BENIGN CONDITIONS

Mallory-Weiss Tears

In 1929, Mallory and Weiss detailed the case histories of 15 patients in whom massive hematemesis developed following severe bouts of vomiting during an alcoholic debauch. Four patients succumbed and at autopsy demonstrated "fissure-like" tears in the mucosa of the gastric cardia, one of which extended across the gastroesophageal junction. They attributed these lacerations to increased intragastric pressure produced as a consequence of vomiting and were able to reproduce the lesions in cadavers by applying pressure to the stomach while occluding both the pylorus and the proximal esophagus. Thereafter, the Mallory-Weiss "syndrome" was considered to be a rare but usually lethal entity. With the advent of the widespread use of fiberoptic endoscopy, however, it is now apparent that the Mallory-Weiss tear is responsible for 5 to 15 per cent of all upper gastrointestinal bleeds and that it is almost always a self-limiting and innocuous condition.

The diagnosis of Mallory-Weiss tears can often be established on historical grounds alone. Vomiting or retching preceding hematemesis is reported in over 50 per cent of instances. Alcohol use and/or abuse is a common accompaniment. Other causes of violent retching can also induce the syndrome: acetylsalicylic acid ingestion, severe hiccupping, cardiopulmonary resuscitation, difficult childbirth, and cancer chemotherapy. Middle-aged adults are those usually afflicted, males more commonly than females. The tears are usually longitudinal and, in approximately 83 per cent of patients, are located on the lesser curvature of the stomach just distal to the gastroesophageal junction. In approximately a third, the gastric tear will extend into the esophageal mucosa. Isolated esophageal tears are distinctly unusual. Many patients will have associated pathologic conditions of the stomach and esophagus, such as hiatal hernia, esophagitis, gastritis, and ulcer disease.

Mallory-Weiss tears develop because of the pressure differentials that occur within the abdominal and thoracic cavities during vomiting. When retching occurs against a closed glottis, the gastric mucosa herniates into the negative-pressure environment of the chest. If intraluminal gastric pressure is simultaneously elevated beyond the tolerable elastic limits of the gastric mucosa and submucosa, a longitudinal tear results. In the absence of gastric mucosal herniation, intraluminal pressure is greatest in the distal esophagus and disruption of esophageal mucosa may occur. At extremely high intraluminal pressure, esophageal circular and longitudinal muscle layers may actually rupture (*Boerhaave's syndrome*, described later).

The bleeding that results from a mucosal tear is most often arterial and is usually unassociated with pain. Early diagnostic endoscopy is highly accurate and can provide valuable information, including the location and length of the laceration and the presence or absence of associated pathology. Further, endoscopic visualization of the tear is of prognostic significance: tears that are actively bleeding or that demonstrate fresh clot may well continue to bleed, although simple mucosal contusions are unlikely to cause the patient any subsequent difficulty. In a few patients, angiography may be required because the magnitude of hemorrhage precludes endoscopic visualization. Angiography has a diagnostic accuracy of approximately 70 per cent in Mallory-Weiss tears, the usual picture being extravasation of the contrast material from the left gastric artery. In the presence of hemorrhage of this magnitude, it is wise to utilize the selectively placed catheter to initiate an immediate trial of angiographic pharmacotherapy using vasopressin. Should this fail, operation can be undertaken. In contrast to endoscopy and arteriography, the use of barium studies as a diagnostic tool in patients with Mallory-Weiss tears is a fruitless exercise having a diagnostic accuracy approaching zero. Furthermore, intraluminal barium precludes the use of diagnostic and/or therapeutic angiography in those rare instances in which this approach is required.

With the recognition that the Mallory-Weiss syndrome is far more common than previously appreciated, its treatment has become much less of a surgical exercise. The initial nonoperative management of afflicted patients is relatively nonspecific, consisting of antacid and cimetidine adminstration, correction of abnormalities in bleeding and clotting function, and administration of transfusions as necessary. In more than 90 per cent of patients, this approach is associated with cessation of hemorrhage, usually within a matter of hours. Rebleeding is uncommon and is usually manifested within 2 to 3 days. In approximately 10 per cent of instances, however, bleeding will continue, necessitating additional therapeutic interventions, usually in patients with severe liver disease. When the rate of hemorrhage exceeds more than 500 ml. every 6 hours, the use of systemic vasopressin is advisable. Vasopressin can also be given selectively if angiographic localization has been required. The success or failure of this approach is usually evident within 1 or 2 hours. Other options include the use of topical norepinephrine, endoscopic electrocautery, and angiographic embolization with gel foam or autologous clot. These may be preferable to the use of vasopressin in patients who have severe cardiovascular or renal disease. Operative therapy should not be delayed once it is clear that alternative approaches have failed. Most lacerations are readily visualized and easily oversewn through a high anterior gastrotomy. Operative mortality is low, although postoperative morbidity can be considerable, especially in cirrhotics. Recurrent bleeding following successful operative repair of a Mallory-Weiss laceration is very uncommon, and the prognosis, especially for non-alcoholic patients, is excellent.

Boerhaave's Syndrome

Occasionally, the forces transmitted to the distal esophageal wall are so great that an emetogenic rupture occurs (Boerhaave's syndrome). In more than 90 per cent of patients, the tears are longitudinal and are located in the left lateral aspect of the distal esophagus. Characteristically, the patient complains of severe epigastric pain shortly after vomiting. Hematemesis is an infrequent accompaniment, but dyspnea is common because of the accumulation of gastric and esophageal content in the pleural space. Mediastinal air may present as palpable crepitus in the suprasternal notch, a sign found in as many as 66 per cent of patients.

Because Boerhaave's syndrome is relatively rare, delay in diagnosis is common. This is an unfortunate circumstance: Survival rates are excellent when patients are operated on within the first 12 hours of rupture; mortality approaches 100 per cent if operation is delayed more than 24 hours. Erect chest films yield the most information because they will demonstrate pleural effusion in 90 per cent of patients, left pneumothorax in 80 per cent, and mediastinal air in 66 per cent. Occasionally, widening of the mediastinum and patchy atelectasis may also be noted. In equivocal cases, an esophagogram using water-soluble contrast material may be helpful in as many as 75 per cent of patients. However, a negative result does not exclude the diagnosis of an emetogenic rupture. In these instances, esophagoscopy should be employed.

Treatment of Boerhaave's syndrome is entirely surgical because nonoperative therapy is uniformly fatal. Specific preoperative measures include the use of antibiotics, correction of volume and electrolyte deficits, and the insertion of a chest tube if pulmonary compromise is evident. Definitive operative therapy consists of débridement and repair of the perforation through a left thoracotomy incision with drainage of the mediastinum and pleural space. The success of such therapy is dependent entirely on the period of time that has elapsed since the rupture occurred.

Menetrier's Disease

Menetrier's disease, first described in 1888, consists of a constellation of findings including enlarged gastric folds, massive protein loss into the gastric lumen, and hypoproteinemia. The etiology of the condition remains obscure. Examination of the gastric mucous membrane reveals a hyperplastic gastropathy that can be broadly classified into three types: (1) *mucous cell*, in which periodic acid–Schiff (PAS)-positive cells predominate and in which hypochlorhydria is the rule; (2) *glandular cell*, in which hyperplasia of both parietal and chief cells is noted; and (3) *mixed mucous glandular*, in which all elements of the gastric mucosa are hyperplastic. The manner in which plasma proteins reach the gastric lumen is unknown, but it may relate either to active secretion of protein via transcellular

routes or passive diffusion of protein through paracellular tight junctions. Regardless of the etiology of the protein loss, it undoubtedly is responsible for the peripheral edema and increased susceptibility to infection commonly seen in afflicted patients.

Epigastric pain, anorexia, nausea, vomiting, and weight loss are common presenting symptoms. Extraintestinal manifestations include peripheral and pulmonary edema, infections, and papillary erythematous rashes. The diagnosis can usually be suspected on clinical grounds and confirmed by radiographic and endoscopic examinations. Both reveal edematous hypertrophic rugae with tenacious intraluminal secretion. These findings, in combination with a decreased serum albumin and total protein, are pathognomonic.

Nonoperative treatment consists of protein repletion and attempts to inhibit gastric secretion using either anticholinergic drugs or cimetidine. Surgical intervention is infrequently necessary, but it may be required in patients who have intractable symptoms or severe and uncontrollable protein loss. Distal gastrectomy with truncal vagotomy has proved beneficial in some instances. On rare occasions, total gastrectomy may be needed.

Acute Gastric Dilatation

Acute gastric dilatation can occur under a variety of circumstances; it is seen most frequently, however, following lengthy operative procedures during which the trachea has been intubated but the stomach has not been decompressed. Its etiology is unclear, but the consequences are certain: increased gastric secretion and diaphragmatic elevation. If acute gastric dilatation is not recognized and treated promptly, cardiovascular and pulmonary compromise may compound an increasing intravascular volume deficit leading to hypotension. The diagnosis is easily made by the finding of a tympanitic fullness over the epigastrium. Abdominal x-rays are rarely required; if obtained, however, they will reveal a massively dilated stomach with a prominent air-fluid level.

Treatment is easy and efficacious: prompt insertion of a nasogastric tube. This is especially important in the unconscious patient in whom vomiting and regurgitation may be the principal signs that the condition exists.

Duodenal Diverticulum

Duodenal diverticulum is a common finding on routine upper gastrointestinal barium studies. For the most part, it is of no clinical consequence whatsoever. Diverticula are almost certainly developmental in origin; 80 per cent are located on the medial wall of the second portion of the duodenum distal to the ampulla of Vater. They are usually solitary and lie in proximity to the pancreas. Although complications are rare, they can occur, especially in diverticula with large sacs and narrow necks. In this circumstance, inflammation, ulceration, and hemorrhage may ensue. On very rare occasions, the diverticulum may actually develop an abscess with internal fistula formation. Diverticula located in the vicinity of the ampulla may cause obstruction of the extrahepatic biliary tree, leading to cholangitis or pancreatitis. The appropriate operative approach to duodenal diverticula depends upon the underlying condition that initially necessitates operation. When bleeding is the principal problem, diverticulectomy is appropriate. When extrahepatic biliary or pancreatic obstruction is the indication, surgical operations include diverticulectomy with sphincteroplasty or bypass of the distal common bile duct.

NEOPLASMS OF THE STOMACH

Benign Tumors

EPITHELIAL POLYPS

Polyps of the gastric mucous membrane are the most common type of benign gastric tumor. Nevertheless, they are unusual pathologic entities, having an overall incidence of less than 1 per cent. In more than 90 per cent of instances, multiplicity is the rule. Two histologic types are distinguished. *Hyperplastic polyps* are the more common and consist of gastric epithelium, which is identical histologically to the morphology of the adjacent normal gastric mucous membrane. Hyperplastic polyps are almost invariably smaller than 2 cm. in diameter and have minimal malignant potential. They tend to be located throughout the entire gastric mucosa and may be associated with polyps elsewhere in the alimentary tract.

In contrast, the *adenomatous polyp* tends to be larger (greater than 2 cm. in diameter), is predominantly antral in location, and develops in gastric mucosa that has undergone intestinal metaplasia. Malignancy has been observed in between 25 and 80 per cent of patients, either within the polyp itself or in the adjacent gastric mucosa. Whether or not adenomatous polyps undergo malignant transformation is currently an unsettled issue. From a clinical perspective, however, adenomatous polyps that are large, sessile, and symptomatic are cause for considerable concern.

Most benign epithelial polyps are completely asymptomatic or associated with extremely vague and nonspecific complaints: discomfort in the epigastrium, a bloating sensation, nausea, and, infrequently, vomiting. On occasion, however, polyps may bleed, leading to hematemesis or melena. If appropriately situated, they may also obstruct the gastric outlet by a ball valve type mechanism. The diagnosis is usually established either by roentgenographic studies or by endoscopy. In any case, gastroscopy should be used for patients with suspicious polyps in order to directly visualize the polyp, remove it, if possible, and perform a biopsy of the adjacent mucosa to determine whether or not a coexisting gastric carcinoma is present. As with colonic polyps, complete removal of the polyp for careful histologic examination is desirable. Should this be unfeasible, operative therapy should be undertaken. The choice of operation depends upon the characteristics, number, and location of the polyp(s). Large, solitary, sessile polyps can be removed by limited local resection. Multiple polyps involving the distal stomach are best treated by antrectomy. If the entire stomach is involved, a distal gastrectomy, combined with polypectomy of the larger polyps in the proximal stomach, is the procedure of choice. Total gastrectomy is rarely necessary.

MESENCHYMAL TUMORS

The stomach can harbor a variety of benign mesenchymal tumors including leiomyomas, fibromas, neurogenic tumors, vascular tumors, and lipomas. By far the most common is the *leiomyoma*. These are invariably located submucosally and are usually well circumscribed. They are usually discovered because of upper gastrointestinal hemorrhage resulting from ulceration of the mucosa overlying the tumor. Leiomyomas are more frequently found near the gastroesophageal junction than are the remainder of the benign mesenchymal tumors, which favor a more distal location in the stomach. The diagnosis is made by the characteristic finding on upper gastrointestinal contrast studies of a circumferential extramucosal defect often in association with an ulcer in the overlying mucosa. Definitive treatment consists of local resection of the involved portion of the stomach if at all possible. Unfortunately, it is often difficult to distinguish benign from malignant lesions histologically, so that not infrequently this distinction is made by the patient's subsequent clinical course.

Malignant Tumors

ADENOCARCINOMA

Although the incidence of gastric adenocarcinoma has been steadily decreasing in the United States over the past several decades, it remains one of the most lethal visceral malignancies. Approximately 23,000 new cases are diagnosed annually. Eighty per cent of patients with this tumor will come to operation; however, only 40 per cent of these tumors are resectable for cure and, of these, fewer than a third of such patients will be alive 5 years later. This unpleasant fact is thought to be a consequence of the advanced stage of the disease in most patients at the time of diagnosis. The experience of the Japanese stands in marked contrast to these dismal statistics. They have initiated massive screening efforts to detect the disease in an early stage because gastric adenocarcinoma is the most common malignancy in that country. In their hands, fully 70 per cent of all gastric cancers are "early" (tumor confined to the mucosa and submucosa, with or without lymph node metastases) and surgical resection is followed by an 80 to 90 per cent 5-year cure rate.

The pathogenesis of gastric adenocarcinoma remains obscure. Several factors have been implicated in its development, however, including (1) atrophic gastritis with anacidity (patients with pernicious anemia have a substantially increased risk of developing gastric malignancy), (2) chronic gastric ulcer (7 per cent of apparently benign gastric ulcers actually harbor adenocarcinoma), (3) epithelial polyps (described earlier), and (4) diet (a higher incidence of malignancy is noted in countries where heavy ingestion of smoked fish and spicy food is popular, e.g., Japan and Finland). Heredity may also play a role.

Pathologically, three variants of gastric adenocarcinoma are encountered. The most common is the *polypoid* and *exophytic* type, seen usually in the distal stomach but also, on occasion, in the region of the gastroesophageal junction. Gastric adenocarcinoma may also present as an *ulcerative lesion* that on occasion can be difficult to distinguish from benign gastric ulcer. The least common but most virulent pathologic variety is the *serous* or *infiltrating type*. The tumor frequently involves the entire stomach, giving it a "leather bottle" appearance because of its impliability. This condition is known as *linitis plastica* and is virtually incurable surgically.

Early symptoms of gastric adenocarcinoma are vague and nonspecific. They include unexplained weight loss, anorexia, early satiety, and, on occasion, mild epigastric discomfort. Dysphagia may also be an early symptom if the malignancy involves the region of the gastroesophageal junction. As the disease progresses, pain becomes a more prominent symptom, vomiting may ensue, particularly if the cancer impinges on the gastric outlet, and the patient may experience melena. Massive hematemesis is distinctly unusual. Rarely, the presenting symptoms may be related to metastatic disease rather than to the gastric primary: abdominal distention as a consequence of malignant ascites, hepatomegaly, jaundice, mechanical small bowel obstruction from peritoneal implants, and difficulty in defecation because of metastatic disease in the pouch of Douglas, the so-called *Blumer's shelf*.

A tentative diagnosis of gastric adenocarcinoma can be made in more than 90 per cent of instances on upper gastrointestinal roentgenographic studies. The diagnosis should be confirmed with endoscopy, employing both biopsy and cytologic evaluation. Computed tomography (CT) may be helpful in staging the disease preoperatively. The finding of hepatic or peritoneal metastases, involvement of the celiac axis nodes with tumor, extensive deposits in neighboring organs such as liver, colon and pancreas, malignant ascites, and extra-abdominal metastatic disease all indicate that the disease is beyond surgical control. Nevertheless, even if it is incurable, most patients will benefit from surgical intervention with palliation in the form of debulking, resections, or bypassses if technically feasible.

Surgery is the only therapeutic modality with potential to cure the disease. The aim of operation is to remove the primary tumor with its primary lymphatic drainage sites. In the stomach they are located above the pylorus in the region of the porta hepatis, below the pylorus in the region of the head of the pancreas, around the origin of the left gastric artery, and in the splenic hilum. The appropriate procedure depends upon the location and extent of the tumor. In general, adenocarcinomas of the distal stomach are best treated by extensive distal gastrectomy with omentectomy. Adequate margins include 5 cm. of disease-free proximal stomach and 1 to 2 cm. of disease-free duodenum. The left gastric artery should be ligated at its origin. Reconstruction is best accomplished as a gastrojejunostomy because symptomatic suture line recurrence is less with this procedure than with a gastroduodenostomy. Some have advocated a more radical approach to include total gastrectomy, distal pancreatectomy, splenectomy, and lesser omentectomy (so-called radical gastrectomy) in an effort to improve overall survivorship. Unfortunately, operative morbidity is the only parameter that increases using this approach.

Adenocarcinomas arising in the body of the stomach are best treated by total extirpation of the organ. The spleen should be included with the specimen as the probability of lymph node metastasis in the splenic hilum with tumors arising in this location is high. Reconstruction is usually accomplished using a Roux-en-Y esophagojejunostomy. Adenocarcinomas of the cardia and fundus present a major technical challenge because of their propensity to spread submucosally into the esophagus. In general, proximal gastrectomy with distal esophagectomy to include at least 3 cm. of disease-free esophageal margin is desirable. Reconstruction is accomplished by esophagoantrostomy to which a pyloroplasty is added because of the high likelihood that the dissection will produce a vagally denervated distal stomach. The appropriate treatment of a patient with linitis plastica involving the entire stomach is controversial. Some feel that a total gastrectomy is appropriate. However, gastric adenocarcinoma of this extent is for all intents and purposes incurable, so that, at best, this major operative procedure can be considered only palliative. For this reason, many surgeons consider linitis plastica involving the entire stomach as an inoperable lesion.

The prognosis of gastric adenocarcinoma is primarily related to the depth of penetration of the gastric wall and to the presence or absence of lymph node metastasis. Tumors confined to the mucosa and submucosa without lymph node metastases are associated with an excellent outlook: a 90 per cent 5-year survivorship. Unfortunately, in the United States, they constitute only 17 per cent of all resectable gastric cancers. Even with lymph node metastases, early cancer patients do extremely well: an 85 per cent 5-year survivorship. As tumors invade the muscularis propria and metastasize to lymph nodes, the prognosis becomes progressively worse so that the overall 5-year survivorship of patients undergoing "curative" resection is 30 per cent or less. The use of adjuvant chemotherapy or radiation has been advocated in the hope that this dismal track record can be improved. Unfortunately, current data indicate that these modalities provide no substantive benefit in terms of prolonging survival.

Gastric Lymphoma

Lymphoma of the stomach may occur either as an isolated entity or as a manifestation of systemic disease. The latter is more common than the former. Even if the lymphoma is apparently isolated, in up to a third of patients systemic manifestations will ultimately develop. Most are histiocytic or lymphocytic in cell type; the Hodgkin's variant is a distinct rarity. The symptomatic presentation of gastric lymphoma is similar to that of gastric adenocarcinoma, although a slightly higher incidence of free perforation is noted. Such an occurrence implies a very poor prognosis. No typical roentgenographic appearance is pathognomonic of the disease. Lymphomas may present as a gastric mass, as large gastric folds, or as multiple ulcerations. Endoscopic biopsy may also fail to provide a definitive diagnosis, since the mucosa is frequently uninvolved. Thus, the true nature of the pathologic process may become apparent only when the specimen is examined postoperatively. Whenever possible, distinction between a primary and secondary lymphoma should be made preoperatively. Disseminated disease mandates chemotherapy and radiation therapy, whereas primary disease is amenable to surgical cure. The surgeon should make every effort to extirpate the disease completely because the prognosis of primary gastric lymphoma is far better than that of gastric adenocarcinoma (40 to 50 per cent 5-year survivorship). In patients in whom tumor is discovered at the resected margin or who demonstrate full-thickness gastric wall involvement associated with positive regional lymph nodes, postoperative radiation therapy appears to have real benefit.

SELECTED REFERENCES

Surgical Anatomy of the Stomach and Duodenum

Griffith, C. A.: Anatomy, *In* Harkins, H. N., and Nyhus, L. M. (Eds.): Surgery of the Stomach and Duodenum. Boston, Little, Brown & Co., 1969, p. 25.

Surgical Physiology of the Stomach and Duodenum

Polk, H. C., Jr., Stone, H. H., and Gardner, B.: Basic Surgery, 2nd ed. Norwalk, Conn., Appleton-Century-Crofts, 1983, pp. 149–164.

Peptic Ulcer Disease

Achord, J. L.: Gastric pepsin and acid secretion in patients with acute and healed duodenal ulcer. Gastroenterology, *81*:15, 1981.

Boey, J., Lee, N. M., Koo, J., et al.: Immediate definitive surgery for perforated duodenal ulcer. Ann. Surg., *196*:338, 1982.

Christiansen, J., et al.: Prospective controlled vagotomy trial for duodenal ulcer: Primary results, sequelae, acid secretion, and recurrent rates two to five years after operation. Ann. Surg., *193*:49, 1981.

Dalton, M. D., Eisenstein, A. M., Walsh, J. H., and Fordtran, J. S.: Effect of secretion on gastric functions in normal subjects and in patients with duodenal ulcer. Gastroenterology, *71*:24, 1976.

Drury, J. K., McKay, A. S., Hutchinson, J. S. F., et al.: Natural history of perforated duodenal ulcers treated by suture closure. Lancet, *2*:749, 1978.

Dwight, R. N., et al.: Controlled study of the surgical treatment of duodenal ulcer. Am. J. Surg., *129*:374, 1975.

Earlham, R.: A computerized questionnaire analysis of duodenal ulcer symptoms. Gastroenterology, *71*:314, 1976.

Elashoff, J. D., and Grossman, M. I.: Trends in hospital admissions and death rates for peptic ulcer in the United States from 1970 to 1978. Gastroenterology *78*:280, 1980.

Greenall, M. J., Gough, M. H., and Kettlewell, M. G. W.: Duodenal ulceration: Is endoscopic biopsy necessary? Br. Med. J., *282*:1061, 1981.

Griffith, W. J., Neumann, D. A., and Welsh, J. D.: The visible vessel as an indication of uncontrolled or recurrent gastrointestinal hemorrhage. N. Engl. J. Med., *300*:1411, 1979.

Hollinshead, J. W., Smith, R. C., and Gillett, D. J.: Parietal cell vagotomy: Experience with 114 patients with pyloric or duodenal ulcer. World J. Surg., *6*:596, 1982.

Hughes, W. S., Synder, N., and Hernandez, A.: Antral gastrin concentration in upper gastrointestinal disease. Am. J. Dis., *22*:201, 1977.

Hughes, W., Van Deventer, G., Shabot, M., and Becker, S.: Antral gastrin concentration in gastric ulcer disease. Dig. Dis. Sci., *25*:568, 1980.

Johnston, D., and Wilkerson, A. R.: Highly selective vagotomy without a drainage procedure in the treatment of duodenal ulcer. Br. J. Surg., *57*:289, 1970.

Jordan, P. H., Jr.: A follow-up report of a prospective evaluation of vagotomy-pyloroplasty and vagotomy-antrectomy for treatment of duodenal ulcer. Ann. Surg., *180*:259, 1974.

Kirkpatrick, P. M., Jr., and Hirschowitz, B. I.: Duodenal ulcer with unexplained marked basal gastric acid hypersecretion. Gastroenterology, *79*:4, 1980.

Malagelada, J. R., et al.: Gastric secretion and emptying after ordinary meals in duodenal ulcer. Gastroenterology, *73*:989, 1977.

McGuigan, J. E., and Trudeau, W. L.: Differences in rates of gastrin release in normal persons and patients with duodenal ulcer disease. N. Engl. J. Med., *288*:64, 1973.

Mulholland, M., et al.: Surgical treatment of duodenal ulcer: A prospective randomized study. Arch. Surg., *117*:393, 1982.

Nielson, H. O., Munoz, J. D., Kronborg, O., et al.: The antrum in duodenal ulcer patients. Scand. J. Gastroenterol., *16*:491, 1981.

Nielson, H. O., Madsen, P. E. R., and Christiansen, L. A.: The parietal cells in duodenal ulcer patients. Scand. J. Gastroenterol., *15*:793, 1980.

Peterson, W. L., Barnett, C. C., Smith, H. J., et al.: Routine early endoscopy in upper gastrointestinal tract bleeding: A randomized controlled trial. N. Engl. J. Med., *304*:925, 1981.

Rotter, J. I., Sones, J. Q., Samloff, I. M., et al.: Duodenal ulcer disease associated with elevated serum pepsinogen I. N. Engl. J. Med., *300*:63, 1979.

Rotter J. I., Peterson, G., Samloff, I. M., et al.: Genetic heterogenicity of hyperpepsinogenemic I and normopepsinogenemic I duodenal ulcer disease. Ann. Intern. Med., *91*:372, 1979.

Smith, M. P.: Decline in duodenal ulcer surgery. J. A. M. A., *237*:987, 1977.

Storey, D. W., Boron, S. G., Swain, C. P., et al.: Endoscopic prediction of recurrent bleeding in peptic ulcers. N. Engl. J. Med., *305*:915, 1981.

Taylor, I. L., Colam, J., Rotter, J. I., et al.: Family studies of hypergastrinemic hyperpepsinogenemic I duodenal ulcer. Ann. Intern. Med., *95*:421, 1981.

Benign Gastric Ulcer

Barr, G. D., et al.: A two-year prospective controlled study of maintenance cimetidine and gastric ulcer. Gastroenterology, *85*:100, 1983.

Davis, Z., Verheyden, C. N., van Heerden, J. A., et al.: The surgically treated chronic gastric ulcer: An extended follow-up. Ann. Surg. *185*:205, 1977.

Duthie, H. L., and Kwong, N. K.: Vagotomy or gastrectomy for gastric ulcer. Br. Med. J., *4*:79, 1973.

Duthie, H. L., Moore, T. H., Bardsley, D., and Clark, R. G.: Surgical treatment of gastric ulcers: Controlled comparison of Billroth I gastrectomy and vagotomy and pyloroplasty. Br. J. Surg., *57*:784, 1970.

Flint, F. J., and Grech, P.: Pyloric regurgitation and gastric ulcer. Gut, *11*:735, 1970.

Johnson, H. D.: Gastric ulcer: Classification, blood group characteristics, secretion pattern and pathogenesis. Arch. Surg., *162*:996, 1965.

Johnson, J. A., and Giercksky, E. K.: Gastric ulcer treated with ulcerectomy, vagotomy and drainage. World J. Surg., *4*:463, 1980.

Jordan, P. H., Jr.: Treatment of gastric ulcer by parietal cell vagotomy and excision of the ulcer. Arch. Surg. *116*:1320, 1981.

Kobayaski, S., Kasugai, J., and Yamazaki, H.: Endoscopic differentiation of early gastric cancer from benign peptic ulcer. Gastrointest. Endosc., *25*:55, 1979.

Kraus, M., Mendeloff, G., and Condon, R. E.: Prognosis of gastric ulcer: Twenty-five year follow-ups. Ann. Surg., *184*:471, 1976.

Oi, M., Oshida, K., and Sugimura, S.: The location of gastric ulcer. Gastroenterology, *36*:45, 1959.

Oi, M., Ito, K., Kumagai, F., et al.: A possible dual control mechanism in the origin of peptic ulcer: A study on ulcer location as affected by mucosa and musculature. Gastroenterology, *57*:280, 1969.

Scheurer, U., Witzel, L., Halter, F., et al.: Gastric and duodenal ulcer healing placebo treatment. Gastroenterology, *72*:838, 1977.

Tedesco, F. S., Best, W. R., Littman, A., et al.: Rate of gastroscopy in gastric ulcer patients. Gastroenterology, *73*:170, 1977.

Stress Erosions and Acute Hemorrhagic Gastritis

Bowen, J. C., Fleming, W. H., and Thompson, J. C.: Increased gastrin release following penetrating central nervous system injury. Surgery, *75*:720, 1974.

Cushing, H.: Peptic ulcers and the interbrain. Surg. Gynecol. Obstet., *55*:134, 1932.

Czaja, A. J., McAlhany, J. C., and Pruitt, B. A.: Acute gastroduodenal disease after thermal injury. N. Engl. J. Med., *291*:925, 1974.

Delaney, J. P., and Michel, H. M.: Hemorrhagic gastritis following operation. In Najarian, J. S., and Delaney, J. P. (Eds.): Critical Surgical Care. Miami, Florida Symposia Specialists, 1977.

Dunn, D. H., Fischer, R. G., Silvis, S. E., et al: The treatment of hemorrhagic gastritis with cimetidine. Surg. Gynecol. Obstet., *147*:737, 1978.

Hubert, H. P., Jr., Kiernan, P. V., Welsh, J. S., et al.: The surgical management of bleeding stress ulcers. Ann. Surg., *191*:672, 1980.

Kwilaalaso, E., Fromm, D., and Silen, W.: Relationship between ulceration and intramural pH of gastric mucosa during hemorrhagic shock. Surgery, *84*:70, 1978.

Lucas, C. E., Sugawa, C., and Riddle, J., et al.: Natural history and surgical dilemma of "stress" gastric bleeding. Arch. Surg., *102*:266, 1971.

Lucas, C. E.: Prevention and treatment of acute gastric erosion and stress-ulceration. In Fiddian-Green, R. C., and Turcotte, J. G. (Eds.): Gastrointestinal Hemorrhage. New York, Grune & Stratton, 1980.

Lucas, C. E.: Stress ulceration: The clinical problem. World J. Surg., *5*:139, 1981.

MacDonald, A. S., Steele, P. J., and Bottomley, M. G.: Treatment of stress induced upper gastrointestinal hemorrhage with metiamide. Lancet, *1*:68, 1976.

McElwee, H. P., Sirinek, K. R., and Levine, B. A.: Cimetidine affords protection equal to antacids in prevention of stress ulceration following thermal injury. Surgery, *86*:620, 1979.

Mengioy, R., Gadacz, T., and Zajtchuk, R.: The surgical management of acute gastric mucosal bleeding. Arch. Surg., *77*:198, 1969.

Richardson, J. D., and Aust, J. B.: Gastric devascularization: A useful salvage procedure for massive hemorrhage gastritis. Ann. Surg., *185*:649, 1977.

Ritchie, W. P., Jr.: Role of bile acid reflux in acute hemorrhagic gastritis. World J. Surg., *5*:189, 1981.

Ritchie, W. P., Jr., McRea, D. B., Jr., and Felger, T. S.: AV acid-base balance during acute gastric mucosal ulcerogenesis. Am. J. Surg., *139*:22, 1980.

Silen, W., Murhaw, A., and Simson, J. N. L.: The pathophysiology of stress ulcer disease. World J. Surg., *5*:165, 1981.

Simonian, S. J., and Curtis, L. E.: Treatment of hemorrhagic gastritis by antacid. Ann. Surg., *184*:429, 1976.

Stother, J. S., Jr., Simonowitz, D. A., Dellinger, E. P., et al.: Randomized prospective evaluation of cimetidine and antacid control of pH in the critically ill. Ann. Surg., 192:169, 1980.

Stremple, J. F., Molot, M. D., McNamara, J. J., et al.: Post-traumatic gastric bleeding: Prospective gastric secretion composition. Arch. Surg., *105*:177, 1972.

Sugawa, C., Werner, M. H., Hayes, D. F., et al.: Early endoscopy: A guide to therapy for acute hemorrhage in the upper gastrointestinal tract. Arch. Surg., *107*:133, 1973.

Williams, J. F., Morrow, A. G., and Braunwald, E.: The incidence and management of "medical" complications following cardiac operations. Circulation, *32*:608, 1965.

Zinner, M. J., Zuidema, G. D., Smith, P. L., et al.: The prevention of upper gastrointestinal tract bleeding in patients in an intensive care unit. Surg. Gynecol. Obstet., *153*:214, 1981.

Zollinger-Ellison Syndrome

Bonfils, S., Mignon, M., and Grotton, J.: Cimetidine treatment of acute and chronic Zollinger-Ellison syndrome. World J. Surg., *3*:597, 1979.

Bonfils, S., Landor, J. H., and Mignon, M.: Results of surgical management in 92 consecutive patients with Zollinger-Ellison syndrome. Ann. Surg., *194*:692, 1981.

Deveney, C. W., Deveney, K. S., and Way, L. W.: The Zollinger-Ellison syndrome—23 years later. Ann Surg., *188*:384, 1978.

Fang, M., Ginsberg, A. L., Glassman, L., et al.: Zollinger-Ellison syndrome with diarrhea as the predominant chemical feature. Gastroenterology, 76:378, 1979.

Gregory, R. A., Tracy, H. J., French, J. M., and Sircus, W.: Extraction of a gastrin-like substance from a pancreatic tumor in a case of Zollinger-Ellison syndrome. Lancet, *1*:1045, 1960.

Isenberg, J. I., Welsh, J. H., and Grossman, M. I.: Zollinger-Ellison syndrome. Gastroenterology, 65:140, 1973.

Majewski, J. T., and Wilson, S. D.: The MEA-I syndrome: An all or none phenomenon? Surgery, 86:475, 1979.

McCarthy, D. M.: The place for surgery in the Zollinger-Ellison syndrome. N. Engl. J. Med., *302*:1344, 1980.

McCarthy, D. M.: Report on the United States experience with cimetidine in Zollinger-Ellison syndrome and other hypersecretory states. Gastroenterology, 74:453, 1978.

Polk, H. C., Jr., Stone, H. H., and Gardner, B.: Basic Surgery, 2nd ed. Norwalk, Conn., Appleton-Century-Crofts, 1983, pp. 149–164.

Reagan, P. T., and Malagelada, J. R.: A reappraisal of clinical, roentgenographic and endoscopic features of the Zollinger-Ellison syndrome. Mayo Clin. Proc., 53:19, 1978.

Zollinger, R. M., and Ellison, E. H.: Primary peptic ulcerations of the jejunum associated with islet cell tumors of the pancreas. Ann. Surg., *142*:709, 1955.

Complications of Gastric Surgery

Amdrup, E., and Jensen, H. E.: One hundred patients five years after selective gastric vagotomy and drainage for duodenal ulcer. Surgery, 74:321, 1973.

Ayulo, J. A.: Cholestyramine in postvagotomy syndrome. Am. J. Gastroenterol., 57:207, 1972.

Becker, J. M.: Complication of gastric surgery. Br. J. Surg. (in press).

Bloom, S. R., Rorpton, C. M. S., and Thomson, J. P. S.: Enteroglucagon release in the dumping syndrome. Lancet, 2:789, 1972.

Bushkin, F. L., and Woodward, E. R.: Postgastrectomy Syndromes. Philadelphia, W. B. Saunders Company, 1976, pp 34-48.

Creaghe, S. B., Saik, R. P., Pearl, J., and Peskin, G. W.: Noninvasive vascular assessment of dumping syndrome. J. Surg. Res., 22:328, 1977.

Domellof, L., and Jananger, K. G.: The risk for gastric carcinoma after partial gastrectomy. Am. J. Surg., *134*:581, 1977.

Eherlein, T. J., Lorenzo, F. V., and Webster, M. V.: Gastric carcinoma following operation for peptic ulcer disease. Ann. Surg., *187*:251, 1978.

Fink, W. J., Heicke, S. T., Gray, T. W., Thompson, B. W., and Read, R. C.: Treatment of postoperative reactive hypoglycemia by a reversed intestinal segment. Am. J. Surg., *131*:19, 1976.

Fromm, D. G.: Complications of Gastric Surgery. New York, John Wiley & Sons, Inc., 1977, pp 7-34, 35-49.

Herrington, J. L., Edwards, W. H., Carter, J. H., and Sawyers, J. L.: Treatment of severe postgastrectomy diarrhea by reversed jejunal segment. Ann. Surg., *168*:522, 1968.

Hocking, M. P., Vogel, S. B., Falasca, C. A., and Woodward, E. R.: Delayed gastric emptying of liquids and solids following Roux-en-Y biliary diversion. Ann. Surg., *194*: 494, 1981.

Jenkins, D. J. A., Gassull, M. A., Leeds, A. R., et al.: Effect of dietary fiber on complications of gastric surgery: Prevention of postprandial hypoglycemia by pectin. Gastroenterology, 72:215, 1977.

Orlando, R., III, and Welsh, J. R.: Carcinoma of the stomach after gastric operation. Am. J. Surg., *114*:487, 1981.

Papachristou, A. N., Agnanti, N., and Fortner, J. G.: Gastric carcinoma after treatment of ulcer. Am. J. Surg., *139*:193, 1960.

Reichle, F. A., Brigman, M. P., Reichle, R. M., and Rosemond, G. P.: The effect of gastrectomy on serotonin metabolism in the human portal vein. Ann. Surg., *172*: 585, 1970.

Ritchie, W. P., and Perez, A. R.: Post-gastrectomy syndromes. *In* Moody, F. C., and Cary, L. C. (Eds.): Surgical Treatment of Digestive Disease. Chicago, Year Book Medical Publishers, 1986.

Ritchie, W. P., Jr.: Alkaline reflux gastritis: A diagnosis in search of a disease. J. Clin. Surg., *1*:414, 1982.

Ritchie, W. P., Jr.: Alkaline reflux gastritis: An objective assessment of its diagnosis and treatment. Ann. Surg., *192*:288, 1980.

Roberts, K. E., Randall, H. T., Farr, H. W., Kidwell, A. P., McNeer, G. P., and Pack, G. T.: Cardiovascular and blood volume alterations resulting from intrajejunal administration of hypertonic solutions to gastrectomized patient: The relationship of these changes to the dumping syndrome. Ann. Surg., *140*:631, 1954.

Sabiston, D. C., Jr.: Textbook of Surgery: The Biological Basis of Modern Surgical Practice. 11th ed. Philadelphia, W. B. Saunders Company, 1977, p. 920.

Sawyers, J. L., and Herrington, J. L., Jr.: Superiority of antiperistaltic jejunal segments in management of severe dumping syndrome. Ann. Surg., *178*:311, 1973.

Silver, D., McGregor, F. H., Jr., Porter, J. M., and Anylan, W. G.: The mechanism of the dumping syndrome. Surg. Clin. North Am., *46*:425, 1966.

Tolin, R. D., Malmud, L. S., Stelzer, F., et al.: Enterogastric reflux in normal subjects and patients with Billroth II gastroenterostomy. Gastroenterology, 77:1027, 1979.

Wang, P. Y., Talamo, R. C., Babiori, B. M., Raymond, G. G., and Colman, R. W.: Kullikrein-kinin system in postgastrectomy dumping syndrome. Ann. Intern. Med., *80*:577, 1974.

Mallory-Weiss Tears

Baum, S., and Nusbaum, M.: The control of gastrointestinal hemorrhage by selective mesenteric infusion of vasopressin. Radiology, 98:497, 1971.

Bubrick, M. P., Lundeen, J. W., Onstad, G. R., and Hitchcock, C. R.: Mallory-Weiss syndrome: Analysis of fifty-nine cases. Surgery, 88:400, 1980.

Curran, D., et al.: Endoscopic application of noradrenaline for Mallory-Weiss bleeding. Lancet, *1*:538, 1981.

Fisher, R. G., Schwartz, J. T., and Graham, D. Y.: Angiotherapy with Mallory-Weiss tears. A. J. R., *134*:560, 1980.

Hastings, P. R., Peters, K. W., Cohn, I., Jr.: Mallory-Weiss syndrome - Review of 69 cases. Am. J. Surg., *142*:560, 1981.

Mallory, E. K., and Weiss, S.: Hemorrhage from laceration of the cardiac orifice of the stomach due to vomiting. Am. J. Med. Sci., *178*:506, 1929.

Michel, L., Serrano, A., and Malt, R. A.: Mallory-Weiss syndrome: Evolution of diagnostic and therapeutic patterns over two decades. Ann. Surg., *192*: 716, 1980.

Rosch, J., Keller, F. S., Kozak, B., Niles, N., and Dotter, C. T.: Gelfoam powder embolization of the left gastric artery in treatment of massive small-vessel gastric bleeding. Radiology, *152*: 365, 1984.

Sugawa, C., Benishek, D., and Walt, A. J.: Mallory-Weiss syndrome: A study of 224 patients. Am. J. Surg., *145*:30, 1982.

Weiss, S., and Mallory, G. K.: Lesions of the cardiac orifice of the stomach produced by vomiting. J. A. M. A., 98:1353, 1932.

Boerhaave's Syndrome

Abbott, O. A., Mansour, K. A., Logan, W. D., Jr., et al.: Atraumatic so-called "spontaneous" rupture of the oesophagus; A review of 47 personal cases with comments on a method of surgical therapy. J. Thorac. Cardiovasc. Surg., *59*:67, 1970.

Callaghan, J.: The Boerhaave syndrome (spontaneous rupture of the oesophagus). Br. J. Surg., *59*:41, 1972.

Campbell, C. T., Andrews, J. L., and Neptune, W. B.: Spontaneous rupture of the esophagus (Boerhaave syndrome): Necessity of early diagnosis and treatment. J. A. M. A., *325*:526, 1976.

Curci, J. J., and Horman, M. J.: Boerhaave's syndrome: The importance of early diagnosis and treatment. Ann. Surg., *183*:401, 1976.

DeLuca, R. F., Tedesco, F. J., Ballan, K., et al.: Esophageal perforation: An unusual presentation with a benign clinical course. Am. J. Gastroenterol., *67*: 362, 1977.

Ivey, T. D., Simonowitz, D. A., Dillard, D. H., Miller, D. W., Jr.: Boerhaave syndrome: Successful conservative management in three patients with late presentation. Am. J. Surg., *141*: 531, 1981.

Landay, M. J., and Berk, R. N.: The radiology corner: Boerhaave's syndrome. Am. J. Gastroenterol., *69*: 212, 1978.

Larrieu, A. J., and Kieffer, R.: Boerhaave syndrome: Report of a case treated non-operatively. Ann. Surg., *181*: 452, 1975.

Patton, A. S., Lawson, D. W., Shannon, J. M., Risley, T. S., and Bixby, F. E.: Reevaluation of the Boerhaave syndrome: A review of fourteen cases. Am. J. Surg., *137*:560, 1979.

Symbas, P. N., Hatcher, C. P., Jr., and Harloftis, N.: Sportaneous rupture of the esophagus. Ann. Surg., *187*:634, 1978.

Menetrier's Disease

Fieber, S. S., and Rickert, R. R.: Hyperplastic gastropathy: Analysis of 50 selected cases from 1955–1980. Am. J. Gastroenterol., *76*: 321, 1981.

Kelly, D. G., Malagelada, J. R., Huizenga, K. A., and Markowitz, H.: Giant hypertrophic gastropathy (Menetrier's disease): Pharmacologic effects on protein leakage and mucosal ultrastructure. Gastroenterology, *83*: 581, 1982.

Menetrier, P.: Des polyadenomes gastriques et de leurs rapports avec le cancer de l'estomac. Arch. Physiol. Norm. Pathol., *1*:32–55, 236–262, 1888.

Myerson, R. M.: Cimetidine in hypertrophic protein-losing gastropathy (Menetrier's disease). Gastroenterology, *84*:201, 1983.

Searcy, R. M., and Malagelada, J. R.: Menetrier's disease and idiopathic hypertrophic gastropathy. Ann. Intern. Med., *100*:565, 1984.

Acute Gastric Dilatation

Schwartz, S. I., Shires, G. T., Spencer, F. C., and Storer, E. H.: Principles of Surgery, 4th ed. New York, McGraw-Hill Book Co., 1984, p. 1136.

Duodenal Diverticulum

Griffen, M., Carey, W. D., Hermann, R., and Buonocore, E.: Recurrent acute pancreatitis and intussusception complicating an intraluminal duodenal diverticulum. Gastroenterology, *81*:345, 1981.

Eggerl, A., Teichmann, W., and Wittmann, D. H.: The pathologic implication of duodenal diverticula. Surg. Gynecol. Obstet., *154*:62, 1982.

Lotveit, T., Osnes, M., and Larsen, S.: Recurrent biliary calculi: Duodenal diverticula as a predisposing factor. Ann. Surg., *196*: 30, 1982.

Manny, J., Muga, M., and Eyal, Z.: The continuing clinical enigma of duodenal diverticulum. Am. J. Surg., *142*: 596, 1981.

Ryan, M. E., Hamilton, J. W., and Morrisey, J. F.: Gastrointestinal hemorrhage from a duodenal diverticulum. Gastrointest. Endosc., *30*:84, 1984.

Thomas, E., and Reddy, K. R.: Cholangitis and pancreatitis due to juxtapapillary duodenal diverticulum: Endoscopic sphincterotomy is the other alternative in selected cases. Am. J. Gastroenterol., 77:303, 1982.

Wells, F.: Pancreatic abscess complicating a perforated duodenal diverticulum. Br. J. Surg., 70:292, 1983.

Yasui, K., Tsukaguchi, I., et al.: Benign duodenocolic fistula due to duodenal diverticulum: Report of two cases. Radiology, *130*:67, 1979.

Benign Gastric Tumors

Bone, G. E., and McClelland, R. N.: Management of gastric polyps. Surg. Gynecol. Obstet., *142*:933, 1976.

Delikoris, P., and Golematis, B.: Smooth muscle neoplasms of the stomach. South. Med. J. 76:440, 1983.

Kamiya, T., Morishita, T., et al.: Histoclinical long-standing follow-up study of hyperglycemic polyps of the stomach. Am. J. Gastroenterol., 75:275, 1981.

King, R. M., van Heerden, J. A., and Weiland, L. H.: The management of gastric polyps. Surg. Gynecol. Obstet., *155*:846, 1982.

Lanza, F. L., Graham, D. Y., et al.: Endoscopic upper gastrointestinal polypectomy: Report of 73 polypectomies in 63 patients. Am. J. Gastroenterol., 75: 345, 1981.

Sabiston, D. C., Jr.: Davis-Christopher Textbook of Surgery: The Biological Basis of Modern Surgical Practice, 12th ed. Philadelphia, W. B. Saunders Company, 1981, p. 947.

Schwartz, S. I., Shires, G. T., Spencer, F. C., and Storer, E. H.: Principles of Surgery, 4th ed. New York, McGraw-Hill Book Company, 1984, Chapter 26.

Stockbrugger, W., Mennon, G. G., Bielby, J. O. W., et al.: Gastroscopic screening in 80 patients with pernicious anemia. Gut, *24*:1141, 1983.

Malignant Gastric Tumors

Antonioli, D. A., and Goldman, H: Changes in the location and type of gastric adenocarcinoma. Cancer, *50*: 775, 1982.

Bizer, L. S.: Adenocarcinoma of the stomach: Current results of treatment. Cancer, *51*: 743, 1983.

Brooks, J. J., and Enterline, H. T.: Primary gastric lymphomas: A clinicopathologic study of 58 cases with long-term follow-up and literature review. Cancer, *51*:701, 1983.

Carter, K. J., Schaffer, H. A., and Ritchie, W. P., Jr.: Early gastric cancer. Ann. Surg., *199*:604, 1984.

Contreary, K., Nance, F. C., and Becker, W. F.: Primary lymphoma of the gastrointestinal tract. Ann. Surg. *191*: 593, 1980.

Fleming, I. D., Mitchell, S., and Dilawari, R. A.: The role of surgery in the management of gastric lymphoma. Cancer, *49*: 1135, 1982.

Fox, E. R., Laufer, I., and Levine, M. S.: Response of gastric lymphoma to chemotherapy: Radiographic appearance. A. J. R., *142*:711, 1984.

Gastrointestinal tumor study group: Controlled trial of adjuvant chemotherapy following curative resection for gastric cancer. Cancer, *49*:1116, 1982.

Kalish, R. J., Clancy, P. E., Orringer, M. B., and Appelman, H. D.: Clinical, endemologic, and morphologic comparison between adenocarcinoma arising in Barrett's esophageal mucosa and in the gastric cardia. Gastroenterology, *486*:461, 1984.

Lavin, P. T., Bruckner, H. N., et al.: Studies in prognostic factors relating to chemotherapy for advanced gastric cancer. Cancer, *50*:2016, 1982.

Moss, A. A., et al: Gastric adenocarcinoma: A comparison of the accuracy and economics of staging by computed tomography and surgery. Gastroenterology, *80*:45, 1981.

Orlando, R., III, Pestuszak, W., Preissler, P. L., and Walsh, J. P.: Gastric lymphoma: A clinicopathologic reappraisal. Am. J. Surg., *143*: 450, 1982.

Papachristou, D. N., and Shiu, M. H.: Management by en bloc multiple organ resection of carcinoma of the stomach invading adjacent organs. Surg. Gynecol. Obstet., *152*:483, 1981.

Shimm, D. S., and Dosoretz, D. E.: Primary gastric lymphoma: An analysis with emphasis on prognostic factors and radiation therapy. Cancer, *52*: 2044, 1983.

Shiu, M. H., Karas, M., et al.: Management of primary gastric lymphoma. Ann. Surg., *195*: 196, 1982.

Weed, T. E., Neussle, W., and Ochsner, A.: A carcinoma of the stomach. Why are we failing to improve survival? Ann. Surg., *193* 407, 1981.

II

Surgical Management of Morbid Obesity

DAVID C. SABISTON, JR., M.D.

Obesity is a common problem in society and is recognized to be associated with a number of other serious medical disorders. There are approximately 12 million citizens in the United States who are obese. Of these, some 3 million are defined as having *morbid obesity,* meaning their weight is at least twice normal.[2] Moreover, the risk of this condition relative to longevity is impressive since there may be as much as a 200 per cent increase in the likelihood of death.[8] The associated disorders that often coexist with morbid obesity include hyperlipidemia, diabetes, cholelithiasis, and hypertension.

There is little doubt that the ideal method of management for these patients is to attain weight loss by *limitation of caloric intake* in the diet. However, the long-term result in the majority of these patients has been repeatedly shown to be poor, since these individuals seem unable to maintain an appropriate diet for a *prolonged* period. Many lose weight by dietary control, only to regain it as they return to a high caloric intake. In carefully controlled studies, only 25 per cent of patients lose as much as 20 pounds on dietary therapy and only 5 per cent lose 40 pounds or more in this way.[7] For this reason, wiring of the teeth to reduce caloric intake has been recommended, inasmuch as such patients can ingest only fluids.[3]

Surgical management of morbid obesity began approximately 25 years ago when it was recognized that either an extensive segmental resection of the small intestine or a bypass procedure designed to exclude most of the small intestine could be effective in achieving weight reduction in massively obese patients.[5] In the meantime, considerable controversy has arisen concerning the wisdom of any type of surgical procedure to control obesity, in large part because of the serious complications that may ensue with the passage of time. *Gastroplastic* operations have been designed to reduce the incidence of these complications.

Surgical procedures that have been attempted with varying degrees of success include three major types:

1. *Jejunal bypass procedures* were originally stimulated by knowledge of the fact that massive small bowel resection usually led to severe weight loss, inanition, and, in extreme cases, death. It is for this reason that bypass of the small intestine was introduced for management of morbid obesity. An end-to-side jejunoileostomy has been performed in many patients as well as end-to-end jejunoileal bypass.[1]

2. *Gastroplastic procedures* are characterized by creating a small pouch of stomach at the esophagogastric junction by placement of sutures or staples across the cardia and leaving only a small channel (1 cm.) (Fig. 1*A* and *B*).[6]

3. *Gastric bypass procedures* are generally characterized by creation of a small proximal gastric pouch together with a Roux-en-Y gastrojejunostomy, again with a channel of about 1 cm. to reduce the reservoir capacity of the proximal gastric pouch (Fig. 1*C*).[6]

Although satisfactory results have been achieved in some patients using these techniques, the complications, both immediate and long-term, are appreciable.[4] Early complications include wound infections, dehiscence, splenectomy for injured spleen at the time of operation, and fluid and electrolyte disturbances. Long-term complications include stomal obstruction, renal stones, cholelithiasis, nutritional deficiency states (vitamin B_{12}), and hepatic insufficiency. If a procedure is to be undertaken, it should be judiciously considered with complete discussion with each individual patient concerning the risks and benefits.

The Task Force of the American Society for Clinical Nutrition has established *guidelines* for appropriate candidates to undergo a surgical procedure.[9] Eligibility includes the presence of extremely severe obesity in patients whose weight exceeds desirable weight by 100 pounds or 100 per cent or in those who have more serious medical conditions related to severe refractory obesity. In addition, the patient should have a history of the following:

1. Having failed repeatedly in previous attempts at weight reduction when on medically acceptable plans.

2. Having been eligible on the basis of weight to be a candidate for the previous 3 to 5 years.

3. Considered capable of tolerating the anesthesia and operative procedure.

4. Having a thorough physical examination to eliminate high-risk categories, including alcoholism, drug addiction, or psychopathology.

This group also recommends that the operations be undertaken only in hospitals making a commitment to surgical management of morbid obesity, including careful postoperative follow-up under the direction of clinical specialists fully familiar with all aspects of the initial and ultimate complications of these procedures. It is emphasized that it is the responsibility of the physician and surgeon to adequately describe to the patient the risks and benefits, presented in understandable terms, as well as the long-term changes in life style.

It is interesting that surgical procedures for morbid obesity are done less frequently today than several years ago.

SELECTED REFERENCES

Alpers, D. H.: Surgical therapy for obesity. N. Engl. J. Med., *308*:1026, 1983.
  This editorial emphasizes the necessity for careful selection of patients undergoing surgical procedures for morbid obesity. The importance of close attention to long-term follow-up, complications, and ultimate results is stressed.

Buchwald, H., and Rucker, R. D.: The history of metabolic surgery for morbid obesity and a commentary. World J. Surg., *5*:781, 1981.
  An excellent historical documentary concerning the development of surgical procedures in the management of morbid obesity.

Griffen, W. O., Young, V. L., and Stevenson, C. C.: A prospective comparison of gastric and jejunoileal bypass procedures for morbid obesity. Ann. Surg., *186*:500, 1977.
  A randomized study comparing the gastric procedure with the jejunoileal bypass procedure is presented. The study indicated significant postoperative diarrhea and the need for continued medication in the jejunoileal patients as well as a high incidence of renal stones and cholecystitis not seen in the gastric procedures. Moreover, fatty hepatic metamorphosis was present in all patients but was more severe in patients with the jejunal bypass procedure.

Van Itallie, T. B., Bray, G. A., Connor, W. E., Faloon, W. W., Kral, J. G., Mason, E. E., and Stunkard, A. J.: Guidelines for surgery for morbid obesity. Am. J. Clin. Nutr., *42*:904, 1985.
  This is a report by a Task Force of the American Society for Clinical Nutrition, prepared by seven authors who are highly knowledgeable in this field. They represent different medical specialties, but each has a role in the diagnosis, management, and long-term follow-up of this challenging group of patients.

REFERENCES

1. Buchwald, H., and Rucker, R. D.: The history of metabolic surgery for morbid obesity and a commentary. World J. Surg., *5*:781, 1981.
2. Griffen, W. O., Jr., Bivins, B. A., Bell, R. M., and Jackson, K. A.: Gastric bypass for morbid obesity. World J. Surg., *5*:817, 1981.
3. Kark, A. E.: Jaw wiring. Am. J. Clin. Nutr., *33*:420, 1980.
4. MacLean, L. D., Rhode, B. M., and Shizgal, H. M.: Nutrition following gastric operations for morbid obesity. Ann. Surg., *198*:347, 1983.
5. Payne, J. H., DeWind, L. T., and Commons, R. R.: Metabolic observations in patients with jejunocolic shunts. Am. J. Surg., *106*:273, 1963.
6. Pories, W. J.: Surgery for morbid obesity. *In* Dudley, H. (Ed.): Rob and Smith's Operative Surgery: Alimentary Tract and Abdominal Wall, 4th ed. London, Butterworth, 1983.
7. Schumacher, N., Groth, B., Kleinsek, J., and Seay, N.: Successful weight control for employees. J. Am. Diet. Assoc., *74*:466, 1979.
8. Sonne-Holm, S., Sorensen, T. I. A., and Christensen, U.: Risk of early death in extremely overweight young men. Br. Med. J., *287*:795, 1983.
9. Task Force of The American Society for Clinical Nutrition—Van Itallie, T. B., Bray, G. A., Connor, W. E., Faloon, W. W., Kral, J. G., Mason, E. E., and Stunkard, A. J.: Guidelines for surgery for morbid obesity. Am. J. Clin. Nutr., *42*:904, 1985.

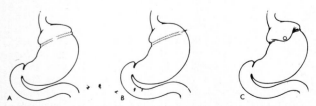

Figure 1. Various types of gastric partition procedures. A, Stapling procedure with central three staples being omitted. B, Omission of staples from short segment along curvatures of the stomach. C, Gastrogastrostomy following complete stapling of the proximal gastric pouch. (From Pories, W. J.: In Dudley, H. (Ed.): Rob and Smith's Operative Surgery: Alimentary Tract and Abdominal Wall, 4th ed. London, Butterworth, 1983.)

SURGICAL DISORDERS OF THE SMALL INTESTINE

BARRY A. LEVINE, M.D. • *J. BRADLEY AUST, M.D., PH.D.*

24

The small intestine includes the duodenum, jejunum, and ileum, encompassing a length of bowel extending from the pylorus to the ileocecal valve. It accounts for the majority of the length of the alimentary tract, and its enormous mucosal surface area is the site of absorption of foodstuffs, water, and minerals that allow normal maintenance, growth, and development. The normal anatomy and physiology of the small intestine as well as pathologic conditions found in this portion of the body are reviewed in this chapter.

ANATOMY

Gross Anatomy

The duodenum is the most proximal portion of the small intestine. It begins at the pylorus and extends approximately 20 to 30 cm. in length distally[10] with a luminal width from 3 to 5 cm. It is fixed, primarily in a retroperitoneal position, in a U shape (Fig. 1). The head of the pancreas is situated in the middle of the U and is applied closely to the medial duodenal wall.

The duodenum is divided into four portions (Fig. 1). The first portion, or *bulb*, is covered almost entirely by peritoneum and is quite mobile. This peritoneum extends cephalad to become the hepatoduodenal and gastrohepatic ligaments. Posteriorly and inferiorly, the peritoneal extension covers the head of the pancreas. The duodenal bulb is the site of approximately 90 per cent of all duodenal ulcers.

The second portion of the duodenum lies in a *vertical line* extending from the apex of the duodenal bulb inferiorly to the horizontal third portion of the duodenum. Its superior portion is at the level of the first lumbar vertebra and extends to the third lumbar vertebra before merging with the third portion of the duodenum. It lies to the right of the midline, has a concavity on its left side, and is adjacent to the head of the pancreas. On the medial wall the common bile duct and major pancreatic duct (Wirsung) enter via the papilla of Vater. The accessory pancreatic duct of Santorini may enter several centimeters proximal to the ampulla. The entire descending duodenum is in a retroperitoneal position.

The third, or *horizontal*, portion of the duodenum extends left from its junction with the distal descending duodenum across the midline at the level of the third lumbar vertebra. It also lies predominantly in a retroperitoneal position. However, there is a peritoneal fold at the junction of the middle and distal thirds of this portion of the duodenum, which forms the root of the mesentery of the small intestine and includes the superior mesenteric artery, vein, and nerves anterior to the duodenum. The inferior vena cava and aorta lie behind this portion of the duodenum.

The fourth, or *ascending*, portion of the duodenum lies to the left and anterior to the aorta. It courses superiorly to the level of the second lumbar vertebra and then turns anteriorly and caudad. At this point, it is fixed by the ligament of Treitz (an extension of the right crus of the diaphragm) and continues as jejunum.

The mucosa of the first part of the duodenum (bulb) differs from that seen in the second, third, and fourth portions. It is smooth with longitudinal folds pointing to the apex. The remainder of the duodenal mucosa forms horizontal ridges, or *valvulae conniventes*, a pattern also seen in the remainder of the small intestine.

The mesenteric small intestine is approximately 20 feet in length, but varies a great deal because of contraction and relaxation, so that it is approximately 10 feet in the natural state. The first 40 per cent comprises the jejunum, the latter 60 per cent the ileum. No definite border exists between the two portions of the small intestine. Rather, a gradual change is seen. The thickness of the intestinal wall decreases the further distal one goes in the bowel. Luminal width follows the same pattern. Therefore, obstruction occurs more easily in the distal ileum than in the proximal jejunum. As previously noted, the mucosa forms transverse folds throughout these portions of the small bowel. Here too, however, differences exist between the jejunum and ileum, since the valvulae conniventes are more prominent, more numerous, and thicker in the jejunum than in the ileum. These differences can be seen on contrast films of the small bowel.

The jejunum and ileum are suspended from a mesentery, the root of which extends approximately 15 cm. from the ligament of Treitz at the level of L2 to the ileocecal valve in the right lower quadrant at the level of L4–5. Therefore, the jejunum tends to lie in the left upper quadrant, and the ileum in the right lower quadrant, of the abdomen. Differences in the mesentery between the proximal and distal small intestine exist. In the jejunal mesen-

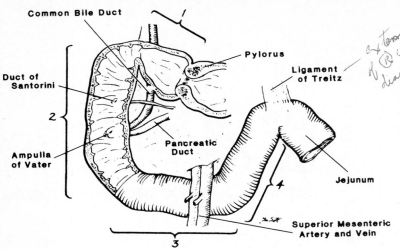

Figure 1. Diagram of the duodenum delineating its four portions and illustrating relation of the duodenum to the common bile duct and pancreatic ducts and to the superior mesenteric artery and vein. (From Haubrich, W. S.: Anatomy of the small intestine, Part I: Gross anatomy. In Bockus, H. L. (Ed.): Gastroenterology, 3rd ed., Vol. 2. Philadelphia, W. B. Saunders Company, 1976.)

tery, the fat contained between the leaves ends well before reaching the border of the bowel, leaving a clear area through which the vessels supplying the jejunum can be seen. Fat in the ileal mesentery extends to the mesenteric bowel wall, thus resulting in poor visualization of vessels.

The vascular supply of the duodenum is provided by two sources: the *celiac artery*, which gives rise sequentially to the hepatic artery, gastroduodenal artery, and superior pancreaticoduodenal artery, and the *superior mesenteric artery*, by its inferior pancreaticoduodenal branch. The two pancreaticoduodenal arteries, superior and inferior, form an anastomosis in the head of the pancreas; this allows a continuing blood supply to the pancreatic head and duodenum even if one of the inflow vessels is narrowed or occluded.

The mesenteric small intestine is supplied entirely by the superior mesenteric artery through the 12 to 15 branches that are given off into the mesentery. These form *arcades*, which in turn give rise to straight arteries that traverse the mesentery directly to the bowel wall. These are end arteries without anastomoses. Therefore, the occlusion of one of these vessels may bring segmental bowel viability into question. The mesenteric arcades differ in the jejunum and ileum. In the former, single arcades exist for the most part which give rise to long, straight arteries to supply the bowel. In the ileum, however, there are more complex tiers of arcades, sometimes three or four in number. The straight arteries rising from these arcades to the bowel wall are much shorter.

The venous drainage of both the duodenum and mesenteric small bowel is into the portal venous system. The duodenum is drained by pancreatic veins entering both the superior mesenteric vein and the portal vein directly. Mesenteric small bowel venous drainage is directly into the superior mesenteric vein.

Microscopic Anatomy

The wall of the small intestine is divided into four layers:

1. *Serosa.* The serosa, or peritoneal covering, is incomplete on the duodenum, where the majority of the second and third portions are without a posterior envelopment.

The serosa is almost complete in the mesenteric small intestine, the exception being a small portion in which the visceral and the mesenteric leaves of the peritoneum join at the edge of the bowel.

2. *Muscularis Propria.* Two coats of nonstriated, smooth muscle compose the muscularis propria of the small intestine. They are thickest in the duodenum and diminish in thickness distally. The outer layer is *longitudinal*; the inner is *circular*. The latter constitutes the bulk of the muscular wall. The myenteric plexus of nerves (Auerbach's) and lymphatic channels lie between the two layers of muscle.

3. *Submucosa.* The submucosa is composed of loose connective tissue that lies between the muscularis propria and the thin layer of muscularis mucosae, which is below the mucosa. Within this space is conducted a network of small blood vessels and lymphatics. In addition, Meissner's neuroplexus is found here.

4. *Mucosa.* The mucosa of the small intestine, except the duodenal bulb, is arranged in circular overlapping folds that interdigitate transversely. Each of these folds is covered with projections, *villi* (Fig. 2).

Both folds and villi are more numerous in the jejunum than in the ileum, thus accounting for the larger absorptive surface in this part of the bowel. Each villus is surrounded at its base by crypts of Lieberkühn, which extend down into the lamina propria. These are mucosal glands lined with columnar epithelium that is divided into *differentiated* and *undifferentiated cells*. The origin of all of these cells is from a junctional area between the crypt and the villus. The differentiated cells become (1) Paneth, (2) goblet, and (3) APUD (amine precursor uptake and decarboxylation) cells. The first two are exocrine in nature.

1. The *Paneth cells* are primarily located at the base of the crypts and contain secretory granules composed mostly of protein-carbohydrate complex.

2. The *goblet cells* are also most numerous at the lower portion of the crypts and secrete mucopolysaccharides.

3. The *APUD cells* are endocrine cells derived from embryonic neural crest and are of three types.[19] The first is the *endochromaffin cell*, which secretes 5-hydroxytryptamine. The two remaining types are the large or *L cells* and the small or *S cells*. The former have been shown to have glucagon-like activity; the latter exist mostly in the duodenum and have been shown to elaborate secretin.

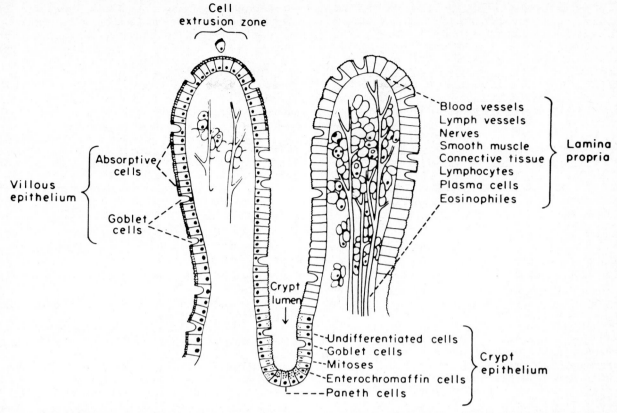

Figure 2. Schematic diagram of two sectioned villi and a crypt illustrates the histologic organization of the small intestinal mucosa. (From Trier, J. S.: Morphology of epithelium of small intestine. In *American Physiological Society: Handbook of Physiology, Section 6, Alimentary Canal. C. F. Code (Ed.): Baltimore, Williams & Wilkins Company, 1968.)*

The intestinal villi are aligned in a single-cell layer of columnar epithelium on a basement membrane. They are also derived from a junctional zone and form the absorptive surface of the intestine. Slips from the muscularis mucosae extend up into each villus and impart to it a contractile property. Blood vessels and lymph channels also extend within the core of each villus. The luminal end of each columnar cell is made up of multiple microvilli known as the *brush border.* New villus-lining cells are formed in the zone of proliferation in the crypts of Lieberkühn and take approximately 2 to 6 days to reach the villus tip and be shed.

Two specialized areas exist in the submucosal level and specific parts of the small intestine:

1. *Peyer's patches* exist mostly in the ileum and are more numerous distally. They consist of aggregates of lymph nodules surrounded by lymphatic plexuses on the antimesenteric surface of the bowel. They are formed during the embryonic period and decrease with age. Both thymus-derived and bursa-derived lymphocytes (T and B cells) are present within the patches.

2. *Brunner's glands* exist almost totally within the duodenum but have been described in the proximal jejunum. They are densest proximally and decrease with age. They consist of multiple acini emptying into tubules that open to either the mucosal surface or the lumen of the crypts of Lieberkühn. No known function for these glands has yet been defined in the human, and their mucinous secretions can be stimulated by glucagon and secretin.

DIGESTION AND ABSORPTION

The major function of the small intestine is to serve as a surface for the movement of nutrients into the internal milieu of the organism in a form capable of use for maintenance of normal function. For most of these constituents, the process involves actions taken upon them within the lumen of the bowel followed by separate processes required for absorption into the villus cells.[1]

Protein

The intraluminal breakdown of both endogenous and exogenous protein in the small intestine is both rapid and efficient.[1, 5] This digestive process is more rapid than the absorption of the products of digestion into the cell, and absorption is therefore the rate-limiting step. Peptidases, secreted as an exocrine function of the pancreas, are channeled into the duodenum via the duct of Wirsung and act to break down the large protein molecules in the duodenum and mesenteric small intestine. Each enzyme acts on specific lengths within the peptide chains, yielding smaller chains and peptide fragments that then undergo further enzymatic breakdown at the brush border of the villus cell. In all, the intraluminal enzymatic action yields approximately 30 per cent free amino acids. The remaining protein is acted upon by the microvillus enzymes at the brush border. Most absorption of exogenous protein occurs in the duodenum and proximal 50 cm. of the jejunum; endogenous protein, the approximately 25 gm. of enzymes secreted per day, is absorbed in the distal jejunum.

The completeness of protein breakdown within the small intestine depends on the amino acid composition of the protein ingested. The pancreas creates two types of peptidases. The first, *endopeptidase*, has a specific affinity for a given peptide bond on the interior of the peptide linkages. The endopeptidases include trypsin, chymotrypsin, and elastase. The products of hydrolysis by these endopeptidases are then acted upon by the second group of pancreatic-derived proteases, *exopeptidase*. These enzymes, carboxypeptidase A and B, each have an affinity for products of a specific endopeptidase and hydrolyze amino acids from C-terminal positions of the protein moiety. The actions of both the exopeptidases and endopeptidases in concert yield a mixture of free amino acids and small peptides ranging from two to six amino acid residues in length.

These products are then presented to the brush border of the cells of the villi. Here they are acted upon by cellular amino peptidases, which are exopeptidase compounds that split amino acids from the N-terminal position of the remaining peptides. The remaining free amino acids and dipeptides are absorbed into the cell by a process of *active transport*. Such transport requires oxidative energy and is coupled to sodium transport as well. Evidence exists that the energy needed is primarily for maintenance for the sodium pump at the cell membrane. Further evidence exists that such transport is carrier-mediated. Specific carriers probably exist for each group of amino acids, and there is competition between amino acids of each group for carriers. Once the amino acids and small peptide fragments are taken into the cell, the latter are further acted on by intracellular peptidases. These are specific for bonds involving given amino acid types. Following this final hydrolysis, the amino acids leave the cell, pass into the venules of the capillary core, and enter the portal venous system.

Carbohydrate

Carbohydrate metabolism depends on the partial breakdown of ingested polysaccharides to disaccharides and oligosaccharides in the lumen of the small intestine.[1, 5] These latter compounds are then hydrolyzed to monosaccharides at the brush border of the intestinal villus cell for absorption into that cell. The partial hydrolysis that occurs intraluminally is dependent on the action of alpha-amylase, secreted by the pancreas and the salivary glands, on ingested carbohydrates. Such carbohydrate is mainly found in the form of starch, which, when processed for human consumption, is broken down into two major components. The first of these is *amylopectin*, which accounts for 80 per cent of ingested starch. It is a water-soluble mixture of glucose unit chains joined by alpha-1,4 bonds. In addition, approximately every 19th to 26th glucose is joined to another chain by an alpha-1,6 linkage. This produces a highly branched molecule. The other form of starch is *amylose*, which is less soluble and simpler than amylopectin. It consists of simple glucose chains joined by alpha-1,4 linkages.

Alpha-amylase hydrolyzes the alpha-1,4 bonds in the interior of the starch molecules. It does not have as great an affinity for alpha-1,6 bonds or alpha-1,4 bonds of either maltose or those that are next to glucoses attached by alpha-1,6 bonds. Thus, the products of amylase action on starches for amylopectin are *maltotriose*, *maltose*, and *al-*

pha-dextrins. The products of amylose hydrolysis are maltotriose and maltose. The rapidity of the actions just described depends upon the amount of pancreatic alpha-amylase secreted as well as the concentration of chloride ion present in the intestinal lumen. Meals containing greater concentrations of starch elicit more potent amylase responses; in addition, the chloride ion appears to increase the activity of a given amount of amylase. The actions of alpha-amylase are usually completed by the time a carbohydrate load reaches the distal duodenum.

The products of alpha-amylase digestion of starch are presented to the brush border of the intestinal villus cell, where enzymes further hydrolyze them to liberate monosaccharides. These enzymes include:

1. *Glucoamylase*, which hydrolyzes maltose and maltotriose to maltose and glucose.

2. *Isomaltase* (dextrinase), which hydrolyzes the alpha-1,6 bonds and yields glucose.

3. *Maltase*, which yields glucose.

4. *Sucrase*, which yields glucose and fructose from sucrose.

5. *Lactase*, which yields galactose and glucose from lactose.

6. *Trehalase*, which hydrolyzes trehalose, a carbohydrate found in mushrooms.

The monosaccharides are then absorbed into the cell. Glucose and galactose enter the cell by a process of active transport that is probably *carrier-dependent*. The requirement for sodium as a cofactor for active transport of these two monosaccharides has been debated. However, it seems that at least small amounts of sodium are needed for transport to take place (Fig. 3). Glucose and galactose compete for the same carrier mechanism. Fructose uptake by the cell is also carrier-dependent but not energy-related. The process by which it absorbs is known as "facilitated diffusion."

Fat

Approximately 60 to 100 gm. of fat are ingested by the average human daily. Assimilation of fat is so complete that only 5 per cent of it is excreted in the stool per day.[1, 5]

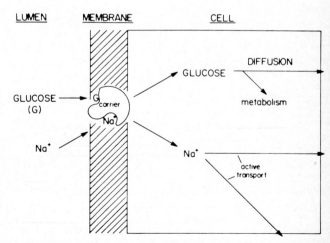

Figure 3. Representation of cotransport of sodium and glucose at the brush border membrane. (From Crane, R. K.: Anatomy of the small intestine, Part III. Carbohydrate assimilation. In Bockus, H. L. (Ed.): Gastroenterology, 3rd ed., Vol. 2. Philadelphia, W. B. Saunders Company, 1976.)

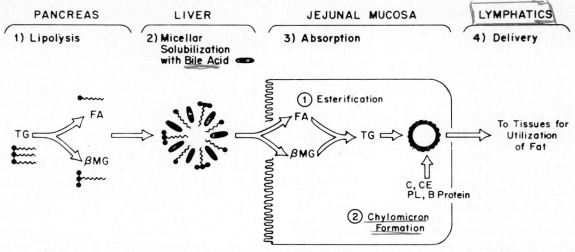

Figure 4. Schematic of lipid assimilation for dietary long-chain triglycerides. (From Rogers, A. I.: Anatomy of the small intestine, Part IV: Fat assimilation. In Bockus, H. L. (Ed.): Gastroenterology, 3rd ed., Vol. 2. Philadelphia, W. B. Saunders Company, 1976.)

Most digested lipid in the diet occurs as triglycerides, compounds in which glycerol, a three-carbon alcohol, is esterified to three chains of fatty acids. The fatty acids in 90 per cent of ingested triglycerides are of the long-chain variety (16 to 18 carbons); 10 per cent are medium-chain (6 to 12 carbons). The assimilation of these compounds can be characterized in four phases: (1) lipolysis, (2) micellarization, (3) absorption, and (4) delivery (Fig. 4).

LIPOLYSIS

Intraluminal lipolysis occurs primarily in the duodenum and requires three requisites for its efficiency. These include (1) the presence of pancreatic lipase, (2) a nearly neutral pH, and (3) a large oil-water interface. The first two of these factors are supplied by the pancreas, which not only secretes the enzyme lipase but also elaborates large amounts of bicarbonate ion to elevate the pH of the acid chyme. The last factor is supplied by emulsification of chyme by bile salts secreted via the biliary tract into the duodenum.

Pancreatic lipase, acting optimally at pH 6.8, cleaves the primary 1- and 3-bonds on triglycerides but leaves the inner bond, which is oriented into the oil phase, intact. Therefore, such hydrolysis yields two fatty acids and a monoglyceride.

MICELLARIZATION

The next intraluminal digestive step, micellarization, also depends on an alkaline pH, the presence of bile salts, and enough ionized fatty acids and monoglycerides. Micelles are aggregates, approximately 50 angstroms in diameter, that coalesce so that the hydrophilic portions all face outward toward the water interface while the hydrophobic portions face inward and are concealed from that interface. The process of micellarization serves to solubilize the fatty acid and monoglyceride fragments of intraluminal lipolysis so that complete digestion and absorption may take place.

Bile salts play a special role in this process. They are amphiphilic and therefore have dual hydrophilic and hydrophobic properties. Fatty acids and monoglycerate, at alkaline pHs, are also amphiphilic. At such pH levels, the bile salts and the products of lipolysis unite to form mixed micelles spontaneously with all their hydrophilic portions facing outward toward the water solution. The fat-soluble vitamins (A, D, E, and K) can also be contained within these micelles.

ABSORPTION AND DELIVERY

The mixed micelles are then brought into contact with the membrane of the cells in the intestinal villus. They then break apart, leaving the bile salts in the lumen. Fatty acids, monoglycerides, and fat-soluble vitamins then cross the brush border into the cytoplasm by a process of diffusion that does not require energy. Once inside the cell, a carrier—fatty acid binding protein (FABP)—is needed to transport these compounds through the hydrophilic cytoplasm to the smooth endoplasmic reticulum. It is here that triglyceride is synthesized by a process known as "re-esterification." Several molecules of the triglyceride then coalesce to form large particles that are then coated with a combination of phospholipid protein and cholesterol to form a *chylomicron*. This chylomicron then passes from the base of the villus cell into the central lacteal and is then transported via the thoracic duct into the systemic venous system. The absorptive process occurs almost entirely in the proximal jejunum.

Medium-chain triglycerides (MCTs) are managed more efficiently and with fewer energy-related processes than are those triglycerides containing long-chain fatty acids. Thirty per cent of the MCTs are absorbed intact. In the other 70 per cent, the pancreatic lipase hydrolyzes all bonds to form three chains of fatty acid. These chains are much more soluble than are the long-chain fatty acids and also form micelles with a greater ease. Once in the cell, MCTs are not re-esterified and enter into the capillary veins and portal system directly.

The bile salts on the cell surface after disaggregation are absorbed in the distal ileum. Their absorption is an active, energy-requiring process against a concentration gradient. Once absorbed, the bile salts enter into the portal venous system and are delivered to the hepatic parenchymal cells where they are taken up and resecreted, a process known as the *enterohepatic circulation*. This process occurs six times within a normal 24-hour period and is 95 per cent effective in its recirculation of secreted bile. Therefore, only approximately 500 mg. of bile salts per day is excreted. This amount is compensated by new synthesis of bile salts in the liver from cholesterol.

Water and Electrolytes

Up to 10 liters of water pass through the lumen of the small bowel per day (Fig. 5).[1, 5] This includes not only the water ingested but water that has been secreted into the lumen of the small bowel as well. Despite the large volume presented to the small intestine each day, only 500 ml. of water passes through the ileocecal valve into the right colon during each 24 hours. Therefore, there is a net absorption of water in the small bowel, but studies have shown that water is constantly moving simultaneously in two directions in relation to the small bowel mucosa. There is movement from lumen to plasma (absorption) while movement from the plasma to the lumen is also in progress (secretion). Water transport in the small bowel is passive, and absorption depends upon the type of mucosa present, the transport of ions and solute, and the osmolality of the luminal contents. Most water absorption occurs within the duodenum and the jejunum. It is postulated that the physiologic membranes of the villus cells are pierced by so-called pores that allow the passage of ions, solute, and water. It has been estimated that the pore size in the duodenum and jejunum approximates 8 angstroms; in the ileum it is only 4 angstroms, which may account for the relatively larger amount of water that can pass through the wall of the jejunum and thus be absorbed.

The amount of sodium presented to the small bowel each day is approximately 500 to 600 mEq. Half of this is from the oral intake of food; the other half is part of

gastrointestinal tract secretions. Since only 4 mEq. of sodium per day is present in the stool, it is evident that absorption of this ion by the gastrointestinal tract is 99 per cent efficient. Most sodium absorption occurs in the jejunum (50 per cent); the ileum (25 per cent) and right colon (25 per cent) account for the remainder. In the jejunum, two mechanisms account for sodium absorption. The first and predominant mechanism is *passive* and secondary to the solvent drag and bulk water flow. Active transport of the hexoses, glucose, and galactose, as well as that of amino acids, stimulates bulk water flow across the pores of the jejunum, a diffusion that follows an osmotic gradient. The dissolved sodium follows this flow passively. The second mechanism involves *active* transport against a modest gradient (13 mEq. per liter) and results in a sodium ion–hydrogen ion exchange. Only minimal amounts of sodium are absorbed by this method in the jejunum. However, this active transport mechanism accounts for all of the absorbed sodium in the ileum. This energy-based transfer is also able to work against a gradient of up to 110 mEq. per liter. In addition, the exchange of bicarbonate ion for chloride ion in the ileum favors net hydrogen secretion into the ileum. This latter secretion allows for easier uptake of sodium ion.

Of the 40 to 60 mEq. of potassium ingested each day, the small bowel absorbs approximately 90 per cent. This is done via passive diffusion and occurs almost entirely in the jejunum. Net secretion of potassium ion occurs in the colon, so that a total of 9 mEq. per day is excreted in the feces.

Chloride is absorbed mostly in the jejunum and is transported passively along with sodium ion, as they are both taken across the membrane pores by solvent drag secondary to the active transport of monosaccharides and amino acids. Electrical neutrality is maintained by the transport of sodium ion and chloride ion together. This occurs via active transport in exchange for bicarbonate ion against a steep gradient of 40 to 50 mEq. per liter. A reciprocal relationship exists between bicarbonate and chloride ions in the ileum. If the bicarbonate concentration in the intraluminal ileal contents falls below 45 mM., chloride ion absorption occurs in exchange for bicarbonate secretion. Once the luminal content concentration of bicarbonate rises above 45 mM., the process is reversed.

Iron absorption in the small intestine is inefficient, since of the 10 to 20 mg. of iron ingested each day, only 10 per cent is absorbed in the steady state. Most of this occurs in the duodenum and proximal jejunum. Iron is released from food in the stomach by the action of acid and pepsin; it is usually in the ferric state and must be converted to the ferrous state by the action of dietary ascorbic acid. While in the stomach, the ferrous iron combines with a mucopolysaccharide macromolecule, secreted by the stomach, that stabilizes the iron to a rising pH. This large complex is displaced in the duodenum, and the ferrous iron complexes again with smaller molecules to form ligands. These include monosaccharides, some amino acids (such as cysteine), ascorbic acid, and citric acid. Iron then crosses the luminal cell membrane as part of these complexes and is released by an enzymatic system within the cell. The iron can then be released to plasma via carrier-related transfer, where it is combined with the compound transferrin. Some of the iron is stored within the cell as *ferritin*, which is lost when the cell is shed into the lumen. A mechanism for control of iron absorption exists such that an increased uptake of iron into the villus cell occurs in states of iron deficiency.

Approximately 1.2 gm. of calcium is presented to the

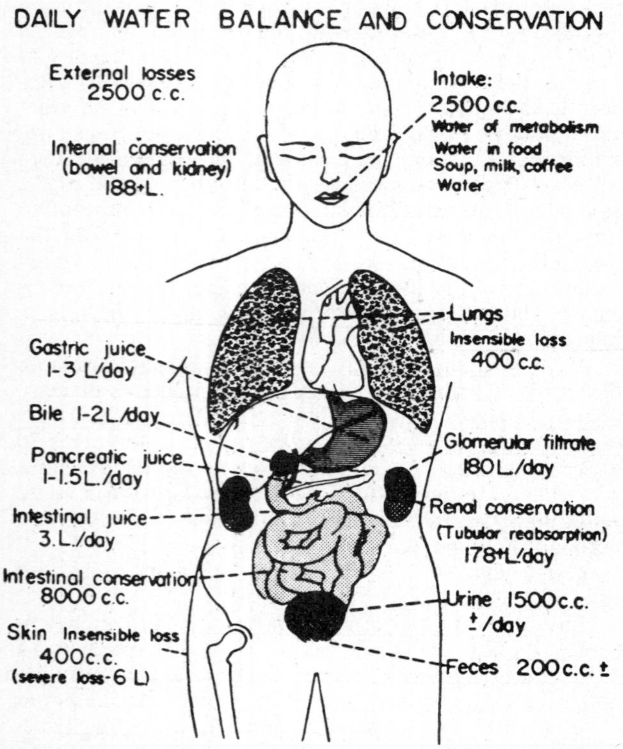

DAILY WATER BALANCE AND CONSERVATION

External losses
2500 c.c.

Internal conservation
(bowel and kidney)
188+ L.

Intake:
2500 c.c.
Water of metabolism
Water in food
Soup, milk, coffee
Water

Lungs
Insensible loss
400 c.c.

Gastric juice
1-3 L/day

Bile 1-2 L/day

Pancreatic juice
1-1.5 L/day

Intestinal juice
3 L/day

Intestinal conservation
8000 c.c.

Skin Insensible loss
400 c.c.
(severe loss-6 L)

Glomerular filtrate
180 L/day

Renal conservation
(Tubular reabsorption)
178+ L/day

Urine 1500 c.c.
±/day

Feces 200 c.c. ±

Figure 5. The gross intake-output record reveals little concerning the tremendous fluid movements that take place within the body continuously. (From Hardy, J. D.: Pathophysiology in Surgery. Baltimore, Williams & Wilkins Company, 1958.)

small bowel each 24-hour period. Of this total, 1 gm. is ingested and 200 mg. represents endogenous secretions (mostly bile). The duodenum and proximal jejunum account for almost all of the absorption of this cation, which approaches 40 per cent of the total calcium load. Calcium compounds are liberated from food in the stomach and ionized by the action of gastric acid. The ionized calcium is actively transported from the intestinal lumen to the serosal side of the villus cell in two steps. Both require the action of 1,2-dihydroxy vitamin D as a cofactor. This latter compound is the active form of intestinally absorbed vitamin D that has been modified by the kidney. The concentration ratio of active to inactive vitamin D depends directly on parathyroid secretory status and inversely on serum phosphorus concentrations. The active form of vitamin D enhances the synthesis of a carrier protein that is necessary for movement of calcium across the brush border into the villus cell by an energy-related mechanism. Once in the cell, the 1,2-dihydroxy vitamin D also assists in the active transport of the calcium ion out of the cell into the plasma. This latter step takes longer than the transport of calcium ion into the cell and is therefore the rate-limiting step in absorption.

Motility

Motility is a function that resides in the muscles of the small bowel, both longitudinal and circular. Motility has a threefold purpose: propelling intestinal contents from the stomach into the colon; mixing the contents of the small intestine with the secretory products of the gastrointestinal tract to permit digestion and absorption; and prevention of bacterial overgrowth by preventing stasis within the small intestine. Such functions result in contractile activity in the small bowel approximately 60 per cent of the time.

The muscular cells of the small intestine are nonstriated. They are approximately 5 x 20 microns in size. They are separate entities with special areas of fusion of the membranes of juxtaposed cells, especially in the circular layer of muscle, which allow several cells to act as a functional unit. Contractile filaments exist within the sarcoplasm of these smooth muscle cells. They are the same size as the actin filaments found in striated muscle, and there is evidence that they are actin. Myosin is also present within the cytoplasm, but not in filamentous form as seen in striated muscle.

The smooth muscle of the small intestine possesses contractile properties not unlike other similar muscles throughout the body. However, contractions are weaker and not as rapid; rather, smooth muscles have the ability to contract over a significant length of bowel. The major difference between the small bowel musculature and other muscles of both striated and nonstriated nature is the presence of a basic electrical rhythm (BER) within the former.[2] This electrical activity or rhythm is initiated within the small bowel muscles of the longitudinal layer and coordinates the rate, frequency, and distribution of contractions throughout the length of the small intestine. Although it does not initiate contractions itself, the BER is responsible for a pattern of control that results in a progression of chyme distally in the intestine. The BER spreads from cell to cell of the longitudinal layer without benefit of neural connection. This is communicated to the circular muscle, also initiating a slow wave, and in turn is responsible for the action potential in circular muscle that

marks the actual contraction of the intestinal wall.[25] In summary, the BER is responsible for establishing a pattern of control so that small bowel contents may progress distally toward the colon. The rate of BER, or slow wave activity, is greatest in the duodenum and proximal jejunum (12 contractions per second) and less in the terminal ileum (8 contractions per second).

The types of contractions initiated by the BER are three. The first is a *segmental contraction*, which involves a short 1- to 2-cm. length of intestine occurring for 2 to 10 seconds. This is a direct response to the slow wave of the BER and results in 10 to 12 such contractions per minute in the upper small bowel. After one has eaten, these segmental contractions may become rhythmic and *sequential*.[13] It is rare for these contractions (also known as *pendular contractions*) to occur in the fasting state. Both segmental and sequential contractions act to mix food and digestive enzymes within a small- to medium-sized area of the small bowel and expose them to mucosal surfaces for digestion and absorption. A third type, or *peristaltic contraction*, consists of muscular contractions passing distally at a rate of 1 to 2 cm. per second through several centimeters of intestine. Occasionally, peristaltic rushes begin in the proximal jejunum and traverse the entire length of intestine to the ileocecal valve.

Control of small bowel contractile function may be modified by both nervous and hormonal mediators. The small bowel has both sympathetic and parasympathetic nerve supply. The splanchnic nerves conduct sympathetic motor neurons to the sympathetic ganglia, which send neurons to the wall of the small bowel. The vagi are the source of parasympathetic preganglionic sensory and motor fibers to the intrinsic nervous plexuses of the bowel wall. Evidence exists for three types of functional nerve fibers acting on small bowel motility. The first of these is the *cholinergic* or *parasympathetic neurons*, which act to facilitate contractions; the *adrenergic* or *sympathetic nerves* seem to inhibit contraction. The third type of nervous connection is the *non-adrenergic inhibitory fiber*, which decreases bowel motility via the release of adenosine triphosphate (ATP).

Effects of hormones on small bowel motility have been studied mainly experimentally using pharmacologic hormonal levels. Although evidence for hormonal control exists, it is not conclusive that such actions occur in the physiologic state. Gastrin, cholecystokinin-pancreozymin, and prostaglandin E all stimulate peristalsis, whereas secretin and glucagon appear to inhibit motility.

Two reflexes in the small bowel are clinically important:

1. The *intestino-intestinal inhibitory reflex* is mediated via the thoracolumbar sympathetic pathways and requires an intact spinal cord below the sixth thoracic vertebra. The reflex itself is stimulated by abnormal distention of a segment of small bowel, resulting in the inhibition of motility in adjacent segments of small bowel. The effects of this are obvious. The adjacent small bowel, without motility itself, becomes distended and triggers the intestino-intestinal inhibitory reflex in even more proximal bowel. Thus, in lesions such as mechanical intestinal obstruction, the distention rapidly spreads proximally from the point of obstruction.

2. The *gastroileal reflex* probably depends on gastrin as its hormonal intermediary. It does not require extrinsic innervation. The reflex itself is a prolonged motor response, and hypermotility in the ileum follows the introduction of food into the stomach.

INTESTINAL OBSTRUCTION

Intestinal obstruction is defined as blockage to the distal passage of intestinal contents. There may be a *mechanical* basis in which a physical block is placed across the intestine, or it may be due to an *ileus*. Ileus is also defined as any type of intestinal obstruction, but the term has come generally to mean an inability of intestinal contents to pass distally secondary to a temporary disorder in motility. It has been estimated that small bowel obstructions account for approximately one fifth of all acute abdominal admissions on surgical services throughout the United States.

Although intestinal obstruction was first described by Hippocrates and treated operatively by other Greeks over 2300 years ago, no truly effective means of therapy was available until the mid-19th century.[23] The reason was twofold: first, there was a lack of understanding of the pathogenesis of bowel obstruction; second, no safe means to counteract or reverse the problem was known. It was not until the 19th century, and the introduction of anesthesia, that operative intervention could reasonably be considered.

In the 20th century, an understanding of the pathophysiology of mechanical bowel obstruction developed, aided by the pioneering work of Hartwell and Hoguet. With this approach came the practical ability to use decompressive gastrointestinal intubation (pioneered by Wangensteen), intravenous replacement therapy, endotracheal anesthesia, and antibiotics. Each allowed the resuscitation of the patient suffering from obstruction as well as safe operations for definitive treatment. Thus, the mortality of 50 per cent for bowel obstruction at the end of the 19th century has decreased today to 1 per cent in simple mechanical obstruction operated on within 24 hours of diagnosis. Challenges still remain in an effort to decrease the 25 per cent mortality associated with *strangulation* and *gangrenous* intestine.

Etiology

Mechanical intestinal obstruction can be divided into three etiologic categories.[17] In order of occurrence, these include (1) extrinsic lesions, (2) intrinsic lesions, and (3) obturation obstruction.

EXTRINSIC LESIONS

Among the extrinsic lesions, adhesions are the most common. These include both those of congenital origin in the pediatric patient (and rarely in the older patient) and are associated with malrotations (Ladd's bands) and a much larger group of acquired adhesions that develop following abdominal operations. Such bands either constrict the bowel or angulate it, producing an obstruction. The second largest category within this group is *hernias*, including inguinal, femoral, umbilical, ventral, incisional, or internal (through a mesenteric defect or the diaphragm). Extraintestinal masses including abscesses, pseudocysts, neoplasms, and hematomas may compress and obstruct the bowel. Intestinal *volvulus* is also included in this group as an additional cause and is produced by a twist in the mesentery of a segment of intestine.

INTRINSIC LESIONS

Lesions intrinsic in the bowel wall may cause mechanical obstruction, and congenital causes include atresias, bowel duplications, and stenoses. In the adult, strictures of the bowel wall may be caused by neoplastic involvement, inflammatory bowel disease, endometriosis, or inflammation secondary to radiation, diverticulitis, or potassium ingestion.

OBTURATION OBSTRUCTION

In children, intussusception, usually of the terminal ileum, as well as meconium plugging is not uncommon. In adults, polypoid tumors (cancers and carcinoids) and gallstones impacted in the terminal ileum are also causes. Impactions secondary to stool, barium, or bezoars are also not uncommon.

The major causes of intestinal obstruction have remained constant over many decades, although their frequency has changed. At the beginning of the century, hernia accounted for approximately 40 per cent of all obstructions, postoperative adhesions 10 to 15 per cent, and malignant neoplasms slightly less. Although carcinoma remains in third place, the relative positions and percentages of hernia and adhesions have changed. This is due to the current practice of routine repair of hernias upon diagnosis as well as the increase in intra-abdominal operative procedures.

Ileus is seen in association with several pathologic states, with the most common being in the postoperative period. Bowel motility does not return to normal for several days after an abdominal operation. This is probably due to the increased inhibitory sympathetic tone to the intestine. Bowel distention is another major cause of ileus and probably follows the previously described intestino-intestinal reflex. Distention of adjacent structures, such as the ureter, may also be associated with ileus. In addition, trauma, spinal fractures, retroperitoneal hemorrhage, hypokalemia, and vascular insufficiency are also associated with ileus. Peritonitis from any cause invariably causes a state of intestinal ileus, and experimental studies have shown this to be of a humoral etiology rather than dependent on a neural etiology.

Idiopathic intestinal pseudo-obstruction is a chronic disorder of unknown etiology. The signs and symptoms of intestinal obstruction are present without demonstration of a physical obstruction in the gastrointestinal tract. Opinion differs on whether there is an abnormality in the intestinal muscle or in the neural plexuses of the intestinal wall. The question of heredity as a predisposing factor has also been considered. In those afflicted, the BER is normal within the duodenum and colon. However, the contractile response of the muscle of the small intestine to distention is absent. Recognition of this disorder is mandatory because treatment is avoidance of operation. When the disorder is present, prolonged intubation with intravenous repletion is the treatment of choice.

Pathophysiology

There are three basic types of mechanical obstruction: (1) simple, (2) strangulated, and (3) closed-loop varieties. Although these share many of the same characteristics, each is different.

SIMPLE OBSTRUCTION

In *simple mechanical obstruction* the problem is secondary to distention of the bowel with fluid and gas. Although it was earlier thought that a toxin elaborated in the obstructed bowel caused the basic derangements, in

1912, Hartwell and Hoguet showed experimentally the primary problem to be the loss of fluid and electrolytes intraluminally. As previously described, the small bowel is the major site for the absorption of both fluid and ions. Approximately 8 to 10 liters of fluid per day, including ingested fluid, saliva, gastric juice, pancreatic and biliary secretions, and small bowel secretions, are absorbed through the small bowel mucosa. The fluid is in constant bidirectional flux across the mucosal surface. Therefore, the net movement of water is the sum of absorption from the lumen and secretion into the lumen. Animal experimentation has demonstrated decreased fluid absorption from the lumen above the point of obstruction but not distal to it. This occurs rapidly after the onset of obstruction, within several hours, while secretions remain normal initially. However, fluid secretion into the lumen increases over the following 24 to 48 hours to yield a net gain of fluid and ions into the bowel. Similar increases in luminal secretions have been shown in man. In addition to this influx of fluid, edema of the bowel wall with exudation of fluid into the peritoneal cavity occurs with further loss of fluid.

The gas present in the small bowel contains 70 per cent nitrogen, approximately 10 per cent oxygen and carbon dioxide, and lesser amounts of methane and hydrogen. The nitrogen represents swallowed air, whereas carbon dioxide is generated within the lumen. Intraluminal gases are absorbed according to their differential concentration gradients in plasma, air, and the lumen. Therefore, carbon dioxide diffuses rapidly out of the bowel lumen, whereas nitrogen remains. Experimental preparations have demonstrated that large amounts of air are present in the bowel following a simple mechanical obstruction, but only one thirtieth (1/30) of that amount is present in the same amount of small intestine in a closed-loop obstruction with no ingress of swallowed air possible. Similarly, in animals with intestinal obstruction with previously placed esophageal fistulas, little gas is seen in the obstructed bowel segment. This evidence has led investigators to conclude that swallowed air accounts for the majority of the gas in distended bowel. A decrease in the amount of swallowed air follows insertion of a nasogastric suction tube.

Soon after the advent of a mechanical obstruction, distention occurs immediately proximal and causes reflex vomiting. After this subsides, peristalsis against the obstruction occurs in an effort to propel the intestinal contents beyond it. Such peristalsis causes crampy, episodic pain with periods of relative relief between episodes. Peristaltic waves are more frequent, occurring every 3 to 5 minutes in the jejunum and every 10 minutes in the ileum. These are probably related to the relative frequency differential in the BER in these parts of the small intestine. Peristaltic activity propels both air and fluid through the loops of bowel, causing the characteristic auscultatory findings heard in mechanical obstruction. With continued obstruction, peristaltic activity becomes less frequent and is finally absent. This is related to the inhibitory intestino-intestinal reflex that follows when the proximal intestine distends with fluid and air. Such distention, and the inhibitory reflex it initiates, forms a vicious circle that proceeds until the entire bowel proximal to the obstruction is involved. As the bowel becomes distended, stasis of intestinal content follows; this sequestration causes rapid bacterial multiplication and overgrowth. In simple obstruction, there are few deleterious effects because the mucosal barrier against such bacteria and their toxins remains intact.

If the obstruction continues and is untreated, vomiting eventually occurs and the onset depends upon the level of obstruction. Obstruction in the more proximal intestine results in earlier vomiting with relatively little bowel distention. In addition to the loss of water, sodium, chloride, and potassium, loss of gastric acid with its high concentration of hydrogen ion results in a metabolic alkalosis. In the more distal small bowel or in colonic obstruction, vomiting may appear late, if at all. When it does occur, losses are usually isotonic with plasma. In summary, the sequelae of a simple mechanical bowel obstruction arise from the loss of extracellular fluid. This results in decreased intravascular volume, hemoconcentration, and oliguria or anuria. If treatment is not instituted in the clinical course, azotemia, decreased cardiac output, hypotension, and shock can result.

STRANGULATED OBSTRUCTION

A strangulated obstruction is a mechanical obstruction with *compromised circulation* to the involved bowel. Such obstructions include volvulus, adhesive bands, hernia, and distention. In addition to the fluid and gas that distend the lumen in simple obstruction, with strangulation there is also movement of blood and plasma into the lumen and wall of the bowel. Plasma may also exude from the serosal aspect of the intestinal wall into the peritoneal cavity. The intestinal mucosa, which normally serves as a barrier to the absorption of bacteria and their toxic products, is the part of the bowel wall most sensitive to changes in blood flow. With prolonged strangulation, ischemia results and the barrier is broken. Bacteria, along with both endotoxins and exotoxins, may pass through the intestinal wall into the peritoneal cavity. In animal studies, this mechanism has been demonstrated to be central to the severe clinical sequelae seen in strangulated obstruction. In addition, the loss of blood and plasma, as well as water, into the bowel lumen quickly produces shock. If these events are not appreciated early, they can lead rapidly to the patient's demise.

CLOSED-LOOP OBSTRUCTION

A closed-loop obstruction occurs when both the ingress and egress of a loop of intestine are obstructed. This type of obstruction holds more danger than most because it progresses to strangulation quickly and before clinical signs and symptoms of obstruction are evident. Causes of closed-loop obstruction include an adhesive band across a loop of bowel, volvulus, or simple distention. In this last situation, secretion into a closed loop can result in a rapid increase of intraluminal pressure, causing obstruction of venous outflow. Such vascular compromise leads to the rapid progression of the sequelae described for strangulated obstruction.

COLON OBSTRUCTION

Colon obstruction is usually less acute (except for volvulus) than is small bowel obstruction. Since the colon is not primarily a fluid-secreting organ and receives only approximately 500 ml. of fluid each day through the ileocecal valve, no rapid accumulations of fluid occur. Therefore, rapid dehydration is not a part of the syndrome associated with colonic obstruction. The most pressing danger in such obstructions is due to distention. If the ileocecal valve is incompetent, the distended colon can decompress into the small bowel. However, if the valve is competent, the obstructed colon forms a closed loop and continued distention causes rupture at the point of widest diameter, usually the cecum. This is based on *Laplace's law*, which defines tension in the wall of a tubular organ at any given pressure to be directly related to the diameter of that tube. Therefore, because the widest diameter of the colon is in the cecum, it is the area that usually ruptures first.

Diagnosis

The diagnosis of intestinal obstruction is not difficult; it is one that should nearly always be made on a clinical basis by the history and physical examination. Reliance upon radiologic examination and laboratory determinations must be seen as confirmatory and should not delay onset of prompt treatment.

Signs and Symptoms

The symptoms of intestinal obstruction are variable in their appearance and severity. They depend upon the level of obstruction as well as when the patient is seen. Symptoms include crampy abdominal pain, vomiting, failure to pass feces or gas, and distention. Abdominal pain is usually rather constant at first and later becomes colicky in nature. It is secondary to the forceful peristaltic contractions of the bowel wall against the obstruction. The frequency of the episodes depends upon the level of obstruction, appearing every 4 to 5 minutes in high jejunal obstruction and every 15 to 20 minutes in low ileal obstruction. The pain from such proximal obstruction is usually localized supraumbilically in the abdomen, whereas those from lower ileal obstructions usually present with intraumbilical pain. With the passage of time, the intestine dilates, motility decreases, and peristaltic waves therefore become less and less frequent until they finally cease. At this point, the pain eases and is replaced by a steady generalized aching over the entire abdomen. Such signs may also be encountered in paralytic ileus. If the abdominal pain becomes well localized, severe, constant, and unremitting, strangulation obstruction should be suspected.

Reflex vomiting is encountered immediately after the onset of obstruction. After this subsides vomiting depends upon the level of obstruction. If the obstruction is proximal, vomiting is seen early in the course and consists of a yellow or green clear liquid. The bowel is decompressed by regurgitation, and therefore no distention is seen. If the obstruction is distal, in the small bowel or colon, vomiting occurs late and after distention has occurred. The vomitus is thick and foul-smelling (feculent) as a result of the overgrowth of bacteria secondary to the stagnation. Because of the length of intestine filled with such contents, vomiting does not totally decompress the bowel above the obstruction.

The failure to pass gas and feces per rectum is also a characteristic feature of intestinal obstruction. After obstruction has occurred, however, the intestine distal to the point must empty its contents before obstipation is noted. Thus, in proximal obstruction a significant length of intestine is left uncompromised distally. The passage of the contents in this part of the distal intestine may require time, and obstipation may not be present, therefore, for several days. In contrast, if the obstruction is in either the distal ileum or colon, obstipation will be noticed earlier. In partial obstruction of the intestine, diarrhea instead of obstipation may be the presenting symptom.

Physical Examination

The physical findings in a patient suffering from intestinal obstruction are variable and depend on examination in the time course. Thus, if the patient is seen within hours to a day following the onset of a simple mechanical obstruction, few signs will be evident. However, if several days are allowed to pass, additional signs become manifest. The reasons for this are based on the pathophysiologic responses to intestinal obstruction. The first finding in examining a patient with suspected intestinal obstruction is the presence of generalized signs of dehydration, including loss of skin turgor as well as a dry mouth and tongue. As more fluid is sequestered in the intestinal lumen, fever, tachycardia, and a decrease in blood pressure may occur.

In examination of the abdomen, attention should be given to the appearance of distention, abdominal scars (suggestive of postoperative adhesions), hernias, and abdominal masses. In thin patients, visible evidence of peristaltic waves may be seen on the abdominal wall and may correlate with the onset of colicky pain. Finally, an attempt should be made to elicit any signs of peritoneal irritation or tenderness, including rebound or involuntary guarding. Such signs, especially in a localized area, more likely indicate a strangulated obstruction. Examination is not complete without auscultation. The classic findings in mechanical intestinal obstruction are the episodic presence of high-pitched metallic tinkles and rushes between quiescent periods. Such rushes coincide with the colicky pain. If the patient has been first seen several days into the course of the illness and the intestine above the obstruction has already dilated, peristaltic activity (and therefore bowel sounds) may be either absent or severely decreased. This lack of bowel sounds may also be found in paralytic ileus or strangulated obstruction.

A final, mandatory part of the examination is the rectal and pelvic examination. These may elicit findings of masses or tumors, and the absence of stool in the rectal vault suggests a proximal obstruction. If either frank blood or guaiac-positive stool is found within the rectum, it is highly likely that the obstruction is based on an intrinsic lesion in the bowel.

Radiologic Examination

X-ray examinations may be very useful in confirming the diagnosis of intestinal obstruction, and a flat and upright film of the abdomen should be the first obtained. If the patient cannot sit upright for the 15 minutes needed prior to taking the film, a film in the left lateral decubitus position is an acceptable substitute.

The presence of distended loops of bowel with air-fluid levels in a stairstep pattern on the upright film strongly suggests intestinal obstruction as the diagnosis (Fig. 6). This is due to the fact that air is not usually seen in the small intestine of adults and is evident only in distended bowel, most often secondary to obstruction of the intestine. Its layering over the fluid phase in the distended bowel is generally pathognomonic of obstruction. Information concerning the level of obstruction may also be gleaned from such films, but it is important to recognize the difference between the pattern of *small intestine* and *colon* when each is distended by air. The small intestine is marked by its position in the central abdomen and, second, by the presence of the valvulae conniventes appearing as lines across the entire width of the lumen (Fig. 7). The colon is identified by its position around the periphery of the abdomen, where it appears to encircle the intestinal contents and is further defined by the presence of the haustral markings that only *partially* cross the luminal diameter.

In advanced simple mechanical obstruction of the small intestine, no gas is seen in the colon. In colonic obstruction

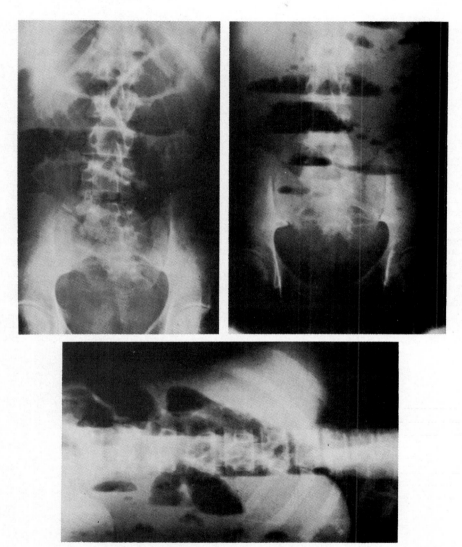

Figure 6. Supine (left upper), upright (right upper), and occasionally lateral decubitus (lower) films usually confirm the diagnosis of acute complete mechanical small bowel obstruction by revealing distended small bowel loops and air fluid levels. (From Jones, R. S.: The small intestine. In Sabiston, D. C., Jr. (Ed.): Textbook of Surgery, 13th ed. Philadelphia, W. B. Saunders Company, 1986.)

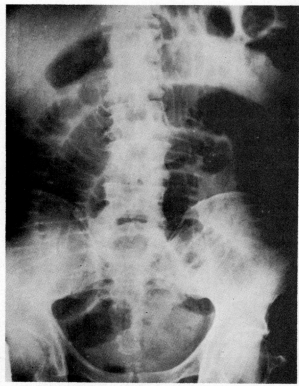

Figure 7. The abdominal film on the top shows the centrally placed bowel loops and depicts the valvulae conniventes, both of which are typical of distended small intestine. The film on the bottom shows gas accumulated in the colon and depicts haustral markings. (From Jones, R. S.: The small intestine. In Sabiston, D. C., Jr. (Ed.): Davis-Christopher Textbook of Surgery, 12th ed. Philadelphia, W. B. Saunders Company, 1981, p. 999.)

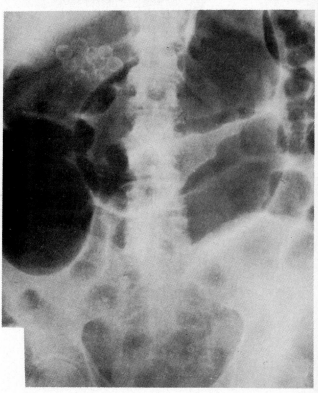

with a competent ileocecal valve, gaseous distention of the colon is the only important finding. If the ileocecal valve is incompetent, distention of the small bowel as well as the colon is present. In the patient with a strangulated obstruction, the clinical course is more rapid and attention is sought earlier. Gaseous distention of the bowel, if present at all, is much less than in simple mechanical obstruction and may be confined to a single loop. Another sign often seen in strangulated obstruction is the pseudotumor or "coffee bean" sign, in which the strangulated, blood-filled intestine is seen as a mass on the abdominal film. In paralytic ileus, the roentgenographic findings may be similar to those seen in simple mechanical obstruction. The gas pattern is not usually one of distention but, rather, is scattered throughout the stomach, duodenum, and small and large intestine.

Contrast studies are sometimes helpful in gaining information concerning intestinal obstruction. The most useful is the barium enema, which defines the point, and at times the etiology, of a colonic obstruction. A bolus of barium, given orally, may assist in more chronic situations in which differentiation of paralytic ileus or partial obstruction from mechanical obstruction is necessary. Finally, an intravenous pyelogram can be useful in detection of renal stones or pyelonephritis, both of which may cause paralytic ileus.

Laboratory Findings

Early in the course of simple mechanical intestinal obstruction, laboratory values are generally within normal limits. With time, more fluid is sequestered in the intestinal lumen and dehydration results. This is reflected by increases in the blood urea nitrogen (BUN), hematocrit, and urine-specific gravity. Decreases in serum levels of sodium, chloride, and potassium are also later manifestations. Also, with severe vomiting in a proximal obstruction (above the pylorus), alkalosis ensues and must be documented by measurements of serum bicarbonate as well as arterial pH. Finally, the white blood cell count (WBC) is usually only moderately elevated in simple mechanical obstruction (15,000 to 20,000). In strangulated obstruction (especially with gangrenous bowel), the WBC may soar to levels between 30,000 and 50,000.

Some regard fever, tachycardia, leukocytosis, and circumscribed abdominal tenderness as being quite significant in differentiating simple mechanical from strangulated obstruction. However, others have noted an overlapping of these signs in patients with either condition and there is no doubt that exceptions do occur. Therefore, the diagnosis of strangulated obstruction (with its attendant high mortality rates) may be overlooked unless operative treatment is performed expediently. With few exceptions, all bowel obstructions should generally be treated rapidly with repletion of fluids and electrolytes and with early operative intervention if continuous objective improvement is not seen.

Therapy

The treatment of mechanical intestinal obstruction usually involves operative intervention. Timing is critical and depends on the type and duration of the obstructive process. Operation is performed as soon as feasible, in view of the patient's overall status. Those with simple mechanical obstruction seen early in the course may be operated on expeditiously. However, older, debilitated patients in shock secondary to strangulated obstruction may benefit from blood, plasma, and crystalloid to improve blood pressure as well as renal function prior to operation.

Along with operative intervention, intravenous repletion of fluid and electrolytes lost into the intestinal lumen, as well as decompression of the gastrointestinal tract by intraluminally placed tubes, are the primary goals of therapy in intestinal obstruction. Infusions of solutions containing sodium, potassium, and chloride are needed in longstanding simple mechanical obstructions or those complicated by strangulation. Attainment of a normal level of hydration and electrolyte concentration may be monitored by observing urinary output, vital signs, central venous pressure, and sequential laboratory determinations. Only as these values approach more normal levels should operation be performed. Bacterial overgrowth, along with the endotoxin and exotoxin products from those bacteria, is primarily responsible for the major morbidity and mortality associated with strangulated obstruction. It has been shown that the placement of antibiotics in loops of intestine affected by this type of obstruction results in an increased survival. Thus, it seems logical that the administration of broad-spectrum antibiotics, with coverage aimed at intestinal flora, should be part of the therapeutic regimen in the treatment of strangulated obstruction. Since it is not always easy to differentiate between simple and strangulated obstruction, antibiotics should be given in all patients with mechanical obstruction.

Tube decompression of the gastrointestinal tract is indicated for two reasons: (1) to decompress the stomach and thereby lessen the chance of aspiration of intestinal contents; and (2) to limit entrance of swallowed air into the digestive tract and thus reduce intestinal distention, which may cause increased intraluminal pressures and possibly vascular compromise. The tubes used for such purposes are divided into two groups: (1) *short*, for the stomach only, and (2) *long*, for intubation of the entire small intestine. The short nasogastric tube (the single-lumen Levin tube or the more efficient double-lumen sump tube) decompresses the stomach and duodenum, which fill from retrograde distention arising from proximal jejunal obstructions. These tubes do not function well for obstructions in the distal ileum. Long intestinal tubes usually have a balloon on the end that may be filled with air or mercury. Once the balloon is beyond the pylorus, peristalsis propels it into the jejunum and distally to the point of obstruction. The long tubes may create problems, including the fact that they are useless in the late obstruction when intestinal motility no longer exists and that they do not decompress the stomach. Therefore, to prevent pulmonary aspiration, a second tube is needed to aspirate gastric contents.

It must be remembered that intestinal intubation is not a substitute for operation. It has been shown that when such patients have been treated with tubes alone, the mortality is higher than in the operated group. In addition, a high recurrent obstruction rate (nearly a third of all patients so treated) occurs in the intubation group. However, decompression of the intestine is recognized as the preferential treatment in several specific instances. These include obstructions seen in the early postoperative period as well as those associated with chronic radiation, metastatic cancer, and regional enteritis. Nonoperative therapy also seems to be of benefit in patients who have undergone previous operations for adhesions and for whom repetitious procedures become more hazardous. Other indications include intussusception in the newborn and sigmoid volvulus. In the former, reduction may be accomplished by the judicious use of hydrostatic pressure generated by a barium enema. In the second case introduction of a sigmoidoscope or rectal tube frequently derotates the volvulus with decompression of the colon.

OPERATIONS

Early operation after decompression with repletion of fluid and electrolytes is done to avoid the complications of sepsis secondary to either strangulation or rupture of the bowel. Therefore, obstructions suspected to be associated with the strangulated, or closed-loop variety, as well as those of the colon, have the highest operative priority. The procedures involved in their operative treatment fall into several categories. These include (1) lysis of adhesive bands or hernia reduction, (2) intestinal bypass, (3) resection with anastomosis, and (4) diversion by stoma with or without resection. Each of these operative maneuvers, other than hernia repair, is usually accomplished through a midline abdominal incision. This facilitates exposure of all parts of the abdominal cavity. Once the abdomen is exposed, note should be taken of the type of fluid encountered. Clear fluid is associated with simple mechanical obstruction, whereas bloody or feculent fluid usually indicates the presence of compromised intestine. The point of mechanical obstruction can usually be found by following the dilated bowel to the juncture where it becomes narrowed and decompressed.

When adhesive bands are found to be the etiologic agent in obstruction, care must be taken that all areas of potential obstruction, other than that primarily responsible, are divided. Intestinal bypass may be used when a chronic inflammatory mass is present, such as in regional enteritis. This may also be a useful technique in avoiding an ileostomy when a large cancer of the right colon is encountered in an elderly debilitated patient. Resection and reanastomosis are most applicable to small intestinal obstruction of the strangulated or closed-loop variety, especially when only a short segment of bowel is involved. Intestinal diversion by placement of an ostomy stoma is most useful in the case of an acutely obstructing carcinoma of the left or transverse colon when no mechanical or antibiotic cleansing of the colon has been possible. Construction of a small bowel ostomy may be the safest procedure when a significant length of strangulated, gangrenous small intestine is resected. If, after release of a vascular obstruction, bowel viability is in doubt, the intestine may be placed in hot packs and re-examined after approximately 15 minutes. If normal color and peristalsis return, the intestinal segment may be left. If doubt exists about the viability of a short segment of bowel, it should be resected. If a significant length of intestine is questionably viable, the use of fluorescein or Doppler techniques may be advisable to determine viability prior to resection. The operative mortality in simple intestinal obstruction (e.g., that related to an adhesive band) is less than 1 per cent. However, when strangulation with necrotic bowel is present, the operative mortality may reach 20 to 30 per cent.

TREATMENT OF ILEUS

Treatment of paralytic ileus is nonoperative and includes intestinal decompression by a long tube as well as intravenous infusion of fluid and electrolytes. Care should be taken that normal levels of serum potassium are attained, as hypokalemia is a common cause of ileus. Even with the above treatment, distention may increase to the point where decompression by operative means is necessary; fortunately, this is not a frequent occurrence.

REGIONAL ENTERITIS

Regional enteritis is an inflammatory disease of the intestinal tract affecting the entire thickness, *transmural*, of the bowel wall.[14] It is chronic in its course with periods of relative quiescence with acute relapses. Although the etiology is unknown, granulomas are found along with the disease in the majority of patients. Any part of the intestinal tract may be affected, but the small bowel and colon are most often involved.

In 1932, Crohn was the first to describe regional enteritis in detail. He and his colleagues integrated the clinical and pathologic data from a group of patients and separated this disorder from other intestinal granulomatous diseases. As a greater understanding of the multiple manifestations of this inflammatory condition has become known, the broader term "regional enteritis" has largely replaced the term "Crohn's disease" for this entity.

Although Crohn was the first to recognize and integrate information that set regional enteritis apart from other diseases, historic evidence exists to suggest that others, beginning with Morgagni in 1769, were aware of this entity. Saunders and Abercrombie, in 1813 and 1828, respectively, each described skip lesions of small bowel and colon of an inflammatory nature. In 1875, Wilks and Moran initially described the *transmural* nature of the inflammatory process. Finally, Moschcowitz and Wilenski recognized the microscopic appearance of granulomas in inflammatory bowel disease in 1923.

Except for peptic ulcer disease, regional enteritis is the most common pathologic entity of the small intestine. Its incidence is highest in the United States, northwestern Europe, and Great Britain. It appears more often in Caucasians than blacks and is said to have an incidence three times higher in Jews. Approximately 60 per 100,000 population are affected in the United States, while the incidence of new cases per year averages between two and four per 100,000. It is a disease primarily beginning in the young, with the average age of onset in the mid-third decade.

Etiology

Although the etiology of regional enteritis is unknown, suggestive evidence exists for both *infectious* and *immunologic* bases.

INFECTION

In the past, the presence of granulomas in the bowel wall led investigators to postulate a role for the tubercle bacillus or sarcoid in the pathophysiology of the disease. However, antituberculous drugs have no effect on the natural course of regional enteritis. Similarly, although noncaseating granulomas with Langhans' giant cells are also found in sarcoidosis, the Kveim test used to diagnose sarcoidosis is not positive in regional enteritis. The granulomatous aspects of regional enteritis have been passed in animal populations by the injection of homogenates of intestine and mesenteric lymph nodes from patients infected with the disease into the intestinal wall and foot pads of the experimental animals. Injection of homogenates from normal persons does not yield these same results. Filtration and purification studies suggest that the active agent in the homogenate may be either a virus or an atypical microbacterium. However, such an agent remains to be isolated.

Immunology

Recently, the most promising research into the etiology of regional enteritis has been an immunologic approach. Such studies have been suggested by the observations that immunologically based extraintestinal phenomena often occur in patients affected with regional enteritis and that exacerbations of the disease are often ameliorated by administration of steroids. It is not clear whether inflammatory bowel disease is a primary immunologic abnormality or involves a defective response to a transmissible agent. Shorter has hypothesized that an immune reaction may be the basis of the inflammation in the bowel wall—with original sensitization in the neonatal period and then re-exposure to the bacteria or virus at a later date in adult life when the mucosal barrier is weakened by a pathologic event. This might lead to a localized immune reaction mediated by both circulating antibody and lymphocytes producing inflammatory lesions. Experimental data both support and contradict such a hypothesis. Thus, circulating levels of several types of immunoglobulins have been demonstrated in patients with regional enteritis. However, circulating lymphocytes in such patients have been demonstrated to be normal in both number and activity. Therefore, it appears that further studies are necessary to clarify an immunologic role.

Heredity

Heredity, or genetic predisposition, has also been hypothesized in the etiology of regional enteritis. This is based on the finding that 10 to 15 per cent of affected patients have relatives who also suffer from the disease. Such a hypothesis has also been strengthened by the finding that the gene-coding frequency for the HLA antigens in regional enteritis patients differs from that seen in the ordinary population. However, it must be stated that at this time no clear inheritance pattern has ever been found for this disease. Although genetic predisposition may play a role, it may be that local factors must come into play before expression of the disease occurs.

Pathology

The lesions of regional enteritis may occur in any part of the gastrointestinal tract, including the esophagus and stomach.[18] However, the highest incidence is found in the small intestine and colon. The terminal ileum is most often involved whether alone or in combination with other parts of the gastrointestinal tract. Therefore, in 75 per cent of patients affected with regional enteritis, there is evidence of the disease in the terminal ileum. In 30 per cent of all affected patients, disease is seen in the small intestine only—with 50 per cent of these instances occurring in the terminal ileum alone. In a minority of patients (15 per cent), the disease is segregated to the colon alone. In the majority of patients (55 per cent), there is both intestinal and colonic involvement. Thus, an overwhelming majority of patients with regional enteritis have evidence of small bowel lesions. Finally, in a small minority (6 per cent), colonic involvement is localized to the rectum only, with or without associated small bowel disease.

Gross Appearance

The gross appearance of the small intestine affected by regional enteritis changes as the disease progresses from acute to more chronic stages. In the *acute stage* the findings may not be severe. They usually include a granular appearance of the serosa with mild hyperemia. In addition, the bowel wall is edematous and softly pliable. The mesentery may be thickened but not firm. Within the mesentery, soft large nodes may be present. When the bowel is opened, the mucosa may also be hyperemic and aphthous ulcers may be present.

When the disease becomes *chronic*, the segmentally affected areas appear dull and dark red, and are thickened and firm with a rubbery, or even leathery, consistency. The serosa is most often granular and off-white in color from dilated lymphatics and granulomas. Mesenteric fat may extend to surround the entire circumference of the affected bowel in the so-called "creeping" manner. The affected intestinal segment may be adherent to normal structures or other involved bowel. These densely adherent masses may include interloop fistulas or abscess cavities. On cut section, the entire bowel wall appears thickened. The majority of this reaction, however, takes place in the submucosa. As a result, the luminal size is compromised to a point where partial obstruction may occur. The mucosa shows varying degrees of destruction with evidence of serpiginous linear ulcers, which may coalesce via transverse ulcers to form a nodular cobblestone appearance. In addition to ulceration, fissures may also be present at various depths through the bowel wall. If they pierce the entire thickness, they may proceed to form contained abscesses or fistulas with other bowel loops. At times they may join other fissures partially through the bowel wall to form intramural fistulas. The small bowel mesentery in chronic disease is foreshortened, firm, and grossly thickened. Lymph nodes within the mesentery are enlarged, firm, and rubbery, reaching 2 to 4 cm. in diameter.

Microscopic Appearance

Like the gross appearance, the microscopic appearance of the small intestine affected by regional enteritis depends on the clinical stage of disease. The basic changes are related to the advance of the inflammatory and cellular response extending through the wall of the bowel.

Early in *acute* disease, this is manifest by edema and lymphangiectasia, most notably seen in the submucosa. The mucosa appears normal with perhaps an increase in the number of goblet cells, and an exudative reaction is seen on the serosa. Granulomas are not found in this early stage. Subacute regional enteritis is characterized by early fibrosis most notably in the submucosal and subserosal layers. Evidence of this is found in the finely fibrillar collagen in these regions along with diffuse plasma cell infiltration, lymphoid follicular hypertrophy, and hyperplasia. In the mucosa, small ulcerations extending to the muscularis mucosae are present. The muscularis propria shows evidence of hypertrophy, fibrosis, and infiltration as well but not to the degree seen in the submucosa and subserosa.

In the advanced, *chronic* form of the disease, fibrosis is more organized and dense. While it occurs mostly in the submucosal and subserosal layers, it extends throughout the wall of the bowel *transmurally*. The mucosal ulcers are larger and deeper and may be confluent and form large denuded areas. Intestinal villi, when present, are blunted, with mucosa resembling that in the colon.

Clinical Presentation

The majority of patients with regional enteritis experience a slow insidious onset of the disease. The symptoms are first short-lived with long periods of well-being, but over a period of time the symptomatic episodes become more frequent with shorter quiescent periods. In general, patients usually experience about 3 years of symptoms before the diagnosis of regional enteritis is confirmed.[21] The symptom complex is varied and depends on the site where the disease begins in the gastrointestinal tract. However, symptoms usually include abdominal pain, diarrhea, weight loss, fever, and anal lesions. In a minority, the onset of regional enteritis is acute. Symptoms include those similar to appendicitis with right lower quadrant pain, tenderness, and fever but usually without nausea and vomiting. The clinical diagnosis is frequently acute appendicitis, and the diagnosis of regional enteritis is made in the operating room.

PAIN

Abdominal pain is the most common symptom described by patients suffering from regional enteritis, occurring with a 95 per cent frequency. The pain patterns follow one of two types. The first of these is episodic and crampy in nature and usually follows ingestion of food. It is most likely secondary to peristalsis against a bowel lumen constricted by an intestinal wall thickened by edema or fibrosis. The lumen of normal bowel may also be compromised when such bowel is adherent to an infected, inflamed loop and can result in a partial bowel obstruction. The second type of pain, aching in nature, is more constant and usually denotes more advanced disease, and it is often associated with a palpable mass and abdominal tenderness. More bowel, both normal and inflamed, is usually involved in such a process, which may also include an enclosed abscess or enteroenteric fistula.

DIARRHEA

Diarrhea, which occurs in 92 per cent of patients with regional enteritis, is the second most common symptom. Patients complain of two to five watery bowel movements per day. However, unlike the diarrhea seen in ulcerative colitis, blood, pus, and mucus are rarely in evidence. In patients with far advanced regional enteritis, diarrhea may be foul-smelling as a result of the associated steatorrhea. The diarrhea of regional enteritis has several interrelated causes.[14]

The first cause is decreased net water absorption secondary to diseased and inflamed mucosa. This is especially true when extensive involvement of the jejunum occurs, because it is where most of the water load is absorbed. Enteroenteric fistulas also cause the intestinal contents to bypass large areas of mucosal surface through which water is normally absorbed. In both of these cases, a greater than normal water load is presented to the right colon, which, even if it is uninvolved in the disease process, cannot reabsorb enough fluid for normal bowel movements to result.

A secondary cause is the presence of partial intestinal obstruction resulting from the inflammatory constriction seen in regional enteritis. The bowel proximal to these involved segments dilates and results in a decreased absorption of fluid. Secretion of fluid into the intestinal lumen remains normal or increases, resulting in an elevated water load delivered through the ileocecal valve.

Partial intestinal obstruction may also be responsible for the overgrowth of bacteria in the stagnant intestinal contents proximal to the involved bowel. The bacterial overgrowth may be partially responsible for a final cause of the diarrhea—nonabsorption of bile salts from the intestine. The abnormal numbers of bacteria that follow overgrowth in the intestinal lumen can deconjugate bile and prevent its absorption in the ileum. Inflammatory disease in the terminal ileum occurs in 75 per cent of patients with regional enteritis and may also be responsible for nonabsorption. When bile salts are not absorbed and pass into the right colon, they inhibit water absorption by the colonic mucosa, which causes watery diarrhea. Also, without reabsorption of bile salts as part of the normal enterohepatic circulation, the bile acid pool is depleted. Since bile acids are integral in the digestion and absorption of ingested fats, fat malabsorption and steatorrhea may result, thus worsening the diarrhea.

FEVER

Fever occurs in slightly more than half of patients with regional enteritis and may be the only symptom. It often antedates abdominal complaints by several years. Therefore, in patients with fevers of unknown origin, regional enteritis should be part of the differential diagnosis. Such fever may be due to abscesses in the bowel walls or between loops of bowel. A fistula may also account for such elevations of temperature.

WEIGHT LOSS AND MALNUTRITION

Weight loss of greater than 5 pounds occurs in over 85 per cent of patients with regional enteritis, but significant weight loss and malnutrition are much less prevalent. Failure to maintain weight is most likely due to a conscious attempt by patients to decrease intake because of the perceived relationship of eating to the onset of symptoms.

MALABSORPTION

Malabsorption of specific nutrients, however, does occur in this disease. In addition to fat malabsorption, the *fat-soluble vitamins* (A,D,E,K) are also not absorbed normally under such conditions. *Protein* malabsorption is well understood and may be secondary to both the hypermotility and the amount of diseased mucosa in the small intestine, so that the ingested protein is not exposed to enough normal mucosa for a sufficient period of time to allow for breakdown to amino acids and dipeptides for absorption. Difficulties in assimilating *carbohydrates* may result from disaccharidase deficiencies in the microvilli of affected bowel mucosa.

Mineral deficiencies may also be seen in advanced regional enteritis. Large amounts of potassium, up to 10 gm. per day, may be lost in diarrhea. Calcium absorption is impaired secondary to fat malabsorption. First it is bound in the nonabsorbed fats intraluminally to form soaps, which are passed unabsorbed in the stool. Second, a deficiency of vitamin D necessary for normal calcium absorption occurs secondary to fat malabsorption. Usually, calcium deficiencies are compensated for by bone resorption. However, serum calcium concentrations may decrease even further secondary to hypoproteinemia and the nonavailability of albumin as a carrier protein for calcium.

ANEMIA

The associated anemias seen in regional enteritis are likely due to several factors, the first being the chronic slow blood loss from the intestinal mucosa involved in the inflammatory process. This loss is not as great as that seen in ulcerative colitis, but it is large enough so that normal iron intake will not compensate. Therefore, if oral iron supplementation is not taken, a chronic microcytic anemia results. Additionally, a megaloblastic anemia may result from vitamin B_{12} deficiency. This vitamin, usually absorbed in the terminal ileum, must be supplemented in patients with a primary disease of that area of the intestine. Derangements in absorption and digestion detailed above may result in growth retardation in pediatric patients with this disease. However, it must be remembered that such retardation can be reversed if repletion and supplementation are initiated via oral or parenteral routes.

ANAL COMPLICATIONS

Anal complications occur in approximately a third of patients with regional enteritis and may precede abdominal complaints by several years.[21] Anal pathology associated with regional enteritis is one-and-a-half to two times more likely if the colon is also involved in the disease. However, approximately a quarter of patients in whom regional enteritis is present in the small bowel alone also show evidence of anal complications. A significant association of anal disease with extraintestinal manifestation of regional enteritis also exists. The anal fissure is the most common lesion, but fistulas and abscesses are also common. The fistulas often do not communicate with any other diseased segment of bowel, and biopsy of perianal lesions often shows granulomas. Care must be taken in the therapy of perianal complications associated with regional enteritis because of a tendency to follow a chronic course of healing postoperatively. Conservative regimens consisting of local drainage combined with oral administration of metronidazole have shown gratifying results, but in some cases severe chronic perianal fistulas cannot be controlled without resection of proximal diseased bowel.

EXTRAINTESTINAL CONDITIONS

Extraintestinal manifestations are seen in approximately a fourth of patients with regional enteritis,[21] and all organ systems are affected. Such manifestations usually are evident only after the clinical onset of bowel disease. They do not follow the episodic nature of the bowel disease, but are constant in their course and are rarely affected by treatment.

Arthritis is present in approximately a third of patients. Fewer show evidence of *skin manifestations* (erythema nodosum and pyrodermic gangrenosum), ocular involvement (uveitis and iritis), or stomatitis.

Hepatic involvement may include fatty infiltration, pericholangitis, and sclerosing cholangitis, and a fourth of patients have evidence of cholelithiasis. The stones are usually cholesterol type because of loss of bile acids that normally serve to solubilize cholesterol in the bile.

Renal manifestations may include hydronephrosis secondary to periureteral fibrosis and nephrolithiasis, with the stones usually composed of oxalate, which is absorbed in greater than normal amounts secondary to impaired calcium absorption and loss through the bowel lumen. Pancreatic fibrosis with secondary amyloid deposition may also occur.

ADENOCARCINOMA

The risk of adenocarcinoma of the small intestine in association with regional enteritis is one hundred times greater than that seen in the normal patient population.[21] However, the problem is not great, since the rate of carcinoma in normals is only 3 per 100,000. Thus, only approximately 62 cases of small bowel adenocarcinoma in association with regional enteritis have been reported. The average age of onset for these tumors is 47 years, 10 years younger than the onset in a normal population. All but one case has occurred in bowel involved in the regional enteritis process, with three quarters of all tumors occurring in the terminal ileum. Approximately a third of all tumors presented in segments that had previously been bypassed surgically. Unlike the case in ulcerative colitis, neither the length of the affected bowel nor the duration of the disease process has been correlated with an increased risk of carcinoma. Prognosis in such cases is dismal, with an average survival of approximately 1 year.

Diagnosis

Since no laboratory tests are diagnostic of regional enteritis, the clinician must have an increased suspicion when a patient presents with a specific history of episodic symptoms, including abdominal pain, diarrhea, fever, and weight loss. The physical examination may be useful in revealing a tender abdominal mass, perianal findings, or one of the extraintestinal manifestations. However, the only truly useful studies in the study of a patient with regional enteritis are intestinal endoscopy with biopsy and radiologic examination of the gastrointestinal tract. Since the esophagus, stomach, and duodenum rarely are involved in regional enteritis, flexible endoscopy of the upper gastrointestinal tract does not usually yield useful diagnostic information. Since the colon and rectum are quite often involved, proctoscopy and flexible fiberoptic colonoscopy can be of great benefit. Examination may reveal hyperemic mucosa, early aphthous ulcers, or the later findings of deeper confluent ulcers and fissures. The finding of a cobblestone mucosa may weigh heavily in the diagnosis of regional enteritis. Inspection may not only serve well in the diagnosis of the disease but may also yield a "baseline" level of findings from which the response to therapeutic measures may be compared. Although the changes of fibrosis and inflammation on microscopic examination may be highly suggestive of a diagnosis of regional enteritis, only the finding of a granuloma is considered pathognomonic of the disease. Since granulomas are present in only 40 to 60 per cent of patients with regional enteritis, it is unlikely that random biopsy will yield this finding. Proctoscopic random biopsy data gathered on 349 patients showed that in only 15 per cent was the microscopic finding of granuloma present. In fact, in only one patient with disease confined to the small intestine alone was there a positive microscopic finding on biopsy.

Radiologic examination of the gastrointestinal tract in regional enteritis is done mainly to determine the changes in mucosal detail seen with this disease. Therefore, a radiologist experienced in double-contrast barium techniques may be extremely helpful in delineating the extent of the disease. The colon and terminal ileum may be examined by barium enema, whereas the upper gastrointestinal tract and small bowel may be delineated by use of swallowed barium along with special air-contrast or clysis techniques. Early in the course of the disease, aphthous ulcers may be evident on the mucosal surface. Later findings include a narrowed lumen, the most extreme example of which is shown by Kantor's "string sign." Additionally, longitudinal ulcers, fissures, and a cobblestone appearance of the mucosa may be evident. Because the wall of the affected bowel as well as the mesentery is grossly thickened, there is an increased space between contrast-filled bowel loops. Bowel dilatation may be demonstrated proximal to areas of luminal narrowing. Finally, masses of inflamed, adherent bowel may displace other contrast-filled intestine. Fistulas, while often present in advanced disease, are difficult to demonstrate.

Treatment

The natural history of regional enteritis is one of remission and exacerbation with much variability from patient to patient. The disease process is episodic, with additional bowel becoming involved in the inflammatory process with time. For this reason, the primary principle of treatment is conservatism with maintenance of bowel length. Unless severe complications ensue, all patients should first be treated medically. Such treatment consists of general support, specific drug therapy directed toward the inflammatory process, nutritional support, and control of diarrhea by the use of diphenoxylate hydrochloride (Lomotil) or atropine. Abdominal pain is treated with analgesics, and, if there is no obstruction, a bland, low-fat diet is prescribed. If obstruction, partial or complete, is present, intestinal decompression by means of nasogastric tube and intravenous therapy is required.

The specific agents used in the treatment of an acute exacerbation of the inflammatory process in regional enteritis are sulfasalazine (Azulfidine), prednisone, and azathioprine. Data concerning each of these drugs were not conclusive until the results of the report of the Cooperative National Crohn's Disease Study were made available in 1979.[21] Over 560 patients were prospectively randomized to each of the drug therapies. Results showed that active exacerbations of disease responded to either prednisone or sulfasalazine. Prednisone was found to be more efficacious in disease primarily located in the small intestine, whereas sulfasalazine was associated with better results in colonic disease. Azathioprine was slightly but not statistically significantly better than placebo in the treatment of regional enteritis. A major point to emerge from this study was that none of these drugs altered the long-term course of the disease. Thus, the length of the quiescent periods between attacks was not increased, nor were the number of recurrent episodes decreased by any of the treatments. Although side effects from sulfasalazine were negligible, those of both prednisone and azathioprine were significant and resulted in either drug removal or significant changes in dosages in large numbers of patients.

Nutritional repletion may be accomplished either orally or parenterally. Orally defined formulas that are low in bulk and without fat are now available. They can be absorbed almost entirely in the upper small intestine, leaving no residue. In the patient with partial obstruction, enteroenteric fistulas, or involvement of large segments of small intestine, total parenteral nutrition may be employed. This includes not only carbohydrate, protein, and fat but also vitamins and minerals, which are malabsorbed in the patient with severe disease. Replacement or supplementation of nutrition is especially useful in the growth-retarded child with regional enteritis who resumes normal growth on such a regimen.

Surgical therapy is reserved for failure of medical management or to treat complications. Even with maximal medical management, the incidence of surgical intervention is approximately 80 per cent after 20 years of symptoms and may approach 100 per cent if the patients are followed long enough. The time from symptomatic onset of the disease to the first operation is shortest in those patients with ileocolic disease, longer in those with disease confined to the small intestine, and longest in those patients with only colonic involvement. It must be stressed that surgical intervention is not a cure for regional enteritis but merely treats specific problems that occur in the course of the disease. Operation does not alter the probability of recurrence or the need for further operative intervention. The indications for operative intervention, in the order of frequency, are intestinal obstruction, enteric fistulas, abscesses, perianal disease, and the failure to ameliorate symptoms on prednisone or sulfasalazine. Some patients undergo operation for gross gastrointestinal hemorrhage or free abdominal perforation, but such instances are rare.

The principle that governs operative therapy in regional enteritis is *conservation* of bowel length. The procedures used include (1) intestinal bypass, (2) intestinal bypass with defunctionalization of the involved segment, and (3) resection with or without reanastomosis. Although bypasses are not generally favored because of unfavorable results, they may still be used in poor-risk patients or those with matted bowel masses obscuring safe dissection of vital structures within the abdomen.

Intestinal resection has become the operation of choice in regional enteritis, and it has been shown that only grossly diseased tissue need be resected without frozen section of resected margins. Only minimal amounts of mesentery should be resected with the bowel in order to maintain vasculature to the remaining intestine. Multiple resections may be performed to remove skip areas of disease. Overall mortality for such operations averages 5 per cent. However, the high incidence of preoperative steroid use in these patients results in a high postoperative morbidity. Such morbidity centers on the intestinal anastomosis, with leaks and fistulas, and sepsis related to intra-abdominal abscesses and wound infections.

A special situation exists in the patient being operated upon with a clinical diagnosis of acute appendicitis who is found to have an inflamed terminal ileum, a thickened mesentery, and firm, enlarged mesenteric lymph nodes. In general, if the cecum is not involved in the process, an appendectomy should be performed and the terminal ileum left undisturbed. In the majority of patients, no further symptoms referable to ileitis will occur.

The outlook for patients with regional enteritis, although not uniformly pessimistic, is associated with significant risks.[20] Patients with a diagnosis of regional enteritis have twice the mortality at any age compared with normals, and this risk is greater in young patients within a few years of diagnosis. The increased mortality seen in these patients is due to causes totally attributable to the regional enteritis or associated complications.

MALABSORPTION SYNDROME

Descriptions of malabsorption have been in evidence since antiquity and first appear in the Ebers papyrus. The first characterizations of sprue appear in the 18th century and the term "steatorrhea" is first seen in the writings of Kunzmann in the early 19th century. Although such descriptions of disease were common in the past, it is only in more recent times, as means for detection and study became more available, that better investigation and definition of malabsorption syndromes have come about. "Malabsorption" defines a diverse group of diseases with differing etiologies that include genetic, metabolic, acquired, post-

TABLE 1. *Classification of Malabsorption Syndromes**

Intraluminal Factors
Decrease in effective length
  Resection of stomach or
    small bowel
  Intestinal fistulization
  Hypermotility
    (hyperthyroidism)
Decreased digestive activity
  Pancreatic juice
    Pancreatitis
    Carcinoma of pancreas
    Pancreatectomy
    Cystic fibrosis
    Pancreatic duct lithiasis
      with obstruction
    Pancreaticocutaneous
      fistula
  Bile
    Hepatitis
    Cirrhosis
    T tube drainage
    Biliary obstruction
    Inadequate resorption
      of bile salts
    Congenital absence of
      bile salts
Changes in microorganism
  population
  Blind loop
  Small intestinal
    diverticula
  Intestinal stasis
    Visceral neuropathy
      (diabetes mellitus)
    Primary neurologic
      diseases
    Scleroderma
    Partial obstruction
  Oral antibiotics
    (neomycin)
  Giardiasis (also
    hookworm, whipworm)
  Acute infectious diarrhea
  Gastric achlorhydria

Changes in Intestinal Wall
  Mucosal epithelial cell
    Celiac disease of
      childhood
    Glutein-induced
      enteropathy

  Tropical sprue
  Disaccharidase deficiency
  Radiation enteritis
  Drug-induced (neomycin,
    etc.)
  Triglyceride enzyme
    deficiency
Ground substance
  Lymphoma, leukemia
  Whipple's disease
  Regional enteritis
  Systemic mast cell disease
  Amyloidosis
  Tuberculosis
  Carcinoma, sarcoma

**Abnormalities in Blood or
  Lymphatic Channels**
Blood
  Arterial or venous
    insufficiency
  Congestive heart failure
  Vasculitis
Lymphatics
  Intestinal
    lymphangiectasis
  Lymphatic obstruction

Indeterminate
Zollinger-Ellison syndrome
Malignant carcinoid
A-beta-lipoproteinemia
Protein-losing enteropathy
Pernicious anemia
Hyperthyroidism
Hypoparathyroidism
Pneumatosis cystoides
  intestinalis
Hemochromatosis
Kwashiorkor
Hypogammaglobulinemia
Adrenal-pituitary
  insufficiency
Tabes mesenterica

*From Johnson, C. F.: Postgrad. Med., *37*:667, 1965.

surgical, and endocrine bases. Several classifications have been devised based on anatomy, etiology, or physiologic abnormality. A comprehensive classification system is shown in Table 1.

Clinical Features

Generally, patients with malabsorption syndromes present with weight loss, diarrhea, and steatorrhea.[16] Each of the three major food constituents that form the basis of nutrition is affected with many of the malabsorption syndromes, but it is digestion and absorption of fat that are involved most frequently. This results in steatorrhea with the presence of light-colored, foul-smelling, bulky, floating stools.

Defects in protein digestion and absorption may become apparent only when severity results in hypoalbuminemia. This leads to a decrease in oncotic pressure in the vascular compartment with loss of extracellular fluid into third spaces. Peripheral edema and ascites are the clinical manifestations that then become apparent. Carbohydrate malabsorption leads to watery diarrhea, flatus, and bloating.

Deficiencies in the fat-soluble vitamins A, D, E, and K also result from steatorrhea. With the loss of vitamin D, hypocalcemia may result and lead to tetany, osteomalacia, and pathologic fractures. Deficiencies in vitamin K may cause hypoprothrombinemia and may produce hemorrhagic diatheses. Reductions in the level of vitamins A and E often result in decreased resistance to infection as well as in anemias caused by a decrease in red blood cell survival.

Finally, chronic anemias may result from the malabsorption of both iron and vitamin B_{12}. Malabsorption of the latter compound may also be associated with a peripheral neuropathy.

Diagnosis

In addition to findings on history and physical examination, the diagnosis of malabsorption should be confirmed by other tests. The stool should be grossly examined to exclude the findings of steatorrhea, and microscopic examination may show the presence of striated muscle fibers, a clue to a decrease in intraluminal digestion. Staining with Sudan III may show a greater than normal number of fat droplets. This qualitative test compares well with the more rigorous quantitative stool fat determination. This latter determination is made after first placing the patient on a diet containing a constant amount of fat. Stools are collected for 3 to 5 days. The total fat content should not exceed 5 to 6 per cent of the dry weight of the collected stool. Serum carotene determinations also may yield evidence of fat malabsorption. Finally, the general absorptive status of the jejunal mucosa may be determined by the use of D-xylose absorption test, xylose being a sugar that is normally absorbed easily through the jejunal mucosa. In the test, 25 gm. of D-xylose is given orally, and urine is collected subsequently for 5 hours. A quantity greater than 5 gm. of xylose should appear in the urine during this period.

Protein malabsorption, like fat malabsorption, may also be diagnosed by determining the quantitative protein content of stool. The patient is placed on a 100-gm. protein diet, and the stool protein is determined. Normal levels should approximate 2.5 gm. per day or less. In addition, a test for protein-losing enteropathies may be done with the use of radiolabeled albumin or other protein macromolecules. They are injected intravenously and stool is then collected for counting of the radioactive tag to determine whether abnormal amounts have been secreted into the bowel lumen.

Carbohydrate malabsorption is tested by the use of the standard oral glucose tolerance test over 3 to 5 hours. Any other compound, such as vitamins or the cations calcium and iron, may be radiolabeled and given orally to determine both uptake and clearance indices. However, this is rarely done. The major exception is the testing for vitamin B_{12} deficiency in the Schilling test. In this test, the urinary clearance of an orally ingested dose of cobalt 57 (^{57}Co)– labeled B_{12} indicates whether normal amounts are being absorbed in the terminal ileum. The amount cleared in the urine should be over 7 per cent of the dose ingested.

SPECIFIC DISORDERS

Postgastrectomy Syndrome

It is not uncommon for patients who have undergone gastric resection to lose at least 10 per cent of their preoperative weight. This may range from approximately a third of patients with small *partial* resections to the majority of patients having *total* gastrectomy. Fortunately, in most cases the weight loss is not severe and does not produce overt malnutrition. Several reasons exist for this decrease in body mass. The first is the occurrence of postoperative anorexia followed by a voluntary decrease in food intake. This may be secondary to alkaline reflux esophagitis symptoms experienced by some patients. However, the loss of part or all of the stomach does result in a decrease in the reservoir and normal mixing capacities of that organ. In addition, an increase in the rate of emptying is seen postoperatively.

Abnormalities in fat, protein, calcium, iron, fat-soluble vitamins, and vitamin B_{12} can all be documented after gastric resection. The magnitude of the malabsorption, however, may depend on the type of reconstruction following the gastrectomy. Billroth I anastomoses (gastroduodenostomies) seem to be associated with a lower rate of clinical malabsorptive abnormalities than do Billroth II reconstructions. This is especially seen in the case of fat malabsorption in which 20 per cent of those reconstructed with a Billroth II anastomosis have clinical steatorrhea, whereas only half that rate occurs in the Billroth I reconstructed group. The increased rate of fat malabsorption in the Billroth II group has several bases. The first is the loss of the duodenal and proximal jejunal mucosal surfaces for absorption. This is the area in which a large percentage of ingested fat is normally absorbed. Second, there is a decreased amount of bile and pancreatic juice secreted in patients with Billroth II reconstructions as opposed those with Billroth I. Since the food does not pass through the duodenal loop in the Billroth II group, the decreased amount of pancreaticobiliary secretions present is not able to thoroughly mix with the foodstuffs. Finally, the possibility exists in the Billroth II group for the formation of a blind loop in which bacteria may proliferate and deconjugate bile, rendering it inactive in the digestion and absorption of fats. Such bacteria may also be factors in decreased vitamin B_{12} absorption. The presence of severe fat malabsorption also decreases the absorption of the fat-soluble vitamins and results in the deficiencies just mentioned. Hypocalcemia may result secondary to steatorrhea. The calcium is bound to the soaps formed intraluminally and passed distally without absorption. In addition, absorption is decreased by the lack of vitamin D.

Finally, anemia may occur in postgastrectomy patients. The megaloblastic variety, caused by deficiency in vitamin B_{12}, is seen only after total gastrectomy in which the source of intrinsic factor, gastric mucosa, is completely removed. Normally, hepatic stores of vitamin B_{12} are depleted in 3 to 4 years and anemia becomes clinically evident. Megaloblastic anemia is not encountered as often as one would expect because patients usually undergo total gastrectomy for malignant disease, and only a minority survive sufficiently long for anemia to occur. The most common type of anemia seen after gastrectomy is due to iron deficiency. This is secondary not only to the decrease in gastric acid seen after operation, but also to the exclusion of the duodenum in Billroth II reconstructed patients from the flow of food. It is in the duodenum that the majority of iron absorption occurs.

→ Need acid to ↓ ferric → ferous for absorption

Most patients suffering various degrees of malabsorption after gastrectomy may be treated by administration of oral diets high in calories. If difficulty in fat and protein digestion and absorption is present, a diet consisting of medium-chain triglycerides and dipeptides may be prescribed. In addition, oral iron, calcium, and vitamin supplements may be needed. In the patient with a Billroth II reconstruction, the use of oral pancreatic enzymatic preparations may be beneficial. Finally, vitamin B_{12} supplementation may be necessary.

Surgical treatment of postgastrectomy syndromes is rarely indicated. In patients with a total gastrectomy, a Roux-en-Y reconstruction may be beneficial in decreasing the alkaline reflux symptoms. Some authors have advocated the creation of a pouch immediately distal to the esophagojejunostomy to restore the reservoir function of the resected stomach. However, there is no conclusive evidence that such a pouch functions as its advocates suggest or that it reverses the weight loss trend.

Vagotomy

In clinical practice, vagotomy is rarely performed without the addition of either a partial gastric resection (antrectomy) or a drainage procedure (pyloroplasty or gastroenterostomy). Therefore, it is difficult to separate the effects of vagotomy alone in the subsequent appearance of malabsorption. It is known from experimental models that sectioning of the vagus nerves does have an effect on small bowel motility, the mixing and reservoir functions of the stomach, and pancreatic and biliary secretions. Approximately a third to half of patients who undergo vagotomy experience postoperative diarrhea. In the overwhelming majority of these patients, the number of stools decreases with time. Thus, only 1 to 2 per cent of patients require long-term treatment of diarrhea severe enough to be associated with continuing weight loss. Although the etiology for postvagotomy diarrhea is unknown, theories concerning stasis and failure of mixing have been expressed. This syndrome is usually treated successfully by the use of antispasmodics such as codeine or diphenoxylate hydrochloride along with dietary manipulation. Surgical intervention is rarely needed for the most severe cases. Improvement has been reported with the use of an interposition of a 10-cm. antiperistaltic loop of small bowel.

Pancreatic Dysfunction

The pancreas is the source of enzymes for intraluminal digestion of carbohydrates, proteins, and fats. In addition, the beta cells in the islets contain insulin needed for carbohydrate utilization by peripheral tissues. The pancreas, like the liver, has a large margin of reserve. However, failure of its function can result in malabsorption, most often of fats, with steatorrhea. The most common cause for pancreatic dysfunction is chronic pancreatitis secondary to either alcoholism or biliary disease. Additionally, pancreatolithiasis, cystic fibrosis, fistulas secondary to trauma or disease, and tumors causing ductal blockage may be etiologic agents. Finally, Billroth II anastomoses after gastric or pancreatic resection for either primary pancreatic or other diseases (e.g., gastric cancer) may also result in decreased pancreatic secretions.

Patients with severe pancreatic dysfunction usually present with weight loss, steatorrhea, and abdominal pain. The clearance of D-xylose is normal in these patients, as the defect is not in the jejunal mucosa. Other evidence strongly suggestive of pancreatic insufficiency includes an abnormal glucose tolerance test, glucosuria, and an abnormally low serum calcium level. However, the confirmatory test for such insufficiency involves the injection of secretin and the sampling of duodenal contents, via a fluoroscopically placed tube, to assay for a stimulated increase in pancreatic enzyme secretion. Failure to discern a secretin-related increase in enzyme levels yields a positive diagnosis.

The treatment of such pancreatic insufficiency varies according to the etiology. Uncomplicated chronic pancreatitis may be treated with administration of oral pancreatic enzymatic extracts alone. When severe abdominal pain is part of the syndrome, however, some attempt should be made to delineate the pancreatic ductal architecture. This may be done either by endoscopic retrograde intubation of the pancreatic duct via the ampulla of Vater (ERCP) or by percutaneous, computed tomography (CT) scan directed, skinny needle puncture of a dilated pancreatic duct. If a ductal obstruction is found, a pancreaticoenteric anastomosis may be performed with reasonable hope of alleviating symptoms. If the ductal system in such a patient is destroyed, pancreatic resection and subsequent replacement with oral enzyme preparations and insulin may be the procedure of choice. In patients with adenocarcinoma of the pancreas, the abdomen should be explored. When the tumor is confined to the pancreas itself, resection should be performed. If the tumor has spread beyond the confines of the gland, various palliative procedures to relieve biliary or gastrointestinal obstruction may be done.

Non–beta cell tumors of the pancreatic islets, such as the Zollinger-Ellison tumor, may also be involved in the etiology of malabsorption. The etiology of the diarrhea seen in this disease is based on the enormous volume of gastric acid hypersecretion caused by the excessive stimulation of the parietal cells by high circulating levels of gastrin; secondarily, this acid also prevents the duodenal luminal contents from reaching the neutral pH level that is normally needed for fat digestion and absorption. Marked steatorrhea results and the management of gastrinomas are discussed in Chapter 23.

Another non–beta islet cell tumor associated with diarrhea and malabsorption elaborates the peptide hormone *vasoactive intestinal polypeptide* (VIP), which acts directly on the small intestine mucosa to greatly increase secretion and thus the water and electrolyte load presented to the colon. The result is intractable diarrhea. The treatment of choice is identification and surgical excision of the tumor.

Hepatobiliary Disorders

The mechanism by which the entities affecting the hepatobiliary tree result in malabsorption is through a decrease in the flow of bile reaching the duodenum. Bile salts are necessary for emulsification of ingested fat as well as micellar formation needed for absorption. If these intraluminal events do not occur, fat is not absorbed and steatorrhea results. Additionally, malabsorption of vitamins A, D, E, and K and calcium is secondary to the steatorrhea.

Decreased bile flow into the duodenum may be the result of primary hepatic disease, obstruction to the flow of bile, or abnormal biliary losses. Hepatitis and cirrhosis are the most common hepatic diseases that result in this syndrome. Obstruction to bile flow may occur within the liver (intrahepatic cholestasis) or may be extrahepatic secondary to biliary stone formation, tumor, or postoperative fibrotic changes caused by scarring. Biliary fistulas may form secondary to trauma or surgical procedures and cause bile to flow elsewhere than into the duodenum.

Therapy for the malabsorption associated with hepatobiliary disease should address the underlying disorder. Therefore, primary hepatic cholestasis, hepatitis, or cirrhosis is best treated by abstinence from any inciting agents (such as alcohol) and support of the compromised liver with high-carbohydrate, high-caloric intake. Steatorrhea may be decreased or controlled by administration of oral bile salts and decreasing the amount of oral fat ingested. In addition, vitamin supplements should be administered. Extrahepatic biliary obstruction should be treated primarily operatively. In patients with biliary fistulas, the goal is to eliminate the fistula so that bile may flow normally into the duodenum. When the fistulous output is less than 200 ml. per day, judicious temporization may be the preferred treatment. However, if the fistula is large or chronic in nature, operative techniques may be needed for its elimination. While the fistula is draining, the bile may be collected and re-fed to the patient. This not only enhances absorption of fat from the intestine but also minimizes losses from the bile acid pool, which even an increased hepatic synthesis cannot replace.

Blind Loop Syndrome

The blind loop syndrome was originally defined as a postsurgical syndrome in which a segment of bowel had been excluded from the caudad progression of the enteric contents. More recently, however, it has become recognized that any process that results in the stasis of small bowel contents may serve as the basis for the blind loop syndrome (Fig. 8). When stasis is present, an overgrowth of bacteria within the intestinal contents follows. This can occur secondary to inflammatory bowel disease, scleroderma, pseudo-obstructive syndromes, or postsurgically.

The abnormally large concentrations of bacteria act to cause malabsorption and diarrhea in two ways. First, they deconjugate bile salts, rendering them ineffective in the intraluminal digestive process for fats. Thus, steatorrhea and malabsorption of fat-soluble vitamins occur. Calcium absorption is also decreased secondary to both its intraluminal binding to soaps and the lack of vitamin D as an absorptive cofactor. Second, deconjugation of the bile salts interferes with their absorption from the terminal ileum for recirculation in the enterohepatic pool. Instead, they pass

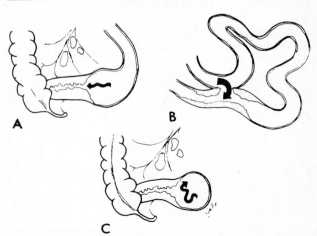

Figure 8. Structural deformities associated with intestinal stasis and the blind loop syndrome. A, *Partial obstruction*. B, *Fistula bypassing a loop of bowel*. C, *Bowel excluded by surgical bypass*. (From Drucker, W. R.: Regional enteritis (Crohn's disease). In Sabiston, D. C., Jr. (Ed.): Davis-Christopher Textbook of Surgery, 12th ed. Philadelphia, W. B. Saunders Company, 1981, p. 1009.)

through the ileocecal valve into the right colon. There, along with the soaps formed by the nonabsorbed fats, they act as an irritant and block normal colonic water absorption. Steatorrhea and watery diarrhea are the clinical results.

The proliferating bacteria in the blind loop syndrome also interfere with vitamin B_{12} absorption. The mechanism by which this is accomplished is not clearly defined. Bacteria either compete themselves for utilization of vitamin B_{12} or elaborate an inhibitory factor that prevents absorption of B_{12} by the terminal ileum. In either case, the result is a megaloblastic anemia.

Patients with the blind loop syndrome present clinically with the symptoms of vitamin deficiency, diarrhea, steatorrhea, weight loss, and anemia. Diagnosis is confirmed by using a three-stage Schilling test. In the first stage, ^{57}Co-labeled vitamin B_{12} is given orally. If less than 6 per cent of the ingested dose appears in the collected urine, vitamin B_{12} malabsorption is diagnosed. However, the etiology of malabsorption can be a blind loop syndrome, disease or absence of the terminal ileum, or lack of gastric intrinsic factor. Thus, in the second stage of the test, another dose of radiolabeled vitamin B_{12} is given along with intrinsic factor. If malabsorption persists, oral tetracycline is added in the third stage. If the percentage of radiolabeled vitamin B_{12} appearing in the urine is raised to a normal level (7 to 25 per cent) by this method, a blind loop syndrome can be diagnosed. Oral dosages of tetracycline should be continued for approximately 3 weeks. The symptoms ordinarily show marked improvement, and only surgical correction of the underlying cause of intestinal stasis will permanently remedy the disorder.

Short Bowel Syndrome

The small intestine is in constant contraction and peristalsis, which renders the length approximately 10 feet. Any significant resection may impair the intraluminal digestive and absorptive function. Normal or near normal function may be maintained if as little as 30 per cent of small bowel length is maintained along with the ileocecal valve. If the ileocecal valve is resected, 50 per cent of small intestinal length must be preserved to obtain the same degree of function. It is generally agreed that, with the ileocecal valve in place, the minimal amount of small intestinal length needed to avoid life-threatening malnutrition is 3 feet. Diseases, both acute and chronic, may lead to the short bowel syndrome. Acutely, vascular insufficiency may compromise not only the viability of the small intestine but that of the patient as well. More chronically, multiple resections for chronic regional enteritis and recurrent bowel obstructions may lead to the same end. The physiologic short bowel syndrome may also occur when an enteroenteric fistula bypasses any significant length of intestine.

Postoperatively, such patients have severe watery diarrhea, dehydration, and electrolyte deficiencies and are unable to maintain weight for several reasons. The first relates to a loss of luminal length and mucosal surface available for digestion and absorption. Also, the shortened bowel length decreases transit time, allowing a shorter exposure of digested foodstuff to the available mucosa for absorption. Loss of proximal jejunum compromises absorption of fats, water, electrolytes, and the cations calcium and iron. Loss of distal ileum compromises the absorption of both bile salts and vitamin B_{12}. The loss of the former results in steatorrhea, watery diarrhea, a decrease in the absorption of fat-soluble vitamins, and hypocalcemia—all by mechanisms described earlier—and loss of vitamin B_{12} results in megaloblastic anemia.

The length of small intestine resected can also be correlated with the degree of postoperative gastric acid hypersecretion encountered. The passage of such an abnormal amount of hydrochloric acid irritates and injures the mucosa of the duodenum and remaining small bowel. The result is an increase in luminal secretion, which causes watery diarrhea. The passage of the acid load also prevents the normally observed rise in duodenal pH that is necessary for digestion and absorption of fats. Fat malabsorption that follows causes steatorrhea, which only intensifies fecal losses and malnutrition.

The steatorrhea, diarrhea, and fluid losses seen with extensive small intestinal resection are worse in the first few weeks following operation. Therefore, it is wise to keep such patients on total parenteral nutrition during this time. Histamine H_2 receptor antagonists, such as cimetidine or ranitidine, should also be given to decrease the volume of gastric acid hypersecretion. Following this recovery period, as well as in patients with less extensive resections, defined formula diets should be administered. The protein content should be by amino acids and dipeptides, while fats may be included as medium-chain triglycerides. Such compounds necessitate less digestive action by the already compromised bowel. Calories can be supplied mostly as carbohydrate. Supplemental vitamins, electrolytes, and fluids should be administered. Antacids and H_2 receptor antagonists should be continued during this initial feeding period. Drugs that decrease intestinal motility, such as diphenoxylate hydrochloride, should be given as part of the regimen. If symptoms remain under control, the diet may be advanced slowly as the intestinal mucosa adapts with villous hypertrophy.

Surgical intervention in short bowel syndrome is rarely undertaken. Some have advocated the use of reversed intestinal segments to slow motility, but this is of questionable value. In the most severe cases, in which patients cannot tolerate oral intake without experiencing life-threatening fecal losses, total parenteral nutrition given via permanent Silastic catheters has become an accepted alternative in selected patients.

NEOPLASMS

Despite the large surface area present in the small intestine, the incidence of both benign and malignant neoplasms is surprisingly low. In fact, carcinomas of the small intestine account for less than 1 per cent of all neoplasms of the gastrointestinal tract.[12] The first malignant tumors of the small intestine were described in the duodenum in the 18th century in reports by Hamburger (1746) and Morgagni (1761). Cruveilhier reported the first benign tumor of the small intestine. It was not until 1932 that Raiford was able to collect 88 cases of small intestinal tumors to form the initial review published on that subject. He reported that most tumors occurred in the terminal ileum.

Neoplasms in the small intestine may arise from all layers of the bowel wall. Although most are of epithelial origin, tumors of smooth muscle, fat, connective tissue, vascular elements, and lymphatics have all been reported. Approximately equal numbers of benign and malignant neoplasms occur in the small intestine as reported in clinical series. In fact, in some, malignancies predominate (Table 2). However, autopsy series show a preponderance of benign over malignant tumors. Most tumors tend to occur in the ileum. However, the highest density of tumors per square area of mucosal surface occurs in the duodenum. In

TABLE 2. Small Bowel Neoplasms*

Type	Duodenum	Jejunum	Ileum	Total
Benign				
Adenomatous polyp	2	3	1	6
Leiomyoma	1	0	2	3
Lipoma	0	1	2	3
Brunner's gland adenoma	3	0	0	3
Villous adenoma	2	0	0	2
Neurofibroma	0	0	1	1
Hamartoma	0	1	0	1
Hemangioma	0	0	1	1
TOTAL	8	5	7	20
Malignant				
Carcinoid	5	7	11	23
Adenocarcinoma	8	2	5	15
Leiomyosarcoma	2	5	1	8
Lymphoma	2	1	4	7
Neurofibrosarcoma	0	1	0	1
TOTAL	17	16	21	54

*From Herbsman, H., et al.: Tumors of the small intestine. *In* Ravitch, M. M. (Ed.): Curr. Probl. Surg., *17*:131, 1980.

addition, the varying histologic tumor types may have different geographic distributions of occurrence within the small bowel.

Symptoms

The symptoms of small bowel neoplasms are nonspecific and may exist for extended periods of time before being brought to the attention of the physician.[12] The two major symptoms are colicky abdominal pain and gastrointestinal hemorrhage. Obstruction occurs most often with tumors of epithelial origin and may be due to one of several differing mechanisms. The first is luminal narrowing by inward growth of a polypoid or circumferential mass. Second, the epithelial mass serves as a lead point for intussusception. These intermittent intussusceptions are different from those found in children. In *adults*, intussusception is associated with a specific lesion in over three fourths of patients; in *children*, a leading point for the intussusception is found only occasionally. Finally, histologically, normal small bowel segments may be involved in fibrosis from local perforation of a tumor in an adjacent bowel loop.

Gastrointestinal hemorrhage occurs in approximately a third of patients with small bowel neoplasms. It is usually occult and episodic in nature. Melena or hematemesis, the latter especially with duodenal lesions, may be occasionally seen. Iron deficiency anemia is common, and approximately 30 per cent of patients present with hematocrit values of less than 30 per cent. Bleeding may be associated with any of the small bowel neoplasms, but it is most often found with hemangiomas and tumors of smooth muscle origin.

A lesser number of patients may present with abdominal masses. These most often occur with tumors of nonepithelial origin, which tend to grow outward from the serosa of the bowel and may attain enormous size. They may outgrow their blood supply as well, resulting in necrosis and cavitation with or without fistulas to other more normal segments of intestine. This may result in fever. Patients with lymphoma may also present with fever of the Pel-Epstein variety. Diarrhea is another less frequent presenting symptom and can be caused by either partial intestinal obstruction or primarily by the actions of hormones elaborated from carcinoid tumors. Finally, patients may present with symptoms of an acute abdomen secondary to perforation of their tumor in the free peritoneal cavity. This last is a rare presentation.

Diagnosis

Since the symptoms associated with small bowel neoplasms allow the lesions to follow an insidious course, they are sometimes difficult to diagnose. Therefore, a careful history plus a physical examination in an attempt to find masses or blood in the stool is mandatory. However, a high index of suspicion on the part of the examining physician is necessary. Establishing an accurate preoperative diagnosis is usually difficult, and only 50 per cent of neoplasms are diagnosed prior to surgical exploration.[12]

Radiologic tests form the primary basis of diagnosis. A plain film of the abdomen may show partial or complete intestinal obstruction with dilated intestinal loops, with or without air fluid levels. Barium studies of the gastrointestinal tract, using the double-contrast technique, may also be of value. A barium enema may be refluxed into the terminal ileum and distal small bowel. Swallowed barium may be followed through the upper gastrointestinal tract, jejunum, and ileum with a progression of films to reveal any masses in these areas. Better delineation may be obtained by using clysis techniques in which fluid is instilled into the small intestine with the barium. An additional finding may be the displacement of small bowel loop by large extramural or mesenteric masses. Patients with signs of mechanical intestinal obstruction should not be given barium orally.

More recently, angiography has been used in the diagnosis of small intestinal lesions. If bleeding is brisk enough, selective injection of the superior mesenteric artery with contrast material may delineate the site of the bleeding lesion. In addition, tumors, especially adenocarcinoma, may distort adjacent vessels. Finally, certain tumors, such as leiomyomas or carcinoids, may be identified by their hypervascular blush. When gastrointestinal hemorrhage is not brisk enough to be identified by angiogram, radionuclide studies utilizing labeled red blood cells injected intravenously may be of value. The patient then undergoes abdominal scanning at intervals up to 24 hours after injection. Several reports show this technique to be highly successful in localizing minimal amounts of gastrointestinal hemorrhage.

Flexible fiberoptic endoscopy may be of limited use and endoscopes normally used in the upper gastrointestinal tract may be advanced to reach through the fourth position of the duodenum into the proximal jejunum. Occasionally, colonoscopes may also be advanced retrograde into the terminal ileum for examination of that portion of the gastrointestinal tract. Flexible endoscopy may also be used intraoperatively. The entire gastrointestinal tract from the ligament of Treitz distally may be telescoped over a colonoscope introduced per anus and advanced retrograde under the direct control of the operating surgeon. This technique has been used to identify lesions not evident by any other mode of examination. Finally, exploratory laparotomy may be necessary to establish a diagnosis.

Benign Neoplasms

Benign neoplasms are reported in clinical series to occur with equal frequency as their malignant counterparts. Anatomically, 40 to 45 per cent are located equally in the duodenum or jejunum. The majority of lesions (55 to 60 per cent) appear in the ileum. Lesions of mucosal origin predominate there, with adenomatous polyps, either single or multiple, accounting for a third of those identified. Extramucosal lesions of various types make up the remainder.

Leiomyomas account for 15 per cent of the total within the gastrointestinal tract. The small intestine is second only to the stomach as a site of frequency for these lesions. Differentiation of benign from malignant leiomyomas is difficult and is usually determined by their clinical behavior as well as the number of mitoses per microscopic field.

Lipomas account for another 15 per cent of tumors. These may appear in either a subserosal or submucosal position and can be single or multiple. In the small intestine, they occur with half the frequency of appearance in the colon and three times the frequency of occurrence in the stomach. They are usually smaller than 4 cm. in diameter, but may achieve large size in the subserosal position.

Hemangiomas, representing 10 per cent of lesions, are often multiple and occur throughout the gastrointestinal tract. There are four types: (1) multiple ectasis, (2) the cavernous variety (the most common), (3) hemangioma simplex, a polypoid lesion projecting into the bowel lumen, and (4) those associated with Rendu-Osler-Weber syndrome, a genetic disorder characterized by multiple telangiectasias of the skin and mucous membranes in addition to those seen in the gastrointestinal tract.

Fibromas make up the last major category (10 per cent). Other neoplasms, seen in much fewer numbers, may include lymphangiomas, hamartomas, and tumors of neural origin.

Treatment of benign small intestinal neoplasms is almost always surgical. Without removal and microscopic examination of the lesion, a definitive diagnosis—and therefore the exclusion of a malignant process—cannot be made. In practice, a local resection of the mass in question is performed with either an enterotomy and polypectomy or a resection of a small segment of intestine. It must be stressed that an extensive search of the entire intestine must be performed to exclude the occurrence of multiple lesions or spread of disease into mesenteric lymph nodes.

Peutz-Jeghers Syndrome

This syndrome, first reported by Peutz in 1921 and confirmed by Jeghers in 1949, consists of the presence of multiple intestinal polyps combined with the appearance of melanin spots on the lips, buccal mucosa, nose, palms of the hands, and soles of the feet.[12] It is inherited as a simple mendelian dominant trait with variable penetrance. Although the control of both aspects of this syndrome has been shown to be located on a single pleiotropic gene, patients have been described in whom either trait has been present without the other.

The jejunum and ileum are the most frequent sites for the intestinal polyps. However, polyps may be found throughout the gastrointestinal tract—with a quarter occurring in the stomach and a third in the colon. The polypoid lesions are actually hamartomas representing adenomas of the mucosa arising in each part of the bowel. Patients with symptoms related to the syndrome present most commonly with colicky pain or anemia. The abdominal pain is due to intermittent intestinal obstruction caused by intussusception of the small intestine with a polyp as the leading point. In most instances, these reduce spontaneously. However, there have been reports of progression to strangulation with dire results. The anemia is secondary to occult gas-

trointestinal blood loss from the polyps. Documentation may be made by stool guaiac determination as well as by radiolabeled red blood cell studies. The hamartomas themselves are benign, but concomitant malignancies have been reported in a small percentage of patients. These have usually occurred in the gastrointestinal tract, but may also appear as ovarian tumors.

Surgical treatment is necessary for symptomatic relief. Local resection of a hemorrhagic polyp or one that is a lead point of an intussusception should be performed. At most, a small segment of affected intestine should be removed. Resection of excessive intestinal length may lead to malabsorption.

Gardner's Syndrome

First described in 1953, Gardner's syndrome is an inherited variant of familial polyposis. Aspects include soft tissue tumors, bone tumors, and intestinal polyps. The desmoids, lipomas, and fibromas that make up the soft tissue tumors appear subcutaneously and are usually multiple. The bone tumors, mostly osteomas, predominantly appear in the mandible but may be evident in the long bones as well. The intestinal polyps are adenomatous and usually begin to appear after the age of 20. They are found most often in the colon but often are identified in the small bowel and duodenum as well. These polyps carry a highly malignant potential. Most malignancies appear in the colon, but several have been reported in the small bowel. These latter tumors usually appear in conjunction with the colonic malignancies. This has led some authors to recommend total colectomy at an early age to lessen the risk of carcinoma formation. Abdominal procedures on patients with Gardner's syndrome should not be undertaken lightly. Healing usually occurs along with an exuberant, desmoplastic reaction that can encase the entire intestinal contents in dense, adherent scar tissue. The result may be acute and chronic intestinal obstruction, which itself may lead to the demise of the patient.

Malignant Neoplasms

Small intestinal malignancies account for less than half of 1 per cent of all deaths from cancer and approximately 2 per cent of gastrointestinal malignancy mortality.[12] Half of these tumors are found in the ileum; the remainder are equally divided between the duodenum and jejunum. *Adenocarcinoma* is the most common malignancy and accounts for 45 per cent of the total. *Carcinoids* rank second at 25 per cent and will be discussed separately below. *Lymphoma* makes up 20 per cent of the total.[22] Most lymphomas originate in nodal tissue. However, the small intestine ranks first as a site of extranodal origination of the disease. Ten per cent of small intestinal malignancies are *sarcomas*, the most common of which is the *leiomyosarcoma*.[4] These tend to metastasize via the bloodstream to more distant organs before local lymph node spread is evident.

The clinical presentation of the patient with a malignancy of the small intestine is the same as that discussed previously. However, in addition, a pronounced weight loss is often present. Symptoms have usually been manifest for approximately 2 years before the patient comes to diagnosis. As a result of the nonspecificity of symptomatology and, therefore, the rather late diagnosis of these malignancies, only 40 per cent are resectable for cure. In such cases, wide resection of the affected intestine along with the lymph node drainage is accomplished. Duodenal malignancies are managed by pancreaticoduodenectomy (Whipple procedure). When there is already significant spread of tumor, especially into the root of the mesentery, resection may not be possible without compromising the vasculature to the remaining intestine. Bypass procedures may be accomplished in such patients to relieve obstructive symptoms. In general, adjunctive therapy for these malignancies is not of benefit. The exception is lymphoma, a situation in which postoperative radiation and chemotherapy have been demonstrated to increase survival.[22] The prognosis for survival from small intestinal malignancies is poor. Overall 5-year survival rates for adenocarcinoma range between 20 to 30 per cent,[11] for lymphoma, 33 per cent,[22] and for leiomyosarcoma 50 per cent.[4]

Carcinoid Tumors

Carcinoid tumors have long been fascinating lesions, no doubt as a result of the link to endocrine-related symptomatology associated with some of these neoplasms. In 1888 Lubarsch first described the multiplicity of ileal carcinoid tumors. In 1907 Oberndorfer introduced the term "karzinoide" to differentiate these lesions from adenocarcinoma and to stress, wrongly as it later became known, their benignity. Masson used specialized silver stains to demonstrate that the tumor originated from the Kultschitzsky cells in the crypts of Lieberkühn. He added the term "argentaffin" to describe the carcinoid tumor. In the 1950s several different groups described the malignant carcinoid syndrome and related the symptoms to the release of 5-hydroxytryptamine (serotonin) from the carcinoid tumors.

As stated earlier, carcinoid tumors are the second most common malignancy found in the small intestine.[9] They may occur in any part of the gastrointestinal tract. The most common site is the appendix (45 per cent), followed by small intestine (30 per cent), rectum (15 per cent), colon (3 per cent), stomach (3 per cent), bronchus (3 per cent), and ovaries (Fig. 9). The overwhelming majority of these tumors must be considered benign, but the potential for malignancy may be predicted from the site of origin as well

Site	Cases	Average % Metastasis	Cases of Carcinoid Syndrome
Esophagus	1	—	0
Stomach	93	23	8
Duodenum	135	20	4
Jejuno-ileum	1,032	34	91
Meckel's diverticulum	42	19	3
Appendix	1,686	2	6
Colon	91	60	5
Rectum	592	18	1
Ovary	34	6	17
Biliary tract	10	30	0
Pancreas	2	—	1
	3,718		136

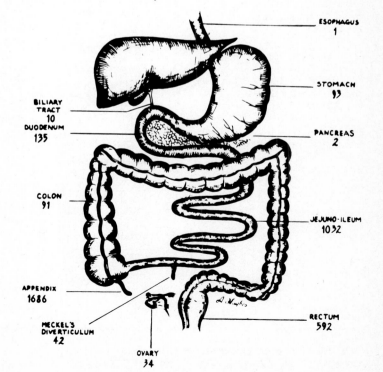

Figure 9. Collected series of carcinoid tumors. (From Wilson, H., Cheek, R. C., Sherman, R. T., and Storer, E. H.: Current Problems in Surgery, November 1970. Chicago, Year Book Medical Publishers, Inc., 1970.)

ESOPHAGUS 1

STOMACH 93

PANCREAS 2

BILIARY TRACT 10

DUODENUM 135

COLON 91

JEJUNO-ILEUM 1032

APPENDIX 1686

MECKEL'S DIVERTICULUM 42

RECTUM 592

OVARY 34

as the size of the primary lesion. Thus, carcinoid tumors of the appendix metastasize in only 2 per cent of cases and those in the rectum are rarely malignant. However, metastases can be found in approximately a third of lesions originating in the small intestine. Over three quarters of carcinoid tumors are smaller than 1 cm. in diameter, and when they are this size, they rarely metastasize. Another 20 per cent are between 1 and 2 cm. in diameter and have a metastatic rate of 50 per cent. The highest malignant potential occurs in those lesions greater than 2 cm. in diameter (5 per cent) in which 90 per cent have evidence of metastatic disease. A primary carcinoid tumor of the gastrointestinal tract rarely attains a diameter greater than 3 cm., but a metastatic lesion may be several times that size. Carcinoids of the small intestine are multiple in a third of patients. Also, additional neoplasms occur in 30 to 50 per cent of patients with carcinoid tumors. Grossly, carcinoid tumors appear submucosally in the bowel wall but may ulcerate as they increase in size. On section, they are firm and yellow or tan in color.

Clinical presentation of patients with carcinoid tumors, to the exclusion of those symptoms related to the *malignant carcinoid syndrome*, is no different from that elaborated for other small intestinal malignancies. The most common presenting symptom is partial or complete small intestinal obstruction. This is not due to obturation of the lumen by the tumor itself but rather by an associated desmoplastic reaction related to the 5-hydroxytryptamine (5-HT) secreted by the carcinoid. Large metastatic deposits may cause the same reaction in the mesentery, with the result that normal small intestinal segments may be drawn into a scarring process, producing multiple areas of obstruction.

This may be similar to that seen in regional enteritis, when radiologic examination of the small intestine is performed with barium. Malignant spread from primary carcinoid lesions is via local mesenteric lymph nodes and into the portal venous system. This progresses to liver metastasis. One third of patients with liver metastasis have evidence of the malignant carcinoid syndrome.

Malignant Carcinoid Syndrome

Malignant carcinoid syndrome is a constellation of cutaneous, cardiopulmonary, and gastrointestinal symptoms that connotes the presence of metastatic carcinoid tumor either in the liver or in other organs draining into the systemic venous system.[12] Approximately 4 per cent of abdominal carcinoids are associated with the malignant syndrome, and most of the primary lesions are in either the ileum or jejunum. The 5-HT that is elaborated from the tumor is metabolized from the ingested essential amino acid tryptophan via the intermediate 5-hydroxytryptophan (Fig. 10). Normally, only 1 per cent of ingested tryptophan is diverted via this metabolic schema. However, in patients with malignant carcinoid syndrome, fully 60 per cent of dietary tryptophan is channeled into this pathway. The resulting 5-HT has been correlated with many of the symptoms found in the malignant carcinoid syndrome. Normally, 5-HT is deaminated in liver and lungs to the inactive metabolite 5-hydroxyindoleacetic acid (5-HIAA), which is subsequently excreted in the urine. It is only when the venous drainage of the tumor bypasses the liver and enters the systemic venous system directly that the active 5-HT is

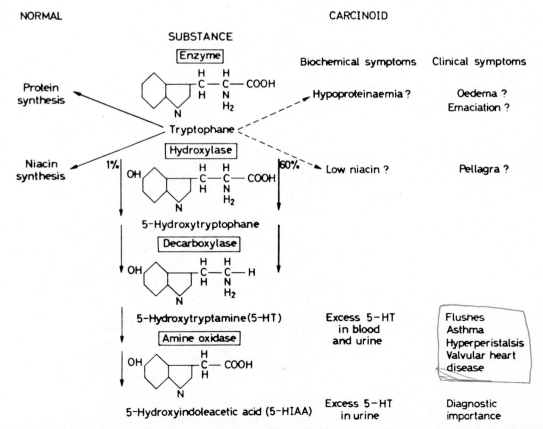

Figure 10. Biochemical explanation of symptoms in carcinoidosis. (From Waldenstrom, J. G.: Carcinoid tumors. In Bockus, H. L. (Ed.): Gastroenterology, 3rd ed. Vol. 2. Philadelphia, W. B. Saunders Company, 1976.)

available to incite symptoms. These tumors have also been shown to elaborate kinins, histamine, and kallikrein—each of which may be responsible for some of the symptoms.

The presenting signs and symptoms of the malignant carcinoid syndrome are episodic and involve several different organ systems. Those most common are related to the skin and are manifested by flushing. This flush may be pink to red but may progress to a bluish hue in more chronic cases. Its basis is a vasomotor instability that, in the most extreme cases, may result in shock. Recent studies have determined that the etiologic agents in this flushing are probably the kinins, and not 5-HT, secreted from the carcinoid tumor. Another cutaneous manifestation found in more chronic cases of the disease is the appearance of rough skin on the lower extremities. The roughness is similar to that found in the skin of patients with pellagra and may be due to the inordinate diversion of ingested tryptophan into 5-HT metabolism. Niacin, a normal tryptophan metabolite, may thus be decreased and result in such a pellagra-like state.

Gastrointestinal symptoms appear in 80 per cent of patients with the carcinoid syndrome and are evidenced by colicky abdominal pain, hyperperistalsis, watery diarrhea, and flatulence. The resulting decrease in transit time for the intestinal contents may cause malabsorption and its sequelae to become evident in more chronic cases. Cardiopulmonary symptoms occur late in the course of the disease. Cardiac manifestations are based on right-sided endocardial thickening and result in stenosis and, later, in insufficiency of the tricuspid and pulmonic valves. This may later lead to hepatic cirrhosis not unlike that seen with chronic right-sided cardiac failure. Asthmatic wheezing may be evident in a quarter of the patients. Both the gastrointestinal and cardiopulmonary symptoms are thought to be caused directly by the increased levels of circulating 5-hydroxytryptamine.

The diagnosis of the malignant carcinoid syndrome can be made presumptively by a history that elicits the above-named symptoms as well as a physical examination demonstrating hepatomegaly with masses. Radiologic studies of the gastrointestinal tract rarely show the small primary lesion. The liver may be scanned using nuclear or computer-assisted tomographic techniques in order to find and delineate metastatic lesions. Confirmation of the diagnosis, however, rests with the demonstration of increased levels of 5-HIAA excreted in the urine. Normally less than 10 mg. per day of this metabolite is excreted. In patients with the malignant carcinoid syndrome, often more than 40 mg. of 5-HIAA is seen in a 24-hour urine specimen. Foods that interfere with the determination of 5-HIAA, such as bananas and pineapple, must be removed from the diet prior to urine collection. Since circulating levels of 5-HT, and therefore urinary levels of 5-HIAA, may be normal between symptomatic episodes, urine collections must be obtained over several consecutive days to ensure a negative result. Finally, tests may be conducted to provoke symptoms of the syndrome. These include injections of small amounts of epinephrine as well as infusions of intravenous calcium. However, since vasomotor responses may be variable and severe, care must be taken when using these tests.

Treatment of carcinoid tumors and the malignant carcinoid syndrome is primarily surgical. If the small intestinal tumor is smaller than 1 cm. in size, and without obvious lymph node metastases, a limited bowel resection or wedge removal of the mass may be performed. When obvious lymph node metastases are present within the bowel mesentery, an en bloc resection of the area of affected bowel along with the subjacent mesentery should be performed. Even when extensive liver metastases are present, subtotal resection of tumor is the treatment of choice. Most often, this results in a decrease in symptomatology that persists for a long period of time. In patients with a large hepatic tumor load, in whom resection cannot be accomplished, hepatic arterial ligation has been advocated.

The bowel symptoms associated with the malignant carcinoid syndrome have been ameliorated by the administration of methysergide and p-chlorophenylalanine. Some relief of flushing has been obtained by the administration of phenothiazines as well as alpha-adrenergic blockers. Postoperative chemotherapy with streptozotocin and 5-fluorouracil has been beneficial. Overall 5-year survival for patients with carcinoid tumors averages 50 to 60 per cent. Those with disease limited to the bowel wall have a 75 per cent 5-year survival, those with mesenteric nodal spread 60 per cent, and those with liver metastases 20 to 35 per cent. Occasional long-term (15 years) survival with known liver metastases is reported.

DIVERTICULA OF THE SMALL INTESTINE

Diverticula of the small intestine are distinctly uncommon. Their incidence is greatest in the duodenum and decreases distally from jejunum to ileum. There is a slight increase again as the terminal ileum is reached. The diverticula may be either acquired or congenital, the most common of the latter being Meckel's diverticulum.

Duodenal Diverticula

Duodenal diverticula existed only as curiosities described at autopsy (100 cases) until the appearance of a report of four patients in 1913. Today, the incidence of duodenal diverticula ranges between 1 and 5 per cent in radiographic studies and 1 and 14 per cent in autopsy studies.[8] The overwhelming majority (95 per cent) project medially from the concavity of the duodenal "C" loop (Fig. 11). Over two thirds originate from the second portion of the duodenum, most within 3 cm. of the ampulla of Vater. In some patients, the ampulla itself is within the diverticulum. Another 20 per cent of diverticula originate from the third portion of the duodenum while a minority (10 per cent) are found in the fourth portion. It is extremely rare for diverticula to be found in the first portion, or bulb, of the duodenum. The diverticula found there are most often pseudodiverticula associated with the scarring of peptic ulcer disease. Although duodenal diverticula have been reported in the pediatric age group, the peak incidence for their occurrence is in the sixth and seventh decades of life. Only one in five patients affected have multiple diverticula.

Duodenal diverticula are usually acquired and are of the pulsion type with mucosa and muscularis mucosae herniating through a defect in the muscular layers of the duodenal wall. This is usually at the site vessels pierce the muscularis propria. Since the diverticulum is not made up of all coats of the duodenal wall, it should be properly termed pseudodiverticulum.

The overwhelming majority of patients with duodenal diverticula are asymptomatic. However, 5 to 13 per cent do have symptoms that may be present over many years and episodic in occurrence. The most common of these is abdominal pain, which may be localized to the epigastrium or right upper quadrant. The pain is usually made worse by eating and is relieved by vomiting. Presentation may be

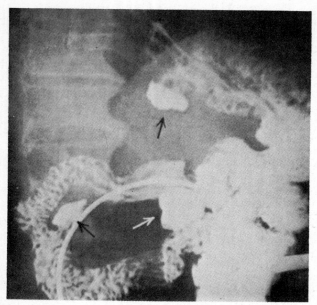

Figure 11. Two diverticula of the duodenum. A medium-sized diverticulum projects from the inner border of the descending duodenum. A second one arises from the ascending duodenum, near the duodenojejunal angle. A third diverticulum projects from the lesser curvature of the stomach. (From Pimparkar, B. D.: Diverticulosis of the small intestine. In Bockus, H. L. (Ed.): Gastroenterology, 3rd ed., Vol. 2. Philadelphia, W. B. Saunders Company, 1976.)

similar to the pain felt and described by patients suffering from peptic ulcer disease with or without gastric outlet obstruction. Additionally, inflammation of the diverticulum may obstruct both the pancreatic and common biliary ducts. This may result in jaundice or acute pancreatitis. Finally, there has been a reported association of duodenal diverticulum with the formation of cholelithiasis, making it difficult to determine which entity is responsible for the symptoms.

The diagnosis of duodenal diverticula depends on demonstration by either radiologic means or endoscopy. Flat and upright plain films of the abdomen may demonstrate an air fluid level in the diverticulum itself. However, an upper gastrointestinal barium contrast study is usually necessary to demonstrate the lesion. If the diverticular neck is narrow, barium may be retained for extended periods of time. More recently, these diverticula have been diagnosed by use of flexible fiberoptic endoscopy. The opening usually can be visualized with ease. Care must be taken not to mistake a wide diverticular opening for a continuation of the lumen, since introduction of the scope into the diverticulum may result in possible perforation.

Major complications of duodenal diverticula include inflammation and hemorrhage. Inflammation, or diverticulitis, may be the result of inspissated food particles, enteroliths, foreign bodies, or ulceration within the lumen of the diverticulum. Such inflammation may lead to perforation of the diverticulum into the retroperitoneal space and can also cause jaundice by pressure on the common bile duct or ampulla of Vater. The ensuing symptoms are acute in onset in the majority of patients and include abdominal pain with accompanying fever. The etiology of these symptoms is recognized preoperatively only rarely (in 6 per cent) and, in a significant number (15 per cent), is not recognized at operation. Operative treatment of this complication should include drainage of the abscess and gastroenterostomy to bypass the affected area. Biliary and

pancreatic diversion may also be necessary. Hemorrhage is a rare complication of duodenal diverticular disease; however, it may be massive and life-threatening in magnitude. Presentation may be with either melena or hematemesis. Bleeding may be brisk enough to cause hypovolemic shock, necessitating immediate resuscitation and emergent operation.

Fortunately, most duodenal diverticula are asymptomatic and need no specific treatment. Surgical intervention is reserved for those with acute complications or with symptoms for which other causes have been excluded. Thus, approximately one in five patients symptomatic from their duodenal diverticulum comes to operation. In the case of acute hemorrhage or chronic symptomatology, direct attack on the duodenal diverticulum is warranted.[8] Resection is preferable to exclusionary procedures. In the diverticulum situated posterior to the pancreatic head, resection and duodenal closure may be performed. For the diverticulum situated within the pancreatic head, invagination and amputation may be accomplished through an anterior duodenotomy. The resulting defect may be closed intramurally. Extirpation may not be possible if the ampulla of Vater lies within the diverticulum. Emergent operative procedures are associated with a significant (30 per cent) mortality rate. Even approached electively, operation for duodenal diverticula is associated with a 5 to 10 per cent mortality rate. Operation for chronic symptomatology should not be undertaken lightly. It has been estimated that only 50 per cent of patients who are operated on for such symptoms experience long-term benefit.

Mesenteric Diverticula

Diverticula of the mesenteric small intestine were first described by Sir Astley Cooper in 1807. They may be found in up to 5 per cent of small intestinal radiographic studies with barium and in up to 1.3 per cent of autopsy studies. Patients over 40 years of age are most often affected (80 to 90 per cent), the highest areas of frequency being in the upper jejunum and lesser areas of frequency being more distally in the small intestine. Diverticula may be found on the mesenteric border of the bowel projecting between the leaves of the mesentery. They are pseudodiverticula consisting of mucosa and muscularis mucosae projecting through weakened areas of the bowel wall—probably in areas where vessels enter. Thus, they are pulsion-type diverticula, the incidence of which has been associated with increased intraluminal pressure, lack of a mesenteric coat in the area of protrusion, and generalized atherosclerosis. Whatever the etiology, it is general in nature. There is an associated increased incidence of diverticula in other parts of the gastrointestinal tract.

Patients with diverticula of the small intestine may be divided into four groups.[24]

1. The majority are asymptomatic.

2. In the second group, chronic nonspecific symptoms of indigestion are present and hyperperistalsis with diarrhea may be evident; other patients may complain of intestinal atony with the resultant constipation. It is rare for abdominal pain to be a problem.

3. The third group may suffer from a blind loop syndrome, resulting from stasis of luminal contents in large diverticula and subsequent bacterial overgrowth. Malabsorption with steatorrhea and megaloblastic anemia may result. Diagnosis of this syndrome may be achieved by the modified Schilling test, as previously described.

4. The minority (10 per cent) have complications related to diverticula.

The first of these complications is *diverticulitis*, which may lead to perforation. It may be difficult to distinguish the symptoms of such perforation from appendicitis or perforated colonic diverticulitis. Equally common as a complication is *intestinal obstruction*. This may be a result of volvulus, adhesions secondary to inflammation of the diverticulum, intussusception with the diverticulum as the leading point, or extrinsic pressure from a distended diverticulum. Obstruction may be diagnosed by the use of the history, physical examination, and plain, supine, and upright films of the abdomen. More chronic, partial obstructions may be diagnosed by the instillation of small amounts of barium, with follow-up films delineating the point of obstruction. *Diverticular hemorrhage* is rare but may be massive and life-threatening with a mortality of 30 per cent in the 77 patients reported. Use of angiography and isotopic studies may be helpful in delineating the site of hemorrhage. Finally, *tumors*, most notably sarcomas and adenocarcinomas, have been reported as rare complications in patients with intestinal diverticula.

In patients with chronic symptoms, causes other than the intestinal diverticula must be sought. If none is found, symptomatic treatment of diarrhea and/or constipation may be initiated. The blind loop syndrome may be treated with oral antibiotics. Operative treatment is reserved for complications, and procedures may range from diverticulectomy to resection of a short segment of small intestine containing several diverticula. Care must be taken not to injure the vascular supply to the surrounding intestine while the mesentery is being dissected. If diverticulosis is widespread throughout the intestine, resection of only those diverticula suspected of being involved should be performed.

Meckel's Diverticulum

Meckel first described the diverticulum that bears his name in 1809, and it is the most frequently encountered congenital gastrointestinal tract anomaly with an autopsy incidence of 0.3 to 3 per cent. All layers of the intestine are found in the wall, making it a true diverticulum. It is usually located approximately 45 to 90 cm. proximal to the ileocecal valve on the antimesenteric border of the bowel. The average length of this wide-mouth diverticulum is approximately 5 cm., and a separate mesentery contains a terminal branch of the ileal artery to supply the diverticulum (Fig. 12). Meckel's diverticulum is the persistence of the omphalomesenteric duct, which in the embryo connects the yolk sac with the primitive midgut. The duct is normally obliterated by the seventh week of embryonic life. Other malformations that may be related to faulty obliteration of the duct are (1) umbilical-ileal fistula, (2) umbilical sinus, and (3) a residual fibrous band between the umbilicus and terminal ileum. Heterotopic tissue is present in over half of Meckel's diverticula. In most cases (85 per cent) this consists of gastric mucosa; however, duodenal mucosa, pancreas, and colonic mucosa have all been described.

The majority of patients with Meckel's diverticulum are asymptomatic. Complications occur in less than 5 per cent—most often in children under the age of 10 years.[6] The most commonly encountered complication, 50 per cent of the total, is intestinal hemorrhage. It is seen most often in children younger than 2 years of age and accounts for half of all lower gastrointestinal hemorrhage seen in the pediatric age group. The bleeding is painless in nature. It is usually the result of acid and pepsin secretion from heterotopic gastric mucosa in the diverticulum which causes peptic ulceration in the surrounding ileal mucosa.

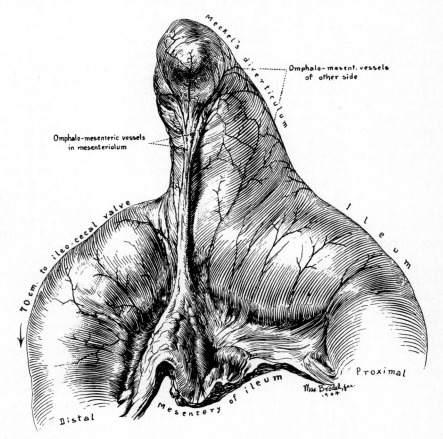

Figure 12. An anatomic example of Meckel's diverticulum. Note the separate blood supply. (From Kelly, H. A., and Huron, E.: The Vermiform Appendix and Its Diseases. Philadelphia, W. B. Saunders Company, 1905.)

Intestinal obstruction is the most common complication seen in adults and represents 25 per cent of the total complication rate. There are several mechanisms responsible for the obstruction, including volvulus of the intestine around a residual fibrous band connecting the diverticulum to the umbilicus, base of the mesentery, or adjacent bowel segment. The diverticulum may also act as a lead point for an ileoileal or ileocolonic intussusception. Such patients often present with classic "currant jelly" stools. Rarely, the diverticulum may incarcerate in an indirect inguinal hernia (Littré) and result in an intestinal obstruction.

Inflammation, which may lead to perforation, accounts for approximately 20 per cent of all complications associated with Meckel's diverticulum. The symptoms are often indistinguishable from those of appendicitis. Often a right lower quadrant incision is made, only to find a normal appendix. The small intestine should then be inspected carefully for the presence of a Meckel's diverticulum.

Radiographic techniques are the basis for diagnosis of the Meckel's diverticulum. In the patient with acute obstruction, a supine and upright plain film of the abdomen, along with a thorough history and physical examination, will often establish the diagnosis. Selective intestinal angiography or isotopic studies with radiolabeled red blood cells may be useful in the patient with an acute diverticular hemorrhage. In the less emergent patient, barium studies of the small intestine may demonstrate the diverticulum. Finally, technetium scanning of the abdomen may be able to highlight the heterotopic gastric mucosa in a diverticulum. Although reports of this last technique are promising, false-positive and false-negative rates limit its usefulness.

Operative treatment of Meckel's diverticulum is indicated only for the complications listed above. Simple wedge resection with oversewing of the defect in the intestinal wall can be performed in patients with simple diverticulitis or obstruction without strangulation. Resection of a segment of small intestine with end-to-end anastomosis to reestablish continuity is more appropriate when an associated ileal ulcer is present. This allows removal of the ulcer and ensures that hemorrhage will not continue in the postoperative period. The operative mortality for resection of Meckel's diverticulum, since most are done under emergent conditions, is 5 to 10 per cent. Finally, incidental removal of an asymptomatic Meckel's diverticulum during an unrelated operative procedure has previously been recommended. However, this practice has been questioned by studies demonstrating that, in the adult population, the morbidity subsequent to diverticulectomy outweighs the risk of diverticular complications. The issue remains controversial.

RADIATION INJURY OF THE SMALL INTESTINE

Ionizing radiation, when directed at living tissue, causes an energy transfer to the cells of that tissue. Excitation and ionization of the intracellular molecules occur and result in a varying degree of damage, which may or may not be irreversible, particularly in the molecular structure of the DNA molecule within the cellular nucleus. This area is especially sensitive and, if affected, can cause mitotic arrest. This characteristic of radiation can be useful when directed against tumors that are especially susceptible because of their high cell turnover or mitotic rate. Although the utility of radiotherapy in treating malignant abdominal neoplasms is great, untoward effects may ensue upon normal tissues and organs. Because the small intestine fills the abdominal cavity and contains a layer (the mucosa) that possesses a high mitotic rate, it is therefore susceptible to radiation injury.

Therapeutic radiation, whether delivered by an external beam or an implanted source, may exert deleterious effects upon the small bowel, causing either acute or chronic injury.[7] Acute injury is proximate to the time of the radiation, localized, and time-limited. It is due to direct mucosal cellular injury and affects mostly the cells of the regenerative zones in the crypts of Lieberkühn. Normally, the villous cells arise from these zones and migrate over a period of 4 to 6 days to the villous tips before they are exfoliated. Radiation causes a decrease in the number of mitoses in the regenerative zone cells as well as frank necrosis, both there and in the cells of the intestinal villus itself, and sloughing of the mucosa may follow. Ultimately, there is a decrease in villous height as well. Symptoms related to such injury include nausea, vomiting, and diarrhea with or without signs of gastrointestinal hemorrhage. Supportive treatment is usually sufficient, and symptoms generally subside within days to a week. Acute radiation injury most often does not result in chronic problems later.

Late injury to the small intestine secondary to radiation is probably due to the effect of such radiation on both the connective tissue and the microvasculature of the intestinal wall. The result is an increased collagen deposition and an aggressive fibrosis seen first in the submucosa. Severe vasculitis characterized by medial widening and endothelial proliferation is also present. Progression of both of these processes is ongoing and inexorable. Eventually, they may lead to a decrease in the blood supply and, therefore, the availability of nutrients and oxygen, to the bowel wall. Necrosis with perforation and abscess formation or fistulization may occur. Alternatively, the mucosa may ulcerate, causing gastrointestinal hemorrhage. Also, a significantly large mucosal area may become compromised so that malabsorption becomes evident. Finally, the aggressive scarring in the bowel wall may lead to luminal narrowing and partial to total intestinal obstruction.

Diagnosis of late radiation injury to the intestine depends on which of the complications has occurred. However, physical examination, a history of therapeutic radiation to the abdomen or pelvis, as well as the judicious use of diagnostic radiologic modalities should suffice to confirm the diagnosis. Involuntary guarding and rebound tenderness may warn of peritonitis secondary to a free perforation. Spiking fever along with an abdominal mass may signal abscess formation. Finally, crampy abdominal pain coupled with the auscultatory finding of episodic high-pitched bowel sounds in the abdomen will yield the diagnosis of intestinal obstruction. Flat and upright plain films of the abdomen, small intestinal contrast studies, and CT abdominal scanning may confirm the diagnoses of obstruction, fistula formation, or abscess, respectively.

Operative treatment for the late intestinal sequelae of radiation therapy is reserved for the complications just listed.[7, 15] Stabilization is achieved by infusions of crystalloid, colloid, or blood products as needed as well as by administration of antibiotics. At operation, the affected bowel may appear thickened, firm, and grayish-white in color. In advanced cases, the intestinal contents may be tightly adherent, forming a firm mass. Ideally, the segment of bowel associated with fistula, perforation, or hemorrhage should be resected and bowel continuity should be reestablished with end-to-end anastomosis of segments unaffected by radiation. In addition, all abscesses should be drained and irrigated. However, such therapy may not always be possible because of the extent of bowel affected by the radiation injury. Thus, if an attempt is made to resect all affected bowel or to dissect the tightly adherent intestinal loops, either a short bowel syndrome or multiple intestinal fistulas will result. In such cases, minimal resections and bypass procedures may be reasonable alternatives.

INTESTINAL BYPASS PROCEDURES

Intestinal bypass, specifically designed to control morbid obesity, was first performed by Varco in 1953. Animal studies documenting the utility of the procedure were done a year later by Kremen. It was Payne who in 1956 initiated the first study of intestinal bypass for morbid obesity in a group of patients specifically selected. It was found that elimination of all but 44 cm. of small intestine (40 cm. of proximal jejunum and 4 cm. of distal ileum) resulted in an appropriate loss of weight. Although greater than three fourths of patients have demonstrated significant weight reduction in several clinical studies since that time, the development of severe complications has led to the gradual abandonment of this procedure. Liver disorders, including cirrhosis and hepatic failure, sometimes leading to death, have occurred in 5 per cent of patients. In addition, diarrhea with malabsorption of fats, proteins, and vitamins as well as severe electrolyte imbalances have occurred rather often. Hair loss, hyperoxaluria with calcium oxalate urinary lithiasis, and polyarthritis are also common complications. As a result, most procedures for morbid obesity are now centered on the stomach (gastric bypass and gastroplasty) and are discussed in Chapter 23.

A modification of the intestinal bypass devised by Varco and Buchwald is still used for treatment of patients with congenital or acquired hypercholesterolemia.[3] Cholesterol has been noted to be one of the risk factors associated with coronary artery disease and it is thought that if serum levels of cholesterol can be lowered, the risk of acquired heart disease will be lessened. Medical trials to attain this goal have centered on manipulation of diet along with the addition of cholesterol-lowering drugs such as cholestyramine, clofibrate, and nicotinic acid. At most, they have resulted in a 12 to 15 per cent decrease in the level of serum cholesterol and have not shown a major effect on the incidence or progression of coronary artery disease. The primary difficulties in these studies is patient compliance with the tedious and sometimes unpleasant drug and dietary regimens. A surgical procedure to achieve the same goal theoretically places the patient in a situation of certain compliance.

According to Buchwald's criteria, eligibility for the ileal bypass operation to control hypercholesterolemia is stringent. Criteria include any adult younger than 60 years of age with a serum cholesterol level of greater than 200 mg. per 100 ml. or two standard deviations greater than normal (age corrected) and with either documented atherosclerotic cardiovascular disease or a strong family history of that disorder. In addition, any child older than 6 years of age is eligible if a history of familial hypercholesterolemia along with a serum cholesterol level of greater than two standard deviations over normal is present.

At operation, the intestine is divided, 40 cm. distal to the ligament of Treitz and 4 cm. proximal to the ileocecal valve. The proximal jejunum is then anastomosed to the remaining distal ileum. The proximal end of the excluded segment is oversewn and tacked to the mesentery, leaving it as a blind pouch. The distal end is anastomosed to the cecum approximately 10 cm. above the stump of the amputated appendix (Fig. 13).

The mechanisms by which this procedure acts are based on the fact that bile acids are an end product of cholesterol metabolism. With removal of the terminal ileum, the area in which bile acids are reabsorbed into the enterohepatic circulation, there is a fourfold increase in fecal bile acid loss. This produces an obligatory diversion of cholesterol by the liver into bile acid synthesis in an attempt to maintain the size of the bile acid pool. In addition, with a decrease in the total amount of bile acids, ingested cholesterol is unable to undergo micellarization in the intestinal lumen. This results in a 60 per cent decrease in the jejunal absorption of ingested cholesterol. Such losses are partially negated by an increase (six times) in hepatic cholesterol synthesis.

Even though the several sequelae following ileal bypass may have opposing effects on the metabolism of cholesterol, the overall summation of changes yields a decrease in serum concentration. The attenuation has averaged 40 per cent in several different clinical series and has remained depressed for up to 18 years of patient follow-up. The procedure has been found to be most effective in patients with Frederickson's hyperlipidemia classification Type II heterozygotes, in whom a greater than 50 per cent decrease in serum cholesterol has been documented. Least affected by the procedure (with a 10 to 15 per cent decrease) are patients with Frederickson's Type II homozygotes. Those with Frederickson's Types III and IV hyperlipidemias also benefit. Postoperatively, clinical improvement in angina has been noted in up to two thirds of affected patients. Also, less

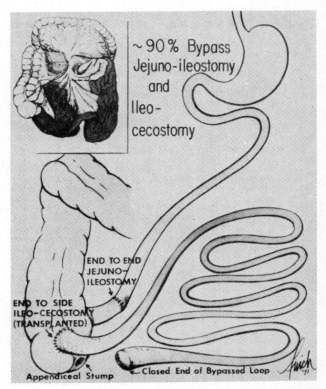

Figure 13. The jejunoileal bypass operation with all but proximal 40 cm. of jejunum and terminal 4 cm. of ileum bypassed. Bowel continuity restored by end-to-end anastomosis, with drainage of bypassed bowel, end-to-side, to cecum. (From Austen, W. G., Scott, H. W., Jr., Fonkalsrud, E. W., and Polk, H. C., Jr.: Current Problems in Surgery, April 1975. Chicago, Year Book Medical Publishers, Inc., 1975.)

progression of coronary artery atherosclerotic changes has been seen in operated patients compared with those not subjected to the procedure. A decrease in the size of or disappearance of xanthomas and xanthelasma has been described by several investigators.

The ileal bypass for hypercholesterolemia seems to have few of the side effects described after jejunoileal bypass for morbid obesity. Weight loss and its associated nutrient malabsorption and electrolyte deficiencies are not seen. Similarly, hepatic decompensation does not occur, but the majority of patients have diarrhea postoperatively. However, within a year, tolerable levels of stool frequency have returned in 90 per cent without the use of medication. Vitamin B_{12} deficiency, with its associated megaloblastic anemia, has been noted after ileal bypass, and it is recommended that parenteral vitamin B_{12} supplementation be given.

VASCULAR LESIONS

There are a number of vascular lesions involving the small intestine, some of which are emergent in nature. These are covered in Chapter 41 (The Arterial System).

Selected References

American Physiology Society: In Code, C. F. (Ed.): Handbook of Physiology, Section 6, Alimentary Canal. Baltimore, Williams & Wilkins Company, 1967–1968.
This five-volume, multiauthored work remains the single most inclusive compendium concerning the various aspects of gastrointestinal physiology. Subjects including digestion, absorption, and motility are exhaustively covered. The references are complete and critically selected.

Herbsman, H., Wetstein, L., Rosen, Y., Orces, H., Alfonso, A. E., Iyer, S. K., and Goodwin, B.: Tumors of the small intestine. *In* Ravitch, M. M. (Ed.): Current Problems in Surgery. Year Book Medical Publishers, Inc., Chicago, 1980, pp. 122–184.
The authors combine their experience at a major teaching institution with that of others in a comprehensive review covering the incidence, presentation, diagnosis, and treatment of both benign and malignant neoplasms of the small intestine.

Losowsky, M. S., Walker, B. E., and Kelleher, J.: Malabsorption in clinical practice. London, Churchill Livingstone, 1974.
This review details the pathophysiology, as well as patient symptomatology and treatment, of most of the malabsorption disorders. The data are presented in a clear, concise manner, and many valuable references are included.

Miller, L. D., Mackie, J. A., and Rhoads, J. E.: The pathophysiology and management of intestinal obstruction. Surg. Clin. North Am., *42*:1285, 1962.
This monograph is directed to the clinical causes of intestinal obstruction. It leads the reader through the pathophysiologic changes produced by obstruction and details the management necessary for their amelioration.

Singleton, J. W.: National Cooperative Crohn's Disease Study. Gastroenterology, *77*:825, 1979.
This issue of Gastroenterology *is devoted entirely to the results of the National Cooperative Crohn's Disease Study. This study has yielded the most current data concerning such topics as presentation of disease and extraintestinal manifestations. Additionally, results of both drug and surgical therapy are detailed.*

REFERENCES

1. American Physiology Society: *In* Code, C. F. (Ed.): Handbook of Physiology, Section 6, Alimentary Canal. Baltimore, Williams & Wilkins Company, 1967–1968.
2. Becker, J. M., Duff, W. M., and Moody, F. G.: Myoelectric control of gastrointestinal and biliary motility: A review. Surgery, *89*:466, 1981.
3. Buchwald, H., Varco, R. L., Moore, R. B., and Schwartz, M. Z.: Intestinal bypass procedures. *In* Current Problems in Surgery. Chicago, Year Book Medical Publishers, Inc., 1975, pp. 1–51.
4. Chiotasso, P. J. P., and Fazio, V. W.: Prognostic factors of 28 leiomyosarcomas of the small intestine. Surg. Gynecol. Obstet., *155*:197, 1982.
5. Davenport, H. W.: Physiology of the Digestive Tract, 2nd ed. Chicago, Year Book Medical Publishers, 1966.
6. DeBartolo, H. M., Jr., and van Heerden, J. A.: Meckel's diverticulum. Ann. Surg., *183*:30, 1976.
7. DeCosse, J. J., Rhodes, R. S., Wentz, W. B., Reagen, J. W., Dworken, H. J., and Holden, W. D.: The natural history and management of radiation induced injury to the gastrointestinal tract. Ann. Surg., *170*:369, 1970.
8. Eggert, A., Teichmann, W., and Wittmann, D. H.: The pathological implication of duodenal diverticula. Surg. Gynecol. Obstet., *154*:62, 1982.
9. Godwin, J. D.: Carcinoid tumors: An analysis of 2,837 cases. Cancer, *36*:560, 1975.
10. Gray, H: Anatomy of the Human Body, 28th ed. *In* Goss, C. M. (Ed.): Philadelphia, Lea & Febiger, 1966.
11. Hartwell, J. A., and Hoguet, J. P.: Experimental intestinal obstruction in dogs with especial reference to the cause of death and the treatment by large amounts of normal saline solution. J.A.M.A., *59*:82, 1912.
12. Herbsman, H., Wetstein, L., Rosen, Y., Orces, H., Alfonso, A. E., Iyer, S. K., and Goodwin, B.: Tumors of the small intestine. *In* Ravitch, M. M. (Ed.): Current Problems in Surgery. Year Book Medical Publishers, Inc., Chicago, 1980, pp. 122–184.
13. Kerlin, P., Zinsmeister, A., and Phillips, S.: Relationship of motility to flow of contents in the human small intestine. Gastroenterology, *82*:701, 1982.
14. Kyle, J.: Crohn's Disease. New York, Appleton-Century-Crofts, 1972.
15. Lillemoe, K. D., Brigham, R. A., Harmon, J. T., Feaster, M. M., Saunders, J. R., and d'Avis, J. A.: Surgical management of small-bowel radiation enteritis. Arch. Surg., *118*:905, 1983.
16. Losowsky, M. S., Walker, B. E., and Kelleher, J.: Malabsorption in Clinical Practice. London, Churchill Livingstone, 1974.
17. Miller, L. D., Mackie, J. A., and Rhoads, J. E.: The pathophysiology and management of intestinal obstruction. Surg. Clin. North Am., *42*:1285, 1962.
18. Morson, B. C., and Dawson, I. M. P.: Gastrointestinal Pathology. Oxford, Blackwell Scientific Publications, Ltd., 1972.
19. Pearse, A. G. E., Polak, J. M., and Bloom, S. R.: The newer gut hormones: Cellular sources, physiology, pathology, and clinical aspects. Gastroenterology, *72*:746, 1977.
20. Prior, P., Gyde, S., Cooke, W. T., Waterhouse, J. A. H., and Allan, R. N.: Mortality in Crohn's disease. Gastroenterology, *80*:307, 1981.
21. Singleton, J. W.: National Cooperative Crohn's Disease Study. Gastroenterology, *77*:825, 1979.
22. Skudder, P. A., and Schwartz, S. I.: Primary lymphoma of the gastrointestinal tract. Surg. Gynecol. Obstet., *160*:5, 1985.
23. Wangensteen, O. H.: Historical aspects of the management of acute intestinal obstruction. Surgery *65*:363, 1969.
24. Williams, R. A., Davidson, D. D., Serota, A. I., and Wilson, S. E.: Surgical problems of diverticula of the small intestine. Surg. Gynecol. Obstet., *152*:621, 1981.
25. Wood, J. D., and Perkins, W. E.: Mechanical interaction between longitudinal and circular axes of the small intestine. Am. J. Physiol., *218*:762, 1970.

SURGICAL DISORDERS OF THE VERMIFORM APPENDIX AND MECKEL'S DIVERTICULUM

DONALD C. McILRATH, M.D.

25

THE APPENDIX

Anatomy and Embryology

The teniae of the cecum, one anterior, one postero-medial, and one posterolateral, originate at the embryologic end of the cecum, which is also the base of the appendix, but which in the adult is often not the lowest part of the cecum. In the fetus the cecum has essentially a conical form, with the appendix representing the apex of the cone. Because the portion of cecum lying between the anterior and posterolateral teniae grows out of proportion to the other segments of the cecum, the original end of the cecum and the attached base of the appendix are carried behind and to the left, with the appendix therefore opening into the posteromedial aspect of the cecum. Because of this the appendix is almost always retrocecal in part,[18] but the term is used to describe an appendix that is turned up behind the cecum and, usually, the ascending colon. Clinically, it usually means one that is fixed in this position, a location that is noted in about 25 per cent of cases. From the fixed base on the posteromedial side of the cecum approximately 2.5 cm. below the ileocecal valve, the appendix may extend in other directions and may be freely movable and hence vary in position with the movements of the intestinal tract. In approximately 50 to 60 per cent of cases it extends to, or over, the pelvic brim. When there is incomplete rotation of the colon, the appendix may be located anywhere within the abdominal cavity.

There is usually a peritoneal fold enclosing the artery to the appendix (mesoappendix) that is attached to the left or posterior side of the mesentery of the terminal ileum, to the cecum, and, for a variable length, to the appendix itself. The appendix is commonly 6 to 10 cm. in length in adults, although ones up to 20 cm. long do occur. Appendicular agenesis is rare and is sometimes associated with cecal hypoplasia. Double appendix and congenital diverticula are very rare, but may be the site of acute inflammation.

The lumen of the appendix is lined by columnar epithelium of colonic type. Lymphoid follicles are present in the submucosa at birth and gradually increase in number to approximately 200 follicles by puberty. Thereafter, there

is progressive reduction in lymphoid tissue until it disappears in the fifth or sixth decade of life. There are two muscular layers in the wall of the appendix. The inner layer (circular) is a continuation of the same muscle of the cecum. The outer layer (longitudinal) is from the coalescence of the three teniae of the cecum. Circular and longitudinal muscle layers are often deficient in some areas, allowing continuity of submucosa and serosa—a fact of importance in acute appendicitis.

Once considered a vestigial structure, the appendix, specifically its submucosal lymphoid follicles, now is considered to play a role in developing and maintaining the immune capability of the host. The precise role of the appendix in this regard remains to be determined.

Pathophysiology

Reginald H. Fitz[3] of Boston presented the classic paper in 1886 entitled "Perforating Inflammation of the Vermiform Appendix with Special Reference to its Early Diagnosis and Treatment." Earlier, the cecum was thought to be the origin of the inflammatory process in the area, and the disorder was called typhlitis or perityphlitis. Fitz considered the cause of acute appendicitis to be due to fecal masses and foreign bodies. This classic concept of etiology—obstruction of the lumen of the appendix and subsequent bacterial inflammation—explains the origin of 70 per cent of cases. Approximately 60 per cent of these are related to hyperplasia of submucosal lymphoid follicles in children, 35 per cent to the presence of a fecolith (particularly in adults), and 5 per cent to foreign bodies or tumors. Etiologic factors postulated to explain appendicitis in the absence of intraluminal obstruction include external compression of the appendix by bands and high intraluminal pressure in the cecum.

Of clinical importance are the different stages of appendicitis. Acute focal appendicitis denotes the early phase of the inflammatory process that is contained within the lumen of the appendix and causes edema in the wall. Acute suppurative appendicitis develops later when bacteria proliferate, form pus in the lumen, and invade the wall of the appendix. As appendicitis progresses further, the blood

461

supply is impaired by bacterial infection in the wall and distention of the lumen by secretion of mucus and formation of pus. This diminution in blood supply results in gangrene of the appendix and the complications of periappendicitis or perforation with localized abscess or generalized peritonitis. The time required for the development of suppurative or gangrenous appendicitis and associated complications is variable, but it may be less than 8 to 12 hours.

The Clinical Problem

Acute appendicitis occurs in approximately 7 per cent of individuals in Western countries and is the most common cause of an acute abdomen requiring surgical intervention. About 200,000 appendectomies are performed annually in the United States. Mortality varies from less than 0.1 per cent in uncomplicated cases to approximately 5 per cent in cases with perforation. The latter figure was five times greater just 25 years ago, so considerable progress has been made in reducing the risk associated with complicated appendicitis. This favorable trend has resulted from improvements in all aspects of preoperative, operative, and postoperative care.

The dominant risk factor that persists today is revealed by the marked difference between 0.1 per cent mortality and 5 per cent mortality associated with uncomplicated and complicated appendicitis, respectively. The obvious challenge in the management of patients with acute appendicitis is to remove the appendix early in the course of the disease.

Recognition of Appendicitis

SYMPTOMS

The classic clinical presentation of acute appendicitis consists of a prodromal phase of diffuse, vague periumbilical pain or discomfort, anorexia, slight nausea, and occasional vomiting. This visceral-type pain, caused by increased pressure in the lumen of the appendix, usually is persistent and continuous, but not severe, and the patient often considers the problem to be "indigestion." After a variable period of time, usually a few hours, the pain shifts to the right lower quadrant of the abdomen (McBurney's point) and becomes more distinct and sharp in character. Typically, this somatic pain caused by contact of the inflamed appendix with the nerve endings in the peritoneum becomes localized and is accentuated by movement or acts such as coughing or sneezing. The patient often prefers to remain motionless in a fetal-type position.

This typical clinical presentation, including the symptoms of both the visceral, or prodromal, phase and the subsequent somatic phase, occurs in approximately 50 per cent of patients who have acute appendicitis.

Recognition of the possibility of acute appendicitis is more difficult when this classic visceral-somatic sequence is altered in any way. Many factors may influence the symptom complex, particularly the location of the appendix, the age and health status of the patient, and the pathologic state of the appendix at the time of examination. The many different combinations or interactions of these basic factors account for the numerous atypical clinical presentations of acute appendicitis and associated complications.

In some patients, the prodromal phase may be minimal or absent and onset of appendicitis is heralded by pain localized in the right lower quadrant of the abdomen.

Conversely, the pain may never become localized and may remain diffuse throughout the preoperative period.

Different possible locations of the inflamed appendix account for some variations in the symptom complex. An example is retrocecal appendicitis, which typically causes pain in the flank with a minimal or absent abdominal component. A long, inflamed appendix that extends into the pelvis may simulate gynecologic or urinary tract pathologies because the symptoms primarily are pelvic in location.

The age of the patient with acute appendicitis may influence the history. Infants and young children are hampered by their inability to verbalize their complaints. Senile patients are limited in a similar way, but even mentally alert elderly patients often do not experience typical symptoms.

Some patients complain of feeling constipated and often take a laxative or an enema. Such measures typically provide no relief. In contrast, the abnormality of bowel function may be diarrhea that suggests gastroenteritis.

Because acute appendicitis is the most common acute surgical condition in the abdomen, the astute physician always entertains the possibility of this entity in the differential diagnosis of acute abdomen. Absence of part of the classic clinical presentation or the presence of bizarre or atypical symptoms does not lessen the possibility of acute appendicitis. Such variations in the symptom complex occur in approximately 50 per cent of patients with acute appendicitis.

PHYSICAL EXAMINATION

The patient with acute appendicitis usually is found lying quietly in bed and gives the general appearance of not feeling well. The ease or difficulty with which movement to the supine position is accomplished may offer the first clue about the presence or absence of peritoneal irritation.

Before abdominal examination is begun, the patient should be asked to point to the area of pain and to demonstrate the amount of finger pressure necessary to produce or aggravate the discomfort. The result of this simple maneuver frequently provides unequivocal evidence of localized peritoneal irritation.

Physical examination of the abdomen always should be performed gently in order to gain the patient's confidence and to allow detection of subtle peritoneal signs. Light palpation of the abdomen from the left side to the right side allows the examiner to appreciate mild involuntary muscle guarding or rigidity. Such gentle palpation does not exacerbate pain in the area of maximal tenderness and does not make the patient apprehensive or resistant to further meaningful examination.

The primary objective of abdominal palpation is to determine whether or not the patient has any peritoneal irritation. The signs of peritoneal irritation are localized tenderness, typically in the right lower quadrant; any degree of muscular guarding or rigidity; and rebound tenderness. The latter is considered to be the most significant peritoneal sign by some physicians, but it is no more meaningful than the other signs in indicating irritation of the anterior parietal peritoneum by an inflamed appendix.

There are a variety of reasons why palpation of the abdomen may not elicit peritoneal signs. Interposition of omentum between the appendix and the peritoneum may account for absence of physical signs. A negative abdominal examination more commonly is due to the fact that the location of the appendix precludes contact with the peritoneum, even when palpation is performed with greater pressure.

When the inflamed appendix is situated in the pelvis, tenderness can be detected by rectal and pelvic examinations. With retrocecal or retroileal appendicitis, the pain may be localized poorly and tenderness absent on abdominal, rectal, or pelvic examination. Tenderness or aggravation of discomfort is found only by palpation or percussion of the right flank or costovertebral angle of the back.

While searching for an area of localized tenderness, one must remember that pathologic conditions other than acute appendicitis may be responsible for the peritoneal sign. Because the other possible causes are numerous, it is helpful to group them into anatomic subdivisions. For example, tenderness in the right lower quadrant of the abdomen suggests an acute pathologic process in the ileum, cecum, or ascending or sigmoid colon as well as in the appendix. When signs are predominantly pelvic in location, major diagnostic considerations include acute conditions of the uterus and adnexa.

Many other acute intra-abdominal or even systemic conditions may mimic acute appendicitis, and sometimes it is not possible to make a specific diagnosis. In such instances the demonstration of localized intra-abdominal tenderness may be the major factor that influences the decision about whether or not surgical therapy is indicated.

Very minimal or absent physical findings in a symptomatic patient suggest the need for careful observation and frequent re-examination. In some cases, significant signs will not become detectable until the third or fourth examination is performed.

LABORATORY TESTS

Laboratory tests for acute appendicitis are nonspecific, and therefore the results cannot be used to either confirm or deny the diagnosis. The value of leukocyte count results from the fact that approximately 90 per cent of patients with acute appendicitis have a leukocytosis greater than 10,000 per microliter, and most also have a shift to the left in the differential count.[2] Consequently, the finding of moderate leukocytosis with an increase in granulocytes is consistent with the diagnosis of acute appendicitis. Undue emphasis on abnormalities of the leukocyte count should be avoided because approximately 5 per cent of patients with acute appendicitis have normal differential and total white blood cell counts.

Most patients with acute appendicitis have less than 30 cells (either white or red) per high-powered field on examination of the urine. A greater number of cells suggests the possibility of primary urologic problems and the need for more specific studies of the urinary tract. An acutely inflamed appendix near or in contact with the ureter may produce a modest increase in these cell counts.

ROENTGENOGRAPHIC FINDINGS

Most cases of acute appendicitis are diagnosed without benefit of the demonstration of radiologic abnormalities. A plain film of the abdomen usually is obtained and may show findings suggestive of acute appendicitis or some other pathologic condition.

The roentgenologic abnormalities suggestive of early acute appendicitis are mild ileus or an appendicolithiasis. As the inflammatory process progresses and complications develop, the plain film may show a soft tissue density in the right lower quadrant, an abnormal right psoas shadow, gas in the lumen of the appendix, and more pronounced ileus.

Some radiologic abnormalities seen on flat films are helpful in evaluating pathologic conditions that mimic acute appendicitis. An example is free intraperitoneal air that documents perforation of a hollow viscus such as the duodenum or colon. Free air is encountered rarely with perforation of the appendix. Other abnormalities evident on flat films are radiopaque stones, foreign bodies, and air-fluid levels in the bowel that are indicative of intestinal obstruction.

For many years barium enema was considered an inappropriate examination for the patient suspected of having acute appendicitis. Conventional teaching emphasized the potential hazard of extrusion of barium into the peritoneal cavity, particularly in the presence of infection. This concern still seems appropriate in cases with free perforation of the appendix. Some reports[8, 15] about the benefit of barium enema have included remarkably few complications. The diagnosis of appendicitis is supported by failure to opacify the appendix, and it is excluded if the organ is opacified. Advocates of barium enema emphasize that the benefits of the examination are greater accuracy in diagnosis, reduction in the number of unnecessary operations, and demonstration of pathologic conditions other than appendicitis. Barium enema examination obviously is unnecessary in most cases of acute appendicitis and perhaps should be reserved for the more complex cases, particularly those in which the risk of operation would be excessive.

Acute Appendicitis in Infants and Elderly Patients

Diagnosis of acute appendicitis in infants, young children, and the elderly often is very difficult. In the early stage of the disease, infants manifest only lethargy, irritability, and anorexia—nonspecific features that fail to alarm parents about a potentially lethal intra-abdominal problem. Unfortunately, the inflammatory process progresses rapidly to serious complications against which the infant's underdeveloped omentum offers minimal defense. In a later stage of appendicitis, the infants may become obviously ill, with vomiting, fever, dehydration, and abdominal distention. The incidence of perforation of acute appendicitis is 90 to 100 per cent in infants and approximately 50 per cent up to age 5.[7, 13] These statistics emphasize the major problem of acute appendicitis in young patients—undue delay between onset of symptoms and surgical treatment.

Early recognition of acute appendicitis in older patients is sometimes difficult because their symptoms often are mild and the physical signs, fever, and leukocytosis are minimal or absent. This paucity of findings in the early stages unfortunately is misleading and causes undue delay in providing appropriate treatment. At least 30 per cent of elderly patients have a ruptured appendix at operation.

It is apparent that further progress in reducing morbidity and mortality associated with acute appendicitis must be made in the management of patients in the younger and older age groups.

Acute Appendicitis and Pregnancy

Appendicitis during pregnancy presents a diagnostic challenge,[5] particularly during the last trimester. One reason is that the enlarging uterus displaces the appendix out of its normal location, usually toward the right upper quadrant. Consequently, localized tenderness is found laterally in the right flank above the umbilicus. The classic findings of anorexia, fever, pain, and leukocytosis are usually present in all three trimesters. Acute cholecystitis and pyelonephritis, common during pregnancy, are major considerations in the differential diagnosis. The rate or occurrence of acute appendicitis is constant throughout the three trimesters of pregnancy and is similar to that in nonpregnant women in the same age groups.

Delay in operation carries serious consequences for both the mother and the fetus, particularly during the late stage of pregnancy, when perforation and peritonitis increase both maternal and fetal mortality. In all trimesters of pregnancy, appendectomy should be performed upon suspicion of the presence of appendicitis.

Perforation of the Appendix—Localized and Diffuse

Patients with perforated appendicitis usually appear toxically ill as a result of dehydration, hyperpyrexia, tachycardia, or even hypotension. Pain is usually severe and is either localized or diffuse, depending on whether the underlying pathology is an abscess or generalized peritonitis from free perforation. A tender mass in the right lower quadrant or pelvis is the significant physical finding in patients with localized perforation. Diffuse abdominal tenderness, distention, hypoactive bowel sounds, and significant muscle guarding and rigidity are physical hallmarks of diffuse peritonitis. Either complication tends to produce marked leukocytosis and a significant shift to the left in the differential count.

Differential Diagnosis

Abdominal pain and other symptoms that mimic acute appendicitis may be caused by numerous pathologic disorders, particularly those involving the gastrointestinal and genitourinary tracts and the gynecologic organs.

The conditions that are most commonly confused with appendicitis are gastroenteritis in adults and mesenteric lymphadenitis in children and young adults. With gastroenteritis, nausea, vomiting, and excessive diarrhea are prominent features, and they characteristically precede the onset of pain, which typically is less well defined or more cramping in character than is the pain noted with appendicitis. The patient's history may reveal that a similar illness is affecting other members of the household, but such a story may be misleading. In most cases, leukocytosis and fever are minimal unless the problem is enterocolitis caused by a specific pathogen such as *Salmonella*.

Other gastrointestinal conditions that may be confused with acute appendicitis are perforated peptic ulcer, colonic diverticulitis, intestinal obstruction, perforated carcinoma of the colon, Meckel's diverticulitis, and regional enteritis. Age of the patient helps reduce the possibilities because diverticulitis and carcinoma of the large intestine are rarely seen in younger patients. Demonstration of free intraabdominal air on upright film of the abdomen is common with perforation of the stomach, duodenum, and colon, but this rarely occurs with ruptured appendicitis. Distinguishing Meckel's diverticulitis from acute appendicitis may be impossible, but failure to do so is not critical because surgical management of the two conditions is similar.

Many gynecologic abnormalities simulate acute appendicitis, particularly when it is located in the pelvis. Ruptured ovarian follicle (mittelschmerz), torsion of an ovarian neoplasm, ruptured ovarian cyst, ectopic pregnancy, and pelvic inflammatory disease, specifically salpingitis with tubo-ovarian abscess, must be considered in the differential diagnosis of right lower quadrant pain in a woman. The relationship of the onset of symptoms to the menstrual period and the character of the pain may be helpful in differentiating one of these pelvic disorders from acute appendicitis. Rupture of an ovarian follicle, cyst, or tubal pregnancy and torsion of ovarian tumor tend to produce sudden onset of pain without a prodromal phase. The patient with mittelschmerz typically does not appear ill, and her pain usually has diminished by the time examination is performed. Twisted ovarian tumors and tubal pregnancies commonly are detected on pelvic examination or documented by ultrasonography. Some patients with ruptured ectopic pregnancy will show signs of hypovolemic shock.

Typically, salpingitis occurs during or just after a menstrual period, mittelschmerz during mid cycle, and ectopic pregnancy after 6 to 8 weeks of amenorrhea with recent vaginal spotting. Pelvic inflammatory disease usually causes high fever and chills, features that are seen quite late in the course of appendicitis. Vaginal discharge and exquisite tenderness on movement of the cervix are prominent signs with salpingitis.

Ureteral or renal calculi rarely are confused with appendiceal disease because the unilateral, colicky back pain that radiates into the groin is difficult to misinterpret. A stone can be demonstrated by plain film of the abdomen or intravenous urogram. Acute pyelonephritis may simulate retrocecal appendicitis because costovertebral angle tenderness may be found with either condition. Chills and high fever are common with pyelonephritis, and pyuria is invariably found.

Preoperative Management

Pain medication and antibiotics should be withheld during the initial phase of evaluation of a patient suspected of having acute appendicitis. Such practice permits more accurate assessment of the patient and avoids possible suppression of clinical symptoms and signs. The interval from admission to operation should be used not only for repeating the physical examination at frequent intervals but also for assessing the status of the patient's general health and the possible coexistence of other diseases, particularly diabetes and cardiac or pulmonary problems in the elderly.

Patients who have gangrenous or perforated appendicitis often are quite ill from sepsis, dehydration, and hyperpyrexia. In such cases, correction of fluid and electrolyte balance and reduction of high fever must be accomplished before anesthesia is considered. Preoperative treatment with nasogastric decompression, intravenous solutions, salicylates, or a cooling blanket usually is effective in less than 2 or 3 hours. Broad-spectrum antibiotics should be started intravenously in large doses to ensure maximal effect preoperatively.

Surgical Treatment

ACUTE APPENDICITIS

Acute appendicitis and associated complications are surgical problems. Exceptions to this general statement are patients who have (1) minimal symptoms or signs that subside rather quickly, (2) coexisting problems of a magnitude that make the risk of operation greater than the risk of observation, or (3) subacute abscess and subsiding symptoms and signs.

Some adult patients with the last complication may be managed expectantly in the hope that the clinical course will continue to improve and the mass will resolve. When this occurs, appendectomy is deferred for several weeks (interval appendectomy). Failure of the problem to resolve or, certainly, re-exacerbation of symptoms demands surgical intervention.

When the preoperative diagnosis is acute appendicitis and tenderness is well localized in the right lower quadrant of the abdomen, either a small transverse or oblique incision provides adequate exposure for appendectomy in most cases (Fig. 1A). The transverse incision (Rockey-Davis) is made 5 to 7 cm. in length in the direction of Langer's lines at about the level of the anterosuperior iliac spine, or 1 to 3 cm. below the umbilicus, and is centered on the midclavicular–mid-iliac line. The external oblique, internal oblique, and transversus abdominis muscles are incised and spread in the direction of their fibers, and the transversalis fascia and peritoneum are divided transversely. The oblique incision (McBurney) is made with one third above and two thirds below a point in a line one third the distance from the iliac crest to the umbilicus.

It is the author's opinion that the transverse incision provides a better cosmetic result, can be enlarged more easily by dividing the anterior rectus sheath, and permits better exposure of a retrocecal appendix. When one is uncertain about the diagnosis of acute appendicitis and anticipates the need for better exposure and more thorough abdominal exploration, a lower midline or right paramedian incision should be made initially.

Gentle palpation of the cecum usually confirms the presence or absence of appendiceal pathology and whether or not localized perforation has occurred. Probing with the index finger will determine the location of the appendix and the ease with which it can be mobilized. When the appendix is in a fixed retrocecal position, the lower part of the ascending colon and cecum must be mobilized in order to reach the appendix. This is done by incising the peritoneum lateral to the colon and reflecting the colon medially and anteriorly.

If exploration reveals no evidence of appendiceal inflammation, a careful search must be made to find an explanation of the signs and symptoms for which operation was performed. Although exploration through a small transverse or oblique type of incision in the right lower quadrant of the abdomen is limited, it usually is possible to examine the cecum, proximal ascending colon, distant

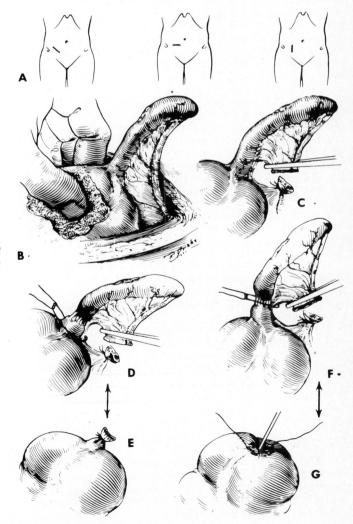

Figure 1. Technique of appendectomy. A, Common incisions, oblique or transverse. B, Delivery of appendix. C, Ligation and division of mesoappendix. D, Ligation of base. E, Residual stump without inversion. F, Removal of appendix with ligation. G, Inversion of unligated stump.

small intestine, and the pelvis. Possible abnormalities in these locations include neoplasms of the intestines, diverticulitis of the colon, Meckel's diverticulitis, Crohn's disease of the terminal ileum, mesenteric adenitis, and a variety of pelvic pathologies. Sometimes it is necessary to enlarge the primary transverse or oblique incision to permit more thorough examination of the abdomen. If the appendix is normal and nothing else is found, appendectomy should be performed. When there is reason to suspect serious pathology other than appendicitis because of abnormal peritoneal fluid, other signs of peritonitis, or palpable abnormalities at a more distant site, the appendiceal incision should be closed and a counter incision made in the midline. Optimal exposure permits complete abdominal exploration, accurate evaluation, and appropriate surgical management of acute cholecystitis, perforated peptic ulcer, pelvic diseases, and other acute abdominal conditions. If the appendix is acutely inflamed (acute focal or suppurative appendicitis), abdominal exploration need not be extended beyond the right lower quadrant.

Appendectomy can be performed in a variety of ways, and there is little evidence that one method is superior (see Fig. 1). After the cecum and appendix have been mobilized adequately, gentle traction on a forceps placed on the free margin of the mesoappendix near the tip of the appendix sets the stage for simple ligation and division of the mesoappendix to the cecum. Special attention should be given to carefully ligating the intramural branch of the appendiceal artery on the surface of the cecum. Some surgeons prefer to crush the base of the appendix with a clamp and apply a ligature to that location before inverting the stump with a pursestring suture or several interrupted sutures in the wall of the cecum. An alternative method is to invert the stump unligated. With either method, the inverted stump should be small so that it will not be confused later with a possible cecal tumor. If a retrocecal or retroileal appendix cannot be mobilized easily, it can be removed retrograde by beginning the dissection at the base of the appendix. Occasionally, the base of the appendix and adjacent cecum are inflamed to the extent that inversion of the stump cannot be accomplished safely. In such instances, it is prudent to doubly ligate the stump or remove it with a cuff of cecum and close the cecal defect with two rows of sutures.

COMPLICATED APPENDICITIS

An intra-abdominal or retroperitoneal abscess is drained via the most direct route, but preferably not through the primary incision. The appendix is removed whenever it is technically possible. Removal of the appendix also is appropriate in cases with diffuse peritonitis. Irrigation of the abdominal cavity with sterile saline solution or one containing antibiotics is appropriate, but there is no evidence that drainage of the abdomen with diffuse peritonitis is beneficial. The presence of a thick-walled abscess or extensive inflammatory reaction localized in the right lower quadrant or the pelvis is an indication for leaving drains.

CLOSURE OF WOUND

The abdominal incision is closed in layers with nonabsorbable suture. Whenever the appendix is gangrenous or perforated and there is gross contamination, the subcutaneous tissue and skin should be packed lightly with running gauze and left open. After several days the pack is

removed, and if the granulation tissue is healthy, the skin margins are approximated with butterfly tapes. A delayed primary closure rarely is necessary. It is the preference of some surgeons to leave a catheter with multiple holes in the subcutaneous space and to close the skin. Suction on the catheter eliminates dead space and collection of fluid in the subcutaneous tissue and provides a route for infusion of antibiotics into the area several times a day for 4 to 5 days. Regardless of which method of wound closure is used in suppurative cases, surgical technique should be meticulous and care should be taken to avoid undue contamination of the wound.

Postoperative Management

Minimal care is required following appendectomy for simple acute appendicitis. Most patients recover rapidly and are ready for discharge from the hospital on the third or fourth postoperative day. In contrast, the patients with suppurative and complicated appendicitis demand intensive care until sepsis, paralytic ileus, and other problems have subsided. Antibiotics begun preoperatively in complicated cases are continued 3 to 10 days after operation, with the duration of treatment adjusted to the magnitude of the intra-abdominal infection.

Postoperative complications develop in approximately 5 per cent of uncomplicated cases and in 20 to 30 per cent of complicated cases. Of major concern are wound infection, intraperitoneal abscesses (pelvic, subphrenic, and subhepatic), and, rarely, fecal fistula, pylephlebitis, and hepatic abscess. Computed tomography or ultrasonography accurately localizes many abscesses, and either procedure can be used to guide percutaneous drainage. When this approach is unsuccessful or inappropriate, prompt surgical drainage is indicated.

Prognosis

The mortality rate is influenced by age of the patient, adequacy of preoperative preparation, and stage of disease at the time of surgical intervention. Uncomplicated appendicitis carries a mortality of less than 0.1 per cent, a figure that reflects the excellent preoperative, operative, and postoperative care available today. The mortality rate with complicated appendicitis has been reduced dramatically to a range of 2 to 5 per cent but remains unacceptably high (10 to 15 per cent) in young children and the elderly. Further reduction in mortality must be accomplished by earlier surgical intervention.

Tumors

Neoplasms of the appendix do not cause a diagnostic problem because most are found incidentally at operation, usually for a pathologic condition other than acute appendicitis. The challenge is to perform the correct operation when one of the malignant tumors is encountered.

CARCINOID

Carcinoid is the most common tumor of the appendix, with an incidence of 0.5 per cent.[4] These tumors account for half of all carcinoids of the gastrointestinal tract. In contrast to the latter, only 2 per cent of the appendiceal variety metastasize to regional lymph nodes. More distant metastases and malignant carcinoid syndrome are extremely rare. Until recently, most surgeons performed simple appendectomy for carcinoids less than 2 cm. in diameter and right hemicolectomy for larger tumors or when metastases were present in regional lymph nodes. Because metastases do occur from tumors 1 to 2 cm. in diameter, right hemicolectomy should be the procedure of choice for appendiceal carcinoids greater than 1 cm. in diameter.

ADENOCARCINOMA

The second most common malignant tumor of the appendix is adenocarcinoma.[22] The propensity of this tumor to metastasize is established by the fact that approximately 10 per cent of patients have widespread disease at the time of operation, and the 5-year survival following right hemicolectomy is only about 60 per cent.

MUCOCELE

Mucocele of the appendix is a confusing term because there are possibly three different types[23]: (1) a true malignant neoplasm (low-grade adenocarcinoma or mucinous cystadenocarcinoma), (2) a benign neoplasm (cystadenoma), and (3) a tumor that is not neoplastic. Mucocele results from chronic obstruction of the proximal part of the appendix and secretion of mucin into the distal part.

Since it is not possible to distinguish one type from another by gross examination, it is fortunate that appendectomy is the appropriate operation for all mucoceles. The critical point is avoidance of rupture of the mucocele and spillage of its contents into the abdominal cavity. When this occurs with the malignant-type mucocele, pseudomyxoma peritonei may result.

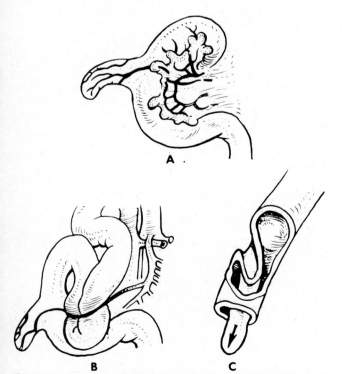

A.

B   C

Figure 2. Meckel's diverticulum and two causes of intestinal obstruction. A, Typical Meckel's diverticulum on antimesenteric border of ileum. B, Volvulus of segment of small bowel beneath mesentery of diverticulum. C, Intussusception with diverticulum acting as leading point.

MECKEL'S DIVERTICULUM

Anatomy and Embryology

Meckel's diverticulum (Fig. 2A) is the most common developmental anomaly of the small intestine, occurring in approximately 2 per cent of the population. Although first reported by Fabricus Hildanus[6] in 1598, it remained for Johann Meckel[10] to describe accurately the anatomic and embryologic features of this distal small bowel diverticulum in 1912. The mechanism responsible for this anomaly is failure of the omphalomesenteric (vitelline) duct, which connects the yolk sac with the foregut during early embryonic life, to become completely obliterated. Normally the obliteration takes place in the fifth to seventh week of gestation and in all but a few individuals undergoes subsequent atrophy. When parts or all of the omphalomesenteric duct and its accompanying vessels fail to become obliterated, the possible anomalies include:

1. A Meckel's diverticulum, when only the umbilical part of the duct closes (Fig. 3A).
2. A fistula between the ileum and the umbilicus, when the entire duct remains patent (Fig. 3B).
3. A Meckel's diverticulum with a band to the umbilicus, when a part of the omphalomesenteric duct or the vessels remain as a fibrous cord (Fig. 3C).
4. A sinus tract, when the duct becomes obliterated except at its umbilical end (in this instance, secretion occurs from the active glandular cells in the mucosa of the open duct) (Fig. 3D).
5. A cyst (enterocystoma), when the proximal and distal ends of the duct close but an opening remains in the middle (Fig. 3E).
6. A fibrous band between the ileum and the umbilicus (Fig. 3F).

Enterogenous cysts or duplications of the alimentary tract occur in the ileum, presenting the two muscular coats of the intestine and often showing no communication with the lumen of the major portion of the intestinal tract. The blood supply is common to the intestinal tract. Diverticula, other than the embryologic type, occur rarely in the terminal ileum and almost always lie in the mesentery in contrast to Meckel's diverticula, which are located on the antimesenteric border and have separate blood supplies reaching them through a small mesentery.

A Meckel's diverticulum occurs in approximately 2 per cent of the population (0.8 to 4 per cent incidence in large autopsy series).[11, 14] The anomaly usually is situated about 90 to 100 cm. from the ileocecal valve and is from 1 to 5 cm. in length.

Heterotopic mucosa may be present in Meckel's diverticulum and is more frequently of the gastric type; less frequently it resembles that of the duodenum or jejunum; sometimes there is heterotopic pancreatic tissue.[16] The gastric mucosa is of both the pyloric and fundic types and occurs in 13 per cent in autopsy series and in 67 per cent of operated cases.[19] The presence of ectopic gastric mucosa with its tendency to cause peptic ulceration is responsible for some of the most common symptoms associated with persistent Meckel's diverticulum.

Complications

Meckel's diverticula are detected during life either as a result of a significant complication (25 per cent) or as an incidental finding at laparotomy (75 per cent). The overall

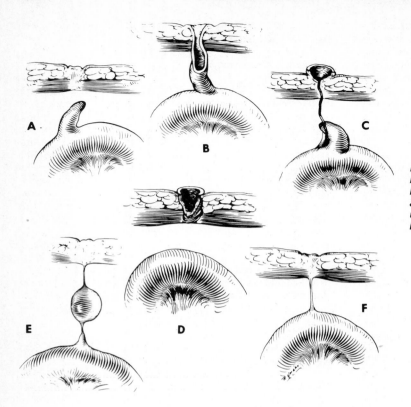

Figure 3. Congenital anomalies related to the omphalo-mesenteric duct. A, Meckel's diverticulum. B, Fistula between ileum and umbilicus. C, Meckel's diverticulum attached to umbilicus by a band. D, Sinus tract at umbilicus. E, Cyst of mid-duct (enterocystoma). F, Fibrous band between ileum to umbilicus.

incidence of complications is considered to be about 3 to 5 per cent,[17, 20] much less than the 25 per cent estimate of Meckel.[10]

Because there are a variety of complications and an age range of occurrence from infancy to old age, the possible clinical presentations are multiple and varied. The most common pathologic problems are ulceration, obstruction, and acute inflammation. Williams[20] summarized the three largest series of clinical cases of Meckel's diverticulum and found the complications were hemorrhage (31 per cent), inflammation (25 per cent), band obstruction (16 per cent), intussusception (11 per cent), hernial entrapment (11 per cent), and miscellaneous (6 per cent).

As mentioned, ulceration of the mucosa of the diverticulum or adjacent ileum is related to ectopic gastric mucosa and is the most common complication of Meckel's diverticulum in children. Peptic ulceration may occur at any age and may lead to secondary complications of bleeding, inflammation, and perforation. Perforation sometimes results from traumatic perforation by a sharp foreign body that lodges in a diverticulum.

Obstruction of the distal small bowel is caused most commonly by torsion of a loop of bowel around a fixed point resulting from a band between the diverticulum and the inferior surface of the umbilicus. Intestinal obstruction also results from kinking of the bowel caused by inflammation or from intussusception (see Fig. 2C). The latter, one of the most serious complications, may occur at any age but is most common in male infants less than 2 years of age. Ectopic tissue, inflammation, stones, or neoplasms within the diverticula may act as the lead point of the intussusception. Other causes of bowel obstruction are volvulus of a segment of intestine around a remnant of the omphalomesenteric vessels and entrapment of a portion of bowel beneath a band extending from the mesentery to the diverticulum (see Fig. 2B).

Although obstruction of the small intestine is one of the two most common complications of Meckel's diverticulum, only a small percentage of small bowel obstructions are caused by this congenital anomaly.

Acute inflammation may result from obstruction of the neck of the diverticulum, but usually it is secondary to peptic ulceration or obstruction of the ileum by one of the causes mentioned previously.

Benign and malignant tumors occur rarely in Meckel's diverticula.[12] Weinstein and co-workers[19] found only ten neoplasms (two leiomyomas, two carcinoids, and six leiomyosarcomas) in 162 diverticula.

Clinical Diagnosis

Meckel's diverticulum is very difficult to diagnose preoperatively because of the many possible clinical presentations and the lack of specific tests. Dr. Charles Mayo[9] said that "Meckel's diverticulum is frequently suspected, often diagnosed, and seldom found." The statement implies that Meckel's diverticulum is seldom diagnosed accurately.

The greatest success in diagnosis occurs with infants or young children who present with rectal bleeding and/or have an umbilical strawberry tumor or sinus tract.

The major types of clinical presentation relate to one or more of the complications: ulceration (bleeding, inflammation, or perforation), obstruction (band, internal hernia, or intussusception), or inflammation (secondary to obstruction and ulceration).

Symptoms and Signs

Rectal bleeding, which may be bright red, maroon, or black, should alert one to the possibility of peptic ulceration associated with ectopic gastric mucosa in a diverticulum. Occult bleeding does occur occasionally and produces iron-deficiency anemia.

Classic symptoms of small bowel obstruction may be the tip-off to the diagnosis of Meckel's diverticulum. In cases with intussusception or volvulus around a band, onset of symptoms may be very acute. At other times the symptoms may come and go over various periods of time as a result of intermittent, incomplete intestinal obstruction.

Sometimes acute inflammation in or about the diverticulum produces symptoms indistinguishable from those associated with acute appendicitis. Nausea, anorexia, and periumbilical pain or discomfort commonly found with acute appendicitis rarely are found in patients with Meckel's diverticulum.

The common physical signs are localized tenderness or a palpable mass in the right lower quadrant of the abdomen, classic signs of intestinal obstruction. None of these signs is specific for Meckel's diverticulum, but any of them should alert the astute examiner to the possibility of this entity or a complication thereof.

Diagnostic Examinations

Plain roentgenograms rarely help except in cases with intestinal obstruction when dilated loops of small bowel containing air-fluid levels are demonstrated. Contrast studies of the small intestine seldom show a Meckel's diverticulum, and for this reason they are no longer in common use in childrens' hospitals.

Abdominal scanning with technetium is a specific test for demonstration of a diverticulum that contains gastric mucosa. This simple, noninvasive test is positive in 85 to 90 per cent of such cases, and the false-negative results are rare.[1, 21]

Surgical Management

The two basic techniques for removing a Meckel's diverticulum are simple excision with transverse closure of the resulting ileotomy and resection of a segment of ileum containing the diverticulum with ileoileostomy (end-to-end).

Diverticulectomy is the procedure of choice in the majority of cases. Diverticula complicated by bleeding or inflammation involving the adjacent ileum or those containing a palpable mass (suggesting ectopic tissue or neoplasm) are managed best by segmental resection of the ileum and primary anastomosis.

In cases with intussusception, an attempt at careful reduction is reasonable and, if successful, will allow simple diverticulectomy. Resection is necessary when reduction of the intussusception is not possible (Fig. 4).

When a malignant tumor arises within the diverticulum, a wedge of the mesentery of the ileum should be

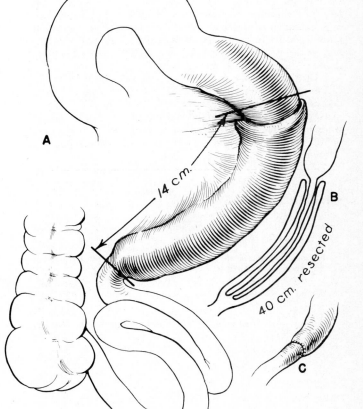

Figure 4. Intussusception of the ileum, a complication of Meckel's diverticula. A, The intussusception. B, Illustration of amount of ileum resected. C, Primary enteroenterostomy (end-to-end).

included in the resection to ensure adequate removal of lymph nodes.

Should a Meckel's diverticulum found incidentally at laparotomy be removed? The question is significant because approximately 75 per cent of diverticula are discovered this way. The conventional answer has been "yes, such diverticula should be excised because the risk of subsequent potentially serious complications is 25 per cent, and the mortality and morbidity rates accompanying diverticulectomy are appreciably greater in nonelective than in elective operations."

Management of a Meckel's diverticulum found incidentally has come under scrutiny because results of more recent studies show that the complication rates are much lower than 25 per cent. Soltero[17] reported a complication rate of 4.2 per cent in infancy, 3 per cent in adulthood, and almost 0.0 per cent in old age. These data were derived from a thorough study of a large population served by one group of hospitals.

The current mortality rates are less than 0.3 per cent with uncomplicated diverticula and approximately 6 per cent with complicated disease. Soltero[17] calculated that with a 6 per cent mortality after surgery for complicated Meckel's diverticula versus essentially no mortality for incidentally removed diverticula one would need to excise 400 normal diverticula to save one life. Such statistical calculations support conservative management of asymptomatic, incidentally found Meckel's diverticula, and they have influenced many surgeons to consider new guidelines of treatment.

Because 50 per cent of complications occur by age 2 and the subsequent chance of trouble decreases with age, perhaps only diverticula found incidentally in the first 2 decades of life should be excised. Williams[20] suggests that it is not rational to excise a wide-mouthed, thin-walled, unattached diverticulum found incidentally in an adult patient. Most surgeons agree that diverticula with narrow necks or those containing a palpable mass suggesting ectopic tissue or neoplasm should be excised.

Until more factual information concerning the complication rates of Meckel's diverticulum become available, the decision about whether to do incidental diverticulectomy will remain a matter of individual judgment. The definitive study necessary to settle the issue would be a careful follow-up of patients in whom diverticula were found but not removed.

SELECTED REFERENCES

DeBartolo, H. M., Jr., and van Heerden, J. A.: Meckel's diverticulum. Ann Surg., *183:*30, 1976.
This is a study of 190 surgically documented cases of Meckel's diverticulum encountered in one medical center over half a century. Clinical features as well as surgical considerations are presented.

Lewis, F. R., Holcroft, J. W., Boey, J., and Dunphy, J. E.: Appendicitis: A critical review of diagnosis and treatment in 1000 cases. Arch. Surg., *110:*677, 1975.
The authors report a retrospective analysis of 1000 consecutive cases of appendicitis operated on during a 10-year period (1963–1973). The study

provides excellent demographic data and discriminates values of various factors that affect diagnosis and treatment.

Stone, H. H., Sanders, S. L., and Martin, J. D., Jr.: Perforated appendicitis in children. Surgery, *69:*673, 1971.
This report concerns a 10-year experience with appendicitis in children 16 years of age or younger and emphasizes the factors that influence development of complications, particularly wound infection and intra-abdominal abscess. Methods of management to reduce morbidity are discussed.

REFERENCES

1. Berquist, T. H., Nolan, N. G., Stephens, D. H., and Carlson, H. C.: Specificity of ^{99m}Tc-pertechnetate in scintigraphic diagnosis of Meckel's diverticulum: Review of 100 cases. J. Nucl. Med., *17:*465, 1976.
2. Bolton, J. P., Craven, E. R., Croft, R. J., and Menzies-Gow, N.: An assessment of the value of the white cell count in the management of suspected acute appendicitis. Br. J. Surg., *62:*906, 1975.
3. Fitz, R. H.: Perforating inflammation of the vermiform appendix; with special reference to its early diagnosis and treatment. Trans. Assoc. Am. Phys., *1:*107, 1886.
4. Glasser, C. M., and Bhagavan, B. S.: Carcinoid tumors of the appendix. Arch. Pathol. Lab. Med., *104:*272, 1980.
5. Gomez, A., and Wood, M.: Acute appendicitis during pregnancy. Am. J. Surg., *137:*180, 1979.
6. Hildanus, F., quoted by Neff, G.: Das Meckelsche Divertikel. Engebn. Chir. Orthop., *30:*227, 1937.
7. Janik, J. S., and Firor, H. V.: Pediatric appendicitis: A 20-year study of 1,640 children at Cook County (Illinois) Hospital. Arch. Surg., *114:*717, 1979.
8. Jona, J. Z., Belin, R. P., and Selke, A. C.: Barium enema as a diagnostic aid in children with abdominal pain. Surg. Gynecol. Obstet., *144:*351, 1977.
9. Mayo, C. W.: Meckel's diverticulum. Proc. Mayo Clin., *8:*230, 1933.
10. Meckel, J. F.: Handbuch der Pathologischen Anatomie, Vol. 1. Leipzig, C. H. Reclam, 1812.
11. Michas, C. A., Cohen, S. E., and Wolfman, E. F., Jr.: Meckel's diverticulum: Should it be excised incidentally at operation? Am. J. Surg., *129:*682, 1975.
12. Moses, W. R.: Meckel's diverticulum: A report of two unusual cases. N. Engl. J. Med., *237:*118, 1947.
13. Savrin, R. A., and Clatworthy, H. W., Jr.: Appendiceal rupture: A continuing diagnostic problem. Pediatrics, *63:*37, 1979.
14. Seagram, C. G. F., Louch, R. E., Stephens, C. A., and Wentworth, P.: Meckel's diverticulum: A 10-year review of 218 cases. Can. J. Surg., *11:*369, 1968.
15. Smith, D. E., Kirchmer, N. A., and Stewart, D. R.: Use of the barium enema in the diagnosis of acute appendicitis and its complications. Am. J. Surg., *138:*829, 1979.
16. Soderlund, S.: Meckel's diverticulum: A clinical and histologic study. Acta. Chir. Scand., Suppl. No. 248, 1959.
17. Soltero, M. J., and Bill, A. H.: The natural history of Meckel's diverticulum and its relation to incidental removal: A study of 202 cases of diseased Meckel's diverticulum found in King County, Washington, over a fifteen year period. Am. J. Surg., *132:*168, 1976.
18. Wakeley, C. P. G.: The position of the vermiform appendix as ascertained by an analysis of 10,000 cases. J. Anat., *67:*277, 1933.
19. Weinstein, E. C., Cain, J. C., and ReMine, W. H.: Meckel's diverticulum: 55 years of clinical and surgical experience. J.A.M.A., *182:*251, 1962.
20. Williams, R. S.: Management of Meckel's diverticulum. Br. J. Surg., *68:*477, 1981.
21. Wine, C. R., Nahrwold, D. L., and Waldhausen, J. A.: Role of the technetium scan in the diagnosis of Meckel's diverticulum. J. Pediatr. Surg., *9:*885, 1974.
22. Wolff, M., and Ahmed, N.: Epithelial neoplasms of the vermiform appendix (exclusive of carcinoid): I. Adenocarcinoma of the appendix. Cancer, *37:*2493, 1976.
23. Woodruff, R., and McDonald, J. R.: Benign and malignant cystic tumors of the appendix. Surg. Gynecol. Obstet., *71:*750, 1940.

DISEASES OF THE COLON AND RECTUM

KENNETH P. RAMMING, M.D.

26

The colon is the terminal portion of the bowel extending from the terminal ileum to the rectoanal junction. It is the site of a number of important and, at times, life-threatening medical and surgical disorders. A wide variety of recently developed diagnostic techniques applicable to diseases of the colon are included in the complete evaluation of a host of inflammatory, vascular, neoplastic, and post traumatic lesions of the colon. These new techniques have recently made it possible to establish an objective diagnosis preoperatively in most patients with these disorders.

ANATOMY AND FUNCTION

The colon is approximately 1.5 meters long and extends from the terminal ileum to the anus. The diameter is greatest (8.5 cm.) in the cecum, diminishing to about 2.5 cm. in the sigmoid, and becoming slightly more dilated in the rectum. The ascending and descending portions are mostly retroperitoneal, whereas the sigmoid and transverse colon have mesenteries and are therefore intraperitoneal. Several external features distinguish the colon from the small intestine, including the presence of three separate longitudinal muscular bands, or teniae coli, that are circumferentially placed around the colon and converge at the base of the appendix. Haustra (sacculations) are present in the colonic wall. The haustra are separated by incomplete internal folds (plicae semilunares), which are transient and depend on the contractile actions of the colon. The serosa of the large bowel has fatty appendages (appendices epiploicae), which are attached to the medial wall of the colon, predominantly in its distal portion. In the sigmoid colon these appear in two rows, one on either side of the anterior tenia. In contrast to the mobile small bowel, the colon is relatively fixed in position because of its retroperitoneal attachments. In addition, the colon is distinguished by the omentum, which is attached to the transverse colon.

The cecum and part of the transverse colon as well as much of the sigmoid colon are completely within the peritoneum, whereas the lower third of the rectum is below the peritoneum and the upper third is extraperitoneal on its posterior surface. The ascending and descending portions of the colon are covered by peritoneum on the anterior surface only.

The wall of the colon is composed of four distinct histologic layers: the serosa, muscularis, submucosa, and mucosa. The outer longitudinal muscle layer is incomplete and forms the three separate teniae, except in the rectum, where it does not appear as separate bands. The ganglion cells of the myenteric (Auerbach's) plexus are located mainly along the external surface of the circular muscle coat (Figs. 1 and 2). The serosa forms the appendices epiploicae, but the distal third of the rectum has no serosal covering. The mucosa is composed of simple columnar epithelium and has no villi, and numerous tubular crypts, which in their lower half have mucus-secreting goblet cells, are present throughout the colon.

Vascular Supply

The blood supply of the colon is primarily through the superior and inferior mesenteric arteries. The superior

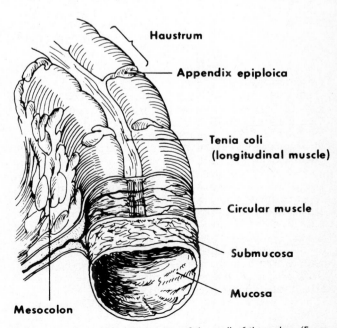

Figure 1. Gross anatomic aspects of the wall of the colon. (From Hardy, J. D. (Ed.): Hardy's Textbook of Surgery. Philadelphia, J. B. Lippincott Company, 1983.)

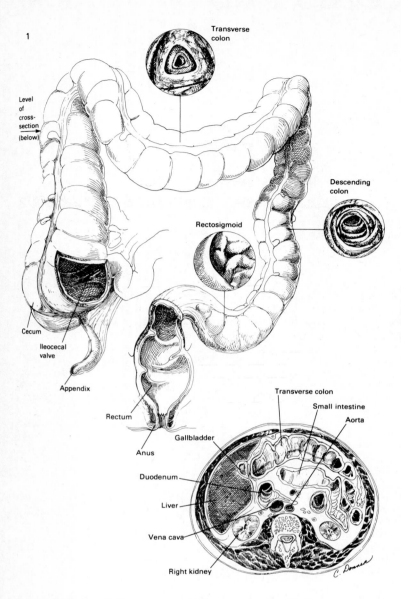

Figure 2. Clinicoanatomic aspects of the colon. Note the representative drawings of endoscopic views at the various levels within the colon. (From Spiro, H. M.: Clinical Gastroenterology. New York, Macmillan Publishing Company, 1983.)

mesenteric artery gives rise to three major branches: (1) the ileocolic, (2) right colic, and (3) middle colic arteries. The inferior mesenteric artery divides into the left colic, the superior hemorrhoidal (rectal), and the sigmoid arteries. Each of these has anastomoses with adjacent arteries, forming a continuous vessel around the entire colon (the "marginal artery" of Drummond). The latter is located about 1 cm. from the margin of the colon, being closest along the descending and sigmoid colon. The rectum is supplied in its upper half by the superior hemorrhoidal artery, which is the terminal branch of the inferior mesenteric artery. The middle hemorrhoidal arteries arise from the internal iliac arteries and provide a less important part of the rectal blood supply. The inferior hemorrhoidal arteries arise from the internal pudendal arteries and supply the lower rectum and anus. All three of these hemorrhoidal arteries anastomose freely with one another.

The venous drainage of the colon parallels the arterial system but does not enter the inferior vena caval system. The superior and inferior mesenteric veins join the splenic vein to form the portal vein and drain into the liver. The rectum contains an extensive plexus of venous anastomoses,

and most of the rectal venous blood drains into the portal system. In the event of increased portal pressure, the venous flow in the rectum is usually reversed, with drainage into the internal iliac veins (Fig. 3).

Lymphatics

The colon is supplied with a rich lymphatic network, and the lymphatic channels follow the regional arteries to the preaortic nodes at the origin of the superior and inferior mesenteric arteries. They then drain into the cisterna chyli, a part of the thoracic duct system, which in turn empties into the venous system at the junction of the left jugular and subclavian veins. Because of this relationship, metastatic carcinoma from the gastrointestinal tract may present in the lymph nodes of the neck (Virchow's node). The rectal lymphatics drain upward along the superior hemorrhoidal vessels, and the lymphatics of the anal canal spread to the internal iliac nodes, whereas the lymphatics of the anus and perineal skin drain into the superficial inguinal nodes (Fig. 4).

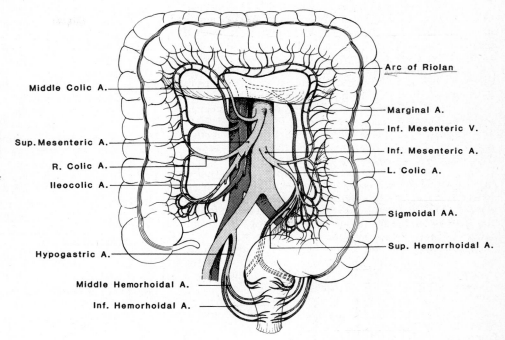

Middle Colic A.

Sup. Mesenteric A.

R. Colic A.

Ileocolic A.

Hypogastric A.

Middle Hemorhoidal A.

Inf. Hemorhoidal A.

Arc of Riolan

Marginal A.

Inf. Mesenteric V.

Inf. Mesenteric A.

L. Colic A.

Sigmoidal AA.

Sup. Hemorrhoidal A.

Figure 3. Vascular supply of the colon. (From Gathright, J. B., and Holmes, J. W. C.: Complications of surgery for colon cancer. In Ferrari, B. T., Ray, J. E., and Gathright, J. B. (Eds.): Complications of Colon and Rectal Surgery: Prevention and Management. Philadelphia, W. B. Saunders Company, 1985, p. 160.)

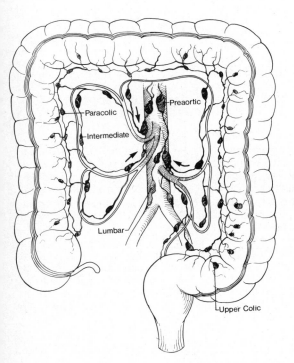

Preaortic

Paracolic

Intermediate

Lumbar

Upper Colic

Figure 4. Lymphatic drainage of the colon. (From Gathright, J. B., and Holmes, J. W. C.: Complications of surgery for colon cancer. In Ferrari, B. T., Ray, J. E., and Gathright, J. B. (Eds.): Complications of Colon and Rectal Surgery: Prevention and Management. Philadelphia, W. B. Saunders Company, 1985, p. 161.)

Innervation

The colon is provided with sympathetic nerve fibers passing from the thoracic and lumbar portions of the spinal cord, through the sympathetic chains, to the preaortic sympathetic ganglia. There they synapse with the postganglionic fibers, which follow the major arteries to terminate in the submucosal (Meissner's) and myenteric (Auerbach's) plexuses. The rectum is supplied by the presacral or hypogastric nerves, which are extensions of the preaortic plexuses and the lumbar splanchnic nerves. The presacral nerve originates below the bifurcation of the aorta and divides to descend on either side of the pelvis, where it joins fibers of the sacral parasympathetic nerves (nervi erigentes) to form two pelvic plexuses, from which fibers go directly to all the viscera of the pelvis. The *parasympathetic innervation* is from fibers of the vagus nerve and the nervi erigentes. The vagus fibers join the sympathetic fibers at the celiac axis and pass with them to the bowel but do not synapse until reaching the plexuses in the bowel itself. This vagus innervation extends distally to the transverse colon. The distal part of the colon is innervated by the second through the fourth sacral segments of the spinal cord through the nervi erigentes passing into the pelvic plexuses. Fibers to the distal transverse colon, descending colon, and sigmoid pass upward through the presacral nerves to join the sympathetics at the inferior mesenteric ganglion, from which they follow the colonic arteries.

Sympathetic activity is mainly inhibitory to the colon and motor to the internal sphincter, whereas parasympathetic activity has the opposite effects. However, the more important control of the bowel is the local reflex activity mediated by the intramural nerve plexuses (Meissner's and Auerbach's) and their interconnections. Thus, even with cord transection or vagotomy, bowel function can continue essentially normally. Conversely, patients lacking these plexuses, e.g., those with Hirschsprung's disease, have abnormal motor activity. If the pelvic autonomics are damaged during rectal procedures, impotence or bladder dysfunction may ensue. The sensory afferent fibers are sympathetic and react to distention, stretching, or spasm. The voluntary muscles, i.e., the levator ani, coccygeus, and external sphincter, are supplied by nerves from the fourth sacral segment.

Physiology

The major functions of the colon are to provide fecal storage and to extract water and electrolytes. The colon receives approximately 1000 ml. of water daily from the small intestine, and all but about 150 ml. is absorbed.

The colon is separated from the small intestine by the ileocecal valve, which prevents the contents of the ileum from refluxing into the cecum. This valve and the relative immobility of colonic contents have been used to explain the marked difference in bacterial ecology between colon and small bowel. The bacterial flora of the small bowel seldom exceeds 10^5 organisms per ml., in contrast to colonic counts of up to 10^{10} organisms per ml.; in fact, one third of the fecal weight in the colon is composed of bacteria.

Potassium is passively diffused from blood to bowel lumen in association with the electrochemical gradient created by active sodium transport. Bile acids are absorbed by passive diffusion. Bacteria in the colon deconjugates bile acids, which, in increasing concentrations, can block sodium and water absorption, leading to diarrhea. The colon normally secretes small quantities of mucus. However, in pathologic states or with mechanical irritation, mucus secretion may increase markedly.

Two motility patterns are observed in the colon. Agitating or segmental contractions knead and mix the fecal mass primarily in the right and transverse colon and appear to aid in water absorption. A second type of contraction, "mass movement," propels the colonic contents distally. These contraction waves do not constitute true peristalsis since there is a simultaneous constriction of long segments of colon. The mass movements empty the contents of the right colon into the sigmoid and upper rectum and can be initiated by food in the stomach (the gastrocolic reflex). True peristalsis, similar to that seen in the small bowel, occurs only rarely in the human colon except in association with the act of defecation. Colonic motility may be altered by a number of stimuli, and the colon is particularly sensitive to paralytic ileus from trauma, infection, or handling at operation. The autonomic nervous system exerts an inhibitory effect on the colon, whereas physical activity increases its motor activity.

Motility patterns demonstrate an increase in intraluminal pressures in those with chronic constipation and in the presence of diverticulosis. Morphine and codeine markedly increase colonic muscle tone and reduce propulsive action. Anticholinergic agents and glucagon are potent inhibitors of colonic motility, whereas the parasympathomimetic drugs, such as neostigmine, increase motor activity.[12, 21]

Rectal Continence and Defecation

The internal anorectal sphincter is an involuntary, circular, smooth muscle, whereas the voluntary muscles are the external sphincter and the anorectal ring, consisting primarily of the levator ani and the puborectalis. Both the internal and external sphincters remain in a state of tonus, and this tone increases in response to an increase in intraabdominal pressure, thus preserving continence. The act of defecation, which results in the expulsion of feces, is a controlled reflex that may be inhibited in the adult until a convenient time.[4,12,23]

The rectum is normally empty, and when mass movements propel feces into the rectum or when intraluminal pressure rises to 20 to 25 cm. H_2O, the desire to defecate becomes manifest. The receptors within the wall of the rectum can usually discriminate between solids, liquids, and gas.

The 75 to 180 gm. of feces (other than bacteria) excreted daily contain 70 per cent water, undigested cellulose, proteins, and fat. Ammonia is produced and absorbed in the colon, principally as a result of bacterial degradation of urea. In the presence of cirrhosis, portal hypertension, and portosystemic shunts, ammonia absorption from the colon may have a significant role in the pathogenesis of hepatic coma.

Gas in the colon is primarily from swallowed air and is chiefly nitrogen, since carbon dioxide and oxygen are rapidly absorbed. Methane and hydrogen are produced by bacterial putrefaction and are present in small quantities. In postoperative patients, the propulsion of gas and the passage of flatus are among the earliest signs of returning bowel function.

DIAGNOSTIC STUDIES IN COLONIC DISEASES

History and Physical and Rectal Examination

An adequate history is mandatory in the diagnosis of colonic disease. Empathy and sensitivity may be required in elucidating a complete and accurate history, since some patients are reluctant to fully volunteer symptoms that may relate to defecation. Careful abdominal examination in a relaxed patient is important, as are visual examination of the anus and a complete digital rectal examination. In performing the rectal examination, the examiner should attempt to mentally visualize the anatomy utilizing a complete tactile evaluation of the area.

Examination of the Stool

Examination of the stool for blood is essential in all patients. Bleeding from the left-sided colonic lesion is often grossly detectable, but bleeding from lesions of the right colon is often occult. Studies for parasites, fat, or unusual bacteria should be done if they are clinically indicated.

Sigmoidoscopy

Sigmoidoscopy allows examination of the lumen at the distal 25 to 30 cm. of the colorectum and is theoretically capable of disclosing as many as 70 per cent of neoplasms of the entire colon as well as sites of hemorrhage and local inflammation. Examination of at least the distal 10 to 15 cm. is easily accomplished and allows detailed inspection of that portion of the colon that yields unreliable roentgenographic results.

An enema given 30 minutes before the examination usually provides a prepared field. The patient is placed in the jackknife position and is constantly reassured by the examiner. After digital examination of the anus, the scope is introduced and, under directed vision, is advanced. The left curve of the sigmoid colon must be passed, and this can be greatly facilitated by insufflation of air. After the instrument has been passed proximally as far as possible, the scope is slowly withdrawn and the entire bowel wall circumference is methodically observed.

Barium Enema

A barium enema is advisable in nearly every patient with suspected colonic disease except in those known to have a perforation or in whom an obstruction is suspected on the plain film. Characteristic mucosal patterns, areas of obstruction, or mass lesions consistent with either inflammatory or neoplastic disease can be identified with the films taken in various positions.

Air Contrast Barium Enema

An air contrast barium study is usually an accurate radiologic study. Barium is introduced, and the colon is then filled with air. The narrow rim of barium on the wall of the bowel greatly facilitates identification of lesions as small as 1.5 cm. in diameter.

Flexible Endoscopy

The advent of fiberoptic instruments that range in length from 85 to 200 cm. permits examination of nearly the entire colon. Indications for colonoscopy include (1) abnormalities in barium x-ray (filling defects, segmental colonic narrowing, and polyps), (2) chronic gastrointestinal bleeding, (3) anatomic abnormalities following colonic procedures, and (4) chronic inflammatory bowel disease in carefully selected patients. Acute inflammatory bowel disease is a contraindication to colonoscopy because of the very real danger of perforation. Flexible colonoscopes can be used effectively for diagnosis or therapy or both. Biopsies may be obtained, and removal or cauterization can be accomplished. Polypoid lesions or lesions greater than 2 cm. in diameter often cannot be removed at colonoscopy, although the use of laser cauterization through such scopes may greatly facilitate resection of these lesions.

Other Diagnostic Tests

Liver function studies and determinations of carcinoembryonic antigen may be of value in patients being evaluated for colonic carcinoma as possible indicators of metastatic disease. The intravenous pyelogram often is helpful in determining the position of the ureters in patients in whom operation is contemplated, since the ureters that are susceptible to iatrogenic injury are close to the dissection plan required for colon resection, particularly if there has been a previous abdominal procedure. Insertion of catheters into the ureters prior to operation in patients who have previously undergone an extensive pelvic procedure is often helpful at the time of operation. Lymphogranuloma venereum can be diagnosed by identifying the virus in the lesion or in the involved lymph nodes by the Frei skin test or by complement fixation. A titer of 1:32 or higher or a rising antibody titer during the active stage is diagnostic.

INTESTINAL ANTISEPSIS

The colon contains numerous bacterial organisms, and adequate preparation of the colon prior to any operative procedure is important. The ideal intestinal antiseptic for controlling bacterial flora in the colon should have (1) rapid, highly bacteriocidal activity against pathogenic organisms in the gastrointestinal tract, (2) the ability to prevent the development or overgrowth of pathogenic organisms, and (3) low toxicity and limited absorption from the intestine. Appropriate antibiotic therapy requires knowledge of the normal bacterial flora and the potentially pathogenic flora (Fig. 5).

The most important aspect of preparation of the colon for elective operations is adequate mechanical preparation, which is the most important aspect of intestinal antisepsis (Table 1). Preparation of the bowel should begin 3 days prior to the scheduled operation and should include mechanical cleansing aided by antibiotic agents. Commonly used antibiotic regimens are given in Table 2. A combination of erythromycin and neomycin has been recommended.

Clinical trials show that many antimicrobial agents used singly or in combination and administered preoperatively are effective in reducing the incidence of postoperative wound and systemic infections. Effective prophylaxis requires *preoperative* administration far enough in advance

TABLE 1. Routine for Bowel Preparation

A laxative is given on the first day.
An elemental diet or a clear liquid diet is begun and continued throughout the preparation period.
Enemas are given daily throughout the preparation period.
The antibiotic of choice is started on the first day, after the laxative has been administered.
The preparation period is 72 hours.

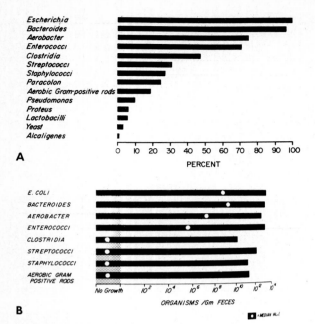

A

B

Figure 5. Incidence of microorganisms (A) and range of bacterial counts (B) in feces of 200 consecutive hospitalized patients. (From Cohn, I., Jr.: Intestinal Antisepsis. Springfield, Ill., Charles C Thomas, 1968.)

such that tissues exposed to a large amount of microorganisms during the operative procedure have adequate protection against microbial colonization. Intraoperative administration of the agent is necessary during long operations to ensure adequate tissue levels throughout this critical period; however, there is no evidence of benefit from administration beyond 24 to 36 hours postoperatively. Limitation of postoperative elective use is important in reducing the possibility of adverse reactions, superinfection, and the masking of signs and symptoms of unrelated infections.

In elective operative procedures on the colon, mechanical bowel preparation is most often accompanied by administration of a nonabsorbable, orally administered antibiotic to control fecal bacteria. In addition, a systemic antibiotic is usually given 12 hours prior to operation and maintained for 24 to 36 hours. Most physicians advocate the copious

irrigation of the peritoneal cavity with 4 to 5 liters of sterile saline at the conclusion of the procedure, particularly if obvious contamination has occurred. Many favor following this with irrigation with 1 liter of saline containing an antibiotic; this solution is also used to irrigate the subcutaneous wound prior to closure.[1, 4, 6]

OPERATIVE CONSIDERATIONS IN COLONIC DISEASE

Improvements in pre- and postoperative care, anesthetic agents and techniques, and instruments (particularly stapling instruments) have greatly facilitated operative procedures involving the colon. In focal disease, the diseased part can be removed and the colon reanastomosed. In patients with neoplastic disease, the lymph nodes that may harbor deposits of tumor cells should also be excised. If the entire colon is removed, an ileostomy is created. The intestinal contents then drain into a plastic bag attached to the skin by a leak-proof adhesion (Figs. 6 and 7). If the anus is removed, as in abdominoperineal resection, the end of the colon is exteriorized as a colostomy and sutured to the abdominal wall. With appropriate irrigation, that is, a daily cleansing enema of the colon with water, usually in the morning, most patients with a colostomy can control bowel movements with relative predictability.

Temporary colostomies may be required in a variety of situations, e.g., to protect an anastomosis that is very low in the pelvis or with temporary diversion of fecal flow while healing occurs. Colostomies are also commonly used when the colon is greatly dilated because of a distal obstructive lesion such as cancer or a diverticular abscess. Resection often cannot be safely performed until the colon is decompressed. Colostomies may also be placed temporarily in patients in whom perforation has occurred; intra-abdominal contamination would place the anastomosis at risk for infection and breakdown.

A colostomy is simply an exteriorization of the colon through the abdominal wall to provide safe diversion of colonic contents. A *loop* colostomy is a loop of bowel

TABLE 2. *Antibiotic Preparations Used Prior to Surgery in the Colon Regimen*

Drug	Dosage
Amphotericin-Neomycin Amphotericin 50 mg. Neomycin 1 gm.	In combination, every hour for 4 hours, then every 6 hours for a total of 72 hours
Bacitracin-Neomycin Bacitracin 40,000 units	In combination, every 6 hours for 72 hours
Kanamycin 1 gm.	Every hour for 4 hours, then every 6 hours for a total of 72 hours
Nystatin-Neomycin Nystatin 250,000 units Neomycin 1 gm.	In combination, every hour for 4 hours, then every 4 hours for a total of 72 hours
Sulfathalidine-Neomycin Sulfathalidine 1.5 gm. Neomycin 1 gm.	In combination, every hour for 4 hours, then every 4 hours for a total of 72 hours
Erythromycin-base 1 gm. Neomycin 1 gm.	One dose at 1:00 P.M., 2:00 P.M., 11:00 P.M. Preop.

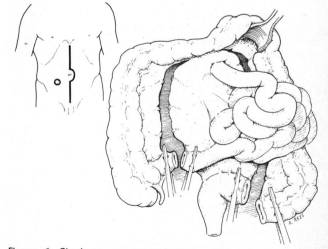

Figure 6. Single-stage protocolectomy. The colon is excised through a midline abdominal incision. The ileum and rectum are divided, and the entire colon is resected. (From Sawyers, J. L.: Granulomatous colitis and ulcerative colitis including toxic megacolon. In Hardy, J. D. (Ed.): Rhoads Textbook of Surgery, 5th ed. Philadelphia, J. B. Lippincott, 1977.)

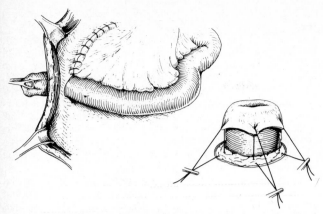

Figure 7. A permanent ileostomy is formed by placing the ileum through a separate opening in the abdominal wall. The mucosa is everted to create a stoma covered by mucosa with a nipple-like configuration to facilitate attachment of a bag to the abdominal wall. (From Sawyers, J. L.: Granulomatous colitis and ulcerative colitis including toxic megacolon. In Hardy, J. D. (Ed.): Rhoads Textbook of Surgery, 5th ed. Philadelphia, J. B. Lippincott Company, 1977.)

delivered through an incision in the abdominal wall placed over a bar or plastic band to prevent return to the peritoneal cavity. The exteriorized loop of bowel is then opened. An *end* colostomy requires division of the colon with delivery of the proximal end through a small incision into the abdominal wall with anastomosis to the skin. The distal end may similarly be brought through the separate opening in the abdominal wall as a mucous fistula, a combination termed a *double-barrel* colostomy (Fig. 8). If there is no obstruction in the distal segment, the open end can be closed and replaced into the abdominal cavity (Hartmann's pouch). This distal rectal segment can be evacuated of any secretions through the anus. At the time of reoperation, the colostomy is removed from the abdominal wall and the two segments are reanastomosed. As in all gastrointestinal procedures, meticulous attention to detail, appropriate antisepsis, and, most important, the maintenance of an adequate blood supply are important.

INFLAMMATORY DISEASES OF THE COLON

Inflammatory bowel disease refers to ulcerative colitis, granulomatous transmural ileocolitis (Crohn's disease), and other less common disorders. The pathologic features of these disorders provide a basis for understanding the clinical manifestations of each. Ulcerative colitis is an inflammatory, ulcerating process primarily involving the *mucosa*, whereas Crohn's disease is a *transmural* granulomatous enteritis that may involve any part of the intestine, primarily the small intestine, but is also found in the colon. Both of these chronic inflammatory disorders are of unknown etiology but share some common clinical, epidemiologic, immunologic, and genetic features, including extraintestinal complications and response to treatment.

Ulcerative Colitis

Ulcerative colitis is a chronic disease characterized by inflammation of the mucosa and submucosa of the colon. The inflammation is variable in the extent and length of colonic involvement. The anatomic extent of the disease may include the entire colon (pancolitis) or a portion, such as proctosigmoiditis, which refers to diseases limited to the rectum or rectosigmoid, or left-sided colitis, which refers to disease of the descending colon.

Ulcerative colitis is estimated to involve 2 to 7 cases per 100,000 population in the United States. Both the incidence and prevalence of ulcerative proctitis are approximately comparable to those for colitis. Although both Crohn's disease and ulcerative colitis are being increasingly *recognized*, there is no evidence that the incidence of ulcerative colitis is *actually increasing*. In the United States, between 200,000 and 400,000 individuals suffer from inflammatory bowel diseases, with some 30,000 new cases diagnosed each year. Ulcerative colitis affects females more often than males and has a bimodal age distribution, with a first peak incidence between the ages of 15 and 20 and a second, smaller peak at age 55 to 60. The incidence of ulcerative colitis in blacks is low and is about one third that seen in Caucasians. The incidence is three to five times greater among Jews than among non-Jews.

ETIOLOGY AND PATHOGENESIS

Despite numerous studies, the etiology of chronic ulcerative colitis remains unknown, and an appropriate experimental animal model of the human disorder has not yet been established. Considerable debate has arisen concerning the role of psychosomatic factors in the initiation and development of ulcerative colitis. When the illness becomes manifest, it is often impossible to distinguish its influences on behavior from the patient's earlier personality. Any illness characterized by severe diarrhea, rectal bleeding, and a variety of constitutional symptoms, especially when occurring in a young and previously healthy patient, constitutes a stressful situation and can undermine a patient's self-confidence. Regressive behavior may ensue, and children with colitis are often compulsively neat, demanding, and immature for their age. During exacerbations

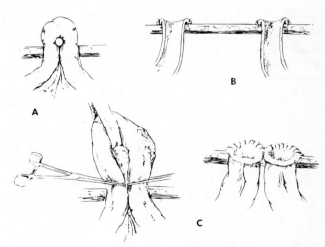

Figure 8. Types of colostomies. A, Loop colostomy (unopened). The colostomy can be opened with a cautery at the bedside after the abdominal wall has become adherent and sealed to the exteriorized loop. B, Divided colostomy. C, Exteriorization of the diseased portion of colon. On the left, the segment of diseased colon (neoplasm) is placed through the abdominal incision. The specimen is removed between clamps, and these clamps are later removed and the two ends of the colon are sutured to the skin. (From Liechty, R. D., and Soper, R. T. (Eds.): Synopsis of Surgery. St. Louis, The C. V. Mosby Company, 1980.)

of the disease, adults may exhibit exaggeration of dependency.

Ulcerative colitis is an inflammatory disease characterized by a tissue reaction in the bowel that resembles that caused by known microbiologic pathogens such as *Shigella*. However, no organism has been reproducibly demonstrated to be responsible for the condition.

Much attention has been given the immunologic phenomena in inflammatory bowel disease, and the frequent personal and family histories of atopic diseases in these patients as well as the concomitant presence of erythema nodosum, arthritis, uveitis, and vasculitis suggest an immunologically mediated pathogenetic mechanism. Circulating anticolon antibodies have been described in ulcerative colitis, but these remain of unknown significance. The beneficial effects of corticosteroid therapy for ulcerative colitis are consistent with this agent's immunosuppressive and anti-inflammatory effects. Some of the extraintestinal manifestations of ulcerative colitis, such as skin rashes, arthritis, and vasculitis, suggest an immune complex deposition. The presense of circulating immune complexes in sera from patients with inflammatory bowel disease has also been inferred from studies indicating that such sera inhibit antibody-dependent, cell-mediated cytotoxicity.

Antilymphocyte antibodies have been found in as many as 40 per cent of patients with ulcerative colitis and as many as 50 per cent of family members and unrelated household contacts of patients with inflammatory bowel disease. In contrast, these antibodies were found in only 4 per cent of family members without the disease.

PATHOLOGIC ASPECTS

The changes seen in ulcerative colitis are nonspecific, and most of the features may be seen in other inflammatory diseases such as shigellosis. However, the chronicity and distribution patterns are characteristic. Ulcerative colitis involves primarily the mucosa, and, unlike the segmental lesions of Crohn's disease, the mucosa is inflamed continuously, occasionally terminating at some point in the colon where the pathologic involvement gradually changes to a normal appearance over a distance of a few centimeters. The involved mucosa is red and granular and bleeds diffusely, and macroscopic lesions may progress from small petechial ulcerations to deeper linear ulcers separated by islands of inflamed mucosa. In severe cases, large areas of the colon may be denuded of mucosa.

Some of the features of ulcerative colitis result from the attempt of the inflamed colon to regenerate or heal the destroyed crypts. Regenerating crypts become diminished in number, distorted, and branching and contain goblet cells. Highly vascular granulation tissue may develop in denuded areas, and collagen may be deposited in the lamina propria with hypertrophy of the muscularis mucosae.

The alternating processes of superficial ulceration and granulation followed by re-epithelialization may lead to polypoid excrescences forming inflammatory polyps (pseudopolyps), which are not neoplastic. Long-standing disease causes hyperplasia of the muscularis mucosae and, when accompanied by postinflammatory fibrosis, shortening of the colon (Fig. 9).

CLINICAL MANIFESTATIONS AND COURSE

The most common symptoms of ulcerative colitis are rectal bleeding, diarrhea, abdominal pain, weight loss, and fever. The patient is usually in the second to fourth decade of life, and the onset of symptoms may follow an emotional experience or an upper respiratory infection.

When signs and symptoms of colonic inflammation, such as malaise, lower abdominal pain, diarrhea, and rectal bleeding, are not marked, a diagnosis of *mild* ulcerative colitis is often made. This form involves about half of all patients with ulcerative colitis and may not be diagnosed for months or years. The mortality is low, and the long-term prognosis for many of these patients is favorable. The incidence of the development of colonic cancer in patients with mild ulcerative colitis is about one seventh of that occurring in patients with the more severe forms of the disease.

Moderate ulcerative colitis defines a more abrupt onset of the disorder, typically associated with several loose and bloody bowel movements daily. In this form, which involves about 30 per cent of patients with ulcerative colitis, abdominal cramps may be severe and may awaken the patient from sleep. Low-grade fever, fatigue, and malaise may be prominent symptoms, as may some of the extracolonic manifestations, including anorexia and weight loss. Some of these patients become worse, with increasingly severe diarrhea, bleeding, and fever, and with progression of the disease the risk of colonic cancer is increased.

Severe (fulminant) ulcerative colitis often presents acutely with profuse diarrhea, rectal bleeding, and fever as high as 39°C. This form occurs in about 15 per cent of patients, and abdominal cramps, rectal urgency, and profound weakness are common presenting symptoms. Intermittent nausea, anorexia, and weight loss may also occur. The physical examination reveals an acutely ill, pale, weak, and febrile patient. Tachycardia, hypotension, and, rarely, shock may be present. Generalized abdominal tenderness with rebound indicates the onset of peritoneal irritation and suggests that the inflammatory process has extended beyond the mucosa. Absence of bowel sounds should

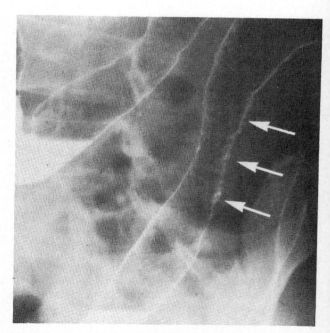

Figure 9. Air contrast barium enema in patient with ulcerative colitis and discrete "collar button" ulcers (arrow) and diffusely granular colon. (From Levin, B.: Ulcerative colitis. In Wyngaarden, J. B., and Smith, L. H., Jr. (Eds.): Cecil Textbook of Medicine, 17th ed. Philadelphia, W. B. Saunders Company, 1985.)

suggest the diagnosis of toxic colonic dilatation, which is a serious complication requiring careful exclusion.

A variety of extracolonic clinical manifestations may be associated with ulcerative colitis, including erythema nodosum, pyoderma gangrenosum, ankylosing spondylitis, peripheral arthritis, a hypercoagulable state, kidney stones, stomatitis, conjunctivitis, iritis, cholangitis, and cirrhosis.

TOXIC DILATATION OF THE COLON (TOXIC MEGACOLON)

In severe ulcerative colitis, the patient may become gravely ill with signs and symptoms of a general toxic state associated with abdominal pain, distention, rebound tenderness, and dilatation of the colon to 6 cm. or greater. In a patient with severe active colitis, toxic megacolon may be precipitated by a barium enema, potassium depletion, or anticholinergic or narcotic medication. Severe inflammation disrupts the neural and muscular elements that maintain normal colonic tone, and this allows the intraluminal pressure to expand the colon well beyond its normal diameter. Bacteria overgrow and are thought to produce toxins that intensify the complication and contribute to the hazard of peritonitis. Absorption of these toxic products into the systemic circulation further augments the toxic state. Clinical signs include fever, tachycardia, dehydration, abdominal distention and tenderness, and loss of bowel sounds. The colon is dilated as demonstrated by a plain film of the abdomen (Fig. 10), and marked leukocytosis, hypokalemia, anemia, and hypoalbuminemia are frequently present. The mortality in toxic dilatation of the colon may be as high as 20 to 30 per cent, and intensive medical therapy with early total colectomy (usually within 24 hours) is mandatory.

TREATMENT

The management of ulcerative colitis requires a comprehensive understanding of the patient's medical, nutritional, and psychological needs. Ulcerative colitis tends to run an acute relapsing course with quiescent intervals, during which the rectal mucosa may appear normal. During remission, therapy is designed to prevent a relapse, whereas with chronic active inflammation therapy is designed to suppress inflammation.

Dietary and nutritional decisions are important, and the fiber content of the diet should be reduced during periods of diarrhea. In patients intolerant to lactose, restriction of lactose intake (avoidance of dairy products) may ameliorate the diarrhea. Alternatively, bacterial lactase is commercially available and may be used to reduce the lactose content of milk to tolerable levels. Nutritionally balanced, minimal residue liquid nutritional formulas are available and are acceptable as supplements to most patients. In the severely ill, catabolic patient, parenteral alimentation may be indicated to place the bowel at rest, especially in preparing patients for colectomy.

The causes of anemia are multiple and include chronic illness, blood loss and resulting iron deficiency, and folate deficiency. Oral iron may be poorly tolerated, necessitating the use of a parenteral preparation. Folate deficiency is associated with *sulfasalazine* therapy as well as inadequate dietary intake owing to reduction in folate-containing foods such as fresh fruits and leafy vegetables.

In the patient with mild or moderate colitis, agents for controlling diarrhea are important and include diphenoxylate with atropine (Lomotil) (2.5 to 5 mg.), codeine (15 to 30 mg.), deodorized tincture of opium (6 to 10 drops), paregoric (4 to 8 ml.), and loperamide (2 to 4 mg.) before

meals and at bedtime. Tincture of belladonna (15 drops) 4 times a day and other anticholinergics may be used to decrease abdominal cramps. Extreme care must be exercised in the use of these medications in the moderately ill patient because of the risk of precipitating toxic dilatation. Other measures include attention to psychological stress, and patients should be encouraged to rest and sleep adequately. As with any other chronic illness, education is important in enabling the patient and the family to understand the nature of the disease and its effects on the individual. Formal psychiatric counseling is useful in appropriate patients.

THERAPY FOR SEVERE ACUTE COLITIS

Early recognition and diagnosis of this condition are important in reducing mortality. A choice between intensive medical treatment and immediate operative intervention may be necessary early in the course of the disease, particularly if there is evidence of perforation or peritonitis or if there is uncontrollable hemorrhage. Toxic dilatation is perhaps the most threatening type of acute severe ulcerative colitis. Failure of toxic dilatation to respond to medical management within 24 hours is ominous, since the mortality is high unless colectomy is performed. Adequate replacement of circulating volume with crystalloid, plasma, and

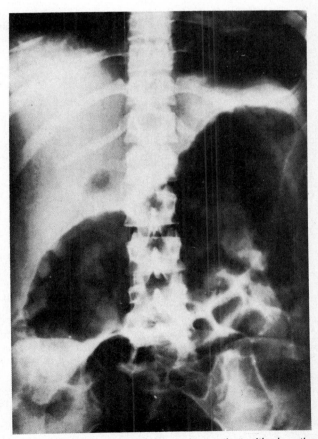

Figure 10. Plain film of the abdomen in a patient with ulcerative colitis and toxic megacolon. Note that the air in the colon silhouettes an irregular colonic mucosa. (From Cello, J. P.: Ulcerative colitis. In Sleisenger, M. H., and Fordtran, J. S. (Eds.): Gastrointestinal Disease, 3rd ed. Philadelphia, W. B. Saunders Company, 1983.)

blood is essential. Broad-spectrum antibiotics should be administered, usually chloramphenicol plus an aminoglycoside or a cephalosporin plus an aminoglycoside in combination with clindamycin. Intravenous corticosteroids are often indicated, and hydrocortisone (300 mg. intravenously daily) is effective but may cause sodium and water retention. Alternatives include intravenous prednisolone, 60 mg. daily, or methylprednisolone, 48 mg. daily, in divided doses.

Successful treatment depends on prompt recognition, early surgical consultation, and intensive resuscitative, antibacterial, and anti-inflammatory therapy. Important measures include administration of intravenous fluids, plasma, blood, antibiotics, and intravenous corticosteroids and nasogastric suction. It is essential that the patient be re-evaluated frequently and that plain abdominal films be obtained twice daily for careful follow-up. Failure to respond to maximal therapy within 24 to 48 hours indicates the need for prompt operative intervention. An abdominal colectomy with ileostomy is usually preferable, leaving the rectum in place for subsequent re-establishment of bowel continuity after recovery if there is no distal involvement.

ULCERATIVE PROCTITIS

Ulcerative proctitis is a form of ulcerative colitis limited to the rectum. Typically the patient presents with mild or moderate rectal bleeding, rectal tenesmus, and diarrhea. Symptomatic episodes recur periodically several times a year. The macroscopic and microscopic features are similar to those seen with ulcerative colitis, although only the distal 3 to 10 cm. of the rectum may be involved. On sigmoidoscopy, there is usually a sharp line of demarcation between the distal inflammatory process and the normal proximal rectal or lower sigmoid mucosa.

Therapy includes the general measures for ulcerative colitis (sulfasalazine, 2 to 4 gm. orally each day) and topical application of corticosteroids. Enemas containing 100 mg. of hydrocortisone or 40 mg. of methylprednisolone administered daily are useful, and steroid suppositories (25 mg. of hydrocortisone) or steroid foam (90 mg. of hydrocortisone per dose) may be inserted rectally once or twice daily. The response to these forms of treatment is usually very satisfactory.

PROGNOSIS OF ULCERATIVE COLITIS

The prognosis for recovery from a first attack of ulcerative colitis is quite good. The mortality, which is about 5 per cent, occurs almost exclusively in those who have a severe form of the disease involving the entire colon. The mortality is higher in patients over 60 (approximately 17 per cent) compared with patients between 20 and 59 (about 2 per cent). Toxic megacolon has a mortality of about 20 per cent, with death generally resulting from the complications of massive hemorrhage, systemic infections, pulmonary embolism, or associated cardiac disorders. Improved medical therapy and earlier colectomy for patients who do not respond to medical therapy have made the prognosis more favorable.

After the first attack, about 10 per cent of patients have a remission lasting up to 15 years or longer. An additional 10 per cent experience continuously active colitis. The remaining 75 per cent have remissions and exacerbations over the years irrespective of the severity of the initial attack. About one fifth of patients require proctocolectomy at some stage in their illness. After the first postoperative year, the long-term prognosis for patients with colectomy

for ulcerative colitis is similar to that of the general population.[9, 12, 14, 23]

Crohn's Disease (Granulomatous Colitis)

Crohn's disease is a granulomatous enteritis of unknown etiology that may involve any part of the intestinal tract. It was first reported as an inflammatory condition of the terminal ileum by Crohn and colleagues in 1932 and was originally called *regional ileitis*. Shortly thereafter, reports of similar transmural granulomatous inflammation of portions of the small and large bowel made the term *regional enteritis* seem more appropriate. A similar granulomatous inflammation of the colon, distinguishable from ulcerative colitis, was subsequently described as ileocolitis with involvement of the distal small bowel and variable segmental involvement of the colon. Ileitis is also a common designation for Crohn's disease confined to the ileum.

EPIDEMIOLOGY

As with ulcerative colitis, Crohn's disease is more common in northern Europe and the United States, less frequent in central Europe and the Middle East, and infrequent in Asia and Africa. Its prevalence is approximately half that of ulcerative colitis. However, its incidence and prevalence are rising, whereas those of ulcerative colitis are stable. Crohn's disease is diagnosed in 2 to 4 patients per 100,000 per year in the United States and northern Europe; in the United States alone it affects 50,000 to 100,000 patients, with 5000 to 10,000 new cases diagnosed each year. The incidence of Crohn's disease is approximately equal in males and females and is uncommon before age 10. The incidence peaks in the next two decades and declines later. Its incidence is low in American blacks, Indians, and Japanese but is six times more frequent in Jewish males and three times more frequent in Jewish females.

PSYCHOGENIC FACTORS

Significant emotional events have often appeared to be temporally related to the onset or exacerbation of inflammatory bowel disease, leading to the hypothesis that psychogenic factors are important in its etiology or pathogenesis. The nervous system may profoundly influence the motor, secretory, vascular, and metabolic functions of the digestive system, but it is difficult to conceive how these variables would lead to the type of segmental involvement of transmural inflammation often seen in Crohn's disease. Psychotherapy, often a most valuable adjunct in the management of patients with these chronic, debilitating, disruptive diseases, has been disappointing as primary or central therapy. It seems most likely that psychogenic factors are important only in their contribution to symptomatic exacerbations.

PATHOLOGY

The most commonly involved part of the intestine is the distal ileum and proximal right colon. The bowel is thickened and hyperemic with serosal fibrin deposition and adhesions between adjacent loops. The adjacent mesentery is commonly thickened with engorgement of the mesenteric lymphatics and enlargement of the lymph nodes. The diseased segments demonstrate a thickened wall, and the mucosa may be nearly normal or only mildly hyperemic, with elongated linear ulcerations usually in the long axis of the bowel. In more advanced disease the mucosal architecture is destroyed by multiple ulcerations, with only small islands of abnormal or regenerating mucosa remaining (see Fig. 11). Deep ulcers or clefts may extend into the thickened and edematous submucosa and sometimes through to the serosal surface.

Fistulas form readily in this setting of a transmural inflammation when deep ulceration and fissures combine with obstruction and stenosis to form a penetrating, pressure-relieving pathway to adjacent and adherent loops of bowel or other viscera and sometimes to the abdominal wall. Ileoileal, ileosigmoid, and ileocecal communications are most common, but communication with other parts of the gastrointestinal tract, including the stomach, duodenum, and gallbladder, has been reported. Fistulas may also occur from the intestine to the urinary bladder, the renal collecting system, and the female genital tract, including the fallopian tubes, uterus, and most often, the vagina.

The inflammatory process involves all layers of the bowel and consists of infiltration of lymphocytes, histiocytes, and plasma cells with characteristic aggregation to form noncaseating granulomas. Focal granulomas are found in about half the patients; in the remainder the inflammation is more diffuse.

These pathologic changes and their progression correlate with many of the important clinical manifestations of Crohn's disease. Abdominal pain and cramps reflect the narrowed lumen and partial obstruction that result from thickening of the bowel wall. Diarrhea may follow disordered mucosal absorptive-secretory function or abnormal intestinal motility. The transmural inflammation increases the adherence of loops of bowel, producing signs of peritoneal irritation and forming abdominal masses.

CLINICAL PRESENTATION

When Crohn's disease affects primarily the distal small intestine (regional enteritis), it often occurs in patients in their teens or twenties with episodic abdominal pain as the presenting symptom. The pain is often periumbilical and is occasionally associated with a low-grade fever and mild diarrhea. Such episodes often subside spontaneously but later recur with increasing frequency and severity, with the pain eventually localizing in the right lower quadrant.

The abdominal pain is often of the same character as that of partial intestinal obstruction, i.e., it is made worse by eating and it responds symptomatically to local heat and fasting. The patient may be aware of tenderness in the right lower quadrant and even a palpable mass in that region. The similarity of this presentation to acute appendicitis commonly results in abdominal exploration, and the diagnosis is made at operation. When involvement is greater, as in the syndrome of jejunoileitis, the presentation may include more diffuse abdominal pain and greater weight loss, growth retardation, and peripheral edema. In children, growth retardation and delayed sexual maturation may be the presenting clinical features in Crohn's disease.

In Crohn's colitis (*ileocolitis*) the presentation is characterized by lower abdominal crampy pain worsened by eating and diarrhea and fever. Crohn's colitis tends to be more subtle in onset than ulcerative colitis and thus may not be diagnosed until anemia or other systemic complications appear.

One third of all patients with Crohn's disease and half of those with Crohn's colitis develop perirectal or perianal fistulas presenting with pain, a mass, purulent drainage,

and fever. Perianal complications may represent communication of a fistulous tract from the small bowel along the presacral gutter to the perirectal area but more commonly are a complication of the deep, penetrating ulceration seen in Crohn's colitis of the lower colon. When drainage is impaired, local abscesses form. Extraintestinal manifestations, such as arthritis, ankylosing spondylitis, and erythema nodosum, may precede or strongly influence the presenting syndrome.

DIAGNOSIS

Crohn's disease should be suspected in patients of any age but particularly in those in the 2nd, 3rd, or 4th decade in whom there is a history of recurrent episodes of abdominal pain worsened by eating and a change in bowel habits with intermittent or persisting diarrhea. Weight loss is common. The presence of pain, tenderness, and a mass in the right lower quadrant should strongly heighten the suspicion of this diagnosis. In addition, unexplained arthritis, perianal disease, recurrent fevers, or, in children, cessation of normal growth should raise the question of Crohn's disease even if gastrointestinal symptoms are minimal.

Peripheral edema may result from protein depletion. The rectum or perianal area may have fistulas or abscess formation, and a purulent vaginal discharge may result from an enterovaginal fistula.

The diagnosis of Crohn's disease depends upon the presence of characteristic radiographic findings in the intestine. The plain film may demonstrate dilated loops of small bowel in the presence of a partial obstruction. The diagnosis depends primarily upon upper and lower intestinal barium contrast studies. Characteristic changes on the small bowel roentgenogram include segmental narrowing, obliteration of the normal mucosal pattern with or without evidence of ulceration, enteroenteric fistula formation, and the classic "string sign" of the contrast medium shown on segmental films of the terminal ileum, particularly when changes are localized to the most distal small bowel and the adjacent right colon. The changes include thickening and edema of the valvulae conniventes in the small bowel and loss of haustral markings of the large bowel. Mucosal ulcers are likely to be longitudinal. When severe ulcerative disease is present, the alternation of ulcers with regenerating mucosa produces a "cobblestone" appearance. As the disease progresses, scar formation becomes more prominent, with loss of mucosal pattern and narrowing of the segments of the involved bowel. The presence of fistulous tracts between segments of bowel can often be demonstrated by careful manipulation during the barium enema. The presence of distinctly narrowed segments of bowel need not be interpreted as clear evidence of cicatricial and irreversible obstruction, as these findings are often manifestations of severe edema and thickening of the bowel. They may improve substantially following treatment (Figs. 11 and 12). Blood studies may show an anemia, and malabsorption and vitamin deficiencies are often present. In contrast to ulcerative colitis, the rectum is involved in less than half of these patients, and proctosigmoidoscopy may reveal only the erythema nonspecifically associated with diarrhea.

TREATMENT

The general treatment of Crohn's disease without complications is directed toward alleviation of symptoms. Symptomatic remissions may occur during therapy or without treatment, but the disease usually persists with remis-

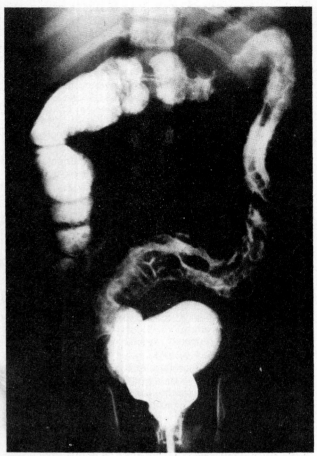

Figure 11. Barium enema in patient with Crohn's disease of the colon with multiple smooth-surfaced, ovoid, and elongated mucosal cobblestones and relatively little involvement of the rectum and right colon. (From Goldner, F. H., and Kraft, S. C.: Idiopathic inflammatory bowel disease. In Stein, J. H. (Ed.): Internal Medicine. Boston, Little, Brown and Company, 1983.)

sions and exacerbations throughout life. Operative management is necessary for the treatment of complications.

Medical Management

Medical management of Crohn's disease requires a comprehensive assessment of the clinical status of the patient. It is particularly important to determine the extent and severity of the disease, largely by radiologic and endoscopic means, and to assess the presence or absence of the complications described previously. Only with this complete information and a knowledge of the patient as an individual can an appropriate program of nutritional, pharmacologic, and supportive therapy be rationally planned.

Nutritional Treatment

Nutritional assessment is based on a careful diet history to determine the extent of caloric insufficiency, documentation of weight loss, and an analysis of nutritional status based on body measurements and laboratory tests. In prepubertal patients, assessment of growth pattern is a critical part of the evaluation. For ambulatory patients, dietary goals should be established that are adequate for the nutritional needs but that minimize stress on the in-

flamed and often narrowed segments of bowel. Evidence of lactose intolerance should be sought by history and, when possible, confirmed by blood or breath test analysis. Removal of lactose-rich foods in the lactase-deficient patient may have a prompt symptomatic benefit. In many patients with cramping and diarrhea, decreasing the intake of fiber-containing foods may be beneficial, and in those with steatorrhea a decrease of fat intake to 70 to 80 gm. per day may substantially improve diarrhea. Attention to restoration of an adequate diet must always accompany these deletions. Anemia and vitamin and mineral deficiencies should be corrected.

Sulfasalazine

Sulfasalazine (3 gm. orally each day) has been established by a national cooperative study as effective treatment for the management of exacerbations of Crohn's disease, particularly when the colon is involved; however, in combination with prednisone it was not more effective than prednisone alone in the treatment of an acute exacerbation of Crohn's disease. The effectiveness of sulfasalazine in Crohn's disease limited to the small intestine is not fully determined. Pharmacologic agents have not been proven to reduce the recurrence of Crohn's disease after clinical remission, whether spontaneous, induced by drugs, or after intestinal resection, but the use of sulfasalazine therapy is often regarded as preferable.

Antimicrobial Therapy

Despite the fact that no specific microbiologic agent has been implicated in the etiology or pathogenesis of

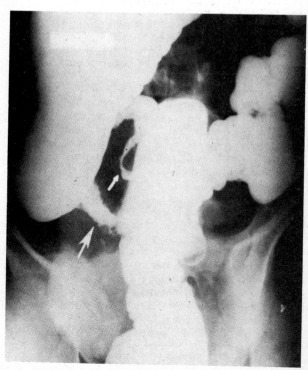

Figure 12. Barium enema in patient with Crohn's disease showing a fistula (larger arrow) between the cecum and the sigmoid colon and an irregularly narrowed distal ileum (smaller arrow). (From Goldner, F. H., and Kraft, S. C.: Idiopathic inflammatory bowel disease. In Stein, J. H. (Ed.): Internal Medicine. Boston, Little, Brown and Company, 1983.)

Crohn's disease, antibiotics are often used empirically. Parenteral antibiotics are commonly given to the acutely ill patient with fever and signs of peritoneal irritation and at times as an adjunct in programs for bowel rest or with corticosteroid therapy. The use of antibiotics in ambulatory patients with Crohn's disease has yielded promising results, but these observations need controlled trials for confirmation.

Corticosteroid Therapy

The rationale for corticosteroid therapy in patients with Crohn's disease, similar to that in patients with ulcerative colitis, is to suppress inflammation as well as the coexisting systemic manifestations of inflammation. The decision to use corticosteroids in Crohn's disease should be made judiciously. Prednisone in doses of 0.25 to 0.75 mg. per kg. for 4 months has been shown to be effective in the treatment of exacerbations of Crohn's disease, but it is questionable whether prolonged corticosteroid use *prevents* exacerbations of the disease. In prepubertal patients, it is particularly important to give corticosteroids on an alternate-day basis if at all possible to reduce growth retardation, and such a regimen should be used when possible in adult patients. The dose of corticosteroids should be steadily tapered as symptoms permit.

Immunosuppressive Therapy

The possible role of immunologic factors in the etiology of Crohn's disease or in the pathogenesis of some of its manifestations and complications has led to the use of immunosuppressive agents. Azathioprine has been used with reportedly encouraging results in the general management of these patients, but such studies have been largely uncontrolled. In Crohn's disease, as well as in ulcerative colitis, daily doses of 1.0 to 1.5 mg. per kg. have permitted the reduction of corticosteroid doses without symptomatic exacerbation in controlled trials. As a single agent, however, azathioprine demonstrated no superiority over placebo in a 4-month trial.

The patient hospitalized with symptomatic exacerbation of Crohn's disease presents a different management problem. More than half of such patients suffer from deficiencies of calories, proteins, certain vitamins, and minerals. They have an inadequate diet limited by the worsening of intestinal symptoms after eating, and the logical approach in such patients is to place the inflamed and narrowed bowel "at rest" by removing the stimulus of food intake on intestinal secretion and motility. Many patients derive symptomatic benefit from partial rather than total bowel rest with the delivery of nutrients enterally in the form of low residue–defined formula diets. Rarely can adequate nutritional maintenance be achieved by the oral intake of formula diets owing to limitations of palatability. The use of small-caliber nasogastric tubes for continuous or intermittent drip provides a well-tolerated alternative means of delivery that is often associated with a marked decrease in bacterial flora, stool frequency, and symptoms. In more severely ill patients and in those who cannot tolerate enteral feeding or who lack adequate intestine for absorption, total parenteral alimentation is being used with increasing frequency.

For the severely malnourished patient, total parenteral nutrition can achieve nutritional repletion during the period of diagnostic testing, to prepare the nutritionally depleted patient for operation, and when necessary for maintenance through the postoperative period. For the patient with a short bowel disability following major intestinal resection, total parenteral nutrition can be used for prolonged nutritional support at home until the adaptive responses permit oral nutritional maintenance. In patients with fistulas, total parenteral nutrition and bowel rest may lead to closure of the fistulas, with sustained remission in 20 to 50 per cent of patients.

In granulomatous colitis, operative therapy is used as conservatively as possible. Unlike ulcerative colitis, in which colectomy with proctectomy and permanent ileostomy are curative, no operation cures granulomatous colitis with certainty. Recurrence following segmental colon resection will occur in about half the patients. The small bowel may be or may become involved, and fistula formation is common. Therefore, operation is reserved for complications such as intestinal obstruction, protracted bloody diarrhea, perforation, or fistula formation. However, the amount of colon resected should be minimal and consistent with achieving the necessary objectives (Table 3).[8, 12]

TABLE 3. *A Comparison of the Clinical and Pathologic Features of Crohn's Granulomatous Colitis and Ulcerative Colitis*

Feature	Crohn's Colitis	Ulcerative Colitis
Intestinal		
Malaise, fever	Common	Uncommon
Rectal bleeding	Intermittent about 50%	Common
Abdominal tenderness	Common	May be present
Abdominal mass	Very common (especially with ileocolitis)	Not present
Abdominal pain	Very common	Unusual
Abdominal wall and internal fistulas	Very common	Rare
Endoscopic		
Rectal disease	About 20%	Almost 100%
Diffuse, continuous symmetric involvement	Uncommon	Very common
Aphthous or linear ulcers	Common	Rare
Friability	Rare	Rare
Radiologic		
Continuous disease	Rare	Very common
Ileal involvement	Very common	Rare
Asymmetry	Very common	Rare
Strictures	Common	Rare
Fistulas	Very common	Rare
Pathologic		
Discontinuity	Common	Rare
Rectal involvement	Rare	Common
Intense vascularity	Rare	Common
Ileal involvement	Common	Nonexistent
Transmural involvement	Common	Rare
Lymphoid aggregates	Common	Uncommon
Crypt abscesses	Rare	Very common
Granulomas	Common	Rare
Linear clefts	Common	Rare
Surgical treatment	Subtotal or total colectomy, rectum frequently preserved	Proctocolectomy with ileostomy

Absolute Indications for Operation in Inflammatory Colon Diseases

Absolute indications for operative treatment include perforation, hemorrhage, obstruction, development of carcinoma, and acute fulminating disease with or without toxic megacolon. Free perforation of the colon usually occurs in association with toxic megacolon and is much more common in patients with ulcerative colitis. Such perforations may be single or multiple, and omentum may be adherent to the colon at the site of an impending perforation and should not be dissected from the bowel wall; rather, the adherent omentum should be resected with the colon. In some patients, the signs and symptoms of colonic perforation are present, but no free perforation can be found at operation. The purulent exudate in the peritoneal cavity is probably secondary to acute, diffuse serosal inflammation developing with granulomatous colitis. Perforating lesions that produce an abscess or fistula are characteristic of granulomatous disease of the colon because of the transmural extension of the process. Fistulas are usually an indication for operative intervention.

Repeat and massive hemorrhage may occur in patients with ulcerative colitis but seldom in patients with granulomatous colitis. It may occur in association with an acute attack and not necessarily in disease of long duration. In most patients, bleeding may be managed by blood transfusions, but when uncontrolled hemorrhage develops, urgent proctocolectomy and ileostomy are necessary.

Obstruction secondary to inflammatory disease of the colon is seldom acute. Chronic obstructive symptoms may develop from stricture formation, which occurs in patients with granulomatous colitis, and a severe stricture causing obstruction arouses suspicion of cancer.

Carcinoma and Inflammatory Colonic Diseases

If carcinoma is present, resection of the tumor is necessary. Studies indicate that the risk of cancer is very low during the first 10 years after the onset of ulcerative colitis but increases thereafter, reaching 40 per cent after 25 years. MacDougall's studies indicate that this high risk of colon cancer is found only in patients with *diffuse* disease involving the entire colon. When ulcerative colitis is limited to the distal end of the colon the risk of cancer is the same as that in the general population.

It has been thought that the incidence of colon cancer in granulomatous colitis is no greater than that in the general population, but in a large series the incidence of colorectal cancer was 20 times greater in patients with Crohn's enteritis than in a control population. All the patients with cancer of the colon in this report had histologically confirmed, coexistent granulomatous colitis, and care was taken by the investigators to exclude any patients with chronic ulcerative colitis.

The onset of ulcerative colitis in childhood is associated with a high risk of later colonic cancer. These younger patients have an opportunity to live long enough to enter the high-risk category of those with disease longer than 10 years. In addition, their disease is more likely to involve the *entire* colon, further increasing the risk. In one study, 46 of 401 children with ulcerative colitis developed carcinoma of the colon (Figs. 13 and 14).

Colon cancer in this situation may be difficult to recognize. The lesions are often multicentric and invade the bowel wall and tend to produce infiltrating lesions that simulate fibrous strictures in the colon. Aggressive surgical

management (proctocolectomy with ileostomy) can lead to long-term survival. Hilton reported a 40 per cent 5-year survival in patients with ulcerative colitis and colon cancer.

Indications for Elective Operative Procedures

Relative indications for surgical treatment include failure to respond to medical management, growth retardation in children, and recurring disease in the elderly.[12] There has been increasing acceptance of permanent ileostomy in the management of symptomatic disease because of improved patient education and availability of trained therapists in managing the ileostomy. The most frequent indication for elective operation is failure of symptoms to respond to medical management. Intractable diarrhea with its restrictions on the patient's occupation and social life and the side effects of anemia, malnutrition, water and electrolyte depletion, and repeated hospitalizations for treatment of exacerbations of disease finally force the patient to seek relief by operative management. Children with intractable colitis have the additional problem of possible growth retardation. Elderly patients (over 60 years of age) have an average annual mortality rate of almost 5 per cent when managed medically. Elective operation in the elderly can reduce the high risk associated with emergency operation and prevent the complications of inflam-

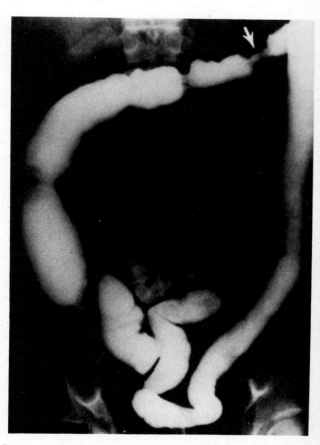

Figure 13. Carcinoma associated with ulcerative colitis. Barium enema showing diminished haustrations, generalized narrowing, and a malignant stricture (arrow) in the distal transverse colon. (From Goldner, F. H., and Kraft, S. C.: Idiopathic inflammatory bowel disease. In Stein, J. H. (Ed.): Internal Medicine. Boston, Little, Brown and Company, 1983.)

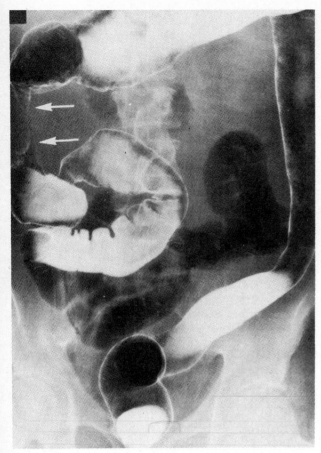

Figure 14. Air contrast barium enema in patient with chronic ulcerative colitis illustrating a haustral, diffuse mucosal granularity and carcinoma in the ascending colon (arrows). (From Levin, B.: Ulcerative colitis. In Wyngaarden, J. B., and Smith, L. H., Jr. (Eds.): Cecil Textbook of Medicine, 17th ed. Philadelphia, W. B. Saunders Company, 1985.)

matory colitis. The choice of the correct operative procedure requires differentiation between ulcerative and granulomatous colitis. Patients with ulcerative colitis can be cured of inflammatory bowel disease by proctocolectomy. Except for possible complications related to the ileostomy, these patients have an excellent prognosis.

Since granulomatous colitis tends to be segmental, the resection of localized disease with end-to-end anastomosis is often possible. It is important that both proximal and distal ends of the bowel be free of gross disease to reduce complications from disruption of the anastomosis. Granulomatous colitis limited to the distal colon and rectum is best managed by abdominoperineal resection and a permanent colostomy. There is risk of producing impotence in males, but this is reduced by maintenance of the dissection close to the bowel wall. Evaluation of surgical therapy is also confused by the variety of operative procedures used in the treatment of granulomatous colitis. Unlike ulcerative colitis, which is cured by proctocolectomy, Crohn's disease may occur in other parts of the gastrointestinal tract after operation for granulomatous colitis. Nevertheless, the prognosis in patients with Crohn's disease limited to the colon (granulomatous colitis) is better than that in patients with regional enteritis. Goligher reported a recurrence rate of 20 per cent after partial colectomy and anastomosis for granulomatous colitis. Most physicians adopt a selective

and conservative approach in the operative treatment of granulomatous colitis and accept the risk of ileal and colonic recurrences. Satisfactory rehabilitation may be anticipated in all survivors after single-stage total proctocolectomy for ulcerative colitis. The formation of a continent ileostomy or the construction of an ileorectal pull-through anastomosis to preserve the sphincter and avoid ileostomy is being done with increasing frequency and improved results.[12, 16, 18]

POLYPS

A polyp is a lesion that arises from the mucosal surface and protrudes into the lumen (Fig. 15). Polyps are usually defined pathologically as overgrowths of epithelial tissue that may be either hyperplastic or neoplastic and benign or malignant. They appear on barium enema as negative shadows in the lumen and can be seen during proctosigmoidoscopy or colonoscopy. Polyps may be single or multiple, *pedunculated* (on a stalk) or *sessile* (flat, without stalk). They may be sporadic in occurrence or part of a dominantly transmitted familial polyposis syndrome. Although polyps may cause symptoms, it is their potential for malignant transformation that is of greatest concern.

Relation of Colonic Polyps to Carcinoma

The evidence that benign adenomas may become malignant is compelling. The epidemiology of adenocarcinomas and adenomas of the colon is similar, and carcinomas occur in the same anatomic distribution as do the adenomas in the colon. The risk for colorectal cancer is high in patients with a prior history of adenomas but is lower if the adenomas are removed. As adenomas grow in size, the frequency of cancer increases. Residual adenomatous tissue can sometimes be found in colorectal cancers on pathologic examination. Finally, the association of cancer and adenomas is particularly high in the heritable disorders of the colon, in which it is clearly established that adenocarcinomas arise from previously benign adenomas. Therefore, it seems likely that in most instances colorectal cancer arises from an antecedent benign adenoma.

The premalignant nature of adenomas is related to both size and histology. The frequency of cancer and adenomas is 1 per cent in adenomas less than 1 cm. in size, 10 per cent in adenomas between 1 and 2 cm., and as high as 50 per cent in some reports of adenomas greater than 2 cm. The relation of cancer to adenomas is much greater with *villous* components. Cancer in adenomas is usually well differentiated and occurs most commonly in the tip of the adenoma without invasion. These are focal cancers (*in situ*) and are not immediately dangerous. Less commonly, cancers in adenomas invade the muscularis mucosae and therefore have the potential to grow down the stalk, invade lymphatics, involve adjacent lymph nodes, and ultimately metastasize.

Clinical Manifestations

Most polyps are usually asymptomatic. When symptoms occur, bleeding is the most frequent, and, when very large, polyps can cause abdominal pain from partial intestinal obstruction. Villous adenomas may occasionally induce watery diarrhea, leading to severe potassium depletion or an excessive secretion of mucus with loss of sufficient protein, producing hypoalbuminemia, a rare cause of pro-

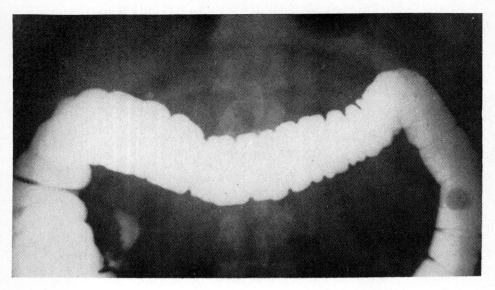

Figure 15. Polyp of the colon showing a filling defect on barium enema. (From Block, G. E., and Liechty, R. D.: Large intestine. In Liechty, R. D., and Soper, R. T. (Eds.): Synopsis of Surgery. St. Louis, The C. V. Mosby Company, 1980.)

tein-losing enteropathy. Since benign polyps retain their potential to become malignant, they should be removed.

Colonoscopic Polypectomy and Excision

Pedunculated polyps of any size and sessile polyps smaller than 2 cm. can usually be removed by cautery snare with the colonoscope. Although larger sessile polyps can be excised segmentally via the colonoscope, this approach is probably not ideal because many already are cancerous and the risk of complications during removal increases significantly. Since there is also risk involved in laparotomy and excision, each patient must be considered individually.

After endoscopic polypectomy, the patient must be followed periodically. Usually repeat colonoscopy is performed 1 year later and then approximately every 3 years thereafter to seek new or additional lesions. If the patient has multiple adenomas, colonoscopy is done annually for several years.

If laparotomy is required for excision, following exposure of the colon, polyps are palpated and the wall of the colon is incised at the site of the polyp. The polyp is then removed and the colotomy closed. Segmental colectomy is rarely necessary, and even when malignant change is found in the tip of a polyp if it has not penetrated the muscularis mucosae no further procedure need be done. If the cancer has penetrated the muscularis mucosae and lymphatic invasion has been demonstrated, if the cancer is poorly differentiated, or if it has extended down to the margin of excision at colonoscopy, follow-up laparotomy with segmental resection as used routinely for adenocarcinomas of the colon is appropriate (Table 4).[20, 25]

HERITABLE DISORDERS

Familial Polyposis

Familial polyposis of the colon is an autosomal dominant trait characterized by multiple adenomas of the large intestine and occasionally the ileum. It occurs approximately once in 8000 births, and hundreds to thousands of polyps develop through the entire colon beginning in childhood. Nearly all patients with familial polyposis develop carcinoma of the colon by age 40, so subtotal colectomy should be performed early in adult life in affected persons. An intensive survey of other family members must be conducted, but a few cases occur without family history and probably represent spontaneous mutations.

Gardner's Syndrome

Gardner's syndrome is a dominantly transmitted disorder characterized by the triad of adenomas of the colon, bone tumors (osteomas), and soft tissue tumors (lipomas, sebaceous cysts, fibromas, fibrosarcomas). Other associated features include retroperitoneal fibrosis, supranumerary teeth, and a tendency toward the development of carcinoma of the thyroid, adrenal gland, and duodenum in the region of the ampulla of Vater. There may be osteosclerosis of the skull in addition to the osteomas of the mandible and the maxillary regions. The colonic polyps resemble those of familial polyposis and have the same high risk for

TABLE 4. *Comparison of Polyps of the Large Bowel*

Type	Frequency	Site	Malignancy	Treatment
Adenomatous	Most common polyp; 10% of all adults; increases with age	Recto-sigmoid 70%	Probable malignant potential	Endoscopy and biopsy excision; excise larger upper colonic polyps
Villous	Relatively common in old age	Recto-sigmoid 80%	About 25% malignant	Total biopsy; radical operation if malignant
Juvenile	Common in first decade; rare in adults	Chiefly rectum	Never	Excise only for bleeding, intussusception, diagnosis
Hereditary familial	Very rare	Scattered	100%	Total or near-total colectomy
Peutz-Jeghers	Very rare	Chiefly small	Very rare	Excise for bleeding or obstruction

malignancy. The treatment is subtotal colectomy and careful survey of other members of the family (Fig. 16).

Turcot Syndrome

Turcot syndrome represents the rare association of adenomas of the colon with a variety of tumors of the central nervous system. The polyps have a high frequency of malignant transformation. The central nervous system lesions have included medulloblastomas, ependymomas, and glioblastomas. The mode of transmission is thought to be autosomal recessive, although this is unclear.

Peutz-Jeghers Syndrome

Peutz-Jeghers syndrome is a rare familial disorder with autosomal dominant transmission characterized by multiple intestinal polyposis and mucocutaneous pigmentation. The polyps, which occur in the small intestine, large intestine, and stomach, are mostly hamartomas rather than true adenomas and as such have a low potential for malignant transformation. It is estimated that 2 to 3 per cent of patients with this syndrome develop adenocarcinoma of the intestinal tract, with the small intestine being more frequently involved than the colon. Pigmentation is particularly marked in the buccal mucosa, the hard and soft palate, the lips, the soles of the feet, the dorsum of the hands, and around the mouth and nostrils. More rarely exostoses, ovarian tumors, and polyps of the bladder occur. Removal of gastric and small bowel polyps is performed only for complications such as bleeding or intestinal obstruction. True adenomas can occur in the colon in this disorder and can usually be removed endoscopically (see Fig. 16).

Juvenile Polyposis

Juvenile polyposis refers to a familial syndrome with autosomal dominant transmission characterized by hamartomatous polyps in the colon and rectum and, to a lesser extent, in the small intestine and stomach. Symptoms usually begin in the first decade of life, with bleeding, diarrhea, and abdominal pain. There are no extraintestinal manifestations. There appears to be an increased incidence of carcinoma in the intestine in families with generalized juvenile polyposis, probably from true adenomas that occur with higher frequencies in these families.

Cronkhite-Canada Syndrome

Cronkhite-Canada syndrome refers to the rare association of generalized intestinal polyposis, dystrophy of the finger nails, alopecia, and cutaneous hyperpigmentation. The polyps are hamartomas, and no familial association has been clearly established.[3, 11, 24]

COLORECTAL MALIGNANCIES

Colorectal cancer is a tremendous health problem in most affluent countries. In the United States it is the second most frequent site for a primary malignant neoplasm, with approximately 140,000 new cases and 60,000 deaths expected in 1986. About 98 per cent of these patients have adenocarcinomas.

Etiology

Numerous studies suggest that the etiology of colorectal cancer is multifactorial, and a two-stage model of carcinogenesis appears applicable. The first step in this model is *initiation* and the second step is *promotion*. Two major views on the morphologic counterparts of this process are currently held. The first suggests that colon carcinoma develops through the stages of adenomatous polyp and noninvasive carcinoma. The second holds that *de novo* dysplastic changes occur in the colon mucosa and that these lead in the later stages to noninvasive and invasive cancers. Whichever model is preferred, both fit well with a multifactorial etiology and with the two-stage model of carcinogenesis. Both models allow for possible genetic susceptibility, and both imply that the factors that alter the risk of colon cancer may differ, depending upon the developmental stage of the process.

At present, little is known about the process of initiation in colon cancer. A viral etiologic basis is possible, given recent results with oncogenes and earlier studies showing cytomegalovirus in malignant colonic tissue. Other possibilities include various protein metabolites, including

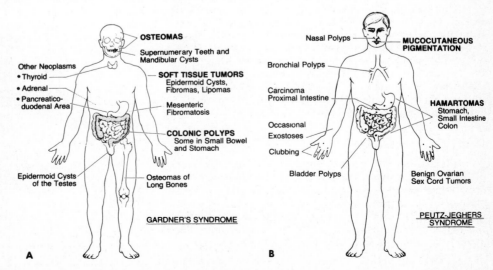

Figure 16. A, Schematic representation of Gardner's syndrome. The triad of colonic polyposis, bone tumors, and soft tissue tumors (heavy print) is the primary feature. Others are shown in lighter print. B, Schematic presentation of the Peutz-Jeghers syndrome. Mucocutaneous pigmentation and benign gastrointestinal polyposis (heavy print) are the primary features. Light print shows the secondary features. (From Boland, C. R., and Kim, Y. S.: Colonic polyps and the gastrointestinal polyposis syndrome. In Sleisenger, M. H., and Fordtran, J. S. (Eds.): Gastrointestinal Disease, 3rd ed. Philadelphia, W. B. Saunders Company, 1983.)

such agents as ammonia, volatile phenols, or tryptophan, and N-nitroso compounds. Carcinogens may also be the result of certain modes of cooking, particularly frying and grilling meat and fish. However, none is well established in humans as a carcinogen.

Much more is known about the process of promotion in colon carcinogenesis. Global epidemiologic studies have revealed that colorectal cancer is much more prevalent in North America and most developed countries than in South American, African, and Asian countries. Studies on migrants have demonstrated that first-generation migrants from low- to high-incidence areas of colorectal carcinoma acquire a higher risk for this disease. This strongly suggests that cancer of the colon is associated with environmental factors. Of the many environmental factors studied to date, those related to diet appear to be the most important. Two major theories of dietary etiology predominate, but neither theory fully explains the available data. The first theory relates to dietary fiber and the second to dietary fat.

DIETARY FIBER

Burkitt supports a strong association between the low incidence of colorectal cancer in the South African Bantu and a diet high in fiber content, which results in rapid transit time and large bulk in the stools. He suggested that a rapid transit time reduces the time the actual carcinogens, or their precursors, are in contact with the colonic mucosa. However, there is little evidence that a decreased transit time reduces bacterial action on colon contents, and studies of populations with widely varying incidences of colon cancer show no differences in bowel transit times. Subsequent epidemiologic studies have been contradictory. For example, Mendeloff concluded that a diet high in fiber appeared to decrease the frequency of cancer, whereas Drasar and Irving found no relationship between dietary fiber and cancer of the colon. Many other studies have been reviewed by Zaridze, who concludes that the true role of fiber in preventing colon carcinogenesis is uncertain.

DIETARY FAT

A correlation between the intake of animal fat and large bowel cancer has been made in several studies and is currently the most widely accepted linkage between diet and cancer. The National Academy of Sciences has recommended that the diet of citizens in the United States be modified to contain less fat as a prudent preventive measure. However, epidemiologic studies have not provided certain support for this association, and most cross-sectional correlation studies, but not all case-control studies, have shown a positive correlation between a high-fat and -meat diet and an increased frequency of colon cancer. Moreover, the best recent studies, using very precise methods for measuring the amount of fat and protein in the diet of study populations, failed to show the expected correlation between colon cancer and fat-protein comsumption.

ALTERATION IN COLONIC MICROFLORA

Hill postulated that the nature of the bacterial flora of the bowel can be determined by the diet and that diet also provides substrate for any bacteria-induced change of normal bowel contents to carcinogens. Since people living in areas with high incidences of colon cancer have high fecal concentrations of bile acids—both normal and degraded—he thought that the capacity of the bacteria to desaturate the bile acid nucleus might be an important factor in carcinogenesis.

Some investigators have noted changes in the microflora of subjects at high risk, whereas others have not found significant differences in fecal microflora of individuals consuming different diets. For instance, Goldberg and coworkers compared the fecal microflora of Seventh-Day Adventists, who have a very low incidence of colon cancer and are often vegetarians, with that of individuals consuming a general Western diet. No statistically significant differences were identified between the fecal microflora of the two groups.

DIETARY SUGAR

The elevated consumption of refined sugar has been noted as a possible etiologic agent in some populations with a high incidence of cancer. However, in Argentina, where the incidence of colon cancer is relatively high, the consumption of refined carbohydrates is low, and a positive correlation between intake of sugar and colon cancer is not uniform on a worldwide basis.

Epidemiology and Biology

Several factors appear to have a significant influence on the incidence of colorectal malignancies and will be discussed separately (Table 5).

AGE

In the general population, the incidence of colon cancer begins to rise significantly after the age of 40 to 45 and increases each decade thereafter by a factor of about two until it peaks at age 75. This may well result from the action of carcinogenic materials on colonic cells over an increasing period. The risk is about the same for males and females over 40 years, and when colon cancer occurs before the age of 40 it is usually in conjunction with some other risk factors, especially familial.

POLYPS

Although the question of whether or not polyps are premalignant is controversial, there is a higher incidence of colon cancer in patients with polyps. It seems logical to consider patients with adenomatous polyps or villous adenomas to be at higher risk for colon cancer, since more evidence suggests that most carcinomas rather than arising *de novo* evolve from adenomatous tissue. (See previous section on polyps.)

TABLE 5. Factors Predisposing to Colorectal Cancer

Family History	Past History	Associated Disease	Age
Juvenile polyps	Colon cancer or polyps	Ulcerative colitis	Over 40
Colon cancer or polyps	Female genital or breast cancer	Granulomatous syndrome	
Familial polyposis syndrome	.	Peutz-Jeghers syndrome	
		Familial polyposis	

HIGH-RISK GROUPS

At Memorial Sloan-Kettering Hospital, the frequency of colorectal cancer patients with previous (3.6 per cent) or simultaneous (1.9 per cent) colon cancer was 5.5 per cent. The annual incidence of multiple primary cancers was 3.5 per 1000. The highest risk for a second colon cancer was a cecal lesion. The presence of adenomatous polyps in the resected specimen increased the risk of future colon cancer to six times that seen in the general population.

Families with a high incidence of carcinoma in other anatomic sites, such as endometrium, ovary, and breast, have a greater than normal risk of malignancy. In addition, the specific risk of cancer of the colon in relatives of patients with colon cancer is three times that seen in the normal population. If a family member has multiple cancers of the colon, the onset of colon cancer in his relatives occurs 5 to 10 years earlier than would be expected.

ASSOCIATED DISEASES AND COLON CANCER

Almost all patients with familial polyposis, a condition with an autosomal dominant mode of inheritance with 80 per cent penetrance, develop colon cancer unless colectomy is performed. Another high-risk group consists of patients with Gardner's syndrome, in whom adenomatous polyps develop in the colon and are associated with soft tissue and lung tumors. Patients with Turcot syndrome (central nervous system tumors) or Oldfield's syndrome (extensive sebaceous cysts) are at high risk to develop colon cancer. Peutz-Jeghers syndrome can occasionally be associated with cancers of the stomach, ileum, and duodenum. Patients with juvenile polyposis are also at high risk for cancer, and their relatives are more likely to develop adenomatous polyps and colon cancer. (See previous section.)

Ulcerative colitis is frequently associated with later development of colon cancer. When age is not considered, the likelihood of developing colon cancer is five to ten times higher in colitis patients than in the general population. The risk begins to rise about 10 years after the onset of the disease, and it is estimated at 20 to 30 per cent at 20 years. The risk doubles in those patients in whom the onset of colitis occurs before the age of 25. In patients who develop colorectal cancers, the average age of onset is earlier and the cancer tends to be multicentric and often highly malignant, developing during an asymptomatic period. Because of this high risk, patients with long-standing ulcerative colitis are usually advised to undergo prophylactic colectomy. For those who refuse colectomy, vigorous surveillance, including periodic rectal biopsies to identify dysplastic changes, is indicated. Granulomatous colitis (Crohn's disease) is also generally thought to be premalignant, especially when the age of onset is before 21 years, but the order of magnitude of risk is less than that in ulcerative colitis.

Pathology and Classification

The vast majority of primary colorectal malignant neoplasms are adenocarcinomas, but other neoplasms rarely may occur. Lymphomas may arise from lymphoid tissue within the alimentary tract and soft tissue sarcomas from mesodermal tissue within the tract. The rare occurrence of squamous cell carcinomas within the colon is less easily explained (Table 6).

In the past, it was stated that half of colorectal carci-

TABLE 6. *World Health Organization Classification of Malignant Neoplasms of the Colon and Rectum**

I. Epithelial Tumors
  A. Benign
    1. Adenoma
      a. Tubular (adenomatous polyp)
      b. Villous
      c. Tubulovillous
    2. Adenomatosis (adenomatous polyposis coli)
  B. Malignant
    1. Adenocarcinoma
    2. Mucinous adenocarcinoma
    3. Signet-ring cell carcinoma
    4. Squamous cell carcinoma
    5. Adenosquamous carcinoma
    6. Undifferentiated carcinoma
    7. Unclassified carcinoma
II. Carcinoid Tumors
  A. Argentaffin
  B. Nonargentaffin
  C. Composite
III. Nonepithelial Tumors
  A. Benign
    1. Leiomyoma
    2. Leiomyoblastoma
    3. Neurilemmoma (schwannoma)
    4. Lipoma
      Lipomatosis
    5. Vascular tumors
      a. Hemangioma
      b. Lymphangioma
    6. Others
  B. Malignant
    1. Leiomyosarcoma
    2. Others
IV. Hematopoietic and Lymphoid Neoplasms
V. Unclassified Tumors
VI. Secondary Tumors
VII. Tumorlike Lesions
  A. Hamartomas
    1. Peutz-Jeghers polyp and polyposis
    2. Juvenile polyp and polyposis
  B. Heterotopia
    1. Gastric
  C. Hyperplastic (metaplastic) polyp
  D. Benign lymphoid polyp and polyposis
  E. Inflammatory polyp
  F. Colitis cystica profunda
  G. Endometriosis
VIII. Epithelial Atypia in Ulcerative Colitis

*From Morson, B. C., et al.: Histological Classification of Tumours. No. 15: Histological typing of intestinal tumours. Geneva, World Health Organization, 1976 and Sobin, L. H., et al.: A Coded Compendium of the International Classification of Tumours, Geneva, World Health Organization, 1978, p. 11.

nomas could be diagnosed by digital examination of the rectum (8 cm.) and two thirds by sigmoidoscopy (25 cm.). In recent years, however, there has been a change in the distribution of colon neoplasms to the more proximal colon. Nevertheless, 70 to 80 per cent of these lesions are still located below the mid-descending colon.

A variety of histopathologic factors may influence prognosis. Annular lesions narrowing the bowel circumference lead to a shorter survival than do lesions that involve only a portion of bowel wall. The shape of the tumor may be significant, and nearly twice as many patients with polypoid or projecting neoplasms survived 5 years as compared with infiltrating growths. In general, the size of the tumor has less bearing on survival than do nodal metastases.

The location of the tumor has been of variable significance, although it is generally thought that those on the right colon have a more favorable prognosis than those on the left colon.

Histologic features related to prognosis include grade of tumor, lymphatic, vascular, and perineural infiltration, and the presence or absence of an inflammatory response. Infiltration of the tumor by eosinophils may represent an especially good prognostic sign. In histologic grading, as in the system of Broders, most observers utilize either a numbering system from 1 to 4, with larger numbers indicating less differentiation, or a series of modifying terms designating tumors as well, moderately, or poorly differentiated. The percentage of cells showing differentiation and the arrangement of cells to form glandular structures or tubules are usually used as criteria of differentiation. Poorly differentiated signet-ring cells and mucinous carcinomas carry a less favorable prognosis than more differentiated neoplasms.

Clinical Features and Diagnosis

The clinical features associated with colorectal carcinomas relate to tumor size and location. Large, exophytic bulky tumors occur more commonly in the right colon, with its large diameter and fluid contents, and result in symptoms of abdominal pain, bleeding, and weight loss rather than obstruction. The pain is vague and dull and may be confused with gallbladder disease or peptic ulcer. Anemia may be present. In the left colon, with its smaller diameter and semisolid or solid contents, tumors are more often infiltrating or annular and cause obstructive symptoms, changes in bowel habits, or bleeding. Gas pains, decrease in stool caliber, and increased use of laxatives are common complaints.

The diagnosis of colorectal carcinomas, as in all malignancies, requires a high index of suspicion and diligent follow-up of all symptoms, especially in high-risk patients.

Test for Fecal Blood

The best test for screening asymptomatic subjects is one using hemoccult guaiac-impregnated paper. It is essential that the patient be on a high-fiber, red meat–free diet for at least 48 hours. Two samples are taken from each of three stool specimens, and the slides are developed within 3 days. If only *one* of the six slides is positive, the patient is evaluated further. The advantages of this test include low cost, ease of performance, and a relatively low false-positive rate (1 per cent).

Proctosigmoidoscopy

This is an important diagnostic aid in the follow-up of lesions seen in other tests and in the symptomatic patient. The cost effectiveness is low in the asymptomatic patient, however, since the results of prospective surveys reveal only about one cancer in every 667 patients examined. However, the routine removal of adenomatous polyps by proctosigmoidoscopy, as indicated earlier, has been shown to decrease the incidence of subsequent cancer. Polyps have been reported in 4 to 9 per cent of patients over 40. Newer flexible instruments have been developed that provide much better patient tolerance and a marked increase in diagnostic accuracy.

Barium Enema

The full-column barium enema examination has been reported to fail to identify one fifth to one fourth of all colon cancers and two fifths of all polypoid lesions. However, the air contrast barium enema will detect almost all colonic lesions of at least 5 mm. in diameter and must be considered the radiologic procedure of choice. Contraindications include acute, severe, inflammatory bowel disease, suspected perforation, and recent bowel wall biopsy.

Colonoscopy

Colonoscopy following air contrast barium enema is frequently used, and lesions can be detected and biopsied or excised or both. The two techniques are complementary and quite useful. Limitations include failure to reach or fully examine the splenic flexure (10 per cent), the hepatic flexure (15 per cent), or the cecum (20 per cent). Asymptomatic patients with well-documented occult blood in the stool and symptomatic patients should have a colonoscopic examination of the entire colon, even with normal sigmoidoscopic findings and normal or equivocal barium enemas. The importance of this is illustrated by the results of a series of colonoscopic examinations performed in 146 patients who had air contrast barium enemas suggesting benign polypoid disease. Thirty-six (25 per cent) did not have a neoplastic lesion at the suspected site. Seven of the 36 (19 per cent) had unsuspected, benign polypoid adenomas elsewhere, and 4 (11 per cent) had benign neoplastic lesions at the suspected area and unsuspected malignant lesions elsewhere. Of the remaining 110 who had neoplastic lesions correctly identified at the suspected site, 17 (15 per cent) were either adenocarcinomas or neoplastic polyps with invasive cancer.

Other Tests

Cytologic techniques on the stool are well developed and accurate. However, the necessity for meticulous, time-consuming bowel preparation and lavage has limited their applicability and probably will continue to do so. Preoperative carcinoembryonic antigen (CEA) values often correlate with tumor burden and prognosis, but the usefulness of this information remains to be determined. Conventional tests, such as complete blood count, blood biochemical panel, chest x-ray, liver scan, and, in selected cases, an intravenous pyelogram, give information concerning the extent of disease that is necessary for appropriate surgical intervention. Other biochemical, immunologic, and radiologic tests are of uncertain value in most cases.

Staging

The early pathologic staging system introduced by Dukes more than 50 years ago divides colorectal malignancies into three groups. Those lesions confined to the bowel wall but not penetrating the muscularis were designated A; lesions penetrating the muscularis into surrounding fat or adventitia were designated B; and lesions with positive lymph node involvement were designated C. Numerous modifications of this system have been published subsequently, including the addition of a so-called Dukes D stage for patients with metastatic disease. Some of these variations are compared in Figure 17. Most cooperative study groups currently use the Aston-Collier modification of the Dukes system.

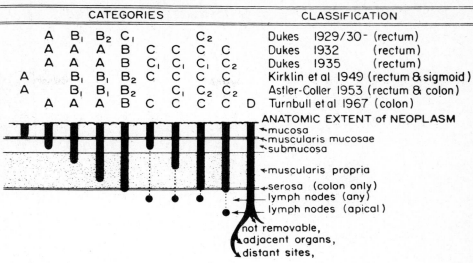

CATEGORIES	CLASSIFICATION
A B₁ B₂ C₁ C₂	Dukes 1929/30⁻ (rectum)
A A A B C C C C	Dukes 1932 (rectum)
A A A B C₁ C₁ C₁ C₂	Dukes 1935 (rectum)
A B₁ B₁ B₂ C C C C	Kirklin et al 1949 (rectum & sigmoid)
A B₁ B₁ B₂ C₁ C₂ C₂	Astler-Coller 1953 (rectum & colon)
A A A B C C C C D	Turnbull et al 1967 (colon)

ANATOMIC EXTENT of NEOPLASM
←mucosa
←muscularis mucosae
←submucosa
←muscularis propria
←serosa (colon only)
←lymph nodes (any)
←lymph nodes (apical)
not removable,
adjacent organs,
distant sites,

Figure 17. The Dukes classification with subsequent systems. All except Turnbull's system are derived from examination of the resected bowel. Not illustrated is the Dukes system that includes both curative and palliative resections, and many of the Class C cases would be qualified as Stage D in Turnbull's system. (From Enker, W. E. (Ed.): Carcinoma of the Colon and Rectum. Chicago, Year Book Medical Publishers, 1978.)

The most recent efforts to develop a universally acceptable staging system for colorectal carcinoma have been those involving the TNM system of the International Union Against Cancer (UICC) and the American Joint Committee on Cancer (AJCC). The TNM system has the advantage of being applicable to presurgical clinical-diagnostic staging as well as postsurgical resection-pathologic staging, and it provides an opportunity to break entirely with the confusion created by the variations in the Dukes A, B, C system. For these reasons, the TNM system proposed by the AJCC will probably become the standard system in the United States in the near future.

Prognosis

The most important guide to prognosis for patients with colorectal carcinoma is the stage of the disease. The survival results from two large surgical series, one using the Dukes system and the other the TNM system of postsurgical resection-pathologic staging, are shown in Table 7. In addition to stage, various histologic factors may be of prognostic importance. The most important of these is tumor grade. In a review of 20,193 patients by the American College of Surgeons, the 5-year survival rate was 57 and 54 per cent for well- and moderately well-differentiated tumors, respectively, but only 35 per cent for poorly differentiated tumors. Overall, females had better survival in this series than did males, and Caucasians survived longer than did blacks.

TABLE 7. Prognosis of Colorectal Carcinoma Based on Postsurgical Resection-Pathologic Staging*

Dukes Stages	Five-Year Survival (%)	TNM Stage	Five-Year Survival (%)
A	81.2	O	75
		I (a and b)	70
B	64.0	II	58
C	27.4	III	25–33
D	14.3	IV	6

*Modified from Zinkin, L.D.: Dis. Colon Rectum, 26:37, 1983. The series by Dukes and Burrey involved 2447 cases and the TNM series 1826 cases.

Median survival time is a more meaningful index of prognosis than 5-year survival rates for patients with advanced disease. Silverman and colleagues have provided guidelines to predict median survival in such patients based on the extent of disease, age, sites of metastases, and treatment performed. Kemeny and Braun have studied the prognosis of patients with metastatic disease. They found that survival was significantly decreased by any of the following: abnormal serum lactic dehydrogenase (LDH), elevated level of CEA, a white blood cell count greater than 10,000 per μl., performance status less than 60 on the Karnofsky scale, and lung as opposed to liver metastasis.[20, 23]

Treatment

The management of primary colorectal malignancies has been almost exclusively surgical. Progressive improvement in surgical skills, aggressiveness, and patient preparation and support have increased operability and resectability, and operative mortality rates have declined. Resectability now approaches 90 per cent, and mortality ranges from 2 to 10 per cent, the lower figure reported by institutions with special interests in colorectal malignancies. As in all applications of operations for malignancy, the key determinant to success is the degree to which disease has spread by the time of operation. A summary of the experience of more than 100 groups by the End Results Group indicates that about 25 per cent of patients with colorectal cancer have distant metastases with little prospect of cure when first seen. In 40 per cent of patients, the tumor is localized in the bowel wall, and in 35 per cent it has spread to the lymph nodes. Since the distribution of these lesions has remained relatively constant, there has been little change in relative survival in the United States following operation in the last two decades. However, in the individual patient, it is the proper application of appropriate surgical judgment and technique that leads to the greatest possibility of cure or the longest and most satisfactory palliation.

OPERATIVE PRINCIPLES

The aims of operation are to excise the primary lesion with adequate margins, to reconstitute continuity of the bowel whenever possible, and to avoid complications. The

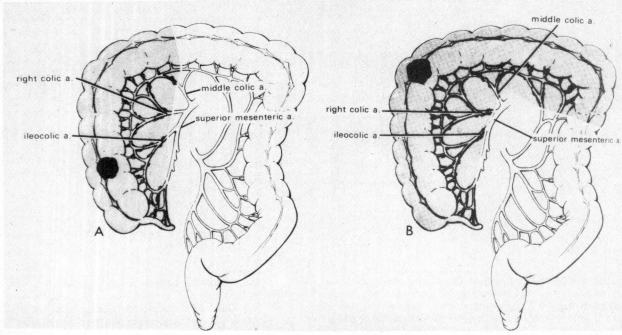

Figure 18. A, Extent of resection necessary for adenocarcinoma of the right colon, as dictated by potential sites of spread via the lymph nodes. B, Extended right colectomy, suitable for lesions in the right colon, hepatic flexure, and transverse colon. (From Grage, T. B., Ferguson, R. M., and Simmons, R. L.: In Horton, J., and Hill, G. J. II (Eds.): Clinical Oncology, Philadelphia, W. B. Saunders Company, 1977.)

various routes of spread must be considered, including mural, venous, implantation, and direct extension. Preoperative preparation includes appropriate clinical staging of the patient and preparation of the bowel with antibiotics and enemas.

Wide removal of the involved segment to include lymphatic drainage areas is imperative. Thus, the standard treatment of neoplasms of the cecum and ascending colon is right colectomy, including a segment of the terminal ileum, the cecum, and the right half of the transverse colon, with removal of the corresponding mesocolon at its base around the superior mesenteric artery to the origin of the middle colic vessels (Fig. 18). Carcinomas of the splenic flexure or the descending or sigmoid colon are treated by excision of the distal transverse, descending, and sigmoid colon together with the associated mesocolon excised to the aorta. For tumors of the sigmoid colon, the proximal resection can be limited and the transverse colon need not necessarily be removed (Fig. 19). For carcinomas in the upper rectum, an anterior resection and reanastomosis can be performed providing a 4- to 5-cm. margin can be achieved. Distal to this the anteroposterior resection generally has provided the best possibility for cure (Fig. 20).

An important surgical principle is the *total excision* of the involved lymphatics as well as adequate surgical margins of the colon. The exception occurs with low anterior colon resection, at which point the distal margin can hardly approximate the proximal margin. It has been shown by the examination of excised specimens that intraluminal spread of cancer is surprisingly short, less than 2 cm. in most instances. Yet, the incidence of suture line recurrence following anterior resection, in which circumstance the well-meaning surgeon may have the inclination to compromise the distal margins in order to preserve rectal function, far exceeds that found in other procedures, and certainly the frequently narrow margin available in the distal specimen must have a direct bearing on this. The choice of operation

for neoplasms of the upper and mid-rectum depends upon the evaluation of the configuration of the pelvis, the size and location of the tumor, and the skill and judgment of the surgeon in these procedures, including familiarity with newer techniques of "pull-through" procedures with ileorectal anastomosis and the transsacral approach for colorectal resection.

A more subjective aspect of the operation, i.e., the aggressiveness of the operative team, has been addressed. An analysis was made of a series in which one group of patients underwent an extremely conservative procedure, often with incomplete removal of all mesenteric nodes. A second group was managed by a moderately aggressive surgical resection, and the third was managed by an extremely aggressive procedure, including initial vascular ligation and wide and even extended resections. When operative mortality, complications, and patient-group characteristics were compared, there was no difference between the groups. However, survival was better in every Dukes category in patients treated by the most aggressive procedure. This correlated best with the operability and resectability rate, which was highest for the most aggressive group. Thus, in this series the more aggressive procedures yielded better results.

ANTERIOR RESECTION AND ABDOMINOPERINEAL RESECTION

Distal intramural spread of rectal cancer is usually restricted, and a margin of 2.5 cm. of grossly normal wall is usually considered adequate. In other studies it has been shown that cancer cells could be found as far as 4 cm. distal to the primary neoplasm in the more advanced cases. Most pathologists agree that a 5-cm. segment of normal rectum distal to the neoplasm is adequate for the margin.

Although Miles reported that lymphatic spread occurred upward, laterally, and downward, subsequent reviews of those with less advanced disease have shown that

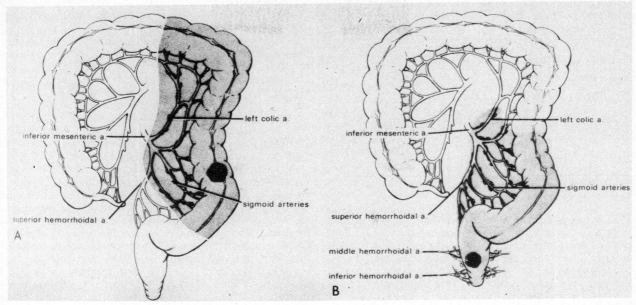

Figure 19. A, Left colectomy, suitable for malignancies involving the sigmoid colon, descending colon, and splenic flexure. B, Extent of combined abdominoperineal resection for tumors of the middle and lower rectum. (From Grage, T. B., Ferguson, R. M., and Simmons, R. L.: Gastrointestinal tract cancer. In Horton, J., and Hill, G. J. II (Eds.): Clinical Oncology. Philadelphia, W. B. Saunders Company, 1977.)

upward displacement is by far the most frequent type of spread. Nodal metastases distal to the primary cancer were noted in only 98 of 1500 abdominoperineal resection specimens. Since most physicians now agree that spread is predominantly upward through superior hemorrhoidal and inferior mesenteric lymphatics, the decision to perform combined abdominoperineal resection or low anterior resection is determined primarily by the distance of the lower border of the cancer from the anus. The lateral pelvic extension of the two operations, both of which remove the upper lymphatic drainage areas, should be essentially the same.

Generally, tumors within 7 to 8 cm. of the anal verge are treated by abdominoperineal resection, whereas those that are 12 cm. or more from the anal verge are adequately managed with anterior resection. Lesions between 7 and 11 cm. from the anal verge require the most judgment, and factors such as pelvis size, size of the lesion, and tumor differentiation must be considered. The narrow pelvis of many males may make low anterior resection in these patients hazardous. If the lesion is easily palpated with the examining finger, abdominoperineal resection is generally indicated. However, if the neoplasm can be delivered to the level of the abdominal incision after mobilization of the rectum from the levator ani, an adequate resection may be performed. The use of the circumferential stapling device greatly facilitates the construction of a low-lying anastomosis (Fig. 21).

Figure 20. The shaded area shows the extent of removal for carcinoma of the upper rectum by abdominoperineal resection (A) and by anterior resection (B). Note the necessity for a 2-inch (5-cm.) margin distal to the lesion in an anterior resection. If this cannot be accomplished, an abdominoperineal excision of the rectum should be performed. (From Butcher, H. R., Jr.: Carcinoma of the rectum. Choice between anterior resection and abdominal perineal resection of the rectum. Cancer, 28:204, 1971.)

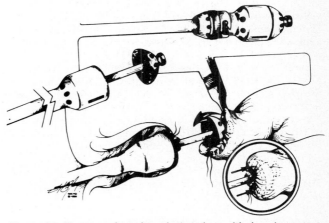

Figure 21. The use of stapling devices has added an important new dimension in intestinal surgery, particularly in the formation of low anastomoses in anterior resections for carcinoma of the colon. The proximal and distal loops are secured around the open stapler. The stapler is closed and then fired. Anastomosis is by a circumferential row of staples to attach the proximal and distal segments. The closed device is then brought out through the anus. (From Beart, R. W., Jr., and Wolff, B. G.: The use of staplers for anterior anastomoses. World J. Surg., 8:525, 1982.)

TABLE 8. *Five-Year Survival in Rectal Cancer: A Comparison of Patients Treated with Anteroposterior Resection and Low Anterior Resection**

Procedure	Dukes Stages	Patients (No.)	Five-Year Survival (No.)	Five-Year Survival (%)
Abdominoperineal resection	A	42	34	81
	B	91	47	52
	C	129	43	33
Total		262	124	47
Anterior resection	A	50	43	86
	B	98	56	57
	C	86	33	38
Total		234	132	56

*From B tcher, H. R.: Cancer, *28*:204, 1971.

If these principles are followed and patients are carefully selected, the survival rates from these operations are generally comparable (Table 8).

In this series, there was no difference in operative mortality between the two approaches. The slight superiority of the anterior resection in every category of the Dukes classification can be attributed to a slightly smaller tumor size among those having anterior resection, together with a slightly greater percentage of Dukes Stages A and B lesions in that group. Local recurrences have ranged from 7 per cent for anterior resection to 18 to 21 per cent for anteroposterior resection. Females have fewer local recurrences in most series, and the more proximal the lesion the less likely is recurrence.[20]

SURGICAL MANAGEMENT OF OBSTRUCTION AND PERFORATION

Complete intestinal obstruction occurs in 8 to 23 per cent of patients with colorectal cancer, and the predominant symptom is abdominal pain. Although a slowly growing annular carcinoma might be expected to cause a gradual onset of symptoms, obstruction frequently appears rapidly without previous warning. Of 1556 cases of colorectal cancer reported from the Massachusetts General Hospital, the median duration of symptoms in obstructed patients was one fourth of that observed in nonobstructed patients. Hypokalemia, hypochloremia, anemia, and hypoproteinemia were uncommon. The median preoperative interval was 12 hours.

Of 124 patients in this series operated on for obstructing carcinoma, the overall mortality was 15 per cent, and the postoperative complication rate was higher than that observed in patients undergoing elective colon procedures. Yet, 40 per cent of those resected for cure survived 5 years or more. When those who survived operation were analyzed by Dukes criteria and compared with patients from the same institution undergoing elective colonic operations, the proportion of patients in the various Dukes categories did not differ significantly. Thus, the most important determinant of survival after successful emergency operation is the pathologic stage of the lesion when first seen, just as in elective operations. This has been observed in other series and is encouraging, since the significant difference between the groups, i.e., the operative mortality, continues to decline each year.

The addition of perforation to acute obstruction of the colon can increase the mortality greatly. Glenn and McSherry reported a 31 per cent operative mortality and a 7 per cent 5-year survival in 29 patients with combined perforation and obstruction. Crowder and Cohn reported

that 42 per cent of patients with proximal perforation of an obstructed colon died, and mortality rates of up to 100 per cent have been reported.

The traditional surgical management of acute obstruction due to cancer has been proximal diversion followed by resection and then cecostomy or a diverting colostomy. Dissatisfaction with cecostomy and a recognition of the greater mortality rates inherent in right-sided obstructions (very thin bowel, leading to a greater degree of distention, perforation, and ischemia) led some authors, including this one, to advocate primary resection of right-sided lesions. However, more than two thirds of obstructing lesions are distal to the transverse colon, and in these instances a three-stage surgical management has predominated. The rationale has been that only one of the three procedures is truly an emergency and that the last two can be done safely and electively on a colon that is prepared, defunctionalized, and empty. However, theoretically, the manipulation of the tumor during operative procedures increases the likelihood of tumor cell invasion of the circulation at a greater rate than after one operation, and the disability from one procedure is much less than that incurred in multiple operations. Fielding and Wells compared the age-adjusted survival in 22 primary resections for obstructing colon cancer with 28 patients who underwent staged resections. The groups were similar in terms of tumor differentiation and Dukes stage. Survival was significantly better in the group who had primary resection. Bose and Sachdeva have advocated emergency hemicolectomy in all cases of perforation, reasoning that the bowel is already decompressed and that management of the complication of peritonitis as well as minimizing potential wound seeding is much better performed by primary resection. This viewpoint has been advocated by others.

The surgical management of either acutely obstructed or perforated carcinoma of the colon or both must rest, as with all things surgical, with the judgment and experience of the surgeon. The dilation and viability of the bowel, the physical status of the patient, and the degree of contamination are all factors. If the diverting colostomy must be used, consideration should be given to placing the colostomy as close to the lesion as possible in order to make the column of stool above the obstruction or leak, which is a source of potential contamination, as short as possible. The use of a cecostomy has been attended by many complications in most series, and, unless absolutely necessary in unique situations, it should be avoided. Although the ideal preoperative randomized series comparing primary resectional therapy with the traditional staged management for obstructing colon cancer has not been (and probably never will be) performed, sufficient evidence in the literature suggests that resectional management should be and will be more widely applied.[20]

EXTENDED SURGICAL PROCEDURES FOR COLON CANCER

Although the number of patients in whom extended surgical procedures might have application is small, several features should be considered when extensive lesions are encountered and wider resections than conventional colectomy are contemplated. It has been established in several series that size of the primary lesion is not a determinant of regional metastases with this lesion. Thus, direct neoplastic extension into an adjacent organ is not statistically a more adverse prognostic sign than are one to five regional lymph node metastases, the latter being a situation in which conventional colectomy is performed uniformly without hesitation. In fact, the seemingly advanced colorectal tumor that has invaded another organ may bear favorable biologic characteristics, such as a tendency to well-differentiated histologic appearance and an inflammatory response around the primary. The finding that the tumor has achieved a large size usually indicates that metastases have not occurred in the relatively long growth period of the tumor required to achieve such size.

Polk reported 24 patients who underwent extended procedures, i.e., colectomy and partial or total excision of at least one invaded organ. There was only one hospital death. Eight patients died of recurrent cancer, with a median survival of 28 months. The patients were alive and well at a median survival of 25 months, and the remainder were alive with disease or dead of other cancers at 33 to 41 months. An aggressive approach to locally advanced disease has been advocated by others. Invasion of the sacrum may not be a contraindication to anteroposterior resection and, when used with an incontinuity sacral resection from the extended lithotomy position, is both feasible and safe. The fact that large, locally advanced tumors may have biologically favorable characteristics, such as slow growth and late metastases, should encourage extended operations with excision of invaded organs when possible.[20]

Suture Line Recurrence

This type of recurrent carcinoma deserves special attention, since if locally recurrent disease is due to judgmental or technical errors during the original procedure the correction of these errors might be expected to lower the recurrence. Conversely, if local recurrence is found prior to the widely disseminated stage, further resection might be curative.

Numerous theories explaining suture line recurrence have been advanced, one being that the intact mucosa normally acts as a barrier to intraluminal tumor cells that are constantly shed from the tumor. As the suture passes through the bowel wall, it breaks this barrier and viable tumor cells are then present in the submucosal and muscularis layers, in which the proper nutritional milieu for tumor cell growth exists. The second theory is similar in that the inverted, raw, viable ends of the cut bowel serve as a hospitable environment onto which shed tumor cells can adhere and grow.

Another theory explains the suture line recurrence as a local metastasis resulting from tumor cells suspended in the fine reticular lymphatic system within the bowel wall. Although most of these cells die, some can become implanted at the site of resection, at which point the lymphatic flow is obstructed. The most easily understood explanation for local recurrence is simply that the margin of resection is inadequate. Manson and colleagues reported that the rate of recurrence is constant until a margin of 7 cm. is reached. They found no recurrence with margins 7 cm. or greater, although 5 cm. is generally accepted as adequate, and other series suggest that a 7-cm. margin is not necessary. It is of interest that two patients in one series failed to develop recurrent cancer, even though the distal margin was involved with tumor.[20]

In experimental models, a number of maneuvers have been devised to lower the incidence of local recurrence. A closed anastomosis, in which sutures do not enter the lumen of the bowel, has been shown to be superior to an open anastomosis. Devitalizing the cut ends of the colon has lowered the incidence of local recurrence. The use of various intraluminal agents to kill viable tumor cells has been accompanied by lessened local recurrence. Cohn carefully analyzed various measures to reduce local recur-

rence in an experimental model in which anastomoses were constructed in bowel that contained intraluminal tumor cells. Tumor implantation was not affected by bacteria in the peritoneal cavity, by use of the automatic stapler, or by irrigation with chlorpactic, dimethyl sulfoxide (DMSO), iodine, mechlorethamine, or saline. Suture line recurrences were reduced by the use of iodized sutures or a closed anastomosis, and peritoneal implants were reduced by irradiation, low-molecular-weight dextran irrigation, and clamping the lumen of the bowel close to the anastomosis.

Clinically, many maneuvers have been suggested to lower the incidence of recurrent cancer. Although few have been universally adopted, it is likely that more emphasis in this area could reduce recurrence. Logical and practical measures include wide local excision, intraluminal irrigation with a cytotoxic agent, avoidance of contamination and hemorrhage, cauterization of freshly cut bowel edges, and, particularly, prevention of laceration or injury to the bowel at any other site during the construction of the anastomosis. The use of iodized sutures has been effective experimentally and clinically in killing cancer cells on contact and requires no modification of technique.

The Second-Look Operation and the Use of Carcinoembryonic Antigen in Diagnosing Recurrence

Local recurrence is an ominous finding, since more than 90 per cent of patients with this finding shortly expired in Welch and Donaldson's experience. Taylor found that 75 per cent of patients with recurrent colorectal carcinoma succumbed from complications of local recurrence. Aware of this, Wangensteen's group systematically reoperated upon patients who were at high risk for recurrence 6 to 9 months after colectomy for colorectal cancer. Forty per cent were found to have recurrence, and 14 per cent eventually were rendered tumor-free. However, the mortality initially reported in this study essentially negated the therapeutic benefit, and the concept of reoperation for all high-risk primary colon cancer patients did not gain wide acceptance.

Mackman and coworkers employed second-look operations to assess the effectiveness of adjuvant 5-fluorouracil (FU) therapy. Recurrence was found in ten of 60 patients, five of whom were made tumor-free by resection. Later recurrence occurred in three of the 50 patients with second-look procedures and in two of the five patients who had been rendered tumor-free by repeated resection. There was no operative mortality. When Gunderson and Sosin analyzed the results of 75 patients who were found at reoperation to have recurrence after presumably curative colectomy, local recurrence or regional lymph node metastases or both were responsible for 50 per cent of recurrences and were a component in 92 per cent.[20]

The use of *immunologic markers of recurrence*, such as the determination of the serum CEA level, may make it possible to choose patients more selectively who would benefit maximally by reoperation. Although it was originally thought to be a relatively specific diagnostic indicator of gastrointestinal tumor, the CEA determination, which presumably measures shed antigen from the tumor itself, has been found to be variably positive in other disease states. Nevertheless, most studies suggest that it can be an important auxiliary means of assessment for recurrent tumor. In general, the CEA usually declines over the first 3 months postoperatively but in the presence of tumor recurrence often rises weeks or months before it is clinically evident. This, of course, is the time when operative intervention is likely to be most beneficial. Although enthusiasm for this test has not been uniform, the CEA level, along with other clinical diagnostic tests, has been instrumental in selecting those patients for reoperation.

A wide variety of potential tumor markers other than CEA are under study, including the measurement of immune complexes, such as Tennessee antigen, alpha$_1$-acid glycoprotein, a variety of other acute-phase reactants, and many other antigens with variable similarities to CEA. None of these markers is currently recommended for routine clinical use.

Several groups are currently studying the use of antibodies to CEA as transmitters of drugs or radioactive chemicals in the diagnosis and treatment of colorectal carcinoma. Antibodies to material other than CEA are also being studied. The terms immunoscintigraphy, radioimmunolocalization, and radioimmunodetection (RAID) have been applied to this methodology, and interest in this subject has been heightened by the availability of monoclonal antibodies to CEA. A variety of technical problems have limited the usefulness of this approach, however, and further work is needed before this approach can be recommended for general use.

OPERATION FOR METASTATIC DISEASE

Although conventional logic might suggest that a localized therapeutic modality such as resection is ill suited for the treatment of disseminated disease, many authors have demonstrated that the judicious application of resection for metastatic colon carcinomas can often prolong life. Foster, in 1970, reported 123 patients from the world literature undergoing liver resection for metastatic cancer. Of 83 patients with colorectal metastases, 47 per cent of the operative survivors lived 2 years and 21 per cent lived 5 years. Wilson and Adson evaluated 60 patients with hepatic resections. Patients with multiple metastases lived 5 or more years, but 15 of 36 patients with resection of solitary lesions lived longer than 5 years, and eight patients were alive 10 years after operation. Fortner and associates reported 23 hepatic resections for colorectal metastases (in a series of 108 resections for primary and metastatic hepatic tumors). Seventy two per cent of the 17 patients undergoing curative resection were alive at 3 years. There were no 2-year survivors of six patients undergoing palliative resection.

In general, the metastasis must be confined to one organ, and single lesions are associated with a better prognosis than are multiple lesions. Smaller lesions are better than larger ones, but a reasonable measure of success accompanies any effort that renders the patient grossly tumor-free. It is not necessary to do a formal anatomic liver resection when removing metastatic disease; rather, the lesion with a margin of uninvolved liver is excised. The use of large liver clamps for such "extended wedge resections" and intrahepatic control of vascular and ductal structures facilitates this.

In *extended resections*, the arteries, extrahepatic ductal systems, portal vein, and hepatic veins are controlled in that order, and the line of hepatic resection is made by finger fracture and electrocautery. T-tube drainage is generally not employed. The size of the lesion is not a contraindication to operation if total excision can be achieved. If this is not feasible, attempts at partial excisions are not indicated.

Isolated pulmonary metastases, without involvement of the liver or other organs, occur in less than 10 per cent of patients with metastases. However, 5-year relapse-free survivals have been reported following pulmonary resection for metastatic colorectal carcinoma when confined to the lungs. All patients considered for these procedures must have negative findings on work-up for hepatic metastases. However, a small laparotomy is advocated with the patient in the lateral position just prior to thoracotomy to eliminate the chance of a false-negative work-up. If intra-abdominal disease is not present, an immediate thoracotomy may be performed. Conventional wedge excision or lobectomy or both are performed as indicated. Median sternotomy for resection of bilateral disease is applicable in some patients.[20]

PALLIATIVE SURGERY FOR COLORECTAL CANCER

In the presence of multiple, unresectable, synchronous metastases found at the time of initial operation, the management of primary colon carcinoma consists of resection of the primary lesion in most patients. Although mortality is determined by progression of the metastases, it has been demonstrated in several series that those who undergo primary resection have a more favorable course. Nielsen and coworkers studied 103 such patients. Fifteen patients who received no operative treatment lived an average of only 6 weeks. Fifty patients who had laparotomy and a bypass procedure lived an average of 20 weeks, whereas those 38 patients who had resection lived an average of 55 weeks. The duration of symptoms had been the same in all three groups. Resection prevented anemia, protein loss, obstruction, and pain but was contraindicated in the presence of ascites. Survival correlated inversely with the extent of metastases. Cady and colleagues also reported longer survival among 269 patients undergoing resection compared with those receiving nonresectional therapy with simultaneous liver metastases.

PATIENT AGE AND SURVIVAL

Advanced age is not a major determinant of survival following resection for colon cancer. Block and Enker reported a survival rate of 57 per cent in all patients older than 70 years following conventional operative procedures, compared with 61 per cent in 1197 patients younger than 70 years from 1950 to 1965. The operative mortality in the octogenarians was 15 per cent greater than that in the younger groups. Most complications were cerebrovascular or cardiovascular in origin. However, if death from operation was excluded, the 5-year survival rate was 67 per cent.

The mean age for the diagnosis of colorectal cancer has been stated to be from 67 to 69 years, although analysis of ongoing studies suggests that the median age of onset might be lower. Certainly, colon cancer in the very young is a worse disease than in the aged. Most of the patients in Block and Enker's series were operated upon 15 to 20 years ago, and it is likely that mortality would be somewhat lower with today's operative management techniques.

Adam and colleagues reported 156 patients more than 80 years of age operated on for colorectal cancer. Twenty two per cent were alive and well at 5 years. Fifty-five per cent of these patients had Dukes Stage C and D lesions. The 5-year survival for patients of all ages undergoing resection for colorectal cancer was 22 per cent during the same period. Thus, although major abdominal procedures are associated with a higher mortality in the older population than in younger patients, the survival rates of those in the older population who recover following surgery are as good as, if not better than, those in the younger population. Advanced age does not justify withholding operative procedures unless specific identifiable contraindications are present.[20]

ALTERNATIVES TO CONVENTIONAL SURGERY

Electrocoagulation

The use of electrocoagulation in the management of carcinoma of the rectum was advocated by Strauss and associates in 1945, and various reports of its use by others, especially Madden, have since appeared. With this approach, the anus is dilated, the lesion is identified, and the entire area is cauterized and usually fulgurated. Ten to 12 days later the procedure is repeated. In a series of 131 patients so treated, Madden and Kandalaft used an average of 3.5 fulguration sessions per patient. Annular lesions were not treated, and only those within 10 cm. of the anus and beneath the peritoneal reflection were considered amenable to cauterization.

The controversy surrounding this form of therapy arises from the claims of some of its advocates that it should be the primary method of treating rectal cancer rather than excision. This position is taken by comparing the 5-year survival rate of patients treated by electrocoagulation with that obtained in larger surgical series of patients undergoing anteroposterior resection. For example, the 5-year survival in the series of Madden and Kandalaft was 78 per cent, which exceeds nearly all conventional surgical series. Moreover, complications and mortality were less. However, these data were based on only 63 of 131 patients treated by cautery; the rest of the patients were not followed.

Since the incidence of local recurrence is relatively low following electrocoagulation, this approach must be considered effective in controlling localized cancer. However, this does not include regional lymph node removal, which is considered to be essential in appropriate cancer treatment. Since the frequency of positive node involvement in large series of patients undergoing anteroposterior resection for rectal cancer is around 45 to 50 per cent, good results from electrocoagulation could be presumed to result from the induction of a systemic response from patient selection factors that are not operative in conventional series. Although it has been suggested that electrocoagulation induces immunologic resistance to tumor, there is little supporting evidence. However, it is likely that the cauterized lesions have more favorable characteristics, such as being smaller, polypoid, noncircumferential, and being detected earlier than those in large surgical series.

Local Excision

Surgical excision with the removal of regional lymph node–bearing tissue remains the treatment of choice for primary cancer of the rectum. However, it is of interest that there are reports in large surgical series that 2 to 3 per cent of patients were treated by cauterization. Although use of cautery as local therapy for advanced symptomatic metastatic or inoperable rectal cancer is clearly useful in selected patients, it is likely that there are only a small number in whom this approach is applicable as the preferred primary treatment. The indications for cautery fulguration include (1) patients who have Dukes Stage A and B carcinoma, i.e., small, superficial lesions, especially when located on the posterior or lateral rectal wall, (2) patients who represent poor surgical risks or who have advanced senility or concomitant serious systemic disorders or both, (3) blind or senescent institutionalized patients who are unable to care for themselves or cannot procure adequate care, (4) patients who have bleeding from inoperable lesions or metastases, and (5) patients who refuse the standard procedures.

The use of local excision rather than conventional colectomy has also been described. Again, it must be emphasized that this alternative to conventional surgery has been applied to very carefully selected patients. For example, at St. Mark's Hospital in London, of 3999 operations done for colorectal cancer, only 143 were local excisions. The selection factors included completeness of excision, depth of spread into the bowel wall, and histologic grade of malignancy. Survival in these carefully selected patients, all of whom were followed for 5 or more years, was excellent.[20]

DIVERTICULAR DISEASE

Acquired diverticula are pulsion-induced outpouchings of the colonic wall developing in a rather classic pattern in two rows between the teniae through defects in the circular musculature at point of entry of blood vessels. Their development is related to localized areas of high intraluminar pressure between haustral contraction rings.

Diverticulosis has a predilection for the sigmoid and distal descending colon in about 80 per cent of patients. It rarely occurs in the rectum and occasionally is observed on the right side. Diverticulosis chiefly afflicts civilized societies, and a lack of dietary roughage may have a causative role. Other factors include aging, obesity, genetic traits, and chronic constipation.

PATHOLOGY

Diverticulosis represents the presence of diverticula in the colon, and the most common pathologic state with this lesion is diverticulitis. This is an inflammatory condition that occurs after obstruction of the neck of the diverticulum by feces and, occasionally, barium. This process causes colonic narrowing and may progress to complete obstruction that simulates the clinical manifestations of carcinoma. Massive lower gastrointestinal bleeding may follow ulceration in the diverticulum. Abscesses, fistulas, or perforation often complicates the course of diverticulitis, often with pericolitis and edema of the mesentery.

CLINICAL PRESENTATION AND DIAGNOSIS

Colonic diverticula are asymptomatic unless complicated by microperforation and infection, diverticulitis, or painless rectal bleeding. Acute diverticulitis follows perforation, and entrapped fecaliths erode the mucosa and allow infection to spread to the adjacent bowel wall.

The clinical manifestations of diverticulitis include abdominal pain and tenderness, constipation, mild distention, fever, and leukocytosis. A mass in the abdomen, rectum, or vagina is usually palpable, and diarrhea may also occur. Symptoms of irritation of the urinary bladder due to pyuria (frequency, dysuria, and urgency) are often caused by the inflammatory mass impinging on the bladder or the development of a fistula into the bladder. Bleeding from the diverticulum presents as sudden passing of bright red or dark red blood from the rectum. It is usually painless or may be associated with mild cramping. Occasionally blood loss may be massive, leading to hemorrhagic shock or death. Fortunately, most of these episodes subside spontaneously. Since such bleeding is rarely occult, blood in the stool should be attributed to diverticula only when all other possible causes, especially carcinoma of the cecum, have been confidently excluded. Diverticular bleeding occurs rarely in association with acute diverticulitis.

The differential diagnosis includes appendicitis, inflam-

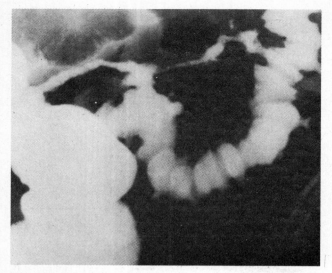

Figure 22. Diverticulitis with linear fistula. This long, linear fistula, sometimes deemed characteristic of Crohn's disease in association with diverticular disease, may be found, as it was in this patient, in the absence of Crohn's disease. (From Spiro, H. M.: Clinical Gastroenterology, 3rd ed. New York, Macmillan Publishing Company, 1983.)

matory adnexal diseases, carcinoma of the ovary, prostatitis, carcinoma of the sigmoid, and the various types of inflammatory, ischemic, and infectious colitis. If the sigmoid colon is redundant and reflects toward the right lower quadrant, diverticulitis in this area can mimic appendicitis.

Barium enema is an essential diagnostic study but is usually deferred during the acute stage. After the acute attack subsides, preparation of the bowel with gentle cleansing enemas rather than with laxatives is accomplished. Radiographic criteria for diagnosis of acute diverticulitis have changed in recent years. Serrated sawtooth patterns with spiked diverticula in luminal narrowing, criteria commonly used in the past, are no longer appropriate evidence of inflammation. Diagnostic criteria for acute diverticulitis are based on perforation of one or more diverticula with small pericolic extravasations. Barium outside the diverticulum indicates that perforation exists, and small abscess formation around the perforation produces an eccentric mass, indenting the lumen of the colon, and is the most common radiographic manifestation of infection (Figs. 22 through 24).

TREATMENT

Severe complications of diverticulitis, including colonic perforation, uncontrolled hemorrhage, fistula, and obstruc-

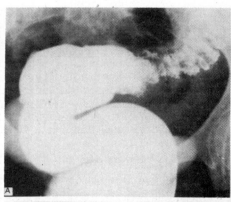

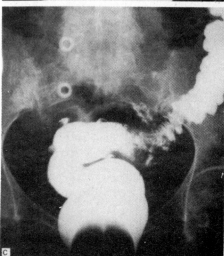

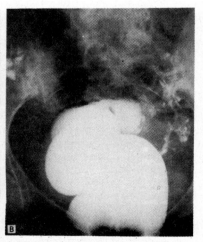

Figure 23. Diverticulitis. When the film was made (A), an area of narrowing and irritability was noted, but no diverticula were seen in this segment. The patient returned 5 months later with intestinal obstruction, and a barium enema at that time (B) showed obstruction to flow of barium with extravasation into the general peritoneal cavity. A diverting colostomy was performed, and 6 months later (C) barium can be seen to pass through the area of diverticulosis and diverticulitis, showing that the diverting colostomy allowed healing. (From Spiro, H. M.: Clinical Gastroenterology, 3rd ed. New York, Macmillan Publishing Company, 1983.)

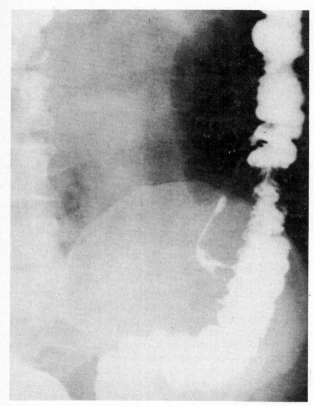

Figure 24. Diverticulitis. This fistulous tract came from a single diverticulum and ended in a simple blind end tract within the abdomen. In a different position, this fistula could have invaded the bladder, uterus, or other abdominal viscus. The photograph emphasizes the isolated nature of the diverticulitis. (From Spiro, H. M.: Clinical Gastroenterology, 3rd ed. New York, Macmillan Publishing Company, 1983.)

tion, are indications for emergent operative intervention. The inflammatory process in acute diverticulitis may be localized by surrounding abdominal peritoneum or may penetrate into an adjacent organ. If the process seems local with no evidence of spreading peritonitis, intensive nonoperative therapy is indicated. Nasogastric suction for distention and intravenous fluids for maintenance of hydration and electrolyte balance are important. Broad-spectrum antibiotics (usually including ampicillin and gentamicin) are administered systemically. The abscess often resolves with such therapy, and laxatives, which absorb water and serve as bulk in the colon, and appropriate diet may prevent further attacks.

Persistence or enlargement of the inflammatory mass with fever, increasing pain and tenderness, leukocytosis, and signs of sepsis necessitates urgent operative intervention. If the inflammatory mass cannot be removed, a diverting colostomy is usually done. This has been the classic management of perforation, and if employed it is probably advisable to place the colostomy as low as possible, preferably in the descending colon or the sigmoid colon to allow evacuation through the colostomy and prevent further inflammation at the site of the abscess. The abscess is also simultaneously drained. Intensive supportive therapy is continued, and resection can be performed electively 6 to 8 weeks later with restoration of continuity. Finally, takedown of the colostomy is performed as the third operation. This is the traditional treatment for perforated

diverticulitis with peritonitis advocated in the past. This approach requires three operations with a prolonged convalescence and increased total mortality. Usually the involved colon is resected with dranage of the abscess and a proximal colostomy with closure of the distal sigmoid colon. An elective reanastomosis of the colon is performed 6 to 8 weeks later. Immediate resection and end-to-end anastomosis without creation of a diverting colostomy has been advocated in selected patients and is an acceptable procedure, particularly in early cases with a minimal peritonitis.

OBSTRUCTION

Obstruction may follow chronic diverticulitis, inflammatory thickening, fibrosis, and pressure from pericolic abscesses. Unless the clinical response to nonoperative therapy is prompt, an operative approach similar to that used for acute diverticulitis with abscess is indicated.

PERFORATION

Perforation of the colon unassociated with abscess is rare but is occasionally seen in association with corticosteroid therapy. The signs of sepsis and shock may be masked temporarily by steroids, and a high index of suspicion is important in making the diagnosis. Immediate excision with a proximal diverting colostomy is the treatment of choice.

BLEEDING

Bleeding from colonic diverticula usually ceases spontaneously and can be managed conservatively with replacement of blood as necessary. Less than 20 per cent of patients with diverticular hemorrhage have a significant persistence or recurrence of bleeding. Although diverticula in the right colon are less frequent than in the left colon, when present they appear to have a greater tendency to bleed. This apparent difference may be due in part to confusion with arteriovenous malformations (AVMs) in the right colon. Since such malformations may be difficult to diagnose by usual means with persistent and unspecified bleeding, arteriography is indicated. Carcinomas of the colon can cause massive bleeding, but such is uncommon.

FISTULAS

Fistulas may develop between hollow viscera, especially the bladder, vagina, and small bowel. Rarely the uterus, adjacent colon, or ureter may be similarly involved. The most frequent internal fistula develops between the sigmoid colon and bladder and is more common in males or those females who have had a hysterectomy. The common genitourinary symptoms are frequency, urgency, and dysuria, usually at the initiation of urination. Pneumaturia, which is interruption of the urinary stream by the passage of gas, is pathognomonic of a vesical fistula. Proctoscopy, barium enema, and cystoscopy may be valuable in diagnosing the opening of the fistula, but the history and physical findings are most useful.

Surgical management consists of identifying the fistula, appropriate resection, and closure. Most fistulas can be managed in one procedure. Should a fistula develop to adjacent bowel, it should be resected with end-to-end anastomosis. Hysterectomy may be indicated if the uterus is involved. With fistulas into the bladder or vagina, resection of the bladder or vagina is usually unnecessary, since prompt healing usually follows closure of the fistula after the adjacent diseased sigmoid colon is resected.[12, 13, 21]

VOLVULUS

Volvulus of the colon is described as the twisting or rotation of a mobile segment of the colon about its mesentery. The degree of rotation can vary from 180 degrees to as many as four to five complete revolutions. Depending on the degree of rotation, partial or complete obstruction is produced, which may advance to bowel ischemia and gangrene. The sigmoid colon is the most common site, constituting about 80 per cent of those involved; the cecum, the next most common site, accounts for about 15 per cent of obstructions. Volvulus is probably the most common cause of strangulated colonic obstruction.

SIGMOID VOLVULUS

Sigmoid volvulus is less common in the United States and Western Europe, where it probably accounts for less than 1 per cent of intestinal obstruction, whereas in Eastern Europe and Africa one fifth of all patients with intestinal obstruction have sigmoid volvulus. One of the reasons proposed for this has been an anatomic difference in the sigmoid, since a long, almost redundant, sigmoid mesentery has been noted in patients from these countries. A high-fiber diet also apparently predisposes to the development of sigmoid volvulus. Neglected bowel habits with chronic constipation, chronic laxative abuse, and pregnancy are also associated conditions. As many as 40 per cent of cases of sigmoid volvulus occur with various diseases of the nervous system, including psychiatric illnesses, chronic brain syndrome, parkinsonism, cerebrovascular accidents, and muscular dystrophy. This condition, therefore, occurs with a surprisingly high incidence in institutions, such as domiciliaries and chronic care institutions for the elderly. Many of the patients in these institutions are also receiving tranquilizers and medications for Parkinson's disease, which may be causative factors.

Clinical Features

Sigmoid volvulus occurs when the sigmoid loop is redundant and has a narrow base, the so-called Omega loop. It is easy for this loop to twist, and when the upper loop descends in front of the lower loop closed obstruction may occur. If the ileocecal valve is competent, a double closed loop obstruction develops. Symptoms are indistinguishable from those of other intestinal obstructions and may be acute or subacute. Acute symptoms are more likely to occur in younger patients. In older persons, a subacute progressive form of the disease may lead to chronic symptoms over a few months and a slowly developing gangrene of the bowel with symptoms suggestive of chronic left colonic obstruction, which is often mistaken for obstructing

carcinoma. Patients with sigmoid volvulus develop marked distention of the abdomen. The sigmoid loop may be palpable and acutely tender, but otherwise there are no significant visible findings. Neither physical examination nor laboratory data ordinarily distinguishes volvulus from other acute abdominal catastrophies, although sometimes the infarcted dilated segment may be palpable as a tympanitic mass.

Diagnosis

Many patients relate previous episodes of abdominal distention that have been relieved by enemas or knee-chest position followed by the passage of large amounts of flatus and stool. The leukocyte count may be normal or moderately elevated in patients without strangulation. Rectal examination usually reveals the bowel to be empty or filled with liquid stool.

Abdominal films are characteristic and show a large dilated loop coursing diagonally across the abdomen from right to left from the pelvis with a bent "inner tube" effect, in which the gas shadow is seen to be bent on itself with two fluid levels, one lying in each limit of the obstructed loop. This will often be sufficient to suggest the diagnosis. However, if necessary, a barium enema should be performed and will show a narrowing at the site of the twist, the so-called bird's beak or ace of spades deformity. Vital signs and clinical parameters, such as the leukocyte count and electrolytes, can vary widely but may be normal, particularly in the absence of sepsis. Sigmoidoscopy should precede barium studies, and often a characteristic twist is seen at the end of the sigmoidoscope (Fig. 25).

Treatment

Sigmoidoscopy should be performed to assess whether strangulation exists. Findings of strangulation include bluish-purple discoloration or hemorrhagic mucosa, bloody fluid in the rectum, and frank ulceration and necrosis of the bowel at the point of the twist. The clinical situation of the patient should also be evaluated. The accurate exclusion of strangulation is not always possible. However, if there is reasonable evidence that it is not present, sigmoidoscopic reduction of the volvulus should be attempted. The sigmoidoscope is advanced to the point of obstruction and gently and carefully passed into the obstructed loop. A massive projectile release of feces and flatus may occur at this time. A lubricated tube is then inserted into the sigmoidoscope and passed into the sigmoid loop. The loop serves as a stent to prevent recurrence of the volvulus and is firmly secured and left in place for several days. Successful sigmoidoscopic reduction of the volvulus can be accomplished in about 80 per cent of patients. Occasionally when

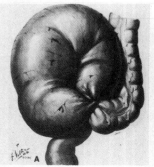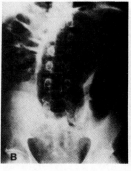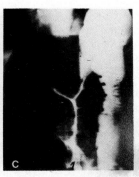

Figure 25. Features of sigmoid volvulus. A, Gross appearance. B, Plain film of abdomen; note "bent inner tube" sign. C, Barium colon examination. Note obstruction of colon, gas-filled loop, and "beak" deformity at end of barium column. (From Hardy, J. D. (Ed.): Hardy's Textbook of Surgery. Philadelphia, J. B. Lippincott Company, 1983.)

sigmoidoscopic reduction is unsuccessful, barium enema may reduce the volvulus and a colon tube should be inserted to prevent recurrence.

If strangulation is suspected or if sigmoidoscopic reduction is not possible, laparotomy should be performed. If strangulation is not present, simple detorsion of the colon is performed. After the loop is untwisted, a colon tube is passed from below and advanced into the sigmoid loop to prevent postoperative recurrence. Mortality from operative reduction of volvulus without gangrene is low, and resection is rarely indicated if the bowel is viable. Some recommend suturing the colon to the posterior peritoneum to prevent further torsion. After decompression of the volvulus by either operative or nonoperative means, the patient should be prepared for elective resection of the redundant sigmoid, usually during the same hospitalization.

If strangulation is encountered at laparotomy, resection of the gangrenous sigmoid loop, accompanied by a double-barrel colostomy or an end colostomy with closure of the rectal stump (Hartmann's pouch), should be performed. Re-establishment of intestinal continuity may be accomplished at a later date. However, the mortality for strangulated volvulus with gangrene is high, being approximately 50 per cent.

CECAL VOLVULUS

Because of poor fixation in 10 to 25 per cent of patients, the cecum and ascending colon are sufficiently mobile to twist on their mesentery and therefore volvulus may result. Torsion is most likely to be in a clockwise direction, obliquely toward the left upper quadrant, and a 360-degree rotation is characteristic. It is usually initiated by sudden distention of the cecum by trauma, pressure, constipation, or obstruction of the colon distal to it.

Diagnosis

Three major complications may ensue. With a sudden tight twisting of the mesentery, volvulus is acute and leads to early gangrene with features no different from any other abdominal emergency. An obstructive type of volvulus without early gangrene may lead to closed loop obstruction characterized by marked distention of the cecum. Finally, intermittent or recurrent volvulus of the cecum and right colon manifests itself by repeated attacks of pain, tenderness, and distention of the right lower quadrant. The patient obtains relief by assuming the knee-chest position or taking an enema. Chronic abdominal pain occurs in a large number of patients because of the tendency of cecal volvulus to resolve spontaneously but then recur in the future. Cecal volvulus can be recognized on abdominal films by the marked distention of the cecum, which classically arises from the right lower quadrant of the abdomen (Fig. 26). A barium enema shows the clinical narrowing at the twist, the so-called bird's beak deformity.

Treatment

Reduction of the volvulus by barium enema and colonoscopy has been reported but involves the risk that the gangrenous bowel will be untwisted. In addition, colonoscopy may be hazardous in distended ischemic bowel. If operation is long delayed, the mortality rate is 30 to 60 per cent; therefore, early operation is generally performed (Fig. 27). The status of the bowel and condition of the patient determine the operative procedure. If the cecum is viable

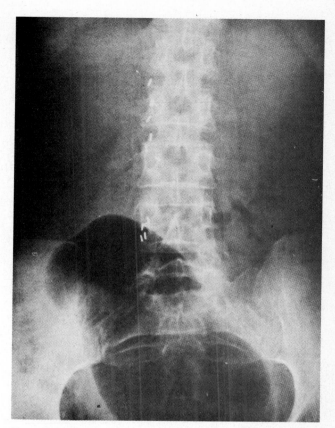

Figure 26. *Cecal volvulus. (From Spiro, H. M.: Clinical Gastroenterology, 3rd ed. New York, Macmillan Publishing Company, 1983.)*

and not tensely distended, detorsion and fixation of the cecum in the lower quadrant may be accomplished. If the cecum is tense and rupture appears imminent, as indicated by serosal tears, decompression by needle or trocar should be performed before detorsion is attempted. If the cecum is gangrenous, right hemicolectomy is necessary.[12, 22]

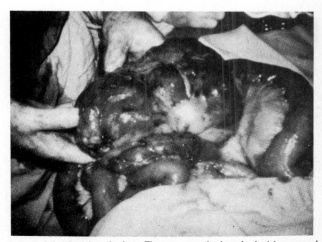

Figure 27. *Cecal volvulus. The surgeon's hands hold a cecal volvulus to emphasize the large size of this hugely distended mass. (From Spiro, H. M.: Clinical Gastroenterology, 3rd ed. New York, Macmillan Publishing Company, 1983.)*

VASCULAR, INFLAMMATORY, AND INFECTIOUS LESIONS OF THE LARGE BOWEL

Ischemic Colitis

Ischemic injury to the colon may be caused by advanced atherosclerosis or interruption of the colonic blood supply during operation, as in resection and grafting of abdominal aortic aneurysms, aortoiliac arterial reconstructions, and abdominoperineal resections in which the inferior mesentery artery is ligated. Ischemic injury may also occur in association with hypercoagulable states, amyloidosis, vasculitis, ruptured aortic aneurysm, colorectal cancer, or the use of oral contraceptive agents. In addition, nonocclusive colonic ischemia may occur in states of low cardiac output or hypoxia, particularly when aggravated by other metabolic conditions, such as diabetic ketoacidosis and dehydration. The syndrome of ischemic colitis may be quite variable in its extent, severity, and prognosis. However, extensive infarction and perforation appear to be infrequent. Localized or segmental ischemia is common, particularly affecting those areas of the colon that lie on the watershed between two adjacent arterial supplies, such as the splenic flexure (superior and inferior mesenteric arteries) and the rectosigmoid (inferior mesenteric and internal iliac arteries). However, evidence of major vessel obstructions is uncommon.

CLINICAL PRESENTATION

Patients over 50 are most often affected and present with abrupt onset of lower abdominal cramping pain, rectal bleeding, and, to a variable degree, vomiting and fever. Some patients have a history of similar symptoms occurring intermittently for weeks to months before presentation. Left-sided abdominal tenderness and peritoneal signs may be present as well as evidence of generalized atherosclerotic disease. This diagnosis should always be suspected in any elderly patient who suddenly develops rectal bleeding and appears to have sudden onset of ulcerative colitis. Indeed, it is likely that a number of elderly patients who have been considered to have ulcerative colitis in fact have had ischemic proctitis.

DIAGNOSIS

The plain abdominal film shows thickening of the bowel wall with edema and fluid. Since the first response of the bowel to ischemia is atonic contraction, the abdominal films may show complete absence of small bowel air if small bowel ischemia is also present. Diffuse abdominal pain may be elicited on physical examination, and signs of peritoneal irritation may be present. Sigmoidoscopy may be normal, may show evidence of mild nonspecific proctitis, or may reveal a spectrum of findings including multiple discrete ulcers, blue-black hemorrhagic submucosal blebs, and an adherent pseudomembrane. Angiography generally has not proved useful in the diagnosis of patients in this setting. The differentiation of ischemic colitis from infections of the colon, diverticulitis, and idiopathic inflammatory bowel disease may be very difficult. Barium enema may show typical narrowing of bowel lumen and thumbprint configuration in the splenic flexure or in the descending colon or the sigmoid. Thumbprinting is the indentation of the barium column due to submucosal hemorrhage and edema. Tubular narrowing and sawtooth irregularities may also be seen (Fig. 28).

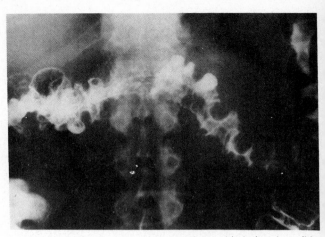

Figure 28. A barium enema in a patient with ischemic colitis showing narrowing and "thumbprinting" (nodular indentations of the bowel wall) in the distal transverse colon. This is one of the watershed areas of the colon between adjacent arterial supplies (superior and inferior mesenteric arteries) where ischemia is likely to develop. (From Grendell, J. H.: Vascular diseases of the intestine. In Wyngaarden, J. B., and Smith, L. H., Jr. (Eds.): Cecil Textbook of Medicine, 17th ed. Philadelphia, W. B. Saunders Company, 1985.)

TREATMENT

Initial management consists of general supportive measures, including antibiotics, together with appropriate fluid management and correction of any underlying medical disabilities, such as low cardiac output, or metabolic abnormalities, such as acidosis or ketoacidosis. Close observation of the patient is necessary. The goals are to restore perfusion to the intestine, reverse the ischemia and tissue hypoxia, and prevent infarction. In patients in whom perforation or infarction of the viscus appears likely, early surgical exploration is indicated. However, most patients will improve without operation. In patients with persistent diarrhea following ischemic injury, codeine can be helpful to mobilize fluid from the colon.

Vascular Malformations

Vascular malformations occur in the gastrointestinal tract in association with diseases involving the skin, such as hereditary hemorrhagic telangiectasis (Rendu-Osler-Weber syndrome), blue rubber bleb nevus syndrome, and the CREST syndrome (calcinosis, Raynaud's phenomenon, esophageal hypomotility, sclerodactyly, and telangiectasia). In addition, vascular malformations may occur as a primary process (angiodysplasia) chiefly involving the colon but also the stomach or small intestine. The latter is being increasingly recognized as a frequent cause of lower intestinal bleeding, particularly in patients over the age of 60.

Angiodysplastic lesions consist of ectatic, tortuous submucosal veins and groups of ectatic mucosal vessels lying under the colonic epithelium or, at times, on the luminal surface unprotected by intestinal epithelium. The etiology of these lesions remains uncertain. One theory suggests that they develop as a result of chronic low-grade obstruction of the submucosal veins as they penetrate the muscularis propria. Another view holds that these lesions develop owing to chronic mucosal ischemia.

Larger vascular malformations, including primary angiodysplastic lesions, may be visualized by selected mesenteric arteriography, although many are small and are best demonstrated by endoscopy. Such lesions are present in a large number of older individuals without apparent gastrointestinal blood loss. For those patients with chronic or recurrent gastrointestinal blood loss without any apparent cause, surgery has been recommended if vascular malformations can be identified and localized, such as right colectomy for lesions in the cecum. This approach is often unsatisfactory, and bleeding may recur either because some lesions in other parts of the gastrointestinal tract may not have been appreciated at the initial evaluation or because new lesions may subsequently develop. However, when there is no other apparent cause of the bleeding and it is life-threatening, selective segmental colectomy at the likely site of bleeding is indicated. Fortunately, nonoperative endoscopic approaches are being developed to obliterate vascular malformations by techniques such as electrocoagulation or photocoagulation. These techniques will probably be the primary therapy for these vascular malformations in the future.[10, 12]

Radiation Colitis

Because of the rapid renewal rate of the epithelial lining, the colon is particularly susceptible to acute radiation injury. In the colon and rectum, mucosal inflammation and atrophy are seen, and symptomatic proctitis and colitis are not rare during acute radiation exposure. The clinical features closely resemble those of idiopathic ulcerative colitis, but the response to treatment with local corticosteroids in the form of enemas or suppositories and sulfasalazine is limited.

Serious radiation enteritis and colitis occur months or several years after radiation therapy has been completed. This delayed lesion results in part from obliterative enteritis of submucosal arterials and appears unrelated to the acute mucosal lesion. Fibrosis and edema of the intestinal colonic wall develop, largely on an ischemic basis, and may produce strictures, obstruction of mucosal lymphatics, and secondary mucosal lesions including ulceration. The threshold tissue dose for the delayed intestinal tissue lesion is in the range of 4000 rads, and the incidence of significant damage rises sharply at doses above 5000 rads. The clinical features of chronic radiation colitis or proctitis resemble those of inflammatory or chronic ischemic disease of the large intestine, with diarrhea, abdominal pain, and hemochezia being prominent symptoms. Stricture formation may produce symptoms of partial colonic obstruction. Barium contrast studies of the colon help characterize the extent of the disease and localize the site of strictures that closely resemble the radiologic features of other inflammatory or ischemic intestinal lesions.

Radiation proctitis is common in patients undergoing pelvic radiation therapy but is seldom serious. Tenesmus, pain, rectal bleeding, and diarrhea may be controlled by low-residue diet, stool softeners, sedation, antispasmodics, and nonabsorbable sulfonamides. Occasionally steroid enemas may be required, and symptoms usually subside after radiation therapy is complete.

Radiation injury to the colon is usually the result of radiation of the cervix, uterus, bladder, or ovaries. Rectal stenosis can occur 6 to 18 months after radiation. Bleeding and diarrhea signal the onset of symptoms. The lesion is almost always in the high rectum about 10 to 14 cm. from the anus. Ulceration of the mucosa is common.

Therapy consists of intermittent dilation, which may relieve symptoms. Progressive obstruction may require diverting colostomy. If possible and if there is no recurrence of pelvic tumor, resection of the stricture with reanastomosis may be performed.

Rectovaginal fistula is most commonly the result of tumor necrosis in patients with recurrent carcinoma of the cervix. Diverting colostomy is the treatment of choice. In patients with biopsy-proven recurrent tumor, this palliative operation is all that is necessary. In patients in whom tumor is cured, attempts should be made to repair the fistula under the protection of the diverting colostomy.[12, 24]

Pseudomembranous Colitis

Pseudomembranous enterocolitis is a severe disease characterized by exudate or plaques on the intestinal mucosa and most commonly involves the colon. It is usually found in association with other conditions, although occasionally it occurs in the healthy patient with no identifiable risk factors. This condition was initially described in the preantibiotic period, when it usually followed intestinal procedures, often in association with shock states. Recognized risk factors include intestinal obstruction, uremia, Hirschsprung's disease, inflammatory bowel disease, shigellosis, intestinal ischemia, and neonatal enterocolitis. During the past three decades the disease has been recognized most frequently as a complication of antibiotic use.

Studies of antibiotic-associated pseudomembranous colitis are divided into two periods with quite different observations. Reports from the 1950s and 1960s indicated that the small intestine usually was involved (enterocolitis), mortality rates were high, and the most frequently implicated drugs were chloramphenicol, tetracycline, and oral neomycin. Staphylococcus aureus was the pathogen in most of those cases. More recent studies of antibiotic-associated pseudomembranous colitis show that the lesions are generally confined to the colon, different antibiotics are usually implicated, and the prognosis is considerably better than previously reported. The more recent work also indicates that Clostridium difficile is the responsible pathogen in the majority of cases.

Nearly all antibiotics with antibacterial spectrum of activity have been implicated; most frequently ampicillin, clindamycin, and cephalosporins. Less frequently implicated are penicillins other than ampicillin, erythromycin, and sulfur drugs. Drugs rarely implicated include tetracycline, chloramphenicol, and enterally administered aminoglycosides.

Clostridium difficile may be found in the colonic flora of 3 per cent of healthy adults and is widely distributed in the environment. Although the mechanism of C. difficile–mediated colitis is not clear, it is a toxin-mediated enteric disease in which there is no microbial invasion of the intestinal mucosa. The integrity of the bowel mucosa is impaired, and its protective effect against bacterial invasion may be diminished. The clinical manifestations consist of fever, abdominal pain and distention, diarrhea, and shock due to fluid loss and bacterial invasion in some patients. The mucosa of the colon is covered with a pseudomembrane of fibrin, mucus, necrotic cells, and leukocytes. Symptoms may begin any time during the course of antibiotic treatment or up to 6 weeks after antibiotics have been discontinued.

DIAGNOSIS

The diagnosis is established by endoscopy. Gross inspection of the colon reveals punctate, raised, yellowish white plaques with skip areas of normal mucosa or mucosa showing erythemia and edema. Microscopic examination shows epithelial necrosis, goblet cells distended with mucus, and infiltration of the lamina propria with polymorphonuclear cells and eosinophilic exudate. The pseudomembrane is attached to the surface of the epithelium and is composed of fibrin, mucin, and polymorphonuclear cells. *C. difficile* is difficult to culture but may be implicated in a tissue culture assay to demonstrate the toxin neutralized by antitoxin to *C. difficile*.

TREATMENT

The most important therapeutic decision is discontinuation of the implicated antibiotic. Patients with severe fluid, albumin, or electrolyte depletion require fluid replenishment and, possibly, hyperalimentation. The role of corticosteroids or attempts to manipulate the flora with oral lactobacilli or enemas, is uncertain, and antiperistaltic drugs are contraindicated. Specific therapy for diarrhea caused by *C. difficile* is the administration of vancomycin. Reports that focus on more seriously ill patients indicate mortality rates of 10 to 30 per cent, but with early institution of vancomycin therapy there is prompt symptomatic response and virtually all patients recover. Vigorous precautions to prevent stool contamination are mandatory. In surgical practice this condition is seen most frequently following an operation in which antibiotics were administered. However, close monitoring is necessary, and a colonic operation may be necessary if perforation occurs or bleeding is uncontrollable.

Amebiasis

Amebae enter the submucosa of the large bowel by excreting a material that allows them to pass between mucosal cells. In the submucosa, the organism releases substances that contribute to tissue anoxia, necrosis, and changes in the environment that render it ideal for replication of the ameba. The ameba then ingests host tissue, particularly red blood cells, to continue its growth. During this process, an ulcer is formed. Since the ulcer is much larger at the base of the submucosa than at the mucosal surface, it appears flask-shaped. The amebic infection may appear as scattered punctate hemorrhagic lesions. Alternatively, when inflammation is marked there is loss of mucosal integrity and the amebic infection appears as large ulcers. Secondary bacterial infections may occur. Ulceration of the bowel may extend through the serosal surface and lead to peritonitis. During the submucosal infection, two other complications may result, the first being a local inflammatory reaction to the combination of ameba and bacteria, causing an intestinal mass ("ameboma").

The second, and most common, complication of amebiasis is the invasion of the vascular system of the bowel with vascular transport to the liver. Amebic infections of the liver appear as progressive necrosis of liver substance in the region of ameba replication. This appears pathologically as a gradually expanding necrotic lesion. The central region of the abscess is filled with debris and end-products of liver necrosis. The liquid has a reddish-brown appearance (anchovy paste). Amebae are seen at the periphery of the abscess at the edge of normal liver tissue. Although referred to as an abscess, this lesion is distinct from the typical inflammatory abscess that requires surgical drainage and represents an area of liver necrosis. Occasionally this enlarging area of liver necrosis may rupture into the perito-

neum, through the diaphragm into the pleural cavity, or into the pericardial sac. Such a rupture is a serious and often fatal complication of amebiasis.

The clinical features of colonic amebiasis range from no symptoms to bloody diarrhea and ulcerative colitis. Amebiasis must be differentiated especially from ulcerative colitis, dysentery, diverticulitis, carcinoma, and even appendicitis. The diagnosis is established by finding the parasites when fresh stool is immediately examined with exclusion of other causes. If no amebae are found but the patient exhibits a liver abscess, serologic tests may be helpful.

Treatment consists of infectious precautions for stools plus appropriate drug therapy. The intraluminal form of the disease is usually treated with Diodoquin and tetracycline and the extraluminal form with Flagyl. Perforation of the colon and, rarely, liver abscesses require operation. However, conservative treatment usually is efficacious.[2, 12]

DISEASES OF THE ANUS AND RECTUM

Hemorrhoids

Internal hemorrhoids are dilated veins of the superior and middle rectal plexuses (Fig. 29) that occur above the dentate line and underlying mucosa. External hemorrhoids are dilated inferior rectal veins that lie below the dentate line and are covered by squamous epithelium. The most common causes that increase pressure in these venous systems are constipation, straining at stool, hereditary varicose tendencies, pregnancy, prolonged upright position, abdominal or pelvic tumors, and portal hypertension (Fig. 30). The usual symptoms are protrusion, bleeding, dull pain, and pruritus. Thrombosis or acute prolapse with edema or ulceration is excruciatingly painful. Internal hemorrhoids are asymptomatic except when they prolapse and become strangulated. The only significant sign caused by internal hemorrhoids is painless bleeding of bright red blood per rectum during or after defecation.

Hemorrhoidal thrombosis is a common event and can occur in the external anal plexus under the squamous mucosa, in the main hemorrhoidal plexus of the submucosa of the upper anal canal, or in both. External anal thrombosis of hemorrhoids is common and is often seen in patients who have no other stigmata of hemorrhoids. The cause is unknown, but it is possibly due to the high venous pressures that develop during excessive straining efforts, which lead to distention and stasis in the veins. The patient notes an acute swelling at the anal verge that may be intensely painful. Pain may continue for several days and then gradually subside spontaneously; however, edema may continue for 3 to 4 weeks. Occasionally the clot wears through the underlying skin and is extruded. Treatment is usually symptomatic, since the condition resolves in a relatively short time. If pain is severe, however, the hemorrhoid should be incised with enucleation of the clot using local anesthesia.

Acute thrombosis of the internal hemorrhoid plexus is a much more unpleasant situation. The patient experiences sudden severe anal pain followed by protrusion of the thrombosed area. The pain can be extremely severe and can last for as long as 1 week. Gradually the edema subsides and the thrombosis is absorbed. Occasionally this process has a therapeutic effect, entirely relieving the patient of previous hemorrhoidal symptoms. If symptoms continue to be severe over several days, surgical treatment may be considered.

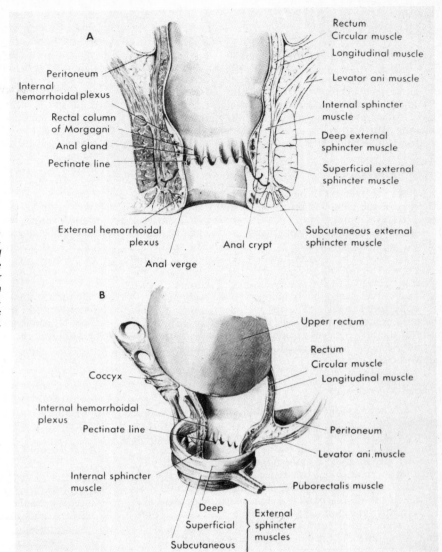

Figure 29. A, *Vertical section of anorectum.* B, *Anorectum. This three-dimensional diagram shows the relationship of external sphincter to internal sphincter. Note that the superficial portion of the external sphincter inserts into both coccyx and pubis. (From Block, G. E., and Liechty, R. D.: Large intestine. In Liechty, R. D., and Soper, R. T. (Eds.): Synopsis of Surgery. St. Louis, The C. V. Mosby Company, 1980.)*

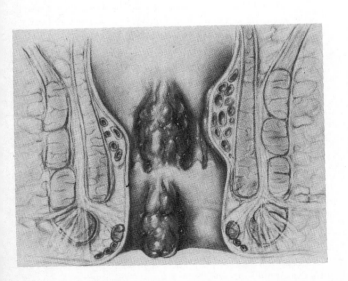

Figure 30. The anatomic location of the internal and external hemorrhoids and their relation to sphincters in the anal rectum. (From Hardy, J. D.: Hardy's Textbook of Surgery. Philadelphia, J. B. Lippincott Company, 1983.)

TREATMENT

Bowel Regulation

In many patients hemorrhoidal symptoms can be relieved by attention to hygiene and avoidance of excessive straining on defecation. Straining causes descent of the pelvic floor, weakening of the sphincter muscles (see Fig. 29), and both rectal and gynecologic prolapse. A firm bulky stool is desirable and can ideally be accomplished by ensuring sufficient fruit and bran in the diet. Use of a bulk laxative is also helpful.

Injection Therapy

Injection therapy of hemorrhoids is designed to cause sclerosis in the surrounding tissue, resulting in fibrosis of these tissues and obliteration of the hemorrhoid. Sclerosing fluids usually contain 5 per cent phenol and a clear vegetable oil or 5 per cent quinine urea hydrochloride. This is injected around the pedicle of each hemorrhoid through a lighted anoscope. The injection is placed in the submucosa of the upper anal canal well above the sensitive squamous mucosa. A fibrous tissue reaction is induced in the submucosa of the upper anal canal and lower rectum, thereby drawing the prolapsed mucosa upward toward its normal site. This form of therapy is effective only in relatively early hemorrhoids and is not appropriate for more severe or prolapsed hemorrhoids.

Rubber Band Ligation

Each hemorrhoid is visualized through a proctoscope, and the upper part above the mucocutaneous line is grasped. A small rubber band is slipped over the hemorrhoid, and the tissue distal to the rubber band undergoes necrosis. Excess mucosa in the upper anal canal is removed, and the lower anal mucosa is reduced by fibrosis, which also causes adherence of the mucosa to the underlying muscle. If the rubber band is too close to the dentate line, pain results and immediate removal and reapplication slightly higher are necessary. In 3 to 5 days the strangulated internal hemorrhoid becomes gangrenous, and 8 to 10 days after ligation the gangrenous hemorrhoid and rubber bands will slough off, leaving a small raw area that will heal in a few days.

Cryotherapy

Another form of therapy involves freezing the hemorrhoidal tissues for a sufficient time to cause necrosis. If carefully used and applied only to the upper part of the hemorrhoidal area at the anal rectal junction, cryotherapy achieves a result similar to that seen with elastic banding, and there is no pain. The cold is induced through a probe from a small machine designed for this process. The procedure is quick and can easily be done in an office or a clinic. The effectiveness of this form of treatment is presently being evaluated. Both ligation and cryosurgery may well come to occupy a position between injection therapy and surgical excision.

Operative Treatment

If permanent descent of the anal mucosa occurs, coupled with more gross hemorrhoidal protrusion at defecation, it is unlikely that any conservative treatment will be useful. The aims of operative correction should be to remove all the vascular hemorrhoidal tissue in the submucosa and to correct the deformities due to mucosal prolapse.

Excision of this tissue must be coupled with the reconstruction of the deformed mucosa of the anal canal. The base of the hemorrhoidal mass just above the dentate line is grasped with a hemostat and retracted from the rectum. A catgut transfixion suture is then placed proximal to the hemorrhoidal plexus. It is important to avoid placing the suture through the internal sphincter muscle. A second hemostat is placed distal to the external hemorrhoids. An elliptical incision is made with the scalpel through the skin and mucosa about the external and internal hemorrhoidal plexuses, which are dissected free from the underlying tissue. The hemorrhoids are excised en masse. When the dissection reaches the catgut transfixion suture, the external hemorrhoids under the skin are excised. After securing hemostasis, the mucosa and anal skin are closed longitudinally with a simple running suture. Usually no more than three groups of hemorrhoids are removed at one time. Rectal stricture can be a catastrophic complication of a too generous excision of rectal mucosa. Therefore, it is better to take too little rather than too much tissue.

Complications include bleeding, which usually is indicative of a technical error in establishing hemostasis. Urinary retention is not uncommon and can be due to spasm, overhydration, excessive sedation, or prostatic obstruction. Fecal impaction may occasionally occur at any time during hospitalization, usually because of the patient's fear of pain on defecation. Ectropion of rectal mucosa can occur if the mucosa is sutured to the lower anal canal of the dentate line. In these patients, part of the anal canal may be covered with rectal mucosa rather than squamous epithelium, resulting in a "wet bottom" and perianal irritation. Surgical revision may be necessary to correct this.[12, 15, 19]

Anal Fissures

Anal fissures are slitlike ulcers in the anal mucosa and commonly arise from (1) trauma, usually from the passage of hard feces, (2) cryptitis, in which the anal crypts become inflamed and subsequently develop a mucosal break extending distally, and (3) ulceration of mucosa covering a thrombosed hemorrhoid. Spasm of the anal sphincters helps sustain anal fissures.

CLINICAL PRESENTATION

Excruciating pain during and after defecation is the most common symptom and may be associated with varying degrees of bleeding. A fissure can usually be seen on general traction on each side of the anus, and anoscopy under local anesthesia confirms the diagnosis.

TREATMENT

Anal phase fissures are treated conservatively by scrupulous anal hygiene, hot sitz baths, and stool softeners. If the fissure does not heal within 3 weeks, sphincter dilation (under anesthesia), fissurectomy, and partial sectioning of the internal sphincter or subcutaneous portion of the external sphincter are the operative options; both relax the sphincter mechanism. Surgical excision is probably the most common method used to manage anal fissures. After satisfactory anesthesia is achieved, the anal canal is gradually dilated. A hemostat is placed in the base of the secondary hemorrhoid, and the posterior midline is pulled out of the rectum. A transfixion suture is placed proximal to the hemorrhoid as described in hemorrhoidectomy. Beginning at the anal verge, an elliptical incision is made about the fissure to include the sentinel pile, anal fissure, papilla,

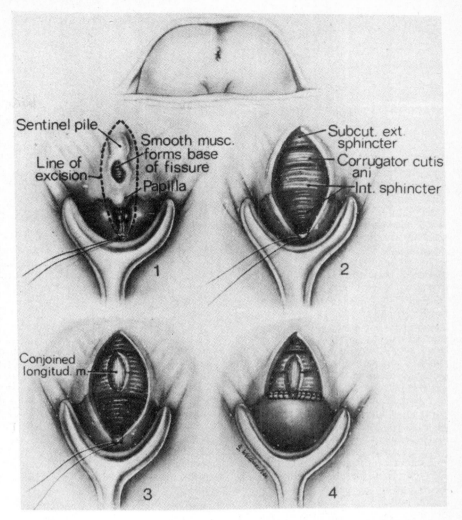

Figure 31. Excision of anal fissure.

1, A submucosal transfixion suture placed proximal to the posterior secondary hemorrhoid. The elliptical incision is illustrated to include "sentinel pile," fissure, papilla, crypts, posterior secondary internal hemorrhoids, and subepithelial tissue.

2, The relationship of the subcutaneous external anal sphincter of the corrugator cutis ani and internal sphincter muscles after en masse excision of the sentinel pile, fissure, papilla, crypts, and subepithelial tissue.

3, The corrugator cutis ani and lower portion of the internal sphincter are severed to the anterior surface of the conjoined longitudinal muscle. The internal sphincterotomy extends cephalad to the level of the dentate line.

4, The rectal mucosa is sutured to the internal sphincter transversely. This increases the diameter of the anal canal. Sutures do not include the skin. The wound distal to the dentate line heals by secondary intention.

(From Hanley, P. H.: Anorectum. In Hardy, J. D. (Ed.): Rhoads Textbook of Surgery, 5th ed. Philadelphia, J. B. Lippincott Company, 1977.)

crypts, and internal hemorrhoid, which are excised en masse. The internal sphincter is divided in the posterior midline to the level of conjoined longitudinal muscle. The upper extension of this incision terminates at the level of the dentate line. The mucosa is dissected from the internal sphincter for a short distance before closing the wound transversely up to the lower edge of the internal sphincter at the level of the dentate line with a running suture. This is tied at the mucocutaneous junction, leaving the external part of the wound open (Fig. 31). Healing may require 3 to 4 weeks.

Anal Abscesses and Fistulas

Perianal abscesses usually result from infected anal glands that erode into underlying tissues. Cultures from anal rectal abscess fistulas show mixed infections with *E. coli* predominating. Chronic use of purgatives and regional enteritis are common causative factors. Uncommon infections, such as actinomycosis, tuberculosis, and other fungal diseases, pelvic inflammatory disease, prostatitis, and cancer may rarely be associated. Common locations of these abscesses are depicted in Figure 32.

Early symptoms of dull rectal aching and mild systemic complaints progress to severe throbbing perianal pain with fever, chills, and malaise. A fluctuant area is not always apparent because of the thick perianal skin. Redness,

tenderness, and generalized protrusion are the usual findings. Prompt incision and drainage without waiting for fluctuation (as in other subcutaneous infections) prevent serious extensions.

It is important to recognize that there is no role for conservative medical treatment of a rectal abscess. Anorectal abscess should be considered a surgical emergency, and delay in operative treatment results in further destruction of tissue. Multilateral extensions can extend into the thighs, scrotum, and even the abdominal wall if operative therapy is deferred.

The surgical principle of treatment is relatively simple. Under anesthesia, with internal and external digital or sigmoidoscopic evaluation, the area of the abscess is drained by simple excision and laying open of the abscess cavity. It is important to digitally vigorously explore the abscess cavity and its surrounding tissue, as fingerlike projections can extend into the surrounding tissue, causing multiple abscesses, all of which must be opened and drained.

Perirectal Fistulas

Probably three of four perirectal abscesses after drainage eventually heal with no sequelae. However, those that fail to heal primarily evolve into fistulas. The external opening may close temporarily, only to reopen when pus accumulates in the tract, and eventually the tract becomes

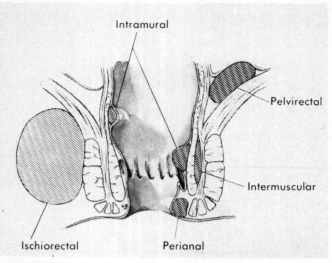

Figure 32. Location of pelvirectal and perirectal abscesses. (From Porter, S. D., and Liechty, R. D.: Anorectum. In Liechty, R. D., and Soper, R. T. (Eds.): Synopsis of Surgery. St. Louis, The C. V. Mosby Company, 1980.)

lined with epithelium. Multiple openings can complicate cases. Extensions into the urinary tract, perineal area, thighs, or bone may occasionally occur.

Usually the fistulous tract follows a variable course, but a few general rules are available for simplification. The primary or internal opening is usually found in one of the anal crypts. Most lie on one side of the posterior midline. If the cutaneous opening is anterior to a transverse line drawn through the anus, the internal opening is on a radial line directly into the anal rectum. If the cutaneous opening is posterior to the line, the internal opening will probably be in a posterior midline (Goodsall's rule) (Fig. 33).

Symptoms are usually confined to intermittent swelling, drainage, pruritus, and varying discomfort. The history of an abscess is of help in the diagnosis.

The cutaneous opening is characteristically a slightly raised, gray-pink papilla of granulation tissue. In time, scarring along the tract becomes palpable. A probe can sometimes be passed through the fistula to the pectinate line. This is ordinarily not painful.

The operative goal is to incise over the fistulous tract, leaving it open to granulate later. This is usually accomplished by placing a probe through both openings of the fistula and cutting down on the probe. If the fistula follows a course that necessitates cutting of the sphincter, the incision must divide the muscle fibers perpendicularly and at only one level. Incontinence may result if the muscle is divided at more than one site (Fig. 34).

If the fistula is the result of carcinoma, tuberculosis, Crohn's disease, or colitis, the primary disease must receive appropriate treatment if the lesion is to heal. Most surgeons are reluctant to perform anorectal operations on patients with inflammatory bowel disease because of local recurrence and failure of wound healing.

Squamous Cell Cancer of the Anus

Squamous cell cancer composes almost 90 per cent of the neoplastic lesions in the skin of the anus. These lesions are generally poorly differentiated, and 20 per cent have a basal cell appearance characterized by small basophilic cells

and are designated *cloacogenic* or *transitional cell* anal tumors, which may have an appearance similar to that of large bowel carcinomas (Fig. 35).

Early squamous carcinoma of the anus often presents as a small nodule resembling a hemorrhoidal tag. As it increases in size, it becomes ulcerated and eventually may become an exophytic mass. Internally, it may extend beneath the intact rectal mucosa and become ulcerated farther above in the form of an apparently separate rectal tumor. Most arise in the anterior or posterior anal quadrants. At the time of initial surgical treatment 28 to 64 per cent of patients are found to have involvement of perirectal or mesenteric nodes, and as many as 27 per cent have inguinal node metastases.

Clinical Features

One of the first symptoms observed is pruritus or bleeding. Tenesmus and pain that are not relieved by defecation may become increasingly noticeable. Constitutional symptoms, including fever, weight loss, anemia, and weakness, are usually absent unless the lesion is far advanced.

Treatment

Surgical excision has been the primary management of anal malignancies. Although there are series reporting 5-year survival rates of approximately 90 per cent with local excision, the marked variability of tumors in this area and the difference in size of lesions operated upon make it difficult to analyze comparative results. Resection should

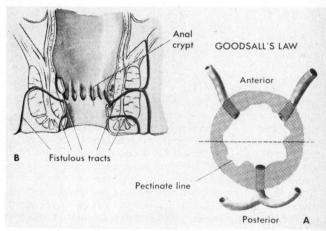

Figure 33. Anorectal fistulas.

A, Location of external fistulous opening is key to position of internal opening.

B, Common courses of anorectal fistulous tracts. Internal (primary) opening is almost always in crypt; fistulas are usually single and involve only portions of sphincter muscles; multiple fistulas or fistulas that involve all external sphincter muscles are less common. Goodsall's rule is that a transverse line divides fistula in ano into two groups: (1) when the secondary opening is anterior to a transverse line bisecting the anal canal to anterior and posterior halves, it is usually connected to the primary opening by a straight fistulous tract; (2) a secondary opening posterior to the transverse line is connected to a primary opening in the midline by a curved fistulous tract that may be horseshoe or semi-horseshoe in pattern.

(From Porter, S. D., and Liechty, R. D.: Anorectum. In Liechty, R. D., and Soper, R. T. (Eds.): Synopsis of Surgery. St. Louis, The C. V. Mosby Company, 1980.)

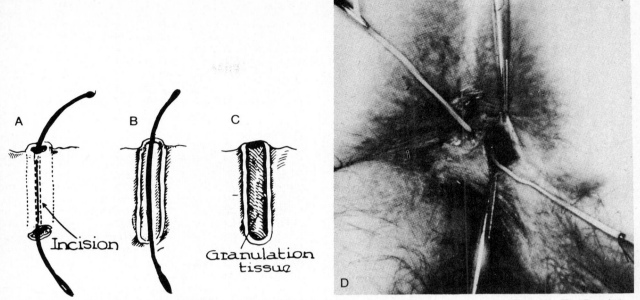

Figure 34. Fistulotomy. A, For superficial subcutaneous fistula in ano. The skin is incised over a probe. B, The skin edges are incised with scissors. C, Granulating wounds heal from within outward. D, Under local anesthesia, a fistulotomy incision is made to the subcutaneous external sphincter muscle. (From Hanley, P. H.: Anorectum. In Hardy, J. D. (Ed.): Rhoads Textbook of Surgery, 5th ed. Philadelphia, J. B. Lippincott Company, 1977.)

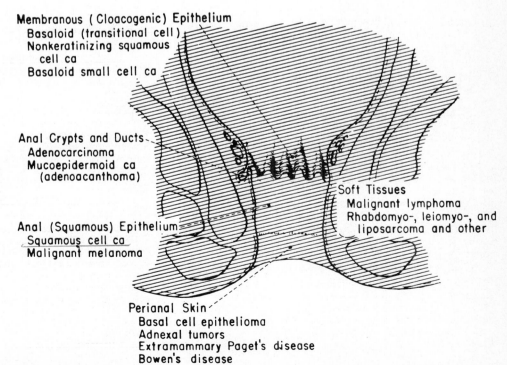

Figure 35. Malignant lesions originating from the various tissues in the area of the anus. (From Harrison, E. C., Jr., Beahrs, O. H., and Hill, J. R.: Dis. Colon Rectum, 9:255, 1966.)

Membranous (Cloacogenic) Epithelium
  Basaloid (transitional cell)
  Nonkeratinizing squamous
    cell ca
  Basaloid small cell ca

Anal Crypts and Ducts
  Adenocarcinoma
  Mucoepidermoid ca
    (adenoacanthoma)

Anal (Squamous) Epithelium
  Squamous cell ca
  Malignant melanoma

Soft Tissues
  Malignant lymphoma
  Rhabdomyo-, leiomyo-, and
    liposarcoma and other

Perianal Skin
  Basal cell epithelioma
  Adnexal tumors
  Extramammary Paget's disease
  Bowen's disease

be sufficient to remove the tumor without entering it and provide wide margins. In general, lesions less than 2 cm. in diameter are treated by local excision, and those larger than 2 cm. in size are best treated with abdominoperineal resection, since considerable local invasion has occurred by the time of treatment.

Although anal lesions drain into the inguinal lymph nodes, there is probably little justification for routine inguinal lymphadenectomy. If the lymph nodes are clinically involved, they are removed, but the prognosis is poor. However, if there is an interval between the time of resection of the primary and the time the node resection is required because of clinical palpable involvement, 5-year survival rates can exceed 60 per cent. The 5-year survival rate of patients treated by combined abdominoperineal resection ranges between 30 and 60 per cent, comparing favorably with patients receiving the same treatment for carcinoma of the rectum.

Radiation therapy is being used more frequently than previously, particularly for early lesions. Both primary radiation and radiation following limited resection have been performed. Cantrell and associates reported on 47 patients, 35 of whom received external radiation therapy alone, which was given as curative treatment. The local control rate was 80 per cent, and the actuarial 5-year survival rate for patients without metastases was 95.6 per cent. The overall survival rate for the entire group was 79.3 per cent. Similar results have been reported by Puthawala and colleagues in 40 patients treated with a combination of interstitial and external beam radiation therapy. These studies indicate the efficacy of radiation therapy in achieving local control of squamous carcinoma of the anus. Judicious use of this modality, perhaps with interstitial implantation of low-energy radiation emitters, may lead to improved cure rates and reduced morbidity.[20]

Prolapse of the Rectum

The three types of rectal prolapse are (1) mucosal prolapse, (2) rectal intussusception, and (3) true prolapse.

Mucosal prolapse occurs with an intact sphincter and evolves in extrusion through the anus of rectal mucosa only. The remainder of the wall is not involved. It becomes symptomatic because of irritation and, occasionally, ulceration of the prolapsed tissue. Soiling results from mucosal secretions. This condition is more common in infants than in the aged. Infant prolapse almost invariably disappears by 5 years of age. In the adult, radial incisions, similar to hemorrhoidectomy incisions, result in scarring, which shrinks and then holds the redundant mucosa in place.

Rectal intussusception involves protrusion of the entire rectal wall without a peritoneal sac. It begins above the pectinate line. The palpable full thickness of tissues in the prolapsed portion and concentric folds distinguish it from mucosal prolapse. This can be considered to be an incomplete prolapse. A sulcus can be palpated along the periphery of the prolapsed part of the anal ring that is not present in true prolapse.

True prolapse occurs by herniation of the pelvic peritoneum through the pelvic diaphragm, the anterior rectal wall, and the anus. The anal sphincter tone is poor. True prolapse occurs mainly in infants, men in their 20s or 30s, and women of any age. In males it probably represents a congenital weakness because the prostate and seminal vesicles lend adequate support anteriorly to prevent herniation. With repeated and prolonged protrusion, the anal sphincter becomes relaxed, progressively stretched, and ultimately paralyzed (Fig. 36).

A variety of surgical procedures have been described to treat rectal prolapse, but no standard or ideal procedure is agreed upon. However, any operation to control this debilitating condition must involve resection of the prolapsing and redundant bowel, reduction in the size of the anus, plastic reconstruction and reinforcement of the perineal floor, transabdominal suspension and fixation of the prolapsed bowel to the pelvis, obliteration of the cul de sac, and/or repair of the perineal sliding hernia.[12, 15, 19]

Pruritus Ani

Pruritus ani is manifest by intense itching of the perianal area and is considered a symptom rather than a disease. It may follow hemorrhoids, fissures, fistulas, prolapse, cryptitis, or neoplasms. Nonsurgical causes include a local dermatitis, fungal lesion, pinworm problem, or antibiotic irritation. Systemic causes include jaundice, diabetes, psoriasis, syphilis, seborrheic dermatitis, and leukemia. Finally, the problem may be idiopathic, including psychosocial problems. Appropriate diagnostic tests to delineate these factors are obvious.

Underlying anatomic factors are treated surgically (fissures, fistulas, hemorrhoids, neoplasm). Systemic conditions such as diabetes or jaundice or local irritants and infestations, such as oral antibiotics, pinworms, or parasites, are specifically treated.

Even after an extensive search, the cause of pruritus ani may remain elusive. Idiopathic pruritus accounts for approximately half the patients seen. Immaculate perianal hygiene alone often relieves the itching. Symptomatic relief may be obtained with locally applied zinc oxide ointment, anesthetic ointment, or corticosteroid cream. Hot sitz baths twice daily followed by careful drying and application of absorbent, nonirritating powder may be helpful. In some patients there is a considerable emotional element to the symptoms, and if present this must be handled appropriately.

Venereal Diseases

Condylomata acuminata, anal venereal warts, apparently are caused by a virus. They occur on the perineum and around the anus, often involving the squamous epithelium of the anal canal. Small warts are usually treated with an application of podophyllin solution, whereas large ones that obstruct the anal canal may be cauterized or excised. Recurrence is frequent, and often in cases with extensive involvement an abdominoperineal resection may be required. Good results have recently been reported following alpha interferon[7] therapy without the need for surgical excision.

Lymphogranuloma venereum is caused by a virus. It is sexually transmitted and primarily involves the genitals and regional lymph nodes. Diagnosis is made by proctoscopy with biopsy of the mucosa as well as the Frei test and complement fixation. Treatment is usually with tetracycline. Late complications may include rectal stricture, rectovaginal or anal fistula, or destruction of the anal canal. Dilatation is sufficient for lesser strictures; advanced cases may require a colostomy and abdominoperineal resection.

Pilonidal Sinus

Although not arising from the anorectum, pilonidal disease often enters the differential diagnosis of anorectal diseases.

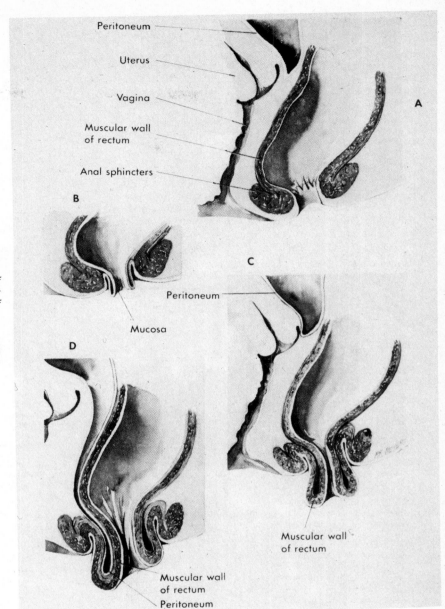

Figure 36. Rectal prolapse. A, Normal. B, The mucosal prolapse is the most common type of prolapse. The mucosa shows radial folds. C, Rectal intussusception, with all layers of rectum prolapsing. The peritoneum is not prolapsed. D, In true prolapse, all layers of rectal wall prolapse and the peritoneum descends as a hernial sac anteriorly. (From Porter, S. D., and Liechty, R. D.: Anorectum. In Liechty, R. D., and Soper, R. T. (Eds.): Synopsis of Surgery. St. Louis, The C. V. Mosby Company, 1980.)

These sinuses appear as small openings commonly found in the intergluteal fold in the sacrococcygeal area, about 3 to 5 cm. posterior to superior to the anal orifice. It is thought that the majority of cases result from hairs penetrating root end first into the dermis and eliciting a foreign body reaction. Some maintain that this condition is congenital in origin.

As the name suggests, a nidus of hair is almost invariably found within these sinus tracts. Almost all the hairs enter the sinus root end first. Hair scales pointing away from the root end apparently are driven inward by a rolling action between the buttocks. Hair follicles or other skin appendages are never found within the sinus walls. These lesions occur in the intergluteal region of young hirsute males and, less commonly, in females. Pilonidal disease is common in young military personnel. It almost never occurs in patients 45 years of age or older.

Infection with rupture through the skin (which forms sinuses), chronicity, and recurrence are the usual findings.

For acutely inflamed sinuses, simple incision and drainage are appropriate. The ideal treatment, when possible, is total excision and primary closure, although many surgeons still prefer to leave the wound open with healing by secondary intention.[12, 15, 19]

SELECTED REFERENCES

Becker, J. M., and Raymond, J. L.: Ileal pouch-anal anastomosis: A single surgeon's experience with 100 consecutive cases. Ann. Surg., *204*:375, 1986.
This is a review of 100 patients undergoing rectal preservation operations for ulcerative colitis and familial polyposis of the colon. The surgical management of these conditions together with the results is admirably reviewed in this paper.

Berk, J. E. (Ed.): Bockus Gastroenterology, Vol. 4, 4th ed. Philadelphia, W. B. Saunders Company, 1985.
This has long been a standard reference for all forms of diseases of the gastrointestinal tract, including fine sections on diseases of the colon and rectum. The student is referred to this source for full details and extensive bibliographies.

Bussey, H. J. R.: Familial Polyposis Coli. Baltimore, Johns Hopkins University Press, 1975.
This is a superb monograph reporting the experience of the surgical staff at St. Mark's Hospital, which is devoted to diseases of the rectum and colon. The genetic, epidemiologic, pathologic, and clinical features of this disorder are included. In addition, the author discusses the experience at St. Mark's Hospital with both Gardner's and Turcot syndromes.

DeVita, V. T., Jr., Hellman, S., and Rosenberg, S. A.: Important Advances in Oncology 1986. Philadelphia, J. B. Lipppincott Company, 1986.
This is a highly commendable monograph on surgical oncology that includes the general principles of the management of malignant neoplasms. The authors are highly knowledgeable and outstanding authorities in the field. The last edition is an update of the most recent work being done at the National Cancer Institute as well as other major clinics around the world.

Goligher, J. C. (Ed.): Surgery of the Anus, Rectum, and Colon. London, Bailliere Tindall, 1984.
This is a world-class reference for all diseases of the anus, rectum, and colon. It is written by an international authority in the field, and details of each of the disorders are admirably presented.

Welch, C. E., Ottinger, L. W., and Welch, J. P.: Manual of Lower Gastrointestinal Surgery. New York, Springer-Verlag, 1980.
This is an excellent reference source for the student seeking superb descriptions and illustrations of the various operative procedures performed on the lower gastrointestinal tract. The authors begin this superb and authoritative atlas with a table of historical landmarks of colorectal surgery, beginning in 1686 with the cure of Louis XIV's fistula in ano by Felix and continuing to the present.

REFERENCES

1. Altemeier, W. A., Burke, J. F., Pruitt, B., and Sandusky, W. R.: Control of Infection in Surgical Patients, 2nd ed. Philadelphia, J. B. Lippincott Company, 1984.
2. Bartlett, J. G.: Pseudomembranous colitis. *In* Wyngaarden, J. B., and Smith, L. H., Jr. (Eds.): Cecil Textbook of Medicine, 17th ed. Philadelphia, W. B. Saunders Company, 1985.
3. Block, G. E., and Liechty, R. D.: Large intestine. *In* Liechty, R. D., and Soper, R. T. (Eds.): Synopsis of Surgery, 4th ed. St. Louis, The C. V. Mosby Company, 1980.
4. Cohn, I., Jr., and Nance, F. C.: Intestinal antisepsis and peritonitis from perforation. *In* Sabiston, D. C., Jr. (Ed.): Davis-Christopher Textbook of Surgery, 12th ed. Philadelphia, W. B. Saunders Company, 1981.
5. Cohn, I., Jr., and Nance, F. C.: Mechanical inflammatory, vascular, and miscellaneous benign lesions. *In* Sabiston, D. C., Jr. (Ed.): Davis-Christopher Textbook of Surgery, 12th ed. Philadelphia, W. B. Saunders Company, 1981.
6. Conte, J. E., Jr., Jacobs, L. S., and Polk, H. C., Jr.: Surgery of the alimentary tract. *In* Antibiotic Prophylaxis in Surgery. Philadelphia, J. B. Lippincott Company, 1984.
7. Gall, S. A., Hughes, C. E., and Trofatter, K.: Interferon for the therapy of condyloma acuminatum. Am. J. Obstet. Gynecol., *153*:157, 1985.
8. Goldner, F. H., and Kraft, S. G.: Idiopathic inflammatory bowel disease. *In* Stein, J. H. (Ed.): Internal Medicine. Boston, Little Brown and Company, 1983.
9. Goligher, J. C.: Treatment of chronic ulcerative colitis. Ann. Probl. Surg., *2*:1, 1965.
10. Grendell, J. H.: Vascular diseases of the intestine. *In* Wyngaarden, J. B., and Smith, L. H., Jr. (Eds.): Cecil Textbook of Medicine, 17th ed. Philadelphia, W. B. Saunders Company, 1985.
11. Grinnell, R. S.: Distal intramural spread of carcinoma of rectum and rectosigmoid. Surg. Gynecol. Obstet., *49*:421, 1954.
12. Hardy, J. D.: The colon, rectum, and anus. *In* Hardy, J. D. (Ed.): Hardy's Textbook of Surgery. Philadelphia, J. B. Lippincott Company, 1983.
13. Labow, S. B., Salvati, E. P., and Rubin, R. J.: The Hartmann procedure in the treatment of diverticular disease. Dis. Colon Rectum, *16*:362, 1973.
14. Levin, B.: Ulcerative colitis. *In* Wyngaarden, J. B., and Smith, L. H., Jr. (Eds.): Cecil Textbook of Medicine, 17th ed. Philadelphia, W. B. Saunders Company, 1985.
15. Liechty, R. D., and Porter, S. O.: Anorectum. *In* Liechty, R. D., and Soper, R. T. (Eds.): Synopsis of Surgery, 4th ed. St. Louis, The C. V. Mosby Company, 1980.
16. Menguy, R. B.: Indications for surgery. *In* Bercovitz, Z. T., Kirsner, J. B., Lindner, A. E., et al. (Eds.): Ulcerative and Granulomatous Colitis. Springfield, Ill., Charles C Thomas, 1973.
17. Minton, J. P., Hoehn, J. L., Gerber, D. M., et al.: Results of a 400-patient carcinoembryonic antigen second-look colorectal cancer study. Cancer, 55:1284, 1985.
18. Oakley, J. R., Jagelman, D. G., Fazio, V. W., Lavery, I. C., Weakley, F. L., Easley, K., and Farmer, R. G.: Complications and quality of life after ileorectal anastomosis for ulcerative colitis. Am. J. Surg., *149*:23, 1985.
19. Polk, H. C., Jr.: Rectal and perianal complaints. *In* Polk, H. C., Jr., Stone, H. H., and Gardner, B.: Basic Surgery, 2nd ed. Norwalk, Conn., Appleton-Century-Crofts, 1983.
20. Ramming, K. P., and Haskell, C. M.: Colorectal malignancies. *In* Haskell, C. M. (Ed.): Cancer Treatment, 2nd ed. Philadelphia, W. B. Saunders Company, 1985.
21. Spiro, H. M.: Structural disorders, diverticular disease. *In* Spiro, H. M.: Clinical Gastroenterology, 3rd ed. New York, Macmillan Publishing Company, 1983.
22. Spiro, H. M.: Structural disorders, cecal volvulus. *In* Spiro, H. M.: Clinical Gasteoenterology, 3rd ed. New York, Macmillan Publishing Company, 1983.
23. Spiro, H. M.: General considerations. *In* Spiro, H. M.: Clinical Gastroenterology, 3rd ed. New York, Macmillan Publishing Company, 1983.
24. Trier, J. S.: Diseases of intestinal absorption. *In* Stein, J. H. (Ed.): Internal Medicine. Boston, Little, Brown and Company, 1983.
25. Winawer, S. J.: Neoplasms of the large and small intestine. *In* Wyngaarden, J. B., and Smith, L. H., Jr. (Eds.): Cecil Textbook of Medicine, 17th ed. Philadelphia, W. B. Saunders Company, 1985.
26. Zinkin, L. D.: A critical review of the classifications and staging of colorectal cancer. Dis. Colon Rectum, *26*:37, 1983.

THE LIVER

DOUGLAS S. REINTGEN, M.D. • DAVID C. SABISTON, JR., M.D.

27

The liver is a remarkably complex organ with a variety of synthetic and degradative metabolic functions. It consists of a complex circulatory system, biliary passages, a collection of reticuloendothelial cells of various types, and the hepatocyte, the metabolic factory of the body. Interference with the functions of one or more of these physiologic-anatomic components can be responsible for the clinical and laboratory abnormalities found in liver and biliary tract disease.

ANATOMY

Many unique anatomic features of the liver enable it to function as a processing area between the digestive system and the remainder of the body. These include a dual blood supply consisting of a portal vein draining absorbed nutrients from the small intestine and a hepatic artery transporting oxygenated blood, specific abilities of the hepatocytes and blood vessels that allow the passive transport of processed nutrients into the bloodstream, and the compartmentalization of the hepatocyte and biliary secretive process.

Gross Anatomy

The liver is a large organ, weighing 1500 gm. It is surrounded by a fibrous capsule called Glisson's capsule and is invested by peritoneum throughout most of its surface. The topographic arrangement of the liver in the right upper quadrant is secured by a number of ligaments. The falciform ligament, the remnant of the obliterated umbilical vein, attaches the liver to the anterior abdominal wall. This ligament resists movement of the liver to the right. The right and left coronary ligaments posteriorly attach the liver to the diaphragm, and the right and left triangular ligaments attach the apex of the left lobe to the diaphragm. The gastrohepatic and hepatoduodenal ligaments contain the important structures in the portal triad, i.e., the hepatic artery, portal vein, and common bile duct.

The liver can be divided into the right and left lobes; the right lobe contains 70 per cent of the liver mass, and each segment of the left lobe makes up 15 per cent. Mays,[6] in a series of innovative studies that involved making corrosion casts of each lobe by injecting the right and left portal veins with vinyl acetate of different colors, demonstrated the true lobar anatomy of the liver, which was found to be quite different from the topographic anatomy (Fig. 1). Thus, the anatomic line of division between the two lobes was drawn between the gallbladder fossa anteriorly and the inferior vena cava posteriorly and superiorly. The right lobe of the liver is divided into anterior and posterior divisions, whereas the left lobe contains the medial and lateral divisions. The line of the falciform ligament divides the left lobe into its medial and lateral segments. The posterior caudate lobe is bounded by the ligamentum teres on the left, gallbladder on the right, and portal triad posteriorly, with most of it being found in the medial segment of the left lobe.

PORTAL VEIN

The portal vein supplies 75 per cent of the hepatic blood, and the hepatic artery supplies 25 per cent. The portal vein is formed behind the head of the pancreas with the components of the splenic and superior mesenteric veins at the level of L1 and L2 (Fig. 2). It then branches into the right and left portal veins at the superior part of the porta hepatis. The portal vein is located posterior to the common bile duct and hepatic artery. Ten per cent of patients have three extrahepatic branches of the portal vein (two right branches). In some instances the portal vein is located anterior to the pancreas and duodenum and, if found, is usually associated with situs inversus. The average length of the main portal vein is 6.5 cm., with a width of 0.8 to 1.0 cm. This vessel receives blood from most of the small intestine, pancreas, and spleen and eventually empties into venules and, later, the hepatic sinusoids.

The portal system is unique in that it has no valves; thus, portal pressure can be measured intraoperatively in a small mesenteric vein. Portal pressure may also be calculated by threading a catheter through the inferior vena cava and wedging it in one of the hepatic veins. This technique is commonly used preoperatively to measure portal pressure and takes advantage of the fact that there are no valves in the system. Venous anatomy is also important in the development of cirrhosis and subsequent portal hypertension and esophageal varices. The main portosystemic anastomosis includes the left gastric or coronary vein, which connects the esophageal venous plexus with the portal vein. With the development of cirrhosis, blood is shunted around the liver and engorges the esophageal venous plexus (Fig. 3). Other portosystemic anastomoses include the short gastric veins, which stimulate the development of gastric and esophageal varices if splenic vein thrombosis occurs. Splenic vein thrombosis is diagnosed most frequently in the

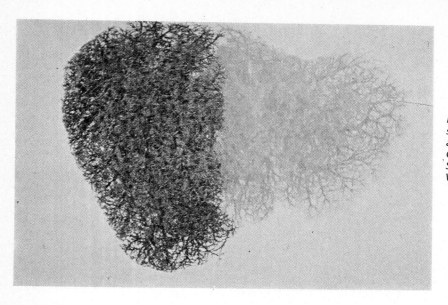

Figure 1. Corrosion cast of the liver demonstrating the anatomic fissure between the right and left lobes of the liver. (From Mays. E. T.: In Calne, R. Y., and Della Rovere, G. Q. D.: Liver Surgery. Philadelphia, Piccis Medical Books, W. B. Saunders Company, 1982, p. 2.)

setting of chronic pancreatitis, and in this situation splenectomy interrupts the shunting pathway through the short gastric veins and alleviates the esophageal varices, reducing their potential for bleeding.

HEPATIC ARTERY

The common hepatic artery arises from the celiac axis and, after contributing the gastroduodenal and right gastric arteries, courses superiorly in the hepatoduodenal ligament to the left of the common bile duct (Fig. 4). The distribution of the hepatic artery accompanies the segmental distribution of the bile ducts into the liver. Fifty per cent of the population have variations in the hepatic artery. For this reason, preoperative arteriography is important in planning hepatic resections. One of the most common variants is the right hepatic artery arising from the superior mesenteric artery (17 per cent). In autopsy dissections, the right hepatic artery crossed ventral to the bile ducts in 24 per cent and dorsal in 64 per cent of patients, and in 91 per cent it crossed ventral to the portal vein. Other variations include the left hepatic artery arising from the left gastric artery

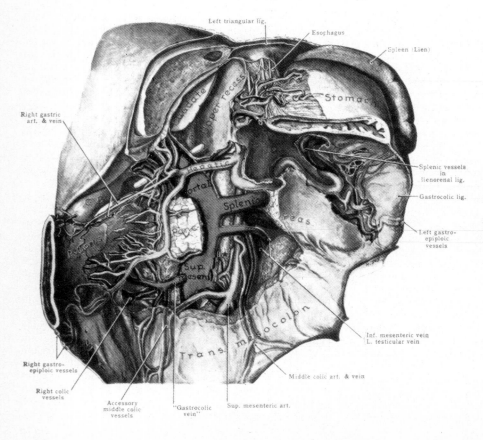

Figure 2. Anatomy of the extrahepatic portal venous system showing the formation of the portal vein by the confluence of the splenic and superior mesenteric vein behind the pancreas. (From Anderson, J. E.: Grant's Atlas of Anatomy, 7th ed. Baltimore, Williams & Wilkins, 1978.)

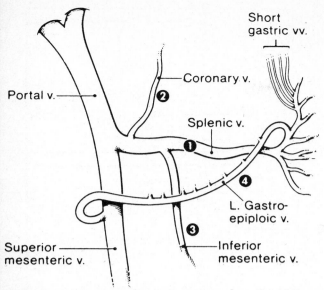

Figure 3. Schematic representation of the venous collateral channels that develop with cirrhosis. The coronary vein (2) feeds the esophageal venous plexus, as does the short gastric vein. (From Henderson, J. T., Millikan, W. J., and Warren, W. D.: World J. Surg., 8:722, 1984.)

(11.5 per cent) and arising partially from the left gastric artery (11.5 per cent). Usually the cystic artery supplying the gallbladder is a branch of the right hepatic artery. The hepatic arteries were originally felt to be end arteries; however, with further experience in anatomic dissection this has not been found to be true.

It is possible to demonstrate at least 26 collateral extrahepatic channels available to supply the liver if the hepatic artery is ligated. Ten collateral routes are derived from accessory or replaced hepatic arteries arising in various ways from the superior mesenteric or left gastric arteries. Ten additional collaterals to the liver arise from arteries not derived from the celiac axis, such as diaphragmatic arterial branches. Most studies have shown that ligation of the proper hepatic artery proximal to the origin of the gastroduodenal artery has no clinical sequelae. Ligation of either the left or right hepatic artery produces liver enzyme elevations but few if any clinical manifestations in 87 per cent of patients.

HEPATIC VEINS

Three short hepatic veins usually drain the liver from the central vein of the liver lobule into the inferior vena cava. The left, middle, and right hepatic veins follow an intersegmental branching course. The right hepatic vein enters the inferior vena cava in its anterolateral portion, and the left and middle hepatic veins enter the inferior vena cava in either a separate or common trunk on its most anterior portion. The hepatic veins are very short and usually the most treacherous and dangerous part of the dissection during hepatic resection. Bleeding from the hepatic veins or retrohepatic vena cava may be difficult to control and, in the trauma setting, is associated with a high mortality.

BILIARY SYSTEM

Biliary canaliculi, which are small channels formed from part of the hepatocyte membrane, drain the bile

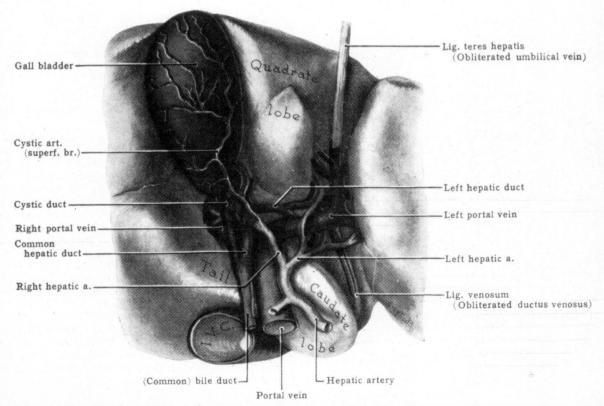

Figure 4. The anatomic relationships of the hepatic artery, common bile duct, and portal vein in the portal triad are demonstrated. (From Anderson, J. E.: Grant's Atlas of Anatomy, 7th ed. Baltimore, Williams & Wilkins, 1978.)

excreted by the liver cell into intrahepatic ducts that follow the segmental anatomy determined by the vascular supply. The right and left hepatic ducts then converge extrahepatically in the porta hepatis and form the common hepatic duct, which usually courses anteriorly in relation to the portal vein and lateral to the hepatic artery (see Fig. 4). The gallbladder is situated in the inferior aspect of the liver to the right of the common bile duct. The common hepatic duct descends in the hepatoduodenal ligament and is joined from the right by the cystic duct. The normal common bile duct is 10 mm. in diameter; however, after cholecystectomy it may increase to 11 to 12 mm. In 90 per cent of the population the major pancreatic duct, the duct of Wirsung, empties into the common bile duct just proximal to the ampulla of Vater. A neuroplexus consisting primarily of sympathetic fibers innervates the hepatic capsule and gallbladder, and pain in this area is usually referred to the right shoulder and scapula via the third and fourth cervical nerves. The lymphatic vessels draining the porta hepatis empty into the cisterna chyli, which eventually drains into the thoracic duct.

Microscopic Anatomy

Studies by Rappaport and others[8] provided a clearer concept of the hepatic functional unit, which is based on the organization of the hepatocytes around the central vein with portal triads in the periphery (Fig. 5). The hepatocytes range in diameter from 18 and 30 microns and are continuous with the sinusoids on all except one side, which is enmeshed in the bile capillaries. Liver cells maintain a constant interchange with the vascular and biliary systems. The microscopic anatomy of the sinusoids, perisinusoidal space of Disse, and hepatocyte reveals the intimate contact

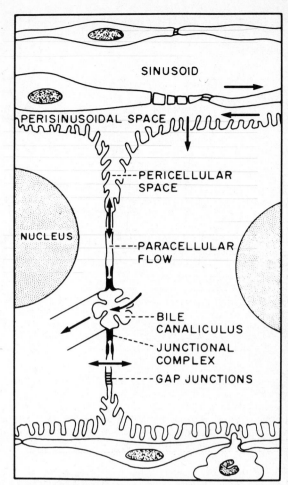

Figure 6. Schematic of the relationship of the hepatocytes, sinusoids, and perisinusoidal space of Disse. Arrows denote direction of fluid movement. (From Arias, I., et al. (Eds.): The Liver: Biology and Pathology. New York, Raven Press, 1982.)

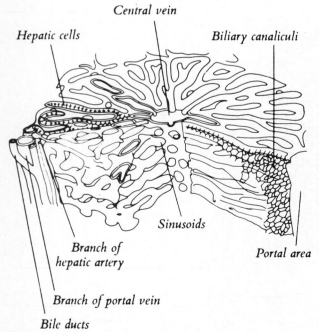

Figure 5. Artist's rendition of the hepatic lobule showing the hepatocytes in close contact with the biliary canaliculi and sinusoids and radiating from the central vein. The portal areas are noted to be in the periphery of the hepatic lobule. (From Evaluation of Liver Function. Indianapolis, The Lily Research Laboratories, 1962.)

of blood flow with the hepatocyte and bile canaliculus (Fig. 6).

The liver lobule is composed of a central vein with hepatocytes radiating from the central vein (see Fig. 5). Blood entering the liver via the portal vein drains into terminal veins and, eventually, the hepatic sinusoids, where the liver cells come in contact with the nutrient-laden blood. The hepatocyte microvilli project through the fenestrations of the endothelial cells of the sinusoids and thus are exposed to the sinusoidal content (Fig. 7). The sinusoids are usually 7 to 15 microns wide with an intraluminal pressure of 2 to 3 mm. Hg. This is an extremely low pressure system; however, pressure is altered with hepatic inflammation, fibrosis, and cirrhosis. Sinusoids are permeable to low- and high-molecular-weight substances, allowing the hepatocyte to take up and process the intestinal effluent. The space of Disse is the area between the vascular endothelium and hepatocyte and is the primary site of lymph formation. The acinar unit has arbitrarily been divided into zones 1, 2, and 3. Zone 1 represents the area nearest the sinusoids, and blood flow in the acinar unit is from zones 1 to 3. Subsequently, zone 3 hepatocytes, located further from the central vein, are less resistant to hepatic toxins since they receive blood of less nutritional value and are the first to show ischemic changes.

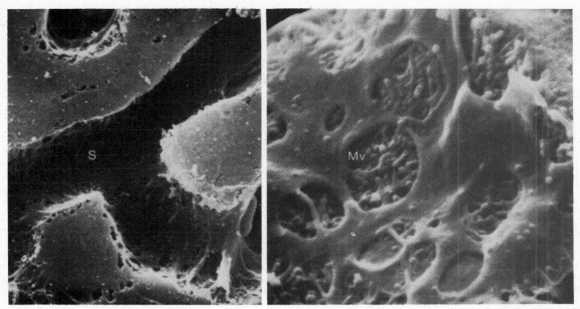

Figure 7. Scanning electron photomicrograph showing the microvilli of the underlying hepatocytes protruding through fenestrations in the endothelial cells. (From Kessel, R., and Hardon, R. H. (Eds.): Tissues and Organs: A Text-Atlas of Scanning Electron Microscopy. New York, W. H. Freeman and Company, 1979.)

Kupffer's cells, the primary phagocytic cells of the liver, are also present in the space of Disse. These cells are part of the reticuloendothelial system and are responsible for the processing of bacteria and foreign antigens by the liver. They are also responsible for the uptake of radionuclides and the image produced with nuclear scans.

PHYSIOLOGY

The liver is a metabolically active organ and accounts for 20 per cent of the body's energy expenditure, while consuming 20 to 25 per cent of the total utilized oxygen. This is despite the fact that it assumes only 4 to 5 per cent of the total body weight. The blood flow to the liver is estimated to be 1500 ml. per min. per 1.73 m.², and about 75 per cent of this flow is derived from the portal vein, with the remainder being derived from the hepatic artery. With a decrease in portal blood flow, such as in Laennec's cirrhosis, there is usually a compensatory increase in arterial flow. However, the opposite is not true; i.e., during ischemic conditions with interruption of hepatic artery flow, there is no corresponding increase in portal venous flow. The normal portal vein pressure is usually 7 to 10 mm. Hg, with the sinusoidal pressure decreasing to the 2- to 4-mm. Hg range. Pressures as high as 40 to 50 mm. Hg are present with portal hypertension.

Bile Formation

Bile is formed in two sites in the liver, one of which is the canalicular membrane. Bile secretion is an active process and is relatively independent of hepatic blood flow. There is an excellent correlation between bile acid output and bile flow so that the term bile acid–dependent flow describes this fraction of bile formation. Secretion of cholesterol and phospholipids is closely linked to the output of bile acid. The other site of bile formation is the bile ductule

itself. This portion is modified by the absorption of water and electrolytes by the epithelial cells. The only function of the gallbladder is to store and concentrate bile, and thus it is expendable. It usually contains 30 to 50 ml. of bile. Cholecystokinin, a gastrointestinal hormone secreted by the mucosa of the small intestine, causes gallbladder contraction and relaxation of the sphinter of Oddi and is important in biliary transport.

Bile flow has been measured in the range of 0.4 ml. per min. with bile acid–dependent production of 0.15 ml. per min. and bile acid–independent production of 0.15 ml. per min. Ductular secretion accounts for another 0.11 ml. per min. The total production of bile by the liver ranges from 600 to 1000 ml. per day. The hormones secretin and glucagon are the primary physiologic stimulators of bile flow. The electrolyte concentration of bile is remarkably similar to that of lactated Ringer's solution, i.e., 140 to 164 mEq. of sodium and 3.8 to 5.8 mEq. of potassium. Thus, Ringer's lactate has been used clinically to replace bile drainage from the biliary fistulas.

The concept of an *enterohepatic circulation* is important in the recirculation of the bile salt pool. The enterohepatic circulation refers to the flow of bile from the liver into the biliary tree and out into the intestine. The size of the bile salt pool and its frequency of cycling may be important in the formation of cholesterol stones. Bile salts are used for micelle formation to increase the solubility of cholesterol and lecithin. When the relative amounts of bile salts and lecithin are insufficient to package all the cholesterol, crystals appear in bile and act as a nidus for stone formation. Eventually, reabsorption of much of the bile salt pool by the terminal ileum occurs with subsequent extraction by the liver. This pool circulates six to ten times daily and produces 2 to 5 gm. of bile salts. It is an efficient circulation in that only 0.2 to 0.6 gm. of bile salts are lost in the stool each day. The liver can remove 80 per cent of the bile salts in a single pass; however, with cirrhosis and portal hypertension the bile salts in the serum increase, causing the pruritus associated with end-stage liver disease. The principal bile acids involved and synthesized by the liver are cholic acid and chenodeoxycholic acid.

Metabolic Processes

The liver is an organ of complex synthetic and degradative metabolic functions and is composed of three major cell types: the hepatocyte, the biliary epithelial cell, and Kupffer's cell. The hepatocyte is the most important cell type. It should be remembered that there is a large reserve capacity of the liver, and mild to moderate injuries may be occult. Liver function tests may be normal in the face of significant injuries. However, some functions are more sensitive to injury than others, but no test effectively measures total liver function.

PROTEIN SYNTHESIS

Albumin is the most important protein synthesized by the liver, and the liver is the *only* site for its production. Albumin has a high molecular weight (66,000) and contains 584 amino acids. Serum albumin provides the best index of the ability of the hepatocyte to perform its function. Normal albumin production is in the range of 120 to 200 mg. per kg. per day. Its half-life is measured from 17 to 20 days. The albumin is synthesized on the rough endoplasmic reticulum, transported to the smooth endoplasmic reticulum and Golgi apparatus, and eventually secreted into the sinusoids. When the liver is damaged, albumin synthesis is affected more than catabolism; however, with the long half-life weeks may elapse before there is a decrease in serum albumin. Thus, serum albumin deficiencies usually denote a chronic process, whereas low serum albumin levels are relatively rare in patients with acute hepatitis. In addition, hypoalbuminemia can be caused by an inadequate amino acid supply and can be seen with either malnutrition or malabsorption. The liver also produces a number of the blood-clotting factors, including fibrinogen, prothrombin, and factors 5, 7, and 10. The half-lives of these factors are shorter than that of albumin and range from 6 hours (factor 7) to 20 hours (prothrombin). The alpha and beta globulins are produced by the liver cell; however, the gamma globulins are produced not only by the reticuloendothelial cells lining the sinusoids but also by the spleen and bone marrow. The technique of protein electrophoresis permits the ready identification of abnormalities of serum protein fractions. For instance, patients with chronic active hepatitis have decreased albumin and increased beta and gamma globulin levels, whereas patients with primary biliary cirrhosis have decreased albumin and increased beta globulin levels.

ENZYME PRODUCTION

With the liver's various metabolic processes, it contains approximately 1000 protein catalysts or enzymes. During significant liver injury there is a leakage of enzymes from the liver cells into the bloodstream, causing elevated serum transaminases. This leakage occurs not only with necrosis but also with changes in the cell permeability (usually caused by ischemia or hypoxia). It should be remembered that there is no direct quantitative correlation between the amount of liver injury and the level of serum enzymes. However, in general, higher levels are associated with more severe injury. In this regard, if the liver function tests are measured after the peak, lower levels may be found as a function of a decrease in liver cell mass. Striking elevations of the serum transaminases are encountered in acute viral

hepatitis, acute drug- or toxin-induced liver damage, and ischemic hepatitis. Rapidly increasing transaminase levels along with a rising bilirubin and prolonged prothrombin time are ominous prognostic signs. With recovery, the transaminase levels return to normal over a course of several months. It is important to remember that significant liver damage may be present with normal transaminase levels.

Some enzymes, such as alkaline phosphatase, are increased in liver disease secondary to an increase in synthesis, *not* an increase in permeability. Alkaline phosphatase is also produced by the bone, placenta, intestine, and kidney, and isoenzyme determination with heat inactivation of the bone alkaline phosphatase is important in differentiating liver disease from other pathologic conditions. Elevations are normal in children with active bone growth and in women in the later stages of pregnancy. Hepatic alkaline phosphatase levels reflect the patency of bile channels and are elevated in 94 per cent of patients with obstruction caused by carcinoma and in 76 per cent with obstruction caused by stones. A related protein, 5' nucleotidase, as with alkaline phosphatase, is elevated with hepatic obstruction. This enzyme is only produced in the hepatic canalicular microvilli and is not found in bone and thus is more specific for biliary obstruction.

AMINO ACID METABOLISM

Amino acid levels in the blood are the direct result of dietary intake, tissue protein catabolism, and amino acid synthesis. There are two principal roots of catabolism of amino acids: oxidative deamination and transamination (the latter being the more important). When the liver is damaged, its utilization of amino acids is impaired and amino acid concentrations in the blood increase.

The liver is also responsible for urea synthesis, which is related to the removal and detoxification of ammonia from the blood. Protein from the diet is a major source of ammonia, and, after digestion, proteins are deaminated by bacterial enzymes. Ammonia is transported via the portal vein and detoxified. However, with chronic liver disease there is an increase in serum ammonia levels. This is caused by a number of mechanisms, the first being a decrease in urea synthesis accounting for a reduced removal of ammonia. Also contributing to the hyperammonia levels is the development of portosystemic shunts seen with portal hypertension, which allows ammonia to escape hepatic detoxification. Thirdly, there is an excessive amount of nitrogenous material in the intestine with any episodes of gastrointestinal bleeding or dietary protein intake, again accounting for increased ammonia levels. All these factors contribute to the increased serum ammonia level and eventual hepatic encephalopathy found with severe liver failure.

LIPID METABOLISM

Five per cent of the weight of the liver is fat, made up of mostly phospholipids, fatty acids, cholesterol, and cholesterol esters. The liver synthesizes lipids, mostly triglyceride, and they are excreted in the blood after combining with protein in the smooth endoplasmic reticulum to form a lipoprotein. Lipids are usually derived from adipose tissue or dietary intake and, in order to be secreted, must be converted into a lipoprotein. Thus, secretion depends on protein metabolism and hepatic cell integrity. Measurement of chylomicrons (nonmigrating lipoproteins), very-low-density (pre-beta) lipoprotein, low-density (beta) lipoprotein, and high-density (alpha) lipoprotein has been useful in evaluating liver injury. Patients with liver disease may exhibit any of the five forms of hyperlipidemia.

The liver is also the major organ involved in the synthesis, esterification, and excretion of cholesterol. Serum cholesterol is the standard for the determination of lipid metabolism. In the presence of liver disease, serum cholesterol is decreased, whereas with biliary obstruction it is increased.

In patients with chronic liver disease there is an increase in fatty deposition in the liver. This is a common finding in patients with alcoholic cirrhosis and is usually considered multifactorial. There is also a decrease in apoprotein synthesis, which is intimately involved in the secretion of fatty acids from the liver, and thus fatty acid concentrations in the liver increase. Malnutrition and starvation, conditions found in the chronic alcoholic, cause increased fatty acid mobilization with an increased flux from adipose tissue. All these mechanisms are important in the transformation from a histologic normal liver to a fatty liver. This transformation may be fairly rapid and may take only 1 to 3 weeks.

CARBOHYDRATE METABOLISM

Glucose is stored in the liver as glycogen and accounts for 5 to 7 per cent of the normal liver weight. The regulation of hepatic glucose output, which maintains blood glucose in the normal range, may be lost with liver cell necrosis or cirrhosis. In cirrhosis there is a decrease in glycogen storage along with a lower liver cell mass, with resultant decreased hepatic production. Thus, the hypoglycemia found in patients with liver disease is usually caused by a decrease in gluconeogenesis. Peripheral insulin resistance is responsible for the hyperglycemia occasionally found in cirrhotics, since serum insulin levels are usually normal.

DETOXIFICATION

The liver is also an important source for detoxification of drugs and other noxious agents. This is done either by the process of conjugation, in which water-insoluble compounds are converted to water-soluble agents and excreted in the bile or urine, or by inactivation of drugs by reduction, oxidation, or hydroxylation. It should be remembered that sedatives and barbiturates are metabolized almost exclusively by the liver; thus, patients with chronic liver disease have a slow metabolism of these compounds. Other drugs, such as phenobarbital and alcohol, stimulate the smooth endoplasmic reticulum of the liver and increase the activity of detoxifying enzymes. This mechanism causes a decrease in serum concentrations of many drugs. The cytochrome P450 system is responsible for the oxidation of a number of drugs and toxins.

VITAMIN METABOLISM

The liver is responsible for the uptake, storage, and mobilization of a number of important vitamins. Vitamin D_3, which is involved in bone metabolism, is hydroxylated in the 25 position in the liver. The hepatocyte is also active in vitamin K metabolism. Two factors contribute to the deficiency of coagulation factors in liver disease. In obstructive jaundice, the bile source required for vitamin K absorption is blocked, and thus there is a decrease in synthesis of factors 2, 7, 9, and 10. The one-stage prothrombin time test performed before and after administration of vitamin K permits differentiation between abnormalities caused by abnormal vitamin K absorption and those due to liver cell

dysfunction. When vitamin K is given parenterally, the prothrombin time returns to normal. Vitamin K has little or no effect on the prothrombin time obtained in patients with jaundice resulting from liver cell damage. A number of chronic liver conditions prolong the prothrombin time because of the effect on vitamin K metabolism. Parenchymal damage causes a decrease in synthesis of prothrombin and is the second factor responsible for coagulation abnormalities found in liver disease.

BILIRUBIN METABOLISM

Seventy-five per cent of derived serum bilirubin originates from senescent red blood cells and is excreted almost entirely in the bile. The bilirubin is conjugated with glucuronide in the hepatocyte, secreted in the intestine in the enterohepatic circulation, and finally excreted as urobilinogen in the urine. Thus, with biliary obstruction there is usually no urobilinogen in the urine. With hepatic cell injury there is decreased removal of bilirubin and, therefore, increased urinary urobilinogen. Recently, it has been shown with high-performance liquid chromatography that all the serum bilirubin in normal patients is unconjugated, and it has been suggested that detection of any conjugated bilirubin is indicative of hepatobiliary disease. The serum bilirubin level has no distinguishing value in differentiating intrahepatic cholestasis from extrahepatic obstruction; however, it may be important in certain conditions, such as alcoholic hepatitis and primary biliary cirrhosis, in which elevations greater than 2.0 mg. per 100 ml. late in the disease process imply a higher mortality. Bilirubin is bound to albumin in the blood, a mechanism that protects tissue from its toxicity.

APPROACH TO THE JAUNDICED PATIENT

One of the most challenging diagnostic problems for physicians is establishing the cause of hyperbilirubinemia in a patient. The question is usually whether the hyperbilirubinemia is of the obstructive type, in which operative therapy has the predominant role, or is secondary to hepatocellular disease. The history and physicial examination are important in initial considerations for the differential diagnosis of jaundice. Clinical manifestations of cirrhosis and portal hypertension are usually readily apparent and should be noted. Liver function tests are also helpful; usually transaminase elevations are exceedingly rare with biliary obstruction. Levels of serum glutamic-oxaloacetic transaminase (SGOT) greater than 300 and most certainly greater than 750 exclude any need for operation, and hepatocellular disease can be assumed. Serum albumin concentration and the resultant hypoalbuminemia give more information about the duration of disease. Elevated alkaline phosphatase and 5'-nucleotidase levels are somewhat nonspecific but provide a means of differentiating biliary obstruction from hepatocellular disease. Prolongation of prothrombin time is involved with abnormal vitamin K metabolism. Injection of vitamin K in a jaundiced patient with a prolonged prothrombin time should return the prothrombin time to normal if the patient has obstructive jaundice.

The initial screening test for patients with obstructive jaundice is either an ultrasound or computed tomographic (CT) scan. With these modalities the liver may be evaluated for the presence of intrahepatic ductal dilation or masses, and the gallbladder, common bile duct, and pancreas may be visualized. More invasive tests, such as the endoscopic retrograde cholangiopancreatography (ERCP), percutaneous transhepatic cholangiography, arteriography, and liver biopsies, can further define borderline cases of hyperbilirubinemia and provide the surgeon with much information about biliary arterial and venous anatomy when an operative approach is indicated.

MAJOR HEPATIC RESECTION

With a better understanding of the anatomy of the liver and the segmental nature of hepatic divisions, coupled with better anesthetic techniques and postoperative care and support, major liver resections can now be done with an operative mortality of 5 to 10 per cent. Basically, four segmental resections of the liver may be performed. A *right hepatic lobectomy* includes removing both the anterior and posterior segments of the right hepatic lobe, whereas a *left hepatic lobectomy* eliminates the medial and lateral segments of the left hepatic lobe. A radical hepatic resection, termed a *right trisegmentectomy,* involves removal of the right hepatic lobe along with the medial segment of the left hepatic lobe. A *left lateral segmentectomy* involves removal of just the left lateral segment and usually does not require hilar dissection.

Longmire[5] has proposed his own technique of liver resection and emphasizes that an adequate abdominal incision with complete exploration and biopsy of the tumor is indicated to confirm that the lesion is confined to an anatomic segment that can be resected and to determine the patency of the inferior vena cava and the portal vein as well as the functional capability of the liver that will be left *in situ*. A thoracic incision extended through the eighth interspace is optional for a right hepatic lobectomy. The lobe to be resected is mobilized by detaching the suspensory ligaments, and a hilar dissection is performed by dividing, in order, the hepatic artery, hepatic bile duct, and portal vein to that lobe being resected. A cholecystectomy is usually also performed. The hepatic veins are approached either retrohepatically or intraparenchymally. Division of the liver parenchyma and ligation of biliary vascular branches are performed either with the newer CUSA instrument or with a finger fracture technique. Postoperative drainage, preferably closed, sterile drainage, is also important.

Other investigators[1, 9] state that it is rare that a thoracic incision is needed and that it only adds to the morbidity and mortality of the procedure. It is also considered much safer to ligate the hepatic veins as they are encountered within the hepatic substance beginning in the anterior inferior position and progressing posterosuperiorly. It is important not only to ligate but to oversew the dissected portions of the portal vein to prevent hemorrhage. Hemoclips are useful for hemostasis. Starzl[11] reports an operative mortality of 3.3 per cent with major hepatic resection and states that the normothermic ischemic time of the human liver is up to 1 hour. This is longer than the previously accepted duration of 15 to 20 minutes. Lin,[4] in an attempt to decrease operative time and transfusion requirements, emphasized the finger fracture technique and the use of a liver clamp as technical improvements in hepatic resection. However, the Lin hepatic liver clamp is bulky and, at times, hard to apply. Hodgson and DelGucicio[2] invented the Cavitron ultrasonic surgical aspirator (CUSA) and with this instrument decreased blood loss to under 1000 ml. for major hepatic resections. The CUSA's tip contains a transducer that oscillates at 23,000 cycles per second (Fig. 8), is irrigated with saline, and contains a suction line to aspirate any of the fragmented hepatocytes. The more fibrous blood vessel walls and biliary ducts are not fragmented by the ultrasound and thus are dissected free and ligated while going through the hepatic parenchyma.

Postoperative Course after Liver Resection

A number of unique clinical situations can present after major hepatic resection, and physicians must be aware of these in caring for patients postoperatively.[12] Hypoglycemia, due to inadequate hepatic gluconeogenesis, is found frequently, and thus infusions of $D_{10}W$ are important in the postoperative period. Hypophosphatemia also occurs as the liver takes up phosphate stores because of increased hepatic adenosine triphosphate (ATP) synthesis and regeneration. Because of decreased synthesis and increased consumption of amino acids along with leakage of albumin from the raw liver edge, hypoalbuminemia is a frequent finding. Thus, it is important to give albumin infusions for the first 7 to 10 days postoperatively. Hyperbilirubinemia also occurs because of increased bile load and decreased number of liver

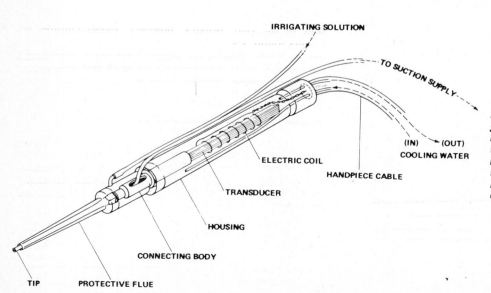

Figure 8. The Cavitron ultrasonic surgical aspiration (CUSA) device has a metal tip that vibrates at a frequency that disrupts the liver parenchyma but leaves biliary and vascular structures intact for ligation. (From CUSA Brochure, Cooper LaserSonics, Santa Clara, Calif.)

cells. Hepatic regeneration starts immediately, and it has been estimated that the liver is functionally normal 2 to 3 weeks after major resection. However, the liver requires 4 to 6 months to regenerate to normal size. In cirrhotics the liver's ability to regenerate is impaired. It is thought that the portal vein contains a factor, called the *hepatotrophic factor*, that is an important nutritional hormone in liver regeneration. This factor has never been discovered and might include any or all of the following: insulin, glucagon, norepinephrine, and somatometrin.

PYOGENIC AND AMEBIC LIVER ABSCESS

The treatment of liver abscesses has dramatically changed since Ochsner and others published their classic series in 1938.[23] Liver abscess is a subtle disease with formidable diagnostic and therapeutic problems. This is emphasized by the fact that pyogenic liver abscesses are the eventual cause of fever of unknown origin in many patients. With the advent of CT and nuclear resonance scanning, mass lesions as small as 1.0 cm. may be localized. In the preantibiotic era the main cause of liver abscesses was from gastrointestinal tract disorders, including ruptured appendicitis. With the development of newer antibiotics, the leading causes of liver abscesses are now complicated biliary tract disease and malignancy. Early drainage of pyogenic liver abscesses continues to be the most important principle of treatment.

Pyogenic Liver Abscess

INCIDENCE AND PATHOGENESIS

The true incidence of liver abscess is not known; however, autopsy studies have estimated an occurrence ranging from 0.3 to 1.47 per cent, and pyogenic abscesses account for approximately 80 per cent of this number. Two conditions are necessary for the development of a liver abscess: the presence of *bacteria* seeding the hepatic substance and the need for a *receptive* liver. These conditions are met in the posttraumatic state when there is either necrotic or injured liver parenchyma with low oxygen tension; this injured parenchyma is an excellent culture medium for septic foci. Also, congenital cysts and obstructive bile ducts are fertile environments for the development of liver abscesses. Any condition associated with immune system suppression, such as chronic granulomatous disease, hepatoma, and tuberculosis, favors the development of pyogenic liver abscess. Those in the transplant population are also at risk.

Infection delivered via the portal vein was the most common cause of liver abscess before the era of antibiotic treatment. In Ochsner's series,[23] 45 per cent of liver abscesses were due to suppuration and seeding of the portal vein, and 34 per cent were caused by appendicitis. With the advent of aggressive treatment for suspected appendicitis and more effective antibiotics, the incidence of appendicitis causing liver abscesses has decreased in frequency, with incidences of 10 to 17 per cent now being quoted. More recently cited series (Table 1) show that the most common causes of pyogenic liver abscesses include malignancy and complex biliary tract disease. This shift in etiology also means a shift in patient population to an older age group with a higher percentage of poor-risk patients. Other common causes of pyogenic liver abscess include hematogenous spread via the hepatic artery, direct exten-

TABLE 1. *Etiology of Pyogenic Liver Abscess in Collected Series**

	Frequency (%)	
	1930–1970* (N = 532)	1970–1984† (N = 367)
Biliary tract	31.6	41.9
Hematogenous via portal vein	21.8	17.9
Hematogenous via hepatic artery	14.5	7.1
Direct extension	5.1	7.1
Cryptogenic	21.9	20.4
Other (traumatic, etc.)	5.1	5.2

*Data from Hill and Laws: Am. Surg., *48*:49, 1982.
†Data from Adams, Butler, de la Maza, Hill, Lazarchick, Ranson, and Wintch.
Reprinted from Ellison, E. C., and Carey, L. C.: *In* Sabiston, D. C., Jr. (Ed.): Textbook of Surgery, 13th ed. Philadelphia, W. B. Saunders Company, 1986, p. 1069.

sion from subhepatic or subdiaphragmatic abscesses, and cryptogenic abscesses with no apparent cause found in 2 to 15 per cent of patients. Traumatic liver abscess and secondary infected congenital cysts or biliary tract instrumentation are rarer causes of pyogenic abscesses.

PATHOLOGY AND MICROBIOLOGY

With a pyogenic abscess, the liver is usually found to be enlarged on physical examination. Grossly, abscesses are readily apparent and are usually multiple. There is a propensity for involvement of the right lobe of the liver because of the laminar flow in the portal vein.[3, 10] With this streaming effect, bacteria are preferentially shunted to the right lobe. Parenthetically, it should be noted that the right lobe constitutes 70 per cent of the liver mass, and an increased incidence of liver abscess would be expected in this lobe. Histologically, the abscess is composed of a thick fibrous capsule with cellular debris in the center. Microbiologic examination shows most liver abscesses to be infected with anaerobes and gastrointestinal flora. *E. coli* or other enteric gram-negative rods are isolated in as many as 50 per cent of patients, whereas streptococcal and staphylococcal species are cultured in some 19 and 11 per cent, respectively. Anaerobic bacteria account for 20 to 40 per cent of the pure isolates; however, mixed cultures are usually found. Candidal hepatic abscesses are rare and are usually found only in the immunosuppressed population. In a recent series managed by percutaneous aspiration,[18] streptococci were cultured in 46 per cent of patients, *E. coli* in 30 per cent, and mixed cultures in the remainder.

NATURAL HISTORY AND COMPLICATIONS

The natural history of untreated pyogenic liver abscess approaches 100 per cent mortality; the cause of death is usually sepsis and multiple organ failure. The complications of liver abscess include rupture into the free peritoneal cavity and rupture into the pleural cavity and lung. Pleural pulmonary complications, however, are less commonly found in pyogenic abscesses than in amebic abscesses.

DIAGNOSIS

Clinical symptoms of pyogenic abscesses include weakness, malaise, and fever in most patients. Nausea, vomiting, and weight loss are also prominent findings. Fever and leukocytosis are usually present with this disease process and signify a toxic state. Underlying conditions are prevalent and include diabetes, biliary tract disease, and immunologic deficiencies. In a recent study,[24] 100 per cent of the patients presented with fever, 81 per cent presented with nonspecific abdominal pain, and 75 per cent had weight loss. Hepatomegaly was present in 94 per cent and jaundice found in less than 50 per cent. Laboratory data included leukocytosis, anemia, and elevated alkaline phosphatase and SGOT levels in over 90 per cent of patients. Elevated bilirubins were found in 69 per cent and hypoalbuminemia in 56 per cent. Differential diagnoses include acute cholecystitis, perforated peptic ulcer, acute alcoholic hepatitis, acute viral hepatitis, and pyelonephritis. With a chronic insidious presentation, malignancy of the liver, biliary tract, or pancreas and cirrhosis are found more frequently on exploration. An occult liver abscess causing fever of unknown origin is responsible for 10 per cent of the abscesses.

Radiologic investigation usually suggests an inflammatory process in the right upper quadrant. Chest films are abnormal in 50 per cent of patients and include an elevated right hemidiaphragm or pleural effusions and atelectasis of the right lower lobe. An ultrasound study is usually the first imaging modality performed and differentiates suspected liver disease from gallbladder problems as well as outlines the pancreas and biliary tree. Radionuclide scan resolution allows the diagnosis of lesions as small as 2.0 cm. and differentiates cystic from solid masses. Halverson and associates[19] report that CT scanning shows a 97 per

cent sensitivity with a false-negative rate of 3 per cent for the diagnosis of pyogenic liver abscess.

The abscess may vary in appearance from a lesion with a smooth margin to a fluid-filled cavity or a poorly defined mass in the liver in 19 per cent of patients. Contrast enhancement is used with CT scanning since the abscess contents will not enhance whereas the surrounding liver will, resulting in rim enhancement (Fig. 9). Fine needle aspiration and drainage have become more important not only in the diagnosis but also in the therapy of liver abscesses.[18] Gram stains of percutaneous aspiration can reveal the predominant organisms in the abscess, and appropriate antibiotic coverage can be instituted quickly. Angiography is also important in differentiating abscess from tumor involvement and in demonstrating the tumor blush if it is hypervascular.

TREATMENT

The treatment of bacterial liver abscesses includes identification of the underlying cause of the abscess, administration of broad-spectrum antibiotics, and early drainage. It has been shown that medical treatment of pyogenic abscesses results in a mortality of 90 to 100 per cent; this has changed little with the advent of newer, more effective antibiotics.[22] The principles of surgical treatment of hepatic abscess with adequate drainage must be emphasized. These include the liberal use of noninvasive diagnostic tests, defining the pathogenesis of the abscess before operation,

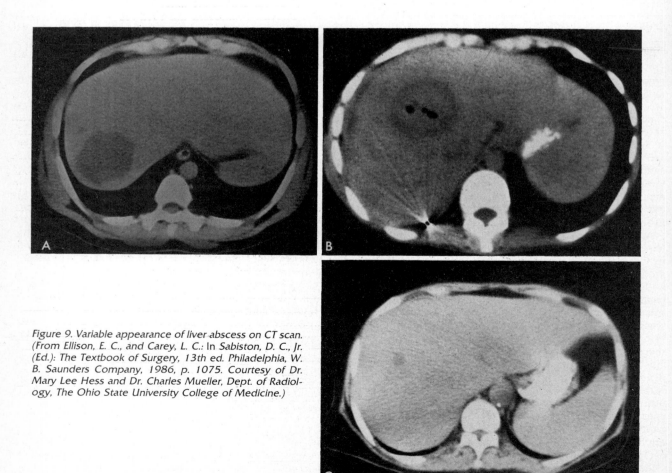

Figure 9. Variable appearance of liver abscess on CT scan. (From Ellison, E. C., and Carey, L. C.: In Sabiston, D. C., Jr. (Ed.): The Textbook of Surgery, 13th ed. Philadelphia, W. B. Saunders Company, 1986, p. 1075. Courtesy of Dr. Mary Lee Hess and Dr. Charles Mueller, Dept. of Radiology, The Ohio State University College of Medicine.)

celiac arteriography for suspected tumors, broad-spectrum antibiotic administration, transperitoneal surgical exploration with intraoperative atraumatic abscess location using the thin needle, and correction of the underlying disease process.

Culture Techniques

Anaerobic culture techniques are important, and multiple abscesses should be excluded. Tubes or soft rubber drains are used, and percutaneous transhepatic drainage is reserved for high-risk patients. The transperitoneal approach permits a thorough exploratory laparotomy with wide exposure of the liver and allows complete examination of the abdominal contents for the septic focus. The origin of the abscess can be removed with this approach.

Antibiotic Administration

Coverage of the patient with broad-spectrum antibiotics is recommended: from 3 weeks for drained abscesses to 4 months if multiple small abscesses that are impossible to drain effectively are found.[22] From these guidelines, the mortality varies from 0 to 59 per cent, depending on the pathogenesis of the abscess. Representative mortality rates include 59 per cent for underlying biliary tract disease causing the abscess, 14 per cent for infected cystic disease, 7 per cent for abscess spread via the portal vein, and 8 per cent for hepatic abscesses caused by contiguous spread. A recent study of 106 patients with liver abscess supports these findings, since patients with complicated biliary tract disease had the highest mortality (59 per cent).[22] The death rates for portal drainage (7 per cent), contiguous spread (8 per cent), infected cysts (4 per cent), and cryptogenic origin (50 per cent) are similar to those of the previous report.

As reported, mortality increases in patients with multiple abscesses or in those who have advanced carcinoma or nonreconstructible biliary disease. This is due primarily to their underlying primary disease and not to the liver abscess *per se*. Retroperitoneal approaches have also been advocated for drainage of liver abscesses that are posterior in the liver, but this technique does not define nor treat the focus of the disease. Long-term broad-spectrum antibiotic administration against both gram-negative rods and anaerobes is recommended for the treatment of hepatic abscesses. Usually metronidazole and an aminoglycoside are administered, since the former also covers *Entamoeba histolytica*.

In the last 5 years a significant advance in reducing the mortality of pyogenic liver abscesses with percutaneous drainage has been reported. Local anesthesia and CT-directed aspiration with an 18-gauge needle are followed by insertion of an 18-French catheter.[25] Relative contraindications to the procedure include the presence of ascites or vital structures near the root of the needle insertion. Advantages were noted and included no significant contamination of peritoneum, the involvement of a closed system that minimizes contamination, and the low cost of the procedure. Percutaneous aspiration is particularly applicable to high-risk patients, and the mortality associated with this procedure was reported as 1.5 per cent with no complications.

Another group headed by Gerzof[18] stressed that true septa were unusual in liver abscesses, and an 89 per cent success rate was reported using percutaneous drainage. Complications occurred in only 2 of 18 attempts and included a perforated gallbladder with spillage of contaminated material into the peritoneal cavity. These investigators suggested that use of this technique resulted in avoidance of a general anesthesia and an operative procedure as well as in provision of a shorter hospitalization time and better patient compliance. They also suggested that percutaneous drainage should precede any operative exploration even if the intra-abdominal focus had been identified. The duration of drainage was in the range of 9 to 38 days. A 9 per cent mortality has been reported with the procedure.[18] However, most believe that this technique is most readily applied to patients with single abscesses or those who have no gastrointestinal source identified as the septic focus.

Amebic Liver Abscess

INCIDENCE AND EPIDEMIOLOGY

Amebic hepatic abscesses are found less frequently than pyogenic abscesses and account for about 20 per cent of all liver abscesses. The incidence varies with the incidence of *E. histolytica* found in the population. The incidence of amebiasis has decreased in the last 30 years; however, the epidemiology is changing from a disease commonly found in the Southeastern United States in native Americans to one occurring in urban immigrant populations.[20] This infection is more common in the tropics, where approximately 10 to 20 per cent of the population harbor the organism in endemic areas. The Centers for Disease Control report 1.3 cases of amebiasis per 100,000 population; in the infested population, liver involvement occurs 2.8 to 25 per cent of the time.

Recently, amebiasis has been reported to be endemic in homosexual communities. The pathogenesis suggests that the cystic form of *E. histolytica* is ingested by humans in contaminated material in water or food. Trophozoites are released from the cyst during the passage through the intestine, and amebic dysentery occurs. At this point the trophozoites invade the mucosa and are absorbed into the portovenous system (Fig. 10). In the liver, the lytic action of the entrapped amebae results in liquefaction necrosis and secondary bacterial infection is common. Untreated amebic abscesses can rupture into other body cavities (Fig. 11). Approximately 3 to 12 per cent of the patients experience pleural pulmonary complications, including empyema, fistula, and lung abscesses. Patients harboring left hepatic lobe abscesses may experience rupture into the peritoneum or through the diaphragm into the pericardium, both situations carrying a high mortality.

DIAGNOSIS

The diagnosis and clinical features of amebic liver abscess are consistent with those of other types of pyogenic liver abscesses and have not changed significantly since DeBakey and colleagues reported their series of amebic abscesses in 1951.[17] Nearly all patients have pain, chills, diarrhea, and fever. However, the amebic fever is marked by a constant course as compared with the picket fence fever curve associated with bacterial abscesses. Usually the patient has right upper quadrant pain, hepatomegaly, and leukocytosis. Stool cultures are positive in only 15 to 20 per cent, and liver function tests are elevated in 25 to 50 per cent. Serologic tests for *E. histolytica* are positive in 90 to 95 per cent of patients. The latex agglutination test is regarded as accurate in nearly all patients.[26] With a clinical syndrome suggestive of a liver abscess, a serologic test for *Echinococcus* should also be done, as special precautions should be taken for drainage of echinococcal cysts. With CT imaging, most patients will have a single abscess of the

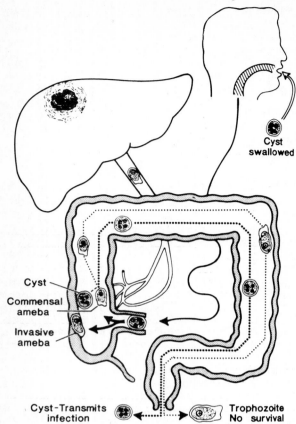

Cyst
swallowed

Cyst
Commensal
ameba

Invasive
ameba

Cyst-Transmits
infection

Trophozoite
No survival

Figure 10. Diagram of colonization, portal vein invasion, and liver abscess formation by E. histolytica. *(From Ellison, E. C., and Carey, L. C.: In* Sabiston, D. C., Jr. (Ed.): The Textbook of Surgery, 13th *ed. Philadelphia, W. B. Saunders Company, 1986, p. 1070.)*

right lobe, although 19 per cent have multiple abscesses and 8.5 per cent have abscesses in the left lobe.

TREATMENT

The role of therapeutic needle aspiration for amebic abscesses is controversial. In areas where *E. histolytica* is endemic, aspiration of abscesses is routinely performed without radiologic guidance. This technique is diagnostic in that it differentiates between pyogenic and amebic abscesses. There are no distinctive radiologic differences between pyogenic and amebic abscesses. The differentiation depends on a positive serologic test for *E. histolytica*.

It is accepted that most amebic abscesses can be effectively treated with chemotherapy, and operation should only be required for ruptured abscesses or for diagnostic purposes. Metronidazole is the drug of choice and has been reported to cure 80 to 100 per cent of amebic abscesses. The dose is usually 500 and 750 mg. three times a day for 10 to 14 days given either by mouth or intravenously. Patients successfully treated with metronidazole have a dramatic clinical response, usually becoming afebrile and free of pain within 24 to 48 hours.

Usually aspiration is unnecessary; however, if symptoms persist longer than 1 week and radiologic imaging shows the continued presence of the cyst after antibiotic treatment, either percutaneous aspiration or surgical drainage may be indicated.[13] This is unusual and could denote

secondary bacterial infection of the amebic abscess. To eradicate the carrier state, it is recommended that diiodohydroxyquinolone, 600 mg., be given three times a day for 20 days to sterilize the gastrointestinal tract of ameba. Recent series[13, 26] from endemic areas, including the San Fernando Valley in the United States, reported that amebic abscesses have been successfully treated with metronidazole in 85 to 94 per cent of patients. Responders usually improve within 72 hours. If there is no response after 72 hours, it is recommended that metronidazole be discontinued and emetine and chloroquine instituted. Thompson and colleagues[26] also recommend that percutaneous drainage be tried after failure of medical treatment. If the abscess ruptures into the peritoneal cavity, open surgical drainage is instituted.

CYSTIC DISEASE OF THE LIVER

It is postulated that congenital cysts of the liver develop when there is an excessive number of hepatic ductules that fail to involute and progressively dilate. These are of little significance, and usually laparotomy is required in only 16 per cent of patients. At operation these are usually single, benign, and lined by biliary epithelium. The male to female ratio is 1:1.4. In one series 54 per cent of patients presented with an abdominal mass, hepatomegaly was present in 40 per cent, and abdominal pain was present in one third of patients. Only 9 per cent presented with jaundice, presumably secondary to compression of the biliary tree by the enlarging cyst. Most hepatic cysts are found incidentally at laparotomy and are quite small. These may be aspirated at the time of operation. Larger cysts may be unroofed and allowed to communicate freely with the peritoneal cavity. If bile is present in the cysts, then they should be drained internally with a Roux-en-Y defunctionalized jejunal limb. Usually cysts less than 8 cm. in diameter can be treated with needle aspiration. Cysts caused by trauma or inflammation are rare and account for only 1 to 2 per cent of cases.

Caroli's Disease

Caroli's disease, another cystic disease of the liver, is a congenital disorder of the intrahepatic bile ducts in which multiple segmental cystic dilations that are in continuity with the bile ducts occur. This condition is distinguished from *polycystic disease* of the liver, in which the cysts do not communicate with the biliary tree. Patients with Caroli's disease are usually susceptible to repeated attacks of jaundice and cholangitis, with the subsequent development of cirrhosis and portal hypertension. Because of impaired normal drainage of bile from the liver and stagnation, intrahepatic biliary calculi form.

The usual treatment of these enlarged dilated intrahepatic bile ducts includes left hepatic lobectomy for extensive involvement of the left lobe and Roux-en-Y drainage of right-sided dilated ducts. Caroli's disease is found more commonly in the Orient, and some reports[16] suggest that it is a premalignant condition, with associated bile duct cancer found in 7 per cent of patients. The interval from the diagnosis of Caroli's disease to the diagnosis of cancer averaged 3.3 years. Cholangiocarcinoma is the histologic pattern most commonly seen. The long-term prognosis in Caroli's disease is poor even without malignant degeneration, in spite of adequate internal drainage by Roux-en-Y hepaticojejunostomy.

Brain abscess
(hematogenous)

Rupture into lung
  (a) Lung abscess
  (b) Broncho-hepatic fistula

Rupture into
pericardium

Rupture into pleural cavity
  (Empyema)
Subphrenic abscess
Rupture externally

Rupture into lung
or pleural cavity

Extension to spleen

Secondary bacterial Infection
  (a) Rupture
  (b) Operative procedure
  (c) Hematogenous

Rupture into
peritoneal cavity
stomach, colon,
kidney or vena cava

Figure 11. Schematic presentation of common complications of amebic liver abscess. (From Ellison, E. C., and Carey, L. C.: In Sabiston, D. C., Jr., (Ed.): The Textbook of Surgery, 13th ed. Philadelphia, W. B. Saunders Company, 1986, p. 1072. Courtesy of Leonard Rosoff, M.D.)

Cystadenomas

Cystadenomas of the liver are rare lesions and are considered precursors of cystadenocarcinoma and thus should be excised. The finding of malignant degeneration of hepatic cystadenomas underscores the principle that biopsies be done for all hepatic cyst walls at the time of exploration to rule out malignancy.

Echinococcal Cystic Disease

Echinococcal cystic disease is an interesting pathologic condition caused by the tapeworm *Echinococcus granulosus.* Hydatid disease has been known from the time of Hippocrates, who referred to the disease as "liver full of water." The disease is endemic in areas where there is a large number of sheep and cattle, such as central Asia, South American, Australia, and central Europe. In the United States it appears most often in the Southeast, Alaska, and the areas that border Mexico.[20]

ETIOLOGY

The definitive host for *E. granulosus* is the dog or associated carnivores, such as the wolf or fox. The small tapeworm is released and is excreted in the feces of these definitive primary hosts. The ova are extremely viable and hardy and can live for months to years outside the body. The intermediate hosts for the ova are hogs, sheep, cattle, and man. With ingestion, the protective membrane of the ova dissolves and the scoleces penetrate the intestinal mucosa. The liver is infested in 60 per cent of cases, whereas the lung harbors disease in 30 per cent. In the liver the scoleces multiply asexually to form a cyst, with the innermost layer forming a germinal epithelium from which the scoleces and daughter cysts arise (Fig. 12). The cyst grows slowly. However, it can assume massive proportions; up to 16 liters of hydatid fluid was reported in one echinococcal cyst. This fluid is highly antigenic and may cause anaphy-

lactic shock if absorbed into the peritoneal cavity during a rupture. The cyst becomes calcified in 25 to 70 per cent of patients (Fig. 13), usually involving the pericyst layer, and this signals the death of the parasite.

CLINICAL PRESENTATION

Symptoms are usually caused by compression by the mass, causing abdominal pain and jaundice, or by localized or systemic reactions to the fluid, including urticaria, pruritus, eosinophilia, anaphylaxis, and shock. The complications of this disease involve contiguous rupture, occurring in about 5 to 10 per cent of patients into the biliary tree, and rupture through the dome of the diaphragm into the lung. Metastatic hydatidosis occurs when the scoleces em-

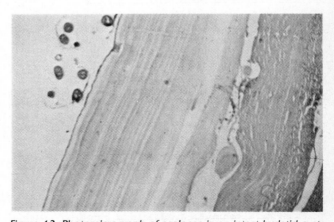

Figure 12. Photomicrograph of scoleces in an intact hydatid cyst wall. The inner pericyst layer is in close contact with but separable from the compressed host tissue. The innermost lining is the germinative membrane from which the scoleces break off to float in the hydatid fluid. (From Calne, R. Y., and Della Rovere, G. Q. D.: Liver Surgery. Philadelphia, Piccis Medical Books, W. B. Saunders Company, 1982, p. 62.)

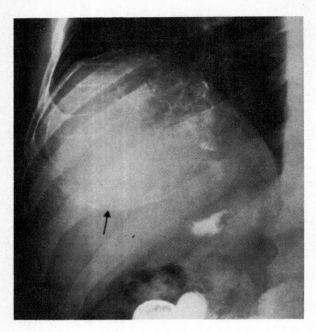

Figure 13. Echinococcal cysts are calcified in as many as 70 per cent of the patients. (From Sherlock, S., and Summerfield, J. A. (Eds.): Color Atlas of Liver Disease. Chicago, Year Book Medical Publishers, Inc., 1979.)

bolize into the inferior vena cava and multiply in the lung or other systemic organs. There is a 10 per cent rate of secondary bacterial infection, and 13 per cent of these cysts communicate with the bile duct.

DIAGNOSIS

Until recently, the primary diagnostic modality was Casoni's skin test, which involved injecting the human hydatid fluid intradermally. Results of this test were reportedly positive in 60 to 70 per cent of the patients with documented disease but a disadvantage was that the test sensitized the host. More recent and sensitive immunoelectrophoretic and enzyme linked–immunosorbent assay (ELISA) tests show sensitivity of up to 93 per cent.

TREATMENT

If an echinococcal cyst is suspected with either positive serologic studies or calcification in the cyst wall on plain radiographs, no percutaneous drainage should be undertaken. In their monograph on liver surgery, Calne and Della Rovere[15] describe the operative treatment for the cyst. It is recommended that the anesthesiologist have pressor agents as well as isoproterenol (Isuprel) and steroids available to relieve any bronchospasm in the event an anaphylactic reaction occurs with manipulation of the cyst. Both preoperative and postoperative steroids have also been found to be helpful. Calne and Della Rovere state that as the cyst enlarges it slowly accumulates an ever-increasing number of scoleces while the surrounding host parenchyma is compressed into a thin fibrous connective tissue. This pericyst layer provides both physical and nutritional support to the scoleces and must be dealt with during operation. They also imply that cysts deep in the liver parenchyma will eventually enlarge and expose themselves in the subcapsular position. At this time they are most amenable to surgical treatment.

Either an abdominal or combination thoracoabdominal incision may be made, depending on the location of the cyst. Technical steps include isolation of the liver with sterile packs and trochar puncture. After puncture, the cyst opening should be enlarged, taking care not to spill any residual contents (Fig. 14). The cyst lining and cyst contents should be removed, followed by instillation of a 0.5 per cent silver nitrate solution to sterilize the cavity of any fertile scoleces. A common bile duct exploration may be needed if a large biliary duct communicates with the cyst to clear the biliary tree of cystic debris. Other agents used to sterilize the cyst cavity include hypertonic saline, chlorhexidine, absolute alcohol, and hydrogen peroxide. Dead space may be obliterated either by suture closure or with a pedicle of omentum.

Lower complication rates are obtained with omentoplasty than with marsupialization and tacking of the cyst edges to the abdominal wall or with tube drainage. Both of these techniques are associated with a high incidence of biliary fistulas. However, with a suppurative secondary infection of the cyst, marsupialization or tube drainage is indicated. Internal drainage may also be used when the cyst communicates with the biliary system.

Belli and others[14] recently reviewed their series of the surgical treatment of hydatid cyst in 42 patients. Single cysts were present in 60 per cent of the cases, and most patients had old, thick, calcified walls. Major hepatic re-

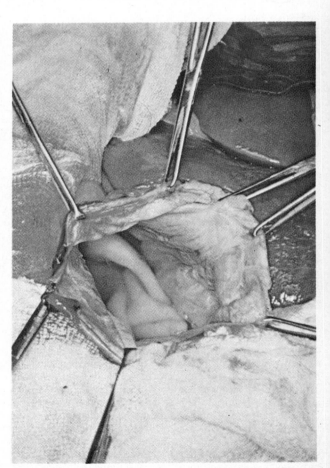

Figure 14. Intraoperative photograph of technique used to treat echinococcal cysts. Note the pack isolation and removal of the pericyst lining from the cavity. (From Calne, R. Y., and Della Rovere, G. Q. D.: Liver Surgery. Philadelphia, Piccis Medical Books, W. B. Saunders Company, 1982, p. 68.)

sections were performed in 18 patients when the majority of the lobe had been destroyed or when prior procedures had failed. Cyst pericystectomy was performed in 15 cases, and marsupialization in 9. There were no deaths or recurrent disease with 1 to 10 years of follow-up. However, the complication rate with marsupialization was 60 per cent, and it was recommended that this procedure be the last resort in treating these patients.

Recently, drug therapy with mebendazole, an anti-echinococcal agent, has been reserved for those patients who are at increased risk for operation or who have known intra-abdominal spillage. A new drug, albendazole (Valbazen), 10 mg. per kg. per day, has been tried as the sole treatment of echinococcal cysts, with a 68 per cent remission rate of cysts documented on CT scan. This drug is also reserved for those patients who are inoperable or who have recurrent multiple cysts or intraoperative contamination.

PORTAL HYPERTENSION

The history of portal hypertension, cirrhosis, and associated jaundice is a fascinating one. The word *cirrhosis* is derived from the Greek word *kirrhos,* which means orange or yellow discoloration. Physicians in the Middle Ages made the association between liver disease and alcoholism. Laennec was responsible for the pathologic identification of the fibrosis found in the liver with chronic alcohol ingestion. Rokitansky postulated that cirrhosis was the response of inflammation caused by direct toxicity of the alcohol. Other investigators prominent in this field included Eck,[77] who performed the first end-to-side portacaval shunt to totally divert portovenous flow. Later the eminent physiologist Pavlov[79] demonstrated that total diversion of the portovenous flow produced encephalopathy in canines. He termed the manifestations "meat intoxication." As we now know, this is the result of hyperammonemia and hepatic coma secondary to dietary intake of protein and shunting of blood around the liver.

Etiology

There are four main pathophysiologic conditions that cause portal hypertension (Fig. 15). The first condition is characterized by an *increase in hepatopedal flow* without any demonstrable obstruction. This is rarely encountered, but conditions characterized by this increased flow include arterial portovenous fistulas as well as splenic arteriovenous fistulas. Massive splenomegaly as well as myeloproliferative disorders may rarely cause portal hypertesion by this mechanism, and splenectomy is usually curative. The second condition causing portal hypertension includes extrahepatic outflow obstruction, termed *Budd-Chiari syndrome,* and has a variety of causes. Anatomically, the hepatic veins constitute the sole efferent vascular drainage of the liver, and endophlebitis or blockage of outflow obstruction causes portal hypertension. This syndrome was originally described by Budd in 1849; the clinical features of hepatomegaly, abdominal pain, and massive ascites were later described by Chiari in 1899. The most common cause is endophlebitis of the hepatic veins. However, in the Japanese a congenital web of the hepatic veins is more commonly found. Clotting disorders found with malignancy or oral contraceptive use have also been associated with Budd-Chiari syndrome. Effective treatment of this condition involves the creation of a side-to-side portacaval shunt, allowing the portal vein to act as an efferent conduit and decompress the liver.

The third condition causing portal hypertension involves *extrahepatic obstruction* to inflow of the portal vein. In this condition the liver function tests and morphology are normal. The most common cause of extrahepatic obstruction includes the cavernomatous transformation of the portal vein. A number of investigators have documented an association between neonatal infection and omphalitis in one third of patients. Other theories suggest that there is a continuation of the embryonic obliteration of the vitelline veins with neonatal thrombosis of the portal vein and recanalization. A disease that is also characterized by a presinusoidal obstruction is schistosomiasis, the most common cause of portal hypertension and variceal bleeding worldwide. This infection causes an intrahepatic presinusoidal obstruction of the portal vein. Hepatic function is normal provided there is no accompanying hepatitis. These patients are younger and healthier than the cirrhotic patient and thus have a better prognosis with the various shunt procedures.

The fourth cause of portal hypertension and the most common is *cirrhosis,* accounting for 90 per cent of the cases. At least three pathologic findings must be present in the liver to make the diagnosis of cirrhosis. Biopsy should show parenchymal necrosis and fibrosis with nodular regeneration of surviving cells. The necrotic cells stimulate a fibroblastic response around the sinusoids. Because of the fibrosis and distortion of the hepatic vascular tree, portal hypertension ensues. The fibrosis and redistribution of blood flow with formation of a basement membrane substance in the space of Disse combine to reduce the metabolic efficiency of the liver. Two different types of nodular regeneration are noted on gross pathologic examination. Micronodular regeneration is characterized by small, regenerating nodules, whereas macronodular regeneration demonstrates a variable nodular size.

Liver failure in cirrhosis is caused by a number of factors. The hepatic fibrosis with resultant compression of the sinusoids by regenerating nodules forms a mechanical obstruction to blood flow. The obstructive microcirculation causes shunts to form that carry blood away from the hepatocyte, escalating deterioration in liver function tests. The increased arterial flow as well as the fatty infiltration and acute inflammation combine to decrease hepatic metabolic capability. The most common causes of cirrhosis are

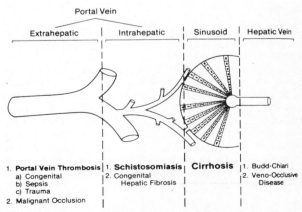

Figure 15. Schematic showing the four categories of portal hypertension. (From Henderson, J. M., and Warren, W. D.: In Sabiston, D. C., Jr. (Ed.): The Textbook of Surgery, 13th ed. Philadelphia, W. B. Saunders Company, 1986, p. 1100.)

alcoholism and viral hepatitis. Other rare causes include biliary, cryptogenic, toxic, nutritional, and congestive cirrhosis. Cirrhosis is the sixth leading cause of death in the United States, and the risk of developing this disease is related to total ethanol consumption. It has been noted that 30 per cent of chronic alcoholics ultimately develop cirrhosis.

Diagnostic Methods

Clinically, cirrhosis may be diagnosed by a triad of physical findings including hepatomegaly, ascites, and spider angiomata. The presence of splenomegaly confirms the diagnosis of portal hypertension. On physical examination one may see spider angiomata, palmar erythema, gynecomastia, and testicular atrophy, all thought to be consistent with an abnormal estrogen metabolism in the cirrhotic patient.

LABORATORY FINDINGS

One may test for subclinical encephalopathy with cognitive as well as motor function tests. Hematologically, the anemia in these patients is multifactorial, with components of gastrointestinal bleeding, hemolysis, and nutrition accounting for the low blood counts. Leukopenia and thrombocytopenia usually denote hypersplenism. Coagulation defects are present with prolongation of the prothrombin time and decreased synthesis of coagulation proteins. Abnormal liver function tests usually suggest severe liver damage. Serum bilirubin is not elevated until late in the disease. An elevation in transaminases usually denotes acute injury and is most commonly seen with viral hepatitis. Decreased serum albumin levels indicate decreased metabolic activity of the liver, since it is the sole source of albumin production.

CHILD'S CLASSIFICATION

Child's classification has been very helpful in categorizing patients with cirrhosis and portal hypertension. The clinical findings of ascites, encephalopathy, and nutritional status do much to predict the clinical prognosis of these patients. Hepatitis screening is also important in a patient presenting with hyperbilirubinemia to exclude a primary hepatocellular process.

LIVER BIOPSY

The definitive diagnosis of cirrhosis is usually achieved with a liver biopsy performed through the eighth or ninth interspace. It is used to identify the pathologic state, the etiology of the pathologic condition, and the stage and activity of inflammation present in the liver. The complication rate for percutaneous liver biopsy has been quoted to be 0.5 per cent. Endoscopy as part of a work-up for gastrointestinal bleeding in this group is important mainly to confirm esophageal varices as a source of bleeding and to exclude other pathologic conditions. Bleeding from esophageal varices accounts for only 50 per cent of the bleeding episodes in the cirrhotic patient, with diffuse gastritis and duodenal ulcer as other principal causes.

RADIOLOGY

Radiologically, the upper gastrointestinal series may show esophageal varices. However, this study is poor in demonstrating gastric varices. The upper gastrointestinal series is helpful in excluding duodenal ulcer. Most recently, endoscopy has supplanted barium studies as the procedure of choice to diagnose esophageal varices. Angiography is important in the evaluation of the cirrhotic patient to visualize the venous anatomy and measure portal pressure. Portal pressure is determined by either direct transhepatic portography or splenoportography or with the hepatic wedge technique. Indirect methods of measuring portal pressure include wedge hepatic vein pressures achieved by threading a catheter into the inferior vena cava and wedging it in the hepatic veins. Since the portal system has no valves, a wedge hepatic vein pressure provides a good approximation of sinusoidal pressure. It should be emphasized that the degree of portal hypertension is not correlated with the risk of bleeding or ascites formation.

Pathophysiology

Hepatopedal flow has been documented in a number of collateral channels even with total portal vein thrombosis. This hepatopedal flow usually does not effectively decompress the portal system and portal hypertension ensues. With a completely occluded 2-cm. portal vein, Poiseuille's law estimates that approximately 4000 collateral veins 0.5 cm wide are needed to effectively decompress the liver, and such are seldom present. Venous phase imaging after splenic artery or superior mesenteric artery (SMA) injection can demonstrate the different collaterals showing hepatofugal flow. The most common portosystemic collateral bed involves the left gastric or coronary vein, which eventually empties into the azygos vein and the superior vena cava (Fig. 16). The coronary vein connects directly with the esophageal venous plexus and delivers blood to the esophageal varices. Other collateral channels that conduct hepatofugal flow include the hemorrhoidal plexus, the

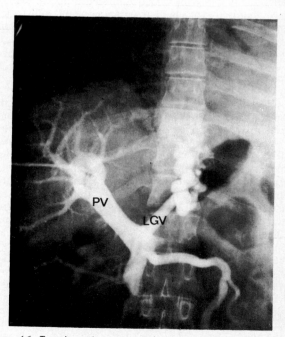

Figure 16. Transhepatic portography in a patient with cirrhosis and portal hypertension. Note the left gastric vein (LGV) feeding the esophageal venous plexus. (From Berk, J. E. (Ed.): Bockus Gastroenterology, 4th ed. Philadelphia, W. B. Saunders Company, 1985, p. 3067.)

retroperitoneal venous channels, and the umbilical vein plexus characterized by a "caput medusae" pattern in advanced cirrhosis.

Hemodynamic studies demonstrate that most cirrhotics have an increase in cardiac output measured in the 20 to 25 per cent range. Because there is an increase in cardiac output with an increase in stroke volume, there must be an accompanying decrease in peripheral resistance. Normally, the portal vein flow is about 1100 ml. per minute, whereas hepatic artery flow is 400 ml. per minute. However, these rates are significantly decreased in cirrhosis and portal hypertension. Attempts have been made to measure portal flow, but most tests are inaccurate. Doppler ultrasonography is a promising technique for measuring portal vein vessel diameter and blood velocity, whereas the galactose elimination test measures the hepatic function directly since normally galactose is almost totally extracted in a single pass through the liver. Serum liver function tests are of limited value in evaluating the stage of cirrhosis. Computed tomography of liver volume can be important in the clinical evaluation of the cirrhotic patient. These tests are used to differentiate patients with large livers, normal hemodynamics, and good hepatocyte reserve from those with end-stage small livers, lost portal perfusion, and minimal residual functional capacity.

Variceal Bleeding

The normal pressure is 5 to 10 mm. Hg in the portal vein and 2 to 3 mm. Hg in the portal sinusoids. Elevated portal pressures usually range from 15 to 40 mm. Hg. Bleeding gastroesophageal varices are the most life-threatening complications of portal hypertension. The most important collateral pathway involves the left gastric or coronary vessel and the short gastric vessels. On endoscopy, varices usually have an overlying mucosa. However, in later stages the mucosa may disappear and the wall of the vein may actually form the lining of the esophagus. Bleeding is precipitated by either an increased pressure within the varix or ulceration secondary to the presence of esophagitis. Bleeding may be anticipated in 30 per cent of cirrhotics with varices, and most episodes occur within 2 years of the diagnosis of esophageal varices. It is reported that 70 per cent of patients die within the first year following the first hemorrhage, with 68 per cent of the patients having re-bleeding episodes.

CONTROL OF ACUTE BLEEDING

An acute bleeding episode requires rapid control to avoid shock and the toxic effects of the absorption of the high protein content of blood from the gastrointestinal tract. The cirrhotic patient may be resuscitated with blood transfusions and fresh frozen plasma to correct coagulation defects and provide platelets. A Swan-Ganz catheter is particularly helpful in monitoring the adequacy of intravascular volume replacement. Cimetidine has been recommended to decrease gastric acid production, and sedation with diazepam (Valium) may be used but caution is necessary owing to the altered liver metabolism of benzodiazepines. With ascites, saline should be avoided. Paracentesis may reduce intra-abdominal pressure and decrease portal pressure. Endoscopy is the diagnostic method of choice not only to confirm the esophageal varices but to exclude other pathologic conditions causing gastrointestinal hemorrhage. Only 50 per cent of the gastrointestinal bleeding in cirrhotic patients can be attributed to varices, with gastritis accounting for 30 per cent and duodenal ulcers another 10 per cent.

PHARMACOLOGIC CONTROL OF ESOPHAGEAL HEMORRHAGE

Vasopressin

Specific measurements may then be taken to control the esophageal hemorrhage. The most commonly used pharmacologic agent for acute variceal bleeding is vasopressin because it is a powerful vasoconstrictor of the splenic and mesenteric arterial systems and produces a decrease in portovenous blood flow of as much as 50 per cent and, thus, a decrease in portal pressure. Reflexly, there is an increase in portovenous resistance, but this may be overcome with vasodilator therapy, specifically nitroglycerin and nitroprusside. The side effects of vasopressin include an adverse action on the heart and systemic circulation with an increase in cardiac afterload and a decrease in coronary flow secondary to the increased peripheral resistance. Cardiac complications ranging from rhythm disturbances to acute myocardial infarctions have been described with vasopressin. Arterial hypertension, stroke, and lower extremity ischemia have also been detailed and are serious consequences.

It has been shown that either intravenous or SMA infusions produce similar changes on portal hemodynamics with equal complication rates, and thus one method has no advantage over the other. Bosch[72] reports that vasopressin controls the bleeding in 50 to 60 per cent of patients; however, the major complication rate, requiring withdrawal of this drug, is about 25 per cent. Hussey[80] notes that three of the four control trials using vasopressin have shown it to be effective; however, the use of vasopressin has not changed the mortality in patients with bleeding esophageal varices (Table 2). The usual dose ranges from 0.2 to 0.8 units per min. IV per kg. per min. Higher doses do not seem to cause any further decrease in portal pressure and may be detrimental owing to the increase in heart rate and cardiac output with the resultant adverse effects on the myocardium. Terlipressin (Glypressin, produced by Ferring in Germany), a new pharmacologic agent, has been shown to be ten times less potent than vasopressin but lacks most of the cardiotoxic effects and is reported to control bleeding in 70 per cent of patients.

Others investigators[76] have used sublingual nitroglycerin to negate the adverse cardiovascular effects of vasopressin. This therapy may concomitantly result in decreased portal pressure. The nitroglycerin may also be delivered via a skin patch. Intravenous nitroprusside[82] has been used to decrease cardiac output and counteract the deleterious cardiac effects of vasopressin, thus returning the preload and afterload levels to normal.

Somatostatin

The gastrointestinal hormone somatostatin has been found to reduce splanchnic blood flow and cause vasoconstriction of the mesenteric artery, which subsequently decreases portal blood flow. Somatostatin causes a prolonged reduction of azygos and, thus, gastroesophageal collateral blood flow and is reported to control bleeding in 53 per cent of patients with no adverse cardiac effects.

Propranolol

Propranolol (Inderal) has been reported to cause a decrease in portal venous pressure in cirrhotic patients.[81]

TABLE 2. Comparison of Controlled Trials of Vasopressin Therapy*

N	60	30	60	38
Dose and route	0.6 units/min. IV	20 units in 20 min. IV	0.05–0.4 units/min. IA	0.2–0.4 units/min. IA
Source of bleeding (%)				
Variceal	55	100	55	33
Other	45	0	45	67
Mortality (%)				
Control group	35	80	56	45
Vasopressin group	27	93	54	44
Duration of therapy (hr.)	24	Variable	Mean, 28; range, 7–74	Mean, 46; range, 1–192
Cessation of bleeding (%)				
without vasopressin	45	0	28	15
with vasopressin	58	50	71	44
p	0.3	*	< 0.001	< 0.05
p				
Transfusion requirements	NS†	Not studied	Units/hr.: < 0.001; total units: NS (> 0.005)	NS*
Mortality	NS	NS	NS	NS

*Modified from Hussey, K. P.: Arch. Intern. Med., *145*:1263, 1985.
†For these comparisons no specific *P* value was given.
Abbreviations: IV = Intravenous; IA = intra-arterial; NS = not significant.

In the initial reports there was a decreased incidence of recurrent variceal hemorrhage, but the reduction of portal vein pressure, caused by a similar decrease in portovenous blood flow, was only in the 10 to 15 per cent range. It has been noted that the azygous venous flow, a direct measure of blood flow in the esophageal variceal system, decreased 32 per cent with propranolol. More important, hepatic artery blood flow was not reduced, and thus liver perfusion was maintained. In one series,[81] 74 patients were given a dose of propranolol sufficient to reduce the resting heart rate 25 per cent. These cirrhotic patients showed a 2-year free-of-hemorrhage survival rate of 90 per cent, with a rate of only 57 per cent reported in control patients (Fig. 17). However, another report demonstrated propranolol to be no more effective than placebo in reducing the rebleeding rate in patients with esophageal varices. However, this study did demonstrate that chronic oral propranolol therapy reduced bleeding from esophageal varices in alcoholic cirrhotics who were in good condition as characterized by clinical Child's A and B classification.

The complications of long-term propranolol therapy involve an increase in arterial ammonia levels in cirrhotics and, thus, an increased rate of encephalopathy. It should be stated that in 25 to 40 per cent of cirrhotics portal pressure failed to be decreased with beta-adrenergic blockade.

BALLOON TAMPONADE

Sengstaken and Blakemore[88] originally reported the technique of *double balloon esophageal and gastric tamponade* in 1950 to control esophageal varices. It has been shown that nearly all blood entering the esophageal varices flows from below the diaphragm through the enlarged coronary vein, and they hypothesized that impaction of the gastric fundus and gastroesophageal junction against the diaphragm with the inflated gastric balloon would decrease flow of blood to the varix and stop the hemorrhage. They designed a double balloon tube that was passed initially into the stomach; the gastric balloon inflated with 250 to

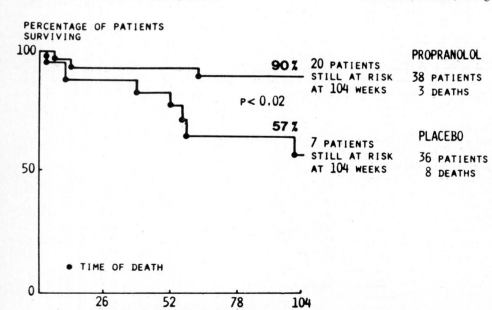

Figure 17. Ninety per cent of the cirrhotic patients treated with propranolol had a period of 2 years free of hemorrhage rate of 90 per cent with only 57 per cent of the control population not rebleeding. (From Lebrec, D.: Hepatology, 4:357, 1984.)

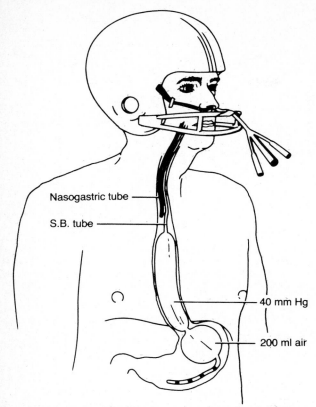

Figure 18. Diagram demonstrating the Sengstaken-Blakemore tube in place with balloons inflated with traction on the proximal tube. (From Bauer, J. J., et al.: Ann. Surg., 179:273, 1974.)

Labels in figure: Nasogastric tube; S.B. tube; 40 mm Hg; 200 ml air

In numerous reports, the hemorrhage has been shown to be controlled in 79 to 92 per cent of patients. Recurrent bleeding after deflation of the balloon occurs in 24 to 42 per cent of patients. The bleeding is not controlled in approximately 33 per cent of patients. The major disadvantage of balloon tamponade is its high complication rate, including pulmonary aspiration, esophageal rupture and erosion, and respiratory obstruction. The mortality reported in a number of series from the literature is in the range of 4 to 22 per cent. However, with proper technique and attention to detail, the Sengstaken-Blakemore tube can be a valuable adjuvant in controlling esophageal bleeding.

Percutaneous Transhepatic Coronary Vein Occlusion

Percutaneous transhepatic coronary vein occlusion involves embolizing the coronary vein with spring coils, absorbable gelatin sponge (Gelfoam), thrombin, or detachable balloons. Another compound used is bucrylate, which totally obliterates the coronary vein. This technique is reported to be successful in the initial control of bleeding in 45 to 90 per cent of patients; however, the rebleeding rate is high (25 to 86 per cent). In reported series, the onset of rebleeding was delayed but there was no difference in mortality rates. Portal vein thrombosis caused by the procedure itself occurs in 20 to 30 per cent of patients. The advantage of this technique is that variceal therapy can usually be done in a single session.

Endoscopic Sclerotherapy

Endoscopic sclerotherapy involves the use of either a rigid or flexible endoscope to directly inject the varices with sclerosing agents. Flexible endoscopes are usually preferred. Although they are less precise in the visualization of the bleeding vessel, they are much safer instruments. Intravariceal or paravariceal injection can be performed (Fig. 19). Paravariceal injection and the resultant inflammatory reaction cause thrombosis of the varix. The keys to success in sclerotherapy are induction of necrosis and stimulation of collagen deposition. Commonly used sclerosants include sodium morrhuate, tetradecasulfate, and absolute alcohol. Protocols for the injection period include treating the acute bleed and then addressing persistent varices with subsequent treatments on the first, fourth, seventh, and fourteenth days. After four treatments, varices should be obliterated.

275 ml. of air. Prior to inflation of the gastric balloon, a plain radiograph of the abdomen was taken to confirm the presence of the lower balloon in the stomach. This is done to prevent esophageal inflation and rupture. Nasal passage is encouraged, and a small amount of traction is placed on the ends of the Sengstaken-Blakemore tube to keep the gastric balloon tightly against the gastroesophageal junction. Initially, only the gastric balloon is inflated to prevent the complications of esophageal balloon inflation, such as airway obstruction and pressure erosion. If this does not control bleeding, the esophageal balloon may be inflated (Fig. 18). After 24 hours the esophageal balloon should be deflated, followed by another 24 hours of observation before the gastric balloon is deflated. After the control of hemorrhage, the tube should be left in place for another 24 hours.

In approximately 75 per cent of patients, control can be achieved using this technique; however, the rebleed rate is 40 to 60 per cent after the initial success. Thus, many investigators recommend repeated injections until all the varices are obliterated, since the rebleeding rate after total

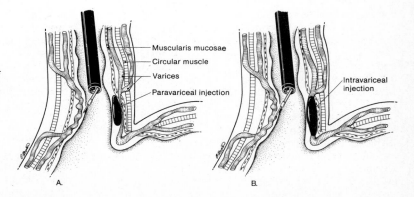

Figure 19. Intravariceal and paravariceal injection of esophageal varices with sclerosant. (From Sabiston, D. C., Jr. (Ed.): The Textbook of Surgery, 13th ed. Philadelphia, W. B. Saunders Company, 1986, p. 1111.)

Labels in figure: Muscularis mucosae; Circular muscle; Varices; Paravariceal injection; Intravariceal injection; A.; B.

obliteration of the varices is only 10 to 30 per cent. The complication rate is 10 to 30 per cent; however, most complications are minor and consist of fever and local discomfort. Mucosal ulcerations, esophageal necrosis, and mediastinitis may ensue and cause significant mortality. Hemorrhage is also possible from esophageal erosion, and strictures occur in 50 per cent of long-term survivors. The strictures usually respond to repeated dilation.

A number of endoscopists have shown that sclerotherapy is more effective than balloon tamponade in controlling variceal hemorrhage.[71, 85] One of the better series using sclerotherapy in over 900 patients reports successful control of the acute bleed in 92 per cent of patients. This is in contrast to the experience with balloon tamponade at this investigator's hospital, where the success rate is only 66 per cent. The rebleeding rates for sclerotherapy and balloon tamponade were 20 and 44 per cent, respectively. The study also reports a decrease in mortality with sclerotherapy. Those patients undergoing endoscopic injection had a mortality rate of 16 per cent, whereas those with balloon tamponade as the initial treatment for variceal hemorrhage had a 1-year mortality rate of 55 per cent. In another series, sclerotherapy was comparable to emergency portacaval shunt in controlling bleeding esophageal varices.[75] A success rate of 57 per cent was reported with sclerotherapy and 58 per cent with portacaval shunt, a 1-year survival of 25 per cent in both groups.

Sclerotherapy costs much less than operative intervention. In a randomized controlled prospective trial comparing sclerotherapy with the performance of a selective distal splenorenal shunt, 36 patients had sclerotherapy. Fifty-three per cent rebled, but with further variceal injections only 31 per cent could not be controlled.[95] The population who continued to bleed after two injections were then placed in the distal splenorenal shunt group. The 2-year survival for the sclerotherapy-only group was 84 per cent. In the 35 patients who underwent distal splenorenal shunt because of variceal bleeding, the rebleeding rate was only 3 per cent. However, the 2-year survival in this latter group was 59 per cent, and it was thought that sclerotherapy better maintained hepatic function and portal perfusion (Fig. 20).

In regard to *chronic sclerotherapy,* 5-year survivals have been noted to be similar in a medically treated and a sclerotherapy-treated group for chronic control of esophageal hemorrhage.[91] The 5-year survival was 35 per cent for both groups. After *obliteration* of the varices there is little chance of recurrent hemorrhage. These data were not substantiated in a randomized trial of sclerotherapy versus medical treatment for the chronic control of esophageal varices.[96] This study showed a 37-month death rate of 32 per cent in the sclerotherapy group and 56 per cent in the chronic medically treated group. The chance of rebleeding in the sclerotherapy group was also lower, 55 per cent compared with 80 per cent.

Prophylactic endoscopy and sclerotherapy can identify those patients with impending hemorrhage.[84] These patients have large varices at endoscopy with demonstrable black points or cherry red spots on the varix or are found to have a prolonged prothrombin time. In a randomized trial, the control group had an 87 per cent bleeding rate, and 64 per cent of the patients died. However, in those patients who were identified to be at high risk for bleeding, prophylactic endoscopic injection resulted in a 9 per cent bleeding rate with only an 18 per cent mortality.

In summary, acute sclerotherapy can control actively bleeding varices in 95 per cent of patients. It seems to be more effective than balloon tamponade or vasopressin therapy, and short-term survival is extended. Long-term

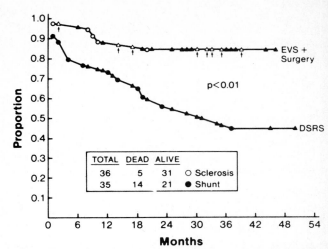

Figure 20. *Actuarial survival curves showing an increased survival in those patients who had endoscopic sclerotherapy and surgical treatment compared with those who had a distal splenorenal shunt. (From Warren, W. D., et al.: Ann. Surg., 203:457, 1986.)*

survival in the number of series seems to be better with chronic sclerotherapy. The concept of prophylactic sclerotherapy is an important one and should be evaluated in further randomized trials.

EMERGENCY SURGERY FOR BLEEDING ESOPHAGEAL VARICES

Many consider a patient (Child's A or B) who is refractory to medical treatment of bleeding varices to be a candidate for operative therapy. It is known that the mortality of patients with bleeding varices is 66 to 73 per cent, and in a number of series the mortality rate for emergency shunts is reported to be around 50 per cent. Orloff and coworkers,[83] in perhaps the literature's best series of emergency portacaval shunts for bleeding esophageal varices, showed an operative survival of 48 per cent and a 7-year survival of 42 per cent if the patient was operated on within 8 hours of the bleed. However, these results have not been repeated in subsequent trials; usually a higher operative mortality rate is reported. The presence of ascites and a Child's C classification reduce the operative survival rate and may contraindicate surgical approaches.

End-to-side portacaval shunts, interposition H grafts between the portal vein and the vena cava as well as between the superior mesenteric vein and vena cava, and distal splenorenal shunts have been advocated for the emergency treatment of bleeding varices. If a patient is not a candidate for a shunt, then other ablative procedures, such as splenectomy, gastric devascularization, or esophageal transection, may be considered. These procedures are usually performed in patients who do not have a portal vein suitable for shunting. Thus, emergency shunts are recommended for patients who are not controlled with more conservative measures such as sclerotherapy, balloon tamponade, and vasopressin therapy and who are not icteric, ascitic, or encephalopathic. It should be remembered that these procedures carry a high operative mortality.

Surgical Approaches for Portal Hypertension

HISTORIC ASPECTS

The portacaval shunt was done experimentally by Eck[77] in 1877. He said "blood of the portal vein, without any danger to the body, could be diverted directly into the general circulation and this by means of a perfectly safe operation." Later, Pavlov disputed this conclusion with meticulous animal data reported in 1893. He showed that portacaval shunting caused the animal to die of "meat intoxication," which clinically is hepatic coma. Blakemore, Whipple, and Liepold reintroduced the concept of portosystemic shunting in the 1940s when newer techniques of venovenous anastomosis showed good patency rates and encephalopathy could be controlled by the restriction of dietary protein. Selective variceal decompression was introduced by Warren and associates[93] in 1966 because of dissatisfaction with total shunting and the high rate of subsequent encephalopathy. The group felt that during the performance of a selective shunt only the gastroesophageal splenic segment was decompressed and portal hypertension and blood flow were maintained, which reduced the rate of encephalopathy. Indeed, this has been the finding in a number of studies.

TOTAL PORTOSYSTEMIC SHUNTS

End-to-Side Shunt

A commonly performed shunt in the United States for control of portal hypertension is the end-to-side portacaval shunt. This method can prevent recurrent esophageal bleeding and reduces portal pressure to the 5 to 10 mm. Hg level. However, it deprives the liver of all portal blood. The procedure is usually performed through a subcostal incision with dissection beginning in the hepatoduodenal ligament. The portal vein, which lies posterior to the common bile duct, is dissected free along its entire course. The inferior vena cava is then dissected from the renal veins inferiorly to the point where the inferior vena cava passes retrohepatically. The portal vein is transected just below its bifurcation and the hepatic end oversewn. A partial occlusion clamp is placed on the inferior vena cava and the anastomosis constructed between the portal vein and inferior vena cava in an end-to-side fashion with the anastomosis being one and one half times as long as the diameter of the portal vein (Fig. 21).

Side-to-Side Shunt

Another popular shunt is the side-to-side portacaval shunt, which provides the additional component of liver

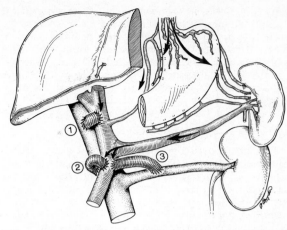

Figure 22. Interposition H-grafts in the (1) portacaval, (2) mesocaval and (3) mesorenal position. (From Henderson, J. M., and Warren, W. D.: In Sabiston, D. C., Jr. (Ed.): The Textbook of Surgery, 13th ed. Philadelphia, W. B. Saunders Company, 1986, p. 1103.)

decompression through the portal vein. It is important to realize that with this shunt prograde flow to the liver is usually not maintained. A shunt large enough to decompress varices converts the portal vein to an exclusive outflow tract. Whether converting the portal vein to an outflow tract is beneficial or harmful is controversial. Some studies suggest that the portal vein, acting as an efferent conduit, may siphon blood away from the liver; however, this shunt relieves ascites in most patients. The 5- to 10-year survival with total portosystemic shunts is 20 to 30 per cent. The operative mortality depends on Child's classification, with the Child's A patient showing little, if any, operative mortality, the Child's B 9 per cent, and the Child's C 53 per cent.

H Graft

An H graft performed with a 14- to 20-mm. Goretex graft between the superior mesenteric vein and the vena cava has also been successful in decompressing esophageal varices (Fig. 22). With the shorter interpositional grafts, there appears to be a higher patency rate. The advantages of this type of graft are that it controls ascites and bleeding and there is an option to ligate the shunt if liver failure ensues. All of the total portosystemic shunts direct blood from the liver. Esophageal variceal decompression is accomplished by relieving portal hypertension at the expense of liver blood flow. Experience indicates that although bleeding is controlled with total portosystemic shunts, survival is not improved. A large number of patients develop hepatic encephalopathy and eventually die of hepatic failure.

Prophylactic Shunting

A number of randomized studies have been performed in an attempt to determine whether prophylactic shunting is beneficial. It was found from these studies that prophylactic shunting reduced bleeding but did not prolong survival, with an operative mortality in the range of 8 to 14 per cent. The 5-year survival in control populations has been reported to be 50 to 60 per cent, whereas 5-year survival in the shunted groups was 35 to 50 per cent. Based on these data, prophylactic shunting should not be considered a viable alternative. In a follow-up of four randomized studies of therapeutic protacaval shunting and medical

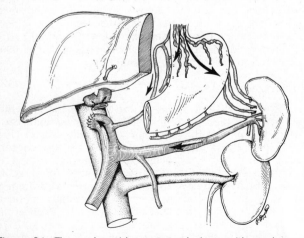

Figure 21. The end-to-side portacaval shunt with total portal diversion. This shunt maintains high sinusoidal pressure. (From Henderson, J. M., and Warren, W. D.: In Sabiston, D. C., Jr. (Ed.): The Textbook of Surgery, 13th ed. Philadelphia, W. B. Saunders Company, 1986, p. 1103.)

therapy, there was no significant increase in survival with portacaval shunting; however, bleeding was controlled more efficiently.[86] Hepatic failure and encephalopathy are accelerated by total portosystemic shunting. Analysis of prerandomization risk factors failed to reveal variables important in the development of encephalopathy in the shunt population or rebleeding in the medically managed patients.

SELECTED VARICEAL DECOMPRESSION

The most physiologic of the surgical procedures for portal hypertension is the distal splenorenal shunt (Fig. 23), since it maintains portal flow and thus decreases hepatocyte damage and liver failure. By sustaining portal hypertension, there is a decreased risk of postoperative hepatic encephalopathy. The distal splenorenal shunt selectively decompresses the esophageal plexus through the short gastric and splenic veins. An oblique subcostal incision is usually used, and the transverse colon and splenic flexure are mobilized and retracted caudad with division of short gastric vessels. One must totally mobilize the pancreas from its bed in order to visualize the splenic vein. By retracting the pancreas cephalad, the splenic vein becomes visible on the posterior aspect of the gland, and dissection should continue directly on top of the splenic vein on its posterior surface.

It is helpful initially to control the splenic vein–portal vein junction. The posterior peritoneum is then incised just medial to the hilum of the left kidney, and the left renal artery and vein are dissected free. The splenic artery is doubly ligated and transected, and the splenic vein is transected as close to the junction of the portal vein as possible. The anastomosis is constructed between the splenic and renal veins in an end-to-side fashion to avoid kinking. Coronary vein disconnection is also an important part of the procedure. To avoid the subsequent development of the pancreatic sump syndrome, all pancreatic branches from the splenic vein should be ligated (Fig. 23). Renal vein hypertension occurs in 20 per cent of patients; however, this usually resolves in 4 to 6 weeks.

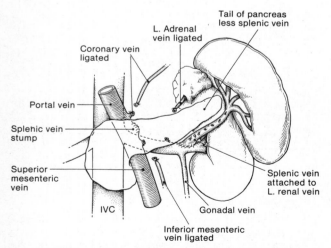

Figure 23. Schematic representation of distal splenorenal shunt. The anastomosis shows the distal end of the splenic vein sutured to the side of the renal vein. Dissection of the splenic vein free of the pancreas prevents development of the pancreatic siphon to provide optimal selective variceal decompression. (From Henderson, J. M., and Warren, W. D.: In Sabiston, D. C., Jr. (Ed.): The Textbook of Surgery, 13th ed. Philadelphia, W. B. Saunders Company, 1986, p. 1109.)

The efficacy of this shunt is supported by a number of nonrandomized and randomized studies. In a summary of nonrandomized studies from 25 centers for the distal splenorenal shunt, a 7 per cent operative mortality and a 90 per cent early patency rate are reported. In 90 per cent of patients bleeding is controlled, with a 5-year survival of 60 per cent. Those patients with nonethanol cirrhosis have a better prognosis than patients with alcoholic cirrhosis. The hepatic encephalopathy rate is remarkably low (reportedly 5 per cent). In the number of randomized trials from Warren[94] and Zeppa's[97] groups it appears that there is no difference in survival between the total shunt and the selective splenorenal shunt. Control of bleeding is similar in the two populations and reportedly 90 per cent. Both studies demonstrate that nonalcoholics have a better prognosis than alcoholics after shunting. The rate of development of encephalopathy with the total systemic shunt group is 35 per cent, whereas only 5 per cent of patients in the distal splenorenal group developed encephalopathy. For this reason, the investigators recommend selected shunts exclusively.

VARICEAL ABLATIVE PROCEDURES

A number of nonshunt surgical procedures have been recommended for the treatment of portal hypertension in those patients who are not shunt candidates. These include total gastric devascularization and esophageal transection procedures. Proponents of these two procedures also recommend them for the elective treatment of portal hypertension.

Gastric Devascularization

Sugiura and Futagawa devised the gastric devascularization technique for the treatment of portal hypertension with the use of a left thoracotomy for esophageal transection and periesophageal devascularization.[90] During the procedure approximately 30 to 50 shunting veins on the esophagus need to be ligated to devascularize 12 to 18 cm. of distal esophagus. The distal esophagus is divided through all layers except the posterior muscle coat and then resutured. The abdominal part of the procedure includes a splenectomy with devascularization of the abdominal esophagus and cardia. The elective operative mortality was 4.5 per cent, which increased to 13.7 per cent for emergency procedures. Ten-year survival was 55 per cent in the emergency population and 72 per cent in the elective population. The rebleeding rate was remarkably low (5 per cent). It is recommended that this procedure be used only on patients who have no vein available for shunting.

Esophageal Transection

The use of the end-to-end anastomosis (EEA) stapler has been recommended for esophageal transection, which makes this part of the procedure technically simpler (Fig. 24). However, 25 per cent of these patients have encountered postoperative dysphagia from esophageal stricture after an EEA-stapled transection. A number of surgeons in the United States have also added an antireflux procedure to the Sugiura operation, since many of these patients have gastroesophageal reflux postoperatively. Spence and Johnson[89] recommend esophageal transection with an EEA stapler only for those patients unsuitable for shunt procedures, such as the elderly, the Child's C patient, the diabetic, and those who have had previous encephalopathy or may later be considered for hepatic transplantation.

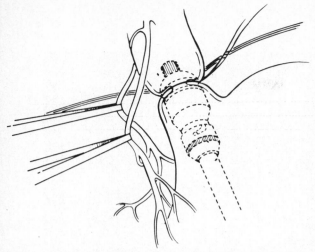

Figure 24. The use of the EEA stapler to divide and restaple the distal esophagus as part of the Sugiura procedure. The stapler is introduced through a separate gastrostomy. (From Mucha, P., and van Heerden, J. A.: Am. J. Surg., 148:399, 1984.)

Portal Hypertension in Children

Extrahepatic presinusoidal obstruction of the portal vein is the most common cause of esophageal varices in children. The clinical manifestations usually involve normal liver function tests, normal liver histology, esophageal varices, and splenomegaly. *Cavernomatous transformation* of the portal vein is the most common cause and is thought to be part of the embryonic obliteration of vitelline veins due to neonatal thrombosis of the portal vein secondary to unbilical cord infections. Indeed, approximately one third of the patients have a neonatal history of omphalitis. There have also been episodes of documented extracellular fluid depletion in the neonatal period.

In a series of 69 patients with cavernomatous transformation of the portal vein, it has been shown that 80 per cent of patients are less than 6 years of age.[78] Fifty-seven per cent of patients in this series presented initially with esophageal variceal bleed as the first clinical sign of portal hypertension. Thirty-eight per cent showed signs of splenomegaly and hypersplenism, with resultant thrombocytopenia occurring in 48 per cent. Because liver function and clotting parameters are normal, these patients usually tolerate the bleeds well. Only 3 per cent of patients die of a hemorrhage, and these patients usually live in remote areas. The bleeding episodes are usually preceded by an upper respiratory infection or a febrile episode with coughing. It is noted that only 24 per cent bleed after the age of 16, and conservative therapy should be instituted prior to this point.

SUPPORTIVE THERAPY

Supportive therapy consists of admission to the hospital and administration of antacids, sedation, vitamin K, and intravenous vasopressin injection (Pitressin). The Sengstaken-Blakemore tube may be used for persistent bleeding. Aspirin should be avoided for the treatment of upper respiratory infections in children with documented cavernomatous transformation. A number of temporizing operative procedures have been recommended; however, experience with these approaches has not shown favorable results. After splenectomy alone, there is a 95 per cent chance of rebleeding with an accompanying mortality from post-splenectomy sepsis in this age group. With operative variceal ligation, rebleeding will occur in 100 per cent of patients; therefore, it has no role in the therapy for these children.

TREATMENT

The elective operative treatment of the pediatric patient with portal hypertension includes creation of a mesocaval shunt, with permanent relief from bleeding in 80 per cent of patients. This shunt should be at least 1 cm. in diameter, and the procedure should be delayed until the patient is at least 8 years old, by which time the mesenteric veins are large enough for the anastomosis. It is essential to perform preoperative venography, since the thrombosis from the portal vein may extend into the inferior vena cava. The post-shunt encephalopathy rate is low and has been reported to be 10 to 15 per cent. The distal splenorenal shunt in the pediatric population can be successful with a decreased rate of encephalopathy.[87] One of the advantages of this procedure in children is that the splenic vein is more caudad in its relationship on the posterior pancreas and thus closer to the renal vein.

HEMOBILIA

Hemobilia has been described as an abnormal connection between blood vessels and bile ducts. It was considered a medical curiosity until Sandblom described the clinical manifestations in 1948.[28] Trauma is the most frequent cause of hemobilia. Traumatic abnormal fistulas should not be unexpected, since bile ducts, hepatic arterioles, and the portovenous system are in close association in the portal triads. Hemobilia arises from the liver parenchyma approximately 50 per cent of the time, from the gallbladder or pancreas 25 per cent of the time, and from the extrahepatic bile ducts 25 per cent of the time. Thrombolysins in the bile may contribute to continual bleeding

Etiology

Trauma is the cause of 50 per cent of the cases reported in the literature, and the mechanisms involved show an equal frequency of blunt, penetrating, and iatrogenic causes.[27, 29] Most of the patients develop symptoms within 1 week to 3 months of the traumatic event. However, there have been reports of patients developing hemobilia 3.5 years after a history of trauma.[29] Usually the bleeding is intermittent in nature; however, the patient may present with massive bleeding acutely. It is important to emphasize that the surgical technique used in handling the original liver injury has much to do with avoiding hemobilia. Mattress sutures used to close liver lacerations are ill advised, and if it is not possible to explore the laceration and oversew bleeders directly, other techniques, such as hepatic artery ligation, should be used. Hemobilia has also been described as a complication after cholecystectomy and with the increased use of percutaneous transhepatic biliary drainage catheters, when the insertion carries a 4 per cent incidence of hemobilia.

Infections cause 28 per cent of the cases of hemobilia and in the Far East are usually caused by the parasites *Clonorchis sinensis* and *Ascaris*. In the United States amebic

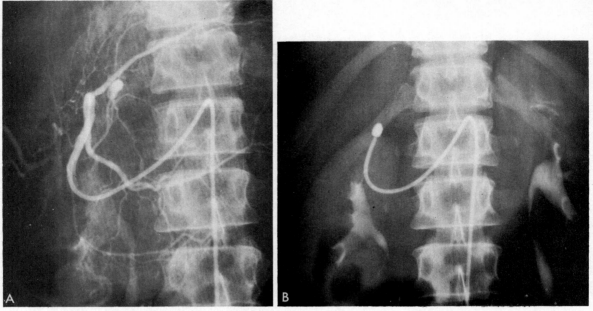

Figure 25. A, Hemobilia complicating percutaneous liver biopsy caused by a traumatic intraparenchymal hepatic artery aneurysm. B, Balloon catheter thrombosis of hepatic artery aneurysm with successful result. (From Dunnick, N. R., et al.: J.A.M.A., 233:2524, 1977.)

abscesses, tuberculosis, and echinococcal cysts are the most frequent infectious causes of hemobilia. Gallstones account for 10 per cent of the cases. Aneurysms cause hemobilia by pressure necrosis, with hepatic artery aneurysms accounting for 7 per cent of reports. Hepatomas are the etiologic agents for hemobilia 5 per cent of the time.

Clinical Presentation

The classic triad of gastrointestinal bleeding, right upper quadrant pain, and jaundice occurs approximately 30 per cent of the time. Bruits are heard over the liver in about 10 per cent of patients. This diagnosis should be suspected in a patient who has gastrointestinal bleeding and is not an alcoholic or does not have peptic ulcer disease. This is especially true if the patient has an antecedent history of trauma. Endoscopy can be helpful if blood is seen coming from the ampulla of Vater. A CT scan is useful to exclude lesions of the pancreas. The definitive diagnostic test is arteriography not only for visualizing the vascular lesion but for possible therapeutic embolization of the bleeding vessel (Fig. 25).

Treatment

Minor gastrointestinal bleeding can be treated expectantly, as the hemobilia in a percentage of these patients will resolve spontaneously. Recurrent bleeding or more vigorous bleeding should be treated surgically, during which time associated conditions, such as liver injuries or biliary tract disease, may also be addressed. Preoperative arteriography is essential, however, in defining the bleeding source. The surgical procedure includes exploring the cavity or liver laceration, ligating the bleeding point, and débridement and drainage. Any deep cavities or hemotomas may be located by palpation and needle aspiration.

ANTIBIOTICS

Antibiotics are an essential part of treatment, since infectious complications are serious. If the control of bleeding is not successful, ligation of one of the hepatic arteries may be performed with relative safety. After this procedure, increases in liver function tests usually develop in these patients, but invariably they return to normal values in 7 to 10 days. Postmortem dissections and arteriograms have shown extrahepatic collateral arterial pathways, and premortem arteriograms have demonstrated interlobar arterial connections, making hepatic artery ligation a less risky procedure.

EMBOLIC THERAPY

Recently, percutaneous angiographic embolization has been recommended as the initial procedure of choice for the treatment of hemobilia.[30] The advantages of embolic therapy include the demonstration of the precise location of the bleeding with the pretherapeutic arteriogram and the avoidance of general anesthesia or exploratory laparotomy in a patient who might be in shock or have obstructive jaundice. It is also apparent that ligation of the hepatic artery in the setting of previous operations is not a straightforward procedure, and this operative approach in itself may not control bleeding because of collaterals. Another advantage is that the patient may have a repeat arteriogram to ascertain if the bleeding has stopped. Embolic therapy is a safe procedure if the patient does not have cirrhosis and if the portal vein is patent.

Infection can be minimized with the use of prophylactic antibiotics. Other complications reported with an incidence of 1 to 4 per cent include embolization of other organs, hepatic abscess, septicemia, and infection of the gallbladder and cholecystitis. Success rates of 85 to 90 per cent have been cited in the literature. Treatment has been described as effective in a number of clinical settings, including false aneurysms of the hepatic artery and its branches, arterial biliary fistulas, arterial hepatic vein fistulas, and true aneurysms of the hepatic artery that rupture into the common bile duct. The advantages of this percutaneous embolic therapy make it the technique of choice in an emergency situation.

MORTALITY

Despite a better understanding in the treatment of liver injury and advances in surgical technique as well as the nonsurgical approach to hemobilia, this condition continues to have a mortality of 10 to 20 per cent. However, this is usually a function of the underlying disease. With a better understanding and awareness of this condition, the mortality should decrease.

PRIMARY AND METASTATIC LIVER TUMORS

Hepatocellular Carcinoma

Hepatomas, or hepatocellular carcinomas, are uncommon tumors in the United States, but they are significant because they are usually lethal. The fatality to case ratio has been estimated to be 0.9. Hepatocellular carcinoma is the most common primary tumor of the liver, accounting for 3000 to 4000 new cases each year, and is 10 to 30 times more frequently diagnosed than cholangiocarcinoma. In 1888, Langenbuch was the first to perform a liver resection for tumor, and in 1911 Wendel performed the first successful resection of a hepatic tumor using the hilar ligation technique.[42, 54] In more recent years, with the advent of better anesthesia, a better understanding of the intricacies of hepatic anatomy as it pertains to liver resection, and better postoperative care, the operative mortality for liver resection has decreased to 5 per cent. With this decrease in operative mortality, the risk-benefit ratio for resection of primary and metastatic liver tumors becomes favorable.

The incidence of hepatocellular carcinoma in the United States varies from one to seven cases per 100,000 population. It is much more frequent in Africa, where the incidence is probably 16 per 100,000, and Nigeria, where the incidence is 164 per 100,000. Throughout the world this is the most prevalent malignant disease. In Africa and Asia hepatocellular carcinoma accounts for 20 to 40 per cent of the cancer deaths; by contrast, in the United States it accounts for only 1 per cent of the cancer deaths. The male-to-female ratio is reported to be 4.9:1, and Orientals outnumber Caucasians 8:1. It is important to note that the incidence of hepatocellular carcinoma in the United States has doubled in the last 20 years.

PATHOLOGY

On gross pathologic examination, two thirds of the cases are of the multinodular form, and a large percentage of these will be in the cirrhotic population. Twenty-five to 30 per cent of patients will present with a large single lesion with satellitosis, and less than 4 per cent will present with the encapsulated type, which usually has a better prognosis. Microscopically, the abnormal hepatocytes vary from well-differentiated cells that are difficult to distinguish from the benign focal nodular hyperplastic lesion and benign adenomas to poorly differentiated histologic types.

The trabecular form of hepatocellular carcinoma is the most common histologic type (Fig. 26). The cells resemble the epithelium of normal hepatic plates. In the center of

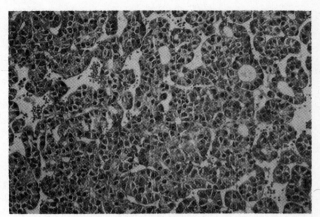

Figure 26. Photomicrograph of the trabecular form of hepatocellular carcinoma. This is the most common histologic type. (From Sherlock, S., and Summerfield, J. A. (Eds.): Color Atlas of Liver Disease. Chicago, Year Book Medical Publishers, Inc., 1979.)

the trabeculum the lumen resembles a bile canaliculus, with occasional bile plugging present. Prominent mitoses and very little intercellular stroma are present. Anaplastic lesions are difficult to differentiate from the more anaplastic metastatic tumors found in the liver. Hepatocellular carcinoma is a very aggressive tumor, and the lesion is confined to the liver in only 11 per cent of patients when diagnosed.

The fibrolamellar variant of hepatomas has a better prognosis. This variant histologically is characterized by parallel bundles of collagen between large and normal hepatocytes with infrequent mitoses, suggesting a less aggressive tumor. It is reported to be androgen responsive. In patients younger than 35, 43 per cent of hepatomas are of the fibrolamellar oncocytic variant. This histologic type of hepatoma is more frequently resectable, with 5 of 10 patients being alive without disease 1.5 to 8 years postoperatively.[36]

NATURAL HISTORY

There are a number of predisposing factors associated with this tumor. Alcoholic cirrhosis, posthepatitic cirrhosis, the use of steroids and birth control pills, aflatoxins, hemochromatosis, and alpha$_1$-antitrypsin disease have each been implicated in the development of a hepatoma. It is estimated that in 3 to 10 per cent of patients with Laennec's cirrhosis hepatomas develop.[32] Further estimates indicate that in 10 per cent of posthepatitic patients, 20 per cent of hemochromatosis patients, and 40 per cent of patients afflicted with alpha$_1$-antitrypsin disease, hepatocellular carcinoma will eventually develop. It is not known whether hepatitis B virus directly causes the hepatoma or whether the resulting cirrhosis and healing are followed by the development of malignancy. In Africa, 70 to 80 per cent of patients with hepatoma show positive results for hepatitis B virus. In contrast, in the United States, only 20 per cent of the hepatoma patients are hepatitis B antigen–positive. Birth control pills have been associated with the development of hepatomas in a small number of cases.[45]

CLINICAL PRESENTATION

In a small percentage of patients, a hepatoma is diagnosed as an asymptomatic lesion. Only 20 per cent of patients are hepatitis B antigen–positive. Palpable abdominal masses are found in 14 per cent of patients, jaundice in 24 per cent, and hepatomegaly in 50 per cent. A bruit is present in 15 to 20 per cent of patients, and 1 to 5 per cent present with an acute abdomen and in shock from rupture into the free peritoneal cavity. Cachexia, wasting, and the sudden development of ascites suggest hepatic vein obstruction. Any rapid deterioration of liver function in a cirrhotic patient should arouse suspicion of a hepatocellular carcinoma. Occasionally, distant metastases are diagnosed, with the lung and bone being the most common sites. Hepatocellular carcinoma is responsible for a number of paraneoplastic syndromes, among which endocrine and coagulation defects predominate. Polycythemia, hypercalcemia, hypoglycemia, hypercalcitonin, and ectopic adrenocorticotropic hormone (ACTH) and gonadotropin production all have been reported. During a metastatic work-up pulmonary metastases are found 36 per cent of the time, with metastases to the great veins, adrenals, and skeleton discovered in 10.4 per cent of patients. Ihde and associates report that 13.4 per cent of patients have secondary malignant tumors associated with hepatomas.[40]

DIAGNOSIS

On physical examination, palpation of a right upper quadrant mass is unusual. Laboratory evaluation shows elevated liver function tests, with increased alkaline phosphatase in 70 to 80 per cent of patients, elevated bilirubins in 43 per cent, and elevated transaminases in 83 per cent. Alpha-fetoprotein (AFP), a normal alpha globulin produced by the embryonic hepatocytes, is elevated in a large percentage of patients.[55] The antigen has been found to be helpful in the preoperative diagnosis of hepatomas as well as in following hepatomas postoperatively. The normal value is less than 10 ng. per ml., and it has been estimated that 75 to 90 per cent of patients with hepatomas will have elevated levels greater than 40 ng. per ml. and usually greater than 400 ng. per ml. A hepatocellular carcinoma should be suspected if the AFP level is greater than 400 ng. per ml.[33] AFP levels are also helpful in screening high-risk populations. Screening populations that were hepatitis B virus antigen–positive detected early hepatomas deemed resectable in 6 of 9 patients.[38] Alpha-fetoprotein screening shows that smaller tumors can be identified.[51] In one series at the time of operation, 34 per cent of the hepatocellular carcinomas were not visible, and intraoperative ultrasound was necessary for localization. Levels of AFP are usually higher in poorly differentiated tumors; however, the serum levels correlate poorly with clinical status.[54] It is also noted that 10 to 15 per cent of hepatocellular carcinoma tumors do not produce detectable AFP. Alpha-fetoprotein levels are helpful, however, in following patients after resection if indeed the level returns to normal postoperatively. A rise in AFP can precede clinical evidence of recurrent disease by 6 months. It has also been found that the AFP serum level correlates with response to systemic chemotherapy; i.e., patients with a good response have falling antigen levels.

Radiologic evaluation starts with abdominal and chest x-rays; however, the abdominal films are usually nonspecific. Calcification is very unusual. A chest x-ray may show an elevated right hemidiaphragm or pulmonary metastases. Liver-spleen scans have not been very helpful, especially in cirrhotic patients, in whom multiple small filling defects are seen normally. With radionuclide scans there is a high false-positive rate, and lesions less than 2 cm. are not imaged. However, a liver-spleen scan using technetium 99m–labeled blood cells may be useful in differentiating hemangiomas from other lesions. In this study the red blood cell flow and blood pool scintiscan show a delayed filling of the mass lesion, suggesting a hemangioma.

Ultrasonography may identify lesions less than 1 cm., despite the fact that 10 to 20 per cent of these studies are judged to be technically inadequate. The advantage of ultrasonography is that the kidney, pancreas, and retroperitoneal area can be examined at the same time for evidence of metastatic disease.

Computed tomography has been helpful in identifying lesions less than 0.5 cm. in size. In conjunction with hepatic-specific intravenous contrast agent, ethiodized oil emulsion,[53] CT improves the detection of focal lesions in the liver with an accuracy rate of 85 per cent.

In a prospective study of hepatic imaging techniques comparing liver scintiscan, CT, and ultrasonography, there is no difference in sensitivity, specificity, or accuracy among the three methods. The combination of the three modalities did not improve the accuracy, and it is recommended that alkaline phosphate, serum glutamic-pyruvic transaminase (SGPT), lactic dehydrogenase (LDH), and carcinoembryonic antigen (CEA) levels be drawn, plus one liver imaging test, to detect liver lesions. Newer magnetic resonance imaging (MRI) scans have not added to the preoperative evaluation of liver masses. Angiography is recommended before major hepatic resections and may show a characteristic vascular pattern, such as the puddling pattern and irregular vessels typical of a hemangioma. CT-directed biopsies of the liver lesion may be indicated if the mass is not suspected to be a hemangioma. Accuracy rates of 90 per cent have been reported, with a complication rate of less than 2 per cent for percutaneous biopsies.

PROGNOSIS

It should be emphasized that the 5-year survival for untreated hepatocellular carcinoma approaches zero. Other studies have shown that 66 per cent of patients are dead within 6 months if no specific treatment is given. Cady states that the length of survival is directly correlated with the percentage of liver involvement.[32] He notes a 16-month survival when less than 25 per cent of the liver is involved with tumor, a 13-month survival when 25 to 50 per cent of the liver is replaced, and an 8-month survival with greater than 50 per cent of the liver involved.

TREATMENT

Surgical Resection

Surgical resection remains the primary treatment with any hope of curing patients with hepatocellular carcinoma; chemotherapy and radiation therapy are palliative treatments at best. The aggressive nature of this tumor is emphasized when studies report that approximately one third of the patients with hepatoma are eventually explored but only one third of these are resectable. A smaller percentage are resected for cure; thus only 3 to 4 per cent of patients are curable when diagnosed. Tumors are unresectable at exploration if there is bilateral lobar involvement or regional lymph node involvement. Encroachment on the hepatic hilar structure and vena cava is a relative contraindication. Invasion of the diaphragm may be treated with en bloc resection.

Most surgeons use a right subcostal incision to expose the lesion and assess resectability. If resection is indicated, the incision may be extended into the right chest or the upper midline through the xyphoid. Hilar control followed by intraparenchymal dissection is recommended to minimize postoperative complications. Both Penrose and closed suction drainage catheters should be used.[39] The operative mortality is about 4 per cent; however, in 8 per cent of patients right subphrenic abscesses that can most often be drained percutaneously develop. These investigators reported a 3-year survival after liver resection for hepatomas of 56 per cent and a 5-year survival of 46 per cent. In the largest series of liver resection for hepatocellular carcinoma reported, there was a 5 per cent operative mortality and a 5-year survival rate of 36 per cent.[31] For 36 patients who underwent hepatic resection for primary liver malignancies, there was a 3-year survival rate of 42 per cent and a 5-year survival rate of 31 per cent after curative resections.[37]

Some favor a thoracoabdominal incision for exposure[43] and report an operative mortality rate of 11 per cent and a 5-year survival of 38 per cent. With the screening of high-risk populations, such as patients with cirrhosis, a positive family history, or a positive hepatitis B–antigen assay, small asymptomatic tumors have been discovered. In a large screening program for detecting alpha-fetoprotein in high-risk populations, 50 per cent of tumors were diagnosed before becoming clinically apparent.[46] Thirty-three per cent of these lesions were smaller than 3 cm., and 61 per cent were resectable. Since 52 of the 60 patients undergoing resection were cirrhotics, this series emphasizes the fact that cirrhotics can tolerate minor and, sometimes, major hepatic resections. Radiation therapy plays a limited role, since the liver is such a radiosensitive organ. One series demonstrated that total liver radiation of 31 patients with a dose of 1000 to 3600 rads showed a median survival of 12 months.[35] These results were thought to be longer than historic controls.

Systemic Chemotherapy

Systemic chemotherapy has been largely ineffective in treating hepatocellular carcinoma. Systemic effusions of 5-fluorouracil (FU) and floxuridine (FUDR) have been shown to result in response rates in the 13 to 37 per cent range. Doxorubicin (Adriamycin) is probably the most effective agent, with a wide range of responses from 13 to 100 per cent noted. The response to chemotherapy seems to depend more on a good performance status of the patient than a more effective chemotherapeutic agent. A median survival of 7 months using an intra-arterial infusion of FUDR has been reported, but 15 to 20 per cent of patients developed biliary strictures, requiring cessation of the infusion.[49]

Hepatic Artery Ligation

Theoretically, hepatic artery ligation is of potential benefit in attempting to decrease the arterial supply to tumor cells. Hepatic tumors derive most of their blood supply from the hepatic artery.[50] It has been shown that dogs survive hepatic artery ligation if protected by antibiotics,[44] and this finding has been applied clinically.[47] The procedure may be safely performed; however, in a matter of months the tumor usually develops collateral arterial flow, and any changes are transient. A study of patients with peripheral embolization of hepatomas with Gelfoam showed that 78 per cent have symptomatic relief with a mean survival of 5 months.[34] Chemoembolization is a possibility for future treatment. A decrease in tumor size to 80 per cent with a 1-year survival of 24 per cent using an infusion of mitomycin C microcapsules into the hepatic artery has been reported.[48] This procedure also decreases the vascularity of hepatocellular carcinoma and perhaps will permit a higher percentage of future resections.

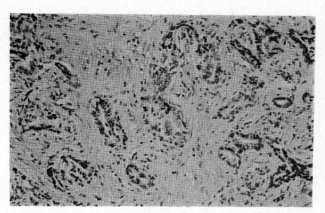

Figure 27. Tubular pattern of cholangiocarcinoma with a moderate amount of fibrous reaction. (From Calne, R. Y., and Della Rovere, G. Q. D.: Liver Surgery. Philadelphia, Piccis Medical Books, W. B. Saunders Company, 1982, p. 255.)

Cholangiocarcinoma

Cholangiocarcinomas arise from the intrahepatic bile ducts in 5 to 30 per cent of patients and are usually solitary lesions, less commonly associated with cirrhosis, and more often resectable. Predisposing factors include cholestasis, cirrhosis, hemochromatosis, and cystic disease of the bile ducts. Ninety per cent of cholangiocarcinomas in Hong Kong are caused by a fluke infection (*Clonorchis sinensis*). The male-to-female ratio is 1:2, and patients usually present with pruritus, pain, cholangitis, and jaundice. Ulcerative colitis is an associated finding in a small number of patients. Microscopically, the tumor is described as a sclerosing adenocarcinoma (Fig. 27). Most frequently cholangiocarcinoma shows a tubular or acinar pattern. There is no bile production by the tumor cells, and most are well differentiated. The amount of fibrous reaction is more prominent with cholangiocarcinoma than with other primary hepatic malignancies. Twenty to 25 per cent of these lesions are resectable, with a 5-year survival reported to be 1 to 25 per cent.

Klatskin tumors are carcinomas involving the *bifurcation of hepatic ducts* and have been found to be resectable in approximately 20 per cent of patients.[41] If unresectable, patients may be palliatively treated by passing Terblanche U-tubes into the right and left hepatic ducts and through the tumor to allow decompression of the liver.

Other less common primary liver tumors include hepatoblastomas, usually found in children, along with primary carcinoids and teratomas of the liver. Angiosarcomas of the liver have been associated with vinyl chloride and thorotrast ingestion. Rhabdomyosarcoma is the most common sarcoma found in the liver and is more prevalent in the pediatric age group.

COLORECTAL LIVER METASTASES

Liver metastases lead directly to death in many patients. Localized metastatic disease to the liver is, however, suitable for resection. In one study of 8455 autopsies on cancer patients, 39 per cent of patients had hepatic metastases. However, only 2.5 per cent were confined to the liver, and only 6 per cent had solitary lesions. Liver metastases are seven times more likely to occur if the primary cancer is drained by the portovenous system. Thus, colorectal cancer is one of the leading tumors that metastasize to the liver. It is estimated that in 1983, 58,000 patients died of colorectal carcinoma, and a large percentage of these deaths were secondary to liver metastases. In 50 per cent of colorectal cancer patients, liver metastases develop some time during their lifetime, and in 15 to 20 per cent of patients synchronous metastases occur. The following discussion is limited to hepatic metastasis from *colorectal* cancer, since there has been a large body of experience in resecting this lesion and the most promising results are obtained with this tumor.

Natural History

To determine whether new therapy is effective in extending survival, there must be an accurate account of historic controls. The average survival from the time of diagnosis of untreated colorectal liver metastases varied from 6 months to 2 years, depending on three conditions.[67] The first was the patient's general physical status, as those patients who were well nourished and without other medical problems had the better survival. The second factor involved the extent of metastatic disease, since patients with solitary metastases lived longer than those with widespread disease. A third prognostic variable involved the presence of extrahepatic tumor. The natural history of colorectal hepatic metastases showed that patients with unresected hepatic metastases lived longer than expected, and those with solitary lesions had a 3-year survival of 21 per cent and a 5-year survival of 3 per cent.[70] Three-year survivals of patients with multiple unilateral lesions and widespread hepatic metastatic disease were 6 and 4 per cent, respectively, with no 5-year survivals in these last two categories (Fig. 28). Thus, any form of therapy must be compared with these historic control groups.

It has also been shown that removal of the primary tumor not only provides palliation but also improves prognosis. The 1-year survival of patients with liver metastases whose primary tumors were removed was 32 per cent, but this decreased to 15 per cent when the primary was left *in situ*. With synchronous liver metastases, survival remains a function of the extent of liver disease. Median survivals of patients with untreated metastasis are 6.1 months. All patients were dead within 36 months with no specific treatment. Patients with metachronous liver metastases had an average survival of 5 months if left untreated. The cause of death in most patients in the United States is liver failure, whereas in Japan the cause of death is usually secondary portal hypertension and bleeding.

In summary, the prognosis for patients with colorectal metastasis to the liver left untreated depends on the extent of liver involvement, but it is reasonable to assume that the 5-year survival approaches 0 to 5 per cent if the lesions are untreated.

Diagnosis

Symptoms of metastatic disease include right upper quadrant pain, weight loss, ascites, and jaundice. Usually the pain is dull, and any episodes of acute pain are likely to represent bleeding into the liver metastases. CEA levels are useful in the postoperative follow-up of patients with colorectal cancer if it is found initially that the tumor secretes CEA and the CEA serum level returns to normal after resection. An increase in CEA levels during the

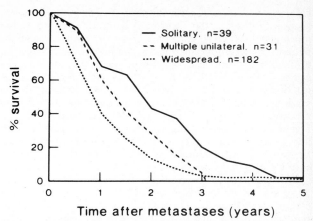

Figure 28. The natural history of patients with untreated liver metastases. (From Wagner, J. S., et al.: Ann. Surg., 199:502, 1984.)

postoperative period may precede the development of hepatic metastases by 3 to 6 months. An increased CEA level postoperatively may be sufficient indication to explore a patient with a second-look operation in the hope of discovering a small volume of recurrent disease. Laboratory data are nonspecific and of little value in diagnosing colorectal liver metastasis. Transaminase and alkaline phosphatase levels are elevated in over 50 per cent of patients. It has been shown[66] that, in combination, elevated alkaline phosphatase and CEA levels give a sensitivity of 88 per cent in diagnosing colorectal metastatic disease, with a false-positive rate of 12 per cent and a false-negative rate of 2 per cent.

Radiologic investigation[52] includes radionuclide liver scanning but has high false-positive and false-negative rates and rarely distinguishes lesions less than 2 cm. When less than 25 per cent of the liver is involved, the radionuclide scan has shown a random correlation with operative findings. Computed tomography and ultrasound examinations have been quoted as being 80 to 85 per cent accurate and show a reasonable resolution with lesions greater than 2 cm. Computed tomography also provides other evidence of tumor spread. Arteriograms are important in the preoperative evaluation of patients for possible hepatic resection. Metastatic lesions are usually hypovascular, except for melanomas, leiomyosarcomas, and metastatic endocrine tumors. At the time of exploration, bimanual examination of the liver has been found to discover 90 to 95 per cent of metastatic disease, and thus with an exploratory laparotomy one may save extensive preoperative evaluations with less than specific imaging modalities.

Treatment

Surgical Resection

Results of surgical treatment of colorectal liver metastases must be compared with the natural history controlling for the extent of liver involvement. Palliative resections are almost never indicated, except perhaps to control disabling symptoms from slow-growing endocrine tumors, such as metastatic insulinomas and gluconomas. Debulking operations in children may also be indicated, since pediatric patients may have an increased response rate to radiation therapy and chemotherapy. Presently, curative resections are performed only for colorectal tumors with localized deposits without other extrahepatic metastatic disease. They cannot be recommended for metastatic disease from the pancreas, stomach, lung, or breast or melanoma secondary to poor survival on initial trials.[61]

In a large series of patients undergoing hepatic resection for colorectal metastases, major resections were performed on 67 per cent of patients, with a 4 per cent operative mortality, and wedge resections on another 74 patients with no operative mortality.[56] There was an overall 5-year survival of 42 per cent and a 10-year survival of 28 per cent in 40 patients. Thus, 7 per cent of all patients are potentially cured from this aggressive posture. If it is estimated that 50,000 patients will be diagnosed as having hepatic metastases each year, 3500 will be helped by hepatic resection. Patients with Dukes' B lesions in whom hepatic metastases developed showed a 5-year survival of 32 per cent compared with an 18 per cent 5-year survival for those with Dukes' C lesions. Females tended to respond better than males, but the presence of extrahepatic metastases had a very unfavorable influence on survival.

It has been shown that colorectal liver metastases are resectable in 30 per cent of patients,[60] with a survival of 66 per cent when the tumor was confined to the resected liver. Levels of CEA returned to normal when all gross disease was resected.[60] Seventeen of the 18 recurrences were within the first 2 years. The prognosis is directly correlated with the stage of liver disease and Dukes' classification of the primary tumor. Among 37 patients with tumor localized to the resected specimen, there was a 3-year survival of 66 per cent, whereas those with inguinal or lymph node spread had a 3-year survival of 55 per cent. Factors not significant in survival were number of metastatic liver nodules, site of the primary colon cancer, age, sex, preoperative liver function tests, and CEA levels. There was no difference in survival between major and wedge resections as long as clear surgical margins were present; nor was there any difference in survival between synchronous and metachronous resections. A collated series from the literature in a recent update on liver resections for colorectal metastasis showed that 5-year survivals have consistently been in the range of 25 per cent, which compares favorably to 0 per cent 5-year survivals with untreated hepatic metastases.

CHEMOTHERAPY

Adjuvant Chemotherapy

The concept of adjuvant chemotherapy is important, since there is a tendency for tumor progression in extrahepatic sites after resection. In one study, a survival rate of 65 per cent was found in patients whose colorectal metastases were resected.[65] However, 10 of 13 patients had recurrences, the lesions were extrahepatic, and most were pulmonary metastases. The patients seemed to be cured of the liver metastases but died of systemic disease. For this reason a regional pulmonary perfusion trial of adjuvant 5-FU therapy through the superior vena cava has been initiated.

Intra-arterial Chemotherapy

The role of systemic 5-FU in treatment has been disappointing. Alone, this agent yields a 15 per cent response rate with objective responses lasting no more than 3 to 6 months. Because of these poor results more specific chemotherapy routes have been investigated. Intra-arterial chemotherapy with the use of the totally implantable In-

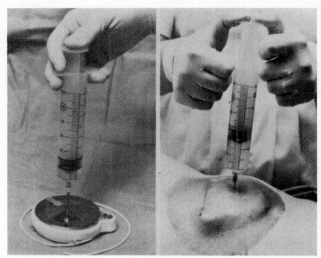

Figure 29. Appearance of the totally implantable Infusaid pump, which is placed subcutaneously and refilled with percutaneous injections. (From Balch, C. M., et al.: Am. J. Surg., 145:285, 1983.)

fusaid pump* (Fig. 29), with catheter placement into the gastroduodenal artery, has its proponents.[57] With this technique, one may selectively infuse the hepatic artery with chemotherapy agents and decrease the systemic toxicity. In one trial there was an 88 per cent response rate and a 1-year survival of 82 per cent versus 36 per cent 1-year survival for historic controls. Fourteen per cent of these patients relapsed, with 54 per cent of the relapses occurring in the lung. Thirty per cent of the patients showed metastatic disease invading the retroperitoneal lymph nodes. A trial of subclavian intravenous infusion and hepatic artery infusion in an attempt to control metastatic disease in the lung and recurrent disease in the liver is being initiated.[57]

A Phase II evaluation of regional FUDR chemotherapy using the totally implantable drug infusion pump has been undertaken in patients with colorectal liver metastases, with an 88 per cent response rate. The criterion for response was an observed fall in serum CEA level.[58] The results of this trial compared with those of a historic control group with liver metastases not treated with regional chemotherapy are shown in Figure 30. Significant increases in survival were obtained (p < 0.0001) in the infusion group. The survival for the regional chemotherapy patients was not influenced by extent of tumor involvement, previous chemotherapy, or systemic disease. It was also encouraging to find that the entire group of regional chemotherapy patients had a greater 1-year survival than a subgroup of control patients who had the most favorable clinical features, including normal liver function test, no symptoms, and unilobar involvement. Since FUDR is extracted by the liver in one pass, systemic toxicity is reduced; however, extrahepatic sites are left untreated. The major cause of death was tumor progression in extrahepatic sites, such as lung and abdominal carcinomatosis.

Other investigators have not been favorably impressed with intra-arterial chemotherapy. Low response rates have been reported, and approximately 33 per cent of the patients could not complete an adequate infusion trial because of technical problems with either vascular access or the development of cholecystitis, gastritis, and chemical

---

*Infusaid Corp., Norwood, Mass.

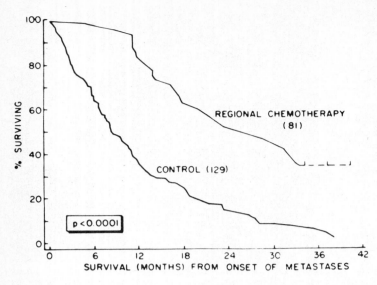

Figure 30. Extended survival in patients treated with continuous intra-arterial infusion of FUDR compared with historic controls. (From Balch, C. M.: Ann. Surg., 198:567, 1983.)

hepatitis. One distressing complication is the development of intrahepatic and extrahepatic bile duct strictures in as many as 20 per cent of those treated (thought to be due to the infusion chemotherapy and possibly confused with earlier reported chemical hepatitis). Other disadvantages are that this approach involves an operative procedure with general anesthesia and has significant financial costs. It has been suggested that this treatment modality be reserved for those with nonresectable liver disease.[59] In a multivariate analysis it was shown that survival is influenced by the extent of metastatic disease. There was no apparent benefit following intrahepatic chemotherapy when greater than 50 per cent of the liver was replaced, if lymph node involvement was present, or if the patient had failed previous chemotherapy trials, which tended to identify those patients who had resistant tumors.

RADIATION THERAPY

Radiation treatment of the liver has been limited because the liver is a very radiosensitive organ. It has been shown that with doses greater than 3000 rads, radiation hepatitis, characterized by injury to the central vein region of the liver lobule, occurs frequently. This causes a Budd-Chiari–like syndrome with outflow obstruction, portal hypertension, and ascites. With lower radiation doses in the 2100- to 2400-rad range, an 89 per cent subjective response rate has been reported with a decrease in pain and liver size and improved liver function tests. One-year survivals are reported to be in the 21 per cent range, and these are usually longer in the patients who respond. Newer techniques include the use of hypoxic cell sensitizer, misonidazole, to increase the relative effectiveness of radiation therapy and decrease the dose. Intra-arterial radiation using utridium 90 microspheres may also be important in the future treatment of these hepatic lesions.

HEPATIC ARTERY LIGATION

Hepatic artery ligation was originally proposed as therapy for hepatic tumors, since a great majority of the primary and secondary cancers derived their nourishment from branches of the hepatic artery even though the initial seeding is via the portal vein.[44] It has been shown that ligation of the hepatic artery may be safely done in those without portal vein thrombosis or cirrhosis. The problem

arises when attempting to permanently exclude arterial blood flow to the liver. It has been demonstrated that after hepatic artery ligation, follow-up angiograms show rapid development of collateral flow to the tumor; thus, minimal effect on survival times has been documented with hepatic artery ligation.

LIVER TRANSPLANTATION

Liver transplantation for colorectal metastatic disease has been tried.[62] Among 24 patients transplanted, the 3- and 5-year survivals were 66 and 57 per cent, respectively. It should be emphasized that this report involved a selected patient population.

Hepatic Tumors in Children

Hepatic tumors are the eighth most common cause of cancer mortality in children younger than 15 years of age. It is possible to remove as much as 85 per cent of the liver in children and expect regeneration in 3 to 4 months. Hepatoblastoma is the most common primary tumor in the pediatric age group and is usually found in children younger than three. It can cause virilization in young males. Pathologically, a pure epithelial pattern or a mixed epithelial and mesenchymal pattern of cellular morphology is demonstrated (Fig. 31). Microscopically, hepatocellular carcinoma in the child appears identical to that seen in the adult and is usually found in children older than five. Pediatric patients present with asymptomatic abdominal masses that most often involve the right lobe of the liver. Abdominal pain, weight loss, and irritability are usual signs of advanced malignancy and are present in less than 25 per cent of patients. Congestive heart failure may also be caused by a large amount of arteriovenous shunting in the tumor, and petechiae from thrombocytopenia are not uncommon. Twenty-five per cent of the children have pulmonary metastases with diffuse liver involvement on presentation.

DIAGNOSIS

Liver function tests are usually normal in this patient population. However, α-fetoprotein, a normal alphaglobulin produced by embryonic hepatocytes, is elevated in two thirds of children with malignant epithelial liver neoplasms.

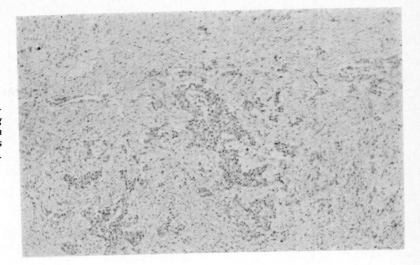

Figure 31. Photomicrograph of hepatoblastoma composed of nests and cords of small cells resembling embryonic hepatocytes. (From Calne, R. Y., and Della Rovere, G. Q. D.: Liver Surgery. Philadelphia, Piccis Medical Books, W. B. Saunders Company, 1982, p. 259.)

Abdominal radiographs may be helpful, but since most abdominal masses in this age group originate in the kidneys, adrenal, or retroperitoneum, the primary screening test is an intravenous pyelogram. Liver-spleen scan, ultrasound, and CT may be helpful in localizing and diagnosing primary malignancy as well as screening for metastatic disease. An angiogram is particularly useful to the surgeon contemplating resection, since it may show abnormal hepatic artery anatomy or a characteristic vascular pattern, such as in the case of a hemangioma.

TREATMENT

Hepatic resection is the only curative treatment in children and is similar to the procedure performed in adults, except for the fact that the extrahepatic veins of children are very short. It is recommended that these structures be approached through the liver substance. A number of the epithelial tumors present as large masses, but up to 85 per cent of the liver may be removed with impunity in children. Hypothermia and total circulatory arrest for up to 60 minutes were helpful in resecting a number of large hepatic epithelial neoplasms in one series.[68] Preoperative chemotherapy may also be useful if the hepatic tumor is bulky or is thought to be unresectable according to radiologic inves-

tigation. In pediatric patients with massive hepatic tumors, preoperative radiation and chemotherapy may shrink the tumor for easier resection.[64] Chemotherapeutic agents used include combinations of Adriamycin, cyclophosphamide, and cis-platinum to achieve higher response rates. The timing of the chemotherapy is crucial, however, in that cytotoxic agents can inhibit normal liver regeneration and have an increased toxicity after liver resection. If the entire tumor can be resected there is a 50 per cent chance of cure in the pediatric population. Other primary hepatic tumors in this age group include rhabdomyosarcomas and benign vascular neoplasms, the most common of which are the hemangioendothelioma and cavernous hemangioma.

Benign Hepatic Neoplasms

ADENOMAS AND FOCAL NODULAR HYPERPLASIA

Focal nodular hyperplasia is thought to represent a hamartomatous malformation or reparative process in an area of focal hepatic injury. Pathologically, these lesions show a central stellate scar that consists of a fibrous core with radiating septa to the periphery (Fig. 32). It often contains lymphocytes and proliferating bile ducts. The

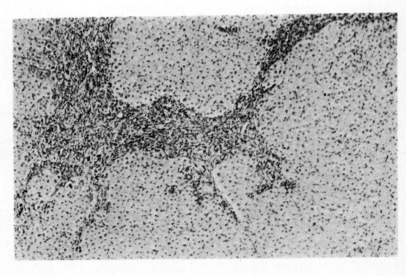

Figure 32. Histologically, focal nodular hyperplasia is characterized by hyperplastic nodules bounded by distinct connective tissue bounds. (From Calne, R. Y., and Della Rovere, G. Q. D.: Liver Surgery. Philadelphia, Piccis Medical Books, W. B. Saunders Company, 1982, p. 267.)

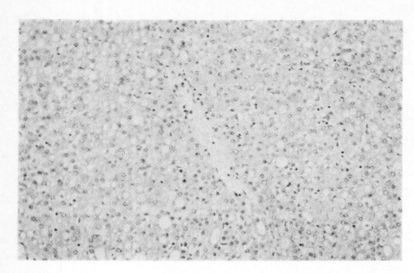

Figure 33. Hepatocellular adenoma demonstrates no true lobular development and vacuolated hepatocytes. (From Calne, R. Y., and Della Rovere, G. Q. D.: Liver Surgery. Philadelphia, Piccis Medical Books, W. B. Saunders Company, 1982, p. 233.)

tumor is found more commonly in females than in males and may or may not be linked with the use of oral contraceptive agents. The clinical course is always benign, and the tumor very rarely undergoes hemorrhagic necrosis and spontaneous rupture. Only 20 per cent of the patients are symptomatic, with two thirds demonstrating abdominal pain or an upper abdominal mass. Focal nodular hyperplastic lesions are usually single and are located in the right lobe of the liver 79 per cent of the time. With liver-spleen scans or angiograms, they are usually hypervascular lesions.

Hepatic liver cell adenomas are almost always seen in females taking *oral contraceptive agents*. These women are between the ages of 20 and 40, and about half have abdominal pain and a mass, whereas one third present with an acute abdomen and shock from spontaneous intraperitoneal hemorrhage. A small percentage of these adenomas are associated with a concurrent pregnancy. Hepatic adenomas are usually encapsulated, soft tan to light brown lesions found in a subcapsular location. Microscopically, it is difficult to differentiate a liver cell adenoma from hepatocellular carcinoma. On pathological examination adenomas show cords of hepatocytes with a vacuolated sinusoidal border but no true lobules (Fig. 33). There is abundant blood supply. The vacuolated appearance of the hepatocytes is due to glycogen deposition, and bile ducts are usually absent. On liver-spleen scan these lesions are usually hypovascular and cold.

In one series adenomas occurred 91 per cent of the time in females, and all used oral contraceptives.[63] Fifty-three per cent of patients had abdominal pain, and 39 per cent presented with hemoperitoneum. Most of the tumors that ruptured were greater than 10 cm. An important aspect of this study was the discovery of hepatocellular carcinoma in 10.5 per cent of the tumors. These lesions can be confused with focal nodular hyperplasia, however, and in 90 per cent of patients the latter tumors are asymptomatic. It was recommended that focal lesions in the liver be explored and adenomas resected to prevent bleeding and potential malignant dedifferentiation. Focal nodular hyperplastic lesions diagnosed by wedge biopsies may be observed, since there is very little chance of spontaneous rupture and no chance of carcinoma dedifferentiation.

The association between ingestion of contraceptives and the development of hepatic adenomas has been found in a number of series. Reports have shown that the average duration of ingestion of birth control pills before the tumor was discovered is 7.8 years. There have been cases of patients with adenomas being observed after discontinuing

oral contraceptive pills and the tumor regressing. For uncomplicated adenomas it might be appropriate to observe the patient off birth control pills, using serial scans to evaluate regression. However, this conservative approach carries with it the chance of spontaneous rupture as well as a 10 per cent chance of hepatocellular carcinoma development. Women who develop hepatocellular carcinoma from adenomas are younger than the total population of patients who develop hepatomas, with an average age of 31 years. This tumor seems to be less aggressive than hepatomas that occur in cirrhotics, with a decreased incidence of metastatic disease and an increased incidence of estrogen receptor–positive tumor cells that may be responsive to anti-estrogen therapy.

CAVERNOUS HEMANGIOMAS

Cavernous hemangiomas are the most common benign tumor found in the liver and occur in 2 per cent of autopsy series. These tumors may be diagnosed with liver-spleen scan and are differentiated from other mass lesions in the liver by blood flow and blood poll scintigraphy using technetium 99m–labeled red blood cells. These studies show a characteristic delayed filling of the tumor, in contrast to the "cold" scan areas found with hepatocellular carcinomas and other primary and metastatic tumors. Transtek and others[69] observed 36 patients with cavernous hemangiomas for up to 15 years, with no need for surgical therapy. There were no deaths, no instances of spontaneous hemorrhage, and no increase in symptoms in these patients. For symptomatic lesions or lesions larger than 4 cm., surgical therapy is indicated, with a low operative mortality but a high morbidity of 31 per cent. Whether these lesions are responsive to radiation or steroid therapy is controversial. Hemangiomas in children have been complicated by anemia, thrombocytopenia, and congestive heart failure, presumably due to the AV shunting. Embolization or hepatic artery ligation is an option if resection is considered technically risky. Tumors found during the first year of life usually involute, and, if possible, nonsurgical therapy is indicated.

Budd-Chiari Syndrome

This condition is a noncirrhotic hepatic venous outflow obstruction of diverse cause, with liver congestion and necrosis. The clinical state is recognized by rapid onset of progressive and refractory ascites and hepatic failure. Various pathologic processes have been discovered to cause this condition, including obstruction of the intrahepatic venule, thrombosis of the hepatic vein, occlusion of the hepatic vein ostia, suprahepatic inferior vena cava occlusion, right atrial myxoma, and constrictive pericarditis. Many patients have an underlying disease process, such as polycythemia, cancer of the kidney or adrenal, primary hepatocellular carcinoma, or myeloproliferative disease. Hepatic vein thrombosis has also been associated with the use of birth control pills. Early liver biopsy, as well as aggressive venography in all patients suspected of having Budd-Chiari syndrome is recommended.[74] Liver biopsies are helpful, since the presence of severe necrosis in zone 3 of the liver lobe is a sign of a failing congested liver (Fig. 34).

These patients need immediate shunting to convert the portal vein to an outflow tract for liver decompression. Since the inferior vena cava is often involved with the disease, it is rare to be able to use the inferior vena cava for a shunt. A mesoatrial graft to decompress the liver is usually performed initially, and if the inferior vena cava becomes recanalized, a side-to-side portacaval shunt may be performed. The operative mortality is about 30 per cent. With the mesoatrial shunt, patients have a tendency to redevelop ascites and thus require another shunt procedure. With patent shunts, the liver architecture often returns to normal. Postoperatively, these patients are placed on Coumadin or aspirin and Persantine. The medical treatment of Budd-Chiari syndrome is associated with a mortality rate of over 80 per cent. However, with surgical treatment and emergency shunting, mortality is decreased to about 30 per cent.[92] A newer approach to this problem involving a trial of streptokinase is occasionally successful in patients with thrombotic occlusion of the hepatic veins. Other investigators have recommended the use of the jugular vein for mesocaval shunt.

Hepatic Coma

Hepatic coma, or ammonia intoxication, is caused by a number of factors involving liver failure. Any esophageal bleeding that results in a large volume of blood in the gastrointestinal tract, with conversion by bacteria, causes increased levels of ammonia in the blood. Absorption of dietary protein and bypass of the liver by portosystemic shunting cause absorbed ammonia to elude the Krebs cycle in the liver. Urea produced in the gastrointestinal tract is also an important source of ammonia. With the portosystemic shunting and the impaired hepatocellular function, hyperammonemia is an inevitable complication. Hepatic coma occurs after portacaval shunt in 11 to 38 per cent of patients. Proponents of the distal splenorenal shunt recommend it on the basis that there is a decreased incidence of postoperative hepatic encephalopathy. Rebleeding and survival rates are similar with total and selective shunting procedures. With the distal splenorenal shunt, hepatic encephalopathy occurs in 5 to 19 per cent of patients, whereas with portacaval shunting 11 to 38 per cent develop hepatic coma postoperatively.

Hepatic encephalopathy usually has three stages of development, depending on the ammonia level and individual sensitivity. An abnormal electroencephalogram (EEG) precedes the clinical symptoms in most reported series and shows progressive slowing of frequency of the normal alpha patterns of 8 to 13 cycles per second to 4 cycles per second. The delirium, or first, stage is marked by mental confusion and exaggerated reflexes and shows the characteristic "liver flap." The second, or stupor, stage is characterized by an increased muscular hypertonicity. With progression of the coma, which is characterized by flaccidity, the third stage is reached. The treatment of hepatic coma includes reduced dietary and protein intake and prompt control of bleeding. The use of enemas and laxatives following gastrointestinal bleeding causes a decrease in ammonia absorption from

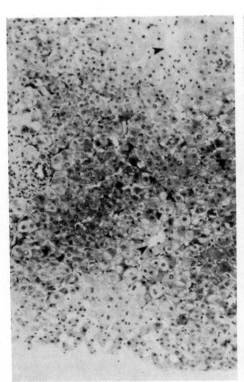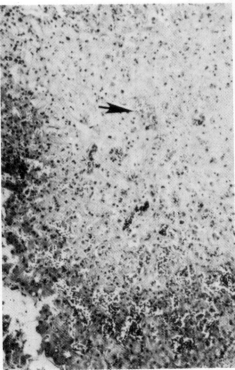

Figure 34. Photomicrographs of the liver preshunting in a patient with portal vein thrombosis. A, Rare extensive hepatocellular loss around the hepatic venule. B, Percutaneous biopsy taken 8 months after successful mesocaval shunt demonstrating lack of congestion with good viability of hepatocytes. (From Cameron, J. L., et al.: Ann. Surg., 198:339, 1983.)

blood loss. Vasopressin, used to control esophageal bleeding, also increases gastric motility and acts as a laxative. Lactulose is used as a mild cathartic but also decreases colonic pH and interferes with ammonia transport. The oral antibiotics neomycin and kanamycin decrease bacterial counts in the intestinal lumen, with a decrease in the reabsorption of ammonia. An increased level of false neurotransmitters is found in the brain with hepatic coma. Chronic L-dopa therapy replenishes the central nervous system stores of norepinephrine and dopamine to normal levels. High concentrations of aromatic amino acids with low levels of branched chain amino acids in the blood are other biochemical abnormalities found in patients in hepatic coma and help explain the deranged neurologic state.

Fulminant Hepatic Failure

This condition occurs with massive hepatic necrosis and is usually caused by acute viral hepatitis. It can also be found in patients with Reye's syndrome and is biochemically associated with high levels of serum transaminase. Treatment of hepatic failure is subjective, and dialysis and plasma exchange decrease toxin levels. The mortality is 85 to 95 per cent and 100 per cent when the stage of flaccidity is reached. Spontaneous recovery occurs in 10 to 20 per cent of patients. Recently a number of patients have been treated with emergency liver transplantation and recovered after 1 month of hepatic failure caused by viral hepatitis.

PERITONEOVENOUS SHUNT FOR REFRACTORY ASCITES

Pathophysiology

Ascites has been described as a pathologic accumulation of fluid in the peritoneal cavity and is found most often with liver disease. A number of theories have been formed as to the mechanism of ascites production, but most likely it involves a combination of the redistribution of fluid between the plasma and extravascular-extracellular space and excessive salt and water retention by the kidneys. Two factors are present in patients with liver disease and portal hypertension that contribute to a decrease in plasma oncotic pressure and account for the movement of fluid from the surface of the liver, bowel, and mesentery: hypoalbuminemia associated with liver disease and sinusoidal hypertension. According to Starling's law, because of low oncotic pressures the intravascular fluid is forced into the extravascular space, the capacity of the lymphatics to remove the fluid is exceeded, and ascites occurs.

A second theory involves the altered renal function present in the cirrhotic. This theory depends on the development of intrarenal shunts that direct blood to the juxtamedullary glomeruli, away from the cortex where most of the functioning glomeruli are found. These juxtamedullary glomeruli have longer loops of Henle and a greater capacity for salt reabsorption than cortical glomeruli. In addition, cirrhotic patients with ascites have a depressed total renal blood flow, which decreases the glomerular filtration rate and thus increases plasma renin, angiotensin, and aldosterone secretion. This has a direct effect on sodium and salt reabsorption in the distal tubule. With liver disease there is also a decrease in inactivation of aldosterone.

A third factor that contributes to the altered renal function in cirrhotics is a vague natriuretic hormone that causes a greatly increased proximal tubular reabsorption of sodium. These three variables account for the movement of fluid from the intravascular space into the peritoneal cavity.

The clinical manifestations of severe ascites include dyspnea, edema of the leg, development of umbilical and groin hernias, and loss of appetite and weight. Another complication associated with ascites in the cirrhotic patient is spontaneous bacterial peritonitis, in which case the ascitic fluid becomes infected without a known source. This occurs in approximately 18 per cent of patients, with gram-negative rods accounting for 70 per cent of the bacterial isolates and pneumococci accounting for 10 to 20 per cent. This condition is most readily diagnosed with ascitic fluid white blood cell counts greater than 250 polymorphonuclear lymphocytes per ml., as only one third of the ascitic fluids are culture positive. The development of ascites in the patient with cirrhosis is an ominous sign and decreases 1-year survival to 83 per cent.

Medical Treatment

Frakes[100] describes a progressive medical regimen that is effective in treating 90 to 95 per cent of cirrhotic patients with ascites. Admission to the hospital is best to permit bed rest, a 20-mEq. sodium diet, and fluid restriction of 1000 ml. per day in an attempt to induce a diuresis of 0.5 to 1 kg. per day. If the patient does not experience this diuresis, spironolactone is given in a dose of 100 to 400 mg. per day, followed by hydrochlorothiazide if diuresis continues to be insufficient. The last addition to the medical treatment is the loop diuretic Lasix, at an initial dose of 40 mg. per day increasing to over 200 mg. per day. This regimen was found to control 95 per cent of patients with intense ascites. The only complications of the therapy noted were those of diuretic therapy and included azotemia, hypokalemia, hyponatremia, and encephalopathy.

Recently, paracentesis, with removal of as much as 4 to 6 liters per procedure, has been tried to control the ascites.[102, 104] This was effective in as many as 80 per cent of patients if certain guidelines were followed, including slow removal of the fluid over 30 to 90 minutes and reinfusion of 40 gm. of albumin as an intravascular expander. It is of interest that hospitalization was much shorter with this modality than with the usual medical diuretic treatment for ascites.

Surgical Treatment

PORTACAVAL SHUNT

Surgical treatment of ascites is indicated in the 5 to 10 per cent of patients who are resistant to in-hospital medical trials. A number of direct surgical procedures, such as portacaval shunting, have been attempted in order to lower pressure in both the splanchnic and intrahepatic portal systems. These procedures usually involve a side-to-side portacaval or mesocaval shunt and are very effective in controlling ascites. However, they may be risky in those patients with a limited hepatic reserve who do not tolerate much blood being shunted away from the liver. Peritoneovenous shunts have been used in an attempt to control ascites by reinfusing peritoneal fluid into the venous system. The LaVeen shunt[103] has a one-way valve that opens with

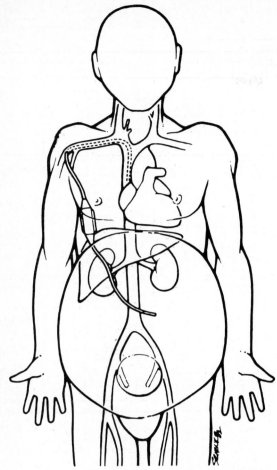

Figure 35. Schematic representation of the Denver shunt with the venous end inserted into the superior vena cava and the pumping chamber located in a subcutaneous position. (From Turner, W. W., and Pate, R. M.: Am. J. Surg., 144:619, 1982.)

3 cm. of water pressure and works on the principle that there is a pressure gradient between the intraperitoneal space and the negative pressure found in the intrathoracic cavity. The venous end of the catheter is placed in either the superior vena cava or right atrium. With the newer Denver shunt and the placement of its valve in the subcutaneous position, there is a possibility of a pumping action (Fig. 35).

PERITONEOVENOUS SHUNT

Placement of a peritoneovenous shunt is a relatively simple procedure. Preoperative evaluation includes initial paracentesis within 2 to 3 days to exclude infection in the ascitic fluid. The patient should be given perioperative antibiotics, and clotting parameters should be normal. The LaVeen shunt is placed deep in the abdominal musculature with the peritoneal side floating free in the abdominal cavity. The venous end is then inserted through either the subclavian or right internal jugular vein and threaded into the superior vena cava. Postoperatively, the patient is encouraged to increase intra-abdominal pressure with breathing maneuvers and an abdominal binder.

The initial results with these shunts are encouraging in that they seem to increase renal blood flow, glomerular filtration rate, and salt and water excretion. However, the morbidity and mortality associated with this procedure are high, with a 26 per cent mortality within the first month.[99] The complication rate was 66 per cent, with a subclinical disseminated invascular coagulopathy occurring in 100 per cent of patients. A consumptive coagulopathy was found in 33 per cent of patients and is probably caused by an activated tissue thromboplastin or bacterial endotoxin. This may be avoided by removing the ascitic fluid at the time of shunt implantation and replacing it with normal saline. Infection is another complication with high mortality, affecting 25 per cent of these shunts.

Early malfunction of the LaVeen shunt has been reported in 20 to 30 per cent of patients. An infection rate of 5 to 10 per cent has also been reported.[98] The 30-day mortality was 7.7 per cent, and the 2-year survival was 43 per cent. Ascites was controlled in 83 per cent of patients at 2 months and 50 per cent at 2 years. There is a significant late malfunction rate of 22 per cent, and late morbidity with a delayed infection appeared in 20 per cent of patients. Delayed variceal bleeding may also complicate long-term follow-up. Varix bleeding was particularly distressing in the series reported by Fulenwilder and associates,[101] occurring on an average of 6 months after shunt insertion and in 30 per cent of the population. Whether insertion of a peritoneovenous shunt is effective in treating hepatorenal syndrome remains controversial.

Another role for peritoneovenous shunting is in the treatment of malignant ascites. This is usually caused by lymphatic blockage, peritoneal inflammation, or secretion of fluid by the tumor. Ascitic fluids with abdominal carcinomatosis have high protein content and are associated with an increased incidence of shunt blockage and failure. Shunt blockage occurring in the first months after insertion is found in about half of the patients, and shunt failure is more likely in patients with positive cell cytology of the ascitic fluid. Tumor embolization has been documented in up to 5 per cent of patients. Because of an overall poor survival, tumor embolization does not seem to have an adverse effect on patient longevity. Approximately 60 per cent of the population have significant palliation, with decreased weight, decreased abdominal girth, and decreased number of paracenteses. Likewise, they usually experience an increasing urinary output and an increase in strength and appetite.

SELECTED REFERENCES

Liver Anatomy and Physiology

Adson, M. A., and Beart, R. W.: Elective hepatic resections. Surg. Clin. North Am., 57:339, 1977.
Longmire, W. P.: Elective hepatic surgery. Ann. Surg., 179:712, 1974.
Starzl, T.: Hepatic trisegmentectomy and other liver resections. Surg. Gynecol. Obstet., 141:429, 1975.
  These three references are authored by leaders in the field of hepatic resection, with detailed descriptions of liver anatomy as it pertains to hepatic dissection along with technical details of the operative procedures.

Pyogenic and Amebic Liver Abscess, Cystic Disease of the Liver

Calne, R. Y., and Della Rovere, G. Q. D.: Liver Surgery. Philadelphia, W. B. Saunders Company, 1982.
  This text on liver surgery is characterized by excellent chapters as well as outstanding illustrations of common liver diseases. The technical features of hepatic resections for various causes are shown in detail.

Ochsner, A., DeBakey, M. E., and Murray, S.: Pyogenic abscess of the liver. Am. J. Surg., *40*:292, 1938.

This classic paper concerns the etiology, pathogenesis, and treatment of liver abscess before the beginning of antibiotic treatment. It makes interesting reading, especially when the data are compared with those of modern series.

Sheinfeld, A. M., Sternei, A. E., Rivkin, L. B., Dernice, R. H., et al.: Transcutaneous drainage of abscesses of the liver guided by computed tomography scan. Surg. Gynecol. Obstet., *155*:662, 1982.

This reference describes the initial report of liver abscesses drained by percutaneous methods. These authors report a relatively high success rate and describe a technique that is particularly useful in treating patients who are a high risk for operative intervention.

Primary Hepatic Tumors

Cady, B.: Natural history of primary and secondary tumors of the liver. Semin. Oncol., *10*:127, 1983.

This excellent article reviews the natural history of both primary and secondary neoplasms of the liver. It emphasizes that some patients, especially those with solitary liver lesions, may live for prolonged periods of time without treatment, and the extent of disease must be controlled when evaluating surgical intervention.

Colorectal Liver Metastases, Hepatic Tumors in Children, Benign Hepatic Neoplasms

Balch, C. M., Urist, M. M., Soong, S. J., and McGuegar, M.: A prospective Phase II clinical treatment of continuous FUDR regional chemotherapy for colorectal metastases to the liver using a totally implantable drug infusion pump. Ann. Surg., *198*:567, 1983.

This reference reviews the initial results of a trail comparing regional FUDR chemotherapy with historic controls. This study showed a marked increase in survival in those who received regional chemotherapy.

Wagner, J. S., Adson, M. A., von Heerden, J. A., Adson, M. H., and Ilstrup, D. M.: The natural history of hepatic metastasis from colorectal cancer. Ann. Surg., *199*:502, 1984.

The natural history of hepatic metastases from colorectal cancer is described in detail from data taken at the Mayo Clinic. It is emphasized that patients with solitary liver lesions may have a reasonable survival period.

Portal Hypertension

Fonkalsrud, E. W.: Surgical management of portal hypertension in children. Long-term results. Arch. Surg., *115*:1042, 1980.

This reference describes the surgical approach to portal hypertension in children and reports excellent results with conservative therapy.

Warren, W. D., Henderson, J. M., et al.: Distal splenorenal shunt versus endoscopic sclerotherapy for long-term management of variceal bleeding. Preliminary report of a prospective, randomized trial. Ann. Surg., *203*:454, 1986.

Warren and his colleagues strongly endorse the distal splenorenal shunt to prevent postoperative encephalopathy by maintaining portovenous flow and hypertension. In this randomized study they have shown quite clearly that the initial treatment for bleeding esophageal varices should be injection sclerotherapy and not emergency shunting. A high percentage of patients with bleeding esophageal varices can be controlled with endoscopic sclerotherapy, which maintains portovenous flow. Significant differences were found in survival, with the endoscopic sclerotherapy group having a better prognosis than the emergency shunt group.

REFERENCES

Liver Anatomy and Physiology

1. Adson, M. A., and Beart, R. W.: Elective hepatic resections. Surg. Clin. North Am., *57*:339, 1977.
2. Hodgson, J. B., and DelGucicio, L. R. M.: Preliminary experience in liver surgery using the ultrasonic scalpel. Surgery, *98*:230, 1984.
3. Kinney, T. D., and Ferrebee, J. W.: Hepatic abscess: Factors determining its localization. Arch. Pathol. Lab. Med., *45*:41, 1948.
4. Lin, T-Y.: A simplified technique for hepatic resection. Ann. Surg., *180*:285, 1974.
5. Longmire, W. P.: Elective hepatic surgery. Ann. Surg., *179*:712, 1974.
6. Mays, E. T.: *In* Calne, R. Y., and Della Rovere, G. Q. D. (Eds.): Liver Surgery. Philadelphia, W. B. Saunders Company, 1982.
7. Michels, M. A.: Newer anatomy of the liver and its variant blood supply and collateral circulation. Am. J. Surg., *112*:337, 1966.

8. Rappaport, A. M., Borowy, Z. J., Lougheed, W. M., and Lotto, W. N.: Subdivision of hexagonal liver lobules into a structural and functional unit. Role in hepatic physiology and pathology. Anat. Rec., *119*:11, 1954.
9. Schwartz, S. I.: Right hepatic lobectomy. Am. J. Surg., *148*:668, 1984.
10. Serege, H.: Contribution a l'étude de la circulation des sang forte dans le foie et des localisation lobaris hépatiques. J. Med. Bord., *31*:208, 1901.
11. Starzl, T.: Hepatic trisegmentectomy and other liver resections. Surg. Gynecol. Obstet., *141*:429, 1975.
12. Stone, H. H., Long, W. D., Smith, R. B. III, and Haynes, C. D.: Physiologic considerations in major hepatic resections. Am. J. Surg., *117*:78, 1969.

Pyogenic and Amebic Liver Abscess, Cystic Disease of the Liver

13. Basile, J. A., Klein, S. R., Worthem, N. J., Wilson, S. E., and Hiatt, J. R.: Amebic liver abscess: The surgeon's role in management. Am. J. Surg., *146*:67, 1983.
14. Belli, L., del Furero, E., Masni, A., and Romani, F.: Resection versus pericystectomy in the treatment of hydatidosis of the liver. Am. J. Surg., *1450*:239, 1983.
15. Calne, R. Y., and Della Rovere, G. Q. D.: Liver Surgery, Philadelphia, W. B. Saunders Company, 1982.
16. Dayton, M. T., Longmire, W. P., and Tompkins, R. K.: Caroli's disease: A premalignant condition? Am. J. Surg., *145*:41, 1983.
17. DeBakey, M. E., and Ochsner, A.: Hepatic amebiasis: A 20-year experience and analysis of 263 cases. Int. Abstr. Surg., *92*:209, 1951.
18. Gerzof, S. G., Johnson, W. C., Robbins, A. H., and Malseth, D. C.: Intrahepatic pyogenic abscesses: Treatment by percutaneous drainage. Am. J. Surg., *149*:487, 1985.
19. Halverson, R. A., Korabkin, M., Foster, W. L., Silverman, P. M., and Thompson, W. M.: The variable CT appearance of hepatic abscess. Am. J. Radiol., *142*:941, 1984.
20. Langer, J. C., Ross, D. B., et al.: Diagnosis and management of hydatid disease of the liver. A 15-year North American experience. Ann. Surg., *199*:412, 1984.
21. Longmire, W. P., Mandiala, S. A., and Gordon, H. E.: Congenital cystic disease of the liver and biliary system. Ann. Surg., *174*:711, 1971.
22. Miedema, B. W., and Dineen, P.: The diagnosis and treatment of pyogenic liver abscess. Ann. Surg., *200*:328, 1984.
23. Ochsner, A., DeBakey, M. E., and Murray, S.: Pyogenic abscess of the liver. Am. J. Surg., *40*:292, 1938.
24. Perera, M. R., Kirk, A., and Moore, P.: Presentation, diagnosis and management of liver abscess. Lancet, *8195*:629, 1920, 1980.
25. Sheinfeld, A. M., Sternei, A. E., Rivkin, L. B., Dernice, R. H., Shemesh, O. M., and Dolberg, M. S.: Transcutaneous drainage of abscesses of the liver guided by computed tomography scan. Surg. Gynecol. Obstet., *155*:662, 1982.
26. Thompson, J. E., Forlenza, S., and Verma, R.: Amebic liver abscess: A therapeutic approach. Rev. Infect. Dis., *7*:171, 1985.

Hemobilia

27. Goodnight, J. E., Jr., and Blaisdell, F. W.: Hemobilia. Surg. Clin. North Am., *61*:973, 1981.
28. Sandblom, P.: Hemorrhage into the biliary tract following trauma—"traumatic hemobilia." Surgery, *42*:571, 1948.
29. Sandblom, P.: Hemobilia (Biliary Tract Hemorrhage). Springfield, Ill., Charles C Thomas, 1972.
30. Vaughan, R., Rosch, J., Keller, F. S., and Antonovic, R.: Treatment of hemobilia by transcatheter vascular occlusion. Europ. J. Radiol., *4*:183, 1984.

Primary Hepatic Tumors

31. Adson, M. A., and Weiland, L. H.: Resection of primary solid hepatic tumors. Am. J. Surg., *141*:18, 1981.
32. Cady, B.: Natural history of primary and secondary tumors of the liver. Semin. Oncol., *10*:127, 1983.
33. Chen, D. S., and Sung, J. L.: Serum alphafetoprotein in hepatocellular carcinoma. Cancer, *40*:779, 1977.
34. Clouse, M. E., et al.: Peripheral hepatic artery embolization for primary and secondary hepatic neoplasms. Radiology, *147*:407, 1983.
35. El-Domeiri, A. A., Huvos, A. G., Goldsmith, H. S., et al.: Primary malignant tumors of the liver. Cancer, *27*:7, 1971.
36. Fahri, D. C., Sheller, R. H., Murari, P. J., and Silverberg, S. G.: Hepatocellular carcinoma in young people. Cancer, *52*:1516, 1983.
37. Fortner, J. G., Kim, D. K., MacLean, B. J., Barrett, M. K., et al.: Major hepatic resection for neoplasia. Ann. Surg., *188*:363, 1978.

38. Heyward, W. L., Lanier, A. P., McMahon, B. J., et al.: Early detection of primary hepatocellular carcinoma. J.A.M.A., 254:3052, 1985.

39. Iwatsuki, S., Shaw, B. W., and Starzl, T. E.: Experience with 150 liver resections. Ann. Surg., 197:247, 1983.

40. Ihde, D. C., Sherlock, P., Winawer, S. J., and Fortner, J. G.: Clinical manifestations of hepatoma—a review of six years experience at a cancer hospital. Am. J. Med., 56:83, 1974.

41. Klatskin, G.: adenocarcinoma of the hepatic duct at its bifurcation within the porta hepatis. Am. J. Med., 38:241, 1965.

42. Langenbuch, C.: Ein Fall von Resection eines linksseintigen Schnurlappens der Leber, Heilung. Berl. Klin. Wochenschr., 25:37, 1888.

43. Longmire, W. P., Jr., Passaro, E. P., and Joseph, W. L.: The surgical treatment of hepatic lesions. Br. J. Surg., 53:852, 1966.

44. Markowitz, J.: The hepatic artery. Editorial. Surg. Gynecol. Obstet., 95:644, 1952.

45. Mays, E. T., Christopherson, W. M., Mahr, M. M., et al.: Hepatic changes in young women ingesting contraceptive steroids. J.A.M.A., 235:730, 1976.

46. Nagasue, W., Yakaya, H., Ogawa, Y., Sasaki, Y., Akamizu, H., and Hamada, T.: Hepatic resection in the treatment of hepatocellular carcinoma: Report of 60 cases. Br. J. Surg., 72:292, 1985.

47. Nilsson, L. A. V.: Therapeutic hepatic artery ligation with surrounding liver tumors. Rev. Surg., 23:374, 1966.

48. Ohnishi, K., Tsuchiya, S., et al.: Arterial chemoembolization of hepatocellular carcinoma with mitomycin-C microcapsules. Radiology, 152:51, 1984.

49. Ramming, K. P.: The effectiveness of hepatic artery infusion in treatment of primary hepatobiliary tumors. Semin. Oncol., 10:199, 1983.

50. Segall, H. N.: An experimental anatomical investigation of the blood and bile channels of the liver. Surg. Gynecol. Obstet., 37:152, 1923.

51. Shen, J. C., Sung, J. L., et al.: Early detection of hepatocellular carcinoma by real-time ultrasonography. Cancer, 56:660, 1985.

52. Smith, T. J., Kemeny, M. M., Sugarbaker, P. H., Jones, A. E., Vermere, M., Shawker, T. H., and Edwards, B. K.: A prospective study of hepatic imaging in the detection of metastatic disease. Ann. Surg., 195:486, 1982.

53. Sugarbaker, P. H., Vermere, M., et al.: Improved detection of focal lesions with computerized tomographic examination of the liver using ethiodized 0.1 emulsion (EOE-13) liver contrast. Cancer, 54:1489, 1985.

54. Wendel, W.: Beitrage zuir Chirurgie du Leber. Arch. Klin. Chir., 95:887, 1911.

55. Wepsic, H. T., and Kirkpatrick, A.: Alpha-fetoprotein and its relevance to human disease. Gastroenterology, 77:787, 1979.

Colorectal Liver Metastases, Hepatic Tumors in Children, Benign Hepatic Neoplasms

56. Adson, M. A., Van Heerden, J. A., Adson, M. H., Wagner, J. S., and Ilstrup, D. M.: Resection of hepatic metastases from colorectal cancer. Arch. Surg., 119:647, 1984.

57. Ansfield, F. J., and Ramirez, C.: The clinical results of 5-FU intrahepatic arterial infusion in the 528 patients with metastatic cancer to the liver. Prog. Clin. Cancer, 7:201, 1978.

58. Balch, C. M., Urist, M. M., Soong, S. J., and McGueger, M.: A prospective Phase II clinical treatment of continuous FUDR regional chemotherapy for colorectal metastases to the liver using a totally implantable drug infusion pump. Ann. Surg., 198:567, 1983.

59. Fortner, J. G., Silva, J. S., Cox, E. B., Golbey, R. B., Gallowitz, H., and MaClean, B. J.: Multivariant analysis of a personal series of 247 patients with liver metastases from colorectal cancer: II. Treatment by intrahepatic chemotherapy. Ann. Surg., 199:317, 1984.

60. Fortner, J. G., Silva, J. S., Golbey, R. B., Cox, E. B., and MaClean, B. J.: Multivariant analysis of a personal series of 247 consecutive patients with liver metastases from colorectal cancer: I. Treatment by hepatic resection. Ann. Surg., 199:306, 1984.

61. Foster, J. H.: Survival after liver resection for secondary tumors. Am. J. Surg., 135:389, 1978.

62. Iwatsuki, S., Gordon, R. D., Shaw, B. W., Jr., and Starzl, T. E.: Role of liver transplantation in cancer therapy. Ann. Surg., 202:401, 1985.

63. Kerlin, P., Davis, G. L., McGill, D. B., Weiland, L. H., Adson, M. A., and Sheedy, P. F.: Hepatic adenoma and focal nodular hyperplasia: Clinical, pathologic and radiologic features. Gastroenterology, 84:994, 1983.

64. Mahour, G. H., Wigue, G. U., Sergil, S. E., and Isaac, H.: Improved survival in infants and children with primary malignant liver tumors. Am. J. Surg., 146:236, 1983.

65. Steele, G., Osteen, R. T., Wilson, R. E., Brooks, D. C., Mayer, R.

J., Zamcheck, M., and Ravikumem, T.: Patterns of failure after surgical care of large liver tumors. Am. J. Surg., 147:554, 1984.

66. Tartter, P. I., Slater, G., Gelernt, I., and Aufses, A., Jr.: Screening for liver metastases from colorectal cancer with carcinoembryonic antigen and alkaline phosphatase. Ann. Surg., 193:357, 1981.

67. Taylor, I.: Colorectal liver metastases—to treat or not to treat? Br. J. Surg., 72:511, 1985.

68. Theman, T., Williams, W. G., Simpson, J. S., et al.: Tumor invasion of the upper inferior vena cava: The use of profound hypothermia and circulation arrest as a surgical adjuvant. J. Pediatr. Surg., 13:331, 1978.

69. Trastek, V. F., van Heerden, J. A., Sheedy, P. F., II, and Adson, M. A.: Cavernous hemangiomas of the liver: Resect or observe. Am. J. Surg., 145:49, 1983.

70. Wagner, J. S., Adson, M. A., von Heerden, J. A., Adson, M. H., and Ilstrup, D. M.: The natural history of hepatic metastasis from colorectal cancer. Ann. Surg., 199:502, 1984.

Portal Hypertension

71. Barsoun, M. S., et al.: The complication of injection sclerotherapy of bleeding esophageal varices. Br. J. Surg., 64:79, 1982.

72. Bosch, J.: Effect of pharmacological agents on portal hypertension: A haemodynamic approach. Clin. Gastroenterol., 14:169, 1985.

73. Burroughs, A. K., Jirrkoris, W. J., Shuback, S., et al.: Controlled trial of propranolol for prevention of recurrent variceal hemorrhage in patients with cirrhosis. N. Engl. J. Med., 309:1539, 1983.

74. Cameron, J. L., Herling, H. F., Sanfey, H., Boitnott, J., Kaufman, S. L., Gott, V. L., and Maddrey, W. C.: The Budd-Chiari syndrome. Am. J. Surg., 198:335, 1983.

75. Cello, V. P., Grendell, J. H., et al.: Endoscopic sclerotherapy vs. portacaval shunt in patients with liver cirrhosis and variceal hemorrhage. N. Engl. J. Med., 311:1589, 1984.

76. Chojkier, M., and Conn, H.: Esophageal tamponade in the treatment of bleeding varices. Digest. Dis. Sci., 25:267, 1980.

77. Eck, N. V.: K Voprosu o perevyazkie votorenois veni. Predvaritelnaye Soobshtshjenye (Ligature of the Portal Vein). Voen. Med. J., St. Petersburg, 130:1, 1877.

78. Fonkalsrud, E. W.: Surgical management of portal hypertension in children. Long-term results. Arch. Surg., 115:1042, 1980.

79. Hahn, M., Mussein, O., Nencki, M., and Pavlov, J.: Die Eck'sche Fistel Zwischen der Unteren Hohlvene und der Pfortader und ihre Folgen fur den Organisms. Arch. Exp. Pathol. Pharmakol., 32:161, 1893.

80. Hussey, K. P.: Vasopressin therapy for upper gastrointestinal tract hemorrhage. Has its efficacy been proved? Arch. Intern. Med., 145:1263, 1985.

81. Lebrec, D.: Propranolol for prevention of recurrent GI bleeding in patients with cirrhosis. N. Engl. J. Med., 305:1371, 1981.

82. Mols, P., et al.: Effects of vasopressin, alone and in combination with nitroprusside, in patients with liver cirrhosis and portal hypertension. Ann. Surg., 199:176, 1984.

83. Orloff, M. J., Bill, R. H., Hyde, P. V., and Skivolocki, W. P.: Long-term results of emergency protocaval shunt for bleeding esophageal varices in unrelated patients with alcoholic cirrhosis. Ann. Surg., 192:325, 1980.

84. Paquet, K. J.: Prophylactic endoscopic sclerosing treatment of the esophageal wall in varices—A prospective controlled randomized trial. Endoscopy, 14:4, 1982.

85. Paquet, K. J., and Feussner, H.: Endoscopic sclerosis and esophageal balloon tamponade in acute hemorrhage from esophagogastric varices: A prospective controlled randomized trial. Hepatology, 5:580, 1983.

86. Reynold, T. B., Donovan, A. J., Mikkelsen, W. P., et al.: Results of a 12-year randomized trial of protocaval shunt in patients with alcoholic liver disease and bleeding varices. Gastroenterology, 80:1005, 1981.

87. Rodgers, B. M., and Talbert, J. L.: Distal splenorenal shunt for portal decompression in childhood. J. Ped. Surg., 14:33, 1979.

88. Sengstaken, R. W., and Blakemore, A. H.: Balloon tamponade in the control of hemorrhage from esophageal varices. Ann. Surg., 131:781, 1950.

89. Spence, R. A. J., and Johnson, G. W.: Results in 100 conservative patients with stapled esophageal transection for varices. Surg. Gynecol. Oncol., 160:323, 1985.

90. Sugiura, M., and Futagawa, J.: Further evaluation of the Sugiura procedure in the treatment of esophageal varices. Arch. Surg., 112:1317, 1977.

91. Terblanche, J., Bornman, P. C., Kahn, D., Jinker, M. A. T., Campbell, J. A. H., Wright, J., and Kirsch, R.: Failure of repeated injection sclerotherapy to improve long-term survival after esophageal variceal bleeding. A five year prospective controlled trial. Lancet, 2:1328, 1983.

92. van Heerden, J. A.: The Budd-Chiari syndrome: Medical and surgical management of 30 patients. Arch. Surg., *120*:657, 1985.
93. Warren, W. D., Zeppa, R., and Foman, J. J.: Selective trans-splenic decompression of gastro-esophageal varices by distal spleno-renal shunt. Ann. Surg., *166*:437, 1967.
94. Warren, W. D., Mittikan, W. J., Jr., Henderson, J. M., et al.: Ten years portal hypertensive surgery at Emory. Ann. Surg., *195*:530, 1982.
95. Warren, W. D., Henderson, J. M., et al.: Distal splenorenal shunt versus endoscopic sclerotherapy for long-term management of variceal bleeding. Preliminary report of a prospective, randomized trial. Ann. Surg., *203*:454, 1986.
96. Westaby, D., MacDougall, R. D., and Williams, P.: Improved survival following injection sclerotherapy from esophageal varices. Final analysis of a controlled trial. Hepatology, *5*:827, 1985.
97. Zeppa, R., Hensley, G. T., Levi, J. U., et al.: The comparative survival of alcoholics versus nonalcoholics after distal splenorenal shunt. Ann. Surg., *187*:510, 1978.

Peritoneovenous Shunts for Refractory Ascites

98. Bernhoff, R. A., Pellegrini, C. A., and Way, L. W.: Peritoneovenous shunts for refractory ascites. Arch. Surg., *117*:631, 1982.
99. Epstein, M.: Peritoneovenous shunt in the management of ascites and the hepatorenal syndrome. Gastroenterology, *82*:790, 1982.
100. Frakes, J. T.: Physiologic consideration in the medical management of ascites. Arch. Intern. Med., *140*:620, 1982.
101. Fulenwider, J. T., Smith, R. B., et al.: Peritoneovenous shunts. Lesions learned from an 8-year experience with 70 patients. Arch. Surg., *119*:1133, 1984.
102. Kao, H. W., Rakov, M. E., Savage, E., and Reynolds, T. B.: The effect of large volume paracentesis on plasma volume—a cause of hypovolemia. Hepatology, *5*:403, 1985.
103. LaVeen, H. H., Christoudias, G., Ip, M., et al.: Peritoneovenous shunting for ascites. Ann. Surg., *180*:580, 1974.
104. Quintiro, E., Arrogo, V., et al.: Paracentesis vs. diuretics in the treatment of cirrhotics with tense ascites. Lancet, *1*:611, 1985.

THE BILIARY SYSTEM

MICHAEL G. SARR, M.D. • JOHN L. CAMERON, M.D.

28

ANATOMY

Embryology

The hepatobiliary tree develops as an endodermal bud off the ventral aspect of the foregut from the region that later becomes the duodenum. The cranial aspect of this bud develops into the hepatic parenchyma and the proximal biliary tree (intrahepatic and common hepatic ducts), whereas the caudal aspect becomes the gallbladder and common bile duct.

Biliary Drainage

Biliary drainage follows the anatomic lobar distribution of the liver and not its gross topographic anatomy. Anatomically, the liver is divided into two lobes, the right and the left, according to the pattern of branching of the hepatic artery, portal vein, and biliary tree. The anatomic right lobe has two segments (anterior, posterior) as does the anatomic left lobe (medial, lateral). The line of division between the right and left lobes is roughly the sagittal plane through the bed of the gallbladder. The topographic quadrate lobe is part of the anatomic left lobe, and the topographic caudate lobe is divided according to its blood supply and biliary drainage between the right and left anatomic lobes. Biliary drainage of the liver occurs in segmental fashion; there is little, if any, interlobar communication. The intrahepatic bile ducts convene into major segmental branches, which join to form the right and left hepatic (lobar) ducts just outside the liver parenchyma in the hepatic hilum (Fig. 1A). The right and left hepatic ducts are short and merge to form the common hepatic duct in the porta hepatis. After a course of 2 to 4 cm. in the anterior aspect of the hepatoduodenal ligament, the hepatic duct accepts the cystic duct from the gallbladder and extends the remaining 8 to 11 cm. into the duodenum as the common bile duct (CBD). Within the hepatoduodenal ligament, the CBD is the most anterior structure, the portal vein lies directly behind and is the most posterior structure, and the hepatic artery is situated medially between these two. The CBD courses medially behind the first portion of the duodenum (retroduodenal portion of CBD) and enters the pancreatic parenchyma (intrapancreatic portion of CBD). The distal CBD extends obliquely within the wall of the duodenum for 10 to 15 mm. (intramural portion of CBD), entering the posteromedial aspect of the second portion of the duodenum at the mucosal papilla of Vater. The intramural portion of the CBD usually accepts the entrance of the major pancreatic duct (duct of Wirsung), forming a "common channel" (Fig. 1B). Occasionally these ducts will join in the intrapancreatic portion of the CBD or, more commonly, may enter separately at the papilla of Vater without a common channel. A common channel is believed important in the pathogenesis of gallstone pancreatitis.

The sphincteric mechanism (sphincter of Oddi) regulating the flow of bile into the duodenum is complex (see Fig. 1B). A separate muscular component (sphincter choledochus of Boyden) is located just proximal to the entrance of the pancreatic duct. Similarly, the separate sphincter ampullae surround the common choledochus in the ampulla of Vater.

Gallbladder

The gallbladder is a reservoir diverticulum off the common duct. The fundus and body lie beneath the anteroinferior aspect of the liver in the gallbladder fossa. The gallbladder drains via the infundibulum, which often forms a redundant pocket called Hartmann's pouch. At the neck of the gallbladder the cystic duct arises and enters the choledochus after a variable length (< 1 to 4 cm.). The cystic duct contains several mucosal folds of doubtful sphincteric function called the valves of Heister.

Histology

The bile ducts are lined with a columnar epithelium with cryptlike formations, within which are interspersed mucous cells. Sparse smooth muscle cells are found in the fibrous wall of the major ducts. The wall of the gallbladder has four layers. The exposed regions of the fundus, body, and infundibulum are covered by serosal peritoneum. The perimuscularis beneath is a layer of connective tissue of variable prominence and is richly endowed with blood vessels and lymphatics. The muscularis contains longitudinally oriented smooth muscle fibers. The mucosa is lined with a high columnar epithelium, which, in the presence of inflammation, may become deeply invaginated to form Rokitansky-Aschoff sinuses. Mucous secretory cells are prominent only in the neck region.

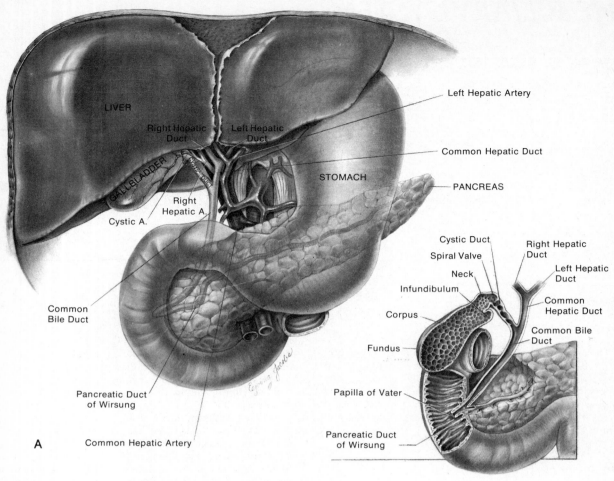

A

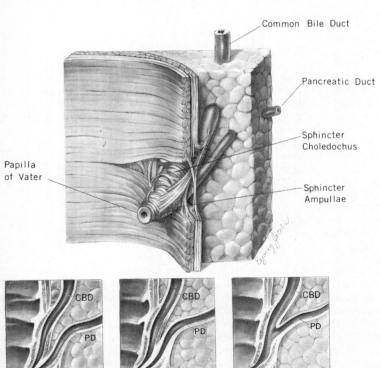

B

Figure 1. A, Biliary anatomy and extrahepatic biliary tree. B, Sphincter of Oddi and papilla of Vater showing common channel. (From Orloff, M. J.: The biliary system. In Sabiston, D. C. (Ed.): Davis-Christopher Textbook of Surgery. Philadelphia, W. B. Saunders Company, 1981, Chap. 36.)

Vascular Supply

The arterial supply to the proximal extrahepatic biliary tree arises from small branches originating from the common and lobar hepatic arteries. The distal common bile duct is supplied by branches from the gastroduodenal and superior pancreaticoduodenal arteries. The cystic artery to the gallbladder usually originates from the right hepatic artery posterior and lateral to the common duct. During cholecystectomy, the cystic artery is found at the base of the cystic duct in the triangle of Calot, the three sides of which are bounded by the common hepatic duct, the cystic duct, and the liver. Venous drainage of the extrahepatic biliary tree and gallbladder is directly into the portal vein.

Lymphatic Drainage

Lymphatic drainage of the hepatobiliary tree is centrifugal. Vessels from the hepatic parenchyma and intrahepatic biliary tree converge at the porta hepatis and course along the common duct in the hepatoduodenal ligament to enter the cysterna chyli and, eventually, the thoracic duct. The gallbladder lymph drains along the cystic duct into this network. With cholecystitis, characteristically enlarged lymph nodes may be found at the neck of the gallbladder (cystic duct node) as well as at the junction of the cystic duct with the choledochus and along the distal supraduodenal portion of the common bile duct.

Innervation of the Biliary System

Autonomic innervation of the biliary tree comprises both parasympathetic (vagal) and sympathetic (thoracic) fibers that follow the vascular supply. Vagal innervation arises from the anterior vagus and appears to be important in maintaining tone and contractility of the gallbladder. Afferent sympathetic fibers mediate the pain of biliary colic. Bile production is, in part, affected by autonomic control.

Anomalies

Anatomic variations of the extrahepatic biliary tree are common. The classic anatomic description of the biliary tree applies to only about one third of individuals. For this reason, an understanding of the common anomalies is of great importance to the surgeon. Accessory hepatic ducts (ducts of Luschka) from the anterior segment of the right hepatic lobe may drain directly into the body or infundibulum of the gallbladder. These are usually small but may rarely be large-caliber communications with the right ductal system and thus require separate ligation during cholecystectomy. Anomalies of the major segmental hepatic ducts are frequent but are important only with the complicated reconstructive procedures performed at the porta hepatis.

Anomalies of the gallbladder are least common (Fig. 2A). The gallbladder may be absent, duplicated, left-sided, or partially or completely intrahepatic and without a serosal surface. The "floating" gallbladder lacks any mesenteric attachment to the undersurface of the liver and is subject to torsion and infarction. Anomalies of the cystic duct are especially important because they may predispose to serious biliary injuries during cholecystectomy (Fig. 2B). The cystic duct may join the choledochus high in the porta hepatis or, more commonly (10 per cent), lower near the duodenum. It often contains a common wall with the choledochus. Less frequently, the cystic duct may drain directly into the anterior segment of the right hepatic duct or, after coursing either anteriorly or posteriorly, into the left side of the common duct.

Anomalous origins and courses of the right and left hepatic arteries are frequent. Variations in the origin and course of the cystic artery are common as well (Fig. 2C). The cystic artery may pass anterior to the common duct after arising from the left hepatic, common hepatic, gastroduodenal, or celiac arteries. Double cystic arteries of various origins also occur.

PHYSIOLOGY

Bile Production

The secretion of bile serves three major functions. First, bile salts, phospholipids, and cholesterol aggregate within the bile to form mixed micelles. By emulsification, this micellar complex allows enteric absorption of ingested fats and the fat-soluble vitamins (A,D,E,K). Absorption of

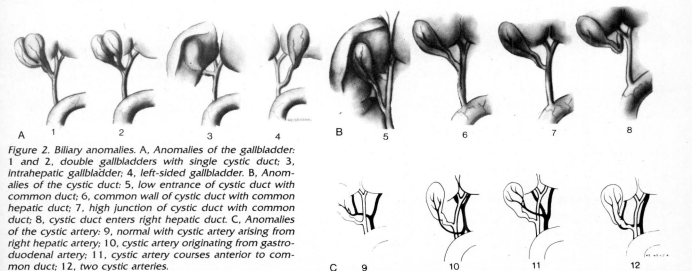

Figure 2. Biliary anomalies. A, Anomalies of the gallbladder: 1 and 2, double gallbladders with single cystic duct; 3, intrahepatic gallbladder; 4, left-sided gallbladder. B, Anomalies of the cystic duct: 5, low entrance of cystic duct with common duct; 6, common wall of cystic duct with common hepatic duct; 7, high junction of cystic duct with common duct; 8, cystic duct enters right hepatic duct. C, Anomalies of the cystic artery: 9, normal with cystic artery arising from right hepatic artery; 10, cystic artery originating from gastroduodenal artery; 11, cystic artery courses anterior to common duct; 12, two cystic arteries.

certain minerals (calcium, copper, iron) is also facilitated. Second, bile serves as the vehicle for enteral excretion of numerous endogenously and exogenously produced substances (such as bilirubin). Third, in part by neutralizing gastric acid, bile helps maintain the proper alkaline environment in the duodenum that, in the presence of bile salts, allows maximal activity of postprandial digestive enzymes.

Normally, the hepatocytes and bile ducts produce 500 to 1500 ml. of bile daily. Bile production is a continuous process that is only partially subject to neural, hormonal, and humoral regulation (Fig. 3). Vagal input acts directly on the bile duct cells to promote secretion of water and electrolytes, whereas splanchnic sympathetic activity tends to inhibit bile production indirectly by decreasing hepatic blood flow. The gastrointestinal hormones cholecystokinin (CCK), secretin, and gastrin augment ductal secretion and bile flow in response to a meal. Bile salts themselves serve as potent choleretics during periods of heightened enterohepatic circulation.

The active secretion of bile salts by the hepatocyte is the primary factor regulating the volume of bile secreted. Water and electrolytes follow passively along osmolar and electrical gradients to maintain neutrality. The excretion of lecithin and cholesterol into the canaliculis to form the mixed micelles is poorly understood and may be coupled with secretion of bile salts across the canalicular membrane. Different and separate active transport systems bring about secretion of bilirubin and other organic anions. Ductular cells augment bile secretion by pumping sodium and bicarbonate into the lumen.

Bile is secreted continuously by the liver into the bile ducts. During fasting, the tonic contraction of the sphincter of Oddi causes bile to reflux into the receptive gallbladder where it is stored and concentrated. Here, bile salts, bile pigments, and cholesterol are concentrated as much as tenfold by the absorption of water and electrolytes. About 50 per cent of the bile salt pool is stored in the gallbladder during fasting. The gallbladder mucosa also secretes a mucus that may serve a protective function. With ingestion of a meal, CCK is released by the fats, and, to a lesser extent, by the amino acids entering the duodenum; CCK stimulates contraction of the gallbladder and relaxation of the sphincter of Oddi. When the pressure in the common duct exceeds the resistance of the sphincteric mechanism (15 to 20 cm. H_2O), bile enters the duodenal lumen. Vagal input facilitates gallbladder tone and contraction; after vagotomy, a relative stasis may occur and predispose to gallstone formation. After cholecystectomy, biliary flow into the duodenum is regulated solely by sphincteric function.

Bile Composition

Bile is a complex aqueous solution containing electrolytes, conjugated bile salts, phospholipids (primarily lecithin), cholesterol, fatty acids, mucin, proteins, and a variety of hepatic metabolites and bile pigments. The electrolyte content and osmolality of bile approach those of plasma.

Bile Salt Metabolism/Enterohepatic Circulation

Bile salts are composed of a steroid moiety synthesized directly from cholesterol. The two primary bile salts, cholate and chenodeoxycholate, are synthesized by the hepatocyte under a poorly understood feedback control. Secondary bile salts, deoxycholate and lithocholate, are formed

in the colon by bacterial degradation of primary bile salts escaping reabsorption in the ileum. Lithocholate is excreted in the stool, but deoxycholate is reabsorbed into the portal blood and, along with the reabsorbed primary bile salts, is extracted by the hepatocyte. These bile salts are conjugated with glycine or taurine and actively secreted into the bile canaliculis as 40 per cent cholate, 40 per cent chenodeoxycholate, and 20 per cent deoxycholate in a total concentration of 10 to 20 mmol.

Because they have both hydrophilic and hydrophobic regions, bile salts function as detergents. They aggregate spontaneously in groups of 8 to 10 molecules to form micelles. The inner hydrophobic core solubilizes the poorly water–soluble lecithin, which itself further augments cholesterol solubilization by expanding the hydrophobic region of the micelle. This bile salt–lecithin-cholesterol complex is called a mixed micelle. The bile salts are further concentrated in the gallbladder to 200 to 300 mmol. The total amount of cholesterol dissolved varies with both the relative ratio of bile salts and lecithin as well as with the total bile salt concentration. These parameters will become important later during discussion of gallstone formation.

After entering the upper small bowel, these mixed micelles markedly potentiate fat absorption by providing both the vehicle and the environment for solubilization, enzymatic hydrolysis, and eventual absorption. The enterohepatic circulation of bile salts is completed when they are enterically deconjugated, reabsorbed in the terminal ileum by an active transport system, and finally extracted from the portal circulation by the hepatocyte (see Fig. 3). The 5 per cent of bile salts that escape reabsorption in the ileum are converted to secondary bile salts in the colon and are partially reabsorbed as deoxycholate. The total bile salt pool of 2.5 to 5 gm. circulates six to eight times a day; the 10 to 20 per cent of the total pool lost daily in the stool is restored by de novo synthesis by the liver.

Biliary Lipids

Lecithin and cholesterol comprise the majority of bile lipids. Lecithin is a phospholipid that is largely insoluble in water. Cholesterol is synthesized by the liver as well as being absorbed by the gastrointestinal tract and, in addition to being used in other intracellular pathways, is either converted into bile salts or excreted directly into the bile. Bile salt micelles markedly increase solubility of these lipids in the bile. However, the mechanism for transport of these intracellular lipids into the bile is poorly understood and may be coupled with the secretion of bile salts across the canalicular membranes. In the intestine, lecithin is hydrolyzed to choline and fatty acids. Cholesterol is reabsorbed into an enterohepatic circulation and serves as a feedback mechanism in the control of cholesterol synthesis in the liver.

Bilirubin Metabolism

As effete red blood cells are degraded in the reticuloendothelial system, hemoglobin is released and metabolized to biliverdin. This pigment is reduced to unconjugated, water-insoluble bilirubin (the "indirect" bilirubin measured by the van den Bergh reaction), carried in the blood bound to albumin, and extracted by the hepatocyte (see Fig. 3). In the cytoplasm, bilirubin is carried by the Y and Z proteins to the endoplasmic reticulum. In the presence of glucuronyl transferase, bilirubin is conjugated with glucuronic acid, and to a lesser extent with sulfate, to form bilirubin glucuronide and bilirubin sulfate. This water-

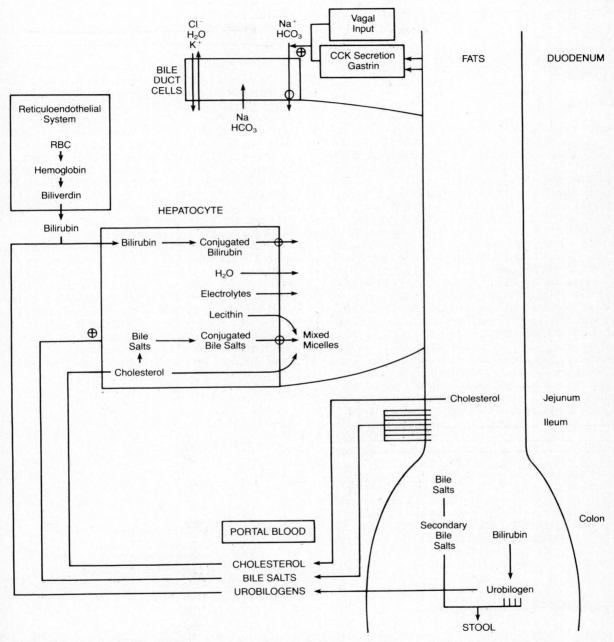

Figure 3. Bile production, bilirubin metabolism, and enterohepatic circulation. (Note: ⟷active transport mechanism; ⊕ positive stimulus to secretion; → passive secretion.)

soluble, conjugated bilirubin ("direct" bilirubin) is then secreted into the bile canaliculis by an active transport mechanism shared by other organic salts but distinct from that of bile salt secretion. The daily load of bilirubin for excretion is about 300 mg. In the gut, intestinal bacteria convert the bilirubin to a class of compounds known as urobilinogens. These urobilinogens are largely excreted in the stool, but a portion is reabsorbed and either extracted by the hepatocyte to enter the enterohepatic circulation or excreted in the urine.

GALLSTONES

Epidemiology

Approximately 16 million people in the U.S. have gallstones, necessitating about 500,000 cholecystectomies a year. Gallstones are directly responsible for about 10,000 deaths a year. The prevalence of gallstones varies with both sex and age. Women with gallstones outnumber men 4 to 1. Women who take exogenous estrogens appear to be at increased risk, further implicating a hormonal basis. With advancing age, this female predominance becomes less marked. Gallstones are unusual in those younger than 20 years old (< 1 per cent), more prevalent in the 40- to 60-year age group (~11 per cent), and found in about 30 per cent of those over 80 years.

Gallstone disease exhibits genetic and environmental variations as well. A tendency to form gallstones may run in families. The Pima Indians, a genetically distinct group in Arizona, have an extremely high prevalence of cholelithiasis affecting 70 per cent of women by age 30 and 70 per cent of the men by age 60. Gallstones are more common in Caucasians than in blacks. Gallstone disease is also prevalent in populations in countries other than the U.S., especially Japan, Chili, and Sweden. Environmental factors also play a role in gallstone formation. The prevalence of gallstones changes with certain racial migrations. Although unusual in the U.S., pigment stones are common in certain parts of the Orient and are believed to be related in part to parasitic and bacterial infections of the biliary tree. There is a well-known association between obesity and increased amounts of cholesterol in the bile. Extensive ileal resections, ileal bypass (as with the jejunoileal bypass operation), or severe ileal disease (as with Crohn's disease), each by interfering with the enterohepatic circulation of bile salts, predisposes to cholesterol stone formation. Patients with hemolytic anemias, such as sickle cell disease and hereditary spherocytosis, manifest a very high prevalence of pigment stones, even as children.

Pathophysiology of Gallstone Formation

CHOLESTEROL STONES

Bile supersaturated with cholesterol accounts for over 90 per cent of gallstones in the Western world. The majority of these stones are mixed cholesterol stones that contain at least 75 per cent cholesterol by weight and varying amounts of phospholipids, biliary pigments, and other organic and inorganic substances. Pure cholesterol stones comprise about 10 per cent of all cholesterol stones. The physiochemical properties of bile vary with the relative concentrations of bile salts, lecithin, and cholesterol. Cholesterol is solu-

bilized in bile within the hydrophobic region of the micelle, and thus its solubility is intimately dependent on the relative amounts of bile salts and lecithin. This can be expressed by a triangular graph (Fig. 4), the coordinates of which are the percentage molar concentrations of bile salts, lecithin, and cholesterol. Bile containing cholesterol entirely within micelles is depicted by the area under the curved line ABC (micellar liquid); however, when the relative concentrations of bile salts, lecithin, and cholesterol fall into the area above line ABC, cholesterol exists in two or more phases (cholesterol crystals and micellar liquid).

The physical process of cholesterol stone formation occurs in three stages: (1) supersaturation of bile with cholesterol; (2) crystallization/precipitation; and (3) growth of the stone by lamellar aggregation/precipitation of cholesterol and other substances that comprise the matrix of the stone. Stone formation is a complicated process in which many poorly understood factors augment each of the three stages of stone formation. Some normal individuals secrete a supersaturated bile, but they never form stones. However, patients with cholesterol gallstones all have a lithogenic bile supersaturated with cholesterol and containing cholesterol crystals. This may occur by hepatic secretion of an already lithogenic hepatic bile or by subsequent conversion to a lithogenic bile secondary to concentration in the gallbladder.

The vast majority of patients with cholesterol stones secrete a lithogenic hepatic bile. Certain groups have a contracted total bile salt pool (1.5 to 2 gm.) that is half the size of normal subjects. This may occur through either an abnormal bile salt feedback with decreased hepatic synthesis of bile salts (as with the Pima Indians) or excessive loss of bile salts in the stool from primary ileal malabsorption or following ileal resection or bypass. Other groups, especially the obese, secrete an excessive amount of cholesterol. Some evidence suggests that dietary intake of cholesterol

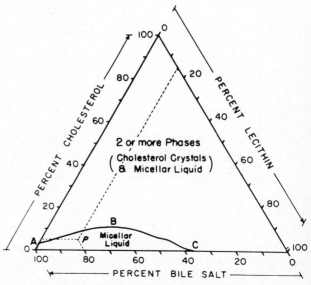

Figure 4. Triangular coordinates depicting physicochemical properties of bile. Area under curved line ABC defines a solution with cholesterol entirely solubilized within micelles. Area above line ABC represents a solution in which cholesterol may exist in several phases. Point P contains 80 mol. per 100 ml. bile salts, 18 mol. per 100 ml. lecithin, and 5 mol. per 100 ml. cholesterol, all of which are in micellar solution. (From Small, D. M.: N. Engl. J. Med., 279:588, 1968.)

and/or the caloric content of the diet may affect cholesterol secretion as well.

Other proposed mechanisms for stone formation implicate dysfunction of the gallbladder. Stasis, either from a mechanical or functional obstruction, may lead to bile stagnation within the gallbladder with excessive water resorption and altered bile constituent solubility. Experimental work suggests that inflammation of the wall may lead to excessive bile salt resorption, alteration in lecithin/bile salt ratio, and secretion of calcium salts, mucoproteins, and cellular organic debris; these changes may convert a normal hepatic bile into a lithogenic bile within the gallbladder. The role of infection in the pathogenesis of cholesterol stone formation is controversial. Although certain enteric organisms may be cultured from the core of cholesterol stones or from the gallbladder wall, the majority of cholesterol stones form in the absence of infection.

Pigment Stones

Pigment stones comprise about 10 per cent of gallstones in this country. There are two forms—the more common pure pigment stones and calcium bilirubinate stones. Pure pigment stones are smaller (2 to 5 mm.), multiple, very hard, and of a green to black appearance. They contain variable amounts of calcium bilirubinate, bilirubin polymers, bile acids, lesser amounts of cholesterol (3 to 26 per cent), and numerous other organic substances. In the Orient, calcium bilirubinate stones predominate and comprise 40 to 60 per cent of all gallstones. These stones are more fragile, brownish to black in color, and often form *de novo* outside of the gallbladder in the common duct or in the intrahepatic bile ducts. Calcium bilirubinate stones are often radiopaque, whereas pure pigment stones may not be radiopaque, depending on their calcium content.

The pathogenesis of pigment stones differs from that of cholesterol stones. Possibilities include the secretion of increased amounts of pigments or elaboration of an abnormal pigment that precipitates in the bile. Cirrhosis and biliary stasis predispose to pigment stone formation. Patients with increased loads of unconjugated bilirubin (hemolytic anemias) commonly form pure pigment stones. Another mechanism less common in the Western world involves the extrahepatic conversion to a lithogenic bile. In the Orient, the high incidence of calcium bilirubinate stones may be related to secondary bacterial invasion of the biliary tree infested with the parasites *Clonorchis sinensis* or *Ascaris lumbricoides. Escherichia coli* makes a B-glucuronidase that is believed to deconjugate bilirubin in bile, which may favor formation of insoluble calcium bilirubinate. The inflamed gallbladder or biliary radicals may play a role by elaborating organic substances, which, by serving as a nidus, may increase the lithogenicity for pigment stones.

Natural History of Gallstones

The natural history of gallstones is still not entirely known. [14]Carbon dating has shown that stones may require as long as 8 years to reach maximal size. Moreover, it may take many years for symptoms to develop after the stones begin to form. Clearly, with the widespread prevalence of gallstones, symptoms that necessitate cholecystectomy never develop in many patients. Only about 30 per cent of patients with gallstones will come to cholecystectomy.

The best means of examining the natural history of gallstones is to divide patients with gallstones into two categories—symptomatic and asymptomatic. Patients with *symptomatic gallstones* constitute a group with a high incidence of future problems. Several large series from Sweden followed over 1300 patients with gallstones from 5 to 20 years. Although over 90 per cent had symptoms at the time of diagnosis, they were not subjected to cholecystectomy. About half of the patients subsequently developed recurrent symptoms or severe complications such as acute cholecystitis, jaundice, pancreatitis, or carcinoma of the gallbladder. Moreover, operative mortality increased with emergency procedures or serious complications. Today, most physicians accept the concept that patients with symptomatic gallstones are candidates for cholecystectomy if they are in reasonable health and have a life expectancy of at least 5 years.

Patients with *asymptomatic gallstones* may well follow a different course. Implications drawn from the above-mentioned studies of symptomatic patients suggest that a high percentage of asymptomatic patients, if followed long enough, would develop symptoms or severe complications. However, the great majority of the symptomatic patients had advanced gallbladder disease at the time of diagnosis and thus do not represent a fair comparison population. Moreover, we know from autopsy studies that many (if not most) patients with gallstones never come to cholecystectomy, and indeed remain asymptomatic. Two good studies have addressed the topic of asymptomatic "silent" gallstones. Gallstones were discovered either incidentally[9] or during a large-scale screening program[12] in 235 asymptomatic patients. Only 15 per cent subsequently developed biliary colic, and only 3 per cent developed a serious complication in long-term follow-up (> 10 yr.).

Today, with our effective diagnostic screening capability (e.g., ultrasonography), many patients with asymptomatic gallstones will be recognized. Within this group, there are certain parameters that might justify "prophylactic" cholecystectomy. Past experience has shown that patients with large gallstones (> 2.5 cm.), a calcified gallbladder, or a nonfunctioning gallbladder or diabetics with gallstones are at increased risk of serious complications related directly to the gallstones; elective cholecystectomy is warranted in these subsets of patients with asymptomatic gallstones.

Dissolution of Gallstones

With a more complete understanding of the formation of gallstones, considerable interest has been generated in the dissolution of gallstones. Feeding of chenodeoxycholate (250 to 1500 mg. per day) or its epimer ursodeoxycholate (the primary bile salt in the bear) expands the bile salt pool and desaturates the bile with respect to cholesterol. Unfortunately, the results of a national cooperative study of gallstone dissolution[21] using chenodeoxycholate were disappointing. In patients with radiolucent stones, only 14 per cent had complete dissolution and 27 per cent partial dissolution. Also, there was no effect on the natural history of the gallstones during the 2-year study in that the same number of patients on placebo or chenodeoxycholate required cholecystectomy. Side effects were common, with diarrhea occurring in 40 per cent and with an appreciable incidence of presumed hepatotoxicity signified by increases in aminotransferases. This oral therapy is ineffective for noncholesterol stones and for patients with nonfunctioning gallbladders. Most important, however, with termination of treatment the bile reverts to its lithogenic state, and gallstones reform. Preliminary results using oral ursodeoxycholate have proved more encouraging and await further evaluation.

DIAGNOSIS OF BILIARY TRACT DISEASE

Disorders of the biliary tree may often be suspected on the basis of history alone. Right upper quadrant pain, fatty food intolerance, fever and chills, and a history of jaundice, dark urine, and light stools are all suggestive of biliary tract disease. In addition, the physical findings of jaundice, right upper quadrant tenderness, and a right upper quadrant mass are very helpful in focusing on the biliary tree. However, these findings are not pathognomonic of biliary disease, and on occasion they may be secondary to diseases in other organ systems. Moreover, because of its anatomic locale, the biliary tree does not lend itself to examination by external palpation (unless the gallbladder is distended). Therefore, unlike many other systems of the body, confident diagnosis of most biliary disorders virtually always requires the aid of laboratory investigations and/or radiographic, sonographic, or radionuclide imaging techniques. These diagnostic tests have been designed primarily to detect the presence of gallstones and/or to determine obstruction or impedance of bile flow, either by chemical analyses of different aspects of hepatic function and bile excretion or by direct visualization of the anatomy of the biliary tree.

Laboratory Tests

Screening for biliary tract disease involves the use of many of the same biochemical tests indicative of hepatocellular dysfunction, i.e., so-called liver-function tests. The *serum bilirubin*, fractionated as the indirect and direct components of the van den Bergh reaction, is by itself very nonspecific. Although elevated serum bilirubin often indicates a hepatobiliary disorder, it may be elevated in the absence of hepatobiliary disease in a wide variety of disorders including significant episodes of intravascular hemolysis and systemic sepsis. More commonly, however, an elevated serum bilirubin will be secondary to intrahepatic cholestasis indicative of hepatic parenchymal dysfunction or extrahepatic cholestasis secondary to biliary obstruction from gallstones, malignancy, or benign pancreatic disease. With complete biliary obstruction, serum bilirubin peaks at 25 to 30 mg. per 100 ml., by which time the urinary excretion of bilirubin equals the daily production. Values greater than 30 mg. per 100 ml. imply concomitant hemolysis or hepatocellular or renal dysfunction. Extrahepatic malignancies most often lead to complete obstruction (serum bilirubin > 20 mg. per 100 ml.), whereas gallstones usually cause a partial obstruction with serum bilirubin rarely exceeding 10 to 15 mg. per 100 ml. *Alanine aminotransferase* (previously called SGOT, serum glutamic-oxaloacetic transaminase) and *aspartate aminotransferase* (previously SGPT, serum glutamic-pyruvic transaminase) are enzymes synthesized in high concentrations in the hepatocyte. Elevations in serum activity are often indicative of hepatocellular disorders; however, elevations of these enzymes (one to three times normal or occasionally quite high but transient elevations) may occur with biliary tract disease, especially biliary obstruction. *Alkaline phosphatase* is an enzyme synthesized in the epithelial cells of the bile ducts. With biliary obstruction, the serum activity increases as the ductal cells increase synthesis of this enzyme. Mark-

edly elevated levels are highly suggestive of biliary obstruction. However, alkaline phosphatase is also found in bone and can be elevated with bony destruction. Although the serum activity can be fractionated into hepatic and bony isoenzymes, this is a tedious endeavor. Similarly, during pregnancy, serum alkaline phosphatase is elevated secondary to placental synthesis. In the presence of bone disease or pregnancy, *leucine aminopeptidase* and *5'-nucleotidase* are synthesized by the biliary ductal cells (but absent in bone and placenta) and behave similarly to alkaline phosphatase in the presence of biliary obstruction.

Radiologic Studies

PLAIN ABDOMINAL RADIOGRAPHS

The plain film may be helpful occasionally but will fail to identify most biliary tract pathology (Fig. 5). Only 15 per cent of gallstones contain sufficient calcium to permit confident identification. Rarely, intense calcification within the wall of the gallbladder (so-called porcelain gallbladder) or the "milk of calcium" bile, in which multiple small calcified stones or organic precipitates are evident within the gallbladder, is indicative of gallbladder disease. Pneumobilia, i.e., the presence of air in the biliary tree or in the lumen or wall of the gallbladder, is abnormal and, in the absence of prior surgery that destroys or bypasses the choledochal sphincter mechanism, is indicative of biliary tract pathology. Air within the wall and lumen of the gallbladder is seen with "emphysematous" cholecystitis, which is secondary to an infection with gas-producing bacteria. The presence of a soft tissue mass indenting the duodenum or the hepatic flexure of the colon may also suggest a distended gallbladder.

BARIUM MEAL

Contrast examination of the stomach and duodenum rarely yields direct information about the biliary tree but may be helpful in a negative sense by excluding disease elsewhere, e.g., duodenal ulcer or gastroesophageal reflux. Reflux of contrast into the biliary tree is always abnormal and carries implications identical to those of pneumobilia in that it suggests an abnormal connection between the biliary tree and intestine, either of spontaneous or postsurgical etiology.

ORAL CHOLECYSTOGRAPHY

The oral cholecystogram, developed by Graham and Cole in 1924, remains the gold standard for diagnosis of gallbladder disease. An iodinated organic agent, usually 6 tablets of iopanoic acid (Telepaque), is administered orally the night before, and the patient is fasted. This drug is absorbed, bound to albumin, extracted by the hepatocyte, secreted into the bile, and concentrated in the gallbladder; opacification of the gallbladder occurs in 8 to 12 hours. Gallstones or tumors appear as filling defects (Fig. 6A). Opacification requires both a patent cystic duct and a functioning gallbladder. Should the gallbladder fail to visualize, the procedure is repeated within 24 hours. Failure of opacification on reinforced or double-dose oral cholecystography is diagnostic of gallbladder disease. The oral cholecystogram is highly sensitive and specific and approaches 98 per cent when used appropriately. The test is unreliable when serum bilirubin is elevated or in the presence of vomiting, diarrhea, or malabsorption.

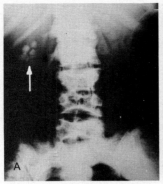
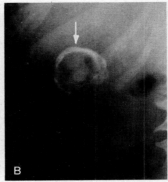
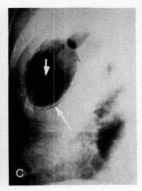

Figure 5. A, Calcified gallstones (arrow). B, Calcified "porcelain" gallbladder (arrow). (From Berk, R. N., and Clement, A. R.: Radiology of the Gallbladder and Bile Ducts. Philadelphia, W. B. Saunders Company, 1977.) C, Emphysematous cholecystitis showing air within the lumen and wall of the gallbladder (arrows). (From May, R. E., and Strong, R.: Br. J. Surg. 58:453, 1971.)

INTRAVENOUS CHOLANGIOGRAPHY

This test was developed in 1954 to allow visualization of the entire extrahepatic biliary tree. However, radiographic resolution is often poor, and the test is unreliable when serum bilirubin exceeds 3 mg. per 100 ml. Moreover, rare but potentially fatal reactions to the intravenous contrast agent have occurred. This test has been supplanted by safer, more reliable investigations and is now a diagnostic anachronism.

ULTRASONOGRAPHY

The development of sophisticated techniques of ultrasonography of the biliary tree has resulted in their replacement of oral cholecystography as the screening test for cholelithiasis. Because ultrasonography is not quite as accurate as oral cholecystography, the oral cholecystogram remains the gold standard in the diagnosis of gallstones. However, ultrasonography is quick, noninvasive, and without radiographic exposure; moreover, it can be used in the jaundiced patient and avoids the vagaries of patient compliance and absorption of oral contrast agents. Thus it is a better screening test. Criteria for diagnosis of cholelithiasis include intraluminal defects that move with changes in patient position and/or produce acoustic shadowing (Fig. 6*B*). When these are present, accuracy approaches 90 per cent. False positives are unusual (1 to 3 per cent), but false negatives occur about 10 per cent of the time secondary to the inability of ultrasonography to detect (1) stones in a gallbladder packed with stones and therefore without a bile/stone interface, (2) very small stones, or (3) a stone impacted in the cystic duct. In certain situations an oral cholecystogram may be required to confirm the presence or absence of gallbladder disease. Recognition of choledocholithiasis is unreliable by ultrasonography.

Ultrasonography is very useful in the jaundiced patient. As a screening technique, not only are intra- and extrahepatic biliary ductal dilatations recognized reliably but other abnormalities in the hepatic parenchyma or the pancreas (such as masses or cysts) may also be evident. In recent years, ultrasonography has clearly become established as the initial screening test when a diagnostic evaluation is being initiated for jaundice. When dilated intrahepatic ducts

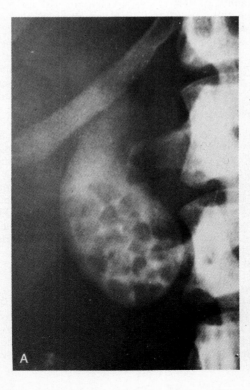
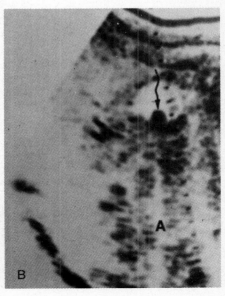

Figure 6. Filling defects. A, Oral cholecystogram showing multiple filling defects. B, Ultrasonography of gallbladder demonstrating acoustically dense filling defect (gallstone) in gallbladder (arrow) and acoustic shadowing (A). (From Berk, R. N., and Clements, A. R.: Radiology of the Gallbladder and Bile Ducts. Philadelphia, W. B. Saunders Company, 1977.)

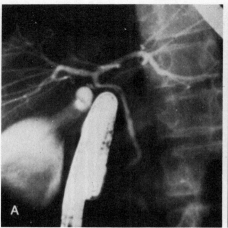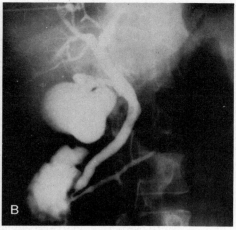

Figure 7. A, Normal endoscopic retrograde cholangiogram. (From Berk, R. N., and Clements, A. R.: Radiology of the Gallbladder and Bile Ducts. Philadelphia, W. B. Saunders Company, 1977.) B, Normal percutaneous transhepatic cholangiogram.

are identified, this establishes the diagnosis of extrahepatic cholestasis (see Obstructive Jaundice hereafter). If no dilated ducts are identified, this suggests intrahepatic cholestasis. The accuracy of ultrasonography in differentiating between intra- and extrahepatic cholestasis is dependent upon the degree and duration of biliary obstruction, but it clearly exceeds 90 per cent. What in the past often took days or weeks to determine with a lesser accuracy can now be determined with a high accuracy within minutes. Gaseous intestinal distention interferes with this investigation.

COMPUTED TOMOGRAPHY (CT SCAN)

The CT scan is very inaccurate in detecting gallstones unless they contain appreciable amounts of calcium. However, with intra-abdominal sepsis believed to be of biliary origin, the CT scan may define intrahepatic, perihepatic, or pericholecystic abscesses. The primary role of the CT scan is in older patients with obstructive jaundice. It is perhaps almost as accurate as ultrasonography in detecting dilated intrahepatic ducts but is far superior in detecting mass lesions in the region of the distal common bile duct and pancreas. However, because the test results in radiation exposure, cannot detect most gallstones, and generally is more expensive, most physicians prefer ultrasonography as the initial screening test.

ENDOSCOPIC RETROGRADE CHOLANGIOPANCREATOGRAPHY (ERCP)

This invasive test involves direct opacification of the biliary tree by endoscopic cannulation of the ampulla of Vater and retrograde injection of contrast agent (Fig. 7A). Excellent radiographs of the biliary (and pancreatic) ductal anatomy are obtained. Moreover, the endoscopist will visualize the duodenum and periampullary mucosa. Aside from pancreatic disorders, ERCP is employed in the mildly jaundiced patient or when nonobstructing lesions such as common duct stones, sclerosing cholangitis, or congenital anomalies, are suspected. The experienced endoscopist can cannulate the bile duct successfully about 90 per cent of the time. Risks of ERCP are essentially those of endoscopy and include a small added incidence of cholangitis in the partially obstructed biliary tree. It should be acknowledged that, with complete biliary obstruction, only the distal extent of the obstruction will be visualized; the anatomy of the proximal biliary tree is usually of more concern in planning surgical therapy, and, therefore, percutaneous

transhepatic cholangiography is often preferable. One advantage of ERCP is that occasionally a therapeutic endoscopic sphincterotomy can be performed simultaneously to allow spontaneous passage of common duct stones or to permit stone removal by retrograde instrumentation of the bile duct (see further). Retrograde insertion of biliary stents or endoprostheses across biliary strictures can also be performed using this endoscopic approach.

PERCUTANEOUS TRANSHEPATIC CHOLANGIOGRAPHY (PTC)

This is an invasive procedure involving percutaneous transhepatic puncture of the intrahepatic biliary ductal system using a "skinny" Chiba needle (21 gauge) and prograde injection of contrast agent. Excellent detail of biliary anatomy is obtained (Fig. 7B). Its primary use is in defining the site and etiology of obstructive jaundice in preparation for surgical intervention. In the presence of ductal dilatation, PTC is successful virtually 100 per cent of the time; without dilatation (as with sclerosing cholangitis or nonobstructing choledocholithiasis), adequate radiographs can be obtained only 60 per cent of the time. Risks of PTC include intraperitoneal bleeding or bile leak from the puncture site (1 to 3 per cent), mild cholangitis (5 to 10 per cent), hemobilia (< 1 per cent), and accidental puncture of a local viscus (gallbladder, pleural cavity).

Interventional radiologists have expanded the concept of PTC by developing a technique of therapeutic percutaneous transhepatic biliary catheterization. This technique allows nonoperative biliary decompression in patients with acute, toxic cholangitis and thus avoids emergency surgery. Percutaneous biliary drainage can be used to prepare patients with obstructive jaundice for surgery by relieving their jaundice and improving hepatic function. Moreover, these percutaneous biliary catheters can be advanced through a malignant biliary stricture into the duodenum and left in place permanently as a means of nonoperative palliation in the poor-risk patient (Fig. 8).

ARTERIOGRAPHY

As a diagnostic test, arteriography has little use in biliary tract disorders. Some surgeons have used arteriography in the preoperative evaluation of patients with biliary tract malignancies. Invasion of major arterial or portal venous structures would preclude resection and direct therapy toward nonoperative palliation via percutaneous transhepatic drainage.

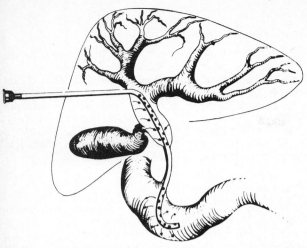

Figure 8. Percutaneous transhepatic internal biliary drainage. The biliary system has been catheterized percutaneously, and the catheter has been advanced through the common duct and into the duodenum, thus allowing prograde internal drainage of bile from the previously obstructed proximal biliary system. (From Pollack, T. W., et al.: Arch. Surg., 114:149, 1979.)

Radionuclide Studies

Technetium 99m–labeled dimethyl iminodiacetic acid (99mTc-HIDA) and parisopropyl iminodiacetic acid (Tc-PIPIDA) are gamma-emitting agents that, when given intravenously, are rapidly extracted by hepatocytes and secreted into the bile. The extrahepatic biliary tree and gallbladder can thus be visualized (Fig. 9A). Their primary use is in diagnosing acute cholecystitis. The pathogenesis of acute cholecystitis involves cystic duct obstruction. Although these radionuclides enter the bile in patients with acute cholecystitis, they do not reach the gallbladder; failure to visualize the gallbladder on scintiscan is virtually diagnostic of cystic duct obstruction (Fig. 9B). Resolution of detail is not adequate to define most other structural abnormalities of biliary anatomy.

Liver Biopsy

In suspected hepatobiliary disorders, liver biopsy can be of use in differentiating intrahepatic from extrahepatic cholestasis. Liver biopsy is not employed as a primary means of diagnosing extrahepatic cholestasis. However, in unusual instances of extrahepatic cholestasis in which ultrasonography does not identify dilated ducts (such as might occur in early obstruction or in sclerosing cholangitis), a liver biopsy might be performed presuming the patient had intrahepatic cholestasis. In such instances, the liver pathologist can usually differentiate intrahepatic and extrahepatic cholestasis. Also, liver biopsy can be helpful in a select group of patients with chronic extrahepatic obstruction because it will define the extent of secondary biliary cirrhosis.

INFLAMMATORY DISEASES OF THE GALLBLADDER

Chronic Cholecystitis

Chronic cholecystitis is the most common symptomatic disorder of the gallbladder and often precedes the development of other complications related to the gallbladder. It represents the most common indication for cholecystectomy and accounts for the majority of cholecystectomies (80 per cent) performed in this country. With approximately 500,000 cholecystectomies performed each year, chronic cholecystitis obviously represents a very prevalent and important health problem.

PATHOPHYSIOLOGY

Chronic cholecystitis is characterized by evidence of gross and histologic inflammatory changes. The gallbladder is often shrunken, scarred, and fibrotic with a thickened wall. Adhesions to the hepatic flexure of the colon or to the duodenum may be evident. Microscopically, the wall of the gallbladder shows chronic inflammatory cells and fibrosis. Rokitansky-Aschoff sinuses, buried crypts of mucosa extending deeply into the wall, are often present as well. These gross and microscopic changes are believed to be secondary to repeated episodes of inflammation.

The pathogenesis of chronic cholecystitis is believed to be related to mechanical and/or chemical irritation of the mucosa. Over 90 per cent of cases are associated with cholelithiasis. Whether gallstones represent the cause or effect remains in dispute. The most likely etiology of mucosal inflammation involves mechanical effects of gallstones, either from repeated bouts of transient cystic duct

Figure 9. A, Normal 99mTc-HIDA scan demonstrating intrahepatic ducts, gallbladder (arrow), and common duct. B, Abnormal scan without filling of gallbladder. (From Schwartz, S. I.: Principles of Surgery. New York, McGraw-Hill Book Company, 1984.)

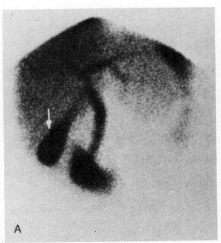

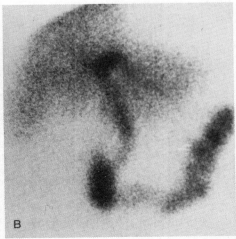

obstruction by the stones or from pressure irritation/necrosis, ulceration, and local reactionary inflammation. Primary bacterial invasion has also been suggested as an etiologic factor. About 15 per cent of the time, enteric organisms (*E. coli, Klebsiella,* enterococcus, and even *Salmonella*) can be cultured from the bile or the gallbladder wall; however, the majority of patients with chronic cholecystitis have sterile bile, and the presence of bacteria probably represents secondary invasion in the presence of inflammation. Some evidence suggests that chronic cholecystitis may in part result from mucosal irritation secondary to bile stasis or stagnation or even perhaps secondary to the presence of pancreatic enzymes that have refluxed up the biliary tree into the gallbladder from the pancreatic duct.

CLINICAL SPECTRUM

Symptomatically, biliary colic is characteristic of chronic cholecystitis. The term biliary colic is a misnomer because it is not a short-lived, cyclical acute spasm, as with intestinal colic. Rather, the pain is of a severe, persistent quality, usually in the right upper quadrant, but often epigastric or referred to the right scapular region. Nausea and vomiting often coexist. The pain is of a crescendo-descrescendo pattern, coming on slowly, lasting for several hours, and slowly relenting over about 30 minutes. It is believed related to intermittent obstruction of the gallbladder from either an obstructing stone in the cystic duct or a gallbladder packed with stones. Biliary colic occurs most commonly 1 to 2 hours postprandially, usually in the evening and almost never in the morning. Biliary colic generally does not occur at night during sleep unless a meal had been taken prior to retiring. There is a prominent relationship of biliary colic to ingestion of fatty foods in many patients (but not all), which is thought to be related to duodenal release of CCK and subsequent gallbladder contraction. The pain of biliary colic may mimic angina or may even stimulate angina; some have even postulated an association between gallbladder disease and angina. Chronic cholecystitis may be heralded by attacks of biliary colic or by a spectrum of nonspecific complaints, including dyspepsia, indigestion, bloating, and belching.

The *physical examination* is unimpressive. During an attack of biliary colic, there is often mild right upper quadrant tenderness. Between attacks, the patient is asymptomatic without any physical findings. Jaundice is absent unless a stone has passed into the common duct; fever is absent as well.

DIAGNOSIS

The differential diagnosis of chronic cholecystitis includes duodenal ulcer disease, pancreatitis, hepatitis, gastroesophageal reflux, irritable bowel disease, renal colic, and angina. The laboratory evaluation is of no help except in a negative sense to exclude hepatocellular disorders. The diagnosis should be suspected by the clinical presentation and can be confirmed easily and rapidly by identifying gallstones on ultrasonography or oral cholecystography. If gallstones are identified, further evaluation in the appropriate clinical setting is rarely necessary, i.e., barium meal, intravenous pyelogram, and so on. The radionuclide scintiscans have no place in the diagnosis of chronic cholecystitis.

TREATMENT

Medical Management

Apart from avoiding ingestion of fatty or fried foods, there is no specific medical management. Prolonged nonoperative management is associated with a 20 per cent incidence of acute cholecystitis or other serious complications. Dissolution therapy of gallstones is currently not feasible and/or practical as discussed earlier (see Gallstones). Unless there is a prohibitive anesthetic risk, all patients with symptomatic chronic cholecystitis with a reasonable life expectancy should be treated surgically.

Surgical Management

With the safety and efficacy of elective cholecystectomy, surgical therapy is appropriate for virtually all patients.[17] Only if a patient has a short life expectancy or if a coexistent severe systemic disease predisposes to a significant anesthetic risk should cholecystectomy not be performed. Operative mortality of cholecystectomy for uncomplicated chronic cholecystitis is about 0.1 per cent, representing essentially the risk of anesthesia. Even with advanced age (> 70 years), elective cholecystectomy is usually warranted when one considers the much higher mortality (increased tenfold) with an acute complication of chronic cholecystitis in this age group.[23]

Cholecystectomy is performed via a right subcostal incision (Kocher's incision) or an upper midline incision. After identifying the cystic duct and its junction with the common hepatic and common bile ducts, the cystic duct is occluded with a noncrushing ligature or vessel loop to avoid pushing a stone out into the common duct during mobilization of the gallbladder. The cystic duct should not be ligated until the gallbladder has been mobilized completely so as to avoid injury to the right hepatic or common hepatic ducts should an anomaly exist. The cystic artery should then be identified, ligated, and divided. The gallbladder is then mobilized from above downward. When the gallbladder has been dissected from the liver bed and the anatomy is absolutely clear, only then is the cystic duct ligated and divided. Many surgeons believe that intraoperative cholangiography should be performed routinely to avoid overlooking an unsuspected common duct stone, which may be present in up to 5 per cent of patients. Others contend that routine cholangiography is not necessary and that if stones are left in the absence of any clinical or laboratory evidence of choledocholithiasis they are invariably small and will pass without sequelae. The indications for common duct exploration are discussed hereafter (see Choledocholithiasis). Most surgeons leave a drain near the bed of the gallbladder to evacuate any bile that may leak from the liver surface; even this traditional practice is currently being seriously challenged as unnecessary.

The morbidity of elective cholecystectomy is minimal. The major complications include wound infection (3 per cent), intra-abdominal abscess, bile peritonitis, major bile duct injury, and serious injury to hepatic blood supply (each < 0.3 per cent).

Acute Cholecystitis

Acute cholecystitis is the most common acute complication of cholelithiasis. About 20 per cent of patients with symptomatic gallstones and chronic cholecystitis will develop acute cholecystitis during the natural history of their disease. Because this entity may progress to serious life-threatening complications, especially in the elderly, its treatment and prevention are important factors in gallstone-related disorders.

PATHOPHYSIOLOGY

Over 90 per cent of patients with acute cholecystitis harbor gallstones. The remaining patients with acalculous cholecystitis have a different pathogenesis and will be discussed separately hereafter (see Acalculous Cholecystitis). Gallstones play a major and perhaps multiple roles in the pathogenesis of acute cholecystitis; it is difficult to reproduce acute cholecystitis in laboratory animals with simple cystic duct obstruction in the absence of gallstones. The factors believed important in the pathogenesis of acute cholecystitis include (1) cystic duct obstruction with gallbladder distention and ischemia, (2) chemical (bile) and/or mechanical (gallstone) injury of the mucosa, and (3) bacterial infection. The initiating event is believed to be impaction of a gallstone in the cystic duct and interference with emptying of the gallbladder, similar to the etiology of biliary colic. However, this must be of a more complete and persistent nature because of the sequelae. Local pressure necrosis from the stone induces ulceration and inflammation. With obstruction, intraluminal pressure in the gallbladder rises, edema forms, venous outflow is impaired, and further ischemia results. Grossly, the gallbladder wall is acutely inflamed, edematous, and indurated. The degree of distention of the gallbladder depends on the amount of pre-existing fibrosis. Patchy hemorrhagic areas are evident externally and are associated with areas of local fibrinous adhesions to surrounding structures.

Mucosal ulceration and patchy necrosis within the gallbladder further stimulate and exacerbate the acute inflammation. The etiology of this mucosal injury is not fully understood. Chemical injury is believed to evolve from the interplay of increased intraluminal pressure, long-standing mucosal changes of chronic cholecystitis, and the presence of bile salts and other constituents of bile. Pancreatic enzymes or lysosomal enzymes released by the injured mucosa (such as phospholipase A) may further exacerbate the inflammatory changes by releasing the locally toxic lysolecithin. Although the inciting pathogenesis of acute calculous cholecystitis is noninfectious, secondary bacterial infection superimposed upon this milieu often occurs; enteric organisms can be cultured from the bile and wall of the gallbladder in 75 per cent of patients with acute cholecystitis. Further effects of bacterial invasion add to local and systemic sequelae.

NATURAL HISTORY

The natural history of acute cholecystitis depends on whether the obstruction is relieved, the degree of bacterial invasion, and certain host factors. Acute cholecystitis resolves spontaneously in 90 per cent; however, 4 to 6 weeks are necessary for the inflammatory changes within the gallbladder wall to resolve. Ten per cent of patients with acute cholecystitis progress to develop a serious complication. Host factors that predispose to complications include diabetes, advanced age (> 65 years), and the presence of early bacterial invasion. Complications include septicemia, abscess formation within the lumen of the gallbladder (empyema of the gallbladder), necrosis with local perforation (pericholecystic abscess), fistulization to another viscus such as the duodenum, stomach, or colon (spontaneous biliary-enteric fistula), and, very rarely, free intraperitoneal perforation (bile peritonitis). In the absence of bacterial infection, persistent obstruction leads to the so-called hydrops of the gallbladder, in which the nonfunctional gallbladder is filled with mucus or "white bile."

CLINICAL SPECTRUM

Although many patients will relate a history of biliary colic, the initial presentation of gallbladder disease with acute cholecystitis is not unusual. *Symptomatically,* the patient describes either the acute or gradual onset of epigastric or right upper quadrant pain similar to biliary colic but not necessarily related to a meal. However, the pain fails to resolve, and right upper abdominal tenderness develops. Unlike the patient with biliary colic who is restless and unable to find a comfortable position, the patient with acute cholecystitis remains still because movement exacerbates the pain. Fever, nausea, and vomiting are common. The presence of a high fever, shaking chills, or severe prostration is not common with acute cholecystitis and should suggest either another diagnosis (such as cholangitis or pyelonephritis) or the development of a serious complication of acute cholecystitis. Rarely, the elderly, diabetic, or immunosuppressed host will present with gram-negative septicemia and septic shock.

On *physical examination,* the patient appears acutely ill. Fever and tachycardia are signs of the underlying inflammatory process. The most prominent finding is the presence of right upper quadrant peritoneal signs. Characteristically, Murphy's sign represents an inspiratory arrest during right upper quadrant palpation. The gallbladder is palpable in up to one third of patients but depends on the distensibility of the gallbladder. Clinically evident jaundice is unusual. Generalized peritonitis or findings of severe sepsis must imply progression to a complication of acute cholecystitis or some other serious disease process.

DIAGNOSIS

The differential diagnosis includes other acute inflammatory disorders such as hepatitis of either viral or alcoholic type, pancreatitis, perforated duodenal ulcer, and appendicitis. Right lower lobe pneumonia, a pulmonary embolus with infarction of a segment of the right lower lobe, or a myocardial infarction may rarely present with symptoms and signs compatible with acute cholecystitis. Laboratory studies are nonspecific and reflect only the underlying inflammatory disorder. A mild leukocytosis is characteristic. The liver function tests may be elevated slightly but in a nonspecific pattern and not to the degree expected with hepatitis. The serum bilirubin may reach levels as high as 4 mg. per 100 ml. in the absence of choledocholithiasis; this is believed secondary to edema and encroachment on the common duct by the inflamed gallbladder. Chest and plain abdominal radiographs are important to exclude other serious conditions but by themselves rarely are diagnostic of acute cholecystitis unless air is noted in the gallbladder wall (emphysematous cholecystitis). The presence of radiolucent gallstones in the appropriate clinical setting would be highly suggestive.

The diagnosis of acute cholecystitis in the past was made on clinical grounds because of the lack of a reliable technique for imaging the gallbladder in an acutely ill patient. Oral cholecystography is unreliable because many other acute conditions will affect not only absorption of the contrast agent but gallbladder function. However, with the introduction of ultrasonography, the rapid, reliable diagnosis of gallstones became possible and, in the appropriate clinical setting, strongly suggests the diagnosis of acute cholecystitis. Radionuclide cholescintigraphy (^{99m}Tc-HIDA scan) demonstrates cystic duct obstruction with a high degree of accuracy in the patient with acute cholecystitis and virtually confirms the diagnosis. This is currently the most accurate test available for making the diagnosis of acute cholecystitis.

Rarely, the clinical situation may dictate use of the more invasive ERCP or PTC. In the jaundiced patient with severe underlying hepatocellular disease, the radionuclide scans are unreliable. If ultrasonography is technically unsatisfactory, these critically ill patients, in whom acute cholecystitis must be differentiated from acute hepatitis, may have to be subjected to either ERCP or PTC to exclude or confirm cystic duct obstruction.

TREATMENT

Interval Cholecystectomy

About 90 per cent of episodes of acute cholecystitis resolve spontaneously over 3 to 7 days. For this reason, some physicians continue to believe that nonoperative therapy is indicated during the acute attack. However, this will require a second hospitalization 6 weeks later for an "interval" cholecystectomy; this prolongs the period until the diseased gallbladder is removed and increases the total number of days of hospitalization and incapacitation. In some instances, an interval cholecystectomy might be desirable. If a patient develops acute cholecystitis early after a myocardial infarction or during evaluation of another acute disorder, delaying cholecystectomy might be in the patient's best interest.

Appropriate nonoperative management should include intravenous hydration, nasogastric intubation to prevent stimulation of the gallbladder and to decompress the stomach when ileus coexists, and parenteral analgesia. Antibiotics are probably unnecessary in mild cases where early clinical improvement is evident. However, with the more ill-appearing patient, most physicians believe that antibiotics are necessary. A second- or third-generation cephalosporin, or in high-risk patients a combination of an aminoglycoside, ampicillin, and either clindamicin or metronidazole, will generally cover the usual spectrum of biliary pathogens.

After resolution of the acute attack, the patient can be discharged with cholecystectomy planned 4 to 6 weeks later when the inflammation has resolved. If gallstones have not been confirmed definitely, ultrasonography or oral cholecystography should be performed during this interval. Prior to the introduction of the newer techniques to image the gallbladder acutely, "interval" cholecystectomy was the accepted management for the patient with presumed acute cholecystitis. Currently, however, this approach is indicated only infrequently.

Early Cholecystectomy

Currently, early cholecystectomy during the acute attack is considered the preferred approach. Cholecystectomy is performed only after achieving the necessary objective evidence of gallstones (ultrasonography) or cystic duct obstruction (^{99m}Tc-HIDA scan). When the patient has been adequately hydrated and parenteral antibiotics have been administered, the cholecystectomy should be performed under semielective conditions within the first 72 hours after the onset of the attack. The local edema often separates

tissue planes and facilitates the dissection. Studies evaluating early surgical therapy of acute cholecystitis have not only shown no differences in mortality or severe morbidity when compared with interval cholecystectomy but also a decrease in total hospitalization and disability time and the prevention of the 15 to 40 per cent incidence of recurrent symptoms or acute complications that occur in patients awaiting interval cholecystectomy.[13] The total cost of medical care is significantly decreased with this approach. Cholecystectomy performed more than 72 hours following the onset of symptoms may be extremely difficult for technical reasons owing to the subacute, established inflammation and severe induration, which may obscure landmarks. In these patients or in selected patients with severe compromising medical problems (CHF, COPD, and so on), an initial nonoperative approach may be the best treatment plan; the medical condition can then be optimized to allow future interval cholecystectomy under elective conditions.

Early cholecystectomy should be differentiated from emergency cholecystectomy. The presence of sepsis, high fever, or generalized peritonitis heralds a complication of acute cholecystitis such as empyema or perforation and necessitates emergency surgical intervention. Similarly, the patient who develops a mass or progressive peritonitis during observation or the elderly or diabetic patient who fails to improve rapidly must be considered to have developed a complication, and emergency cholecystectomy should be planned.

COMPLICATIONS OF ACUTE CHOLECYSTITIS

Serious complications requiring emergent surgical intervention occur in approximately 10 per cent of patients with acute cholecystitis. These acute complications are more common in the elderly, especially diabetics. The acute inflammatory process may involve a virulent, gas-forming organism (emphysematous cholecystitis) or may progress to suppuration (empyema of the gallbladder) or perforation in an area of localized gangrene. Clinically, the patient either fails to improve or visibly worsens in spite of aggressive, supportive therapy. In each case, successful treatment requires emergency surgery. If possible, cholecystectomy should be performed without delay; occasionally the patient is too sick to undergo the trauma of a general anesthetic, and tube decompression of the gallbladder (cholecystostomy) can be performed under a local anesthetic, thereby draining the area of sepsis and temporarily relieving the acute problem.

Emphysematous Cholecystitis

This is an unusual form of acute cholecystitis involving invasion with a virulent, gas-forming organism, usually a clostridial, coliform, or anaerobic streptococcal species. Unlike most forms of cholecystitis, the incidence in men outnumbers that in women 3 to 1. Diabetics are especially prone to this complication. Clinically, emphysematous cholecystitis is generally of a more sudden onset. Patients appear quite toxic with a high fever and often with a right upper quadrant mass. Diagnosis is made by abdominal radiography, which reveals air in the lumen of the gallbladder or outlining the wall of the viscus (see Fig. 5C). Because stones are absent in one third of cases, some have suggested that an ischemic etiology predisposes to a primary, bacterial cholecystitis. Free perforation occurs in 20 to 40 per cent of patients. The mortality is high and reflects both the virulence of the infection and the generally poor underlying condition of the patient.

Empyema of the Gallbladder

Local suppuration leads to an empyema (gross pus in the gallbladder) in 5 per cent of patients with acute cholecystitis. These patients may be quite ill and may present a clinical picture of an undrained source of infection. A palpable gallbladder is usually present. At surgery, the gallbladder is filled with pus; stones are virtually always present. Following cholecystectomy or cholecystostomy, recovery is usually rapid.

Perforation of the Gallbladder

Gangrenous changes within the wall of the gallbladder progress to perforation in 5 per cent of cases of acute cholecystitis. Perforation is of one of three types: (1) localized, (2) free, or (3) into a surrounding viscus. *Localized perforation* is the most common form and leads to a pericholecystic abscess. The intense acute inflammation induces adherence of surrounding organs and the omentum in the area of the inflamed gallbladder; this local reaction effectively walls off the area of perforation in the gallbladder wall. The development of a mass during treatment for acute cholecystitis should alert one to the possibility of this complication. *Free intraperitoneal perforation* is much less common. This complication occurs early in the course of acute cholecystitis, usually within the first 48 hours before local inflammatory adhesions develop. Clinically, patients may decompensate acutely with a change from localized right upper quadrant pain to generalized peritoneal signs. Depending on the extent of bacterial invasion, these patients may develop a severe, generalized bile peritonitis. Surgical intervention must be undertaken immediately. Mortality is high (20 to 40 per cent). *Spontaneous cholecystoenteric fistulas* may occur when acute inflammation of the gallbladder causes intimate serosal adherence to a surrounding hollow viscus, most commonly the duodenum or colon. Acute gangrenous changes (or chronic pressure necrosis from gallstones) eventuate in a controlled perforation into the lumen of the adherent viscus. With acute cholecystitis, decompression of the gallbladder usually leads to spontaneous resolution of the symptoms. Later complications such as gallstone ileus may occur (see Biliary-enteric Fistula later).

Acalculous Cholecystitis

Between 5 and 10 per cent of all cases of cholecystitis are not associated with gallstones. The acalculous type has a different pathogenesis from that of calculous cholecystitis and is a distinct clinical entity. Two different clinical presentations occur—chronic and acute acalculous cholecystitis.

CHRONIC ACALCULOUS CHOLECYSTITIS

This entity in many ways resembles chronic calculous cholecystitis. However, the pathogenesis differs and still is not completely understood. Intermittent cystic duct obstruction may occur from anatomic kinking of the cystic duct or, perhaps in some instances, a functional obstruction. Others have postulated an underlying chronic ischemia with reactionary inflammation or infection. Pathologically, many cases of chronic acalculous cholecystitis are classified among the hyperplastic cholecystoses. These include a spectra of benign, degenerative changes in the mucosa and submucosa that may be either the cause or the result of recurrent inflammation. Adenomyomatosis represents a spectrum of proliferative mucosal and submucosal tissues with distorted glandular elements and polyplike mucosal formations. Cholesterolosis involves areas of submucosal macrophages packed with cholesterol crystals, which, on gross examination, have a reticularlike pattern of yellow dots within the red mucosal background—the so-called strawberry gallbladder.

Clinically, the symptoms of chronic acalculous cholecystitis closely resemble those of the calculous form, except that discrete episodes of biliary colic are less common and the more nonspecific complaints predominate. Diagnosis usually requires oral cholecystography to reveal either small, mucosal-based filling defects or nonopacification of the gallbladder. Ultrasonography may show a thickened wall or suggest an area of exaggerated mucosal polyp formation, but stones will not be seen. Cholecystectomy usually relieves the symptoms.

ACUTE ACALCULOUS CHOLECYSTITIS

Acute acalculous cholecystitis occurs in a distinctly different clinical setting from acute calculous cholecystitis.[11] Several separate clinical forms have been recognized. Postoperative acute acalculous cholecystitis has been described following many procedures unrelated to the biliary tree, most commonly after major cardiac and aortic surgery or renal transplantation. Posttraumatic acute acalculous cholecystitis tends to occur in the acutely ill patients with sepsis after multiple organ trauma or major burn injury. A distinct form of acalculous cholecystitis has been described in the patient on prolonged total parenteral nutrition. In each of these forms, an element of gallbladder stasis has been incriminated, possibly from a combination of decreased oral intake, lack of endogenous release of CCK from the duodenum, and/or exacerbation by narcotic administration. Stasis may lead to overconcentration of bile, mucosal irritation, inflammation, and ischemia. Multiple blood transfusions may contribute by increasing the biliary clearance of hemoglobin pigments. The role of cystic duct obstruction in this entity is unknown. Several other forms of acalculous cholecystitis include primary Salmonella infection, an ischemic variety associated with the collagen vasculitides, and a poorly understood childhood form associated with unrelated acute illnesses.

The diagnosis of acute acalculous cholecystitis remains primarily a clinical diagnosis and requires a high index of suspicion. The patients are often acutely ill and unable to relate a good history. The physical findings are not pathognomonic and, many times, vague. An objective diagnosis is difficult to obtain. Ultrasonography may reveal a dilated, rounded gallbladder without stones or a thickened wall but with evidence of biliary "sludge"; ^{99m}Tc-HIDA scan many times will not visualize the gallbladder. Successful treatment necessitates emergent surgical intervention. The increased mortality (10 to 25 per cent) is related to delayed diagnosis, the compromised medical condition of the patient, and the increased incidence of associated complications, including perforation and complete gangrene of the gallbladder.

Choledocholithiasis (Common Duct Stones)

Ten to 15 per cent of patients undergoing cholecystectomy for gallstones will harbor stones in the common bile duct as well. Conversely, almost all patients with choledocholithiasis have concomitant gallstones in the gallbladder. The incidence of choledocholithiasis at the time of cholecystectomy increases with age, being approximately 3 per cent between the ages of 20 and 40 and increasing to 25 per cent between the ages of 60 and 80.

Common duct stones are classified as primary and secondary. The latter are far more common and reach the common duct by migrating through the cystic duct after having formed in the gallbladder. Primary stones form within the intrahepatic or extrahepatic biliary tree.

Common duct stones may pass asymptomatically into the duodenum or may remain in the biliary tree for months or even years without causing symptoms. However, choledocholithiasis is often the source of very serious problems because of the potentially life-threatening infectious and mechanical complications. Common duct stones are associated with bacterobilia in over 75 per cent of patients, and, in the presence of biliary obstruction, acute cholangitis can occur. Severe episodes of acute cholangitis can result in liver abscesses. Migration of a small gallstone through the ampulla of Vater when a common channel exists between the distal common bile duct and the pancreatic duct can result in gallstone pancreatitis. Impaction of a gallstone in the ampulla will result in obstructive jaundice. Chronic subclinical biliary obstruction may eventuate in secondary biliary cirrhosis.

The seriousness of the clinical presentation is determined by the degree and duration of biliary obstruction and the extent of secondary infection. Although choledocholithiasis is frequently asymptomatic, when symptoms do occur the biliary colic of choledocholithiasis is often indistinguishable from that of cholecystolithiasis. However, spiking fevers, chills, and jaundice suggest the presence of common duct stones and acute cholangitis. Jaundice is characteristically transient and episodic. Choledocholithiasis generally does not result in complete obstruction. Gallstone pancreatitis will be discussed hereafter.

DIAGNOSIS

The diagnosis of choledocholithiasis usually involves the differential diagnosis of jaundice. The serum bilirubin is usually less than 10 mg. per cent and may fluctuate. An elevated alkaline phosphatase level characteristically out of proportion to the liver enzymes is suggestive of extrahepatic cholestasis as opposed to intrahepatic cholestasis. Screening tests include ultrasonography and computerized tomography to detect coexistent gallstones within the gallbladder and/or intrahepatic and extrahepatic ductal dilatation. Although on occasion the diagnosis of a common duct stone may be highly suggested by the clinical presentation, many surgeons believe that an objective preoperative diagnosis is imperative to exclude other possible etiologies. This can be accomplished by percutaneous transhepatic or endoscopic retrograde cholangiography (Fig. 10). These techniques (1) exclude biliary tract or periampullary malignancies as a cause of the obstructive jaundice; (2) diagnose sclerosing cholangitis, (3) avoid the time delay of intraoperative cholangiography, and (4) produce superior radiographs to those obtained at surgery. With this approach, the surgeon can avoid discovering a tumor or an inflammatory or congenital abnormality at exploration that he may not be prepared or qualified to deal with at that time.

MANAGEMENT

The patient should be prepared for cholecystectomy and/or common duct exploration, preferably under elective conditions. In the patient who has had a previous cholecystectomy, surgery may be avoided by endoscopic sphincterotomy. This technique involves cutting the sphincter at the ampulla of Vater through an endoscope. The stones will

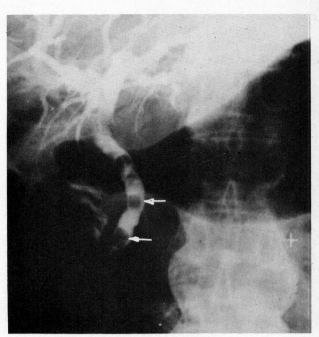

Figure 10. Cholangiogram showing multiple filling defects (gallstones) within the common bile duct (arrows).

then generally pass spontaneously. If they do not, the stones can be removed under endoscopic control using a balloon-tipped catheter or a stone-retrieving basket.

COMMON DUCT EXPLORATION

Operative mortality is increased four- to ten-fold with the addition of common duct exploration at the time of cholecystectomy. Absolute and relative indications for common duct exploration have been enumerated.[25] Absolute indications include a palpable stone in the common duct, radiographic visualization of a stone either preoperatively or intraoperatively, a significantly dilated common duct (> 15 mm.), and the presence of jaundice. In addition, if a patient is being explored as an emergency in the presence of cholangitis or gallstone pancreatitis, common duct exploration, or at least choledochal decompression with a T-tube, will be indicated. Relative indications include a mildly dilated common duct (10 to 15 mm.), a recent history of jaundice, a single faceted stone or multiple small stones in the gallbladder, and a history of cholangitis or pancreatitis. Most surgeons will perform operative cholangiography for the relative indications rather than proceeding with routine common duct exploration.

At the time of cholecystectomy, all patients should be evaluated for the possible presence of choledocholithiasis by a review of clinical parameters and liver function tests and/or by intraoperative cholangiography. In the absence of a suggestive history and in the presence of normal liver function tests, most studies have suggested that the likelihood of a common duct stone is remote. The introduction of intraoperative cholangiography via the cystic duct stump has decreased the incidence of common duct exploration from 65 to 25 per cent and has increased the incidence of a positive exploration (i.e., finding stones) from 23 to 66 per cent. This technique has proven most useful in patients with relative indications for duct exploration. Many surgeons subject all patients undergoing routine, uncomplicated cholecystectomy to intraoperative cholangiography, although choledocholithiasis is not suspected. Advocates argue that unsuspected stones are found in 5 per cent of patients. Opponents of routine intraoperative cholangiography maintain that unsuspected stones are small, remain silent, and usually pass without sequelae; the potential morbidity of common duct exploration can thus be avoided.

The biliary tree is explored through a longitudinal incision on the anterior surface of the common bile duct. Numerous common duct instruments have been developed for retrieving stones, including special forceps, scoops, irrigating catheters, and balloon-tipped catheters. Endoscopic visualization of the lumen of the biliary tree and retrieval of stones are also possible utilizing a choledochoscope. After the surgeon is satisfied that all stones have been removed, a T-tube is inserted, the duct is closed, and a completion cholangiogram is obtained through the T-tube. If stones are still present, the duct is immediately reexplored. Occasionally a stone impacted at the ampulla of Vater will prove impossible to extract from above via the choledochotomy. In this situation, a duodenotomy and sphincterotomy of the ampulla of Vater will be necessary to remove the stone.

A T-tube cholangiogram is performed 5 to 7 days postoperatively. If no stones are present, the T-tube is clamped, the patient is discharged, and the T-tube is removed 2 to 4 weeks later.

RETAINED COMMON DUCT STONES

At the time of T-tube cholangiography 1 week after surgery, retained common duct stones are found despite a normal, intraoperative completion T-tube cholangiogram in 5 to 10 per cent of patients undergoing primary choledocholithotomy. Some have suggested that the routine use of choledochoscopy may decrease this incidence. The approach to the treatment of a retained stone depends upon whether the patient is symptomatic. If the T-tube can be clamped without causing pain, fever, or an abnormality in liver function tests, the patient can be discharged. Approximately 20 per cent of stones smaller than 1 cm. will pass spontaneously, and no further treatment will be necessary; the T-tube can then be removed. If the stone(s) remains asymptomatic but is still present at 6 weeks, attempts at percutaneous instrumental removal through the now matured tract of the T-tube are warranted (Fig. 11). Under fluoroscopic control, the T-tube is removed, and a "steerable" catheter is guided into the common duct via the T-tube tract.[4] A stone basket is inserted, and the stone is captured and removed in retrograde fashion. The T-tube tract can also be instrumented with a flexible choledochoscope and the stone either removed or crushed and washed out through the ampulla under direct vision. If the T-tube tract is too small (a T-tube less than 14 French size having been used) or too circuitous (because of the course of the T-tube through the abdominal wall) to allow for instrumentation, the biliary tree can be entered percutaneously via the transhepatic approach; stones can then be crushed, washed, or extruded through the ampulla from this transhepatic approach. Successful nonoperative stone removal approaches 95 per cent without mortality or serious morbidity.

If the retained stone(s) is large (> 1 cm.) and/or symptomatic, one may not be afforded the opportunity of waiting the necessary 6 weeks for the tract to mature to allow attempts at percutaneous extraction. If the stone is a

cholesterol stone, attempts at dissolution using the cholesterol solvents sodium cholate or monooctanoin perfused into the common duct via the T-tube can be successful in 55 to 85 per cent of patients in 3 to 14 days. If stone dissolution fails, another option in the immediate postoperative period is endoscopic sphincterotomy. Following enlargement of the ampullary opening, the stone(s) will often pass spontaneously or can be removed with endoscopic techniques using stone-retrieving baskets or balloon-tipped catheters passed retrograde. Endoscopic sphincterotomy is successful in approximately 90 per cent of patients. However, it carries a 1 to 2 per cent mortality and a morbidity of 8 to 10 per cent that includes bleeding, pancreatitis, cholangitis, and duodenal perforation.

PRIMARY COMMON DUCT STONES

Primary common duct stones are gallstones that form *de novo* in the bile ducts. By convention, stones found in the common duct less than 2 years following cholecystectomy are usually considered as retained secondary stones. Primary stones are usually soft, crumbly, and "earthy." They tend to conform to the shape of the duct and are often associated with "biliary mud" or sludge. They tend to form either in lithogenic bile and have a high cholesterol content or in the presence of stasis, chronic biliary obstruction, or chronic infection and have a high content of pigment residues. Primary choledocholithiasis is prominent in the Orient and is believed to be associated with *Chonorchis silensis* or *Ascaris* infestation.

Patients with primary common duct stones usually present with jaundice and often with cholangitis. They are generally a decade older than patients with secondary common duct stones. Preoperative diagnosis may be delayed because the physician assumes that biliary stone disease is unlikely with a surgically absent gallbladder. Diagnosis generally is made by endoscopic retrograde or percutaneous transhepatic cholangiography. Often, the extrahepatic biliary tree is dilated out of proportion to the only slightly elevated serum bilirubin. The common duct may be packed with stones and sludge.

Appropriate treatment of primary choledocholithiasis differs from that of secondary common duct stones. Because stasis is believed to play a dominant role in pathogenesis,

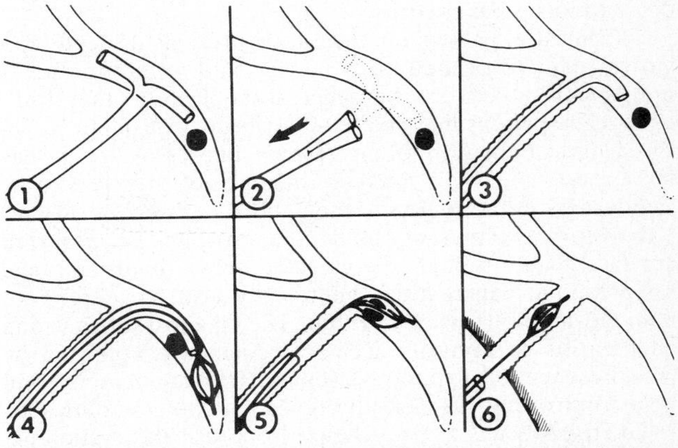

Figure 11. Percutaneous stone extraction. 1, Retained stone present after T-tube tract has matured (approximately 6 weeks). 2, T-tube removed. 3, Steerable catheter introduced into duct fluoroscopically. 4, Stone basket guided past stone. 5, Stone captured. 6, Stone extracted through T-tube tract. (From Burhenne, H. J.: Am. J. Roentgenol., 117:388, 1973.)

simple common duct exploration and removal of all stones does little to treat the underlying problem, and recurrent stone formation may follow. Transduodenal sphincteroplasty or biliary bypass via side-to-side choledochoduodenostomy or choledochojejunostomy will promote biliary drainage, prevent stasis, and allow any stones or sludge left behind (or formed in the future) to pass unimpeded by the ampullary sphincter.

Gallstone Pancreatitis

Acute pancreatitis is thought to be secondary to biliary tract disease in 25 to 75 per cent of patients depending on the patient population. In the inner city hospital, alcohol remains the most common etiology of pancreatitis, whereas in the suburban hospital gallstone pancreatitis is more prevalent. The etiology is believed to be related to the migration of a small gallstone through the ampulla of Vater. Halsted and Opie, at the turn of the century, were the first to postulate the common channel theory of gallstone pancreatitis. While performing an autopsy on a patient who had died with acute pancreatitis immediately after being operated upon by Halsted, Opie recognized a gallstone impacted at the ampulla. Halsted and Opie proposed that a stone might obstruct the "common channel" part of the distal bile duct, encourage bile reflux into the pancreatic duct, and thereby lead to pancreatitis. This theory remained in doubt for many years because only rarely was a stone found impacted at the ampulla at the time of surgery in a patient with acute pancreatitis. However, in 1974, Acosta and Ledesma[1] rekindled and confirmed the common channel theory by finding small gallstones in the stool in 34 of 36 patients with a clinical diagnosis of gallstone pancreatitis. Further support for this theory is a functional common channel at the time of intraoperative cholangiography in two thirds of patients with presumed gallstone pancreatitis but in only about 20 per cent of those patients undergoing cholecystectomy for symptomatic chronic cholecystitis. Exactly how a small gallstone migrating through this common channel causes pancreatitis is unknown. Some investigators believe that bile refluxes into the pancreatic duct and induces pancreatitis. Others believe that pancreatitis may be related to partial and transient pancreatic ductal obstruction. Interestingly, the vast majority of gallstones that become impacted in the distal bile duct and cause jaundice do not induce pancreatitis.

Clinically, gallstone pancreatitis presents as acute epigastric pain associated with nausea and vomiting and is indistinguishable from the pancreatitis of most other etiologies. The patient may relate a past history of biliary colic. Physical examination often reveals impressive epigastric tenderness, but only rarely is the patient grossly icteric. Tenderness in the region of the gallbladder may be absent. Laboratory evaluation usually demonstrates an elevated amylase level, often greatly elevated above the usual range for alcoholic pancreatitis. There may also be a transient mild elevation in serum bilirubin. The diagnosis of gallstone pancreatitis is primarily a clinical diagnosis supported by the presence of hyperamylasemia. Ultrasonography will help confirm the diagnosis by revealing cholecystolithiasis. ^{99m}Tc-HIDA scans are not helpful because the cystic duct is usually patent, and a normal examination does not exclude a biliary etiology for the pancreatitis.

TREATMENT

Treatment of gallstone pancreatitis involves initial conservative management with intravenous hydration and withholding of oral intake until symptoms subside. The timing of cholecystectomy is somewhat controversial. Classically, surgery has been delayed to allow the pancreatitis to resolve fully, and an interval cholecystectomy is performed 6 weeks later. However, many patients (up to 30 per cent) will develop recurrent symptoms during this 6-week interval. Therefore, many surgeons presently advocate early cholecystectomy after resolution of the symptoms of pancreatitis (usually within 4 to 7 days) seen during initial admission. There has been no increase in morbidity or mortality, and total hospitalization has been decreased. A few investigators have advocated immediate cholecystectomy, common duct exploration, and sphincteroplasty within 72 hours of admission for gallstone pancreatitis.[2] This course has been suggested as a means of decreasing the severity and duration of the attack of pancreatitis. Others have suggested endoscopic sphincterotomy and stone retrieval to serve the same purpose. Most studies have demonstrated, however, that in almost all instances the stone will rapidly pass spontaneously (unlike Halsted and Opie's patient), and that immediate intervention with common duct exploration is unnecessary.

Spontaneous Biliary-Enteric Fistulas and Gallstone Ileus

Biliary-enteric fistulas are spontaneously occurring communications between the biliary tree and the gastrointestinal tract. Since most of these fistulas are caused by gallstones, this entity is primarily a disease of elderly females, often in association with underlying medical disorders such as diabetes. Occasionally, gallstones will pass into the intestinal tract through the fistula and cause a mechanical small bowel obstruction (so-called gallstone ileus).[10] Internal biliary fistulas have also been recognized to communicate with viscus cavities other than the gastrointestinal tract, such as the pleura, pericardium, tracheobronchial tree, or intra-abdominal hollow viscera (bladder, uterus).

ETIOLOGY

The etiology of biliary-enteric fistulas is related primarily to gallstones, but occasionally trauma, neoplasms, or a perforating duodenal ulcer may be responsible. Gallstones may effect a biliary-enteric fistula in two ways: (1) a large stone can result in chronic pressure necrosis and erosion into adjacent bowel, or (2) an episode of acute cholecystitis can result in localized, gangrenous perforation into bowel adherent secondary to the inflammatory response. These fistulas are most common between the gallbladder and the duodenum. They may also occur between the gallbladder and the colon, stomach, or jejunum or, rarely, between the common duct and the duodenum. In the absence of distal biliary obstruction (either cystic duct obstruction or distal common bile duct obstruction), some of these fistulas may close spontaneously.

CLINICAL PRESENTATION

Clinically, patients with biliary-enteric fistulas may remain asymptomatic. Specific symptoms directly referable to the fistula, such as cholangitis or biliary obstruction, are unusual. More commonly, patients come to evaluation because of symptoms related to chronic cholecystitis, such as biliary colic. In these patients, the fistula may be recognized only incidentally at the time of cholecystectomy. Another group of patients present with symptoms of subacute, intermittent partial small bowel obstruction—gallstone ileus. It is believed that the offending intraluminal gallstone intermittently impacts and disimpacts, thus causing a so-called tumbling, partial obstruction. However, when it becomes impacted (usually in the distal ileum), it causes the clinical picture of a complete small bowel obstruction. About 30 to 50 per cent of these patients relate a past history indicative of gallbladder disease, but less than 25 per cent manifest a recent episode suggestive of acute cholecystitis.

DIAGNOSIS

The diagnosis of a biliary-enteric fistula is often not made preoperatively. The presence of air in the biliary tree (pneumobilia) or the reflux of orally ingested contrast agent into the biliary tree is virtually pathognomonic of a fistula in the absence of previous surgery on the sphincter of Oddi. The diagnosis of gallstone ileus requires a high index of suspicion and should always be entertained in the elderly patient with intestinal obstruction in the absence of previous abdominal surgery (Fig. 12). The presence of pneumobilia (40 per cent) or an ectopic gallstone (20 per cent) will confirm the diagnosis.

TREATMENT

The treatment of biliary-enteric fistulas depends on the clinical situation. When found incidentally at the time of cholecystectomy, the fistula is simply closed. When associated with cholangitis, the cholangitis is treated medically.

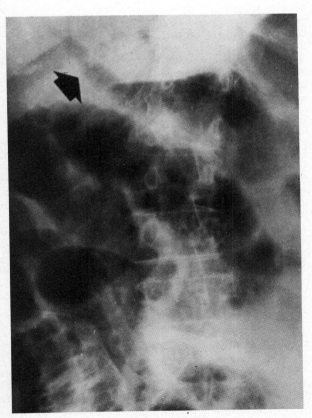

Figure 12. Gallstone ileus. Air is present in the biliary tree (arrow) in presence of dilated small bowel characteristic of small intestinal obstruction. (From Berk, R. N., and Clements, A. R.: Radiology of the Gallbladder and Bile Ducts. Philadelphia, W. B. Saunders Company, 1977.)

After resolution of the acute symptoms, preoperative evaluation for biliary pathology is then undertaken, usually via endoscopic retrograde or percutaneous transhepatic cholangiography. Definitive therapy involves cholecystectomy, closure of the fistula, and treatment of associated biliary pathology.

Treatment of gallstone ileus requires a different approach. Since most of these patients are elderly and further stressed by the pathophysiology of intestinal obstruction, appropriate therapy includes adequate preoperative rehydration. At the time of surgery, the impacted gallstone is either milked into the colon (if possible), to be passed spontaneously, or extracted by enterotomy. A diligent search for other stones proximally in the gut should be undertaken because the incidence of recurrent gallstone ileus has been as high as 5 to 9 per cent. In most elderly patients, simultaneous cholecystectomy and closure of the fistula should be postponed to a later date under elective conditions. In the younger or healthy patient, arguments can be made for simultaneous cholecystectomy or cholecystostomy with removal of any remaining stones in the gallbladder. The need for future cholecystectomy is controversial. Several groups maintain that these fistulas often close, and recurrent symptoms of gallbladder disease occur in only one third of patients; thus cholecystectomy might be deferred in these elderly patients until symptoms recur. Others have noted a small association with carcinoma of the gallbladder and a significant incidence of recurrent, serious complications of cholecystitis, and thus they advocate routine interval cholecystectomy. Treatment must be tailored to the individual patient.

INFLAMMATORY DISEASES OF THE BILE DUCTS

Acute Cholangitis

Acute cholangitis refers to an invasive bacterial infection of the biliary tree with systemic sequelae, such as bacteremia or septicemia. Classically, two forms have been described, differing only in degree of severity. Acute cholangitis, formerly termed "nonsuppurative" cholangitis, is usually associated with a partial biliary obstruction in which the biliary symptoms predominate in the symptomatology; treatment with parenteral antibiotics usually allows the cholangitis to resolve. In contrast, toxic cholangitis, in the past called "suppurative" cholangitis, is a life-threatening disease often associated with pus in a completely obstructed biliary tree. With toxic cholangitis, systemic signs of sepsis may overshadow biliary symptoms. Treatment may necessitate direct emergency biliary decompression; antibiotics alone may be unsuccessful in resolving the cholangitis and the systemic sequelae.

PATHOGENESIS

To develop cholangitis, two factors must be present: (1) the intraductal pressure in the biliary tree must be increased (partial or complete biliary obstruction), and (2) the bile must be infected. Obstruction is related to choledocholithiasis (most commonly) or a benign biliary stricture following previous biliary surgery or biliary trauma or associated with chronic pancreatitis. Less commonly, malignant strictures of the biliary tree (pancreatic carcinoma, cholangiocarcinoma) will lead to cholangitis. Unusual entities, such as sclerosing cholangitis, oriental cholangiohepatitis, and fibrosis of the sphincter of Oddi (see further), may present with cholangitis. Biliary stasis, as occurs with congenital biliary anomalies such as Caroli's disease and choledochal cysts, may also be associated with cholangitis. Not uncommonly, transient cholangitis occurs during or immediately after radiographic opacification of the biliary tree by percutaneous transhepatic, endoscopic retrograde, or T-tube cholangiography. This is thought to be secondary to a transient increase in intraductal pressure that often occurs during cholangiography.

Besides an increase in intraductal pressure, the bile must be infected. Acute cholangitis will not develop with infected bile in the absence of an increase in intraductal pressure (relative biliary obstruction) or with obstruction in the absence of infected bile. Patients may have bile colonized chronically with bacteria, but in the absence of obstruction they remain asymptomatic. For instance, following biliary-enteric bypass or sphincteroplasty, all patients have free reflux of intestinal content into the biliary tree and thus have bacterobilia, but without anastomotic stricture and obstruction, cholangitis does not develop. However, with relative biliary obstruction, pressure within the biliary tree increases above the physiologic 6 to 12 cm. H_2O and may reach 30 cm. H_2O, equaling the maximal hepatic secretory pressure. In the presence of bacterobilia, the increased biliary pressures allow reflux of bacteria into the lymphatic channels and also into the blood, probably at the hepatic sinusoids, resulting in a bacteremia. In the presence of total or near total obstruction, the infected bile may progress to gross suppuration and lead to toxic cholangitis. Liver abscesses develop in approximately 15 per cent of patients with toxic cholangitis.

CLINICAL PRESENTATION

The classic symptoms of acute cholangitis (Charcot's triad) include fever and chills, jaundice, and right upper quadrant abdominal pain or biliary colic. Although all three components of this triad usually are present some time during the course of acute cholangitis, only 50 per cent of patients will have all three at the time of admission. With toxic cholangitis, the systemic sequelae of life-threatening septicemia, such as mental obtundation, septic shock, and hypothermia, may completely overshadow the biliary symptoms. Physical examination usually reveals fever and often right-sided, upper quadrant abdominal tenderness. The tenderness, however, is often mild and may be absent. The presence of marked right upper quadrant pain, tenderness, and peritoneal signs should alert the physician to the possibility of another intra-abdominal process such as acute cholecystitis, pancreatitis, or a perforated duodenal ulcer. Clinically evident jaundice is usually, but not invariably, present. Routine laboratory evaluation reveals leukocytosis, hyperbilirubinemia, and an elevated alkaline phosphatase level. In the elderly, leukopenia may be found. The liver enzyme levels are also mildly to moderately elevated and reflect an element of secondary hepatic parenchymal injury. The serum amylase will be elevated in about one third of patients, emphasizing choledocholithiasis as the most common underlying pathology.

DIAGNOSIS

The diagnosis often requires a high index of suspicion. Acute cholangitis should always be considered in the patient with fever and jaundice, even in the absence of other findings. In this clinical setting, the presence of bacteremia is quite suggestive of cholangitis. A screening abdominal radiograph to detect air within the biliary tree should be obtained. Objective evidence of biliary pathology (stones, ductal dilatation, hepatic abscess) may be obtained with ultrasonography or computerized tomography. However, these noninvasive tests may be nondiagnostic, and a clinical diagnosis must suffice. Invasive diagnostic procedures to visualize the biliary tree (PTC, ERCP) should be postponed whenever possible until the cholangitis has resolved.

TREATMENT

Acute cholangitis in the past was considered to be a surgical emergency. However, with appropriate antibiotic therapy, most episodes of acute cholangitis can be controlled, thereby allowing diagnostic work-up after symptoms abate. Eventual surgical correction can then be undertaken under elective conditions.[19] The bacteriology of acute cholangitis is of enteric origin. Mixed infections are quite common; anaerobes are present in at least 20 per cent, and greater than 50 per cent of bile cultures yield more than one organism. *E. coli* and *Klebsiella* are the predominant gram-negative organisms. The gram-positive enterococcus is the third most commonly cultured organism. The predominant anaerobic organisms are *Bacteroides fragilis* and clostridial species. For this bacteriologic spectrum, when faced with an episode of severe sepsis, an appropriate choice of antibiotics for acute cholangitis would include an aminoglycoside or a third-generation cephalosporin, ampicillin (to cover *Enterococcus*), and clindamycin or metronidazole. With milder episodes of acute cholangitis, many physicians prefer using only a single antibiotic (a second-generation cephalosporin) such as cefoxitin.

The patient who presents with a clinical picture of toxic cholangitis and fails to improve rapidly with intravenous antibiotic administration requires emergent decompression of the obstructed biliary tree. Until recently, this meant an emergency operation to insert a T-tube. Any instrumental manipulation within the choledochus was minimized for fear of further bacteremia and the risk of a liver abscess. Hospital mortality for these critically ill patients undergoing emergency surgery is in the range of 50 per cent. Definitive surgical correction was necessarily postponed to a later date.

With the development of percutaneous, transhepatic biliary intubation and external biliary drainage, emergency surgical intervention can often be avoided. The biliary tree is intubated and decompressed, and the patient is treated aggressively with high-dose parenteral antibiotics. Definitive surgical correction can thus be postponed until the patient has recovered from the life-threatening sepsis and a satisfactory diagnostic work-up can be completed. Less commonly, emergency endoscopic sphincterotomy and endoscopic removal of common duct stones have been similarly employed to assure biliary decompression and to avoid emergency surgery. In the patient with an isolated hepatic abscess and cholangitis, percutaneous drainage can also be performed under sonographic or CT guidance.

Sclerosing Cholangitis

Sclerosing cholangitis is a chronic idiopathic disorder characterized by a progressive, obliterative inflammatory fibrosis and stricturing of the intra- and extrahepatic biliary tree.[26] This disorder demonstrates a clear male predominance (70 per cent), with the majority of patients developing symptoms before the age of 40. An association exists with inflammatory bowel disease (50 per cent), especially ulcerative colitis, chronic pancreatitis (15 per cent), and rarely with Riedel's thyroiditis, retroperitoneal/mediastinal fibrosis, and scleroderma.

PATHOLOGY

The obliterative biliary fibrosis and stricturing involve a chronic inflammatory infiltrate of the walls of the major intra- and extrahepatic bile ducts, leading to progressive thickening of the wall with obliteration of the lumen. The area of the hepatic duct bifurcation is often the site of most severe disease. This process notably spares the gallbladder, and gallstones are usually not present. Nonspecific, periportal reactive lymphadenopathy can be quite prominent. The liver biopsy is nonspecific early in the course of the disease. Later, pericholangitis or triaditis becomes evident, and bile stasis is often present. With time, changes of secondary biliary cirrhosis appear with the potential sequelae of portal hypertension, bleeding esophageal varices, and hepatic failure.

ETIOLOGY

The disorder is idiopathic without evidence of heredity. Numerous etiologies have been proposed. Perhaps the most attractive is the concept of portal vein bacteremia. Experimental evidence supporting this theory relates to work in animal models demonstrating a histologic picture of pericholangitis after portal vein bacteremia. Moreover, patients with ulcerative colitis have a high incidence (up to 25 per cent) of recurrent portal bacteremia. Chronic, recurrent bacterial infection of the biliary tree seems unlikely because bile cultures are usually sterile, and systemic symptoms of cholangitis are distinctly unusual until the patient has undergone biliary tract surgery. Thereafter, the bile is often infected and episodes of fever and chills are common. A viral etiology has been inferred from the reactive plasma lymphocytosis and local lymphadenopathy that often coexist; however, efforts to culture an agent, demonstrate viral inclusion bodies histopathologically, or transmit the disease have been unsuccessful. Recurrent trauma from choledocholithiasis is unlikely because stones are not present in most patients. An autoimmune phenomenon is another possibility despite the absence of serologic markers such as antinuclear antibody, antimitochondrial antibody, the hepatitis antigen, or characteristics of the collagen vascular disorders. The significance of increased hepatic copper levels that occur in this disorder is unknown, but they probably represent a result rather than a cause of the disorder. Although the association with inflammatory bowel disease might be expected to differentiate a subgroup, no distinguishing clinical or histologic features in these patients can be recognized.

CLINICAL PRESENTATION

Sclerosing cholangitis presents with the gradual onset of painless jaundice and pruritus. The jaundice is episodic at first, and intervals of months or even years may separate episodes. The disease is progressive, however, and eventually most, if not all, patients will develop secondary biliary cirrhosis, persistent jaundice, and hepatic failure. Despite the name sclerosing cholangitis, the presence of fever and chills, suggestive of bacterial cholangitis, is unusual in the absence of previous biliary intubation or surgery. Malaise, anorexia, and weight loss are common. As stated previously, sclerosing cholangitis is associated with inflammatory

bowel disease, primarily chronic ulcerative colitis, in approximately 50 per cent of cases and may predate the onset of symptomatic inflammatory bowel disease. Apart from the findings of jaundice, the physical examination is nonspecific. Hepatomegaly may be present. Routine laboratory investigation is indicative of extrahepatic biliary obstruction. Serum bilirubin averages 4 to 6 mg. per cent but may reach much higher levels late in the course. The alkaline phosphatase is markedly elevated and often disproportionate to the serum bilirubin. The hepatic enzymes are mildly to moderately elevated. Notably absent are the serologic markers of autoimmune disease.

DIAGNOSIS

The diagnosis of sclerosing cholangitis is one of exclusion and follows the routine approach to the jaundiced patient. The lack of dilatation of the biliary tree on screening ultrasound may delay the diagnosis. The liver biopsy may be nonspecific. The gold standard for diagnosis is cholangiography. In the past, most cholangiograms were obtained intraoperatively at the time of exploration. With the advent of percutaneous transhepatic cholangiography (PTC) and endoscopic retrograde cholangiography (ERC), the diagnosis can be made in most patients preoperatively. In spite of the biliary obstruction and jaundice, PTC may be unsuccessful owing to the characteristic lack of intrahepatic ductal dilatation secondary to ductal fibrosis; ERC is the preferred initial approach in the patient suspected of having sclerosing cholangitis.

Cholangiographically, the findings are those of diffuse intra- and extrahepatic involvement with multiple areas of stricturing, beading, and narrowing (Fig. 13). The biliary tree often has a "pruned-tree" appearance.[8] The hepatic duct bifurcation is especially prone to involvement and is the area of dominant obstruction in two thirds of patients. Although the disease may rarely be limited to either the intra- or extrahepatic ducts or to the hepatic duct bifurcation alone, the vast majority of patients (> 90 per cent) have evidence of both intra- and extrahepatic involvement. Characteristically, the intrahepatic ducts are not dilated in spite of distal obstruction; this is probably a consequence of the diffuse ductal fibrosis. Occasionally, differentiation from sclerosing cholangiocarcinoma of the biliary tree may be difficult or impossible.

TREATMENT

The natural history of sclerosing cholangitis is not well defined. The course is one of an episodic but chronically progressive disorder that terminates in biliary cirrhosis, portal hypertension, and hepatic failure. Mean survival from the time of diagnosis is approximately 5 years, but the course may occasionally be prolonged over 10 years.

Medical treatment is of unproven efficacy. Various agents have been used, including steroids, immunosuppressants, antibiotics, cholestyramine, and cholecystagogues to "thin" the bile. However, there is no objective evidence to support their use.

Surgical treatment offers potential benefit to selected patients. In the past, when the diagnosis was made at the time of exploration, a T-tube was often placed and left to external drainage for weeks, months, or even years. This treatment probably had little if any effect on the course of the disease. Moreover, such biliary intubation set the stage for superinfection in the still-obstructed biliary tree. Recently, several groups have suggested an aggressive ap-

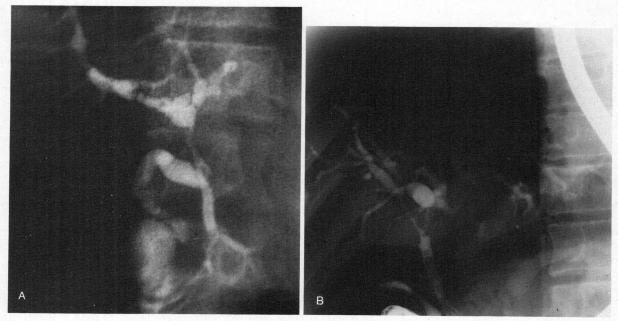

Figure 13. Sclerosing cholangitis. A, Percutaneous transhepatic cholangiogram showing diffuse intra- and extrahepatic biliary changes of sclerosing cholangitis with segmental strictures and beading. B, Endoscopic retrograde cholangiogram showing diffuse intra- and extrahepatic biliary involvement but with the most severe stricturing at the bifurcation of the hepatic duct. (From Cameron, J. L., et al.: Ann. Surg., 200:54, 1984.)

proach to the patient with an area of relatively isolated, dominant stenosis. If feasible, resection, biliary bypass, and/or insertion of transhepatic biliary stents to maintain prograde biliary drainage have yielded encouraging preliminary results.[7] Other groups adamantly avoid surgery on the biliary tree with the belief that hepatic transplantation offers the best overall approach to this disease; prior biliary surgery clearly decreases the success rate of a hepatic transplant. As experience with hepatic transplantation improves, this probably will prove the best approach. When inflammatory bowel disease coexists, resection of the involved bowel offers little if any benefit to the biliary pathology.

Oriental Cholangiohepatitis

Oriental cholangiohepatitis, also called *recurrent pyogenic cholangitis,* is a chronic, recurrent bacterial cholangitis that occurs in patients having lived in the coastal areas from Japan to Southeast Asia.[22] It is endemic in areas where parasitic infestation of the biliary tree occurs with *Clonorchis sinensis* and *Ascaris sp.* In these areas, cholangiohepatitis represents the most common cause for emergent biliary surgery and is the third most common abdominal emergency.

In contrast to gallstone disease and cholecystitis in the West, Oriental cholangiohepatitis is a primary disease not of the gallbladder but of the bile ducts. Most cases are believed to be related to ascending parasitic infestation, irritation of the biliary tree, reactionary mucosal inflammation, and secondary enteric bacterial infection. Chronic, recurrent cholangitis leads to segmental intrahepatic biliary strictures, areas of ductal ectasia, and pericholangiolar abscesses. Primary ductal stones form in both the intra- and extrahepatic tree and are the soft, muddy, pigment stones of calcium bilirubinate believed to be related to the

chronic bacterial cholangitis. Cholecystolithiasis occurs in only 15 to 20 per cent of patients, lending further support to the hypothesis that this is not a disease that occurs secondary to stone formation in the gallbladder. Indeed, ductal changes and episodes of cholangitis may occur before ductal stones have formed.

CLINICAL PRESENTATION

Clinically, patients usually present in the third or fourth decade, and, unlike gallstone disease, there is an equal sex distribution. Symptoms are primarily those of cholangitis, with fever and chills, jaundice, and prominent right upper quadrant abdominal pain. There may be a long past history of recurrent episodic pain. Pancreatitis occurs in about 1 per cent of patients, and hemobilia is not uncommon, occurring in up to 10 per cent. The laboratory findings are those of acute cholangitis. Diagnostic evaluation with ultrasonography, computerized tomography, or direct biliary visualization studies (PTC, ERC) reveals segmental ductal ectasia, strictures, intra/extrahepatic stones, and often pericholangiolar abscesses.

TREATMENT

Although antibiotics are necessary, primary treatment is surgical and is often required on an emergent basis. Surgical objectives include acute and adequate biliary drainage, removal of stones and debris, and provision of an improved communication between the common duct and the intestine, not only to promote drainage but to allow recurrent stones to pass. Surgical treatment includes cholecystectomy, common duct exploration, and either choledochoduodenostomy, sphincteroplasty, or choledochojejunostomy. It is often impossible to remove all the intrahepatic stones. With high biliary strictures at or just above the hepatic bifurcation, use of a long-term transhepatic biliary stent (see Biliary Strictures) has been suggested, to both assure prograde biliary drainage and permit percutaneous access to the intrahepatic biliary tree for future instrumental manipulation of recurrent stones or strictures. The left hepatic duct appears more susceptible to stenosis just above the hepatic bifurcation with resultant saccular cholangiectasis, multiple intrahepatic stones, and associated abscesses; left hepatic lobectomy may be justified. Recurrent symptoms and episodic cholangitis occur in 15 to 75 per cent of patients depending on the extent and severity of anatomic ductal destruction. With end-stage disease, sepsis, liver failure, or cholangiocarcinoma may occur.

BENIGN BILIARY STRICTURES

Benign strictures of the biliary tree develop after trauma or iatrogenic injury to the extrahepatic bile ducts or are found in association with chronic pancreatitis. Sclerosing cholangitis is a benign condition causing multiple segmental biliary strictures and is described separately (see Inflammatory Diseases of the Bile Ducts).

Etiology

The vast majority (95 per cent) of benign biliary strictures are iatrogenic and follow previous biliary surgery. Most occur after cholecystectomy, but occasionally biliary injury is incurred during a common duct exploration, gastric resection, or periampullary pancreatic surgery. As might be expected, the region most often injured during cholecystectomy is at or near the junction of the cystic duct with the common hepatic duct. Only about 10 per cent of iatrogenic strictures occur at or above the hepatic bifurcation. Retroduodenal and intrapancreatic choledochal injuries are most common after gastric and pancreatic surgery. Other unusual causes of benign biliary strictures include external trauma, gallstone migration or penetration, and chronic pancreatitis. Strictures from pancreatitis characteristically involve the intrapancreatic portion of the distal common duct. Reversible biliary obstruction may occur from acute pancreatitis, extrinsic pressure from a pseudocyst, or a periampullary duodenal diverticulum either acutely inflamed or filled with an enterolith and distorting the entrance of the distal common bile duct. Another cause of benign biliary stricture is stenosis of a previously performed biliary-enteric anastomosis. This may result from a technically unsatisfactory anastomosis constructed under too much tension or in the presence of severe fibrosis or ischemia. In the past, the gallbladder was used as a conduit for biliary-enteric bypass for benign disease (e.g., cholecystojejunostomy). Many of these anastomoses subsequently strictured, probably related to inflammation in the gallbladder wall; we now know that this is an unsatisfactory technique for long-term reconstruction.

Most commonly, biliary strictures follow technical mishaps during cholecystectomy. Several factors have been identified as being associated with an increased risk of ductal injury during cholecystectomy. Hemorrhage controlled by the blind application of hemostats, ligaclips, or suture ligatures may result in ductal injury. Similarly, with acute inflammation, the plane between the cystic duct and the common hepatic duct may be obscured, and dissection or ligation of what is believed to be the "cystic" duct may injure the common duct. Also, in an overzealous attempt to ligate the cystic duct flush at its insertion into the common duct, too much tension may be placed on the cystic duct, thereby tenting up the common duct and leading to the inclusion of the lateral wall of the common duct within the ligature with the subsequent development of a localized stenosis.

Probably the majority of ductal injuries occur from inadequate knowledge of the common anatomic anomalies that occur in the biliary tree and from incomplete dissection and identification of the cystic, common hepatic, and common bile ducts. The biliary stricture may develop in several ways. The bile duct may have been ligated directly, especially the common hepatic duct or the right hepatic duct when the cystic duct originates from the right hepatic ductal system. Traumatic contusion or devascularization of the duct may lead to necrosis, local inflammation, fibrosis, contraction, and subsequent cicatrix. Transection or laceration may lead to a biliary fistula, which then may heal with a stricture. Finally, the duct may be compressed extrinsically, as occurs with fibrosing chronic pancreatitis.

Clinical Presentation

About 15 per cent of iatrogenic biliary injuries are recognized immediately at the time of injury and are dealt with appropriately. More commonly, the injury goes unnoticed, often following a seemingly uncomplicated cholecystectomy. The biliary stricture or injury may present within the first few postoperative days heralded by excessive drainage of bile from the wound or the drains or by the onset of jaundice, cholangitis, or bile ascites. Biliary strictures may remain asymptomatic for several months or years, only to present later as episodic cholangitis, jaundice, hepatic abscess, biliary fistula, or, rarely, biliary cirrhosis and its sequelae of portal hypertension, bleeding esophageal varices, and hepatic failure. Physical findings may include jaundice, hepatomegaly, or a biliary-cutaneous fistula. Routine laboratory evaluation reveals hyperbilirubinemia, elevated alkaline phosphatase, mildly elevated liver enzymes, and, in the presence of cholangitis, a leukocytosis.

Diagnosis

Diagnosis requires direct radiographic visualization of the biliary tree. Percutaneous transhepatic cholangiography is generally preferred to endoscopic retrograde cholangiography. Opacification of the dilated proximal biliary tract provides the surgeon with more important and useful information than demonstrating only the distal collapsed biliary system. In addition, simultaneous percutaneous biliary intubation may be employed for biliary decompression, especially in the presence of cholangitis. Occasionally a sinogram performed through an external, biliary-cutaneous fistula will provide valuable information concerning biliary anatomy and pathology. *De novo* benign biliary strictures are extremely unusual, and although they may occur, an isolated biliary stricture found in the absence of previous surgery must be considered malignant until proven otherwise in any age group.

Treatment

If a biliary injury is manifest in the immediate postcholecystectomy period, the first priorities are to treat cholangitis and to drain any intra-abdominal bile collections or abscesses present. When the patient has been stabilized and the biliary anatomy adequately defined, the timing of definitive repair can be planned. Because of the option of temporary percutaneous transhepatic biliary drainage to decompress the obstructed biliary tree, the timing of repair of most benign strictures can be entirely elective. If a patient presents months or years after cholecystectomy with repeated bouts of cholangitis secondary to a benign stricture, surgical repair will almost always be indicated. Despite the fact that antibiotic administration might be effective in treating and/or controlling recurrent cholangitis, surgical correction is generally indicated for fear of the development of secondary biliary cirrhosis or hepatic abscess.

Nonsurgical Management

One nonoperative technique of management that has proved successful in selected patients with biliary strictures is balloon dilatation. This can be performed either via a percutaneous, transhepatic approach or endoscopically via retrograde transampullary cannulation of the biliary tree. Balloon-tipped catheters, similar to those developed for balloon angioplasty, are positioned across the stricture and forcibly inflated. Results have been most successful with strictured biliary-enteric anastomoses and less successful with *in situ* strictures within the biliary tree.

Surgical Management

The surgical techniques utilized to deal with benign biliary strictures include resection of the stricture and anastomosis of the proximal biliary segment with the distal bile duct, duodenum, or, most commonly, a Roux-en-Y jejunal loop.[6] Most surgeons feel the use of a biliary stent is also indicated. Techniques of repair as well as the prognosis vary with the site of stricture, condition of the duct and mucosa, amount of surrounding fibrosis, and the number of previous repairs.

Stricture resection and end-to-end choledochocholedochostomy (Fig. 14A) theoretically would seem to be ideal because it preserves the integrity of the distal sphincter mechanism. Although this is occasionally applicable with limited injuries to the common duct that are noted immediately at the time of injury, most established biliary strictures are not suitable for this repair for several reasons: (1) discrepancy in size between the dilated proximal obstructed duct and the distal collapsed duct, (2) inability to reapproximate the proximal and distal ductal segments without tension, and (3) a diseased, fibrosed proximal duct obviating a satisfactory mucosa-to-mucosa anastomosis. Past experience with duct-to-duct anastomoses has repeatedly proved unsatisfactory with recurrence rates over 50 per cent.

Choledochoduodenostomy (Fig. 14B) would seem a better choice since concern about size discrepancy is avoided. However, at times it is difficult to perform the anastomosis without tension; in addition, if one develops an anastomotic leak, which is common, one not only has a biliary-cutaneous fistula but also the much more serious problem of a duodenal-cutaneous fistula.

By far the best and safest approach utilizes an anastomosis between the proximal biliary segment and a defunctionalized Roux-en-Y jejunal limb. The benign stricture is excised, and the distal common duct is oversewn. Depending on the proximal extent of the stricture, the anastomosis is accomplished by an end-to-side choledochojejunostomy or hepaticojejunostomy (Fig. 14C). The proximal extent of the anastomosis has little effect on outcome provided that a relatively normal, pliable biliary duct wall is available for a tensionfree, biliary mucosa-to-intestinal mucosa anastomosis. If a satisfactory mucosa-to-mucosa anastomosis can be performed, most surgeons do not believe that long-term stenting is necessary. With the more unusual distal common duct strictures, as might be associated with chronic pancreatitis, a side-to-side choledochoduodenostomy may be possible; results are excellent.

High strictures at or near the hepatic duct bifurcation represent a problem of a different magnitude. With these strictures, the proximal common hepatic duct or the right and left hepatic ducts may be involved in severe surrounding fibrosis, and an adequate length of "normal" duct may not be available for a satisfactory mucosa-to-mucosa anastomosis. Under these conditions, an anastomotic stricture is inevitable unless the anastomotic lumen is stented on a long-term basis with a biliary stent. In the past, stents were often made of latex rubber and were fashioned as Y or T tubes. More recently, stents have been positioned transhepatically (Fig. 15A), which allows for easy future replacement on a regular basis using a modification of the Seldinger technique. In addition, the transhepatic biliary stents are made of Silastic, which allows for wound healing and maturation with a minimum of foreign body reaction. If the stent is left *in situ* for a 12-month period, scar contracture and maturation develop over the large-bore Silastic stent such that when the stent is removed later, a stable, large-lumen anastomosis is present.

Occasionally, operative dissection at the liver hilum is technically impossible because of severe inflammation and fibrosis from multiple previous attempts at surgical correction of the high biliary stricture. Often in these instances, secondary biliary cirrhosis and portal hypertension are present, making the dissection even more hazardous. In this situation, several procedures have been developed to isolate a dilated intrahepatic duct for anastomosis. The Longmire procedure (Fig. 15B) involves a distal left hepatic lobectomy and intrahepatic cholangiojejunostomy; this per

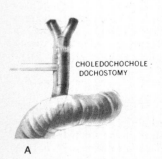

CHOLEDOCHOCHOLE-
DOCHOSTOMY

A

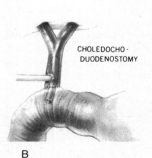

CHOLEDOCHO -
DUODENOSTOMY

B

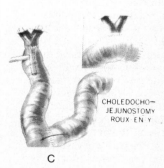

CHOLEDOCHO—
JEJUNOSTOMY
ROUX-EN-Y

C

Figure 14. Techniques used in the repair of benign biliary strictures. A, Resection of stricture with end-to-side choledochocholedochostomy. B, Resection of stricture with end-to-side choledochoduodenostomy. C, Resection of stricture with end-to-side choledochojejunostomy to a Roux-en-Y limb. Transanastomotic T-tubes are optional. (Adapted from Orloff, M. J.: The Biliary System. In Sabiston, D. C. (Ed.): Davis-Christopher Textbook of Surgery. Philadelphia, W. B. Saunders Company, 1981.)

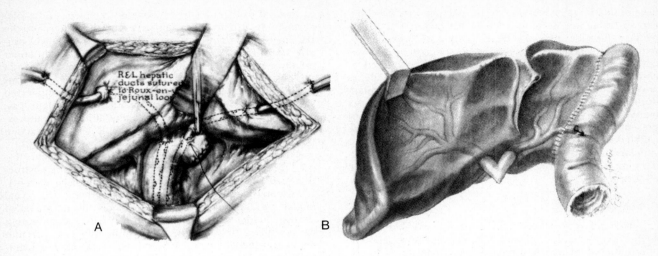

INTRAHEPATIC
CHOLANGIOJEJUNOSTOMY

Figure 15. Repair of complicated benign hilar strictures. A, Hepaticojejunostomy to a Roux-en-Y limb with a transhepatic biliary stent. (From Cameron, J. L., et al.: Surgery, 94:324, 1983.) B, Longmire procedure: distal left hepatic lobectomy with intrahepatic cholangiojejunostomy to Roux-en-Y limb. (From Orloff, M. J.: The biliary system. In Sabiston, D. C. (Ed.): Davis-Christopher Textbook of Surgery. Philadelphia, W. B. Saunders Company, 1981, Chap. 36.)

mits retrograde biliary decompression. Similarly, the anterior segment of the left hepatic duct can be isolated within the hepatic parenchyma by following the round ligament into the liver; intrahepatic cholangiojejunostomy is then performed.

SURGICAL RESULTS

Benign biliary strictures carry a formidable morbidity and mortality that vary with the complexity of the stricture. With present techniques, 80 to 90 per cent of patients experience a good result without further biliary sequelae. However, recurrent anastomotic stricture and cholangitis still recur in about 10 per cent. Operative mortality may be as high as 5 per cent with complicated hilar strictures.

NEOPLASMS OF THE BILIARY SYSTEM

Benign Neoplasms

GALLBLADDER

Benign neoplasms of the gallbladder are unusual and include polyps, adenomatous hyperplasia, adenomas, papillomas, myomas, lipomas, and fibromas. Most of these lesions are discovered as filling defects or mass lesions in patients being screened for suspected gallbladder disease. Most commonly, what appears as a *polyp* on both cholecystography and gross examination actually is not a true neoplasm but rather a mucosal projection of a localized cholesterol deposit. Microscopically, this localized form of cholesterolosis is composed of a cluster of lipid-filled macrophages. *Adenomatous hyperplasia* may represent a form of hamartoma, often called adenomyomatosis, cholecystitis glandularis proliferans, and diverticulosis of the gallbladder. This localized proliferation of the glandular elements occurs most commonly in the fundus. It extends through the submucosa but also projects into the lumen and appears as a convex indentation with central umbilication on cholecystography. True *adenomas* of the gallbladder usually appear as single pedunculated polyps. Histopathologically, they may contain papillary or nonpapillary elements. Up to 20 per cent of these adenomas may harbor a focus of carcinoma-in-situ and may behave as precursors in the development of carcinoma of the gallbladder. The relationship of these benign neoplasms to the development of symptoms suggestive of gallbladder disease is uncertain. However, with a filling defect seen on cholecystography and symptoms suggestive of gallbladder dysfunction, cholecystectomy is usually warranted.

BILE DUCT

Benign neoplasms of the bile ducts are distinctly unusual with only about 100 cases reported to date. These lesions are either cystadenomas or papillomas and usually present with jaundice or hemobilia. They are often multiple and probably reflect an underlying neoplastic tendency of the ductal epithelium. Recurrence after local excision is common, and treatment may necessitate an extended resection of the involved ductal area.

Malignant Neoplasms

CARCINOMA OF THE GALLBLADDER

Carcinoma of the gallbladder is a tumor of the elderly and predominates in women (80 per cent). Cholelithiasis is associated with over 90 per cent of cases and has been strongly implicated in the pathogenesis. The chronic mucosal irritation related to cholelithiasis and cholecystitis is believed to be important in the malignant degeneration of the mucosa. The duration of cholelithiasis is also believed to be of importance in this process. Some have used this association as an indication for routine cholecystectomy in all patients with asymptomatic as well as symptomatic gallstones. However, the risk of developing carcinoma with asymptomatic gallstones has been estimated to be 1 per cent or less in long-term follow-up (> 25 years). Carcinoma of the gallbladder may also develop in up to 15 per cent of patients with persistent nonoperated, spontaneous biliary-enteric fistulas. Again, this is believed to be related to chronic mucosal irritation. Carcinoma of the gallbladder is also associated with calcification of the wall of the gallbladder—the so-called porcelain gallbladder (see Fig. 5*B*). As many as 15 to 25 per cent of these patients at the time of presentation either harbor a simultaneous carcinoma of the gallbladder or will develop carcinoma in the future if the gallbladder is not removed. Therefore, a calcified gallbladder is an indication for cholecystectomy even in the absence of symptoms.

Pathology

The majority of carcinomas of the gallbladder are adenocarcinomas, but adenosquamous, squamous, and undifferentiated anaplastic carcinomas occur in up to 15 per cent of cases. Three types of adenocarcinoma predominate: scirrhous, papillary, and mucinous. Scirrhous carcinomas are most common and spread rapidly, with early obliteration of the lumen of the gallbladder and direct local invasion of the liver. Their surrounding fibrous reaction is characteristic. Papillary carcinomas are more slow-growing and appear as polypoid filling defects. Mucinous carcinomas are the least common and are evident by the production of a soft, gelatinous substance that fills the gallbladder.

Carcinoma of the gallbladder characteristically spreads early in its course, not only along lymphatic drainage channels to involve the periportal and periduodenal nodes but also hematogenously via the portal system to involve the liver with metastatic deposits. The tumor also spreads contiguously to directly involve the right and left anatomic lobes of the liver that comprise the bed of the gallbladder. Extension down the cystic duct, in conjunction with periportal nodal metastases, may lead to obstructive jaundice. By the time symptoms related directly to the carcinoma and not to associated gallstone disease have developed, the tumor has usually disseminated.

Clinical Presentation

Carcinoma of the gallbladder is distinctly unusual in patients below the age of 50 years. Symptoms are often indistinguishable from the cholelithiasis-cholecystitis spectrum, and, indeed, many patients are operated on with the preoperative diagnosis of chronic cholecystitis. Pain related to the carcinoma is of a more constant nature and usually lacks the episodic biliary colic so characteristic of gallstone disease. The presence of gallstones complicates the clinical picture; the preoperative symptoms in some patients are wholly, or in part, related to the gallstones and not the tumor. Weight loss is a frequent complaint; cholangitis is unusual.

By the time of presentation, over 50 per cent of patients are jaundiced. A mass in the right upper quadrant may be palpable and is often confused with the palpable gallbladder of acute cholecystitis. In the absence of jaundice, the laboratory evaluation is unremarkable. When jaundice is present, the findings are indicative of extrahepatic biliary obstruction with an elevated serum bilirubin and alkaline phosphatase; the liver enzymes are usually only slightly elevated.

Diagnosis

Because most patients carry a clinical diagnosis of gallstone disease, work-up proceeds with attention directed to the gallbladder. In the absence of jaundice, oral cholecystography usually fails to opacify the gallbladder, and the patient is prepared for surgery. Ultrasonography will usually reveal gallstones but may also distinguish a right upper quadrant mass that may or may not be distinguishable from the obstructed gallbladder of acute cholecystitis. With this finding, the astute clinician may suspect a more complicated situation, especially in an elderly patient with weight loss, a palpable right upper quadrant mass, and a clinical presentation not characteristic of acute cholecystitis to explain the palpable gallbladder.

With jaundice, the diagnostic evaluation should proceed as in any patient with suspected extrahepatic obstruction (see Diagnostic Evaluation of the Jaundiced Patient). Ultrasonography or computerized tomography will reveal dilated intrahepatic biliary ducts. A mass in the region of the gallbladder may also be apparent. Direct visualization of the biliary tree can then be accomplished by percutaneous transhepatic or endoscopic retrograde cholangiography. Most commonly, obstruction of the common hepatic duct will occur near the entrance of the cystic duct. The absence of filling of the gallbladder is suspicious of carcinoma of the gallbladder. In spite of these indirect findings suggestive of carcinoma of the gallbladder, the preoperative diagnosis is made firmly in only about 20 per cent of patients.

Treatment

When carcinoma of the gallbladder is evident preoperatively in an elderly patient with obstructive jaundice, surgery has little to offer. The patient has advanced disease, and palliation is best achieved by relieving the jaundice with placement of a percutaneous internal biliary drainage catheter. However, more commonly, the diagnosis is not made preoperatively, and the patient comes to surgical exploration. Unfortunately, few patients benefit from surgery. Radiotherapy and chemotherapy are also of little benefit.

At the time of exploration, three situations can exist. First and most frequently, advanced disseminated disease may be found with direct and metastatic liver involvement, lymphatic spread to the periportal nodes, or peritoneal metastases. The surgeon has little to offer except to attempt to relieve the jaundice by stenting the biliary obstruction if possible. Cholecystectomy offers no benefit unless local sepsis is present (pericholecystic abscesses). Operative mortality is high.

Occasionally (up to 25 per cent of patients), the carcinoma appears grossly to be localized to the area of the gallbladder. Under these circumstances, radical resection has been of some benefit in a small percentage of patients.[3] Cholecystectomy with en bloc wedge resection of the liver bordering the gallbladder bed and lymphadenectomy along the common duct from the porta hepatis to pylorus can be warranted in selected patients. Formal hepatic lobectomy affords no additional benefit to these patients.

The third situation involves the incidental discovery of carcinoma of the gallbladder either intraoperatively at the time of elective cholecystectomy for symptomatic cholelithiasis or postoperatively by pathologic examination of the resected specimen. These patients comprise the vast majority of long-term survivors with carcinoma of the gallbladder and represent a compelling justification for routine examination of the lumen of the gallbladder at the time of surgical removal. Should a small localized tumor be recognized intraoperatively, one might consider wedge resection of the liver and lymphadenectomy. If the lesion is discovered postoperatively by the pathologist, cholecystectomy alone is adequate treatment if the malignancy is localized to the mucosa and submucosa. Should the tumor extend into or through the muscularis, consideration in selected patients should be given to early reoperation for wedge resection of the liver and lymphadenectomy.

Survival

Carcinoma of the gallbladder is an aggressive disease, and extended survival is unusual. Most patients die within the first year of biliary obstruction, liver failure, and/or biliary sepsis. The 5-year survival remains less than 5 per cent; most of these patients are found only incidentally to have carcinoma of the gallbladder at the time of elective cholecystectomy for cholelithiasis. When the tumor is confined to the mucosa and submucosa, 5-year survival approaches 60 per cent.

CARCINOMA OF THE BILE DUCTS (CHOLANGIOCARCINOMA)

Malignant tumors of the bile ducts currently occur more commonly than carcinoma of the gallbladder. They are often slow growing and late to metastasize. However, they often extend into or arise in the porta hepatis and by the time of diagnosis frequently have involved local structures and thus are difficult lesions to treat surgically. Carcinoma of the biliary tree is a disease of the elderly and is somewhat more common in the male than the female. The highest incidence occurs in the Japanese, the Israelis, and the Southwestern American Indians. Its association with gallstones is of uncertain importance; concomitant cholelithiasis is present in 20 to 40 per cent of patients, but choledocholithiasis is unusual.

Certain conditions are associated with an increased incidence of cholangiocarcinoma. Patients with Oriental cholangiohepatitis are at increased risk of developing bile duct tumors as are patients with Caroli's disease or choledochal cysts who have undergone biliary-enteric anastomosis without cyst excision. Stasis leading to chronic biliary irritation, metaplasia, and subsequent malignant degeneration is believed to be the mechanism by which these patients develop cholangiocarcinoma. Recently, both chronic ulcerative colitis and polyposis coli/Gardner's syndrome have been linked to cholangiocarcinoma. Of interest is that the severity or duration of the colonic disease, the response to medical therapy, or even surgical excision of the entire colon does not appear to affect the occurrence of bile duct cancer. Moreover, in this select group, the onset of cholangiocarcinoma occurs in a much younger age group (the third and fourth decades).

Pathology

These tumors are often small and produce symptoms early by obstructing the bile duct. They can arise anywhere along the course of the biliary tree. The incidence of distal versus proximal cholangiocarcinomas varies in different centers. In some series, the majority of bile duct tumors occur in the common hepatic and proximal common bile ducts, whereas in other reports tumors arising in the porta hepatis at the bifurcation of the hepatic ducts (Klatskin tumors) have been recognized with increasing frequency and predominate in incidence. Many distal bile duct tumors have probably been overlooked as such and have been categorized as carcinomas of the head of the pancreas or ampulla of Vater.

The vast majority of these carcinomas are adenocarcinomas with varying degrees of differentiation and scirrhous reaction. Rarely, squamous cell carcinomas occur in the biliary tree and may possibly be related to the malignant degeneration of squamous metaplasia secondary to chronic irritation. Three histopathologic forms of adenocarcinoma exist. By far the most common is the scirrhous variety, which is characterized by an intense desmoplastic reaction involving the bile duct(s). This is especially common with tumors at the hepatic duct bifurcation. Tissue diagnosis is often difficult prior to resection because of the paucity of tumor cells in biopsy or cytologic specimens. The second, less common form is a diffuse medullary carcinoma. This is an especially virulent, rapidly growing tumor that extends throughout much of the extrahepatic biliary tree, filling the ducts with sheets of tumor cells. The third form is the rare papillary carcinoma. This soft, fleshy tumor extends into the biliary lumen and may exhibit multicentricity. Cholangiocarcinomas tend to metastasize to the liver and to surrounding periportal lymph nodes, but this usually occurs late in the course. Direct invasion into the portal vein, hepatic artery, and liver parenchyma is common. Cholangiocarcinomas tend to cause death not by distant metastases but by causing biliary obstruction, ultimately leading to liver failure and/or biliary sepsis.

Clinical Presentation

Malignant biliary tumors usually present with the onset of jaundice and pruritus. Initially the jaundice may fluctuate but soon becomes relentless. Weight loss and vague, nonspecific upper abdominal pain may occur; biliary colic is notably absent. Unlike gallstone disease, symptoms of cholangitis prior to biliary instrumentation are quite unusual. Physical examination is unimpressive except for icterus. There may be hepatomegaly secondary to biliary obstruction, but a palpable tumor mass is virtually never present. If the tumor occurs in the distal bile duct, a palpable gallbladder may be appreciated. Routine laboratory evaluation reveals findings of extrahepatic biliary obstruction with an elevated alkaline phosphatase and a raised serum bilirubin, often greater than 15 mg. per 100 ml., signifying complete ductal obstruction.

Diagnosis

The diagnostic evaluation should proceed along the same lines as for all patients with obstructive jaundice (see Diagnostic Evaluation of the Jaundiced Patient). The oral cholecystogram is not helpful because of the raised serum bilirubin. Ultrasonography or computerized tomography will show dilated intrahepatic biliary ducts. With proximal biliary tumors, the common hepatic and common bile ducts will not be dilated, which should immediately raise the suspicion of a Klatskin tumor. Because many of these lesions are small, a mass is usually not evident on ultrasonography or computerized tomography. Distal bile duct tumors are indistinguishable from cancer of the head of the pancreas.

The next step is direct visualization of the biliary tree. The preoperative diagnosis of cholangiocarcinoma is a radiographic diagnosis. The finding of a stricture or blockage in the biliary tree with proximal dilatation and distal collapse in the absence of prior biliary surgery is virtually pathognomonic of a biliary tumor (Fig. 16). Endoscopic retrograde cholangiography may be attempted, but if the duct is completely obstructed, the proximal extent of the biliary obstruction will remain undefined. Percutaneous transhepatic cholangiography is a better option because the proximal biliary tree will be visualized, and one will be able

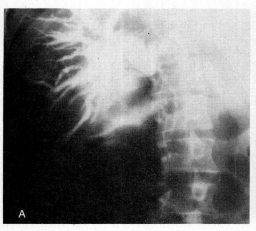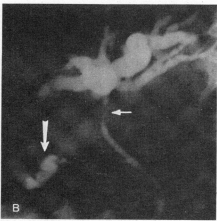

Figure 16. Carcinoma of the bile ducts. A, *Percutaneous transhepatic cholangiogram (PTC) showing complete biliary obstruction at the hepatic duct bifurcation.* B, *PTC showing narrowing of common hepatic duct (small arrow) with proximal biliary dilatation and normal distal ducts with collapsed gallbladder (large arrow). (From Broe, P., and Cameron, J. L.: Management of proximal biliary tract tumors.* In *MacLean, L. D. (Ed.): Advances in Surgery, Vol. 15. Chicago, Year Book Medical Publishers, 1981.)*

to determine whether or not the hepatic duct bifurcation is obstructed. The radiologic picture may resemble that of sclerosing cholangitis when extensive ductal involvement occurs. At the time of transhepatic cholangiography, percutaneous biliary drainage catheters can be placed to relieve the often severe jaundice in preparation for surgical intervention. Bilateral biliary drainage catheters are often necessary when the tumor is located at the hepatic bifurcation.

Preoperative attempts to obtain a tissue diagnosis are usually futile, and the preoperative diagnosis of cholangiocarcinoma depends on the radiologic picture. Recently, increased success (approximately 80 per cent) has been obtained with radiographically directed percutaneous skinny-needle biopsy techniques. Biliary cytology is only occasionally successful in demonstrating malignant cells. Some groups routinely screen patients for resectability with splanchnic arteriography to detect tumor encasement of vessels in the porta hepatis.

Treatment

Carcinoma of the bile ducts should be approached more aggressively than carcinoma of the gallbladder.[5] In the patient with obvious proximal extension of the tumor up into the hepatic parenchyma (on cholangiography), with local extension into the hepatic artery or portal vein (on angiography), or in the presence of proven metastatic disease, primary nonoperative palliation should be undertaken by insertion of percutaneous transhepatic biliary drainage catheters. However, unlike carcinoma of the gallbladder, aggressive attempts at tumor resection are warranted in many patients. Even if not fully resectable, operative palliation is excellent and can be combined with postoperative radiotherapy. Extended survival is not uncommon with residual gross and/or microscopic disease.

At the time of exploration, all gross disease should be resected whenever possible. Between 15 and 50 per cent of tumors, depending on location, prove resectable. If unresectable disease is found, palliation (relief of jaundice) should be undertaken by either proximal biliary-enteric bypass for distal ductal tumors or intraoperative biliary ductal dilatation with insertion of permanent indwelling Silastic transhepatic biliary stents for proximal biliary tumors. Biliary-enteric bypass or transhepatic biliary stents serve to maintain long-term biliary decompression and eliminate the risk of early demise of the patient from liver failure and/or biliary tract sepsis.

In the patient with localized, resectable disease, a major resection can be justified. The type of procedure varies with the location of the tumor. Distal bile duct tumors (which may be indistinguishable from carcinoma of the head of the pancreas) require a pancreaticoduodenectomy (Whipple resection). Tumors of the midportion of the common duct are managed by en bloc excision of the extrahepatic biliary tree and a proximal hepaticojejunostomy. Proximal biliary tumors at or near the hepatic duct bifurcation should be treated by resection of the extrahepatic biliary tree and the hepatic duct bifurcation. Reconstruction is accomplished with individual hepaticojejunostomies over Silastic transhepatic biliary stents to each of the major hepatic ducts. Attempts to add hepatic lobectomy to resection of a proximal biliary tumor that involves primarily the right or left hepatic duct have generally resulted in hospital mortality rates unacceptably high for a disease in which extended survival is often achievable merely by biliary intubation.

Whether the cholangiocarcinoma is resectable or not, many physicians believe that radiotherapy offers potential benefit. This can be delivered by standard external beam therapy or, if the patient has transhepatic biliary stents,[192] Iridium seeds can be passed through the stents to deliver local, high-dose irradiation directly to the region of the tumor. Chemotherapy is ineffective.

Survival

Cholangiocarcinomas are often relatively slow growing, and survivals of 2 to 3 years are achievable if biliary decompression can be performed even without curative resection. Curative resections of distal bile duct tumors yield 5-year survivals of between 30 and 40 per cent. Prolonged survival of patients following resection of proximal bile duct tumors and adjuvant radiotherapy is not as favorable but may be as high as 10 to 25 per cent. However, if the biliary obstruction can be relieved, survival is extended, and the metabolic and infective sequelae of chronic biliary obstruction are avoided.

CARCINOMA OF THE AMPULLA OF VATER

Ampullary carcinomas are uncommon malignancies. They are best considered bile duct tumors, tend to cause symptoms early, and spread primarily locally with distal metastases occurring late. They are often confused with carcinoma of the head of the pancreas because of their location; however, differentiation from pancreatic cancer is very important because of their markedly different biologic behavior.

Clinical Presentation

As many as 25 per cent of patients will describe intermittent episodes of jaundice due to tumor obstruction, tumor necrosis, and subsequent relief of the obstruction. Chills and fever, an unusual presenting feature of cancer of the head of the pancreas, is occasionally seen with ampullary cancer because of the incomplete and often intermittent nature of the biliary obstruction. Weight loss and pain are less prominent with ampullary cancer than with pancreatic cancer and may be a distinguishing feature in the jaundiced patient with a mass in the head of the pancreas. The physical examination is significant only for the rather common finding of occult blood in the stool. Laboratory evaluation is consistent with extrahepatic biliary obstruction.

Diagnosis

The diagnosis of ampullary carcinoma is often delayed for several reasons. First, these tumors may be small, and the routine screening tests (ultrasonography and computerized tomography) may fail to show a mass despite dilated biliary ducts. Second, intermittent jaundice may delay aggressive diagnostic evaluation; moreover, biliary ductal dilatation may be absent on routine screening tests. Barium swallow may reveal a duodenal mass in the region of the ampulla, but with small tumors the study is more often normal. In the absence of jaundice, both the oral cholecystogram and ultrasonogram are normal. Objective diagnosis is best obtained by gastroduodenoscopy with special attention and biopsy directed at the region of the ampulla. When jaundice is present, attempts at endoscopic retrograde cholangiography are usually unsuccessful, but the diagnosis should be suspected by visualization of the ampullary tumor mass. Percutaneous transhepatic cholangiography often reveals a pathognomonic tapered obstruction distally at the ampulla (Fig. 17) and not in the intrapancreatic portion of the common bile duct, which is characteristic of a pancreatic lesion.

Treatment and Prognosis

With the preoperative diagnosis of carcinoma of the ampulla of Vater, every attempt at curative resection should be undertaken. Even the presence of local nodal metastases within the field of resection should not discourage aggressive surgery. Although several instances of local transduodenal resection have been reported (including one by Halsted in 1899), most authorities advocate radical pancreaticoduodenectomy (Whipple resection).[24] Five-year survival is between 30 and 40 per cent.

CONGENITAL ANOMALIES OF THE BILIARY SYSTEM

Congenital anomalies are very common in the biliary tree and its vascular supply, some of which are so common as to be considered normal variants (see Anatomy). Major congenital anomalies have fascinated and challenged surgeons for decades in both their pathogenesis and treatment. These include the spectrum of biliary atresia and congenital cystic dilatation of the biliary tree.

Biliary Atresia

Biliary atresia can be considered as a spectrum of disorders ranging from segmental or generalized biliary hypoplasia and atresia to complete obliteration of intra- or extrahepatic biliary ducts. This disorder presents as persistent jaundice in the newborn; the differential diagnosis involves the often difficult distinction between biliary atresia and neonatal hepatitis related to various infectious, inflammatory, or metabolic disorders. Biliary atresia complicates approximately 1 in every 20,000 births. It affects both sexes equally and has occasionally been recognized as a familial disorder. About 25 per cent of patients have other congenital anomalies, especially those involving the cardiovascular system. (See also Chapter 33, Pediatric Surgery.)

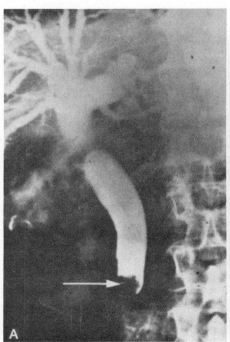
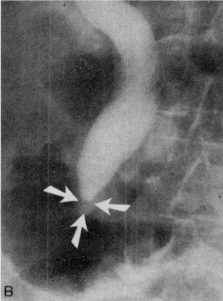

Figure 17. Carcinoma of the ampulla of Vater. A, Complete distal common bile duct obstruction with terminal filling defect (arrow). B, Distal common bile duct obstruction at ampulla (arrow) without a mass evident (patient had a small, 1-cm. obstructing tumor). (From Berk, R. N., and Clements, A. R.: Radiology of the Gallbladder and Bile Ducts. Philadelphia, W. B. Saunders Company, 1977.)

PATHOLOGY

In biliary atresia, the bile ducts are not absent but can be recognized microscopically as fibrous cords obliterated to a variable extent by surrounding fibrosis and inflammation. Biliary hypoplasia is a nonsegmental, generalized defect in which the intra- and extrahepatic biliary system, although completely patent, is small and hypoplastic. At the other extreme, biliary atresia involves an atresia of the extrahepatic bile ducts, often with complete obliteration of the lumen. Biliary atresia has been classified in the past as "correctable" and "noncorrectable" atresia. Although this nomenclature is outdated today, the so-called correctable form unfortunately accounts for only 15 per cent of cases; the proximal most extrahepatic ductal system is spared, and the atresia involves primarily the distal choledochus. Far more common is the so-called uncorrectable biliary atresia, where the atretic process involves the porta hepatis. Although the right and left hepatic ducts and the proximal common hepatic duct may appear only as obliterated remnants, microscopically patent biliary channels that communicate with the intrahepatic biliary system are usually found within this fibrous tissue and can serve as biliary conduits to allow effective biliary drainage. This more common form of biliary atresia has been further classified into three types. Type I has biliary channels of greater than 150 microns and carries the best prognosis. Type II is the most common, with the biliary channels less than 150 microns but still recognizable microscopically. Prognosis in Type II is intermediate. In Type III, no channels are recognizable, and the prognosis is dismal.

PATHOGENESIS

The pathogenesis of biliary atresia is unknown. Originally, the consensus was that this disorder represented a congenital defect of development. Embryologically the bile ducts develop from a solid anlage by vacuolization and eventual coalescence to form a lumen. An arrest at some stage in this development might lead to biliary atresia. However, recent evidence suggests that biliary atresia may be an acquired disorder involving a dynamic inflammatory process that arises peripartum and continues after birth. Some investigators have even been suggested that neonatal hepatitis, biliary atresia, and choledochal cyst may represent a spectrum of inflammatory disorders. Similarly, biliary hypoplasia, with its patent biliary tree, may not be a developmental disorder at all but rather a consequence of hepatic disorders of cholestasis and low bile flow with a resultant disuse-hypoplasia of the biliary system.

CLINICAL PRESENTATION AND DIAGNOSIS

Biliary atresia presents in the neonate. These infants are usually full-term babies of normal birth weight. They appear healthy and continue to gain weight normally over the first month. However, by the first or second week, jaundice becomes more noticeable and continues relentlessly, reaching markedly elevated levels by the second or third week. Hepatomegaly and, rarely, ascites develop. The child becomes irritable, ill-appearing, and fails to gain weight.

By this stage, the diagnostic evaluation should be well underway. The differential diagnosis involves distinguishing neonatal hepatitis from biliary atresia and choledochal cyst. This distinction is often difficult. Liver function tests usually are not helpful because they are abnormal in all groups. Ultrasonography should detect patients with choledochal cysts. Liver biopsy, although usually able to identify neonatal hepatitis, may also prove nonspecific. Radionuclide biliary excretion tests likewise may be inconclusive. The early diagnosis of biliary atresia is of considerable importance. When definitive treatment is delayed beyond 2 to 3 months, operative results are markedly worse owing to the progressive and irreversible hepatic damage prior to surgery. When differentiation of biliary atresia from neonatal hepatitis is impossible, the patient should undergo exploratory celiotomy.

TREATMENT AND PROGNOSIS

If undertaken within the first 2 months of life, surgical therapy can be expected to allow prolonged survival (? cure) in over one third of patients with biliary atresia, even in some with the so-called uncorrectable form. Exploration is performed initially through a limited incision. When a normal gallbladder is found, a cholangiogram is obtained; if normal, neonatal hepatitis is confirmed, a liver biopsy is obtained, and the procedure is terminated. However, if the cholangiogram shows an atretic proximal biliary tree or if the gallbladder is absent or atretic, biliary atresia is confirmed, and the incision is extended. In those few patients with a relatively normal proximal biliary tree ("correctable" biliary atresia), proximal bypass by hepaticojejunostomy is performed with full expectation of normal survival.

The majority of patients will have the so-called uncorrectable biliary atresia with fibrosis and obliteration of the entire extrahepatic biliary tree. In 1959, Kasai first described the procedure of portojejunostomy in an attempt to allow biliary drainage. His theory was that although no grossly recognizable ductal lumen was present, microscopic biliary channels could be recognized within the fibrous cord in the porta hepatis, and with time these channels may grow and effect adequate biliary drainage. Although there were many skeptics, his results and those of others have proven very encouraging. Many modifications have been introduced. Presently, many pediatric surgeons use a double Roux-en-Y portojejunostomy (Fig. 18), which incorporates an external vent to minimize the incidence of ascending cholangitis.[14] Prognosis for prolonged survival depends on the size of the biliary channels as mentioned previously. Currently, biliary atresia represents one of the most common indications for liver transplantation. As liver transplantation becomes safer and more widely available, this may offer the best option for selected patients with the severe form of biliary atresia.

Cystic Dilatation of the Biliary Tree

Congenital cystic dilatation of the biliary system includes a spectrum of disorders either limited to the extrahepatic biliary tree (choledochal cysts), involving primarily the intrahepatic bile ducts (Caroli's disease), or involving both intra- and extrahepatic ducts. These disorders are believed to represent congenital anomalies of biliary development and may represent the various clinical extremes in this spectrum.

CHOLEDOCHAL CYSTS

Choledochal cysts are localized or generalized saccular or fusiform dilatations of the extrahepatic biliary tree and can vary in size from 3 to 25 cm. in diameter. The walls are comprised of fibrous tissue with interspersed sparse

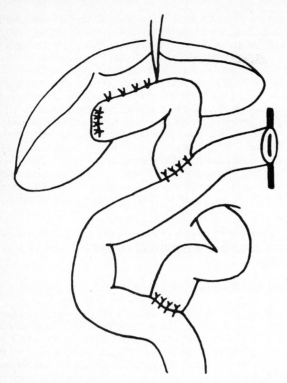

Figure 18. Double Roux-en-Y portojejunostomy for patients with biliary atresia. (From Kasai, M., et al.: World J. Surg., 2:571, 1978.)

muscle fibers. The lining is usually of a columnar epithelium, but when stasis, chronic irritation, and cholangitis coexist, no recognizable mucosal lining may be evident. The presence of coexisting gallstones is unusual. Cholan-

giocarcinoma arising from the wall of the cyst is estimated to occur in 3 to 5 per cent of patients when the cyst is left *in situ* or at the time of presentation in the adult. Sixty per cent are diagnosed in the first decade of life; occasional patients will remain asymptomatic until adulthood. Females outnumber males 4 to 1.

In recent years, an abnormal junction of the pancreatic and common bile ducts has been noted in patients with choledochal cysts. The pancreatic duct often joins the common bile duct not only more proximally than normal, resulting in a long "common channel," but also at right angles as opposed to the more normal acute angle. Some have suggested that this abnormal junction may represent the congenital abnormality in patients with choledochal cysts. Cystic dilatation in the biliary tree may actually occur secondary to this anomaly, possibly related to this long "common channel" with reflux of pancreatic digestive enzymes into the proximal biliary tree.

Classification

Numerous classifications of choledochal cysts have been proposed, but the following is the simplest and most practical. Type I cysts are by far the most common and are fusiform or saccular dilatations of the common hepatic or proximal common bile ducts or both (Fig. 19). The cystic duct often drains directly into the cyst. Type II cysts are diverticula that arise laterally from the wall of the choledochus. Type III choledochal cysts, also called choledochoceles, involve a localized dilatation of the intraduodenal portion of the common bile duct, occasionally including the orifice of the pancreatic duct. The most unusual variety in this country, Type IV, includes multiple areas of cystic dilatation along the choledochus and has been referred to as polycystic biliary disease or diverticulosis of the common duct.[15] Recent series from Japan suggest that as many as 70 per cent of patients with extrahepatic choledochal cysts

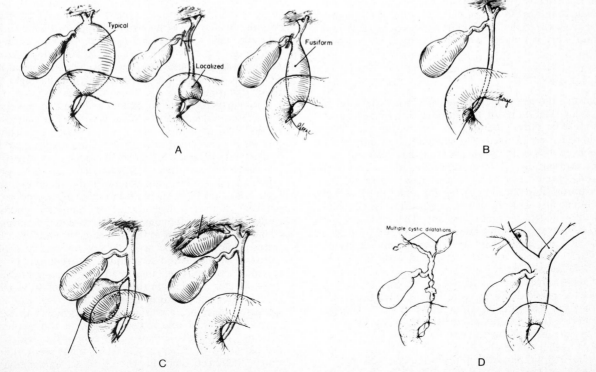

Figure 19. Choledochal cysts. A, Type I, three forms. B, Type II, two forms. C, Type III. D, Type IV, two forms. (From Longmire, W. P., Mandiola, S. A., and Gordon, H. E.: Ann. Surg., 174:711, 1971.)

have concomitant saccular or cystic dilatation of the intra-hepatic biliary tree.

Clinical Presentation

In the neonate, choledochal cysts usually present as persistent jaundice, often with a palpable right upper quadrant mass. In children and adults, a more common presentation is fever and chills (cholangitis) and jaundice. Laboratory findings are consistent with cholangitis and suggest a biliary obstructive disorder with elevated serum bilirubin and increased alkaline phosphatase. On occasion, patients may present with pancreatitis and hyperamylasemia.

Diagnosis is usually immediately evident on screening with either ultrasonography or computerized tomography. In the older child or the adult, direct biliary visualization by percutaneous transhepatic cholangiography or endoscopic retrograde cholangiography is requisite to define the proximal extent of the cystic changes and plan the appropriate surgical procedure.

Treatment

In the past, patients with choledochal cysts were treated by a cystointestinal bypass to decompress the cystic dilatation. Both cystoduodenostomy and cystojejunostomy were utilized; however, results were often unsatisfactory and were characterized by a significant incidence of anastomotic stricture and recurrent, episodic cholangitis. More recently, most authorities advocate complete excision of the cyst with restoration of biliary-intestinal continuity with a hepaticojejunostomy. This eliminates the risk of a subsequent malignancy developing in the cyst and permits biliary-enteric anastomosis to a healthy duct. Type II cysts are treated by excision of the choledochal diverticulum. Type III choledochoceles can often be treated by a long transduodenal sphincteroplasty but may on rare occasions require excision with reconstruction of both biliary and pancreatic drainage. With complete excision, the prognosis in patients with choledochal cysts is excellent, and long-term morbidity is limited to that of a biliary-enteric anastomosis.

CAROLI'S DISEASE

Caroli's disease is a congenital disorder characterized by saccular dilatations of the intrahepatic biliary ducts.[27] This should be differentiated from Oriental cholangiohepatitis, in which similar areas of ductal dilatation and stricture are believed to occur on an acquired basis secondary to parasitic infestations and recurrent cholangitis. Two forms of Caroli's disease exist. One is associated with congenital hepatic fibrosis and portal hypertension and usually presents in the infant first with the sequelae of portal hypertension. Renal tubular ectasia is also present. The more common form is not associated with hepatic fibrosis and presents in adolescents or young adults with jaundice and/or cholangitis. Caroli's disease may be associated with an extrahepatic choledochal cyst.

Diagnosis becomes evident on screening tests by the presence of marked intrahepatic biliary dilatation, often with saccules. This ductal dilatation is of an asymmetric nature and is thus differentiated from the symmetric dilatation of extrahepatic obstruction of other causes. Percutaneous transhepatic cholangiography or retrograde endoscopic cholangiography will confirm the diagnosis.

Treatment has been unsatisfactory. Episodic cholan-gitis is treated with antibiotics. Surgical therapy has usually included not only intraoperative removal of stones, sludge, and debris from the intrahepatic bile ducts but attempts to promote internal drainage of the intrahepatic tree via choledochoduodenostomy or choledochojejunostomy to a Roux-en-Y, defunctionalized limb. The results have generally been poor with recurrent cholangitis, liver failure, and death. If the disease is limited in extent to one lobe of the liver (often the left lobe), hepatic resection is indicated. Recently, several patients have been treated by insertion of bilateral Silastic transhepatic biliary stents to assure biliary decompression of the intrahepatic ducts. The results have been encouraging with less episodes of cholangitis. Patients with Caroli's disease, as are patients with choledochal cysts, are prone to develop cholangiocarcinomas.

MISCELLANEOUS DISORDERS OF THE BILIARY SYSTEM

Biliary Dyskinesia

Biliary dyskinesia remains an unusual and controversial spectrum of disorders. One form incriminates an abnormality in coordinated contraction of the gallbladder. A better documented form involves an abnormality in the motor function of the distal biliary sphincter mechanism (sphincter of Oddi) such that the flow of bile into the duodenum is impeded. This spectrum of disorders is presumably a functional disorder of motor coordination, possibly due to a denervation phenomenon with spasm or an abnormality in frequency or orchestration of phasic contractions.

Clinically, patients present with episodic biliary colic–like pain precipitated by eating. Nausea and vomiting may be present. The physical examination is unremarkable. Associated elevations of serum bilirubin and alkaline phosphatase or other objective findings are unusual. By history, these patients have rather classic biliary colic, but the routine evaluation with ultrasonography or oral cholecystography fails to reveal gallstones or gallbladder dysfunction. Even patients subjected to routine endoscopic retrograde cholangiography are found to have a normal biliary tree. These patients are often recorded as having a "functional disorder."

Nevertheless, in the patient believed to have biliary dyskinesia, objective evidence supporting the diagnosis can be obtained in several ways. After routine oral cholecystography, persistence of contrast within the gallbladder 24 hours later or failure of the gallbladder to contract by 50 per cent or more after CCK administration, with precipitation of biliary-like pain, supports the diagnosis. Cholecystectomy has been successful in relieving symptoms in 80 per cent of these selected patients. Similarly, endoscopic retrograde cholangiomanometry has revealed abnormalities of motor coordination at the sphincter of Oddi in a highly select group of patients who did not respond to cholecystectomy. Sophisticated techniques are required but have revealed a nonphasic, abnormally high basal pressure in the sphincter mechanism (basal pressures of 40 to 60 mm. Hg with normal pressures being 15 mm. Hg). Endoscopic sphincterotomy has abolished this abnormality in baseline pressure and has relieved symptoms in the majority of patients. Although there is some supportive evidence for the existence of biliary dyskinesia, many authorities are still unconvinced, and this should be an uncommon diagnosis not made hastily.

Hemobilia (Hematobilia)

Hemobilia is an uncommon condition involving an arteriobiliary fistula, i.e., arterial hemorrhage into the biliary tree.[20] Such communications might be expected because of the anatomic proximity of the hepatic arterial system and the biliary tree in their intra- and extrahepatic locations. Lesions causing hemobilia are about evenly divided between intra- and extrahepatic origin. Blunt, penetrating, or operative trauma accounts for a large percentage of cases. Central hepatic injuries with associated intrahepatic hematomas or liver lacerations closed superficially by the surgeon prior to adequate control of bleeding or adequate debridement may rupture into the biliary tree as they expand intrahepatically. An increasingly common etiology, which in many hospitals today is the most common, involves iatrogenic injury by needle biopsy of the liver, percutaneous transhepatic cholangiography, or transhepatic biliary catheterization by the interventional radiologist. Many of these injuries involve hepatic artery–portal venous fistulas that communicate with the biliary tree as well. An injury to the hepatic arterial tree unrecognized during biliary surgery may lead to a pseudoaneurysm that ruptures into the biliary system. Other primary hepatic causes include liver tumors and hepatic abscesses. Primary biliary etiologies of hemobilia include gallstone disease with mucosal or transmural erosion, hemorrhagic cholecystitis, and suppurative cholangitis, especially in Oriental cholangiohepatitis. The last common etiology includes rupture of primary hepatic arterial aneurysms into a bile duct.

Clinically, hemobilia presents with the triad of gastrointestinal bleeding (usually not massive), intermittent jaundice, and colicky right upper abdominal pain. A common setting occurs several days to several weeks following abdominal trauma with hepatic injury. Diagnosis requires a high index of suspicion. Hepatic arteriography is the best diagnostic evaluation and will show either a direct biliary communication or evidence of a hepatic artery aneurysm. Computed tomography and ultrasonography may show an intrahepatic defect (hematoma). Cholangiography often reveals irregular filling defects (blood clots) within the ducts. Upper gastrointestinal endoscopy is important to exclude the presence of other causes of hemorrhage; moreover, the endoscopist may see blood coming from the ampulla of Vater.

Treatment depends on the etiology. Hepatic lesions with significant intrahepatic hematoma require operative intervention with drainage and debridement; direct vascular ligation of the bleeding site may be required. Lobar hepatic artery ligation or even major liver resection is occasionally necessary. With biliary etiologies, ductal exploration, stone extraction, and antibiotic treatment are usually successful. Currently, experience with nonoperative angiographic embolization of bleeding sites or angiographic thrombosis of hepatic artery aneurysms has proven successful in controlling hemobilia, and either is the procedure of choice in most cases of iatrogenic hemobilia following needle biopsy or transhepatic biliary catheterizations.

Duodenal Diverticula

Duodenal diverticula are quite common and when looked for carefully can be found in up to 20 per cent of the population. These diverticula are wide-mouthed, thin-walled sacs composed of mucosa and submucosa. They occur on the medial side or inner aspect of the duodenum in intimate contact with the posterior head of the pancreas; 80 per cent occur within 2 cm. of the ampulla of Vater (so-called peri-Vaterian diverticula). The vast majority are asymptomatic. Rarely they may ulcerate and bleed, or they may become inflamed and perforate. However, in most instances symptoms result because of their adjacency to the distal common bile duct and pancreatic duct. As these diverticula fill, they are believed to extrinsically compress the distal bile duct and/or pancreatic duct, causing a partial obstruction. The patient may present with acute symptoms of upper abdominal pain accompanied on occasion by elevation of the liver function enzymes or hyperamylasemia. In addition, a duodenal diverticulum can lead to a relative, chronic biliary stasis and predispose to gallstone formation. Direct excision of the duodenal diverticulum can be hazardous because of its proximity to both the distal bile duct and the pancreatic duct. When resection is necessary, it should be done with a catheter in the common duct and with the duodenum opened so that injury to the sphincter of Oddi mechanism is avoided. If the common duct is dilated, a proximal side-to-side choledochoduodenostomy may be preferred. When cholelithiasis is present, cholecystectomy alone may result in recurrent primary common duct stones, necessitating future resection or bypass of the duodenal diverticulum.

Postcholecystectomy Syndrome

Approximately 95 per cent of patients undergoing cholecystectomy are relieved of their preoperative symptoms. In a small percentage, symptoms suggestive of biliary tract disease either persist or develop following cholecystectomy; these patients have been designated as having the "postcholecystectomy syndrome." Symptoms may be attributable to biliary disease, such as a retained stone, stricture, biliary dyskinesia, or ampullary stenosis. Others have suggested that stenosis of the pancreatic duct orifice, secondary to stone passage, is the cause. Some investigators have suggested that an abnormally long cystic duct remnant may enlarge, form stones, and cause symptoms much as does the gallbladder. It is up to the surgeon to exclude a biliary cause.

Extrabiliary disorders, such as peptic ulcer disease, gastroesophageal reflux, or the irritable bowel syndrome, may have led the patient's original complaints to be attributed to gallbladder disease. This is especially common when the symptoms were of the so-called nonspecific variety such as dyspepsia, nausea, belching, or bloating and not classic biliary colic. Many times the etiology of the patient's complaints defies explanation, and they are considered functional.

Fibrosis/Stenosis of Sphincter of Oddi and Papillitis

Some investigators believe that stenosis of the sphincter of Oddi may occur from idiopathic fibrosis or recurrent irritation/inflammation secondary to passage of common duct stones or may be directly related to surgical trauma. Papillitis is a proposed benign inflammatory and fibrous process involving the ampulla of Vater. These disorders purportedly have been associated with recurrent right upper quadrant abdominal pain and occasionally are associated with ductal dilatation, pancreatitis, and transient elevations of liver function tests. Objective evidence for these diagnoses is hard to obtain and requires either sophisticated preoperative endoscopic retrograde biliary manometry, intraoperative manometry of the sphincter, or biopsy of the ampulla. Successful results have been claimed, with relief of pain, following sphincteroplasty or biliary-enteric bypass. Whether or not these two entities actually exist is not clear, and if they do their incidence is not known.

OBSTRUCTIVE JAUNDICE

Diagnostic Evaluation of the Jaundiced Patient

Many factors must be considered when evaluating the patient who presents *de novo* with jaundice. The clinical presentation, severity of the jaundice, and patient's age are all important factors that must be considered in the initial evaluation. In addition, the liver function tests are of great value and in some instances will be diagnostic. However, in many patients the clinical and biochemical information will not be sufficient to accurately differentiate intrahepatic cholestasis (hepatocellular disease) from extrahepatic cholestasis (obstructive jaundice). Because this differentiation often dictates whether the patient will be operated upon, it must be made with absolute accuracy.

The approach to the jaundiced patient has changed markedly over the last decade with the introduction of sophisticated but readily available noninvasive diagnostic techniques. In the recent past, differentiation of intrahepatic and extrahepatic cholestasis was made solely on the basis of temporal changes in the liver function tests. Patients were often followed for several weeks while their liver function tests were monitored in an attempt to determine whether surgical intervention was indicated. Today this differentation can be made with a high degree of accuracy within 24 hours of hospital admission.[18] Patients can be screened with ultrasonography or CT scan on the day of admission (Fig. 20A). By identification of dilated intrahepatic ducts in the patient with extrahepatic cholestasis, either test can differentiate intrahepatic from extrahepatic cholestasis with an accuracy of over 90 per cent (Fig. 21). In the absence of biliary ductal dilatation, intrahepatic cholestasis (primary hepatocellular disease) is virtually assured, and a liver biopsy can be performed if indicated. With this approach, the diagnosis of obstructive jaundice can be made within 24 hours. There are two groups of patients in whom this approach may lead to an error in diagnosis: (1) those patients with acute onset of jaundice (< 3 days) who may not have had sufficient time for biliary dilatation to occur; and (2) patients with sclerosing cholangitis with obstructive jaundice in whom biliary dilatation often fails to occur because of ductal fibrosis.

Diagnostic Evaluation of Obstructive Jaundice

Once the diagnosis of obstructive jaundice is made by identifying dilated intrahepatic ducts, the next step involves identifying the level of the obstruction and the etiology. Obviously, the clinical presentation and the patient's age play a role in determining the diagnostic approach. Obstructive jaundice in the neonate or child is most likely from a congenital anomaly, whereas the threat of a malignant obstruction increases markedly in the elderly population.

INITIAL SCREENING TESTS

The initial screening tests (ultrasonography or CT scan) used to differentiate obstructive jaundice (extrahepatic cholestasis) from hepatocellular disease (intrahepatic cholestasis) also may add considerable etiologic information. In the child, the characteristic dilatation of a choledochal cyst may be evident. In the adult, the presence or absence of a pancreatic mass may determine the subsequent diagnostic approach (see Fig. 20B). For instance an elderly patient who presents with weight loss, anorexia, and obstructive jaundice and who has a large mass in the head of the pancreas and evidence of liver metastases almost certainly has carcinoma of the pancreas. This patient is not a candi-

date for curative pancreatic resection, and a nonoperative approach to treatment (percutanoeus transhepatic biliary drainage) can be undertaken after the diagnosis has been confirmed by percutaneous biopsy of the liver metastases or the pancreatic mass. In contrast, the patient with a pancreatic mass without evidence of metastatic disease and the patient without a pancreatic mass both require further diagnostic evaluation. The presence of gallstones in the gallbladder is of little diagnostic benefit in determining the etiology of obstructive jaundice; the prevalence of gallstones in the older population is well known, and although their presence makes the possibility of obstructing choledocholithiasis more likely, their presence may be coincidental.

OPACIFICATION

The next step in the diagnostic evaluation of the patient with obstructive jaundice involves direct opacification of the biliary system, either by endoscopic retrograde cholangiopancreatography (ERCP) or by percutaneous transhepatic cholangiography (PTC).[16] There are advantages to each technique. ERCP, in addition to opacifying the biliary tree, also permits simultaneous gastroduodenoscopy. This can be helpful for periampullary tumors and may afford biopsy and a tissue diagnosis. Pancreatography, when successful (85 per cent), is the most sensitive test for pancreatic cancer. Moreover, if obstructing gallstones are found, a therapeutic endoscopic sphincterotomy can be performed simultaneously in selected patients. In *incomplete* biliary obstruction (bilirubin < 5 mg. per 100 ml.), ERCP is preferred. However, with *complete* biliary obstruction (serum bilirubin > 10 mg. per 100 ml.), opacification of the proximal, dilated biliary tree will be impossible by injection of contrast from below (ERCP), and the crucial information the surgeon needs, i.e., the proximal extent of the biliary obstruction, will not be obtained. Use of PTC may be preferred not only because the proximal biliary tree will be seen but because a transhepatic biliary drainage catheter can be placed simultaneously, either for short-term decompression in preparation for surgery or for long-term palliation of the biliary obstruction in patients who are not operative candidates.

ETIOLOGY

With adequate opacification of the biliary tree, both ERCP and PTC usually provide important information as to the etiology of the biliary obstruction. The most common benign etiologies include gallstones, postoperative biliary strictures, pancreatitis, sclerosing cholangitis, and choledochal cysts. Each has its characteristic, distinguishing features. In contrast, malignant lesions are usually evident by their location and tapered appearance. Biliary tumors commonly involve the more proximal biliary tree at or near the hepatic duct bifurcation, pancreatic lesions obstruct the common bile duct in its retroduodenal portion, and ampullary, duodenal, or distal bile duct lesions are usually evident as obstructions at the distal intraduodenal common bile duct. Use of ERCP and PTC may also help to define potential resectability. For instance, with proximal biliary tumors, if the obstruction extends well up into the right and left hepatic ducts, the lesion is unresectable, and the patient should be treated nonoperatively.

The evaluation of the patient with obstructive jaundice is an orderly process that should be directed by the clinical presentation. Not all patients need *all* tests. Screening with either ultrasonography or CT scan is usually sufficient. In an older patient in whom a pancreatic malignancy is likely, the CT scan would be more appropriate since it provides a

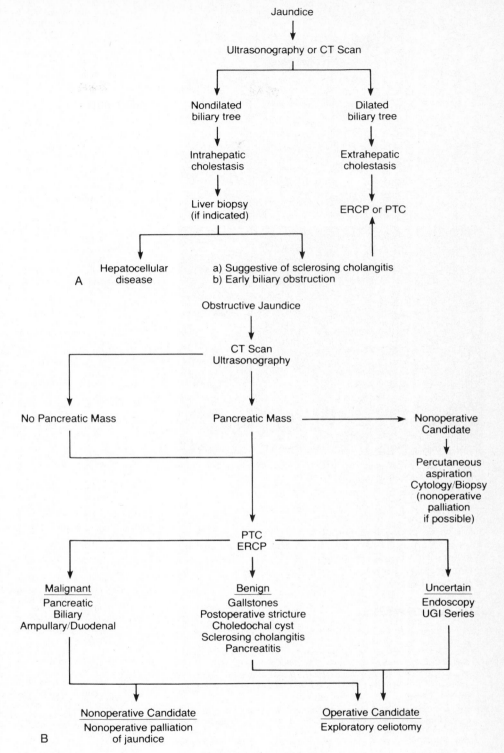

Figure 20. A, Evaluation of the jaundiced patient to differentiate hepatocellular disease from obstructive jaundice. B, Diagnosis of etiology of obstructive jaundice and approach to management in the adult.

better, more reliable image of the pancreas. In contrast, in the younger patient with a history suggestive of biliary colic, ultrasonography is preferred. Ultrasonography is less expensive than a CT, is without risk, and is far superior to the CT scan in detecting gallstones. Preoperative cholangiography is indicated in virtually all patients with obstructive jaundice, even when the diagnosis of choledocholithiasis seems evident. The risks of cholangiography are minimal, and this approach will almost always provide an accurate diagnosis. This approach avoids the possibility of

exploring a patient with a presumed benign etiology and finding another condition that might require a high-risk, major resection for appropriate treatment. In the patient with a periampullary malignancy evident on CT scan and PTC, no further evaluation may be needed. Routine use of gastroduodenoscopy, ERCP, or upper gastrointestinal series may be unnecessary, as these tests may add no additional information that will affect therapy.

Thus, diagnosis of biliary obstruction can be made with a high degree of accuracy within hours of admission, and

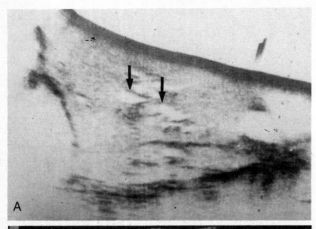

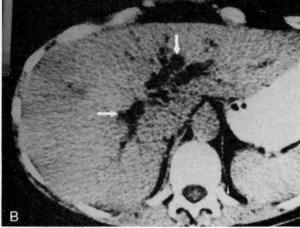

Figure 21. Obstructive jaundice with dilated intrahepatic bile ducts (arrows). A, Ultrasonography. B, CT scan.

cholangiography can define the site and etiology of the obstruction the following day. Just a decade ago the diagnostic work-up of jaundice took days, even weeks, and was often inaccurate. Today virtually all patients with obstructive jaundice coming to surgery do so with the surgeon having accurate knowledge as to the exact site and cause of the jaundice.

SELECTED REFERENCES

Blitzer, B. L., and Boyer, J. L.: Cellular mechanisms of bile formation. Gastroenterology, 82:346, 1982.
The authors are pre-eminent investigators in the field of bile physiology. This discussion centers on state-of-the-art cellular and subcellular mechanisms of bile acid–dependent and bile acid–independent biliary secretion. The article focuses on the physiology of bile production without discussing pathophysiology.

Broe, P., and Cameron, J. L.: Management of proximal biliary tract tumors. *In* MacLean, L. D. (Ed.): Advances in Surgery, Vol. 15. Chicago, Year Book Medical Publishers, 1981.
This article reviews the diagnosis and management of proximal biliary tract malignancies. These tumors require complicated biliary reconstructions at the porta hepatis. Options in operative techniques are well described with emphasis on transhepatic biliary stents.

Matolo, N. M., LaMorte, W. W., and Wolfe, B. M.: Acute and chronic cholecystitis. Surg. Clin. North Am., 61:875, 1981.
This reference concentrates on the pathogenesis of acute and chronic cholecystitis with a brief but concise discussion of diagnosis and treatment options.

Shaffer, E. A., and Small, D. M.: Gallstone disease: Pathogenesis and management. Curr. Probl. Surg., 13(7):1, 1976.
The differences between cholesterol and pigment stones and the underlying factors predisposing to stone formation are amply discussed. The primary emphasis centers on cholesterol stone formation.

Tompkins, R. K., and Pitt, H. A.: Surgical management of benign lesions of the bile ducts. Curr. Probl. Surg., 19:321, 1982.
The authors are well known in the field of biliary surgery. They present a concise but in-depth review of the diagnosis, preoperative preparation, and operative techniques employed in the treatment of lesions or conditions involving primarily the bile ducts, such as choledocholithiasis, cholangitis, biliary strictures, and selected congenital lesions.

References

1. Acosta, J. M., and Ledesma, C. L.: Gallstone migration as a cause of acute pancreatitis. N. Engl. J. Med., 290:484, 1974.
2. Acosta, J. M., Pellegrini, C. A., and Skinner, D. B.: Etiology and pathogenesis of acute biliary pancreatitis. Surgery, 88:118, 1980.
3. Adson, M. A.: Carcinoma of the gallbladder. Surg. Clin. North Am., 53:1203, 1973.
4. Burhenne, H. J.: Non-operative retained biliary tract stone extraction: A new roentgenologic technique. Am. J. Roentgenol., 117:388, 1973.
5. Cameron, J. L., Broe, P., and Zuidema, G. D.: Proximal bile duct tumors: Surgical management with silastic transhepatic biliary stents. Ann. Surg., 196:412, 1982.
6. Cameron, J. L., Gaylor, B. W., and Zuidema, G. D.: The use of Silastic transhepatic stents in benign and malignant biliary strictures. Ann. Surg., 188:552, 1978.
7. Cameron, J. L., Gaylor, B. W., Herlong, H. F., and Maddrey, W. C.: Sclerosing cholangitis: Biliary reconstruction with Silastic transhepatic stents. Surgery, 94:324, 1983.
8. Cameron, J. L., Gaylor, B. W., Sanfey, H., Milligan, F., Kaufman, S., Maddrey, W. C., and Herlong, H. F.: Sclerosing cholangitis: Anatomic distribution of obstructive lesions. Ann. Surg., 200:54, 1984.
9. Comfort, M. W., Gray, H. K., and Wilson, J. M.: The silent gallstone: A 10- to 20-year follow-up study of 112 cases. Ann. Surg., 128:931, 1948.
10. Day, E. A., and Marks, C.: Gallstone ileus: Review of the literature and presentation of 34 new cases. Am. J. Surg., 129:552, 1975.
11. Glenn, F., and Becker, G. G.: Acute acalculous cholecystitis: An increasing entity. Ann. Surg., 195:131, 1982.
12. Gracie, W. A., and Ransohoff, D. F.: The natural history of silent gallstones: The innocent gallstone is not a myth. N. Engl. J. Med., 307:798, 1982.
13. Jarvinen, H. J., and Hastbacka, J.: Early cholecystectomy for acute cholecystitis: A prospective randomized study. Ann. Surg., 191:501, 1980.
14. Kasai, M., Suzuki, H., Ohashi, E., Ohi, R., Chiba, T., and Okamato, A.: Technique and results of operative management of biliary atresia. World J. Surg., 2:571, 1978.
15. Longmire, W. P., Jr., Mandiola, S. A., and Gordon, H. E.: Congenital cystic disease of the liver and biliary system. Ann. Surg., 174:711, 1971.
16. Matzen, P., Haubeck, A., Holst-Christensen, J., Lejerstofte, J., and Juhl, E.: Accuracy of direct cholangiography by endoscopic or transhepatic route in jaundice—a prospective study. Gastroenterology, 81:237, 1981.
17. McSherry, C. K., and Glenn, F.: The incidence and causes of death following surgery for nonmalignant biliary tract disease. Ann. Surg., 191:271, 1980.
18. O'Connor, K. W., Snodgrass, P. J., Swonder, J. E., Mahoney, S., Burt, R., Cockerill, E. M., and Lumeng, L.: A blinded prospective study comparing four current non-invasive approaches in the differential diagnosis of medical versus surgical jaundice. Gastroenterology, 84:1498, 1983.
19. Saharia, P. C., and Cameron, J. L.: Clinical management of acute cholangitis. Surg. Gynecol. Obstet., 142:369, 1976.
20. Sandblom, P.: Hemobilia. Surg. Clin. North Am., 53:1191, 1973.
21. Schoenfield, L. J., and Lachin, J. M.: Chenodiol (chenodeoxycholic acid) for dissolution of gallstones: The national cooperative gallstone study. A controlled trial of efficacy and safety. Ann. Intern. Med., 95:257, 1981.
22. Seel, D. J., and Park, Y. K.: Oriental infestational cholangitis. Am. J. Surg., 146:366, 1983.
23. Sullivan, D. M., Hood, T. R., and Griffen, W. O., Jr.: Biliary tract surgery in the elderly. Am. J. Surg., 143:218, 1982.
24. Walsh, D. B., Eckhauser, F. E., Cronenwett, J. L., Turcotte, J. G., and Lindenauer, S. M.: Adenocarcinoma of the ampulla of Vater: Diagnosis and treatment. Ann. Surg., 195:152, 1982.
25. Way, L. W., Admirand, W. H., and Dunphy, J. E.: Management of choledocholithiasis. Ann. Surg., 176:347, 1972.
26. Weisner, R. H., and LaRusso, N. F.: Clinicopathologic features of the syndrome of primary sclerosing cholangitis. Gastroenterology, 79:200, 1980.
27. Witlin, L. T., Gadacz, T. R., Zuidema, G. D., and Kridelbaugh, W. W.: Transhepatic decompression of the biliary tree in Caroli's disease. Surgery, 91:205, 1982.

THE PANCREAS

DANA K. ANDERSEN, M.D.

29

ANATOMY AND HISTOLOGY

The pancreas is a soft, yellowish, fleshy (Greek: *pan*—all; *kreas*—flesh), finely lobulated organ that lies behind the posterior peritoneal membrane and extends from the concavity of the duodenum to the hilum of the spleen at the level of the second lumbar vertebra (Fig. 1). It is generally 15 to 20 cm. in length and weighs from 75 to 100 gm. The regions of the pancreas are described as the *head* (and uncinate process), which is bordered by the duodenal C-loop; the *neck*, which overlies the superior mesenteric vessels; and the remaining distal portion of the gland, which is divided into the *body* and *tail*. The head is the thickest part of the organ (3 to 3.5 cm.), and the gland tapers progressively toward the tail. The neck, therefore, divides the pancreas into sections of approximately equal mass.

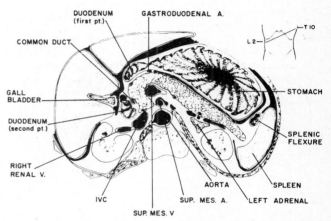

Figure 2. Cross-sectional relationship of the pancreas to other abdominal structures in an oblique plane through the long axis of the pancreas extending from the level of L2 on the right to T10 on the left. (From Mackie, C. R., and Moossa, A. R.: Surgical anatomy of the pancreas. In Moossa, A. R. (Ed.): Tumors of the Pancreas. Baltimore, Williams & Wilkins, 1980.)

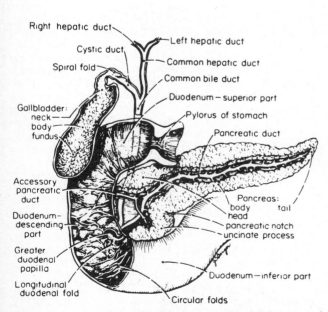

Figure 1. Relationship of the pancreas to the duodenum and extrahepatic biliary system. (From Woodburne, R. T.: Essentials of Human Anatomy. New York, Oxford University Press, 1973.)

Relationship to Other Structures

The peritoneum covering the neck, body, and tail forms the posterior floor of the lesser sac; anterior to these regions lies the posterior wall of the stomach (Fig. 2). Behind the pancreatic head are the inferior vena cava, the renal veins, and the right renal artery. The medial portion of the uncinate process lies just anterior to the aorta, below the origin of the superior mesenteric artery. The body of the pancreas lies just anterior to the left adrenal gland, and the tail ends in the lower splenic hilar area. Whereas the splenic artery is usually slightly superior to the posterior surface of the pancreatic body and tail, the splenic vein generally lies within an actual groove along this posterior surface of the gland and receives many delicate pancreatic branches.

The common bile duct descends behind the upper duodenum, then passes into the posterior surface of the pancreatic head before ending jointly with the main pancreatic duct at the ampulla of Vater in the medial wall of the duodenum. The complexity of these anatomic relation-

587

ships indicates how pancreatic disorders may easily involve other organ systems and how trauma or manipulation of these adjacent structures may easily result in pancreatic injury.

Surgical Anatomy

EMBRYOLOGY

During early fetal development, the pancreas originates from two primordial structures, a *ventral* bud or outpouching arising from the hepatic diverticulum, and a *dorsal* portion arising directly from the developing duodenum (Fig. 3). At about the fifth week of life, the ventral pancreatic bud and biliary duct rotate clockwise behind the duodenum until the ventral structures fuse with the dorsal pancreatic tissue. Each of these pancreatic structures contains ductular elements. As the ventral portion forms the head and uncinate process of the gland, its duct becomes the duct of Wirsung, or main pancreatic duct. This duct fuses with the ductular portion of the dorsal portion and usually becomes the predominant ductular system for the entire gland. The proximal duct of the dorsal portion becomes the duct of Santorini, or lesser duct, and usually persists, complete with a lesser or accessory papilla lying just proximal to the main papilla of Vater. The separate embryologic origins of the pancreatic head and body are reflected in certain anatomic and functional properties of the endocrine elements of the gland. Abnormalities in the proper rotation or fusion of the developing pancreas may result in specific congenital disorders, which are reviewed later.

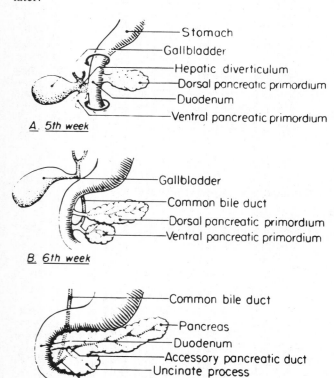

A. 5th week

— Stomach
— Gallbladder
— Hepatic diverticulum
— Dorsal pancreatic primordium
— Duodenum
— Ventral pancreatic primordium

B. 6th week

— Gallbladder
— Common bile duct
— Dorsal pancreatic primordium
— Ventral pancreatic primordium

C. 7th week

— Common bile duct
— Pancreas
— Duodenum
— Accessory pancreatic duct
— Uncinate process
— Pancreatic duct

Figure 3. Embryologic development and fusion of the dorsal and ventral portions of the pancreas. (From Woodburne, R. T.: Essentials of Human Anatomy. New York, Oxford University Press, 1973.)

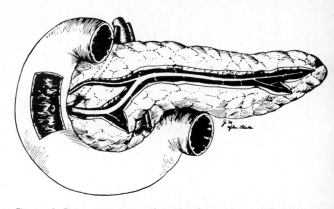

Figure 4. Pancreatic ducts, showing the major papilla (of Vater) draining the duct of Wirsung and the common bile duct and the lesser papilla draining the duct of Santorini. (From Rienhoff, W. F., Jr., and Pickrell, K. L.: Arch. Surg., 51:205, 1945.)

PANCREATIC DUCTS

The main pancreatic duct (duct of Wirsung) begins at the tail of the gland and passes through the center of the gland toward the head (Fig. 4). It may reside somewhat anteriorly or posteriorly but is nearly always midway between the superior and inferior borders of the body and tail. After passing the neck of the gland, the main duct turns inferiorly and dorsally and joins the distal common bile duct at the ampulla of Vater. Generally, the pancreatic duct enters the region of the ampulla inferomedially and often appears as a separate orifice on the distal medial wall of the common bile duct. Occasionally, the pancreatic duct retains its own identity all the way out to the tip of the ampulla and runs parallel to the distal common duct without actually joining it. When the common bile duct and pancreatic duct join together prior to entering the ampulla, a short *common channel* results (Fig. 5).

The lesser pancreatic duct (duct of Santorini) generally drains the head of the pancreas and enters the duodenum through a smaller accessory papilla located 2 to 2.5 cm. proximal and slightly anterior to the papilla of Vater. The lesser duct usually joins the main duct at the level of the head or neck of the pancreas, but this is not a consistent finding. Several variations exist on the degree of development of the lesser duct, the presence or patency of the lesser papilla, and the degree of communication with the main duct. Rarely, the lesser duct is the principal route of drainage of the body and tail owing to incomplete fusion of the ventral pancreatic duct with the dorsal duct during fetal development. This anomaly is referred to as *pancreas divisum* and is seen in 5 per cent of patients.

The main pancreatic duct varies in diameter from 2 to 3.5 mm. as it courses through the body of the gland and from 1 to 2 mm. in the region of the tail of the pancreas. Approximately 20 secondary branches drain into the duct throughout the body and tail, and the delicate patterns of these secondary ducts, and the tertiary ductules which form them, form an important radiologic criterion for the diagnosis of disease.

The sphincter of Oddi represents a complex set of muscular fibers surrounding the common bile duct, pancreatic duct, and the common channel of both ducts within the ampulla of Vater. This sphincter, which is regulated by neural and hormonal factors, controls the output of pancreatic and biliary secretions and serves to prevent reflux

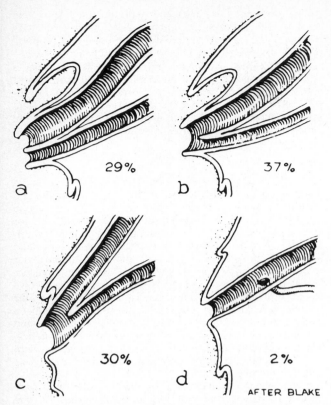

Figure 5. Variations in the relationship between the intrapancreatic portion of the common bile duct and the main pancreatic duct at the ampulla of Vater. A common channel (C) is found in almost one third of subjects. (From Rienhoff, W. F., Jr., and Pickrell, K. L.: Arch. Surg., 51:205, 1945.)

of duodenal contents into these ductular systems. In addition, individual sphincter fibers around the distal pancreatic duct serve to prevent the reflux of bile from the distal common duct into the pancreatic duct. Normal fasting common duct pressure has been found to range from 7 to 17 mm. Hg, whereas main pancreatic duct pressure ranges from 15 to 30 mm. Hg.

ARTERIAL SUPPLY

The pancreas receives a vigorous blood supply from a variety of major arterial sources (Fig. 6). Both the celiac and mesenteric arterial trunks supply branches to the pancreas, and numerous communications exist within the gland between the arteries arising from these two systems. The head of the pancreas is supplied superiorly by the anterior and posterior superior pancreaticoduodenal arteries, which generally arise from the gastroduodenal artery. Inferiorly, the head is supplied by the anterior and posterior inferior pancreaticoduodenal arteries, which originate from the superior mesenteric artery. The splenic artery gives rise to several arterial branches to the body and tail of the pancreas, including the dorsal pancreatic artery, the inferior pancreatic artery, and the artery pancreatica magna. In addition, numerous smaller branches arising from the splenic, hepatic, and gastroduodenal arteries provide blood flow to the gland.

The network of arteries serving the head of the pancreas also provides the arterial supply to the duodenum. Therefore, it is not possible to resect the entire pancreatic head without causing severe ischemia to the duodenum. Several anomalies of the splanchnic arterial system are known to occur in up to 20 per cent of patients and may result in variations from the normal pattern of pancreatic blood flow. The common hepatic, right hepatic, or gastroduodenal arteries may arise from the superior mesenteric

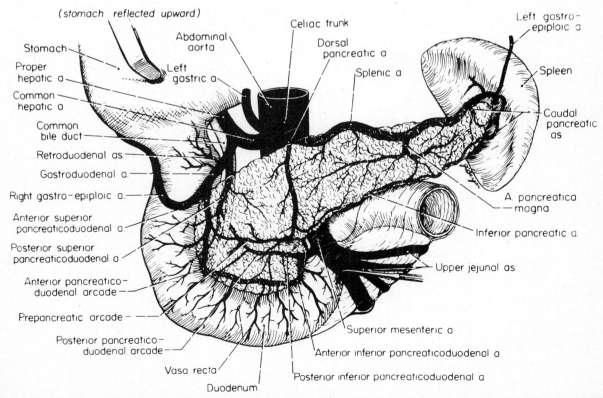

Figure 6. Arterial supply to the pancreas. (From Woodburne, R. T.: Essentials of Human Anatomy. New York, Oxford University Press, 1973.)

artery and can pass anterior or posterior to the pancreatic head or, very rarely, directly through the pancreatic head.

VENOUS DRAINAGE

Venous blood flow from the pancreas ultimately drains into the portal vein, and the relationship of the portal and superior mesenteric veins to the pancreas is surgically most important. The pancreatic veins generally follow the arterial pattern, with the individual veins lying superficial to the arteries. As with the arterial system, the pancreatic venous pattern exhibits frequent anomalies. Consistently, however, major venous drainage areas are comprised of the suprapancreatic portal vein, the retropancreatic portal and splenic veins, and the infrapancreatic superior mesenteric vein (Fig. 7).

The venous drainage of the head of the pancreas is directed superiorly through the anterior and posterior superior pancreaticoduodenal veins, which enter the suprapancreatic portion of the portal vein directly. These veins lie adjacent to their corresponding arteries and receive branches from the pancreas and duodenum. Venous drainage of the head is directed inferiorly through the anterior inferior pancreaticoduodenal vein and the right gastroepiploic vein, which generally combine with the right colic vein to form a common venous trunk (called the *gastrocolic* or *Henle's trunk*) before entering the superior mesenteric vein at the inferior border of the neck of the pancreas. The posterior inferior pancreaticoduodenal vein empties directly into the superior mesenteric vein or joins with the first jejunal vein.

The splenic vein receives many small pancreatic branches from the posterior surface of the pancreas as well as the inferior pancreatic vein, the caudal pancreatic vein, and the great pancreatic vein arising from the body of the gland. The inferior mesenteric vein may also receive small pancreatic venous branches and may join the splenic vein directly, the superior mesenteric vein directly, or may combine with each of these major veins to form a "tripod" origin of the portal vein behind the neck of the pancreas.

Several small pancreatic veins enter the lateral surfaces of the retropancreatic superior mesenteric and portal veins. Seldom are there any branches entering the portal or superior mesenteric vein directly anteriorly, however, and this fact allows relatively safe dissection of the neck of the pancreas from these underlying venous structures.

LYMPHATIC DRAINAGE

The lymphatic drainage of the pancreas resembles the vascular system of the organ in that it is abundant and diffuse (Fig. 8). The predominant lymphatic groups receiving drainage from the pancreas are the celiac and superior mesenteric nodes, but other regional lymphatic groups include the splenic, transverse mesocolic, subpyloric, and hepatic lymph nodes. In addition, lymph nodes in the lesser gastric omentum, along the greater curve of the stomach, and in the jejunal and colonic mesentery may also receive lymph drainage from the pancreas or may be sites for lymphangitic spread of pancreatic malignancy. It has been documented that the surgically resectable region around the entire pancreas contains roughly 70 lymph nodes, whereas resection of the head of the pancreas together with the duodenum (Whipple procedure) removes about one half that number.[5]

The pancreatic lymphatic system is made even more diffuse by the absence of a peritoneal barrier on the posterior surface of the gland. Direct lymphatic connections between intrapancreatic lymphatics and retroperitoneal tissues occur, and there are intrapancreatic lymph nodes as well. The interconnection of these lymphatic channels and the absence of any single nodal drainage area for specific

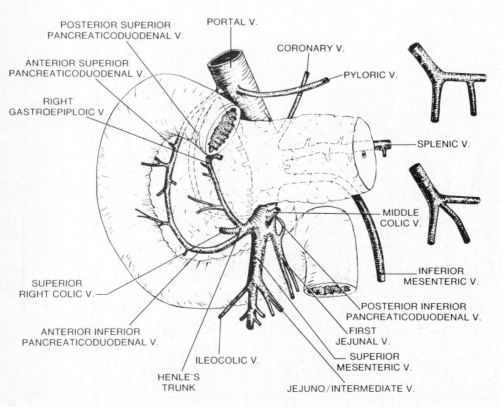

POSTERIOR SUPERIOR PANCREATICODUODENAL V.

PORTAL V.

CORONARY V.

PYLORIC V.

ANTERIOR SUPERIOR PANCREATICODUODENAL V.

RIGHT GASTROEPIPLOIC V.

SPLENIC V.

MIDDLE COLIC V.

SUPERIOR RIGHT COLIC V.

INFERIOR MESENTERIC V.

POSTERIOR INFERIOR PANCREATICODUODENAL V.

ANTERIOR INFERIOR PANCREATICODUODENAL V.

FIRST JEJUNAL V.

SUPERIOR MESENTERIC V.

HENLE'S TRUNK

ILEOCOLIC V.

JEJUNO/INTERMEDIATE V.

Figure 7. Venous drainage of the pancreas. Variations in the relationship of the portal, splenic, superior mesenteric, and inferior mesenteric veins are shown to the right. (From Mackie, C. R., and Moossa, A. R.: Surgical anatomy of the pancreas. In Moossa, A. R. (Ed.): Tumors of the Pancreas. Baltimore, Williams & Wilkins, 1980.)

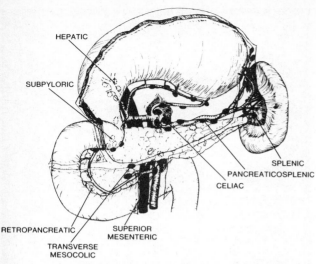

Figure 8. Lymph node groups receiving drainage from the pancreas. (From Mackie, C. R., and Moossa, A. R.: Surgical anatomy of the pancreas. In Moossa, A. R. (Ed.): Tumors of the Pancreas. Baltimore, Williams & Wilkins, 1980.)

regions of the pancreas are major contributing factors to the observed high incidence of recurrent malignancy after apparently curative resections of even small pancreatic carcinomas.

INNERVATION

The pancreas receives both sympathetic innervation via the splanchnic nerves and cholinergic innervation via the vagal fibers. The splanchnic nerves travel in the para-aortic area and send predominantly sympathetic fibers to the pancreas along the celiac axis and splenic artery. Vagal fibers traverse the lesser gastric omentum and innervate the area of the duodenum and pancreatic head, after which they communicate with all regions of the gland.

Intrapancreatic fibers of both sympathetic and cholinergic origin give rise to periacinar plexuses, which, in turn, send neural fibers to the base of acinar cell groups. Similar plexuses exist around the pancreatic islets, and terminal fibers form a particularly rich network that innervates the islet and communicates directly with the endocrine cells.

Afferent sensory fibers travel from the pancreas to the celiac plexus, then accompany the sympathetic para-aortic fibers before reaching the afferent neuronal cell bodies in the dorsal root ganglia of T5 to T12. Thus, intrinsic pancreatic pain may be noted in the epigastrium, may be felt in the right or left hypochondrium, or may present as lower thoracic backache.

Benign or malignant disease may result in chronic, severe pancreatic pain. Ganglionectomy or celiac ganglion blockade may be performed either operatively or percutaneously in an effort to interrupt these somatic fibers, but good results have been reported only after combined bilateral thoracic sympathectomy and celiac ganglionectomy.[21]

Structure of the Exocrine Pancreas

ACINI

The elements of the exocrine portion of the pancreas comprise 80 to 90 per cent of the total volume of the gland

and are divided into the acinar and ductular systems. Twenty to 40 acinar cells form the functional unit called the *acinus*, and from each acinus emerges a small *intercalated duct* (Fig. 9).

The pyramid-shaped acinar cells are oriented with their apex facing the lumen of the acinus. The luminal membrane contains numerous microvilli, and large, darkly staining zymogen granules are seen in the apical portion of each cell; the large nucleus resides in the central or basilar portion. An elaborate network of endoplasmic reticulum and microtubules supports the vigorous synthetic and secretory functions of these cells. The *centroacinar cells* line the lumen of the acinus and extend to the epithelium of the intercalated duct. Centroacinar cells are smaller than acinar cells and contain microvilli but not zymogen granules. These cells contain specific enzymes, such as carbonic anhydrase, that are required for bicarbonate and electrolyte transport and are specifically responsible for fluid and electrolyte secretion by the pancreas.[12]

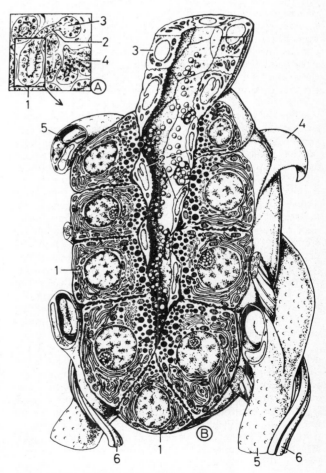

Figure 9. Histologic anatomy of the acinus.

A, Lower magnification view of a portion of the pancreas. 1, A single acinus; 2, intercalated duct; 3, intralobular duct; 4, centroacinar cells.

B, Higher magnification view of a single acinus. 1, Acinar cells releasing contents of zymogen granules into the acinar lumen; 2, centroacinar cells; 3, intercalated duct cell; 4, acinar basement membrane; 5, capillary; 6, periacinar neural fibers.

(From Krstić, R. V.: Die Gewebe des Menschen und der Säugetiere. Berlin, Springer-Verlag, 1978.)

Ducts

The intercalated ducts from several acini combine to form *interlobular ducts*, which combine to form secondary ducts leading to the main ductular system of the pancreas. As the duct size increases, the ductular cells become more cuboidal and contain only a small rim of cytoplasm. Although the secondary ducts and main ducts may contribute a small amount of water and electrolyte secretion, this function is performed primarily by the centroacinar cells and interlobular ducts.

Structure of the Endocrine Pancreas

Islet Cells

The islets of Langerhans form the endocrine, or ductless, portion of the pancreas and comprise only 2 to 3 per cent of the total volume of the gland. The islets are heterogeneous nests of cuboidal cells and measure 100 to 600 μm. in diameter. They are scattered uniformly throughout the pancreas. It has been estimated that the adult pancreas contains roughly one million islets, although this number varies considerably. Islets normally contain four specific cell types, alpha, beta, delta, and PP cells, which contain the hormones glucagon, insulin, somatostatin, and pancreatic polypeptide, respectively. Although the islets themselves are present uniformly throughout the pancreas, the distribution of the individual hormone-containing cells varies from one area of the pancreas to another.[24] The insulin-containing beta cells are most prevalent throughout the pancreas and comprise 70 to 75 per cent of all endocrine cells. They are present in higher numbers in the dorsal portion (body and tail) than in the ventral portion (head and uncinate process) of the gland. The glucagon-containing alpha cells comprise roughly 10 to 12 per cent of all endocrine cells throughout the pancreas but are found almost exclusively in the dorsal portion. Conversely, the pancreatic polypeptide–secreting cells are found almost exclusively in the ventral portion of the pancreas but still comprise 15 to 20 per cent of the total endocrine cells present in the entire pancreas. The somatostatin-containing cells are distributed uniformly throughout the pancreas and comprise approximately 5 per cent of all endocrine cells (Fig. 10). The arrangement of the hormone-secreting cells within each islet is also specific; beta cells occupy the central portion of each islet, and nonbeta cells are present around the periphery of the islet.

In addition to the well-established hormone-producing cells described here, immunohistochemical studies suggest that small numbers of additional hormone-containing cells are present in the islets. These include D_1 cells, which contain the hormone vasoactive intestinal polypeptide (VIP), and enterochromafin (EC) cells, which contain numerous amines including 5-hydroxytryptamine (5HT), or serotonin. The presence of occasional gastrin-containing G cells has been proposed by some studies, but their presence in normal islets remains unconfirmed.

Vascular Pattern

The distribution of blood flow within the pancreas provides arterial supply to the islets preferentially. Histologic studies indicate that the majority of the arterioles communicate directly with the islets, whereas a minority supply the acinar tissue directly. The collecting vessels draining all but the largest islets also perfuse the acinar tissue, allowing endocrine regulation of the exocrine pan-

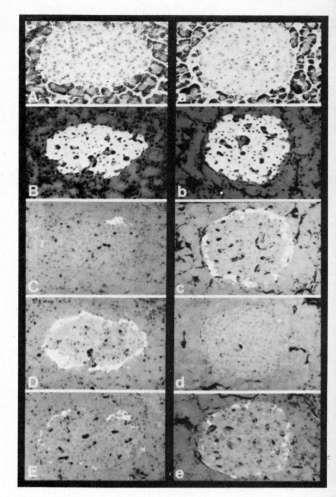

Figure 10. Histologic anatomy of the islet. Serial sections of a representative islet found in the ventral (A to E) and dorsal portion (a to e) of the pancreas. A,a, Stained with hematoxylin-eosin. B,b, Beta cells immunohistochemically stained with anti-insulin antisera. C,c, Alpha cells stained with antiglucagon antisera. D,d, PP cells stained with antipancreatic polypeptide antisera. E,e, Delta cells stained with antisomatostatin antisera. (Adapted from Orci, L.: Diabetes, 31:538, 1982.)

creas, but this "insuloacinar portal system" may also result in the exocrine pancreas being more susceptible to ischemia than the endocrine portion of the gland. The arteriolar distribution of the islets themselves is also organized in a specific pattern. Rather than provide a nonspecific "glomerular" network of arterial supply to the entire islet, arterioles appear to enter each islet directly into the beta cell mass, after which collecting venules supply the non–beta cell mantle or periphery of the islet.[3] This pattern of distribution of blood flow allows insulin secretion to modulate other endocrine cell populations and reduces the influence of the peripheral hormone-secreting cells on the responses of the beta cells.

PANCREATIC PHYSIOLOGY AND BIOCHEMISTRY

Exocrine Function

Pancreatic juice contains two major components, alkaline fluid and digestive enzymes. Between 500 and 800 ml. per day is secreted into the duodenum, and the high levels of bicarbonate serve to neutralize gastric acid and regulate the pH of intestinal contents. The enzymatic portion of this juice contains the necessary enzymes for digestion of carbohydrates, proteins, and fats. The products of digestion and the action of these enzymes on intestinal peptides and hormones also serve to regulate pancreatic secretion in a negative feedback fashion.

BICARBONATE SECRETION

Fluid secreted by the centroacinar cells and ductular epithelium contains 20 mM. bicarbonate in the resting state and as much as 150 mM. under maximal stimulation. The pH of this fluid ranges from 7.6 to almost 9.0. Sodium and potassium concentrations in pancreatic fluid remain relatively constant and reflect their concentration in the plasma. As bicarbonate secretion increases, the concentration of the other major anion, chloride, decreases. The total concentration of anions, therefore, remains constant, and the osmotic pressure of the pancreatic fluid remains the same as that of plasma. The exchange of bicarbonate and chloride occurs in the intercalated and interlobular ducts, with almost no secretion or exchange occurring in the main ducts.[6] The precise mechanism by which bicarbonate secretion is regulated remains controversial. The ubiquitous presence of carbon dioxide in the pericellular fluid, however, the formation of carbonic acid, and the specific presence of carbonic anhydrase associated with the centroacinar and ductular epithelial cells allow the constant formation and secretion of bicarbonate.

The major stimulus for the secretion of bicarbonate is the activation of intracellular cyclic adenosine monophosphate (AMP) formation by the presence of the hormone secretin. Secretin is secreted by specific cells located throughout the duodenal mucosa and is present in highest concentrations in the duodenal bulb. The secretin-containing cells release this peptide into the bloodstream in response to acid entering the duodenum in direct proportion to the amount of acid presented. When the pH is above 3.0, secretin release decreases; when the pH reaches 4.5 to 5.0, it ceases entirely. Therefore, the secretion of bicarbonate is particularly responsive to any stimulus that results in acid delivery to the duodenum. The presence of nutrients *per se* in the duodenal lumen may also result in a small increase in plasma secretin levels, although this finding has been difficult to confirm.

Cholecystokinin (CCK), also produced by specific duodenal mucosal cells, greatly augments the action of secretin but alone is a weak stimulant of bicarbonate secretion. Other peptides with a structure similar to CCK, such as gastrin, are also weak agonists of bicarbonate secretion and augment the effect of secretin. In contrast to the minimal response of secretin to ingested nutrients, CCK release occurs promptly after the entry of fatty acids or protein into the duodenum. Because of the ability of CCK to augment the bicarbonate response to even low levels of secretin, the interaction of these hormonal stimuli may provoke bicarbonate secretion despite the absence of marked duodenal acidification. Although acetylcholine is a poor stimulant of bicarbonate secretion, pancreatic cholinergic innervation plays a permissive role; bicarbonate secretion is inhibited by atropine and is reduced by up to 90 per cent following truncal vagotomy.

The fluid and bicarbonate content of pancreatic juice is probably most important as a vehicle for pancreatic enzyme secretion and a mechanism for preventing the activation of proteolytic enzymes until they are delivered to the intestinal lumen. The maintenance of a high pH in the pancreatic duct fluid prevents premature proteolysis of the pancreatic tissues. A major digestive disturbance occurs not as a result of the loss of pancreatic fluid or bicarbonate secretion alone but as a consequence of absent enzyme secretion.

ENZYME SECRETION

Pancreatic juice contains three major enzyme groups: amylases, lipases, and proteases. These enzymes are secreted by the acinar cells in multiple forms called *isoenzymes* together with a small amount of electrolyte-containing fluid.

Human pancreatic *amylase* is an α-amylase, which splits the α-1,4-glycosidic bond of starches to produce glucose, maltose, maltotriose, and a mixture of dextrins. Amylase is secreted in the active state and is stable over a relatively wide range of pH.

At least three *lipolytic enzymes* are secreted by the acinar cells. Lipase hydrolyzes insoluble esters of *glycerol* with the help of emulsifiers such as bile salts and colipase, which is also secreted in pancreatic juice. Another lipase hydrolyzes *alcohol esters*, such as those of cholesterol, and also requires bile salts as a cofactor. A third lipase hydrolyzes *water-soluble esters*. Phospholipase A is also secreted and is activated by trypsin to catalyze the hydrolysis of lecithin to lysolecithin. Lipases function optimally in a pH range of 7.0 to 9.0. Therefore, gastric hypersecretory states that result in duodenal and jejunal acidification may result in inadequate fat digestion and absorption and, thereby, produce steatorrhea.

Proteolytic enzymes are secreted by the acinar cells in an inactive precursor form. When activated, they form trypsin and several chymotrypsins. Trypsinogen is activated to form trypsin either through its own dissociation, which occurs as the pH falls to 7.0 or below, or through the action of enterokinase. Enterokinase is an enzyme located on intestinal mucosal cells that resists digestion by the secreted proteases owing to its heavy polysaccharide content. Enterokinase specifically converts trypsinogen to trypsin, whereupon the trypsin further activates the chymotrypsins, phospholipase, carboxypeptidases, and elastase, which are also secreted in precursor form. Although gastric pepsin contributes to protein digestion, its presence is not essential. The activated proteases of pancreatic juice are capable of complete protein digestion in the absence of gastric secretion.

In addition to the *nucleolytic enzymes* ribonuclease and deoxyribonuclease, the acinar cells also synthesize a small amount of trypsin inhibitor. This *antiproteolytic enzyme* binds directly with trypsin and inactivates it. It is thought to protect the pancreatic tissue from the effects of trypsin, which may become activated in small amounts within the duct fluid, but the concentration of trypsinogen greatly exceeds that of the trypsin inhibitor protein. When full activation of the trypsinogen occurs, the relatively small quantity of inhibitor becomes ineffective and is itself digested.

Upon synthesis within the endoplasmic reticulum of the acinar cells, the enzyme precursors are packaged within the zymogen granules seen in the apical portion of these cells. After release into the lumen of the acinus, the zymogen granules remain intact until the pH of the duct fluid rises above 7.0 as a consequence of bicarbonate secretion. At this pH, the granules dissolve, discharging the enzyme precursors into the duct fluid. With sustained stimulation of the acinar cells, enzyme synthesis and secretion continue without demonstrable granule formation. The secretion of these enzymes, however, does not occur in an absolutely fixed ratio. Specific stimulants may result in only one form of enzyme secretion; the intestinal peptide chymodenin, for example, stimulates the release of chymotrypsinogen without causing release of other enzymes. Furthermore, long-term alterations in the dietary composition of nutrients may result in corresponding changes in the relative amounts of amylase, lipases, and proteases being secreted. Recently, it has been shown that specific nutrients (glucose or amino acids) can alter the immediate response of stimulated acinar cells and result in a corresponding shift toward predominantly amylytic or proteolytic enzyme secretion. This specific regulation of enzyme secretion may be mediated through the release of corresponding islet hormones (insulin or glucagon) via the insuloacinar portal system.[25] These findings demonstrate, however, that pancreatic enzyme secretion is a rather finely regulated process.

Hormonal and neural factors serve as the principal stimuli to enzyme secretion. Cholecystokinin stimulates the acinar cells by binding with specific membrane-bound receptors, which results in the transport and accumulation of cytoplasmic calcium and the intracellular production of cyclic guanosine monophosphate (GMP). Acetylcholine is also a major stimulant of the acinar cells and is released from postganglionic fibers of the pancreatic plexus. Acetylcholine and CCK act synergistically, and pancreatic enzyme secretion may be reduced as much as 50 per cent after truncal vagotomy.[13] Secretin and vasoactive intestinal polypeptide are also capable of stimulating acinar cells and serve to augment the responses to CCK and acetylcholine by increasing intracellular cyclic AMP production.

Endocrine Function

INSULIN

In 1890, Von Mering and Minkowski demonstrated that the pancreas is essential to normal glucose metabolism. In 1921, Banting and Best isolated insulin, first called isletin, from canine pancreas and successfully reversed diabetes by administering insulin to animals. The amino acid sequence was determined by Sanger in the 1950s and consists of a 21-amino acid A chain connected to a 30-amino acid B chain by two disulfide bridges. The molecule is synthesized as an 81-amino acid precursor peptide called *proinsulin*, from which a 30- to 35-amino acid connecting peptide, or *C-peptide*, is cleaved. This cleavage occurs in the secretory granules of the beta cell, and the C-peptide fragment is secreted together with insulin on an equimolar basis. Proinsulin is occasionally secreted intact, and its concentration in the blood is elevated in chronic renal failure and cases of insulin-secreting tumors. The structure of insulin varies slightly from species to species, and administration of insulin preparations can, therefore, provoke the development of antibodies. The investigation of this antibody formation to insulin led Berson and Yalow in 1959 to develop the radioimmunoassay (RIA) method for measuring circulating levels of the hormone. This technique revolutionized the study of all endocrine systems.

Insulin binds to specific receptor proteins on cell membranes and promotes the transport of glucose into cells. Only beta cells, hepatocytes, and cells of the central nervous system do not require insulin for this purpose. The interaction of insulin with its receptor sites is a dynamic process; when insulin concentrations change over a prolonged period of time, the availability of receptor sites and their binding

affinity for the molecule compensate to allow continued stable rates of glucose transport. When receptor number or affinity decreases, *insulin resistance* results. This compensatory relationship is an ubiquitous characteristic of endocrine systems.

Insulin Metabolism

Insulin is metabolized primarily by the liver, and 40 to 50 per cent of the insulin entering the portal system is metabolized on its passage through the liver. Insulin regulates hepatocyte function by suppressing glycogenolysis and accelerates nucleic acid formation and protein synthesis. Insulin is also antilipolytic in that it prevents the breakdown of fatty acids and therefore inhibits the formation of ketones produced by fatty acid oxidation. For this reason, severe insulin deficiency results not only in the progressive accumulation of glucose in the blood but the appearance of ketone formation, which results in *diabetic ketoacidosis*. Insulin excess or an exaggerated hepatic or peripheral effect of insulin results in hypoglycemia.

Insulin Secretion

The secretion of insulin is regulated by the concentration of glucose presented to the beta cell and, therefore, by the rate of intracellular glucose metabolism. Insulin release is also stimulated, but to a lesser degree, by the presence of other nutrients such as amino acids and free fatty acids. Hormonal and neural factors also mediate the beta cell, and intestinal hormones that are released by feeding, such as gastric inhibitory polypeptide (GIP), enhance the insulin response to glucose. This regulatory effect of the gut on beta cell function is termed the *enteroinsular axis*. Cholinergic stimulation augments insulin release, whereas sympathetic stimulation (via the α-adrenergic system) inhibits insulin secretion. In the normal pancreas, considerable functional reserve of insulin secretion is present; destruction or removal of over 80 per cent of the beta cell mass is required before diabetes mellitus becomes clinically apparent.

GLUCAGON

In 1923, Murlin and co-workers identified a factor in pancreatic extracts that caused hyperglycemia, and in 1949 Sutherland and associates purified this hyperglycemic-glycogenolytic factor (HGF) from both insulin preparations and gastric mucosa. Renamed *glucagon*, the structure was determined to be a 29 amino acid peptide similar in amino acid composition to secretin. Multiple forms of glucagon exist in the gastrointestinal tract, and larger glucagon-like peptides in the small intestine are called enteroglucagon. Unger and co-workers first developed an RIA for detecting glucagon in 1961, but the presence of multiple circulating forms has made it difficult to measure pancreatic glucagon specifically *in vivo*.

Glucagon Metabolism

Pancreatic glucagon functions essentially in a reciprocal fashion to insulin. Its release from the alpha cell is stimulated by hypoglycemia and suppressed by hyperglycemia and hyperinsulinemia. Glucagon activates the breakdown of glycogen through the dephosphorylation of glucose-1-phosphate and accelerates gluconeogenesis, thereby causing endogenous glucose production to increase and plasma glucose levels to rise. In situations of physiologic stress or increased metabolic demands, this process is beneficial and serves to provide additional metabolic fuel for all tissues. Glucagon secretion increases during acute stress, along with cortisol, growth hormone, and catechols. When these "stress hormones" are stimulated by hypoglycemia, they are referred to as "counterregulatory hormones," as they cause a reversal of the decline in plasma glucose.

Glucagon Secretion

Secretion of glucagon is also stimulated by amino acids, particularly arginine and alanine, and by norepinephrine. Free fatty acids inhibit glucagon release. A true hormonal stimulant for glucagon release has yet to be confirmed.

In normal man, carbohydrate feeding or a mixed meal results in a modest decline in glucagon levels as insulin release occurs. In patients with diabetes mellitus, however, the glucagon response to these nutrients is paradoxically increased, which contributes to the resulting hyperglycemia. Glucagon is lipolytic and accelerates fatty acid mobilization. Through this process, glucagon contributes to ketoacidosis in uncontrolled diabetes. In pharmacologic doses, glucagon demonstrates an inotropic effect on the heart, slows gastric and duodenal peristalsis, and relaxes the sphincter of Oddi. Metabolism of glucagon occurs in the kidney and, to a lesser degree, in the liver.

SOMATOSTATIN

In 1973, after prolonged investigation of the factors regulating the release of growth hormones, Brazeau and colleagues isolated a hypothalamic peptide that inhibited the release of growth hormone. Because of its antisomatotropin action, this 14-amino acid peptide was named *somatostatin*. Alberti and associates quickly demonstrated that in man somatostatin is a potent and reversible inhibitor of the release of insulin. Subsequently, many investigators demonstrated that this peptide inhibits the release of virtually all known pancreatic and intestinal peptide hormones as well as gastric, pancreatic, and biliary secretion. Somatostatin inhibits the release of pituitary hormones such as thyroid-stimulating hormone (TSH) but does not inhibit prolactin secretion or adrenal cortisol release.

With the development of specific antisera to somatostatin, immunohistochemical studies demonstrated the presence of somatostatin within the previously known but functionally obscure pancreatic delta cell. The release of somatostatin by the isolated pancreas and the demonstration of a nutrient-induced rise in somatostatin levels in pancreatic venous blood *in vivo* confirmed its role as an islet hormone. Somatostatin was also localized to specific cells in the gastric fundus and, to a much lesser extent, is present throughout the gastrointestinal tract.

Because of its presence in both the central nervous system (CNS) and the intestinal tract, somatostatin is a prime example of a hormonal link between these diverse organ systems. This relationship, referred to as the "brain-gut axis," includes several hormones known to interact with, or reside within, the pancreas. These include vasoactive intestinal polypeptide and serotonin.

Despite its inhibitory effect on insulin release, pancreatic somatostatin probably influences beta cell function to a minor degree, as its secretion into the vascular bed of the islet is "downstream" of the majority of islet cells. Studies of islet cell changes in diabetes demonstrate an increase in the number of somatostatin-containing delta cells, along with an increase in the number of alpha cells.

The pathogenic significance of this finding remains unclear. Although it is thought that somatostatin must exert a modulating role on pancreatic and gastrointestinal functions, the extent of this function is still under investigation.

PANCREATIC POLYPEPTIDE

This 36-amino acid polypeptide was originally isolated as a contaminant of insulin preparations in 1974 by Chance and colleagues and, independently, by Kimmel and co-workers. It was subsequently localized to an islet cell distinct from alpha, beta, or delta cells, now referred to histologically as the pancreatic polypeptide (PP) cell. The specific distribution of PP cells has been reviewed previously, and the localization of PP to the pancreas is specific; following total pancreatectomy, plasma levels of PP in man are undetectable.

The physiologic role of PP is unclear. There is wide experimental evidence that PP inhibits pancreatic enzyme and bicarbonate secretion as well as choleresis and gallbladder emptying. Other studies suggest the involvement of PP in nutrient or glucose homeostasis. Examination of the responses of PP to different stimuli are provocative, however. Carbohydrates, proteins, and fats stimulate PP release when ingested but not when administered intravenously. Therefore, the release of PP is thought to result from one or more intestinal signals. Cholecystokinin appears to best fulfill the role of a hormonal stimulant of PP, and vagal innervation is crucial to PP release. Pancreatic polypeptide responses are markedly reduced after vagotomy as well as antrectomy. Circulating levels of PP are increased in diabetes, and hyperplasia of islet PP cells has been documented in diabetic subjects. Levels of PP also increase with normal aging, which suggests a compensatory response to changes in nutrient metabolism or other hormonal functions.

DIAGNOSTIC PROCEDURES

Tests of Exocrine Function

SECRETIN TEST

The standard provocative test of pancreatic fluid volume and bicarbonate and enzyme secretion is the secretin test. Although overall exocrine function may be diminished as a consequence of a variety of pancreatic diseases, this test has been employed to attempt to distinguish benign conditions (e.g., chronic pancreatitis) from malignancy. After an overnight fast, a double lumen tube is passed to the second portion of the duodenum under fluoroscopic control. After a 20-minute basal collection period in which duodenal fluid is aspirated and collected on ice, secretin (1 clinical unit/kg.) is given intravenously. Repeated aspirations from four subsequent 20-minute periods are obtained, and the total volume, bicarbonate, and enzyme (usually amylase) output are determined. Normal responses are 2 to 4 ml. per kg. of volume output, 90 to 130 mEq. per liter of bicarbonate secretion, and 6 to 18 units per kg. of amylase secretion.[8]

Results from a large series of patients studied by Dreiling and Wolfson are presented in Table 1. There is considerable overlap in the results observed in different clinical groups. In general, however, moderately advanced chronic pancreatitis is associated with decreased bicarbonate secretion, whereas pancreatic carcinoma is associated with decreased volume secretion. The selective deficiency

TABLE 1. *Characteristic Results of Secretin Testing: Flow, Bicarbonate, and Enzyme Changes Observed in Patients with Various Pancreatic and Other Disorders**

Disorders	Pattern	Flow Rate	Maximum HCO₃ Concentration	Enzyme Secretion
End-stage pancreatitis, advanced pancreatic cancer	Total insufficiency	Decreased	Decreased	Decreased
Chronic pancreatitis	Qualitative insufficiency	Normal	Decreased	Normal
Pancreatic cancer	Quantitative insufficiency	Decreased	Normal	Normal
Malnutrition†	Isolated enzyme deficiency	Normal	Normal	Decreased
Hemochromatosis, Zollinger-Ellison syndrome, various cirrhoses	Hypersecretion	Increased	Normal	Normal

*From Dreiling, D. A., and Wolfson, P.: New insights into pancreatic disease revealed by the secretin test. *In* Berk, J. E. (Ed.): Developments in Digestive Diseases, Vol. 2. Philadelphia, Lea & Febiger, 1979, pp. 155–170.
†Sprue, ulcerative colitis, and regional enteritis.

of bicarbonate secretion in chronic pancreatitis is thought to result from stasis within a dilated ductular system, which allows prolonged equilibration between chloride and bicarbonate ions. The selective deficiency of volume secretion in carcinoma is thought to result from the replacement of an otherwise normal exocrine cell mass with neoplasm.

Efforts to improve the specificity and accuracy of the secretin test have included collection of pancreatic fluid directly through endoscopically guided catheterization of the ampulla and the use of an augmented secretin dose or the addition of CCK to the stimulus. Expertise with the procedure and the establishment of locally prevailing standards are essential for useful interpretation of results.

LUNDH TEST

A test meal provides an endogenous stimulus for the secretion of pancreatic enzymes. Aspiration of four 30-minute fluid samples from the intubated duodenum is analyzed for trypsin content following ingestion of a meal containing 18 gm. of corn oil, 15 gm. of casein, and 40 gm. of glucose dissolved in 300 ml. of water. The output of enzyme activity correlates well with frank pancreatic insufficiency, but discrimination between benign and malignant conditions is difficult. Results are subject to error by the presence of delayed gastric emptying or intestinal mucosal abnormalities.

PABA TEST

The orally administered synthetic peptide N-benzoyl-L-tyrosyl-para-aminobenzoic acid (BT-PABA) was shown by Imondi and associates to be cleaved by chymotrypsin to form PABA, which is then absorbed in the small intestine and excreted in the urine. This process has been applied clinically as a test of exocrine function[2]; 1 gm. of BT-PABA (containing 340 mg. PABA) in 300 ml. of water is administered and urine collections are obtained for 6 hours. Between 60 and 95 per cent of the ingested PABA is excreted in normal subjects, whereas patients with chronic pancreatitis excrete less. The test is attractive because of its noninvasiveness, but its sensitivity in cases of mild to moderate dysfunction awaits confirmation.

DIMETHADIONE (DMO) TEST

With the finding that the pancreas has the capacity to demethylate the anticonvulsant drug tridione (3,5,5-trimethyl-2,4-oxazolidine dione) and secrete the product dimethadione (5,5-dimethyl-2,4-oxazolidine dione, or DMO), a new clinical test of exocrine function has been intro-

duced.[18] Patients are first given 0.45 gm. of tridione three times daily for 3 days, after which a duodenal tube is placed and secretin administered. The duodenal output of DMO, when corrected for circulating plasma levels of DMO, appears to offer a good index of exocrine function and may discriminate even mild cases of disease.[17] The procedure is cumbersome, however, and further clinical verification is required.

FECAL FAT TEST

The quantitation of unabsorbed fat excreted in feces is the standard index of lipase deficiency and, therefore, exocrine dysfunction. Unfortunately, an elevated 24-hour fecal fat content (greater than 20 gm.) occurs only after lipase secretion is reduced by 90 per cent or more and gross steatorrhea is present. Steatorrhea in the presence of low levels of fecal fat usually indicates intestinal dysfunction or malabsorption and therefore the test is a better index of enteric disease than of pancreatic dysfunction (Table 2). It is a useful guide, however, in pancreatic enzyme replacement therapy of patients with exocrine deficiency.

TRIOLEIN BREATH TEST

In an effort to assess fat digestion noninvasively with a recoverable, absorbable marker, ^{14}carbon-labeled triglycerides may be administered orally, and the excretion of $^{14}CO_2$ in the breath can be quantified. Twenty five gm. of corn oil containing 5 μCi. of ^{14}C-triolein is administered, and breath samples are obtained 4 to 6 hours later in a liquid vehicle and radioactivity determined. Normal subjects exhale greater than 3 per cent of the ^{14}C-triolein dose given per hour, whereas patients with disorders of fat digestion or absorption exhale less. Discrimination between pancreatic insufficiency and enteric dysfunction is possible by repeating the study after oral pancreatic enzyme replacement; patients with exocrine deficiency usually increase their $^{14}CO_2$ excretion rate by 500 per cent or achieve normal levels, whereas patients with enteric disorders remain essentially unchanged.[11] The simplicity of the test is attractive, and its use is increasing.

Tests of Endocrine Function

ORAL GLUCOSE TOLERANCE TEST (OGTT)

The OGTT is the most commonly performed test thought to assess insulin responsiveness. Unfortunately, it is also most prone to errors in performance or interpretation because of several factors:

TABLE 2. Differential Diagnosis of Intestinal and Pancreatic Steatorrhea*

Parameter	Intestinal Steatorrhea	Pancreatitis
Fecal fat	<20 gm. mono- and diglycerides, soapy consistency	>20 gm. triglycerides, oily seepage
D-xylose	Low	Normal
Secretin test	Normal	Abnormal
Small bowel series	Abnormal	Normal
Small bowel biopsy	Abnormal	Normal
Lundh meal	Normal	Abnormal
PABA test	Normal	Abnormal
Alkaline phosphatase	Normal or high (bone)	Normal or high (liver)
Vitamin B_{12} and folate	Low	Normal
Treatment with pancreatic enzymes	No change	Improvement

*From Brandt, L. J.: Gastrointestinal Disorders of the Elderly. New York, Raven Press, 1984, p. 470.

1. The test measures glucose appearance and disappearance rather than the response of insulin *per se*.

2. The dose of glucose administered is usually not corrected for body mass.

3. The absorption rate of glucose is affected by gastric and intestinal factors.

4. The effect of enterally absorbed glucose on insulin release is mediated by the integrity of the enteroinsular axis as well as the response of the beta cell to glucose.

5. Several clinical factors may temporarily or permanently affect the OGTT, including antecedent diet, exercise, drug use, and age of the patient.

This test is frequently used as an index of endocrine pancreatic function, however, since relative or absolute insulin deficiency results ultimately in diabetes mellitus. The recommended technique for performing the 2-hour OGTT, as advised by the National Diabetes Data Group[16] is as follows: 75 gm. of glucose (or 40 gm. glucose/meter[2] body surface area), dissolved in at least 4 ml. of water per gm., is taken orally over 10 minutes after two fasting blood samples are obtained. Blood samples are then drawn at 30-minute intervals for 2 hours. The interpretation of the glucose values obtained is reviewed in Table 3. The diagnosis of diabetes mellitus must be based upon either (1) the presence of classic symptoms of diabetes together with gross and unequivocal elevation in plasma glucose, or (2) *repeated* or confirmed "diabetic" interpretation on testing as noted in Table 3.

INTRAVENOUS GLUCOSE TOLERANCE TEST (IVGTT)

The measurement of the disappearance or disposal of plasma glucose that is acutely elevated by an intravenous infusion eliminates the influence of gastrointestinal factors on glucose metabolism. The resulting glucose disappearance rate, or K value, reflects more directly the secretion of insulin but is also a product of the sensitivity or resistance

to insulin at its target tissues. Doses of glucose used vary, but 0.5 gm. of glucose per kg. administered over 2 to 5 minutes with plasma glucose measured every 5 to 10 minutes for 1 hour normally results in a K value (per cent glucose disappearance per minute) of 1.5 or greater. A major factor that influences the interpretation of this test is the age of the patient; there is a progressive age-related decline in IVGTT performance, as with OGTT performance, and the results should therefore be evaluated with age-adjusted criteria.[1]

TOLBUTAMIDE RESPONSE TEST (TRT)

The sulfonylurea tolbutamide is a potent stimulant for the release of insulin and has been employed as a diagnostic test of glucose intolerance as well as a provocative test in cases of suspected hyperinsulinism. One gm. of sodium tolbutamide is given intravenously over 2 minutes, and frequent blood samples are obtained for 1 hour or longer. Blood glucose falls at about 30 minutes to a nadir, which is normally between 50 and 75 per cent of the fasting value. Analysis of the glucose response using appropriate criteria[1] provides an index of glucose intolerance. Sustained hypoglycemia together with an exaggerated insulin response suggests the presence of a beta cell tumor. The TRT is also used as a provocative test for delta cell tumors, as somatostatin release is also provoked by tolbutamide.

ARGININE TEST

The amino acid arginine serves as a potent stimulus for the release of several hormones. A 30-minute infusion of 0.5 gm. of arginine per kg. (up to a maximum of 30 gm.) results in an immediate or progressive release of the islet cell hormones as well as growth hormone. Quantitation of the hormone, particularly glucagon, is useful in the diagnosis of hormone-secreting tumors.

TABLE 3. Interpretation of Oral Glucose Tolerance Test Results*

Interpretation	Fasting Glucose Value (mg./100 ml.)		Intermediate Glucose Value (mg./100 ml.)		Two-Hour Glucose Value (mg./100 ml.)	
Normal	<115	and	All	<200	and	<140
Impaired glucose tolerance	<140	and	Any value	≥200	and	140–199
Diabetic Or	≥140		(Glucose tolerance test not necessary)			
	<140	and	Any value	≥200	and	≥200
Nondiagnostic	Any combination of glucose values that does not fit into another category					

*Adapted from National Diabetes Data Group: Diabetes, *28*:1039, 1979.

Calcium Infusion Test

Many peptide hormones respond to intravenous calcium infusion, and the hypersecretion of insulin, gastrin, and serotonin to this challenge provides a diagnostic test for suspected hormone-secreting tumors. A 30-minute infusion of 4 mg. of calcium per kg. min. $^{-1}$ is given, during which multiple blood samples are obtained. The test must be performed under electrocardiographic monitoring as serious arrhythmias occasionally occur. Other hormonal stimuli may be used in the diagnosis of specific islet cell tumors and are reviewed in that section.

Anatomic Studies

Sonography

The least invasive and safest method of assessing pancreatic anatomy is (ultra)sonography. The image produced is based on the degree of reflectance or scatter of acoustic pulses, which are transmitted by a transducer placed on the skin. Each sonographic scan reflects the pattern of tissues within a specific plane. Multiple scans are obtained in horizontal, vertrical, or oblique planes to produce a complete image of the area of the pancreas. An interface with intervening gas is a relative obstacle for the detection of the sound waves reflected, and therefore the presence of overlying bowel gas may result in an unsuccessful attempt to visualize the pancreas. Because of its noninvasive nature, sonography is particularly useful as a screening study, and its application has dramatically increased the understanding of the evolution of inflammatory disorders of the pancreas.

Dilated, fluid-filled ducts, pancreatic cysts and pseudocysts, and increased interstitial edema associated with pancreatitis are all distinguished with this technique. Tumors are detected as focal enlargements in the pancreatic mass or as discrete echodense lesions within the pancreas. Resolution of pancreatic anatomy is generally quite adequate for a screening technique, although further radiologic studies are usually required for more precise definition of pathology.

Computed Tomography (CT)

In addition to sonography, the development of CT scanning has been the major advance in improved methods of imaging the pancreas. Hundreds of transverse radiograms are obtained around a 360-degree sweep within a few seconds and are reconstructed by computer to reveal a cross-sectional image of the entire body. The pancreas is usually clearly defined in relation to its surrounding structures from upper abdominal scans obtained in 0.5- 1.0-cm. increments. The differentiation of duodenum and stomach is augmented by the simultaneous ingestion of dilute contrast material. Intravenous contrast infusion further enhances the discrimination between various structures or results in the identification of hypervascular or hypovascular tissue masses. Obstructed ductular systems, cystic lesions, and the relationship of vascular structures to the pancreas are well visualized (Fig. 11). CT scanning is particularly advantageous to the surgeon, as it defines not only the structure and location of pancreatic tissue but the relationship of the pancreas to other abdominal structures.

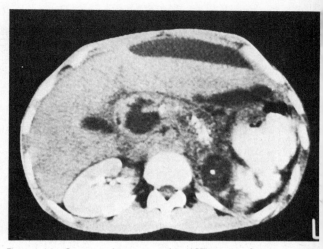

Figure 11. Computed tomographic (CT) scan of patient with chronic pancreatitis. Pancreas demonstrates calcification throughout the body of the gland, with pseudocyst in the head and pseudocyst of the tail (white marker). Also shown is loculated fluid surrounding the left lobe of the liver. Lucent areas to patient's right of the pseudocyst in the pancreatic head represent the intrapancreatic common bile duct (small lucency) and the gallbladder (large lucency). Compare these findings with those shown in Figure 2. (Courtesy of Dr. S. Glanz, Department of Radiology, State University of New York Health Science Center at Brooklyn.)

Upper Gastrointestinal Series

Although cross-sectional imaging techniques such as sonography and CT scanning have become favored methods for pancreatic visualization, pancreatic disease may be diagnosed from characteristic abnormalities seen during upper gastrointestinal contrast studies. Scout films of the abdomen may reveal pancreatic calcification indicating chronic pancreatitis, adynamic ileus or ileus of a segment of small bowel ("sentinel loop") associated with acute pancreatitis, a distended ascending or proximal transverse colon that ends abruptly in the region of the pancreas ("colon cut-off sign"), indicating peripancreatic inflammation, or speckled gas collections in the region of the pancreas suggestive of a pancreatic abscess. The contrast study may reveal displacement or extrinsic compression of the stomach or duodenum due to acute inflammation (phlegmon) or pseudocyst in acute pancreatitis or destruction or invasion of duodenal mucosa by a malignancy in the region of the pancreatic head. Papillary edema ("Poppel's sign") may indicate pancreatitis, an impacted common bile duct stone, or duodenal ulcer. Contrast studies of the upper gastrointestinal tract are, therefore, particularly valuable in differentiating pancreatic disease from other upper abdominal abnormalities (Fig. 12).

Arteriography

Angiographic visualization of the pancreas provides useful information in the diagnosis and management of neoplastic lesions. Percutaneous catheterization of the celiac axis and superior mesenteric artery allows the arterial supply to be delineated precisely, and, from venous-phase exposures, the pattern of contrast-filled major veins can provide useful information regarding vascular involvement by certain malignancies. Hypervascular lesions of the pancreas, such as islet cell adenomas, are frequently seen

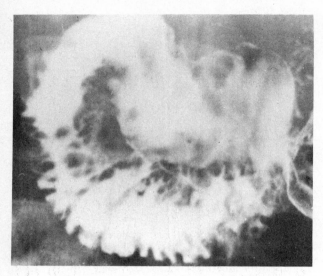

Figure 12. Upper gastrointestinal contrast study. Close-up duodenal C-loop showing polypoid appearance of pancreatic adenocarcinoma arising near the ampulla of Vater. (Courtesy of Dr. J. Farman, Department of Radiology, State University of New York Health Science Center at Brooklyn.)

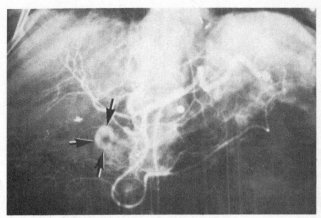

Figure 13. Celiac arteriogram of patient with suspected islet cell tumor. Arrows show hypervascular "blush" of the tumor located in the pancreatic head. (From Mackie, C. R., Moossa, A. R., and Frank, P. H.: The place of angiography in the diagnosis and management of pancreatic tumors. In Moossa, A. R. (Ed.): Tumors of the Pancreas. Baltimore, Williams & Wilkins, 1980.)

arteriographically when other imaging techniques fail to visualize them (Fig. 13). Selective catheterization of specific pancreatic arteries or branches of the major arterial vessels may reveal subtle arteriographic findings of neoplasia, such as increased tortuosity and neovascularity. Larger hypovascular lesions are delineated because of the findings of displacement, absence, or encasement of regional blood vessels. The management of pancreatic malignancy is facilitated by angiographic studies not only by the clarification of the location and probable resectability of the lesion but by the finding of angiographically demonstrable metastatic lesions, which may elude standard radiographic techniques.

ENDOSCOPIC RETROGRADE CHOLANGIOPANCREATOGRAPHY (ERCP)

A major advance in the diagnosis of upper gastrointestinal illness in general, and pancreatic disease in particular, has been the application of fiberoptic endoscopy for the purpose of cannulation and radiographic delineation of the ducts leading to the ampulla of Vater. ERCP is performed by advancing a side-viewing endoscope to the level of the ampulla, followed by cannulation of the papilla and gentle infusion of contrast material. The biliary and pancreatic ducts may be visualized separately or together at the time of contrast infusion. This technique has resulted in an improved understanding of both normal pancreatic duct anatomy and anomalies as well as the early and late ductular abnormalities associated with pancreatic disease. Pancreatic duct stenosis or obstruction (associated with benign or malignant disease), distal ductular dilatation or ectasia (associated with chronic pancreatitis), and pseudocysts or cystic dilatation of the ductular system (so-called retention cysts) are all frequently delineated by ERCP (Fig. 14).

Complications of ERCP are rare but include transient hyperamylasemia or frank pancreatitis; the presence of acute pancreatitis is therefore a relative contraindication to the procedure. In addition, the technique of endoscopic cannulation of the papilla may also be used to obtain samples of pancreatic fluid for cytologic studies.

PERCUTANEOUS TRANSHEPATIC CHOLANGIOGRAPHY (PTC)

An alternative method to ERCP for obtaining radiographic studies of the biliary ducts involves the transhepatic puncture of a dilated intrahepatic biliary duct, followed by instillation of a contrast agent that fills both the intra- and extrahepatic biliary systems. Potential complications of the procedure, such as bleeding and bile leak from the hepatic

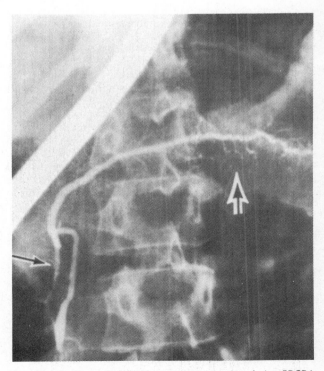

Figure 14. Radiograph following contrast injection during ERCP in normal subject. Shown are the main pancreatic duct (large arrow) and lesser pancreatic duct (small arrow). (From Kollins, S. A.: Diagnostic procedures. In Cooperman, A. M., and Hoerr, S. O. (Eds.): Surgery of the Pancreas. A Text and Atlas. St. Louis, C. V. Mosby Co., 1978.)

surface, have been greatly reduced through the use of small-gauge, "skinny" needle techniques. PTC is particularly useful for determining the extent and probable etiology of lesions of the head of the pancreas. Obstructive jaundice may be caused by fibrosis, inflammation, or neoplasm of the pancreatic head as well as primary biliary tract disease. Although PTC does not usually visualize the pancreatic duct, the findings of altered anatomy of the common duct, together with the results obtained from other studies, greatly facilitate operative planning and management of pancreatobiliary tract disease.

Percutaneous Transhepatic Venous Sampling (PTVS)

This method is an application of the PTC technique and provides information to help localize hormone-secreting tumors of the pancreas. The transhepatic needle is advanced into a branch of the portal venous system, as verified by a fluoroscopically observed test injection of contrast material. A catheter is then passed in a retrograde manner into the portal vein, and blood samples are obtained from various locations along the portal, splenic, and superior mesenteric veins and their pancreatic venous tributaries. The samples are then assayed for the hormone under question, and the location of the hormone-secreting tumor, or the presence of diffuse hypersecretion from the pancreas, may be identified. The technique is tedious, and great care is required for its successful completion. The results may be invaluable, however, in the identification of a small lesion that may otherwise elude radiologic or even surgical detection.

Operative Pancreatography

The most invasive but also the most definitive procedure for the delineation of pancreatic duct anatomy is achieved by intraoperative contrast radiography following direct puncture or cannulation of the pancreatic duct. The technique is frequently required in cases of chronic pancreatitis, where the proximal pancreatic duct may be occluded by stricture or calculus formation, which prevents successful ERCP, and where the choice of an appropriate surgical procedure rests upon a precise knowledge of the ductular lesion(s) (Fig. 15). A dilated pancreatic duct may be identified as an area of palpable fluctuance or distention in the midpancreas ("Cattell's sign"), but even a 2- 3-mm. duct may be entered by direct puncture. The risk of pancreatic fluid leak is minimized through the use of a small (22 or 23 gauge) needle, and care must be taken to avoid any unnecessary manipulation of the gland.

PATHOLOGIC DISORDERS

Congenital Disorders

Anular Pancreas

A ring or collar of pancreatic tissue that completely encircles the second portion of the duodenum is thought to result from abnormal embryologic fusion of dorsal and ventral pancreatic segments. This condition usually results in stenosis of the duodenum, and complete duodenal obstruction is the usual presentation of anular pancreas in the neonate. Half of the reported cases of anular pancreas have been adults, however, with some remaining undiagnosed until the eighth decade of life. Peptic ulcer disease

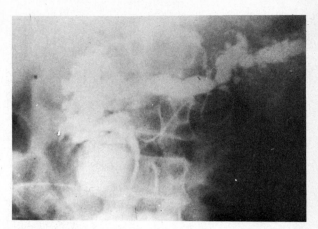

Figure 15. Operative pancreatogram. Contrast medium was gently infused into main pancreatic duct after direct puncture. Shown is a massively dilated pancreatic ductal system, with compression and displacement of duct in pancreatic head by a contrast-filled pseudocyst.

occurs in one fifth of adults with this lesion, probably as a consequence of duodenal stasis. The autopsy incidence of the condition is about 1 in 7000. Bypass of the stenotic or obstructing segment is the treatment of choice, and direct surgical attack on the pancreatic tissue is to be avoided. Duodenojejunostomy or gastrojejunostomy is usually performed.

Ectopic Pancreas

The presence of pancreatic tissue that lacks anatomic or vascular continuity with the main body of the pancreas is called ectopic pancreas. It is also referred to as aberrant pancreas or heterotopic pancreas. It is a relatively common finding, occurring in 1 to 5 per cent of autopsies, and is noted in about 1 of every 500 upper abdominal operations. The lesion may cause no symptoms or may result in recurrent pain. It is usually seen as a button of tissue, 1 to 4 cm. in diameter, present on either the mucosal or serosal surface of the stomach or duodenum, or may present as a pedunculated duodenal polyp. When ectopic pancreatic tissue occurs in the distal small bowel, it is usually present in the fundus of a Meckel's diverticulum of the ileum. Histologically, ectopic pancreatic tissue contains normal elements of acinar, ductular, and islet tissue. Rare instances of malignancy have been documented, and there is a higher than expected association with islet cell adenomas, including insulinoma and gastrinoma (Zollinger-Ellison syndrome). Surgical excision is usually curative in symptomatic lesions.

Pancreas Divisum

As discussed in the section on Embryology earlier, failure of fusion of the main and lesser pancreatic ducts, with persistence of primary ductular drainage of the pancreas through the lesser papilla, is referred to as pancreas divisum. It is a relatively common finding, occurring in about 5 per cent of patients, and is usually of no clinical consequence. The incidence of pancreas divisum among patients with pancreatitis, however, is 10 to 15 per cent. When the lesser papilla becomes obstructed or stenotic, persistent symptoms may occur. Because the ampulla of Vater is not involved and appears normal, the presence of the lesion may be overlooked. ERCP usually reveals a shortened duct of Wirsung that drains only the uncinate process of the gland. The lesser papilla must be sought in order to document the cause of symptoms, and a sphincterotomy or sphincteroplasty of the lesser papilla may be necessary to relieve the obstruction.

Acute Pancreatitis

GENERAL DESCRIPTION

Acute pancreatitis is one of the most common abdominal disorders accounting for hospital admission. Acute inflammation of the pancreas occurs in all socioeconomic and age groups. It is a disorder marked by a wide spectrum of clinical severity ranging from a mild, self-limited, transient disorder to a fulminating, progressive, unremitting process and has an overall mortality rate of 10 per cent. Although multiple etiologies are known or suspected, the disease develops when metabolic or mechanical factors cause a disruption of the physiologic mechanisms that normally protect against intrapancreatic activation of proteolytic enzymes (Fig. 16).

ETIOLOGY AND PATHOPHYSIOLOGY

Multiple metabolic, vascular, or mechanical factors can result in acute inflammation of the pancreas.

Alcohol

The majority of patients with acute pancreatitis have a history of heavy alcohol ingestion or recent significant alcohol abuse. Large-scale studies indicate that 55 to 65 per cent of acute pancreatitis is associated with alcoholism, but this factor varies depending on the location and population characteristics that prevail. It has been stated that 10 to 15 per cent of alcoholics have evidence of pancreatitis. The pathophysiology of alcohol-induced pancreatitis remains unclear. Sarles demonstrated the development of increased pancreatic protein secretion following chronic ethanol administration and noted the development of protein precipitants in the pancreatic ducts, which may result in ductular obstruction.[23] Other possible mechanisms include the development of increased permeability of ductular epithelium following ethanol ingestion, allowing efflux of pancreatic enzymes into the surrounding parenchyma,[9] and the effect of chronically elevated levels of secretory hormones stimulated by alcohol, which result in persistent hypersecretion of the acini and eventual ductal injury. Once acute pancreatitis has occurred, repeated episodes of alcohol-associated pancreatitis are common if total abstention is not achieved.

Gallstones

The second most common cause of acute pancreatitis is biliary tract disease. Calculus formation may result in an impacted common duct stone at the level of the ampulla, thereby resulting in trauma or obstruction of the main pancreatic duct, or regurgitation of bile into the pancreas due to an obstructed "common channel."

The association between pancreatitis and an obstructed common channel was first described in detail by Opie in 1901 and was initially thought to be the major cause of pancreatitis. Biliary disease is found in 5 to 50 per cent of North American series of acute pancreatitis but varies

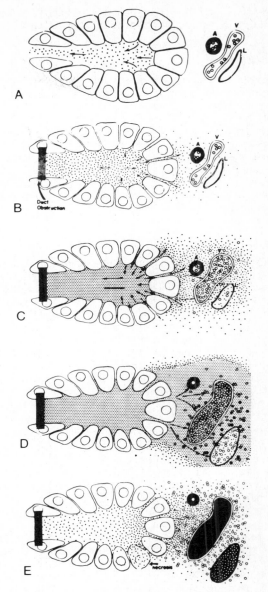

Figure 16. Schematic representation of the development of severe acute pancreatitis due to obstruction of pancreatic duct.

A, Normal acinar secretion with adjacent artery, vein, and lymphatic duct.

B, Duct obstruction results in dilated acinar lumen with pericellular leak of secretory products into interstitial tissues.

C, Increased secretion from acinar cells, with increased interstitial extravasation, edema, and venous engorgement.

D, Massive interstitial edema, arterial spasm, local hemorrhage, and engorged veins.

E, Cellular necrosis, hemorrhage, thrombosis of vessels, and extravasation of blood and secretory products into lymphatic ducts.

(From Anderson, M. C., et al.: Surg. Clin. North Am., 47:127, 1967.)

considerably depending on the socioeconomic characteristics of the population studied. In patients who recover from acute pancreatitis associated with cholelithiasis, the risk of subsequent episodes of pancreatitis ranges from 36 to 63 per cent if the cholelithiasis is allowed to persist. Following cholecystectomy, however, the risk of repeated attacks has been noted to fall to 2 to 8 per cent, thereby strongly implicating calculous disease as the etiologic factor.[19]

Hyperlipidemia

There is a strong association of hyperlipidemia with the development of pancreatitis, and patients with the most common form of the disorder, Type IV or hypertriglyceridemia, have about a 15 per cent incidence of pancreatitis. The pathophysiologic mechanism is unclear, but it has been suggested that pancreatic lipases may convert increased tissue levels of triglycerides into free fatty acids, which may then cause ductular or parenchymal injury. Although the severity of pancreatitis associated with hyperlipidemia is usually of a mild degree, severe, chronic, or even fatal episodes have been observed.

Trauma

External accidental trauma represents an important mechanical cause of pancreatitis and is reviewed elsewhere. Operative trauma also constitutes a significant cause of acute inflammation, and pancreatitis occurs following gastric or biliary procedures in a small percentage of cases. The insult is usually not noticed at the time of surgery and may result from direct blunt or sharp injury or trauma to the region of the ampulla. A related cause of pancreatitis is that seen rarely following ERCP and may involve ductular trauma or innoculation of the duct with contaminated material.

Drugs

A number of drugs have been implicated in the development of acute pancreatitis, but none has been proven to cause the disease. Steroid administration, particularly in children or young adults, has been associated repeatedly with pancreatitis, but frequently the condition for which the steroids are administered is also a possible factor. Diuretics, azathioprine (Imuran), azulfidine, L-asparaginase, and estrogen preparations have all been reported to be possible etiologic factors, although the mechanisms responsible are unknown. The combined use of steroids and azathioprine following renal transplantation may account for the relatively high incidence of pancreatitis in that setting.

Infection

Viral infections have been associated with acute pancreatitis, particularly mumps and Coxsackie infection, and a transient elevation in serum amylase is not unusual during mumps infection. Other viral illnesses, such as mononucleosis and cytomegalovirus disease, have been suspected but not proven as etiologic factors.

Vasculitis and Vascular Insufficiency

Ischemia is an established experimental model of acute pancreatitis and is thought to result in the disorder clinically in cases of atherosclerotic disease of the pancreatic vessels as well as systemic vasculitis. Arterial insufficiency due to low cardiac output or as a consequence of cardiopulmonary bypass is also thought to result in acute pancreatitis postoperatively in as many as 1 to 2 per cent of patients undergoing these procedures.

Miscellaneous Causes

Hypercalcemia due to hyperparathyroidism has been suggested as a cause of pancreatitis, and the sting of a particular species of scorpion endemic to Trinidad and Venezuela, *Tityus trinitatis*, is frequently followed by acute pancreatitis. The precise etiology related to these factors is unknown. Hereditary factors may also be involved in the development of the disease, as several clusters of pediatric and adult cases of pancreatitis have occurred within single families. Finally, a significant number of acute, even severe, episodes of pancreatitis occur idiopathically and are associated with none of the above.

CLINICAL PRESENTATION AND DIAGNOSIS

The diagnosis of acute pancreatitis is made on the basis of clinical findings and frequently involves the exclusion of other possibilities. No single finding is pathognomonic of the disease, and laboratory data should be regarded as supportive or confirmatory, but not as conclusive proof of the presence or absence of the disorder.

Symptoms

Pain is nearly always the presenting complaint and may be epigastric, lower abdominal, or localized to the posterior thoracic or lumbar area. The pain may be noted in the right or left hypochondrium or may be diffusely present throughout the entire abdomen. The pain may be mild or severe but is usually *steady* and not cramping in nature. *Nausea* and *vomiting* frequently occur, and *anorexia* is common. Low-grade *fever* may accompany these symptoms, and mild *hypertension* is commonly seen unless dehydration or hypovolemia is present. Frequently, these symptoms have occurred 1 to 3 days after heavy alcohol ingestion.

Physical Findings

The patient is frequently uncomfortable in the supine position and prefers to sit up or lie on one side. Midepigastric tenderness is usually present, and a mass effect may be palpable within the upper abdomen. Bowel sounds are quiet or hypoactive, and jaundice is occasionally present. Signs of peritonitis are usually absent but may occur. The patient may appear dehydrated and hypotensive. Diffuse abdominal fullness or mild distention is frequently present.

Laboratory Findings

The most commonly observed abnormality is hyperamylasemia, but this is neither a specific nor a sensitive finding. Large-scale studies have shown that 20 to 30 per cent of patients with otherwise documented acute pancreatitis have normal amylase levels, and 35 per cent of patients with hyperamylasemia have an illness other than pancreatitis. Alternative causes of elevated serum amylase include bowel obstruction, bowel infarction, ectopic pregnancy, renal failure, and hepatic disorders as well as the normal variant of macroamylasemia. Urinary amylase levels are usually elevated for 2 to 5 days after hyperamylasemia subsides and therefore also should be determined. The excretion of amylase depends on the glomerular filtration rate, however, and the relationship of the urinary clearance of amylase to the urinary clearance of creatinine is the best assessment of increased amylase secretion. A spot urine sample, or 24-hour collection, is assayed for both amylase and creatinine. A simultaneous blood sample is likewise assayed, and the amylase-creatinine clearance ratio (C_{am}/C_{cr}) is calculated as (urine amylase/serum amylase) x (serum creatinine/urine creatinine) $\times$ 100. A C_{am}/C_{cr} greater than 5 per cent is very specific for acute pancreatitis; a value of 4 per cent or greater is highly suggestive.[14]

In addition to amylase, serum lipase levels also rise during acute pancreatitis, and recent studies suggest this may be a more specific test for the disorder. Other laboratory findings may include an elevated white blood cell count, a hemoglobin or hematocrit that is either elevated (due to volume contraction) or low (due to retroperitoneal hemorrhage), an increased blood urea nitrogen and creatinine, elevated hepatic enzymes and bilirubin, and a metabolic acidosis or mixed metabolic and respiratory acidosis associated with hypoxia. Plasma glucose levels may be elevated owing to loss of insulin-secreting ability but are rarely at the diabetic ketoacidosis level. Plasma calcium may be low owing to sequestration of calcium by fat necrosis with saponification, and hypocalcemia may result in signs of tetany. Plain roentgenograms, sonograms, and CT scans of the abdomen may also indicate an enlarged, edematous pancreas as well as signs of ileus, abscess, or cyst formation.

CLINICAL COURSE AND COMPLICATIONS

Pathologic changes in acute pancreatitis range from interstitial edema with mild inflammatory cell infiltrates surrounding intact ductular and parenchymal tissue, to necrosis of acinar elements, focal hemorrhage, and massive edema, to extensive coagulation necrosis of whole areas of the gland with necrosis of peripancreatic tissues and blood vessels resulting in massive retroperitoneal hemorrhage. The most common cause of morbidity and mortality is *sepsis,* as areas of necrosis become secondarily infected with bacteria. In addition to abscess and pseudocyst formation and the development of pancreatic fluid extravasation, several other complications occur as the pathologic changes progress. Adjacent structures including the stomach, duodenum, and biliary ducts may become involved in regional edema and necrosis, resulting in obstruction or local hemorrhage. Splenic or portal vein thrombosis may occur and may result in variceal hemorrhage when antecedent portal hypertension has existed. Pulmonary insuffi-

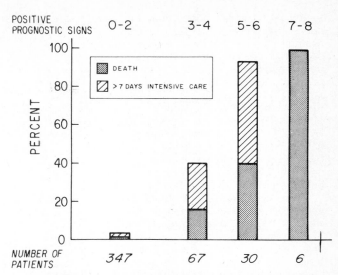

Figure 17. Mortality and morbidity of acute pancreatitis compared with number of positive prognostic signs (see Table 4). (From Ranson, J. H. C., Rifkind, K. M., and Roses, D. F.: Surg. Gynecol. Obstet., 139:69, 1974.)

ciency is a common sequela of pancreatitis and may involve only pleural effusion and atelectasis, pneumonia, or florid adult respiratory distress syndrome. Oliguria, azotemia, or renal vein thrombosis may result in renal failure, and disseminated intravascular coagulation, pericardial effusion, or refractory circulatory collapse may occur.

In order to distinguish those patients with a "mild" form of the disease, and are therefore likely to recover, from those patients with "severe" pancreatitis who are at high risk for the development of one or more of the previously mentioned complications, a method of clinical evaluation has evolved. After careful review of multiple laboratory and clinical findings in patients with acute pancreatitis, Ranson and colleagues[20] determined five criteria seen at the time of initial diagnosis and six criteria based upon the clinical course of the patient in the subsequent 48 hours that correlate particularly well with the ultimate risk of morbidity and mortality (Table 4). It is to be noted that the presence or degree of hyperamylasemia is *not* a useful index of the severity of the disease. The correlation between the number of positive criteria and the mortality and morbidity of the patients was linear and dramatic; patients with three or more positive signs (defined as "severe" pancreatitis) had an average mortality of 28 per cent (Fig. 17).

TREATMENT

In 75 to 80 per cent of patients, acute pancreatitis is "mild" (less than three criteria positive), and a successful outcome is usually achieved with nonoperative supportive therapy. Surgical intervention is indicated only when a definitive diagnosis of pancreatitis has not been made but signs of an upper abdominal catastrophe persist, when pancreatic abscess is suspected or proven, or when complications or etiologic factors require operative intervention.

Supportive Therapy

The first priority is to *put the gland at rest.* The patient is given *nothing by mouth,* and a *nasogastric tube* is strongly recommended. The removal of gastric acid and the elimi-

TABLE 4. *Early Objective Findings that Correlate with the Risk of Major Complications or Death in Acute Pancreatitis**

At Admission or Diagnosis
1. Age over 55 years
2. White blood cell count over 16,000/cu. mm.
3. Blood glucose level over 200 mg./100 ml.
4. Serum lactic dehydrogenase (LDH) concentration over 350 I.U./liter
5. Serum glutamic oxaloacetic transaminase (SGOT) over 250 Sigma-Frankel units/100 ml.

During Initial 48 Hours
6. Hematocrit decrease greater than 10 per cent points
7. Blood urea nitrogen increase more than 5 mg./100 ml.
8. Serum calcium level below 8 mg./100 ml.
9. Arterial P_{O_2} below 60 mm. Hg
10. Base deficit greater than 4 mEq./liter
11. Estimated fluid sequestration (IV fluid replacement requirement) more than 6000 ml.

*Modified from Ranson, J. H. C., Rifkind, K. M., and Roses, D. F.: Surg. Gynecol. Obstet., *139*:69, 1974.

nation of gastric distention reduce the neural and hormonal stimulation of the exocrine pancreas and help prevent aspiration due to vomiting. *Analgesics* are prescribed, both for patient comfort as well as to reduce stress-induced neural stimulation of gastric and pancreatic secretion. *Meperidine* (Demerol) is used in place of morphine, as the latter may induce spasm of the sphincter of Oddi. Additional agents that are intended to reduce pancreatic stimulation, such as anticholinergics (atropine or glycopyrrolate [Robinul]), trypsin inhibitors (aprotinin), or hormones that have been shown experimentally to inhibit exocrine secretion (glucagon or somatostatin), have not been found to be useful in large-scale studies or require further evaluation before their routine use can be recommended.

The second priority of supportive therapy is to prevent potential complications of pancreatitis. Since the major cause of death is sepsis, *antibiotics* are usually prescribed. Their routine application has not been shown to be statistically significantly beneficial, however, although clinical series usually contain only a small number of patients with "moderate" or "severe" pancreatitis in whom the risk of sepsis is high. *Antacids* are usually prescribed to reduce both gastric acid output to the duodenum and the risk of bleeding secondary to gastritis or duodenitis. In all but the mildest forms of pancreatitis, retroperitoneal fluid sequestration and hypovolemia occur and require *intravenous fluid administration*. Fluid losses from anorexia, vomiting, and retroperitoneal inflammation and hemorrhage may necessitate massive fluid replacement if renal failure and circulatory collapse are to be avoided. Hypocalcemia and other ion deficiencies require intravenous replacement, and nutritional support usually requires *parenteral alimentation* with careful monitoring of blood glucose levels. Ventilatory support is frequently needed, and the common occurrence of hypoxia and pulmonary infiltrates usually requires mechanical ventilatory assistance with positive end-expiratory pressure (PEEP) for successful management.

Surgical Intervention

In addition to the establishment of the diagnosis, surgical treatment can provide additional support to reduce retroperitoneal inflammation. Peritoneal lavage has proven to be an effective measure that frequently results in dramatic clinical improvement in the symptoms and signs of "moderately severe" pancreatitis. The risk of subsequent sepsis remains high in these patients, however, and the overall time course of the illness is relatively unchanged.[19] Careful attention must be given to possible septic complications, and early refeeding of the patient with apparent resolution of symptoms is to be avoided.

More extensive drainage of the peripancreatic tissues is hazardous in milder forms of acute pancreatitis and may actually contribute to increased morbidity and mortality. In severe pancreatitis, however, extensive lavage and sump drainage of the region of the pancreas may improve survival and should be considered if the disease becomes progressively more severe and retroperitoneal necrosis is present. In cases of advanced pancreatic necrosis, resection or debridement of the necrotic gland with extensive drainage of the region may offer the only hope of survival.

Operative therapy may be required in cases of acute pancreatitis associated with biliary calculous disease. If cholecystitis or common duct obstruction does not respond to conservative management during the first 48 hours, cholecystostomy, cholecystectomy, or common duct decompression may be required to reverse a progressively

deteriorating clinical course. Frequently, the coexistence of gangrenous cholecystitis or cholangitis is difficult to exclude in these cases, and early surgical intervention may be required. In general, however, conservative management is advised until the pancreatitis has resolved, whereupon necessary biliary tract procedures may be undertaken with a greater margin of safety. Surgical treatment of complications such as abscess and pseudocyst formation is reviewed in subsequent sections.

Chronic Pancreatitis

GENERAL DESCRIPTION

Recurrent episodes of acute pancreatitis or persistent inflammation within the pancreas may ultimately result in a chronic disorder characterized by fibrosis, calculus formation, and cystic changes within the gland. Chronic pancreatitis usually presents in males between the ages of 35 to 50 but may occur in patients of either sex from the second to the eighth decade of life. The disease is usually progressive, and although symptoms may be controlled by medical therapy or, in selected cases, resolved by surgical treatment, the histologic changes within the gland are irreversible.

ETIOLOGY AND PATHOPHYSIOLOGY

The usual etiologic factor associated with the development of chronic pancreatitis is alcohol abuse, but chronic inflammation and fibrosis may result from a variety of factors including trauma, biliary tract disease, and hypercalcemia. Alcoholism is the most common cause of "calcific" pancreatitis, in which calcium carbonate calculi form within the ducts, and ductular and parenchymal calcium deposits are seen. These changes occur in one third of patients with advanced chronic pancreatitis.

Progressive fibrosis leads to distortion of the parenchyma, with loss of acinar tissue, a reduced number of islets, disruption of normal vascular supply, and distortion or obliteration of various portions of the ductular system. Ductular pathology occurs in several forms and may include proximal (periampullary) obstruction due to stricture or stone formation with resultant distal duct dilatation, intermittent areas of stenosis and dilatation throughout the ductular system ("chain of lakes" appearance), or complete stenosis or sclerosis of the ducts, with or without parenchymal cyst formation. Fibrosis may involve adjacent structures such as the distal common bile duct or duodenum, and low-grade obstructive jaundice is frequently seen.

The loss of acinar tissue results in clinically apparent exocrine insufficiency when enzyme secretion falls to less than 10 per cent of normal capacity. Similarly, the progressive loss of islet tissue results in a steady deterioration of glucose tolerance, and clinically demonstrable diabetes mellitus is seen in as many as one third of patients with chronic pancreatitis. Laennec's cirrhosis is seen in patients with a history of alcoholism, but the coexistence of chronic pancreatitis and severe cirrhosis is less than might otherwise be expected and occurs in only a minority of patients.

CLINICAL PRESENTATION AND DIAGNOSIS

Patients present with persistent abdominal *pain*, which is usually localized to the midepigastrium and may penetrate through to the posterior thoracolumbar region. The pain is usually *steady,* and it may be exacerbated by eating or may occur as separate crises of severe pain associated with heavy alcohol ingestion. Although nausea and vomiting may occur, there is less hemodynamic instability than is seen in acute pancreatitis. Abdominal examination usually reveals moderate tenderness in the midepigastrium, and upper abdominal fullness or a palpable mass may be present. Frequently there is evidence of malnutrition, and jaundice may be present. The patient may relate a history consistent with steatorrhea, although demonstrable exocrine deficiency may be present in patients who report unremarkable bowel function.

Laboratory studies usually reveal normal or only modestly elevated serum amylase levels and white blood cell counts. Hyperglycemia is common, as are low-grade elevations of bilirubin and alkaline phosphatase. Liver enzyme elevations are frequently seen, as are laboratory parameters of malnutrition. The diagnosis is usually confirmed by characteristic findings on radiologic studies such as plain roentgenograms of the abdomen (which may reveal diffuse calcification in the region of the pancreas), sonograms and CT scans (which demonstrate ductular dilatation, cyst disease, and calcification), or ERCP (which shows ductular distortion, dilatation, stenosis, or obstruction). Functional tests of exocrine function (secretin test, Lundh meal, PABA test, or DMO test) or endocrine function (oral glucose tolerance test) provide additional support for the diagnosis of chronic pancreatic disease.

CLINICAL COURSE AND COMPLICATIONS

The natural history of chronic pancreatitis is that of persistent pain associated with progressive signs and symptoms of exocrine and endocrine (insulin) insufficiency. Acute exacerbations of severe pain are associated with increased duct obstruction and cyst formation. It has been shown that when intraductular pressure rises 15 to 20 cm. of H_2O above normal, pain usually occurs or increases. Patients demonstrate progressive malnutrition and general debilitation and frequently exhibit heavy dependence on analgesics.

Complications of associated splanchnic and gastrointestinal involvement by progressive inflammation include biliary tract disease (with calculus formation or common duct stenosis), portal hypertension, splenic vein thrombosis, gastritis, duodenitis, and complications of pseudocyst disease. Sepsis may occur but is relatively infrequent.

TREATMENT

Nonoperative Therapy

Supportive therapy during episodes of acute exacerbation of chronic disease is similar to that of acute pancreatitis, with the addition of enteral pancreatic enzyme replacement. The medical therapy of progressive chronic pancreatitis includes the removal of precipitating factors, such as alcohol, drugs, or hypercalcemia, together with appropriate treatment of pain, steatorrhea, weight loss, and diabetes. The management of the patient with "pancreatogenic" diabetes is directed toward the control of blood glucose levels, but with particular attention to the avoidance of hypoglycemia. Patients with chronic pancreatitis frequently manifest a "brittle" form of diabetes in which even modest doses of insulin may result in profound lowering of blood glucose. This effect may be secondary to the loss of pancreatic secretion of the counterregulatory hormone glu-

cagon or the increased number and affinity of insulin receptors due to chronic hypoinsulinemia.

Surgical Therapy

Although nonoperative therapy may control the exocrine and endocrine deficiency, the persistence of severe pain or jaundice is usually regarded as an indication for surgical therapy. No single operation is advocated for patients with chronic pancreatitis, and the choice of a suitable surgical procedure depends upon the specific anatomic considerations in each patient. Biliary and pancreatic ductular anatomy is carefully evaluated by CT scanning and ERCP to determine the location and extent of the disease process. When ERCP is unsuccessful, cholangiography and operative pancreatograms form the basis for surgical decision making.

Biliary tract procedures may be required to treat cholelithiasis or choledocholithiasis, and stenosis or stricture of the ampulla of Vater is carefully sought. In a minority of cases, significant stenosis or obstruction of the ampulla will respond to *sphincteroplasty,* in which the ampulla of Vater is enlarged and the sphincter of Oddi sewn open to prevent obstruction. This maneuver has been advocated for the pancreatic duct sphincter as well but is seldom indicated.

More commonly, the predominant ductular pathology consists of either generalized dilatation behind a proximal obstruction in the region of the head or uncinate process or diffuse sclerosis of the ductular system. A dilated, obstructed pancreatic duct is best treated with internal drainage into a Roux-en-Y loop of jejunum, and a number of procedures have been advocated to achieve this decompression (Fig. 18). The earliest attempts at pancreatic duct decompression included the creation of an external pancreatostomy performed by Link in 1911. Modern procedures designed to allow internal drainage of the ductular system include the distal (caudal) pancreaticojejunostomy advocated by Zollinger and by DuVal in 1954 and the side-to-side pancreaticojejunostomy described by Puestow and Gillesby in 1958. Both of these procedures require splenectomy and resection of the pancreatic tail and have been supplanted by the Partington and Rochelle modification of the Puestow procedure described in 1960. In this procedure, a long (10 to 12 cm.) longitudinal opening of the anterior aspect of the pancreatic duct is anostomosed to a similar longitudinal enterotomy in a Roux-en-Y limb of jejunum. The operative morbidity and mortality are generally low, and 70 to 80 per cent of patients report good to excellent pain relief following this procedure.

When the main pancreatic duct is not dilated but is sclerotic, a decompression procedure is infeasible. Resection of most or all of the diseased portion of the gland may then offer relief of pain. In 1944, Priestly and Claggett first performed resection in treatment of chronic pancreatitis, and there has been continued debate regarding the benefit of partial (40 to 80 per cent) distal pancreatectomy, subtotal (95 per cent) distal pancreatectomy (Child's procedure), partial proximal pancreatectomy (Whipple procedure), or total pancreatectomy in the treatment of this disorder. In general, the procedure that offers the best likelihood of pain relief with the lowest risk of operative or postoperative morbidity and mortality is preferred. Each resectional procedure carries specific disadvantages, however. Although partial distal pancreatectomy is usually the safest procedure to perform, it is also associated with only a 50 to 60 per cent incidence of prolonged pain relief. Conversely, al-

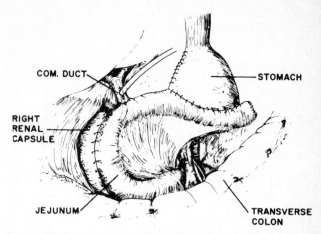

Figure 19. Total pancreatectomy. The pancreas, spleen, gastric antrum, duodenum, and distal common bile duct have been removed and a gastrojejunostomy and choledochojejunostomy performed. A T-tube drains the common bile duct and stents the anastomosis. (From Moossa, A. R. In Maingot, R. (Ed.): Abdominal Operations. Norwalk, Conn., Appleton-Century-Crofts, 1980.)

Pancreatic Pseudocysts

GENERAL DESCRIPTION AND PATHOPHYSIOLOGY

A *pseudocyst* is a collection of fluid that, unlike a true cyst, has no epithelial lining. The wall of the pseudocyst is composed of the inflammatory reaction (granulation tissue and fibrosis) that forms around the perimeter of the fluid. Pseudocysts are a particularly common finding in patients with either acute or chronic pancreatitis and are thought to arise from a loss of continuity or leak from the ductular

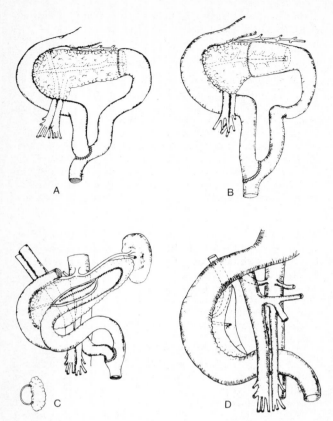

Figure 18. Surgical approaches to chronic pancreatitis. A, Caudal pancreaticojeunostomy, after Duval. B, Caudal longitudinal pancreaticojejunostomy, after Puestow and Gillesby. C, Side-to-side longitudinal pancreaticojejunostomy, after Partington and Rochelle. D, Ninety-five per cent distal pancreatectomy, after Child. (Adapted from Brooks, J. R.: Chronic pancreatitis. In Surgery of the Pancreas. Philadelphia, W. B. Saunders Company, 1983.)

though subtotal distal resection and total pancreatic resection (Fig. 19) provide improved pain relief, they are invariably accompanied by severe exocrine deficiency and a particularly brittle form of diabetes mellitus. Proximal pancreatectomy (and duodenectomy) (Fig. 20) is indicated only in the unusual situation of severe sclerotic disease limited to the head of the pancreas and carries a high risk of perioperative morbidity and mortality. Therefore, resectional procedures are embarked upon only with considerable caution and only in carefully selected cases. Demonstrated failure of aggressive nonoperative management of chronic pancreatitis is an absolute prerequisite before these procedures are performed.

Recent attempts have been made to reduce or eliminate the obligatory endocrine disease that accompanies subtotal or total pancreatectomy by means of isolated autologous islet transplantation performed at the time of resection.[15] Technical problems have limited its success owing to poor islet yields from the resected portion of pancreas, failure of the isolated islets to function when implanted into the liver via intraportal infusion, and portal hypertension secondary to intrahepatic portal congestion. The method offers considerable promise, however, and clinical experience with these techniques continues to grow at a number of specialized surgical centers.

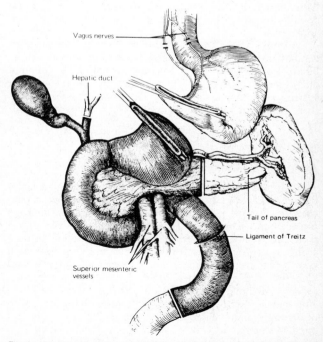

Figure 20. Pancreaticoduodenectomy (Whipple procedure). The tissues shaded are resected en bloc. Reconstruction is illustrated in Figure 22. (From Frey, C. F.: Surg. Tech. Illus., 4:96, 1977.)

elements of the gland. Pseudocysts may be completely surrounded by pancreatic parenchyma or may extend beyond the confines of the gland. They may occur in any region of the pancreas, and recent studies indicate that approximately 1 in 7 patients with pseudocyst disease harbors multiple pseudocysts.

CLINICAL COURSE AND COMPLICATIONS

The routine use of serial sonograms during the course of acute pancreatitis reveals that 30 to 40 per cent of acute pseudocysts resolve spontaneously and require no surgical therapy. When a pseudocyst persists for 4 to 6 weeks or shows evidence of steady enlargement, surgical decompression is indicated to avoid subsequent complications. Pseudocysts produce symptoms by virtue of displacement of the pancreas or surrounding structures, by free intraperitoneal rupture, by penetration or perforation into adjacent organs, by erosion into the blood vessels with intracystic hemorrhage, or by becoming secondarily infected, at which time they are indistinguishable from abscesses.[22]

TREATMENT

Decompression can be achieved by either internal or external drainage. Internal drainage into the gastrointestinal tract is preferred, as external drainage usually results in persistent pancreaticocutaneous drainage for 3 to 6 weeks and a 20 to 30 per cent incidence of pseudocyst recurrence. Internal drainage of a pseudocyst may be accomplished by creation of a cystoenteric anastomosis to either an adjacent portion of stomach (cystogastrostomy) or duodenum (cystoduodenostomy) or to a Roux-en-Y limb of jejunum. The presence of multiple pseudocysts does not alter this general treatment plan, and multiple cystoenteric anastomoses may be performed. At the time of operative drainage, a biopsy of the wall of the pseudocyst is also usually obtained to confirm the diagnosis. Occasionally other cystic lesions of the pancreas, such as cystadenomas and cystadenocarcinomas, may resemble pseudocysts but require resection rather than decompression.

In severe chronic pancreatitis, pseudocysts are frequently accompanied by generalized dilatation of the main pancreatic duct, and both lesions may be decompressed using the Puestow method of a single longitudinal pancreaticojejunostomy. Although simple aspiration of pseudocysts has been attempted by some, the recurrence rate following this maneuver is high and varies from 20 to 80 per cent. Accordingly, patients who are poor surgical risks, and who may therefore be chosen as candidates for percutaneous decompression of pseudocysts, should be treated with prolonged catheter drainage rather than simple aspiration.

When a pseudocyst becomes secondarily infected, the resulting pancreatic abscess carries a substantially greater risk of morbidity and mortality. For this reason, radiographic delineation of pseudocysts by noninvasive means, such as sonogram and CT scanning, is generally preferred to invasive techniques such as ERCP. The suspicion of pseudocyst disease is therefore a relative contraindication to ERCP unless immediate subsequent surgical decompression is planned.

Pancreatic Abscess

GENERAL DESCRIPTION AND PATHOPHYSIOLOGY

The development of a pancreatic abscess represents a severe, life-threatening complication for the patient with pancreatitis. The mortality rate for pancreatic abscesses that are *not* treated by operative drainage is virtually 100 per cent, and the most successful series of surgical treatment still demonstrate a 30 to 50 per cent mortality. Pancreatic abscess can accompany acute pancreatitis caused by virtually any etiologic factor or can occur as a complication of chronic pancreatitis accompanied by ductular obstruction or pseudocyst disease.

The etiology of the infection is thought to be due to either the reflux of enteric flora into the pancreas or hematogenous seeding of a pancreatic phlegmon during a septic episode. Bacteria isolated from pancreatic abscesses include a wide range of organisms but are predominantly gram-negative enteric species. The septic state resulting from a pancreatic abscess is particularly severe owing to the relatively unconfined retroperitoneal location of the abscess, the exuberant vascular and lymphatic supply to the area, and the accompanying tissue damage and necrosis that result from the liberation of proteolytic enzymes in the area.

CLINICAL PRESENTATION

The diagnosis is usually made when the clinical course of the patient fails to reveal significant improvement during supportive therapy and when physical and laboratory parameters are consistent with possible sepsis. Noninvasive radiologic studies, such as sonograms and CT scanning, may then reveal a heterogeneous mass in the region of the pancreas with evidence of entrapped air or liquified debris. Occasionally, such clear-cut radiographic findings are not evident, and the decision to proceed with surgical intervention must be made on purely clinical grounds.

TREATMENT

The treatment of a pancreatic abscess should provide thorough drainage and débridement of necrotic debris. Multiple sump and irrigation drains are inserted into the abscess and brought out of the abdominal cavity at various sites. Despite this vigorous approach, several reoperations may be required to maintain adequate drainage, and clinical signs of progressive or recurrent sepsis are indications for re-exploration. Some authors recommend débridement and open packing of pancreatic abscesses, leaving the abdominal wound open to allow frequent removal and replacement of the packing material.[7] This procedure is called *marsupialization* of the pancreas, and, despite its seemingly radical nature, the beneficial results obtained with the technique warrant its use in selected cases when pancreatic necrosis is widespread. The clinical course of the patient with a successfully treated pancreatic abscess is still protracted and frequently complicated. Aggressive and meticulous attention to the metabolic and nutritional needs of the patient is essential for a satisfactory outcome.

Pancreatic Ascites and Hydrothorax

GENERAL DESCRIPTION AND PATHOPHYSIOLOGY

The free intraperitoneal rupture of a pancreatic duct or pseudocyst may result in the general accumulation of pancreatic fluid within the abdomen. When this process occurs in the absence of surrounding inflammation, the fluid collection does not become encapsulated but merely drains into the peritoneal cavity. This is referred to as *pancreatic ascites*. When the leak of pancreatic fluid occurs in the retroperitoneal tissues, the fluid may track into the mediastinum, forming a mediastinal pseudocyst. A *pancreatic pleural effusion,* or hydrothorax, can occur when pancreatic fluid penetrates into the pleural cavity from a mediastinal collection or traverses the diaphragm directly from an intraperitoneal collection. Because of their common etiology, pancreatic ascites and pancreatic pleural effusions are referred to as internal pancreatic fistulas.

CLINICAL PRESENTATION

Nearly 80 per cent of patients with pancreatic ascites have a history of alcoholism, whereas trauma accounts for the etiology in 10 per cent.[4] Frequently, the ascites is initially thought to be the result of alcoholic cirrhosis, and many patients lack any history of antecedent acute pancreatitis. Patients with posttraumatic pancreatic ascites usually have a history of posttraumatic pancreatitis, followed by the development of ascites within 1 to 5 weeks. The clinical presentation of pancreatic ascites usually consists of increasing abdominal girth together with mild abdominal pain. Patients with pancreatic pleural effusions have large unilateral or bilateral hydrothorax accompanied by respiratory compromise. Unlike the small spontaneously resolving pleural effusion associated with acute pancreatitis, pancreatic pleural effusions persist and recur rapidly after initial thoracentesis. Pancreatic ascites and hydrothorax occasionally occur simultaneously. Paracentesis or thoracentesis reveals elevated levels of amylase and albumin in the fluid, and the diagnosis is confirmed by ERCP or operative pancreatograms that demonstrate pancreatic fluid extravasation.

TREATMENT

Patients are initially treated nonoperatively, and the goals of supportive therapy are to reduce pancreatic secretion, remove pancreatic fluid, and support the nutritional status of the patient in the hope that spontaneous closure of the fistula will occur. Patients are given nothing by mouth, nasogastric drainage is maintained, and anticholinergics and carbonic anhydrase inhibitors are administered. Paracentesis or thoracentesis or tube thoracostomy drainage is performed, and patients are given parenteral hyperalimentation. In a significant number of patients, fluid collections will resolve on this regimen, and in some, permanent resolution will be shown. If nonoperative therapy does not result in resolution in 2 weeks, surgical correction is accomplished. Long-term nonoperative management has been associated with a significant incidence of sudden death in these patients, and therefore the trial of supportive therapy is intentionally limited.[4]

Operative therapy is dependent upon the etiology of the pancreatic leak. In the case of an anterior pancreatic duct disruption, a Roux-en-Y pancreaticojejunal anastomosis may establish internal drainage (Fig. 21). Leakage from a pseudocyst may be controlled by a cystoenteric anastomosis or resection of a small distal pseudocyst with oversewing of the proximal pancreatic stump. In the case of a pancreatic pleural effusion, attention is also directed to the pancreas, and ligation of the retroperitoneal sinus tract together with resection or drainage of the site of duct or cyst disruption results in resolution of the fistula. In all cases of internal pancreatic fistulas, careful delineation of the pancreatic ductular anatomy is essential for successful treatment.

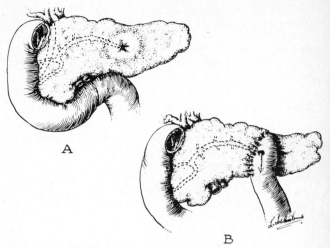

Figure 21. Treatment of pancreatic duct leak from anterior surface of gland. A, Operative findings after exposure of the fistula. B, Internal drainage via Roux-en-Y pancreaticojejunostomy. (From Cameron, J. L., et al.: Ann. Surg., 170:668, 1969.)

Pancreatic Neoplasms

GENERAL DESCRIPTION

Tumors of the pancreas represent a wide spectrum of diagnostic and therapeutic challenges. The most common malignancy, ductular adenocarcinoma, is a particularly insidious disease and continues to carry a poor prognosis with an overall 5-year patient survival rate of less than 1 per cent. The rare islet cell tumors can be treated successfully and have contributed greatly to an understanding of endocrine physiology through documentation of the effects of their excessive hormone secretion. The distinction between the benign and malignant histologic status of various pancreatic neoplasms is frequently unclear, and the early diagnosis of potentially curable pancreatic malignancy remains largely an unfulfilled goal.

EXOCRINE TUMORS

Benign Tumors

Benign tumors of exocrine cell origin are rare and include *acinar cell* and *ductular cell adenomas* and connective tissue tumors such as *hemangiomas, lymphangiomas,* and *dermoid* tumors. *Serous cystadenomas* (arising from acinar cells) and *mucinous cystadenomas* (arising from ductular cells), although histologically benign, are thought to have the capacity to degenerate into cystadenocarcinomas. Large, cystic lesions may resemble pseudocysts and are detected by their increasing size. Smaller lesions are diagnosed on the basis of investigation of complaints of vague or intermittent abdominal discomfort or when the lesion arises near the ampulla or distal common bile duct and results in obstructive jaundice. This general pattern occurs for all exocrine neoplasms and accounts for the relative failure to diagnose these tumors at an early stage of their development, except when they arise in the head of the pancreas. When a tumor has been identified by radiologic studies or at the time of surgery, it is usually impossible to discriminate between the rare benign exocrine tumors and their more common malignant counterparts, and resection is therefore the treatment of choice when feasible.

Malignant Tumors

Malignant exocrine tumors include a wide spectrum of ductular, acinar cell, and connective tissue tumors, but over 90 per cent present as *ductular adenocarcinoma*. The etiology of this malignancy remains obscure, and the incidence rises progressively from the third decade of life. Multiple intrapancreatic foci of carcinoma are seen in 10 to 20 per cent of patients, and the malignancy is characterized by an aggressive pattern of regional and distant metastasis.

Diagnosis. Although the diagnosis is usually made from histologic examination of a biopsy or surgically resected specimen, attempts have been made to identify specific *tumor markers* that may provide an early indication of the presence of the disease. A variety of proteins are secreted by various malignancies of gastrointestinal and pancreatic origin, and, although the synthesis of these proteins by normal tissues may occur embryologically, they are usually detected in adult life only in very low circulating levels. Occasionally their synthesis is activated by the malignant process, and these proteins are referred to as *oncofetal antigens* or oncofetal proteins. *Carcinoembryonic antigen* (CEA) is the most widely studied, and, although plasma levels of CEA rise in cases of ductular adenocarcinoma, the lack of sensitivity and specificity of this marker for pancreatic cancer *per se* precludes its use as a reliable marker. *Pancreatic oncofetal antigen* (POA), described by Banwo and colleagues in 1974, is seen in highest levels in patients with pancreatic adenocarcinoma, but the presence of modestly elevated levels of POA can occur in a variety of benign and malignant conditions. Elevations in CEA or POA levels that occur after surgical resection of a malignancy, however, can be useful indicators of the presence of recurrent or metastatic disease.

Clinical Presentation. Patients with pancreatic adenocarcinoma usually manifest symptoms of weight loss and vague abdominal discomfort and may present with obstructive jaundice if the tumor arises in the head of the pancreas. Pain penetrating into the back is frequently noted, and there is a greater than expected association with psychiatric disturbances such as depression and psychosis. When distal common bile duct obstruction occurs, a dilated palpable gallbladder may be present ("Courvoisier's sign"). The presence of the tumor may be confirmed by contrast or scanning radiography, and evidence of metastatic disease is present in more than half of all patients with adenocarcinoma. When the tumor is well localized by ERCP or other studies and when metastatic disease is not detected, arteriography is frequently employed to determine potential resectability. The findings of *encasement* or obliteration of major vessels or of angiographically demonstrable metastases assist in the identification of those patients in whom surgical attack on the lesion is unwarranted. The angiographic finding of *compression* or mild displacement of the superior mesenteric or portal vein is not a consistent sign of the lack of resectability, however, as edema and inflammation around the tumor, rather than the tumor itself, may produce these findings. Final assessment of resectability is by surgical exploration, and approximately 20 per cent of patients are found to have a lesion that can be successfully resected in hope of cure or long-term survival.

Surgical Therapy. Surgically resectable adenocarcinomas are usually located in the head of the pancreas, since distal lesions almost always demonstrate metastases by the time the diagnosis is made. The most widely performed procedure is the *pancreaticoduodenectomy*, or Whipple procedure (Fig. 22). Total pancreatectomy is advocated by some authorities but is generally avoided owing to the great degree of postoperative morbidity secondary to the metabolic and nutritional abnormalities that accompany this operation.

In less than 10 per cent of patients with resectable exocrine malignancy, the lesion is found to be a *cystadenocarcinoma* of the *papillary* or *serous* type. This lesion is less aggressive in its capacity to metastasize early compared with ductular adenocarcinoma, and therefore surgical resection is associated with a significant 5-year survival in the range of 10 to 20 per cent. The tumor is frequently found to arise in the body or tail of the pancreas, and a *subtotal*

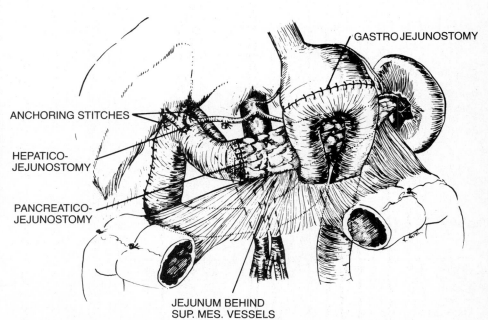

Figure 22. Pancreaticojejunostomy (Whipple procedure). The surgical reconstruction is shown following en bloc resection of the pancreatic head and neck, gastric antrum, and duodenum. (From Moossa, A. R.: In Maingot, R. (Ed.): Abdominal Operations. Norwalk, Conn., Appleton-Century-Crofts, 1980.)

GASTROJEJUNOSTOMY

ANCHORING STITCHES

HEPATICO-JEJUNOSTOMY

PANCREATICO-JEJUNOSTOMY

JEJUNUM BEHIND SUP. MES. VESSELS

distal pancreatectomy may then be performed. Absolute exocrine and endocrine deficiency is usually avoided if 10 to 20 per cent of the pancreatic mass is preserved.

Other malignancies of non-endocrine origin that may occur include lymphomas, various sarcomas, and tumors whose origin lies in the duodenal or biliary duct epithelium of the ampulla. Well-localized lesions, particularly in the region of the ampulla, are resected as described previously, and significant albeit modest rates of long-term survival may be achieved.

ENDOCRINE TUMORS

Benign lesions of islet cell origin include disorders of *hyperplasia* and *adenoma* formation. *Islet cell tumors* have now been described for each of the four principal islet cell types as well as a variety of additional hormone-secreting tumors of pancreatic origin. Islet cell tumors (adenomas or adenocarcinomas) may be "nonfunctional" and associated with no detectable elevation of known hormones but frequently secrete at least one hormone product in sufficient excess to cause significant signs and symptoms. Occasionally, these tumors are *pleuripotential* and secrete more than one hormone either simultaneously or sequentially over a period of months to years. Rarely, islet cell adenomas (particularly those that secrete gastrin) are associated with hyperplasia or adenomatosis of other endocrine tissue such as the parathyroids, pituitary, and adrenals and may therefore form part of the Type I *multiple endocrine neoplasia* (MEN) syndrome[10] (Table 5). The histologic differentiation of adenoma from adenocarcinoma is frequently difficult in these lesions, and the designation of malignancy is often dependent upon the presence of grossly apparent metastases.

Islet Hyperplasia and Nesidioblastosis

Islet cell *hyperplasia* occurs in a variety of conditions including obesity, following oral hypoglycemic agent therapy, and in some cases of hypergastrinemia (Zollinger-Ellison syndrome) and secretory diarrhea (Verner-Morrison syndrome). Very rarely, the hypersecretion of insulin or vasoactive intestinal polypeptide (VIP) associated with diffuse islet cell hyperplasia may warrant subtotal or even total pancreatectomy to control the resulting disease.

A related disorder is *nesidioblastosis*, in which islets become hyperplastic or adenomatous and tufts of islet cells develop around the ductular epithelium. Although this

TABLE 5. *Islet Cell Tumor Syndromes*

Syndrome	Excess Hormone	Cell Type	Signs and Symptoms*	Diagnostic Studies†
Insulinoma	Insulin (+ proinsulin C-peptide)	Beta	*Hypoglycemia* *Altered mental status* Syncope Dizziness	72-hr. fast Tolbutamide test Calcium infusion
Gastrinoma (Zollinger-Ellison)	Gastrin	Gamma	*Gastric acid hypersecretion* *Peptic ulceration* Diarrhea (steatorrhea) Weight loss	Secretin test Calcium infusion Test meal Evidence of MEN-1‡
Glucagonoma	Glucagon	Alpha	*Hyperglycemia* *Diabetes mellitus* *Skin rash (MNE§)* *Glossitis* Thrombophlebitis Weight loss	Skin biopsy Arginine infusion
Somatostatinoma	Somatostatin	Delta	*Diabetes mellitus* *Gallstones* *Hypochlorhydria* Steatorrhea Weight loss	Test meal Tolbutamide test
WDHA (Verner-Morrison)	VIP (or PGE₁)	Delta₁	*Watery diarrhea* *Hypokalemia* *Achlorhydria* Dehydration Psychosis	Improvement in symptoms with trial of prostaglandin-synthesis inhibitor (indomethacin) or steroid therapy
Carcinoid	Serotonin (substance P)	EC	*Flushing* *Diarrhea* Tachycardia Abdominal pain	Calcium infusion Pentagastrin test
PP-OMA	Pancreatic polypeptide	PP	*Weight loss* Abdominal discomfort Diarrhea	Evidence of MEN-I‡

*Signs and symptoms that occur in greater than two thirds of cases are italicized.

†In addition to documented elevated levels of hormone, CT scanning, arteriography, and, in selected cases, transhepatic portal venous sampling.

‡Multiple endocrine neoplasia Type I—pituitary, parathyroid, and/or adrenal cortical adenomas.

§Migratory necrolytic erythema.

appearance is occasionally noted incidentally in pancreatic tissue resected from adults, it can cause a life-threatening illness in infants. *Neonatal hyperinsulinism* due to nesidioblastosis may result in profound hypoglycemia and may require pancreatic resection for control. This etiology of hyperinsulinism is characterized by a marked sensitivity of the beta cells to infusion of *leucine,* and a dramatic rise in insulin following such a challenge suggests this histologic abnormality.

Insulinoma

The largest number of islet cell tumors reported to date are those of beta cell origin associated with hyperinsulinism and hypoglycemia. The classic triad, described by Whipple in 1935, of *neurologic dysfunction,* documented fasting *hypoglycemia,* and *reversal of symptoms* following *glucose* administration, still stands as a hallmark of the disease. Patients commonly describe a prolonged history of vague or nonspecific symptoms, including altered mental status, prior to the documentation of hypoglycemia. Since a number of conditions may result in hypoglycemia, however, specific studies are required for the diagnosis of insulinoma. They include:

1. The response to a *72-hour* fast (which reveals inappropriately elevated levels of insulin occurring during hypoglycemia).

2. A *tolbutamide response test* or calcium infusion test (which demonstrates exaggerated insulin release and hypoglycemia).

3. Elevated circulating levels of *proinsulin* or *C-peptide.*

4. Identification of a *tumor mass* (by CT scanning or arteriography).

5. Localization of a *focus of excess insulin secretion* by percutaneous transhepatic venous sampling.

Factitious hypoglycemia due to exogenous insulin or sulfonylurea administration should be excluded and can be identified by the presence of low levels of C-peptide, detectable levels of anti-insulin antibodies, or the presence of sulfonylurea compounds in blood or urine.

The majority of beta cell tumors are smaller than 2 cm. in diameter, and radiologic studies may fail to reveal them. Surgical exploration is, therefore, frequently required for definitive localization. About 80 per cent of insulinomas are single, benign adenomas that allow surgical cure in the majority of cases by either resection or "shelling out" of the small encapsulated tumor.

Gastrinoma

The next most widely reported islet cell tumor, but probably the most frequently occurring, is that originally described in 1955 by Zollinger and Ellison. Histologically distinct gamma or G cells are rarely identifiable in normal islets but under pathologic conditions may comprise a pancreatic or peripancreatic adenoma or adenocarcinoma characterized by a high rate of gastrin secretion. Hypergastrinemia, in turn, results in dramatic hypersecretion of gastric acid and subsequent peptic ulceration of the upper gastrointestinal tract. Gastrinomas have been detected in patients of all ages but are most commonly seen in patients in the third to fifth decade. Persistent and complicated ulcer disease that is refractory to normal therapy is found in a majority of patients, but as many as one third of all cases may demonstrate a relatively unremarkable history of peptic disease. Five to 10 per cent of patients have a familial incidence of the disease or manifest evidence of the MEN syndrome. Gastric hypersecretion may result in diarrhea or steatorrhea (due to mucosal injury and digestion of exocrine enzymes by the increased acid production), and significant weight loss is commonly reported.

Diagnosis. The diagnosis rests on the documentation of plasma levels of gastrin, which are elevated two- to one hundredfold and which respond paradoxically to feeding (in which the elevated basal levels of gastrin remain unchanged) or intravenous *secretin* administration (in which the plasma gastrin rises abruptly to levels that are at least twice basal). The tumor may be localized by the radiologic means described for insulinoma, and metastatic disease is often apparent.

Treatment. Although the majority of gastrinomas are malignant, the tumor is typically a slow-growing one, and the principal cause of morbidity and mortality, other than the progression of the malignancy itself, is related to the complications of the resulting peptic ulcer disease. Treatment is therefore directed toward the absolute prevention of gastric acid secretion. This may be accomplished surgically by removing a solitary resectable tumor or, in the vast majority of cases in which the tumor is irresectable, by performing a total gastrectomy together with a Roux-en-Y *esophagojejunostomy.* This procedure is generally well tolerated by patients with gastrinoma whose disease has been brought under control preoperatively through the use of Type II histamine (H$_2$) receptor antagonists (e.g., Cimetidine or Ranitidine). An alternative albeit controversial approach is to maintain these patients on long-term H$_2$ receptor antagonist therapy indefinitely. The ultimate safety and success of this nonsurgical approach are currently under study.

Glucagonoma

Although patients with diabetes mellitus frequently exhibit paradoxical elevations in fasting or postprandial levels of glucagon, the diabetic state is occasionally the direct consequence of excess production of glucagon by an alpha cell adenoma or adenocarcinoma. These patients may appear essentially indistinguishable from those with common forms of diabetes unless they demonstrate the characteristic dermatologic finding of *migratory necrolytic erythema.* This circular, reddish, occasionally psoriatic-appearing rash may be present over the trunk and limbs and in intertrigenous areas. Other manifestations of hyperglucagonemia include glossitis, anemia, hypoaminoacidemia, and repeated episodes of thrombophlebitis.

A skin biopsy frequently reveals the characteristic dermatologic pathology, and elevated levels of glucagon that are at least three to five times normal strongly suggest the presence of this pancreatic lesion. The tumor is usually localized through radiologic scanning studies and arteriography, and surgical excision is attempted when widespread metastatic disease is not apparent. Frequently, these lesions are diagnosed rather late in their course, and the disease is usually at a metastatic level when the diagnosis is made.

In cases in which a high index of suspicion suggests the presence of a glucagonoma, the diagnosis may be confirmed through the use of provocative testing, such as the *arginine infusion test,* or with localization procedures, such as percutaneous transhepatic *portal venous sampling.*

Somatostatinoma

With the elucidation of the presence and physiologic properties of somatostatin in the early 1970s, numerous investigators sought to identify a delta cell adenoma or adenocarcinoma secreting excess quantities of the hormone. This was first documented by Larsson and colleagues in 1977, and subsequent reports have verified that this lesion is usually associated with both diabetes (owing to inhibition of insulin secretion) and gallstones (owing to cholestasis). The finding of a pancreatic tumor in association with these common conditions is an indication for determination of plasma levels of somatostatin. Provocative studies that may demonstrate exaggerated secretion include the *tolbutamide response test* as well as a *test meal* study. Localization procedures as described for other islet cell tumors may then be performed in the hope of defining a resectable lesion, although these tumors are also frequently metastatic at the time of diagnosis.

WDHA Syndrome

Three years after Zollinger and Ellison described the gastrinoma syndrome, Verner and Morrison reported a syndrome associated with islet cell tumors that consisted of watery diarrhea, hypokalemia, and achlorhydria (WDHA). The profuse secretory diarrhea of greater than 3 liters per day suggested the alternative name of *pancreatic cholera*, and led to both severe potassium loss and dehydration, frequently resulting in renal failure. Histologically, the islet cell adenoma associated with the syndrome was found to be distinct from that which secretes gastrin, and two hormones have been identified as causative agents in the development of the WDHA syndrome. The most frequently documented hormonal product is *vasoactive intestinal polypeptide* (VIP). VIP was isolated and characterized by Said and Mutt in 1970 and is found in gastrointestinal and neural tissues throughout the abdomen. VIP-containing cells are extremely scarce in normal pancreas, but these cells, identified as delta$_1$ cells, may form the adenoma that results in the WDHA syndrome. Occasionally, the WDHA syndrome may occur in patients with normal VIP levels, and in 1977 Jaffe and colleagues demonstrated that prostaglandin E$_1$ (PGE$_1$) may also mediate the syndrome when secreted in excess by an islet cell tumor. These adenomas are frequently less than 1 cm. in diameter and may elude standard radiologic imaging techniques. They may be localized by portal venous sampling studies but are frequently identified at the time of careful surgical exploration of the pancreas. Because these lesions are usually solitary and benign, surgical resection commonly results in relief from all symptoms.

Carcinoid Syndrome

The majority of carcinoid tumors are found in the distal small intestine and colon, but these lesions may arise as rare islet cell tumors as well. Through the effects of excess secretion of *serotonin* (5-hydroxytryptamine) and other neuropeptides such as *substance P,* these tumors produce their characteristic syndrome of *diarrhea*, cutaneous *flushing, tachycardia,* and *abdominal discomfort.* High plasma levels of serotonin may be measured directly or may be implied by excess urinary excretion of the serotonin metabolite *5-hydroxyindoleacetic acid* (5-HIAA). Provocative studies, such as calcium or pentagastrin infusion, may cause exacerbation of symptoms and an abrupt increase in the levels of serotonin. Although localization studies are of help in planning treatment, islet cell carcinoid tumors are frequently metastatic when first diagnosed. Surgical resection of the tumor, or "debulking" of the metastatic tissue, provides the best likelihood of cure or control of symptoms.

Miscellaneous Syndromes

A variety of other peptide hormone products are associated with islet cell tumors and non–islet cell tumors of the pancreas. *Pancreatic polypeptide* may be secreted in excess by islet cell tumors and provides a useful marker for an otherwise occult pancreatic tumor. Elevated levels of PP may be the only indication of an islet cell tumor arising as part of the multiple endocrine neoplasia (MEN) Type I syndrome and should be documented in patients with these disorders.[10] A variety of pituitary hormones may be secreted by pancreatic tumors, including adrenocorticotropic hormone (ACTH), melanocyte-stimulating hormone (MSH), and antidiuretic hormone (ADH), and related releasing factors. The tremendous potential for peptide secretion by adenomas or adenocarcinomas of the pancreas underscores the complex regulatory role of this organ.

SELECTED REFERENCES

Texts

Brooks, J. R. (Ed.): Surgery of the Pancreas. Philadelphia, W. B. Saunders Company, 1983.
  This text represents the contribution of 27 authors in the areas of pancreatic anatomy, physiology, pathology, diagnostic approaches, and surgical disease. It is a clearly worded and well-illustrated book and is also concise and relatively complete. The sections on radiology of the pancreas, acute pancreatitis, chronic pancreatitis, and carcinoma of the pancreas are particularly well organized.

Cooperman, A. M., and Hoerr, S. O.: Surgery of the Pancreas: A Text and Atlas. St. Louis, The C. V. Mosby Company, 1978.
  This is an especially useful atlas of surgical procedures on the pancreas, superbly illustrated by R. M. Reed. Important technical features are clearly emphasized, and the principles of each procedure are carefully outlined in a concise text that accompanies the illustrations.

Moossa, A. R. (Ed.): Tumors of the Pancreas. Baltimore, Williams & Wilkins Company, 1980.
  The senior editor has combined his own extensive experience with the contributions of 26 other authorities in this excellent reference that focuses on pancreatic neoplasms. Introductory chapters detail relevant surgical anatomy and its abnormalities as they may affect the interpretation of diagnostic studies or the approach to resection of the pancreas. Emphasis is placed on experimental studies on pancreatic cancer as well as clinical considerations of exocrine and endocrine tumors and their treatment.

Articles

Banting, F. S., and Best, C. H.: The internal secretion of the pancreas. J. Lab. Clin. Med., 7:251, 1922.
  This classic paper describes the meticulous studies conducted by the student, Charles Best, and his mentor, surgeon Frederick Banting, that led to the establishment of insulin as the hormone responsible for glucose homeostasis. The details of their studies in dogs reveal the methods by which these investigators established their important discovery within a few weeks' time during the summer of 1921.

Bradley, E. L. III, and Clements, J. L.: Spontaneous resolution of pancreatic pseudocysts: Implications for timing of operative intervention. Am. J. Surg., 129:23, 1975.
  The careful use of serial examinations with ultrasonography in patients with acute pancreatitis revealed the high incidence of pseudocyst formation in this disease and a 40 per cent incidence of spontaneous regression of the pseudocysts. This study further demonstrated that pseudocysts that persist for 6 weeks are likely to require surgical decompression, since the spontaneous regression rate beyond this period is minimal.

Comfort, M. W., Gambill, E. E., and Bagenstoss, A. H.: Chronic relapsing pancreatitis: A study of 29 cases without associated disease of the biliary or gastrointestinal tract. Gastroenterology, 6:239, 1946.
  This study represents a milestone in the understanding of chronic pancreatitis. On the basis of meticulous examination of diseased glands, the authors documented that the changes within the pancreas are remarkably variable and include ductular changes of dilatation or sclerosis as well as focal areas of stenosis in addition to the formation of calculous and cyst disease. These findings provide the basis for the importance of careful delineation of the individual changes present in each patient in order to determine the correct operative procedure.

Kelly, T. R.: Gallstone pancreatitis: The timing of surgery. Surgery, *88:*345, 1980.

The difficult clinical situation of acute pancreatitis accompanied by biliary calculous disease is addressed in this study of 172 patients. "Early" (within 72 hours), "delayed" (within 5 to 7 days) and "elective" (during a subsequent hospitalization) operations were evaluated, with delayed cholecystectomy resulting in the lowest mortality and avoidance of recurrent episodes of pancreatitis. The findings of this study form the basis for a sound approach to the management of a frequently difficult clinical problem.

Opie, E. L.: The etiology of acute hemorrhagic pancreatitis. Bull. Johns Hopkins Hosp., *12:*182, 1901.

The autopsy findings and experimental data presented in this landmark article established the validity of the pathophysiology of "gallstone pancreatitis." Clinical data are presented to support the hypothesis of the "common channel theory" of pancreatic duct obstruction, and further studies in dogs demonstrated the reproducible induction of pancreatitis after infusion of bile into the pancreatic duct.

Pearse, A. G. E., and Polak, J. M.: Neural crest origin of the endocrine polypeptide (APUD) cells of the gastrointestinal tract and pancreas. Gut, *12:*783, 1971.

This histologic study of the embryologic origin of peptide hormone–containing cells demonstrated the likely common development of hormone-secreting cells and tissues derived from the fetal neural crest. These findings demonstrate that peptide hormone cells of the pancreas not only share specific biochemical properties (including the process of amine precursor uptake and degradation, from which the acronym APUD is derived) but also share a possible common developmental origin. The study provides a basis for the clinically observed association of adenomas that arise in multiple endocrine organs.

Puestow, C. B., and Gillesby, W. J.: Retrograde surgical drainage of pancreas for chronic relapsing pancreatitis. Arch. Surg., *76:*898, 1958.

The authors carefully review their rationale for the development of a new approach to the surgical treatment of chronic pancreatitis and describe the evolution of the operative approach that has become a standard in the treatment of this disease. Written during a period in which pancreatic resection was a popular treatment for this disease and when drainage procedures on the pancreas frequently failed, the description offers an interesting insight into the authors' ability to solve technical problems in order to establish an important principle in the surgical treatment of this disease.

Ranson, J. H. C., Rifkind, K. M., Roses, D. F., et al.: Prognostic signs and the role of operative management in acute pancreatitis. Surg. Gynecol. Obstet., *139:*69, 1974.

This paper represents the original series of observations from a group of authorities who have contributed greatly to the care of patients with acute pancreatitis. The determination through careful retrospective analysis of the prognostic criteria, now known simply as "Ranson's criteria," which allow clinical assessment of the severity of the disease within the first 48 hours of hospitalization, provided a major advance in the approach to acute pancreatitis.

Sankaran, S., and Walt, A. J.: The natural and unnatural history of pancreatic pseudocysts. Br. J. Surg., *62:*37, 1975.

A superbly detailed evaluation of the clinical course of 131 pseudocysts in 112 patients is provided in this study. One third of the pseudocysts were seen to result in significant morbidity or mortality, and therefore this series provides useful information regarding the likelihood of specific complications and the rationale for the treatment of persistent pseudocysts.

Skandalakis, J. E., Gray, S. W., Rowe, J. S., and Skandalakis, L. J.: Anatomical complications of pancreatic surgery. Parts I and II. Contemp. Surg., *15:*17, 21, 1979.

Far more than a review of surgical complications, this concise pair of articles provides a wealth of detailed anatomic information for the student and surgeon alike. A careful discussion of ductular and vascular anomalies provides an excellent review of the surgical anatomy of the gland.

Stefanini, P., Carboni, M., Patrassi, N., and Basoli, A.: Beta–islet cell tumors of the pancreas: Results of a study on 1,067 cases. Surgery, *75:*597, 1974.

This paper represents one of the largest single reports on the clinical manifestations, diagnosis, and treatment of a surgical disease. Although many of the cases reviewed had been incompletely documented or investigated, the authors have assembled a relatively definitive clinical summary of the disease and its outcome. Since many of the patients represented in this report were operated upon several years earlier, the reported success of surgical treatment seriously underestimates current expectations. The article stands, however, as a valuable summary of insulinoma.

Verner, J. V., and Morrison, A. B.: Islet cell tumor and a syndrome of refractory watery diarrhea and hypokalemia. Am. J. Med., *25:*374, 1958.

The authors describe the clinical and pathologic findings of two patients of their own, plus seven others from the literature, to formulate the pathophysiology of the entity now known as the WDHA syndrome. The relationship of this islet cell tumor to others known at that time and the elucidation of the chemical basis for the clinical aspects of the disease are clearly outlined in this fascinating description of the previously unrecognized syndrome.

Whipple, A. O., Parson, W., and Mullins, S.: Treatment of carcinoma of the ampulla of Vater. Ann. Surg., *102:*763, 1935.

The original description of the clinical and technical concerns that led to the development of pancreaticoduodenectomy are found in this classic paper. Despite the fact that the duodenum had been thought to be an essential part of the gastrointestinal tract and that pancreatic secretions had likewise been regarded as indispensable, Whipple and coauthors combined their knowledge of laboratory studies, which refuted the previous tenets, with their prodigious technical skill and designed a two-stage operation for the resection of tumors in the region of the ampulla. Although Trimble and others subsequently performed the first one-stage pancreaticoduodenectomy, the undeniable contribution of Whipple's surgical courage and determination makes this paper a landmark in the surgical attack on pancreatic neoplasms.

Zollinger, R. M., and Ellison, E.: Primary peptic ulceration of the jejunum associated with islet cell tumors of the pancreas. Ann. Surg., *142:*709, 1955.

The modern era of surgical endocrinology began with the publication of this description of the syndrome that bears the authors' names. The perception of a hormonal cause for the intense acid peptic disease seen in these patients led ultimately to the isolation and characterization of the hormone gastrin and to the development of the surgical approach of removal of the target organ (gastrectomy) in the treatment of the disease.

REFERENCES

1. Andres, R., and Tobin, J. D.: Endocrine systems. *In* Finch, C. E., and Hayflick, L. (Eds.): Handbook of the Biology of Aging. New York, Van Nostrand Reinhold, 1977, pp. 357–378.
2. Arvanitakis, C., and Greenberger, N. J.: Diagnosis of pancreatic disease by a synthetic peptide: A new test of exocrine pancreatic function. Lancet, *1:*663, 1976.
3. Bonner-Weir, S., and Orci, L.: New perspectives on the microvasculature of the islets of Langerhans in the rat. Diabetes, *31:*883, 1982.
4. Broe, P. J., and Cameron, J. L.: Pancreatic ascites and pancreatic pleural effusions. *In* Bradley, E. L. (Ed.): Complications of Pancreatitis—Medical and Surgical Management. Philadelphia, W. B. Saunders Company, 1982, pp. 245–264.
5. Cubilla, A. C., Fortner, J. C., and Fitzgerald, P. J.: Lymph node involvement in carcinoma of the head of the pancreas area. Cancer, *41:*880, 1978.
6. Davenport, H. W.: Pancreatic secretion. *In* Physiology of the Digestive Tract, 5th ed. Chicago, Year Book Medical Publishers, Inc., 1982, pp. 143–154.
7. Davidson, E. D., and Bradley, E. L.: "Marsupialization" in the treatment of pancreatic abscess. Surgery, *89:*252, 1981.
8. Dreiling, D. A., and Wolfson, P.: New insights into pancreatic disease revealed by the secretin test. *In* Berk, J. E. (Ed.): Developments in Digestive Diseases, Vol. 2. Philadelphia, Lea & Febiger, 1979, pp. 155–170.
9. Farmer, R. C., Maslin, S. C., and Reber, H. A.: Acute pancreatitis—role of duct permeability. Surg. Forum, *34:*224, 1983.
10. Friesen, S. R.: The multiple endocrine adenopathy, type I, syndrome. *In* Brooks, J. R. (Ed.): Surgery of the Pancreas. Philadelphia, W. B. Saunders Company, 1983, pp. 334–347.
11. Goff, J. S.: Two-stage triolein breath test differentiates pancreatic insufficiency from other causes of malabsorption. Gastroenterology, *83:*44, 1982.
12. Gorelick, F. S., and Jamieson, J. D.: Structure-function relationship of the pancreas. *In* Johnson, L. R. (Ed.): Physiology of the Gastrointestinal Tract. New York, Raven Press, 1981, pp. 773–794.
13. Konturek, S. J., Becker, H. D., and Thompson, J. C.: Effect of vagotomy on hormones stimulating pancreatic secretion. Arch. Surg., *108:*704, 1974.
14. Levitt, M. D., Rapoport, M., and Cooperband, S. R.: The renal clearance of amylase in renal insufficiency, acute pancreatitis, and macroamylasemia. Ann. Intern. Med., *71:*919, 1969.

15. Morrow, C. E., Cohen, J. I., Sutherland, D. E. R., and Najarian, J. S.: Chronic pancreatitis: Long-term surgical results of pancreatic duct drainage, pancreatic resection, and near-total pancreatectomy and islet autotransplantation. Surgery, *96:*608, 1984.

16. National Diabetes Data Group: Classification and diagnosis of diabetes mellitus and other categories of glucose intolerance. Diabetes, *28:*1039, 1979.

17. Noda, A., Hayakowa, T., Kondo, T., Katada, N., and Kameya, A.: Clinical evaluation of pancreatic excretion test with dimethadione and oral BT-PABA test in chronic pancreatitis. Dig. Dis. Sci., *28:*230, 1983.

18. Noda, A., Hayakawa, T., Nakajima, S., Suzuki, T., and Toda, Y.: Pancreatic excretion of 5,5-dimethyl-2,4-oxazolidinedione in normal subjects. Am. J. Dig. Dis., *20:*1011, 1975.

19. Ranson, J. H. C.: Acute pancreatitis. *In* Brooks, J. R. (Ed.): Surgery of the Pancreas. Philadelphia, W. B. Saunders Company, 1983, pp. 146–181.

20. Ranson, J. H. C., Rifkind, K. M., and Roses, D. F.: Prognostic signs and the role of operative management in acute pancreatitis. Surg. Gynecol. Obstet., *139:*69, 1974.

21. Sadar, E. S., and Cooperman, A. M.: Bilateral thoracic sympathectomy-splanchnicectomy in the treatment of intractable pain due to pancreatic carcinoma. Clev. Clin. Q., *41:*185, 1974.

22. Sankaran, S., and Walt, A. J.: The natural and unnatural history of pancreatic pseudocysts. Br. J. Surg., *62:*37, 1975.

23. Sarles, H.: Chronic calcifying pancreatitis-chronic alcoholic pancreatitis. Gastroenterology, *66:*604, 1974.

24. Stefan, Y., Orci, L., Malaisse-Legae, F., Perrelet, A., Patel, Y., and Unger, R. H.: Quantitation of endocrine cell content in the pancreas of non-diabetic and diabetic humans. Diabetes, *31:*694, 1982.

25. Tseng, H. C., Grendell, J. H., and Rothman, S. S.: Regulation of digestion: II. Effects of insulin and glucagon on pancreatic secretion. Am. J. Physiol., *246:*G451, 1984.

THE SPLEEN

TERUO MATSUMOTO, M.D., PH.D. • MORTON H. PERLMAN, M.D.

30

HISTORIC ASPECTS

Splenectomy for the treatment of trauma was reported as early as 1549, but probably followed splenic evisceration in battle rather than a planned incision. The first formal splenectomy was unsuccessfully performed by Quittenbaum in 1826, and it was not until 1887 that Wells operated to relieve massive splenomegaly and reported a series of splenectomies. For the next 50 years, splenectomy was performed primarily for trauma, massive enlargement, twisted pedicles, and cysts. Later splenectomy was done to alleviate a variety of hematologic disorders.

FUNCTIONS OF THE SPLEEN

The spleen has multiple functions, primarily directed toward removal of abnormal cells or invading microorganisms (Table 1). *In utero*, the human spleen is a site of hematopoiesis, but this function ceases at about 6 months' gestation. The stem cells necessary for blood formation remain and can be reactivated, as occurs in agnogenic myeloid metaplasia. Although the daily blood flow through the human spleen is 350 liters, the organ does not store blood volume or red blood cells, as it has a blood content of less than 50 ml. and contains only 20 to 40 ml. of red cells. However, platelets may be stored in the spleen, since about 30 per cent of the platelets in the circulation are present in the spleen.

Erythrocyte Interaction

Normal red blood cells are biconcave discs and are easily deformed, behaving more like fluid droplets than particles. This enables easy passage through the microcirculation, especially that of the splenic pulp pores, which are less than 3 mm. in diameter. Some abnormal red cells have impaired deformability; others are coated with "sticky" material. Passage of these abnormal cells through the microcirculation is impaired and can impede and even occlude flow. The spleen recognizes and sequesters these abnormal cells. Cells not easily able to become deformed cannot readily pass through the pores in the splenic pulp, and cells with membranes that contain glycoproteins or that are coated with antibody complexes are recognized and

TABLE 1. Functions Attributed to the Spleen

Erythrocyte maturation and repair
Removal of aged and damaged blood cells
Removal of particulate matter from the blood,
    including bacteria and other microorganisms
Production of lymphocytes, monocytes, and
    plasma cells
Synthesis of antibodies and other factors used in
    immunologic defect
Hematopoiesis
Storage of blood and blood elements

adhere to specialized cells in the pulp. Depending upon the cause of the abnormality, the spleen repairs or destroys these impaired red cells.

Erythrocyte Maturation

The spleen serves as a site for maturing immature red cells, which contain nuclear remnants (Howell-Jolly bodies), denatured protein (Heinz bodies), iron granules (Pappenheimer bodies), and iron-protein particles (siderocytes) or have excessive or pitted cell membranes. These defects decrease deformability and lead to sequestration. In addition, these cells may be "sticky" owing to the coat of transferrin acquired during iron uptake. Immature cells with these inclusions are "pitted" on removal; cells with excessive or pitted membranes are "molded." After completion of these processes, the cells are released to the circulation, where they function normally. Although the bone marrow usually retains red cells until maturation is complete, sequestration, pitting, and molding after premature marrow release are functions unique to the spleen.

Erythrocyte Removal

The spleen sequesters and removes senescent erythrocytes. After circulating for about 100 days, erythrocytes begin to show the effects of aging and such cells develop enzyme deficiencies. These apparently lead to defective membranes that are less pliable and may have "sticky" spots and therefore cannot readily escape the spleen. Delaying the passage of cells with an already deficient enzyme system through the anoxic splenic environment further aggravates the injury. This process hastens the eventual removal of these cells by entrapment and phagocytosis.

The recognition and removal of aged cells is not unique to the spleen, since all parts of the reticuloendothelial system can perform this function. Since sequestration of senescent red cells can be assumed by other parts of this system, splenectomy has no measurable effect on red cell kinetics in the hematologically normal human. In addition to aging, injury by chemical and physical agents, microorganisms, and immunologic activities and coating by antibody complexes can render red cells abnormal, and the spleen also sequesters and destroys these cells.

Destruction of the red cell by this means is actually a type of hemolysis that occurs intracellularly within the splenic or reticuloendothelial phagocyte. Under normal circumstances its products are easily handled within the iron-porphyrin cycling mechanisms. Release of excessive quantities of the products of red cell destruction can lead to jaundice, gallstone formation, and other disorders but does not create an immediate threat to life with intravascular hemolysis.

Leukocyte Removal

The spleen removes circulating leukocytes. As a quasi-lymphoid organ, the spleen produces lymphocytes, monocytes, and plasma cells. It also synthesizes tuftsin, an opsonin facilitating polymorphonuclear phagocytosis, as well as properdin, also an opsonin and a component of the alternate pathway of complement activation. In addition, the white pulp produces antibodies.

As a part of the reticuloendothelial system, the spleen also serves as a filter by trapping and removing foreign particulate substances. The liver also has this ability to filter blood-borne microorganisms; however, the spleen is more efficient. This is especially true in regard to bacteria with which the body has had no prior exposure, and therefore an intact spleen is necessary for optimal protection.

BASIC SCIENCE ASPECTS

Gross and Developmental Anatomy

The *normal* spleen weighs 150 to 250 gm. and is about the size of an adult fist. It is suspended by ligaments attaching in the left upper quadrant of the abdomen and is protected from injury by the ribs. It is shaped somewhat like a lima bean with two sides and four edges; the anterior side is mildly indented, similar to the hilus of the bean. Its smooth and convex lateral surface is immediately adjacent to the diaphragm and left lower rib cage and can be lacerated by trauma, including compression and fracture of the ninth and tenth ribs. The medial surface is concave. The spleen receives its blood supply primarily in its central portion, termed the *hilum*, which is bordered by the greater curvature of the stomach and the tail of the pancreas (Fig. 1*A*). The pancreas is often quite closely related to the spleen and may be injured during splenectomy. The superior edge of the spleen lies against the diaphragm; the posterior edge relates to the left kidney and the inferior surface against the colon (Fig. 1*B*). The anterior edge is indented, and this indentation is exaggerated by splenomegaly to form the "splenic notch," which can, at times, be felt on physical examination.

In early *embryologic development*, mesodermal swellings appear beneath the epithelial surface of the dorsal mesogastrium. These rapidly coalesce into a group with a single blood supply, the rudimentary spleen, which is at first lobulated. By the end of the third intrauterine month, the lobulations have disappeared and the spleen has assumed an adult form (Fig. 2).

As development proceeds, the dorsal mesogastrium folds to the left with the spleen at its apex. Except at its lateral portion, where it reflects from the left kidney as the splenorenal ligament, the most dorsal half, containing the splenic artery and vein, becomes adherent to the left posterior abdominal wall as a retroperitoneal structure. The ventral half of the dorsal mesogastrium, containing the short gastric branches of the splenic vessels, forms the gastrosplenic ligament. There are two other major ligaments: the splenophrenic to the posterior diaphragm and the splenocolic to the splenic flexure of the colon. These two ligaments, and the lateral leaf of the splenorenal, are usually avascular. Incising them to open the retroperitoneal fusion plane recreates the mesenteric spleen of early fetal life and permits easy exposure. However, in the congestive splenomegalies, such as portal hypertension, these ligaments can become extremely vascular as pathways of portosystemic return.

ACCESSORY SPLEENS

Accessory spleens occur commonly and are of physiologic and therapeutic significance. Most are located near the spleen in the hilar region or along the splenic ligaments or greater omentum. Their origin represents a failure of coalescence of the splenic buds. The incidence of accessory spleens varies in different series. In a series of splenectomies for trauma, the incidence is low and under 10 per cent, whereas for hematologic disorders the incidence is 25 to 30 per cent. In postmortem studies the incidence is usually between these figures. The lower figures found in trauma series undoubtedly reflect an incomplete search at the time of operation. However, there is evidence that the incidence of accessory spleens in hematologic disorders is actually increased above normal, probably the result of stimulation of growth of otherwise unrecognized microscopic sites of splenic tissue.

The spleen is quite vascular and may be regarded as a specialized "noncapillary" bed interposed between the splenic artery and the portal vein, and its immunologic and hematologic functions reflect this specialized histology. The organ is covered by a 2- to 3-mm. thick fibrous capsule that imparts a feeling of firmness, masking the softness of the parenchyma contained within. As the vessels enter at the hilus, they are accompanied into the spleen by extensions of connective tissue, the *trabeculae*. The trabeculae form a framework dividing the organ into small compartments containing the parenchyma, or, as it is called, the "splenic pulp." The major blood supply is via the splenic artery and vein, the splenic artery being one of the three major branches of the celiac artery. It courses along the upper border of the pancreas, giving rise to pancreatic and short gastric branches before entering the halves of the spleen. Several venous tributaries exit the hilus and promptly coalesce to form the splenic vein, which courses medially partially within the posterior surface of the distal pancreas just below its superior margin. Along its course it receives short gastric and pancreatic tributaries as well as the inferior mesenteric vein. The splenic vein joins the superior mesenteric vein to form the portal vein (Fig. 3).

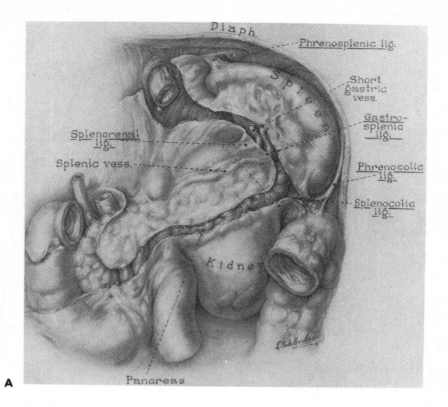

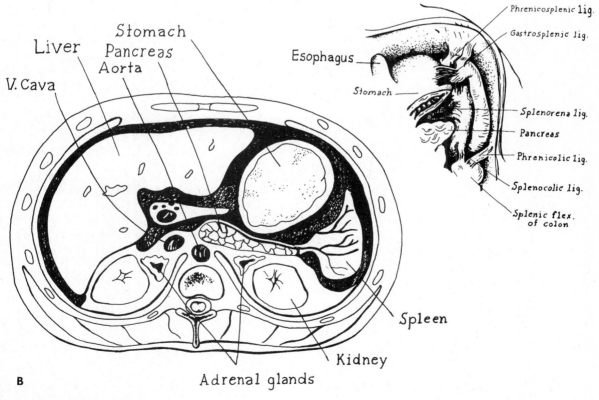

Figure 1. Anatomy of the spleen.
   A, *Suspensory ligaments of the spleen. (From Ballinger, W. F., and Erslev, A. J.: Splenectomy. In Ravitch, M. M., et al. (Eds.): Curr. Probl. Surg. Chicago, Year Book Medical Publishers, 1965.)*
   B, *Sagittal section and anterior view of the body in relation to the spleen and other organs.*

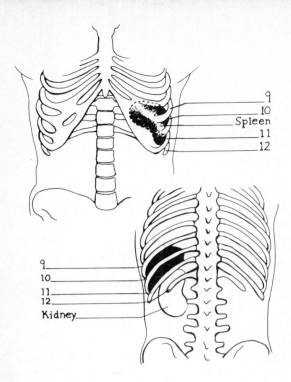

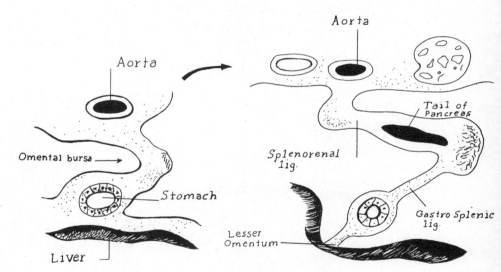

Figure 2. Anterior and posterior anatomy in relation to the location of the spleen.

Figure 3. Development of the spleen.

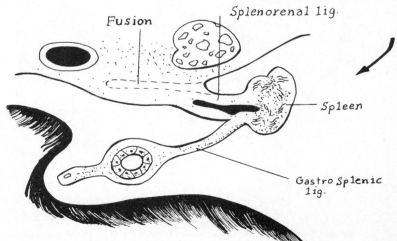

SPLENIC ARTERY

The main branches of the splenic artery subdivide into trabecular arteries. These continue their branchings as they course within the trabeculae into the organ. At the ends of the trabeculae they continue into the pulp as central arteries. The fibrous tissue of the trabeculae continues into the pulp as a delicate open reticular meshwork that supports the cords and sinuses. The splenic veins also follow the course of the trabeculae as they leave the parenchyma. The spleen has only efferent lymphatics, and these are confined to the fibrous tissue of the pulp and capsule.

SPLENIC PULP

The splenic pulp is composed of vascular components and lymphoid and reticuloendothelial cells. The three areas include the white pulp, the marginal zone, and the red pulp. The white pulp is an aggregation of lymphoid tissue within the reticular mesh sheathing the central arteries as they exit the trabeculae. The elements of the white pulp can also be arranged as follicles in the form of germinal centers of "malpighian bodies." The sheathing lymphocytes are primarily of the T cell type, whereas the follicles are composed predominantly of B-lymphocytes and plasma cells. The central arteries of the white pulp give rise to arterioles, which penetrate it at right angles (follicular arteries). This arrangement is conducive to removal of plasma, which is rich in antigens, and its selective direction to the antibody-producing lymphoid tissue of the white pulp.

The marginal zone is a poorly defined region surrounding the white pulp with a varying size and an indefinite structure. The zone can be considered a vascular space within a reticular network. It can, in certain disorders, sequester and contain plasma, cellular elements, and foreign materials. The size of the marginal zone depends on the quantity of material retained.

The red pulp is composed of the cords and sinuses. The cords are rows of interconnected reticuloendothelial cells lying on the reticular meshwork in the pattern of an irregular honeycomb. The sinuses are branching blood-filled spaces lying between the cords that are several hundred microns in length and about 40 microns (μ.) in diameter that drain into the splenic venous system. The central arteries diminish in size as they traverse the white pulp, becoming arteriolar on entry into the red pulp, where they are termed *penicillar arteries* (Fig. 4).

MICROCIRCULATION

Although much is yet to be discovered about the microcirculation of the spleen, it is known that blood can take several pathways, each of which favors certain splenic functions. Some penicillar vessels directly enter the sinuses, and some appear to reach the veins through capillary networks sheathed with specialized cells. Some penicillar arteries open directly into the cords, and the blood then enters the sinuses through small pores between the reticuloendothelial cells. The blood then rejoins the vascular system by entering the venules that drain the sinuses. This pathway is known as the "open circulation of the spleen," and approximately 90 per cent of the splenic flow follows this route directly into the substance of the cords.

The pores allowing passage from the cords into the sinuses are about 3 μ. in diameter, a narrower diameter than some of the formed elements of the blood. Since normal red cells are quite pliable, they can readily enter this passage into the sinuses and venules. Aged and damaged red cells are not readily deformed and cannot easily pass into the sinuses. Cells coated with "sticky" materials, such as immature red cells and antibody-coated cells, can be trapped through adherence to the cells and other structures of the cords.

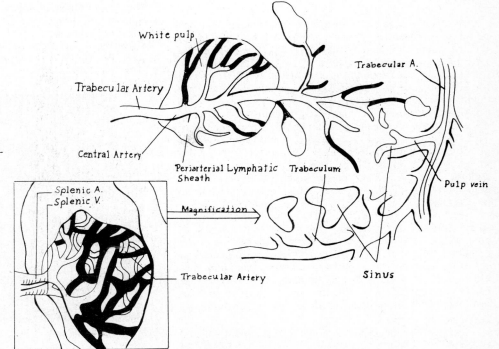

Figure 4. Gross and simplified microcirculation of the spleen.

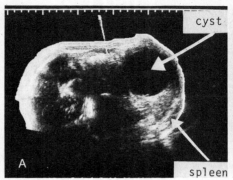

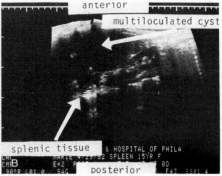

Figure 5. Ultrasonography.

Clinical Evaluation

Symptoms directly attributable to the spleen include a sense of upper fullness in the presence of an enlarged spleen and left upper quadrant or pleuritic pain caused by an inflammatory reaction such as splenic infarct or abscess. Pain may also be felt in the left shoulder as a result of diaphragmatic irritation and is often caused by the blood from a ruptured spleen.

Palpation for splenomegaly should be done with the patient in both the supine and right decubitus positions. The normal spleen is palpable in less than 3 per cent of the population, and therefore spleens that can be palpated should be investigated. The considerably enlarged spleen is notched on its anterior palpable edge, distinguishing it from other upper abdominal masses. As the spleen enlarges, it can be percussed before it can be palpated. The splenic outline is sufficiently distinct on supine roentgen films to allow an assessment of splenic size. When the borders are not distinct, splenic enlargement is suggested by displacement of the stomach medially and the splenic flexure of the colon posteroinferiorly.

Imaging the Spleen

Ultrasonography is a noninvasive technique that can be used to accurately assess splenic size, especially in nondistended individuals (Fig. 5). It can also delineate intrasplenic cysts and collections.

The *computed tomography (CT) scan* is quite accurate for evaluation of splenic size and location (Fig. 6). It can demonstrate small defects, such as lacerations and collections, and the use of concurrently administered contrast material increases the interpretability of the examination. The CT scan is a sensitive test even in the presence of obesity or abdominal distention. It is especially useful for the rapid evaluation of trauma victims in showing intraabdominal bleeding and splenic injury. It is of value in demonstrating splenic, hepatic, and retroperitoneal node involvement.

Technetium radionuclide ⁹⁹ᵐTc-sulfur scanning of the spleen and liver depends upon the ability of the organs to phagocytize colloid (Fig. 7). The technique is of great value in delineating liver and spleen size and position and in detecting the presence of intrinsic nonfunctional abnormalities, such as lacerations and hematoma. However, the results are devoid of specificity, and adjunctive gallium scanning has been utilized to demonstrate inflammatory processes.

The spleen can also be imaged with heat-damaged chromium-51–tagged erythrocytes, which are sequestered by the spleen. The test can be used in qualitative fashion to demonstrate the role of the spleen in the hemolytic anemias and is also utilized to ascertain the presence and location of accessory spleens.

The use of *arteriography* and *splenoportography* (Fig. 8) in the evaluation of isolated splenic disorders is not as widespread as it was in the past, but arteriography is frequently employed in the evaluation of portal hypertension when an operative procedure is planned. It may also be indicated in the evaluation of splenic and other left upper quadrant masses.

Assessment of Splenic Function

Routine blood count, reticulocyte count, peripheral blood smear, and plasma bilirubin studies can be affected by disorders characterized by altered splenic function. Other more specialized examinations of blood formation and behavior, such as bone marrow aspiration, the Coombs' test, the sickle cell preparation, and hemoglobin electrophoresis, may also be useful.

The destruction of red cells within the spleen can be quantitated by transfusion requirements or by determination of the longevity of readministered tagged red cells. These methods may not be valid, however, because of the assumption that destruction occurs primarily in the spleen. A more direct assessment is derived from studies of the radioactivity accumulated by the spleen and liver after administration of the tagged red cells.

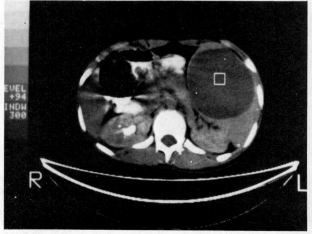

Figure 6. Computed tomography scan of large posttraumatic splenic cyst.

Left Lateral   Anterior

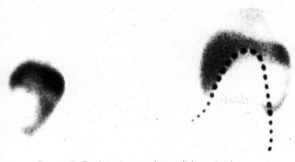

Figure 7. Technetium radionuclide scanning.

HYPOSPLENISM

Until recently, diminished splenic function or even complete absence of the spleen was felt to have few, if any, significant consequences. It is now apparent that impaired splenic function can be severe and even fatal. Agenesis of the spleen is rare, and the commonest cause of asplenism is splenectomy for trauma or splenic disorder or as an incidental part of another operation. Splenic function can be depressed even when the spleen is normal or enlarged, and this dysfunction occurs in sickle cell disease, sarcoidosis, and amyloidosis. Atrophy of the spleen occurs rarely with ulcerative colitis, celiac disease, Graves' disease, and lupus erythematosus.

Asplenism results in several characteristic hematologic findings as a result of permanent loss of the ability to mature, mold, and pit red blood cells. These findings include reticulocytes, Howell-Jolly bodies, Heinz bodies, siderocytes, and target cells appearing in the peripheral blood.

Splenectomy

Loss of the spleen does not cause a noticeable change in red cell kinetics or red cell survival, and the number of circulating erythrocytes remains the same. After splenectomy a transient moderate leukocytosis lasting several weeks occurs. The lack of change in red cell kinetics and the slight change in the leukocyte count may reflect the absence of a splenic reservoir for red cells and the presence of a small splenic pool of leukocytes.

Splenectomy is followed by an immediate and often significant rise in the platelet count, and moderate elevation often persists indefinitely. At times this is preceded by an elevation to very high levels with counts above 1,000,000 per mm.[3] and creates the danger of thromboembolic complications. It most often occurs in patients with active erythropoietic tissues, such as is seen in the hemolytic anemias and with the myeloproliferative disorders.

An unproven theory to explain this rebound thrombocytosis is that splenectomy removes a platelet-inhibiting factor secreted by the spleen. A better theory, which explains the persisting mild elevation to levels one third above normal, is that the splenic reservoir has been removed. The total amount remains constant, so that more are in the circulating pool.

Postsplenectomy Sepsis

The previously described hematologic effects of splenectomy do not usually produce symptoms. However, a serious problem may ensue as the result of a loss of filtering ability and is manifested by an increased susceptibility to rapidly fatal infection by encapsulated bacteria, especially *Pneumococcus*. The problem is not an inability to synthesize substances such as IgM, properdin, or tuftsin but the inability to filter virulent organisms that have invaded the bloodstream and with which there is no prior immunologic experience. Not only is the hyposplenic individual more susceptible to infection, but the established infection is refractory to treatment, with fatality rates being 30 to 50 per cent.

Children are significantly more susceptible to postsplenectomy sepsis than are adults, and the risk varies with the circumstances of the splenectomy. Splenectomy for trauma is followed by the least risk, and splenectomy for congenital hereditary spherocytosis carries slightly more risk. For idiopathic thrombocytopenic purpura, the risk is still higher. Splenectomy for staging of Hodgkin's disease or for the treatment of thalassemia major has a quite significant risk.

A more conservative attitude toward splenectomy is currently advocated, especially in children, and it has been shown that the presence of a splenic laceration does not necessarily mandate splenectomy or even laparotomy. If blood loss is not excessive and there is little likelihood of another intra-abdominal injury, careful observation may allow spontaneous stabilization and healing of the injury. Even if operation to control splenic bleeding becomes necessary, repair of the spleen (splenorrhaphy) may be feasible. If 50 per cent or more of the spleen is intact, competence is maintained. There have been attempts to achieve protection with smaller splenic fragments or with implanted fragments of spleen in the peritoneal cavity. Synthesis of opsonins and trapping of red cells have been demonstrated, but there is no clear evidence that the filtering function is sufficient. If splenectomy must be per-

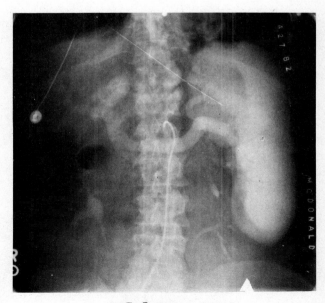

Spleen
Portal Hypertension
Figure 8. Angiography.

formed, the patient should be inoculated with pneumococcal vaccine. Prophylactic antibiotics have been advised for children and others at high risk. The patient, parents, and physicians must be alert until adulthood and act rapidly if signs of sepsis occur.

OPERATIVE PROCEDURES

Preoperative Aspects

Most splenic operations are performed as emergencies for trauma. Preoperative preparation consists primarily of replacement of lost blood volume. If pneumothorax or hemothorax is present on the chest film, a chest tube should be inserted. Nasogastric intubation and evacuation of the stomach to prevent aspiration are also important.

Elective operations on the spleen are undertaken only after meticulous diagnosis and evaluation. Anemias should be corrected to a hematocrit level in the 25 to 30 range, and, when possible, existing infections should be eradicated. Appropriate antibiotics should be administered when the procedure is performed in the presence of active infection or in an immunologically compromised patient. The need for corticosteroid administration should be ascertained, since many patients undergoing splenectomy have a history of having received corticoids. Sufficient time should be allowed to have blood and any necessary blood elements available in adequate amounts, since it should be emphasized that hematologic disorders are often associated with difficulties in cross-matching.

Technical Aspects

Operations on the spleen are usually performed with the patient under general endotracheal anesthesia. Spinal anesthesia has several disadvantages; a high level of anesthesia is necessary, and this increases the risk of postoperative respiratory complications. Intrathecal bleeding is a possibility if a coagulopathy exists, and, in addition, spinal anesthesia may increase splenic blood flow and size.

The spleen can be approached through vertical, midline, or abdominal incisions or by a left subcostal approach. Midline incisions are generally preferred when exploration is being done for trauma, in situations in which the spleen is likely to be mobile, with severe thrombocytopenia, in patients with massively enlarged spleens, and for staging lymphomas. A left subcostal incision is often preferred for obese patients or when the splenic disorder is apt to be associated with adherence to structures in the left upper quadrant. Occasionally, a thoracic or thoracoabdominal approach is indicated.

BASIC TECHNIQUES

There are two basic techniques for splenectomy. In the first, the spleen is mobilized and delivered from the abdomen before the vascular pedicle is divided. The avascular portion of the splenorenal ligament is incised, and the phrenosplenic and splenocolic ligaments are divided. The retroperitoneal fusion plane over the kidney is opened, and the spleen is mobilized by rotating it anteromedially. The short gastric and splenic vessels are then dissected and divided, usually from the posterior side of the pedicle, with care taken to avoid injury to the tail of the pancreas. This technique is rapid and is utilized in trauma and when the spleen is small and nonadherent (Fig. 9, upper portion).

In the presence of *very large spleens* and those attached to the abdominal wall by vascular adhesions, it may be advantageous to secure the vascular pedicle prior to mobilizing the spleen. The lesser omental sac is entered through the gastrocolic ligament, and the stomach is dissected from the anterior aspect of the distal pancreas, demonstrating its superior border and the splenic artery and vein. These are then isolated, ligated, and divided. With the major vessels

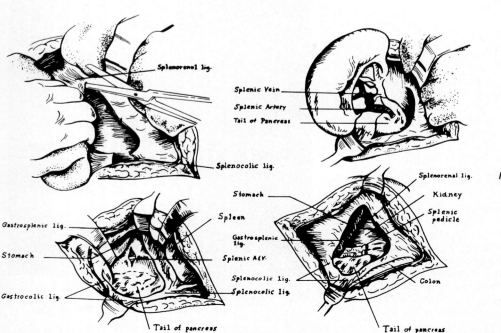

Figure 9. Operative technique.

controlled, the short gastrics can be divided and the spleen mobilized and removed (Fig. 9, lower portion). In hematologic disorders, including idiopathic thrombocytopenic purpura and congenital hemolytic anemia, accessory spleens should be sought and removed. Drainage of the splenic bed is usually unnecessary for simple splenectomy; however, if the pancreas has been injured, adequate drainage is indicated.

SPLEEN-SPARING TECHNIQUES

In the past, splenectomy was the only operation performed on the spleen. Recently it has been shown that the absence of a spleen can be associated with a threat of severe sepsis. Consequently, techniques have been developed to repair injuries and to resect only portions of the spleen. These techniques entail the use of bolstered suturing methods, meshes, and microfibrillar collagen as hemostatic agents. With the use of these methods, the spleen can be spared in most patients with iatrogenic injury and, in many instances, those with penetrating and nonpenetrating trauma. When splenectomy is indicated for hypersplenism but the risk of open splenectomy is unacceptable, transcatheter embolization by a retrograde percutaneous technique can be employed.

Complications

The complications of operations involving the spleen include bleeding, atelectasis, subphrenic collections, and thrombocytosis. Significant bleeding may occur even if the splenectomy is not done for a bleeding disorder. If transfusions are required for maintenance of the hematocrit level and if the abdominal girth is increasing, reoperation should be performed. Even if no obvious bleeding point is found, there is usually no recurrence after evacuation of the hematoma and application of warm packs and hemostatic agents.

Atelectasis of the left lower lobe is the most common complication of splenectomy, and the use of nasogastric suction, analgesics, early mobilization, and respiratory therapy minimizes the risk of its occurrence. Pleural effusion may be a complication of atelectasis or an indication of an underlying subphrenic collection or abscess. Postoperative fever usually results from atelectasis, wound infection, subphrenic collection, or the underlying disorder. Ultrasound imaging and CT scanning are of great value in ascertaining the presence of intra-abdominal collections. They have also been utilized in the treatment of these collections by enabling percutaneous catheter insertion and drainage.

The presence of postsplenectomy thrombocytosis can present problems. A rise in the platelet count is common after splenectomy for trauma or spherocytosis, but is usually mild and not associated with thromboembolic phenomena. The thrombocytosis associated with splenectomy for myeloid metaplasia is more marked and is often associated with thrombotic episodes. Platelet count elevations of less than 800,000 per mm.[3] usually cause no difficulties. With more extreme elevations, therapy directed toward interfering with platelet activity, impeding the coagulation mechanism, or impairing platelet production is indicated. Aspirin and similar drugs are used, and intravenous heparin is indicated in the presence of a severe risk of thrombosis. If the thrombocytosis is severe and expected to be prolonged, suppression of formation with antimetabolites can be considered.

SPLENOMEGALY AND HYPERSPLENISM

Splenomegaly

The fact that a spleen cannot be palpated does not mean it is not enlarged. In many individuals the protected position of the spleen prevents palpation despite mild enlargement. Additionally, the fact that a spleen is not enlarged does not mean it is functioning normally, since apparently normal spleens can hyperfunction, as occurs in idiopathic thrombocytopenic purpura. Finally, the fact that a spleen is enlarged does not mean it is not functioning normally, since mildly enlarged spleens are normal functionally and histologically.

The spleen is anatomically and functionally complex and is affected by a multitude of disorders, many of which do not directly injure it but exert their effects from a distance. Disorders affecting the spleen often are manifest only in certain population groups or geographic areas.

Mild to moderate splenomegaly has many specific causes, and they can be grouped into seven categories (Table 2).

1. *Congestive splenomegaly secondary to venous hypertension.* Portal hypertension caused by diseases obstructing the portal vein, including Laennec's and postnecrotic cirrhosis, cavernous degeneration of the portal vein, neoplastic compression of the portal vein, and schistosomiasis of the liver, regularly produces splenic enlargement. The most common cause of splenomegaly in the United States is the venous congestion associated with liver disease.

TABLE 2. *Causes of Splenomegaly and Hypersplenism*

Primary Hypersplenism
Hereditary spherocytosis
Hereditary elliptocytosis
Thalassemia
Sickle cell disease
Pyruvate kinase deficiency
Porphyria erythropoietica
Acquired autoimmune hemolytic anemia
Idiopathic thrombocytopenic purpura
Thrombotic thrombocytopenic purpura
Primary splenic neutropenia
Primary splenic pancytopenia
Secondary Hypersplenism
Cirrhosis of the liver
Portal vein obstruction
Splenic vein obstruction
Congestive heart failure
Infectious mononucleosis
Felty's syndrome
Subacute bacterial endocarditis
Typhoid fever
Tuberculosis
Abscess
Leishmaniasis
Malaria
Schistosomiasis
Echinococcal cyst
Sarcoidosis
Gaucher's disease
Niemann-Pick disease
Amyloidosis
Hyperlipidemia
Malignant lymphomas
Leukemias
Primary neoplasms
Agnogenic myeloid metaplasia

2. *Hypertrophy as a response to an infectious or inflammatory disorder*. Characterized by lymphoid hypertrophy, this may represent an immune response to infection or inflammation in the body, the spleen reacting as a giant lymph node. Examples include the splenomegaly associated with infectious mononucleosis, Felty's syndrome, and subacute bacterial endocarditis.

3. *Work hypertrophy secondary to red cell sequestration and destruction*. The spleen, faced with increased quantities of abnormal red cells, enlarges to accomplish the task. Disorders leading to this response include hereditary spherocytosis, thalassemia major, and the early phase of sickle cell disease.

4. *Myeloproliferative disorders with splenic hematopoiesis*. Rests in the spleen are activated and enlarged, assuming the role of the marrow. At the same time, the spleen may be involved in fibrosis, infiltrative processes, and increased destruction of blood elements. Examples include agnogenic myeloid metaplasia and chronic myeloid leukemia.

5. *Infiltrative disease of the spleen*. The spleen is infiltrated with granulomatous tissue, amyloid, lipid, and so on. The site of deposition may be the marginal zone, as in the storage diseases. Examples include sarcoidosis, Gaucher's disease, and amyloidosis.

6. *Infections of the spleen*. Although infections of the spleen occur, they are uncommon in the United States. They include splenic abscess, tuberculosis of the spleen, malaria, and leishmaniasis. In some parts of the world, these are common causes of splenomegaly.

7. *Neoplastic infiltrations, primary or secondary*. Although frequently greatly enlarged by involvement with leukemic and lymphomatous infiltrations, the spleen is not often a site for massive metastases of intra-abdominal adenocarcinoma. Adenocarcinomas metastasize to the spleen, but the deposits usually remain small.

Miscellaneous causes include echinococcal and nonparasitic cysts.

At times more than one of the preceding conditions combine to cause splenic enlargement. *Giant splenomegaly* denotes massive enlargements of more than 2000 gm., and some spleens weigh 5000 gm. or more. In the United States giant splenomegaly is associated with only a few diseases, and its usual causes are agnogenic myeloid metaplasia, chronic myelogenous leukemia, hairy cell leukemia (leukemic reticuloendotheliosis), and Gaucher's disease. In the late stages of chronic lymphocytic leukemia and thalassemia, the spleen can also attain huge proportions.

In giant splenomegaly, the increased blood flow to the spleen can result in increased flow into the portal venous system and an induced portal hypertension. The portal vascular space is increased. This may result in a dilutional anemia and a significant thrombocytopenia resulting from an increased space for platelet pooling.

Hypersplenism

Hypersplenism denotes overactivity of the spleen in its sequestration and destruction of formed blood elements so that the quantity in circulation is reduced. The disorder may involve only erythrocytes or platelets, or it may involve all three elements. This definition is a deviation from the classic one, which required splenomegaly, any combination of element deficiency, compensatory marrow hyperplasia of that element, and improvement after splenectomy. This stricter definition does not allow the inclusion of such disorders as idiopathic thrombocytopenic purpura and agnogenic myeloid metaplasia.

Hypersplenism is classified as primary or secondary. In *primary hypersplenism* the problem begins in the cells. The originally normal spleen is presented with an excessive work load of abnormal cells and responds with great efficiency, removing the cells so rapidly that the marrow cannot maintain normal circulating levels. Splenic hypertrophy and splenomegaly are not necessary for this to occur. Splenomegaly is common in the hemolytic anemias with hypersplenism, but is absent in idiopathic thrombocytopenic purpura. Disorders associated with primary hypersplenism that have operative significance are listed in Table 2.

Secondary hypersplenism follows involvement of the spleen by a primary process, nearly always producing splenomegaly. The enlarged spleen sequesters or destroys more than the required amounts of formed blood elements. In secondary hypersplenism the blood cells do not have to be abnormal for removal. Congestive splenomegaly, as occurs in the portal hypertension of Laennec's cirrhosis, is the most common cause of secondary hypersplenism in the United States. In this type of hypersplenism, the cytopenia affects all elements. Not all the sequestered cells are destroyed; some are merely pooled in the enlarged splenic bed. Inflammatory, infiltrative, and neoplastic involvements of the spleen, such as sarcoidosis, Gaucher's disease, and lymphoma, can cause secondary hypersplenism. Secondary hypersplenism also may occur as a complication of primary hypersplenism, when the work-hypertrophied spleen autonomously begins the sequestration of uninvolved cells.

SPLENECTOMY FOR HEMATOLOGIC DISORDERS

The following is a general grouping of the indications for splenectomy.

Injury to the Spleen. Trauma or major vascular accident can mandate splenectomy, but a committed attempt should always be made to preserve the spleen or to save as much as is safely possible.

Hematologic Syndromes. These include the hemolytic anemias and purpuras, either primary or secondary. For splenectomy to be of value, the spleen must play a major role in the sequestration and destruction of the blood elements involved.

Splenic Enlargement. The enlarged spleen can cause discomfort, can impair other activities, and carries the threat of rupturing.

Miscellaneous Splenic Diseases. Included in this group are splenic cysts, neoplasms, and abscesses.

Splenectomy as Part of Other Procedures. At times splenectomy is a part of an operative procedure, as in some types of splenorenal shunts and some operations for cancer of an adjacent organ.

Although several of these indications would not suffice if considered alone, when combined they may justify operation.

Splenomegaly is usually present when spleens are removed for those indications other than trauma. Several disorders characterized by splenomegaly in which splenectomy may be of value are Gaucher's disease, sarcoidosis, Felty's syndrome, and cirrhosis with portal hypertension. Other causes of splenomegaly for which splenectomy may be of value are covered in subsequent sections.

Gaucher's Disease

Gaucher's disease is a familial disorder usually found in Ashkenazic Jews. It is characterized by accumulation of glucocerebroside lipids in the reticuloendothelial system because of deficiency of the degrading enzyme. The spleen, liver, and lymph nodes are enlarged, and bone lesions are present. The most virulent forms occur in childhood and also affect the nervous system. The adult form is chronic.

Splenomegaly is frequently the presenting complaint, especially in adults, and the spleen often reaches the giant splenomegaly level. Pain and disability from the bony involvement are frequent. The acute neurotrophic form is destructive and becomes manifest in early infancy and leads to death in early childhood. The symptoms of nervous system involvement in the juvenile form appear later but are slowly progressive. Hypergammaglobulinemia may be present, and acid phosphatase of the nonprostatic type is elevated. The diagnosis is suspected if Gaucher foam cells are present in marrow aspirates and confirmed by the demonstration of decreased glucosylceramide-B-D-glucosidase activity in cell culture.

Many of these patients develop hypersplenism, and all cell lives may be involved, with platelet depression usually being the most prominent. The bone marrow is usually normal or hypercellular. Some aspects of the cytopenia, especially the thrombocytopenia, appear to be dilutional and related to pooling in an expanded portal system associated with the flow-induced portal hypertension of massive splenomegaly. Splenectomy is indicated to alleviate the discomfort of the huge spleen or to control hypersplenism. It may accelerate the development of the bone lesions in the juvenile form.

Sarcoidosis

Sarcoidosis mostly affects young adults. Common symptoms are fatigability, low-grade fever, night sweats, and shortness of breath. Generalized lymphadenopathy is common, and hepatomegaly and splenomegaly occur in 25 per cent of cases. In one fifth of those with splenomegaly, hypersplenism may follow, usually producing thrombocytopenic purpura. Splenectomy may be indicated to control the hematologic abnormality or to prevent splenic rupture.

Felty's Syndrome

Felty's syndrome is a hematologic complication of rheumatoid arthritis. In rheumatoid arthritis, splenomegaly occurs in 5 to 10 per cent of cases. In about 1 per cent, the full triad of Felty's syndrome is present: rheumatoid arthritis, splenomegaly, and neutropenia. The cause of the neutropenia is unclear; antineutrophile antibody production, marrow suppression by a splenic factor, and splenic pooling and sequestration have each been proposed as etiologic mechanisms.

The major problem and the usual cause for diagnosis is that the patient has symptoms in addition to arthritis and an increased susceptibility to infections. Leg ulcers and hepatomegaly are frequent, and the spleen is universally enlarged, the amount of enlargement varying. The hematologic findings show neutropenia with anemia in 80 per cent and thrombocytopenia in 20 per cent. Examination of the marrow shows hyperplasia of the erythroid and usually the myeloid elements. The rheumatoid factor is present, and antinuclear factors are usually present. Treatment is designed to lessen the impact of infection, and corticosteroids are of little benefit. Splenectomy does improve, at least temporarily, the hematologic status as well as the resistance to infection, and leg ulcers and chronic infections often heal.

Cirrhosis of the Liver

In about 60 per cent of those with cirrhosis splenomegaly develops. One tenth of these, or about 5 per cent of the total, evidence hypersplenism, but it is generally quite mild. All the decompressive procedures performed for esophageal variceal bleeding, if successful, will improve the anemia and thrombocytopenia and reduce the size of the spleen. Thus, the presence of hypersplenism is not usually a factor in the choice of a decompressive procedure. It should be considered, however, if a devascularization operation is comtemplated. In the uncommon situation in which thrombosis of the splenic vein results in esophageal variceal bleeding, splenectomy is indicated.

The Hemolytic Anemias

There are a group of primary disorders of the blood and blood-forming organs in which splenectomy may be indicated (Table 3), but the frequency with which it is necessary to perform splenectomy for these disorders varies widely. At times, splenectomy affects the disease process itself and it may be necessary to remove the spleen solely because of the physical problems caused by its size. Most often, splenectomy is directed toward excising an organ that is performing its function of removing abnormal cells from the blood.

The hemolytic anemias for which splenectomy is performed are characterized by excessive splenic sequestration and destruction of erythrocytes, and the cause lies in the cells rather than the spleen. They are abnormal because of an intrinsic defect or damage by an external factor. The hemolytic anemias can be classified as congenital or ac-

TABLE 3. Hematologic Disorders in Which Splenectomy Is Utilized

The hemolytic anemias
  Hereditary spherocytosis
  Hereditary elliptocytosis
  Pyruvate kinase deficiency
  Thalassemia
  Sickle cell disease
  Porphyria hematopoietica
  Autoimmune hemolytic anemia

The purpuras
  Idiopathic thrombocytopenic purpura
  Thrombotic thrombocytopenic purpura

Splenic neutropenia and splenic pancytopenia

Felty's syndrome

Myeloproliferative disorders
  Agnogenic myeloid metaplasia
  Chronic myeloid leukemia

Lymphoproliferative disorders
  Chronic lymphatic leukemia
  Hairy cell leukemia

quired. In the congenital group, hereditary genetic factors are responsible for the development of an intrinsic defect in the cell membrane, cellular enzymatic activity, or hemoglobin structure or synthesis. The acquired group of hemolytic anemias are associated with red cells that begin life normally but that are damaged as the result of the action of extrinsic factors, such as dyplastic alteration during formation, alteration or damage to the cell after release by immunologic agents, chemicals, parasitization, or physical trauma. The acquired hemolytic anemia for which splenectomy is, at times, indicated is the autoimmune hemolytic anemia of the warm agglutination type.

The defective red cells in the congenital anemias are not capable of the deformation required to allow passage through the spleen. They show changes of internal shape and constituency, membrane abnormalities, or assumption of an abnormal nonmoldable shape. The cells altered by antibody in the autoimmune hemolytic anemias adhere to phagocytes in the splenic pulp and reticuloendothelial tissues. The spleen recognizes these abnormal cells and removes them from the circulation.

The hemolytic anemias share several common clinical features, and anemia is always present, the magnitude depending upon the rate of red cell destruction and replacement. The erythrocyte survival time is decreased; plasma bilirubin, especially the direct fraction, is elevated; and jaundice is often present. Reticulocytosis and polychromatophilia in the peripheral blood smear and erythroid hyperplasia on marrow biopsy provide evidence of increased hematopoietic activity. There is usually splenomegaly of the work-hypertrophy type at some time during the course of the disease. This can progress to a secondary hypersplenism, aggravating the hemolysis. The Coombs' test is negative in the congenital anemias.

Thrombocytopenia

The role of splenectomy is associated with thrombocytopenia. Thrombocytopenia is present when the platelet count is below 100,000 per mm.[3]. Platelet counts above 50,000 per mm.[3] are usually not associated with significant bleeding. Counts in the 20,000 to 50,000 per mm.[3] range evidence prolonged bleeding after injury, and counts below 20,000 per mm.[3] are associated with spontaneous bleeding and the threat of gastrointestinal hemorrhage or central nervous system hemorrhage, especially if fever and anemia coexist. Thrombocytopenia results from four mechanisms: decreased or inefficient platelet production, diminished platelet survival due to increased destruction or consumption, sequestration, and intravascular dilution.

Splenectomy has a role in the treatment of only a few types of purpuras and then only in specific circumstances. These are idiopathic thrombocytopenic purpura, thrombotic thrombocytopenic purpura, the thrombocytopenia due to hypersplenism, and, possibly, immune thrombocytopenia associated with HTLV-III infection. Of these, only idiopathic thrombocytopenic purpura is a purely hematologic disorder.

Myeloproliferative Disorders

The myeloproliferative disorders are a group of diseases in which the marrow cells, and at times the extramedullary stem cells, proliferate in a self-perpetuating fashion more or less in mass. Included in this group of hematologic disorders are chronic myelogenous leukemia, agnogenic myeloid metaplasia, polycythemia vera, and "essential" polycythemia. In each of these, although one cell type predominates, there is often evidence of proliferation of the rest at some time in the course. All can involve the spleen as well as the marrow. Most show fibrous tissue increase in areas of hematopoiesis. Splenectomy is helpful in many patients with agnogenic myeloid metaplasia, but indications for its use in chronic myeloid leukemia are rare.

Hereditary Spherocytosis

This disorder is also known as *congenital hemolytic jaundice* or *familial hemolytic anemia* and is transmitted as an autosomal dominant trait. Although its occurrence is universal, the incidence is highest in those of northern European extraction. A cellular membrane defect is present that allows increased permeability to sodium and water and alters glucose metabolism. The red blood cells are spheroidal in shape, smaller than usual, and demonstrate increased osmotic fragility. The abnormal cells cannot change shape readily and are susceptible to splenic trapping and destruction.

DIAGNOSIS

Hereditary spherocytosis is usually diagnosed by the third decade of life. In addition to a suggestive family history, its clinical manifestations include anemia, jaundice, and splenomegaly. The anemia is usually not severe, the hemoglobin being in the 9- to 12-gm. range. Hematologic findings include spherocytosis, reticulocytosis, increased mean corpuscular hemoglobin concentration, increased osmotic fragility, a positive autohemolysis test partially corrected by glucose, and a shortened red cell life span with splenic sequestration.

In childhood, "aplastic" crises can occur with decreased marrow activity and worsening of the anemia and are usually associated with infections. In later life as the spleen enlarges, an increased hemolysis occurs owing to an element of secondary hypersplenism. Cholelithiasis is present in about half the patients, its incidence becoming significant in the teen years. In fact, biliary symptoms may be the presenting complaint.

TREATMENT

Splenectomy is the treatment for hereditary spherocytosis and is recommended for all patients. Splenectomy does not correct the erythrocyte defect but rather removes the site of cell trapping and destruction. In nearly all patients, this results in freedom from hemolysis, and postsplenectomy sepsis has a low incidence in this disorder. When the disease is diagnosed early in life, splenectomy should be deferred to late childhood to balance the prevention of hematologic and biliary tract problems with freedom from sepsis. Operation should not be performed during a crisis. Prior to operation the biliary tract should be evaluated so that concomitant cholecystectomy and bile duct exploration can be performed if indicated.

Sickle Cell Disease

Occurring predominantly in blacks, but also occasionally seen in those of Mediterranean ancestry, sickle cell disease is the most important of a group of inheritable hemoglobinopathies. There is replacement of the normal hemoglobin, Hb A, with a sickle hemoglobin, Hb S, containing a structurally abnormal β-globin chain. When exposed to low oxygen tension, Hb S assumes a deoxy configuration in which its molecules can aggregate. This may result in a characteristic deformation or "sickling" of the cell. Restoration of oxygenation can reverse the process unless damage to the membrane has occurred. With damage, the cell remains deformed. Sickled cells are caught in the microcirculation, impairing flow. The resultant hypoxia promotes further sickling. If occlusion is sufficient, the microvessels thrombose and the resultant ischemia leads to necrosis and infarction. Eventually there is fibrosis of tissues.

Sickled cells in the general circulation are sequestered by the spleen. Early in the course the spleen is enlarged through work hypertrophy. It then undergoes "autosplenectomy" through a prolonged series of painful infarctions, and hyposplenism ensues. Before the spleen involutes, it can manifest secondary hypersplenism and may be involved in hemolytic crises.

Factors promoting sickling include high concentrations of Hb S in the red cell hemoglobin, hypoxia, dehydration with increased corpuscular hemoglobin concentration, stasis, acidosis, and admixture of Hb C or D with the Hb S. Admixture of Hb F is protective.

If inheritance is from one parent, the sickle cell trait (Hb SA) exists and few, if any, symptoms occur. However, there is damage to the hyperosmolar renal medulla with loss of concentrating power. In the presence of severe hypoxia, vaso-occlusive crisis may occur. For the complete syndrome, the individual must be homozygous, i.e., must have Hb SS. Combinations of Hb S with other abnormal hemoglobins, such as Hb C or the thalassemia hemoglobin, produce clinical manifestations combining features of both.

CLINICAL PRESENTATION

The major aspects of the clinical profile of sickle cell disease result from vessel occlusion and hemolysis. Episodic crises are characteristic, and the predominant type is the vaso-occlusive crisis resulting from increased sickling in the microcirculation. Although often spontaneous, these attacks can be precipitated by infection, dehydration, hypoxia, or acidosis. Bone and joint pain is common and occurs in the absence of physical signs. Acute chest crisis can mimic pulmonary infarction. Abdominal pain can simulate intra-abdominal disease requiring operation, and often results from splenic infarcts. Hepatic crisis with hyperbilirubinemia can be confused with calculous biliary tract disease. Convulsions and hemiparesis can result from central nervous system involvement. Acute renal papillary infarct can occur as can priapism.

The anemia of sickle cell disease is chronic and usually compensated, the hemoglobin being from 7 to 10 gm. Sickle cells are present in blood preparations for sickling. After autosplenectomy, Howell-Jolly bodies appear in blood smears. Two types of crisis have been described as causing increased anemia. One, acute splenic sequestration, occurs in young patients prior to their expected autosplenectomy. The second, hypoplastic crisis, occurs as a result of bone marrow depression, often precipitated by infection.

The findings in sickle cell disease include growth retardation, ocular disturbances from retinal vessel occlusion or rupture and retinal detachment, degenerative joint disease, leg ulcers, and cholelithiasis. Hyposthenuria is universal

and is the result of vaso-occlusive damage to the renal medulla induced by the high osmolarity. There is also decreased resistance to infection. The diagnosis is established by the familial incidence and the presence of sickle cells and confirmed by hemoglobin electrophoresis.

MANAGEMENT

General methods of management include prevention of sepsis and maintenance of hydration. Crises are treated with oxygen, hydration with alkaline hypotonic fluids, and analgesics. Transfusions, exchange transfusions, and infusion of blood treated extracorporeally with sodium cyanate have been employed. Splenectomy is of value in young patients with enlarged spleens with significant secondary hypersplenism. The incidence of postsplenectomy sepsis is greater in those undergoing splenectomy for sickle cell disease than in those undergoing splenectomy for trauma or congenital spherocytosis.

Severe β-Thalassemia

This disorder, also known as Mediterranean anemia, Cooley's anemia, or erythroblastic anemia, is transmitted as a dominant autosomal trait and occurs most frequently in people of southern European ancestry. A deficiency in the synthesis of the β-globin chain of Hb A results in the hemoglobin molecule containing excessive amounts of A2-globin, and the cell formed is physically abnormal. It interferes with the erythrocyte marrow cycle, has a retarded release from the marrow, tends to die before leaving the marrow, and exhibits membrane damage, making it prone to splenic sequestration. As in sickle cell disease, but to a lesser extent, there is impairment of its passage through the microcirculation.

THALASSEMIA MAJOR

Homozygous individuals develop severe β-thalassemia, which occurs as two variants: (1) the devastating thalassemia major and (2) a lesser thalassemia intermedia. The defect produces ineffective hematopoiesis and severe anemia with stimulation of erythroid hyperplasia and extramedullary hematopoiesis. The enlarged erythroid tissue mass results in bony deformities, pathologic fractures, and spinal cord compression. Severe thalassemia becomes manifest in infancy as the hemoglobin changes from Hb F to Hb A, a process that is complete at the end of the first year of life. Clinical features include a pallid, muddy complexion; enlargement of the head; retarded, deformed body growth; isothenuria; hepatosplenomegaly; and recurrent infections. Gallstones are frequent. The diagnosis is made by family history, with both parents having the trait, and the presence of a hypochromic microcytic anemia with characteristic target and fragmented cells. Hemoglobin electrophoresis shows decreased Hb A, increased Hb A2, and persistence of Hb F in abnormal amounts. Reticulocytosis and leukocytosis are present with a normal platelet count. The red cells exhibit decreased osmotic fragility.

The severity of the disease, as evidenced by the need for blood transfusion, separates thalassemia major from thalassemia intermedia. In the major form, without transfusion death occurs in infancy or early childhood. Regular transfusion therapy decreases the drive on the marrow, diminishes the deformity, and corrects growth retardation. Difficulty from hemosiderosis, usually in the form of cardiomyopathy, occurs in the teen years as a complication of the hypertransfusion regimen. A chelating agent, deferoxamine, is of benefit in its amelioration.

THALASSEMIA INTERMEDIA

Patients with thalassemia intermedia have fairly normal growth and development and can survive into adulthood. A hemoglobin of 6 to 7 gm. can be maintained without transfusion. Difficulties arising from extramedullary sites of erythropoiesis can be controlled by local radiotherapy. Iron retention can cause problems. Transfusions are eventually required. The usual heterozygote manifests only a mild asymptomatic anemia compatible with a normal life and is said to have thalassemia minor. Splenectomy is of palliative benefit in selected patients. Indications are splenomegaly causing symptoms because of the physical effects of the huge spleen and splenic overactivity, resulting in an excessive need for transfusions. Although it does not affect the basic process, splenectomy may decrease hemolysis and prolong the period between transfusions.

Miscellaneous Congenital Hemolytic Anemia

HEREDITARY ELLIPTOCYTOSIS

Hereditary elliptocytosis, also known as *ovalocytosis*, usually occurs in the innocuous trait form. The abnormal cells have defective membranes that are more permeable, exhibit increased osmotic fragility, and have oval and rod shapes. These properties make them more susceptible to sequestration and destruction in the spleen. In the vast majority, only 10 per cent of the cells are abnormal and red cell survival is not shortened. In a few, 50 per cent or more of the cells can be abnormal, causing a picture similar to that seen in hereditary spherocytosis. If the patient is symptomatic, splenectomy should be performed; the abnormal cells are not changed but hemolysis ceases. As in spherocytosis, attention should be given to the biliary tract.

The enzyme deficiencies causing hemolytic anemias involve the Embden-Meyerhof pathway of glycolytic metabolism or the hexose monophosphate shunt. There is impairment of energy production and in membrane deformity, and the red cells are more susceptible to stress and hemolysis. However, osmotic fragility is normal. Pyruvate kinase (PK) deficiency is the major glycolytic pathway defect; glucose-6-phosphate dehydrogenase (G-6-PD) deficiency is the prime shunt defect. Specific tests of enzyme function are available to differentiate the disorders.

PYRUVATE KINASE DEFICIENCY

Pyruvate kinase deficiency usually manifests itself in early childhood, and infant mortality is increased. Anemia and jaundice may occur, and the spleen in often enlarged. The smear is often normal except for some crenated cells. The autohemolysis test findings are positive and are not corrected by glucose addition. Assays show a decrease in pyruvate kinase activity and an increase in 2,3-diphosphoglycerate (DPG) quantity. Many patients maintain an adequate hemoglobin level and have few symptoms of hemolysis. In patients with sequestration in the spleen, and marked anemias requiring frequent transfusion, splenectomy is helpful. Cholelithiasis may also be present.

PORPHYRIA ERYTHROPOIETICA

Porphyria erythropoietica is a rare disorder of erythrocyte pyrrole synthesis, and the cells are susceptible to premature splenic sequestration and destruction. There is hemolysis with excessive blood cell production, and porphyrins are deposited in the skin, where they can precipitate severe photosensitivity and bullous dermatitis. When the disease is complicated by hemolysis or splenomegaly, benefit in all aspects may be achieved by splenectomy.

Autoimmune Hemolytic Anemia

Hemolytic anemias are caused by autoimmune processes with antibodies being formed that react with previously normal red cells. In many of the autoimmune anemias, intravascular hemolysis occurs or the entire reticuloendothelial system traps and destroys cells. In some, however, the destruction is primarily in the spleen.

CLASSIFICATION

Two forms exist. The *cold agglutination type* usually involves IgM globulin and occurs in the elderly as a chronic form associated with lymphoma and after infections such as infectious mononucleosis and *Mycoplasma pneumoniae* infections, which are often self-limited. The symptoms are related to chilling, the spleen size is variable, and splenectomy is of little or no benefit.

Autoimmune hemolytic anemia of the *warm agglutination type* is usually associated with an IgG globulin acting in conjunction with complement. The disorder usually occurs in or after midlife in women. In one third, no other disease is evident; in two thirds there is an underlying disease, typically chronic lymphocytic leukemia, lymphoma, or systemic lupus erythematosus. The course of the disease varies, and it may be quite mild or severe. Pallor, anemia, and possible jaundice are present. Splenomegaly is usually present with reticulocytosis and spherocytosis, and products of cell destruction are present in the blood, urine, and stool. The direct Coombs' test is positive. The marrow is hypercellular with a predominance of erythroid precursors. Gallstones occur in 25 per cent of patients.

CLINICAL PRESENTATION

In most patients the course is prolonged with remissions and exacerbations. The severe form can produce acute crises with chills, fever, back pain, hemoglobinuria, and renal failure from intravascular hemolysis. This form of the disease is associated with a mortality of 40 to 50 per cent. Corticosteroids are the primary treatment, an initial favorable response being obtained in about two thirds of patients. However, only about 25 per cent can be easily withdrawn from steroids without exacerbation. If steroids have no effect or must be discontinued, immunosuppression or splenectomy controls the disease in most patients. Immunosuppressants are indicated in older patients, whereas splenectomy is usually preferable in the younger group. The overall splenectomy response is in the 60 per cent range and is higher if there is evidence of significant splenic sequestration.

Idiopathic Thrombocytopenic Purpura

The thrombocytopenic purpuras are difficult to classify and have been divided into primary, or idiopathic, and secondary types. The secondary types include thrombocytopenia complicating infections such as infectious mononucleosis, the use of certain drugs, disseminated lupus erythematosus, and the lymphoproliferative disorders. Recently, immune thrombocytopenia has been associated with HTLV-III infection. The term "idiopathic thrombocytopenic purpura" (ITP) should be reserved for patients without other evident cause of thrombocytopenia. Since IgG antibody has been found in 85 per cent of patients, it has been suggested that the term "autoimmune thrombocytopenic purpura" be substituted.

PRIMARY THROMBOCYTOPENIC PURPURA

Thrombocytopenia and an often otherwise normal blood smear are present. The bleeding time is increased, the clotting time is normal, but clot retraction is poor. Capillary fragility (the Rumpel-Leede test) is increased, and the platelet survival time is decreased. There may or may not be a marrow megakaryocyte response, but even if the number of megakaryocytes is normal, their morphology is not. The spleen in ITP sequesters and removes platelets and may also contribute to antibody production. Some have suggested that it elaborates a factor suppressing marrow megakaryocyte maturation and release, but this is questionable. Idiopathic thrombocytopenic purpura is not associated with splenomegaly.

Clinical Presentation

Idiopathic thrombocytopenic purpura occurs in two forms, acute and chronic. The acute form is most common in children, occurring most frequently in those under 8 years and with no sex predominance. There has usually been an antecedent upper respiratory tract infection, suggesting that it may be a response to a viral condition. It is characterized by spontaneous and significant bleeding, and the skin is involved with petechiae and purpura. Bleeding occurs from the gums, gastrointestinal tract, vagina, and urinary tract. Central nervous system bleeding is present in 2 to 4 per cent of cases and is especially likely to occur if the platelet count is below 20,000 per mm.[3] If intracranial bleeding is imminent, it usually occurs early in the course and is an indication for emergency splenectomy.

Treatment

Splenectomy has long been known to be helpful in ITP. Although corticosteroids have lessened the need for its use, definite indications remain. The response to steroids does not correlate with the response to splenectomy, and splenectomy may succeed when steroids fail. The spleen is not enlarged, and therefore splenectomy is technically relatively easy. Accessory spleens must be sought, and all splenic tissue must be removed. Bleeding is usually not a significant problem, and it has long been held that during splenectomy for ITP platelet concentrates should be given only when definitely indicated and only after the spleen has been removed. The incidence of postsplenectomy sepsis is mild. Lack of response or recurrence following splenectomy-induced remission raises a question as to the presence of accessory splenic tissue. Scanning with technetium or radiochromatized red cells is of value in establishing a diagnosis.

In patients under 16 with ITP, there is an 80 per cent chance of spontaneous complete recovery within 6 weeks. Corticosteroids usually make up the initial therapy, and some physicians treat all patients irrespective of the severity for the first 4 weeks. If full remission is not attained in several months, recovery is unlikely and a decision must be made whether to continue steroids or resort to splenectomy. Corticoids are often utilized in adults, whereas splenectomy is usually favored in children.

SECONDARY THROMBOCYTOPENIC PURPURA

Immune thrombocytopenia has recently been described as part of the clinical syndrome of HTLV-III–associated disease. Thrombocytopenia may represent an alternative response to infection with HTLV-III or may be a prodromal state of the more severe manifestations of the acquired immune deficiency syndrome (AIDS). The sustained response rate to steroid therapy is poor, and there is a high incidence of steroid-related side effects, prednisone being reserved for patients with acute significant bleeding episodes. Responses to splenectomy are similar to results obtained in patients with classic immune thrombocytopenia. However, the long-term effects of splenectomy in this cohort are unknown. There has been a low incidence of life-threatening bleeding events reported in these patients, and expectant therapy is considered an alternative in AIDS-related immune thrombocytopenia.

Agnogenic Myeloid Metaplasia

Myeloid metaplasia or extramedullary hematopoiesis refers to blood element formation in organs and tissues not usually involved in adult hematopoiesis. This can occur in response to severe hemolytic anemias, with lymphomas, and in marrow replacement by tumor or fibrous tissue, as occurs in metastatic malignancy, chronic granulocytic leukemia, polycythemia vera, and tuberculosis. When without cause and associated with varying degrees of marrow fibrosis, it is known as agnogenic myeloid metaplasia. Other terms are myelofibrosis with myeloid metaplasia and myelofibrosis with extramedullary hematopoiesis.

The major sites of extramedullary hematopoiesis are the liver and the spleen. The predominant symptoms are caused by the anemia and the splenomegaly, but in about 30 per cent of cases these are not significant. Later manifestations include spontaneous bleeding, infections, bone pain, and splenic infarcts. Hyperuricemia and gouty attacks are common. The splenomegaly can become quite massive, and hepatomegaly occurs in 75 per cent of cases. Overt portal hypertension occurs even with portal obstruction as a result of the increased splenic flow, and secondary hypersplenism with hemolytic anemia and thrombocytopenia is common.

Splenectomy is of definite value in certain circumstances. Indications include massive splenomegaly, severe anemia, and thrombocytopenia due to hypersplenism and portal hypertension. Study of splenic red cell sequestration is of value in quantifying the role of the spleen in the anemia. If portal hypertension is present, it should be evaluated to ascertain the proper management. It should be noted that the so-called rebound thrombocytosis is especially prone to occur following splenectomy for this disorder and can be quite severe, leading to major occlusions and hemorrhage. Ordinarily, splenectomy is not performed unless the platelet count is under 100,000 per mm.[3]

Chronic Myeloid Leukemia

Splenectomy has been advocated to temper the effect of the enlarged spleen and to allow more intensive therapy. The operation has a significant complication rate, and there is little evidence to support the latter claim. It should be reserved for selected chronic-phase patients in whom it is necessary to palliate a massively enlarged spleen or control secondary hypersplenism.

Lymphoproliferative Disorders

The role of splenectomy in myelogenous leukemia also applies to chronic lymphatic leukemia. Hairy cell leukemia, or leukemic reticuloendotheliosis, is an uncommon form of chronic leukemia. The spleen becomes massively filled with cells so that blood cells cannot traverse it, leading to their sequestration and resultant pancytopenia. Bacterial infections are common and appear to be linked to the granulocytopenia. Splenectomy is currently the preferred management for this disorder; however, recent reports of therapy with alpha interferon have been encouraging.

MISCELLANEOUS LESIONS OF THE SPLEEN

Splenic Cysts

Rarely, cysts occur in the spleen and are classified as parasitic or nonparasitic. Nonparasitic cysts are classified as either true cysts, lined by epithelium, or pseudocysts, without a lining. Most are pseudocysts and probably represent the resolution of a previous splenic infarct or hematoma. Although they can be painful, splenic cysts usually present as an incidental left upper quadrant mass. Some advocate aspiration for diagnosis and treatment, but splenectomy is probably preferable.

The only parasitic cyst occurring in the United States is caused by the *Echinococcus* parasite. Two per cent of *Echinococcus* infestations are associated with splenic cysts and are usually asymptomatic until rupture. Echinococcal cysts may present as a mass on routine physical examination or are first evident on x-ray or CT scan. If an echinococcal cyst is suspected, diagnosis can be confirmed by serologic testing. Echinococcal cysts of the spleen should be treated by splenectomy.

Splenic Tissue Outside the Spleen

Accessory spleens are rarely symptomatic. When present, symptoms are usually the result of torsion of a pedicle. The clinical significance of an accessory spleen lies in its ability to perpetuate a hematologic condition for which splenectomy has been performed.

An ectopic spleen is one that is in an abnormal position because of a very long pedicle. The spleen may be mobile and is referred to as a "wandering spleen." Ectopic spleens may present as asymptomatic mobile masses or with pain caused by acute torsion of the pedicle, a situation warranting laparotomy and splenectomy.

Splenosis refers to the autotransplantation of fragments of splenic tissue in other parts of the abdomen following trauma and splenic rupture, and it is usually asymptomatic. When symptoms occur, they are secondary to bowel obstruction or torsion of a pedicle. These transplanted fragments are competent to maintain, at least partially, the immunologic functions of the spleen.

Vascular Problems Involving the Spleen

The vascular problems associated with the spleen include (1) aneurysm of the splenic artery, (2) splenic arteriovenous fistula, and (3) infarction.

Splenic aneurysm is second only to aortic aneurysm as the most common intra-abdominal aneurysm and occurs in two forms and in two age ranges. One occurs primarily in older males and represents a manifestation of generalized atherosclerosis. The other form occurs primarily in women in the child-bearing ages. Such aneurysms are probably congenital but have a propensity to rupture during pregnancy, especially in the last trimester. Both types are usually calcified. Symptoms, when present, often consist of abdominal pain and/or evidence of intra-abdominal bleeding. Asymptomatic aneurysms are usually found as typical round, calcified masses on x-rays of the abdomen. Operation should be performed in the younger group, whereas, in the older group, the aneurysms can be closely observed if they are small (under 2 cm.) and asymptomatic.

Splenic arteriovenous fistulas usually are associated with splenic aneurysm but may follow trauma or splenectomy. Bruits are usually present. The spleen, if present, is usually enlarged. The large quantities of blood delivered to the portal system may cause portal hypertension, and the presence of a fistula should be suspected when portal hypertension is accompanied by a left upper quadrant bruit. Selective angiography is diagnostic, and treatment consists of splenectomy and excision of the fistula. Alternatively, in poor-risk groups, fistulas have been successfully controlled by catheter occlusion.

Splenic infarction is common in disorders such as sickle cell disease. However, these infarcts are relatively small and resolve spontaneously. Major infarcts requiring splenectomy are rare and usually embolic.

Neoplasms of the Spleen

Primary splenic tumors are rare and have been classified as arising from the fibrous tissue of the capsule and trabecular framework, the lymphoid elements, vascular and sinus tissue, and other rare types such as embryonic inclusion tumors. The usual type arises from lymphoid elements. Symptoms are usually caused by the large size achieved by the tumor. Despite this, therapeutic efforts have resulted in 5-year survivals of 30 per cent. In appropriate types of tumors, resection is indicated.

The spleen is a common site for metastases, but they usually remain small and are only rarely symptomatic.

Splenic Abscess

Splenic abscesses occur as a result of direct extension from adjacent intra-abdominal sepsis or of infection of a pre-existing infarct or hematoma by the bloodstream, and as a manifestation of generalized sepsis. The latter is the usual cause, and splenic involvement is a terminal event.

Splenic abscesses can be single or multiple. The presenting manifestations include pain and tenderness in the left upper quadrant, splenomegaly, and signs of continued sepsis. Atelectasis of the left lower lobe and pleural effusion are commonly found, and gas may be present in the splenic area. Ultrasonography and CT scanning are the most useful diagnostic tests. These abscesses should be treated by splenectomy and drainage of the splenic bed after appropriate antibiotic preparation.

Rupture of the Spleen

Rupture of the spleen by penetrating or nonpenetrating trauma is discussed in Chapter 13. Iatrogenic injuries, usually occurring during the performance of an abdominal operation, were once responsible for 20 per cent of all splenectomies. This high incidence of incidental splenectomy has been greatly reduced by both avoidance of injury and the development of techniques to repair the injury so as to preserve the spleen for its immunologic function. Iatrogenic injury usually occurs during gastric procedures or mobilization of the splenic flexure during colostomy. It usually occurs during retraction, causing avulsion of the capsule or short gastric vessels.

Spontaneous rupture of the normal spleen is rare, but it may occur in the absence of evidence of trauma. Spleens involved in pathologic processes are often enlarged and susceptible to injury. In some disorders, the spleen may be fragile and spontaneous rupture can occur. For example, patients with infectious mononucleosis have a significant incidence of spontaneous splenic rupture. Sarcoidosis, the lymphomas and leukemia, and the hemolytic anemias have also been known to lead to rupture, as may also occur with malaria and typhoid fever. Anticoagulant therapy is another recognized cause of this complication.

LAPAROTOMY AND SPLENECTOMY IN MALIGNANT LYMPHOMA

Basic Considerations

The malignant lymphomas, of which Hodgkin's disease and non-Hodgkin's lymphoma are the major types, are neoplasms of the reticuloendothelial system. They involve primarily lymph nodes but can invade other reticuloendothelial organs, such as the spleen and liver. Over the past several decades advances in the methods of management of the lymphomas have produced a more than fivefold improvement in survival, and over 85 per cent of those afflicted with Hodgkin's disease currently survive beyond 5 years. Of major significance in the achievement of these results has been the development of classifications of the disease based on natural history that can be closely correlated with therapeutic choices.

CLASSIFICATION

The Rye Classification is a widely accepted classification of Hodgkin's disease according to histopathologic type, with listings in ascending order of virulence (Table 4). Lymphocyte-predominant Hodgkin's has the best prognosis, and lymphocyte-depleted disease the worst. Non-Hodgkin's lymphomas are more difficult to differentiate, and again there is considerable difference in aggressiveness among the various types. The *nodular* form of non-Hodgkin's lymphomas proceeds slowly and may be widespread and yet without significant symptoms. Contrarily, the *diffuse* type spreads rapidly and is usually fatal within 3 years.

Hodgkin's disease almost always begins in a group of lymph nodes, usually in the cervical or mediastinal region. Spread occurs in a stepwise fashion to contiguous nodes, and the rate of spread is dependent upon the histopathologic type. After reaching the lower mediastinal nodes, the disease traverses the diaphragm and involves the celiac nodes. Since the abdominal nodes are in the form of a T, spread next involves the nodes at the hilus of the liver and the spleen as well as the contiguous paraortic group. The spleen is also often involved at this time. If the disease initially involves the inguinal or pelvic region, spread of the process is reversed.

CLINICAL PRESENTATION

Hodgkin's disease remains confined to the lymph nodes for considerable periods before extranodal spread. The organs first involved are those containing reticuloendothelial tissue, such as the liver and the bone marrow. At the time of initial presentation, about 20 per cent of patients with Hodgkin's manifest extranodal involvement. Weight loss, fever, and night sweats, the factors responsible for classification in the "B" stage, correlate with widespread disease and often indicate extranodal involvement.

DIAGNOSIS

Lymphangiography and CT scanning are helpful in establishing a diagnosis. Lymphangiography reveals greater detail of the abnormality, whereas the CT scan covers a wider field. Liver-spleen scans may also be indicated. Among patients with extensive adenopathy, anemia, and bony involvement, bone biopsy is indicated. Liver biopsy should be considered if clinical findings or scans suggest involvement. Laparoscopy has been used to clarify equivocal findings, especially in non-Hodgkin's A-12 lymphoma, in which there is little need for staging laparotomy. Pathologic staging of the abdomen by laparotomy and splenectomy may be indicated.

Unlike Hodgkin's disease, non-Hodgkin's lymphoma is usually systemic at the time of presentation, with more than 40 per cent of patients already having extranodal involvement. Non-Hodgkin's lymphoma frequently presents with parenchymatous organ involvement. Although it may be widespread at the time of diagnosis, the nodular type has a relatively long natural history, whereas the diffuse type is more often characterized by a rapid course.

Management of Lymphomas

The diagnosis of a lymphoma is usually confirmed by biopsy of an involved node, an *excisional* biopsy being preferred. Enough tissue is needed for complete recognition of the architecture and pathologic process. At biopsy, touch imprints should be made on slides, and after confirmation of diagnosis, the lymphoma should be staged. The Ann Arbor Classification developed at the University of Michi-

TABLE 4. *Histopathologic Types of Hodgkin's Disease in Rye Classification*

Type	Incidence (%)
Lymphocyte predominant	5
Nodular sclerosis	40–50
Mixed	40–50
Lymphocyte depleted	5

gan has been the most widely used (Table 5). Although most relevant to Hodgkin's disease, it is used in all lymphomas. The clinical staging of a lymphoma includes:

1. Thorough history and physical examination
2. Complete blood count, urinalysis, multiphase screen (SMA-12)
3. Chest roentgenography, possibly chest tomography
4. Bipedal lymphangiography
5. Computed tomography

Radiotherapy is an effective means of therapy and can help in controlling nodal disease and in completely eradicating the disease even when used as the sole method of treatment. For success of this therapy, the disease must be confined to the nodes treated without massive involvement of any group. The usual dose is 3500 to 4500 rads, with the field of radiotherapy limited to the area involved. Extended field treatment covers the involved area plus the immediately adjacent noninvolved site. Total nodal fields cover all nodal areas, and if present the spleen may also be included. Extended fields commonly employed are the "mantle"and "inverted Y" (Fig. 10). The total nodal field is the mantle plus the inverted Y.

Lymphomas also respond to antimetabolite *chemotherapy*, and the response is often complete if multiple agents are used. *Multiple* drug regimens are currently utilized in most patients when chemotherapy is given. Several widely accepted regimens are listed in Table 6. If bulky disease is present in a region, the involved field is also treated with radiotherapy.

Although the management of lymphomas is still in transition, in the non-Hodgkin's lymphomas treatment depends upon the histopathologic type. If the disease is of low grade and limited to nodes, persistent responses have occurred with limited radiotherapy. If it is of very low grade and extranodal, one-drug chemotherapy has been advocated. Moderate- and high-grade lymphomas are best managed with chemotherapy.

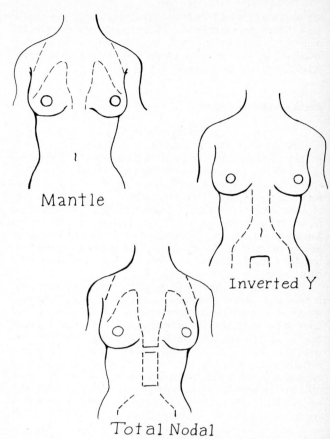

Figure 10. Radiation fields used in treating malignant lymphomas.

The treatment of Hodgkin's disease is evolving, but with some exception it is preferable to use either irradiation or chemotherapy. Radiotherapy is advocated for Stages IA and IIA, and some advocate its use for Stages IB, IIB, and IIIA. Controversy arises concerning the use of total nodal irradiation or a mantle or inverted Y technique. Chemotherapy is used by all for Stage IV and by most for IIIB. In patients with bulky involvement but still Stage II disease, chemotherapy with added involved field radiotherapy is being advocated.

Laparotomy for Staging

Although all lymphomas cannot be unequivocally staged by noninvasive clinical means, the staging laparot-

TABLE 5. Ann Arbor Classification for Staging of Malignant Lymphomas

Stage	Characteristic
Stage I	Involvement of single region of nodes
IE	Involvement of single extranodal organ
Stage II	Involvement of two or more nodal regions on same side of diapharagm
IIE	Involvement of single extranodal organ and contiguous node regions on same side of diaphragm
Stage III	Involvement of nodal regions on both sides of diaphragm
IIIA1	Only upper abdominal nodes and spleen involved
IIIA2	Both upper and lower nodes involved
IIIE	Involvement of a single extranodal site or organ in addition
IIIS	Involved organ is spleen
Stage IV	Disseminated or diffuse involvement of multiple organs and sites

Notes: Suffix "A" or "B" indicates the presence or absence of the symptomatology of generalized disease: A, no symptoms of generalized disease; B, symptoms of generalized disease: unexplained loss of over 10 per cent of body weight, unexplained fever of over 103°F., night sweats.
Organ suffixes: N = nodes, P = pleura, O = bone, H = liver, S = spleen, D = skin, M = marrow, L = lung.

TABLE 6. Chemotherapy Regimen for Malignant Lymphoma

MOPP	Nitrogen mustard (Mustargen)
	Vincristine (Oncovin)
	Procarbazine
	Prednisone
ABVD	Adriamycin
	Bleomycin
	Vinblastine
	Dacarbazine (DTIC)
BCVPP	Carmustine (BCNU)
	Cyclophosphamide
	Vinblastine
	Procarbazine
	Prednisone

omy was developed to provide the necessary precision. This is not a simple cursory exploration of the abdomen but rather a meticulous search for involvement. The procedure includes (1) exploration of the abdomen through a generous midline incision; (2) biopsy of both lobes of the liver; (3) usually splenectomy, including the hilar nodes; (4) biopsy of the abdominal nodal areas in sequential fashion from the T-shaped upper abdominal area to include the pelvic nodes along the ilea; and (5) in the female, medial fixation of the ovaries if radiation is contemplated.

During the operation, lymphangiograms and CT scans are obtained together with intraoperative radiograms, and biopsies of suspicious sites are made. Laparotomy represents a precise method for evaluating the upper abdominal nodes and spleen, which is an area somewhat difficult to thoroughly evaluate by CT scanning and lymphangiography. The use of staging has decreased in recent years as a result of several factors. Although the procedure itself has a low morbidity and mortality, postsplenectomy sepsis does occur, and some have attempted to avoid this complication by doing only a partial resection of the spleen. It is also an invasive procedure associated with postoperative pain. Increased knowledge, much of which has been derived from its use, and a tendency to use total nodal irradiation or chemotherapy have decreased the indications for its use.

Staging laparotomy should be utilized only when the information it provides will influence the selection of therapy. This includes situations in which CT scanning or lymphangiography is equivocal or when questionable liver or splenic areas cannot be assessed percutaneously; different treatments would be selected for different results. The other indication for this procedure is when radiotherapy is to be employed when it is desirable to preserve ovarian function.

SELECTED REFERENCES

Annotated References

Ballinger, W. F., and Erslev, A. J.: Splenectomy: Indications, technique and complications, *In* Current Problems in Surgery, Vol. 2, Chicago, Year Book Medical Publishers, 1965.
The operative technique, anatomy, and management of splenectomy are detailed.

Dameshek, H. L., and Ellis, L. D.: Hematologic indications for splenectomy. Surg. Clin. North Am., 55:253, 1975.
This is written from the viewpoint of a hematologist. Some of the ideas expressed about immune etiologic factors are now accepted as fact.

Eichner, E. R.: Splenic function: Normal, too much and too little. Am. J. Med., 66:311, 1979.
This short review addresses the salient features of splenic physiology, especially in the area of resistance to infection. Hyposplenism is well defined.

Koller, C. A.: Immune thrombocytopenic purpura. Med. Clin. North Am., 64:761, 1980.
The thrombocytopenic purpuras are reviewed briefly, and each variant is considered from diagnostic and management points of view.

Oishi, N.: The malignant lymphomas. *In* Kahn, S. B., et al. (Eds.): Concepts in Cancer Medicine. New York, Grune & Stratton, 1983.
This text is written for medical students. The chapter on lymphomas includes incidences and etiologic aspects written concisely and with sections on radiotherapy and chemotherapy.

Schwartz, S. I.: Splenectomy for hematologic disease. Surg. Clin. North Am., 61:117, 1981.
The hematologic disorders for which splenectomy is done are reviewed from the standpoint of a surgeon.

Wyngaarden, J. B., and Smith, L. H. (Eds.): Cecil's Textbook of Medicine, 16th ed. Philadelphia, W. B. Saunders Company, 1982.
Since the disorders for which splenectomy is done are frequently medical, an inclusive reference of this type is essential. The descriptions of the pathophysiology of the disorders are well written and complete, and the treatment options are current.

General References

Breitfeld, V., and Lee, R. E.: Pathology of the spleen in hematologic disease. Surg. Clin. North Am., 55:233, 1975.
Chabner, B. A., et al.: Staging of non-Hodgkin's lymphoma. Semin. Oncol., 7:285, 1980.
Chen, L.: Microcirculation of the spleen: An open or closed circulation? Science, 201:157, 1978.
Chun, C. H., et al.: Splenic abscess. Medicine, 59:50, 1980.
Das Gupta, T., et al.: Primary malignant neoplasms of the spleen. Surg. Gynecol. Obstet., 120:947, 1965.
DiFino, S. M., et al.: Adult thrombocytopenic purpura: Clinical findings and response to therapy. Am. J. Med., 69:430, 1980.
Fleming, C. R., et al.: Splenosis: Autotransplantation of splenic tissue. Am. J. Surg., 81:414, 1976.
Goldstone, J.: Splenectomy for massive splenomegaly. Am. J. Surg., 135:385, 1978.
Golumb, H. M., et al.: Hairy cell leukemia. A clinical review based on 71 cases. Ann. Intern. Med., 89:677, 1978.
Grieco, M. B., and Cady, B.: Staging laparotomy in Hodgkin's disease. Surg. Clin. North Am., 60:369, 1980.
Hess, C. E., et al.: Mechanism of dilutional anemia in massive splenomegaly. Blood, 47:629, 1976.
Jones, S. E.: Importance of staging in Hodgkin's disease. Semin. Oncol., 7:126, 1980.
Laszlo, M. D., et al.: Splenectomy for Felty's syndrome: Clinicopathologic study of 27 patients. Arch. Intern. Med., 138:597, 1978.
Laws, H. L., et al.: Splenectomy for hematologic disease. Surg. Gynecol. Obstet., 149:509, 1979.
Leonard, A. S., et al.: The overwhelming postsplenectomy sepsis problem. World J. Surg., 4:432, 1983.
Morgenstern, L., and Shapiro, S. J.: Techniques of splenic conservation. Arch. Surg., 114:449, 1979.
Olsen, W. R., and Beaudoin, D. E.: Increased incidence of accessory spleens in hematologic disease. Arch. Surg., 98:762, 1969.
Picozzi, V. J., et al.: Fate of therapy failures in adult thrombocytopenic purpura. Am. J. Med., 69:690, 1980.
Rutkow, I. M.: Thrombotic thrombocytopenic purpura (TTP) and splenectomy: A current appraisal. Ann. Surg., 188:701, 1978.
Salky, B., et al.: Splenectomy for Gaucher's disease. Ann. Surg., 190:592, 1979.
Schwartz, S. I.: Myeloproliferative disorders. Ann. Surg., 182:464, 1975.
Schwartz, S. I., et al.: Splenectomy for thrombocytopenia. Surgery, 88:499, 1980.
Webb, A. B., et al.: Splenectomy and splenomegaly in sarcoidosis. J. Clin. Pathol., 32:1050, 1979.
Westcott, J. L., and Ziter, F. M.: Aneurysms of the splenic artery. Surg. Gynecol. Obstet., 136:541, 1973.
Wolf, D. J., et al.: Splenectomy in chronic myeloid leukemia. Ann. Intern. Med., 89:684, 1979.

THE LYMPHATIC SYSTEM

RICHARD L. McCANN, M.D.

31

HISTORICAL ASPECTS

Although lymphatics were observed centuries earlier, Gasparo Aselli (1581–1626) is credited with first recognizing that these structures were vessels rather than cords and that they conducted a fluid distinct from blood. In 1651, Pecquet described the *cysterna chyli* and from dissection of a dog correctly deduced that the thoracic duct emptied into the venous system. Bartholin first applied the term "lymphatics" to these vessels and recognized their wide distribution in the body. A century later Mascagni injected mercury into the lymphatics of a human cadaver to enhance visualization. William Hunter, in the mid-18th century, espoused that the lymphatic system had the function of fluid absorption throughout the body and the transportation of this volume into the vascular compartment.

In the late 19th century, Starling proposed a concept of capillary fluid filtration and reabsorption that remains nearly intact today. This theory for the first time gave a satisfactory explanation for lymph formation and led the way for investigation of diseases of the lymphatic system. Visualization of lymphatic vessels in living subjects was not achieved until 1930, when Hudack and McMaster injected patent blue violet dye and observed its absorption by dermal and subcutaneous lymphatics. The next important step was the direct cannulation of lymphatic vessels and injection of radiopaque contrast media for the radiographic study of lymphatic anatomy. This was achieved by Glenn in 1948 in animals and rapidly led to the development of the clinical techniques of lymphangiography in use today.[2]

ANATOMY

The lymphatic network is composed of three major compartments. Lymphatic capillaries are the site of lymph absorption throughout the body. These empty into the collecting vessels that traverse the extremities and body cavities, eventually emptying into the venous system via the thoracic duct. The collecting vessels are periodically interrupted by the lymph nodes, which filter the lymph and serve primarily an immunologic function.

Lymphatic capillaries are similar to blood capillaries, except that the basement membrane is much less well defined. Large gaps between adjacent lymphatic endothelial cells have been identified so that particles as large as red blood cells and lymphocytes have been observed passing through them. Certain tissues are notable for the absence of lymphatic capillaries. The entire epidermis, the central nervous system, the coats of the eye and muscle, cartilage, and tendon do not have lymphatic vessels. The dermis is richly supplied with lymphatics that are easily identified by intradermal injection of certain dyes. These valveless vessels communicate with the collecting vessels of the dermal-subcutaneous junction. The superficial lymphatic vessels of the extremities consist of several valved channels that pass primarily on the medial aspect of the limb toward the groin or axilla, where they end in one or more lymph nodes. These vessels maintain a uniform caliber as they ascend and frequently communicate with each other through transverse branches. A separate deep system of lymphatic vessels also exists in the extremities. This network closely follows the main vascular pathways deep to the muscular fascia. In the normal individual, there is little, if any, communication between the two systems.

Lymph vessels have a structure similar to blood vessels with well-defined adventitia, a media containing smooth muscle cells, and an intima. These vessels are also innervated, and spasm as well as natural rhythmic contractions have been observed.

Lymph nodes are periodically interposed throughout the course of collecting lymphatic channels. Each may have several afferent channels entering through the capsule. Lymph then enters the sinuses, bathes the cortical and medullary areas, and exits via a single efferent channel. Cortical areas contain predominantly lymphocytes, which are arranged in follicles separated by trabecular extensions of the capsule. Within the follicles are discrete germinal centers. The medulla may contain macrophages and plasma cells as well as lymphocytes, and these cells are thought to be in dynamic equilibrium within the node. Each node also has a separate vascular and nervous supply, and it is now known that lymphatic-vascular interaction may occur within the node.

Visceral and lower extremity lymphatic channels coalesce to form the cysterna chyli adjacent to the aorta in the upper abdomen. The latter structure passes through the diaphragm to become the thoracic duct. Within the chest the duct receives the intercostal and thoracic visceral lymph vessels and finally enters the venous system by joining the left subclavian vein. A separate right lymphatic duct drains the right upper extremity and neck and enters the right subclavian vein.

PHYSIOLOGY

Lymph circulation is a complex and incompletely understood process. One major function of the lymphatic system is to participate in the continuous exchange of interstitial fluid. Starling hypothesized that interstitial fluid was a filtrate of plasma across the capillary wall and the rate of its formation was dependent upon the pressure gradient across this membrane. Pappenheimer and Soto-Rivera[5] contributed the concept that the capillary pores were small and only partially permeable to large molecules such as plasma proteins. These large molecules trapped within the capillaries exert an osmotic effect tending to keep fluid volume within the capillary space. Thus, the exchange of fluid between the capillaries and interstitial space is dependent upon four factors: the hydrostatic pressure within the capillary and within the interstitial space and the osmotic pressure within these two compartments. The oncotic pressure of normal plasma is about 25 mm. Hg while the oncotic pressure of interstitial fluid approximates only 1 mm. Hg. The hydrostatic pressure at the arteriolar end of a capillary is estimated to be 37 mm. Hg and at the venous end 17 mm. Hg. The hydrostatic pressure of the interstitial fluid varies in different tissues being -2 mm. Hg in subcutaneous tissue and $+6$ mm. Hg in the kidney. There is a net flux of fluid out of the capillary into the interstitial space at the high pressure arteriolar end of a capillary and a net flux inward at the venular end (Fig. 1). Net efflux normally exceeds net influx, and this extra fluid returns to the circulation by way of the lymphatics. Normal lymph flow is 2 to 4 liters per day. The rate of flow is greatly influenced by a number of local and systemic factors, including protein concentration in plasma and interstitial fluid, local arterial and venous pressure relationships, and capillary pore size and integrity.

Lymph propulsion is also a complex process. At rest the intrinsic rhythmic contraction of the walls of the collecting ducts is thought to propel lymph toward the thoracic duct in a peristaltic fashion. Active skeletal muscle contraction compresses the lymphatic channels, and because

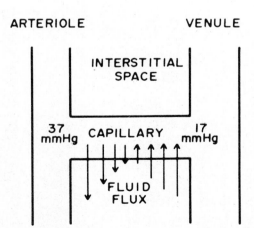

ARTERIOLE   VENULE

INTERSTITIAL SPACE

37 mmHg   CAPILLARY   17 mmHg

FLUID FLUX

Plasma oncotic pressure = 25 mmHg
Interstitial oncotic pressure = 1 mm Hg

Figure 1. Fluid flux across the capillary is dependent upon the net hydrostatic and oncotic pressure gradient. This is positive near the arteriolar end leading to outflow of fluid and negative near the venular end, where most of the fluid returns to the capillary lumen.

of the presence of competent valves in the lymphatic channels, lymph is propelled cephalad. Increased intra-abdominal pressure, as from coughing or straining, also compresses the lymphatic vessels accelerating the flow of lymph upward. The phasic changes in intrathoracic pressure associated with respiration establishes another pumping mechanism to propel lymph through the mediastinum. The rapid flow of blood in the subclavian vein may exert a siphon effect on the thoracic duct.

A second function of the lymphatic system is to return macromolecules from the interstitial space to the vascular system. These large molecules cannot be readily reasborbed in vascular capillaries because of the small pore size in the latter structures. Actual gaps between endothelial cells of the terminal lymphatics, however, readily admit these large molecules. It is estimated that 50 to 80 per cent of the total intravascular protein circulates in this manner each 24 hours. The protein concentration of lymph depends greatly upon the tissue being drained. In extremity lymph, protein concentration may be as low as 0.5 gm. per 100 ml., while liver lymph may contain 6 gm. per 100 ml. Lymph draining the intestine following a meal will be opalescent in color as a result of the content of fat in the form of chylomicrons.

An additional function of the lymphatic system that has surgical implications is that of filtration and immunologic protection. Bacteria, foreign bodies, and malignant cells are known to be collected by the lymphatic system and transported to the regional nodes where concentrations of macrophages, plasma cells, and lymphocytes can interact with them, initiating an immune response.

LYMPHEDEMA

The delicate homeostatic mechanism controlling interstitial fluid volume can fail if an abnormality develops in any of its components. A local or generalized accumulation of excessive interstitial fluid is called *edema*. Severe hypoproteinemia reduces plasma oncotic pressure and decreases the reabsorption of fluid from the venous end of the vascular capillary. This results in generalized interstitial fluid accumulation. Venous hypertension caused by local obstruction or cardiac failure may result in local or generalized edema, respectively, by similarly reducing reabsorption of fluid by the distal capillary. When edema is due to an abnormality in lymph transport, it is called lymphedema. The accumulation of interstitial fluid with increasing protein concentration initiates a vicious circle because the increased interstitial fluid oncotic pressure draws even more fluid into the extracellular space. Over a long period of time and by mechanisms that are poorly understood, the protein-rich fluid initiates a reaction that results in irreversible fibrosis of the subcutaneous tissue.

Patient Evaluation

Although there are many causes of extremity edema, it is usually not difficult to establish whether the swelling is due to a systemic disorder, to disease in the venous system, or to an abnormality of the lymphatic system. Systemic disorders that result in edema include heart failure, many forms of renal disease, cirrhosis of the liver, and hypoproteinemia. These should be apparent from an initial clinical evaluation. *Acute deep venous thrombosis* as a cause of edema can often be diagnosed by the clinical setting, by noninvasive Doppler examination, and plethysmography, or, if necessary, by phlebography. *Chronic deep venous insufficiency,* the post-phlebitic syndrome, can be recognized by the characteristic eczema and stasis pigmentation with or without skin ulceration and can be confirmed by noninvasive vascular laboratory studies or phlebography.

Other causes of extremity swelling such as *arteriovenous fistula* or allergic disorders should be considered as well.

Classification

Lymphedema may be due to a primary or acquired defect in lymph transport. The primary lymphedemas may be classified by (1) mode of onset and (2) lymphangiographic appearance.

MODE OF ONSET

Lymphedema congenita is apparent at birth or during early infancy. The condition most frequently involves the lower extremities, and the right side is affected twice as frequently as the left. In 25 per cent of cases, the condition is bilateral. In a minority of cases, there is a familial history. Milroy's disease refers to an uncommon sex-linked form of lower extremity lymphedema. Congenital lymphedema may be associated with other conditions such as Turner's syndrome (gonadal dysgenesis), distichiasis, and lymphangioma.

Lymphedema praecox is the most common form of primary lymphedema, accounting for more than 80 per cent of the cases. In these patients, swelling appears about the time of adolescence. Lymphedema praecox occurs more often in females with a female-to-male ratio of 3:1. It is thought that most of these patients also have a congenital defect of the lymphatic vessels. If the lymphatic vessels are marginally adequate at birth, the lymph transport system may decompensate later, particularly with the increased demands associated with puberty, and edema may then appear.

Lymphedema tarda is a classification that was added later to apply to cases of lymphedema that do not appear until after age 25 to 30.

LYMPHOANGIOGRAPHIC APPEARANCE

More recently, lymphatic diseases have been classified on the basis of lymphangiographic appearance. This examination is performed by first identifying the lymphatics on the dorsum of the foot by injecting a blue dye subcutaneously. A vessel outlined by the blue dye is then cannulated after directly exposing it with a cutdown under local anesthesia. These vessels are often extremely small, and optical magnification is frequently helpful. Once the vessel is successfully cannulated, ethiodized oil contrast medium is slowly injected and the transit of the dye is observed by serial roentgenograms over 24 or more hours. Because the dye eventually enters the venous circulation, it is trapped in pulmonary capillaries. Previous pulmonary radiation may allow the oil to pass through the lungs and enter the systemic circulation. This could result in cerebral oil embolism, and a history of previous pulmonary irradiation is a contraindication to lymphangiography. Other complications of lymphangiography include allergic reactions and symptomatic pulmonary oil embolism if excessive volumes of dye are injected. If no lymphatics are found in the foot, an inguinal lymph node can be injected directly to visualize the pelvic lymphatic vessels.

Normal lymphangiographic anatomy will demonstrate several parallel channels coursing on the medial aspect of the limb. These often branch and intercommunicate, but the diameter remains relatively constant as the vessels ascend. Small ampullae will be demonstrated every several millimeters, representing the site of the valves. The deep lymphatics are only rarely seen with a dorsal pedal injection. Normal lymph nodes have a uniform ground glass appearance and may remain opacified for weeks.

Several lymphangiographic patterns can be observed in patients with lymphedema. The most commonly observed pattern is *hypoplasia,* seen in over 90 per cent of cases of primary lymphedema (Fig. 2). In these patients, the lymph vessels are small and few in number. Usually less than five trunks will enter the inguinal region. The vessels present may be discontinuous. In severe cases, no major lymphatic trunks may be identified (aplasia). Hypoplasia may be limited to the distal portions of the limb, in which case the limb swelling is usually mild and nonprogressive. Hypoplasia of the proximal lymphatic system in the pelvis usually results in a more severe clinical picture, with swelling of the entire limb that is often progressive. In this condition, "dermal backflow" is frequently seen in which there is abnormal movement of dye out of the lymphatic channels into the dermal plexus.

The second major lymphangiographic pattern seen in lymphedema is *hyperplasia* (Fig. 3). It is thought that this pattern results from lymphatic obstruction at the level of the cysterna chyli or thoracic duct and thus the disease is always bilateral. Numerous mildly dilated vessels are usually demonstrated in both legs. This condition is distinct from a rarer unilateral form of hyperplasia termed *megalymphatics.* In the latter condition, varicose, valveless lymphatic vessels are seen, usually in only one limb, and it is frequently associated with cutaneous angiomas. Chylous reflux may be prominent and may present as chylometrorrhea, chylous skin vesicles, or chyluria.

Secondary Lymphedema

Secondary lymphedema is due to acquired lymphatic obstruction. Obstruction may be produced by tumor infil-

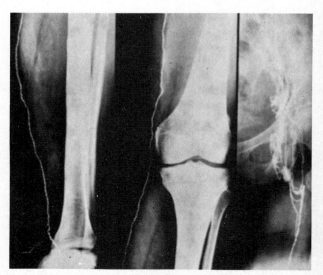

Figure 2. Lymphangiogram in a 43-year-old woman with lymphedema of feet and ankles. A single lymphatic channel is demonstrated below the groin, but pelvic lymphatics are normal. This is an example of distal hypoplasia. (From Kinmonth, J. B., and Eustace, P. W.: Ann. Roy. Coll. Surg. Engl., 58:278, 1976.)

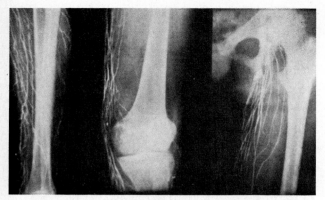

Figure 3. Lymphangiogram demonstrating hyperplasia with multiple channels of normal caliber and with competent valves. (From Gough, M. H.: Br. J. Surg., 53:917, 1966.)

tration of regional nodes, by surgical extirpation of regional nodes, by fibrosis resulting from radiation therapy, or by a number of infectious and inflammatory processes. In many tropical countries, *Wuchereria bancrofti* is endemic. The adult nematode lodges in lymph nodes and vessels and results in a severe lymphedema. Tuberculous lymphadenitis may also be a cause in areas where this disease remains common. In the Western world, most cases of lymphedema result from lymph node dissections for malignant disease. Lymphedema is particularly prone to develop if lymph node dissection is either combined with radiation therapy or complicated by infection.

Treatment of Lymphedema

CONSERVATIVE THERAPY

In the majority of patients with lymphedema, a conservative program of meticulous skin hygiene, external support garments, and extremity elevation will maintain a functional extremity. Avoiding skin and nail infections includes daily use of mild antiseptic soap and careful nail trimming. Care should be taken to keep the web spaces dry, and use of an antifungal powder may be helpful. An emollient cream may be used to keep the skin soft and to avoid cracks or fissures. If eczema appears, short courses of a steroid-containing cream may be used, but these should not be employed for long periods. Ulceration as observed in deep venous insufficiency is rarely seen in lymphedema. If cellulitis does occur, it should be treated promptly with systemic antibiotics and bed rest with elevation of the involved extremity.

External compression is the most useful method of controlling excessive fluid volume in the lymphedematous limb. Several brands of elastic stockings are commercially available. The most effective garments are those that are custom-manufactured and designed with a built-in pressure gradient from the toe to the groin. The lighter mass-produced garments may be more cosmetically pleasing but are much less effective. It should be remembered that the elastic in these garments will stretch with use, and the garments should be replaced every 3 to 4 months if they are to maintain their effectiveness. Also available are pneumatic compression devices that contain several compartments incorporated into a sleeve fitted over the affected limb. The compartments are serially inflated to induce lymphedema fluid to migrate cephalad. These may be applied several times daily or may be used at night while

sleeping. Diuretics are of little use in controlling lymphedema fluid because they do not act on the specific pathogenetic mechanisms involved.

SURGICAL THERAPY

Surgical treatment is indicated if swelling compromises function of the extremity, if recurrent cellulitis occurs, or in carefully selected cases for cosmetic reasons. Three approaches to the surgical treatment of lymphedema have been described. Most attempts to improve lymphatic drainage by *pedicle transfer* of lymphatic-bearing omentum, skin, or defunctionalized bowel have met with disappointment. An unacceptably high incidence of complications has followed these procedures, and they cannot be recommended at this time.

Simple excision of lymphedematous tissue has been employed since the turn of the century. In the Charles procedure, the entire skin and subcutaneous tissue are removed and the surface is then covered with full- or split-thickness skin grafts (Fig. 4). Although the cosmetic result is marginal and the grafts may subsequently suffer from eczema, this may be the operation of choice for advanced cases in which severe skin changes are present. In less

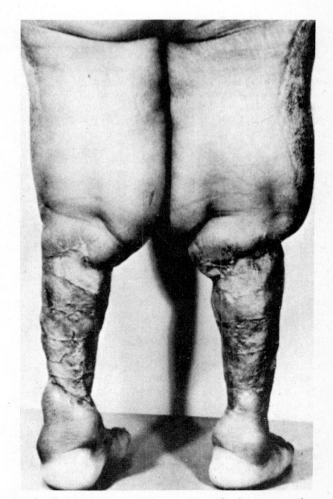

Figure 4. Long-term result after excision of subcutaneous tissue and skin and skin grafting. Note the pantaloon appearance. (From Bunchman, H. H. II, and Lewis, S. R.: Plast. & Reconstr. Surg., 54:64, 1974.)

severe cases in which the skin is still adequate, simple staged excision of the thickened fibrotic subcutaneous tissue beneath 1- to 2-cm. thick skin flaps may be the best procedure. The medial side is usually done first, followed in 3 to 4 months by the lateral side. It is interesting to note that lymph drainage, as measured by clearance of subcutaneously injected radioactive albumin, increases twofold after this procedure.[3]

Recently, increasingly encouraging results have been reported with *microscopic surgical repair* of obstructed lymphatics. In these procedures, patent lymphatic vessels or lymph nodes distal to a lymphatic blockage are anastomosed using microvascular techniques to local veins, providing a means of egress of lymph from a lymphedematous extremity. As many as two thirds of patients may show long-term benefit. The procedure is more successful in cases of secondary lymphedema, and particularly good results have been reported in women suffering from arm lymphedema following treatment for breast cancer.[4] This treatment must still be considered experimental, however, until larger series with long-term follow-up are available.

LYMPHATIC TUMORS AND MALFORMATIONS

Lymphangiomas

Lymphangiomas are congenital malformations of the lymphatic vessels that usually are apparent in infancy. Although malignant potential is thought to be low, the lesions often increase in size and may cause symptoms by compression of adjacent structures. The lesions may consist of masses of small capillary-size lymphatic channels *(lymphangioma simplex)*, dilated lymphatic vessels *(cavernous lymphangioma)*, or endothelium-lined cysts *(cystic hygroma)*. They may be located anywhere in the body, but larger cystic lesions are usually found in the neck or axilla. Treatment is surgical excision with preservation of surrounding vital structures (Fig. 5). If possible, operation is delayed until the child is 2 to 3 years of age to minimize the risk of injury to adjacent tissues. Lymphangiomas may require staged excision.[1]

Chylous Syndromes

Chyle is formed in the lacteals of the small intestine by absorption of the products of fat digestion. Chyle is normally transported to the cisterna chyli and thence to the thoracic duct. Chyle may be found outside of the normal channels if there is an acquired or congenital block of the thoracic duct or incompetence of the lymphatic valves. Fistulization may occur into the peritoneal, pleural, or pericardial cavities. Chylous ascites and chylothorax may respond to treatment with a medium-chain triglyceride diet. These fats are transported directly to the liver via the portal venous system, thus decreasing chylomicron formation and intestinal lymph volume. Occasionally, direct suture closure of a chylous fistula is indicated if conservative measures fail. Chylous ascites developing spontaneously in an older patient is nearly always due to an underlying malignancy, and this should be sought prior to initiating therapy.

Lymphangiosarcoma

Lymphangiosarcoma is a rare lesion that may develop in a lymphedematous extremity regardless of cause. It

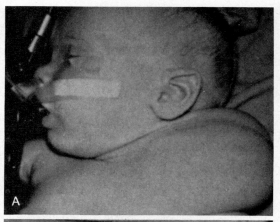
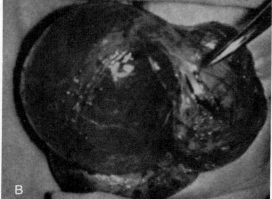

Figure 5. Cystic hygroma. A, Gross appearance in a 5-month-old boy. B, Appearance at surgery. Clamp points out spinal accessory nerve. (From Fonkalsrud, E. W.: Am. J. Surg., 128:152, 1974.)

appears first as purple-red nodules in the skin. Although a very unusual event, it is a rapidly fatal lesion.

SELECTED REFERENCES

Kinmonth, J. B.: The Lymphatics: Surgery, Lymphography and Diseases of the Chyle and Lymph Systems, 2nd ed. London, Edward Arnold, 1982.
This volume summarizes a lifetime of work and interest with diseases of the lymphatic system. A large clinical experience is discussed. Lymphangiography is particularly well illustrated.

Wolfe, J. H. N.: Diagnosis and classification of lymphedema. *In* Rutherford, R. B. (Ed.): Vascular Surgery, 2nd ed. Philadelphia, W. B. Saunders Company, 1984.
This chapter is an excellent summary of the clinical approach to the patient with limb edema. The modern classification of congenital lymphedema is succinctly illustrated.

REFERENCES

1. Fonkalsrud, E. W.: Surgical management of congenital malformations of the lymphatic system. Am. J. Surg., *128*:152, 1974.
2. Glenn, W.: The lymphatic system, some surgical considerations. Arch. Surg., *116*:989, 1981.
3. Miller, T. A.: Surgical management of lymphedema of the extremity. Plast. Reconstruct. Surg. 56:633, 1975.
4. O'Brien, B. M., and Shafiroff, B. B.: Microlymphaticovenous and resectional surgery in obstructive lymphedema. World J. Surg., *3*:3, 1979.
5. Pappenheimer, J. R., and Soto-Rivera, A.: Effective osmotic pressure of the plasma proteins and other quantities associated with the capillary circulation in the hindlimbs of cats and dogs. Am. J. Physiol., *157*:471, 1948.

HERNIAS

WARREN J. KORTZ, M.D. • DAVID C. SABISTON, JR., M.D.

A protrusion of any viscus from its proper cavity is
termed a hernia.

Sir Astley Cooper, 1804

32

The word *hernia* essentially means "a protrusion of a
sac of peritoneum, an organ, or preperitoneal fat through
a congenital or acquired defect in the musculoaponeurotic
parietes of the abdominal wall, through which they do not
normally pass."[10] Hernias are common conditions seen by
all physicians; therefore, a general knowledge of their
clinical manifestations, physical findings, and management
is essential.

Whereas in years past many hernias were treated by
trusses, this is rare today, and nearly all hernias are
corrected surgically unless there is a significant overriding
contraindication. Hernias occur in approximately 1.5 per
cent of the general population in the United States,[19] and
537,000 hernias were surgically repaired in 1980.[20] The vast
majority of hernias occur in the inguinal region, with
approximately 50 per cent of these being *indirect* and 25
per cent being *direct* inguinal hernias. Incisional hernias
(including ventral hernias) make up about 10 per cent of
all hernias, femoral hernias approximately 5 per cent, and
umbilical hernias 3 per cent; rare hernias account for the
remainder. Whereas recurrence following surgical correction was a problem in the past, this is now quite rare, with
the exception of recurrent or large hernias requiring the
use of prosthetic materials.

HISTORIC ASPECTS

Inguinal hernias were described in the records of
ancient civilizations. However, centuries elapsed before a
clear understanding of the *anatomy* of hernias was appreciated. Despite the advances and descriptions of human
anatomy in the 1800s, hernias were managed at that time
primarily by observation or application of a truss, since the
surgical results were very poor. For example, in 1891 Bull
reported the results of hernia repair in the United States;
there was a recurrence rate of 30 to 40 per cent at 1 year
and 100 per cent by 4 years. In 1889, Bassini was the first
to report consistently successful results with surgical repair
of inguinal hernias.[2] He utilized a careful dissection with
high ligation of the hernial sac and meticulous anatomic
approximation of the conjoined fascia of the internal
oblique and transversus abdominus muscles to the inguinal
(Poupart's) ligament. The recurrence rate among his first
251 patients was only 3 per cent.

Halsted, unaware of Bassini's contribution since it was
published in an obscure Italian journal, independently
described a similar procedure in 1889. Halsted's procedure
also consisted of suturing the internal oblique and transversus abdominis fascia to the inguinal ligament. In his first
procedure, Halsted transplanted the spermatic cord above
the closure of the external oblique fascia (Halsted I). Later,
he did the same procedure but allowed the spermatic cord
to remain in its normal position beneath the external
oblique fascia (Halsted II). The Bassini and Halsted procedures represented *major* advances and an era of widespread surgical management of inguinal hernias began.[17]

Since their pioneering work, a number of technical
variations have been introduced along with new concepts
in an effort to decrease an already low recurrence rate.
McVay popularized the technique of approximating the
conjoined tendon of the internal oblique and rectus abdominis muscles to Cooper's ligament, an operation originally
described by Lotheissen in 1898.[11] Shouldice introduced the
concept of opening the inguinal floor and imbricating transversalis fascia with a continuous suture technique. Today,
the operations described by these pioneers are primarily
used in correcting inguinal hernias.

ANATOMY

A clear understanding of the normal and abnormal
anatomy of the inguinal region is essential to comprehend
the principles underlying direct inguinal herniorrhaphy.[13, 15]
This area of the body is one of the most complex with
regard to anatomy, as several different layers of the abdominal wall converge and terminate in the groin. The student
should not become frustrated in initial attempts to understand the anatomic features of the inguinal region, since it
is only after exposure in the operating room that one can
fully comprehend this complex subject. The pertinent anatomic structures found in the inguinal region are depicted
in Figures 1 and 2. For details, the classic anatomic studies
of Anson and McVay are recommended.[14]

INGUINAL HERNIA

Indirect hernias are *congenital* in origin and are caused
by a failure of obliteration of the processus vaginalis (hernia
sac) as it descends into the scrotum. The resultant sac may
extend along the inguinal canal; if it extends into the
scrotum it is termed a *complete* hernia. Since the processus

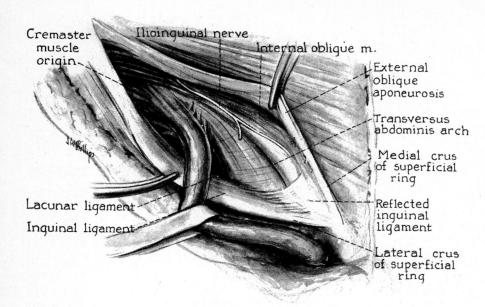

Cremaster muscle origin

Ilioinguinal nerve

Internal oblique m.

External oblique aponeurosis

Transversus abdominis arch

Medial crus of superficial ring

Reflected inguinal ligament

Lateral crus of superficial ring

Lacunar ligament

Inguinal ligament

Figure 1. The external oblique aponeurosis has been opened widely, and the spermatic cord has been mobilized by transection of many of its areolar (cremasteric fascia) attachments to the walls of the inguinal canal. (From Condon, R. E.: In Nyhus, L. M., and Harkins, H. N.: Hernia. Philadelphia, J. B. Lippincott Company, 1964.)

vaginalis is within the spermatic cord, it is surrounded by the cremaster muscle and is made up of the pampiniform plexus of veins, the spermatic duct, and the spermatic artery. The important point in anatomic definition is that the internal opening into the peritoneal cavity is always *lateral* to the deep epigastric artery in the presence of an *indirect* inguinal hernia, whereas the internal opening is *medial* to this vessel when the hernia is *direct*.

Inguinal hernias occur most often in males and are more frequent on the right side than the left side. Increases in intra-abdominal pressure from a variety of causes, including sudden straining, heavy exercise, obesity, chronic cough, ascites, straining at stool, pregnancy, and the presence of a large abdominal mass, predispose the patient to the development of a hernia.

Clinical Manifestations

The majority of hernias are asymptomatic, and many are found on routine physical examination by palpation of a bulge at the external inguinal ring or a sac at the level of the internal inguinal ring. The latter is made more prominent when the patient coughs. One of the first signs of a hernia is the presence of a mass in either the inguinal region or the upper portion of the scrotum. With the passage of time, some hernias descend into the scrotum as they enlarge. Patients with hernias often complain of an aching discomfort in the region, which can be relieved by manual reduction of the hernia into the peritoneal cavity. However, upon standing or especially with exercise the hernia usually reappears.

Figure 2. Posterior (internal) view of the right groin following removal of the peritoneum, the preperitoneal fat and lymphatics, and the iliacus fascia. The spermatic cord has been transected just internal to the deep inguinal ring. The structures of the transversus abdominis lamina are well shown. The inferior epigastric vein is more frequently a double channel where it lies upon the rectus abdominis, and its junction with the external iliac vein is often a little more proximal.

This drawing also exemplifies the difficulties of drawing medical illustrations of the groin region, problems similar to those faced by the cartographer in attempting to depict a curved surface on a flat plane. In order to present a drawing with no discontinuities, distortion and exaggeration must be increasingly introduced as one proceeds from the central focus to the margins of the picture. The geographic exaggerations of a world map drawn on Mercator's projection are analogous to those of this figure.

(From Condon, R. E.: In Nyhus, L. M., and Harkins, H. N.: Hernia, Philadelphia, J. B. Lippincott Company, 1964.)

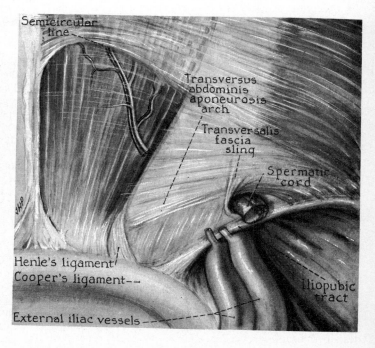

Semicircular line

Transversus abdominis aponeurosis arch

Transversalis fascia sling

Spermatic cord

Henle's ligament

Cooper's ligament

Iliopubic tract

External iliac vessels

Physical Examination

The inguinal area is first examined by inspection. Frequently a bulge appears in the groin and is quite obvious. The index finger is then placed on the lateral aspect of scrotal skin and invaginated along the spermatic cord until the fingertip reaches the internal inguinal ring (Fig. 3). A sac that is accentuated by coughing can usually be felt at this point. If the finger cannot be passed into the internal inguinal ring owing to the presence of mass, the presence of a hernia is generally indicated. A hernia is also indicated when one feels tissue moving down into the inguinal canal along the examining finger during coughing.

Although there are suggestive signs indicating whether the hernia is indirect or direct, this is generally of little importance, since both usually require surgical management and the exact anatomic diagnosis can be made conclusively at the time of operation. Features favoring the presence of an *indirect* hernia include descent into the scrotum, often found in an indirect hernia but uncommon in the direct form. A direct hernia is more apt to appear as a mass located at the *external inguinal ring*, and the mass can usually be replaced into the peritoneal cavity, especially while the patient is in the recumbent position (Fig. 4). In general, with the examining finger in the inguinal canal, an indirect inguinal hernia advances down the canal against the side of the finger, whereas a protrusion directly forward on the finger is characteristic of a direct hernia.

The *differential diagnosis* of inguinal hernias includes other masses in the groin such as lymphadenopathy, varicocele, undescended testis, lipoma, and hematoma.

Surgical Management

With only rare exceptions, inguinal hernias should be corrected surgically to prevent subsequent incarceration, intestinal obstruction, and, finally, infarction of the bowel.

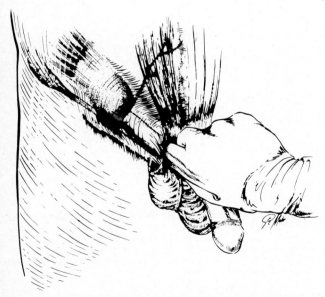

Figure 3. Upon digital examination, the indirect inguinal hernia can be seen to protrude through the abdomen at the internal ring, lateral to the deep inferior epigastric artery. The floor of Hesselbach's triangle is intact. (From Ponka, J. L.: Hernias of the Abdominal Wall. Philadelphia, W. B. Saunders Company, 1980.)

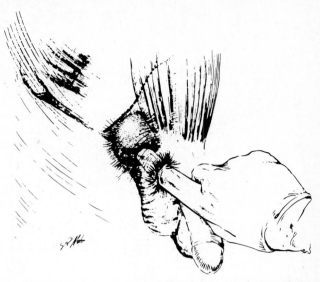

Figure 4. In a direct inguinal hernia, the mass protrudes directly through the floor of Hesselbach's triangle, medial to the deep inferior epigastric vessels. The weak inguinal floor may permit palpation of Cooper's ligament. (From Ponka, J. L.: Hernias of the Abdominal Wall. Philadelphia, W. B. Saunders Company, 1980.)

The potential complication of infarction of the intestine may be quite serious. Since inguinal hernias do not resolve spontaneously but usually continue to enlarge and lead to complications, they should be corrected surgically. Hernias in infants and children present special problems and are separately described in Chapter 33, "Pediatric Surgery."

If the patient presents with incarceration of the hernia, it can be manually reduced in many instances, thus allowing the operation to be done electively. Gentle pressure on the hernial mass toward the inguinal ring, usually with the patient in the head-lowered (Trendelenburg) position is generally effective. If the mass is tender and the pressure causes pain, appropriate analgesic agents can be administered to relieve discomfort and the procedure repeated. Although gangrenous bowel can rarely be reduced by this method, it is quite uncommon, and such patients can be followed for the development of peritoneal signs. However, it should be emphasized that manual reduction should not be traumatic; if this technique is not successful shortly after trial, it should be abandoned and immediate operation undertaken.

The first principle of the operation is careful dissection and identification of the hernial sac. The skin incision should be properly located to avoid injury to the iliohypogastric and ilioinguinal nerves, which are important in their cutaneous innervation of the skin of the lower abdomen, penis, and scrotum (Fig. 5). The incision should be placed as shown in Figure 6. The sac is dissected free of surrounding structures and is opened to reduce its contents back into the peritoneal cavity (Fig. 7). The neck of the sac is closed at its peritoneal origin, and the excess sac is excised. This procedure alone is sufficient for correction in infants and young children. However, in the adult the floor of the inguinal canal is reconstructed by one of several techniques.

The *Bassini* procedure is quite often used for straightforward indirect hernias with approximation of the conjoined tendon of the transversus abdominis and internal oblique muscles to the inguinal (Poupart's) ligament. The principles of the Bassini operation are illustrated in Figures 8 through 14.

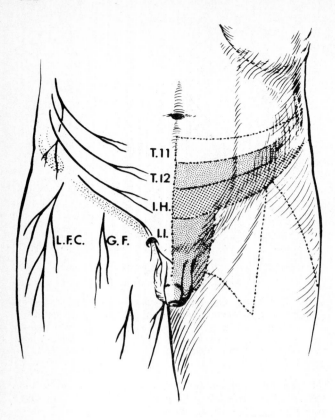

T.11

T.12

I.H.

L.I.

L.F.C.   G.F.

Figure 5. Cutaneous nerve distribution to the lower abdomen and upper thigh. I. H. = Iliohypogastric nerve; I.I. = ilioinguinal nerve; G.F. = genitofemoral nerve; L.F.C. = lateral femoral cutaneous nerve. (From Ponka, J. L.: Hernias of the Abdominal Wall. Philadelphia, W. B. Saunders Company, 1980.)

Figure 6. The skin incision is made approximately 2 cm. above the inguinal ligament in a gentle curve following Langer's lines. (From Ponka, J. L.: Hernias of the Abdominal Wall. Philadelphia, W. B. Saunders Company, 1980.)

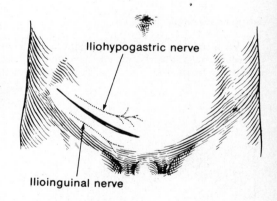

Iliohypogastric nerve

Ilioinguinal nerve

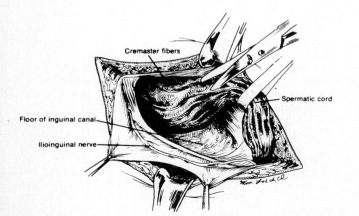

Cremaster fibers

Spermatic cord

Floor of inguinal canal

Ilioinguinal nerve

Figure 7. The external oblique aponeurosis has been opened. The cord is freed from the inguinal floor. The freed ilioinguinal nerve is seen overlying the retracted lower leaflet of the external oblique aponeurosis. The cremaster muscle is being dissected free of the cord. (From Ponka, J. L.: Hernias of the Abdominal Wall. Philadelphia, W. B. Saunders Company, 1980.)

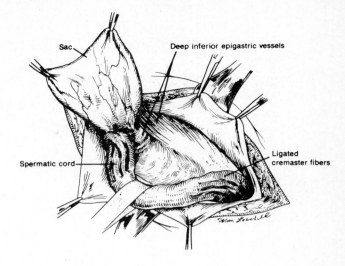

Figure 8. The peritoneal sac must be dissected free of the cord and the abdominal wall at the internal abdominal ring. (From Ponka, J. L.: Hernias of the Abdominal Wall. Philadelphia, W. B. Saunders Company, 1980.)

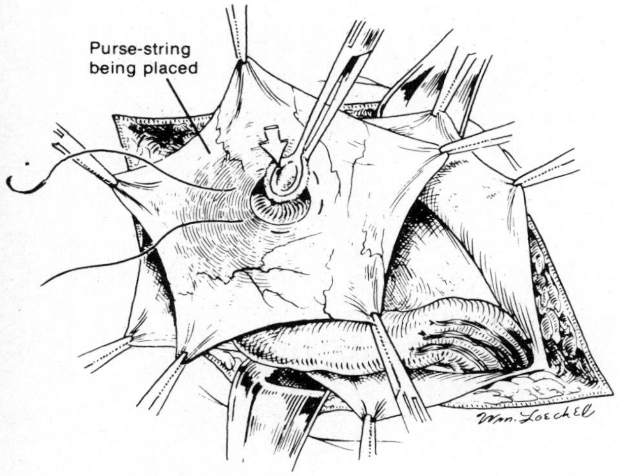

Figure 9. The technical detail of high ligation of the sac is important in an orderly repair. The peritoneum must be freed of omentum, and adherent viscera must be detached. Appendices epiploicae or omentum must not be caught in the closure. (From Ponka, J. L.: Hernias of the Abdominal Wall. Philadelphia, W. B. Saunders Company, 1980.)

Figure 10. The components of the transversus abdominis lamina must be accurately identified and closed at the internal ring. Triangulation of the transversalis fascia (shown here) is a useful detail to help achieve accurate closure at the internal ring. (From Ponka, J. L.: Hernias of the Abdominal Wall. Philadelphia, W. B. Saunders Company, 1980.)

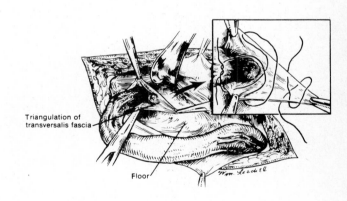

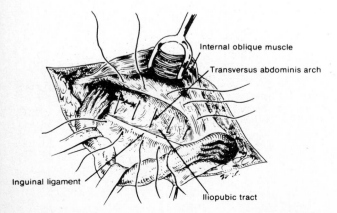

Figure 11. The transversus abdominis arch is sutured to the iliopubic tract and inguinal ligament. (From Ponka, J. L.: Hernias of the Abdominal Wall. Philadelphia, W. B. Saunders Company, 1980.)

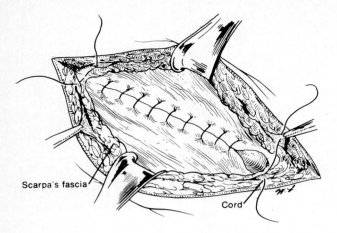

Scarpa's fascia

Cord

Figure 12. The external oblique aponeurosis is closed over the spermatic cord. Slight imbrication of this structure gives an excellent closure. Scarpa's fascia is then closed with interrupted sutures of number 3–0 plain catgut. (From Ponka, J. L.: Hernias of the Abdominal Wall. Philadelphia, W. B. Saunders Company, 1980.)

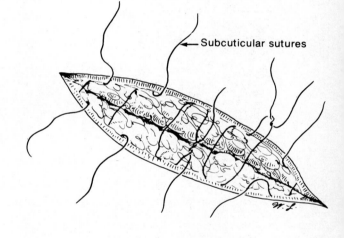

← Subcuticular sutures

Figure 13. Subcuticular sutures of number 4–0 synthetic absorbable material bring the margins of the wound together. (From Ponka, J. L.: Hernias of the Abdominal Wall. Philadelphia, W. B. Saunders Company, 1980.)

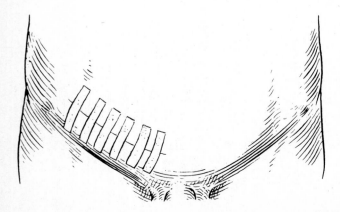

Figure 14. Small strips of adhesive nonallergenic microporous paper are used to tape together the epidermal edges. (From Ponka, J. L.: Hernias of the Abdominal Wall. Philadelphia, W. B. Saunders Company, 1980.)

The *Halsted* procedure is also quite effective, and the principles of this operation are illustrated in Figures 15 and 16. However, for large indirect hernias, the *McVay* repair may be indicated, with suture of the conjoined tendon to Cooper's ligament. The McVay operation is shown in Figure 17. For direct inguinal hernias, particularly large ones, and recurrent hernias in the groin, the McVay repair is generally preferable. Some advocate the *preperitoneal approach*; in this procedure the inguinal region is exposed between the transversalis fascia and peritoneum by low incision in the abdomen. This approach has not been as popular as other procedures.

The *Shouldice* repair is also used. In this procedure the incision is made in the groin and the operation is characterized by two primary components. The first involves the technique employed at the internal inguinal ring and is associated with correction of an indirect inguinal hernia. The second concerns the use of the posterior inguinal wall and is the main objective in the cure of a direct inguinal hernia. Since it is a comprehensive operation, it is applicable to the cure of both indirect and direct inguinal hernias. Closure is achieved with continuous monofilament sutures of stainless steel wire. Prosthetic materials are not used, and the authors report a low mortality in the long-term follow-up period.

Today, inguinal herniorrhaphies are often being performed as outpatient procedures. The patient arrives in the morning at the Ambulatory Surgical Unit and is given premedication. Either local or general anesthesia may be used, followed by the operation. The patient remains until sufficiently recovered and is discharged later the same day. Although some patients involved in minor activity can return to work earlier, most, and certainly those involved in heavy labor, should be restricted for approximately 6 weeks to permit proper healing.

Postoperative Complications

Complications occur in approximately 10 per cent of patients undergoing inguinal herniorrhaphy.[4, 22] Rarely, inadvertent placement of sutures on the external iliac or

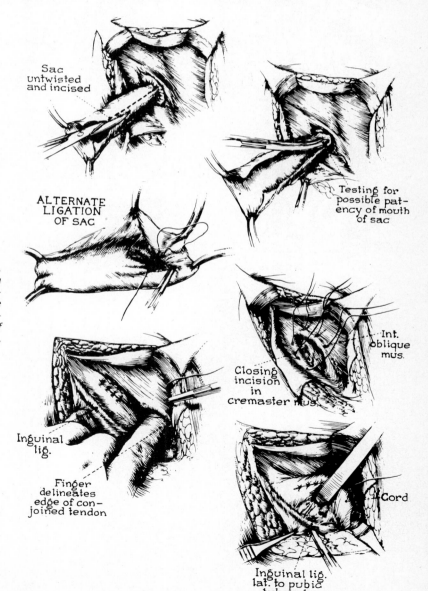

Figure 15. The classic Halsted-Ferguson operation. The anterior approach has reached the stage of high ligation of the peritoneal sac. The arch of the transversus abdominis aponeurosis (frequently called the conjoined tendon) is delineated as well as the inguinal ligament. (From Ravitch, M. M.: Repair of Hernias. Chicago, Year Book Medical Publishers, 1969.)

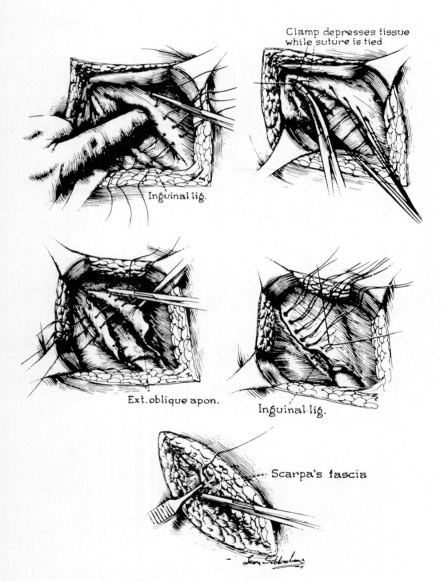

Clamp depresses tissue
while suture is tied

Inguinal lig.

Ext. oblique apon.

Inguinal lig.

Scarpa's fascia

Figure 16. The classic Halsted-Ferguson operation. The arch of transversus abdominis is joined to the inguinal ligament from the tubercle of the pubis medially to near the internal ring laterally. Note that the spermatic cord has not been displaced and will lie beneath the joined tissues except for its exit at the superior edge of the pubis. The aponeurosis of the external oblique is imbricated with the medial flap overlapping as demonstrated. The free medial flap of aponeurotic fascia is then sutured to the lateral flap. (From Ravitch, M. M.: Repair of Hernias. Chicago, Year Book Medical Publishers, 1969.)

Large Indirect Inguinal Hernia   Direct Inguinal Hernia

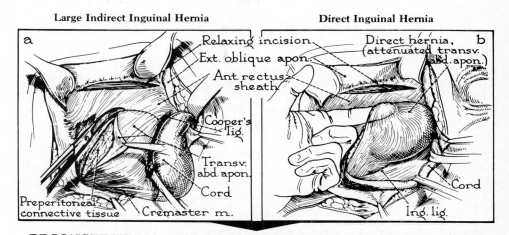

RECONSTRUCTION OF THE POSTERIOR INGUINAL WALL

Figure 17. Hernioplasty for large indirect and direct inguinal hernias. a, Cutting out the attenuated portion of the posterior inguinal wall in a large indirect inguinal hernia. b, Attenuated posterior inguinal wall that is to be removed in a direct inguinal hernia. c through f, Successive steps in the reconstruction of the posterior inguinal wall. Hernioplasty for both large indirect and direct inguinal hernias. (From McVay, C. B.: In Davis, L. (Ed.): Christopher's Textbook of Surgery, 9th ed. Philadelphia, W. B. Saunders Company, 1968.)

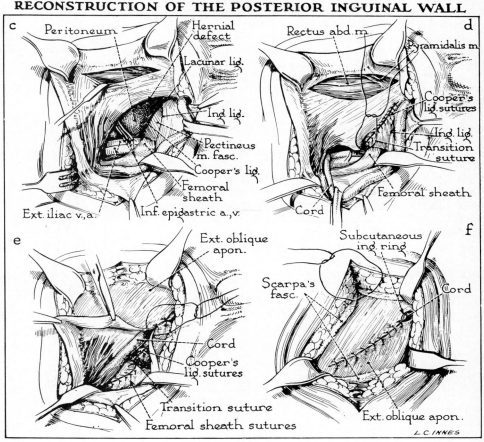

femoral vessels has been reported. The ilioinguinal and iliohypogastric nerves can be injured, followed by numbness and paresthesias over the area of skin. Rarely, the spermatic artery is compromised, resulting in ischemic orchitis and testicular atrophy. If the vas deferens is injured during operation, an end-to-end anastomosis should be performed. Injuries to the intestine, bladder, and ureter are rare but can be serious.

Postoperatively, urinary retention may be a problem, and catheterization be required. Scrotal bleeding may occur, and reoperation may be necessary for control. However, the hematoma is most often self-limited and subsequently will be reabsorbed. Wound infection occurs in approximately 2 per cent of patients following herniorrhaphy. The systemic complications in a large series of hernia repairs are listed in Table 1, and the local complications are listed in Table 2.

FEMORAL HERNIA

A femoral hernia in the groin is a protrusion of a peritoneal sac underneath the inguinal ligament between the lacunar ligament medially and the femoral vein laterally. Patients with femoral hernias often complain of pain without a palpable swelling in the groin. Incarceration occurs in approximately 25 per cent of patients (Fig. 18).

Cystograms demonstrating the urinary bladder in a femoral hernia before and after herniorraphy are shown in Figure 19. The neck of the sac is narrow, and in the presence of an incarcerated hernia it may be necessary to divide the inguinal ligament transversely to permit effective exposure and reduction. The inguinal ligament need not be resutured because it does not contribute to the overall repair of a femoral hernia. In this type of hernia, it is essential to approximate the transversalis fascia to Cooper's ligament to close the femoral triangle, since it lies *beneath* the inguinal ligament (Figs. 20 and 21). In other words, a repair to the inguinal ligament would be inappropriate, since it would not adequately close the femoral hernial defect. Although femoral hernias are much more common in males than in females, they account for approximately one third of all hernias in females.

BILATERAL INGUINAL HERNIA

Bilateral inguinal hernias, either direct or indirect, occur frequently. Their repair may involve correcting both sides simultaneously or as two separate procedures. If the

TABLE 1. Systemic Complications in Adults following Inguinal Hernia Repair (961 Operations)*

Complication	Number	Per Cent
Cardiovascular-pulmonary	39	4.1
Atelectasis, pneumonitis	(24)	(2.5)
Thrombophlebitis	(13)	(1.4)
Coronary occlusion	(2)	(0.2)
Urinary retention (requiring TUR)	10	1.0
Urinary infection	5	0.5
Miscellaneous	12	1.3
Total	66	6.9

*From Rydell, W. B., Jr.: Arch. Surg., 87:493, 1963.
Abbreviation: TUR = Transurethral resection.

TABLE 2. Local Complications in Adults following Repair of 1053 Hernias*

Complication	Number	Per Cent
Wound	21	2.0
Major infection	(14)	(1.3)
Hematoma	(7)	(0.7)
Scrotal and cord (924 male hernias)	62	6.7
Marked swelling	(24)	(2.6)
Testicular atrophy	(16)	(1.8)
Postoperative hydrocele	(5)	(0.5)
Ilioinguinal neuritis	(14)	(1.5)
Cut vas deferens	(3)	(0.3)
Total	83	8.7

*From Rydell, W. B., Jr.: Arch. Surg., 87:493, 1963.

hernias are large and extensive dissection (and resulting tension of the suture line) is needed, one hernia should probably be done at a time. However, it is usually possible to do both sides simultaneously with good results. The appropriate operation depends upon the nature of the hernia (i.e., direct, indirect, recurrent, or femoral).

UMBILICAL HERNIA

Umbilical hernias are generally congenital in origin and are fascinating, since most spontaneously close by the age of 4. However, when the hernia persists beyond that

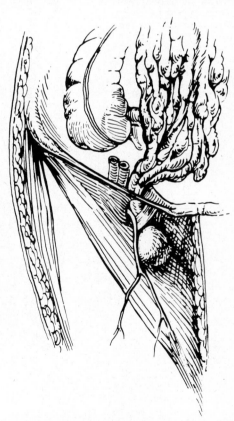

Figure 18. If a small femoral hernia protrudes through the fossa ovalis and remains unchanged for some time, it may lead to the diagnosis of inguinal lymphadenopathy. (From Ponka, J. L.: Hernias of the Abdominal Wall. Philadelphia, W. B. Saunders Company, 1980.)

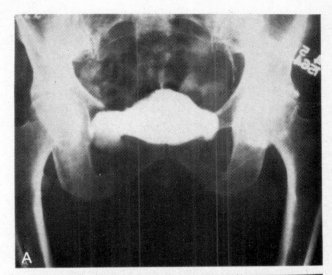
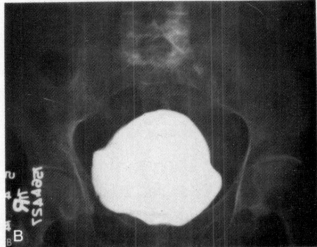

Figure 19. A, Bilateral femoral hernias are demonstrated in the cystogram. The patient was operated upon by Dr. Gomez of the Henry Ford Hospital staff. B, The bladder appears normal in the postoperative cystogram following repair of both femoral hernias via the preperitoneal approach. (From Ponka, J. L.: Hernias of the Abdominal Wall. Philadelphia, W. B. Saunders Company, 1980.)

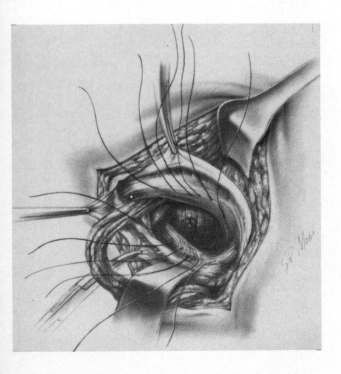

Figure 20. The hernial sac has been eliminated. Cooper's ligament is clearly identified, and sutures are placed between the transversus abdominis arch and Cooper's ligament. The lateralmost stitch (transition suture) includes transversus arch, femoral sheath, and Cooper's ligament. (From Ponka, J. L.: Hernias of the Abdominal Wall. Philadelphia, W. B. Saunders Company, 1980.)

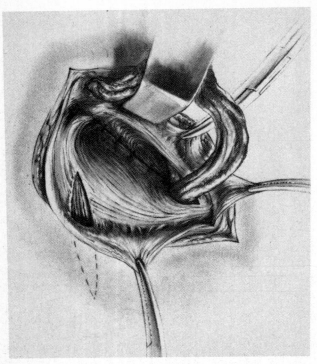

Figure 21. The Lotheissen-McVay repair to Cooper's ligament has been completed. The transversus abdominis lamina at the internal ring must be precisely closed. Note the relaxing incision. (From Ponka, J. L.: Hernias of the Abdominal Wall. Philadelphia, W. B. Saunders Company, 1980.)

age, it is generally wise to advise surgical correction, since it may become incarcerated if it persists. Occasionally, the umbilical defect will be so large before the age of 4 that the family insists upon operation for cosmetic reasons to remove an unsightly bulge. This is an appropriate indication for surgery. In adults, umbilical hernias may be caused by a number of potential predisposing factors, including pregnancy, abdominal distention due to ascites or large abdominal masses, and obesity. The closure of umbilical hernias is straightforward, generally employing a transverse curved subumbilical incision with exposure of the edges of the defect and direct closure with nonabsorbable sutures (Fig. 22). Recurrence is quite rare.

VENTRAL HERNIA

Most ventral hernias are the result of previous surgical incisions that did not initially heal correctly or that have separated owing to abnormal strain. The defect allows a protrusion of a hernia, and operation is generally recommended. If the defect is of small or moderate size, the procedure is relatively straightforward, and an excellent result and low recurrence rate can be expected. However, large ventral hernias of considerable size with poor fascial tissues do not have such favorable prognoses. In general, it is preferable to mobilize the tissues very carefully to achieve a primary direct closure if possible. At times, the use of some type of prosthetic mesh, such as Marlex, or fascia lata is indicated (Fig. 23).[14, 21] Relaxing incisions on either side of the repair are helpful to prevent tension on the suture line. A barium enema demonstrating incarcera-

Figure 22. The important detail in repair of an umbilical hernia. A, Skin incision. B, Dissection of the peritoneal sac. C, Opening of the peritoneal sac. D, Excision of the sac. E, Closure of the peritoneum. F, Placement of sutures through the aponeurosis. G, Tacking down the free aponeurotic edge. H, Placement of the subepidermal sutures. I, Gauze pledgets are cut to fit the umbilical depression. J, Epidermal edges are held in place with strips of adhesive. (From Ponka, J. L.: Hernias of the Abdominal Wall. Philadelphia, W. B. Saunders Company, 1980.)

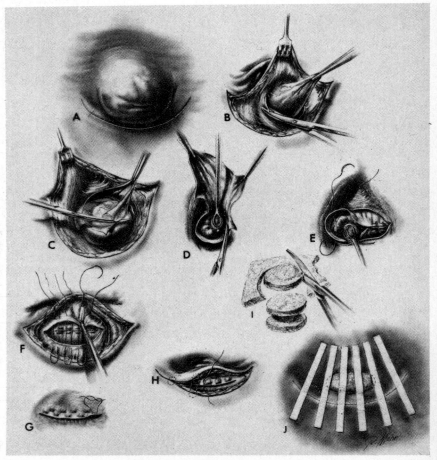

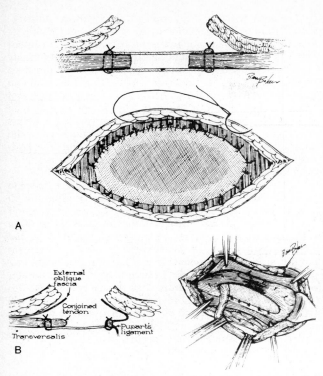

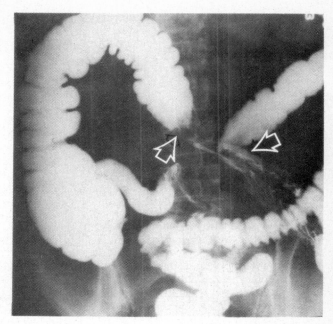

Figure 24. This barium enema examination in a patient with a large incisional hernia shows partial obstruction of the ileum and transverse colon. Arrows show the site of constriction at the point of herniation. (From Ponka, J. L.: Hernias of the Abdominal Wall. Philadelphia, W. B. Saunders Company, 1980.)

A

B

External oblique fascia
Conjoined tendon
Transversalis
Pupart's ligament

Figure 23. A, Repair of incisional hernia using two layers of Marlex mesh to bridge the defect. B, Repair of inguinal hernia using a single layer of mesh to bridge the defect. (From Usher, F. C.: Surg. Gynecol. Obstet., 131:525, 1970.)

tion of the transverse colon in a ventral hernia is shown in Figure 24.

SLIDING INGUINAL HERNIA

Particular anatomic knowledge and special attention are required for surgical reconstruction of the sliding inguinal hernia because the *neck* of the sac is partially formed by a segment of bowel or urinary bladder (Fig. 25). On the right, the cecum commonly comprises a portion of the sac of the indirect inguinal hernia. Particular care must be taken not to open the bowel or devascularize the area during dissection and ligation of the sac. Until the sac is actually entered, it is difficult to be certain whether or not a sliding hernia is present; therefore, it should be opened on its anterior medial border. In the left inguinal region, the sigmoid colon is commonly involved and must be similarly protected. After appropriate dissection and ligation of the neck of the sac, a standard inguinal herniorrhaphy is performed. Although sliding hernias are uncommon, the surgeon must be quite familiar with the anatomic problems presented so as to correctly interpret them and repair the hernia appropriately.

INCARCERATED AND STRANGULATED HERNIA

An incarcerated hernia is one that cannot be reduced into the abdominal cavity. Another term for an incarcerated hernia is *irreducible* hernia. This situation can be prevented by elective surgical correction. Once a hernia is incarcerated, strangulation is possible because a progressive swell-

ing of the incarcerated contents may occur as a result of venous and lymphatic obstruction at the neck of the sac. This contributes to further edema; eventually the pressure is such that arterial inflow is compromised and may progress to severe ischemia and gangrene of the incarcerated bowel. Therefore, if the hernia is not reduced in time, strangulation

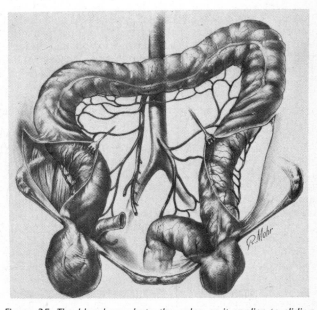

Figure 25. The blood supply to the colon as it applies to sliding hernias. On the left side, the inferior mesenteric artery, by means of its sigmoid branches, supplies that portion of colon found in a sliding hernia. On the right side, the ileocolic artery and ileal branches are of major concern. (From Ponka, J. L.: Hernias of the Abdominal Wall. Philadelphia, W. B. Saunders Company, 1980.)

is followed by gangrene, which may be perilous, and immediate operation may be mandatory.

In a review of a series of patients with strangulated hernias, 40 to 50 per cent of the hernias were inguinal, 30 to 35 per cent were femoral, 10 to 15 per cent were umbilical, and the remainder were incisional or epigastric. Ten per cent of all inguinal hernias presented as incarcerated hernias, whereas 20 to 25 per cent of femoral hernias presented as incarcerations.[1]

Diagnosis

The diagnosis of an incarcerated or strangulated hernia is usually obvious. A mass in the region of a previously recognized hernia is frequently firm, painful, and tender. There may be some erythema of the overlying skin. An incarcerated *femoral* hernia is the most difficult to diagnose, since the hernia may be very small and the mass may not be detected on physical examination. In addition, patients frequently complain of nausea and vomiting if small bowel obstruction is present. There may also be fever and chills.

Physical Examination and Treatment

Pertinent aspects on physical examination include vital signs, fluid status, signs of peritoneal irritation and distention, and inspection of the incarcerated hernial site. The hernia itself may be extremely tender, preventing detailed evaluation.

If the patient is hemodynamically unstable, this condition takes precedence. In such a case, appropriate hemodynamic monitoring is instituted, a catheter is inserted in the urinary bladder, adequate fluids and electrolytes are administered, and pharmacologic support of the arterial pressure is given if needed.

If the patient is not in septic shock or in need of emergent fluid or other resuscitative measures, a more detailed examination of the incarcerated hernia can be performed. Reduction of the hernia by manual palpation should be attempted.[5] Since tenderness is a difficult obstacle during attempted reduction, adequate analgesia and sedation should be given, and the patient is placed in a moderate Trendelenburg position with a cold pack placed on the mass. With the head and thorax lower than the abdomen, gravity tends to draw the hernia back into the peritoneal cavity. After the patient is as comfortable as possible, reduction can be attempted. One hand is placed over the anatomic neck of the hernia sac to guide the direction of the hernia contents, and the other hand provides pressure to the hernia sac as the contents are pressed back through the fascial defect. Thirty to 50 per cent of incarcerated hernias can be reduced in this manner, thus preventing the need for an emergency operation.

If the patient is hemodynamically stable and the hernia can be reduced by the closed technique, admission to the hospital is probably the best course, with later plans for a semi-elective herniorrhaphy. During this time, the patient should receive appropriate fluids and electrolytes. If closed reduction is not possible, then emergency operation is required to prevent complete strangulation and ultimate tissue gangrene of the involved bowel. The patient should receive adequate fluid and electrolyte resuscitation and broad-spectrum antibiotics preoperatively.

The surgical approach to an incarcerated hernia under emergency conditions is similar to that under elective circumstances. Once the hernia sac is identified and dissected free, it is opened and the contents examined. If there is nonviable intestine present, resection is performed. Small intestine and omentum are the most commonly incarcerated tissues. If there is doubt about the presence of gangrene, a warm, moist pad is placed on the bowel and allowed to remain for about 20 minutes. Color of the bowel as well as the presence of arterial pulsations in the small mesenteric arteries is noted. If the incarcerated contents are viable, they may be reduced by incising the neck of the hernia sac, allowing the contents to retract into the peritoneal cavity. The remainder of the hernia repair is similar to that described in previous sections.

The results of surgical correction of incarcerated and strangulated hernias point to the necessity of repairing all hernias on an elective basis. If intestinal resection is required, the mortality is further increased. This is often secondary to the eventual septic shock produced by the gangrenous tissue. Such data also emphasize the emergent nature of an incarcerated hernia. The mortality is about 8 per cent in patients with incarcerated femoral hernias operated on within 24 hours, but mortality increases to nearly 50 per cent if more than 24 hours have elapsed between incarceration and surgical repair.[18] The morbidity is also increased, and wound infection is the most common complication postoperatively, occurring in 5 to 10 per cent of patients with incarcerated or strangulated hernias.

RARE HERNIA

Epigastric Hernia

Epigastric hernias occur through a defect in the linea alba between the umbilicus and the xiphoid process.[12] They are more common in males than in females and are usually asymptomatic. Some patients complain of a mass and pain on palpation. Twenty per cent of patients have multiple hernias in the epigastrium. These hernias should be repaired if they are symptomatic or if the fascial defect is 1 cm. or more in diameter. A vertical incision is used to dissect the linea alba in search of additional epigastric hernias. The fascial edges are freed from the hernia sac and the defect repaired by direct suture. The falciform ligament and omentum are the two most common contents found in the hernia. Ten per cent of epigastric hernias recur, probably owing to a missed second epigastric hernia or secondary to a pre-existing weakness in the linea alba.

Parastomal Hernia

A hernia through the same fascial opening created for a colostomy or ileostomy is designated a *parastomal hernia*.[9, 16] These hernias occur more commonly in the obese and in those in whom a colostomy is placed lateral to the rectus muscle or through the incision of the initial operation. Insofar as hernia prevention is concerned, the ideal site for a colostomy is through the rectus muscle. The indications for repair of a parastomal hernia include (1) an unsatisfactory stoma needing placement at another site, (2) stricture or prolapse of the stoma, (3) large size of the hernia, (4) presence of a small fascial defect surrounding the hernia, (5) incarceration or strangulation of the hernia, and (6) cosmetic repair.

The preferred reparative technique for parastomal hernias begins with preoperative preparation of the large bowel. The original incision is then reopened, and the colostomy moved to a new site. A defect through the rectus muscle barely admitting two fingers is created for the new colostomy. The fascial defect of the original colostomy is then closed from within the peritoneal cavity. The hernia sac should be dissected free from the subcutaneous tissue and removed prior to closure of the fascial defect. The midline wound is closed with packing of the residual subcutaneous space from the previous colostomy.

Richter's Hernia

Richter's hernia occurs when only a portion of the bowel wall is entrapped in the hernia orifice.[6] It most commonly involves the antimesenteric border of the small intestine (Fig. 26). When two thirds or more of the circumference of the small bowel is involved, intestinal obstruction may occur. Richter's hernias constitute about 15 per cent of all incarcerated hernias, and 80 to 90 per cent of these are femoral hernias. Because of the anatomic location of the femoral canal and the small segment of intestine incorporated in Richter's hernia, the preoperative diagnosis can

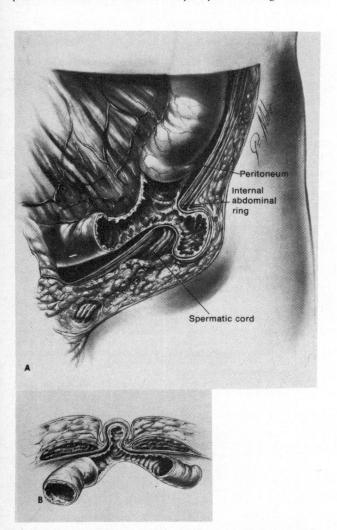

Figure 26. The internal ring may be the site of a Richter's type hernia in the presence of a small, constricted orifice at this site. (From Ponka, J. L.: Hernias of the Abdominal Wall. Philadelphia, W. B. Saunders Company, 1980.)

be difficult. There may be swelling or tenderness over the hernial site, and routine hernia repair with open reduction of the incarcerated small bowel is required for operative correction. If necrotic intestine is present as a consequence of Richter's hernia, intestinal resection must be performed. Since most of these hernias are femoral, a separate abdominal midline incision is often required for intestinal resection.

Littre's Hernia

The presence of Meckel's diverticulum in a hernia sac is defined as Littre's hernia.[23] The majority of Littre's hernias are inguinal or femoral and are also frequently incarcerated. The clinical presentation and surgical management are identical to those of inguinal and femoral hernias.

Spigelian Hernia

The semilunar line is the site where the transversus abdominis muscle becomes an aponeurosis. It is an outwardly curved line extending from the midportion of the costal margin to the pubic tubercle. This line is lateral to the lateral edge of the rectus muscle, and the space between the semilunar line and the lateral edge of the rectus muscle is the *Spigelian fascia*. A hernia through this fascia can be called a Spigelian hernia,[3, 24] but most commonly this hernia occurs through the Spigelian fascia inferior to the semicircular line of Douglas. The posterior rectus fascia is present above the semicircular line, but there is no fascia posterior to the rectus muscle below. Patients complain of pain, and sometimes an abdominal mass is located inferior to the umbilicus and lateral to the rectus muscle. Such patients are frequently obese, and the preoperative diagnosis is correct in only 50 per cent of patients. These hernias should be corrected when diagnosed.

A transverse incision over the site of the hernia is made, and the hernia is exposed beneath the external oblique fascia, which must be divided in the direction of its fibers for proper exposure of the hernia. The hernia sac frequently contains small bowel or omentum and should be dissected and either removed or invaginated through the fascial defect. The defect in the transversus abdominis aponeurosis and the internal oblique muscle is then repaired with interrupted sutures and the external oblique closed. Recurrence is rare after surgical repair.

Obturator Hernia

Obturator hernias pass through the obturator canal in the pelvis.[7, 8] The hernia sac exits at the site of the obturator vessels and nerve and pierces the obturator membrane to course through the obturator foramen. These hernias are difficult to diagnose, and the patients are usually elderly females and frequently thin. They may present with abdominal symptoms, including nausea, vomiting, and abdominal pain, suggestive of small bowel obstruction. They may also have pain along the distribution of the obturator nerve, which supplies sensation to the upper medial aspect of the thigh (Howship-Romberg sign). These hernias are frequently incarcerated with strangulated bowel at the time of presentation. The patient should be stabilized preoperatively with fluids and electrolytes and then explored through a lower midline incision. The hernia can be seen to exit through the pelvic sidewall and should be reduced into the abdomen and any gangrenous intestine resected. The small defect in the obturator foramen is then closed with interrupted sutures.

LUMBAR (DORSAL) HERNIA

Lumbar or dorsal hernias can occur in the lumbar region through the posterior abdominal wall. The most common sites are the superior and inferior lumbar triangles. The superior triangle (Grynfelt's) is the larger and more frequently involved, whereas the inferior triangle (Petit's) is less involved. A mass in the flank is a common complaint and may be associated with a feeling of discomfort. The mass is usually reducible, but incarceration and strangulation occur in approximately 10 per cent of patients. The differential diagnosis includes soft tissue tumors, hematomas, abscess, and herniated muscle. Correction is accomplished by approximation of the fascial edges with direct repair.

SCIATIC HERNIA

A *sciatic* hernia consists of intra-abdominal contents passing through the greater sciatic foramen. The diagnosis is usually not made until the hernia has become incarcerated. The operation is usually through an abdominal approach. The hernia sac and its contents are reduced with resection of any potential necrotic bowel and closure with a segment of nearby fascia.

PERINEAL HERNIA

A protrusion through the muscles of the fascia of the perineal floor represents a *perineal hernia*. Although it can be primary, it may also be acquired following perineal procedures, such as abdominoperineal resection, pelvic exenteration, and prostatectomy. In general, these hernias present few, if any, symptoms, although sitting may be painful and those located anteriorly may cause dysuria. Correction is by a combined abdominoperineal approach with fascial closure.

SELECTED REFERENCES

McVay, C. B.: Anson and McVay's Surgical Anatomy, 6th ed. Philadelphia, W. B. Saunders Company, 1984.
This is the key reference for surgical anatomy, including anatomy of the inguinal region. Dr. McVay is an international authority on hernia anatomy and surgical correction.

McVay, C. B., Reed, R. C., and Ravitch, M. M.: Inguinal hernia. Curr. Probl. Surg., Oct. 1967.
This reference provides considerable detail of the classic Halsted-Ferguson procedure as well as the McVay procedure.

Nyhus, L. M., and Condon, R. E. (Eds.): Hernia, 2nd ed. Philadelphia, J. B. Lippincott Company, 1978.
This is an extensive and detailed monograph relating to all forms of hernias. For the student seeking details as well as descriptions of the rarer hernias, this is a valuable resource.

Ponka, J. L.: Hernias of the Abdominal Wall. Philadelphia, W. B. Saunders Company, 1980.
The author presents a wide spectrum of hernias together with their diagnosis and treatment. There are many excellent illustrations.

Usher, F. C.: The repair of incisional and inguinal hernia. Surg. Gynecol. Obstet., *131*:525, 1970.
This is one of the classic references in the literature concerning the use of prosthetic materials in hernial repair.

REFERENCES

1. Andrews, N. J.: Presentation and outcome of strangulated external hernia in a district general hospital. Br. J. Surg., 68:329, 1981.
2. Bassini, E.: Nuovo metodo per la cura radicale dell'ernia. Atti Cong. Ass. Med. Ital. (1887), 2:179, 1889.
3. Bertelsen, S.: The surgical treatment of Spigelian hernia. Surg. Gynecol. Obstet., 122:567, 1966.
4. Condon, R. E., and Nyhus, L. M.: Complications of groin hernia and hernia repair. Surg. Clin. North Am., 51:1325, 1971.
5. Kauffman, H. M., and O'Brien, D. P.: Selective reduction of incarcerated inguinal hernia. Am. J. Surg., 119:660, 1970.
6. Keynes, W. M.: Richter's hernia. In Nyhus, L. M.: Hernia, 2nd ed. Philadelphia, J. B. Lippincott Company, 1978.
7. Kozlowski, J. M., and Beal, J. M.: Obturator hernia: An elusive diagnosis. Arch. Surg., 112:1001, 1977.
8. Kwong, K. H., and Ong, G. B.: Obturator hernia. Br. J. Surg., 53:23, 1966.
9. Lesli, D.: The parastomal hernia. Surg. Clin. North Am. 64(2):407, 1984.
10. Ljungdahl, I.: Inguinal and femoral hernia. Personal experience with 502 operations. Acta. Chir. Scand., (Suppl.):1, 1973.
11. Lotheissen, G.: Zur Radikaloperation der Schenkelhernien. Zentralbl. Chir., 25:548, 1898.
12. McCaugham, J. J.: Epigastric hernia. In Nyhus, L. M., and Condon, R. E. (Eds.): Hernia, 2nd ed. Philadelphia, J. B. Lippincott Company, 1978.
13. McVay, C. B.: The anatomic basis for inguinal and femoral hernioplasty. Surg. Gynecol. Obstet., 139:931, 1974.
14. McVay, C. B.: Anson and McVay's Surgical Anatomy, 6th ed. Philadelphia, W. B. Saunders Company, 1984.
15. McVay, C. B., and Anson, B. J.: A fundamental error in current methods of inguinal herniorrhaphy. Surg. Gynecol. Obstet., 74:746, 1942.
16. Prian, G. W., Sawyer, R. B., and Sawyer, K. C.: Repair of peristomal colostomy hernias. Am. J. Surg., 130:694, 1975.
17. Read, R. C.: The development of inguinal herniorrhaphy. Surg. Clin. North Am., 64(2):185, 1984.
18. Rogers, F. A.: Strangulated femoral hernia: A review of 170 cases. Ann. Surg., 149:9, 1959.
19. U.S. Department of Health, Education and Welfare: National Health Survey on Hernias. Series B, No. 25, Dec. 1960.
20. U.S. Department of Health and Human Services, Public Health Service, National Center for Health Statistics: National Health Survey: Utilization of Short-Stay Hospitals, Annual Summary for the United States, 1980. Series 13, No. 64. Washington, D.C., U.S. Government Printing Office, March 1982.
21. Usher, F. C.: The repair of incisional and inguinal hernias. Surg. Gynecol. Obstet., 131:525, 1970.
22. Wantz, G. E.: Complications of inguinal hernia repair. Surg. Clin. North Am., 64(2):287, 1984.
23. Weinstein, E. C., and Remine, W. H.: Littre's hernia: Review of the Mayo Clinic experience. Am. J. Surg., 108:870, 1964.
24. Weiss, Y., Lernan, O. B., and Nissan, S.: Spigelian hernia. Ann. Surg., 180:836, 1974.

PEDIATRIC SURGERY

JAMES L. TALBERT, M.D.

33

The special challenge in pediatric surgery is the recognition and correction of a spectrum of unique anatomic and physiologic conditions that occur in a rapidly growing and relatively vulnerable patient. Because of constraints imposed by the small size and immaturity of these patients, preciseness and constant vigilance are essential requirements for successful treatment. Concomitantly, the resilience of these children is remarkable, and, with appropriate management, the special reward of the health professionals involved in their care is the pleasure and pride derived from following their subsequent emergence as healthy and productive adults.

NEONATAL SURGICAL EMERGENCIES

These considerations are epitomized in the treatment of the newborn infant, in whom miniature structures, immature physiologic responses, and associated anomalies often exaggerate the hazards. This risk is compounded further by the frequent occurrence of neonatal surgical emergencies in premature newborns (less than 37 weeks' gestation) in whom there is an increased morbidity and mortality, even in the absence of congenital malformations or other complicating conditions.

As a consequence, complex neonatal surgical emergencies are best treated in a regional center specifically equipped and staffed to manage the total spectrum of unusual and challenging conditions that may be encountered in these infants. Indeed, one of the first responsibilities of the primary physician is to determine whether adequate care can be rendered by locally available facilities and personnel or whether initial efforts should be directed toward resuscitation and rapid transfer of the patient to a recognized center.

Early diagnosis is obviously desirable in these circumstances, and the increasing availability of *maternal sonography* for monitoring pregnancy has provided a new method for detecting abnormalities in the fetus from the 12th week of gestation onward.[22] In some instances, the delay necessitated for transport of a sick neonate can be completely obviated when antepartum diagnosis allows the mother to be delivered in a regional perinatal center, where immediate availability of optimal surgical care can be ensured for the newborn infant. The list of conditions that can be successfully diagnosed before birth by maternal ultrasound has expanded rapidly and includes intestinal atresia, gastroschisis, omphalocele, sacrococcygeal teratoma, conjoined twins, intra-abdominal cysts, and diaphragmatic hernia.

At the time of birth, the finding of a single umbilical artery may indicate the presence of other anomalies, whereas the identification of specific abnormalities suggests potential associations, such as the frequent occurrence of esophageal atresia with vertebral, anal, cardiac, tracheoesophageal, renal, and limb anomalies (VACTERL syndrome), duodenal atresia with Down's syndrome, and gastroschisis with intestinal atresia or stenosis. The diagnosis of meconium ileus may also be suggested by a family history of siblings affected by cystic fibrosis.

Special Considerations in Management

Seemingly trivial details, which assume importance only in complicated problems in older children, demand routine attention in the pre- and postoperative care of neonates. The margin for error at this age is limited, and the physician must maintain constant vigilance to detect those subtle signs that may portend serious alterations in homeostasis. In these circumstances, continuous monitoring of respiratory, cardiocirculatory, and metabolic function is imperative.

RESPIRATORY FUNCTION

Adequate ventilation in an infant may be impaired by an immaturity of the pulmonary tissues as well as by the tiny air passages that are easily occluded by edema or secretions. As a consequence, monitoring of arterial oxygen levels represents an important aspect of management.

One of the significant physiologic differences between neonates and older children and adults is the increased oxygen demand required for their relatively high metabolic rate (oxygen consumption in the neonate is 6 ml. per kg. per minute versus 3 ml. per kg. per minute in the adult). Concomitantly, the process of pulmonary alveolar maturation is not complete until 8 to 10 years of age, and the number of saccules and primitive alveoli in the lung of a newborn infant is only 8 per cent of the number of alveoli in an adult.[5] Therefore, to satisfy the increased oxygen demand, alveolar ventilation must be twice that of the adult (100 to 150 ml. per kg. per minute versus 60 ml. per kg. per minute). The neonate adjusts to this need primarily by maintaining a high respiratory rate.

CARDIOCIRCULATORY FUNCTION

Time devoted to the preoperative preparation of the critically ill infant can provide important benefits, both during and following the surgical procedure. However, such efforts must be accomplished quickly. A satisfactory circulating blood volume is the most important factor in determining whether an operation can be undertaken safely, and in the absence of cardiac failure, an infant will tolerate rapid infusion of 20 to 25 ml. per kg. of whole blood or plasma without ill effect. The blood volume of a newborn infant approximates 10 per cent of the total body weight, and a minimal deficit of 25 per cent can be anticipated in the presence of acute hypovolemic shock. Normally, the hematocrit is also high in the first few days of life (>50 per cent) and lower levels, which are acceptable in older infants, may signify blood loss or anemia. When blood replacement is required, a transfusion of 10 ml. per kg. is approximately equivalent to the administration of a single unit of whole blood to a 70-kg. adult. When the preoperative hematocrit is especially high, plasma infusion may be preferred to decrease blood viscosity. Intraoperatively, the limited blood volume of the newborn infant also creates a special threat, since the seemingly innocuous quantity of blood lost in a few saturated sponges may prove sufficient to precipitate shock (as much as 20 ml. of blood may be absorbed by a single surgical sponge).

FLUID AND ELECTROLYTE REGULATION

Although newborn infants possess a proportionally greater reservoir of total body water and extracellular fluid than do adults, a considerably higher rate of water excretion renders them more sensitive to the large losses that may be incurred by conditions such as intestinal obstruction, peritonitis, and gastroschisis. In these circumstances, deficits can ensue rapidly and the maximal fluid loss that can be tolerated at this age is equivalent to 20 per cent of the total body weight. Especially difficult to assess in the postoperative patient are "hidden losses," which may result from sequestration of fluids in traumatized tissues, intestines, and body cavities.

Renal immaturity in the newborn, especially premature infants, may be reflected by an inability to concentrate and conserve fluid and electrolytes. As a consequence, urine specific gravity may remain low (frequently resulting in a maximal specific gravity of 1.015 in the premature versus a specific gravity of 1.035 in the older child) even in the presence of significant fluid deficits. Concomitantly, congestive failure may ensue rapidly when overhydration occurs, since a decreased glomerular filtration rate may also limit renal excretion.[7] In no instance should large volumes of intravenous fluid be suspended without interposition of a small plastic reservoir in the connecting line, to ensure that the fluid is administered in small aliquots and to guard against accidental flooding by an uncontrolled infusion. Utilization of constant infusion pumps also allows small volumes of fluid to be administered over protracted periods.

Maintenance fluid requirements are diminished during the first few days of life as a consequence of the relative excess of total body water, but they can be subsequently calculated at 100 ml. per kg. per 24 hours (for patients weighing less than 10 kg.) and administered as 10 per cent dextrose. Three to 4 mEq. of sodium and 2 to 3 mEq. of potassium should be included with each 100 ml. of fluid infused. Normal urinary output in the adequately hydrated infant should approximate 1 to 2 ml. per kg. per hour.

Serial measurements of arterial gases allow an assessment of the effectiveness of alveolar ventilation and acid-base equilibrium and provide important assistance in the resuscitation of a critically ill infant. An elevation in arterial PCO_2 may indicate a need for endotracheal intubation and mechanical ventilation; a decrease in arterial PO_2 may reflect impaired ventilation perfusion as a consequence of pulmonary parenchymal disease or right to left shunting. Base deficits calculated on the basis of serum pH and PCO_2 by utilizing the standard Siggaard-Andersen nomogram also provide an accurate guide for correcting metabolic acidosis through infusion of sodium bicarbonate.

METABOLISM AND THERMAL REGULATION

Newborn infants are potentially *thermolabile* as a consequence of an increased body surface area relative to weight, limited stores of insulating fat, and immature thermal regulatory mechanisms. Premature newborns and infants compromised by sepsis and shock are especially vulnerable to this threat. These natural deficiencies are compounded by any alteration in environmental temperature, as may be induced by administration of cold intravenous solutions or blood, exposure in air-conditioned rooms, or application of cold or highly volatile surgical preparatory solutions. Continuous temperature monitoring should be provided in these circumstances by placement of a thermister probe in the axilla or esophagus. A warm environment must also be maintained during all phases of preoperative, intraoperative, and postoperative treatment by regulation of room temperature and utilization of isolettes, overhead radiant heaters or lights, or warm-water heating pads.[5]

A host of metabolic derangements may occur in the newborn stressed by surgical trauma or disease. Because of a deficiency of glycogen storage, impaired gluconeogenesis, and difficulties with insulin regulation, hypoglycemia often ensues. As a consequence, these infants should be routinely maintained on intravenous solutions containing 10 per cent glucose, with a need for higher concentrations determined by frequent monitoring of blood levels. Subsequent development of hypoglycemia in a previously stable patient may also portend the onset of sepsis or hypothermia. Hypocalcemia is commonly encountered at this age, especially in premature infants, and calcium supplementation is often necessary in neonates undergoing complex operative procedures. Hyperbilirubinemia also occurs frequently in newborns and may be exaggerated by the same conditions, such as intestinal obstruction, which necessitate surgical intervention. Accordingly, serial monitoring of serum bilirubin levels is required in these circumstances.

NUTRITION

Because of the limited caloric reserves and the heightened demands imposed by rapid growth and maturation, maintenance of adequate nutritional support is of paramount importance to achieving successful convalescence of the neonatal surgical patient. The advent of techniques for delivering increased calories and essential substrates by the central venous or peripheral venous route has proved especially beneficial and has allowed pediatric surgeons to overcome a major source of postoperative morbidity and mortality.[1, 5, 9, 19] With this approach, adequate quantities of glucose, protein hydrolysates or amino acids, lipids, minerals, and vitamins can now be administered parenterally to sustain growth, even in the rapidly developing infant.

More dilute solutions can be administered via peripheral vein, whereas infusions containing carbohydrate concentrations greater than 15 gm. per 100 ml. require delivery directly into the superior vena cava by means of a central catheter, inserted via cutdown on a neck vein or percutaneous puncture of a subclavian vein (Fig. 1).

INFECTION

Although evidence suggests that phagocytosis intracellular killing of bacteria is normal in the stable premature infant, with the added stress of sepsis or operation there is a significant decrease in bactericidal activity, possibly as a consequence of an immunosuppressive effect of operation and anesthesia. By far, the most serious infections, and the most difficult to identify and treat, involve gram-negative septicemias. Whereas the mature newborn may respond with an anticipated elevation in temperature, sepsis, especially in *premature* infants, is frequently heralded by the onset of lethargy and hypothermia, which may quickly progress to severe acidosis and circulatory collapse. Because of this increased susceptibility and because of the rapidity with which life-threatening complications may ensue, broad-spectrum antibiotic coverage is usually indicated when complex surgical procedures are performed in neonates.

Neonatal Respiratory Emergencies

FACTORS IN SUSCEPTIBILITY

A number of unique anatomic and physiologic factors render the newborn infant especially susceptible to respiratory distress.[5, 7] At birth, initiation of ventilation may require transient increases in intrapulmonary pressure as high as 40 to 80 cm. H_2O to overcome the viscosity of fluid in the airway and the forces of surface tension as well as to stretch the pulmonary parenchyma. This process of inflation may progress unevenly, and if excessively high pressures are selectively maintained in the aerated alveoli as a consequence of persistent obstruction and/or atelectasis elsewhere in the lung, spontaneous rupture, pneumomediastinum, and pneumothorax may ensue. The potential for significant impairment of air flow through the tiny tracheobronchial passages is readily evident, and the risk is magnified by any further compromise of lumen diameter. These young patients also rely primarily on diaphragmatic excursions to achieve air exchange, in contrast to adults and older children, who preferentially utilize the rib cage and chest wall musculature for breathing. As a consequence, abdominal distention and impaired diaphragmatic function may produce significant respiratory distress.

Finally, newborn infants are especially susceptible to alterations of intrapleural pressure. In the adult, any unilateral increase in intrapleural pressure is buffered by a stable mediastinum, but in the neonate the mediastinum is relatively mobile and can be readily displaced by an expanding intrapleural lesion or increasing tension. Accordingly, conditions such as *tension pneumothorax* represent a special threat to these patients because of the potential for compressing both the contralateral and the ipsilateral lung. The flail mediastinum may also exaggerate any inadequacy of diaphragmatic function, as induced by unilateral phrenic nerve palsy, and may prohibit effective air exchange.

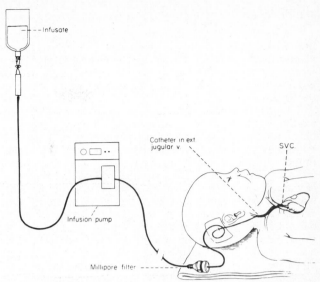

Figure 1. System for long-term central venous parenteral hyperalimentation. A small Silastic catheter is introduced into the superior vena cava via a cutdown on the external jugular vein and tunneled cephalad to exit the skin immediately posterior to the ear. When the external jugular vein proves excessively small, as may occur in premature infants, the facial vein or internal jugular vein may be utilized as alternate routes for cannulation. The position of the catheter tip at the junction of the superior vena cava and the right atrium must always be confirmed by anteroposterior and lateral chest roentgenograms. The catheter is connected to an infusion system that includes a millipore filter for removing any particulate matter, bacteria, or fungi. Incorporation of a continuous pump and a calibrated buret into the system ensures uniform, hourly flow rates. (From Holder, T. M., and Ashcraft, K. W. (Eds.): Pediatric Surgery. Philadelphia, W. B. Saunders Company, 1980, p. 37.)

EVALUATION

Evaluation of a neonate in respiratory distress should include passage of a size No. 8 or No. 10 French catheter via the nares, pharynx, and esophagus into the stomach, thereby excluding the presence of either choanal or esophageal atresia. Anteroposterior and lateral chest roentgenograms must be obtained immediately and should also demonstrate the neck and abdomen, since conditions causing respiratory distress at this age may originate above the thoracic inlet as well as below the diaphragm.

EXTRATHORACIC CONDITIONS

Choanal Atresia

Choanal atresia is the most common anomaly of the nasopharynx, and since the newborn infant is a mandatory nasal breather, bilateral obstruction may rapidly result in asphyxia. Initial management requires insertion of an oral airway and supportive treatment until a pattern of mouth breathing can be established.

Micrognathia

Mandibular hypoplasia may be associated with the *Treacher-Collins syndrome* (mandibulofacial dysostosis) or the *Pierre-Robin syndrome*. The latter condition is frequently accompanied by cleft palate. In both instances, airway obstruction results from glossoptosis, which, when severe, may necessitate insertion of a tracheostomy.

Tumors of the Head and Neck

A variety of tumors may produce respiratory obstruction in the newborn as a consequence of either direct involvement of the wall of the oropharynx, larynx, and trachea or compression of the cervical airway. Cystic hygromas, teratomas, and congenital goiters are included in this group.

Cystic Hygroma. This lesion is a congenital malformation of the lymphatic system that is usually evident at birth. Cystic hygroma occurs predominantly in the neck, but it may also present in the axilla or groin and within the thorax. Although cystic hygromas are usually unilocular and located posterior to the sternocleidomastoid muscles, in some instances the lesion may present as a multilocular mass with a dramatic, beardlike configuration resulting from extensive involvement of the larynx and pharynx, tongue, parotid gland, and soft tissues of the lower face and neck (Fig. 2). Successful treatment entails staged, surgical resection, often with tracheostomy and gastrostomy to facilitate feedings and to maintain a patent airway.[21] Since the process is histologically benign and since eventual satisfactory removal usually proves feasible, every effort should be di-

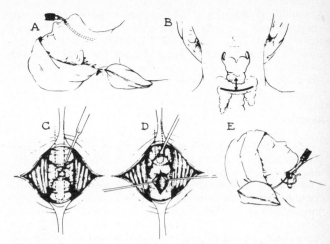

Figure 3. Tracheostomy technique for infants and children.

A, Following insertion of endotracheal tube, the patient is positioned with neck extended.

B, A transverse skin incision at level of thyroid isthmus has proved preferable for use with Silastic tubes.

C, The strap muscles are separated vertically by blunt dissection, and the thyroid isthmus is reflected cephalad after division of the pretracheal fascia. The anterior tracheal wall is then incised vertically, dividing the second, third, fourth and, if needed, fifth tracheal cartilages in the midline. No transverse counterincision is employed, and no tracheal flap or window is ever removed in infants or small children.

D, The endotracheal tube is then withdrawn into the proximal trachea, the tracheostomy margins are reflected laterally by small hooks, and an appropriate sized Silastic tube is inserted.

E, The tube is tied securely in place with neck flexed, in order to ensure snugness and to guard against accidental dislodgment. (From Haller, J. A., Jr., and Talbert, J. L.: Surgical Emergencies in the Newborn. Philadelphia, Lea & Febiger, 1972, p. 20.)

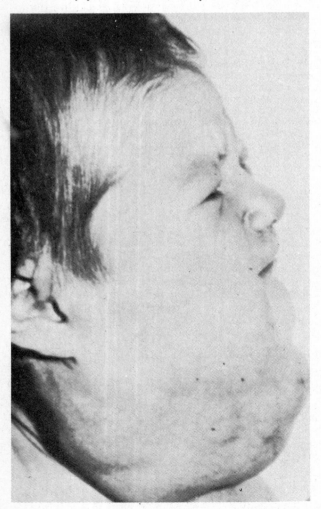

Figure 2. A massive cystic hygroma in the newborn infant, which was eventually treated successfully by staged resection, following temporary insertion of a tracheostomy and gastrostomy to relieve airway obstruction and to facilitate feeding. (From Haller, J. A., Jr., and Talbert, J. L.: Surgical Emergencies in the Newborn. Philadelphia, Lea & Febiger, 1972, p. 38.)

rected toward preservation of functional tissue, including the nerves and vascular structures, which are frequently intertwined.

Hemangioma. Hemangiomas can occur in the head and neck and may produce airway obstruction when they involve the larynx or trachea. Characteristically, these tumors enlarge rapidly during the first few months of life, but eventually they undergo spontaneous involution. Accordingly, treatment should be primarily supportive, with insertion of a tracheostomy when the airway is unduly compromised (Fig. 3). Systemic administration or direct injection of corticosteroids has been utilized in some instances to hasten the process of spontaneous regression.

Teratoma. Teratomas of the neck are rare, but may arise in association with the thyroid gland and produce airway obstruction as a consequence of tracheal compression. Roentgenographic identification of calcification within a neck mass in a neonate suggests either this diagnosis or that of a cervical *neuroblastoma*, with the latter tumor usually located more laterally and posteriorly.

Laryngeal and Tracheal Obstruction

Stridor or impaired phonation suggests an anatomic or functional abnormality of the upper trachea or larynx, as may result from laryngeal web, laryngotracheoesophageal cleft, subglottic stenosis, laryngomalacia, vocal cord paralysis, hemangioma, or lymphangioma. Differentiation of this group of lesions is largely dependent on direct laryngoscopy and bronchoscopy, with treatment often entailing tracheostomy.

Laryngotracheoesophageal Cleft. This is an unusual anomaly reflecting a failure of normal separation of embryonic foregut into the trachea and esophagus, resulting in a common channel that may be limited to the larynx or may extend the entire length of the trachea and adjacent esophagus (an esophagotrachea). As a consequence of this persistent communication between the esophagus and trachea, aspiration and respiratory distress are inevitable.

Subglottic Stenosis. This may be congenital in origin or may follow prolonged endotracheal intubation in newborn infants requiring mechanical ventilation. If treatment is initiated early, serial dilations of the trachea are usually effective often with an associated tracheostomy. In severe cases, cryosurgery or laser therapy may also be required for resection of the subglottic scar.

Laryngomalacia and Tracheomalacia. An exaggeration of the normal flexibility of these cartilaginous structures in the young infant may produce varying degrees of airway collapse and obstruction. Ordinarily, this condition resolves spontaneously with growth and maturation; rarely, however, a tracheostomy may be required for temporary relief when the obstruction is severe.

INTRATHORACIC CONDITIONS

Esophageal Atresia and Tracheoesophageal Fistula

The diagnosis of esophageal atresia is usually associated with respiratory distress as a result of overflow of secretions from the blind, proximal esophageal pouch with passage into the adjacent trachea, and, when combined with a distal tracheoesophageal fistula, from reflux of acidic gastric contents into the bronchopulmonary tree. The resultant threat of airway obstruction and contamination is compounded by a high incidence of prematurity and by the frequent occurrence of other serious congenital anomalies. Significant cardiovascular defects are especially noteworthy and in combination with respiratory embarrassment can prove extremely hazardous.

The most frequently encountered form of this anomaly, occurring in approximately 87 per cent of patients, consists of a proximal, blind esophageal pouch in association with a distal tracheoesophageal fistula that communicates with the stomach.[5] Rarely, a fistula may also link the upper trachea with the proximal esophageal pouch. Complete esophageal atresia, without an associated fistula, is found in approximately 8 per cent of patients; an isolated H- or N-type tracheoesophageal fistula, without associated esophageal atresia, occurs in 4 per cent (Fig. 4).

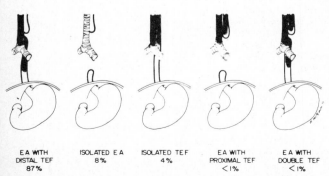

| EA WITH DISTAL TEF 87% | ISOLATED E A 8% | ISOLATED TEF 4% | EA WITH PROXIMAL TEF <1% | E A WITH DOUBLE TEF <1% |

Figure 4. Types of esophageal atresia (EA) and tracheoesophageal fistula (TEF) with relative frequencies. (From Holder, T. M., and Ashcraft, K. W.: Surg. Clin. North Am., 61:1051, 1981.)

The presence of esophageal atresia is suggested at birth by maternal hydramnios, excessive oropharyngeal secretions, respiratory distress, and choking with feedings. The diagnosis can be confirmed by failure of a No. 10 French catheter to pass via the mouth and esophagus into the stomach. A roentgenogram of the chest, obtained with the catheter inserted, shows the exact level of proximal esophageal obstruction. Careful instillation of a small amount of contrast media via the catheter clearly identifies the rare associated fistula between the proximal esophageal pouch and upper trachea. The initial chest roentgenogram must include the upper abdomen, since demonstration of air in the stomach confirms the presence of a distal tracheoesophageal fistula, whereas absence of air effectively excludes this diagnosis (Fig. 5). Clarification of the presence of a fistula has important connotations in management, since in complete atresia without a tracheoesophageal fistula the extent of absent esophagus usually precludes early transthoracic correction. At the same time, placement of a gastrostomy in these patients permits feedings to be started immediately. In those patients with distal tracheoesophageal fistulas who represent a special risk because of complicating factors (such as prematurity, associated anomalies, or pneumonia), immediate insertion of a gastrostomy will also facilitate decompression of the stomach and will prevent reflux of gastric juice into the tracheobronchial tree. Concomitantly, secretions in the proximal blind esophageal pouch can be cleared by continuous suction and nutrition maintained by parenteral alimentation, thereby allowing definitive surgical repair to be delayed until the patient's condition has been optimally stabilized.

To minimize the threat of anastomotic leakage and consequent empyema, an extrapleural approach is frequently utilized when dividing the distal tracheoesophageal fistula and performing the esophageal anastomosis. In those patients in whom an excessively short upper pouch and consequent absent long segment of esophagus are encountered, circumferential myotomies can be employed to achieve additional length of the upper pouch without compromising the blood supply. Patients with complete atresia without fistula are characteristically associated with absence of long segments of esophagus, but occasionally primary anastomosis may be performed by combining the technique of circular myotomy with preoperative bougienage and dilation of the upper pouch. However, primary anastomosis often proves unfeasible and establishment of gastrointestinal continuity is best done at about 1 year of age. At that time, the esophageal defect is bridged by interposition of a segment of colon or gastric tube. In the interim, decompression of the proximal pouch can be achieved via cervical esophagostomy and the patient can be maintained safely at home with gastrostomy feedings.

The rare instance of an isolated H- or N-type congenital tracheoesophageal fistula without associated esophageal atresia may produce immediate symptoms of airway congestion and choking with feedings, or it may become apparent later, with recurrent bouts of pneumonia. Confirmation is provided by cine-esophagograms (Fig. 5). When a suspected H-type tracheoesophageal fistula cannot be successfully demonstrated roentgenographically, rigid bronchoscopy and esophagoscopy with a fiberoptic lens system may prove especially helpful. This technique may also facilitate exposure of the fistulous tract at the time of operation by allowing preoperative insertion of a loop of catheter via the trachea and esophagus to serve as a marker. In contrast to the characteristic intrathoracic position of most tracheoesophageal fistulas associated with esophageal atresia, the

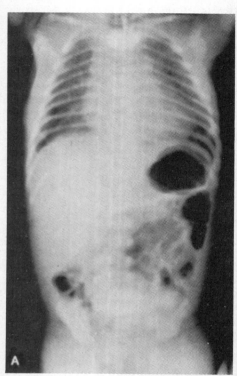

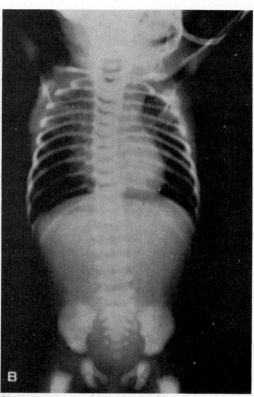

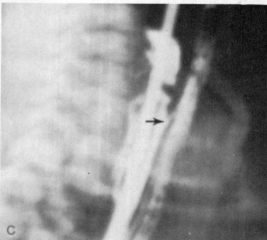

Figure 5. Chest roentgenogram in esophageal atresia and/or tracheoesophageal fistula.

A, Instillation of a small amount of contrast media via an oropharyngeal tube confirms a blind upper pouch, while air in the stomach indicates a distal tracheoesophageal fistula.

B, Catheter coiled in the upper esophagus confirms a blind pouch, while absence of air in the stomach suggests an isolated atresia without distal tracheoesophageal fistula.

C, Injection of contrast media via a catheter into the normally patent esophagus confirms an N-shaped fistula, leading upward from the esophagus into the trachea. (Grosfeld, J. L. (Ed.): Symposium on pediatric surgery. Surg. Clin. North Am. 61:1053, 1054, 1981.)

(C is from Holder, T. M., and Ashcraft, K. W. (Eds.): Pediatric Surgery. Philadelphia, W. B. Saunders Company, 1980, p. 273.)

isolated N- or H-type fistula is ordinarily located in the lower neck.

Vascular Rings

Vascular rings are the most common cause of compression and obstruction of the intrathoracic airway in the newborn. Although the exact configuration varies, the trachea and esophagus are compressed by embryonic aortic arches (Fig. 6). The characteristic symptoms are inspiratory stridor and suprasternal retraction. The most common anomaly is either a double aortic arch or a right aortic arch in association with a persistent ligamentum or ductus arteriosus. The diagnosis is confirmed by a barium esophagogram, demonstrating an indentation of the posterior wall of the esophagus.

Mediastinal Masses

Mediastinal masses may also cause obstruction and are discussed in Chapter 44.

Intrapleural Tension Problems

With the relative instability of mediastinal structures early in life, any expanding intrapleural process not only threatens the ipsilateral lung, but also, through shifting of the mediastinum, compresses the contralateral lung and impedes venous return to the heart. In such circumstances, prompt recognition and early treatment are imperative.

Frequent roentgenographic evidence of minor degrees of mediastinal emphysema and/or intrapleural air in newborn infants attests to the high incidence of spontaneous alveolar rupture as a consequence of the unique mechanical stresses that are exerted during the process of clearing the airway and initiating ventilatory exchange. Such leaks may be intensified by resuscitative efforts entailing mechanical insufflation, with the resultant *tension pneumothorax* producing severe respiratory distress (Fig. 7). Prompt insertion of a thoracoscopy drainage tube is curative. Rarely, *congenital chylothorax* or a *tension hydrothorax* produced by extravasation of fluid from a central venous hyperalimentation catheter may simulate this condition.

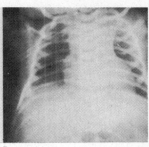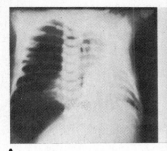

A **B**

Figure 7. A, Tension pneumothorax in a newborn infant, producing marked mediastinal shift with compression of both lungs. B, Immediate restoration of normal anatomy following insertion of a thoracostomy tube. (From Haller, J. A., Jr., and Talbert, J. L.: Surgical Emergencies in the Newborn. Philadelphia, Lea & Febiger, 1972, p. 51.)

Congenital Diaphragmatic Hernia

The sequence of mediastinal displacement and consequent compression of both ipsilateral and contralateral lungs may also be induced by herniation of intra-abdominal contents through the *congenital posterolateral diaphragmatic defect of Bochdalek*. Since this is a congenital malformation developing in utero, significant *pulmonary hypoplasia* may ensue. Symptomatic hernias are most commonly encountered on the left (5:1), whereas the presence of the liver also tends to limit the extent of visceral herniation and pulmonary compression on the right. Following delivery, the degree of mediastinal shift is accentuated and cardiorespiratory function further compromised by entrapment of ingested air in the intrathoracic intestine. Any newborn infant presenting with a clinical picture of respiratory distress in association with a scaphoid abdomen should be suspected of having a congenital diaphragmatic hernia. Immediate chest and abdominal films confirm this diagnosis by demonstrating air- and fluid-filled loops of intestine in the affected hemithorax with a relative absence of gas-filled bowel in the abdomen (Fig. 8).

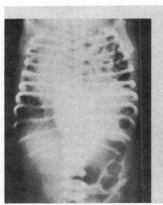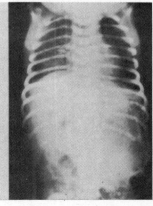

A **B**

Figure 8. Diaphragmatic defect. A, Typical roentgenogram of a newborn with a left posterolateral diaphragmatic defect of the Bochdalek type as manifested by air- and fluid-filled loops of intestine in the left hemithorax and a relative absence of gas-filled loops in the abdomen. A marked shift of the mediastinum to the right has resulted in distortion of the tracheobronchial tree and compression of the right lung. B, Postoperative chest roentgenogram in the same patient confirming closure of the diaphragmatic defect, realignment of the mediastinum in a normal position, and re-expansion of the right lung. (From Haller, J. A., Jr., and Talbert, J. L.: Surgical Emergencies in the Newborn. Philadelphia, Lea & Febiger, 1972, p. 53.)

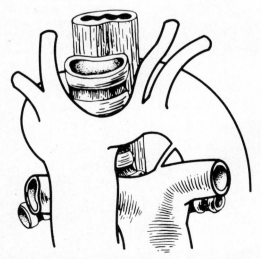

Figure 6. A double aortic arch vascular ring anomaly encompasses the esophagus and trachea and may produce symptoms of stridor and dysphagia. (From Holder, T. M., and Ashcraft, K. W. (Eds.): Pediatric Surgery. Philadelphia, W. B. Saunders Company, 1980, p. 190.)

Patients with Bochdalek hernias are nearly always symptomatic and may have a poor prognosis because of *associated* severe pulmonary hypoplasia. Preoperative correction of acidosis, hypercarbia, and hypoxia appears to improve survival, and recent techniques for support of infants by extracorporeal membrane oxygenation (ECMO) may be important in future improvement in this difficult group of patients.[22]

Closure of the diaphragmatic defect by direct suture or by insertion of a prosthesis may be accomplished either through the chest or abdomen. Most favor the abdominal approach because it offers a capability for correcting the intestinal malrotation that frequently accompanies extra-abdominal displacement of the viscera. If necessary, this incision can be closed with creation of a ventral hernia by approximating only the skin and subcutaneous tissue (Fig. 9). While 60 to 70 per cent of infants with this condition

survive, others become affected with progressive pulmonary hypertension, which often ends fatally.

Eventration of the Diaphragm

Unilateral eventration or paralysis of the diaphragm may be poorly tolerated in infancy as a consequence of the mediastinal instability, which allows a to-and-fro, pendulum-like motion, occurring synchronous with movement of the normal diaphragm and impeding effective air exchange. Although a comparable circumstance in older infants and children may be well tolerated, young infants are frequently symptomatic and death may ensue unless diaphragmatic plication is performed. The resultant fixation of the diaphragm also stabilizes the mediastinum and improves ventilation.

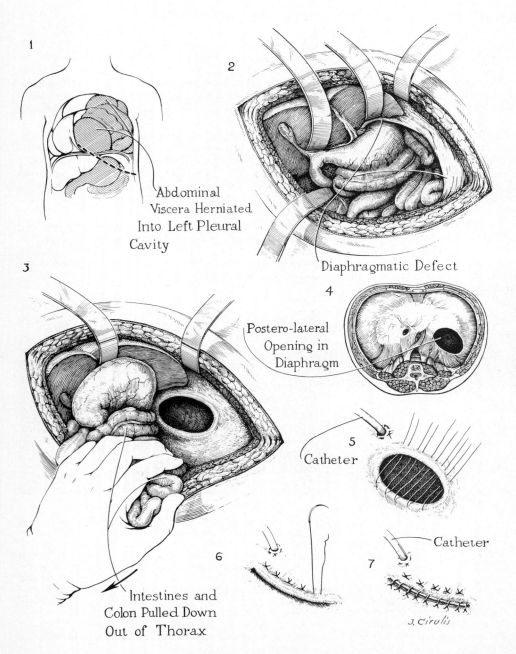

Abdominal Viscera Herniated Into Left Pleural Cavity

Diaphragmatic Defect

Postero-lateral Opening in Diaphragm

Catheter

Catheter

Intestines and Colon Pulled Down Out of Thorax

J. Cirulis

Figure 9. Repair of a congenital diaphragmatic defect of the Bochdalek type via an abdominal approach by reduction of the intrathoracic viscera and closure of the posterolateral opening in the diaphragm. (From Gross, R. E.: An Atlas of Children's Surgery. Philadelphia, W. B. Saunders Company, 1970, p. 61.)

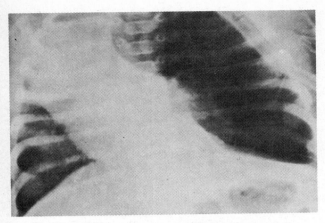

Figure 10. Intralobar emphysema resulting from bronchial obstruction by an inspissated mucous plug. (From Haller, J. A., Jr., and Talbert, J. L.: Surgical Emergencies in the Newborn. Philadelphia, Lea & Febiger, 1972, p. 57.)

Intrapulmonary Space-Occupying Lesions

Expanding intrapulmonary lesions may produce anatomic and physiologic changes identical to those associated with increased intrapleural tension. Although staphylococcal pneumonia may occasionally produce large pneumatoceles, the most commonly encountered congenital problem is *lobar emphysema.*

Congenital Lobar Emphysema. Congenital lobar emphysema follows progressive hyperinflation of the upper or middle lobe of the lung, occurring spontaneously or as a consequence of an anatomic abnormality of the bronchus. The latter is present in 50 per cent of cases. In infants maintained on prolonged endotracheal intubation and mechanical ventilatory support, this condition is similar to mucous obstruction of bronchial segments. As a result of air trapping and progressive hyperinflation of the affected lung in lobar emphysema, the sequence of mediastinal displacement and bilateral pulmonary compression may be initiated and demand emergency thoracotomy and lobectomy. The chest roentgenogram demonstrates this condition, and it can be differentiated from congenital lung cysts and pneumothorax by the identification of bronchovascular markings in the affected area (Fig. 10).

Adenomatoid Malformation of the Lung (Congenital Cystic Disease). Adenomatoid lung malformation is characterized by the presence of multiple cysts, which impart a honeycomb appearance to the affected lung, most frequently the lower lobe. The resultant roentgenographic appearance may be confused with congenital diaphragmatic hernia, but the presence of normal air-filled intestine beneath the diaphragm in congenital cystic disease provides a distinctive clue.

Neonatal Gastrointestinal Emergencies

NEONATAL INTESTINAL OBSTRUCTION

The presenting signs and symptoms of neonatal intestinal obstruction include maternal hydramnios, excessive gastric aspirate, bilious vomiting, abdominal distention, and obstipation.

The development of *maternal hydramnios* frequently indicates obstruction of the proximal gastrointestinal tract in the fetus, since during gestation amniotic fluid is continually ingested and absorbed from the intestine. Normally, this fluid is transferred to the maternal circulation via the placenta and is partially excreted in the urine of the mother. In the presence of upper gastrointestinal obstruction, however, this cycle is interrupted and amniotic fluid accumulates. A mechanism is thereby provided for alerting the obstetrician and pediatrician either during the course of the pregnancy or at the time of delivery. A nasogastric tube should be inserted in these circumstances, and aspiration of more than 15 to 20 ml. of fluid, especially when bile-stained, further substantiates the possibility of intestinal obstruction.

The observation of *bilious vomiting* is also highly significant, since healthy, full-term newborn infants frequently "spit up" small amounts of feedings but rarely vomit bile.

Abdominal distention may appear as ingested gas accumulates within the blocked intestine, and the consequent configuration of the protruding abdominal wall may suggest the level of obstruction (i.e., prominence of the epigastrium occurs with obstruction of the stomach or duodenum, while generalized abdominal distention, which is usually delayed in onset until 12 to 24 hours after birth, may signify obstruction of the distal gastrointestinal tract). Failure of an apparently healthy full-term neonate to pass meconium stool by 24 hours also suggests some form of intestinal obstruction, although passage of a small inspissated stool does not necessarily exclude the presence of an obstructing lesion in the proximal gastrointestinal tract.

Abdominal films will usually provide confirmatory evidence of intestinal obstruction, and in some instances may prove pathognomonic (i.e., duodenal obstruction, where a "double bubble" results from distention of the duodenum and stomach). *High intestinal obstruction* is manifested by distended air-filled loops of jejunum and an absence of gas in the distal bowel (Fig. 11). The exact level of a *low intestinal obstruction* may be difficult to define because of similarities in the roentgenographic appearance of distended large and small intestine at this age. In meconium ileus, the abdominal film may demonstrate minute bubbles of gas that intermingle with the meconium within the intestinal lumen and produce a granular "ground glass" appearance. The presence of intraperitoneal and/or scrotal calcifications suggests an antenatal perforation with consequent meconium peritonitis (Fig. 12). Insufflation of air into the stomach via a nasogastric tube may assist in radiographically defining "high" forms of obstruction, but administration of other contrast media is rarely required in these circumstances. A barium enema may demonstrate an unused *microcolon* in low forms of obstruction, or it may confirm intestinal malrotation by identifying the cecum in the upper abdomen. In questionable cases of *intestinal malrotation,* an upper gastrointestinal roentgenographic series confirms downward displacement of the duodenojejunal junction and positioning of the jejunal loops on the right side of the abdomen. In *meconium ileus,* administration of a meglumine diatrizoate (Gastrografin) enema under fluoroscopic monitoring may prove both diagnostic and therapeutic.

Gastric Obstruction

Gastric obstruction is rarely encountered at birth, since the onset of symptoms with *hypertrophic pyloric stenosis* is usually delayed until after the first week of life, and complete or partial blockage by a *congenital pyloric membrane* is exceedingly unusual. The possibility of a gastric obstruction, however, is suggested by nonbilious vomiting and by gaseous distention localized to the stomach.

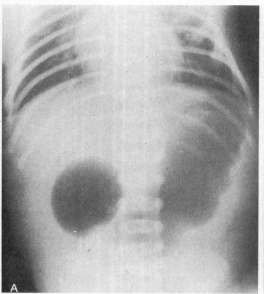
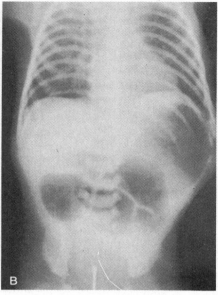

Figure 11. Roentgenographic findings in intestinal atresia. A, The classic "double bubble" sign produced by gaseous distention of the duodenum and stomach and pathognomonic of duodenal atresia. B, Jejunal atresia suggested by multiple loops of air-filled, distended intestine, which are limited to the upper abdomen. (From Haller, J. A., Jr., and Talbert, J. L.: Surgical Emergencies in the Newborn. Philadelphia, Lea & Febiger, 1972, pp. 87, 88.)

Duodenal Obstruction

Duodenal obstruction in the newborn may be produced by congenital duodenal atresia or stenosis, annular pancreas, or lateral peritoneal bands (Ladd's bands) in association with intestinal malrotation. Bilious vomiting characterizes each of these entities, since even in those circumstances where the ampulla of Vater drains distal to the obstruction, accessory ducts usually allow bile flow into the proximal duodenum. *Annular pancreas* is frequently associated with prematurity; *duodenal atresia* occurs with Down's syndrome in 25 to 30 per cent of patients.[7] Other anomalies, especially cardiac, are also frequent in Down's syndrome.

In most patients with duodenal obstruction from atresia, stenosis, or annular pancreas, operative correction can be achieved by performing a direct anastomosis between the proximal and distal duodenal segments with avoidance of injury to the pancreas and to the biliary ducts. A gastrostomy also facilitates management of these patients, providing a reliable mechanism for decompressing the stomach and safe administration of postoperative feedings.

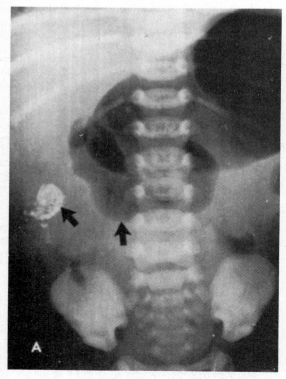
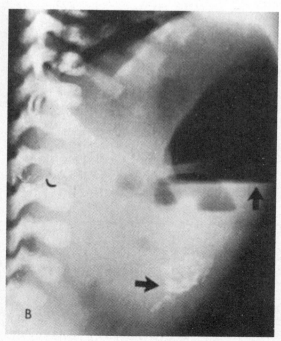

Figure 12. Abdominal roentgenograms in a newborn demonstrating calcifications, which suggest meconium peritonitis as the etiology of the associated intestinal obstruction. (From Holder, T. M., and Ashcraft, K. W. (Eds.): Pediatric Surgery. Philadelphia, W. B. Saunders Company, 1980, p. 368.)

Intestinal Malrotation

Intestinal malrotation may produce partial obstruction as a consequence of extrinsic compression of the distal duodenum by fibrous bands that attach the malpositioned cecum to the lateral peritoneal wall and liver. Relief of obstruction is achieved by division of these bands in concert with mobilization of the duodenum and small intestine to the right, and the cecum and large bowel to the left of the abdomen *(Ladd's procedure)*. An appendectomy should be performed because of the diagnostic confusion that may arise later as a consequence of the distorted anatomy.

Embryologically, intestinal malrotation reflects events occurring at the tenth week of gestation when the midgut returns to the abdominal cavity from a prolapsed position within the umbilical cord (Fig. 13). In the course of this process, the cecum and duodenum undergo a counterclockwise rotation around the superior mesenteric artery, eventually resulting in the broad mesenteric attachment of the small bowel, which ordinarily extends downward and obliquely from the ligament of Treitz to the right lower quadrant. If this process is interrupted, however, and the cecum remains positioned high in the upper abdomen, the entire midgut is suspended by only a narrow vascular pedicle, which may readily twist and thereby produce a volvulus with consequent intestinal ischemia. This catastrophe should be suspected in any newborn who presents a clinical picture of duodenal obstruction, abdominal distention, palpable abdominal mass, and bloody stools. In these circumstances, peritonitis and shock may ensue rapidly. Because of the threat of impending intestinal infarction, immediate diagnosis and surgical intervention are imperative. *Indeed, the possibility of midgut volvulus must always be given first consideration in any neonate who vomits bile because of the irreparable and frequently lethal damage that may ensue if treatment is delayed.*

At operation, the volvulus can be relieved by rotation of the intestine in a counterclockwise manner, following which the underlying intestinal malrotation is corrected by Ladd's procedure (Fig. 14). Any necrotic intestine should be resected. However, if the extent of nonviable bowel appears incompatible with long-term survival, resection may be deferred for 24 to 36 hours, at which time re-exploration for a "second look" allows any gangrenous segments to be clearly defined.

Intestinal Atresia

Intestinal atresia is the most frequent congenital cause of newborn intestinal obstruction, with the ileum affected in approximately 50 per cent of patients, followed by the duodenum, jejunum, and colon in order of occurrence. Jejunal and ileal atresia has been confirmed by antenatal experiments in puppies to be a consequence of occlusion of the fetal mesenteric blood supply, with the resultant intestinal infarction producing a spectrum of deformities, varying from localized webs to extensive defects in both intestine and adjacent mesentery. Successful surgical correction is often complicated by the challenge of anastomosing a markedly distended, proximally obstructed segment to a minute distal lumen.[1, 15] In those instances when stretching of the wall of the proximal bowel has been so great as to impede effective peristalsis, resection of the affected segment or temporary decompression via an enterostomy may be required. Eventual end-to-end or end-to-oblique anastomosis is usually preferred in these cases, with tapering of the proximal bowel sometimes required to facilitate establishment of a functional union (Fig. 15). Because of the possibility of associated distal stenoses, which may not be readily evident on inspection of the intestine, bowel patency must be confirmed prior to performing the anastomosis by intraoperative injection of saline or preoperative roentgenographic contrast studies.[1]

Meconium Ileus

Meconium ileus occurs in approximately 10 per cent of neonates with cystic fibrosis. As a consequence of the absence of pancreatic enzymes, the meconium is poorly dissolved and accumulates as thick, tenacious concretions that plug the distal ileum and cecum (Fig. 16). Passage of stools following birth is delayed, and the irregular rubbery masses of meconium can often be palpated in the obstructed bowel. Intestinal atresia and stenosis may also accompany this condition as a consequence of an antenatal volvulus or perforation of the distended bowel.

Diagnosis of meconium ileus is aided by demonstration of the characteristic ground glass appearance on abdominal roentgenogram. In these circumstances, a contrast enema confirms a distal unused microcolon with obstruction of the cecum and terminal ileum by inspissated meconium. If the

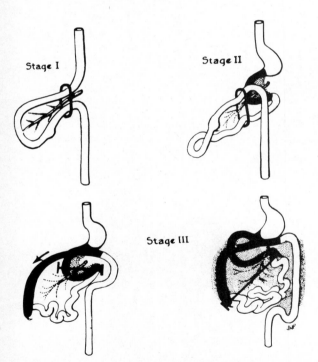

Figure 13. The embryology of intestinal rotation and normal fixation.

Stage I *depicts protrusion of the midgut into the base of the umbilical cord.*

Stage II *represents withdrawal of the duodenum within the abdomen, followed by rotation and eventual placement of the duodenojejunal junction below and to the left of the superior mesenteric vessels.*

Stage III, *indicating completion of intestinal rotation by withdrawal of the remaining midgut and colon within the abdomen and passage of the cecum above the superior mesenteric vessels, downward and to the right. Eventual fixation of the cecum in the right lower quadrant stabilizes the intestinal mesentery along a broad base which extends upward and medially to the ligament of Treitz.*

(From Holder, T. M., and Ashcraft, K. W. (Eds.): Pediatric Surgery. Philadelphia, W. B. Saunders Company, 1980, p. 347.)

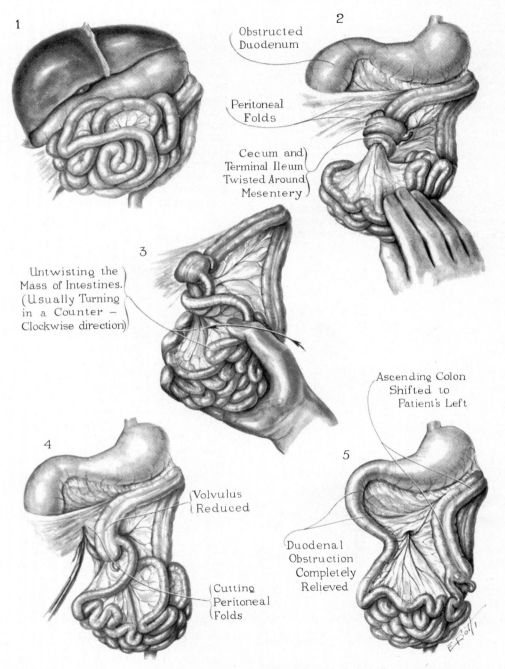

1

2

Obstructed
Duodenum

Peritoneal
Folds

Cecum and
Terminal Ileum
Twisted Around
Mesentery

3

Untwisting the
Mass of Intestines.
(Usually Turning
in a Counter –
Clockwise direction)

Ascending Colon
Shifted to
Patient's Left

4

5

Volvulus
Reduced

Duodenal
Obstruction
Completely
Relieved

Cutting
Peritoneal
Folds

Figure 14. Intestinal malrotation with obstruction produced both by duodenal bands and by midgut volvulus. The volvulus is corrected by untwisting the mass of intestine in a counterclockwise direction, while the duodenal compression and obstruction are relieved by dividing the lateral peritoneal bands. The operation is completed by a Ladd's procedure, in which the duodenum and jejunum are positioned to the right of the abdomen and the cecum and ascending colon to the left of the abdomen, thereby preventing subsequent recurrence of either duodenal obstruction or midgut volvulus. (From Gross, R. E.: An Atlas of Children's Surgery. Philadelphia, W. B. Saunders Company, 1970, p. 19.)

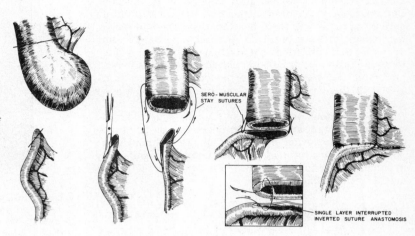

Figure 15. Surgical correction of intestinal atresia. The distended and atonic proximal pouch is resected back to relatively normal bowel. An anastomosis is then performed to the tiny distal lumen in an end-to-oblique manner, utilizing a single layer of interrupted, inverted fine suture. (From Holder, T. M., and Ashcraft, K. W. (Eds.): Pediatric Surgery. Philadelphia, W. B. Saunders Company, 1980, p. 342.)

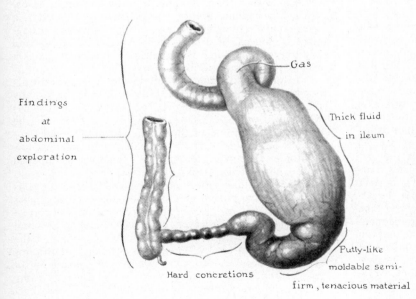

Figure 16. Meconium ileus. A depiction of the characteristic findings at abdominal exploration, with marked distention of the proximal bowel and blockage of the distal ileum and cecum by hard meconium concretions. (Modified from Gross, R. E.: An Atlas of Children's Surgery. Philadelphia, W. B. Saunders Company, p. 23.)

study is performed with meglumine diatrizoate under fluoroscopic monitoring, it may not only prove diagnostic but may also assist in mobilizing the inspissated meconium and inducing its passage. This procedure may need to be repeated on several occasions until complete evacuation of the meconium is achieved. When an associated anatomic obstruction is identified, or when the meglumine diatrizoate enemas are ineffectual, surgical exploration is indicated. Intraoperative evacuation of the meconium and performance of a primary intestinal anastomosis are often feasible, but in some instances a staged approach involving creation of temporary diverting enterostomies with subsequent cleansing of the intestine and delayed anastomosis may be preferable. Supplementation of pancreatic enzyme is required in these patients following resumption of regular feedings.

The eventual outcome in meconium ileus is largely dependent on the severity of the underlying cystic fibrosis and its accompanying pulmonary disease, although the potential for long-term survival has improved significantly in recent years as a consequence of advances in the overall management of this condition.

Meconium Plug Syndrome

Meconium plug syndrome connotes localized obstruction of the distal colon by a tenacious mass of inspissated meconium in the absence of cystic fibrosis. In most instances, digital examination of the rectum and/or barium enema will induce spontaneous passage of the obstructing cast of meconium with subsequent complete relief of symptoms. However, *Hirschsprung's disease* should be suspected as a possible underlying etiology in all infants affected by the meconium plug syndrome.

Hirschsprung's Disease (Congenital Megacolon)

Hirschsprung's disease characteristically occurs in male infants as a consequence of a congenital absence of myenteric parasympathetic ganglia in the rectum and colon, with this deficiency almost always beginning in the anus and extending proximally in the bowel wall for variable distances. Rarely, the process may involve the entire colon and even the small intestine. The functional obstruction that is produced by abnormal innervation of the distal bowel is usually manifested by chronic constipation dating from birth. Passage of the first meconium stool is delayed beyond 24 hours, and persistence of obstruction may require performance of an emergency colostomy. This characteristic onset of symptoms in early infancy is an important clue in distinguishing congenital megacolon from the acquired megacolon that may ensue later, often at the time of toilet training. Hirschsprung's disease may also be manifested by alternating constipation and diarrhea, or even diarrhea alone, in association with failure to thrive. Of special note is the potential for affected infants to develop a fulminant enterocolitis that is usually preceded by explosive diarrhea, in association with massive fluid, electrolyte, and protein losses, with rapid progression to sepsis and shock. Enterocolitis represents a grave complication of Hirshsprung's disease with a high mortality rate.

The diagnosis of Hirschsprung's disease is suggested by a barium enema, performed on unprepared bowel and demonstrating the dilation and hypertrophy of the proximal normally innervated colon, which develops in response to the distal functional obstruction (Fig. 17). Twenty-four hour follow-up roentgenograms are especially helpful in confirming the delay of normal emptying and in defining the exact

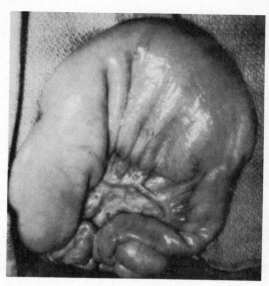

Figure 17. Hirschsprung's disease. At operation, the relatively collapsed, aganglionic bowel contrasts with the normally innervated, proximal colon, which has become markedly dilated and hypertrophied in response to the distal, functional obstruction. (From Holder, T. M., and Ashcraft, K. W. (Eds.): Pediatric Surgery. Philadelphia, W. B. Saunders Company, 1980, p. 389.)

level of obstruction. However, roentgenographic diagnosis may be unreliable in a newborn infant because of insufficient time for significant dilation and hypertrophy to evolve in the proximal bowel.

Definitive diagnosis of Hirschsprung's disease is provided by a full-thickness biopsy of the rectal wall, which confirms absence of ganglion cells in the myenteric plexus. A valuable modification of this technique, which offers a safe, reliable screening method, involves obtaining a fragment of mucosa and submucosa by suction biopsy and histologically verifying the presence or absence of ganglion cells in the submucosal plexus.

In the young infant presenting with intestinal obstruction and/or fulminant enterocolitis, a diverting colostomy should be established immediately. After the patient has grown to a weight of 10 kg., definitive correction can be performed using one of three standard pull-through procedures (Swenson, Duhamel, or Soave) to create a low anastomosis between the normally innervated proximal bowel and the anus. Although the specific technical details of these operations differ, in experienced hands the results with each have proved good and the long-term prognosis for patients who have undergone successful surgical correction is excellent.[24] However, early recognition and prompt intervention are clearly essential in this condition if the complications of growth retardation and fatal enterocolitis are to be avoided. *As a consequence, the possibility of Hirschsprung's disease must always be considered in any infant who presents with chronic constipation, persistent diarrhea, alternating constipation and diarrhea, and/or failure to thrive.*

Imperforate Anus (Anal Atresia)

Although abnormalities of the anal orifice should be readily evident at birth, they may be overlooked in the absence of a careful examination of the perineum. Functionally, patients with imperforate anus may be divided into two major groups:

1. Those with an absent anus but with adequate decompression of the gastrointestinal tract achieved via an external fistulous tract.

2. Those with an absent anus and with no fistula or an inadequate tract for egress of stool (Fig. 18).

The first group involves predominantly female infants who present with relatively large rectovaginal or rectofourchette fistulas through which, often with the assistance of dilations, adequate temporary decompression of the intestine can be achieved. In the second group, the absence of any mechanism for achieving spontaneous decompression of the colon demands some form of immediate surgical intervention. Such patients may be further classified into two anatomic subgroups:

1. A low-lying rectal pouch allows a satisfactory anoproctoplasty to be readily accomplished via a transperineal operative approach.

2. A high-lying rectal pouch, positioned cephalad to the puborectalis sling and urogenital diaphragm and almost always associated with a fistulous connection to the urethra, bladder, or upper vagina, prohibits operative access via the perineum.

The second subgroup group includes the majority (60 per cent) of male infants with imperforate anus who are best managed initially by construction of a diverting abdominal colostomy. Since identification of a fistula to the urinary tract in males almost always signifies a high-lying rectal pouch, it is essential that samples of all voidings be examined for the presence of meconium in the urine. Roentgenograms of the abdomen and pelvis may also confirm a fistulous communication to the urinary tract by demonstrating air in the bladder. In patients with perineal or vaginal fistulae, passage of a small catheter via the fistulous tract and injection of contrast media will clearly define the anatomy of the defect and facilitate planning for subsequent surgical correction. In the absence of a demonstrable fistula, Wangensteen-Rice "upside down" roentgenographic studies of the abdomen and pelvis have been utilized in the past to clarify the level of the blind rectal pouch. Unfortunately, this technique may prove misleading, especially in the first few days of life, since air may not have had adequate opportunity to traverse the entire intestine or may be prevented by the tenacious meconium from filling the distal pouch. In some instances, pelvic sonography may assist in identifying the pouch and in guiding transperineal insertion of a needle through which contrast media can be injected to define the exact anatomic position of the pouch.

In general, the accepted plan for successfully managing a patient with imperforate anus is to proceed with a proximal diverting colostomy whenever the possibility of a high-lying rectal pouch cannot be excluded by preoperative studies, since an unsuccessful attempt to perform a transperineal anoproctoplasty may seriously jeopardize any future capability for achieving an adequate repair. In infants who have fistulous communications to the urinary tract, a diverting colostomy not only ensures adequate decompression of the obstructed intestine but also protects against urinary contamination, infection, and potentially serious renal damage.

The majority of female infants (70 per cent) with this defect have a low-lying rectal pouch, which is usually associated with a rectovaginal or rectofourchette fistula. Fistulas to the urinary tract are almost nonexistent in females because of the protection provided by the interposed reproductive organs.

Imperforate anus is associated with other congenital anomalies in a high percentage of patients. Because of the high frequency of urologic abnormalities, an intravenous pyelogram should be obtained in all patients. Spinal anomalies are also frequent, and roentgenographic screening of the lumbosacral spine is especially indicated.

A transperineal approach for correction of a low rectal pouch is feasible in approximately 40 per cent of males and 70 per cent of females and can achieve a high level of functional success because of relatively normal anatomy and sphincteric musculature in such patients. In those with a perineal or vaginal fistula sufficiently patent to maintain interim decompression of the intestinal tract, definitive correction can be deferred until 3 to 6 months of age. When a temporary colostomy is required for initial management of a high type of rectal pouch, a definitive pull-through procedure may be postponed until the patient's weight approximates 10 kg. Classically, an abdominosacroperineal approach is employed to facilitate identification and division of the fistula and to ensure optimal utilization and preservation of the levator ani muscle and its component puborectalis sling. However, a persistently high incidence of postoperative fecal incontinence and anal mucosal prolapse has led Pena and deVries to advocate a posterior sagittal approach with division of the levator ani and external sphincter muscles in the midline to facilitate mobilization of the proximal rectal pouch and division of any associated fistula.[2] Following transposition of the pouch to the perineum, the pelvic structures are precisely reconstructed. Initial results with this procedure have proved encouraging, although further follow-up is required to determine the exact level of success in achieving long-term fecal continence.

NEONATAL INTESTINAL PERFORATION

Because fetal intestinal contents are sterile and remain so during the first few days of life, perforation during this period produces only a reactive form of peritonitis. If leakage occurs later, however, the usual pattern of bacterial peritonitis ensues.

Antepartum perforation may occur during fetal development following intrauterine intestinal obstruction or ischemia and result in a sterile *meconium peritonitis*, which may be demonstrated roentgenographically by intra-abdominal or scrotal calcifications if the peritoneal spillage precedes closure of the processus vaginalis (see Fig. 12). In some instances, persistent leakage will lead to formation of a large *meconium cyst*, which may occur in the newborn as

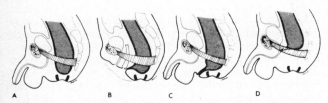

Figure 18. Major types of imperforate anus. A, A low pouch anomaly in a male, with the rectum passing through the puborectalis sling and no fistula. B, A low pouch anomaly in a female, with the rectum passing through the puborectalis sling and a fistula communicating with the vaginal fourchette. C, A low pouch anomaly in a male, with the rectum passing through the puborectalis sling and a fistula communicating to the perineum. D, A high pouch anomaly in a male, with the rectum positioned cephalad to the puborectalis sling and a fistula communicating to the urethra. (From Leape, L.L., and Holder, T. M.: Pediatric surgery. In Sabiston, D. C., Jr. (Ed.): Davis-Christopher Textbook of Surgery, 12th ed. Philadelphia, W. B. Saunders Company, 1981, p. 1378.)

A   B   C   D

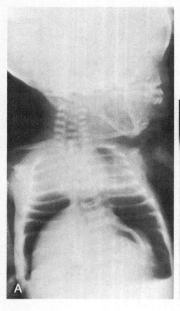
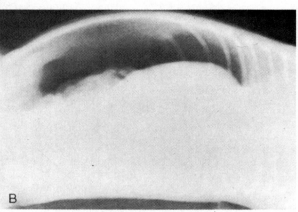

Figure 19. Tension pneumoperitoneum in a 2-day-old infant resulting from spontaneous gastric perforation and confirmed by (A) upright and (B) lateral decubitus abdominal roentgenograms demonstrating the classic "saddle bag" appearance produced by the accumulation of free air anterior and lateral to the abdominal viscera. (From Haller, J. A., Jr., and Talbert, J. L.: Surgical Emergencies in the Newborn. Philadelphia, Lea & Febiger, 1972, p. 108.)

an abdominal mass and which may be associated with intestinal obstruction.

Postpartum perforation is usually signified by pneumoperitoneum and may follow an iatrogenic injury, or perforation of an ischemic, inflamed or obstructed segment of bowel. These conditions result in peritoneal contamination by intestinal contents and must be differentiated from the occasional occurrence of *spontaneous pneumoperitoneum* in newborn infants who are maintained on mechanical ventilation and in whom air extravasated into the mediastinal and intraperitoneal tissues may eventually dissect into the peritoneal cavity. Potential souces of *iatrogenic injury* include colonic perforation by a thermometer that may be inadvertently inserted beyond the confines of the short rectal canal of a newborn infant or by penetration of the proximal gastrointestinal tract, most often the duodenum, by a feeding catheter.

Spontaneous Gastric Perforation

Spontaneous gastric perforation represents an unusual condition that characteristically appears within the first week of life in an infant who, after an initial period of mild distress, subsequently does well until massive abdominal distention develops following initiation of feedings (Fig. 19). The resultant tension pneumoperitoneum may produce severe cardiorespiratory embarrassment and require prompt decompression. At exploration, a tear can usually be identified along the greater curvature of the stomach; however, the etiology remains obscure in most instances. The possibility of its being caused by a nasogastric tube or from high intragastric pressure following resuscitation must be considered.

Neonatal Necrotizing Enterocolitis

Neonatal necrotizing enterocolitis (NEC) represents an unfortunate sequel to the advent of sophisticated techniques for supporting premature infants and indeed is now the most commonly encountered acquired form of neonatal gastrointestinal emergency.[12] Although the overall incidence approximates 2 per cent of all admissions to neonatal intensive care units, the frequency is inversely proportional to gestational age, with as many as 12 per cent of low-birth-weight infants affected.

Characteristically, this entity presents between the third and tenth day in premature stressed infants following the initiation of formula feedings. They develop lethargy, bilious vomiting, abdominal distention, and bloody stools. Although the diagnosis may be suspected on the basis of the characteristic clinical presentation, confirmation is dependent on the roentgenographic demonstration of *pneumatosis intestinalis* or intrahepatic gas (Fig. 20). The terminal ileum and ascending colon are affected primarily, and histologic examination in these instances reveals intramural hemorrhage and necrosis in association with subserosal and submucosal gas.

Although the etiology remains obscure, hypotheses have focused increasingly on three possible causes, either separately or in combination: (1) intestinal ischemia, (2) abnormal bacterial colonization by highly pathogenic flora, and (3) accumulation of an excess of protein substrate in the intestinal lumen.[13] Intestinal ischemia may follow vasospasm, vascular thrombosis, or reduced cardiac output. Vasospasm may represent a recognized physiologic response to asphyxia, the so-called "diving reflex," by which blood flow is selectively diverted to the brain and heart at the expense of other organs, whereas thrombosis may follow microemboli or hypertonic solutions infused through umbilical vessel catheters. The emergence of pathogenic flora has been attributed to a delay in colonization, fostered by maintenance of these infants in a relatively sterile environment (the neonatal intensive care unit), and an absence of immunoprotective factors in commercial formula.

Medical treatment of NEC includes nasogastric decompression, maintenance of adequate hydration with vascular expansion, ventilatory support, and parenteral administration of broad-spectrum antibiotics. Frequent roentgenographic monitoring for the appearance of pneumoperitoneum or other serious complications should be maintained every 6 hours during the acute phase. Although surgical intervention is clearly demanded in the presence of intestinal perforation, as signaled by the appearance of pneumoperitoneum, other indications may include persistence of a palpable abdominal mass (usually

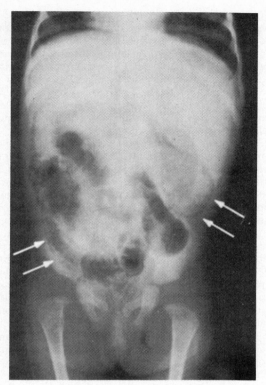

Figure 20. Necrotizing enterocolitis as confirmed by pneumatosis intestinalis. (Arrows outline linear strips of intramural gas in the bowel wall.) (From Leape, L. L., and Holder, T. M.: Pediatric surgery. In Sabiston, D. C., Jr. (Ed.): Davis-Christopher Textbook of Surgery. 12th ed. Philadelphia, W. B. Saunders Company, 1981, p. 1385.)

located in the right lower quadrant), repeated roentgenographic demonstration of a dilated loop of bowel, erythema of the abdominal wall, severe gastrointestinal hemorrhage, and/or failure to respond to medical therapy as manifested by progressive thrombocytopenia, acidosis, and shock. Paracentesis has proved to be a valuable technique, especially in the presence of ascites, for confirming bowel necrosis by providing brown-stained peritoneal fluid in which bacteria can be identified by Gram's stain and culture.

A special challenge for the surgeon at the time of exploration for NEC may be the differentiation of potentially salvageable bowel from that in which complete transmural necrosis has occurred. If it is feasible, gangrenous segments should be resected and defunctionalizing enterostomies constructed. Rarely, in patients with localized necrosis, resection and primary anastomosis may be achieved. However, when the gangrenous process appears so extensive that resection of all involved bowel will be incompatible with long-term survival, a repeat second-look laparotomy in 24 hours may assist in more clearly defining the limits of injury.

The surgical mortality in NEC has been reported at 20 to 40 per cent. The major long-term complications include (1) stricture formation in 10 to 40 per cent and (2) "short gut" syndrome in 10 per cent of survivors. With the high frequency of strictures, roentgenographic contrast studies of the distal bowel must be obtained prior to operative closure of diverting enterostomies and reanastomosis of the intestine. Although NEC represents a clinically frustrating and, potentially, highly dangerous condition, the long-term follow-up of infants who have been successfully treated has been encouraging, since growth and development have appeared comparable with matched controls.

NEONATAL GASTROINTESTINAL BLEEDING

Neonatal gastrointestinal bleeding of surgical significance usually accompanies those conditions such as *volvulus, intussusception,* or *NEC* in which mucosal erosion and ulceration occur as a consequence of intestinal ischemia and/or congestion. Rarely, *a stress ulcer* of the stomach or duodenum may develop at this age and requires surgical exploration and direct suture ligation of a bleeding vessel in the base to control rapid exsanguination.

Abdominal Wall Defects

Congenital full-thickness abdominal wall defects pose a lethal threat to the newborn infant as a consequence of exposed viscera and the potential for bacterial contamination. The two most common of such defects are *gastroschisis* and *omphalocele*, with the latter usually distinguished by an intact sac of peritoneum covering intra-abdominal viscera that are herniated into the base of the umbilical cord (Fig. 21). In gastroschisis, there is no evidence of a peritoneal sac and the viscera freely extrude through a full-thickness defect in the abdominal wall, which is often relatively small and is usually located lateral and to the right of an intact umbilical cord. The exposed loops of bowel often have a characteristic dark, thickened, foreshortened, and matted appearance as a consequence of

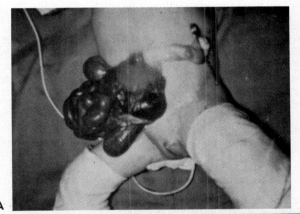

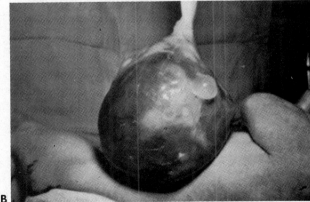

Figure 21. A, A typical gastroschisis defect of the abdominal wall, located immediately to the right of the umbilicus, and through which thick, dark, matted, and foreshortened intestine is freely extruded. B, A giant omphalocele characterized by a large, intact peritoneal sac located at the base of the umbilicus and containing liver and intestine. (From Grosfeld, J. L., Dawes, L., and Weber, T. R.: Symposium on pediatric surgery. Surg. Clin. North Am. 61:1038, 1939, 1981.)

their intrauterine exposure to amniotic fluid. In most instances, the limited size of the gastroschisis defect allows evisceration of only stomach and intestine and may pose a threat of compression and occlusion of the mesenteric vessels in the presence of intestinal distention. This potential is confirmed by the frequent finding of intestinal atresia and stenosis in this condition.

The incidence of omphalocele has been reported between 1:3000 and 1:10,000 live births, whereas the incidence of gastroschisis has undergone a remarkable change over the past two decades, with an increase in frequency from 1:150,000 live births in the 1960s to an experience today which, in some centers, is comparable to that with omphalocele. Gastroschisis tends to occur in babies of young primigravida mothers, and with a high incidence of prematurity (60 per cent). Other anomalies are encountered in 15 to 20 per cent of gastroschisis patients and are usually limited to the gastrointestinal tract. In contrast, the majority of omphaloceles are found to have associated anomalies, with an especially high frequency of cardiovascular and gastrointestinal defects as well as an occurrence of Beckwith-Wiedemann syndrome and a variety of chromosomal abnormalities (Table 1).

The exact etiology of gastroschisis remains unclear, although it has been hypothesized to represent an intrauterine rupture of the amniotic membrane at the base of the umbilical cord. The embryologic etiology of omphalocele has been thought to be a failure of fusion of the cephalic, caudal, and lateral abdominal wall folds, with a central defect resulting from inhibition of the lateral wall folds and epigastric and low midline omphaloceles resulting, respectively, from an interruption in migration of the cephalic and caudal folds. Epigastric omphaloceles may be associated with defects of the lower sternum, diaphragm, and heart, whereas caudal omphaloceles may be accompanied by genitourinary and gastrointestinal anomalies, including cloacal exstrophy (vesicointestinal fissure).

Preoperative preparation of the patient with a congenital abdominal wall defect must focus immediately on the prevention of hypothermia, hypovolemia, acidosis, bacterial contamination, and vascular compromise of the eviscerated bowel. The intact sac of an omphalocele provides some degree of protection for the contained viscera, but in gastroschisis the exposed intestine represents a source of significant evaporative water loss and rapid body cooling. Accordingly, the patient must be placed in a heated environment immediately. The exposed organs must also be covered by sterile, moist saline dressings and protected by enclosing them within a plastic wrap or by inserting the distal two thirds of the infant's body into a sterile "bowel bag." An orogastric tube must be passed to decompress the proximal gastrointestinal tract, and in those instances in which an excessively tight defect presents a significant threat to mesenteric blood flow in the contained bowel, it should be enlarged immediately by incising the margin. Intravenous fluids and broad-spectrum antibiotics should be given and metabolic acidosis should be corrected.

Intra-abdominal reduction of the exposed viscera and primary closure of skin, or even fascia, will usually prove feasible in gastroschisis, after the intestine has been adequately decompressed and the peritoneal cavity enlarged by manual stretching of the abdominal wall. When intestinal atresia is identified, primary anastomosis or, more frequently, temporary diverting enterostomy is required. If primary closure of the gastroschisis proves unfeasible or appears to produce an intolerable level of intra-abdominal pressure, a staged closure may be achieved by constructing a prosthetic pouch (a Silastic "silo" or "chimney") within which the exposed viscera can be contained. The protruding silo is progressively shortened over the next 7 to 10 days, as spontaneous stretching of the abdominal wall muscles and decompression of the intestine gradually allow the contained viscera to be replaced within the peritoneal cavity. Fascial and/or skin closure can then be accomplished (Fig. 22). Since prolonged intestinal malfunction frequently ensues, the advent of improved techniques for parenteral nutrition and mechanical ventilation has contributed importantly to the recent dramatic improvement in the mortality rate, which has decreased from levels of 80 per cent in the 1950s and 1960s to only 10 per cent today.

The frequent association of other serious anomalies and/or large size of the omphalocele present special challenges in the successful management of this entity. Unless antenatal rupture of the sac has occurred, the contained bowel is protected from contact with amniotic fluid and, accordingly, escapes the characteristic changes observed with gastroschisis. The techniques described for correction of gastroschisis are usually successful in achieving closure of an omphalocele, but nonoperative management has also been advocated in the presence of an intact sac, when there is a giant defect exceeding 8 cm. in diameter or when there are associated life-threatening anomalies that demand immediate correction. This approach has been utilized most often in European centers. The omphalocele sac is coated with a bacteriostatic agent to prevent infection and is covered by sterile dressings until closure is achieved by a gradual ingrowth of epithelium from the margins of the defect. The resultant ventral hernia can then be closed later electively.

In contrast to the dramatic improvement in survival of patients with gastroschisis that has occurred over the past 2 decades, the overall mortality for patients with omphaloceles has remained relatively stable at 20 to 30 per cent, largely as a consequence of the frequent association of other serious life-threatening anomalies.[16] Accordingly, concise preoperative evaluation is imperative, and the exact form of surgical management must be individualized.

TABLE 1. *Syndromes Commonly Associated with Omphalocele**

Pentalogy of Cantrell (Defect in Cephalad Embryonic Fold)
1. Upper midline omphalocele
2. Anterior diaphragmatic hernia
3. Sternal cleft
4. Ectopia cordis
5. Intracardiac defects

Lower Midline Syndrome (Defect in Caudal Embryonic Fold)
1. Bladder or cloacal exstrophy
2. Imperforate anus
3. Colonic atresia
4. Vesicointestinal fissure
5. Sacral vertebral anomalies
6. Meningomyelocele

Beckwith-Weidemann Syndrome
1. Gigantism
2. Macroglossia
3. Omphalocele or umbilical hernia
4. Pancreatic islet cell hyperplasia

Trisomy Syndromes
1. Trisomy 13–15
2. Trisomy 16–18

*Modified from Grosfeld, J. L.: Surg. Clin. North Am. *61*:1039, 1981.

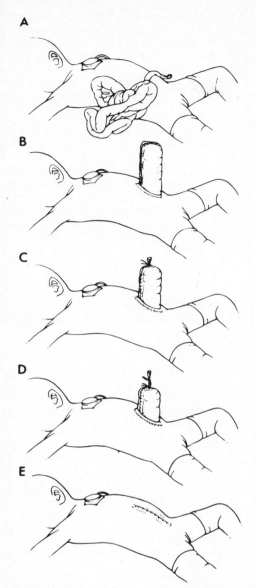

Figure 22. Staged closure of a gastroschisis defect of the abdominal wall utilizing a Dacron-reinforced Silastic "silo." The extruded viscera are encompassed within the silo and are gradually reduced into the abdominal cavity over the subsequent 7 to 10 days, until complete wound closure can be achieved. (From Grosfeld, J. L. (Ed.): Symposium on pediatric surgery. Surg. Clin. North Am. 61:1041, 1981.)

Neonatal Jaundice

Although transient jaundice occurs relatively often within the first few weeks of life, subsequent persistence or onset of jaundice may signify the presence of biliary obstruction produced either by *atresia of the biliary tract* or by a *congenital choledochal cyst*. The latter condition is encountered most frequently in young female infants in whom a palpable right upper quadrant abdominal mass is associated with hyperbilirubinemia. Most other causes of jaundice occurring in infants beyond 2 weeks of age can be identified on the basis of history and appropriate laboratory studies, but differentiation between neonatal hepatitis and atresia of the biliary tract can prove especially difficult. The urgency of promptly establishing the diagnosis of biliary

atresia is reflected by the fact that surgical correction undertaken by 8 weeks of age results in a relatively high success rate, whereas any delay beyond 12 weeks is fraught with a dismal prognosis.[5, 8] Radioactive nuclide scanning of the liver has proved to be the most helpful method for confirming patency of the bile ducts, and appearance of the isotope in the gastrointestinal tract effectively excludes the presence of complete biliary obstruction. The diagnostic accuracy of this technique may be enhanced by pretreatment of the infant with phenobarbital. In those patients in whom the isotope is concentrated in the liver but in whom none is excreted in the intestine, and in whom the diagnosis of biliary atresia cannot be excluded, a limited laparotomy with liver biopsy and operative cholangiogram is indicated. When the cholangiogram confirms patency of the biliary tract and the liver biopsy shows hepatitis, no further surgery is required. When the gallbladder is absent or the cholangiogram demonstrates obstruction of the common bile duct, surgical exploration of the extrahepatic biliary tract should be undertaken. In approximately 10 per cent of such cases, a favorable anatomic configuration is encountered that will permit anastomosis of a hepatic or common bile duct to a Roux-en-Y limb of jejunum with a high probability of success. In the remaining patients, a fibrous remnant of common duct should be carefully dissected into the porta hepatis where transection and histologic examination will often confirm persistence of microscopically patent biliary channels (Fig. 23). In this circumstance, a modified Kasai hepatoportoenterostomy offers an excellent possibility of relieving the biliary obstruction and jaundice. In this procedure, an isolated limb of jejunum is anastomosed at the porta hepatis to the fibrous remnant containing the rudimentary bile ducts and is drained externally through a distal enterostomy (Fig. 24). Postoperative cholangitis with con-

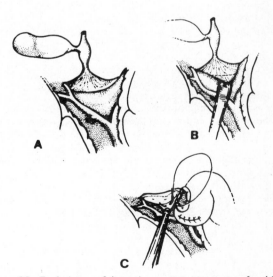

Figure 23. Technique of hepatic portoenterostomy for biliary atresia. A, The rudimentary extrahepatic biliary tract, including the gallbladder, has been isolated, transected distally, and reflected upward. B, The underlying portal vein and hepatic arteries are reflected downward, exposing the fan-shaped web of fibrous tissue at the base of the obliterated extrahepatic biliary tract, which is then transected (dotted line) and examined histologically for microductules. C, Following confirmation of rudimentary bile ducts, an isolated limb of jejunum is meticulously anastomosed to the transected fibrous stump at the porta hepatis. (From Grosfeld, J. L. (Ed.): Symposium on pediatric surgery. Surg. Clin. North Am. 61:1084, 1981.)

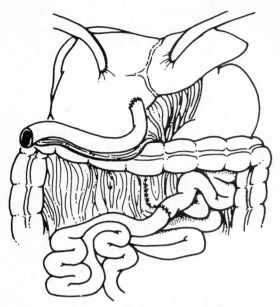

Figure 24. Completion of the Kasai portoenterostomy (Sawaguchi modification). Following completion of the proximal anastomosis at the porta hepatis, the isolated limb of jejunum is drained distally via a cutaneous enterostomy, allowing collection and refeeding of the excreted bile. After 18 to 24 months, the enterostomy can be taken down and internal drainage of bile established by direct anastomosis and drainage of the jejunal limb into the intestinal tract. (From Weber, T. R., and Grosfeld, J. L.: Symposium on pediatric surgery. Surg. Clin. North Am., 61:1085, 1981.)

sequent progressive fibrosis represents a significant long-term threat to infants who have undergone successful portoenterostomy, but the frequency and severity of this problem can be reduced by external venting of the biliary conduit and by prophylactic antibiotics during the first 2 and 3 years of life. In patients in whom adequate bile flow has been maintained for 18 to 24 months, the diverting enterostomy can be subsequently closed and internal drainage achieved by anastomosis to a Roux-en-Y limb of intestine. Present experience indicates that if hepatoporto-enterostomy is performed prior to 3 months of age, an immediate restitution of bile flow can be anticipated in approximately two thirds of patients, with a third of all patients eventually achieving a good, long-term result. Although this experience emphasizes the serious morbidity that continues to accompany biliary atresia, it contrasts dramatically with data reported prior to the advent of the Kasai hepatoportoenterostomy, when only 5 per cent of patients were successfully salvaged over the long term.

Despite significant improvements in operative management, the majority of patients with biliary atresia eventually require liver transplantation for correction of the disorder, and the capability for successfully performing this procedure in children has been enhanced by an immunosuppressive drug regimen incorporating cyclosporine and low-dose steroids.[10, 15, 22] With this approach, the infectious complications that have previously represented a major source of morbidity and mortality following liver transplantation have become less frequent. Other complications previously incurred by the use of "high-dose" steroids, such as growth retardation, Cushing-like features, and bone disease, have also been minimized. The 1-year postoperative survival rate has increased to 65 per cent, and the young age of a patient no longer represents a contraindication to hepatic trans-

plants.[10] In those children who have undergone successful hepatoportoenterostomy, transplantation should be deferred until progressive cholestasis, hepatocellular decompensation, or severe portal hypertension supervenes. However, multiple attempts at hepatoportoenterostomy or surgical portosystemic venous shunting may render eventual transplant surgery technically more difficult and should be avoided.

Ambiguous Genitalia

Ambiguous genitalia, although rarely associated with life-threatening conditions, represent a neonatal surgical emergency because of the importance of achieving immediate evaluation and appropriate gender assignment in order to prevent crippling social and emotional sequelae.[9] In most instances, gender assignment can be accomplished within the first few days of life and surgical repair completed prior to 1 year of age.

SPECIAL PROBLEMS IN INFANTS AND CHILDREN

Foreign Body Aspiration

A frequent cause of respiratory distress in older infants and children that demands prompt diagnosis and surgical treatment is foreign body aspiration. The majority of instances occur in patients between 6 months and 3 years of age and are characterized by a clinical triad of choking while eating, coughing, and wheezing.[17] The diagnosis is initially overlooked in many instances, but a positive history of aspiration can be elicited in over two thirds of patients. This etiology should also be considered in any patient with persistent or recurrent pneumonia and/or atelectasis. A frequent physical finding in foreign body aspiration is wheezing localized to its anatomic site. Confirmation of air trapping and obstructive emphysema by inspiratory and expiratory chest films is also highly suggestive.

Although preoperative physiotherapy and postural drainage have been advocated in an attempt to achieve spontaneous expulsion of the foreign body, this is followed by a low success rate and may prove hazardous. In contrast, endoscopic extraction of the foreign body can be accomplished safely and expeditiously, especially when performed in centers that manage such children routinely and are specifically equipped with pediatric bronchoscopes incorporating telescopic lens systems and optical forceps.

Hypertrophic Pyloric Stenosis

Hypertrophic pyloric stenosis represents a dramatic example of a serious problem in young infants that can be rapidly and safely corrected by surgical intervention. Gastric outlet obstruction develops between 2 weeks and 2 months of age as a consequence of progressive narrowing of the pyloric channel by hypertrophied muscle.

The exact etiology remains unclear, although the feeding of formulas that result in formation of milk curds may potentiate the obstruction and intensify the resultant pyloric spasm and edema. The condition also occurs four times more frequently in males than females, with an incidence of 1:200 live births in Caucasians and 1:2000 live births in blacks. There is a positive family history of pyloric stenosis in 6.9 per cent, and an affected mother has a four times greater chance of transmitting congenital hypertrophic pyloric stenosis to her offspring than does an affected father.

Characteristically, the onset of symptoms in the first few weeks is heralded by nonbilious vomiting, which becomes progressively more frequent and then projectile. This is followed by constipation, emaciation, and dehydration. The stomach becomes large and hypertrophied, and visible peristaltic waves are seen traversing the upper abdomen following feedings. Physical examination often reveals a thin, hungry infant who may also appear dehydrated. The hypertrophic pylorus can usually be defined by deep palpation in the right upper abdomen and is characterized by a firm, mobile, and somewhat elongated "olive." Identification of an "olive" is sufficient indication for surgical intervention. However, when this mass cannot be confirmed by physical examination, an abdominal sonogram or upper gastrointestinal roentgenographic series demonstrating a stringlike narrowing of the pyloric channel will provide a definitive diagnosis.

Preoperative preparation of the patient includes hydration and correction of the hypochloremic, hypokalemic alkalosis that frequently ensues as a consequence of the loss of hydrogen and chloride ions in the vomitus and compensatory excretion of potassium in the urine. Accordingly, adequate fluid resuscitation includes repletion of potassium and chloride deficits by administration of saline solution containing added potassium.

Operative correction of hypertrophic pyloric stenosis is achieved by a pyloromyotomy (Fredet-Ramstedt operation) in which the seromuscular layer is incised longitudinally and spread bluntly to the submucosal base, allowing the underlying mucosa to bulge through the defect (Fig. 25). In the absence of accidental perforation of the duodenal or gastric mucosa, feedings can be instituted within 8 to 12 hours following operation with a normal schedule rapidly being resumed over the next few days.

Gastroesophageal Reflux

Gastroesophageal reflux (GER) or "chalasia" has been previously recognized as a relatively common disorder in infancy, resulting from an incompetence of the lower esophageal sphincter that usually resolves spontaneously with maturation and growth. However, the potential for this problem to produce malnutrition, growth retardation, recurrent aspiration with pneumonia and asthma, esophagitis, esophageal stricture, and even episodes of apnea and sudden death (SIDS) has been emphasized increasingly during the past decade.[3, 22] The clinical features are characterized by persistent postprandial, nonbilious vomiting that fails to respond to thickening and decreased volume of feedings and to placing the infant at a 60-degree upright position.

The association of vomiting in a young infant with failure to thrive, significant respiratory symptoms, or episodes of apnea represents a special indication for intensive evaluation and possible surgical intervention. There is also increasing recognition of clinically significant GER following repair of congenital esophageal atresia and tracheoesophageal fistula. A barium esphagogram may confirm the diagnosis of GER and may also identify a hiatal hernia, which sometimes accompanies this condition in older infants and children and results in esophagitis and stricture formation. However, 24-hour esophageal pH monitoring, utilizing miniaturized equipment, represents the most accurate method for verifying the presence of GER as well as for evaluating the postoperative result. Esophagoscopy and

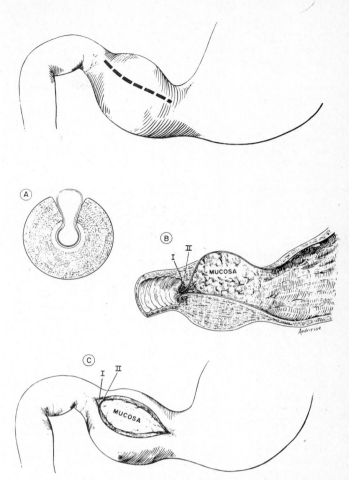

Figure 25. Fredet-Ramstedt pyloromyotomy. The seromuscular layer of the pyloric "olive" is incised longitudinally and spread bluntly down to the submucosal base. A, The underlying mucosa bulges through the resultant defect, effectively relieving all obstruction. B and C, Complete division of the constricting muscle fibers is most difficult to achieve distally, where the pylorus protrudes into the duodenum (II) much as the cervix protrudes into the vagina. As a consequence, inadvertent perforation of the overlapping duodenal mucosa (I) can occur relatively easily and must always be excluded by inflating the stomach and duodenum with air. (From Holder, T. M., and Ashcraft, K. W. (Eds.): Pediatric Surgery. Philadelphia, W. B. Saunders Company, 1980, p. 320.)

biopsy can assist in confirming the presence and extent of the esophagitis that may accompany GER in older patients. Approximately 50 per cent of patients with symptomatic GER also have associated gastric dysmotility, and radionuclide studies with technetium colloidal sulfur in semisolid feedings have been utilized to determine the magnitude of postprandial gastric retention and to identify those children who may require performance of pyloroplasty in concert with an antireflux procedure.[3]

If the symptoms of GER fail to respond to conservative management or appear to represent a significant health threat, following confirmation of the diagnosis surgical correction should be undertaken. A transabdominal gastroesophageal fundoplication (Nissen "wrap") has been employed in most instances. Because of the frequent association of esophageal dysmotility in infants and children requiring this procedure, it is important that constriction of the gastroesophageal junction be avoided and that the Nissen wrap be relatively loose. In young children, concomitant insertion of a temporary gastrostomy can assist in preventing postoperative "gas bloat" and in administering initial feedings. Because of the frequent occurrence of GER in brain-damaged children, with consequent aspiration and growth failure, a simultaneous fundoplication has been recommended whenever inserting a feeding gastrostomy in such patients.

Symptomatic GER that is unresponsive to medical therapy has been recognized increasingly in infants younger than 1 year of age, and currently more than 50 per cent of the antireflux procedures performed in children involve this group. The excellent clinical results that are achieved by fundoplication in more than 95 per cent of cases, with repeated verification of an extremely low operative morbidity and mortality, amply justify early performance of this procedure in infants and children with symptomatic GER.

Intussusception

Intussusception is a condition in which a proximal segment of bowel (intussusceptum) invaginates into a distal segment (intussuscipiens) and is then propelled distally by intestinal peristalsis. Sixty-five per cent of cases occur in infants younger than 1 year of age, with a peak incidence between the fifth and ninth month of life.[9, 19] Although the condition may occur postoperatively, involving only the small bowel in 86 per cent of such patients, or may result in older children when a lesion such as a polyp or a Meckel's diverticulum serves as the lead point, there is usually no recognized cause in the infant. In children under 4 years old, 95 per cent of intussusceptions begin at, or near, the ileocecal valve. As a consequence of the telescoping of the proximal intestinal segment into the distal bowel, venous engorgement ensues, initially resulting in intestinal obstruction and passage of a dark, bloody, mucoid ("currant jelly") stool and eventually progressing to intestinal ischemia, infarction, and perforation. Classically, the onset of intussusception is characterized by increasingly frequent attacks of abdominal colic, with subsequent appearance of abdominal distention, vomiting, fever, lethargy, and eventually, passage of the typical "currant jelly" stool. During the early phase, abdominal examination may prove uninformative unless an elongated mass can be defined in the right upper quadrant or epigastrium in the absence of a palpable cecum in the right lower quadrant (Dance's sign). Later in the course, signs of peritonitis and shock may ensue. Rarely, the intussusceptum may present as a mass, prolapsing from the anus or palpated by an examining finger on rectal examination.

In the uncomplicated case, hydrostatic barium enema reduction, as described by Ravitch, represents the accepted method both for confirming the diagnosis and for initiating treatment.[19] However, this procedure should be performed only with joint participation of the radiologist and surgeon, since failure of hydrostatic reduction or inadvertent perforation of bowel requires an immediate abdominal exploration. Concomitant with the roentgenographic procedure, the surgeon should accomplish gastrointestinal decompression and fluid resuscitation and should alert the operating room. In the presence of an intussusception, barium outlines the invaginated segment of bowel and produces a typical "coiled spring" appearance. With the level of gravity pressure limited to no more than 3½ feet, successful reduction can be achieved in approximately two thirds of cases and will be confirmed by free reflux of contrast media into the ileum as well as by immediate symptomatic improvement in the patient. Unfortunately, use of this technique does not enable detection of intussusceptions limited to the small bowel and should not be attempted in the presence of signs that suggest intestinal necrosis or peritonitis.

In those instances in which barium enema reduction proves unsuccessful or equivocal, immediate abdominal exploration is undertaken through a right lower quadrant transverse incision and reduction by retrograde compression and milking of the bowel, beginning distally at the leading aspect of the invaginated mass to induce its proximal extrusion (Fig. 26). Traction should never be utilized to separate the proximal and distal bowel because of the potential for disruption. When gangrenous changes are identified, resection and primary anastomosis can usually be performed. With prompt recognition, the treatment and results in this condition are excellent and an extremely low level of morbidity and mortality can be anticipated.

Meckel's Diverticulum and Other Vitelline (Omphalomesenteric) Duct Vestiges

Normally, the embryonic omphalomesenteric duct involutes, but its rare persistence may be evidenced in the newborn infant by passage of meconium from an umbilical sinus (Fig. 27). A sinogram confirms the diagnosis by reflux of contrast media into the small bowel. In other patients, partial involution may be manifested by a residual fibrous band that links the ileum to the umbilicus and presents a potential focus for subsequent internal hernia or volvulus. The most common remnant of the omphalomesenteric duct, however, is a Meckel's diverticulum, which occurs as an antimesenteric outpouching of the terminal ileum in approximately 1.5 to 3 per cent of the general population.[9, 19] These diverticula usually remain asymptomatic, but they may serve as a lead point for an intussusception or as a site for inflammation, perforation, or bleeding, with the last complication related to the frequent presence of ectopic gastric mucosa, which can produce peptic ulceration of the adjacent ileum. Sixty per cent of those patients who manifest symptoms do so within the first 2 years of life. Boys are affected more often than girls.

The most frequent clinical presentation is painless rectal bleeding, often significant in amount and occasionally requiring transfusion. These episodes tend to be repetitive; when they are persistent, or when the amount of contained gastric mucosa is sufficient to allow demonstration by ^{99m}technetium radioisotope scan, surgical resection should be performed (Fig. 28). Unfortunately, barium contrast studies of the gastrointestinal tract seldom confirm the presence of a Meckel's diverticulum. Inflammation and/or perforation of the Meckel's diverticulum may also mimic appendicitis, and the possibility of this entity must be excluded whenever a normal appendix is identified in the course of surgical exploration for lower abdominal pain.

Appendicitis

The diagnosis of appendicitis presents a challenge in the infant or very young child because of its relatively rare occurrence, the inability of these patients to verbalize their symptoms, the unanticipated high anatomic position of the cecum and appendix, and the limited capability of the poorly developed omentum to localize an intra-abdominal inflammatory process. As a consequence, perforation and generalized peritonitis are frequent complications and a high level of suspicion must be maintained by the examiner

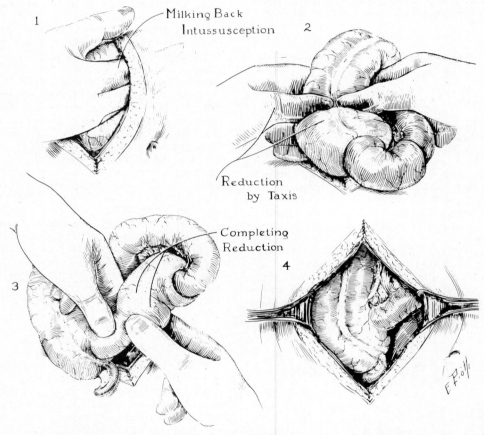

Figure 26. Operative reduction of intussusception. Reduction is accomplished by gently milking the distal intussuscipiens to produce proximal extrusion of the intussusceptum. Traction on the proximal and distal bowel should be avoided because of the potential for disrupting the edematous, friable intestine. Manual reduction should not be attempted in the presence of gangrenous changes. (Modified from Gross, R. E.: An Atlas of Children's Surgery. Philadelphia, W. B. Saunders Company, 1970, p. 29.)

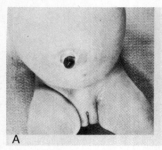
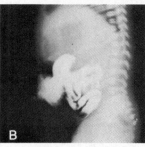

Figure 27. Persistent omphalomesenteric duct in a newborn infant. A, Manifested by a draining umbilical sinus which (B) by sinogram, communicates via a patent duct and cyst with the distal small intestine. (From Haller, J. A., Jr., and Talbert, J. L.: Surgical Emergencies in the Newborn. Philadelphia, Lea & Febiger, 1972, p. 143.)

if early diagnosis and treatment are to be achieved. This problem is discussed further in Chapter 25.

Hernias

Umbilical hernias are rarely symptomatic in infants and young children, and they usually close spontaneously by 5 years of age; however, *inguinal hernias* are fraught with an especially high frequency of incarceration at this age. Strangulation of the entrapped intestine clearly represents a threat in these circumstances, but a more frequent complication is damage sustained by the testicle as a consequence of congestive infarction if reduction is delayed. Accordingly, in the absence of some medical contraindication, identification of an inguinal hernia in an infant or young child signifies the need for prompt surgical repair. In the majority of instances, an incarcerated hernia can be reduced by manual compression with surgical repair performed within the next few days as an elective procedure after the

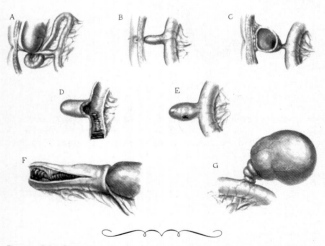

Figure 28. Complications of vitelline duct vestiges. A, Intestinal obstruction resulting from a persistent band linking the tip of a Meckel's diverticulum to the umbilicus. B, Persistent omphalomesenteric duct. C, Persistent cyst beneath the umbilicus. D, Ulceration and bleeding produced by ectopic gastric mucosa within a Meckel's diverticulum. E, Diverticulitis. F, A Meckel's diverticulum serving as a lead point for an intussusception. G, Torsion and infarction of a Meckel's diverticulum. (From Gross, R. E.: An Atlas of Children's Surgery. Philadelphia, W. B. Saunders Company, 1970, p. 172.)

patient has been optimally prepared for operation. Exposure of the hernial sac in the inguinal canal with high ligation and excision of the sac is generally sufficient in infants, and a formal hernia repair is not necessary.

Accidental Injury

Not only does trauma account for half of all childhood deaths in the United States, but at least one in every five children is hospitalized each year for treatment of an accidental injury.[4] Infants and older teenagers are most prone to injury, and boys suffer mishaps more often than girls. Approximately two thirds of all accidents involving preschool children occur at home, whereas lethal injuries are usually related to motor vehicles, fires, falls, and poisoning. A large proportion of these accidental injuries are avoidable, and it is estimated that the incidence of childhood deaths from trauma can be reduced by as much as 29 per cent annually through implementation of twelve currently available prevention strategies.[20]

Successful treatment of serious injuries in infants and young children frequently demands a level of skill and experience best provided in a center staffed by multidisciplinary teams of child health care specialists. Blunt trauma is encountered most often, and surgical management of injuries of the spleen, the most frequently ruptured intraabdominal viscera, emphasizes some of the contrasts in treating children and adults. Although *splenectomy* has been generally accepted as appropriate for handling splenic injuries in older patients, *salvage of the spleen* has proved feasible in 90 per cent of children. Preservation of the spleen has also been demonstrated to be especially important in this age group because of the significant risk of postsplenectomy sepsis with its attendant threat of a fulminant, frequently lethal, infection.[5] For this reason, it is quite appropriate to follow a patient with suspected splenic injury carefully in the hope that operation may be unnecessary.

CHILD ABUSE

Child abuse is a unique form of trauma that most often involves children under 3 years of age. Physicians must maintain a high index of suspicion, since failure to recognize this entity often results in repetitive injuries, serious emotional and physical crippling, or even death.[11] Each year more than one million children in the United States are seriously abused by their parents, guardians, or other individuals, and 2000 to 5000 die as a consequence of these injuries. Physicians and other professionals providing services to children are required by state law to report suspected incidents of child abuse and neglect and, as mandated reporters, are afforded legal immunity.

POISONING AND CAUSTIC INGESTIONS

Poisoning represents a major source of accidental injury in children. Injuries involving caustic ingestion require immediate surgical attention because of the potential for producing serious damage to the airway and the upper gastrointestinal tract.[23] The agents most frequently involved are alkaline caustics (lye), acid or acid-like corrosives, and household bleaches. However, severe localized esophageal burns can also result from ingestion of Clinitest tablets, which are used for testing sugar in the urine and contain significant amounts of anhydrous sodium hydroxide, or from swallowing small, disc-shaped (button) alkaline batteries, which may become entrapped in the esophagus of a young child and subsequently leak their highly corrosive contents.

The most important element in the successful management of a corrosive burn of the esophagus is immediate verification of the etiologic agent and accurate assessment of the depth and extent of injury. Induced vomiting and gastric lavage are contraindicated because of the dangers of compounding the original injury and of potentially inducing laryngeal damage. Substernal and back or abdominal pain and rigidity are suggestive of mediastinal or peritoneal perforation; hoarseness, stridor, and dyspnea characterize laryngeal injury.

The absence of any visible evidence of oropharyngeal burns does not exclude the possibility of esophageal injury, and it is essential that esophagoscopy be performed within the first 12 to 24 hours to confirm the extent and severity of the burn. The only exception to this rule are those patients in whom esophageal or gastric perforation or impending airway obstruction is evident. The goal of the endoscopist is simply to confirm the presence or absence of a caustic burn, and it is essential that no attempt be made to pass the esophagoscope beyond the proximal point of injury. The status of the distal esophagus can be subsequently assessed by cine-esophagograms.

When a caustic esophageal burn has been verified, the patient should be placed on a 3-week course of therapy with steroids and antibiotics in an effort to prevent stricture formation through pharmacologic modification of wound healing. At the end of 3 weeks, the steroid dosage should be tapered and ultimately discontinued, since prolongation of treatment beyond this time appears to simply postpone stricture formation and does not alter the eventual outcome.

If evidence of stricture formation develops during the course of steroid treatment, the regimen is abandoned and esophageal bougienage is instituted. If the stricture proves refractory to bougienage, some form of esophageal reconstruction must be considered, most frequently involving interposition of a segment of colon or a reversed antiperistaltic gastric tube, based proximally on the greater curvature of the stomach and receiving its blood supply from the left gastroepiploic artery.[9] Either of these methods provides excellent long-term function and allows normal growth and development. Late complications of corrosive burns of the esophagus include development of a hiatal hernia as a consequence of esophageal scarring and contraction and a thousand-fold increase in the frequency of esophageal cancer as a consequence of malignant degeneration in the previously injured tissues.

Tumors

The relative significance of tumors as a source of morbidity and mortality in children is emphasized by the fact that although accidental injury is the primary cause of death, cancer now leads all other diseases and accounts for 11 per cent of the overall mortality between ages 1 and 15 years. Almost half of these deaths result from leukemia and lymphoma, whereas solid tumors comprise the remainder. Despite these seemingly grave statistics, however, multidisciplinary management, in which surgery often plays a key role, has produced dramatic improvements, and excellent survival can be expected in the treatment of many childhood malignancies.[5, 18, 22]

Although it is necessary to be familiar with a spectrum of neoplasms that may present in a variety of anatomic sites, *the most frequent differential diagnosis involves the child who presents with a palpable abdominal mass.* Such masses may represent either cystic or solid tumors and often arise from the genitourinary system. Urinalysis and contrast studies of the kidney, excretory system, and bladder have been considered essential to achieving an accurate diagnosis. More recently, abdominal sonograms and computed tomographic (CT) scans have been utilized with increasing frequency. Occasionally, roentgenographic studies of the gastrointestinal tract and angiograms are also required.

ABDOMINAL MASSES OF GENITOURINARY ORIGIN

Renal Masses

Renal masses at this age most often present as (1) benign cysts, (2) hydronephrosis, (3) renal vein thrombosis, and (4) Wilms' tumor.

Benign Cysts. *Infantile polycystic disease* of the kidneys is manifested at birth by bilateral renal enlargement and almost always leads to early death or stillbirth. A more favorable lesion, the unilateral *multicystic kidney*, may be seen in the newborn, often caused by atresia of the ureter. This diagnosis is suggested by a normal urinalysis, the presence of a unilateral flank mass (which may be ectopic in location), and absence of function in the affected kidney on intravenous pyelography.

Hydronephrosis. *Unilateral hydronephrosis* may result from congenital stenosis of the ureteropelvic junction or extrinsic compression by an aberrant vessel; *bilateral hydronephrosis* suggests obstruction of the urethra or bladder neck.

Renal Vein Thrombosis. Acute renal vein thrombosis in the newborn may accompany maternal diabetes and may appear as a flank mass in association with hematuria and thrombocytopenia.

Wilms' Tumor. Wilms' tumor comprises approximately 6 per cent of all malignant neoplasms in childhood, with highest incidence in the first 2 years of life. Although bilaterality occurs (in 5 per cent), the usual presentation is that of a unilateral flank mass, often surprisingly large, which is detected incidentally by the mother or a physician in the course of examining the infant or child for another condition.[18] In other patients, the tumor may become manifest by abdominal pain, fever, hematuria, hypertension, or dyspnea due to pulmonary metastases. In fact, 20 per cent of patients have pulmonary metastases at the time of initial diagnosis. Metastases to the liver, brain, and bone are less frequent.

Preoperative diagnostic studies include a thorough abdominal evaluation by sonography and intravenous pyelography and/or CT scan, together with chest films and CT scan of the chest. The diagnosis of Wilms' tumor is established by demonstration of a solid intrarenal mass that distorts the caliceal system (Fig. 29). Rarely, the tumor may invade the renal pelvis and produce complete ureteral obstruction with nonvisualization by pyelograms.

The advances that have been achieved in recent years through the coordinated treatment of childhood cancer by a multidisciplinary approach encompassing the medical oncologist, radiotherapist, and surgeon are epitomized by the results in Wilms' tumor, with cure being achieved in more than 90 per cent of patients without metastatic disease. The basis of successful therapy is complete removal of the tumor mass by radical nephrectomy together with dissection of the adjacent hilar and periaortic lymph nodes. Rupture and spillage of the tumor should be carefully avoided, and the contralateral kidney should always be

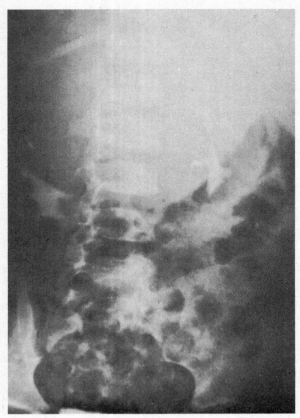

Figure 29. Wilms' tumor of the right kidney. Characteristic distortion and displacement of the caliceal system by an intrarenal mass, as demonstrated by intravenous pyelography. (From Haller, J. A., Jr., and Talbert, J. L.: Surgical Emergencies in the Newborn. Philadelphia, Lea & Febiger, 1972, p. 133.)

examined for evidence of involvement. All patients should receive postoperative chemotherapy, primarily actinomycin-D and vincristine, with the period of treatment dependent on the stage of disease. Radiation therapy should be given patients with demonstrable lymph node metastases and significant tumor extension or spillage. Pulmonary metastases often respond to chemotherapy administered together with surgical resection or pulmonary irradiation.

The microscopic appearance is an especially significant prognostic factor because anaplastic and sarcomatous tumors, although representing a relatively small number, contribute heavily to the overall recurrence rate and mortality. Although the period of maximal risk for recurrence or metastasis of Wilms' tumor is in the first 2 years following initial treatment, the importance of long-term follow-up of pediatric cancer patients has been increasingly emphasized to facilitate early detection and possible correction of adverse sequelae of therapy.

Although malignant Wilms' tumor is the most common solid renal neoplasm in children, a benign hamartomatous variant—the *mesoblastic nephroma*—occurs most often in infants under 1 month of age and requires only wide excision for adequate treatment.

Abnormalities of the Distal Genitourinary System

Abdominal masses may also arise as a consequence of abnormalities of the distal genitourinary system. Since the space in the pelvis is limited at this age, rapidly expanding cystic or solid masses either are displaced intra-abdominally or involve adjacent structures and may protrude into the perineum (Fig. 30). A *distended bladder* can be confused with a pelvic tumor and can result from any form of outlet or urethral obstruction, as may be produced by congenital urethral valves. In the female, an *imperforate hymen* or *vaginal atresia* may be manifest, either in the newborn period or following menarche, as a consequence of retained secretions or menstrual flow within the obstructed uterus and vagina, producing a *hydrometrocolpos* or *hematometrocolpos*.

Ovarian Neoplasms

Ovarian neoplasms comprise 1.5 percent of all childhood tumors and frequently present as abdominal masses, most often representing *simple cysts* in newborns or *benign cystic teratomas* in older girls. However, with the exception of neonates, there is a significant incidence of ovarian cancer that is inversely proportional to the age of the patient (i.e., 82 per cent of ovarian tumors are malignant in girls under 9 years of age). Bilateral involvement also occurs frequently, with both benign and malignant ovarian neoplasms. Occasionally, an endocrinologically active tumor may be manifested by precocious puberty, vaginal bleeding, or masculinization, and assays of blood and urine samples confirm hormonal activity. Elevations in the plasma levels of human chorionic gonadotropin (HCG) and alpha fetoprotein (AFP) may also signal the presence of *malignant germ cell tumors,* such as the endodermal sinus tumor (yolk sac tumor), embryonal carcinoma, and choriocarcinoma. There is a 10 to 30 per cent incidence of malignancy in ovarian neoplasms in children, and prompt diagnosis and treatment are imperative.

Rhabdomyosarcoma

Rhabdomyosarcoma is an embryonic tumor that may arise throughout the body, either from striated muscle or a variety of mesenchymal tissues, and comprises 4 to 8 per cent of all childhood malignancies. A bi-peaked occurrence is seen with tumors of the bladder, prostate, vagina, and head and neck, presenting most frequently within the first 4 years of life, whereas those involving paratesticular, uterine, extremity, and trunk sites usually appear after 5 years of age, reaching a peak incidence at approximately 15 years. With vaginal origin, the neoplasm may protrude as a multilobulated, grapelike cluster of tissue, the *sarcoma*

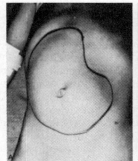
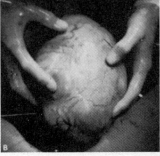

Figure 30. Ovarian tumor. A and B, A large, benign cystic teratoma presenting as an intra-abdominal mass in an 11-year-old girl. (From Holder, T. M., and Ashcraft, K. W. (Eds.): Pediatric Surgery. Philadelphia, W. B. Saunders Company, 1980, p. 1012.)

botryoides. The major histologic types of rhabdomyosarcoma are *embryonal* and *alveolar,* with most deaths confined to the latter category even though it represents only 20 to 25 per cent of the total group.

Patients in whom the primary tumor can be excised, with or without microscopic residual, have a much better prognosis than patients in whom gross tumor remains. Postoperatively, therapy consisting of vincristine, actinomycin-D, and cyclophosphamide (VAC) is ordinarily administered for 2 years. If microscopic foci remain after operation or if lymph nodes are involved, local radiotherapy is indicated. Patients in whom the tumor has been grossly excised have survival rates approximating 75 per cent. Metastatic spread primarily occurs in regional lymph nodes and in the lungs.

Although surgical extirpation and precise staging remain important in successful treatment, attention has focused recently on preservation of function. As an example, avoidance of pelvic exenteration in infants and children with this lesion has proved increasingly feasible and, together with regimens employing chemotherapy and radiotherapy, salvage of the bladder has been achieved in as many as 50 per cent of patients. With appropriate management, patients with vaginal, paratesticular, and orbital tumors have an extremely favorable response (80 to 90 per cent survival); those with neoplasms in other locations on the head and neck have a 50 per cent survival. Among all major sites, rhabdomyosarcomas of the extremities and trunk are the most difficult to manage, probably because 50 per cent of these tumors are of the *alveolar* type.

Neuroblastoma

Neuroblastoma comprises approximately 7 to 8 per cent of all malignant neoplasms in childhood and arises from the adrenals or the paravertebral sympathetic ganglia. The mean age at diagnosis is 2½ years, with 40 per cent of lesions appearing within the first year of life. The majority of neuroblastomas occur in the abdomen; other sites include the mediastinum, pelvis, and neck in order of frequency. Autopsy findings in stillborns suggest that the incidence of neuroblastoma may be many times higher in the newborn than is subsequently manifest clinically.

Histologically, neuroblastoma varies from an undifferentiated, highly malignant form to a more mature lesion and has been observed rarely to evolve into a benign ganglioneuroma. With origin from the neural crest, these tumors frequently produce catecholamines and the metabolites—vanillylmandelic acid (VMA), homovanillic acid (HVA)—can be identified in the urine. The screening of urine samples for these substances in suspected patients assists in confirming the diagnosis and also provides means for monitoring the therapeutic response and identifying recurrence.

Neuroblastoma is a non-encapsulated tumor that spreads by direct extension into adjacent tissues and metastasizes through lymphatic channels and bloodstream to the skeleton, retroorbital area, liver, and subcutaneous tissues. Unlike that of Wilms' tumor, metastatic spread to the pulmonary parenchyma is rare. Bony metastases may be confirmed by bone scans, skeletal roentgenograms, and bone marrow aspiration. Detection of bone involvement implies a poor prognosis, whereas liver and skin metastases in an infant younger than 1 year of age with a localized primary tumor (Stage IV-S) (Table 2) often prove compatible with eventual cure, either as a consequence of spontaneous regression or as a response to therapy.

TABLE 2. Staging Classification of Neuroblastoma*

I	Tumor confined to organ of origin
II	Tumor extends beyond organ of origin, but does not cross midline (regional nodes may be involved)
III	Tumor extends beyond midline
IV	Distant metastases (skeleton, organs, soft tissues, distant lymph node groups)
IV-S	Localized primary (Stage I or II) with remote disease limited to liver, skin, or bone marrow (no evidence of bone metastases)

*From Randolph, J.: World J. Surg., 4:1, 1980.

Although the most common initial finding is a palpable mass, these patients frequently manifest symptoms of fever, diarrhea, anorexia, weight loss, and bone pain, with the last reflecting metastatic involvement. Abnormal physical findings include lymphadenopathy, subcutaneous nodules, hepatomegaly, proptosis, Horner's syndrome, and paraplegia.

As a consequence of their frequent intra-abdominal presentation, the differential diagnosis involves Wilms' tumor of the kidney. Neuroblastoma is distinguished by its tendency to infiltrate midline structures; by its firm, finely nodular consistency; by the identification of calcification on roentgenograms; by its characteristic spread to bone and liver; and by the detection of VMA and HVA in the urine. Roentgenographic demonstration of extrinsic displacement of the kidney, usually laterally and inferiorly, also contrasts with the intrinsic caliceal distortion classically observed with Wilms' tumor (Fig. 31). Occasionally, a neuroblastoma may extend through an adjacent intervertebral foramen into the intrathecal space, producing compression of the spinal cord and paraplegia. Fortunately, the response of these "dumbbell" tumors to therapy is quite good and function is frequently restored in the affected extremities.

The overall probability of success in treating a neuroblastoma is related to the site of origin, stage of disease, age of patient, and degree of cellular maturation. The outlook is especially favorable in those neoplasms that are localized and can be surgically removed, with survival rates exceeding 90 per cent. Such tumors are frequently encountered in the mediastinum, neck, and pelvis. Unfortunately, more than half of children with neuroblastoma (55 to 60 per cent) have disseminated disease at the time of initial presentation. In this group, as well as in patients with intra-abdominal tumors that have invaded adjacent structures, the mortality exceeds 90 per cent. The age of the patient is also an important prognostic factor, since the prospect for survival is good in patients under 1 year of age (74 per cent), somewhat less favorable in patients between 1 and 2 years of age (43 per cent), and poor in older children (14 per cent). Although adjuvant radiotherapy and multidrug chemotherapy have been utilized when complete excision is not possible, the long-term effects of these agents have not been clearly established and the results have not been as dramatic as those for some other childhood neoplasms.

Teratoma

Teratomas are congenital neoplasms made up of derivatives of all three germinal layers—ectoderm, mesoderm, and endoderm—with variable degrees of histologic differentiation and malignant potential. These tumors are usually located near the midline and may be found in the sacrococcygeal and retroperitoneal areas, the gonads, the anterior mediastinum, the thyroid, and the nasopharynx. Intra-abdominal teratomas usually occur as encapsulated, upper midline neoplasms in which bony elements or teeth may be seen roentgenographically.

Sacrococcygeal teratoma is the most frequently encountered form of this neoplasm and may present primarily as a presacral or pelvic mass or, more often, may protrude from the buttocks and coccygeal area (Fig. 32). In some instances, the large size of the tumor may impede delivery of the fetus, and prenatal detection by maternal sonography is helpful. Despite their grotesque appearance, complete excision of even huge sacrococcygeal teratomas can nearly always be accomplished in continuity with a coccygectomy. An excellent cosmetic result can be expected with reapproximation of the pelvic tissues and closure of the defect by skin flaps. When pelvic extension of the tumor has occurred, a combined abdominosacral approach may be required. A rare, often familial form of presacral teratoma may also be associated with anorectal stenosis or atresia that requires concomitant surgical correction.

The majority of sacrococcygeal teratomas are benign, but the potential for malignant degeneration is high. After the second month of life, many tumors contain malignant components with a mortality of 55 per cent in patients who

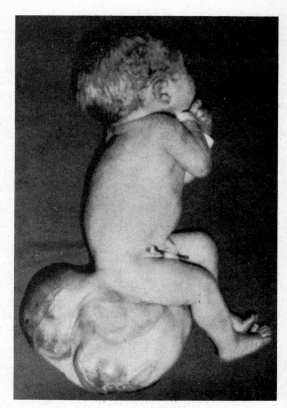

Figure 32. Sacrococcygeal teratoma. Despite the large size and grotesque appearance of these congenital neoplasms, successful surgical excision can almost always be accomplished in continuity with a coccygectomy. In the newborn infant, an excellent cosmetic and functional result can be anticipated, with minimal potential for malignancy. (From Holder, T. M., and Ashcraft, K. W. (Eds.): Pediatric Surgery. Philadelphia, W. B. Saunders Company, 1980, p. 964.)

are older than 2 years of age at the time of treatment. Accordingly, early identification and prompt surgical intervention are essential and can usually be accomplished within the first few days of life, when the incidence of malignancy is rare, without damaging the adjacent rectum or genitourinary structures.

HEPATOBILIARY TUMORS

Hepatobiliary tumors of infants and children include a variety of cystic and solid lesions. Large *solitary cysts of the liver* occur rarely and require treatment by excision of the involved segment or by marsupialization and external drainage, depending on size and anatomic location. A *congenital choledochal cyst* may also present as a right upper quadrant abdominal mass, occurring predominantly in females (4:1) and associated with jaundice, depending on the severity of the accompanying anatomic obstruction to extra-hepatic biliary drainage (Fig. 33). When feasible, excision of the cyst or stripping of the lining is warranted because of a documented malignant potential, with drainage of the proximal hepatic ducts established by anastomosis to a Roux-en-Y loop of jejunum. Confirmation of the diagnosis of choledochal cyst is facilitated by liver scan, abdominal ultrasonography, or CT scan. Excellent results can be anticipated with surgical correction.

Benign solid neoplasms of the liver that may present in infants and children include *hamartomas*, *adenomas*,

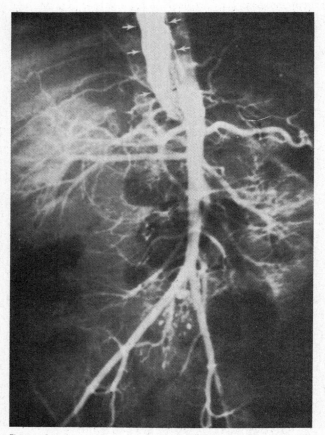

Figure 31. Neuroblastoma. Myelogram and arteriogram in an infant presenting with a right flank mass and paraplegia. The right kidney is displaced laterally by the tumor, which is located immediately inferior to the renal artery. The myelogram (arrows) confirms intraspinal extension of the "dumbbell" tumor, which is obstructing the subarachnoid space. Following treatment, the patient regained normal motor activity in her legs and has shown no evidence of tumor recurrence over the subsequent 15 years. (From Haller, J. A., Jr., and Talbert, J. L.: Surgical Emergencies in the Newborn. Philadelphia, Lea & Febiger, 1972, p. 133.)

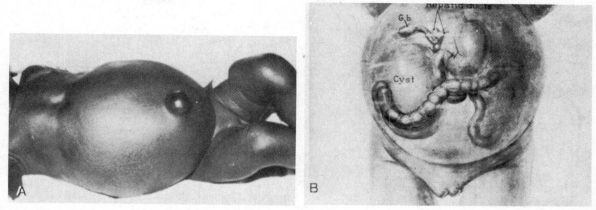

Figure 33. Congenital choledochal cyst. A, This 3-month-old female infant presented with jaundice and a large, palpable abdominal mass. B, Preoperative studies confirmed the mass to represent a huge choledochal cyst containing over 500 ml. of fluid, and subsequent surgical correction was successfully achieved. (From Haller, J. A., Jr., and Talbert, J. L.: Surgical Emergencies in the Newborn. Philadelphia, Lea & Febiger, 1972, p. 141.)

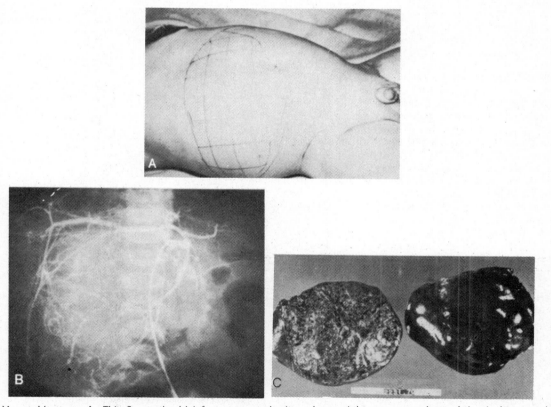

Figure 34. Hepatoblastoma. A, This 3-month-old infant presented with a large, right upper quadrant abdominal mass which (B) on arteriogram, was demonstrated to represent a solid tumor arising in the right lobe of the liver. C, The neoplasm was completely resected in continuity with the entire right lobe and medial segment of the left lobe of the liver and was confirmed histologically to be a hepatoblastoma. (From Haller, J. A., Jr., and Talbert, J. L.: Surgical Emergencies in the Newborn. Philadelphia, Lea & Febiger, 1972, p. 140.)

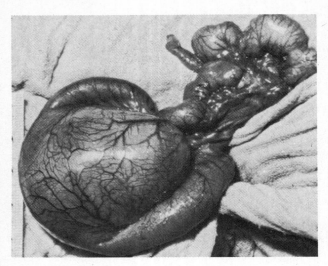

Figure 35. This duplication cyst of the ileum was producing partial intestinal obstruction by extrinsic compression of the intestinal lumen. (From Haller, J. A., Jr., and Talbert, J. L.: Surgical Emergencies in the Newborn. Philadelphia, Lea & Febiger, 1972, p. 142.)

lymphangiomas, and *hemangiomas.* Hemangiomas elsewhere characteristically follow a benign course of progressive enlargement during the first year of life, with subsequent gradual involution, but hemangiomas of the liver may be life-threatening because of associated major intrahepatic arteriovenous communications that can produce high-output cardiac failure refractory to medical management. Although nonoperative treatment is associated with 90 per cent mortality, hepatic artery ligation or embolization provides a reliable technique for dramatically controlling the cardiac failure with negligible side effects.

Primary malignant tumors of the liver comprise 1.2 per cent of malignant neoplasms in childhood, the most common being *hepatoblastomas,* which are usually unicentric in origin and occur predominantly in infants, and multicentric *hepatomas (hepatocellular carcinoma),* which usually present in older children. The detection of alpha fetoprotein in the serum of patients with hepatoblastoma provides a useful biologic marker, both for diagnosis and for monitoring of the postoperative response. In addition to the usual measures for assessment of abdominal masses, selective arteriography is useful in defining the anatomic location of the intrahepatic tumor and planning its successful surgical extirpation (Fig. 34). Survival exceeding 90 per cent has been reported in Stage I hepatoblastoma when complete surgical removal has been followed postoperatively by multidrug chemotherapy. However, as a consequence of its frequent multicentric origin, the results in hepatocellular carcinoma are less favorable.

Hepatomegaly also occurs as a consequence of metastatic involvement by *neuroblastoma,* but spread to the liver in patients under 1 year of age does not necessarily connote a poor prognosis.

MISCELLANEOUS BENIGN ABDOMINAL MASSES

Gastrointestinal duplication cysts are most commonly found in the terminal ileum and cecum but may also occur in the duodenum and colon. These lesions may produce intestinal obstruction as a consequence of compression of the adjacent bowel or intestinal bleeding as a result of peptic ulceration induced by contained gastric mucosa. In the latter instance, a ⁹⁹ᵐtechnetium scan may prove helpful in confirming the presence of gastric mucosa. Characteristically, duplications arise as cystic masses within the mesentery and share a common wall with the adjacent bowel (Fig. 35). Treatment may entail excision of a localized cyst in continuity with the intestine, or with more extensive, tubular-shaped cysts, multiple enterotomies with mucosal stripping or marsupialization by windowing into the contiguous bowel wall may be required.

Omental and mesenteric cysts may result from anomalous lymphatic development and may contain either serous or chylous fluid.

Urachal cysts represent a persistent remnant of the urachus that during fetal development provides a free communication between the bladder and the abdominal wall and exits adjacent to the omphalomesenteric duct. Persistent patency of this tract following birth is signaled by drainage of urine from the umbilicus or, as a consequence of partial obliteration, by the appearance of an extraperitoneal cystic mass within the lower abdominal wall between the bladder and the umbilicus.

SELECTED REFERENCES

Holder, T. M., and Ashcraft, K. W. (Eds.): Pediatric Surgery. Philadelphia, W. B. Saunders Company, 1980.
This highly readable text on pediatric surgery provides an excellent, current reference source for health professionals or students seeking a more extensive discussion of general areas or individual subjects encompassed within this specialty.

Welch, K. J., Randolph, J. G., Ravitch, M. M., O'Neil, J. A., Jr., and Rowe, M. I. (Eds.): Pediatric Surgery, 4th ed. Chicago, Year Book Medical Publishers, Inc., 1986.
This two-volume "encyclopedia" of pediatric surgery represents the definitive reference source when a comprehensive presentation of a specific topic is required.

REFERENCES

1. Coran, A. G., Behrendt, D. M., Weintraub, W. H., et al: Surgery of the Neonate. Boston, Little, Brown and Company, 1978.
2. deVries, P. A.: The surgery of anorectal anomalies: Its evolution, with evaluations of procedures. In Ravitch, M. M., Steichen, F. M., Austen, W. G., et al. (Eds.): Current Problems in Surgery, vol. XXI. Chicago, Year Book Medical Publishers, Inc., 1984.
3. Fonkalsrud, E. W., Ament, M. E., and Berquist, W.: Surgical management of the gastroesophageal reflux syndrome in childhood. Surgery, 97:42, 1985.
4. Gallagher, S. S., Finison, K., Guyer, B., et al: The incidence of injuries among 87,000 Massachusetts children and adolescents: Results of the 1980–81 statewide childhood injury prevention program surveillance system. Am. J. Public Health, 74:1340, 1984.
5. Grosfeld, J. L. (Ed.): Symposium on pediatric surgery. Surg. Clin. North Am., 61:995, 1981.
6. Gross, R. E.: An Atlas of Children's Surgery. Philadelphia, W. B. Saunders Company, 1970.
7. Haller, J. A., Jr., and Talbert, J. L.: Surgical Emergencies in the Newborn. Philadelphia, Lea & Febiger, 1972.
8. Hays, D. M., and Kimura, K.: Biliary atresia: New concepts of management. In Ravitch, M. M., Steichen, F. M., Austen, W. G., et al. (Eds.): Current Problems In Surgery, vol. XVIII. Chicago, Year Book Medical Publishers, Inc., 1981.
9. Holder, T. M., and Ashcraft, K. W. (Eds.): Pediatric Surgery. Philadelphia, W. B. Saunders Company, 1980.
10. Iwatsuki, S., Shaw, B. W., and Starzl, T. E.: Liver transplantation for biliary atresia. World J. Surg., 8:51, 1984.
11. Kempe, C. H., Silverman, F. N., Steele, B. F., et al.: The battered-child syndrome. J.A.M.A., 181:17, 1962; reprinted 251:3288, 1984, with commentary by Heins, M.
12. Kliegman, R. M., and Fanaroff, A. A.: Necrotizing enterocolitis. N. Engl. J. Med., 310:1093, 1984.

13. Kosloske, A. M.: Pathogenesis and prevention of necrotizing entero-colitis: A hypothesis based on personal observation and a review of the literature. Pediatrics, *74*:1086, 1984.

14. Leape, L. L., and Holder, T. M.: Pediatric surgery. *In* Sabiston, D. C., Jr. (Ed.): Davis-Christopher Textbook of Surgery, 12th ed. Philadelphia, W. B. Saunders Company, 1981, p. 1351.

15. Liver transplantation. Consensus conference. J.A.M.A., *250*:2961, 1983.

16. Mabogunje, O. A., and Mahour, G. H.: Omphalocele and gastroschisis: Trends in survival across two decades. Am. J. Surg., *148*:679, 1984.

17. Moazam, F., Talbert, J. L., and Rodgers, B. M.: Foreign bodies in the pediatric tracheobronchial tree. Clin. Pediatr., *22*:148, 1983.

18. Randolph, J. (Ed.): Progress in the treatment of malignant tumors of childhood. World J. Surg., *4*:1, 1980.

19. Ravitch, M. M., Welch, K. J., Benson, C. D., et al. (Eds.): Pediatric Surgery, 3rd ed. Chicago, Year Book Medical Publishers, Inc., 1979.

20. Rivara, F. P.: Traumatic deaths of children in the United States: Currently available prevention strategies. Pediatrics, *75*:456, 1985.

21. Rodgers, B. M., Rooks, J. J., and Talbert, J. L.: Pediatric tracheostomy: Long-term evaluation. J. Pediatr. Surg., *14*:258, 1979.

22. Shaw, A. (Ed.): Frontiers in pediatric surgery. Pediatr. Ann. *11*:877, 1982.

23. Talbert, J. L.: Corrosive strictures of the esophagus. *In* Sabiston, D. C., Jr. (Ed.): Davis-Christopher Textbook of Surgery, 12th ed. Philadelphia, W. B. Saunders Company, 1981, p. 834.

24. Talbert, J. L., Seashore, J. H., and Ravitch, M. M.: Evaluation of a modified Duhamel operation for correction of Hirschsprung's disease. Ann. Surg., *179*:671, 1974.

OTOLARYNGOLOGY

JOSEPH C. FARMER, JR., M.D.

34

THE EAR

Historic Perspectives

In the field of otology, Meniere described the labyrinthine origin of episodic vertigo and deafness in 1861, and von Helmholtz described the theory of the middle ear transformer in 1868. Simple mastoidectomy for the treatment of mastoiditis was introduced by Schwartze in 1873, followed by the radical mastoid operation, introduced by Zaufal in 1890. Although less frequently needed as a result of the effectiveness of antibiotics and the use of tampanostomy tubes, these procedures are still used to treat acute and chronic mastoiditis and otologic cholesteatoma. In 1922, the binocular operating microscope was introduced by Holmgren. In 1953, Rosen first described stapes mobilization for the management of otosclerosis, and stapedectomy was introduced by Shea in 1958. In 1961, von Bekesy received the Nobel Prize for his revealing studies of the physiology of the middle and inner ear.

Functional Anatomy of the Organs of Hearing and Balance

The evolution of the ear canal and middle ear transformer, the full development of which is seen in man, has resulted in a structure that efficiently overcomes, to a remarkable degree, the impedance mismatch of sound transmission from air to fluid. The human ear is basically a pressure transducer, capable of responding to extremely small changes in atmospheric pressure on the order of 2×10^{-4} dynes per cm.[2] The amplitude of vibration of the eardrum at the threshold of hearing is approximately 10^{-9} cm., or about one tenth the diameter of a hydrogen atom[3] (Fig. 1). The acoustic impedance matching of the middle ear is achieved by two mechanical advantages: (1) the relatively large ratio (17:1) of the vibrating area of the tympanic membrane to the area of the stapes footplate, and (2) a lesser contribution from the ratio (1.3:1) of the lengths of the long processes of the malleus and incus from the common axis of rotation. Also, the tympanic membrane protects the round window; if sound arrives at the round and oval windows with the same intensity and phase, displacement of inner ear fluids will not occur. The overall result is that acoustic energy is transformed into wave forms of higher pressure density and lesser volume displacement.

The combined external and middle ear structures have a broad resonating effect that enhances auditory thresholds in the midfrequencies (1000 to 3000 Hz.) (Fig. 2).[7]

Movement of the stapes footplate results in similar motion of the incompressible inner ear fluids, with pressure release being accomplished through opposite phase motion of the round window membrane. Rapid movements at the frequencies within the auditory range (100 to 10,000 Hz.) result in a traveling wave propagated from the cochlear base to the apex with displacement of the organ of Corti, alteration of the tectorial membrane–hair cell relationship, depolarization of the hair cells, and the generation of an alternating electrical current, the cochlear microphonic, which faithfully follows the wave form of the acoustic stimulus and can be recorded by an electrode on the round window membrane[7] (Figs. 3 and 4).

FREQUENCY AND INTENSITY DISCRIMINATION

The basilar membrane is relatively narrow at the cochlear base and widens progressively to the apex (Fig. 4). Higher frequency signals result in maximal basilar membrane displacement and neuronal discharge closer to the base; conversely, lower frequency signals result in maximal discharge of neurons located in the upper turns. This tonotopical relationship is maintained in the auditory division of the eighth cranial nerve, central auditory pathways, and the auditory cortex. Other factors involved in frequency discrimination include different neuronal firing rates for low-frequency signals and groups of neurons firing in synchronous volleys for frequencies above the maximal neuronal discharge rate (1000 Hz.). Intensity discrimination probably occurs in the cochlea, where variations in the width of basilar membrane deflection and hair cell displacement are detected. These variations depend upon the intensity of the sound. High-intensity sounds stimulate all four rows of hair cells; low-intensity sounds stimulate hair cells in the three outer rows with lesser effects on inner row hair cells. An efferent neuronal system originates from centers in the olivary complex and innervates cochlear hair cell–dendritic junctions. The exact function of this system is unknown but is felt to involve fine tuning of the acoustic signal and/or suppression of undesired acoustic sounds.

METABOLIC ACTIVITY

The saccule communicates with the cochlear duct by the ductus reuniens and with the utricle and endolymphatic

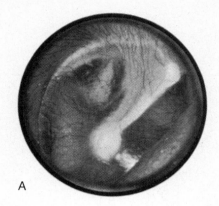

A

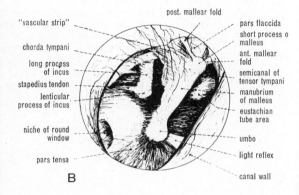

B

"vascular strip"

chorda tympani

long process
of incus

stapedius tendon

lenticular
process of incus

niche of round
window

pars tensa

post. mallear fold

pars flaccida

short process o
malleus

ant. mallear
fold

semicanal of
tensor tympani

manubrium
of malleus

eustachian
tube area

umbo

light reflex

canal wall

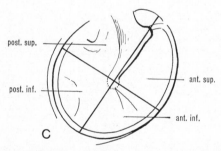

post. sup.

post. inf.

ant. sup.

ant. inf.

C

*Figure 1. The normal right eardrum. A, Otoscopic view. B, Land-
marks. C, Anatomic quadrants. (From Buckingham, R. A.: In Becker,
W. et al.: Atlas of Otorhinolaryngology and Bronchoesophagos-
copy. Philadelphia, W. B. Saunders Company, 1969, p. 20)*

VESTIBULAR END-ORGANS

The utricle and saccule each have a flat, ovoid sensory area (macula) containing sensory receptors and hair cells. The hairs project into a membrane composed of crystals of calcium carbonate, otoconia, which are denser than the surrounding endolymph and thus respond to gravity and linear acceleration. The macula of the saccule lies in a vertical plane and is perpendicular to the macula of the utricle, which lies in a horizontal plane.

The three semicircular canals are oriented in perpendicular planes and have an enlargement at one end, the ampulla, containing a transverse ridge of tissue, the crista, with hair cells and the dendrites of the primary vestibular neurons. The hairs project into a gelatinous cupula extending from the crista to the roof of the ampulla so that movement of endolymph moves the cupula and bends the hairs. The density of the cupula is the same as that of the surrounding endolymph; thus, the semicircular canals respond to angular acceleration with an inertial movement of endolymph toward the ampulla in one canal and away from the ampulla in the canal oriented in the same plane in the opposite inner ear. Thus, the resting discharge rate of the neuroepithelium in one crista is increased, whereas the rate on the other side is decreased.

BALANCE AND SPATIAL ORIENTATION

With continued movement at a steady velocity, endolymph moves at the same speed as the semicircular canal walls and there are no cupula deflections, with a return to the resting discharge rate. During deceleration, the inertial lag of the endolymph causes opposite cupular deflections and alterations in the neuronal discharge rate. These increases and decreases in discharge rates are transmitted over the primary vestibular neurons in the vestibular division of the eighth cranial nerve to the vestibular nuclei in the brainstem, the major way stations. From these nuclei, sensory input from the vestibular end-organs is integrated with visual and proprioceptive inputs to maintain balance and spatial orientation. The ocular motor nuclei move the eyes to maintain the field of last gaze. The anterior horn cells in the spinal cord adjust the trunk and limb muscles. The cerebral cortex interprets the sensory input as a particular position or motion of specific direction and speed. The cerebellum adjusts muscle tone to compensate for motion, acceleration, and position alteration and modulates the firing rates in the brainstem vestibular nuclei by selective inhibition.[15]

Clinical Evaluation of Otologic Symptoms

EAR PAIN (OTALGIA)

Pain sensory receptors are quite dense in the external ear canal, eardrum, and middle ear; thus, pain resulting from disease in these structures can be quite intense. Otalgia can also represent referred pain from disease in the pharynx, maxillary sinuses, teeth, temporomandibular joints, or parotid or submaxillary glands.

HEARING LOSS

Any process that increases the impedance of the sound conduction system—the external auditory canal, the eardrum, or the ossicular chain—results in a conductive hearing loss. These include a complete seal of the canal, masses

duct by the ultriculosaccular duct; the utricle communicates with the semicircular canals by direct connections. Communication between the utricle and saccule is limited by an intraductal fold, the endolymphatic valve of Bast. The endolymphatic duct connects with the endolymphatic sac, which lies within the posterior fossa dura and is felt to reabsorb endolymph, which is thought to be formed by the stria vascularis in the cochlear and vestibular portions of the membranous labyrinth. Some reabsorption of endolymph is also felt to occur within the stria vascularis. Metabolic activity and active transport within the stria vascularis and Reissner's membrane maintain the high-potassium and low-sodium concentrations of endolymph. These electrolyte differences account for a resting direct current potential difference between endolymph and perilymph of 80 mV.[7]

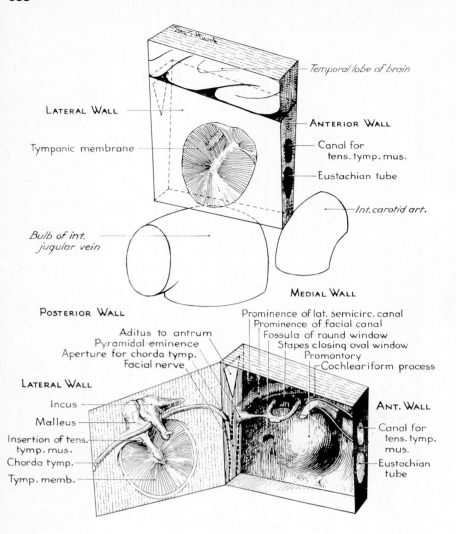

LATERAL WALL

Tympanic membrane

ANTERIOR WALL

Canal for tens. tymp. mus.

Eustachian tube

Int. carotid art.

Temporal lobe of brain

Bulb of int. jugular vein

MEDIAL WALL

POSTERIOR WALL

Aditus to antrum
Pyramidal eminence
Aperture for chorda tymp.
Facial nerve

LATERAL WALL

Incus

Malleus

Insertion of tens. tymp. mus.

Chorda tymp.

Tymp. memb.

Prominence of lat. semicirc. canal
Prominence of facial canal
Fossula of round window
Stapes closing oval window
Promontory
Cochleariform process

ANT. WALL

Canal for tens. tymp. mus.

Eustachian tube

Figure 2. Diagrammatic relationships of the right tympanic membrane, middle ear, and adjacent structures. (From Adams, G. E., et al.: Boies's Fundamentals of Otolaryngology, 5th ed. Philadelphia, W. B. Saunders Company, 1978, p. 162.)

Figure 3. The osseous and membranous labyrinths. (From Adams, G.L., et al.: Boies's Fundamentals of Otolaryngology, 5th ed. Philadelphia, W. B. Saunders Company, 1978, p. 167.)

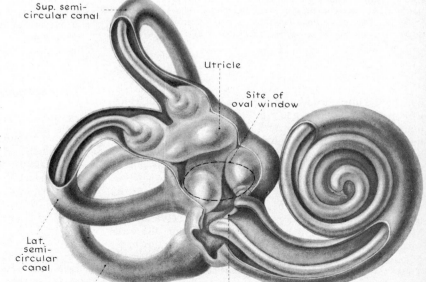

Sup. semi-circular canal

Utricle

Site of oval window

Lat. semi-circular canal

Inf. semicircular canal

Ductus reuniens

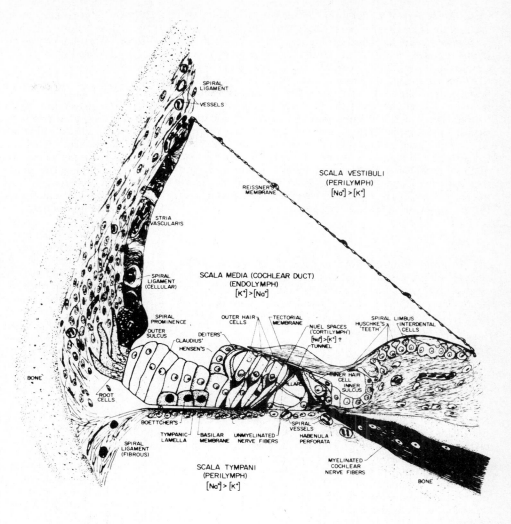

Figure 4. Midmodiolar cross section of the cochlear duct. (Reprinted with permission of Joseph E. Hawkins, Jr., Kresge Hearing Research Institute.)

such as cerumen lying against the eardrum, inflammation of the eardrum and middle ear mucosa, middle ear effusions or exudates, pressure differentials across the eardrum, ossicular fixation, tympanic membrane perforations, and interruption of the ossicular chain. Conductive hearing losses are associated with the sensation of a blocked ear, one's voice sounding louder, and mild tinnitus, since sounds initiated within the skull are more easily heard because of a decrease in the masking effect of omnipresent ambient noise.

Diseases in the inner ear, the primary auditory neurons (auditory division of the eighth cranial nerve), or the brainstem cochlear nuclei cause sensorineural nerve deafness and include arterial occlusive disease, tumors, trauma, perilymph fistulas from labyrinthine window ruptures, alterations in inner ear fluid physiology such as endolymphatic hydrops, inflammatory disease such as labyrinthitis or meningitis, idiopathic degenerative diseases such as presbycusis, and excessive noise or ototoxic drug exposure.

Mixed hearing losses are seen with pre-existing middle ear or inner ear disease and the development of additional disease in the other area. Such can occur with temporal bone fractures, middle and inner ear otosclerosis, or inflammatory middle and inner ear disease.

Tuning fork tests can frequently differentiate a *conductive* from a *sensorineural* hearing loss. Tuning forks (512 and/or 1024 Hz.) should be used in quiet surroundings. Lower-frequency forks may elicit a response to vibration.

Weber Test. The stem of a struck tuning fork placed in a midline position on the forehead or the upper incisor teeth results in vibration of the skull and equal stimulation of both inner ears. In the presence of a conductive hearing loss, the patient perceives the sound as louder in the involved ear; with a sensorineural hearing loss, the patient perceives the sound as louder in the uninvolved ear.

Rinne Test. Hearing by air conduction and bone conduction is compared. With normal hearing, mild conductive hearing loss, or a pure sensorineural hearing loss, air-conducted sound from a vibrating tuning fork placed about 2 inches from the ear is heard with greater intensity and duration than bone-conducted sound from the base of the fork placed against the mastoid tip. With a moderate or severe conductive hearing loss, bone-conducted sound is equal to, or louder and longer lasting than, air-conducted sound.

Schwabach Test. The bone conduction of the examiner, known by prior audiometry, is compared with that of the patient. The patient is instructed to signal the examiner when the sound of a vibrating tuning fork placed on the mastoid tip is no longer heard. The stem of the tuning fork is then immediately placed on the examiner's mastoid tip. If the sound is heard by the examiner, an elevated bone conduction threshold of the patient is suggested.

The complete evaluation of suspected hearing loss is best accomplished by certified audiologists using sound-proof booth audiometry with calibrated electronic devices to determine auditory thresholds, speech discrimination, sites of auditory pathway lesions, and middle ear impedance. Impedance audiometry involves the measurement of sound reflected from the eardrum to assess the compliance of the middle ear transformer, middle ear pressures, and the stapedius reflex threshold. It is useful in detecting middle ear effusions, ossicular dislocation or fixation, and the site of lesion in facial nerve palsy.

TINNITUS

Tinnitus resulting from disease of the inner ear or central auditory system is usually nonpulsatile and can present as low-pitched, high-pitched, or diffuse noise, depending upon the location of the lesion or the neuronal elements involved.

VERTIGO AND NYSTAGMUS

Sudden unilateral disease affecting the end-organ, primary vestibular neurons, or brainstem vestibular nuclei results in unequal resting firing rates in the central vestibular system, which is programmed during the first year of life to associate these signals with linear and angular acceleration. The cerebral cortex interprets this as vertigo, with pitching, yawing, or rolling. A rotational component usually predominates because of the greater innervation from the semicircular canals than from the otolithic organs. The eyes are deviated to maintain the field of last gaze during the perceived rotation. This is the slow component of nystagmus and is in a direction toward the hypofunctioning, diseased side. The patient may describe subjective vertigo, i.e., the sensation of turning in an opposite direction from the slow component of nystagmus or away from the hypofunctioning side, or objective vertigo, i.e., the sensation of the surroundings turning in the same direction as the slow component or toward the hypofunctioning side.

At the limits of ocular rotation, reticular inhibitory neurons block the incoming impulses from the vestibular nuclei, and reticular activating neurons direct opposing ocular motor neurons to quickly rotate the eyes in the opposite direction, producing the fast component of nystagmus. Staggering and ataxia occur in an attempt to adjust limb and trunk muscles for the perceived motion. Nausea and vomiting plus pallor and sweating occur from stimulation of the dorsal efferent nucleus of the tenth cranial nerve and hypothalamus. The cerebellum responds by inhibiting the firing rates of the vestibular nuclei on the hyperactive or uninjured side (the cerebellar clamp); thus, if the patient lies still with eyes closed, the magnitude and intensity of the symptoms decrease.

Equilibrium can be restored over a period of time after acute end-organ vestibular injury in two ways: (1) the return of the affected end-organ to its previously healthy state (this frequently does not occur); and (2) the appearance over 4 to 6 weeks of a new resting electrical activity in the ipsilateral brainstem vestibular nuclei that balances the contralateral, initially hyperactive side. This central compensation accounts for the gradual disappearance of the vertigo and gaze nystagmus after permanent unilateral vestibular end-organ injury. With disease affecting the central vestibular system, this compensation may be prolonged or absent.[15]

EVALUATION OF THE DIZZY PATIENT

The major goal is to determine whether a patient's dizziness is related to secondary vestibular system dysfunction or to disease in the inner ear or central nervous system. A detailed history and review of systems is essential, since most human maladies and many medications are associated with dizziness. The first step is to determine the onset, duration, and type of dizziness. Vertigo must be differentiated from unsteadiness, lightheadedness, and presyncopal symptoms. If a patient does not have vertigo, the dizziness is unlikely to be related to primary vestibular disease. Exceptions are individuals with slowly expanding intracranial lesions, who usually describe continuous, progressive unsteadiness with brief and mild vertiginous components; also, patients with bilateral end-organ disease caused by ototoxic drug exposure who have nonvertiginous unsteadiness that becomes quite severe with the loss of sensation from a second balance system input, such as decreased vision in dark surroundings.

The next step is to determine the relationship of the dizziness to position, activity, time of day, and other symptoms. Vertigo with head turning or lying in a specific position may indicate inner ear disease. Dizziness occurring upon arising from a sitting or supine position commonly reflects postural hypotension. Dizziness related to time of day may be due to hypoglycemia. Dizziness occurring with physical exertion may indicate respiratory or cerebrovascular insufficiency. Associated otologic symptoms, such as hearing loss, tinnitus, or otorrhea, suggest possible inner ear origin. Associated neurologic symptoms, such as visual disturbances, motor or sensory alterations, or aphasia, suggest a central nervous system cause.

Once the history indicates that a patient's dizziness is likely to be due to primary vestibular system disease, the next step is to determine whether the pathology is located in the vestibular end-organ or the central vestibular system by physical examination and appropriate tests. Accompanying neurologic signs usually point to a central lesion. Signs or symptoms of disease in the tympanic membrane or middle ear would suggest an end-organ origin. The presence of vertical gaze nystagmus usually indicates central pathology. Horizontal gaze nystagmus is also seen with central disease or in the acute phase of end-organ disturbances. Further objective testing should include electronystagmography, audiometry, and temporal bone and skull radiography.

Diseases of the External Ear and External Auditory Canal

CONGENITAL DEFORMITIES

Protruding pinna, or lop ear, is caused by a lack of development of the pinna antihelix. Surgical correction involves creating an antihelical fold by weakening the spring of the cartilage. It is optimally performed when the child is 5 or 6, when the ear has reached at least 75 per cent of adult size, but before the child enters school to lessen ridicule by peer groups.

Partial or complete absence of the pinna and the frequently accompanying ear canal and middle ear atresia can be associated with anomalies of the mouth, palate, tongue, mandible, salivary glands, urinary tract, eyes, and skeleton. If most of the pinna cartilage is absent, cosmetic surgical reconstruction is a repetitive, long-term process and rarely produces a satisfactory result; thus, an artistic prosthesis is the best solution.

Surgical procedures to correct conductive hearing losses caused by *ear canal and middle ear atresias* can be hazardous because of an abnormally located facial nerve and possible inner ear injury. With unilateral defects and normal hearing in the other ear, surgery is not recommended. With bilateral defects, bone conduction hearing aids should be fitted soon after birth. Evoked response audiometry should be done to determine cochlear function, since congenital malformations of the inner ear with sensorineural hearing losses may be present. If adequate cochlear function is found, surgical correction should be considered at age 4 to 6 after radiographic studies of the temporal bone. In general, less severe middle ear anomalies are found with the presence of a normal tragus.[19]

Pre- and infra-auricular cysts and sinus tracts may be present. Recurrent infection and/or drainage is an indication for surgical excision; however, the surgeon should be prepared to undertake a facial nerve exploration, since these sinus tracts may lie close to this nerve.

TRAUMA

Subperichondrial hematomas of the pinna result from blunt trauma and may cause avascular necrosis of the cartilage. Treatment involves incision with through-and-through drainage and dressings that approximate the skin and perichondrium to the cartilage. Lacerations of the pinna are managed by suturing and external splinting with cotton dressings. Suturing of the cartilage should be avoided. Keloids of the pinna are best treated by excision. Some have advocated keloid injections of triamcinalone. Pinna frostbite is best managed by slow and gradual warming, using dry heat at 100 to 110°F.

Foreign bodies, insects, and cerumen impactions of the external auditory canal are common problems. Cerumen may be removed by irrigations with water warmed to body temperature to avoid vertigo from a caloric response. If an eardrum perforation or retraction pocket is present, irrigation should be avoided and the material carefully removed by suction or instruments. Large impacted foreign bodies, particularly in children, usually require general anesthesia and surgery.

INFLAMMATORY DISEASES

Perichondritis of the pinna is usually a complication of trauma. The accumulation of pus between the perichondrium and cartilage results in cartilage necrosis and requires débridement of necrotic cartilage, surgical drainage, and antibiotic therapy.

Otitis externa (swimmer's ear) is a common condition in warm humid environments and in individuals engaging in aquatic activities. Optimal conditions for ear canal skin infections by *E. coli*, Pseudomonas, *Proteus*, and staphylococcal organisms are created by moisture that macerates the canal wall skin and removes the water-soluble fatty acids of cerumen with a shift to an alkaline pH. Insertion of cotton-tipped applicators or other objects into the canal disrupts the normal self-cleansing function of the canal and predisposes to this condition. Examination shows marked tenderness with an inflamed, swollen external auditory canal plus possible pinna erythema and cervical lymphadenitis.

Treatment involves gentle cleansing of the ear canal followed by administration of topical antibiotics and steroids. Significant canal swelling requires the use of a wick of twisted cotton or cellulose sponge. Topical medications are instilled onto the wick, which is removed in 3 to 4 days. After recovery, prophylaxis is best achieved by instilling drops of 2 per cent acetic acid into the ear canal after swimming or showering.

Furuncles of the hair-bearing area of the external auditory canal, the outer one third, are usually caused by *Staphylococcus aureus*. These may drain spontaneously; incision is occasionally needed. Topical antibiotics are indicated; with inflammation of the pinna or cervical adenitis, systemic antibiotics are also needed. Primary fungal infections of the external auditory canal usually occur after prolonged use of topical antibiotics and are best treated with 0.5 per cent acetic acid drops.

NEOPLASIA

Sun exposure predisposes to the most common neoplasms of the pinna, squamous and basal cell carcinomas. Although some advocate the treatment of such lesions with radiation or cautery and curettage, cartilage invasion occurs and requires surgical excision with microscopic control of the margins. Squamous cell and basal cell carcinomas also arise in the external auditory canal. Surgical resection is the treatment of choice and requires en bloc removal of the entire canal. Invasive squamous cell carcinomas of the anterior canal wall may spread to the parotid gland and upper jugular lymph nodes, necessitating a radical neck dissection and parotidectomy with exposure and sparing of the facial nerve if not involved.

Ear canal squamous cell carcinomas affecting the middle ear require a temporal bone resection and consideration of postoperative radiation therapy and chemotherapy. Melanomas may arise on the pinna. The best treatment is wide local excision with careful histologic examination of the specimen. Deeper invasion may require regional node dissections. Cerumenomas arising from the cerumenous glands in the outer third of the ear canal appear benign histologically; however, they behave in a malignant manner and should be widely excised. Other neoplasms, such as rhabdomyosarcoma, may arise in the external auditory canal, the pinna, or the adjacent scalp. These are more common in younger children.

Diseases of the Tympanic Membrane and Middle Ear

INFLAMMATORY DISEASES

Serous and Secretory Otitis Media. Eustachian tube obstruction caused by nasal inflammatory disease, nasopharyngeal masses, or cleft palate results in negative middle ear pressure, eardrum restriction, middle ear mucosal edema, transudation of amber, serous fluid, and a conductive hearing loss, usually without ear pain. A mucoid effusion (secretory otitis media) frequently occurs with incomplete resolution of an acute otitis media. Management involves appropriate treatment of factors causing eustachian tube obstruction, such as adenoidectomy in children or medical and surgical treatment of chronic rhinosinusitis. An examination of the nasopharynx to exclude tumor is indicated in adults. Unresponsive serous or mucoid otitis

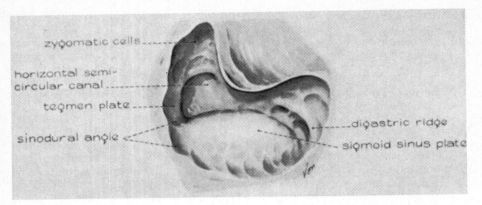

Figure 5. Complete, simple mastoidectomy; right ear, surgeon's view posteriorly. The osseous posterior external canal wall is intact; the tegmen plate is the floor of the middle fossa; the attic and ossicles are not visible in this view but are located just anterior to the indicated prominence of the horizontal semicircular canal. (From Shambaugh, G., and Glasscock, M.E.: Surgery of the Ear. Philadelphia, W. B. Saunders Company, 1980, p. 44.)

necessitates an anterior myringotomy with aspiration of fluid and insertion of a tympanostomy tube to maintain the opening and ventilate the middle ear cleft.

Acute Otitis Media and Mastoiditis. Eustachian tube obstruction predisposes to viral and bacterial infections of the middle ear and mastoid spaces. Presenting signs include a purulent exudate, positive pressure, bulging eardrum, ear pain, and occasional eardrum rupture and otorrhea. Common bacteria include Group A β-hemolytic streptococcus, *Streptococcus pneumoniae*, *Staphylococcus aureus*, and *Hemophilus influenzae*. These infections are seen more frequently in infants and children than adults. Treatment includes an appropriate antibiotic given in adequate doses for 12 to 14 days. Incomplete resolution requires tube myringotomy. The complications of acute otitis media include mastoid abscesses with bone breakdown, labyrinthitis, petrositis with sixth cranial nerve palsy (Gradenigo's syndrome), facial paralysis, and meningitis. Less common intracranial complications include epidural or subdural abscesses, brain abscess, lateral sinus thrombosis, and otitic hydrocephalus. Mastoid x-rays in acute otitis media show increased density in the mastoid air cells because of effusion and mucosal inflammation. With bone breakdown, indistinct bony septae and increased density (coalescence) are seen and intracranial complications are more likely. Drainage and exenteration of the mastoid air cell system (mastoidectomy) and ventilation of the middle ear by myringotomy are indicated (Fig. 5).

Chronic Otitis Media and Mastoiditis. Chronic otitis media is associated with repeated otorrhea, eardrum perforation, middle ear scarring (tympanosclerosis), conductive hearing loss, and a thin flaccid drum that invaginates into the middle ear and attic, forming a squamous epithelium-lined sac, or *cholesteatoma*. Keratinized debris collects in the sac, providing a culture medium for microorganisms; infection results in erosion of the ossicles, labyrinth, facial nerve canal, and the floor of the middle cranial fossa. A cholesteatoma should be suspected with any chronic draining ear, particularly with a marginal or attic perforation. Management includes temporal bone radiography and surgery to remove or widely exteriorize the sac.

Chronic tympanic membrane perforation and conductive hearing loss can be surgically repaired by tympanoplasty. Ossicular continuity, or a columella between the stapes footplate and reconstructed eardrum, is created by using the patient's own ossicles, homograph ossicles, or alloplastic materials.[11] A radical mastoidectomy is required for middle ear cholesteatoma, which cannot be excised, and involves removal of the posterior external ear canal wall, malleus, and incus. The mastoid cavity, attic, middle ear, and ear canal become one cavity. Hearing may be preserved when the cholesteatoma sacs are small and can be removed completely without sacrificing the ossicles or posterior external auditory canal wall. For cholesteatoma that can be removed from the middle ear but not the attic, a modified radical mastoidectomy sparing the tympanic membrane remnants and part of all of the ossicular chain may be performed, with preservation of hearing.

OTOSCLEROSIS

Otosclerosis involves the otic capsule with foci of irregular, immature vascular formations of bone, a histologic appearance similar to that seen in Paget's disease, and tends to occur in a familial pattern, being more common in women than men. Studies of temporal bones have revealed otosclerotic foci in approximately 10 per cent of the Caucasian population, 1 per cent of whom have a normal eardrum with a clinical conductive hearing loss from fixation of the stapes footplate.[10] Foci adjacent to the scala media or semicircular canals can result in sensorial deafness or loss of vestibular function. The conductive hearing loss can be treated surgically by stapes fenestration or complete stapes removal and insertion of a prosthesis from the incus to a tissue graft (vein or fascia) placed over the oval window. The complication of sensorineural hearing loss occurs in 2 to 4 per cent of patients.[24] Patients with bilateral conductive hearing losses who decline a surgical approach frequently benefit from a hearing aid.

MIDDLE EAR NEOPLASIA

Glomus tumors are vascular, slow-growing, nonchromaffin paragangliomas that arise from glomus bodies in the jugular bulb or in Jacobson's nerve on the middle ear promontory. Clinical signs include pulsatile tinnitus, facial nerve paralysis, otorrhea, ear hemorrhage, vertigo, and cranial nerve palsies. Otoscopy reveals a reddish mass that blanches upon increasing ear canal pressure. The diagnosis and extent of involvement are revealed by radiographic examinations, including arteriography and venography. Treatment consists of surgical excision, which may not be feasible for large lesions with intracranial involvement. Palliative benefit with radiotherapy can be obtained owing to a reduction in the vascularity because the tumor cells are relatively radioresistant.

Other rarely seen middle ear tumors include neuromas of the seventh and eighth cranial nerves, cylindromas, dermoid cysts, squamous cell carcinomas, sarcomas, adeno-carcinomas, and meningiomas.

MIDDLE EAR BAROTRAUMA

Middle ear barotrauma following diving or flying is due to inadequate pressure equilibration during descent. The subsequent negative middle ear pressure results in vascular congestion, rupture of vessels in the eardrum and middle ear mucosa, bleeding into the middle ear (hemotympanum), and tympanic membrane rupture. Explosive ruptures of the round or oval windows with inner ear injury can also occur.[9] Patients without signs of inner ear injury are treated with topical nasal decongestants and the avoidance of altered ambient pressure exposure until the process has cleared.

PERIPHERAL FACIAL NERVE PARALYSIS

Sudden, unilateral peripheral facial paralysis without identifiable cause is termed *Bell's palsy*. The suspected pathogenesis is a neurotropic viral infection with inflammation in the temporal bone facial canal, compression of the blood supply, degeneration of the myelin tubes surrounding each axon, and a conduction block, neurapraxia. With continued pressure, axonal death (axonotmesis) or disruption of perineurium, myelin tubes, and axons (neurotmesis) occurs. With disappearance of inflammation, axonal regeneration and recovery of function can occur. Misalignment of myelin tubes inhibits regenerating axons or results in growth to different or multiple facial muscles, with dyskinesis or synkinesis.

Approximately 85 per cent of patients with Bell's palsy will completely recover over a 3- to 4-week period. Another 5 to 10 per cent have partial recovery. Ten to 14 days of corticosteroid therapy begun soon after the onset of paralysis is felt to improve the chances for complete recovery. If recovery has not begun within 3 weeks after paralytic onset, some advocate facial nerve decompression. If tearing is preserved, decompression of the horizontal and vertical portions can be done by a mastoidectomy approach. With absent or decreased tearing, decompression proximal to the geniculate ganglion by a middle fossa intracranial procedure must be considered.

There are many other causes of peripheral facial nerve paralysis. Congenital origins include aplasia and Melkersson's syndrome (furrowed tongue, facial paralysis, and faciolabial edema). Trauma following facial crush or lacerations, basilar skull fractures, penetrating injuries into the middle ear, or birth forceps injury can result in facial nerve paralysis. Central nervous system disease, e.g., Guillain-Barré syndrome, multiple sclerosis, brainstem cerebrovascular accident, or cerebropontine angle tumors, can cause facial nerve paralysis. Neoplastic causes include seventh nerve neuroma and tumors of the internal auditory canal, middle ear, external auditory canal, and parotid gland. Iatrogenic causes include local anesthetic agents and parotid, middle ear, and mastoid surgery. Inflammation and infection, such as are seen in malignant otitis externa (osteomyelitis of the temporal bone in elderly diabetic patients), otitis media with a dehiscent horizontal facial canal, herpes zoster oticus (Ramsay Hunt syndrome), cholesteatoma, encephalitis, mumps, and meningitis, can also lead to facial nerve paralysis.

Diseases of the Inner Ear and Retrocochlear Region

INFLAMMATORY DISEASE

Labyrinthitis usually occurs as a complication of inflammation or infection in adjacent regions. It is the most common complication of otitis media and occurs with meningitis, trauma with labyrinthine hemorrhage, and labyrinthine window fistulas. Labyrinthitis can also be seen with syphilis, tuberculosis, and herpes zoster infections (Ramsay Hunt syndrome). Recent evidence suggests that the inner ear may be a site of autoimmune disease.

LABYRINTHINE TRAUMA

Approximately 80 per cent of temporal bone (basilar skull) fractures are longitudinal (parallel) and 20 per cent are transverse (perpendicular) to the petrous pyramid. Longitudinal fractures frequently involve the middle ear and external auditory canal, with disruption of the ossicular chain and conductive hearing loss. Approximately one third of longitudinal fractures also have a sensorineural hearing loss, and 15 per cent result in a facial paralysis. Transverse fractures usually extend across the cochlea or internal auditory and facial canals to produce a sensorineural hearing loss and facial paralysis.[24] Temporal bone fracture should be suspected in patients with head injury involving bleeding in the middle ear or external auditory canal, ecchymosis around the ear, disruption of the tympanic membrane, a step-off deformity of the external auditory canal, nystagmus, sensorineural hearing loss, peripheral facial nerve palsy, or cerebrospinal fluid otorrhea. Appropriate management includes evaluation of auditory, vestibular, and facial nerve function as soon as feasible in addition to radiographic studies to evaluate skull and intracranial injury. After the patient has been stabilized, definitive treatment of the otologic problem may be undertaken. Ossicular chain disruption may require future surgery. Facial nerve exploration and reanastomosis should be considered for facial nerve palsy of immediate onset.

NOISE INDUCED HEARING LOSS

Common sources of loud noise that cause injury to cochlear hair cells and sensory deafness include engines, i.e., chain saws, aircraft, snowmobiles, construction and industrial machinery, as well as loud music, gunfire, explosions, jack hammers, and rivet guns. The degree of hearing loss is related to the intensity and duration of the exposure. The loss of hearing occurs first at 4000 Hz. and, with repeated exposures, involves other frequencies. Protection from excessive noise exposure may be obtained by the use of solid, sealing ear canal plugs or special head set devices. However, gunfire and explosive noise may produce such intense peak sound levels that adequate protection cannot be obtained.

INNER EAR INJURY DUE TO BAROTRAUMA

Inner ear injury with nerve deafness, tinnitus, and/or vertigo due to labyrinthine window ruptures or inner ear membrane breaks occurs in association with middle ear barotrauma in divers and flyers. Initial treatment includes bed rest, elevation of the head, and maneuvers to avoid increases in intracranial pressure. With deterioration or no improvement in 24 to 72 hours, middle ear exploration for repair of a possible labyrinthine window rupture should be considered. Inner ear decompression sickness occurs as an isolated injury or with other signs of skin, musculoskeletal, or central nervous system decompression sickness. Isolated inner ear decompression sickness is less common in sport scuba divers, being seen more often in deeper, mixed-gas, commercial diving. Treatment includes prompt recompression.[9]

DEGENERATIVE DISEASE

Progressive sensorineural hearing loss and tinnitus with aging is termed presbycusis. The pathologic changes begin at around age 20 and include atrophy of the organ of Corti and auditory nerves, with degeneration of hair cells, spiral ganglia, and brainstem cochlear nuclei.[20] The hearing loss is usually not noted until the fifth and sixth decades, with 4000 to 8000 Hz., being initially involved. The speech frequencies, 500 to 2000 Hz., become affected in the sixth and seventh decades. Suspected etiologies include excessive noise exposure and atherosclerosis. Patients who have adequate discrimination of amplified speech may benefit from a hearing aid.

ACOUSTIC NEUROMAS

Neuromas of the eighth cranial nerve arise from Schwann cells in the vestibular division twice as often as from the auditory division and account for 7 per cent of all intracranial tumors. Symptoms include progressive tinnitus, nonvertiginous dysequilibrium, and/or nerve deafness. Continued growth results in expansion of the internal auditory canal and extension into the cerebropontine angle with involvement of the fifth and seventh cranial nerves, brainstem, or cerebellum. The most consistent audiometric test for diagnosis of an acoustic neuroma is the brainstem evoked response, in which the fifth peak latency on the involved side is increased. Electronystagmography may show a unilateral weakness or central signs if brainstem or cerebellar involvement is present. Radiographic studies include polytomography, computed tomography, and myelography of the posterior fossa. *Nuclear magnetic resonance imaging* is also useful. With no useful hearing, a translabyrinthine microsurgical approach has been advocated for small tumors.[12] For preservation of remaining hearing, a middle cranial fossa approach is suggested. For large tumors, an occipital craniotomy or combined occipital and translabyrinthine approach offers the best chance of removal.

MENIERE'S DISEASE

Meniere's disease is characterized by recurrent, unpredictable episodes of vertigo, sensorineural hearing loss, roaring tinnitus, ear fullness, nausea, and vomiting, usually lasting 3 to 12 hours. In the early stages, only vestibular or auditory symptoms may be present, and inner ear function usually returns to normal between attacks. As the disease progresses, a fluctuating low tone followed by a constant, flat sensorineural hearing loss develops. Sixty to 70 per cent of the patients have unilateral involvement; patients who develop bilateral involvement usually exhibit signs or symptoms in the opposite ear within 2 to 3 years. Temporal bone pathology has demonstrated endolymphatic hydrops with generalized dilatation of the endolymphatic space and membranous ruptures and healing, changes also seen as the pathologic sequelae of other inner ear diseases, such as labyrinthitis, syphilitic otitis, cochlear otosclerosis, and head trauma.[20]

The etiology is unknown; future studies will possibly demonstrate specific abnormalities of production and/or reabsorption of endolymph. Numerous medical treatments, such as the use of vasodilators, diuretics, and salt restriction, have been tried without well-documented benefit. Diazepam is helpful in reducing the severity of the vertigo.

Corrective procedures include transcanal or transmastoid labyrinthectomy or posterior fossa sectioning of the vestibular nerve or the entire eighth cranial nerve. Potentially less destructive procedures include the insertion of a tack through the stapes footplate so that the saccule is ruptured with distention and procedures to drain the endolymphatic sac interior into the subarachnoid or mastoid spaces. Schuknecht has described the creation of a permanent fistula between the perilymphatic space, the scala media of the cochlear basilar turn, and the saccule by placing a 3-mm. right angle pick in a superior direction through the round window membrane. This procedure can cause further loss of hearing but has been effective in relieving vertigo and dysequilibrium in approximately 70 per cent of patients.[21]

OTOTOXIC DRUG EXPOSURE

The aminoglycoside antibiotics (neomycin, streptomycin, kanamycin, gentamycin, and tobramycin) damage sensory and hair cells in the auditory and/or vestibular organs to varying degrees. The extent of damage is directly related to blood levels. Since almost all ototoxic drugs are excreted through the kidneys, renal impairment increases the chance of ototoxic blood levels. Neomycin and kanamycin, the most ototoxic antibiotics, given orally, by colonic irrigation, or used in wound irrigations, have caused irreversible deafness. Ethacrynic acid and furosemide cause either transient or permanent hearing loss, especially in combination with other ototoxic drugs. Ototoxic cancer chemotherapeutic agents include cis-platinum. Salicylates and quinine cause reversible ototoxicity.

If ototoxic drug treatment is required, pretreatment audiometric levels and measures of renal function should be obtained. Doses of the drugs should be monitored by peak and trough blood levels so that ototoxic levels may be avoided and bactericidal levels maintained. The first signs of ototoxicity are high-frequency tinnitus and hearing loss; however, these cannot be relied upon for warning, since further hearing loss can develop after the drug is discontinued. Also, vertigo and nystagmus do not usually occur since both vestibular end-organs are destroyed equally. The hearing disability in older individuals who suffer ototoxicity is usually greater because of a reduced number of hair cells and neural elements owing to presbycusis.

VESTIBULAR NEURONITIS

Vestibular neuronitis is thought to be related to a neurotropic virus and is characterized by sudden attacks of vertigo without auditory or other neurologic symptoms. The first attack usually lasts several days and then subsides; subsequent attacks then occur with decreasing frequency and usually disappear after 1 to 2 years. Some patients will have a history of a viral-like illness several weeks prior to the onset of the vertigo. Electronystagmography usually demonstrates a reduced caloric response in the involved ear. Recovery is related to central vestibular compensation. Management includes the exclusion of other otologic or central nervous system disease, supportive therapy during the attacks, and head movement exercises after the acute phase to stimulate compensation.

IDIOPATHIC SUDDEN DEAFNESS

Sudden sensorineural deafness occurring in the absence of vestibular or central nervous system symptoms, trauma, or other otologic disease has been termed idiopathic sudden deafness. Numerous medical therapies, including vasodilating agents, anticoagulation with heparin, superior sympathetic ganglion block, and steriods, have been tried without proven benefit. A viral etiology is suspected; indeed, this entity may be the auditory equivalent of vestibular neuronitis. Approximately one third of patients experience complete recovery of hearing over 1 to 3 weeks, one third have partial recovery, and one third have no recovery regardless of treatment.

BENIGN POSITIONAL VERTIGO

Episodic vertigo related to specific head position lasting 2 to 3 weeks in the absence of other otologic or central nervous system symptoms has been termed benign positional vertigo, or cupulolithiasis. Once the eliciting head position is assumed, there is a latent period of several seconds before the onset of the vertigo. Also, the vertigo can be suppressed by visual fixation and is noted to be less intense or fatigable with repeated assumption of the position. Schuknecht[20] has found granular basophilic masses on the cupula of the posterior semicircular canal and suggests that these deposits represent calcium carbonate crystals from the utricle otoliths that have fallen into the ampulla as a result of degeneration, labryrinthine concussion, or labyrinthitis.

CONGENITAL INNER EAR MALFORMATIONS

Congenital inner ear malformations with sensorineural deafness may be inherited or acquired *in utero* (rubella, Rh incompatibility, toxemia). The inner ear is derived from neural ectoderm, the middle ear from first and second branchial arch tissue. Inner ear malformations may occur with or without external and middle ear anomalies. Associated anomalies commonly include deformities of the skeletal, urologic, and gastrointestinal systems. Early diagnosis utilizing a high index of suspicion and routine screening audiometry in premature and newborn nurseries is important, since the best development of communication and learning skills is seen with early (within 6 months of age) amplification of residual hearing plus special parental counseling and childhood deaf education.

THE NOSE AND PARANASAL SINUSES

Historic Perspectives[24]

In 1882, Ingals introduced nasal septal surgery, followed by Killian, who pioneered surgical procedures for frontal sinus infections. In 1900, Joseph developed the principles and techniques of modern rhinoplasty. A notable achievement was accomplished in 1900 when Caldwell in New York and Luc in Paris first described an operation for maxillary sinusitis (Caldwell-Luc procedure). This was followed by the development of osteoplastic obliteration for chronic frontal sinusitis in the 1950s.

Functional Anatomy

The nose and paranasal sinuses cleanse, filter, humidify, and warm the inspired air for physiologic gas exchange in the lung alveoli. The mucosal lining—pseudostratified, ciliated, columnar epithelium—secretes about 1 liter of mucous per day in the adult; one half is evaporated by the inspired air stream, and the remaining half is swept by the cilia to the nasopharynx and swallowed. The mucous blanket has an electrostatic charge and contains immunoglobulins and lysozymes; it efficiently collects small particles and defends against microorganisms.

On the side of each nasal passageway are the very vascular inferior, middle, and variable superior turbinates (Fig. 6). The lamina propria of the turbinate mucosa contains large, thin-walled vascular spaces that empty and fill with alterations in temperature, humidity, and emotional stimuli such as fear, anger, grief, and sexual arousal. Inspiration of cold air with a low water vapor pressure results in increased nasal blood flow, mucous production, and congestion; inspiration of warm humid air has the opposite effects. The paranasal sinus ostia open into the middle meatus, beneath the middle turbinate, except for the ostia of the sphenoid sinus and posterior ethmoidal cells, which open into the posterior aspect of the superior meatus. It is likely that the paranasal sinuses provide an increased surface area for mucous production. The nasal olfactory epithelium lies in the superior portions of the septum and the roof of the nasal cavity and sends olfactory fibers through the cribriform plate. Lacrimal secretions are collected via the nasolacrimal duct, which opens into the anterior inferior meatus.

Because the anterior nasal opening (naris) is smaller than the posterior opening (choana), the inspired air stream passes superiorly in a wide curve to the olfactory epithelium, and eddy currents are produced over the anterior inferior turbinates and along the upper posterior wall of the nasopharynx. On expiration, eddy currents fill the nasal cavity. These nasal air flow patterns play a role in olfaction as well as respired air conditioning.[17]

Congenital Nasal Malformations

Choanal atresia involves mucous membrane and bone in 90 per cent of the patients and mucous membrane in 10 per cent of the patients. The unilateral form results in chronic unilateral nasal discharge and obstruction and is frequently not diagnosed until childhood or adolescence. Bilateral choanal atresia is usually diagnosed as neonatal respiratory distress, since newborn infants are obligatory nose breathers. Treatment is by prompt insertion of an oral airway with careful nursing over the next 2 to 3 weeks until mouth breathing develops. The diagnosis can be confirmed by gently insufflating each nasal passageway with an anterior nares tube, by failing to pass a small tube into the oropharynx, by lateral x-rays with the nasal instillation of radiopaque drops, and by computed tomography (CT) techniques. Perforation of the atretic area and insertion of polyethylene tubes for stenting may be attempted; however, stenosis often occurs. A transpalatal surgical repair at age 3 to 5 years is more definitive.[24]

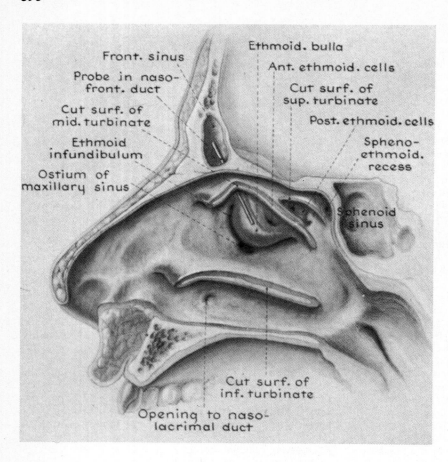

Figure 6. Lateral nasal wall with turbinates removed showing the ostia of the paranasal sinuses and nasolacrimal duct. (From Adams, G. L., et al.: Boies's Fundamentals of Otolaryngology, 5th ed. Philadelphia, W. B. Saunders Company, p. 292.)

Nasal meningoceles and encephaloceles are pale, polyp-like masses found in the upper nasal cavity presenting through defects in the cribriform plate and are differentiated from allergic nasal polyps, which arise in the middle meatus. Nasal gliomas and dermoids occur on the nasal dorsum or intranasally and may also have intracranial connections, which can be demonstrated by CT. These lesions should be excised, using a nasal approach with frontal craniotomy, if intracranial connections are present.[24]

Inflammatory Disease of the Nose and Paranasal Sinuses

RHINITIS AND RHINOSINUSITIS

Acute rhinitis and rhinosinusitis are caused by bacteria, viruses, and, rarely, fungi. They usually occur secondarily to other factors that alter the protective nasal physiology. Many patients have mild chronic problems and secondary infection develops with exposure to cold dry air in the winter. The underlying factors include the following:

1. *Allergic rhinitis and rhinosinusitis*. Symptoms may be seasonal or perennial and include obstruction, sneezing, watery rhinorrhea, and, occasionally, anosmia. Bronchitis and asthma are frequently present. Examination reveals pale congestion and swelling of the membranes and turbinates. Pale, gray nasal polyps may occur in the more severe cases, particularly with secondary infections. Treatment includes desensitization of allergens identified on skin testing plus topical intranasal steroids, systemic decongestants, nasal saline irrigations, and cold weather precautions. Sur-

gery is indicated for removal of polyps, relief of nasal obstruction, and improved sinus ventilation to decrease secondary infection.

2. *Chronic nasal irritation*. This may result from smoking, excessive use of topical nasal adrenergic agents, and industrial fume exposure.

3. *Mechanical nasal obstruction*. This is usually due to external and internal nasal deformities and, less frequently, polyps or neoplasia. In children, adenoidal hypertrophy is a common cause.

4. *Vasomotor rhinitis*. Nonallergic vascular engorgement of nasal mucosa with sneezing and watery discharge can be due to increased parasympathetic stimulation from emotional stress or medications such as adrenergic blocking agents. Conservative treatment is usually indicated.

Less common primary causes of *chronic rhinitis or rhinosinusitis* include:

1. *Primary infections* (e.g., syphilis, tuberculosis, rhinoscleroma, or leprosy).

2. *Mycotic infections* (e.g., *Aspergillus* or *Mucor* infestations, both usually seen in patients debilitated from other systemic diseases such as uncontrolled diabetes).

3. *Biochemical disorders* (e.g., cystic fibrosis).

4. *Microstructural anomalies* (e.g., Kartagener's syndrome [situs inversus and chronic polypoid rhinosinusitis], syndromes with immotile cilia that lack dynen arms on electron microscopy).

5. *Idiopathic causes* (e.g., (1) Wegener's granulomatosis (granulomas of the nose, lung, and renal glomeruli), (2) necrotizing vasculitis, (3) periarteritis nodosa, (4) lethal midline granuloma, (5) relapsing polychondritis, (6) lupus erythematosus, and (7) sarcoidosis).

SINUSITUS

Acute sinusitis is usually related to nasal or dental infections and develops with obstruction of the ostia, absorption of oxygen with a negative pressure, and sinus mucosal congestion followed by bacterial invasion, infiltration of leukocytes, pus formation, and positive pressure. Symptoms include purulent nasal discharge and pain. Treatment includes the use of decongestants (topical and systemic), warmth, humidification, and appropriate antibiotics for 10 to 14 days.

Virulent sinus infections or an infected mucocele (a mucous retention cyst) in the frontal or ethmoid sinuses can result in osteomyelitis or bone erosion with spread of infection to the orbit or intracranium. Acute ethmoid sinusitis is particularly associated with orbital inflammation, which presents with cellulitis of the eyelid, proptosis, and displacement of the globe laterally and inferiorly, followed by limitations of extraocular motion, orbital abscesses, and blindness. Treatment includes parenteral antibiotic therapy. Drainage and orbital decompression by an external ethmoidectomy through a medial orbital incision are needed before complete losses of extraocular motion and vision occur. Frontal sinus abscesses are drained by trephination of the inferior medial wall. Mucoceles or other frontal sinus lesions may be approached with an osteoplastic flap of the anterior wall through an eyebrow incision or a scalp incision behind the hairline. The mucous membrane and other lesions are removed and the cavity is obliterated by a fat graft from the abdominal wall.

Chronic maxillary sinusitis usually responds to an intranasal antrostomy placed through the lateral nasal wall beneath the inferior turbinate. Severe maxillary sinusitis may require removal of diseased mucosa or polyps via a Caldwell-Luc operation, which allows exposure of the entire sinus cavity through an upper sublabial incision and osteotomy of the anterior wall. Intranasal surgery for chronic ethmoid sinusitis carries an increased risk of intracranial or orbital injury; an external ethmoidectomy is safer. The sphenoid sinus is optimally exposed via an external ethmoidectomy or a transseptal approach using the operating microscope and intraoperative fluoroscopic control.

Nasal Fracture

Nasal fractures are usually associated with breaks of the nasal lining and epistaxis. Septal hematomas may occur. The immediate soft tissue swelling may obscure the bony deformity; diagnosis is established by gentle nasal palpation that demonstrates step-off deformities, instability, or crepitus. X-rays may not reveal the nasal fracture but are needed to evaluate other facial fractures that may be present. Cerebrospinal fluid rhinorrhea may occur but usually subsides spontaneously with prophylactic antibiotics, bed rest, head elevation, and the avoidance of nasal blowing to prevent intracranial pneumatocele. Reduction of nasal fractures should occur within 10 days, before fibrosis and displaced fixation occur, and is accomplished by manipulation externally by the fingers and internally by elevators. Unstable fractures are splinted both internally and externally. If significant septal deformity remains after closed reduction, septoplasty may be required. Septal hematomas must be drained to prevent abscess, necrosis of the septal cartilage, and subsequent saddle nasal deformity.

Internal and External Nasal Deformities

Nasal septal deformities result from developmental anomalies or trauma at birth or later in life and produce nasal obstruction with sinusitis and/or chronic eustachian tubal obstruction with middle ear disease. Correction is by septoplasty in which the deviated cartilage and bone are exposed and remodeled. Septal deformities are often associated with external nasal deformities; thus septoplasty and external nasal reconstruction or rhinoplasty may be needed for physiologic as well as cosmetic reasons.

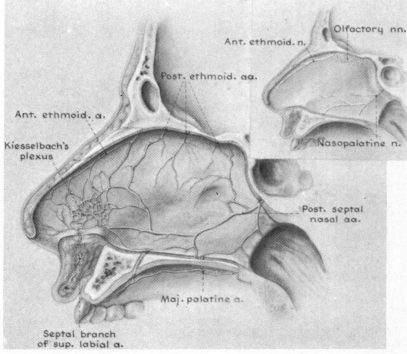

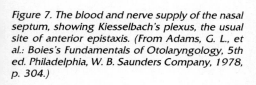

Figure 7. The blood and nerve supply of the nasal septum, showing Kiesselbach's plexus, the usual site of anterior epistaxis. (From Adams, G. L., et al.: Boies's Fundamentals of Otolaryngology, 5th ed. Philadelphia, W. B. Saunders Company, 1978, p. 304.)

Nasal Foreign Bodies

Nasal foreign bodies are particularly common in children and should be suspected with a history of chronic, unilateral purulent discharge and/or obstruction. Removal usually requires general anesthesia using topical nasal vasoconstrictors and intranasal approaches.

Epistaxis

Epistaxis is a hazardous clinical problem, particularly when originating posteriorly. Predisposing factors include hypertension, arteriosclerosis, chronic irritation from smoking, cold dry air exposure, and rhinitis. Neoplasia, coagulation deficits, and hereditary telangiectasia are less common predisposing factors. Ninety per cent of spontaneous epistaxis is from a plexus of superficial vessels in the anterior, inferior septum (Fig. 7) and is more easily managed than posterior epistaxis, which occurs in 10 per cent of patients from vessels in the lateral nasal wall close to the nasopharynx and has been associated with a 4 to 5 per cent mortality.[24]

Anterior epistaxis is treated by pinching the anterior nose for 5 to 10 minutes with the patient sitting and the head tilted forward. Bleeding not controlled by this method requires visualization of the bleeding point, application of topical anesthetics, and cautery with silver nitrate or electrocautery. If this is unsuccessful, bilateral packing using 0.25- to 0.5-inch bacitracin-impregnated gauze strips is inserted for 2 to 4 days. Nasal packing causes obstruction of the paranasal sinus ostia; thus, prophylactic antibiotics should be used.

The control of posterior epistaxis utilizes the principle of tamponade obtained by obstruction of the posterior choanae with a Foley catheter balloon or posterior nasal pack and the nares by anterior packs. Posterior packs are rolls of 4 × 4 inch gauze (2 × 2 inch gauze for children) to which are tied two strands of #2 black silk or umbilical tape. Topical anesthesia is applied, and a catheter is passed through the nose and brought out the mouth, where two ends of one strand are tied. The catheter and ties are then withdrawn, and the pack is guided into the nasopharynx. The ties are held tautly while an anterior pack is inserted and are tied over a roll of 4 × 4 inch gauze at the anterior nares. The two ends of the other strand are either trimmed just below the level of the soft palate or are brought out through the mouth and taped to the side of the cheek so that they are available for pack removal. Both anterior nares should be packed to avoid significant septal deflection. With severe bleeding, bilateral posterior packs are usually required (Fig. 8).

The packs are left in place for 4 to 5 days; prophylactic antibiotics, supplemental humidified oxygen by mask, replacement of blood loss, and close monitoring of vital signs plus fluid and electrolyte balance are required. Posterior epistaxis may also be treated angiographically by catheterization and embolization of the internal maxillary artery and its branches. Silver clip occlusion of these vessels in the pterygomaxillary space via a Caldwell-Luc approach with removal of the posterior maxillary sinus wall is also used.[5] Superiorly located bleeding points may require ligation of the anterior ethmoidal artery through a medial orbital incision.

Neoplasia

Benign tumors arising in the nose and paranasal sinuses include squamous papillomas, osteomas, ossifying fibromas, hemangiomas, neurofibromas, neurilemmomas, and plasmacytomas. Inverting papillomas are pale, polypoid lesions that usually arise in the middle meatus from the lateral nasal wall. Malignant degeneration to squamous cell carcinomas occurs in 10 per cent of patients. Local invasion of the orbit, ethmoid and maxillary sinuses, and intracranium is seen. Treatment requires surgical resection, which may be extensive.[4]

Squamous cell carcinoma is the most common malignant tumor arising in the nose and paranasal sinuses and is

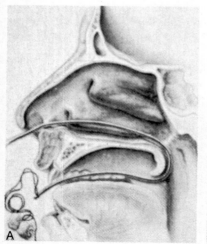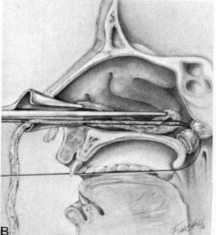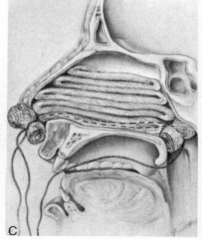

Figure 8. Anterior and posterior nasal packs for posterior epistaxis. A, Two strands of one tie are secured to the oral end of a rubber catheter passed through the nose and out the mouth. B, The catheter has been withdrawn from the nose, and the pack is secured in the posterior choana. Bilateral anterior packing is layered into position. C, The two anterior strands are tied over a rolled 4×4 inch gauze. The posterior one or two strands facilitate pack removal and are loosely secured to the face. (From Adams, G. L., et al.: Boies's Fundamentals of Otolaryngoogy, 5th ed. Philadelphia, W. B. Saunders Company, 1978, p. 369.)

most frequently seen in the maxillary sinus. Late diagnosis with spread to the nose, ethmoid sinuses, orbit, or anterior face is not uncommon. Treatment requires surgical excision, a partial or total maxillectomy, and pre- or postoperative radiation therapy. Involvement of the orbit requires orbital exenteration; ethmoid involvement requires a combined removal of the floor of the anterior cranial fossa, ethmoids, and maxilla to obtain an en bloc resection.[22] Spread to the pterygomaxillary space, posterior ethmoids, or sphenoid sinuses cannot be removed en bloc. The addition of multiagent chemotherapy after surgery and radiation for advanced lesions may result in improved response rates.[13]

Lymphomas are treated by radiation therapy and/or chemotherapy. Sarcomas, particularly rhabdomyosarcoma in children, are treated by surgical removal of the bulk of the lesion followed by prolonged multiagent chemotherapy.

THE PHARYNX

Functional Anatomy

The pharynx is bounded from the base of the skull to the opening of the esophagus by constrictor muscles, which insert posteriorly into a midline raphe. The functions of the pharynx are speech articulation, respiratory passage, and deglutition. A circumferential band of lymphoid tissues, Waldeyer's ring, contains the adenoids on the posterior wall of the nasopharynx, the palatine tonsils, and the lingual tonsils on the base of the tongue. The pharynx is divided into the nasopharynx, oropharynx, and hypopharynx. The anterior boundaries of the nasopharynx include the nasal choanae and the dorsal surface of the soft palate. The cartilaginous eustachian tubes project from the posterolateral wall at a 45-degree angle. The inferior limit is an imaginary plane extending posteriorly from the plane of the hard palate. The oropharynx begins at the level of the anterior tonsillar pillars and extends posteriorly to the pharyngeal wall. The lateral wall contains the tonsillar fossae, and the inferior extent includes the vallecula and the base of the tongue. The hypopharynx can be imagined as an inverted funnel with the narrow portion at the cricopharyngeal sphincter and the superior opening at the level of the hyoid bone and epiglottis. The pyriform sinuses lie on each side, and the posterior pharyngeal wall forms the posterior boundary. The larynx projects from the anterior hypopharynx.

Inflammatory Disease of the Pharynx

ADENOIDITIS AND TONSILLITIS

Hyperplasia of the adenoids, palatine tonsils, and lingual tonsils usually occurs during childhood. Involution during adolescence may be limited by fibrous tissue resulting from previous infections. Surface clefts or crypts that collect debris may become sites of chronic infection. Adenoidal enlargement or chronic adenoiditis may result in nasal obstruction with mouth breathing, hyponasal voice, rhinorrhea, eustachian tube obstruction with acute or chronic otitis media, or frequent upper respiratory infections.

Depending upon the severity, frequency, and refractiveness to medical management, adenoidectomy may be indicated. The adenoidal tissue is removed superficial to the fascia of the superior constrictor muscle, using a curette or an adenotome, with the patient under general orotracheal anesthesia. Chronic cryptic tonsillitis is characterized by a history of sore throat and findings of white, cheesy, foul-tasting material in tonsillar crypts, asymmetric tonsillar enlargement, and persistent upper cervical lymphadenitis. Recurrent acute tonsillitis (three or more times per year), peritonsillar abscess, and airway obstruction due to massive tonsillar enlargement are indications for a tonsillectomy. Using general orotracheal anesthesia, the capsule of the tonsil is exposed through an incision close to the edge of the anterior tonsillar pillar, and the tonsil is removed by an extracapsular dissection superficial to the superior constrictor muscle. The most common complication of tonsillectomy is bleeding (seen in 1 to 2 per cent of patients), which may occur within the first 24 hours or 7 to 14 days later, when the healing crusts slough. Exposure and control of the bleeding site with cautery or suture ligatures, usually with the patient under general orotracheal anesthesia, are required. Because of the greater risk of blood loss in small children, tonsillectomy is best deferred until the growing child attains a weight of 40 pounds.

THE PHARYNGEAL-RELATED ABSCESSES

Abscesses in the retropharyngeal, parapharyngeal, or peritonsillar spaces occur secondary to acute pharyngitis, tonsillitis, adenoiditis, dental infections, and, less commonly, sinusitis.

Retropharyngeal abscesses are most common in infants and young children and occur in the space between the muscular pharyngeal constrictors and the prevertebral fascia. Clinical presentation includes fever, toxicity, stridor, neck hyperextension to maintain an airway, and anterior displacement of the posterior pharyngeal wall. Lateral neck and skull x-rays reveal widening of and/or air in the retropharyngeal space. Care should be taken in the physical examination to avoid rupturing the abscess, with possible aspiration of the contents. Treatment requires parenteral antibiotic therapy and drainage by vertical incision of the posterior pharyngeal wall mucosa with the patient under general orotracheal anesthesia in the Trendelenburg position. Retropharyngeal abscesses, once drained, tend to remain empty by the action of swallowing.

Parapharyngeal abscesses result from infection in lymph nodes lateral to the superior pharyngeal constrictor muscles and adjacent to the carotid sheath. Presenting signs usually include trismus, drooling, dysphasia, swelling in the anterior cervical triangle, and medial displacement of the tonsil and soft palate. Treatment includes administration of parenteral antibiotics and drainage of fluctuant swelling via an external neck incision along the anterior border of the sternocleidomastoid muscle; transoral drainage is not done because of the proximity of the vessels of the carotid sheath. Smears and cultures for bacteria, acid-fast bacilli and fungi are obtained. A drain is sutured into position and left in place until drainage ceases.

A *peritonsillar abscess* occurs between the capsule of the tonsil and the superior constrictor muscle from spread of acute tonsillitis, most commonly after puberty. Presenting signs include fever, dysphagia, foul-smelling breath, trismus, medial displacement of the tonsil, and inflammation of the adjacent soft palate and uvula. An abscess cavity may be detected by careful aspiration using a syringe and needle inserted no more than 2.5 cm. into the most swollen tissues superior to the tonsillar capsule. If pus is encountered, the abscessed cavity is drained using local anesthesia and a curvilinear incision along the course of the anterior tonsillar pillar. Repeated swallowing keeps the cavity empty; however, the incision site can seal and may require reopening. A tonsillectomy is performed about 3 to 4 weeks later.

Pharyngeal Neoplasia

JUVENILE ANGIOFIBROMA OF THE NASOPHARYNX

Juvenile angiofibromas are vascular tumors arising in pubescent males, usually from the nasopharyngeal vault. Involvement of the paranasal sinuses, orbit, skull base, or intracranial cavity may occur. Some involution after puberty occurs. The common presenting symptoms include nasal obstruction, epistaxis, which may be massive, and purulent discharge. Radiographic studies may reveal erosion of the bony walls of the sinuses, orbit, and intracranial cavity plus widening of the pterygomaxillary fissure with extension into the infratemporal fossa. Arteriography shows a vascular pattern with blood supply from branches of the internal maxillary, middle meningeal, and internal carotid arteries. If feasible, the treatment involves surgical removal using a transpalatal or lateral rhinotomy approach and preparations for rapid, massive blood replacement. Preoperative estrogen treatment and embolization of major feeding arteries may reduce blood loss. Newer techniques of surgical approach to the skull base may offer some advantages. Because of moderate radiosensitivity, radiation therapy, either preoperatively or in lieu of surgery, is feasible for massive tumors.[25]

MALIGNANT TUMORS OF THE NASOPHARYNX, OROPHARYNX, AND HYPOPHARYNX

Ninety per cent of tumors in these regions are squamous cell carcinomas and lymphoepitheliomas commonly related to tobacco use, excessive alcohol consumption, and the use of betel nuts. The remaining 10 per cent include minor salivary gland malignancies, lymphomas, melanomas, and sarcomas. The evaluation of all head and neck cancer patients should include staging using the TNM system.[1] Only in this manner can the extent of the cancer be adequately assessed and appropriate treatment and prognosis determined.

Carcinoma of the Nasopharynx

Of all malignant tumors in males, nasopharyngeal carcinoma ranks thirty-third in frequency in the United States and first in the Far East. A genetic predisposition has been suggested. Elevated levels of IgG and IgA antibodies to Epstein-Barr virus (EBV) have been noted in patients with these carcinomas. The etiologic relationship to the virus is unknown; IgA antibodies to the EBV-viral capsid antigen appear to be the most sensitive for monitoring the disease.[16] There are three histologic types of nasopharyngeal carcinomas: (1) undifferentiated carcinoma (lymphoepithelioma and lymphopenic types), (2) nonkeratinizing carcinoma, and (3) squamous cell carcinoma. Lymphocytes occur predominantly in Type 1; they are probably not neoplastic, since they occur in all three types. Type 1 tumors are the most radiosensitive.[2]

Patients with nasopharyngeal carcinomas present with obstruction, rhinorrhea, epistaxis, eustachian tube obstruction with middle ear effusion, cervical mass caused by regional node spread, mass or ulcer in the nasopharynx, or bulging and paralysis of the palate. The tumor spreads along the skull base to the foramen lacerum, the middle cranial fossa, the cavernous sinus, and the jugular foramen, causing multiple cranial nerve palsies. Biopsies of neck masses may not be necessary and may result in the implantation of tumor into the skin and other tissues, making subsequent en bloc resection by radical neck dissection difficult; thus, neck biopsies should be deferred until after examination and biopsies of the nasopharynx, hypopharynx, and larynx to search for a primary lesion. Radiation therapy is the primary treatment for nasopharyngeal carcinomas. Radical neck dissection is used to control residual neck disease if radiation therapy controls the primary lesion. The overall 5-year survival rate, combining all stages, is 35 to 40 per cent.[6]

Carcinoma of the Oropharynx

Squamous cell carcinoma of the tonsil accounts for 1.5 to 3 per cent of all cancers and is the second most frequent upper respiratory cancer after laryngeal carcinoma. Cancers of the soft palate and tongue base are less common. Sore throat, referred pain to the ear, and a metastatic mass in the neck are the most common presenting factors. The rate of regional metastasis ranges from 40 per cent for the soft palate to 70 per cent for the tongue base. Management includes radiography of the chest and head and neck, including computed tomography (CT) scans, followed by panendoscopy and biopsy of suspicious pharyngeal or laryngeal lesions. Concurrent second primary cancers are found in 10 per cent of patients. Surgery alone, radical radiation alone, or combined therapy is advocated. For Stage I and II disease, radical radiation of the primary lesion and neck with or without primary resection seems to be the best treatment. For more extensive Stage III and IV operable cancers, combination therapy with pre- or postoperative radiation appears to offer increased local and regional node control. Multiagent chemotherapy given before or after surgery and radiation therapy may offer additional control for Stage III and IV disease, particularly when chemotherapy is given when fewer residual tumor cells are present.[13] High-risk factors, such as smoking and alcoholic beverage intake, must be discontinued to lessen the risks of radionecrosis, poor wound healing, and new primary cancers.

Carcinoma of the Hypopharynx

Carcinomas of the pyriform sinus, postcricoid area, and posterior pharyngeal wall often do not cause symptoms until advanced and have a high incidence (40 to 70 per cent) of regional cervical node metastasis, which may be bilateral. The initial presentation includes a neck mass, sore throat, referred ear pain, dysphagia, and hoarseness. Treatment of pyriform sinus lesions includes laryngopharyngectomy and neck dissection. Postoperative radical radiation therapy after tumor resection seems to result in the best survival (64 per cent).[8] Lesions of the postcricoid or cervical esophagus require a total pharyngectomy and reconstruction by gastric pull-up, tubed pedicle flaps, or intestinal free grafts with microvascular anastomosis. Posterior pharyngeal wall cancers are surgically resected through an extended lateral pharyngotomy with postoperative radiation therapy. Postcricoid cancers carry the worst prognosis because of mediastinal node involvement.

Other Pharyngeal Diseases

PHARYNGEAL FOREIGN BODIES

Foreign bodies of the pharynx are likely to be found in the palatine and lingual tonsils, the valleculae, and the pyriform sinuses and include fish bones and other sharp, irregular animal bones. Impaction of poorly chewed food occurs at the cricopharyngeal sphincter, particularly in edentulous elderly people. Management of pharyngeal foreign bodies involves a lateral x-ray, barium swallow, and endoscopy. Foreign bodies in the palatine tonsil may be removed by direct vision and a hemostat.

TORNWALDT'S CYST OF THE NASOPHARYNX

A pit or cyst in the posterior midline of the upper nasopharynx exists in approximately 3 per cent of individuals and is thought to represent a persistence of the communication of the anterior end of the embryonic notocord and the pharyngeal roof.[24] Infection usually presents in the second and third decades of life, with tenacious and purulent postnasal drainage, occipital headache, sore throat, unpleasant taste, or halitosis. Nasopharyngoscopy reveals a smooth, submucosal midline cyst, frequently with a central dimple or opening. Lateral x-rays demonstrate the mass. Treatment is by marsupialization. These cysts should be differentiated from pituitary remnants in Rathke's pouch, which are located more superiorly in the roof of the nasopharynx, and smaller mucous gland cysts, which are frequently multiple, more lateral, and superficial to the superior constrictor muscle.

VELOPHARYNGEAL INSUFFICIENCY

Speech and deglutition require closure of the velopharyngeal sphincter by contraction of the palate and superior constrictor muscles. Closure can be impaired in patients with palatal clefts and paralysis or hypoplasia after palatal resection for neoplasia. Symptoms include hypernasal speech and nasal regurgitation during deglutition. Speech cinefluoroscopy demonstrates the insufficient closure; surgical management includes pharyngeal flaps and palatal pushback procedures.

HYPOPHARYNGEAL DIVERTICULA

Pulsion or Zenker's diverticula occur, usually in older individuals, through the posterior hypopharyngeal wall in a weak triangle formed by the oblique fibers of the inferior constrictor and the transverse fibers of the cricopharyngeus muscles (Killian's dehiscence). Hiatal hernia and reflux esophagitis with subsequent spasm and incomplete relaxation of the cricopharyngeal sphincter during deglutition may play etiologic roles. The diverticulum fills during eating and empties upon lying down, with regurgitation and possible aspiration. Barium swallow radiography demonstrates the pouch lying on the left side, between the esophagus and vertebrae. Treatment is by excision through an anterior neck approach and cricopharyngeal myotomy.

THE LARYNX

Functional Anatomy

The larynx is a specifically structured, mucosal-lined tube of cartilage and muscle connecting to the trachea inferiorly and projecting into the hypopharynx anteriorly. The extrinsic strap muscles and the thyrohyoid membrane connect the larynx to the sternum and hyoid bone, which is suspended from the floor of mouth and skull by the myelohyoid, geniohyoid, digrastic, and stylohyoid muscles (Fig. 9). The shield-shaped thyroid cartilage has superior and inferior cornua, the latter articulating with the ring-like cricoid cartilage. The arytenoid cartilages articulate with the posterosuperior cricoid ring in a synovial joint that allows the arytenoids to glide, rotate, and tilt. The anterior vocal process of the arytenoids anchors the posterior ends of the true vocal cords; most of the intrinsic laryngeal muscles insert onto the posterior muscular process. The arytenoid cartilages are rotated about a superoinferior axis by the lateral cricoarytenoid muscles for vocal cord adduction and by the posterior cricoarytenoid muscles for vocal cord abduction. Contraction of the cricothyroid muscles, innervated by the superior laryngeal nerves, causes the cricoid and the attached arytenoids to tilt posteriorly with tightening of the vocal cords (Fig. 10). Superior laryngeal nerve paralysis results in a loose vocal cord with preservation of abduction and adduction. Paralysis of the recurrent laryngeal nerves that innervate the other intrinsic muscles results in the loss of abduction and adduction, with the vocal cords fixed in a paramedian position.

Anatomically, the larynx is divided into three regions:

1. The *supraglottis* (epiglottis, aryepiglottic folds, false vocal cords, roof and lateral walls of the laryngeal ventricles).

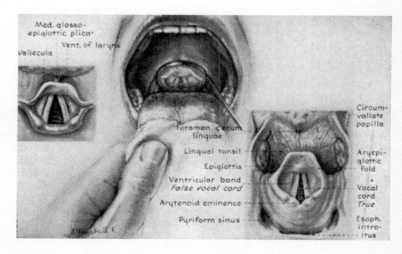

Figure 9. The anatomy of the laryngopharynx as viewed by mirror, indirect laryngoscopy. (From Adams, G. L., et al.: Boies's Fundamentals of Otolaryngology, 5th ed. Philadelphia, W. B. Saunders Company, 1978, p. 23.)

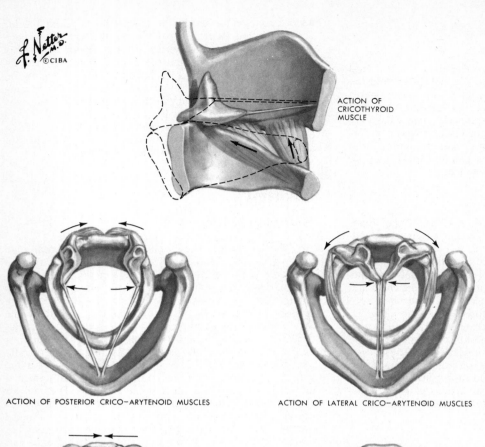

ACTION OF
CRICOTHYROID
MUSCLE

Figure 10. Action of the intrinsic laryngeal muscles. (From Saunders, W. H.: The Larynx. Copyright 1964, CIBA Pharmaceutical Company, Division of CIBA-GEIGY Corporation. Reprinted with permission from Clinical Symposia, illustrated by Frank H. Netter, M.D. All rights reserved.)

ACTION OF POSTERIOR CRICO-ARYTENOID MUSCLES

ACTION OF LATERAL CRICO-ARYTENOID MUSCLES

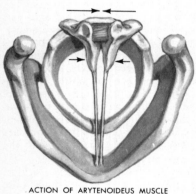

ACTION OF ARYTENOIDEUS MUSCLE

ACTION OF VOCALIS AND THYRO-ARYTENOID MUSCLES

NS-3-64 – CLINICAL SYMPOSIA – ACTION OF THE INTRINSIC MUSCLES – DR. SAUNDERS

2. The *glottis* (true vocal cords, vocal processes of the arytenoids, anterior and posterior commissures).

3. The *subglottis* (the conus elasticus, extending 10 mm. below the free edge of the vocal cords).

The larynx primarily is a sphincter used for closure of the false and true vocal cords and posterior deflection of the epiglottis during deglutition to prevent aspiration. The sphincteric action also serves as a respiratory outlet valve to increase intratracheal, thoracic, and abdominal pressures during coughing, defecation, and parturition and as an inlet valve to limit chest expansion and stabilize the thorax and

shoulder girdle when lifting heavy objects or climbing. Vocal cord abduction during inspiration and adduction during expiration are thought to help maintain blood carbon dioxide levels and regulate acid base balance. Speech evolved later than the sphincteric functions and is produced by vocal cord vibrations, which break exhaled air into fundamental frequencies, about 125 Hz. in adult males and 250 Hz. in adult females, and harmonic frequencies, which are modulated by the pharynx, palate, tongue, cheeks, teeth, and lips. Vocal cord inflammation results in alterations of the fundamental and harmonic frequencies and a raspy, coarse voice. Lesions such as polyps, nodules, and neoplasia plus vocal cord paralysis interfere with smooth vocal cord approximation and result in a breathy voice.[24]

Congenital Malformations of the Larynx

Respiratory obstruction in newborns may be congenital or acquired. Inspiratory stridor that worsens in the supine position with a normal or slightly muffled cry suggests a supraglottic obstruction. A hoarse cry with predominantly inspiratory stridor unaffected by position change indicates a glottic lesion. A subglottic or tracheal obstruction usually produces both inspiratory and expiratory stridor with an unaltered cry.

Laryngotracheomalacia caused by immature cartilaginous support is the most common cause of neonatal airway obstruction and results in the indrawing of the epiglottis and aryepiglottic folds plus collapse of the trachea on inspiration. Laryngeal clefts are rare and result from incomplete fusion of the laryngotracheal septum, with respiratory distress owing to aspiration. Congenital supraglottic disorders may be caused by cysts, which are immediately relieved by aspiration and marsupialization. Glottic disorders may be related to bilateral vocal cord paralysis from birth trauma, Arnold-Chiari malformation, meningomyeloceles, or hydrocephalus. Congenital glottic anomalies include stenosis or webs, most often in the anterior two thirds of the vocal cords. Congenital subglottic obstruction is caused by stenosis and hemangiomas. Acquired subglottic stenosis is usually related to prolonged endotracheal intubation. Tracheal obstruction may be caused by congenital stenosis, absent tracheal ring development, or extrinsic compression from vascular rings or tumors of adjacent structures.

The management of neonatal respiratory obstruction involves diagnosis by direct laryngoscopy, monitoring, and preparations for intubation and/or tracheostomy. Since many forms of congenital stridor, particularly laryngotracheomalacia, improve with time, conservative management should be attempted if respiratory exchange is adequate. If not, intubation or tracheostomy may be needed; however, tracheostomy in the newborn is associated with management problems and a high incidence of complications.

Laryngeal Inflammatory Disease

The most common causes of laryngeal obstruction in infants and children are viral laryngotracheobronchitis (croup) and epiglottitis due to *Haemophilus influenzae*, type B infections. *Laryngotracheobronchitis* presents with a croupy cough and hoarse voice; epiglottitis presents with a muffled voice and difficulty with oral secretions. Upper respiratory obstruction with inspiratory stridor may develop rapidly with both diseases. Patients with *epiglottitis* have a cherry red epiglottis at the base of the tongue and an enlarged epiglottis on lateral neck x-ray; with croup, subglottic edema may be seen on a posteroanterior neck x-ray.

The immediate problem is management of the respiratory obstruction, the severity of which is evaluated by the volume of ventilatory exchange, degree of stridor, rates of respiration and pulse, and patient fatigue. Cyanosis or apparent relaxation with decreased respiratory effort, pulse rate, and ventilation volume is a late sign and indicates impending cardiac arrest and death. Children with significant airway obstruction should be promptly intubated with an endotracheal tube small enough to avoid laryngotracheal injury yet of sufficient size to ensure adequate gas exchange. Ideally intubation should take place in the operating room with endoscopy, anesthesia support, and tracheostomy preparation. Airway management should not be delayed to obtain radiographic and blood gas studies; these studies may increase anxiety and respiratory obstruction and rarely provide information that alters the need for prompt intubation. Oro- or nasotracheal intubation can be performed and tracheostomy avoided in most cases. Intensive care of the entotracheal tube, intravenous antibiotics using drugs effective against *Hemophilus*, steroid therapy, and humidification are needed. After 48 to 72 hours, the patient is electively returned to the operating room, the endotracheal tube removed under anesthesia, and endoscopy repeated. Persistent or recurrent respiratory obstruction requires reintubation and tracheostomy.

Juvenile laryngotracheal papillomatosis is suspected to be of viral etiology and consists of exuberant growths of multiple papillomas in the supraglottis, glottis, trachea, and bronchi. Clinical presentation frequently occurs between ages 1 to 3 with acute respiratory obstruction. Treatment is removal of papillomata using microscopic endoscopy and laser with the patient under general anesthesia. Vigorous removal in the anterior third of the supraglottis or glottis results in laryngeal stenosis. Current studies suggest that interferon therapy may lessen papilloma recurrence.[18]

Vocal Abuse

Loud or prolonged speech produces acute and chronic inflammation of the vocal cords, polyps of the vocal cords, or nodules at the junction of the anterior third and posterior two thirds of the vocal cords. Presenting symptoms include chronic hoarseness and/or breathy voice. Treatment includes voice restraint. Significant lesions, particularly in patients whose voice quality is professionally important, necessitate removal of polyps or stripping of chronically inflamed mucosa by microscopically directed laryngoscopy with the patient under general anesthesia. Postoperative voice rest, alteration of vocal habits, and removal of irritative factors such as smoking are important; otherwise, the lesions may recur. Contact vocal ulcers over the arytenoid vocal process also result from vocal abuse and cause painful phonation, hoarseness, and coughing. Direct laryngoscopy and biopsy are performed to exclude carcinoma. Prolonged voice rest is required for healing.

Laryngeal Trauma

Blows to the anterior neck can impinge the larynx against the cervical vertebrae, with subsequent fractures of the hyoid bone and thyroid or cricoid cartilages, dislocation of the arytenoid cartilages, disruption of the thyrohyoid and cricothyroid membranes and suprahyoid muscles, and/or subglottic transection of the trachea. These injuries occur with automobile accidents or a fall against bicycle handlebars or when riding a horse or bicycle against a tight line. Symptoms include hoarseness, dysphonia or aphonia, cough, hemoptysis, neck pain, and painful swallowing. Stridor may initially be absent, only to occur later upon swelling and ecchymosis of the laryngopharynx. Physical examination reveals neck tenderness and swelling with alterations in the normal contour and/or subcutaneous emphysema. Indirect or fiberoptic laryngoscopy reveals a distorted glottis with mucosal lacerations, exposed cartilage, and limited vocal cord motion. Lateral neck x-rays, polytomography or CT scans, and barium swallow studies are obtained to evaluate possible fractures and dislocations of the cervical spine and the integrity of the laryngopharynx.

The initial management includes ensuring an adequate airway and stabilizing the neck. Immediate tracheostomy may be needed. Evaluation of laryngeal injuries should proceed once the airway and cardiovascular system are stabilized; delays longer than 7 to 10 days can result in laryngeal stenosis. Surgical repair is accomplished through a transverse neck incision and midline division of the thyroid cartilage (laryngofissure) to expose the larynx. A lower tracheostomy is inserted, cartilages are realigned, mucosal lacerations are repaired, and a solid mold is used for internal splinting for 6 weeks.

Tracheostomy

The indications for tracheostomy are upper respiratory obstruction, difficulties with lower or upper respiratory secretions, and ventilatory insufficiency in patients requiring prolonged (greater than 5 to 7 days) nasal or orotracheal intubation. Tracheostomies are not simple surgical procedures. Bleeding from midline external jugular veins and the thyroid isthmus can be encountered. Other complications include pneumomediastinum, pneumothorax, and injury to the recurrent laryngeal nerves and esophagus, particularly in children. Late complications include massive hemorrhage from cuff or tube erosions through the anterior tracheal wall into the innominate artery, tracheal stenosis, and tracheoesophageal fistula.

Tracheostomy is best performed electively in the operating room with oro- or nasotracheal intubation and anesthesia support. Intubation with tubes that are too large or rigid and excessive or prolonged cuff inflation must be avoided. The technique for performing tracheostomy is shown in Chapter 44 in the section on "Physiologic Aspects of Respiratory Function in Surgical Patients." Posttracheostomy care includes ultrasonic humidification, regular wound and tube cleaning, avoidance of tube twisting by respirator connections, deflation of cuffs when not needed for ventilatory assistance or prevention of aspiration, and minimal cuff inflation to maintain an adequate seal with a small air leak.

Acute upper airway obstruction due to large tumors, inflammatory distortion, or foreign bodies may preclude prompt orotracheal intubation. In these patients, an emergency cricothyroidotomy can be employed. However, a lower, elective tracheostomy with removal of the cricothyroidotomy should be performed as soon as feasible to prevent subglottic stenosis.

Laryngoceles

Increased laryngeal pressures encountered in glass blowers and wind instrument musicians can result in herniation of the laryngeal ventricular mucosa into the false cord (internal laryngocele) or through the thyrohyoid membrane, presenting as a mass in the neck (external laryngocele). These diverticula may become infected. Radiographic examinations reveal air- and/or fluid-filled cysts in the region of the false cord or lateral to the thyroid cartilage. Symptomatic external laryngoceles are excised through a transverse cervical incision with repair of the mucous membrane. Internal laryngoceles require further dissection into the larynx through a partial removal of the thyroid alar.

Laryngeal Neoplasia

Benign neoplasms of the larynx include papillomas, fibromas, myxomas, chondromas, neurofibromas, and hemangiomas. The most common malignant lesion is squamous cell carcinoma, which accounts for approximately 2 per cent of all cancer mortalities. The male:female ratio is about 7:1, with a peak occurrence in the fifth and sixth decades. Smoking and excessive alcoholic beverage intake are predisposing factors. Squamous cell carcinoma occurs in the supraglottic, glottic, and subglottic larynx. The most common site is the glottis. The early presenting symptom is hoarseness lasting longer than 2 weeks. Stridor, pain, dysphagia, hemoptysis, and a neck mass are late symptoms. Initial evaluation requires direct laryngoscopy and biopsy of suspicious primary sites. Biopsy of neck masses is rarely needed and may seed the skin or deeper tissues, making subsequent en bloc removal of lymphatic metastases more difficult. Laryngeal and all head and neck cancers should be staged using the TNM classification.[1]

Early *glottic lesions* (T1, T2) can be treated by surgery; however, radiation therapy results in equal cure rates and is chosen to preserve voice quality; surgery is reserved for salvage. T3 and T4 glottic lesions require total laryngectomy with en bloc neck dissection for clinically palpable nodes. Five-year survival rates for glottic lesions vary and range from 70 to 96 per cent for T1 and T2 cancers and 0 to 59 per cent for T3 and T4 cancers.[14]

Supraglottic carcinomas tend to be more extensive on initial diagnosis with a high incidence of cervical node metastasis (55 per cent). The best 5-year survival rates are obtained with combination surgery and radiation therapy either pre- or postoperatively. For early lesions, a supraglottic laryngectomy with some preservation of voice and sphincter function in combination with an en bloc radical neck dissection is performed. More advanced lesions require a total laryngectomy. The incidence of postoperative wound healing problems is higher in patients who have had previous radiation therapy, particularly in patients who have undergone a subtotal laryngectomy. The 2-year disease-free survival of supraglottic cancer is about 70 per cent, with lower survival for more extensive lesions.[23]

Subglottic cancer occurs primarily or by extension of glottic tumors and is associated with a high rate (50 per cent) of cervical node metastasis. Appropriate treatment involves total laryngectomy and en bloc radical neck dissection with ipsilateral thyroid lobectomy. Overall survival rates vary widely from 40 to 70 per cent.[14] Because of increased postoperative complications after radiation therapy and the greater effectiveness of radiation and chemotherapy against fewer tumor cells, treatment of advanced laryngeal cancers with surgery followed by radiation therapy and multiagent chemotherapy is recommended.[13]

Foreign Bodies of the Larynx, Tracheobronchial Tree, and Esophagus

Aspirated foods, usually a bolus of meat, are the most common *laryngeal foreign body* and are frequently fatal. Such episodes commonly occur in restaurants (cafe coronaries) and are distinguished from a myocardial infarction by signs of upper respiratory obstruction. Techniques for aiding choking individuals, such as pounding on the back, finger probing of the throat, or turning a choking child upside down, are dangerous and may result in further impaction and total obstruction. If airway obstruction is unrelieved by the patient's own reflexes, the *Heimlich maneuver* should be attempted by placing the arms around the person from behind, grasping both hands, and applying brisk, subxiphoid pressure to the diaphragm. The resulting increased intrathorax pressure may expel the foreign body. However, if this maneuver fails, an emergency cricothyroidotomy should be performed to prevent death.

Tracheobronchial foreign bodies are usually smooth objects—seeds, nuts, and toys—that most commonly lodge in the right bronchus because of its larger size and more direct relationship to the trachea. The initial coughing spasms usually subside after 20 to 30 minutes. One-way valve bronchial obstruction with distal lung emphysema may develop; this is detected by careful chest auscultation and expiratory chest x-ray, which reveals a relatively radiolucent lung and a contralaterally shifted mediastinum. Complete bronchial obstruction results in rapid distal lung atelectasis with an ipsilateral mediastinal shift and compensatory emphysema in the normal lung. Tracheobronchial foreign bodies must be promptly removed by bronchoscopy and special forceps with the patient under general anesthesia. Persistent foreign bodies produce pneumonitis, bronchiectasis, lung abscess, and empyema. Vegetable foreign bodies, especially peanuts, cause a severe local inflammatory reaction and tracheobronchitis.

Most *esophageal foreign bodies* lodge at or just below the cricopharyngeal sphincter; the gastroesophageal junction and the esophageal indentations from the aortic arch and left bronchus are less frequent sites. Dysphagia and substernal pain with swallowing are the usual presenting symptoms. Radiopaque foreign bodies are visible on neck and chest x-rays; radiolucent objects may be demonstrated by barium esophagogram using barium-soaked, small cotton pledgets, which hang on sharp foreign bodies. Treatment involves removal by esophagoscopy (with the patient under general anesthesia) using special forceps and techniques to avoid esophageal perforation by sharp edges.

SELECTED REFERENCES

Ballantyne, J., and Groves, J.: Scott-Brown's Diseases of the Ear, Nose, and Throat, 4th ed. Boston, Butterworth, Inc., 1979.
This is a well-written, four-volume text with excellent sections on auditory physiology and otolaryngologic pathology.

Paparella, M. M., and Shumrick, D. A.: Otolaryngology, 2nd ed. Philadelphia, W. B. Saunders Company, 1980.
This complete three-volume text has fine presentations and descriptions of the basic sciences (Volume I) and diseases and surgical procedures (Volumes II and III).

Shambaugh, G. E., and Glasscock, M. E.: Surgery of the Ear, 3rd ed. Philadelphia, W. B. Saunders Company, 1980.
This is an outstanding and comprehensive otologic text with emphasis on historic development and surgery.

Snow, J. B.: Introduction to Otorhinolaryngology. Chicago, Year Book Medical Publishers, Inc., 1979.
This is a superb one-volume introductory text that highlights basic concepts. It is strongly recommended for the physician's quick reference library.

Suen, J. Y., and Myers, E. N.: Cancer of the Head and Neck. New York, Churchill Livingstone, Inc., 1981.
This is a complete current text on the pathology, epidemiology, and management of head and neck neoplasia.

REFERENCES

1. American Joint Committee for Cancer Staging and End-Results Reporting: Staging of Cancer of the Head and Neck Sites and of Melanoma. Chicago, 1980.
2. Batsakis, J. G., Solomon, A. R., and Rice, D. H.: The pathology of head and neck tumors: carcinoma of the nasopharynx. Part II. Head Neck Surg., *3*:511, 1981.
3. Bekesy, G. V., and Rosenblith, W. A.: The mechanical properties of the ear. *In* Stevens, S. S. (Ed.): Handbook of Experimental Psychology. New York. J. Wiley & Sons, 1951.
4. Calcaterra, T. C., Thompson, J. W., and Paglia, D. E.: Inverting papillomas of the nose and paranasal sinuses. Laryngoscope, *90*:53, 1980.
5. Chandler, J. R., and Serrins, A. J.: Transantral ligation of the internal maxillary artery for epistaxis. Laryngoscope, *75*:1151, 1965.
6. Choa, G.: Cancer of the nasopharynx. *In* Suen, J. Y., and Myers, E. N. (Eds.): Cancer of the Head and Neck. New York, Churchill Livingstone, Inc., 1981.
7. Davis, H., and Silverman, S. R.: Hearing and Deafness, 4th ed. New York, Holt, Rinehart, and Winston, 1978.
8. Donald, P. J., Hayes, J. R., and Dhaliwal, R.: Combined therapy for pyriform sinus cancer using postoperative irradiation. Otolaryngol. Head Neck Surg., *88*:738, 1980.
9. Farmer, J. C.: Diving injuries to the inner ear. Ann. Otol. Rhinol. Laryngol., *86*:Supplement 36, 1977.
10. Guild, S.: Histologic otosclerosis. Ann. Otol., *53*:246, 1944.
11. Hough, J. V. D.: Tympanoplasty with interior fascial graft technique and ossicular reconstruction. Laryngoscope, *80*:1385, 1970.
12. House, W. F.: Transtemporal bone microsurgical removal of acoustic neuromas. Arch. Otolaryngol. *80*:601, 1964.
13. Huang, A. T., Cole, T. B., Fishburn, R., and Jelovsek, S. B.: Adjuvant chemotherapy after surgery and radiation for Stage III and IV head and neck cancer. Ann. Surg. *200*:195, 1984.
14. Lawson, W., and Biller, H. F.: Cancer of the larynx. *In* Suen, J. Y., and Myers, E. N. (Eds.): Cancer of the Head and Neck. New York, Churchill Livingstone, Inc., 1981.
15. McCabe, B. F.: Vestibular physiology: its clinical application in understanding the dizzy patient. *In* Paparella, M. M., and Shumrick, D. A. (Eds.): Otolaryngology, Vol. I. Basic Sciences and Related Disciplines. Philadelphia, W. B. Saunders Company, 1980.
16. Neel, H. B., Pearson, G. R., Weiland, L. H., Taylor, W. F., Goepfert, H. H., Pilch, B. Z., Goodman, M., Lanier, A. P., Huang, A. T., Hyams, V. J., Levine, P. H., Henle, G., and Henle, W.: Application of Epstein-Barr virus serology to the diagnosis and staging of North American patients with nasopharyngeal carcinoma. Otolaryngol. Head Neck Surg., *91*:255, 1983.
17. Proetz, A. W.: Applied Physiology of the Nose. St. Louis, Annals Publishing Co., 1953.
18. Robbins, K. T., and Woodson, G. E.: Current concepts in the management of laryngeal papillomatosis. Head Neck Surg., *6*:861, 1984.
19. Sando, I., and Wood, R. P.: Congenital middle ear anomalies. Otolaryngol. Clin. North Am., *4*:291, 1971.
20. Schuknecht, H. F.: Pathology of the Ear. Cambridge, Mass., Harvard University Press, 1974.
21. Schuknecht, H. F.: Cochleosacculotomy for Meniere's disease: Theory, technique, and results. Laryngoscope, *92*:853, 1982.
22. Sisson, G. A., and Becker, S. P.: Cancer of the nasal cavity and paranasal sinuses. *In* Suen, J. Y., and Myers, E. N. (Eds.): Cancer of the Head and Neck. New York, Churchill Livingstone, Inc., 1981.
23. Snow, J. B., Gelber, R. D., Kramer, S., Davis, L. W., Marcial, V. A., and Lowry, L. D.: Evaluation of randomized preoperative and postoperative radiation therapy for supraglottic carcinoma. Ann. Otol. Rhinol. Laryngol., *87*:686, 1978.
24. Snow, J. B.: Introduction to Otorhinolaryngology. Chicago, Year Book Medical Publishers, Inc., 1979.
25. Standefer, J., Holt, G. R., Brown, W. E., and Gates, G. A.: Combined intracranial and extracranial excision of nasopharyngeal angiofibroma. Laryngoscope, *93*:772, 1983.

THE HEAD AND NECK

JOHN J. COLEMAN III, M.D. • M. J. JURKIEWICZ, M.D.

35

EPIDEMIOLOGY OF HEAD AND NECK CANCER

Epidermoid or squamous cell carcinoma of the mucosa of the upper aerodigestive tract occurs in the Western world primarily in men between the ages of 50 and 70, with a mean age of 58. In the United States in 1983, there were 18,700 new cases of carcinoma of the oral cavity and pharynx in men with 6400 deaths, and 9300 new cases of carcinoma of the larynx in men with 3100 deaths. The incidence and mortality for women in the United States and the Western world in 1983 are somewhat lower, with 8800 new cases of oral cavity and pharynx cancer and 2950 deaths and 1800 new cases of larynx cancer and 650 deaths.

The age range and geographical frequency are similar for both incidence and mortality from site to site throughout the upper aerodigestive tract, except for carcinoma of the nasopharynx, which is seen in somewhat younger patients and is endemic to Southern China. Overall, carcinomas of the upper aerodigestive tract make up approximately 4 per cent of the new cancers in American men yearly and 2 per cent in women, with 3 and 1 per cent of the mortalities respectively.[7] The predominance in males is largely a function of their increased use of tobacco and alcohol.

Although only 5 per cent of the total carcinomas of the head and neck occur in American patients below the age of 45, there appears to be a greater risk of early onset and late-stage disease at presentation among black patients. This group of young black males has a poorer overall survival than age-matched Caucasian patients.

Worldwide Incidence

The worldwide incidence of cancer of the upper aerodigestive tract varies greatly. In no other neoplasm except lung cancer is the relationship to tobacco as clear. There are endemic areas of cancer of the oropharynx and oral cavity in India and Southeast Asia, where uncured tobacco, bidi, is smoked or added to a concoction of betel nut and lime and placed in the gingivobuccal fold. In Bombay, India, where this betel nut–tobacco-lime mixture is common, 50 per cent of new cancers occur in the buccal cavity. Carcinoma of the hard palate is rare in most of the world but is endemic in areas of India, Venezuela, and Panama where the custom of smoking lighted cigarettes with the burning end inside the mouth persists. Snuff use among Southern women has resulted in an increase in buccal cancer in the area adjacent to the snuff. In South Africa, the Bantus inhale snuff made with local tobacco heavily contaminated with nickel and chromium, resulting in a high incidence of carcinoma of the nasal cavity.[13]

In the United States and the Western world, there is a clear association between lung cancer and inhalation of tobacco smoke. This risk is mirrored in carcinoma of the larynx. In most other areas of the upper aerodigestive tract, the oral cavity, oropharynx, and hypopharynx, there is a dual association with tobacco and alcohol. The risk of the development of malignancy is both time- and dose-related with both factors (Fig. 1). Therefore, although chronic use of cigarettes alone places the public at high risk of developing lung cancer, the risk of oral cancer is low unless there is concomitant use of alcohol. Similarly, heavy alcohol use slightly increases the risk of oral cancer, but not nearly as much as the combination of excessive alcohol and tobacco.[23]

Etiology

An understanding of the theory of cocarcinogenesis in chemical carcinogenesis is important in considering the etiology of head and neck cancer in the Western world. In

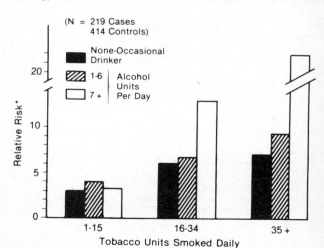

Figure 1. Relative risk of laryngeal cancer for male smokers according to amount of cigarettes smoked and alcohol consumed. (*Relative risk of 1.0 for nonsmokers who never or only occasionally drank alcohol.)

cocarcinogenesis, there are two steps in the production of neoplasia in the cell or organ.[9] *Initiation* is defined as some change in the cell or tissue that allows the later expression of malignancy. Initiation is a permanent change but does not render the cell malignant nor change the cell so that it is recognized as foreign or neoplastic by the host. Initiation probably involves a change in deoxyribonucleic acid (DNA) at either a structural or regulatory segment of the strand. This DNA change may be fixed within the chromosome by a round of cell proliferation, making it a permanent, irreparable part of the now abnormal but not neoplastic cell. The specific carcinogenic agent in tobacco is not known. As with many carcinogens, it may first be metabolized either systemically or locally from its procarcinogen state to an active state. This transformation is supported epidemiologically by the observation that in areas, such as the United States, where inhalation of tobacco smoke is the major form of use, head and neck cancer is most frequently found in the lateral tongue floor of the mouth area, where saliva pools, rather than over the entire mucosal surfaces of the oral cavity, oropharynx, nasal cavity, and nasopharynx, through which the smoke travels on its route to and from the lungs. Therefore, there is probably some change rendered in the procarcinogen to make it most active in these areas.

In chemical carcinogenesis, the *promoting substance* may act on the surrounding cells to allow expression of the initiated cell. The *sine qua non* of promotion is cell proliferation. Proliferation may be induced by local injury with attempts at repair, by direct mitogenic effect of the promoting substance, or by the creation of a regional environment where normal cells are less successful in their attempts at growth than are abnormal cells, e.g., continued cell injury where the chronically inflamed oral mucosa reacts less vigorously, allowing the initiated cell preferential expression. Frequent alcohol use causes intense local injury to the oropharyngeal and hypopharyngeal mucosa. This chronic effect may promote expression of the localized change rendered by tobacco. Localized proliferative or neoplastic lesions may progress to invasive cancer or may regress or remodel because of inadequate neoplastic potential or organism surveillance mechanisms (Fig. 2).

Field Cancerization

Although the floor of the mouth and lateral tongue are the most common sites of neoplasm (Fig. 3), it is obvious that the entire mucosa of the upper aerodigestive tract is at risk of damage by tobacco and alcohol through either their local or systemic effects. Furthermore, the nature of heavy tobacco and alcohol abuse is chronic and repetitive, providing long-term exposure to both initiating and promoting factors. For these reasons, the concept of *field cancerization* is important. Since the entire mucosal surface is at risk, there is a high probability that adjacent to the tumor will be areas of dysplasia and cancer *in situ*. Synchronous squamous cell carcinomas are found in as many as 20 per cent of patients, and obviously the risk of metachronous primary cancers is also high. Synchronous and metachronous primary cancers have been found in lung, esophagus, oral cavity, oropharynx, and hypopharynx, in that order of frequency.[16] The risk of metachronous cancers of the upper aerodigestive tract is thought to be approximately 6 per cent per year.

HISTOLOGIC CONSIDERATIONS

The upper aerodigestive tract consists of adjacent connected cavities lined with respiratory epithelium or squamous epithelium. The cavities, in addition to their lining surfaces, contain minor salivary glands, predominantly mucus secreting, that drain through short ducts. Localized aggregations of lymphoid tissue in the pharynx and base of the tongue make up the tonsils. The mucosal surfaces of the upper aerodigestive tract are modified in some areas to aid in special sensations and functions. Thus, the circumvallate papillae, while lined with stratified squamous mucosa like the rest of the oral cavity, have surrounding crevices that increase surface area and provide the subjacent taste buds, specialized neuroepithelial cells, more intimate contact with ingested food.

The basic unit of organization in the upper aerodigestive tract is repeated throughout the entire digestive tract. An epithelial lining, the mucous membrane with its immediately subjacent lamina propria or basement membrane, is the most superficial layer. Beneath this lies a submucosal layer of connective tissue varying in thickness and holding the specialized invaginations of the epithelium, the glands. Within this layer there frequently course neurovascular structures. The next layer is one of mesodermal structures, either muscle or periosteum and bone, depending on the site. There is no serosal layer in the upper aerodigestive tract; this is not present until the stomach and peritoneal cavity are reached.

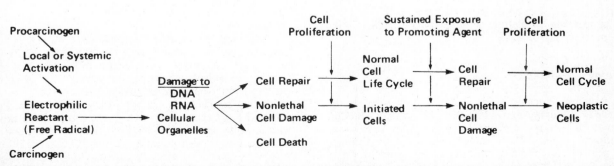

Figure 2. Chemical cocarcinogenesis. In squamous cell carcinoma of the head and neck, the initiating agent is thought to be tobacco and the promoting agent alcohol. Initiation usually involves a change in DNA. Promotion may affect DNA, membrane structure and function, cellular enzyme system, or other processes. (Adapted from Farber, E.: N. Engl. J. Med., 305:1379, 1981.)

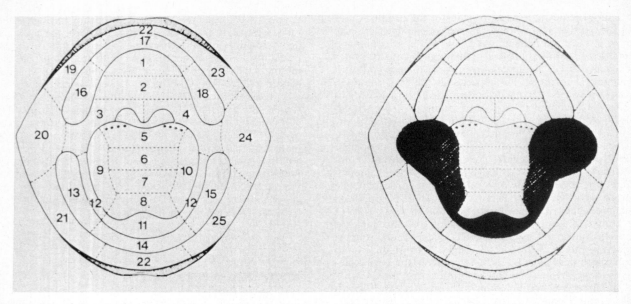

Figure 3. Schematic representation of oral cavity with 25 subdivisions. Shaded areas are most frequent sites of oral cancer. These are areas with prolonged exposure to pooled saliva. (From Baker, H. W.: Diagnosis of oral cancer. In Baker, H. W., Rickles, N. H., Helsper, J. T., Jesse, R. H., Stark, R. B., Osterkamp, R. W., and Whitten, J. B. (Eds.): Oral Cancer. American Cancer Society Professional Education Publication, 1973, pp. 2–10. (Courtesy of Condict Moore, M.D.)

Squamous Epithelium

Aberrations of cellular growth occur in all parts of the upper aerodigestive tract. Thus, lymphomas may arise in the lymphoid aggregates of the tonsils, adenomas or adenocarcinomas may arise from the salivary glands, and various sarcomas may arise from the muscle, bone, nerve, lymphatic, and blood vessels.

By far the most common abnormality is neoplastic change in the squamous epithelium. Stratified squamous epithelium undergoes an orderly progression from its growth area, the basal layer adjacent to the basement membrane, to the surface of the cavity. The cells of the basal layer are cuboidal with regularly organized nuclei, and there is a gradual progression through several irregular layers of polyhedral cells, the prickle cell layer, with less prominent nuclei, to successive layers of flattened cells with no apparent nuclei. On the skin, this stratified squamous epithelium is keratinized, that is, covered by a thick layer of dead enucleated cells. On the oral mucosa, there is no keratinized surface, although the progression from cuboidal cells to flattened enucleated cells occurs. Respiratory epithelium or pseudostratified columnar epithelium consists of layers of irregular cuboidal cells that do not pass through the progression of flattening and loss of nucleus from bottom to surface (Fig. 4).

Histologic Response

Because chemical carcinogenesis is thought to be important in the upper aerodigestive tract, an understanding of the normal response of the mucosal surface to irritation and injury is crucial. The histologic response of the stratified squamous epithelium to injury is usually some form of squamous cell hyperplasia or overgrowth. There is an increase in the number of squamous cells at all layers. In *papillary hyperplasia* or *papillomatosis,* not only does the

mucosa proliferate outward but the ridges or papillae project downward further into the underlying submucosal layer, the appearance of which is similar to the rete ridges of the skin rather than the more blunted interface of mucosa and submucosa seen in the mucous membranes. A more exuberant and disorganized form, *pseudoepitheliomatous hyperplasia,* may be mistaken for cancer.

In addition to the increase in the number of cells as a response to injury, there is usually a loss of the normal progression of nucleated squamous cells at the basal layer to enucleated cells at the surface. The appearance of nuclei in the most superficial layers of the mucosa with decreasing thickness of the basal and granular layers is known as *parakeratosis* or *orthokeratosis.*

Lesser cellular forms of response to injury include thickening of all layers of the epithelium, or acanthosis, and presence of an abnormally thick enucleate layer similar to the stratum corneum of the skin, known as *keratosis* or *hyperkeratosis.* These responses to injury preserve normal individual cellular morphology and do not extend deep to the basement membrane and are therefore benign.

Clinical Presentation

The clinical manifestation of these histologic changes is sometimes called *leukoplakia* or white patch. Although in the past leukoplakia was thought to be a premalignant entity, it is now felt to be a less serious sign of chronic irritation found most often in men over 40 years of age. According to Batsakis, leukoplakia is most often found histologically to consist of (1) simple keratosis or acanthosis without inflammation, (2) combinations of hyperkeratosis, parakeratosis, and acanthosis with submucosal infiltration of chronic inflammatory cells, plasma cells, and lymphocytes, and (3) combinations of hyperkeratosis and cellular hyperplasia with or without dysplasia. Leukoplakia as a clinical entity is more important as a concomitant of cancer

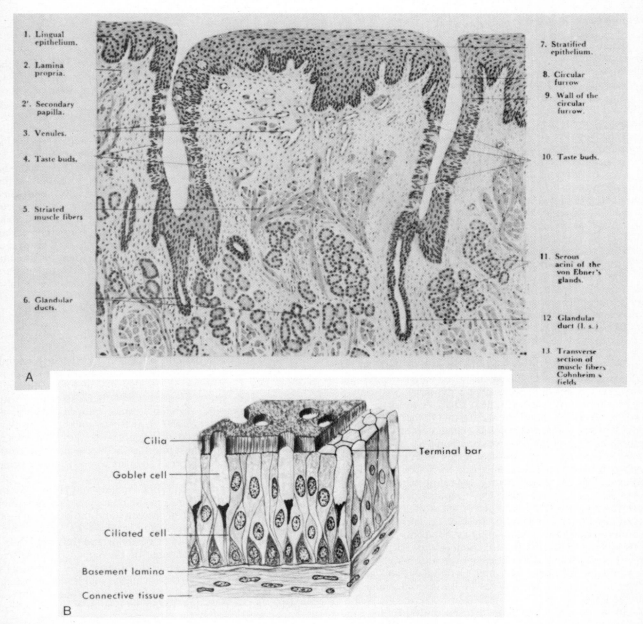

Figure 4. Normal epithelium.

A, Stratified squamous epithelium of the oral cavity and pharynx. Note relatively blunted rete ridges and orderly progression of horizontally oriented cells from basement membrane to mucosal surface without keratinization. The submucosal layer contains muscle, blood vessels and glands, and specialized sensory structures. (From Di Fiore, M. S. H.: An Atlas of Human Histology. Philadelphia, Lea & Febiger, 1957.)

B, Pseudostratified columnar ciliated (respiratory) epithelium. Notice the vertical orientation of cells, nuclei at irregular intervals, distinct basement membrane without rete ridges, and ciliated surface cells. (From Bloom, W., and Fawcett, D. W.: A Textbook of Histology, 9th ed. Philadelphia, W. B. Saunders Company, 1968.)

than a precursor. Numerous studies have shown that leukoplakia alone usually consists of epithelial changes having no dysplastic components and is thus unlikely to be premalignant.[15]

Premalignant Changes

There are, however, definite premalignant changes in the epithelium of the upper aerodigestive tract. At the cellular level there is an increase in the size of nuclei, hyperchromatism, frequent mitotic figures, basophilic cytoplasm, and irregular cell shapes, or pleomorphism. These cellular changes are known as *atypia*. The increase in number of cells seen as a response to injury, known as hyperplasia, when combined with cellular atypia becomes *atypical hyperplasia* or *dysplasia*. More extensive loss of normal cellular stratification with replacement of the keratinocytes by atypical and immature cells but with preservation of an intact basement membrane is known as squamous cell *carcinoma in situ* or *intraepithelial carcinoma*. Unlike the changes that constitute leukoplakia, dysplasia and carcinoma *in situ* show little keratin production. Exfoliation of the epithelium of carcinoma *in situ* produces cells that are indistinguishable on cytologic examination from those of invasive cancer.

The clinical appearance of these abnormalities is varied, but they frequently present as *erythroplakia* or red patch, an entity of considerable importance. Mashberg's close examination of a veteran population has demonstrated that 98 per cent of patients with asymptomatic early malignancies had an erythroplakic component and only 5 per cent had a leukoplakic component alone. This is consistent with the data of Waldron and Shafer, who found that of all leukoplakic lesions, 92 per cent were benign or moderate dysplasia, 4.5 per cent were severe dysplasia, and only 3 per cent were invasive carcinoma. Changes consistent with erythroplakia are therefore significant in themselves and should prompt a search of the remainder of the upper aerodigestive tract for invasive carcinoma.

The histologic and clinical changes of leukoplakia and erythroplakia may be reversible if the irritating stimulus is removed. There is controversy regarding whether carcinoma *in situ* is reversible. The preponderance of data, however, suggests that carcinoma *in situ* of the oral mucosa, if not treated, progresses to invasive cancer. There is a common association of immediately adjacent or synchronous invasive cancers with carcinoma *in situ*. Furthermore, intraepithelial carcinomas elsewhere in the body, such as Bowen's disease of the skin and erythroplasia of Queyrat of the glans penis, often progress to invasive squamous cell carcinoma.

In a disease that is thought to be caused by ingested carcinogens, the concept of field cancerization must be considered. This states that, although some areas of mucosa may be at higher risk, the entire upper aerodigestive tract is likely to be affected. Erythroplakia and, to a lesser degree, leukoplakia in one area may be signs of invasive cancer at another site in the upper aerodigestive tract.

Dysplasia and carcinoma *in situ* are the most important early changes of squamous cell carcinoma seen in the United States. However, in Asia, another premalignant entity is associated with chronic irritation of the upper aerodigestive tract. *Submucous fibrosis* presents clinically as diffuse blanching of the oral mucosa with palpable fibrous bands. There is atrophy of the mucosa and replacement of the submucosal layer with dense connective tissue. This is thought to be a hypersensitivity response to the commonly ingested irritants, such as betel nut, chili, and tobacco, that is promoted by dietary deficiency of iron, B_{12}, or folate. Submucous fibrosis is felt to be analogous to the sideropenic dysphagia called Plummer-Vinson syndrome commonly seen in Scandinavian women.

Invasive Cancer

The hallmark of invasive cancer is spread beyond the epithelial confines or through the basement membrane to the underlying structures. In invasive squamous cell carcinoma, also known as *epidermoid carcinoma,* there is cellular pleomorphism, loss of stratification and maturation of cells, and infiltration of abnormal cells into the underlying submucosa or muscle. As in other cancers, some elements of normal function may persist despite deranged structure. In squamous cell carcinoma, therefore, *keratin pearls* may be found at various depths in the cell layers, representing the normal tendency of maturing squamous cells to produce keratin. The degree of cellular derangement of the cancer characterizes the aggressiveness of the tumor. In well-differentiated tumors there are relatively normal-appearing cells that may produce keratin. *Verrucous carcinoma* is a special form of squamous cell carcinoma found most commonly on the buccal mucosa. It is exophytic with papillary projections of malignant cells and considerable keratin production. There is usually a dense inflammatory cell infiltrate. Invasion through the basement membrane is variable.[4]

Attempts have been made to predict the aggressiveness of squamous cell carcinoma by tumor markers, subcellular characteristics, and patterns of response of the surrounding tissue to the tumor. Excessive prostaglandin E_2 production[2] and a low percentage of lymphocytes in Ficoll-Hypaque gradient white cell suspensions[8] have been associated with poor prognosis and aggressive tumor behavior. Holm reported that increased DNA content as measured by flow cytometry is correlated with poor prognosis. Histologic studies of the tumor-host interface have revealed that cordlike invasion by tumor cells signifies a much poorer prognosis than the more well-defined pressing invasive borderline.[24] Although these and other methods of study may be of considerable importance in the biology of this and other tumors, at present light microscopy and the determination of histologic grade as suggested by Broders[6] are the standards for determining tumor behavior and thus prognosis.

Squamous cell carcinoma of the upper aerodigestive tract spreads along the path of least resistance. This usually involves downward growth into muscle and frequently along the potential spaces next to motor and sensory nerves. Fascia and periosteum serve as temporary barriers but ultimately become involved. Local invasion of blood vessels is an indication of an aggressive tumor. Emboli of tumor pass through the efferent lymphatics to lymph nodes.

ANATOMY

The head and neck comprise an intricate juxtaposition of skeletal structures, fixed and mobile with their attached muscles, and several series of interconnected mucosa-lined cavities with adjacent glands that are dedicated to the vegetative functions of alimentation and respiration and their more specialized subfunctions of mastication, deglutition, and phonation. Although a complex synergy char-

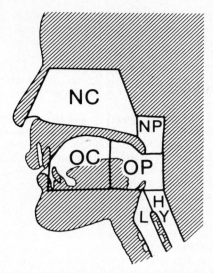

Figure 5. Schematic representation of upper aerodigestive tract cavities. NC = Nasal cavity; NP = nasopharynx; OC = oral cavity; OP = oropharynx; H = hypopharynx; L = larynx.

acterizes the whole area, the dominant function of each anatomic part is reflected by the histology of the mucosa. Therefore, the nasal cavity (beyond the vestibule), the nasopharynx, the paranasal sinuses, the glottic and infraglottic larynx, and the trachea, all of which primarily effect the delivery of moisturized air to the lungs, are lined with pseudostratified ciliated columnar epithelium, respiratory epithelium. The lips, oral cavity, oropharynx, hypopharynx, and cervical esophagus, all of which serve to propel food into the stomach, are lined with stratified nonkeratinizing squamous epithelium. The accessory salivary and mucous glands to both series of mucosa-lined cavities are similarly specialized for either respiration (mucous glands) or alimentation (serous glands).

The predominant neoplasm in this area is *squamous cell carcinoma*, and its behavior is somewhat more aggressive and thus more morbid than that of its counterpart on the keratinizing squamous epithelium of the skin. The morbidity and ultimate mortality of this disease are usually a direct function of their local effects on the site of origin or locoregional effects in the neck, the primary site of lymphatic drainage. Because of this indolent nature and localized morbidity, a detailed knowledge of the anatomy of the head and neck is necessary to understand and treat this disease. The specific functions of each area will be discussed with the anatomy. Further exploration of functional anatomy will be made when the derangements caused by the cancer and its therapy are examined.

The upper aerodigestive tract consists of ten mucosa-lined areas and their accessory structures (Fig. 5). Five of these areas—the oral cavity, the oropharynx, the supraglottic larynx, the hypopharynx, and the cervical esophagus—are designed specifically for alimentation. The other five, the nasal cavity, the paranasal sinuses, the nasopharynx, the larynx, and the trachea, are concerned with respiration. These areas overlap somewhat but possess anatomically and functionally different elements and are considered distinct.

Oral Cavity

The oral cavity extends from the vermilion of the lips to the anterior tonsillar pillar. The overwhelming orienta-

tion of this area is to prepare food and drink for delivery around the larynx and into the esophagus. The oral cavity is divided into (1) the lips, (2) the labial and buccal mucosa (the oral vestibule), (3) the gums (the mandibular and maxillary alveoli), (4) the floor of the mouth (alveololingual sulcus), (5) the mobile tongue, (6) the retromolar trigone, (7) the anterior tonsillar pillar, and (8) the hard palate. The oral cavity can be viewed as the first in a series of muscular tubes that make up the entire alimentary tract.

LIPS

The lips begin with the white line or vermilion border, the junction between keratinizing and nonkeratinizing squamous epithelium, and the oral cavity begins with the labial mucosa. The orbicularis oris muscle creates the main oral sphincter. The orbicularis oris and its numerous connecting muscles, the depressor labii inferioris, depressor anguli oris, mentalis, risorius, zygomaticus, and quadratus labii superioris, are supplied by the marginal mandibular and buccal branches of the facial nerve and in large part are responsible for facial expression. Sensation to the lower lips occurs via the mental nerve, the termination of the inferior alveolar branch of the third division of the trigeminal nerve. The mucosa of the upper lip receives its sensory innervation from the terminations of the infraorbital nerve, a branch of the second division of the trigeminal nerve. As in all areas of the upper aerodigestive tract, there is a marked interplay between sensory and motor activity in normal function. Surgical manipulations in this area may cause microstomia, oral incontinence, or interference with the production of labial consonants during speech.

ORAL VESTIBULE

The oral vestibule consists of the labial and buccal mucosa and the alveololabial and alveolobuccal sulci. The buccal mucosa covers the buccinator muscle, which courses horizontally from the pterygomandibular raphe posteriorly to the orbicularis oris muscle anteriorly and the buccal fat pad and masseter muscle more posteriorly, making up the internal lining of the cheek. The parotid duct, Stensen's duct, opens into the oral cavity through the buccal mucosa just opposite the upper second molar tooth, supplying some of the components of saliva to the cavity. The oral vestibule serves as a capacitance area before swallowing and helps stabilize the food bolus for the tongue and teeth. Tumor or surgical extirpation of this area may result in disturbance of parotid gland function, facial nerve weakness and asymmetry of smile, decreased orbicularis oris function, and decreased volume of the oral cavity.

GINGIVA

The gingiva (gums) are the mucosal coverings of the mandibular and maxillary alveoli. They separate the oral vestibule from the hard palate superiorly and the floor of the mouth inferiorly. The alveolar portion of the mandible primarily functions to stabilize the teeth. The mandible itself, with its numerous muscular attachments, provides a framework to maintain the volume of the oral cavity, to provide an area of attachment for the tongue, and to mediate chewing against the fixed maxilla. In addition to the insertion of several muscles of facial expression, three major muscle groups attach to the mandible, the genioglossus muscle, the depressors of the mandible (elevators of the larynx), which form the floor of the mouth, and the muscles of mastication.

The *genioglossus muscle* arises from the superior genial tubercle at the mandibular symphysis and attaches to the base of the tongue and the hyoid bone. It lends stability to the tongue and a fixed focus for traction on the hyoid bone as well as support for the internal musculature of the tongue. Loss of the central segment of the mandible prevents elevation of the larynx and protrusion of the tongue. The *depressors of the mandible* (or elevators of the larynx) act on the anterior mandible and the hyoid bone and form the floor of the mouth. The mylohyoid muscles spread inferiorly and laterally from the mylohyoid groove of the mandible to the medial hyoid bone, forming a cup-shaped cavity that, when lined with mucosa, constitutes the floor of the mouth. The anterior belly of the digastric and the geniohyoid muscles similarly pull on the anterior mandible through their attachments to the hyoid bone. Since the anterior bellies of the digastric and mylohyoid muscles function to depress the mandible, they can be considered *muscles of mastication* and are therefore supplied by the motor branch of the trigeminal nerve at its termination, the mylohyoid nerve.

The most powerful of the mandibular muscles are the *elevators* of the mandible, the masseter, temporalis, and pterygoid muscles. These pull from several various attachments on the skull to raise the mandible against the fixed maxilla to protrude and retract it, thereby grinding food between the teeth. Again, as muscles of mastication, they are powered and innervated by the motor branch of the trigeminal nerve. Resection of the lateral body or ramus of the mandible may interfere with their function. Because these muscles pull on several distinct axes to cause elevation, protrusion, and retraction of the mandible, paralysis, resection, or detachment from the mandibular insertions may result in *malocclusion* of the teeth, or misalignment of the normal bite. Infiltration by tumor from the oral cavity or oropharynx deep to these muscles results in *trismus*, characterized by muscle spasm, pain, and inability to open the jaws.

The maxillary alveolus, or gum, is less frequently involved with carcinoma. The maxilla, which is primarily responsible for midfacial appearance and vertical elongation of the face, is fixed to the cranium at several suture lines. The palatine bone provides the bony separation between the oral cavity, the nasal cavity, and paranasal sinuses. Loss of the barrier function of the palate results in nasal regurgitation of food, disturbances in inspiration, and hypernasality of speech as air resounds through the nasal cavity as well as the oral cavity during phonation.

Tongue

The predominant structure of the oral cavity is the tongue. At rest, the tongue fills most of the oral cavity and a large portion of the oropharynx. Formed mostly of voluntary skeletal muscle, it is covered by a mucous membrane of squamous epithelium interspersed with mucous glands and a few serous glands. The tongue extends anteriorly from the lingual frenulum and medially from the mucosa of the floor of the mouth posteriorly to the epiglottis and lateral pharyngeal walls. The ventral surface of the tongue is lined with glistening mucosa and the dorsal surface with taste buds and various papillary projections, the filiform, fungiform, and foliate papillae, all of which provide friction for the manipulation of food throughout the oral cavity. The anterior two thirds of the tongue, the mobile tongue, is visible in the oral cavity on simple inspection and is the most common site of carcinoma of the oral cavity

in the United States. The posterior one third of the tongue begins at the anterior tonsillar pillar. The superficial landmark for this separation is the circumvallate papillae. The surface of the posterior one third of the tongue, or base of the tongue, is studded with lymphoid follicles, or lingual tonsils. This area is not visible on simple inspection; a mirror and light source, e.g., indirect laryngoscopy, are needed for thorough examination.

The bulk of the tongue is made up of an intricate synthesis of muscle. Four intrinsic muscles allow the tongue to change its shape readily, and the superior and inferior longitudinal muscles shorten the tongue and raise and lower the tip. The verticalis muscle flattens the tongue, and the transversalis muscle narrows and elongates the tongue. The complex synergy of tongue motion with jaw, pharyngeal, and laryngeal movements in phonation and deglutition is effected by the extrinsic muscles of the tongue. The genioglossus is the main attachment of both the anterior two thirds and posterior one third of the tongue to the anterior mandible and is primarily responsible for protrusion and retraction of the tongue. The hyoglossus and geniohyoid connect the tongue to the hyoid bone for elevation of the larynx; the palatoglossus and syloglossus attach the tongue to the base of the skull and soft palate and serve as a part of the constrictor mechanism of the alimentary tube.

Motor innervation to the intrinsic muscles and most of the extrinsic muscles of the tongue is from cranial nerve XII, the hypoglossal nerve. The close relationship in function of the tongue and the larynx can be seen by the fact that the depressors of the larynx receive their motor innervation from the ansa hypoglossi, which carries both branches of the twelfth cranial nerve and the cervical plexus.

The tongue contains sensory nerve fibers for both general (pressure, pain, heat, cold, and so on) and specialized sensation. General sensation in the anterior two thirds of the tongue is carried by the fifth cranial nerve, the lingual nerve. Specialized sensation, taste, travels in fibers of the seventh cranial nerve, which course in the lingual nerve as the chorda tympani. In the posterior one third of the tongue, the base of the tongue, general sensation and specialized sensation are carried by the ninth cranial nerve, the glossopharyngeal nerve. Around the vallecula, the area between the base of the tongue and lingual surface of the epiglottis, there is considerable overlap in general sensation between the glossopharyngeal nerve IX and the vagus nerve X, the internal branch of the superior laryngeal nerve. These rich sensorineural anastomoses are particularly important when we are considering pathways of referred pain, an important symptom in head and neck cancer.

Salivary Glands

Salivary secretion is a complex and intricately regulated phenomenon that occurs predominantly in the oral cavity. There are three pairs of major salivary glands: the parotid glands, the submaxillary glands, and the sublingual glands. The salivary secretions of the parotid and submaxillary glands are mostly serous, rich in enzymes, electrolytes, and antibodies. The sublingual gland produces mucus, as do the accessory, or minor, salivary glands, which are plentiful within the lip, buccal mucosa, and tongue. The parotid duct empties into the oral cavity, piercing the buccal mucosa via Stensen's duct. The submandibular duct enters the sublingual caruncle just lateral to the lingual frenulum, and the sublingual gland sends a series of orifices into the mucosa of the floor of the mouth. The enzymatic, lubricative, and antibiotic properties of saliva facilitate transport and digestion of food.

Pharynx

As a functional anatomic unit, the pharynx serves two purposes. First, it continues the muscular propulsion of food down the alimentary canal. Second, it separates the respiratory and digestive tracts during the act of swallowing. It extends from and attaches to the base of the skull at the sphenoid bone anteriorly and the occiput posteriorly to the postcricoid area at the level of the sixth cervical vertebra.

Axially, the *nasopharynx* extends from the base of the sphenoid sinus to the nasal soft palate (C2); the oropharynx extends from the oral soft palate to the epiglottis (C2 to C3, C4); and the *hypopharynx* or *laryngopharynx* extends from the epiglottis to the postcricoid esophagus (C3, C4 to C6). The nasal cavity, oral cavity, and larynx are related anteriorly and the spine lies posterior to the nasopharynx. The soft tissues of the neck, particularly the carotid sheath, lie lateral to the pharynx. Since the nasopharynx is primarily a part of the respiratory system, it will be described with the nasal cavity.

Oropharynx

The *oropharynx* consists of four basic muscular units and their investing mucosa and fascia: (1) the velar or soft palate structures, (2) the tonsillar or faucial structures, (3) the constrictors of the pharynx, and (4) the base of the tongue. Although all are intimately connected both structurally and functionally, accounting for the synergy in this area, consideration of each of these units separately simplifies the complex anatomy and function.

The *soft palate* is a synthesis of two groups of muscles with opposite function. The muscles that raise the soft palate to close off the connection between the nasal and oral cavities are attached to the base of the skull and posterior nasal spine. They are the tensor veli palatini, the levator veli palatini, and the uvula. Fibers from these muscles are interwoven with the palatoglossus and palatopharyngeus muscles, which arise from the tongue and lateral pharyngeal wall and pull the soft palate inferiorly to close the oral cavity and open the nasopharynx. The palatoglossus muscle forms the anterior tonsillary pillar and shares connections in the tongue with the styloglossus muscle, which is attached posterosuperiorly to the styloid process at the base of the skull. The palatopharyngeus muscle forms the posterior tonsillar pillar, coursing inferiorly from the soft palate to the lateral pharyngeal wall and receiving fibers from the superolaterally based stylopharyngeus muscle. Between the tonsillar pillars rests a collection of lymphoid tissues, the palatine tonsil. The contraction and relaxation of these axially directed tonsillar muscles narrow and widen the area between the oral cavity and oropharynx and act with the palatine group to open and close the oral cavity.

The posterior and inferolateral aspect of the oropharynx is formed by the confluence of the three *constrictors of the pharynx*. The fibers of these three muscles overlap at the extremes, and they form the transverse muscular layer of the pharynx, the antecedent of the circular muscle layer of the esophagus, stomach, and bowel.

1. The *superior constrictor* has fixed attachments to the pharyngeal tubercle of the occipital bone and the medial pharyngeal raphe, a condensation of fascia coursing inferiorly along the midline of the vertebral bodies. This thin muscle extends laterally around the pterygoid plate to the pterygomandibular raphe, where it terminates as a line between the pterygoid hamulus and the angle of the mandible, serving as the posterior limit of the oral sphincter, which is made up of the lips and buccinator muscles. The constriction and relaxation of the superior constrictor and the elevation and depression of the soft palate control the opening between the oropharynx and nasopharynx. Caudally the superior constrictor interdigitates with the middle constrictor.

2. The *middle pharyngeal constrictor* again attaches to the medial pharyngeal raphe into the hyoid bone and stylohyoid ligament laterally and anteriorly. Through the numerous muscular attachments of the hyoid bone to the mobile tongue and the base of the tongue, the middle constrictor coordinates the motion of the midoropharynx and the base of the tongue.

3. Intermingling with the fibers of the middle constrictor at the pharyngeal raphe and extending caudad to it is the *inferior constrictor* of the pharynx. This long segment consists of two basic parts, the oblique portion, which arises from the lateral thyroid cartilage and inserts on the medial raphe, and the most inferior portion, the cricopharyngeus, which courses in a complete circle not attached to the raphe and is continuous with the circular muscle of the esophagus. In addition to continuing the propulsion of food toward the stomach, the inferior constrictor, particularly the cricopharyngeus, prevents air from entering the digestive system during respiration, serving as the final valve before the esophageal phase of swallowing.

The complex motor function of the oropharynx results in an intricate and remarkable synergy that effects swallowing. Most of the motor fibers of this area are carried by the vagus nerve, cranial nerve X, although they probably arise from the eleventh cranial nerve. Sensation to the area travels through both the glossopharyngeal nerve IX and the vagus nerve X. Both motor and sensory nerves arise from the pharyngeal plexus. There is considerable sensory overlap in the oropharynx between cranial nerves IX and X.

Larynx

The larynx is part of the respiratory system, the aditus to the lower respiratory tract. Its detailed interplay with the pharynx structurally and functionally necessitates consideration of its anatomy with that of the oropharynx. To simplify the difficult anatomy of the larynx, the organ consists of a relatively fixed cartilaginous exoskeleton and an internal group of mobile cartilages and ligaments. The exoskeleton is composed of the hyoid bone, thyroid cartilages, and cricoid cartilage connected in series by the thyrohyoid and cricothyroid membranes. The internal structure consists of the mucosa-lined epiglottis, arytenoid cartilages, and vocal cords (vocal ligaments). The epiglottis lies at the most inferior aspect of the base of the tongue. This broad cartilage is covered by mucosa on both its lingual and laryngeal surfaces and is attached by several ligaments to the hyoid bone, the base of the tongue, lateral pharynx, and thyroid cartilage. Its attachment to the thyroid cartilage, to which it is relatively fixed, by the thyroepiglottic ligament provides a focal point.

Elevation and depression of the rest of the larynx about this point are effected by the extrinsic muscles of the larynx, the elevators, mylohyoid, stylopharyngeus, digastric, and so on, and the depressors, the omohyoid, sterno-hyoid, and sternothyroid. These motions allow the epiglottis to open and close the aditus of the larynx during swallowing, respiration, and phonation.

Sensation to the larynx derives from the internal branch of the superior laryngeal nerve, a termination of the vagus nerve. The external branch of the superior thyroid provides motor innervation to the inferior pharyngeal constrictor, including the cricopharyngeus, and the cricothyroid muscle. The remainder of the laryngeal muscles are supplied by the recurrent laryngeal nerve. Injury to the recurrent laryngeal nerve paralyzes the ipsilateral vocal cord in the paramedian position. Injury to the superior laryngeal branch results in early fatigue of the voice secondary to paralysis of the cricothyroid and, more importantly, the loss of sensation to the area, increasing the likelihood of aspiration of saliva and food. For clinical consideration, the larynx is divided into the supraglottic, glottic, and infraglottic larynx. The supraglottic larynx consists of the epiglottis and false cords, the glottic larynx of the true cords, and the infraglottic larynx of the cricoid and trachea.

Nasal Cavity, Nasopharynx, and Paranasal Sinuses

The remainder of the upper airway consists of the nasal cavity, nasopharynx, and paranasal sinuses. The ciliated pseudostratified columnar epithelium, respiratory epithelium, and interspersed mucous glands moisten, clean, and warm the air on its passage to the lungs. These cavities, except for the nasopharynx and sometimes the sphenoid sinus, are paired.

The *nasal cavity* arises at the nasal vestibule, the skin-lined opening of the nares, and is divided into two sections. The bony septum creates the posterior division and is made up of the vomer, an extension of the sphenoid bone, which attaches to the posterior palatine bone, and the perpendicular plate of the ethmoid bone, which connects to the vomer inferiorly. The anterior midline division of the nasal cavity is effected by the cartilaginous septum, which extends from the bony septum to the nasal bones. The lateral wall of the nasal cavity is formed by mucosa-lined projections of the facial bones, the conchae or turbinates. All the paranasal sinuses open into the nasal cavity through holes in the lateral nasal wall. The posterior nasal cavity communicates with the nasopharynx through the choanae. Important anatomic relationships to the nasal cavity are the orbits, which lie superolateral, and the cribriform plates, which separate the nasal cavity from the cranial cavity and contain the nerve endings of the olfactory nerve responsible for the special sensation of smell. The floor of the nasal cavity consists of the hard palate, which is made up of the palatine bone and the palatine projections of the maxilla.

The *paranasal sinuses* are extensions of the nasal cavity hollowed out of the adjacent facial and cranial bones. The largest sinuses are the maxillary sinuses, which are lateral to the main nasal cavity. The ethmoid sinuses consist of a group of air cells superior to the nasal cavity. The frontal sinuses lie in the frontal bone and the sphenoid sinuses in the sphenoid bone. Occlusion of the orifices of the paranasal sinuses results in infection and possibly abscess formation. The proximity to the cranial cavity is important in the natural history of both infection and tumor.

The *nasopharynx* is more functionally related to the nasal cavity than to the remainder of the pharynx. Its superior boundary is the base of the skull and its inferior boundary the nasal side of the soft palate and the superior pharyngeal constrictor.

Sensory innervation to the nasal cavity, the nasopharynx, and the paranasal sinuses derives from the maxillary and ophthalmic branches of the trigeminal nerve.

The Neck

In regard to cancer of the head and neck, the anatomy of the neck is important for two main reasons: (1) as it affects the functions of the respiratory and alimentary tracts, i.e., the character of its muscles and nerves, and (2) as a repository for the lymphatic drainage of the upper aerodigestive tract.

MUSCULATURE

The muscle groups of the neck have three main functions: (1) movement of the skull around the axis of the spine, (2) flexible connection of the skull to the trunk, and (3) facilitation of action of the structures of the oral cavity, pharynx, and larynx. The axial musculature of the neck, the paravertebral muscles, the rectus capitis, longus capitis, longus colli, and scalenes, serves to flex the neck, elevate the shoulders, and stabilize the skull. The trapezius and sternocleidomastoid muscles are responsible mainly for rotation around the vertical axis as well as some flexion and elevation. The strap muscles, the omohyoid, sterno-thyroid, and sternohyoid muscles, serve to depress the larynx. The thyrohyoid, mylohyoid, stylohyoid, and digastric muscles are elevators of the larynx and, as previously discussed, help form the floor of the mouth.

LYMPHATIC DRAINAGE

Of considerably more importance in the natural history and evaluation of head and neck cancer is the role of the neck as a lymph node station for the upper aerodigestive tract. The parotid lymph node group drains the scalp, lateral orbit and eye, nasal vestibule, and ear. The remainder of the upper aerodigestive tract drains through the neck. Knowledge of the lymphatic anatomy of the neck allows prediction of the site of primary disease on the mucosal surfaces.

The basic pattern of lymph flow in the head and upper aerodigestive tract is from the apex of the skull downward to the thoracic duct and accessory thoracic duct and the supraclavicular fossae. Although there are numerous nodes throughout the area, the main clusters are associated with the jugular vein and its tributaries and several nerves of the neck. Discrete anatomic areas contribute the majority of their lymphatic channels to lymph nodes at specific stations along the pathway of flow toward the thoracic duct. In addition to receiving afferent lymphatic vessels from the skin, soft tissue, and mucosa, distal lymph nodes receive vessels from more proximal stations along the lymphatic chain. The surface anatomy of the neck is characterized by several triangles formed by the intersection of the sterno-cleidomastoid, omohyoid, and trapezius muscles (Fig. 6). The lymph nodes of the neck are all present in a distinct fascial compartment lying between the superficial cervical fascia (the platysma and its condensations) and the prevertebral fascia, which envelops the axial muscles of the neck. This is of considerable importance in radical neck dissection.

The posterior scalp is drained by the *occipital lymph nodes*, which are associated with the greater occipital nerve and lie on the medial aspect of the trapezius muscle in the posterior triangle of the neck. They drain to the supracla-

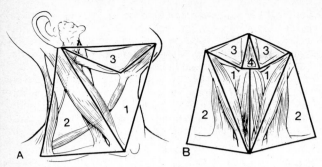

Figure 6. A and B, Anatomic triangles of the neck. 1 = Anterior triangle; 2 = posterior triangle; 3 = submaxillary triangle; 4 = submental triangle.

vicular area along the spinal accessory nerve. The back of the ear is drained by postauricular nodes, which are less constant in location and may drain either medially to the jugular nodes or laterally down the spinal accessory chain to the supraclavicular fossa. These two lymph node groups are important in the consideration of malignant melanoma of the scalp or the occasional squamous cell carcinoma of the skin that metastasizes via the lymph nodes. They are also occasionally involved in tumor metastasis from the upper aerodigestive tract when previous therapy, such as radiation or radical neck dissection, has interrupted the lymph flow.

The skin and mucosa of the medial lip and anterior floor of the mouth drain to the *submental lymph nodes*, which lie in a triangle bounded by the hyoid bone inferiorly and the anterior bellies of the left and right digastric muscle to their insertion at the symphysis of the mandible. These nodes have numerous interconnections with the more lateral *submandibular lymph nodes*, which lie in the triangle bounded by the digastric muscle and the lower border of the mandible. These nodes are intimately associated with the submandibular salivary gland, the mandibular branch of the facial nerve, and the ascending branch of the facial artery. They receive, along with the adjacent group of *facial lymph nodes*, lymphatic vessels from the submandibular gland, lower and upper lips, anterior oral cavity, nasal fossa, and medial orbital structures.

An important confluence of lymphatics occurs just below the posterior belly of the digastric muscle at the base of the skull. Here, adjacent to the jugular foramen where the jugular vein and tenth and eleventh cranial nerves exit the skull and the hypoglossal nerve passes, lies the *jugulodigastric lymph node group*. This group of nodes receives efferent vessels from the retropharyngeal lymph nodes, the submandibular lymph nodes, and the postauricular and parotid lymph nodes. In addition, the jugulodigastric nodes directly drain most of the surface of the pharynx, a large part of the tongue, the hard and soft palates, the tonsils, the external canal of the ear and the middle ear, the hypopharynx and larynx, and the parotid and submandibular glands. Naturally, this is an important site in metastasis from head and neck cancer and is the most frequent site of presenting metastasis when the site of primary malignancy cannot be determined (Fig. 7).[5]

The main lymphatic drainage of the neck is by way of the *jugular chain*, and the next dominant lymph node station is the midjugular group. These nodes lie medial to the jugular vein and generally present medial to the anterior edge of the sternocleidomastoid muscle. The predominant primary drainage site for this group of nodes is the larynx, although there are also efferent vessels from the base of the tongue and hypopharynx as well as receiving connections from the more medial thyroid chain. The posterior group, lying in the posterior triangle of the neck, is the major drainage site for lymphatic efferents from the nasopharynx but also receives vessels from the hypopharynx and thyroid areas.

The most medial neck contains the *anterior cervical nodes*, which consist of a minor group of superficial nodes accompanying the anterior jugular chain and the more important juxtavisceral nodes including the prelaryngeal, pretracheal, and recurrent laryngeal nerve groups. Efferent lymphatics from this group of nodes drain directly to the supraclavicular confluence of the jugular nodes and also to the superior mediastinum. This group serves as the main drainage of the thyroid gland and also receives vessels from the hypopharynx and infraglottic larynx.

The spinal accessory chain, the jugular chain, and the anterior cervical chain of the lymph nodes all converge at the supraclavicular fossa near the confluence of the jugular vein and the subclavian vein. This area also serves as a major drainage site for neoplasms arising in the breast and lung. Therefore, isolated supraclavicular adenopathy is less likely to be a sign of head and neck cancer than of metastasis from the more common cancers of the lung, breast, and gastrointestinal tract (Virchow's node).

NATURAL HISTORY OF HEAD AND NECK CANCER

Squamous cell carcinoma is a "solid tumor" and as such can be simplistically considered to develop locally, probably in some malignant form, to grow locally, invading the lymphatics and sending tumor emboli through the lymphatics into the regional lymph nodes, and ultimately to spread either from its local or locoregional origin to distant areas. Among solid neoplasms, squamous cell carcinoma is a relatively indolent tumor. First, the premalignant and early primary phases of the disease are probably of long duration; second, the locoregional phase of the disease is more prominent than that of other tumors such as carcinoma of the breast and colon and melanoma and sarcoma.

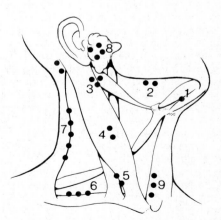

Figure 7. Lymph node stations of the neck. 1 = Submental; 2 = submandibular (submaxillary); 3 = jugulodigastric; 4 = midjugular; 5 = jugulo-omohyoid (lower jugular); 6 = posterior triangle (transverse cervical); 7 = spinal accessory; 8 = parotid; 9 = juxtavisceral.

Metastasis

Squamous cell carcinoma originates in the mucosa of the upper aerodigestive tract either as progression in the pathway of neoplasia from a premalignant lesion or *de novo* from normal tissue. Unless treated, the malignancy invades locally, involving subjacent muscle, cartilage, and bone and proceeding in three dimensions. Gross morphology describes the tumors as either exophytic, projecting outward into the lumen, or infiltrative, extending into the underlying tissues, and frequently having an ulcer with necrotic tumor at the epicenter of the mass. As the squamous cell carcinoma increases in size, not only is its local effect more deleterious but the likelihood of regional lymphatic metastases and distant metastases is increased. Microscopic evidence of blood vessel invasion indicates a particularly aggressive tumor that is capable of penetrating the normal elastin barrier of blood vessels.

Among squamous cell carcinomas, *size* is the most important clinical characteristic of the primary tumor in determining its ultimate behavior and the patient's progress. The site of origin of squamous cell carcinoma is also important in determining prognosis. Collected experience has shown survival by *site* to decrease in roughly the following order: lip, glottic larynx, oral cavity, nasopharynx, oropharynx, supraglottic larynx, and hypopharynx. Multivariate analysis of grouped sites has shown both oral cavity and oropharynx cancers to have a poorer prognosis than lip lesions, but no significant difference has been found between oral cavity and oropharynx carcinomas.

The mucosa, submucosa, and muscle of the upper aerodigestive tract are richly supplied by lymphatics. The afferent and efferent pathways of lymphatic drainage toward the thoracic duct have been described previously. The normal progression of squamous cell carcinoma is to metastasize via lymphatics to the first station of lymph nodes draining the primary site. When the primary site is well lateralized, such as on the buccal mucosa, tonsil, lateral tongue, or floor of the mouth, the lymph node metastases are to the ipsilateral neck. Progression of the disease at the primary site or in the draining lymph nodes results in further extension of lymph node metastases to the secondary drainage areas, usually in orderly fashion. Bilateral or contralateral lymph node metastases may occur when the primary tumor is located in an area with crossing afferent lymphatics and bilateral representation, such as the anterior floor of the mouth and the central base of the tongue. This may be the result of a small, centrally placed tumor or of the enlargement of an initially lateralized tumor. This may also occur when there is no distinct midline, as in the epiglottis and supraglottic larynx. Another cause of bilateral or contralateral metastasis is obstruction of collateral lymphatic flow by tumor bulk in the lymph nodes or previous therapy with surgery or irradiation. Complete obstruction of the lymphatic flow may result in spillage of tumor emboli into the skin and soft tissue and extensive local tumor infiltration of the neck.

The volume of metastasis to the lymph node is assessed clinically by site. Micrometastases to the lymph nodes may be undetectable by physical examination but are of importance in prognosis. There is a precipitous decrease in survival rate with locoregional disease, that is, primary tumor with lymph node metastases, compared with patients with local disease alone. A manifestation of aggressiveness of the squamous cell carcinoma in the neck is *extracapsular spread*. As the size of the metastatic node increases, the likelihood of disruption of the capsule and tumor growth into the soft tissue also increases. Even in patients with a small number and size of lymph node metastases, extension of the tumor through the capsule of the node markedly decreases survival. Johnson and others[12] suggest that this extracapsular spread is a more important prognosticator than the presence of lymph node metastases. In their study, there was no difference in survival between patients having no cervical lymph node metastases and those having metastases where tumor was confined to the lymph node. There was, however, a marked decrease in survival in those patients with spread of tumor beyond the confines of the node.

Locoregional Disease

Unlike other solid tumors, such as those of colon and lung cancer, in which 30 per cent or more of patients may present with distant metastases, most patients with head and neck cancer present with locoregional disease. The incidence of distant metastases in squamous cell carcinoma varies in studies from 1 to 47 per cent, depending on numerous factors. A number of studies using patients with comparable treatment and data collection have placed the number at around 12 per cent over the course of the disease. This relatively low incidence may be a function of the high morbidity and mortality caused by local and locoregional disease.

The most common sites of distant metastases from squamous cell carcinoma of the head and neck are the lungs, bone, liver, skin, and brain, in descending order. In the past, distant metastases were rare unless local or locoregional recurrence was present. Recent experience with multimodality therapy has, however, changed this. Probert[19] showed that 51 per cent of patients with distant metastases had local control of tumor. In untreated patients, the risk of distant metastases increases with size of primary tumor volume and extent of metastasis to the neck.

There is considerable variability in the risk of distant metastasis depending on the site of the primary tumor. Probert demonstrated distant metastases in a collected series of squamous cell carcinomas from different sites in the head and neck in the following sequence: nasopharynx 22.1 per cent, hypopharynx 14.6 per cent, oral cavity 13.8 per cent, supraglottic and subglottic larynx 12.3 per cent, oropharynx 11.1 per cent, and glottic larynx 1.4 per cent. When distant metastasis occurs, 1-year survival is approximately 20 per cent.

Just as untreated squamous cell carcinoma progresses locally and locoregionally, so treatment failure is usually at the primary site or in the neck. Distant metastasis as the sole site of progression or treatment failure is relatively unusual. Progression and treatment failure are a function of extent of disease at presentation. In a 5-year collected series of all sites in the head and neck from Memorial Sloan-Kettering Cancer Center, Strong[22] reported that, in patients with recurrent squamous cell carcinoma of the upper aerodigestive tract, 54.3 per cent demonstrated recurrence within 6 months, 74.9 per cent within 12 months, 82.7 per cent within 18 months, and 89.7 per cent within 24 months (Fig. 8). Therefore, disease-free survival of 2 or more years gives a 90 per cent likelihood of cure.

Prognosis

Platz and others,[18] in a European multi-institutional retrospective study of patients with squamous cell carcinoma of the oral cavity and oropharynx, examined 18

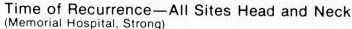

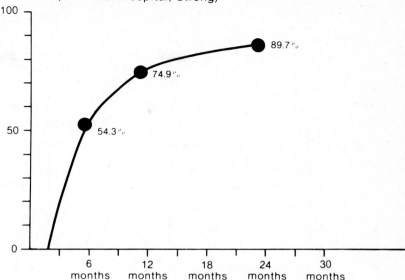

Figure 8. Most recurrences in head and neck cancer are prompt, so that survival beyond 2 years is a good prognostic sign.

criteria for survival with both univariate and multivariate analysis. The prognostically relevant factors were primary tumor size, primary tumor infiltration into subjacent muscle or other structures, histologic degree of differentiation, site of primary tumor, presence of palpable lymph nodes, fixation of cervical lymph nodes to underlying tissue, evidence of distant metastases, and age of the patient. Factors that were not found to be independent predictors of the outcome included mobility of the primary tumor, location of the primary tumor within the oral cavity or oropharynx, laterality of the primary tumor, number of metastatic cervical lymph nodes, laterality of lymph node metastases, anatomic level of lymph node metastases, and sex.

APPROACH TO THE PATIENT

Squamous cell carcinoma most commonly presents as an immediate problem in a patient with numerous underlying subacute medical disorders. Because the treatment of the disease may cause derangements in physiology and function, not only in the upper aerodigestive tract but elsewhere, careful evaluation of the entire patient is of paramount importance.

Despite the relatively indolent nature of this disease and the accessibility of its primary sites, most patients with squamous cell carcinoma of the head and neck present with advanced disease. Barkley[17] and others[3] found that, of 568 patients presenting with cancer of the oropharynx, only 202 had tumor confined to the primary site without regional lymph node invasion. The late presentation of these patients is undoubtedly multifactorial. In the oral and respiratory mucosa chronically injured by tobacco and alcohol, the primary cancer is usually not painful until it has invaded sensory nerves, periosteum, or skin. Some of the sites of origin of squamous cell carcinoma are beyond easy examination. Many of the symptoms are nonspecific. Probably most important, however, is the epidemiologic fact that the majority of these patients are abusers of tobacco and alcohol, generally of rather stoical personality using consid-

erable denial in their approach to problems and unlikely to seek medical attention until late in the natural history of the disease. Furthermore, they are often outside the populations that are amenable to screening programs by dental examination or other means. Limited screening can be done by recognizing those patients at high risk for the disease and performing a comprehensive physical examination of the upper aerodigestive tract as has been advocated by Mashberg and colleagues in the veteran population.[15]

History and Physical Examination

The diagnosis of the primary disease begins with a thorough history and physical examination. Important historic data include intensity and duration of tobacco and alcohol consumption and previous malignancy of the upper aerodigestive tract. Frank pain is not a frequent complaint, but tumor growth may interfere with the complicated relationships of swallowing and respiration and may produce a description of "tickling in the throat," gagging or choking on food, or being awakened at night by coughing secondary to aspiration of saliva. Increasing bulk of the tumor may result in dysphagia, pain on swallowing, or obstruction to the passage of solid food. Symptoms of airway obstruction are usually self-evident, but a history of wheezing should be carefully investigated to exclude upper airway obstruction by tumor and stridor. Hoarseness or change in voice strength or quality may be caused by invasion of the recurrent laryngeal nerve or direct infiltration of the larynx. Because of the variable sensory distributions of the vagus, glossopharyngeal, and trigeminal nerves in the head and neck, referred pain can be an important symptom of primary squamous cell carcinoma. Owing to the proximity of afferent pathways, ear pain may be the presenting symptom in patients with lesions in the pyriform sinus (CN 10), base of the tongue (CNS 9, 10), or floor of the mouth (CN 5). Because otitis media is a relatively uncommon disease in adults, patients with ear pain, particularly those in high-risk groups, should have thorough evaluation of the oral cavity, oropharynx, hypopharynx, nasopharynx, and larynx, as well as otoscopy.

Physical examination of the head and neck requires a systematic approach and familiarity with the use of the laryngeal mirror (Fig. 9). The mucosa-lined surfaces can best be inspected with a head lamp or other independent light source and tongue blades to expose the tissues of the oral cavity. Gentle traction of the tongue and use of the laryngeal mirror will allow examination of the oropharynx, nasopharynx, hypopharynx, and larynx in more than 90 per cent of patients without the need for topical anesthesia. In most cases, squamous cell carcinoma will be visible as either an exophytic papillary erythematous lesion projecting from the normal glistening mucosa or an erythematous infiltrative lesion with raised telangiectatic edges and an ulcerated center with or without necrotic debris. Palpation of the lesion usually reveals relatively painless induration with irregular margins. Palpation is of particular importance in lesions of the base of the tongue, where the normal papilliform projections of the lingual tonsils may obscure a malignancy.

Differential diagnosis of primary nodular lesions consists mainly of benign tumors of minor salivary gland origin and various inflammatory disorders such as necrotizing sialometaplasia, herpes simplex, medial rhomboid glossitis, pyogenic granuloma, and mucocele. Bony exostoses and tori of the mandible and palate may produce submucosal masses.

Examination of the neck is an integral part of the evaluation of the patient with squamous cell carcinoma of the upper aerodigestive tract. Lymph node metastases from mucosal primaries present as firm nodules, usually in the lateral neck. As nodal disease increases, it may become fixed to the underlying soft tissues or carotid artery or may ulcerate through the overlying skin. The location of a dominant nodule may point to the location of a small primary malignancy that is difficult to locate by indirect laryngoscopy. Approximately 3 to 4 per cent of all malignancies present as metastatic lymph nodes with no apparent primary site, and the head and neck account for two thirds of these unknown primaries. Most important, however, is the fact that one fourth of patients with cancer of the oral cavity and oropharynx, one fourth of patients with carci-

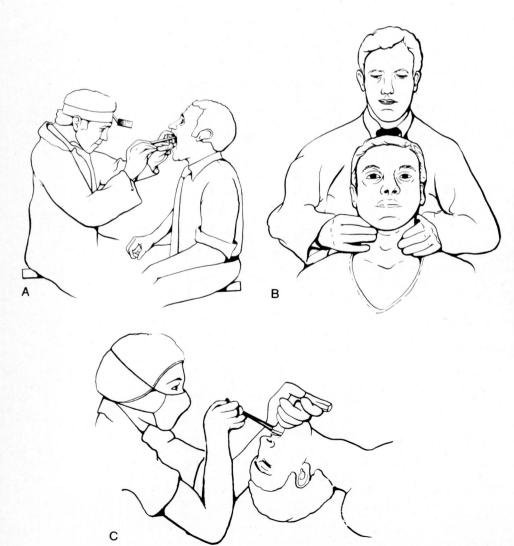

Figure 9. Physical examination of the head and neck. A, Systemic examination of the oral cavity with a light source and laryngeal mirror for indirect laryngoscopy. B, Palpation of the neck is best performed from behind the patient with both sides of the neck palpated simultaneously. C, Direct laryngopharyngoscopy, bronchoscopy, esophagoscopy, and biopsy should be performed to obtain histologic diagnosis and exclude synchronous neoplasms of the upper aerodigestive tract.

noma of the thyroid, and one half of patients with cancer of the nasopharynx present with the initial complaint of a mass in the neck. The great majority of these lesions are easily localized by appropriate physical examination. In the adult, the differential diagnosis of isolated firm neck masses overwhelmingly favors metastatic carcinoma (90 per cent), with 90 per cent of these originating in the upper aerodigestive tract. Other significant possibilities include inclusion cysts and branchial cleft cysts, nonspecific benign lymphadenitis, low-lying parotid gland tumors, prominent carotid bulb, carotid body tumors, neurofibromas, and other neural tumors and primary lymphomas. Any patient over 40 years old presenting with a firm mass in the neck should be assiduously evaluated for squamous cell carcinoma of the upper aerodigestive tract.

The concept of field cancerization must be addressed in the evaluation of the patient with carcinoma of the upper aerodigestive tract. Examination of the mucosal surfaces of the bronchi and cervical and thoracic esophagus is an important part of the work-up and post-therapy follow-up. Bronchoscopy and esophagoscopy with either rigid or fiberoptic endoscopes can be performed under general or local anesthesia. To provide the detailed anatomic information concerning primary extent necessary for treatment, direct laryngopharyngoscopy is often essential. The additional knowledge obtained from triple endoscopy has resulted in the discovery of synchronous tumors in 4 to 20 per cent of patients with head and neck cancers.

Associated Diseases

Associated diseases must be considered in the patient with squamous cell carcinoma of the upper aerodigestive tract.

DENTAL DISEASE

Serious dental disease, including periodontitis, caries, mucositis, and other oral infections, is a logical concomitant of the substance abuse characteristic of this group of patients. These problems must be addressed early, since they may interfere with either surgery or radiotherapy. Tooth restoration, peridontal treatment, or extractions should be accomplished before radiotherapy, since the risk of osteoradionecrosis of the mandible is significant in those patients who develop dental abscesses or require extractions after radiotherapy. The mandible is within the field of irradiation of most upper aerodigestive tract tumors. Osteoradionecrosis or osteomyelitis is difficult to treat in such a setting and may necessitate surgical resection of the mandible despite cure of the tumor.

PULMONARY DISEASE

Another obvious problem in this group of patients is pulmonary disease. Prolonged tobacco use results in chronic obstructive pulmonary disease. The presence of an upper aerodigestive tract tumor may result in aspiration of saliva or food of acute or chronic duration, further insulting the lower respiratory tree. For these reasons and to exclude metastasis to the lung, careful examination of the chest and chest x-ray are important. In patients who are to undergo major surgical procedures, pulmonary function tests are frequently indicated. Preoperative vigorous pulmonary toi-

let will decrease the risk of complications during the sometimes prolonged resection and reconstruction. Temporary derangement of function of the oropharynx and larynx after surgery and radiation further insults the lungs and must be considered before pneumonitis occurs.

GASTROINTESTINAL DISEASE

Other potential major problems in patients with head and neck cancer lie in the gastrointestinal system. Chronic alcohol abuse may result in cirrhosis or acute alcoholic hepatitis. Portal hypertension, hypoalbuminemia, anemia of chronic disease, and ascites are sequelae that may interfere with planned therapy. Diabetes mellitus may be seen with chronic pancreatitis and complicates wound healing and the already difficult nutritional maintenance of these patients. Severe malnutrition of both protein and calories has been found in 40 per cent of patients with head and neck cancer and good nutrition in only 20 per cent. This malnutrition has been associated with a higher incidence of major and minor surgical complications and mortality and obviously makes the feeding problems attendant to radiation therapy more severe. Immunologic incompetence, a logical concomitant to malnutrition, has been identified in 50 per cent of head and neck cancer patients. Numerous series have shown that these patients have a deficient cell-mediated immunological state, as documented by skin testing, in vitro T lymphocyte function tests, and lymphocyte count at the time of presentation. This immunologic state is further compromised by operation or general anesthesia and even more potently by radiation therapy. Correction of malnutrition and immune deficits is usually possible by pretherapy hyperalimentation, usually by inserting a nasogastric feeding tube and discontinuing alcohol. The obvious dangers of the numerous alcohol withdrawal syndromes must be carefully considered.

Diagnostic Studies

Work-up of the head and neck cancer patient requires relatively little other than careful history and physical examination. Plain roentgenograms of the head are useful in certain instances to either detect disease or to document the extent of spread. Because the paranasal sinuses are not readily accessible to visualization, sinus films may aid in investigating an occult primary or evaluating symptoms in that area. Mandibular films may reveal invasion by malignancy in the floor of the mouth or tongue.

Radionuclide bone scans with technetium-99 can also be effective in determining mandibular invasion by tumor. Tomograms of the base of the skull may reveal invasion by cancer of the foramen ovale by extension up the trigeminal nerve. Computed tomography gives excellent imaging of the bony structures and some soft tissue areas, such as the infratemporal fossa, and may be helpful in staging the disease. Soft tissue is best evaluated by physical examination, but the development of magnetic resonance imaging (MRI) may improve the ability to assess mucosal and submucosal spread of squamous cell carcinoma.

In patients with no major systemic problems or symptoms suggestive of metastasis to bone, a chest roentgenogram and serum alkaline phosphatase level will be adequate laboratory study. In the absence of symptoms and with normal serum alkaline phosphatase levels, bone and liver scans are unlikely to contribute significantly to the diagnosis.

Clinical Staging

When the physical examination and collection of appropriate data are complete, it is essential that the clinical information be compiled and an overall assessment of the extent of disease be made. The upper aerodigestive tract is a compact area with intricate anatomy and sometimes confusing nomenclature. It is, therefore, of paramount importance that an accurate reproducible description of the primary tumor, the regional spread, and the presence or absence of distant metastases be stated. Clinical staging of the disease accomplishes this.

By convention of the American Joint Committee on Cancer (AJCC), the primary tumor is staged by size and involvement of adjacent structures. For staging purposes, the upper aerodigestive tract is divided into four sites: the oral cavity, the pharynx, the larynx, and the paranasal sinuses. The symbol for extent of primary disease is T (tumor). In the oral cavity and pharynx, T_1 tumors are less than 2.0 cm. in diameter, T_2 tumors are 2.0 to 4.0 cm., T_3 tumors are greater than 4.0 cm., and T_4 tumors have invaded soft tissues other than the site of origin. In the paranasal sinuses, nasopharynx, and larynx, the involvement of more than one distinct anatomic area increases the T stage.

Regional disease is assessed by N (node) staging. Increasing size of individual lymph nodes, increasing number of lymph nodes, and bilaterality or contralaterality are the parameters that increase N stage. The presence or absence of distant metastasis is the sole determinant of M (metastasis) stage in head and neck cancer. As in all solid tumors, accurate TNM staging in head and neck cancer is essential. First, the approach to cancer treatment is multidisciplinary. To make treatment planning most effective, it is important that practitioners with different backgrounds have the same understanding of the anatomy, site, and extent of the disease at the time of presentation and at any point later in the course of the disease. Second, accurate prognosis depends on a clear conception of how advanced the cancer is; the higher the stage the poorer the prognosis. Third, evaluation of the efficacy of treatment regimens relies completely on the retrospective analysis of results in well-defined disease states. What is effective treatment for Stage 1 disease may be ineffective for Stage 3 disease. With inaccurate assessment of disease stage, important information can be overlooked. The accurate staging of squamous cell carcinoma of the upper aerodigestive tract, preferably using the AJCC diagrams, is of obvious import (Fig. 10).

THERAPY OPTIONS

At the present time, therapy of squamous cell carcinoma of the upper aerodigestive tract consists of surgical extirpation of tumor and its regional metastases, irradiation of the tumor and the neck, or both. In treating the patient with squamous cell carcinoma of the upper aerodigestive tract, as in any therapeutic approach to any patient, there is a hierarchy of priorities. This decision-making process is of particular importance when there is more than one type of treatment to be chosen with relatively equivalent results.

Of primary significance is *survival*, which implies control of the disease. A second consideration is restoration or avoidance of interference with *function*. The second consideration is particularly cogent in squamous cell carcinoma of the upper aerodigestive tract because of the intricate mechanical relationships in this area that control

our important vegetative functions, respiration and alimentation, and the specialized functions, speech and swallowing. Advances in surgical technique have allowed much closer attention to the restoration of function by sophisticated reconstructive techniques. The third consideration, and one that is particularly germane to head and neck cancer patients, is preservation or restoration of *physical appearance*. When possible, efforts to avoid disfiguring operations or restore normal facial stucture should be considered. Fourth, attention must be paid to the *efficiency of therapy*. Because most patients with squamous cell carcinoma present with advanced disease, there is a high therapeutic failure rate. Recurrent carcinoma sometimes can be ameliorated, but cure is unusual. Since 90 per cent of recurrences present within 2 years of diagnosis and survival following recurrence is frequently brief, the treatment regimen should be structured to restore the patient to function in a relatively short period of time. Prolonged courses of treatment or reconstruction should be avoided whenever possible in favor of one- or two-stage therapies with equivalent success.

Although radiation therapy and surgery are the mainstays of treatment for squamous cell carcinoma of the upper aerodigestive tract, trials of chemotherapy and immunotherapy have presented varying results and should be examined.

Immunotherapy

Investigation of immunocompetence in patients with squamous cell carcinoma of the upper aerodigestive tract reveals numerous abnormalities. With the high incidence of protein malnutrition, alcohol abuse, and other chronic diseases, it is not surprising that immunity is depressed in general. Numerous studies have identified deficient *cell-mediated immunity*, as demonstrated by T lymphocyte function *in vitro*, skin testing to dinitrochlorobenzene (DNCB) and other antigens, and absolute T lymphocyte counts in peripheral blood.

In most cases, the incidence of depressed cell-mediated immunity is a function of the stage of the disease. Patients with Stage 1 and Stage 2 cancers demonstrate a depressed function in 15 to 40 per cent of cases tested. Those with Stage 3 cancers demonstrate variations, with from 71 to 85 per cent showing depressed function. Immunocompetence appears to be restored with control of the disease and appears to deteriorate with progression of the disease. Although it is intellectually attractive to consider immunodeficiency to be the cause or at least a promoting factor for the occurrence of squamous cell carcinoma, the epidemiologic evidence favors the converse, i.e., the squamous cell carcinoma itself, although local or locoregional, is a systemic immunodepressant. Of further significance is the fact that one of the main therapeutic modalities for squamous cell carcinoma, radiation therapy, is a very potent depressant of immune function.

Immunostimulation

Given the data that squamous cell carcinoma is associated with a relatively high incidence of immune incompetence, particularly when compared with adenocarcinoma, melanoma, and sarcomas of similar stage, that immunocompetence decreases as stage of disease increases, and that control of progression of disease is directly reflected by changes in the immune system, it seems likely that manip-

Figure 10. American Joint Committee on Cancer staging sheet for pharyngeal cancer. Text and diagrams facilitate accurate storage of data. (From the American Joint Committee for Cancer Staging and End Results Reporting: Manual for Staging of Cancer, 1977.)

DATA FORM FOR CANCER STAGING

Patient Identification   Institutional Identification
Name _____   Hospital or Clinic _____
Address _____   Address _____
Hospital or Clinic Number _____
Age _____ Sex _____ Race _____

ONCOLOGY RECORD

Anatomic Site of Cancer _____   Histologic Cell Type _____
                                         Grade _____
Time of Classification*   cTNM ____ sTNM ____ pTNM ____ rTNM ____ aTNM ____
Date of Classification _____

SITE-SPECIFIC INFORMATION — PHARYNX
Status Before Treatment Anywhere — Primary Tumor

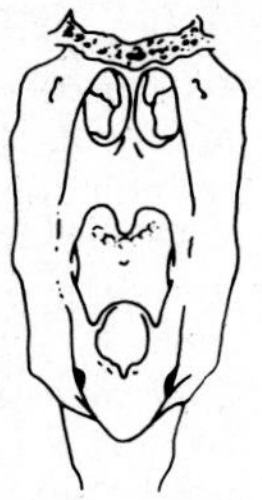

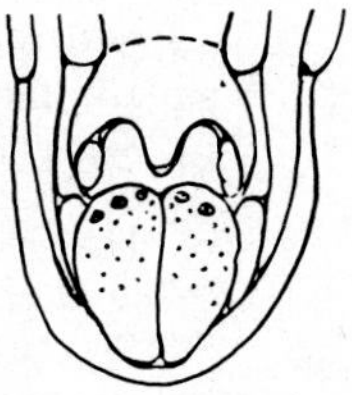

Location of Tumor	Site of origin (check one)	Site(s) also involved	Anatomic extent
Nasopharynx			
Posterosuperior wall	_____	_____	T1 _____
Lateral wall	_____	_____	T2 _____
			T3 _____
			T4 _____
Oropharynx			
Faucial arch	_____	_____	T1 _____
Tonsillar fossa, tonsil	_____	_____	T2 _____
Base of tongue	_____	_____	T3 _____
Pharyngeal wall	_____	_____	T4 _____
Hypopharynx			
Pyriform fossa	_____	_____	T1 _____
Postcricoid area	_____	_____	T2 _____
Posterior wall	_____	_____	T3 _____
			T4 _____

Characteristics of Tumor (check one)
Superficial   _____
Exophytic   _____
Moderate infiltration _____
Deep infiltration   _____

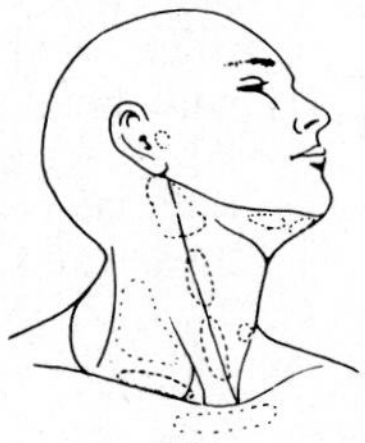

Regional Lymph Nodes (check one only; diagram)
N0 _____   N3a _____
N1 _____   N3b _____
N2a _____   N3c _____
N2b _____
If bilateral nodes present, stage each side separately.
Right _____   Left _____
Distant Metastasis
MX _____   M0 _____   M1 _____   Specify _____
Sites: Lung _____   Bone _____   Liver _____   Other _____
Classification
T _____   N _____   M _____
Stage _____
Residual Tumor
R _____

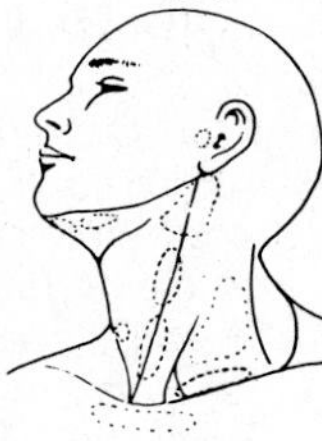

Host — Performance Status (H)
H _____ Scale used: AJC _____ Zubrod _____ Karnofsky _____
*cTNM, clinical-diagnostic; sTNM, surgical-evaluative; pTNM, postsurgical treatment-pathologic; rTNM, retreatment; aTNM, autopsy.

ulation of cell-mediated immunity might be profitable in the therapy of these patients. As in other solid tumors, changes in *humoral* immunity do not appear to be as dramatic. Squamous cell carcinoma is difficult to grow in tissue culture and, when grown, is not very antigenic. Specific immunity, either by vaccine or sensitized lymphocytes, is, therefore, impossible at present. Further refinements in tissue culture technique may change this. Nonspecific immunostimulation has been utilized in this group of patients. Most immunopotentiators, such as interferon, bacille Calmette Guérin (BCG), levamisole, and thymosin, work indirectly on the lymphocyte through the macrophage. Several studies have shown restoration or improvement of *in vitro* tests of cell-mediated immunity with thymosin and levamisole. In preliminary clinical studies, there has been a suggestion that adjuvant use of levamisole may lengthen disease-free intervals in patients with successfully resected carcinoma of the oral cavity.

IMMUNE SYSTEM MANIPULATION

Another approach to immunotherapy lies in the somewhat controversial theory that malignancy arises and progresses because of deficits in the immune surveillance system. Suppression of the immune surveillance system may come from excessive prostaglandin synthesis by tumor cells or by native suppressor lymphocytes. In addition, it appears that some prostaglandins directly stimulate tumor growth. Several investigators have demonstrated regression of tumor by the use of the prostaglandin synthetase inhibitor indomethacin. Improvement of *in vitro* tests of lymphocyte function has been associated with this tumor regression. Manipulation of the immune system in the therapy of head and neck cancer is a promising avenue of approach, although at present it is at best experimental and should be subjected to controlled clinical trials when favorable laboratory data are obtained.

Chemotherapy

Control of local and locoregional disease has been the primary consideration in cancer of the head and neck because most of the morbidity and mortality of the disease is locoregional. There are, however, numerous problems that make chemotherapy a desirable adjuvant to surgery and radiation therapy. A significant number of patients develop distant metastases even with control of the primary tumor. There is a high failure rate of the definitive therapy, i.e., surgery, radiation, or both. A decrease in the size of the primary tumor before surgery or irradiation might make the definitive therapy less functionally devastating and thus more effective.

In addition to systemic administration of chemotherapy by the intravenous route, the patient with head and neck cancer can be treated with regional infusion of the agent through the external carotid artery, delivering a higer dose with less systemic toxicity. For these reasons, as well as the general enthusiasm for chemotherapy of solid tumors, many regimens have been examined.[10]

The response rate (the relative number of patients who demonstrate measurable shrinkage of their tumor to 50 per cent of original volume) of squamous cell carcinoma of the upper aerodigestive tract is respectable. *Methotrexate* has been the most active single agent, giving response rates of greater than 50 per cent in numerous studies. As a single agent given in a low dose, it has been shown to be more effective than several combination regimens and a high-dose, more toxic methotrexate schedule. Other particularly active single agents are *cis*-platinum and bleomycin, both with somewhat lower response rates than methotrexate. Combinations of bleomycin and *cis*-platinum have given response rates as high as 90 per cent in several studies. A recent regimen of *cis*-platinum and 4-day infusion of 5-fluorouracil has given a complete response (disappearance of all measurable tumor) in 20 per cent of patients and a total response rate of 90 per cent. Although better mechanisms of delivery are being studied, intra-arterial infusion chemotherapy does not seem to show a major advantage over systemic intravenous therapy.

Despite the encouraging response rate seen with chemotherapy in squamous cell carcinoma of the upper aerodigestive tract, the contribution to survival in this cancer, as in most solid tumors, has been modest, if present at all. The responses to chemotherapy are, in general, of short duration in a disease characterized by relatively slow growth. Small tumors are most likely to respond, and larger tumors with lymph node metastases are less likely to respond either at the primary site or in the neck. The toxicity of the most active agents, including nausea and vomiting, stomatitis, esophagitis, and diarrhea, add to the pre-existing disturbances in alimentation caused by tumor or underlying malnutrition. Patient compliance is a problem in a subset of patients in whom substance abuse is prominent. A recent randomized controlled study by the National Cancer Institute compared patients undergoing the standard therapy for Stage 3 cancer of the oral cavity, hypopharynx, and larynx (surgery followed by adjuvant irradiation) with a second group treated with two preoperative courses of *cis*-platinum and bleomycin followed by standard therapy and with a third group treated with both preoperative chemotherapy and a postirradiation course of chemotherapy. There was no improvement in disease-free survival in either of the groups treated with chemotherapy.

Chemotherapy may ultimately play a role in the treatment of squamous cell carcinoma of the upper aerodigestive tract, particularly in those patients with late-stage disease and those with recurrent disease after definitive therapy. At present, however, its role as an adjuvant to surgery and radiation is questionable, and its role as sole treatment of these cancers is nonexistent.

RADIATION THERAPY

Delivery of ionizing radiation to the area of squamous cell carcinoma is one of the two major forms of therapy for this disease. Depending on several factors involving the stage of the tumor and the patient, radiation therapy may stand alone or be used in combination with surgery. Like surgery, radiation is a local treatment. Eradication of malignant cells is limited to those areas where the radiation therapy is delivered. Ionizing radiation is toxic or lethal to both benign and malignant cells and when delivered to an area contacts all of the cells and cellular organelles within its field. At dosage levels used in clinical cancer treatment, the mechanism of cell kill thought to be of primary importance is the conversion of intracellular H_2O molecules into electron-positive free radicals. This transformation requires that free oxygen be available in the cytoplasm of the cell. The electron-positive free radicals of peroxide and superoxide react with DNA, causing disruption of the strand. Although most cells contain mechanisms for the repair of

DNA strand breaks, tumor cells appear to be less efficient than normal cells at this reparative function. The ultimate effect of ionizing irradiation occurs when DNA replication commences and is ineffectual or abnormal. Although the ionizing irradiation contacts cellular organelles other than the chromosome, the biochemical dysfunction caused to these organelles at clinically safe doses is minimal.[1]

Radiosensitivity

The lethal effect of radiation depends on the presence of intracellular oxygen (Fig. 11). As tumor volume increases, a greater amount of the neoplasm is relatively avascular, having outgrown its blood supply, and contains, therefore, hypoxic cells. These cells are radioresistant. The size of the primary tumor is, therefore, a major factor in selection of therapy. For T1 and T2 squamous cell carcinomas (1.0 to 4.0 cm.), eradication of the cancer is usually possible with radiation alone, making it equivalent to surgery in therapeutic success. In tumors larger than 4.0 cm. in diameter (T3 or T4), there is considerably less likelihood of cure, and combined therapy with surgery is more likely to be successful. Although larger lesions can be treated successfully with higher doses of irradiation, normal tissue complications increase greatly with escalating doses and the overall benefit to the patient decreases.

Histology

Although most squamous cell carcinomas behave similarly, with a gradual increase in risk of treatment failure from well-differentiated to poorly differentiated, the histologic subtype of squamous cell carcinoma plays some role in the radiosensitivity. Radiocurability, like survival, is more a function of stage of disease than of histology. Lymphoepithelioma is a squamous cell carcinoma with a pronounced lymphocytic infiltrate. Lymphoepitheliomas occur most frequently in areas with normal lymphatic tissue, such as the tonsils, base of the tongue, and nasopharynx, and are more radiosensitive than other squamous cell carcinomas. Verrucous squamous cell carcinomas appear to be less radiosensitive.

Site of Origin

The site of origin of the squamous cell carcinoma does not appear to affect its sensitivity to irradiation. Variability in control rates at different sites, although not great, is probably related to the difficulty in delivery of irradiation rather than any inherent property of the area. Absorption or scattering of irradiation by adjacent bone or cartilage may decrease the absorbed dose. Obviously, site of origin has a major influence on selection of therapy. Surgical extirpation of a T1 tumor of the larynx usually results in a more serious functional deficit than does irradiation.

The same principles and predictors of success that apply to regional cervical disease also apply to the primary site in the upper aerodigestive tract, except that the neck appears to require larger doses for control. Radiation therapy provides excellent cure rates in clinically negative necks, i.e., those with presumed micrometastases. The ability to eradicate lymph node metastases greater than 2.0 cm. in diameter is limited, and there is considerable controversy over success rate with smaller lymph nodes. Most patients presenting with clinically positive neck nodes require either surgery or combined therapy.

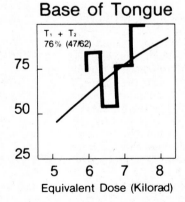
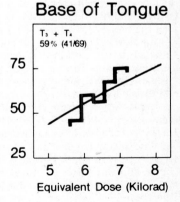
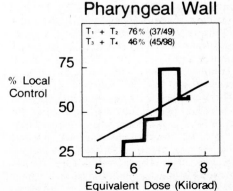

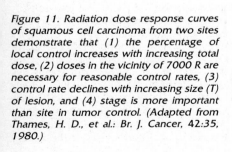

Figure 11. Radiation dose response curves of squamous cell carcinoma from two sites demonstrate that (1) the percentage of local control increases with increasing total dose, (2) doses in the vicinity of 7000 R are necessary for reasonable control rates, (3) control rate declines with increasing size (T) of lesion, and (4) stage is more important than site in tumor control. (Adapted from Thames, H. D., et al.: Br. J. Cancer, 42:35, 1980.)

Delivery of Irradiation

Radiation therapy is delivered in intervals that are designed to maximize the tumoricidal effect yet allow adjacent normal tissues to recover to some extent. The total dose (R) of irradiation delivered depends to some degree on the size and site of the tumor but in the head and neck region generally ranges between 5500 and 7500 R (see Fig. 11). These doses are delivered usually in 200-R fractions five times per week for 6 to 8 weeks. The field or portal is designed to treat a wide area around the tumor as well as the lymphatic drainage of the primary site. The neck is usually treated to 5000 R. Using the shrinking field technique,[17] higher doses may be delivered to a very small area near the epicenter of the tumor to increase tumoricidal effect in the hypoxic central area while avoiding surrounding tissue damage. The radiation energy in the form of gamma rays, electrons, or photons is usually transmitted to the field of treatment on the patient through a tube connected to the energy source. In some instances, however, direct implantation of radioactive seeds into the tissues or tubes perforating the tissue will give a higher radiation dose over a limited area. Interstitial implantation of radiation sources is useful in massive lymphadenopathy secondary to metastasis and in some intraoral cancers.

Side Effects

The toxic effect of radiation on tumor cells is also active on normal cells. The cellular events are represented on the gross scale by changes in the tissues of the upper aerodigestive tract. These changes are dose-dependent and are both acute and reversible and chronic and progressive. The dose-dependent effects are cumulative not only to the area of treatment but to the surrounding areas as well. For this reason, when an area of the head and neck is treated with radiation, it is dangerous to treat any other area in the region a second time with irradiation.

Acute complications of radiation therapy include desquamation of the skin and mucositis. Cheilitis, stomatitis, and esophagitis can all interfere with alimentation during therapy. Interrupting the course or decreasing the absorbed dose usually results in improvement. Occasionally edema of the larynx or tongue secondary to the radiation effect of tumor kill may cause upper airway obstruction. Curative doses of radiation may interfere with postoperative wound healing, giving a higher risk of surgical complications. Very high doses of radiation rarely cause acute necrosis of skin, bone, and cartilage.

The chronic effects of radiation on normal tissue or the treated aerodigestive tract may also be problematic. Loss of salivary secretion from the major and minor salivary glands occurs at curative doses. The numerous functions of saliva include lubrication of the oral cavity to facilitate the movement of food through the pharynx and hypopharynx, digestion (with its minor enzymatic contribution), and an immunologic response, with its antibiotic action mediated through immunoglobulins. The discomfort of xerostomia is added to the decrease in oral hygiene attendant on the loss of saliva. The vasculitis and endarteritis of chronic radiation effect may cause relative ischemia of bone, increasing the risk of osteomyelitis and osteoradionecrosis with dental disease or extraction. Stricture of the hypopharynx and esophagus is also seen after curative doses of irradiation. Transverse myelitis may occur either acutely or late because of radiation injury to the blood supply of the cervical spinal cord.

Advantages and Disadvantages

There are several advantages of radiation therapy over surgery in the treatment of squamous cell carcinoma. Although loss of salivary function and structure certainly result in disability, in general there is less interference with function after irradiation alone than after major surgery. This is particularly true in the hypopharynx and larynx; voice quality is almost always better after irradiation than after conservative surgery of the larynx, and speech is almost always better after irradiation than esophageal speech after total laryngectomy. When the lesion involves visible tissue, physical appearance is usually better after radiation. Avoidance of a major operation is sometimes of benefit in patients with serious associated systemic diseases. Recurrent disease after radiation therapy is more likely to be treated successfully by surgery than is recurrence after surgery to be salvaged with irradiation.

There are several disadvantages of radiation therapy that are, conversely, advantages of surgery. A wide area of tissue other than the site of treatment is exposed to irradiation. Definitive therapy cannot be repeated, unlike surgery, which can be performed as many times as necessary in this disease characterized by recurrence. An implicit disadvantage of the one-time nature of radiation therapy is that it requires more prolonged cooperation on the part of the patient. The treatment regimen usually lasts from 5 to 8 weeks, with daily doses. Interruption of this schedule by patient noncompliance severely jeopardizes a successful outcome. Submucosal extension of disease in the head and neck is a common problem. Although this characteristic is addressed to a certain degree by planning the original portals of treatment, there is no accurate pathologic evaluation of the extent of tumor at the primary site or of involvement of lymph nodes in the neck to aid in planning adjuvant therapy. There is evidence that radiation at high or low dose is carcinogenic over long periods of time.

SURGICAL THERAPY

The principle underlying successful surgical treatment of squamous cell carcinoma of the upper aerodigestive tract is identical to that governing treatment of all solid tumors: the entire mass of malignant cells must be removed. To accomplish this, the treatment plan must take into consideration the stage of the disease (for local disease, whether it is primary or recurrent). The visible, palpable tumor, along with an appropriate margin of normal tissue (usually 2.0 cm. to address the problem of microscopic submucosal extension), is excised. If there is regional disease in the neck or if the primary tumor is so large that there is a high risk of subclinical metastasis to the neck, a radical neck dissection is performed simultaneously. Whenever possible, an *en bloc* or *composite* resection is performed, leaving the primary tumor site attached to the structures of the neck.

Technique

Squamous cell carcinoma tends to spread in a radial fashion, but tumor growth may be blocked or redirected by fascial planes, perichondrium, or periosteum. There is, however, ultimately invasion of adjacent structures. In oral cancer the mandible is frequently invaded. In laryngeal cancer the thyroid cartilage may be involved. To adequately remove the primary tumor, adjacent structures, such as a

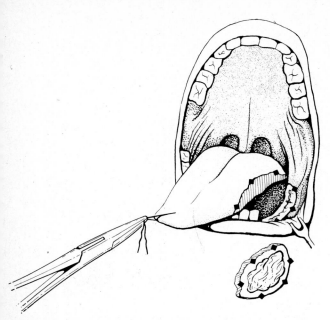

Figure 12. The primary cancer is excised with a 2-cm. margin of normal tissue. Multiple specimens (diamonds) are sent for frozen section to exclude submucosal involvement. These sections may be taken from either the excised tumor or the edges of the resection.

segment of mandible or the extrinsic larynx, may be sacrificed. A clear margin is essential to the eradication of the disease (Fig. 12). At the time of surgical removal, the surgeon sends the specimen or pieces of tissue from the three-dimensional borders of the defect for immediate pathologic analysis, i.e., frozen section (see Fig. 12). If these specimens show no evidence of tumor, the likelihood of cure is higher. Extension of the tumor to the edge of the resected specimen decreases the likelihood of cure. If extension is detected at the time of operation, further tissue should be excised. If detected in the permanent section of the specimen, reoperation should be considered or adjuvant radiotherapy contemplated. Although pathologic examination of the margins is not infallible, it is important. Looser and coworkers[14] showed that patients with positive margins at the time of resection have a local recurrence rate of 71 per cent as opposed to 32 per cent in those with negative margins. They suggest that adjuvant radiotherapy is not particularly useful in decreasing this high risk of failure, implying that reoperation may be more appropriate.

Although in many cases it is adequate to remove a 2.0-cm. margin of normal tissue around the neoplasm, it is sometimes necessary to remove the entire structure. Total laryngectomy and total glossectomy may be necessary in the surgical treatment of cancer of the larynx or extensive neoplasms of the base of the tongue. Whenever a firm mass in the neck is present simultaneously with a squamous cell carcinoma of the upper aerodigestive tract, an approach to the neck must be included in the treatment plan. Like the regional lymphatic stations in the axilla and groin, the lymph nodes of the neck lie between two distinct fascial planes and can therefore be removed as a unit, including the jugular vein and sternocleidomastoid muscle. Radical neck dissection removes the lymphatic drainage of the primary tumor and, therefore, any tumor metastases that may be present. Whenever possible, the contents of the neck are left attached to the primary tumor to include any draining lymphatics between the primary and the first

station of lymph nodes. The surgical principle of *en bloc* resection requires removal of the primary tumor and its cervical metastases wtihout cutting across tumor. This dictum is satisfied by therapeutic neck dissection (see Fig. 12).

As the primary tumor increases in size, the likelihood of lymph node metastases becomes greater. Surgical decisions depend on the physical examination; the accuracy of physical examination in the neck is higher than that in the axilla or groin. False-negative rates vary from 10 to 50 per cent, whereas false-positive rates vary from 10 to 15 per cent. Micrometastases to the neck that are not clinically apparent may manifest later if untreated. Jesse and others[11] have demonstrated that occurrence of subclinical disease in the neck varies with the primary site: oral tongue 34 per cent, floor of mouth 29.5 per cent, mandibular alveolus 18.5 per cent, and buccal mucosa 9 per cent. In general, in patients presenting with T2 or greater carcinomas of the floor of the mouth or mandiubular alveolus, hypopharynx, or supraglottic larynx, neck dissection should be performed even in the absence of palpable nodal metastases. Elective or prophylactic neck dissection or elective irradiation of the N0 neck is an important concept in the treatment of cancer of the upper aerodigestive tract.

The classic radical neck dissection for removal of lymphatic metastases to the neck has remained relatively unchanged since Crile's description in 1906. The lymph nodes of the neck lie in a compartment that is enveloped by distinct fascial layers, allowing removal of the compartment as a single unit and thereby satisfying those dictates of cancer surgery that prohibit cutting across tumor. The platysma muscle and its extensions form the superficial fascia of the neck. The deep fascia of the neck has two leaves; the superficial leaf is the investing fascia and lies on top of the sternocleidomastoid and trapezius muscles and extends to the carotid sheath. The deep layer of the deep cervical fascia lies on the axial muscles of the neck, the scalenes, the levator scapulae, and the splenius capitis muscles. In removing the contents of this fascial envelope, the sternocleidomastoid and omohyoid muscles, the cutaneous branches of the cervical plexus, and the accessory nerve and internal jugular vein with its major tributaries are all removed.

To remove a cancer in the upper aerodigestive tract, proper exposure is necessary. Approach to the pharynx or larynx and oral cavity can be made through the neck when accompanied by radical neck dissection. The floor of the mouth or pharyngeal constrictors are incised, the tumor is visualized, and an adequate margin of normal tissue is resected. This approach lends itself well to *en bloc* resections. If the lesion is small and lies in the anterior or anterolateral portion of the oral cavity or oropharynx, adequate exposure may be obtained through the mouth. Most cancers of this region are large and require a more expansive approach involving division of the lip and mandible whether or not this area is to be resected. This technique allows adequate visualization for safe and accurate resection of the tumor.

After resection and reconstruction, the mandible and lip are reapproximated with little loss of function. If the operative procedure is extensive and there is a high probability of postoperative edema with danger of upper airway obstruction, tracheostomy is performed at the beginning of the operation. This assures an adequate airway independent of the operative manipulations and facilitates the administration of anesthesia without interfering with surgery. After wound healing and re-establishment of a satisfactory airway, the tracheostomy tube can be removed and the stoma will usually close spontaneously.

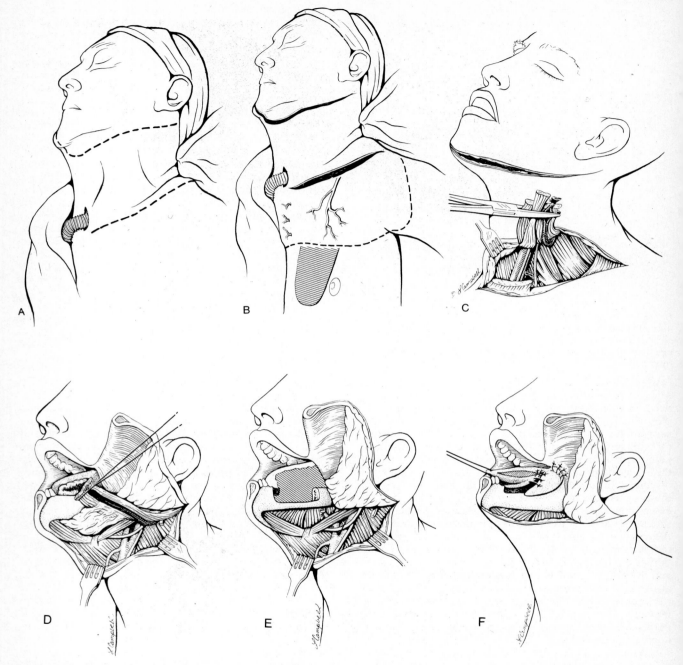

Figure 13. This patient has a T2N1M0 carcinoma of the floor of the mouth that appears to be attached to the mandible.

A, Resection of the primary tumor and segmental mandibulectomy with incontinuity radical neck dissection and reconstruction are planned. Preoperative tracheostomy is performed and McFee skin incisions for radical neck dissection are marked.

B, The deltopectoral flap receives its blood supply from perforating vessels from the internal mammary artery that pass through the second, third, and fourth intercostal spaces. The pectoralis major musculocutaneous flap (shaded) is supplied by the thoracoacromial artery and vein. Either or both of these flaps may be used for the ultimate reconstruction of the defect.

C, The radical neck dissection is begun through the inferior incision. Sternocleidomastoid and omohyoid muscles and internal jugular vein are divided and retracted upward.

D, The radical neck dissection is continued through the upper incision. The contents of the neck, including the cervical lymph nodes, are left in continuity to the tumor in the submandibular area. The upper incision is extended through the midline of the chin and lip to allow development of a cheek flap and exposure of the oral cavity.

E, The defect includes the mucosa and muscle of a portion of the lateral tongue and the alveolingual sulcus as well as a segment of the mandible and the soft tissue of the neck. There are many ways to reconstruct this defect, each with inherent advantages and problems. Three of the most appropriate methods will be demonstrated.

F, A tongue flap can be created by splitting the tongue. The blood supply comes in through the base of the tongue. This is a quick and reliable method of providing a lining similar to that removed. There is usually significant tethering of the tongue that may interfere with speech and swallowing. The amount of tissue available is limited.

Illustration continued on opposite page

Numerous incisions are available for neck dissection. The McFee incision consists of parallel incisions, the superior one in the submandibular skin fold extending from the trapezius border to the midline of the neck and the inferior one just cephalad to the clavicle (Fig. 13*A*). The flap is raised between these incisions in either the subcutaneous or subplatysmal layer. Both heads of the sternocleidomastoid muscle are divided at the origin and insertion. Inferomedially, the jugular vein is identified and divided, exposing the vagus nerve and carotid sheath (Fig. 13*B*). Below the deep layer of the cervical fascia lies the phrenic nerve just superficial to the anterior scalene muscle. This is preserved as dissection proceeds from medial to lateral, dividing the omohyoid muscle, transverse cervical vessels, and connective tissue and fat of the posterior triangle to the margin of the trapezius muscle.

Moving to the origin of the sternocleidomastoid on the mastoid process, the distal portion of the occipital artery is divided, and the internal jugular vein is identified at its exit from the base of the skull by retracting the posterior belly of the digastric muscle cephalad. At the jugular foramen, in proximity to the internal jugular vein, lie the spinal accessory nerve, vagus and hypoglossal nerves. The spinal accessory nerve is usually sacrificed when the jugular vein is ligated and transected. The vagus and hypoglossal nerves can usually be preserved.

Attention is now turned to the submandibular triangle. The tail of the parotid gland is transected and the posterior facial vein divided. The marginal mandibular branches of the facial nerve are identified and retracted cephalad, and the ascending branches of the facial artery and vein are divided. Division of the superficial fascia along the mandible opens the submandibular triangle; dissection along the lateral border of the anterior belly of the digastric and myohyoid further opens this interval.

DISSECTION

At this point, dissection is begun from lateral to medial commencing at the border of the trapezius muscle. Progression along the deep cervical fascia continues until the cutaneous branches of the cervical plexus C2-3 and C3-4 are transected. With further movement medially, the carotid sheath inferiorly and the facial artery superiorly are encountered. Division of the facial artery allows exposure of the deep surface of the submandibular gland. The superficial investing fascia connecting the sternocleidomastoid muscle to the medial strap muscles and digastric muscle is divided at the medial margin, and the anterior belly of the omohyoid muscle is divided at the hyoid bone.

If an *incontinuity dissection* is to be performed, the intraoral resection can be begun with the contents of the

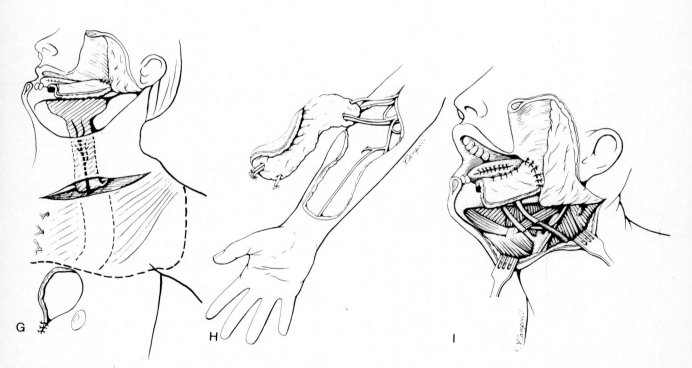

G   **H**   **I**

Figure 13. Continued

G, *The pectoralis musculocutaneous flap provides well-vascularized muscle and ample skin for lining in the oral cavity. It is relatively easy to raise, leaves a minimal functional deficit, is reliable, and provides coverage of the carotid vessels with its muscular pedicle, which is tunnelled under the neck skin flaps. The skin paddle can be tailored to the size of the mucosal defect. Disadvantages are mainly due to its bulk, particularly if the mandible is left intact. Gravitational pull may interfere with mobility of the tongue and larynx.*

H, *The radial forearm skin flap can be raised on the radial artery and its venae comitantes and also the cephalic vein. The donor site is skin grafted.*

I, *Using microvascular technique, the radial artery is anastomosed to the superior thyroid artery and the cephalic vein to the external jugular vein, which has been preserved during the radical neck dissection. The skin is sutured to the lateral tongue and cheek mucosa and draped over the mandible, providing a relatively thin covering that recreates the sulci. There is minimal bulk and gravitational effect and, thus, little disturbance of tongue mobility. Disadvantages are the length of operation and the need for microvascular equipment and expertise.*

neck attached. In *discontinuous dissection*, the submandibular ganglion and the submaxillary duct are divided superficial to the hypoglossal and lingual nerves, and the contents of the neck are removed. Closure of the McFee incisions completes the neck dissection, and the carotid artery is at minimal risk of exposure in the event of suture line breakdown.

In selected patients, the neck dissection may be altered in an attempt to decrease the morbidity of the procedure. These modified or functional neck dissections may preserve the spinal accessory nerve, the internal jugular vein, or the sternocleidomastoid muscle and are of use primarily in elective neck dissection.

In very advanced cases of squamous cell carcinoma, the patient may be considered to have surgically unresectable disease. This occurs usually when the tumor has extended up into the base of the skull along the jugular vein or one of the cranial nerves. If the tumor is fixed to the prevertebral fascia or has penetrated the deep cervical fascia to the scalene muscles, it is unlikely that surgical resection will be possible. Lymphatic metastases fixed in the supraclavicular area are another manifestation of extensive disease. Rarely, unresectable disease may be rendered operable by chemotherapy or radiotherapy, but the prognosis remains grave.

Complications

Complications of surgery consist mainly of problems with wound breakdown, although functional disturbances are another group of undesirable sequelae. The environment of the upper aerodigestive tract is hostile to wound healing, primarily because of its varied and virulent bacterial flora. Concentrations of aerobic and anaerobic bacteria in the range of 10^8 per ml. of saliva may retard wound healing. Fortunately, the head and neck are well supplied with blood through an extensive collateral network between the internal and external carotid arteries bilaterally. This blood supply may, however, be attenuated by vasculitis attendant on radiation therapy. Several studies have demonstrated a higher risk of wound complications and mortality when major surgery is performed after irradiation. Other factors that increase the risk of wound complications are malnutrition, immunodeficiency as demonstrated by anergy to skin testing, anemia, and diabetes mellitus.

Breakdown of the skin suture line is usually not a serious problem unless the patient has been irradiated and the wound exposes the carotid artery. Because of the obliteration of the small vasa vasorum coursing in the adventitia of the carotid secondary to surgery and irradiation, the exposed irradiated carotid artery is at high risk of infection and rupture with catastrophic hemorrhage. Selection of the McFee parallel skin incisions minimizes the chance of exposure of the carotid in the event of wound breakdown. The exposed irradiated carotid artery should be covered with well-vascularized tissue, such as the pectoralis major muscle, to prevent rupture.

Breakdown of the intraoral suture lines can result in exposure of the mandible. If the breakdown is extensive, an orocutaneous fistula will result. Again, if irradiation has not been given previously, débridement of necrotic tissue and conventional wound care will usually allow contraction and epithelialization to resolve the problem. Further operation is sometimes, but not usually, necessary. If, however, the tissue has been irradiated, the risk of osteomyelitis or osteoradionecrosis is great. Occasionally local procedures are adequate to cover exposed irradiated bone or to close fistulae in an unirradiated field, but more frequently provision of well-vascularized tissue from outside the head and neck will be required. The thoracic musculocutaneous flaps are ideal for this problem.

Functional complications of extirpative surgery in the head and neck are numerous. Derangements in speech and swallowing, oral incontinence, aspiration, and other disabilities are seen after interruption of sensory and motor nervous pathways and removal of mobile, specialized muscle cartilage and bone. Transection of the spinal accessory nerve in radical neck dissection results in weakness in elevation of the shoulder. Much improvement may be made with physical therapy, and time alone may result in adaptation. Refinements in reconstruction in the head and neck are directed toward minimizing functional disturbances after curative surgery. In procedures in which the risk of functional disturbance is high, tracheostomy and tube gastrostomy may be used as temporary or permanent methods of facilitating respiration and alimentation.

RECONSTRUCTION

Reconstruction of the defect resulting from extirpative surgery for cancer of the head and neck is an essential part of restoring the patient to a state of health. In the past, there was considerable sentiment for delayed reconstruction, reasoning that better detection of recurrent tumor would be possible if the site of the resected primary could be closely observed. The resultant distress of the patient left with a large pharyngostome or other enterocutaneous communication may have been justified by the lack of safe and effective methods of reconstruction available at that time. This reluctance gradually ceded to a working philosophy that the extirpative and reconstructive operations should be done by two different surgeons, presumably so that the margins of tumor resection would not be slighted in deference to considerations of ease of reconstruction. Again, as there has been improvement in abilities to perform more radical procedures and in maintenance of patients through difficult operations and recovery periods and advances in reconstruction itself, this philosophy has given way to one that identifies the surgeon as planner and performer of the most appropriate procedure for cure and the best available single- or multistage reconstruction as either a single- or multiteam effort.

Methods of Reconstruction

The methods of reconstruction are many. The goal is to restore the patient to the best function and appearance in as short a time as possible. Squamous cell carcinoma of the upper aerodigestive tract presents as late stage disease in many cases. The recurrence and ultimate failure rates are high, and 90 per cent of recurrences manifest within 2 years of initial therapy. For these reasons, *efficiency* of surgical reconstruction is important. Courses of reconstruction requiring five or six major operations over a 6-month period are less desirable than single-stage reconstructions or one major procedure and one or two minor refinements. Fortunately, in the past 10 years, the improvements in technology permitting microvascular tissue transfers and the elucidation of the anatomy of the numerous musculocutaneous units of the body have given the surgeon ample opportunity to resolve these difficult problems.

Reconstruction after surgery for cancer of the upper aerodigestive tract has a number of goals specific to the region of the head and neck. First is *restoration of continuity of the alimentary and respiratory tracts*, with the corollary function of preventing spillage of oronasal secretions to the outside. Second is *separation* of the highly colonized *bacterial flora* of the mucosal surfaces from the important structures exposed during surgery, such as the cranial cavity with its meningeal linings, the carotid artery, and the facial bones. *Restoration of the specialized functions* of speech and swallowing is a third important consideration. Finally, the *preservation or restoration of* as normal an *appearance* as possible is crucial in this area, which characterizes the human being more than any other anatomic area.

In choosing one of the methods of reconstruction for the head and neck there are two major, closely related considerations: *risk of infection* and *availability of blood supply*. The upper aerodigestive tract above the larynx has a high concentration of mixed aerobic and anaerobic flora. Loculation of these bacteria in a closed space, such as a surgical incision, provides the ideal environment for anaerobic proliferation, abscess, and wound breakdown. The luxuriant vascular supply of the head and neck counteracts this to a certain degree, particularly if supplemented by antibiotic therapy. In the irradiated field, however, the native blood supply is less generous, and methods of reconstruction that provide their own blood supply are more reliable. Because squamous cell carcinoma grows in a radial fashion and patients present at late stage, the defect may involve both the mucosal surface and external skin. The reconstruction, therefore, must address restoration of both internal lining, mucosa, and external coverage, skin.

PRIMARY CLOSURE

The simplest form of reconstruction in the upper aerodigestive tract is primary closure, the direct apposition of mucosal, muscular, and skin surfaces by suture. This is frequently appropriate in the lip, pharynx, and buccal mucosa, where there is redundant tissue and closure can be performed without tension. When primary closure requires approximation of a mobile structure, such as the tongue, to an immobile structure, such as the mandibular alveolar mucosa, it interferes with function and is inappropriate.

ADVANCEMENT FLAPS

Mobilization of local tissue in the form of advancement or rotation flaps is frequently adequate to close small defects in the oral cavity and oropharynx. Division of the tongue or a small portion of it allows rotation in several directions to cover defects of the tonsillar pillar, palate, lateral pharynx, or floor of the mouth (Fig. 13*F*). Similarly, buccal mucosa rotation flaps can be used to provide lining in reconstruction of the lip or buccal area. The size of these flaps is limited, but a major advantage is that they provide normal specialized tissue to replace the deficit.

FREE TISSUE TRANSPLANTATION

Transplantation of autogenous tissue to the defect is an important method of reconstruction in this area. Because the free tissue transplant must derive its blood supply from the area of reconstruction, the success of these grafts depends on the presence of a well-vascularized recipient bed. Their use is, therefore, limited in the irradiated patient. Split-thickness skin grafts provide an excellent choice for lining the buccal mucosa, pharyngeal mucosa, and lateral tongue. The keratinized epithelium functions well in the upper aerodigestive tract. Despite the heavy bacterial flora in the oral cavity, these grafts have a high success rate. Reconstruction of the mandible or other bony structures of the head and neck can be achieved with free grafts of bone from the rib, iliac crest, or calvarium. Osteocytes from the adjacent bone eventually repopulate the bony matrix of these grafts after ingrowth of blood vessels from the surrounding tissue. These grafts are less hardy than skin grafts and require complete separation from the mucosal cavities to prevent infection. The bed into which they are placed must have an adequate blood supply and must be relatively free of scar. Composite free grafts of skin and cartilage can be taken from the ear to replace three-dimensional loss of the nasal alae.

SKIN FLAPS

Since surgical removal of a massive tumor frequently leaves a large and complex defect, reconstruction may require more tissue than is available locally. Importation of tissue, usually skin, from distant sites, such as the arm and thorax, is an important recent method of head and neck reconstruction.

Construction of skin flaps is based on the principle that the circulation of a segment of skin lies in the subdermal plexus. Attachment of that skin to the site of reconstruction will ultimately provide connections between the vascular system of tissue surrounding the defect and that of the flap. After the flap has parasitized its new environment, it is separated from its original blood supply and the reconstruction is completed. The development of a *random pattern* skin flap depending solely on the native subdermal plexus requires numerous stages before transfer to the head and neck defect.

The relative deficiencies of blood supply in the recipient area jeopardize the success of transfer. McGregor, Bakamjian, and others discovered areas of the skin where a large axial blood vessel could be incorporated into the flap to increase the reliability of its blood supply and, therefore, its length. The forehead flap of McGregor and the deltopectoral flap of Bakamjian have become the major methods of reconstruction of the oral cavity and pharynx, replacing, for the most part, the tubed random pattern flaps and cervical skin rotation flaps previously used. Other arterialized flaps useful in the head and neck are the nasolabial fold, the supratrochlear flap, and the temporal island flap.

A disadvantage to all skin flaps is that the blood supply to the skin is relatively tenuous, particularly when compared with that of muscle, and is subject to more circulating humoral regulation. Furthermore, skin flaps almost always must ultimately derive their blood supply from the surrounding tissue, which is frequently irradiated, scarred, or chronically infected and may, therefore, have a limited blood supply.

MUSCULOCUTANEOUS FLAPS

In the past 10 years, another aspect of the blood supply to the skin has emerged. Much of the body's cutaneous covering is supplied not only by the subdermal plexus and a few large axial cutaneous arteries but by vessels perforating through the underlying muscles to the subdermal plexus.

In many areas these muscles are supplied by large axial blood vessels coursing on their undersurface. The muscle and its overlying skin can be defined as a single unit based on its dominant axial blood supply.

The musculolcutaneous flap has several advantageous characteristics. The blood flow to muscle is high and relatively constant, thereby providing insurance against infection and local tissue ischemia. A large mass of well-vascularized tissue can be transposed at a single operation, contributing both lining and coverage and decreasing the number of operations necessary to transfer tissue. Because of their bulk and vigorous blood supply, these flaps may be turned and rotated into several planes to satisfy three-dimensional defects. Finally, there are a large number of suitable areas in the body to provide musculocutaneous flaps with relatively little donor site morbidity.

For replacement of large defects in the head and neck, the pectoralis major musculocutaneous flap (Fig. 13B) is most commonly used, being both reliable and relatively easy to transfer with minimal morbidity. It is particularly useful in the oral cavity and pharynx. The trapezius musculocutaneous unit can be transferred to the midface or scalp area and may be used as an osteomusculocutaneous flap if a piece of the scapular spine is included. Based on the thoracodorsal vessels arising in the axilla, the latissimus dorsi musculocutaneous flap can provide a massive amount of tissue if necessary. Occasionally the sternocleidomastoid muscle and a segment of overlying skin are useful. In cases where a thin lining must be restored, the platysma muscle and an overlying paddle of skin can be transposed on the facial artery to provide a functional reconstruction. The ready availability of these thoracic and cervical musculocutaneous units has improved efficiency in head and neck surgery and has permitted a more aggressive surgical approach to definitive therapy for cure and to surgical palliation of recurrent disease.

FREE FLAPS

It has recently become possible to transfer segments of tissue supplied by an artery and vein of 1.0 mm. or greater in diameter to distant areas of the body by microvascular anastomosis to local arteries and veins. This has been of major consequence in the rehabilitation of patients with squamous cell carcinoma of the upper aerodigestive tract.

The free flap has several potential benefits in head and neck reconstruction:

1. It can transport either a large or small amount of tissue as needed for the appropriate reconstruction; this relative independence from local anatomy is of great advantage when recreating function.

2. Composite flaps of skin, muscle, and bone can be transferred to replace a similarly complex defect.

3. Bowel, which has similar properties to the mucosa of the upper aerodigestive tract, can be interposed.

4. The blood supply is independent of local tissue conditions.

Reconstitution of the alimentary canal from the base of the tongue to the cervical esophagus is nicely effected by the interposition of a segment of jejunum or colon with its mesenteric vessels anastomosed to a branch of the external carotid artery and the external jugular or transverse cervical vein. Replacement of a segment of mandible in an irradiated patient with a free bone graft carries a high risk of failure. The iliac crest area with overlying transversus abdominis muscle and skin is supplied by the deep circumflex iliac artery and vein. This bone can be fashioned to various shapes as necessary and after anastomosis of its blood supply in the neck serves as an excellent and reliable replacement as a single-stage procedure. In reconstruction of the lateral pharyngeal wall or floor of the mouth, where bulky tissue may interfere with the mobility of the larynx or the tongue, the appropriate thin tissue can be obtained by using a patch of bowel or the dorsal radial forearm flap of skin and connecting the blood supply of the flap to the neck (Fig. 13H). The numerous donor sites for tissue throughout the body make free tissue transfer an attractive method for reconstruction of head and neck cancer defects.

Restoration of Function

As the skill of the surgeon has increased and methods of reconstruction have become more numerous, closer attention to restoration of function has been emphasized. Refinements should allow not only the restoration of vegetative function but a simulation of the normal state.

In some patients, the size and location of the defect, underlying poor health, or simple volition may militate against surgical reconstructive effects. In these patients and others, *prosthetic rehabilitation* is useful. Defects of the hard palate are amenable to obliteration by dental prostheses. External defects in the midface, particularly of the nose and malar area, can be covered by plastic recreations attached to eyeglasses. Various prosthetic and mechanical devices have been used in the production of artificial speech to the great benefit of the disabled patient.

CARCINOMA OF THE ORAL CAVITY

The Lip

Carcinoma of the lip is the most common malignancy of the mucosa of the head and neck in North America. It is predominantly a disease of men, with a 20:1 male:female ratio. Although tobacco smoking is common among patients with cancer of the lip, the previously accepted causative relationship to pipe smoking is of less importance than is the exposure of the lower lip to solar ultraviolet radiation. Like skin cancer, lip cancer occurs frequently in fair-skinned individuals chronically exposed to the sun. Squamous cell carcinoma accounts for 95 per cent of all cancers of the lip, and they are usually on the lower lip. Basal cell carcinomas account for approximately 4 per cent and occur most frequently on the upper lip. The relationship of lip cancer to chronic trauma is possible but unclear. Most lip cancers are well differentiated, and in collected series 70 to 80 per cent of patients present with localized Stage I disease T1M0M0. Nodal metastases, usually to the submaxillary or submental nodes, are present initially in about 10 per cent of patients. Survival rate, as in all oral cancers, is stage dependent but is better in lip cancer stage for stage than in cancer anywhere else in the upper aerodigestive tract. Localized disease has an 87 per cent cure rate and locoregional disease a 60 to 73 per cent cure rate. Both radiation and surgery are effective in local disease. Wedge resection of small lesions may be amenable to primary closure. Larger defects (greater than one third the total width of the lip) require reconstruction with a cross lip flap or cheek flap. Since the entire mucosa is at risk, leukoplakia or chronic actinic changes should be removed by excision of the vermillion border and lip skin and advancement of the labial mucosa forward to the skin edge. Lip shave or vermillionectomy can be performed as a preventive procedure as well. Preservation or restoration of oral continence is the primary consideration in reconstruction of the lip.

The Gum (Mandibular Alveolus), Floor of the Mouth, Retromolar Trigone, and Oral (Mobile) Tongue

Cancers in these areas share common epidemiologic factors and account for a large percentage of upper aerodigestive tract tumors in the United States. Direct irritative effects, e.g., from jagged teeth and from chewing tobacco, may play a role in the development of leukoplakia, erythroplakia, and malignancy in these areas, but the most likely reason for the high incidence of these cancers is the pooling of saliva with high concentrations of tobacco and alcohol derivatives.

Prognosis and treatment are dependent on stage. Five-year survival ranges from 50 to 65 per cent for localized disease and 25 to 35 per cent for locoregional disease. In a collected series, well over half the patients present with Stage II or III disease, with at least half of the total series of patients having lymph node metastases, or Stage III disease. The proximity of these mucosal sites to the mandible results in a high likelihood of bony invasion. This poses specific therapeutic problems. The incidence of osteoradionecrosis and osteomyelitis after definitive radiation therapy rises with the size of the primary tumor. In a collection of patients presented in 1971, the risk ranged from 15 per cent in patients with T1 lesions to 50 per cent in patients with T3 tumors. More modern radiotherapy techniques should ameliorate these undesirable sequelae. When the periosteum of the mandible has not been invaded by tumor, surgical extirpation may require only adequate soft tissue resection. If, however, there is bony invasion, the segment of mandible involved must be removed in continuity with the primary lesion and the neck dissection if there are lymph nodes (see Fig. 12). This may require only segmental or sagittal mandibulectomy or complete hemimandibulectomy depending on the extent of invasion. Because of the high likelihood of cervical micrometastases in the clinically negative neck, malignancies in this area staged N2N0, T3N0, or T4N0 should be treated with resection and elective neck dissection.

Provision of a water-tight oral cavity is the prime consideration in reconstruction. Integrity of the mandible and mobility of the tongue are of obvious importance in the maintenance of good speech and alimentation. In this regard, considerable attention should be given to reconstruction. Providing independently vascularized bone for mandible reconstruction, as in osteomusculocutaneous microvascular transfer, may bypass problems with bone grafts in a scarred or irradiated area. The remaining tongue after partial glossectomy should be left as mobile as possible and should not be tethered to relatively fixed structures or bulky flaps.

Hard Palate

In the United States, the mucosa of the hard palate is the only area in the upper aerodigestive tract where squamous cell carcinoma is not the most common histologic type of malignancy. Neoplasms, both benign and malignant, of the minor salivary glands predominate in this area. In India and Sri Lanka, however, squamous cell carcinoma of the hard palate is common, probably because of the custom of smoking cheroots with the lighted end inside the mouth.

Squamous cell carcinoma of the hard palate occurs predominantly in elderly men. The relative fixation of the mucosa to the subjacent bone increases the risk of osteoradionecrosis and other healing problems after radiation therapy. Operative resection of the malignancy and the underlying bone, if invaded, is the treatment of choice. Maxillectomy is occasionally indicated. In the consequent oronasal or oroantral fistula, dental obturators are frequently useful for reconstruction. Separation of the oral and nasal cavities is an important consideration in speech and alimentation and can be effected with prosthesis or vascularized tissue.

Stage of tumor again is the most important prognosticator. Ratzer and associates[20] reported that lesions greater than 3.0 cm. in diameter showed only 16 per cent 5-year survival as opposed to 54 per cent in lesions less than 3.0 cm. Cervical metastasis reduced 5-year survival to 8 per cent. The disproportionately low survival may be due, in part, to the older age of patients with this neoplasm.

The Buccal Mucosa

In the United States, this form of oral cavity carcinoma is most frequently associated with the use of snuff by elderly women in the Southeastern states. In parts of India, buccal carcinoma is the most common presenting malignancy, again associated with a tobacco concoction. There is a higher than usual percentage of verrucous carcinomas arising in this area, and, therefore, the prognosis is somewhat better. Buccal cancers account for 30 to 50 per cent of total oral cavity verrucous carcinomas. Lymph node metastases are less common with buccal cancers than primaries arising in other oral cavity sites. Ulceroinfiltrative squamous cell carcinoma on the buccal mucosa may extend posteriorly into the masseteric region to cause trismus. Deep invasion into the buccal fat and cheek skin requires full-thickness resection of mucosa and skin. Multifocal lesions have been identified in 31 per cent of patients.

There is some speculation that irradiation of verrucous carcinoma may be dangerous or ineffective. For other cancers of the buccal mucosa, radiation is useful, as is operative intervention. Five-year survivals are in the vicinity of 65 per cent for local disease and 32 per cent for locoregional disease.

Reconstructive considerations are totally a function of the thickness of excision necessary in carcinoma of the buccal mucosa. Superficial defects can be covered with a split-thickness skin graft or platysma musculocutaneous flap. Full-thickness excision usually requires a musculocutaneous flap from the thorax or a cervical or deltopectoral axial skin flap to provide both coverage and lining.

CARCINOMA OF THE PHARYNX

Squamous cell carcinoma of the oropharynx presents almost invariably as late stage disease. The inaccessibility to physical examination, the luxuriant lymphatic supply with frequent bilateral representation, and the confluence of anatomic structures allow primary tumors to develop without symptoms. Otalgia representing referred pain and a firm mass in the neck are common first manifestations in this group of cancers. The usual risk factors of tobacco and alcohol predominate in this patient population.

Pharynx and Soft Palate

The mucosal surfaces of the soft palate and the lateral posterior pharyngeal walls are connected by the palato-pharyngeus muscle or faucial arch. Lesions arising in the soft palate have a lower likelihood of early neck metastasis. Advanced lesions spread circumferentially to involve the hard palate, lateral pharynx, and tonsil. Surgical resection of the soft palate results in oronasal incontinence, which greatly interferes with speech and allows regurgitation of food and liquid from the oral cavity to the nasal cavity. This can be circumvented by reconstructing the defect with a superiorly based pharyngeal flap. Approach to the soft palate and posterolateral pharynx can be made transorally or by median labioglossotomy. Radiation therapy is effective for small lesions, but combined surgery and radiation is necessary to achieve 5-year survival rates of approximately 50 per cent in advanced lesions.

Base of the Tongue

The posterior one third of base of the tongue is one of the most difficult areas of the upper aerodigestive tract to treat. In some series, up to 70 per cent of patients present with cervical metastastases and up to 40 per cent with bilateral nodes. There is controversy over whether the lesions in the base of the tongue are more anaplastic than tumors at other sites in the head and neck. The high percentage of poorly differentiated cancers may be inherent to the area or may be a function of late stage. Because the primary extent of tumor is frequently across the midline of the tongue, adequate resection often requires sacrifice of both lingual arteries and, therefore, total glossectomy. The intimate anatomic functional relationship of the base of the tongue with the larynx necessitates consideration of this structure in treatment planning. Resection of a major portion of the base of the tongue interferes with movement of the larynx and may result in aspiration. Occasionally, resection of the uninvolved larynx is necessary to avoid the inevitable aspiration pneumonitis in the already debilitated patient. Reconstruction of the base of the tongue with pendulous flaps may interfere with its motion and again cause aspiration as well as interference with speech.

The invasion of these tumors into the pre-epiglottic space, anterior two thirds of the tongue, tonsil, and pharynx makes determination of adequate treatment volume for external beam radiation therapy difficult. The use of interstitial radiation has been of some benefit in carcinoma of the base of the tongue, but, as with external beam radiotherapy, residual disease is the most common problem. The large doses required for tumor control and the central location of the base of the tongue increase the risk of radiation sequelae, such as osteoradionecrosis of the mandible and carotid artery rupture.

Combined operative and radiation therapy yields 5-year survival rates in the range of 45 to 60 per cent for localized disease and 10 to 40 per cent for locoregional disease.

The Tonsil

Carcinoma of the tonsil is the most common malignancy of the oropharynx. A disease of elderly men, it is again characterized by late-stage presentation. A histologic variant of squamous cell carcinoma, lymphoepithelioma, comprises 10 to 20 per cent of the tumors in this area. These poorly differentiated lesions are characterized by diffuse lymphocyte infiltration. The abundance of lymphocytes is a function of the location in Waldeyer's ring, and the mesodermal elements, the lymphocytes, are not a part of the malignant process. Lymphoepitheliomas are exquisitely radiosensitive, but, like all squamous cell carcinomas of the upper aerodigestive tract, survival is based primarily on the stage of the disease. Most tonsillar cancers are moderately or poorly differentiated squamous cell carcinomas.

Pathways of spread of primary cancer of the tonsils are inferior to the base of the tongue, superior to the soft palate, posterior to the pharynx, and anterior to the retromolar trigone and mandible. Extension beyond the tonsil is apparent in 50 per cent of primary tumors. Metastasis to the neck is present in 50 per cent of patients at the time of presentation.

Localized T1 and T2 lesions are well treated with radiation therapy alone. More advanced local cases or patients with cervical metastases will require operative resection and postoperative irradiation. Five-year survival rates for localized disease range from 50 to 90 per cent and for locoregional disease from 10 to 60 per cent.

CARCINOMA OF THE HYPOPHARYNX

The area known as the hypopharynx lies behind and lateral to the larynx and consists of the pyriform sinuses, the posterior pharyngeal wall, and the postcricoid cervical esophagus. Like the oropharynx, it is relatively inaccessible to the usual physical examination, and symptoms of neoplasm may be undramatic, consisting mainly of mild sore throat, referred pain to the ear, or, with more advanced disease, dysphagia and hoarseness. Carcinoma of the hypopharynx in women may be associated with Plummer-Vinson syndrome, a premalignant condition consisting of iron-deficiency anemia, gastric achlorhydria, and atrophy of the mucosa of the tongue.

The lymphatic network in this area is conducive to early lymph node metastasis. Many patients present with cervical metastases. In those patients with clinically negative necks, 69 per cent had micrometastases when evaluated by elective neck dissection. Forty per cent of T1 lesions had cervical metastases. Pyriform sinus primaries are the most common of the hypopharyngeal tumors, comprising about 61 per cent of lesions according to Batsakis. Postcricoid esophagus cancers make up 24 per cent and posterior pharynx 15 per cent of hypopharyngeal tumors. Radiation alone is ineffective in these cancers. In the occasional early lesion, surgical approach to the tumor can be made through the neck with a transhyoid or transthyroid pharyngotomy. Large pyriform sinus lesions may invade through the medial wall of the sinus into the larynx, producing cord fixation.

Appropriate therapy requires laryngopharyngectomy. Because of the large amount of mucosa resected, reconstruction with distant tissue is often necessary. Microvascular anastomosis of a jejunal segment or the radial forearm skin free flap, transposition of the deltopectoral skin flap, and rotation of the pectoralis major musculocutaneous flap are all effective methods of restoration of the alimentary canal. Combined surgery and irradiation results in 5-year survivals in the range of 40 to 50 per cent for local disease and 5 to 20 per cent for locoregional disease.

CARCINOMA OF THE LARYNX

The embryologic origin of the various parts of the larynx determines the epidemiology, natural history, prognosis, and treatment choice of squamous carcinomas arising in this area. The supraglottic larynx from the epiglottis to the ventricle of the larynx arises from the pharyngobuccal anlage, and the glottic larynx arises from the tracheobronchial anlage.[21] Although malignancies in both areas are almost exclusively squamous cell carcinomas, they behave quite differently.

Carcinoma of the *supraglottic larynx* has risk factors similar to those of carcinoma of the oral cavity and oropharynx, occurring in patients who are heavy users of alcohol and tobacco. The early cancers arise at the junction of the epiglottis and false cords and may invade downward to become *transglottic cancers* (involving two segments of larynx) or outward through the thyrohyoid membrane to the pre-epiglottic space. Local disease is frequently extensive at presentation, and there is a high likelihood of ipsilateral and bilateral cervical lymph node metastasis at relatively early primary size. Consequently, the prognosis in supraglottic larynx cancer is poor irrespective of therapy.

Glottic cancers arise primarily in the anterior portion of the vocal cords. They are associated, like lung cancer, with tobacco smoking and somewhat less intimately with alcohol use. Early primary stage presentation, well-differentiated histology, and a low incidence of cervical lymph node metastases are characteristic of glottic laryngeal lesions. The local disease tends to spread across the anterior commissure of the larynx to the other cord. Extension into the surrounding tissues is late. Vocal cord fixation results from infiltration of the thyroarytenoid muscle. Invasion through the cricothyroid membrane usually precedes lymph node metastasis. Prognosis is more favorable in these cancers.

Subglottic lesions arising below the cords account for 4 to 6 per cent of laryngeal neoplasms. They are usually not discovered until fairly late in their course and metastasize to paratracheal lymph nodes.

The importance of speech influences the *treatment* of squamous cell carcinoma of the larynx. Radiation therapy usually results in voice quality superior to that following conservation surgery or esophageal speech after total laryngectomy. T1N0 lesions of the supraglottic larynx and T1N0 and T2N0 lesions of the glottic larynx are usually treated by radiation therapy. Because of the anatomic distinction between the supraglottic and glottic larynx, the supraglottic larynx alone can be removed in some lesions, preserving speech. Similarly, in glottic tumors confined to one cord, vertical hemilaryngectomy, leaving one vocal cord intact, can result in a satisfactory quality of speech and higher rates of cure. T3 and T4 tumors and those with lymph node metastases are usually treated by total laryngectomy with irradiation as adjuvant, but in some centers irradiation is used primarily, with surgery reserved to salvage recurrences. Five-year survival rates from collected series utilizing various therapies reflect the difference in the natural history of these laryngeal lesions: supraglottic, local 75 to 82 per cent, locoregional 9 to 49 per cent; glottic, local 58 to 95 per cent, locoregional 9 to 59 per cent; subglottic 40 per cent.

CARCINOMA OF THE NASOPHARYNX

Although carcinoma of the nasopharynx is rare in the United States, comprising only 0.3 per cent of new malignancies, it is a very common malignancy in South China and Malaysia, accounting for 14 per cent of cancers in Indonesia, 18 per cent in Hong Kong, and 21 per cent in Taiwan. The predilection of this tumor for Southeast Asians holds true among groups migrating to other areas. Chinese in California, even after several generations, have a much higher risk of development of nasopharyngeal cancer than the remainder of the population.

The etiology of the disease is unknown. Inhalation of smoke or perhaps some carcinogenic plant substance has been implicated. The usual association with tobacco and alcohol is not as dramatic as in other upper aerodigestive tract tumors. Epstein-Barr herpes virus may play a role in the initiation of the disease. The virus is found in patients with cancer of the nasopharynx, and antibody titers to the virus rise in proportion to tumor load. Whether the virus is causative or merely a tumor marker is as yet uncertain. There is speculation that Orientals may have genetic susceptibility to the oncogenic potential of this virus.

The nasopharynx lies at the base of the skull behind the nasal cavity and superior to the oropharynx. This area can be examined with the mirror and light source, but symptoms are unlikely to present until the disease has progressed considerably. Cancer of the nasopharynx invades the bone of the base of the skull and the cavernous sinus. Invasion in this area causes involvement of cranial nerves III, IV, and VI, resulting in various oculomotor signs. Invasion anteriorly into the nasal cavity may cause nasal stuffiness. The most common presentation, however, is a node in the neck with no obvious primary site. Greater than 50 per cent of patients with nasopharyngeal tumors present with either jugulodigastric or posterior triangle nodes, making careful examination of the nasopharynx an obviously important part of the evaluation of any suspicious neck nodes.

Squamous cell carcinoma of the nasopharynx tends to be nonkeratinizing or poorly differentiated. Like the tonsil, the nasopharynx is part of Waldmeyer's ring of lymphatic tissue. There is, therefore, a high incidence of lymphoepithelioma (up to 20 per cent). Distant metastases are more common from nasopharyngeal primaries than from any other upper aerodigestive tract primary site.

Primary site disease is usually treated with radiotherapy. Cervical metastases from the nasopharynx are more radiosensitive than other head and neck metastases and may be controlled with radiation. If the neck disease does not resolve with radiation, radical neck dissection can be employed. Surgery is occasionally helpful in dealing with primary site disease. Survival is again stage dependent, with 5-year rates ranging from 40 to 55 per cent for local disease and 12 to 25 per cent for locoregional disease.

NEOPLASMS OF THE SALIVARY GLANDS

Although the natural history of salivary gland tumors is considerably different from that of squamous cell carcinoma of the mucosa of the upper aerodigestive tract, these tumors comprise an important segment of head and neck cancers.

The major salivary glands are the parotid gland, the submaxillary gland, and the sublingual gland. Numerous minor salivary glands arise in the mucosal surfaces of the upper aerodigestive tract, with high concentrations in the hard palate, maxillary sinus, and base of the tongue.

Benign Lesions

Most salivary gland neoplasms are benign, and by far the most common site for neoplasia is the *parotid gland*. The "rule of 80s" concerning the parotid gland states that 80 per cent of parotid neoplasms are benign, of which 80 per cent are pleomorphic adenomas (benign mixed tumors) and 80 per cent are located in the superficial (lateral) lobe. The ratio of benign to malignant lesions is somewhat lower in the submaxillary and sublingual glands, approaching 50:50. Other benign neoplasms of the salivary glands include Warthin's tumor (papillary adenocystoma lymphomatosum), oncocytoma, and monomorphic adenoma.

Malignant Lesions

The most common malignant tumor of the parotid gland is the *mucoepidermoid carcinoma*, which histologically resembles the less frequently seen squamous cell carcinoma of the parotid gland. This tumor occurs in a low grade form that usually remains localized. High-grade mucoepidermoid cancers metastasize to cervical lymph nodes and, hematogenously, to the lungs. Adenoid cystic carcinoma, or cylindroma, is an insidious form of salivary gland cancer with a propensity for invasion along nerves. It is characterized by high rates of local recurrence and extension along the facial and trigeminal nerves to the base of the skull. Hematogenous metastases to the lung are prominent and can be present for years without symptoms. Other salivary gland cancers include adenocarcinoma, acinic cell carcinoma, and malignant mixed tumor.

The position of the facial nerve between the superficial and deep lobes of the parotid gland makes it an important consideration in both the presentation and therapy of the parotid gland. Facial nerve weakness is never seen in association with benign tumors of the parotid gland, even if they grow to massive size. Weakness of the facial nerve in association with a mass in the parotid is a sign of malignancy and occurs in 8 to 33 per cent of parotid cancers, according to Batsakis. Another important consideration in the diagnosis of malignancy is the presence of pain.

Treatment

The treatment of salivary gland tumors is by surgical resection of the gland. Benign parotid gland tumors may be treated by superficial lobectomy or total parotidectomy with preservation of the facial nerve, depending on whether they are present in the superficial or deep lobe of the gland. Enucleation of the lesion should not be considered. Malignant tumors that do not involve facial nerve necessitate total parotidectomy with preservation of the facial nerve. If the main trunk or any peripheral branches are involved by tumor, they should be included in the resection. Reconstruction of the nerve can be performed by an interposition nerve graft. Adjuvant radiotherapy is frequently useful in malignant tumors of the salivary glands.

Like the remainder of the head and neck, the parotid and submaxillary glands send their efferent lymphatic drainage to the neck. The histologic types of malignancy occurring in the salivary glands are, however, less likely to metastasize early. Any patient presenting with cervical lymphadenopathy must be considered for neck dissection as well as resection of the primary tumor.

Adequate resection of benign salivary gland lesions provides a 97 to 98 per cent control rate. Low-grade mucoepidermoid cancers of the salivary glands and acinic cell carcinomas are very curable. Squamous cell carcinoma, malignant mixed tumors, and high-grade mucoepidermoid cancers are less curable, with 5-year survivals in the range of 50 per cent. Adenoid cystic cancer is more indolent, but the overall 10-year survival is low (10 to 25 per cent).

CARCINOMA OF THE NASAL CAVITY AND PARANASAL SINUSES

Carcinoma of the nasal cavity and paranasal sinuses is rare in the United States and accounts for approximately 0.3 per cent of all malignancies. The majority of these tumors are squamous cell carcinomas, although minor mucous and salivary gland adenocarcinomas constitute about 20 per cent of the total. Epidemiologic data demonstrate an increased risk for adenocarcinoma of the maxillary sinus among furniture workers, possibly from the chronic inhalation of wood dust. Cancer of the nasal cavity is endemic among the Bantus of South Africa, probably because of their lifelong habit of sniffing tobacco.

Squamous cell carcinoma of the maxillary sinus is by far the most common of the neoplasms of the paranasal sinuses, accounting for about two thirds of the cases. Nasal cavity primaries and ethmoid sinus primaries together make up the remainder, with frontal sinus and sphenoid sinus malignancies a rarity. Although these tumors metastasize to cervical lymph nodes in only 15 per cent of cases, they are locally advanced at the time of presentation. Early symptoms, if any, are nondescript, usually nasal stuffiness or unilateral nasal discharge. Extension downward may cause pain, loosening of the teeth, and, ultimately, oroantral fistula. Superior invasion into the orbit may cause proptosis, diplopia, or anesthesia over the distribution of the infraorbital nerve. Extension anteriorly into the skin may cause pain and bulging in the midface area. Massive tumors may invade the middle cranial fossa, causing meningitis or central nervous system symptoms, or extend into the infratemporal fossa, precipitating trismus.

Irradiation alone provides poor survival and palliation; combined therapy is somewhat more successful. A major improvement in 5-year survival (from 5 to 10 to 35 to 50 per cent) resulted from Ketcham's introduction of the combined intracranial-extracranial approach to these tumors. With this technique, the neurosurgeon approaches the cribriform plate through the anterior cranial fossa while the oncologist approaches through the midface. Precise osteotomies allow *en bloc* resection of the tumor and decrease the risk of inadvertent entry of the dura. Total resection of early disease by maxillectomy is successful. In tumors in this area, the operative defect frequently includes the fistula between the oral cavity and the nasal cavity or maxillary antrum. Prosthetic obturation of this defect with dentures may restore function with relative ease. More extensive defects can be reconstructed with microvascular free tissue transfer.

SELECTED REFERENCES

Batsakis, J. G.: Tumors of the Head and Neck: Clinical and Pathological Considerations, 2nd ed. Baltimore, Williams & Wilkins, 1979.
This hallmark text covers all aspects of head and neck disease, with an emphasis on natural history, epidemiology, and histology. Careful and detailed attention is given by the author to both benign and malignant neoplasms not only of the mucosal surfaces but of all structures in the head and neck. The chapters on salivary gland neoplasia and premalignant mucosal lesions are excellent. For the student or physician with a detailed interest in cancer of the head and neck, this book is essential.

Netter, F. H.: The CIBA Collection of Medical Illustrations. Vol. 3. Digesive System, Part I: Upper Digestive Tract. New York, R. R. Donelly and Sons Company, 1959.
The functional anatomy of the head and neck is superbly depicted in this portion of Netter's collection. Anatomic detail is shown in sagittal, coronal, transverse, and cut-out views that emphasize the interrelationship of the various structures in the upper aerodigestive tract. The artistic portrayal of the physiology of swallowing and the paintings of the disorders of the upper aerodigestive tract are particularly useful to the student in clarifying these complex problems.

Platz, H., Fries, R., Hudec, M., Tjou, A. M., and Wagner, R. R.: The prognostic relevance of various factors at the time of the first admission of the patient. Retrospective DOSAK Study on carcinoma of the oral cavity. J. Maxillofac. Surg., *11*:3, 1983.
Although this is a retrospective study examining the natural history of squamous cancer, it is the best discussion of the real risk factors in this group of cancers. With its tabular supplement it shows how sophisticated multivariate and univariate analyses of risk factors may differ and assigns relative importance to tumor size, degree of infiltration, degree of histologic differentiation, site of primary tumor, fixation of regional lymph nodes, age, and the presence of distant metastases. These findings suggest the data base necessary for prospective studies and for a general approach to the patient.

Silverman, S., Jr.: Oral Cancer. New York, American Cancer Society, 1981.
This professional education publication of the American Cancer Society is a 124-page monograph on cancer of the oral cavity. The subject matter is heavily weighted toward nonsurgical therapy. There are a large number of excellent clinical and histologic photographs that nicely represent the natural history of neoplasia from the premalignant to the advanced stages. The discussion of prosthetic rehabilitation is informative. The monograph is available at no cost from the American Cancer Society.

REFERENCES

1. Archambeau, J. O., and Shymko, R. M.: The role of radiation in the treatment of cancer: Radiobiologic and cell kinetic concepts. Curr. Prob. Cancer, VII(13):1, 1984.
2. Balch, C. M., Dougherty, M. S., and Tilden, A. B.: Excessive prostaglandin E_2 production by suppressor monocytes in head and neck cancer patients. Ann. Surg., *196*(6):645, 1982.
3. Barkley, H. T., Fletcher, G. T., Jesse, R. H., and Lindberg, R. D.: Management of cervical lymph node metastases in squamous cell carcinoma of the tonsillar fossa, base of tongue, supraglottic larynx and hypopharynx. Am. J. Surg., *124*:462, 1972.
4. Batsakis, J. G.: Tumors of the Head and Neck, Clinical and Pathological Considerations, 2nd ed. Baltimore, Williams & Wilkins, 1979.
5. Batsakis, J. G.: The pathology of head and neck tumors: The occult primary and metastases to the head and neck. Part 10. Head Neck Surg., *3*:409, 1981.
6. Broders, A. C.: Carcinoma. Arch. Pathol., *2*:376, 1926.
7. Cancer Statistics, 1984. Ca-A Cancer J. Clin., *34*(1):1984, Published by American Cancer Society.
8. Check, I. J., et al.: Prediction of survival in head and neck cancer based on leukocyte sedimentation in Ficoll-Hypaque gradients. Laryngoscope, *90*:1281, 1980.
9. Farber, E.: Chemical carcinogenesis. N. Engl. J. Med., *305*:1379, 1981.
10. Hong, W. K., and Bromer, R.: Chemotherapy in head and neck cancer. N. Engl. J. Med., *308*:75, 1983.
11. Jesse, R. H., Barkley, H. W., Jr., Lindberg, R. D., and Fletcher, G. H.: Cancer of the oral cavity. Is elective neck dissection beneficial? Am. J. Surg., *120*:505, 1970.
12. Johnson, J. T., Barnes, L., Myers, E. N., Schramm, V. L., Jr., Borochovitz, D., and Sigler, B. A.: The extracapsular spread of tumors in cervical node metastasis. Arch. Otolaryngol., *107*:725, 1981.
13. Keane, W. M., Atkins, J. P., Jr., Wetmore, R., and Vitas, M.: Epidemiology of head and neck cancer. Laryngoscope, *91*:2037, 1981.
14. Looser, K. G., Shah, J. P., and Strong, E. W.: The significance of "positive" margins in surgically resected epidermoid carcinomas. Head Neck Surg., *1*:107, 1978.
15. Mashberg, A., and Garfinkel, L.: Early diagnosis of oral cancer: The erythroplastic lesion at high risk sites. American Cancer Society, 1978.
16. McGuirt, W. F.: Panendoscopy as a screening examination for simultaneous primary tumors in head and neck cancer: A prospective sequential study and review of the literature. Laryngoscope, *92*:569, 1982.
17. Million, R. R., and Cassini, N. M.: Management of Head and Neck Cancer: A Multidisciplinary Approach. Philadelphia, J. B. Lippincott Company, 1984.
18. Platz, H., Fries, R., Hudec, M., Tjoa, A. M., and Wagner, R. R.: The prognostic relevance of various factors at the time of the first admission of the patient. Retrospective DOSAK study on carcinoma of the oral cavity. J. Maxillofac. Surg., *11*:3, 1983.
19. Probert, J. C., Thompson, R. W., and Bagshaw, M. A.: Patterns of spread of distant metastases in head and neck cancer. Cancer, *33*:127, 1974.
20. Ratzer, E. R., Schweitzer, R. J., and Frazell, E. L.: Epidermoid carcinoma of the palate. Am. J. Surg., *119*:294, 1970.
21. Silver, C. E.: Surgical management of neoplasms of the larynx, hypopharynx and cervical esophagus. Curr. Probl. Surg., *14*:2, 1977.
22. Strong, E. W.: Sites of treatment failure in head and neck cancer. Cancer Treat. Symp., *2*:5, 1983.
23. Wynder, E. L., Mushinski, M. H., and Spivak, J. C.: Tobacco and alcohol consumption in relation to the development of multiple primary cancers. Cancer, *40*:1872, 1977.
24. Yamamoto, E., Miyakawa, A., and Kohama, G.-I.: Mode of invasion and lymph node metastasis in squamous cell carcinoma of the oral cavity. Head Neck Surg., *6*:938, 1984.

THE MUSCULOSKELETAL SYSTEM

JAMES R. URBANIAK, M.D.

36

Dramatic and explosive achievements in the diagnosis and management of injuries and diseases of the musculoskeletal system have occurred in the past decade. The innovations in noninvasive and invasive diagnostic studies including computed tomography (CT) and magnetic resonance imaging (MRI) have allowed earlier and exact diagnosis. Technologically, advancements in the instrumentation, internal and external fixation devices, and joint replacement have provided methods of restoring useful function and relieving pain in severely traumatized and diseased bone and joints of the limbs and spine. Refinements in operative arthroscopy have provided superior methods of reconstructing injured joints with minimal surgical trauma. The attainment of proficiency in microsurgery has made it possible to successfully reattach completely amputated limbs and transfer vascularized tissues from one part of the body to another in order to reconstruct lost or injured portions of the musculoskeletal system.

Because of rapidly advancing knowledge and technological developments in the treatment of the musculoskeletal system, the surgical speciality of orthopedic surgery has become fragmented with subspecializations in several areas such as joint reconstruction, sports medicine, oncology, pediatric surgery, hand surgery, spine surgery, foot surgery, and others. It has become mandatory for practicing surgeons to actively participate in continuing education in order to stay abreast of these rapid advancements in the subspecialty areas. Since current knowledge about the numerous diseases and injuries in the musculoskeletal system is massive, the introduction to this chapter attempts to provide a basic core of information in this field. Basic concepts, anatomy, pathogenesis, diagnosis, surgical treatment, and rehabilitation of the more common injuries and diseases of the musculoskeletal system will be presented. Only the pertinent and readily accessible references are listed at the end of each section for more detailed information on these specific subjects.

The majority of diagnoses of problems with the musculoskeletal system can be made by obtaining a complete and pertinent history and performing a thorough physical examination of the extremities and spine. In all diseases of the musculoskeletal system, the physician must obtain a detailed history about the patient's injury or disease. This should include information regarding age, occupation, previous injury, or related diseases. If trauma has been involved, the history should include details about the date and time of injury, time elapsed from injury to initial treatment, place of injury, mechanism of injury, and conditions at the time of injury (e.g., whether the wounds are clean or dirty)—information that is helpful in determining the amount of contamination or blood loss. If no trauma has been involved, information about pain, swelling, sensory changes, weakness, functional impairment, diurnal variations of symptoms with relation to work, recreation, and other forms of activity are important. A complete review of past history is essential.

The physician who deals with the musculoskeletal system must be able to perform a thorough physical examination of the extremities and spine, including gait analysis, muscle testing, and neurologic and vascular status of the extremities. Pertinent history and physical findings will be discussed under each section that follows.

I

The Hand and Wrist

JAMES R. URBANIAK, M.D.

The human hand is an exquisitely designed organ that basically performs the functions of grasp, pinch, and prehension. Because of its sensitivity and intricate and precise connections with the cerebral cortex, the hand is capable of performing a wide range of tasks, such as manipulating rough and heavy tools, performing a concert on a piano, stroking an infant to sleep, or conveying an emotional message. Although more hours of productivity are lost from injuries of this structure compared with any other area of the body, the hand has a remarkable capacity to heal its own injuries. No prosthetic device, no matter how cleverly designed, can adequately substitute for the lost hand or portions of it.

The study of hand function and disabilities is enjoyable and stimulating because of the ingeniously designed anatomy of the smooth gliding tendons, critically positioned pulley system, and small intrinsic muscles and ligaments that move the multiple small joints. The patterns of digital excursion, sensitivity response, and coordinated hand activity are all related to the peripheral nerves and vessels, which generally follow a reproducible pattern. The diagnosis of hand injuries and diseases can often be established by astute observation and understanding the surface and functional anatomy of this structure. Treatment—both operative and nonoperative—of the hand must be exact and at times is difficult, but a thorough understanding of the functional anatomy and healing potential is essential for achieving optimal recovery. The recent advancements in hand surgery have been dramatic with the development of artifical silicone tendons, joint replacements, vascularized tissue transfers (e.g., toe to thumb), and replantation of amputated parts.

PERTINENT ANATOMY

To provide pleasurable reading and to prevent needless repetition, most of the anatomy will be described and correlated with the specific diseases or injuries of the hand. The physician who is equipped with a thorough knowledge of the anatomy of the hand, especially the functional anatomy, and who obtains an appropriate history can diagnose most hand problems. The terminology of the surface and skeletal anatomy is universal and should be mastered by all students of medicine (Fig. 1). The digits and hand have *dorsal* and *volar* (*palmar*) surfaces and *radial* and *ulnar* borders. The digits are the thumb, index, middle (long), ring, and little fingers. Each finger has three joints: the metacarpophalangeal (MCP), proximal interphalangeal (PIP), and distal interphalangeal (DIP) joints. It is important to appreciate that the distal palmar crease is at the level of the MCP joints and the palmar digital creases and finger webs are over the middle section of the proximal phalanges. The palm comprises three areas: thenar, hypothenar, and midpalm. The thenar area covers the thumb

metacarpal and the intrinsic muscles of the thumb; the hypothenar area covers the little finger metacarpal and the intrinsic muscles of this digit.

HAND EVALUATION

History and General Information

Before the hand is examined, a careful history of the presenting problem must be obtained. The history should include the suggestions described in the introduction of the muscloskeletal section. When the patient with a hand problem is first seen, the physician should be certain that there are no serious life-threatening problems for which immediate attention is required. The patient should be made comfortable and the entire upper extremity exposed.

A few basic tools are necessary for adequate assessment of the hand. These include a goniometer, a pinch dynamometer, a grip dynamometer, a two-point caliper (a bent paper clip will suffice), and a tape measure. It is helpful to draw a diagram of the hand (a photograph is even more useful). The unaffected side should be compared. The skin should be examined for appearance, color, pseudomotor function, temperature, swelling, atrophy, and continuity.

The *posture* of the hand at rest and in active function should be observed.

The *range of motion* of the involved digits or hand is recorded. The standard terminology for motion of the hand and digits is illustrated in Figure 2. The individual joint motion is measured for the involved digits, as shown in Figure 3.

Nerves

INNERVATION

The hand is innervated by three major nerves: the median, the ulnar, and the radial. All three nerves are involved in the motor and sensory function of the thumb, fingers, and wrist.

Median Nerve. The median nerve innervates the muscles for precision grip, and the sensory branches provide the most useful sensitivity for hand function. The median nerve enters the forearm between the two bellies of the pronator teres muscle and innervates the muscles illustrated in Figure 4*A*. It enters the hand through the carpal tunnel with the thumb and finger flexor tendons.

The *sensory branches* supply the volar surfaces of the thumb, index, middle, and radial half of the ring finger (Fig. 5*A*).

Ulnar Nerve. The ulnar nerve innervates the muscles necessary for a power grip and a strong pinch. Its sensory

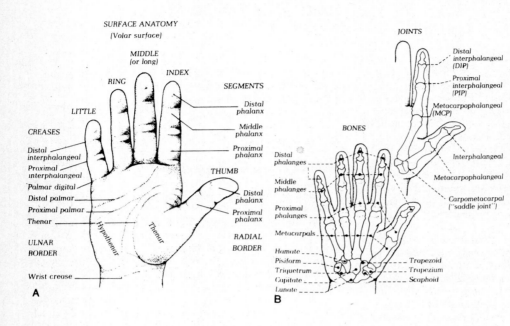

Figure 1. A, *Surface anatomy of the hand.* B, *Skeleton of the hand and wrist. (Reproduced with permission from the American Society for Surgery of the Hand: The Hand: Examination and Diagnosis. New York, Churchill Livingstone, 1983, pp. 4, 5.)*

Figure 2. A, B, *Terminology of hand and digit motion (Reproduced with permission from the American Society for Surgery of The Hand: The Hand: Examination and Diagnosis. New York, Churchill Livingstone, 1983, pp. 8, 9.)*

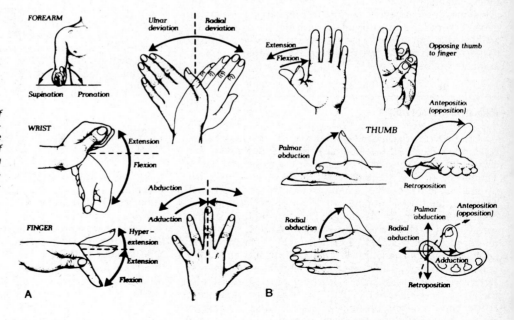

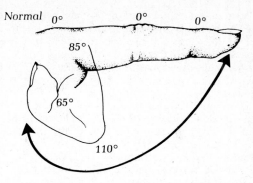

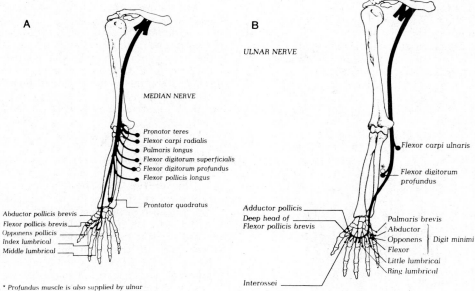

A

MEDIAN NERVE

Pronator teres
Flexor carpi radialis
Palmaris longus
Flexor digitorum superficialis
* Flexor digitorum profundus
Flexor pollicis longus

Prontator quadratus

Abductor pollicis brevis
Flexor pollicis brevis
Opponens pollicis
Index lumbrical
Middle lumbrical

* Profundus muscle is also supplied by ulnar
nerve (see text)

B

ULNAR NERVE

Flexor carpi ulnaris

* Flexor digitorum
profundus

Adductor pollicis
Deep head of
Flexor pollicis brevis

Palmaris brevis
Abductor
Opponens } Digit minimi
Flexor
Little lumbrical
Ring lumbrical

Interossei

* Profundus muscle is also supplied by
median nerve (see text)

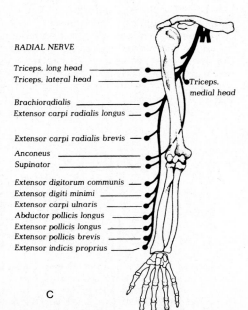

RADIAL NERVE

Triceps, long head
Triceps, lateral head
                                        Triceps,
                                        medial head
Brachioradialis
Extensor carpi radialis longus

Extensor carpi radialis brevis

Anconeus
Supinator

Extensor digitorum communis
Extensor digiti minimi
Extensor carpi ulnaris
Abductor pollicis longus
Extensor pollicis longus
Extensor pollicis brevis
Extensor indicis proprius

C

Figure 4. Muscles innervated by nerves in the forearm and hand. A, Median nerve. B, Ulnar nerve. C, Radial nerve. (Reproduced with permission from The American Society for Surgery of the Hand: The Hand: Examination and Diagnosis. New York, Churchill Livingstone, 1983, pp. 33, 34, 37.)

contribution to the hand is less important than that afforded by the median nerve. It enters the forearm in the cubital tunnel (posterior to the medial epicondyle of the elbow) and passes through the flexor carpi ulnaris muscle. The *motor* branches innervate the muscles illustrated in Figure 4*B*. The ulnar nerve enters the hand through Guyon's canal at the wrist.

The *sensory* branches innervate the skin over the palmar and dorsal surface of the ulnar half of the hand and the palmar surface of the ulnar side of the ring finger and entire little finger (Fig. 5).

Radial Nerve. The radial nerve is primarily a motor nerve that is responsible for wrist, finger, and thumb extension. It does *not* innervate any of the intrinsic muscles of the hand. The *motor* contributions of radial nerve to the upper extremity are illustrated in Figure 4*C*. The *sensory* branches of the radial nerve innervate only the dorsum of the radial half of the hand (Fig. 5).

NERVE TESTING

If a nerve or muscle injury is suspected, the individual muscles must be examined and rated by having the patient actively move the extremity to the positions illustrated in Figure 2. The examiner must know the muscles used to

achieve the posture and then attempt to overcome (or "break") the assumed hand or digit position.

The standard muscle grading system is as follows: 0, no muscle contraction; 1, trace of flicker of contraction; 2, active motion, gravity eliminated; 3, active motion against gravity; 4, active motion against some resistance; and 5, normal muscle power.

Grip and pinch strength should be tested with appropriate dynamometers and recorded. Deep tendon reflexes are tested if a proximal lesion is suspected.

The sensory examination should *not* begin with a sharp pin, for this frequently frightens the patient, especially a child. The appreciation of soft touch is important.

A paper clip that has been opened and bent serves as a good caliper for testing two-point discrimination on the digits. The two points are spread apart and applied to the radial and ulnar sides of the digit in a longitudinal position. The points of the clip (or caliper) are gradually approximated until the patient perceives them as one point. Normal two-point discrimination for the finger pulp is 6 mm. or less.

Examination of the skin for *sweating* is useful, since sympathetic disruption results in sweat loss. Percussion of the nerve pathway may produce sensitivity (or dysesthesias) over the area of abnormal or regenerating axons (*Tinel's sign*). Since this provides some indication of growing or disturbed axons, a reducing Tinel's sign at the injury site and an increasing Tinel's sign distally are good prognostic indicators.

Tendons and Joints

Flexor Tendons. The function of the *flexor digitorum profundus* (FDP) must be distinguished from that of the flexor digitorum superficialis (FDS). Since the FDP inserts on the base of the distal phalanx, the examiner tests the tendon by stabilizing the PIP joint in extension and asking the patient to "bend your fingertip" (Fig. 6*A*). The examiner tests the FDS by stabilizing in extension all of the joints on the uninvolved digit and asking the patient to "bend your middle joint of the finger" (Fig. 6*B*). Since the thumb has only one extrinsic flexor, the flexor pollicis longus (FPL), the examiner tests this tendon by asking the patient to flex the tip of the thumb.

Extensor Tendons. The extensor tendons are evaluated by asking the patient to extend the MCP joints with the PIP joints held in flexion. This test is valid because the extensor tendons actually extend only the MCP joints and the intrinsic muscles (lumbricals and interossei) extend the PIP and DIP joints.

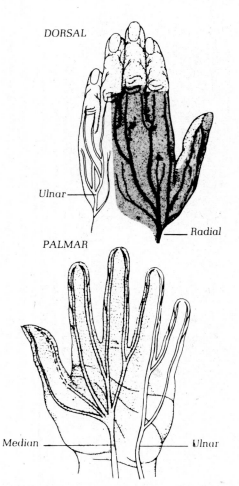

DORSAL

Ulnar

Radial

PALMAR

Median   Ulnar

Figure 5. Distribution of major nerves innervating the hand for sensory function. (Reproduced with permission from the American Society for Surgery of the Hand. The Hand: Examination and Diagnosis. New York, Churchill Livingstone, 1983, p. 38.)

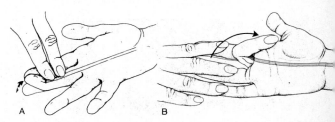

A   B

Figure 6. Testing for musculotendinous function. A, Flexor digitorum profundus. B, Flexor digitorum superficialis. (Reproduced with permission from the American Society for Surgery of the Hand: The Hand: Examination and Diagnosis. New York, Churchill Livingstone, 1983, pp. 14, 15.)

Joints. The joints should be tested for capsular and ligamentous stability or laxity.

Circulation

The radial and ulnar arteries are the major vessels that supply blood to the hand. The ulnar artery, which is dominant in most individuals, supplies the hand via the superficial palmar arch, and the radial artery, via the deep palmar arch. The proper digital vessels accompany the digital nerves to each side of the digit. In the digit, the nerves are more volar, so that when an artery is severed through a palmar laceration the nerve is usually also severed. The major blood supply to the thumb is the *princeps pollicis,* which usually comes from the first metacarpal artery branch of the deep palmar arch. Vascular variations are more common than nerve anomalies in the hand.

The circulation of the hand is evaluated by observing the color, temperature, and turgor of the finger pulp. Capillary refill or blanching is best examined by applying and releasing pressure in the area between the volar finger pulp and the lateral nail plate.

The *Allen test* is used to determine the patency of the radial and ulnar arteries at the wrist as follows:

1. To test the ulnar artery patency, both the ulnar and radial arteries are occluded by the examiner and the patient "opens and closes" the hand three times.

2. The radial artery is released. If the hand pinks ("flushes") immediately or within 6 seconds, the ulnar artery is patent. If no "refilling" occurs, the ulnar artery is partially or totally occluded (or absent).

3. The procedure is reversed to test the patency of the radial artery.

GENERAL PRINCIPLES OF SURGERY

For any surgical treatment of the hand, the patient should be comfortable in a supine position with the involved hand on a hand table. The surgeon should be seated in a comfortable position with good lighting. Operating loupes (2.5 to 4.5 magnification) are essential for careful atraumatic technique required in hand surgery. Appropriate refined and delicate hand instruments are mandatory. A pneumatic tourniquet over a well-padded (cast padding) upper arm must be used on all patients undergoing surgery of the hand. The upper extremity is exsanguinated by elevation for 1 minute or by the use of a rubber Esmarch wrap. The pneumatic cuff should be inflated to 100 mm. Hg above the systolic pressure. Penrose drains or rubber bands around the base of the digits should be *avoided.*

In most operative procedures on the hand, local or regional block anesthesia can be employed. Xylocaine (1 or 2 per cent *without* epinephrine) can be injected for a metacarpal block. The injection of 3 to 4 cc. of lidocaine (Xylocaine) into the web space or through the dorsal skin just proximal to the web space into the areas of the digital nerve is the safest and most comfortable method. Piercing the sensitive palm with a needle is painful, and more distal injections are potentially hazardous to the vascular flow of the digit.

In acute open injuries of the hand, the wound must be assessed for the degree of contamination, tissues involved, and depth of wound. Under tourniquet ischemia, adequate exposure of all potentially injured tissues is essential.

If the wound is tidy, the primary repair of all injured structures is acceptable and often preferred by the well-trained and experienced hand surgeon. However, the urgency of repair is necessary only for bone stabilization and for vessels if the area is avascular. Bone stabilization may even be delayed a few days if immediate fixation is not feasible. Although most hand surgeons currently prefer primary repair of the tendons and nerves, delayed repair of 3 days to 3 weeks will achieve comparable results. In general, in tidy sharp wounds, primary or immediae repair of all structures is indicated. In untidy wounds or avulsed or "mangled" injuries, delayed repair of the tendons and nerves is safer. Thorough débridement and irrigation are essential, and skin closure should be performed for only the tidy wounds of the hand.

As a general rule a well-padded (not constricting) dressing should be used with the wrist at neutral, the MCP joints in 60 to 90 degrees of flexion, and the PIP and DIP joints in extension. A dorsal plaster splint is applied usually to include the elbow to prevent slippage of the dressing. The extremity should be elevated during the early postoperative days.

SKIN INJURY

The glabrous palmar skin is thick, moist, and irregular and provides durability and traction. To prevent *longitudinal* restricting palmar scars, operative incisions in the palm should not cross the flexion *creases.* The incisions should be designed to transgress the different palmar areas subdivided by the creases by oblique incisions at the corners of the crease or Z-type incisions as shown in Figure 7.

The skin on the dorsum of the hand is thin and mobile and permits joint excursion. Since most of the venous and lymphatic drainage is dorsal, this is a common site for edema. Small, innocuous-appearing wounds in the skin may be associated with severe underlying damage. With any type of puncture wound, the examiner must always suspect a foreign body or damage to deep vital structures.

Coverage

When an extensive amount of skin has been lost, the surgeon must determine the optimal method of coverage. Factors influencing the selection are exposed tissues, tissues to be reconstructed, and the potential function, sensibility, and cosmetic result.

Early coverage is necessary for certain structures to prevent necrosis or loss of function. They are joint surfaces, tendons without paratenon, bone without periosteum, nerves, and vessels. If the hand is thoroughly and properly débrided, even large wounds with only muscle or subcutaneous tissue exposed will granulate and re-epithelialize spontaneously.

As previously emphasized, primary or delayed primary closure of the hand wound should be performed only when the wound is tidy. Undermining the skin to advance the edges for approximation must be avoided in attempting direct closure since skin necrosis will surely ensue.

Split-thickness skin grafting (with or without meshing) or full-thickness skin grafts may be used to cover clean subcutaneous tissue, vascular adipose tissue, muscle, and intact tendons with paratenon. If further reconstruction—such as tendon grafting or transfers, nerve, bone and

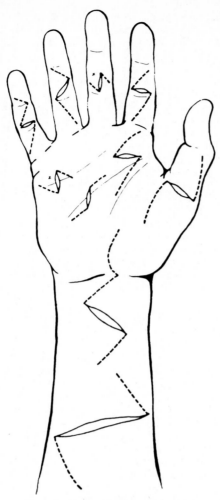

Figure 7. Acceptable surgical incisions on the palmar surface of the hand and forearm. (Reproduced with permission from Milford, L.: The hand. In Edmonson, A. S., and Crenshaw, A. H. (Eds.): Campbell's Operative Orthopaedics. St. Louis, C. V. Mosby, 1980.)

joint repair—is planned, the injured hand must be covered with a thick flap that contains skin and subcutaneous tissue. In these situations, flaps from a distance, such as a groin flap or a free vascularized tissue transfer, are selected.

Since the palmar surface of the digits is a sophisticated organ of touch, skin with neurovascular structures may have to be transferred to damaged vital functioning areas, such as the thumb and index palmar surfaces. Appropriate donor site selection for skin color, texture, and hair distribution is necessary for an acceptable cosmetic result.

Dupuytren's Disease

In 1932, Dupuytren of France described a "permanent retraction of the fingers produced by an affliction of the palmar fascia." This common problem is a disease primarily of the palmar aponeurosis and its digital prolongations. Pathologic changes in the fascia result in the formation of nodules in the palm and contractures in the digits. Similar changes of fibromatosis may occur in other areas, such as dorsal knuckle pads (Garrod's nodes), dorsum of the penis (Peyronie's disease), and plantar fascia (Ledderhose's disease). Although the exact etiology is unknown, it is a genetic

disease and has a frequent association with other diseases such as epilepsy, alcoholism, and diabetes.

Dupuytren's disease usually appears after the age of 40, more frequently in males than females (7:1). Bilateral involvement is frequent (over 50 per cent), and it usually begins at the base of the ring and little finger. Progression is usually slow, but may vary. A flexion contracture is most common at the MCP joint and PIP joints, with the DIP joint rarely involved. The nodules are usually not painful, and full active flexion is usually possible.

There is no successful nonoperative treatment. Indications for excision of the diseased fascia are: (1) bothersome contracture, (2) MCP contracture of 30 degrees or more, and (3) PIP contracture of 15 degrees or more, because of the difficulty of obtaining correction of the severely flexed PIP joint.

Operative correction of Dupuytren's contracture necessitates expertise in hand surgery, since the digital nerves may be entrapped by the proliferating aponeurosis, skin healing is a frequent problem, and recurrence rate is high. The most common operation presently is a regional fasciectomy in the palm and an extensive fasciectomy in the digits. The skin may be managed by leaving the wound open, Z-plasty closure, or coverage by skin grafting.

VASCULAR DISORDERS

Acute Injuries

Lacerations or amputations of the hand rarely present with life-threatening hemorrhage. Major vessels that have been completely transected will usually retract, restrict, and clot. However, partial transections of major vessels may result in persistent and profuse bleeding. The management of bleeding vessels should never involve blind clamping, since important nerves may be seriously damaged. Direct compression is usually successful, and tourniquet control is seldom indicated. Vascular repair distal to the elbow must be performed by microsurgical methods, utilizing an operating microscope, microinstruments, and microsuture material.

Although repair of a single lacerated major vessel in the forearm is recommended, only about 50 per cent of these anastomosed vessels remain patent. If both the radial and ulnar arteries are severed, both should be repaired. In the hand, a single lacerated digital vessel does not necessitate repair if the contralateral digital vessel is intact and good capillary refill is present in the fingertip. If the hand or forearm has been avascular for more than 4 hours, forearm *fasciotomy* must be performed after the revascularization procedure to prevent a compartment syndrome from the increased tissue pressure secondary to reperfusion and edema.

Chronic Injuries

Traumatic false aneurysms and arteriovenous fistulas occur in the hand. The diagnosis of these vascular injuries is frequently delayed because they are not suspected. A palpable and audible bruit over the mass is usually present, and the definitive diagnosis is made by arteriography. Resection plus direct vascular repair or interpositional vein grafting by microsurgical technique is the treatment of choice.

Occlusive Diseases

The radial or ulnar arteries may be acutely occluded in the wrist or hand by emboli from the heart or subclavian artery. Direct drug injections and coagulopathies are other common causes. Local repetitive trauma is a frequent cause of *ulnar artery thrombosis*. The superficial palmar arch is incomplete in 20 per cent of human hands. If the ulnar or radial artery is occluded in an individual with an incomplete arch, vascular insufficiency of the hand is likely. Even if the arch is complete, vascular compromise may occur in some hands.

Ulnar artery thrombosis characteristically occurs in males in the fifth decade of life who have an occupational predisposition, such as hammering with the hypothenar area. The symptoms include pain, cold intolerance, numbness, and ulceration of the ulnar digits. The diagnosis is suspected by a lack of flow through the ulnar artery by the Allen test and is confirmed by angiography. Excision of the thrombosed segment and reconstruction by interpositional vein grafting by microsurgical methods is presently the most popular treatment.

Vasospastic Disorders

Raynaud's phenomenon is pallor of the digits with or without cyanosis on exposure to cold. *Raynaud's disease* is an entity in which the phenomenon occurs without a demonstrable associated disease. It is characterized by bilateral gangrene or trophic changes in the distal digital skin, in young women with absence of clinical occlusion of peripheral arteries, and absence of an organic disease as a cause of vasospasm. *Raynaud's syndrome,* or secondary Raynaud's phenomenon, is the phenomenon in association or caused by a disease, e.g., connective tissue or arterio-occlusive disorders.

When the phenomenon has failed to respond to various methods of conservative management, including protection from cold, discontinuance of smoking, psychotherapy, biofeedback, and vasodilator drugs, digital sympathectomy may be helpful. This surgical procedure involves a sectional adventeciectomy of the common digital arteries in the distal palm. Oftentimes the beneficial effects are temporary because of the progressive nature of the underlying systemic disease.

PERIPHERAL NERVE INJURY

Peripheral nerves may be injured by open or closed trauma or compressed by local entrapment in specific areas of the upper limb. Seddon described three grades of nerve injuries:

1. *Neurapraxia.* The nerve is contused or compressed, but there is no interruption of continuity.

2. *Axonotmesis.* The axon is disrupted, but the epineural sheath is intact.

3. *Neurotmesis.* The peripheral nerve is completely severed.

Surgical repair of the severed nerve stumps is required for neurotmesis; neurapraxia and axonotmesis will heal spontaneously or with decompression and neurolysis when indicated.

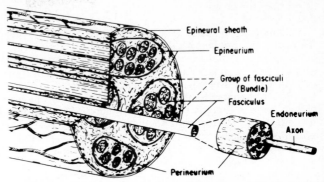

Figure 8. The basic structures of a peripheral nerve. (Reproduced with permission from Urbaniak, J. R.: Clin. Orthop., 163:57, 1982.)

Repair of Peripheral Nerves

The essential components that must be understood for repair of the injured peripheral nerve are illustrated in Figure 8. The *nerve fiber*, composed of the axon and sheath, is the smallest functional unit of a peripheral nerve. It is encased by endoneurium. The *fasciculus* (fascicle, funiculus) is a group of nerve fibers and is the smallest unit that can be surgically repaired. The *perineurium* encases each fasciculus. *Group fasciculi* (bundles) are arranged individually or in groups as they proceed through the peripheral nerve. The *epineurium* is areolar tissue that separates the fasciculi and generally accounts for 30 to 75 per cent of the cross section of a nerve. The *epineurial sheath* is the condensed sheath of epineurium that encases the nerve.

PHYSIOLOGY OF NERVE REGENERATION

Metabolic changes occur in the central cell body (located in the spinal cord or dorsal root ganglia) when the peripheral nerve is injured. Hypertrophy of the cell body occurs about 4 to 20 days after nerve injury, and neuronal regeneration follows. *Wallerian degeneration* is the process of Schwann cells digesting the fragmented myelin in the endoneurial tubes. The debris is removed within 2 to 8 weeks, and shrinkage of the cross-sectional area of the fasciculi occurs. Shrinkage may reach a maximum by 3 months, and by 2 years the fascicular cross section may be only 1 per cent of normal. This is the primary rationale for early repair of severed nerves.

Axonal budding from the proximal stump begins about 4 days after injury, but may be delayed up to 21 days in a severe crushing injury. The goals of the surgeon in aiding a physiologic repair are to minimize scarring and the appropriate capture of sprouting axons in the distal tubules (geographic alignment of the severed fascicles). The rate of peripheral nerve regeneration is 1 to 3 mm. per day. In calculating the expected date of distal recovery, the clinician must also include the 4 to 21 days before axonal sprouting, 30 days for the axons to cross the suture line, and additional delays occur at the motor end plates and sensory receptor organs.

TIMING AND CHOICE OF REPAIR

The type of wound, associated injuries, and location of the nerve injury influence the timing of the repair. In general, tidy, sharply severed nerves should be primarily repaired, but there is no substantial proof that the results of primary repair are better than delayed repair within the first 2 months.

Some advantages of *primary repair* are as follows: (1) the dissection is quicker and easier; (2) only one procedure is necessary; (3) fascicular orientation is easier; (4) stump retraction is minimal; and (5) secondary exploration may endanger previously repaired neighboring vessels.

Some advantages of *secondary repair* are as follows: (1) the surgeon is better prepared; (2) there is less potential for infection; (3) the thickened epineurium is easier to grasp; (4) the cell body is more "primed" for regeneration; and (5) in an avulsion or gunshot injury normal fasciculi are easier to identify.

The surgeon has several choices of repair. Use of microsurgical principles with atraumatic 8–0 to 11–0 monofilament nylon or prolene increases the potential for optimal nerve recovery. Nerves should not be repaired under tension. Both stumps must be sharply resected until normal pouting fascicles or groups of fascicles are visualized under magnification. After geographic alignment is ascertained, the nerves are joined by one of the following methods:

1. *Epineurial repair,* the placement of interrupted sutures through the epineurial sheath. This is the most universal type of repair; most nerves can be repaired by this method, especially if they are pure motor or pure sensory nerves.

2. *Group fascicular repair (bundle repair),* the alignment of groups (bundles) of fasciculi and placement of sutures in the epineurium surrounding each bundle. This method is useful for partially severed nerves or mixed (motor and sensory) nerves.

3. *Fascicular repair,* the placement of sutures through the *perineurium* that surrounds the individual fascicle. This type of repair is reserved for partially severed nerves when individual fascicles can be identified and matched.

4. *Interfascicular nerve grafting,* the bridging (grafting) of groups of fascicles (bundles) with small cutaneous nerves. This method is most beneficial when a large gap (usually 3 cm. or greater) is present. It has the advantage of allowing early joint motion since the repaired nerve is under no tension.

Entrapment Neuropathies

There are a number of locations in the upper extremity in which peripheral nerves may be entrapped by a variety of causes. These include normal or abnormal anatomic structures, postural compression, inflammation (especially tenosynovitis), metabolic changes (e.g., pregnancy), trauma, and iatrogenic provocation (e.g., injections, casts, or dressings). A thorough understanding of upper extremity anatomy in conjunction with elicitation of a good history and a complete examination will result in an accurate diagnosis in greater than 95 per cent of the presentations. The most common entrapment syndromes will be presented in this section.

MEDIAN NERVE

Carpal Tunnel Syndrome

Compression of the median nerve at the wrist is by far the most common entrapment neuropathy in the upper limb. The nerve is compressed by the transverse carpal ligament. The most common cause is tenosynovitis of the digital flexors; other causes are pregnancy, occupational

trauma, benign tumors, and abnormal muscles. The symptoms are numbness in the thumb, index, middle, and ring fingers; nocturnal burning pain; and clumsiness, weakness, and pain on using the hand (e.g., driving).

The physical findings are diminished sensitivity and sweating over the thumb, index, middle, and radial one half of the ring finger; thenar atrophy; weakness of thumb abduction and opposition; and a positive percussion test over the median nerve at the wrist (Tinel's sign). Holding the wrist in full flexion (Phalen flexion test) or full extension may produce numbness in the digits innervated by the median nerve. Inflation of a blood pressure cuff around the upper arm to above the venous pressure may also result in numbness in the median nerve distribution of the hand. Normal sensitivity is present in the proximal palm, which is innervated by the palmar cutaneous branch of the median nerve, which passes superficial to the transverse carpal ligament.

Electrodiagnostic studies and wrist roentgenographs, including carpal tunnel views, are recommended. Conservative treatment with a wrist splint and a steroid injection into the carpal tunnel (*not* the nerve) will cure the mild syndrome in less than 50 per cent of presentations. Release of the transverse carpal ligament is necessary in severe cases or when conservative measures fail.

Pronator Teres Syndrome

The pronator teres syndrome occurs when the median nerve is compressed in the proximal forearm by the lacertus fibrosus, pronator teres, or proximal arch of the flexor digitorum superficialis. The symptoms are pain in the volar forearm that increases with activity and numbness in the radial three-and-one-half digits. Physical findings are similar to those of carpal tunnel syndrome, except that the percussion test is positive in the proximal forearm and flexion and extension tests are negative. Pain may be elicited by pronation against resistance or resistance to isolated flexion of the PIP joint of the long and ring fingers.

Electrodiagnostic studies confirm the diagnosis. Conservative treatment consists of rest and splinting for 4 to 6 weeks. Injection is not advised. Surgical decompression to release the pronator teres, lacertus fibrosus, or arch of the FDS is usually necessary.

ULNAR NERVE

Cubital Tunnel Syndrome

Ulnar nerve entrapment occurs more often at the elbow level than at the wrist. Compression of the ulnar nerve at the elbow, the *cubital tunnel syndrome,* is common. Signs of ulnar nerve irritation include compression between the ulnar and humeral origins of the flexor carpi ulnaris, direct trauma, a hypermobile ulnar nerve, bony spurs secondary to arthritis, swelling, and abnormal bone or muscles. The symptoms are pain and numbness of the ulnar forearm and ring and little fingers, weakness of the ulnar innervated intrinsic muscles, and, less frequently, the FDP of the ulnar digits and the flexor carpi ulnaris. The physical findings include a positive percussion test at the cubital tunnel, positive elbow flexion test, anesthesia or hypesthesia in the ulnar nerve distribution, and intrinsic atrophy of the hand. Electrodiagnostic studies are helpful.

Conservative treatment consists of a padded extension splint at night, rest, and avoidance of activity that provokes the symptoms. Operation is advisable if the symptoms persist, and the choice of procedure depends to an extent on the pathologic conditions found at exploration. The nerve must be decompressed by dividing the aponeurosis between the two heads of the flexor carpi ulnaris and division of the intermuscular septum above the elbow. The nerve may be transferred anteriorly from the cubital tunnel to a less restricting position.

Ulnar Tunnel Syndrome

Compression of the ulnar nerve at the wrist is less common than compression of the ulnar nerve at the elbow or the median nerve at the wrist, since the ulnar nerve passes into the hand through *Guyon's canal*, which does not contain synovium. Ulnar tunnel syndrome is characterized by symptoms of dyesthesias and pain in the ulnar one half of the ring finger and the little finger, with weakness and possibly atrophy of the intrinsics. Physical examination reveals insensitivity over the ulnar one-and-a-half digits, intrinsic atrophy and weakness, positive percussion test over Guyon's canal, and possible positive wrist flexion and extension tests.

Causes of this syndrome are ulnar artery lesions, ganglia, anomalous muscles, and repetitive trauma. Treatment consists of splinting, rest, and avoidance of repetitive trauma. Steroid injections are to be avoided since there is no synovial tissue present. Surgical decompression is usually necessary.

Other relatively common but less frequent upper extremity entrapment syndromes include compression of the radial nerve at the distal third of the humerus, the posterior interosseous branch of the radial nerve in the forearm, the anterior interosseous branch of the median nerve in the forearm, and the superficial branch of the radial nerve at the wrist. Spinner has given an excellent description of all of these entrapment syndromes.

TENDONS

Flexor Tendons

TENDON HEALING

There are nine extrinsic flexor tendons to the digits, one to flex each interphalangeal joint. Division of any one of these tendons may result in a serious hand disability, although an isolated FDS severance may be well tolerated.

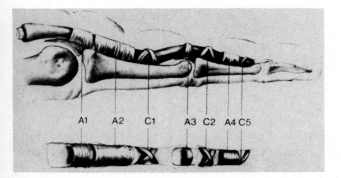

Figure 9. The flexor pulley system of the finger. A = Annular, C = cruciate. (Reproduced with permission from Doyle, J. R., and Blyth, W.: The Finger Flexor Tendon Sheath and Pulleys: Anatomy and Reconstruction. American Academy of Orthopaedic Surgeons Symposium on Tendon Surgery in the Hand. St. Louis, C. V. Mosby, 1975, p. 81.)

Even with excellent treatment, functional motion may be limited. The *problem area* for flexor tendon reconstruction is the digital sheath section, which extends from the distal palmar crease to the middle of the middle phalanx (Zone II or "no man's land"). There are basically four annular ligaments (pulleys) for each finger (Fig. 9). The tendon sheath (fibro-osseous tunnel) begins with the A1 pulley and ends with the A4 pulley. Full excursion of the flexor tendons in these tunnels is necessary for functional range of motion of the fingers. If one of the tendons is severed or scarred or more than two annular ligaments are divided, tendon amplitude will be seriously limited. Reconstruction of the injured flexor tendon system in this region is a difficult challenge for the surgeon in an effort to restore useful function.

Although flexor tendons are relatively avascular, they receive their blood supply from four major sources: (1) the musculotendinous junction in the wrist, (2) the mesotendon in the palm, (3) the vincula in the digital sheath, and (4) insertion into the distal phalanx. In addition to these blood vessels, there is good evidence that the tendon is nourished by synovial-like fluid in the sheath.

A completely severed flexor tendon in the digital sheath will not heal unless the divided ends are united by surgical methods. Healing of the repaired flexor tendon in the fibro-osseous tunnel appears to be dependent upon a combination of extrinsic vascular ingrowth into the repair site as well as intrinsic fluid nourishment. The actual surgical repair is not difficult, but the dilemma is the tendon healing process, which frequently results in multiple adhesions from the sheath to the tendon substance, which restricts tendon excursion.

SURGICAL REPAIR

The surgeon has several repair options: (1) primary repair, (2) delayed primary repair, (3) secondary repair, and (4) tendon graft, which consists of a one-stage free tendon graft or a two-stage graft with a silicone rod.

There is no universal agreement among hand surgeons on the timing of flexor tendon repair in fibro-osseous sheath (Zone II). Some stress that the repair should be performed within a few hours after injury (*primary repair*). Others advise repair within a few days (*delayed primary repair*); yet evidence is available to show that repair 7 to 21 days after injury (*secondary repair*) does not compromise the result.

If a digital flexor tendon has not been repaired within 2 months after injury, a free tendon graft is usually necessary because proximal tendon retraction will not permit coaptation of the two ends. A free tendon graft is also chosen if there is moderate scarring in the digital sheath. If the scarring is extensive and multiple pulleys have to be reconstructed, the two-stage tendon graft method is often used. This technique involves excision of scar tissue, pulley reconstruction, and insertion of a temporary silicone rod in the sheath. For a postoperative period of at least 6 to 8 weeks, the digit is passively flexed and extended to allow a smooth sheath to form about the silicone rod. The rod is subsequently removed and replaced with a free tendon graft. The most common sources for free tendon grafts are the palmaris longus, long toe extensors, plantaris tendon, or discarded flexor superficialis tendon.

Tendon reconstruction should be done with magnification and the atraumatic technique. The tendons are exposed through palmar zigzag or midlateral incisions. All pulleys must be preserved, and gentle tendon retrieval is

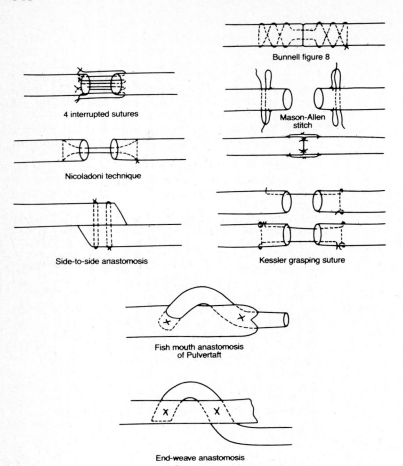

4 interrupted sutures

Nicoladoni technique

Side-to-side anastomosis

Bunnell figure 8

Mason-Allen stitch

Kessler grasping suture

Fish mouth anastomosis of Pulvertaft

End-weave anastomosis

Figure 10. Common methods of tendon repair. The three types on the upper right provide greater strength of union than the three on the left. The lower two methods provide the greatest repair but are too bulky to be used in the flexor sheath of the digit. (Reproduced with permission from Urbaniak, J. R., Cahill, J. D., Jr., and Mortenson, R. A.: Tendon Suturing Methods: Analysis of Tensile Strengths. American Academy of Orthopaedic Surgeons Symposium on Tendon Surgery in the Hand. St. Louis, C. V. Mosby, 1975, p. 71.)

important to diminish scarring. Nonabsorbable suture such as nylon (4–0 or 3–0) is used for the repair. A minimal amount of suture material should be exposed on the tendon surface. Many types of repairs have been proposed, but the most common types are the Kessler "grasping suture" and the Bunnell "figure of 8," or slight modification of them (Fig. 10). Repair of the digital sheath with fine 6–0 or 7–0 nylon suture remains controversial.

The postoperative management of repaired flexor tendons is just as important as the operative procedure. The repaired tendon has regained some tensile strength by 3 weeks to withstand mild resistance and by 6 weeks to withstand moderate resistance. It requires 6 to 8 months for the repair process to result in normal strength. After the tendon is repaired, the hand is splinted with the wrist and MCP joints in flexion to relieve the tension at the suture line. The PIP joints are positioned in extension to prevent joint contractures at this level. Based on the strength-duration healing curve, many surgeons do not begin active motion for 3 to 5 weeks. Conversely, in order to prevent tendon adhesions, others stress early controlled active or passive motion under the supervision of hand therapists. Good results of flexor tendon repair outside of Zone II are usually anticipated; however, within this area the functional results are less certain.

Extensor Tendons

The superficial position of the extensor tendons on the dorsum of the hand allow them to be divided by closed trauma over the digits or superficial lacerations over the digits and dorsum of the hand. It is therefore wise to explore seemingly minor lacerations for possible tendon injury. Extensor tendon injuries should be regarded with the same respect as flexor tendon injuries; however, there is no digital sheath and pulley system on the dorsum of the digits to cause the problems in excursion. Over the fingers the tendon is thin and friable so that suture retention is difficult. Also, there is a tendency for the tendon scar tissue to adhere to bone, especially if the periosteum has been violated.

The thinner and flatter extensor tendons over the digits are best repaired by a horizontal mattress suture (e.g., Nicoladoni type) (Fig. 10). On the dorsum of the hand and wrist, the tendons have an oval structure similar to that of the flexors and may be repaired with a similar suture method.

A *mallet finger* (baseball finger, drop finger) is due to a disruption of the extensor tendon from its insertion on the distal phalanx. It may be secondary to a fracture or a laceration. If the injury is open, the tendon should be operatively repaired. Usually, a small Kirschner wire is placed across the DIP joint to act as an internal splint for 3 to 6 weeks. Most of the injuries are secondary to closed trauma and operative intervention is not indicated. The DIP joint is splinted in full extension with the PIP remaining free. Healing (even with a fracture) will usually occur after 8 weeks of splinting. Chronic injuries of 6 months to 1 year may be successfully managed by this splinting method.

A *boutonnière deformity* (Fig. 11) can result from either a closed or open injury to the central slip attachment of the extensor tendon on the base of the middle phalanx.

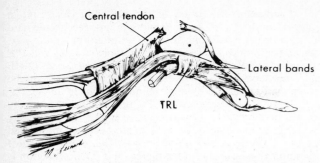

Figure 11. Pathomechanics of the boutonnière deformity. The central tendon is severed from its insertion on the middle phalanx. The lateral bands are displaced volar to the axis of the rotation of the PIP joint. In this position, the lateral bands flex the PIP joint, rather than extending it, and cause hyperextension at the DIP joint. TRL = Transverse retinacular ligament. (Reproduced with permission from the American Society for Surgery of the Hand: Regional Review Courses in Hand Surgery. Aurora, Colo., 1984, p. 50.)

The deformity occurs because the central extensor mechanism is disrupted, and the lateral bands, which are normally dorsal to the axis of rotation of the PIP joint, slip volar to the axis. These bands, which normally extend the PIP joint, now act as paradoxical flexors of the PIP joint. Additionally, the DIP is hyperextended by the shortened extensor mechanism.

Management of the acutely disrupted central slip is by operative repair if the injury is an open one. A closed injury is best treated by splinting the PIP joint in extension and allowing the DIP joint to be free for active flexion to prevent shortening of the extensor mechanism. Eight weeks of splinting is suggested. The treatment of the chronic boutonnière deformity by any method is difficult, and the results are frequently less than desirable.

Severed extensor tendons on the dorsum of the hand (especially the extensor pollicis longus, since it is independent) may retract several centimeters. Adequate incisions must be planned to retrieve the divided tendons. After repair, the wrist and MCP joints are splinted in extension for 4 weeks; the PIP and DIP joints may be free to move. The wrist is then held in extension for another 3 weeks, and MCP motion may begin.

FRACTURES AND DISLOCATIONS

As in other areas of the skeleton, fractures of the hand are classified as *open* or *closed* and by the *type* and *site* of the fracture line (Fig. 12). In addition, the fracture should be labeled as intra-articular or extra-articular if a joint is involved. In a growing child a description of the epiphysis may need to be included. If a fracture or dislocation is suspected, the physical examination should include a description of local swelling and tenderness, range of motion, rotational and angulatory alignment, and neurovascular status.

Phalanges and Metacarpals

The diagnosis of a fracture or dislocation of a phalanx or metacarpal may be suspected if there is an obvious rotatory or angulatory deformity of the digit. The deforming forces of the musculotendinous units acting across the fracture site contribute to the bony deformity and must be

considered in the management. Necessary roentgenograms include an anteroposterior and lateral view of the *isolated digit*, an oblique view if the fracture is close to a joint, and a post-reduction view. Most of the hand fractures can be treated by local or regional anesthetic blocks.

TREATMENT OF EXTRA-ARTICULAR FRACTURES

If the fracture is stable, the involved digit may be splinted with the MCP joint in flexion (60 to 90 degrees) and the PIP joint in slight flexion (10 to 15 degrees) for 4 weeks. Frequently taping the fractured digit to the adjacent digit ("buddy taping") will suffice. The roentgenogram needs to be repeated in 1 week to assess alignment and stability.

Unstable fractures, such as oblique, angulated, or rotated fractures, can often be treated by closed reduction under digital or wrist block anesthesia. Longitudinal traction is applied to restore length, and manipulation is then performed to correct rotation and angulation. The plane of the finger nails is observed for rotational alignment, and the flexed digits should point to the scaphoid tubercle if the radial and ulnar alignment is correct. If a satisfactory reduction is confirmed by radiographs, the digit(s) may be immobilized with a splint, cast, or percutaneous pinning.

The cast or splint should immobilize the wrist in moderate dorsiflexion (30 degrees), the MCP joints in 60- to 90-degree flexion and the PIP joints in nearly full extension. For fractures of the proximal phalanx with volar angulation and fractures of the volar base of the middle phalanx, flexion of the PIP joint is required to achieve and maintain reduction. Phalangeal fractures are immobilized for 3 weeks, metacarpal fractures for 4 weeks. Since it may take 2 to 4 months for healing to be apparent on radiographic studies, motion should begin at the 3- to 4-week period.

Percutaneous pinning with small Kirschner wires (0.35 to 0.45) is not easy. At least two pins are required for fixation, and a motorized pin driver and imaging radiogra-

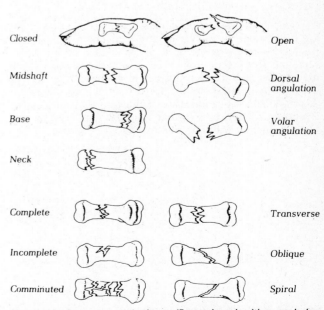

Figure 12. Fracture terminology. (Reproduced with permission from the American Society for Surgery of the Hand: The Hand: Examination and Diagnosis. New York, Churchill Livingstone, 1983, p. 54.)

phy are mandatory. Some indications for percutaneous pinning are metacarpal fractures with angulation and spiral fractures of the proximal phalanx. It is difficult to use this method on a transverse fracture through the shaft of a bone. In this instance, a longitudinal intramedullary pin is suggested.

Open reduction and internal fixation (ORIF) is indicated if the fracture cannot be reduced and stabilized by closed methods. Currently, there is a greater tendency to treat many of the small bone fractures with ORIF in order to begin immediate or early motion of the digits; however, this approach is not necessarily the best. The fracture may be fixed with a number of devices, including K-wires, tension band wiring, interosseous wiring, and miniscrews with and without miniplates.

Some common complications of closed reduction are inadequate anesthesia, rotational and angulatory malalignment, displacement of the fracture, and soft tissue interposition. In the ORIF method, the technique must be precise because the fragments are so small, and operative exposure increases the soft tissue trauma, which may cause formation of more adhesions.

TREATMENT OF INTRA-ARTICULAR FRACTURES

The nondisplaced stable fracture may be treated with a splint or the buddy-taping method. Again, radiographs are necessary at 1 week. In general, ORIF is necessary in most displaced intra-articular fractures to achieve joint congruity. In some instances, closed reduction with percutaneous K-wire stabilization may be chosen. Specific fractures for which internal fixation is required include the following:

1. A fracture dislocation of the base of the first metacarpal (Bennett's fracture) (Fig. 13).
2. An injury similar to the base of the fifth metacarpal.
3. Avulsed collateral ligament fracture of the metacarpal neck.
4. Displaced condylar fracture.

DISLOCATIONS OF THE PHALANGES AND METACARPALS

Dislocations are most common at the PIP joints. They are usually dorsal, are stable after reduction, and may be treated by buddy taping or a splint. Volar dislocations are rare, but they may be open injuries and operative repair may be needed. The central extensor mechanism may be damaged with the potential for a boutonnière deformity. A rotational dislocation usually indicates that the condyle is entrapped between the lateral band and central slip. Open reduction with internal fixation is necessary.

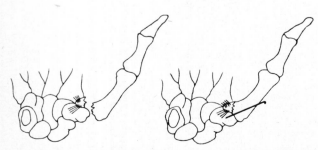

Figure 13. Bennett's fracture, a fracture dislocation of the base of the thumb metacarpal, is best treated by reduction and pin fixation. (Reproduced with permission from Swanson, A. B.: Surg. Clin. North Am., 1(2):26, 1970.)

A fracture dislocation of the PIP joint can result in almost total loss of joint motion if not recognized and treated promptly. Extensor block splinting (preventing extension beyond 30 to 40 degrees but encouraging full PIP active flexion) is the preferred method of treatment. ORIF may be necessary, but is usually difficult because of the fragmentation of the base of the middle phalanx.

Usually, a dislocated MCP joint can be reduced by closed manipulation. Occasionally, a closed reduction may be impossible because the volar plate becomes interposed in the joint (complex dislocation). This injury is most commonly seen in the index finger, and open reduction is required. Following reduction, the MCP joint is splinted in flexion for 2 to 3 weeks.

A *gamekeeper's thumb (skier's thumb)* is an injury that involves a tear of the ulnar collateral ligament of the MCP joint of the thumb. If this injury is left untreated, a severe disability weakness of pinch and grip occurs. If stress is applied in a radial direction and the ulnar side of the MCP joint opens more than 35 degrees or 15 per cent more than the contralateral thumb, operative repair is usually indicated because the torn ligament frequently becomes located outside the adductor aponeurosis (Stener lesion), where healing cannot occur. The MCP joint should be stressed with the joint in full extension and at 35-degree flexion.

Carpal Bones

The most frequently fractured carpal bone is the *scaphoid* (Fig. 14; see also Fig. 1*B*). This injury most commonly occurs in the young adult (under 30 years) as a result of a fall on the outstretched upper limb. Localized tenderness is present in the "anatomic snuff box," the area over the radial aspect of the wrist between the first dorsal compartment (abductor pollicis longus and extensor pollicis brevis tendons) and the second dorsal compartment (extensor pollicis longus tendon). The patient experiences pain on radial deviation. A high index of suspicion is necessary, for if the diagnosis is made immediately, more than 95 per cent of the fractures will heal with proper casting. Delayed treatment may lead to avascular necrosis of the scaphoid, non-union, and multiple surgical procedures. Required roentgenograms are anteroposterior, lateral, oblique, and scaphoid views (wrist in ulnar deviation). If the radiographic findings are normal at the time of injury, the wrist should be placed in a short arm cast or splint and the roentgenograms should be repeated in 10 to 14 days when the fracture line may be apparent because of increased calcification.

Seventy per cent of the fractures occur through the waist (middle one third) of the scaphoid (Fig. 14). This locus is significant because most of the blood supply of the scaphoid enters the bone through the dorsal radial surface and the blood flow to the proximal pole may be disrupted with the development of avascular necrosis of the proximal fragment.

Early diagnosis and treatment with a below-elbow cast that includes the thumb will result in over a 95 per cent success rate of healing. Some physicians prefer to include the elbow in the cast for the first 4 to 6 weeks. Open reduction with internal fixation of the acute injury is necessary only when malalignment of the fracture fragments exists.

If non-union or prolonged avascular necrosis occurs, numerous operative methods have been devised for healing. The most popular current methods are bone grafting with or without a compression screw. If healing does not occur, degenerative arthritis of the wrist joint is a certain sequela.

FRACTURE LOCATION BLOOD SUPPLY

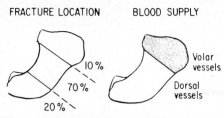

Figure 14. Scaphoid fractures. (Reproduced with permission from the American Society for Surgery of the Hand: Regional Review Courses in Hand Surgery. Aurora, Colo., 1984, p. 130.)

The second most common injury to the carpal bones is a dislocation of the lunate (see Fig. *1*B). This occurs from hyperextending the wrist in a fall on the outstretched forearm with a volar dislocation of the lunate. The physical examination reveals swelling and tenderness over the mid-volar aspect of the wrist with limited and painful wrist motion. A frequent occurrence is *compression of the median nerve* by the dislocated lunate, which produces numbness in the median nerve distribution of the hand, especially the index and middle fingers.

The diagnosis is confirmed by anteroposterior and lateral roentgenograms. Usually, reduction can be accomplished by closed manipulation; however, anatomic reduction is essential. Open reduction is necessary if the reduction is inadequate or if median nerve symptoms do not improve within 24 hours.

A similar mechanism of injury can produce a *perilunate dislocation*, in which the lunate remains colinear with the radius but the other carpal bones are dorsally dislocated. Multiple complexities of these dislocations are possible because of the eight carpal bones with their numerous ligamentous attachments. Immediate ORIF with accurate anatomic reduction, ligamentous repair, and K-wire fixation is necessary in these situations if normal or near-normal wrist function is to be achieved.

Other relatively common carpal bone problems include *Kienböck's disease* of the lunate, or avascular necrosis of this bone. The etiology is thought to be trauma-related. Spontaneous healing rarely occurs, and current operative treatments include steps to decrease the longitudinal compressive forces in the lunate (e.g., shortening of the radius or lengthening of the ulna). Chronic *carpal instability* secondary to trauma most commonly affects the scapholunate joint. Although numerous methods of stabilizing the bones have been designed, reliable operative procedures for correction are nonexistent; therefore, early diagnosis and treatment of acute instabilities or dissociations of the carpal bones are critical.

Distal Radius and Ulna

The distal radius and ulna are frequently fractured when the patient falls on the upper extremity. In the growing child, the *distal radial epiphysis* is likely to be dislocated. The diagnosis is confirmed by roentgenography, and closed reduction is usually easily achieved under a local block or no anesthesia. A long arm cast is applied for 3 weeks, and a short arm cast is applied for an additional 3 weeks.

The most common distal radial fracture is the *Colles fracture,* a transverse fracture of the distal radius and ulna with dorsal and radial displacement of the distal fragments.

The apex of the fracture is volar. This injury is most common in elderly individuals. The *Smith fracture,* in which the distal fragment is displaced volarly with apex of the fracture being dorsal, is less common.

Examination reveals local tenderness, swelling, limited motion, possibly crepitus, and median nerve compression. The roentgenograms identify the derangement of the articular surface of the radius.

Most fractures of the distal radius and ulna can be managed by local or regional anesthesia and closed manipulation and casting. It is essential to restore the normal length and distal inclination of the radius to achieve a good functional wrist. The Colles fracture is reduced by applying longitudinal traction to disimpact the fracture and then volar flexing the wrist at the fracture site. Accurate reduction can usually be determined by dorsal palpation with experienced hands. The post-reduction radiographs should show the articular surface of the distal radius angulating 15 to 30 degrees ulnarly (the radial styloid more distal than the ulnar styloid) and at least a 10-degree volar tilt.

The wrist is mobilized in 20 degrees of flexion and 30 degrees of ulnar deviation with a "sugar tong" splint (volar and dorsal foreman splint that incorporates the elbow but allows elbow flexion and extension). As in all upper limb casts that include the hand, it is important that the volar distal portion of the cast stop at or proximal to the *distal palmar crease* to allow full active flexion of the MCP joints. The hand should be elevated for 48 hours, and early finger motion should be encouraged to diminish edema and prevent joint stiffness.

Less than 5 per cent of Colles fractures are unstable, and stabilization by pins, screws and plates, or external fixators is required. A frequent complication of distal radial fractures is median nerve compression. If the nerve symptoms do not improve in 24 to 48 hours after injury, operative exploration is indicated. The incidence of reflex sympathetic dystrophy can be diminished by careful application of well-padded splint or casts, frequent examinations, elevation, preventing and alleviating pain (change the cast if painful), and encouraging early finger, elbow, and shoulder motion.

INFLAMMATORY DISEASES

Inflammatory diseases of the hand are common. There are four major categories: (1) tenosynovitis, (2) infections, (3) rheumatoid arthritis, and (4) osteoarthritis. The most common entities under each of these categories will be emphasized.

Tenosynovitis

Inflammatory processes of hand tendon sheaths are common. Although the etiology is frequently unknown, repetitive stress (overuse) or trauma is often a contributory factor. An underlying systemic disease, such as rheumatoid arthritis or gout, must be suspected. The diagnosis is made by careful examination, which will reveal a localized area of tenderness and possibly crepitus, swelling, and redness. Radiographic calcification may be present when the wrist flexors or extensors are involved, but it is usually not observed in other areas. Most of these inflammatory lesions will respond to splinting, limitation of activity, anti-inflammatory agents, and local steroid injections. Surgical intervention is usually not necessary.

Stenosing Tenosynovitis of the Digital Flexor Sheath

"Triggering" can occur in any location where there is a restraining retinacular system such as the flexor tendon sheaths or dorsal wrist compartments. It occurs most commonly in the flexor tendons of the thumb ("trigger thumb") and long and ring fingers ("trigger finger"). The condition is caused by inflammation of the synovium, which results in a size discrepancy between the tendon and annular ligament. At operation both a nodule in the tendon and a thickened synovial sheath are usually seen.

The patient complains of "locking" or triggering of the digit, which is caused by the nodule of the tendon "jamming" beneath the pulley, usually the A1 pulley (see Fig. 9), when the patient attempts to extend the digit from the flexed position. The maneuver may be painful. The nodule is usually palpable proximal to the A1 pulley or over the MCP joint in the thumb. Usually, the condition will respond to steroid injection into the sheath, and splinting, rest, and anti-inflammatory agents. Occasionally operative intervention is necessary to release the proximal pulley.

De Quervain's Stenosing Tenosynovitis

De Quervain's stenosing tenosynovitis of the first dorsal extensor compartment (which contains the extensor pollicis brevis and abductor pollicis longus tendons) is most common in women (ages 30 to 50 years) and is painful on thumb activity. Tenderness, crepitus, and swelling are present over the first dorsal extensor compartment. A positive *Finklestein's test* is pathognomonic for this entity. This is produced by having the patient grasp the thumb in the palm (flex the thumb) and ulnar deviate the wrist. Pain in the first dorsal extensor compartment, produced by tethering the enclosed extensor tendons, is a positive test. The treatment is the same as for other forms of stenosing tenosynovitis.

Infections

Most hand infections necessitate incision and drainage and, frequently, débridement. The history should include inquiry about mechanism of injury, prior systemic infections, diabetes, gout, drug or alcohol abuse, and coagulopathies. The examination must include the entire upper limb for lymphangitis and adenopathy. Gram-positive staphylococci and streptococci are the most common organisms cultured, but gram-negative organisms, anaerobes, mycobacteria, certain viruses, and fungi are not infrequently encountered. Appropriate antibiotic therapy is always used as an adjunct to operation. For infections involving tendon sheaths, joints, bone, and deep spaces of the hand, hospitalization for operation, elevation, rest, and intravenous antibiotics are required.

Paronychia

The paronychia is the most common infection of the finger. It involves the periungual tissues (Fig. 15) and is usually caused by *Staphylococcus aureus*. It may spread to involve the entire eponychial area or even into the pulp space. An early paronychia with cellulitis and no abscess is treated with soaks and antibiotics.

An abscess must be drained by elevating the nail margin and removing the part of the nail plate on the involved side. If both sides of the nail margin are involved, the entire nail should be removed. A small wick is inserted

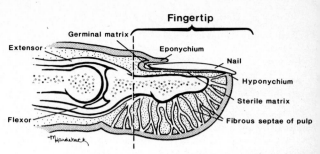

Figure 15. Anatomy of the fingertip. (Reproduced with permission from the American Society for Surgery of the Hand: Regional Review Courses in Hand Surgery. Aurora, Colo., 1984, p. 191.)

for drainage, and the nail bed is covered with a nonadherent gauze. An appropriate antibiotic, usually a synthetic penicillin, is given. The operative procedure may be performed under metacarpal block anesthesia.

Felon

A felon is a deep infection of the pulp space of a digit. There is frequently a history of a puncture wound, and the patient complains of an intense throbbing pain. The finger pulp is tense, swollen, and tender, and *staphylococcus aureus* is usually the causative organism. The infection is contained in the vertical fibrous septa of the pulp (Fig. 15). The abscess must be drained and cultured. The most common incision is a unilateral longitudinal incision near the nail skin margin. The septa must be divided. If the abscess points more toward the midpulp, a palmar midline longitudinal incision is made in the pulp. Care must be taken not to cross the flexion crease at right angles and to avoid the digital nerves. The wound is left open with a wick inserted for drainage. A synthetic penicillin or cephalosporin is administered while the culture report is being awaited.

Web Space Infection

Web space infections usually begin subcutaneously in the palm from a puncture and extend through the fascia to the dorsum of the web space *(collar button abscess)*. Swelling and erythema are present in the web space, and incision and drainage are necessary.

Acute Suppurative Tenosynovitis

Infection of the digital tendon sheath presents as Kanavel's four cardinal signs: (1) swelling, (2) flexed position of the digit, (3) pain on passive extension, and (4) tenderness over the flexor tendon sheath. The infection may extend to the thenar, hypothenar, or midpalmar spaces. A *horseshoe abscess* occurs when there is a coalescence of infection in the radial and ulnar bursae (e.g., from the little finger to the thumb). Drainage is always necessary, and there are two common methods. The first is by a midlateral incision along the entire tendon sheath and leaving the wound open. The second approach involves two limited incisions into the sheath, one over the middle phalanx and one in the distal palmar crease. A silicone catheter is inserted in one of the incisions, and every 2 hours the sheath is irrigated with 50 cc. of sterile saline. The catheter may be removed at 2 days and early motion instituted.

Even with early surgical treatment, full functional range of motion of the digit may not be achieved. A palmar zigzag incision is to be avoided for this problem.

HUMAN AND ANIMAL BITES

Human bites frequently occur over the dorsum of the MCP joint as a result of striking a tooth in a fight. Although the wound may initially appear to be benign, the joint is usually inoculated by oral bacteria. Prompt treatment of wound excision and drainage, and leaving the wound open, is mandatory. Puncture wounds from animal bites warrant the same management—wound excision and open treatment. Human bites inoculate a mixture of potent flora, including *Eikenella corrodens* (sensitive to penicillin). *Pasteurella multocida* (sensitive to penicillin) is present in more than half of dog and cat bites.

HERPETIC WHITLOW

Herpetic whitlow appears as small vesicles on the fingertips, usually in medical personnel who care for the orotracheal area. It is caused by the herpes simplex virus, which is confirmed by culture. Operative intervention is *not* indicated, and the infection usually subsides in 10 to 14 days with splinting and elevation.

Rheumatoid Arthritis

The primary target of rheumatoid arthritis is the *synovium.* The proliferative synovitis is usually initially manifested by swollen and stiff wrist and finger joints. As the disease progresses, the synovitis may result in increased joint pressure, distention, and disruption of the capsule and ligaments. Subluxation of the MCP joints and the development of the classic ulnar drift often occur. Hyperextension or flexion deformities may develop in the PIP joints of the fingers, MCP, and IP joints of the thumb. Tenosynovitis, trigger finger, rupture of the tendons, and carpal tunnel syndrome are common. Further synovial proliferation, with the release of collagenases and production of lysozymes by the phagocytes, cause articular and periarticular erosion and the formation of cysts and spurs with eventual destruction and collapse of the joints.

RADIOGRAPHIC CHANGES

Early roentgenographic changes are periarticular porosis and erosions, especially in the metacarpal heads. Later changes include loss of the articular surface, subluxation, and joint collapse.

INDICATIONS FOR SURGERY

The indications for operative intervention include (1) failure to halt the progression of the disease with a sound medical regimen, (2) severe pain, (3) nerve entrapment, (4) tendon ruptures, and (5) deformities that impair hand function. The goals of operation are to relieve pain, correct the deformity, and restore function.

OPERATIVE PROCEDURES

Early Phase. In the early phases of the disease, numerous procedures are utilized for pain relief and to preserve function. These include tendon and joint synovectomy, nerve decompression (especially of the median and ulnar nerves at the wrist), and trigger finger releases.

After the deformities have occurred, the operative procedures must be more extensive. Soft tissue reconstruction to restore alignment and function is accomplished by releasing and plicating collateral ligaments and by performing tendon repairs, grafts, and transfers.

Late Phase. After joint destruction has occurred, function and alignment may be restored by reconstructive arthroplasty or arthrodesis. Joint resection and reconstruction with interpositional silicone or silicone-dacron implants in the MCP and PIP joints frequently achieve the operative goals of pain relief and functional restoration. The destroyed wrist joint may be reconstructed by a fusion, a hinged silicone implant, or an articulated metal and plastic prosthesis that is stabilized with bone cement (polymethyl methacrylate). Most surgeons prefer not to insert polymethyl methacrylate into the small bones of the hands.

Osteoarthritis

Osteoarthritis, or degenerative arthritis of the hand, is very common (35 per cent of elderly patients). It is more common in men under 45 years of age and in women over 45 years of age. The most commonly involved joints are the DIP joints and carpometacarpal joints of the thumb. The PIP joints are also involved, and the MCP and wrist joints are less commonly afflicted. The etiology is unknown, but chronic loading on the joint surfaces is a factor.

The marginal osteophytes at the DIP joints are called *Heberden's nodes,* and those at the PIP joints *Bouchard's nodes. Mucous cysts* are ganglion cysts that frequently develop from degenerative changes at the DIP joints. A groove may appear in the nail.

Osteoarthritis of the carpometacarpal of the thumb is most common in women over 50 years of age and is manifested by weakness of pinch, pain, and a "lump" at the base of the thumb. A positive "grind test" elicited by a compressive load on this joint is usually diagnostic. The radiographic findings vary from a decreased joint space to complete joint destruction and displacement.

Initially, a small splint, aspirin, anti-inflammatory agents, and steroid injections into the joint are all frequently beneficial. If the condition progresses and pain and diminished function persist, surgery is indicated. The DIP joints may be treated by excision of the cysts and osteophytes, but often arthrodesis is recommended. The PIP joints are managed by silicone interpositional arthroplasty or arthrodesis.

The carpometacarpal (CMC) thumb arthritis is treated with splinting, anti-inflammatory agents, and local steroid injection in the early stages. Involvement of this joint is the most common indication for surgery in osteoarthritis of the hand. Multiple procedures are used, including (1) resection of the trapezium and replacement with soft tissue, (2) resection of the trapezium and replacement with a silicone implant, (3) coverage of one joint surface with a silicone implant (hemiarthroplasty), and (4) arthrodesis of the CMC joint.

COMMON BENIGN TUMORS

Malignant tumors occur rarely in the hand and will not be described in this section, except to mention that skin cancers (basal cell, squamous cell, and malignant melanoma) are the most frequently occurring malignant types.

Ganglion

The ganglion is the most common soft tissue mass in the hand. Ganglia are more common in women (3:1) and most often occur in young adults. These soft tissue cysts have a smooth capsule, contain viscous mucin, and are fixed to a deep structure. The most common sites are (1) the dorsal carpal (scapholunate) joint, (2) the volar carpal (scaphotrapezium) joint, (3) the palmar digital crease (between A1 and A2 pulleys), and (4) the DIP joint (mucous cysts).

About half of these cysts are asymptomatic, and no treatment is needed other than reassurance. Symptomatic cysts may be treated by aspiration and local steroid injection, but most treated in this manner will recur. Excision necessitates the use of magnification and tourniquet ischemia, and excision of a small portion of the involved joint capsule is required. If the capsular defect is closed, the recurrence rate is high.

Giant Cell Tumor of the Tendon Sheath

The second most common tumor of the hand is the giant cell tumor of the tendon sheath (*xanthoma*). There is no sexual predilection, and most xanthomas occur between the ages of 40 to 60 years in the volar surface of the digits. The nodules vary in size, are firm, usually nontender, and may be mobile. Since they are near the small joints, digital function may be impaired. Gross inspection reveals an encapsulated yellow-brown nodule, which contains varying numbers of giant cells. Treatment is excision with a portion of the sheath or capsule. Xanthomas may recur if they are incompletely excised.

Epidermoid Cysts

Epidermoid cysts (inclusion cysts) are common, painless, slow-growing keratinizing cysts that are caused by a penetrating injury that embeds keratin-producing epithelium into the subcutaneous tissue. They are most common on the finger pulp, are painless, and are firm. Treatment is complete excision.

Enchondroma

The enchondroma is the most common primary bone tumor of the hand. It occurs in the young (10 to 40 years), most often in the proximal phalanx, and is usually asymptomatic until a fracture occurs through the lesion. Roentgenograms reveal a radiolucent lesion in the diaphysis and metaphysis with a thin cortex and flecks of calcium. This benign cartilage tumor is managed by curettage with bone graft replacement. Recurrence is rare.

AMPUTATION AND REPLANTATION

Amputation of fingers occurs commonly, and inappropriate management may lead to significant disability. Restoration of function is of prime importance, but cosmesis should not be ignored because the hand is the only exposed portion of the body visualized throughout the day. The general principles are to (1) preserve functional length, (2) minimize scar and adjacent contractures, (3) maintain mobility and sensibility, (4) prevent painful neuromas, and (5) shorten morbidity. Important considerations include age, sex, hand dominance, occupation, avocations, future reconstruction, prosthetic fitting, and patient attitude about amputation.

Fingertip Injuries

Fingertip injuries are the most common hand injuries. The fingertip is the portion of the digit distal to the insertion of the flexor and extensor tendons (Fig. 15).

If the nail matrix has been damaged, it must be cleansed and meticulously repaired with 6-0 or 7-0 suture to allow a normal contour of the regenerating nail plate. If the germinal matrix has been avulsed, it must be resutured in place if nail regeneration is to occur. The avulsed or removed nail plate should be cleansed and resutured in place. Lacerations of the eponychium should be repaired.

If the tissue loss of the finger pulp is 1 cm. or less, treatment by wound cleansing and dressing only is recommended. The area will epithelialize with a good functional and aesthetic result. In children, even larger defects will heal with excellent results.

Larger defects may be covered with split-thickness grafts obtained from the hypothenar area. The split-thickness graft will contract better than a full-thickness graft and will provide a better result. If there is loss of soft tissue and bone, or if bone is exposed, the wound may be closed by rongeuring exposed bone and applying a split-thickness graft. Occasionally, a local advancement flap (V-Y flap) (Fig. 16) is advisable. This is accomplished by incising only

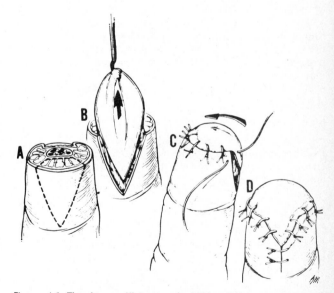

Figure 16. The Atasoy-Kleinert volar V-Y technique is applicable to distal tip injuries with bone exposed and where the distal injury is either transverse or oblique sloping from volar-distal to dorsal-proximal. In injuries where there is more volar pad loss, there is usually insufficient skin for this technique to be used. (Reproduced with permission from Louis, D. S.: Amputations. In Green, D. P. (Ed.): Operative Hand Surgery. New York, Churchill Livingstone, 1982, p. 59.)

through the dermis and carefully separating the septa from the phalanx just enough to allow advancement of the flap and still retain its blood supply. If the flap is not properly mobilized, necrosis will ensue.

Levels of Amputation

At each level of amputation in the hand the basic concepts are similar:
1. Contour the articular condyles, volar and lateral.
2. If the tendon insertion site is absent, sever the tendon and allow it to retract.
3. Do *not* suture flexors to extensors.
4. Freely dissect the nerves, gently pull and sharply transect them, and allow them to retract.
5. A volar skin flap is preferred.

Distal Phalanx. If the amputation occurs proximal to the base of the nail, bone shortening and primary closure are usually indicated. Amputation at the DIP joint should be managed by contouring the bone and primary closure with no fixation of the tendons.

Middle Phalanx. The bone should be shortened and contoured, the FDS insertion preserved and primary closure performed.

Proximal Phalanx. Frequently, a dorsal flap is needed for closure. The intrinsics will control the flexion. Ray resection (i.e., amputation through the base of the metacarpal) should be considered only for the index finger because the long and ring fingers should be preserved to prevent a gap and the little finger should be preserved for grip strength.

Thumb. The thumb should be reattached when possible. The bone should not be shortened. Coverage with durable and sensate skin is the goal.

Wrist. There is no value in preserving the carpal bones. In general, a wrist disarticulation is favored over a more proximal revision in order to preserve forearm pronation and supination and to provide better prosthetic suspension.

Replantation

Replantation utilizing microvascular techniques is an effective method of reconstructing the upper limb that has sustained a complete or incomplete amputation. Most replantations are performed in centers with experienced microvascular teams. Essential instruments include an operating microscope and ultrafine needles (50 to 100 microns) and suture material (8-0 to 11-0 nylon).

PREPARATION OF THE AMPUTATED PART

Devascularized tissue will survive about 6 hours of warm ischemia. Since cooling diminishes the metabolic needs of the tissue, an amputated part may be successfully replanted 12 hours after severance if it is cooled. Because digits have no muscle tissue, proper cooling will allow successful restoration as long as 30 hours after amputation.

Two basic methods are used to preserve the amputated part: (1) immersion of the part in Ringer's lactate solution in a plastic bag and placement of the bag on ice, and (2) wrapping the part in a cloth moistened with Ringer's lactate solution and placement into a plastic bag on ice. Care must be taken to prevent freezing of the part. The vessels should not be ligated or perfused because initimal damage may result.

PATIENT SELECTION

Candidates for replantation are selected according to the following priorities: (1) thumb, (2) multiple digits, (3) palmar amputations, (4) most body parts in a child, (5) wrist or forearm, (6) elbow or proximal (only if sharply severed), and (7) individual digit distal to the FDS insertion. This listing is not a strict order of preference, however, and if other factors are favorable, replantation should be attempted.

Contraindications for replantation include (1) severely crushed or mangled parts, (2) multiple-level amputations, (3) amputation in patients with serious injuries or diseases, (4) arteriosclerotic vessels, (5) mentally unstable patients, and (6) an individual finger in an adult proximal to the FDS insertion.

OPERATIVE TECHNIQUE

It is not within the scope of this chapter to detail the meticulous technique of replantation, and only the surgical sequence of events will be outlined. One member of the team takes the amputated part immediately to the operating theater to begin the débridement and dissection. Other members of the team prepare the patient, and, when possible, the operation is performed under axillary block anesthesia. The steps are to (1) isolate and tag the vessels and nerves, (2) débride, (3) shorten and stabilize the bone, (4) repair extensor tendons, (5) repair flexor tendons, (6) anastomose arteries, (7) repair nerves, (8) anastomose veins, and (9) obtain skin coverage.

None of the structures, especially the vessels and nerves, should be repaired under tension. Vein grafts may be necessary for ease of vessel approximation. In major limb replantation (proximal to the wrist), *temporary* vascular shunts of silicone tubes may be necessary initially to provide early revascularization of the amputated part.

Postoperative management includes the use of anticoagulants, vasodilators, a warm environment, and close monitoring of the perfusion of the replanted part.

RESULTS

The Duke Orthopaedic Replantation Team has attempted revascularizations of over 1200 amputations or partial amputations since 1973. Ninety-four per cent of partial amputations have been successfully revascularized, and 81 per cent of complete amputations have been successfully replanted. The sensibility recovery is similar to the results achieved in repair of isolated injury to a peripheral nerve. The arch of motion in a replanted digit is about 50 per cent of normal. Pain is not a problem, but cold intolerance persists for 1 or 2 years, then subsides. Replantation of amputated thumbs and hands at the wrist (Fig. 17) provides the best functional results in terms of grip, grasp, and aesthetic recovery. Replantation of fingers at the base (proximal to the FDS insertion) provides good sensibility but poor excursion. Our experience has shown that it is worthwhile to replant many severely avulsed parts, not just the guillotine-type of deletion.

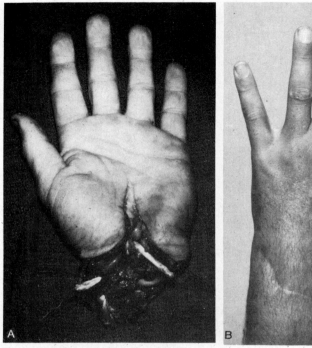

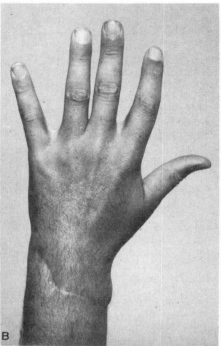

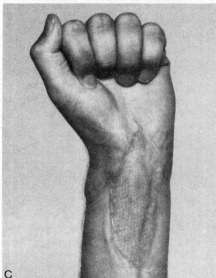

Figure 17. A, *A completely amputated hand of a 22-year-old male. B and C, One year after replantation the patient has nearly full flexion and extension of the fingers. Intrinsic function has returned to the thenar and hyperthenar muscles. He has protective sensibility but no tactilognosis. (Reproduced with permission from Urbaniak, J. R., and Porubsky, G. L.: Digital and limb transplantation. In Flye, M. W. (Ed.): Principles of Organ Transplantation, Philadelphia, W. B. Saunders Company, in press.)*

SELECTED REFERENCES

Annotated References

Green, D. P. (Ed.): Operative Hand Surgery. New York, Churchill Livingstone, 1982.

This textbook on hand surgery is already a classic. Every section of hand surgery is covered in detail, yet is easy to read and understand. The illustrations are excellent and clearly labeled in bold type. Each area of hand surgery is covered by an international expert on the subject. The individual authors review the current concepts and management and conclude by describing their preferred technique.

Urbaniak, J. R., and Strickland, J. W. (Eds.): Regional Review Course in Hand Surgery. American Society for Surgery of the Hand. Aurora, Col., 1984.

A well-illustrated study guide of 23 lectures on various areas of hand surgery. Controversy is minimized, and emphasis is placed on the functional anatomy, pathomechanics, and basic principles of evaluation and management of hand injuries, diseases, and deformities. Each section contains abridged references that are current and readily accessible.

General References

American Society for Surgery of the Hand. The Hand: Examination and Diagnosis, 2nd ed. New York, Churchill Livingstone, 1983.

American Society for Surgery of the Hand. The Hand: Primary Care of Common Problems. Aurora, Col., 1985.

Coleman, S. S., and Anson, B. J.: Arterial patterns in the hand based upon a study of 650 specimens. Surg. Gynecol. Obstet., *113*:409, 1961.

Green, D. P. (Ed.): Operative Hand Surgery. New York, Churchill Livingstone, 1982.

Koman, L. A., and Urbaniak, J. R.: Diagnostic studies of vascular lesions. Hand Clinics, *1*:217, 1985.

Lister, G.: The Hand: Diagnosis and Indications. New York, Churchill Livingstone, 1977.

Omer, G. E., and Spinner, M. (Eds.): Management of Peripheral Nerve Problems. Philadelphia, W. B. Saunders Company, 1980.

Urbaniak, J. R.: Replantation. *In* Green, D. P. (Ed.): Operative Hand Surgery. New York, Churchill Livingstone, 1982, pp. 811–827.

Urbaniak, J. R., and Roth, J. H.: Office diagnosis and treatment of hand pain: Symposium on office orthopedic practice. Orthop. Clin. North Am., *13*:477, 1982.

II

Musculoskeletal Trauma: General Principles

JOHN M. HARRELSON, M.D.

In an age of high-speed vehicles and increasing emphasis on athletics and physical fitness, injury to the musculoskeletal system is common and accounts for approximately 80 per cent of the general practice of orthopedics. Injuries may be acute from a single traumatic event, or they may be chronic from the cumulative effect of repeated episodes of lesser trauma. Although fractures are the most obvious example of musculoskeletal trauma, injury to ligaments, tendons, joints, and muscle account for a major portion of the problems seen in routine practice.

STRAINS, SPRAINS, AND DISLOCATIONS

Injury to ligaments, those fibrous structures that provide joint stability, result from force applied to the joint in an abnormal plane or excessive force in the plane of motion of the joint. A mild injury in which the ligament is stressed but remains intact is called a *strain*, and the patient will usually recover with rest. *Sprains* result when ligament fibers are torn and may be classified as mild (a few fibers), moderate (50 per cent of the fibers), or severe (complete disruption). Sprains produce bleeding, and the clinical signs of abrupt swelling and ecchymosis aid in diagnosis. The treatment of sprains depends on the severity and location of the injury. Rest may be required for a mild ankle sprain; brace or cast immobilization, for moderate knee ligament sprain; or operative repair, for complete knee ligament disruption.

When sufficient force is sustained to produce complete ligament disruption, *dislocation* or *subluxation* (partial dis-

location) of the joint may occur. In this type of injury, reduction is required for restoration of anatomic position; as in a sprain, immobilization or repair, depending on the severity of the injury and joint involved, may also be necessary. Specific treatments of sprains and dislocations will be discussed in the sections on the upper extremity, lower extremity, and spine.

FRACTURES

By definition, a fracture is a disruption in the continuity of a bone. However, trauma sufficient to cause a fracture almost inevitably produces soft tissue injury. Thus, for both the assessment of acute fractures and the rehabilitation after fracture, a knowledge of the muscular, vascular, and neurologic components of injury is needed. Further, many fractures result from violent trauma, and neurologic, respiratory, circulatory, abdominal, and genitourinary evaluation is frequently a component of complete care.

Classification

When a single fracture line is produced, a *simple* fracture exists. Multiple fracture lines and bone fragments constitute a *comminuted* fracture. Either of these injuries may be nondisplaced (in anatomic position) or displaced. A wound communicating with the fracture may result from external penetrating injury or from fracture fragments piercing the skin in the course of the injury. Thus, fractures are described as simple or comminuted, displaced or non-displaced, and open or closed. These distinctions are important because they influence treatment and prognosis.

The pattern of fracture is governed to some extent by the nature of the force applied. A bending movement applied to a long bone produces a simple transverse or oblique fracture; a direct blow or crushing force usually produces a comminuted fracture; torque or twisting forces often produce a spiral fracture; and axial compression may produce an impacted fracture. Traction force at the point of attachment of tendons may produce an avulsion fracture with a fragment being displaced by violent muscle contraction.

Chronic, repetitive trauma may also result in fracture. In an athlete who is performing daily excessive exercise, *fatigue* or *stress* fractures in the lower extremity may result. In the elderly patient with osteoporosis, routine daily activity, either repetitive (walking) or sudden (lifting an object) may result in an *insufficiency* fracture. Nontraumatic fractures in the presence of metastatic deposits or infection are referred to as *pathologic* fractures.

Evaluation of Acute Injury

When a fracture occurs, local bleeding produces an enlarging hematoma that envelops the fracture site. Pressure on local nerves and vessels may result from the hematoma or from displacement of the fracture by contraction of those muscles crossing the fracture site. Careful neurologic and vascular evaluation is required. Nerve or vessel injury may result from penetration by sharp fracture fragments. Bleeding into anatomic compartments, such as the anterior compartment of the leg or the volar compartment of the forearm, may also produce acute neurologic and vascular deficit necessitating decompressive fasciotomy. Adjacent organ injury may occur with certain fractures. Bladder injury with pelvic fractures, liver, spleen, or lung injury with rib fractures, and spinal cord injury with spinal fractures must all be considered. With pelvic and femoral fractures or with multiple fractures, hemorrhage at the fracture site(s) may be sufficient to produce hypovolemic shock.

In a small number of patients, usually those who have experienced hypovolemic shock, the syndrome of *fat embolization* may occur. This respiratory complication is first recognized by a rising pulse rate, falling hemoglobin, and falling arterial P_{O_2}. Mental confusion, petechiae on the chest and abdomen, free fat particles in the urine, and a patchy infiltrate on the chest film complete the clinical picture. Early recognition is essential to avoid rapid deterioration and death. Large doses of corticosteroids and oxygen administered by mask, intubation or tracheostomy will usually result in reversal of the process in 4 to 5 days.

Principles of Fracture Treatment

REDUCTION

Restoring anatomic alignment to the fractured bone is termed *reduction*. Obviously, no reduction is required for nondisplaced fractures and inherently stable impacted fractures. Displaced fractures result from the etiologic trauma and the pull of those muscles crossing the fracture site. Reduction necessitates restoration of length and correction of angular and rotational deformity. *Manipulative* reduction can usually be performed in fractures of the distal extremities (hand, wrist, foot, leg) where muscle spasm is not excessive. More proximally, because of the pull of the quadriceps and hamstrings in femoral fractures and the biceps and triceps in humeral fractures, the application of continuous *traction* may be required to overcome these more powerful muscles and achieve reduction. Traction may be applied either by adhesive felt strips on the skin or by inserting a transverse pin through bone distal to the fracture. Certain fractures may not be appropriate for manipulative or traction reduction, in which case operative *open reduction* is performed. Open reduction is usually accompanied by some form of internal fixation with plates, pins, rods, or screws.

In specific circumstances, it may be desirable to remove a portion of bone rather than attempt reduction. Comminuted fracture of the patella or radial head, where disruption of the articular surface precludes anatomic reduction, is most appropriately treated by removal of the patella or radial head. Fractures of the neck of the femur in elderly patients are often slow to heal, and the patient may be more rapidly rehabilitated by removal of the femoral head and replacement with a prosthesis. Specifics of operative fracture care will be covered in other sections of this chapter.

IMMOBILIZATION

When reduction has been achieved, *immobilization* of the fracture site is required until sufficient healing has occurred. A variety of techniques are used for immobilization, depending on the fracture. Impacted fractures of the proximal humerus are inherently stable, and only a sling or soft dressing is required. Similarly, compression (impaction) fractures of the vertebrae are appropriately treated with a corset or brace. Fractures for which open operative reduction is required are usually immobilized with internal hardware, and external immobilization is not normally necessary. Most fractures of the extremities can be immobilized with a plaster or fiberglass cast or with commercially available braces. Familiarity with plaster technique is essential because improperly applied casts may produce damaging neural, vascular, or skin pressure. For extremity fractures, immobilization of the joints above and below the fracture site is usually necessary to eliminate force transmission to the fracture. For example, a long arm cast immobilizing both the elbow and the wrist is necessary for a forearm fracture. When the cast is applied, the patient is cautioned to watch for progressive pain, and numbness or pallor, which are signs of continued swelling within the rigid confines of the cast. Should these symptoms occur, it is necessary to split the cast to relieve pressure. All fracture patients are seen the following day for neurologic and vascular assessment.

When traction is utilized for reduction, it also serves as a means of immobilization with the limb supported on the bed or on splints until reduction is achieved. Traction is then continued until there is sufficient healing so that the patient can be transferred to a cast or brace.

OPEN FRACTURES

An open fracture is an emergency. Wound débridement is required in the operating room when other injuries have been evaluated and the patient is medically stable. Open fractures may be graded according to the size of the wound and degree of contamination. All devitalized tissue is removed, with special attention paid to nonviable muscle.

Macerated skin edges are sharply débrided, vessels and nerves are preserved, and bone ends, which may contain embedded dirt, paint, or other debris, are débrided with rongeurs. Deep cultures are taken, and the wound is thoroughly irrigated with antibiotic solution. Immediate repair of nerves or tendons is not necessary and may be performed only in clean wounds. Arterial repair may be required if the limb is in jeopardy. When the fracture wound is small (less than 1 cm.) and contamination is minimal, wound closure may be appropriate. For more extensive wounds, the wound is dressed open, the fracture immobilized with a cast, splint or by traction, and delayed primary closure is performed in 3 to 5 days if suppuration is not present. Generally, the insertion of internal fixation in an open fracture at the time of débridement is not advised. Where extensive skin loss prevents closure, splint skin or pedicle skin grafts may be required.

FRACTURE HEALING

Within the hematoma that envelops the fracture site and the adjacent edema from venous congestion, initially a sterile inflammatory reaction occurs. Primitive mesenchymal cells from the adjacent periosteum, endosteum, and fascial planes begin to differentiate into osteoblasts, and granulation tissue invades the hematoma. These changes, appreciable at 2 to 3 days microscopically, produce the "fracture callus," which becomes radiographically evident at 12 to 14 days when mineralization in primitive osteoid occurs. The fracture callus bridges the gap between fragments and gradually matures into lamellar bone. The rate at which fractures heal is influenced by age, site, and local physical forces on the fracture. If compression of the fracture ends is present (compression plate, weight bearing in lower extremity fractures), maturation of the fracture callus is accelerated. If motion is present, the primitive mesenchymal cells may differentiate into cartilage rather than bone. If motion is not excessive, cartilage calcification followed by endochondral ossification results in ultimate healing. With continued excessive motion, however, a cleft develops in the cartilaginous callus, producing a *pseudoarthrosis*. Excessive distraction at the fracture site may produce fibrous tissue rather than bone and a resulting *fibrous non-union*. Fracture healing is also affected by available blood supply. Metaphyseal fractures thus heal more rapidly than diaphyseal fractures, and fractures with more overlying muscle (femur) heal more predictably than fractures in which the bone is subcutaneous (tibia).

REHABILITATION

When solid bony union has occurred, rehabilitation is largely a matter of soft tissue recovery. Contracted ligaments, muscles, and joint capsules restrict joint motion when the cast or splint is removed. These limitations are more evident in fractures close to joints than in the midshaft of long bones. Physical therapy for active and passive motion and muscle strengthening is advised. Stasis edema, present after cast removal, gradually diminishes with the return of motion and muscle tone.

LATE COMPLICATIONS

Non-union subsequent to excessive motion or distraction may necessitate operative intervention for bone grafting or may be successfully treated by electrical stimulation. *Malunion* occurs when there is excessive rotary or angular malalignment that is allowed to heal. Malunion may produce functional or cosmetic problems that are unacceptable, and osteotomy and repositioning may be needed. *Posttraumatic arthritis* may occur when the fracture extends through a joint surface and healing results in joint irregularity. For intra-articular fractures, operative treatment is usually necessary for accurate reduction. *Avascular necrosis* of bone may result in certain fractures in which the blood supply to a portion of bone is interrupted. Most often, this complication is seen in the femoral head with femoral neck fractures and in the carpal scaphoid bone. The development of avascular necrosis leads to joint surface collapse and results in the need for prosthetic arthroplasty. *Shortening* of an extremity after fracture is a frequent occurrence. In the upper extremity, shortening is normally not noticed and is not a functional problem. In the lower extremity, a shoe lift may be needed for shortening of greater than one-half inch.

FRACTURES IN CHILDREN

Skeletal maturity is reached at approximately age 13 in girls and age 16 in boys. Fractures prior to these ages deserve special considerations. Bone is under the influence of growth hormone throughout these years, and fractures tend to heal more rapidly and predictably than in adults. Non-union is rare. Furthermore, the skeleton is constantly enlarging and changing shape to accomodate changes in body size, habitus, and activity. This potential for accommodation is observed in fracture remodeling in children. Angular malunion can remodel to an amazing degree, particularly when in the plane of motion (flexion, extension) of an adjacent joint. There is less remodeling potential when there is malposition at right angles to adjacent joint motion (varus, valgus) and no potential for remodeling of rotary malalignment. The younger the child, the greater the potential for remodeling. As the child approaches skeletal maturity, malposition is less acceptable.

The preceding guidelines apply particularly to diaphyseal fractures. For fractures involving the physeal growth plate, other concerns are raised. Injury to the physeal plate may result in total growth arrest of that plate with future shortening of the limb or in partial arrest with subsequent angular growth and deformity. Salter has classified physeal plate fractures according to their potential for growth disturbance.

Type I fractures are through the physeal plate only, involve no adjacent bone, and have the least potential for growth arrest after anatomic reduction.

In *Type II* injuries, the fracture line extends partly through the physeal plate and exits through the adjacent metaphysis.

Type III injuries involve the physeal plate and adjacent epiphysis.

In *Type IV* injuries, the fracture line extends from the metaphysis across the physeal plate and into the epiphysis.

Type V injuries involve an axial force that crushes the physeal plate and is associated with a high incidence of growth arrest.

Physeal plate injuries necessitate anatomic reduction and may require operative intervention. If internal fixation is required after reduction, a smooth pin is used and is removed as soon as the fracture is stable.

III

Fractures of the Upper Extremity

ROBERT D. FITCH, M.D.

DISLOCATION OF THE SHOULDER

The anatomic features of the shoulder, an unconstrained joint, allow a remarkable range of motion but also render it susceptible to traumatic dislocation. The humeral head articulates with a shallow articular disc of the scapula termed the *glenoid*. The glenoid is anteverted approximately 20 degrees, which in part accounts for the more frequent occurrence of anterior versus posterior dislocations. Joint stability is primarily provided by the glenoid labrum, joint capsule, and rotator cuff musculature.

An anterior shoulder dislocation is caused by forced abduction and external rotation of the shoulder. With this mechanism the anterior labrum and capsule is torn (*Bankhardt lesion*[2]) and the humeral head is levered over the anterior rim of the glenoid, which can cause a groove in the posterior aspect of the humerus (*Hill-Sachs' lesion*).[9] This injury occurs most commonly in young, active adults. A similar mechanism in children and young adolescents is more likely to result in a fracture of the proximal humerus, usually through the growth plate.

Evaluation

Clinical examination of the patient with an acute dislocation of the shoulder will reveal the arm splinted at the side. An obvious indentation in the soft tissue is usually seen just beneath the acromion. Physical examination should include a thorough neurologic and vascular evaluation because injury to the axillary nerve and artery can occur. The diagnosis is confirmed by radiographs, including anteroposterior and tangential scapular views.

Treatment

Treatment should be prompt, since the longer the shoulder remains unreduced the more difficult it is to obtain a reduction because of progressive muscle spasm. The reduction should be done in a gentle manner, and sedation is usually required. Occasionally, general anesthesia is needed. Reduction is usually achieved by gradual longitudinal traction on the arm with countertraction applied to the axilla. Alternatively, the patient can be placed in the prone position with the arm allowed to extend off the table. With sedation and gradual traction, reduction usually occurs spontaneously within 15 to 20 minutes (*Stimson method*).[18] Postmanipulation radiographs are obtained to confirm reduction and to exclude an associated fracture of the greater tuberosity. The arm is then immobilized at the side in a sling in internal rotation for about 3 weeks. Progressive range of motion exercises are then begun. Recurrent anterior dislocation is common, particularly in the younger age group, and reconstruction may be needed.[1, 8, 15]

FRACTURES OF THE PROXIMAL HUMERUS

Fractures of the proximal humerus usually result from a fall on the outstretched arm, causing forced abduction, extension, and external rotation. This injury may also occur from a direct blow to the lateral aspect of the proximal humerus. Because of the occurrence of osteoporosis in the elderly, fractures in the proximal humerus are frequent in this age group and are usually a result of relatively minor trauma. When fractures of the proximal humerus occur in young adults, severe trauma is usually involved.

Neer has proposed a classification based on the observation that fractures in this region occur between all four of its major components: the articular segment, the greater tuberosity, the lesser tuberosity, and the metaphyseal region or surgical neck. The fracture is identified as having one, two, three, or four parts, depending upon how many fracture segments are displaced or angulated (Fig. 1).[14]

Evaluation

Clinical examination should include evaluation of the vascular supply to the limb as well as a thorough neurologic examination to exclude an associated brachial plexus injury. Radiographic evaluation includes an anteroposterior and

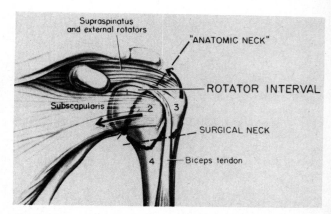

Figure 1. The proximal humerus is divided into four parts. 1, Articular segment; 2, lesser tuberosity; 3, greater tuberosity; 4, proximal humerus. Neers' classification of fractures is dependent upon recognition of fracture lines and displacement of the various parts.

transcapular lateral view to document the fracture, the number of fracture fragments, and the degree of displacement.

Treatment

Nondisplaced fractures can be treated by immobilization of the arm in a sling and swath for 2 to 3 weeks followed by a range-of-motion exercise program. Displaced surgical neck fractures are usually treated successfully without surgical intervention by manipulation of the distal fracture fragment into position followed by a similar period of immobilization as described earlier. If there is an associated greater tuberosity fracture that cannot be reduced closed and is displaced more than 1 cm., open reduction with internal fixation is indicated since malunion in a displaced position will interfere with a functional range of motion of the shoulder. For displaced three-part fractures of the humerus, open reduction with some form of internal fixation is usually required. Fractures involving the anatomic neck, as in four-part fractures are managed by open reduction or acute prosthetic replacement of the articular segment. A prolonged postoperative rehabilitation program is usually required to obtain a functional range of shoulder motion following severe trauma.

FRACTURES OF THE SHAFT OF THE HUMERUS

Humeral shaft fractures are usually caused by direct trauma or fall on the arm. Direct blows or lateral bending movements usually cause a transverse fracture, whereas indirect torsional forces result in oblique spiral fractures. In complete fractures, displacement usually results because of muscles acting on the separate fracture fragments. The proximal fragment is usually abducted by the deltoid muscle, whereas the distal fragment is shortened and adducted by the pull of the biceps, triceps, and coracobrachialis. The radial nerve is in proximity to the humerus in the middle and distal thirds of the humeral diaphysis. With fractures in this location, direct contusion or laceration can occur.[17]

Evaluation

Clinical examination should include assessment of radial nerve function. Pain and swelling in the region of the fracture are noted, and motion at the fracture site is usually clinically detectable. Anteroposterior and lateral radiographs of the humerus will identify the fracture location, pattern, and degree of comminution.

Treatment

Nondisplaced fractures can be treated by immobilization of the humerus against the chest in a sling and swath manner for 2 to 3 weeks and protected activities for about 8 to 10 weeks. When the fracture is displaced, gentle repositioning of the arm will usually align the fragments adequately. A coaptation splint,[5] a sugar tong plaster splint applied from the axilla around the elbow to the level of the proximal humerus laterally, is adequate to maintain an acceptable reduction. Occasionally, a hanging arm cast is utilized.[4] In this treatment modality, a light cast is applied above the elbow to the level of the fracture site. A sling is applied to the cast, and the fracture alignment can be changed by the location of the sling attachment to the cast.

The radial nerve, if injured prior to fracture manipulation, is usually not operatively explored, since gradual return of radial nerve function can be expected. However, if radial nerve function is present initially and subsequently lost following manipulation or if there has been no evidence of radial nerve recovery after 8 to 12 weeks, exploration of the radial nerve should be performed. Only rarely, as in the case of vascular compromise or nerve repair, are open reduction and internal fixation of this fracture indicated, because most can be expected to unite with nonoperative treatment. In established non-unions, open reduction and internal fixation with plates or intramedullary devices and bone grafting are necessary.

SUPRACONDYLAR AND INTERCONDYLAR FRACTURES

Supracondylar fractures of the humerus account for 50 to 60 per cent of all fractures about the elbow. This is a common injury in children, and management is fraught with complications unless careful consideration is given the injury. In the child, radiographic evaluation is difficult because many of the secondary ossification centers about the elbow may not yet be ossified. In adults, these fractures tend to be comminuted and involve the articular surface of the distal humerus and may lead to permanent joint incongruity and stiffness. Injury to the brachial artery or median nerve by direct laceration or compression is not uncommon in this injury. If arterial inflow is disrupted by a displaced fracture or edema, the severe complication of a Volkmann's ischemic contracture may result.[12]

There are two types of supracondylar fractures, depending upon the mechanism of injury. The most common type is the *extension injury*. This is a result of a fall on the outstretched arm with subsequent posterior displacement of the distal fragment with varying degrees of anterior angulation at the fracture. Loss of the normal 20-degree anterior tilt of the distal humerus is evident on radiographs. The *flexion type* of supracondylar fracture occurs less frequently. This is a result of a fall on a flexed elbow with the compression and flexion forces resulting in anterior displacement of the distal fragment with a resultant posterior angulation at the fracture site.

Evaluation

Clinical examination will reveal pain and varying degrees of swelling in the region of the distal humerus and elbow. Neurovascular status must be carefully assessed because of the frequent association with arterial or nerve injury. Anteroposterior and lateral radiographs of the distal humerus are evaluated to determine the location of fracture, amount of displacement, and degree of comminution. In children, comparison radiographs of the uninvolved distal humerus are important in assisting in interpretation of fractures about the elbow. The subtle x-ray findings of rotary malalignment and varus impaction should be carefully assessed, and Baumann's angle is a useful measurement to avoid varus malposition.[6]

Treatment

Immobilization with the elbow flexed to 90 degrees for approximately 3 weeks is required for nondisplaced fractures. What may appear to be a nondisplaced fracture initially on the radiograph may in fact be a varus impacted fracture, and if it is not reduced, this will lead to loss of the normal carrying angle of the arm and cubitus varus. A varus impacted fracture should be manipulated, and this usually can be performed under sedation. Disimpaction of the varus angulation is followed by immobilization of the elbow in a posterior plaster splint. For the displaced fractures without neurologic deficit or vascular compromise, closed reduction under anesthesia is indicated. Reduction is performed by gradual gentle traction with the arm slightly flexed. When the fracture fragments are disimpacted, manual flexion of the distal humerus is performed and medial or lateral displacement is corrected at this time. The elbow is then flexed to 90 degrees, and the stability of the fracture is assessed. If the fracture is not stable with the elbow flexed to 90 degrees, percutaneous pinning of the fracture is recommended. When the supracondylar fracture is associated with severe edema, preliminary side arm or overhead traction is useful. When properly applied, this type of traction can also be used to achieve a gradual reduction of the fracture.[6] This can be performed with the use of skin traction or skeletal traction by placement of a pin through the olecranon. If the fracture cannot be adequately reduced with traction, closed reduction with anesthesia with or without percutaneous pinning can be performed after the swelling has subsided.

A variation of the supracondylar fracture seen in children is a transepiphyseal fracture Salter-Harris Type I or II. In young children this condition may not be diagnosed or may be confused with a dislocation of the elbow. Careful radiographic evaluation of the relationship between the distal humerus, capitellum, and proximal radius will be necessary to identify this injury. With a displaced transepiphyseal fracture, the metaphysis of the distal humerus is displaced relative to the capitellum while the capitellum and proximal radius and ulnar maintain their normal anatomic relationship.

A lateral condyle fracture in a child may appear radiographically to be a minor injury but may lead to significant deformity if not diagnosed and properly managed. This type of fracture occurs by a fall on the outstretched arm with the forearm forcefully abducted, imparting a valgus and compressive force to the distal humerus. This is an intra-articular fracture, usually a Salter-Harris Type IV injury. Unlike most fractures in children, there is a significant propensity for this fracture to eventually result in non-union.[7] Furthermore, if union occurs in a malreduced position, because of its intra-articular nature this will lead to an incongruous joint. Radiographs of the distal humerus must be closely inspected in regard to this injury. In young children, the only sign of this injury may be slight malposition of the capitellum ossific nucleus compared with the contralateral side or the presence of a small metaphyseal fragment (*Thurston Holland sign*).[10]

Nondisplaced fractures can be managed by immobilization of the arm at 90 degrees flexion for approximately 3 weeks. However, one must be careful to evaluate radiographs to be certain that there is no significant displacement and that there is no rotary malalignment. Displaced lateral condyle fractures require open reduction and anatomic restoration of position as well as pin fixation to diminish the likelihood of malunion or non-union.

FRACTURE OF THE OLECRANON

The olecranon is subject to fracture because of its subcutaneous location and susceptibility to direct trauma. The olecranon forms the ulnar articulation at the elbow and is the point of insertion for the triceps tendon.

Evaluation

Physical examination will show swelling and pain in the region of the proximal ulna and, if displaced, the fracture line should be palpable and crepitance may be noted. Anteroposterior and lateral radiographs of the elbow will determine the location of the fracture, the amount of displacement, and the degree of comminution.

Treatment

For displaced fractures, open reduction and internal fixation are necessary so that the articular surface can anatomically be maintained and the triceps extensor mechanism of the elbow can be restored. Internal fixation is usually performed by a modified tension band wiring technique or a single intramedullary screw. Nondisplaced fractures can be treated by immobilization of the elbow at about 60 degrees of flexion for 3 weeks. Rigid internal fixation of displaced fractures will allow early active motion and decrease the late complication of elbow stiffness.

FRACTURE OF THE RADIAL HEAD

Radial head fractures are common in both adults and children. Such fractures usually occur as the result of a fall on the outstretched arm, which may impart a valgus compressive stress to the proximal radius. Impaction of the radial head against the capitellum may lead to fracture. In children, this mechanism may cause an epiphyseal fracture or a compression fracture distal to the epiphysis in the metaphyseal region. In adults most fractures are intra-articular and treatment depends on the amount of displacement and angulation as well as the amount of articular surface damage.

Evaluation

Physical examination will reveal tenderness in the region of the radial humeral joint and proximal radius, and forearm rotation (pronation and supination) will be painful and limited. Radiographic evaluation is necessary to determine the location of the fracture, the amount of displacement, and the degree of comminution.

Treatment

Treatment depends upon the severity of the injury. Most epiphyseal injuries can be reduced by manipulation and treated nonoperatively. Metaphyseal compression fractures in children should also be reduced if the angular deformity is greater than 30 degrees. If closed reduction cannot be obtained, open reduction may be necessary. In adults with minimally displaced fractures, only temporary immobilization is required for pain to subside; however, if the fracture involves more than 50 per cent of the articular surface and is comminuted, primary radial head excision may be the treatment of choice. Articular fractures involving less than a third of the articular surface should be treated by temporary immobilization and early range of motion exercises.

SHAFT FRACTURES OF THE RADIUS AND ULNA

The two bones of the forearm, radius and ulna, share a complex relationship. Proximally, the radius and ulna articulate with one another and with the distal humerus. Distally, the radial-ulnar articulation at the wrist is maintained by the triangular fibrocartilage complex. The shafts of the radius and ulna are connected by a fibrous interosseous sheath. Any distortion of the anatomy in the forearm will alter its biomechanical function and limit the ability of the forearm to undergo pronation and supination.

One or both bones of the forearm may be fractured. A fracture of the proximal one third of the ulna associated with radial head dislocation is termed a *Monteggia fracture*.[3] A fracture of the middle or distal one third of the radius can be associated with the disruption of the distal radial ulnar joint (*Galeazzi*[16] or *Piedmont*[11] *fracture*). Most commonly, however, both forearm bones are fractured.

Evaluation

Evaluation of a patient with both bone forearm fractures will show obvious deformity of the forearm with angulation. Early assessment of the neurovascular condition of the extremity is important because swelling within the forearm muscle compartments can lead to a *compartment syndrome* and decompression may be required. The forearm findings associated with a compartment syndrome include increased tissue pressure upon palpation of the forearm musculature. One of the early sensitive physical findings is that of pain on passive extension of the fingers. Loss of radial pulse and loss of median and ulnar nerve sensation in the hand are late findings.

Radiographs of forearm injuries will define the location of the fracture and the pattern of injury and should include the elbow and wrist to identify associated radial head displacement or disruption of the radial-ulnar joint.

Treatment

In adults, displaced both bone fractures of the forearm should be treated by open reduction and internal fixation with compression plating.[13] Anatomic alignment between the radius and ulna must be restored to allow recovery of pronation and supination. Monteggia fractures should be treated by stabilization of the ulnar fracture and reduction of the radial head dislocation. Fractures of the distal third of the radius with or without radial-ulnar joint disruption (Piedmont fracture) should be treated by open reduction and internal fixation. Unlike the treatment in adults, most

of the time, management of these fractures in children can be accomplished by closed reduction and casting. Occasionally, a Monteggia fracture must be treated by open reduction if the radial head dislocation cannot be managed or if there is a persistent angular displacement of the ulna.

The serious complication of compartment syndrome, which can lead to *Volkmann's ischemic contracture,* must be avoided. Early recognition and surgical decompression will prevent this severe deformity.

FRACTURES OF THE HAND AND WRIST

Fractures of the hand and wrist have been described in the first section of this chapter.

SELECTED REFERENCES

Ogden, J. A.: Skeletal Injury in the Child. Philadelphia, Lea & Febiger, 1982, pp. 228–229.
Rockwood, C. A., and Green, D. P.: Fractures. Philadelphia, J. B. Lippincott Co., 1984.

REFERENCES

1. Bankart, A. S. B.: Dislocation of the shoulder joints. *In* Robert Jones' Birthday Volume: A Collection of Surgical Essays. London, Oxford University Press, 1928.
2. Bankart, A. S. B.: Pathology and treatment of recurrent dislocation of the shoulder joint. Br. J. Surg., *26*:23, 1939.
3. Bryan, R. S.: Monteggia's fracture of the forearm. J. Trauma, *11*:992, 1971.
4. Caldwell, J. A.: Treatment of fractures of the shaft of the humerus by hanging cast. Surg. Gynecol. Obstet., *70*:421, 1940.
5. Charnley, J.: The Closed Treatment of Common Fractures. Baltimore, Williams & Wilkins, 1961.
6. Dodge, H. S.: Displaced supracondylar fractures of the humerus in children: Treatment by Dunlop's traction. J. Bone Joint Surg., *54A*:1408, 1972.
7. Flynn, J. C., and Richards, J. F., Jr.: Nonunion of minimally displaced fractures of the lateral condyle of the humerus in children. J. Bone Joint Surg., *53A*:1096, 1971.
8. Heflet, A. J.: Coracoid transplantation for recurring dislocation of the shoulder. J. Bone Joint Surg., *40B*:198, 1958.
9. Hill, M. A., and Sachs, M. D.: A groove defect of the humeral head. A shoulder joint. Radiology, *35*:690, 1940.
10. Holland, C. T.: Radiographic note on injuries to the distal epiphyses of radius and ulna. Proc. World Soc. Med., *22*:695, 1929.
11. Hughston, J. C.: Fracture of the distal radial shaft: Mistakes in management. J. Bone Joint Surg., *39A*:249, 1957.
12. Lipscomb, P. R., and Burlson, R. J.: Vascular and neural complications in supracondylar fractures of the humerus in children. J. Bone Joint Surg., *37A*:487, 1955.
13. Muller, M. E., Allgower, M., and Willenegger, H.: Manual of Internal Fixation: Technique Recommended by the AP-Group. New York, Springer-Verlag, 1970.
14. Neer, S., II: Displaced proximal humeral fractures: Part I. Classification and evaluation. J. Bone Joint Surg., *52A*:1077, 1970.
15. Osmond-Clarke, H.: Habitual dislocation of the shoulder. The Putti-Platt operation. J. Bone Joint Surg., *30B*:19, 1948.
16. Range, M.: Anthology of Orthopaedics. Edinburgh, E. & S. Livingstone, 1968.
17. Seedon, H. J.: Nerve lesions complicating certain closed bone injuries. J.A.M.A., *135*:691, 1947.
18. Stimson, L. A.: An easy method of reducing dislocations of the shoulder and hip. Med. Rec., *57*:356, 1900.

IV

Pelvic and Lower Extremity Fractures

JOHN M. HARRELSON, M.D.

PELVIC FRACTURES

The pelvis is composed of the ilium, ischium, and pubis sacrum, and coccyx. Dense ligamentous attachments at the pubis anteriorly, and the sacroiliac joints posteriorly create a rigid ring. For practical purposes, fractures of the pelvis may be divided into stable, unstable, and acetabular fractures. The treatment and prognostic implications are different for each type.

Stable Fractures

Stable pelvic fractures are injuries that do not violate the bony ring of the pelvis or do so at only one site. Common examples of stable pelvic fractures are shown in Figure 1A. The fractures are through the pubic and/or ischial ramus in only one plane, and the bony ring remains stable. The two common sites of avulsion fractures at the point of insertion of major muscle groups, forceful contraction of which may avulse a fragment of bone, are shown in Figure 1B. Stable pelvic fractures normally result from moderate trauma and are appropriately treated by bed rest for 2 to 3 weeks followed by gradual mobilization. Crutches may be required in the early phase of rehabilitation.

Unstable Fractures

Unstable pelvic fractures are injuries that violate the pelvic ring in two or more places with loss of stable continuity between the two sides of the pelvis. The points of violation of the pelvis ring need not be fracture lines but may be disruption of the symphysis pubis or sacroiliac joint (Fig. 2). These injuries result from violent trauma and, as a result, are often associated with other fractures and injury in other tissue systems (pulmonary, visceral, head). The most life-threatening aspect of pelvic fracture is hemorrhage. Hypovolemic shock is not uncommon. A rising pulse rate, falling blood pressure and falling central venous pressure must be countered with rapid volume replacement. If bleeding persists and cardiovascular stability cannot be maintained, arteriography should be performed. Often, disruption of vessels in the hypogastric distribution can be identified and controlled by catheter injection of absorbable gelatin sponge (Gelfoam), autogenous clot, or metal coil. Rarely, disruption of the common or external iliac arteries may necessitate open operative control.

Direct injury to adjacent organs may also occur with displaced pelvic fractures. If displacement is present at the symphysis pubis, rupture of the bladder and rupture of the membranous urethra (in males) must be excluded. A retro-grade urethrogram is first obtained. The catheter is advanced into the bladder for cystography only if results are negative. Otherwise, direct catheterization may convert a partial urethral tear into a complete tear. If findings from both studies are negative but hematuria is present, an intravenous urogram should be obtained to determine ureteral or renal injury.

Since displaced fracture of the sacrum is rare, injuries to the rectum are uncommon. Similarly, vaginal injury is infrequently seen. Nonetheless, rectal and vaginal examination for bleeding, defects, and prostatic displacement should be performed. If findings are positive, further evaluation is required. When the fracture line traverses the sacrum or violates the sciatic notch, neurologic injury may be present; therefore, careful motor and sensory examination of the lower extremities is necessary.

Displacement in pelvic fractures results from both the etiologic trauma and the pull of muscles across the fracture. Treatment varies with the degree of displacement and the experience of the surgeon. When there is minor displacement, reduction may not be needed. Opening of the pelvis anteriorly may be reduced with a pelvic sling. When there is cephalad displacement of one half of the pelvis, heavy skeletal traction on the displaced side may be necessary. Operative reduction with internal fixation is usually not advised unless the acetabulum is involved and the surgeon has considerable experience, since the incidence of hemorrhage and postoperative infection is high. Traction and bed rest are maintained for 8 to 12 weeks or until fracture callus is evident. Gradual rehabilitation is then begun.

Acetabular Fractures

Acetabular fractures may be stable or unstable, depending on associated injury. The most common acetabular fracture is at the posterior rim and is associated with posterior dislocation of the hip. With this injury, the blood supply to the femoral head is disrupted and avascular necrosis may ensue. Dislocation of the hip is an emergency requiring prompt reduction and usually requiring spinal or general anesthesia. Open reduction is advised if (1) the hip is unstable after reduction, (2) a large displaced posterior rim fragment is present, or (3) the hip cannot be reduced by manipulation.

For central fractures of the acetabulum that distort the articular surface, open reduction is often required in an attempt to minimize the likelihood of future post-traumatic arthritis. This is particularly true when the superior weight-bearing portion of the acetabulum is involved. This procedure is difficult, is associated with a high morbidity, and is best performed by a surgeon with wide experience. In the older patient, later treatment by hip arthroplasty may be preferable to attempted open reduction.

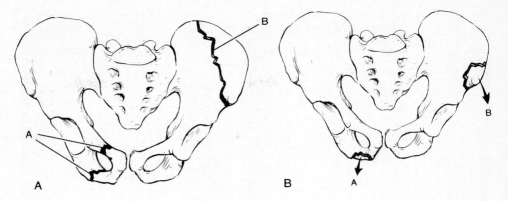

Figure 1. Pelvic fracture. A, Examples of stable pelvic fractures through the ischial and pubic ramus (A), which violates the pelvic ring at only one site, and through the iliac wing (B), which does not violate the pelvic ring. B, Examples of avulsion fractures of the pelvis at the site of attachment of the hamstrings (A) and the rectus femoris (B).

PROXIMAL FEMORAL FRACTURES

Fractures of the proximal femur are commonly referred to as "hip" fractures. Although most commonly encountered in the elderly female with osteoporosis, sufficient trauma may produce these fractures at any age. Proximal femoral fractures are classified anatomically (Fig. 3).

Femoral Head Fractures

Fractures of the femoral head are rare and are normally seen in association with dislocation of the hip joint. A portion of the femoral head is left in the acetabulum with the hip dislocation. These fragments are usually best removed, since reduction is difficult, blood supply is marginal, and healing unpredictable.

Femoral Neck Fractures

Fractures of the femoral neck may occur in the subcapital, midcervical, or basal regions. The femoral neck is within the joint and thus lacks periosteum. Accordingly, accurate reduction and bony apposition are necessary for endosteal healing to occur. The blood supply to the femoral head is primarily from the femoral side, and there is a 20 to 25 per cent risk of avascular necrosis in any femoral neck fracture. Increased age, displacement of the fracture, and length of time from injury to treatment all increase the likelihood of avascular necrosis.

Subcapital fractures are usually impacted and minimally displaced in valgus. Although they may be initially stable, resorption at the fracture site often results in displacement with conservative treatment. Internal fixation with threaded pins can be accomplished under fluoroscopy with minimal morbidity and allows more rapid rehabilitation. *Transcervical* and *basilar neck fractures* are usually displaced and are inherently unstable. Displacement may further compromise blood supply by injury to capsular vessels. In the young patient, prompt reduction and internal fixation are advised. In the elderly patient, general debility and the increased risk of avascular necrosis make replacement of the femoral head with a prosthesis more appropriate. Since fracture healing is no longer a factor, prosthetic arthroplasty allows more rapid mobilization and diminishes the morbidity associated with prolonged bed rest in the elderly. Hip prostheses eventually produce acetabular wear or loosen with time (events that require further operative procedures) and should be avoided in the young or active patient.

Intertrochanteric Fractures

Fractures of the intertrochanteric region of the femur are common. Avascular necrosis is not a threat, since the hip capsule and its vessels remain intact. Intertrochanteric

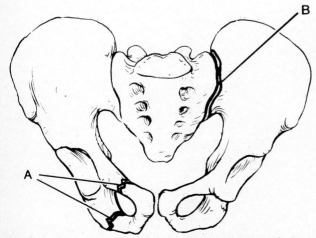

Figure 2. Example of an unstable pelvic fracture with violation of the pelvic ring at two sites (A and B).

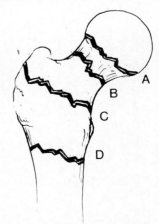

Figure 3. Examples of common proximal femoral fractures through the subcapital region (A), the midcervical region (B), the intertrochanteric region (C), and the subtrochanteric region (D).

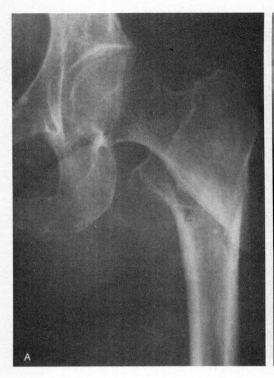
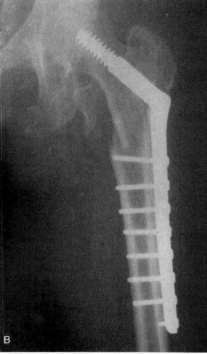

Figure 4. These radiographs demonstrate a preoperative intertrochanteric fracture (A) and postoperative fixation (B) with screw and side plate.

fractures are best treated operatively to avoid the 12 to 14 weeks of immobility required for conservative treatment. Particularly in the elderly, the morbidity of operative treatment is less than that associated with prolonged conservative care. Since these fractures usually occur in the elderly, careful preoperative evaluation is necessary.

Intertrochanteric fractures are classified by the location of the fracture line(s) and degree of comminution (Boyd). A *Type I fracture* is a single fracture along the intertrochanteric line. It can be reduced by longitudinal traction and internal rotation and is immobilized by insertion of a screw and side plate device (Fig. 4). *Type II fractures* are comminuted and may be more difficult to reduce. Fixation is with a screw and sideplate but repositioning of the proximal (head and neck) fragment in valgus may be necessary to achieve medial bone contact and stability.

Type III and IV fractures occur in the *subtrochanteric* region of the femur and are inherently unstable. These fractures may not be adequately supported by a conventional screw and side plate and the use of an intramedullary rod in conjunction with a femoral neck nail (Zickel) provides better stability (Fig. 5).

FEMORAL SHAFT FRACTURES

Fractures of the femoral shaft occur from major trauma, and associated injuries are common. Hemorrhage into the thigh from femoral fracture may approach 1500 to 2000 ml., and hypovolemic shock may ensue. When the fracture is open, prompt débridement, irrigation, and an-

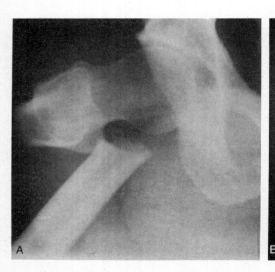
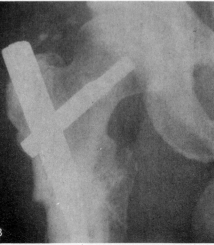

Figure 5. These radiographs demonstrate a subtrochanteric fracture fixed with an intramedullary nail (A) and femoral neck nail (Zickel) (B).

tibiotics are indicated followed by conservative management in traction with delayed wound closure. When associated injuries are present, reduction and immobilization by traction are also appropriate until the patient's condition is stable. Indeed, in decades past, skeletal traction for 5 to 6 weeks followed by immobilization in a spica cast from nipples to toes was standard treatment. Disadvantages of traction and spica cast management include joint stiffness, imperfect reduction, a higher incidence of malunion and non-union, and the increased cost of prolonged hospitalization.

Today, there are three basic methods of treating femoral shaft fractures: cast, brace, intramedullary nails, and plate fixation.

Cast Brace

Cast brace immobilization employs a total contact cast applied over an elastic stocking with minimal or no padding. The fracture is first reduced by skeletal traction for 10 to 14 days or until swelling and tenderness have subsided. Hinges connect the thigh portion of the cast to the below-knee portion and allow knee motion to be maintained. Crutch walking with partial weight bearing is allowed when sufficient fracture callus is present. This technique results in minimal shortening, allows better joint motion than spica casting, and avoids the risks of operative intervention. However, experience is important and careful monitoring of the fracture by x-ray is needed to avoid loss of reduction. Cast bracing is best suited for midshaft and distal shaft fractures. When the cast brace is used for upper shaft fractures, an attached pelvic band and hip hinge are required.

Intramedullary Nails

Intramedullary nailing of femoral shaft fractures was introduced by Küntscher. As originally described, the fracture site and proximal end of the femur were exposed, the fracture fragments were reamed to uniform internal diameter, and the intramedullary nail was driven from the greater trochanter across the reduced fracture. The development of newer nails and instruments and the availability of intraoperative fluoroscopy have popularized the "closed nailing" technique, in which the fracture is reduced under fluoroscopy and all reaming and nailing are performed through a single incision over the greater trochanter. Intramedullary nailing is best suited for simple fractures at the isthmus (junction of proximal and middle thirds) of the femur but may be used for more proximal or distal fractures. In comminuted fractures, transverse interlocking screws may be fixed to the intramedullary nail and bone for added stability. Operation is undertaken only when the patient is medically stable and any open wounds have been satisfactorily managed. The advantages of intramedullary nailing include early ambulation, preservation of joint motion, and reduced hospital stay. The disadvantages include the risks of anesthesia and infection. Severe comminution may preclude intramedullary fixation because stable fixation, the goal of the operation, cannot be achieved.

Plate Fixation

Plate fixation of femoral shaft fractures is not commonly employed but may be considered for comminuted fractures in which intramedullary nailing is contraindicated and reduction cannot be achieved or maintained by traction and cast management. The degree of stability achieved by plating is less than with intramedullary fixation, and supplementation with a cast brace is often necessary.

SUPRACONDYLAR FEMORAL FRACTURES

Fractures in the *supracondylar* region of the femur may be simple transverse injuries or may be comminuted, dividing the condyles (Fig. 6). These fractures are generally unstable, with the forces of the quadriceps, hamstrings, and gastrocnemius causing extension at the fracture site. Undisplaced fractures may be satisfactorily treated by cast immobilization. However, satisfactory reduction by traction is difficult to achieve when displacement is present. Deformity and limited motion at the knee often result from closed treatment. Accurate reduction of the articular surface is mandatory. Operative reduction with internal screw and plate fixation produces better overall results.

FRACTURES OF THE PATELLA

The patella is most frequently injured by violent contact with a dashboard or by a fall on a hard surface. Violent contraction of the quadriceps may produce an avulsion fracture. By whatever mechanism, there is usually an associated tear of the retinaculum of the knee joint when the fracture fragments separate. Since the entire dorsal surface of the patella is articular, any treatment that leaves the fragments unreduced is unacceptable. When comminution is not excessive, surgical reduction, wire or screw fixation, and retinacular repair constitute the preferred treatment. When comminution is extensive and reduction cannot be achieved, patellectomy may be required to obtain adequate knee function. If comminution is present only at the superior or inferior pole, partial patellectomy may produce good results. Postoperatively, the knee is immobilized for 2 to 3 weeks before motion exercises are begun.

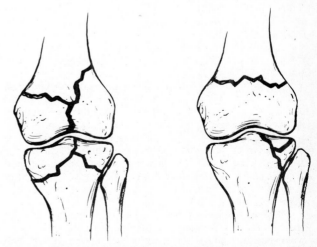

Figure 6. These drawings demonstrate common patterns of fractures of the distal femur and proximal tibia. When there is displacement of these fracture fragments, open reduction and internal fixation are usually required.

FRACTURES OF THE UPPER TIBIA

The upper tibial articular surface is basically a flat plane or *plateau* on which rest the two rounded condyles of the femur. Bending, twisting, or axial trauma to this area may produce a variety of fractures of the *tibial plateau*. In the simplest of these injuries, the femoral condyle is driven into the underlying tibia, producing a central, depressed, articular fracture. More frequently, the trauma is sufficient to produce comminution, which extends to the tibial metaphyseal cortex. One or both condyles may be involved with loss of congruity of the upper tibial articular surface (Fig. 6). Tomograms are required for complete delineation of these injuries.

When only central depression is present and the amount of displacement is less than 5 mm., conservative treatment is sufficient. Immobilization with cast or brace until effusion and tenderness have resolved, crutches to avoid weight bearing, and gradual mobilization are appropriate. When articular depression is greater than 5 mm. or when comminution results in angular displacement of the condyles, operative restoration of tibial articular congruity is required. For isolated central depression, arthrotomy to visualize the defect, reduction by prying the fragment into position through a hole placed in the tibial cortex, and bone grafting are performed. The graft and fracture fragment are further supported with transverse pins or screws. Extensive comminution with condylar displacement requires a buttress plate for adequate support.

FRACTURES OF THE TIBIAL SHAFT

The tibia is exposed to a wide variety of vehicular, industrial, and athletic trauma. Because the anterior surface of the tibia is subcutaneous throughout its length, tibial fractures are often open injuries. Also because of its subcutaneous location, the blood supply to the tibia is less than for other bones and infection, and delayed union and non-union are more common.

For *closed tibial shaft fractures,* reduction is accomplished manually under general or spinal anesthesia and immobilization provided by long leg cast. Fluoroscopy aids in achieving reduction. The goal of reduction is to regain length and correct rotary and angular alignment. With satisfactory reduction, weight bearing can be started in 3 to 4 weeks or when adequate fracture callus is present. Solid healing may occur as early as 12 to 14 weeks in young patients, but delayed union up to 6 months is not uncommon.

For *open tibial shaft fractures,* prompt débridement, irrigation, and antibiotics are required. Primary wound closure is usually not indicated. Skin loss is not uncommon with violent trauma, and delayed closure with split-thickness grafts, full-thickness grafts, or rotational muscle flaps may be required. These demands for wound care may make cast management difficult. Fixation can be accomplished with transverse skeletal pins above and below the fracture attached to an external frame that allows access to the wound (Fig. 7).

Surgical fixation of tibial fractures is indicated when adequate reduction cannot be achieved or maintained by closed methods and when overall care of the patient will be facilitated by early ambulation. Both plates and intramedullary nails have been used for internal fixation. Operative intervention for closed fractures introduces the risks

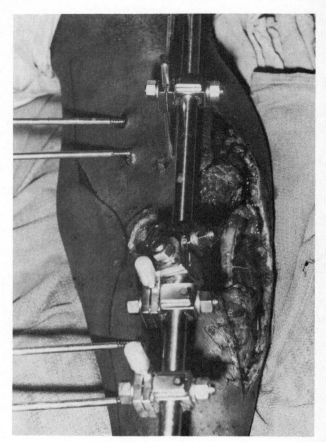

Figure 7. This surgical photograph demonstrates external fixation of an open tibial fracture with transverse pins and an external metal frame. This technique allows access for wound management.

of infection and must be weighed against the risks of closed treatment. Since the patient with a tibial fracture can be mobilized on crutches promptly, there is less to recommend operative intervention.

FIBULAR FRACTURES

Isolated fractures of the upper two thirds of the fibula are uncommon and of little clinical consequence. Fractures in the distal fibula affect ankle stability and will be considered under ankle fractures. When an apparent isolated fibular fracture is seen, careful attention should be given to the tibia to exclude occult fracture and to the medial ankle ligaments, which may be injured in association with proximal spiral fractures of the fibula. Fractures at the fibular neck may be associated with injury to the adjacent peroneal nerve. A protective cast and crutches for 2 to 3 weeks until tenderness resolves are usually sufficient as treatment.

ANKLE FRACTURES

In contrast to the hip and knee, the ankle joint depends on bony congruity for much of its stability. Small alterations in alignment of the articular surfaces can result in future post-traumatic arthritis. Accordingly, accurate reduction of fractures involving the ankle is mandatory. Operative internal fixation is most often employed. Fracture of the distal tibial or fibula usually results from a combination of abduction or adduction stress combined with some degree of internal or external rotation.

Abduction and/or *external rotation stress* may tear the medial deltoid ligament or produce an avulsion fracture of the medial malleolus. Laterally the fibula may sustain a spiral or transverse fracture, usually above the level of the ankle joint, and may be displaced laterally by tearing of the interosseous membrane. Further displacement may fracture the posterior portion of the tibia (the posterior malleolus). Thus, abduction external rotation stress may produce (1) a medial malleolar fracture, (2) a medial malleolar fracture with spread of the tibiofibular interval, (3) a bimalleolar fracture, (4) a bimalleolar fracture with spread of the tibiofibular interval, or (5) a trimalleolar fracture (Fig. 8).

Adduction and/or *internal rotation injury* to the ankle most often causes a sprain of the lateral ligaments. Greater force, however, may produce an avulsion fracture of the fibular malleolus at the joint level and a shearing injury of the medial malleolus, which usually extends above the joint line (Fig. 9).

Medial and posterior malleolar fractures are fixed with a cancellous screw. Fibular fractures are best controlled with a semitubular plate. For spread of the tibiofibular interval in abduction/external rotation injuries, a screw from the fibula into the tibia may be required for anatomic reduction. This screw should be removed at 6 weeks before weight bearing is begun. Postoperative care involves 6 weeks in a short leg cast without weight bearing. Thereafter, 4 weeks in a walking cast is required, by which time complete union is usually present.

In a high-speed vehicular accident, axial force to the foot may so severely comminute the distal tibia that anatomic reduction cannot be achieved by any means. Post-

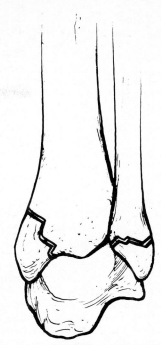

Figure 9. A common pattern of adduction internal rotation fracture of the ankle with an avulsion fracture of the fibula at the joint line and an oblique fracture of the medial malleolus.

traumatic arthritis usually ensues, and ankle fusion is required for salvage.

FRACTURES OF THE FOOT

Calcaneal Fractures

Fracture of the *calcaneus* is a common injury usually resulting from falling or jumping from a height. For practical purposes, these injuries may be classified as extra-articular and intra-articular.

Extra-articular fractures in the body or tuberosity of the calcaneus do not communicate with the subtalar joint. Displacement is usually minimal, and treatment by cast immobilization and gradual weight bearing produce good results with minimal residual disability or deformity. When displacement of a tuberosity fracture is excessive or when an avulsion fracture at the attachment of the Achilles tendon is present, reduction and screw fixation may be required to achieve healing and avoid deformity.

Intra-articular fractures of the calcaneus are more frequent, and because of extensive comminution they involve depression of the subtalar articular surface, loss of height of the calcaneus due to flattening, and varus malposition of the posterior portion of the calcaneus. Treatment of this injury by cast immobilization often results in disability from post-traumatic arthritis. There has been a renewed interest in open reduction and internal fixation of comminuted intra-articular calcaneus fractures prompted by more accurate preoperative assessment by computed tomography. For operative reduction to be accomplished, a medial exposure is required to reduce the varus component and restore the height of the calcaneus and a lateral exposure with arthrotomy of the subtalar joint is needed to reduce the articular fragment and to add bone graft beneath it for support.

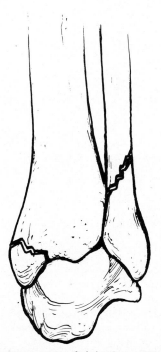

Figure 8. A common pattern of abduction external rotation fracture with a fracture of the fibula above the level of the ankle joint and an avulsion fracture of the medial malleolus.

Fixation is done with pins and staples. Cast immobilization and non–weight bearing are maintained for 6 to 8 weeks. Operative reduction restores the anatomic relationship between the calcaneus and talus and diminishes the likelihood of future post-traumatic arthritis. When post-traumatic arthritis does occur, it produces disability and pain. Arthrodesis of the subtalar, talonavicular and calcaneocuboid joints (triple arthrodesis) will relieve pain and improve function.

Talar Fractures

Fracture of the talus is uncommon and involves some of the problems encountered in hip fractures. These injuries, when displaced, may interrupt the blood supply to the body of the talus with resulting avascular necrosis. *Talar neck fractures* are usually vertical and result from acute dorsiflexion (foot on the brake pedal in a head-on collision). When the fracture is undisplaced, treatment by cast immobilization with non–weight bearing for 8 to 10 weeks is adequate and non-union and avascular necrosis are rare. When there is displacement at the fracture site, anatomic reduction is mandatory. Although this can sometimes be accomplished with closed reduction, open reduction with internal fixation is often necessary. Avascular necrosis is more frequent with displaced fractures and is virtually certain to occur when there is associated dislocation of the tibiotalar joint. Avascular necrosis is seen on post-treatment radiographs as relative increased density of the body of the talus. Although a few patients may regain a blood supply subsequently, the usual course is one of collapse of the talus with secondary arthritis of both the ankle and subtalar joints requiring ankle and triple arthrodesis for relief.

Midtarsal Fractures

Fractures of the midtarsal bones are uncommon and usually result from either a direct crushing injury or a fall from a height. These fractures can usually be managed conservatively by manual reduction and cast application. Only when manual reduction cannot be achieved and significant comminution and displacement are present is operative intervention entertained. Dislocation at the tarsometatarsal level may occur at one or more of the tarsometatarsal joints. In its severest form, this plantar flexion injury results in a spread between the first metatarsal and lateral metatarsals and may result in disruption of the dorsalis pedis artery. Manual reduction is attempted, but if it is unsuccessful it should be followed by open reduction. Excessive bleeding from the torn dorsalis pedis artery can produce massive dorsal swelling with ultimate compression of the posterior tibial artery and a risk of forefoot gangrene. Decompression and ligation of the dorsalis pedis artery may be required in this injury.

Metatarsal and Phalangeal Fractures

Fractures of the metatarsals may occur at any level within the bone and are usually the result of direct blows or falls. When the fracture is isolated to one metatarsal, operative treatment is rarely indicated. Manual reduction can usually be achieved and anatomic reduction is not necessary, since the foot is supported by the remaining metatarsals. Whe multiple fractures occur involving all metatarsals, forefoot instability may make it desirable to perform open reduction and internal intramedullary fixation with Kirschner wires.

For fractures of the phalanges, only manual reduction and taping to an adjacent sound toe are required.

V

Fractures of the Spinal Column

JAMES R. URBANIAK, M.D.

If a patient complains of neck or back pain or of tenderness after an accident, a fracture of the spine must be suspected. A thorough neurologic examination is necessary, since the early neurologic state influences the management and prognosis. Since more than 90 per cent of spinal fractures do not involve the neural structures, the institution of appropriate treatment provides an excellent prognosis. An understanding of spatial relationships of the contents of the neural canal and the skeletal structures is necessary for the management of these injuries. In the cervical and thoracic areas, the spinal cord occupies 50 per cent of the spinal canal. The spinal cord terminates at L2, and in the lumbar area there is a capacious space about the cauda equina.

CERVICAL SPINE

If the patient complains of neck pain, stiffness, or tenderness after an accident, a careful history and neurologic examination are important. Cervical spine roentgenograms, including anteroposterior, lateral, open-mouth odontoid, and oblique views, are necessary. The cervical spine should be immobilized until the radiographic studies are obtained. If these findings are negative, supervised gentle lateral flexion-extension views of the cervical spine should be obtained. Tomograms and computed tomography (CT) scans are often necessary to delineate the injury.

Fractures of the Atlas

The atlas is most often fractured through the arches by axial loading on the top of the head (Fig. 1*A*). Fracture of the ring of C1 is termed a *Jefferson fracture*. Since the fragments usually spread and enlarge the neural canal, the spinal cord is rarely injured. If the neurologic examination is normal, the injury can be treated with a neck and chin brace (four-poster brace). If motion (flexion-extension) radiographs demonstrate instability, a halo-vest brace is recommended.

Fractures of the Odontoid

Fractures of the odontoid (dens) are frequent and occur at two anatomic regions—the waist and the base of the odontoid (Fig. 1*B*). The fracture may be difficult to visualize on routine films, and tomograms of the odontoid are helpful. The dens, spinal cord, and empty space all occupy a third of the spinal canal at the level of the arch of the atlas ("rule of thirds"). This free space may be compromised by a rupture of the transverse or alar ligaments or by an unstable fracture of the dens. Immediate or delayed myelopathy may result from ligamentous injury of odontoid fractures.

Fractures through the base of the dens involve cancellous bone and will usually unite in 3 months in a four-poster brace. Fractures through the waist of the dens are more common and more difficult to manage. Reduction is necessary by traction with a halo or tongs attached to the skull. If union does not occur after 3 months of immobilization in a halo-vest brace, the posterior cervical fusion of C1 to C2 is indicated.

Fractures of the Pedicle of the Axis

A fracture through the pedicle of C2 results from a severe extension injury of the neck. It has been called the *hangman's fracture*, since autopsy studies have demonstrated that hanging by a rope will produce this fracture. The body of C2 becomes displaced anteriorly on C3, and the neural arch is usually enlarged; cord compression is therefore rare. The fracture is treated by a four-poster brace and union usually occurs in 3 months.

Fractures and Dislocations of the Lower Cervical Spine

Fractures and dislocations of the C3 to C7 vertebrae are common. Motor vehicular accidents are the most common cause, but many of these injuries occur from diving into shallow water and from sports injuries. If a cervical spine injury is suspected, the C7 vertebra must be visualized on the lateral radiograph. If it is not, the patient's shoulders must be pulled caudad for clear views of the lower cervical spine. These fractures may be stable or unstable, depending on the mechanism of injury and the structures involved.

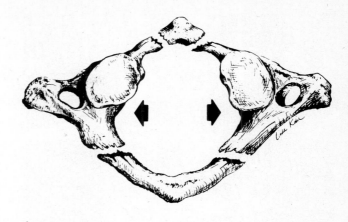

A

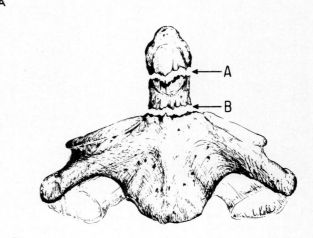

B

Figure 1. A, Jefferson fracture. Fracture of the arches of C1 secondary to an axial load. The result of the forces, indicated by the arrows, produces the fracture at the thinnest areas of the arch. B, A fracture of the odontoid may occur at the waist (A) or at the base (B). The fracture at the base is more stable and usually heals with immobilization. A fracture in the waist of the odontoid is less stable, and surgical fusion may be required for stabilization. (From Urbaniak, J. R.: Fractures of the spine. In Sabiston, D. C., Jr. (Ed.): Davis-Christopher Textbook of Surgery. Philadelphia, W. B. Saunders Company, 1977, p. 1528.)

A *compression fracture* of the vertebral body secondary to a flexion force is usually not severe. This fracture is stable if there is no comminution of the body, no facet dislocation, and no tearing of the posterior longitudinal ligament. Since neurologic involvement is unusual, minimal bracing is necessary.

In contrast, the *burst* or *tear drop fracture* of the body is usually catastrophic with a high incidence of spinal cord damage. The fragments of the body may be posteriorly displaced to impact the spinal cord. The fracture is extremely unstable and cervical skeletal traction, cervical fusion, and halo-vest immobilization are usually required for 3 to 4 months. Another method of management is anterior resection of the fragments and disc material and interbody arthrodesis with a bone graft.

Dislocations of the Lower Cervical Spine

Dislocations of the lower cervical spine are caused by flexion-rotation forces with dislocations of the facet and

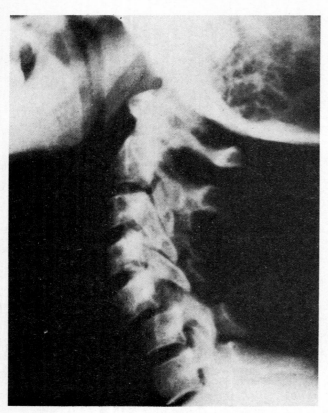

Figure 2. A dislocation of the cervical spine. This injury may or may not produce cord or nerve root damage. Reduction is usually achieved by relaxation and skull traction with tongs or a halo. Surgery is sometimes necessary to achieve reduction and stabilization.

disc and tearing of the posterior longitudinal ligaments. One or both facets may be jumped and locked. Associated fractures may occur. The neurologic involvement ranges from none to complete quadriplegia. A lateral roentgenogram demonstrates the forward dislocation of the vertebral body and the jumped facet or facets (Fig. 2).

Fracture and dislocations of the cervical spine are managed in a similar fashion to fracture and dislocations of other parts of the skeleton; the fragments are realigned and the dislocation reduced. Most dislocations can be reduced by skeletal traction and manipulation; in some cases, operative reduction is required. When there is neurologic involvement, the reduction is more urgent.

After the diagnosis and neurologic status are determined, skeletal traction (tongs or halo) is applied. With the use of serial radiographs, the initial weight of 15 to 20 pounds is gradually increased over a few hours by 5-pound increments with the patient awake. If reduction is achieved, immobilization in a halo-vest is maintained for 3 months. If closed reduction is not possible, operative reduction with posterior cervical fusion is performed. Fusion is also indicated if the reduction is unstable.

THE THORACOLUMBAR SPINE

In the thoracic area, the spinal cord occupies nearly half of the spinal canal; however, in the lumbar area—since the spinal cord usually terminates at L2—the neural canal has considerable free space. Consequently, for fractures or dislocations in the lumbar area more displacement is needed to produce neurologic damage than for fractures in the thoracic spine. Also, fractures below L2 will involve only the roots and not the spinal cord.

If a spinal injury is suspected, the patient should be examined in the position initially found. After a brief neurologic examination to determine the motor and sensory status, the clothing should be removed for a detailed inspection. The patient may be gently manipulated to a lateral position to palpate each vertebra for tenderness. A complete neurologic examination is essential prior to radiographic studies. Motor, sensory, and reflexes as well as intercostal and abdominal muscle function are tested. The anal sphincter tone and bulbocavernosus reflexes as well as perianal sensation are important. The *bulbocavernosus reflex* usually recovers during the first 24 hours after injury. Recovery of the reflex in the presence of complete anesthesia (including the perianal region) and paralysis is definite evidence that the paralysis of the lower extremities will be permanent. Also, complete loss of motor and sensory function, including *perianal sensation*, during the first 24 hours after injury indicates complete cord injury.

Following routine roentgenographs of the suspected area of injury, tomograms, myelogram, and CT scans are frequently indicated, especially if there is neurologic involvement.

For purposes of management, it is practical to classify spinal fractures as stable or unstable. In a *stable* fracture, the fragments are not likely to move and cause neural damage during the healing phase. In an *unstable* fracture, movement and neural damage are likely. The instability may be acute or chronic. The goal is to achieve or maintain spinal stability to establish a painless, functional back.

Stable Injuries

FLEXION

Flexion injuries that result in wedge compression fractures of the thoracolumbar spine are common and stable (Fig. 3A). Neurologic loss is uncommon. These injuries are painful, and treatment consists of hospitalization for a few days of bed rest and observation for paralytic ileus secondary to involvement of the sympathetic ganglia. If the wedging is greater than 50 per cent, a brace or cast in extension is suggested. Otherwise, analgesics, a corset, and early ambulation are recommended. Prolonged discomfort is not uncommon.

LATERAL BENDING AND EXTENSION

Lateral bending (Fig. 3B) and extension injuries are uncommon in the thoracolumbar area. These injuries are stable, and neurologic deficit is rare. Treatment for comfort (analgesics and corset) is all that is necessary.

VERTICAL COMPRESSION

Axial forces cause compression fractures of two types: (1) protrusion of the disc into the vertebral end-plate and (2) the "burst" fracture (Fig. 3C). The former occurs in the young patient with protrusion of the nucleus through the vertebral end-plate into the softer cancellous bone. These are stable fractures, and neurologic deficit does not occur. Treatment includes analgesics, a few days of bed rest, and a corset for a few weeks.

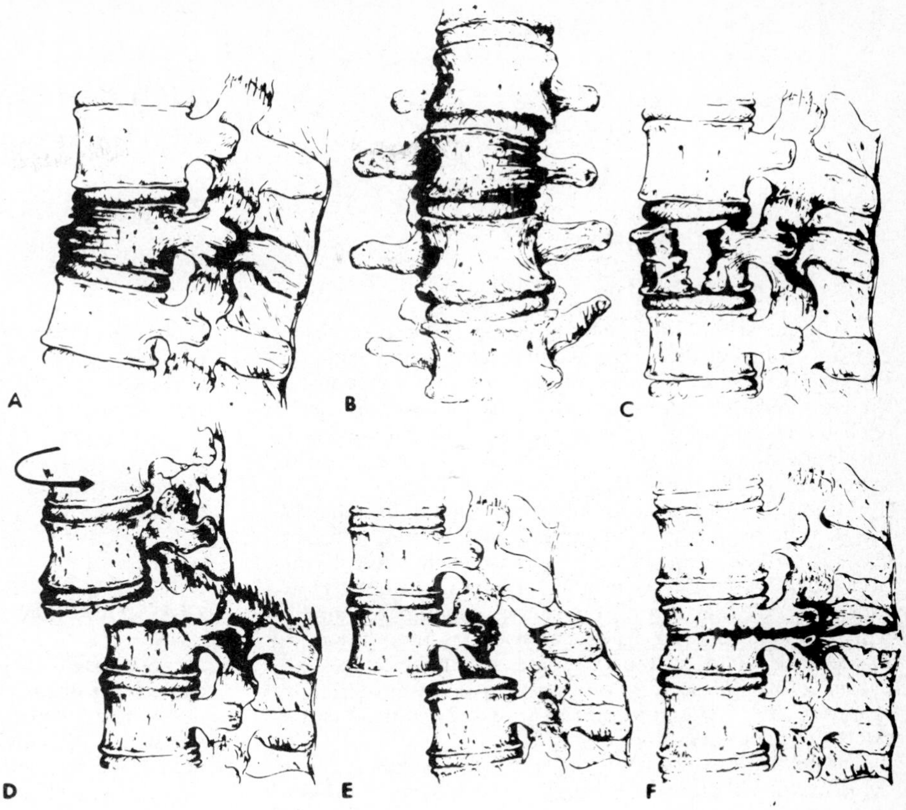

Figure 3. Stable and unstable injury.
A, A wedge compression fracture of the dorsolumbar spine. The posterior elements and ligaments remain intact. This fracture is stable, and neurologic loss is uncommon.

B, A lateral wedge compression fracture of the vertebral body is a stable fracture and usually without neurologic loss.

C, "Burst" fracture of the lumbar vertebral body. These fractures are usually stable, but neurologic loss may result from posterior displacement of the fragments into the spinal cord or roots.

D, Unstable flexion-rotation injury of the dorsolumbar spine. Neurologic loss is uncommon with this injury and reduction and stabilization by surgery are usually indicated.

E, The anteroposterior "shear" fracture of the lumbar spine. This fracture is generally stable above T10, but unstable below this level.

F, A "Chance fracture" is a horizontal splitting of the neural arch and vertebral body. It is secondary to a flexion-distraction force and may or may not be stable.

(From Urbaniak, J. R.: Fractures of the spine. In Sabiston, D. C., Jr. (Ed.): Davis-Christopher Textbook of Surgery. Philadelphia, W. B. Saunders Company, 1977, p. 1533.)

Although the "burst" fracture is quite stable, neurologic involvement may occur because of encroachment of the fragments into the spinal canal. The CT scan provides most valuable radiologic information in the injury. If no neurologic involvement is present, the patient is managed by bed rest until the acute symptoms subside. A brace or plaster jacket to hold the spine in extension for 3 or 4 months is recommended.

When neurologic involvement exists, the fragments must be removed from the neural canal. The approach may be anterior, lateral, or posterior. Stabilization by wire rods, plates, or bone grafts is necessary to prevent instability after the decompression.

Unstable Injuries

ROTATION-FLEXION INJURY

The combination of flexion and rotation can result in a fracture-dislocation with a very unstable spine (Fig. 3D). Since these injuries are so unstable, the patient must be handled with care to protect the spinal cord and roots. These fracture-dislocations most often occur at the transitional area of T10 to L1 and are associated with a high incidence of neurologic loss.

After accurate radiographic assessment (especially a CT scan), decompression by removal of the displaced elements and spinal stabilization by various metallic devices are indicated.

SHEAR FRACTURES

A vertebra may be displaced in an anteroposterior or lateral direction (Fig. 3E) by severe trauma. The pedicles or articular processes are usually fractured. If the injury occurs in the thoracic region, complete paraplegia results.

Although the fracture is very unstable in the lumbar area, neurologic sparing is common because of the large free space in the lumbar neural canal. These fractures are managed the same as the flexion-rotation injuries.

FLEXION-DISTRACTION INJURY

The *Chance fracture* (Fig. 3F) occurs from a flexion-distraction force such as a seat belt injury. A horizontal splitting results, and the fracture is usually unstable. Surgical stabilization is recommended.

SELECTED REFERENCES

Annotated References

Denis, F.: Spinal instability as defined by the three-column spine concept in acute spinal trauma. Clin. Orthop. Relat. Res., *189*:65, 1984.
This article presents the currently accepted classification of spinal fractures in the thoracolumbar area. This classification, based on the anterior, middle, and posterior columns, provides a practical categorization for treatment selection.

Rockwood, C. A., Jr., and Green, D. P. (Eds.): Fractures in Adults, 2nd ed. Philadelphia, J. B. Lippincott Co., 1984.
A complete text for thorough description of all fractures of the extremities and spine. In each section, different methods of treatment are discussed and each author emphasizes a preferred method.

General References

Bohlman, H. H., and Eismont, F. J.: Surgical techniques of anterior decompression and fusion for spinal cord injuries. Clin. Orthop. Relat. Res., *154*:57, 1981.
Flesch, J. R., Leider, L. L., Erickson, D. L., Chou, S. N., and Bradford, D. S.: Harrington instrumentation and spine fusion for unstable fractures and fracture-dislocations of the thoracic and lumbar spine. J. Bone Joint Surg., *59A*:143, 1977.
Holdsworth, F. W.: Fractures, dislocations and fracture dislocations of the spine. J. Bone Joint Surg., *52A*:1534, 1970.
McAfee, P. C., Yuan, H. A., and Lasda, N. A.: The unstable burst fracture. Spine, *7*:365, 1982.

VI

Introduction to Pediatric Orthopedics

ROBERT D. FITCH, M.D.

Musculoskeletal disorders affecting children represent a wide variety of diseases affecting the growing skeleton. Because of the growth plate of the axial and appendicular skeleton, a different response to injury and disease can be expected compared with that seen in the adult. In addition, congenital and developmental anomalies as well as a wide variety of genetic disorders must be considered.

Because pediatric orthopedics is such a broad field, this section, by necessity, must be limited to selected topics, chosen for their frequency and significance in clinical practice. Not covered in this section is pediatric trauma. However, the physician caring for children should be familiar with the Salter-Harris classification of fractures involving the growth plate. Although some specific fractures are discussed in the section on upper and lower extremity fractures, the reader is referred to excellent texts extensively covering this subject.[3, 4]

Osteomyelitis, pyarthrosis, and other pediatric musculoskeletal infections are causes of significant morbidity and can lead to permanent disturbance of growth with secondary deformity. The reader is referred to excellent discussions of this topic in the basic pediatric orthopedic texts.[2, 5]

Neuromuscular conditions in children are associated with many skeletal abnormalities. For diagnosis and treatment of these conditions, an understanding of the pathophysiology as it relates to the musculoskeletal system is often required. These disorders include paralytic conditions such as poliomyelitis, myelodysplasia, cerebral palsy, arthrogryposis, and the muscular dystrophies.[1]

The topics covered in this section are outlined to emphasize the clinical and radiographic features of the disorders. Treatment modalities are discussed; for the reader who desires in-depth coverage of treatment, pertinent references are provided.

REFERENCES

1. Drennan, J. C.: Orthopedic Management of Neuromuscular Disorders. Philadelphia, J. B. Lippincott Co., 1983.
2. Lovell, W. B., and Winter, R. B.: Pediatric Orthopedics. Philadelphia, J. B. Lippincott Co., 1978.
3. Ogden, J. A.: Skeletal Injury in the Child. Philadelphia, Lea & Febiger, 1982.
4. Rockwood, C. A., and Green, D. P.: Fractures. Philadelphia, J. B. Lippincott Co., 1984.
5. Tachdjian, M. O.: Pediatric Orthopedics. Philadelphia, W. B. Saunders Company, 1972.

1 • SCOLIOSIS

Scoliosis, derived from a Greek word meaning curvature, implies a pathologic condition. The cervical, thoracic, and lumbar vertebrae form a vertical column with the center of the vertebrae representing the midline. Any lateral deviation of the vertebrae from the midline constitutes scoliosis. Although a frontal plane deformity is always considered abnormal, spinal curvature in the sagittal plane is physiologic. These spinal contours are termed *kyphosis* and *lordosis*. The thoracic spine normally has a gentle kyphotic contour, and the cervical and lumbar spine are lordotic.

CLASSIFICATION

Scoliosis can be *structural* or *functional*; a structural curve lacks normal flexibility, whereas a functional curve is not a fixed deformity. An example of a functional (or *nonstructural*) scoliosis is that secondary to a limb length discrepancy. In order for the trunk to be centered over the pelvis, it must assume a scoliotic posture. Paravertebral muscle spasm as seen with a herniated nucleus pulposus may also lead to a nonstructural scoliosis. Occasionally, a hysterical conversion reaction may present as scoliosis.

Structural scoliosis may be divided into three major categories: congenital, neuromuscular, and idiopathic. Congenital scoliosis is that secondary to abnormal vertebral development. The anomalies may be due to partial failure of formation of vertebra. The most common anomaly in this category is the hemivertebra. Vertebral malformations may be due to failure of segmentation, the most significant of which is the unilateral unsegmented bar. These vertebral anomalies may lead to significant structural scoliosis early in life. The unilateral unsegmented vertebral bar, in particular, is at risk for rapid curve progression. Congenital scoliosis may be associated with congenital anomalies of other organ systems, particularly renal and cardiac. Other skeletal abnormalities frequently associated with congenital scoliosis include Sprengel's deformity, Klippel-Feil syndrome, and radial dysplasia (radial clubhand).[10, 11]

ETIOLOGY

Scoliosis is seen as a complication of many neuromuscular diseases. Up to 80 per cent of patients with myelomeningocele have some form of scoliosis either secondary to paralysis or that due to congenital vertebral anomalies.[8] In virtually all children with Duchenne's muscular dystrophy, scoliosis develops at about age 8 to 10 years, which is coincidental with loss of ability to walk.[1] There is a high incidence of scoliosis associated with cerebral palsy, particularly in children with total body involvement, spastic quadriplegia.[3, 7] Other neurologic conditions frequently associated with scoliosis include spinal muscular atrophy, Friedreich's ataxia, poliomyelitis, and arthrogryposis.

IDIOPATHIC SCOLIOSIS

In most patients with structural scoliosis, there is no known obvious associated abnormality. These patients are categorized as having *idiopathic scoliosis*. Although the etiology of idiopathic scoliosis has not been defined, recent evidence points to subtle abnormalities in vestibulo-ocular and posterior column function.[12] The category of idiopathic scoliosis is further subdivided:

1. *Infantile scoliosis* is a spinal curvature developing from birth to 3 years of life.

2. *Juvenile scoliosis* has an onset of from 3 to 10 years.

3. If onset of scoliosis occurs after 10 years of age, the patient is said to have *adolescent idiopathic scoliosis*.

PHYSICAL FINDINGS

The physical findings seen in scoliosis are a manifestation of a three-dimensional deformity. Findings are due to a combination of lateral deviation of the spine and rotational deformity of the vertebral bodies and chest wall. As lateral deviation of the spine occurs, the vertebrae rotate around their long axes. Curves convex to the right demonstrate a varying degree of rotation, which causes the right transverse processes, ribs, and paraspinal muscles to be displaced posteriorly (Fig. 1). It is this rotational deformity that causes the rib hump and paralumbar prominence.

When the patient is viewed from the back, examination may reveal lateral deviation of the spinous processes from the midline. Scapular asymmetry may be a manifestation of scoliosis, and one should observe variation in height of the distal tip of the scapula and any prominence of one scapula to the other. Lateral deviation of the trunk or trunk shift is best observed by comparing the triangle formed by the arm, trunk, and pelvis right and left. A right thoracic scoliosis with a trunk shift to the right will lead to an enlargement of the right triangle and the right upper extremity will hang further away from the pelvis than the left (Fig. 2A). Spinal decompensation, a deformity in which the head and neck are not centered over the pelvis, can be

determined by dropping a plumb bob from the spinous process of C7. Normally, the plumb line is continuous with the gluteal cleft. Lateral deviation of this line from the gluteal cleft is measured in centimeters.

After the patient has been viewed from the back in the standing upright position, the *forward flexion test* is performed (Fig. 2B). In the forward flexed position rotational deformity can be most easily observed and rib hump or paralumbar prominence can be detected. Minor curves are often most easily detectable by their rotational component. In general, as lateral deviation of the spine increases, so does the rotational deformity; however, this relationship is not linear, and many minor curves demonstrate significant rotation whereas some moderate or severe scoliotic deformities show only a milder rotational component. When the patient is viewed from the front, breast and chest wall asymmetry may be seen.

EVALUATION

Examination of patients with scoliosis must include observation for congenital skeletal anomalies. A thorough neurologic examination must be performed to exclude an associated neurologic condition. The skin should be inspected for café au lait spots seen in neurofibromatosis or any cutaneous manifestations of spinal dysraphism (hairy patch, sacral dimple).

Patients with evidence of structural scoliosis should have posteroanterior and lateral radiographic evaluation for congenital vertebral anomalies, posterior element defects, evidence of interpediculate widening, diastematomyelia, infection, or tumor. The radiographic measurement of scoliosis is determined by the *Cobb method*. The Cobb angle is measured by drawing a line perpendicular to the superior end plate of the uppermost vertebra in the curve and a perpendicular line from the inferior end plate of the most caudal vertebra. The intersection of these lines forms an angle that is measured (Fig. 3). Other useful information obtained by the radiograph includes the appearance and excursion of the iliac apophysis.[9] This and the ring apophysis of the vertebra provide information regarding the degree of skeletal maturity. In patients with infantile scoliosis, the rib-vertebral angle described by Mehta is a useful measurement in determining the prognosis of progression.[6]

TREATMENT

Whether treatment will be required for a scoliotic curve is dependent upon many factors, including etiology, skeletal age, curve magnitude, and evidence of progressive deformity. Successful treatment, in part, is dependent upon early detection of scoliosis. Screening programs are commonplace throughout the American school systems, and many adolescent and preadolescent patients are referred for evaluation. It is estimated that 5 to 10 per cent of children screened will have some spinal asymmetry. Fortunately, in adolescent idiopathic scoliosis most curves are mild and not progressive. Therefore, routine treatment of mild curves without evidence of progression is not indicated. The *mild curve* is classified as a curve under 25 degrees; a *moderate curve* is one that measures 25 to 40 degrees, and a *severe curve* is angled at greater than 40 degrees. In a patient who presents with a moderate scoliosis and is skeletally immature, there is a high risk for progression of the curve; in contrast, in a patient with the same curve who is skeletally

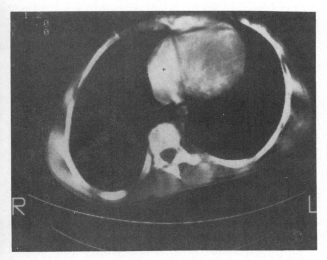

Figure 1. CT scan section through the apical vertebra of a patient with idiopathic scoliosis demonstrates the rotational deformity of the vertebral body, transverse processes, and ribs.

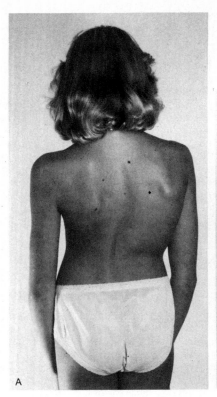
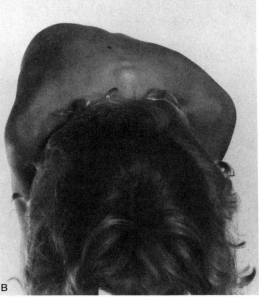

Figure 2. A, Right thoracic scoliosis. The clinical findings of right scapular elevation and asymmetry of the triangles formed by the arms and trunk are shown. B, The forward flexion test is used to demonstrate the rib deformity, often the earliest clinically detectable physical finding.

mature, there is an extremely low risk of progression.[4] Treatment is needed for curves in the moderate range that are progressive. One must realize that the goal of treatment in moderate curves is to deter progression of the deformity.

Currently, there are no nonoperative treatment methods available that offer permanent correction of the spinal deformity present at the institution of therapy. Therefore, treatment of a 30-degree scoliosis in a skeletally mature patient would not be beneficial, since it is unlikely that progression will occur and no permanent correction of deformity can be obtained.

Braces

The standard care for moderate curves in idiopathic scoliosis has been brace treatment, and spinal orthoses have been utilized for centuries. The modern era of brace treatment began with the development of the Milwaukee brace, designed by Blount and Schmidt in 1946. Since then, other thoracolumbosacral orthoses have been effectively utilized in controlling these spinal deformities.

Braces provide corrective forces through a combination of active distraction and passive correction with padding localized over the appropriate areas of the spine. A brace is utilized for patients who are skeletally immature and who demonstrate a progressive curve in the 25- to 40-degree range. The brace should be worn for 16 to 23 hours a day and must be worn until skeletal maturity, which is usually 14 years in females and 16 years in males. At skeletal maturity, the patient is gradually weaned from the brace. Periodically during brace treatment, radiographs of the spine are obtained to document the efficacy of treatment. Despite bracing, approximately 15 to 20 per cent of patients treated will show significant curve progression.

Surgery

Bracing is generally not effective for curves of a magnitude greater than 40 degrees. In general, when a curve reaches this severity or greater and the patient is

Figure 3. The Cobb angle is a useful means of measuring the lateral plane deformity in scoliosis.

60°

skeletally immature, operation is recommended. In addition, in the adult, operation is recommended if the curve is greater than 45 to 50 degrees. Curves of this magnitude have been shown to progress gradually over time even in adulthood. The goal in the operative treatment of scoliosis is to correct the deformity and maintain the correction until fusion of the spine occurs. It is the surgical technique of fusion that provides long-term spinal stability. Prior to the advent of the Harrington rod, correction of the spinal deformity was obtained through complicated casting techniques. In 1960, Harrington reported the use of stainless steel distraction rods for the correction and stabilization of spinal deformities.[2] This instrumentation has become the mainstay of surgical treatment of scoliosis.

Spinal Instrumentation

Segmental spinal instrumentation, introduced by Luque, has been developed for the management of spinal deformities and is particularly useful in complex cases such as patients with insensitive skin, spasticity, or respiratory compromise.[5] The stability achieved by this instrumentation is usually sufficient so that no external support by cast or brace is required.

The Cotrel-Dubousset instrumentation has recently been developed in France and is segmentally attached to the spine by a multiple hook fixation technique. It provides strong fixation like the Luque system and is effective in partially correcting the rotational deformity (Fig. 4).

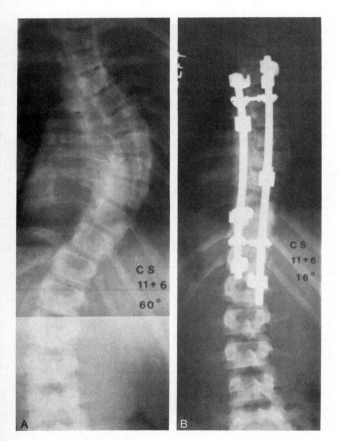

Figure 4. Progressive idiopathic right thoracic scoliosis. A, Sixty-degree curve. B, Treatment by fusion and correction with Cotrel-Dubousset instrumentation.

SELECTED REFERENCES

Moe, J. H., Winter, R. B., and Bradford, D. S.: Scoliosis and Other Spinal Deformities. Philadelphia, W. B. Saunders Company, 1978.
Winter, R. B.: The spine. In Lovell, W. B., and Winter, R. B. (Eds.): Pediatric Orthopedics. Philadelphia, J. B. Lippincott Co., 1978.

REFERENCES

1. Gibson, D. A., Koreska, J., Robertson, D., Kahn, A., and Albisser, A. M.: The management of spinal deformity in Duchenne's muscular dystrophy. Orthop. Clin. North Am., 9:437, 1978.
2. Harrington, P. R.: Treatment of scoliosis: Correction and internal fixation by spine instrumentation. J. Bone Joint Surg. 44A:591, 1962.
3. Lonstein, J. E., and Akbarnia, B. A.: Operative treatment of spinal deformities in patients with cerebral palsy or mental retardation. J. Bone Joint Surg., 65A:43, 1983.
4. Lonstein, J. E., and Carlson, M. J.: The prediction of curve progression in untreated idiopathic scoliosis during growth. J. Bone Joint Surg., 66A:1061, 1984.
5. Luque, E. R.: The anatomic bases and development of segmental spinal instrumentation. Spine, 7:256, 1982.
6. Mehta, M. H.: The rib-vertebral angle in the early diagnosis between resolving and progressive infantile scoliosis. J. Bone Joint Surg., 54B:230, 1972.
7. Palmer, G. A., and MacEwen, G. D.: The incidence and treatment of scoliosis in cerebral palsy. J. Bone Joint Surg., 52B:134, 1970.
8. Schafer, M. F., and Dias, L. S. Myelomeningocele: Orthopaedic Treatment. Baltimore, Williams & Wilkins, 1983.
9. Urbaniak, J. R., Schaefer, W. W., and Stelling, F. H.: Iliac apophysis. Clin. Orthop., 116:80, 1976.
10. Winter, R. B., Moe, J. H., and Eilers, V. E.: Congenital scoliosis: A study of 234 patients treated and untreated. J. Bone Joint Surg., 50A:15, 1968.
11. Winter, R. B., Moe, J. H., and Lonstein, J. E.: Posterior spinal arthrodesis for congenital scoliosis: An analysis of the cases of 290 patients, five to nineteen years old. J. Bone Joint Surg., 66A: 1188, 1984.
12. Yamada, K., Yamamoto, H., Nakugawa, Y., Tezuka, A., Tamura, T., and Kawata, S.: Etiology of idiopathic scoliosis. Clin. Orthop., 184:50, 1984.

2 • CONGENITAL DISLOCATION OF THE HIP

With the early detection of congenital dislocation of the hip (CDH), simple, safe, and effective treatment can be expected. It is during the first week of life that detection is most easily made. If the infant with CDH is not diagnosed during this period, successful nonoperative treatment becomes less likely and the complications of treatment increase considerably. The complications of avascular necrosis and inadequate reduction have further serious impact on the long-term prognosis of the hip.[1, 4] Therefore it is the orthopedist, pediatrician, and general practitioner's responsibility to be aware of physical findings that establish the diagnosis in the neonatal period.

There is a spectrum of pathology involved in CDH that ranges from subluxation to true dislocation. The incidence of hip dysplasia in the United States is approximately ten cases per 1000 live births. Most of these, however, are milder forms of hip dysplasia, with the incidence of true dislocation approximately one case per 1000. The incidence of CDH is much higher in females than males, with a risk ratio of 6:1. Additional risk factors include breech presentation, positive family history, firstborn child, and oligohydramnios. Furthermore, there is a definite association with muscular torticollis, positional calcaneovalgus feet, and metatarsus adductus. Thus, the classic profile of a child with CDH is the firstborn female with breech presentation and associated congenital or developmental anomalies.

The *typical* CDH must be distinguished from the teratologic hip dislocation. The distinguishing factor in the teratologic hip is the time at which the dislocation occurs. For the typical CDH, dislocation occurs in the perinatal period, at the time of birth or shortly thereafter. The teratologic hip dislocates antenatally, at some time during the fetal period. The distinguishing features in the teratologic hip are the presence of an unreducible hip at birth, secondary soft tissue contracture, and specific radiographic features, which will be discussed.

DIAGNOSIS

The importance of neonatal recognition has been emphasized. Successful diagnosis depends on familiarity with physical findings of CDH in the newborn. These findings are a manifestation of joint laxity and instability of the femoral head within the acetabulum. All infants should be examined in the newborn period for hip instability, with follow-up examinations performed at 1 and 3 months of age. For hip dysplasia to be detected by the Ortolani and Barlow maneuvers, the infant should be relaxed, preferably sleeping or feeding. If the infant is crying or otherwise agitated, these subtle physical findings will not be detectable.

The *Ortolani test* is a gentle manipulation of a dislocated hip into the acetabulum (reduction test). This maneuver is performed by examination of the hip in flexion. As traction is applied to the femur, the hip is gently abducted while pressure is applied to the trochanter posteriorly, encouraging the femoral head to slip over the rim of the acetablum obtaining a reduced position. This maneuver, when positive, is associated with a palpable "clunk" and feeling of migration of the proximal femur.

The *Barlow* or *provocation dislocation test* is a manifestation of the hip being translocated from a reduced position within the acetabulum to a subluxated or dislocated position. This test is performed in a manner similar to the Ortolani test except that the traction force is replaced by compression force applied to the femur. Simultaneously, the hip is adducted and an outward force is applied to the proximal femur by the thumb. Again, motion in the proximal femur is detected as the femoral head slips out of the acetabulum (Fig. 1).

These findings are usually present up to about 3 to 4 months of age. About this time, these physical findings are replaced by secondary findings, which are a manifestation of soft tissue shortening and contracture. As the hip remains in a dislocated position, the hamstrings and iliopsoas, which are already tight, become further contracted. In addition, the adductor muscles develop secondary shortening and the soft tissue contracture replaces the Barlow and Ortolani test findings by limited hip abduction and apparent femoral shortening (positive *Galeazzi's sign*) (Fig. 2). Other findings include asymmetric skin folds and elevation of the trochanter above an imaginary line drawn from the ischial tuberosity to the anterior superior iliac spine (*Nelaton's line*).

Radiographs in the newborn period are generally not helpful except to exclude other conditions such as congenital short femur or proximal femoral focal deficiency. However, as contractures develop, secondary radiographic findings become evident. There is a delay in the appearance of the ossific nucleus of the capital femur, Shenton's line is disrupted, there is lateral displacement of the proximal femoral metaphysis, roentgenographic signs of acetabular dysplasia become evident, and the development of a false acetabulum becomes visible (Fig. 3).[2] The latter finding may be present at birth in a teratologic hip dislocation.

TREATMENT

The goal of treatment is to obtain and maintain a concentric reduction of the hip dislocation without the complication of avascular necrosis. The safest and most effective method of treatment in the infant younger than 6 months of age is the Pavlik harness (Fig. 4).[3, 6] This device allows the proximal femur to be placed and maintained in flexion and moderate abduction, which positions the femoral head toward the center of the acetabulum. This is a "dynamic" splint, in that the infant can actively kick and exercise the extremities, which promotes a guided and gradual reduction of the hip dislocation without force. A mild degree of soft tissue contracture of the adductors will be treated with this device. The anterior straps allow positioning of the hips in flexion, and the hips should be flexed 90 to 110 degrees. The posterior straps limit adduction but should not be tightened to the extreme of passive abduction. The harness is 85 to 95 per cent successful when used in infants under 6 months of age and is associated with an extremely low incidence of avascular necrosis.

In children over 6 months of age or in whom treatment with the Pavlik harness has failed, traction is utilized prior to attempted closed reduction to decrease the risk of

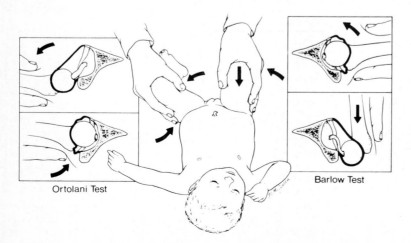

Ortolani Test

Barlow Test

Figure 1. On the left, the Ortolani (reduction) test is demonstrated. The Barlow (provocation dislocation) test is shown on the right. These tests must be performed on a relaxed infant.

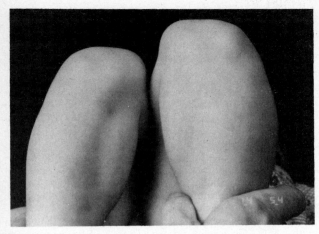

Figure 2. The Galeazzi test is performed by comparison of the relative height of the femoral condyles by holding the hips in flexion. The right femur appears shorter because of a right hip dislocation. This test is usually not helpful in the case of bilateral hip dislocations.

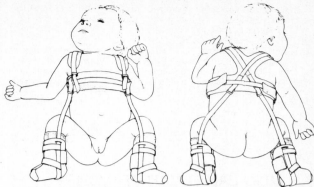

Figure 4. The Pavlik harness positions the hips in flexion and moderate abduction and is a safe and effective method of treatment for congenital hip dislocation in the infant under 6 months of age.

avascular necrosis. Traction is usually performed in the hospital, and the patient is placed in skin traction with adhesive wraps applied to both lower extremities. Generally, 2 to 3 weeks of traction are required to diminish soft tissue contracture, particularly the contracted adductors and hamstrings, and then under general anesthesia the dislocated hip is reduced. Oftentimes the quality of reduction is assessed by hip arthrography.[7] If an adequate reduction is obtained, the child is placed in a double hip spica cast with the hips in flexion and moderate abduction similar to the position desired with the Pavlik harness avoiding forced abduction.

If the hip cannot be reduced, if the reduction is poor as determined by arthrography, or if the reduction is extremely unstable and excessive abduction is required, open reduction is indicated.[9, 10] With surgical reduction, the main obstruction to reduction (hourglass constriction of capsule, transverse acetabular ligament, iliopsoas tendon, pulvinar, hypertrophied ligamentum teres) can be relieved.

In the older child beyond 2 years of age, secondary reconstructive procedures are often utilized to achieve improved stability of the hip at the time of operation. There are many procedures performed on the acetabulum to improve lateral coverage or redirect the acetabulum.[8] An alternative to traction in the older child beyond 2 years of age is primary femoral shortening.[5] This is done in the subtrochanteric region at the time of operation to achieve relaxation of the soft tissues. This procedure has the same beneficial effect as preliminary traction in terms of reducing the incidence of redislocation and avascular necrosis.

In conclusion, the importance of early detection of congenital dislocation of the hip is emphasized. The primary care physician must be familiar with the physical findings in the newborn. If there is any question that the hip is unstable, referral to a pediatric orthopedist is mandatory. The Pavlik harness is the most accepted method of treatment for infants under 6 months of age, and the old method of triple diapers is not acceptable. Finally, the forms of treatment discussed are widely accepted because they have been shown to reduce the serious complication of avascular necrosis of the femoral head.

SELECTED REFERENCES

Coleman, S.: Congenital Dysplasia and Dislocation of the Hip. St. Louis, C. V. Mosby Co., 1978.
Hensinger, R. H.: Congenital Dislocation of the Hip. N. J., CIBA Pharmaceutical Co., Vol. 31, No. 1, 1979.
Tachdjian, M. O.: Congenital Dislocation of the Hip. New York, Churchill Livingstone, 1982.

REFERENCES

1. Buchannan, J. R., Greer, R. B., and Colter, J. M.: Management strategy for prevention of avascular necrosis during treatment of congenital dislocation of the hip. J. Bone Joint Surg., 63A:140, 1981.
2. Caffe, J.: Pediatric X-Ray Diagnosis. Chicago, Year Book Medical Publishers, 1950.
3. Filipe G., and Carlioz, H.: Use of the Pavlik harness in treating congenital dislocation of the hips. J. Pediatr. Orthop. 2:357, 1982.
4. Gage, J. R., and Winter, R. B.: Avascular necrosis of the capital femoral epiphysis. J. Bone Joint Surg., 54A:373, 1972.
5. Klesic P., and Jankovic, L.: Combined procedures of open reduction and shortening of the femur in treatment of congenital dislocation of the hips in older children. Clin. Orthop., 119:60, 1976.

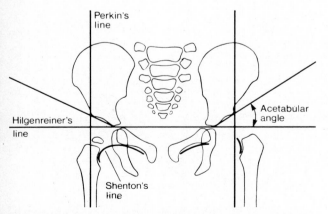

Figure 3. Radiographic features of congenital dislocation of the hip (left hip dislocated, right hip normal). There is a delay in ossification of capital femoral epiphysis. Shenton's line, a smooth continuation of an imaginary line drawn along the femoral neck and superior margin of the obturator foramen, is disrupted. The acetabular angle is increased usually greater than 30 degrees. The proximal medial margin of the femoral metaphysis is displaced lateral to Perkin's line, a line drawn from the lateral margin of the acetabulum perpendicular to Hilgenreiner's line.

6. Mubaruk, S., Garfen, S., Vance, R., McKennon, B., and Sutherland, D.: Pitfalls in the use of the Pavlik harness for treatment of congenital dysplasia, subluxation, and dislocation of the hip. J. Bone Joint Surg., *63A*:1239, 1981.

7. Race, C., and Herring, J. A.: Congenital dislocation of the hip: An evaluation of closed reduction. J. Pediatr. Orthop. *3*:166, 1983.

8. Salter, R. B.: Role of innominate osteotomy in the treatment of congenital dislocation and subluxation of the hip in the older child. J. Bone Joint Surg., *48A*:1413, 1966.

9. Scaglietti, O., and Calandriello, B.: Open reduction of congenital dislocation of the hip. J. Bone Joint Surg., *44B*:257, 1962.

10. Somerville, E. W., and Scott, J. C.: The direct approach to congenital dislocation of the hip. J. Bone Joint Surg., *32B*:623, 1957.

3 • LEGG-CALVÉ-PERTHES DISEASE

In 1909 and 1910, 15 years after the discovery of x-rays by Röntgen, the entity known as Legg-Calvé-Perthes disease was established. Waldenström,[15] in 1909, thought that the condition represented a benign form of tuberculous involvement of the hip. Later that year, Legg presented his paper at the American Orthopedic Association meeting, and in 1910 independent papers by Legg,[4] Calvé,[2] and Perthes[6] were published.

Although the etiology of this disease is obscure, the pathologic events are due to avascular necrosis of the capital femoral epiphysis. The process of infarction and subsequent repair is responsible for the syndrome known as Legg-Calvé-Perthes disease.[8, 9]

The blood supply to the proximal femur is derived from the medial femoral circumflex artery.[14] This vessel forms an anastomotic ring at the base of the femoral neck. From this ring, the posteroinferior and posterosuperior retinacular arteries traverse the femoral neck to supply the secondary ossification center of the capital femoral epiphysis. A branch of the lateral femoral circumflex artery supplies the region of the greater trochanter. Partial or total occlusion of this group of vessels leads to a varying degree of necrosis of the secondary ossification center.

When ischemia leads to bone infarction, the normal growth of the bony epiphysis temporarily ceases; however, the cartilage, which derives its nutrition from diffusion from the synovial fluid, continues to grow. A small area of cartilage adjacent to the bony epiphysis, which relies on the intact blood supply to this area, undergoes necrosis.

Blood flow eventually becomes re-established to the bony epiphysis. During this revascularization phase children usually become symptomatic. As granulation tissue invades the necrotic bone, the dead trabeculae undergo *creeping substitution* (a gradual replacement of dead bone with viable bone). During this healing phase, the bony epiphysis and overlying cartilage are susceptible to deformation and loss of sphericity, particularly if there is an abnormal distribution of the transarticular forces at the hip.

The onset of disease is generally from age 4 to 10 years, but children as young as 2 and as old as 13 can be affected. Boys are affected four times as often as girls, and the overall incidence in the United States is about one case per 1200 children. The disease is bilateral in approximately 20 per cent of patients. Legg-Calvé-Perthes disease must be differentiated from other conditions, including Meyers' disease, which is a benign irregular ossification of the capital femoral epiphysis in young children. In bilateral cases this disease can be confused with epiphyseal dysplasia. Also one must consider aseptic necrosis secondary to some underlying disease, such as the glycogen storage diseases and hemoglobinopathies, particularly sickle cell disease.

SIGNS AND SYMPTOMS

The most common presenting complaint is that of a limp. Usually, this is of insidious onset and is noted especially after physical activity and upon arising in the morning. In the younger patient, pain may be a minor symptom but appears to be more significant in the older age group. Pain may be located in the groin or anterior thigh, but it also can be referred to the knee. There are two forms of presentation of pain: (1) acute onset of pain, usually associated with fracture of the subchondral plate of the bony epiphysis, and (2) chronic, low-grade discomfort aggravated by activity. Stiffness is a significant component of the symptomatology and is particularly noted upon arising from bed in the morning.

Physical examination will show an antalgic gait, often with a knee-flexed gait pattern. There will be moderate to severe loss of range of motion of the affected hip, and the child usually guards the hip, resisting passive range of motion. Significant loss of abduction and internal rotation is common.

Radiographs are mandatory in evaluation of the child with a painful hip and anteroposterior pelvis, and frog lateral views are needed to assess the stage and degree of involvement of this disease.

Sommerville has classified the radiographic evolution of the disease into four stages.[13] The initial phase is the *ischemic stage*, followed by *fragmentation, healing*, and a final phase of *remodeling*. The earliest radiographic findings present prior to radiographic signs of bony infarction are loss of epiphyseal height and apparent widening of the joint space, which may be due in part to synovitis but is mostly due to loss of endochondral ossification within the bony epiphysis and continued growth of the unossified cartilage. In the necrotic phase the bony epiphysis appears radiodense and sclerotic. This is due to relative osteopenia of the

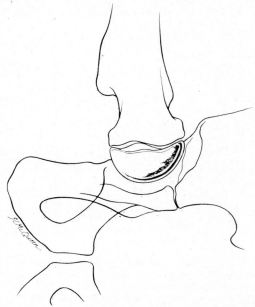

Figure 1. The subchondral fracture line, or Caffey's sign, is an early transient finding that is best seen on the lateral radiograph of the hip. This precedes the onset of epiphyseal fragmentation. The extent of the line correlates with the amount of epiphysis involved.

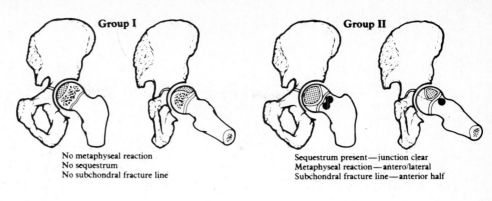

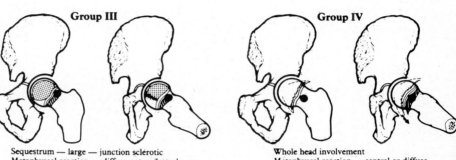

Figure 2. The Catterall classification of Legg-Calvé-Perthes disease is demonstrated. Radiographic features are divided into four groups, depending upon the amount of femoral head involved.

Group I

No metaphyseal reaction
No sequestrum
No subchondral fracture line

Group II

Sequestrum present—junction clear
Metaphyseal reaction—antero/lateral
Subchondral fracture line—anterior half

Group III

Sequestrum — large — junction sclerotic
Metaphyseal reaction — diffuse antero/lateral area
Subchondral fracture line — posterior half

Group IV

Whole head involvement
Metaphyseal reaction — central or diffuse
Posterior remodelling

metaphysis from disuse as well as true increase in bone deposition at the beginning of revascularization. At this time the subchondral fracture line, or *Caffey's sign,* can be seen (Fig. 1).[1, 12] This is best observed on the frog lateral view and gives a radiographic indication of the degree of epiphyseal involvement. During the fragmentation phase, the revascularization process is well under way and the bone is undergoing creeping substitution. During this fragmentation phase, deformation of the epiphysis can occur. Toward the end of the fragmentation phase, the bony epiphysis becomes reconstituted by woven bone and subsequent trabecular bone. The final phase of remodeling will continue until skeletal maturity.

Catterall has recognized that there is a spectrum of involvement of the femoral head and that prognosis is related to the amount of epiphysis involved. He has divided patients into four groups, depending upon the radiographic findings (Fig. 2).[3] Patients with more than 50 per cent head involvement are noted to have a significantly worse prognosis. Other risk factors include sex (females have a worse prognosis than males), age at onset of disease (the older patient has a worse prognosis), and loss of containment of the femoral head within the acetabulum (lateral subluxation).

TREATMENT

Treatment should be divided into two phases. The first goal of treatment should be to re-establish a satisfactory range of motion of the hip. This is accomplished by bed rest, traction, and salicylates. The next step is to identify those patients for whom the prognosis is poor. As mentioned, this includes patients with greater than 50 per cent head involvement and patients with the other associated risk factors. These patients should be treated long-term

with the principle of "containment." Containment refers to maintaining congruous contact of the femoral head within the acetabulum and ensures an even distribution of weight-bearing forces across the hip, thereby maintaining a spherical shape to the femoral head. On the other hand, if the femoral head migrates partially lateral within the acetabulum, the asymmetric weight-bearing forces cause flattening of the lateral portion of the femoral head with resultant loss of sphericity and congruency between the femoral head and acetabulum. Containment can be achieved by various methods, including an abduction weight bearing cast (Petrie cast),[7] bracing,[10] innominate osteotomy,[11] or varus osteotomy[5] of the proximal femur.

SELECTED REFERENCES

Catterall, A.: Legg-Calvé-Perthes Disease. New York, Churchill Livingstone, 1982.
Stulberg, S. D., Cooperman, D. R., and Wallensten, R.: The natural history of Legg-Calvé-Perthes disease. J. Bone Joint Surg., *63A*:1095, 1981.

REFERENCES

1. Caffey, J.: The early roentgenographic changes in essential coxa plana: Their significance in pathogenesis. Am. J. Roentgenol., *103*:620, 1968.
2. Calvé, J.: Sur une forme particulière de pseudo-coxalgia greffée sur des déformations caracteristiques de l'extrémité supérieure du fémur. Revue de Chirurgie, *30*:54, 1910.
3. Catterall, A.: The natural history of Perthes' disease. J. Bone Joint Surg., *53B*:37, 1971.
4. Legg, A. T.: An obscure affection of the hip joint. Boston Medical and Surgical Journal, *162*:202, 1910.
5. Lloyd-Roberts, G. C., Catterall, A., and Salaman, P. B.: A controlled study of the indications and results of femoral osteotomy in Perthes' disease. J. Bone Joint Surg., *58B*:31, 1976.
6. Perthes, G. C.: Über Arthritis Deformans Juvenilis. Deutsche Zeitschrift fur Chirurgie, *107*:11, 1910.

7. Petrie, J. G., and Bitenc, I.: The abduction weight-bearing treatment in Legg-Perthes disease. J. Bone Joint Surg., *53B*:54, 1971.

8. Phemister, D. B.: Repair of bone in the presence of aseptic necrosis resulting from fractures, transplantations, and vascular obstruction. J. Bone Joint Surg., *12*:769, 1930.

9. Ponseti, I. V.: Legg-Perthes disease: Observation on pathological changes in two cases. J. Bone Joint Surg., *38A*:739, 1956.

10. Purvis, J. M., Dimon, J. H., Meehan, P. C., and Lovell, W. W.: Preliminary experience with Scottish Rite Hospital abduction orthoses for Legg-Perthes disease. Clin. Orthop. *150*:49, 1980.

11. Salter, R. B.: Legg-Perthes disease: Treatment by innominate osteotomy. American Academy of Orthopedic Surgeons, Instructional Course Lectures *22*:309, 1973.

12. Salter, R. B., and Thompson, G. H.: Legg-Calvé-Perthes disease: The prognostic significance of the subchondral fracture and two-group classification of the femoral head involvement. J. Bone Joint Surg., *66A*:479, 1984.

13. Sommerville, E. W.: Perthes' disease of the hips. J. Bone Joint Surg., *53B*:639, 1971.

14. Trueta, J.: The normal vascular anatomy of the femoral head during growth. J. Bone Joint Surg., *39B*:358, 1957.

15. Waldenström, H.: Der Obere Tuberkulose Collumherd. Zeitschrift für Orthopädische Chirurgie, *24*:487, 1909.

4 • SLIPPED CAPITAL FEMORAL EPIPHYSIS

The most common hip disorder in children aged 9 to 15 is slipped capital femoral epiphysis. Although the precise etiology of this disease is not known, chronic trauma to the growth plate of the proximal femur and some subtle endocrine abnormalities are thought to play a role.[6] The end result is that of a disorganized growth plate with disruption of the orderly columns of chondrocyte proliferation as well as changes in the cartilage matrix.[5] There is a gradual posterior migration of the bony epiphysis relative to the femoral neck. This deformity usually occurs very gradually, and symptoms are insidious and present for several weeks to months. This form of slip (*chronic slip*) must be separated from the *acute slip*, in which symptoms are sudden and severe and usually related to trauma to the extremity.[1] The acute slip in most cases represents an epiphyseal fracture through the growth plate with displacement.

SIGNS AND SYMPTOMS

The most frequent patient complaint is that of vague knee pain. This is particularly important to recognize, since attention may be focused to the knee rather than the hip and there may be a delay in diagnosis. It should be emphasized that children and adolescents with hip disorders frequently complain of knee pain. Other complaints include vague thigh and hip pain and a limp. Physical examination invariably will show limitation of motion, particularly loss of internal rotation. A helpful maneuver is to take the hip through a range of motion from extension to flexion. As the hip is flexed, the leg will assume an increasing external rotation position with flexion. There may also be an associated loss of range of motion secondary to muscle spasm.

The diagnosis is confirmed by good anteroposterior and lateral radiographs of the proximal femur. The posterior migration of the femoral head relative to the femoral neck is best seen on the frog lateral x-ray whereas in mild cases the diagnosis can be overlooked on an anteroposterior radiograph. Other findings include widening of the epiphysis and metaphyseal irregularity. Normally, a line drawn up the lateral and anterior margin of the femoral neck should intersect the lateral portion of the bony epiphysis.

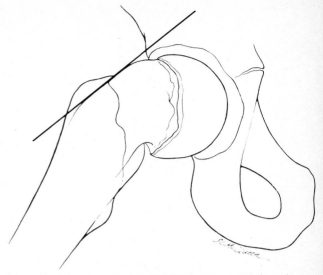

Figure 1. Slipped capital femoral epiphysis is most reliably seen on the lateral radiograph. Posterior migration of the femoral head relative to the neck is seen. A line drawn up the anterior or lateral margin of the femoral neck does not intersect the epiphysis.

With a slipped epiphysis, this line no longer will cross a portion of the femoral head (Fig. 1).

TREATMENT

Initial treatment should be focused upon synovitis and muscle spasm. This consists of bed rest and traction. The long-term treatment principle is to prevent further slippage of the femoral head. Stabilization of the head can be accomplished by *in situ* pinning,[9] open bone grafting,[3] or closed bone grafting.[2] Attempt at manipulative reduction of the slip should not be performed unless there is clear evidence that the slip is acute. Manipulation is associated with a high incidence of subsequent avascular necrosis of the femoral head. In mild slips the most accepted treatment is *in situ* pinning. In more severe slips the technique of pinning becomes much more difficult and open bone grafting should be considered. Some authors recommend intracapsular or extracapsular osteotomy of the proximal femur to realign the femoral head.[7] This should not be performed as an initial procedure, since some remodeling of the femoral head and neck will occur subsequent to pinning. Repositional osteotomies should be performed only in patients who have reached skeletal maturity and have persistent severe abnormality in range of motion.

COMPLICATIONS

Avascular necrosis of the femoral head can occur as a result of compromised blood flow to the capital femoral epiphysis in acute slip, or it can occur as a result of corrective osteotomy if the blood supply is damaged. Segmental avascular necrosis can also occur if multiple pins are stacked too closely in the weight-bearing area of the femoral head.

A severe complication of slipped epiphysis is *chondrolysis*.[4] Although the etiology is not known, a combination of mechanical and autoimmune factors may play a role in destruction of the articular cartilage. The presence of chondrolysis must be suspected if the patient's range of motion does not improve quickly with bed rest and traction and if radiographs show narrowing of the joint space. Blacks appear to be more predisposed to the development of chondrolysis, and this complication is often seen in chronic untreated cases. Chondrolysis may also be a secondary complication of fixation pins placed into the joint space.[8]

Treatment of chondrolysis is aimed at removal of the inciting agent if pins are protruding. The hip should be maintained in a functional position, and general range of motion exercises and salicylates may be helpful. Ankylosis of the hip in a nonfunctional position is to be avoided.

SELECTED REFERENCES

Lovell, W. B., and Winter, R. B.: Pediatric Orthopedics. Philadelphia, J. B. Lippincott Co., 1978.
Tachdjian, M. O.: Pediatric Orthopedics. Philadelphia, W. B. Saunders Company, 1972.

REFERENCES

1. Fahey, J. J., and O'Brien, E. T.: Acute slipped capital femoral epiphysis; review of the literature and report of ten cases. J. Bone Joint Surg., 47A:1105, 1965.
2. Heiple, K., and Shirreffs, T. G.: Extra-articular epiphysiodesis for slipped capital femoral epiphysis. Proc. A.A.O.S., 36, 1983.
3. Howorth, B.: The bone-pegging operation for slipping of the capital femoral epiphysis. Clin. Orthop., 48:79, 1966.
4. Mauer, R. C., and Larsen, I. J.: Acute necrosis of cartilage in slipped capital femoral epiphysis. J. Bone Joint Surg., 52A:39, 1970.
5. Mickelson, M. R., Ponseti, I. V., Cooper, R. R., and Maynard, J. A.: The ultrastructure of the growth plate in slipped capital femoral epiphysis. J. Bone Joint Surg., 54A:1076, 1977.
6. Ogden, J., and Southwick, W.: Endocrine dysfunction and SCFE. Yale J. Biol. Med. 50:1, 1977.
7. Southwick, W.: Osteotomy through the lesser trochanter for slipped capital femoral epiphysis. J. Bone Joint Surg., 49A:807, 1967.
8. Walters, R., and Simon, S. R.: Joint destruction: A sequel of unrecognized pin penetration in patients with slipped capital femoral epiphysis. Proc. Hip Soc., 1980, pp. 145–164.
9. Zahrawi, F. B., Stephens, T. L., Spencer, G. E., and Clough, J. M.: A comparative study of pinning *in situ* and open epiphysiodesis in 105 patients with slipped capital femoral epiphysis. Clin. Orthop., 177:161, 1983.

5 • CLUBFOOT

Talipes equinovarus, or clubfoot, is a common congenital anomaly. The estimated incidence of this disorder is one case per 1000 live births. Males are affected more commonly than females in a ratio of 2:1. Although the etiology is unknown, there is a frequent association of this deformity with neurologic conditions, such as arthrogryposis and myelodysplasia. Most often, however, this condition occurs unassociated with other identifiable neurogenic abnormalities. The inheritance pattern is multifactorial, indicating a complex genetic and environmental interaction. Wynne-Davies has shown that the incidence of this deformity in a first-degree relative with clubfoot is 20 to 30 times the incidence in the normal population, and if the parents are involved the risk may be as high as 25 per cent.[6]

ETIOLOGY

Several theories have been proposed to explain the occurrence of talipes equinovarus. Although a primary myogenic or neurogenic etiology has been considered, pathologic studies have not supported these theories.[2] It has been proposed that this condition is due to an arrest of normal embryologic development of the foot *in utero*. Between the fourth and eighth weeks of fetal development, the foot is normally in marked equinus with severe adduction and varus of the foot. During the third month, the foot begins to derotate and there is a gradual resolution of equinus supination and adduction. However, most authors currently believe that the congenital clubfoot represents a primary germ plasm defect (a limb bud–deficient foot), and this is supported by the pathologic anatomy.

PATHOLOGY

Fetal dissections have shown the talus anlage to be abnormally formed and positioned. The talar neck is shortened, plantar flexed, and medially deviated. The axis of the talus from body to talar head is medially rotated relative to the tibia. The articular surface of the subtalar joint is inclined medially, and the calcaneus is secondarily positioned in varus. In addition, there is a rotational abnormality of the calcaneus with the anterior aspect of the calcaneus displaced medially, the posterior portion lateral. The navicular is displaced medial on the talar head and may be so displaced as to articulate with the medial malleolus. There is contracture of the posteromedial ligament and tendon complex, and this includes the ankle and subtalar joint capsule, Achilles' tendon, and calcaneofibular ligament posteriorly. The deltoid ligament, tendon sheaths, and medial tendons as well as the spring ligament and talonavicular joint capsule are all contracted.

CLINICAL FINDINGS

There is a spectrum of severity in this disorder and the foot position will show varying degrees of (1) equinus, varus, and internal rotation of the hindfoot and (2) adduction, supination, and cavus of the forefoot. The diagnosis is easily made at birth by observation of these deformities (Fig. 1). However, the true limb bud–deficient talipes equinovarus must be differentiated from the positional variety associated with conditions such as spinal dysraphic states, primary congenital peroneal nerve palsy, and that associated with spastic static encephalopathy.

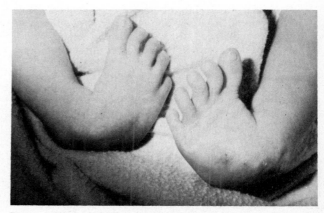

Figure 1. Bilateral clubfeet in the neonate demonstrate the typical hindfoot and forefoot deformities.

The physical findings show fixed hindfoot equinus and internal rotation of the foot relative to the knee. This internal rotation is not due to an abnormal torsion of the tibia but rather to internal rotation distal to the ankle mortise. The navicular can often be palpated in a medially displaced position adjacent to the medial malleolus. The talar head is palpable laterally and is uncovered. The normal indentation of the sinus tarsi is not present. On the medial aspect, there may be a deep medial crease opposite the talonavicular joint and the forefoot shows the typical adduction deformity with a varying degree of cavus.

Although 30 to 50 per cent of all cases of clubfoot will respond well to adequate nonoperative treatment, the severity of the deformity at birth is not a good predictor of the outcome. However, the presence of a deep medial crease, a posterior transverse crease, a hypoplastic calcaneus, or severe forefoot adduction and cavus is more likely to be associated with the intrinsic type of foot that is not likely to respond to nonoperative treatment.

RADIOGRAPHIC EVALUATION

Anteroposterior, lateral, and stress dorsiflexion lateral radiographs should be obtained.[4] This serves to exclude other conditions such as tibial dysplasia and establishes the relationship of the tibia, talus, and calcaneus at the initiation of treatment. Subsequent radiographs will confirm the success or failure of treatment. On the anteroposterior radiograph, *Kite's angle* is measured. This is the angle formed between lines drawn down the long axis of the talus and the calcaneus. The normal angle measures from 20 to 40 degrees. If the angle is less than 25 degrees, as it should be in clubfoot deformity, this indicates hindfoot varus. If the angle is greater than 40 degrees, excessive heel valgus is expected.

On the lateral radiograph with the foot in maximal dorsiflexion, the relationship between the talus and calcaneus is observed. With dorsiflexion, the axis of the calcaneus and talus should be convergent anteriorly. The angle formed by lines drawn down the long axis of these two bones is termed the *lateral talocalcaneal angle* and should measure at least 30 degrees. The clubfoot will show a relative parallelism between these two lines. With successful treatment this parallelism should be gradually improved or diminished (Fig. 2).

TREATMENT

All patients with clubfoot deformities should be given a trial of nonoperative treatment.[3] About 30 to 50 per cent of clubfoot deformities will resolve if early manipulation and plaster treatment are initiated and performed properly. Casting should be initiated as soon as possible after birth, and casts should be changed at a 1- to 2-week interval. Manipulation is an important part of the management and the foot should be gently repositioned, correcting first the internal rotation deformity, supination, and forefoot adduction. The posterior aspect of the calcaneus is tightly contracted against the fibula, and an attempt should be made to rotate the posterior aspect of the calcaneus medial as the remainder of the foot is rotated lateral. After adequate derotation of the foot, the foot is manipulated out of equinus with care being taken not to cause a breach at the midtarsal joint level creating a "rocker bottom" deformity.

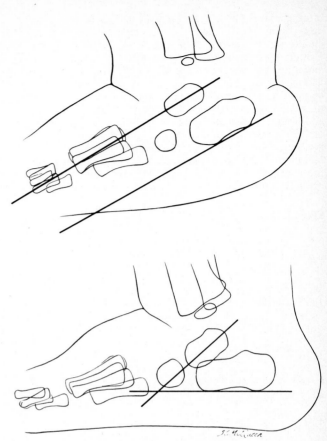

Figure 2. The lateral talocalcaneal angle in an untreated clubfoot will demonstrate parallelism (top). Following treatment, this angle should approach normal or 30 to 50 degrees (bottom).

OPERATIVE TREATMENT

For those feet that do not respond to a 3- to 4-month trial of serial manipulation and casting followed by a splinting program, operative intervention should be considered. Many operative procedures have been described.[1, 5] The most successful procedures are ones that deal with the entire deformity in a one-stage correction. The contracted ligaments are sectioned, and the appropriate tendons are lengthened. For this procedure, an extensive posterior, medial, and lateral release is required. The older patient with a failed previously treated clubfoot or a patient with an untreated deformity may require a salvage procedure such as multiple osteotomies or triple arthrodesis.

SELECTED REFERENCES

Turco, V. J.: Clubfoot. New York, Churchill Livingstone, 1981.

REFERENCES

1. Goldner, J. L.: Congenital Talipes Equinovarus—Fifteen Years of Surgical Treatment: Current Practice in Orthopedic Surgery. St. Louis, C. V. Mosby Co., 1969.
2. Irani, R. N., and Sherman, M. S.: The pathological anatomy of clubfoot. J. Bone Joint Surg., *45A*:45, 1963.
3. Kite, J. H.: Conservative treatment of the resistant recurrent clubfoot. Clin. Orthop., *70*:93, 1970.

4. Simons, G. W.: Analytical radiography and the progressive approach in talipes equinovarus. Orthop. Clin. North Am., *9*:187, 1978.
5. Turco, V. J.: Surgical correction of the resistant clubfoot—one-stage posteromedial release with internal fixation: A preliminary report. J. Bone Joint Surg., *53A*:477, 1971.
6. Wynn-Davies, R.: Family studies and the cause of congenital clubfoot: Talipes equinovarus, talipes calcaneovalgus, and metatarsus varus. J. Bone Joint Surg., *46B*:445, 1964.

6 • TORSIONAL DEFORMITIES OF THE LOWER LIMBS

Lower extremity posture is a frequent concern of parents of infants and young children. In pediatric clinics many children are seen for evaluation of "toe-in" or "toe-out" gait and for angular deformities (bow legs, knock knees). For most patients, however, these positional variations do not represent a deformity but rather fall in the physiologic range of normal. There is a broad spectrum of normal lower extremity positions in infants and children and an expected change in rotational and angular position as children grow.

ETIOLOGY

The typical position of the lower extremities in the newborn is secondary to multiple factors, the most significant of which is intrauterine positioning. In the newborn period, the hips are usually positioned in external rotation secondary to contracture of the posterior hip capsule and external rotators of the hip. The legs, however, are usually positioned in internal rotation secondary to excessive internal rotation at the knee and medial torsion of the tibia. As the external rotation contracture of the hip begins to resolve during the first 12 to 18 months, internal rotation of the limbs is evident secondary to internal tibial torsion. If external rotation contractures of the hips remain present at walking age, the lower limbs appear to be bowed secondary to the combination of these two factors. From age 2 to 8, excessive femoral anteversion may lead to an in-toeing gait pattern.

ANATOMIC VARIATIONS

After walking age, the most common parental concern regarding gait is an in-toeing pattern. This can be secondary to three anatomic variations: femoral anteversion, internal tibial torsion, and metatarsus adductus.

Femoral Anteversion

Version of the long bone refers to the angular difference between the axis of the ends of the long bone. For the femur, *anteversion* represents the anterior angulation of the femoral head and neck with reference to the transcondylar axis of the distal femur.[2] In infants anteversion is normally 30 to 40 degrees; in adults it gradually decreases to an angle of approximately 15 to 20 degrees (Fig. 1). When the external rotation contracture at the hips resolves, the excessive femoral anteversion will manifest itself by increase in internal rotation of the hips relative to external rotation. This results in an in-toeing gait pattern.

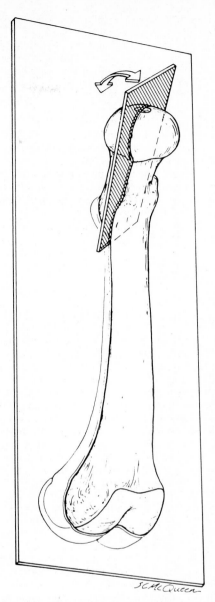

Figure 1. *Femoral anteversion is the angle formed by the plane of the femoral head and neck and the transcondylar axis of the distal femur. This angle gradually decreases from 30 to 40 degrees in the infant to approximately 15 degrees in the adult.*

When the posterior hip capsular contractures resolve in the infant, femoral anteversion can be implicated as a cause of in-toeing if clinical examination shows that the hips rotate internally considerably more than they rotate laterally. This, again, is a normal finding in children from about 18 months to 5 years. By age 5 internal and external rotation of the hips should be approximately symmetrical.

The way to evaluate hip rotation is by placing the patient in the prone position. The hips are held in an extended position; the knees are flexed, the hips are sequentially rotated medially and laterally, and the resultant arc of motion of the limb is recorded.

Radiographic documentation of degree of femoral anteversion is possible with biplane radiographic techniques or a computed tomography (CT) scan, but in general these diagnostic modalities are not indicated since clinical examination is sufficient to pinpoint the diagnosis.

As stated, the natural history of excessive femoral anteversion is spontaneous correction with growth. Derotation of the femoral head and neck relative to the transcondylar axis of the distal femur occurs gradually in almost all children. With the natural history, one realizes that there should be no treatment for excessive femoral anteversion because spontaneous correction can be expected. Furthermore, special shoes, twister cables, or orthotics have not been shown to have any significant effect on the resolution of femoral anteversion.

In the rare individual in whom excessive femoral anteversion persists and is severe enough to create both functional and cosmetic deformity, surgical derotation of the proximal femur can be performed. This is usually done just prior to skeletal maturity to allow maximal physiologic spontaneous correction.

Internal Tibial Torsion

The most common cause for internal rotation of the lower limbs in infants and children is internal tibial torsion. Like the femur, the tibia at birth is rotated medially relative to its long axis. Spontaneous derotation is expected to occur rapidly during the first 12 months and somewhat more slowly thereafter to about age 5. Children beyond walking age with persistent medial version or excessive but resolving medial torsion will have an in-toeing gait pattern.[10]

In the infant and child younger than age 3, the way to assess tibial torsion clinically is to compare the flexion extension axis of the knee relative to the transmalleolar axis of the ankle. This is done by flexing the knee 90 degrees facing the patella and tibial tubercle forward and by palpating the midportion of the medial malleolus and lateral malleolus. Normally, in the adult the fibular malleolus lies about one finger breadth, or 20 degrees, posterior to the medial malleolus. With increasing degrees of internal tibial torsion, the fibula will be palpated more parallel or occasionally even anterior to the medial malleolus. In the child beyond 3 years of age, the degree of tibial torsion can be assessed by measuring the thigh-foot axis (Fig. 2).

Although persistent internal tibial torsion is a frequent cause of in-toeing in children, it rarely requires treatment. Spontaneous resolution is the rule. However, the parents must be warned that correction will be gradual, particularly if there is persistent internal tibial torsion beyond walking age.

A wide variety of orthotics and "corrective" shoes have been advocated for the treatment of internal tibial torsion. However, none of these has been shown to have any definite effect on the natural history of the deformity. It is likely that most of the corrective forces applied by these devices exert their force at the knee and ankle, dissipating any true corrective forces for the tibia.

Rarely, in patients with severe deformities that have failed to improve adequately by age 8 to 10 years, corrective rotational osteotomies of either the proximal or distal tibia can reliably correct the deformities.

Metatarsus Adductus

Metatarsus adductus was first described in 1863 by Henke of Germany.[3] Many terms have been used to describe this deformity, some descriptive and some with

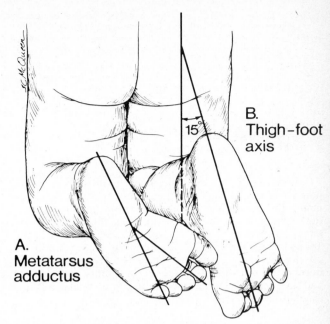

Figure 2. The heel bisector line is utilized in determining the severity of metatarsus adductus (A). Deviation of the forefoot causes this line to extend lateral to the second toe. The deviation of the forefoot causes the lateral border of the foot to be convex and the medial border to be concave. The thigh-foot axis (B) is used to determine tibial version. The normal thigh-foot axis is external 15 degrees as demonstrated.

reference to the pathologic anatomy. This foot disorder has been referred to as *metatarsus adductus, metatarsus varus*, "one-third of a clubfoot," and *skewfoot*. A wide variation of deformity is seen within the spectrum of this disorder. In general, this condition is characterized by a varying degree of the following: forefoot adduction with supination; cavus; hindfoot position of neutral or valgus; and occasional abnormal posterior tibial or anterior tibial tendon insertion (Fig. 2A). It is useful to think of this disorder in terms of the typical (positional) variety and to separate those from other less common forms (such as that associated with clubfoot) or the teratologic category (as seen with spina bifida and arthrogryposis).

The positional metatarsus adductus is a common congenital foot condition that appears to have increased significantly in incidence since World War II. The positional group is usually associated with medial rotation of the tibia and/or persistent medial deviation of the talus at the ankle joint. This leads to an increase in the in-toeing pattern if it persists beyond walking age. The teratologic category seen with or without an associated neurologic condition, in general, is rigid and therefore more resistant to nonoperative treatment. In examination of children with a forefoot abnormality, a number of disorders must be excluded. These include *metatarsus primus varus*,[6] in which the first ray is adducted but there is no other associated metatarsal deformity. This condition is strongly hereditary and is more common in females. Unlike metatarsus adductus, it is associated with the development of hallux valgus deformities in bunions in adolescence or adulthood. Other conditions that need to be excluded include *hallux varus* and other torsional deformities of the lower limb. Hallux varus is an abducted position of the great toe that is usually due to overactivity of the abductor hallucis muscle. This is a dynamic deformity and resolves without treatment.

The association of metatarsus adductus and hip dysplasia should be mentioned. Jacobs reported a 10 per cent incidence of hip dysplasia as determined by an abnormal acetabular index.[5] The incidence of clinically significant hip dysplasia is probably in the region of 1 to 2 per cent as documented by MacEwen, which is considerably higher than the 0.15 per cent incidence of persistent hip instability in the general population.[7]

The natural history of this disorder is spontaneous resolution in most patients.[9] Certainly passively correctable deformities will improve without treatment. Ponseti found that of 379 patients only 11 per cent required corrective plaster treatment.

Bleck has classified metatarsus adductus into three categories: (1) mild, (2) moderate, and (3) severe.[1]

Treatment is not required for mild metatarsus adductus, since gradual spontaneous resolution can be expected. In the moderate grouping, there is some degree of cavus and passive correction of the deformity is usually limited to about neutral position. This deformity will usually resolve spontaneously; however, resolution will take longer than that for Group I, and in some patients a mild deformity may persist. Plaster treatment is utilized in this group, since it will guarantee a good result if treatment is initiated prior to 6 to 8 months of age.

In the severe category, the crease on the medial side of the foot is deeper and the forefoot cannot be passively corrected to neutral position. The heel may be in neutral or valgus position and there is excessive cavus and supination of the forefoot. Patients in this group require plaster manipulation and casting every 2 to 4 weeks for 4 to 6 months.

If severe metatarsus adductus remains untreated or if significant deformity persists after treatment, operative intervention is recommended and is best performed at approximately 2 years of age. Most deformities can be corrected by wedge osteotomies through the cuboid and cuneiforms,[8] with tarsal-metatarsal joint release[4] or metatarsal osteotomies being reserved for the severe teratologic limb bud-deficient foot.

SELECTED REFERENCES

Gross, R. H.: Common angular and rotational problems of early childhood. Orthop. Surg. Update Series, Vol. 3, No. 39, 1985.

Scoles, P. V.: Pediatric Orthopedics in Clinical Practice. Chicago Year Book Medical Publishers, Inc., 1982.

REFERENCES

1. Bleck, E. E.: Metatarsus adductus: Classification and relationship to outcomes of treatment. J. Pediatr. Orthop., 3:2, 1983.
2. Fabry, G., MacEwen, G. D., and Shands, A. R.: Torsion of the femur. J. Bone Joint Surg., 55A:1726, 1973.
3. Henke, W.: Contractur des Metatarsuz. Z rat. Med., 17:188, 1863.
4. Heyman, C. H., Herndon, C. R., and Strong, J. M.: Mobilization of the tarsometatarsal and intermetatarsal joints for the correction of resistant adduction of the forepart of the foot in congenital clubfoot or congenital metatarsus varus. J. Bone Joint Surg., 40A:299, 1958.
5. Jacobs, J. E.: Metatarsus varus and hip dysplasia. Clin. Orthop., 16:203, 1960.
6. Kite, J. H.: Congenital metatarsus varus. J. Bone Joint Surg., 49A:388, 1967.
7. Kumar, S. J., and MacEwen, G. D.: The incidence of hip dysplasia with metatarsus adductus. Clin. Orthop., 164:234, 1982.
8. Lincoln, C. R., Wood, K. E., and Bugg, E. I.: Metatarsus varus corrected by open wedge osteotomy of the first cuneiform. Orthop. Clin. North Am., 7:795, 1976.
9. Rushforth, G. F.: The natural history of hooked forefoot. J. Bone Joint Surg., 60B:530, 1978.
10. Staheli, L. T., and Engel, G. M.: Tibial torsion: A method of assessment and a survey of normal children. Clin. Orthop. 86:183, 1972.

VII

General Orthopedics

JOHN M. HARRELSON, M.D.

INFECTIONS

Infections in the musculoskeletal system may develop in one of two ways. Blood-borne bacteria from a preexisting focus of infection (upper respiratory infection, genitourinary infection, furuncle) may lodge in bone, synovium, or extremity soft tissue and establish an abscess. Bacteria may also reach the musculoskeletal system from the external environment (penetrating wounds, surgical incisions, open fractures). *Hematogenous infection* is more commonly encountered in childhood, whereas *exogenous infection* is more frequently encountered in adults exposed to trauma. Continued development of effective antibiotics has greatly reduced the incidence of both hematogenous and exogenous infections, compared with the preantibiotic era, with a concomitant reduction in both mortality and morbidity.

Osteomyelitis

Hematogenous osteomyelitis is a disease of childhood occurring most commonly between the ages of 5 and 15 years of age. Males are more frequently affected than females (3:1). The metaphyseal ends of long bones are the sites of predilection for hematogenous osteomyelitis, with the distal femur, proximal tibia, and proximal humerus most frequently affected. The predisposition for infection in the metaphysis is thought to be related to the pattern of blood flow at the level of the metaphyseal physeal plate junction. Sluggish blood flow through efferent veins at this level provides a site for bacterial seeding. The epiphyses of long bones have a separate blood supply and are rarely involved with acute osteomyelitis. With maturation, there is total ossification of the physeal plate and the characteristics of sluggish blood flow are eliminated. Accordingly, hematogenous osteomyelitis in the adult is an uncommon event.

The abscess cavity formed by bacterial multiplication and leukocyte invasion produces interstitial edema and increasing pressure within the bone. Thrombosis of local vessels produces an infarct which extends the infection. Increased local pressure and hyperemia result in localized pain over the area of infection without radiographic changes. As the process continues, the abscess cavity enlarges until it reaches the cortical surface of the bone where purulent material percolates through the overlying cortex and elevates the surrounding periosteum. By this time (usually 10 to 12 days) radiographs will show a central area of increased density (infarcted bone) surrounded by a zone of relative radiolucency (granulation tissue) and associated periosteal elevation. Without therapeutic intervention, this process continues until the periosteum is stripped circumferentially, resulting in cortical infarction.

CLINICAL COURSE

The *clinical course* of osteomyelitis usually begins with the rapid onset of localized pain, generalized malaise, fever, and chills. A history of preceding infection is obtained in approximately 50 per cent of patients. Generalized swelling in the area of the infection is usually accompanied by erythema. Proximal lymph node enlargement may be present. Laboratory examination reveals a leukocytosis, mild to moderate anemia, and an elevated erythrocyte sedimentation rate (ESR). Because radiographic signs of osteomyelitis are not evident for approximately 10 days, the diagnosis is usually made on clinical grounds alone in acute cases. Blood cultures should be obtained and will be positive in approximately 50 per cent of patients. *Staphylococcus aureus* is the most frequent offending organism. In infants and neonates, *Streptococcus* may produce the same clinical picture. Gram-negative organisms may also be etiologic, although they generally produce a less fulminating course than described. In particular, salmonella osteomyelitis involving the diaphysis of long bones may be a complication of sickle cell anemia.

Exogenous osteomyelitis most frequently follows contaminated open fractures. Any organism may be involved. Infection is usually limited to the site of injury, and because the periosteum has been disrupted, periosteal elevation and extension of infection are not seen. If the wound has been closed, continued bacterial multiplication may cause spontaneous dehiscence with purulent drainage.

DIFFERENTIAL DIAGNOSIS

Other diseases may mimic acute osteomyelitis. Acute juvenile rheumatoid arthritis, acute rheumatic fever, leukemia, acute septic arthritis, scurvy, and Ewing's sarcoma may all present a similar clinical picture. Careful examination of the extremity is required to localize pain at the metaphyseal versus the joint level in distinguishing metaphyseal osteomyelitis from acute pyogenic arthritis. In acute

rheumatic fever and juvenile rheumatoid arthritis, multiple joints may be involved. Hematogenous osteomyelitis in the adult is uncommon and produces a less dramatic clinical picture than described above. In children who have been treated with antibiotics for a preceding soft tissue infection, the clinical course of osteomyelitis may also be less aggressive.

TREATMENT

Acute hematogenous osteomyelitis must be treated promptly. In the days prior to antibiotics, the mortality of this disease was as high as 50 per cent. Blood cultures are obtained and intravenous antibiotics are started without awaiting the results of culture. Since *Staphylococcus* is the most frequent offending organism, the antibiotic selected should have an antistaphylococcal spectrum. If blood cultures are subsequently negative, subperiosteal aspiration or intramedullary aspiration of the involved bone may be required. The patient is placed at bed rest, fluid and electrolyte balance is maintained, antipyretics are administered for fever, and the limb is immobilized in bi-valved plaster, which allows daily inspection. Clinical improvement is usually seen within 24 hours after institution of antibiotic therapy. If deterioration occurs, operative intervention is required.

The surgical treatment of osteomyelitis is incision and drainage. The surgical approach depends on the location and extent of infection and should allow for subsequent dependent drainage of the wound if possible. The cortex overlying the intramedullary abscess in windowed, and necrotic debris is removed by manual curettage and pulse lavage irrigation. Care is taken to avoid the adjacent physeal plate. The wound is dressed open to allow drainage and the extremity immobilized in plaster. Intravenous antibiotics are continued for a minumum of 2 weeks and may be required for as long as 6 weeks, depending on the organism and its susceptibility to antibiotic therapy. The wound is dressed at regular intervals and allowed to heal by secondary intention or covered with a split-thickness skin graft when adequate granulation tissue has developed. When the acute process is under control, daily physical therapy for range of motion is instituted. The resumption of full activity depends on the amount of bone involved. In extensive infection, subsequent weakening resulting from bone loss may result in pathologic fracture.

Exogenous osteomyelitis is treated in a similar manner. The organism is usually identified by wound cultures rather than blood cultures. Adequate wound débridement is necessary, as is antibiotic therapy selected on the basis of bacterial sensitivities. In some cases, the extent of disease and the virulence of the organism involved preclude ultimate eradication of the infection. Chronic draining sinus tracts may develop, and chronic osteomyelitis may persist for years. There may be periods of quiescence with exacerbations of drainage, fever, and swelling. Chronic osteomyelitis that is not adequately controlled by antibiotics and produces significant disability for the patient may be best treated by amputation of the extremity and fitting with a prosthesis.

Pyogenic Arthritis

Acute pyogenic arthritis, like osteomyelitis, may occur from hematogenous seeding, penetrating injuries, or the extension of adjacent osteomyelitis. *Staphylococcus* is the most common organism recovered, although *Streptococcus*, pneumococcus, and gonococcus are frequently seen. Pyogenic arthritis is usually monarticular, which helps distinguish it from acute rheumatic fever and acute juvenile rheumatoid arthritis. Most frequently affected is the hip joint, followed by the knee and wrist.

CLINICAL ONSET

The clinical onset of pyogenic arthritis is similar to that of acute osteomyelitis, with pain, fever, chills, and localized swelling with overlying erythema. Careful physical examination helps distinguish this from metaphyseal osteomyelitis. Patients with acute pyogenic arthritis usually have a tense joint effusion and will not tolerate even slight amounts of joint motion. Laboratory studies show an elevated ESR and elevated white blood cell count. Aspiration of the involved joint under sterile conditions will produce cloudy synovial fluid with a cell count ranging from 50,000 to 200,000 cells per cubic centimeter. A differential count will show 80 to 90 per cent polymorphonuclear leukocytes and Gram stain will demonstrate the organism in approximately 50 per cent of cases. A large-bore needle should be used for joint aspiration, since proteinaceous debris and synovial edema may make it difficult to obtain fluid. Radiographs in cases of acute pyogenic arthritis generally show only soft tissue swelling with no underlying bony changes. Widening of the joint space may be seen if the effusion is under pressure, and in severe cases pathologic dislocation of the joint may occur.

TREATMENT

The continued proliferation of bacteria within a joint produces increasing pressure and a rising amount of lysozomal enzymes, both of which can destroy articular cartilage. For these reasons, pyogenic arthritis is treated as an emergency with intravenous antibiotics administered when the joint has been aspirated and without awaiting the results of culture. An antibiotic with antistaphylococcal activity is best selected. The affected joint is put at rest with gentle longitudinal skin traction, which diminishes pressure on the articular cartilage. In the early stages, the joint fluid will be serosanguinous with a lower cell count. In this situation it is acceptable to irrigate the joint with saline and observe the patient during the first 24 hours of antibiotic therapy. If the fever diminishes and ESR declines, antibiotics and daily joint aspirations for cell count and culture are continued.

If improvement fails to occur with this regimen or if the initial joint aspirate is thick and turbid with a high cell count, antibiotic therapy alone will not be successful. Surgical drainage of the joint is indicated with the incision placed to allow dependent drainage if possible. Pyarthrosis of the hip in children often fails to respond to antibiotic therapy alone, and surgical drainage should be considered as initial therapy. The wound is left open, the dressings are changed daily, and the wound allowed to heal by secondary intention. Physical therapy for active and passive motion is begun as soon as the infection is clinically under control.

Skeletal Tuberculous Infections

Tuberculous osteomyelitis and *tuberculous pyarthrosis* have undergone a steady decline with the advent of effective antituberculous medications. Skeletal infection with tuber-

cle bacilli results from hematogenous seeding from a pre-existing pulmonary or gastrointestinal focus. The intervertebral discs of the lower thoracic and upper lumbar spine are most frequently involved, with the hip and knee being the next most common. Adjacent bone involvement most often results from a pre-existing tuberculous joint infection. The tubercle bacillus is a more indolent organism than are pyogenic bacteria. Accordingly, the clinical onset of tuberculous skeletal infection is more insidious, usually beginning with dull aching in the area of the affected joint.

SYMPTOMS AND SIGNS

Because of visceral infection, the patient will often appear debilitated. A history of weight loss, fever, and easy fatigability are common. Diminished motion of the affected joint with protective muscle spasm may be present. Exquisite pain like that elicited in pyogenic arthritis is usually lacking. Examination of the involved joint will reveal mild synovial thickening, effusion, and increased local heat. Erythema is uncommon. Muscle atrophy and proximal nodal enlargement may also be encountered.

CLINICAL FINDINGS

The white blood cell count is normal or slightly elevated, the ESR is usually elevated, and a mild anemia may be present. The tuberculin skin test will be positive. Synovial fluid aspirated from the joint will show moderate turbidity with an elevated white blood cell count and an increased number of mononuclear cells. Examination of joint fluid sediment for acid-fast bacilli and culture of the joint fluid should be obtained. Radiographic changes in skeletal tuberculosis are similarly slow to develop. The most striking feature is osteoporosis about the joint. In early cases there will be preservation of joint space and distention of the joint capsule. Later bone erosion at the point of synovial attachment produces a characteristic defect at the margin of the joint.

TREATMENT

Skeletal tuberculosis is treated by appropriate antituberculous medications. In the past, arthrodesis of affected joints was performed to salvage function but is less frequently required today. During the early phases of antimicrobial treatment the joint should be protected. In cases of spinal tuberculosis, bed rest, and a plaster cast or rigid corset are recommended. Extremity infections are managed by traction or bivalved plaster. Range of motion and gradual resumption of activity are allowed as healing occurs. Arthrodesis is required only if there is extensive joint destruction.

SKELETAL NEOPLASMS

The mature skeleton is composed of bone, fibrous tissue, and cartilage. From these cells or the primitive mesenchymal tissue from which they originate may develop benign or malignant primary skeletal neoplasms. Malignant disease may also be of marrow cell origin (lymphoma, multiple myeloma). The majority of malignant lesions seen in bone (70 per cent) are metastatic lesions usually from carcinoma, although sarcoma may be seen. For a rational approach to the patient with a skeletal neoplasm, an

TABLE 1. Common Skeletal Neoplasms

	Cartilage	Bone	Fibrous
Benign	Osteochondroma Enchondroma Chondroblastoma	Osteoid osteoma Osteoblastoma	Nonossifying fibroma Giant cell tumor Desmoplastic fibroma
Malignant	Primary chondrosarcoma Secondary chondrosarcoma	Osteosarcoma Periosteal osteosarcoma	Fibrosarcoma Fibrous histiocytoma

understanding of the biologic behavior of skeletal tumors, the diagnostic staging studies required, the techniques and risks of biopsy, and the treatment modalities employed are necessary. The most common benign and malignant primary skeletal neoplasms are outlined in Table 1.

Classification

BENIGN NEOPLASMS

Benign skeletal neoplasms are graded according to their aggressiveness and tendency to destroy local bone. In the system proposed by Enneking, *Grade I* lesions are inactive and tend to remain static or regress, *Grade II* lesions are active with a potential for continued local growth, and *Grade III* lesions are aggressive with potential for rapid growth and further bone destruction. Aggressiveness is primarily a radiographic assessment. Most of the benign lesions in Table 1 are Grade I or Grade II. The exceptions would be giant cell tumor and desmoplastic fibroma, which are aggressive lesions (Grade III) with a potential for further destruction.

MALIGNANT NEOPLASMS

For staging of *malignant primary skeletal neoplasms*, accurate information on anatomic location and histologic aggressiveness is required. Radionuclide scanning, CT scan, magnetic resonance imaging (MRI), and angiography are usually required to determine the anatomic extent of a malignant lesion. It must be determined whether the lesion is contained completely within bone (intracompartmental) or has invaded adjacent tissues (extracompartmental) and whether metastases are present. This anatomic information must be obtained before biopsy is performed for histologic grading. Table 2 shows the staging system proposed by Enneking and the Musculoskeletal Tumor Society. In this system, intracompartmental lesions are designated by the letter A, extracompartmental lesions by the letter B, histologically low-grade lesions by the number I, and high-grade lesions by the number II.

Biopsy is performed to establish the histologic grade of the lesion. For practical purposes, skeletal malignancies may be divided into *low-grade* (Broders' 1, 2) or *high-grade* (Broders' 3, 4) lesions. Several important factors must be understood before biopsy is undertaken. Many skeletal tumors do not have a uniform histologic appearance, and the biopsy specimen must be sufficient to provide representative material for histologic evaluation. Needle biopsy, therefore, is used only in those lesions that are difficult to approach surgically. For many skeletal neoplasms, *wide local excision* is needed for cure. Because of possible contamination of the biopsy tract, surgical planning for future treatment should be completed before biopsy is undertaken. The incision should be placed in a position that allows its complete extirpation at the time of definitive treatment. Further, hematoma emanating from a biopsy incision can contaminate tissue planes. Meticulous hemostasis is mandatory before the biopsy incision is closed. Careless placement of a biopsy incision or extensive hematoma following a biopsy may necessitate amputation where limb salvage might have been possible.

Treatment

The treatment of primary skeletal neoplasms is based on their *biologic behavior*. All neoplasms, whether benign or malignant, tend to grow by peripheral expansion and create a reactive capsule of compressed normal tissue about their margins. For benign or low-grade lesions, this pseudocapsule represents the maximal extent of the disease. However, high-grade malignancies have the potential to invade local blood vessels and lymphatics and extend their sphere of influence beyond the pseudocapsule. In this manner, malignant lesions may produce not only distant metastases (lungs, lymph nodes, liver), but also satellite lesions within the antomic compartment of origin.

Four basic surgical procedures may be used to treat primary skeletal neoplasms.

1. *Intralesional resection* involves invasion of the lesion and removal by a curette or other instrument.

2. *Local resection* involves removal of the lesion intact through the pseudocapsule or reactive tissues about its margins.

3. *Wide local excision* involves removal of the entire neoplasm with a margin of normal tissue and the biopsy tract.

4. *Radical excision* involves removal of the entire anatomic compartment of origin of the lesion. Radical excision frequently necessitates amputation.

Grade I benign skeletal neoplasms are usually asymptomatic and clearly benign by radiographic evaluation. As such, treatment is required only if symptomatic and intralesional removal is appropriate. Grade II benign lesions are defined as active, with a potential for further bone destruction. They may be treated by intralesional removal, but there is some chance of local recurrence. Local recurrence is diminished by local resection around the reactive capsule of the lesion. Grade III benign lesions, lesions with a potential for rapid growth and aggressive destruction of bone, are most appropriately treated by wide local excision.

For many years, the treatment of malignant primary skeletal neoplasms was by surgery alone. Progress in radiotherapy techniques and chemotherapeutic agents, in some

TABLE 2. Staging of Malignant Skeletal Neoplasms

	Low Grade	High Grade
Intracompartmental	Stage IA	Stage IIA
Extracompartmental	Stage IB	Stage IIB

Stage III = any grade, any site with metastases

instances, has led to a modified operative approach to malignant skeletal neoplasms. When surgery alone is utilized, Stage IA (low-grade, intracompartmental) lesions are adequately treated by wide local excision. Stage IB (low-grade, extracompartmental), IIA (high-grade, intracompartmental), and IIB (high-grade, extracompartmental) lesions usually necessitate radical excision. In the case of skeletal malignancy, radical excision (removal of the entire anatomic compartment of origin) often means amputation. In recent years pretreatment with radiotherapy or chemotherapy has allowed wide local excision for some high-grade tumors and limb salvage is a possibility. The decision to attempt limb salvage is based on the original staging studies and restaging after pretreatment with chemotherapy or radiotherapy. The extent of the tumor within bone, the extent of soft tissue extension of tumor, and the relationship of tumor to major neural and vascular studies must all be defined.

Osteosarcoma and *fibrous histiocytoma* are the most frequent *high-grade primary skeletal neoplasms*. These lesions tend to destroy surrounding trabecular bone, to permeate through the cortex and invade adjacent soft tissues, and to demonstrate early vascular invasion. Since lymphatics in bone are sparse, lymph node metastases are rarely seen; however, pulmonary metastases from vascular invasion are common. Historically, patients with osteosarcoma had an 80 per cent mortality rate at 5 years with radical surgery alone. Currently, patients with osteosarcoma treated by preoperative chemotherapy and limb salvage or by radical excision and postoperative adjuvant chemotherapy have a 55 per cent 5-year survival. *Chondrosarcomas* and *fibrosarcomas* are *low-grade lesions*. There is no established role for chemotherapy or radiotherapy in these tumors. Wide local excision remains the treatment of choice.

Metastatic carcinoma and *multiple myeloma* represent the majority of malignant lesions in bone. In these diseases the orthopedic surgeon has no curative role. Rather, attention is directed toward palliation by maintenance of skeletal stability, reduction of pain, and maintenance of mobility. Not infrequently, the initial diagnosis of carcinoma or multiple myeloma is made from presenting complaints of skeletal pain. This is particularly true of renal cell carcinoma and thyroid carcinoma, which often produce painful metastases before producing local symptoms at the primary site.

Skeletal metastases and *lesions of myeloma* represent a potential threat for pathologic fracture. When the lesion is greater than 3 cm. in diameter or when there is greater than 50 per cent cortical destruction, pathologic fracture is likely. If the prognosis for survival is greater than 3 months and the patient is medically able to undergo surgery, prophylactic fixation of long bone lesions is indicated. For prophylactic fixation and pathologic fractures, many of the techniques utilized for fixation of traumatic fractures may be employed. Because there is often permeative destruction of bone extending beyond the margins of radiographically definable tumor, plate fixation is seldom used. The quality of bone is not sufficient to hold the screws and plate in place, and failure of the fixation device occurs. Wherever possible, it is preferable to use intramedullary fixation as described in previous sections. In many instances, bone loss results in poor fixation, even with intramedullary techniques. Methylmethacrylate, a plastic polymer, may be used to provide added stability and maintain skeletal length. Successful treatment of skeletal metastatic disease increases patient comfort and reduces medical costs by shortening the hospitalization that would be required for more conservative management.

ARTHRITIS

Classification

There are over one hundred different clinical types of arthritis. Collectively, these joint afflictions affect tens of millions in the United States and cause more lost man-hours of work than any other disease. Each form of arthritis is distinguished by clinical features, radiographic appearance, and laboratory tests. The etiology of most types of arthritis is unknown. Four basic pathologic patterns of joint destruction are seen in arthritis, and from the point of view of treatment it is helpful to consider arthritis in these terms.

1. *Inflammatory arthritis* is primarily a disease of the synovial membrane. Synovial proliferation and inflammation with release of lysozomal enzymes eventually produces erosion first at the margin of the affected joint and later at the weight-bearing surface. *Rheumatoid arthritis* is the classic example of inflammatory arthritis. Psoriatic arthritis, infectious arthritis, and Reiter's syndrome are other examples.

2. *Degenerative arthritis* is primarily a disease of the articular cartilage. Loss of joint space resulting from cartilage erosion and the formation of osteophytes at the joint margin are the radiographic hallmarks. Degenerative arthritis may be hereditary (osteoarthritis), may follow joint injury (post-traumatic arthritis), or may be seen after preexisting inflammatory joint disease.

3. *Metabolic arthritis* occurs in response to deposition of crystals in the articular cartilage and synovium. The radiographic changes have features of both inflammatory and degenerative disease plus the deposition of mineral in the joint. Gout, pseudogout, and ochronosis are the most common examples of metabolic arthritis.

4. *Neurotrophic arthritis* occurs in response to loss of sensation in the joint. Neurosyphillis was the classic example described by Charcot. Today diabetes mellitus and alcoholic neuropathy are more frequently etiologic. Painless joint destruction with marked fragmentation of the articular bone and cartilage, gross joint instability, and subluxation or dislocation are the radiographic and clinical features of neurotrophic arthropathy.

Treatment

The primary treatment for all types of arthritis is medical, whether directed toward the underlying etiology (metabolic, neurotrophic, infections) or at the symptoms in idiopathic arthritis. Nonsteroidal anti-inflammatory drugs, physical therapy, and bracing are the primary therapeutic tools. When medical treatment fails to relieve pain or when progressive joint deformity produces mechanical disability, surgery may be indicated.

SYNOVECTOMY

Synovectomy may be of benefit in the early phase of inflammatory arthritis. With newer medications and better medical control of synovitis, synovectomy is used only in selected cases today. Removal of proliferative synovium reduces or delays destruction of articular cartilage by reducing the inflammatory by-products and mechanical effects of excessive synovium. The effect is temporary and does not eliminate the need for continued medical treatment. Synovectomy is not helpful in degenerative, metabolic, or neurotrophic arthritis.

ARTHRODESIS

Arthrodesis (fusion of a joint) may be required when severe destruction from inflammatory or neurotrophic arthritis is present. Widely in use prior to the evolution of *prosthetic arthroplasty*, arthrodesis today is used mainly for the small joints (interphalangeal, wrist, foot), spine, and infected major joints for which a prosthetic implant is contraindicated. The damaged joint surfaces are débrided to the level of bare bone, the joint is placed in the position of function, and internal or external immobilization is applied until union occurs.

RESECTION ARTHROPLASTY

Resection arthroplasty for relief of arthritic pain involves removal of one or both articular surfaces. The joint is immobilized without bony apposition until fibrous scar fills the defect and then motion exercises are begun. Today, resection arthroplasty is most commonly employed at the metatarsophalangeal joints (metatarsal head resection) for rheumatoid arthritis, the radial head for comminuted fracture, and the hip (femoral head resection) for chronic infection.

OSTEOTOMY

Osteotomy (division and realignment of bone) at the hip and knee was also widely used prior to prosthetic arthroplasty. Primarily used for degenerative arthritis, osteotomy allows realignment of deformity and moves undamaged cartilage into the weight-bearing area. Occasionally, severe deformity may require realignment by osteotomy in preparation for prosthetic arthroplasty.

PROSTHETIC ARTHROPLASTY

In the same way by which improved medical management has resulted in reduced frequency of synovectomy, prosthetic arthroplasty has led to reduced use of arthrodesis, resection arthroplasty, and osteotomy. The first prostheses were designed to replace only one side of a diarthrodial joint (hemiarthroplasty). Advances in materials technology and surgical techniques have led to replacement of both joint surfaces (total joint replacement). Hemiarthroplasty is still useful in the non–weight-bearing upper extremity (proximal humerus, radial head, distal radius) but is of more limited use in the lower extremity. Total joint replacement is of primary benefit in the hip and knee and of more limited use in selected cases for the elbow and ankle.

Active or chronic infection is a contraindication to prosthetic arthroplasty. The implantation of a foreign object only exacerbates and perpetuates the problem. Similarly, the development of postoperative infection after arthroplasty may necessitate removal of the prosthetic components and salvage either by resection arthroplasty (hip, elbow) or arthrodesis (knee, ankle).

Total joint arthroplasty may ultimately fail as a result of loosening of the components within bone. The standard method of component fixation is to embed the prosthesis in methylmethacrylate. The interface between bone and methacrylate is the weak link in the system. Greater strength and activity make loosening a more common problem in the young patient than in the elderly. Thus, prosthetic arthroplasty is not advised for the vigorous patient and other conventional surgical solutions (arthrodesis, osteotomy) should be considered. Current evaluation of *noncemented prostheses* is under way. These devices allow bone ingrowth into the prosthesis and, if successful, may offer new alternatives for the active patient.

SURGICAL DISORDERS OF THE SKIN

P. MICHAEL OLMSTEAD, M.D. • WILLIAM P. GRAHAM III, M.D.

37

The integument is one of the most important systems in the body, both to the surgeon and the patient. The surgeon must consider the skin or mucosa in almost every operative procedure, and the resultant scar often attests to the success of the operation.

NORMAL HISTOLOGY AND ULTRASTRUCTURE

The skin is divided into two principal layers, the epidermis and dermis. These two layers are functionally related in terms of development and disease processes. Although the two layers are intimately associated, they are interdependent throughout prenatal and postnatal life. The *epidermis* contains a heterogeneous population of cells of different types, function, and developmental origin. The *dermis* is a dense fibroelastic connective tissue stroma that contains extensive vascular and neural networks as well as specialized glands and appendages derived from the epidermis. Beneath the dermis is a subcutaneous layer of variable thickness composed predominantly of *fat cells*.

Embryology

The development of the skin is unique in that it must grow dramatically in size to maintain a covering for the entire body. It is exposed to many internal and external environmental changes throughout every phase of growth. Despite all the regionally specific influences that affect the skin throughout development, there is a similarity in the ontogenetic pattern and in the ultimate differentiation end product of the skin from any part of the body.

During the first 3 weeks of fetal life, the epidermis consists of only a single layer of undifferentiated glycogen-filled cells. By 4 to 6 weeks, two layers of cells are observed; by 8 to 11 weeks, a middle layer begins to form. At this time, collections of primitive mesenchymal cells can be observed to have focal collections and subsequently downward protuberance of the epidermis, which will become the *hair follicle*. Three buds come from the hair follicle, which are the future *sebaceous gland and duct*, the *apocrine gland and duct*, and the *arrector pilar muscle*. The *eccrine sweat glands* begin developing at about 9 weeks and become fully developed by 14 to 15 weeks. They develop from a separate primitive epidermal bud.

Melanocytes originate in the neural crest and migrate to the epidermis during fetal life. These early melanocytes

do not produce pigment before 4 to 6 months' gestation, but dopa-positive melanocytes can be demonstrated earlier.

The dermis is formed by mesenchymal cells migrating from the mesodermal areas. These mesenchymal cells give rise to the blood and connective tissue cells, including fibroblasts and mast cells of the dermis and the fat cells of the subcutaneous tissue.

Epidermis

The epidermis is composed of several layers of keratinocytes and other resident cells, such as melanocytes and Langerhans' cells. There are nerve processes that extend focally into the epidermis, but there are no blood or lymphatic channels. There are essentially four layers of keratinocytes in the epidermis. The combined basal, spinous, and granular layers are termed collectively the *malpighian layer*. The basal layer of keratinocytes is the layer adjacent to the dermis and is composed of cuboidal cells that are very basophilic as a result of the high content of ribosomes and other organelles. The basal cells have a modified type of desmosome called the half desmosome, or *hemidesmosome*. This will be discussed later with the *basement membrane*.

The next layer is the spinous layer (stratum spinosum). These cells are more abundant and have more eosinophilic cytoplasm because of a higher keratin content. The spinous cells are so named because of the intracellular connections called *intercellular bridges*. These are not really "bridges" but are the site of cell-to-cell contact seen ultrastructurally as desmosomes. Ultrastructurally, the spinous cells show numerous tonofilaments. There are stellate masses of keratohyalin beginning to form in this layer, but they are much more prominent in the next layer, the granular layer (stratum granulosum). The keratohyalin accrues progressively among the filaments to form larger and larger dense masses enclosing the filaments. In the granular layer the development of an ultrastructural lamellar granule with an internal laminated structure is noted. These structures are present both in the cytoplasm and in the extracellular space.

The most dramatic change occurs in the most superficial layer, the stratum corneum. This layer is associated with the degradation of mitochondria and ribosomes, disappearance of the nuclear envelope, and ultimate disappearance of the nucleus. The cells become flattened and filled with keratohyalin masses and filaments. At this stage of keratinization, a dense marginal band adjacent to the inner face of the plasma membrane appears. This creates the thickened cell envelope of the cornified cell. The stratum corneum consists of 15 to 20 layers of flat anucleate cells, which are thin squames of a thickness approximating 0.5 μm. and a width of 30 to 40 μm. One squame in the stratum corneum covers approximately 25 basal cells.

Langerhans' cells can be seen on routine sections stained with hematoxylin and eosin (H&E) as clear cells with small dark nuclei located in the higher levels of the epidermis. The Langerhans' cells are dendritic cells that stain with gold chloride, and by electron microscopy they have distinct cytoplasmic organelles that are shaped like tennis rackets and are called *Langerhans'* or *Birbeck granules*. These cells can also be recognized by specific immunologic and histochemical methods. Langerhans' cells show positive staining by monoclonal antibodies to primitive thymic antigens (OKT6), human leucocyte antigens (HLA), and immune response gene-associated antigens (Ia). Langerhans' cells stain positively for alkaline phosphatase.

Melanocytes are located in the basal layer. They have clear cytoplasm and small, dark nuclei pushed to one side of the cell. There are dendritic processes that extend from the main body of the melanocyte between adjacent keratinocytes. Each melanocyte produces and supplies melanin to 10 to 30 keratinocytes. The association of the melanocyte with keratinocytes is called the *epidermal melanin unit*. The melanocytes contain specific organelles called *melanosomes*, which can be demonstrated by electron microscopy. These are membrane-bound ellipsoidal structures having internal concentric lamellae of constant periodicity. The density of melanocytes varies in different parts of the body, with the highest concentration in sun-exposed areas of the head and neck and the genital and intertriginous areas.

Basement Membrane

At the boundary between the epidermis and underlying dermis is a supporting structure called the basement membrane. By light microscopy there is a periodic acid-Schiff (PAS)–positive membrane zone. This zone represents a high concentration of carbohydrate-rich mucopolysaccharides in the papillary dermis and does not correspond to the basement membrane seen with the electron microscope. Ultrastructurally, there is a clear zone immediately beneath the plasma membrane of the basal keratinocyte called the *lamina lucida*. Beneath the lamina lucida is a dense homogenous layer, the *lamina densa*, or *basal lamina*. Anchoring the basal keratinocyte to the dermis is a special type of desmosome, the *hemidesmosome*. The tonofilaments of the keratinocyte extend into the hemidesmosome plate. Located between the hemidesmosome and the basal lamina are small *anchoring filaments*. Below the basal lamina, small structures, the *anchoring fibrils*, are seen. These structures serve as an attachment plate to the dermis.

Dermis

There are two easily recognizable levels in the dermis (Fig. 1). The thin, superficial portion is called the *papillary dermis*, and the deeper area, composed of thick collagen bundles, is the *reticular dermis*. Both of these areas of the dermis have cellular, fibrous, and ground substance elements. The cellular elements of the dermis are fibroblasts, histiocytes, endothelial cells, pericytes, and mast cells. The fibrous component consists of collagen, reticulin, and elastic fibers. The collagen furnishes tensile strength, and the elastic fibers give flexibility to the skin. The dermal papilla is composed of collagen, elastic fibers, and a superficial capillary venule.

The *vascular supply* of the skin is very rich. There is a deep and superficial plexus of arteries and veins, and the superficial plexus is located in the high reticular dermis near the junction of the reticular and papillary dermis. A superficial capillary venule arises from the superficial plexus. These vessels are very labile and help control temperature. Special vascular regulatory shunts are controlled by groups of smooth muscle cells called *glomus bodies*. Lymphatics are numerous throughout the dermis and can be differentiated from veins because they lack pericytes.

There are many nerve fibers (free and encapsulated, myelinated and unmyelinated) in the skin, particularly in the areas of touch. There are three distinctive types of receptors: the *pacinian corpuscles*, *Meissner's corpuscles*, and *Merkel's cells*. The motor fibers of the skin are autonomic. Adrenergic fibers control the contraction of arrector pilar smooth muscle, the smooth muscle of arterial walls, the glomus body, and apocrine gland myoepithelial cells. The cholinergic fibers supply the eccrine glands.

The hair arises from hair follicles, which consist of specialized epidermal invagination associated with a specialized dermal structure, the *hair papilla*. The hair papilla controls the growth and maintenance of the hair follicle. For example, the mechanism of permanent hair removal is to cauterize the hair papillae, which then no longer can produce hair. The hair is also associated with melanocytes, sensory nerves, the arrector pilar muscle, sebaceous glands, and sometimes apocrine glands. There are three phases of hair growth: the anagen (growth) phase, the catagen (involution) phase, and the telogen (resting) phase.

The sebaceous glands are associated with almost all hair follicles except those on the lip, prepuce, labia minora, and eyelids (meibomian glands), and secrete a substance rich in triglycerides and lipids by holocrine processes. This secretion is mediated by hormonal factors and is important in the pathogenesis of acne. The *apocrine glands* are associated with some hair follicles and are present in the axillae, genital and perinal areas, areolae, periumbilical areas, external ear canal (ceruminous glands), and the eyelids (Moll's glands). The apocrine gland is composed of a coiled tubular, glandular structure located in the deep dermis or subcutis. A relatively straight duct leads to the hair follicle or directly to the skin surface. The apocrine material is secreted by so-called apocrine or *cytocrine secretion*. Apocrine gland secretion is regulated by adrenergic nerves and consists of an odorless, milky fluid that when contaminated by bacteria produces strong odors.

The *eccrine glands* are distributed over the palm, sole, and axilla. Only the lips and portions of the genitalia are free of eccrine glands. Each gland consists of a coiled tubular, glandular structure located at or near the junction of the dermis and subcutis. A relatively straight duct extends from the gland through the dermis into the epidermis. The intraepidermal portion of the duct courses a spiral tract through the epidermis. The gland is lined by two types of cells on the luminal surface, which are dark cuboidal cells rich in neutral polysaccharides and cells with clear cytoplasm rich in glycogen. The most external layer is composed of myoepithelial cells. The eccrine section is a thin, watery fluid and is secreted by the *merocrine process*. Secretion is controlled by cholinergic autonomic nerves; it is easily blocked and is the cause of heat rash *miliaria*. Occasionally, a patient will have severe hyperactivity, resulting in hyperhidrosis.

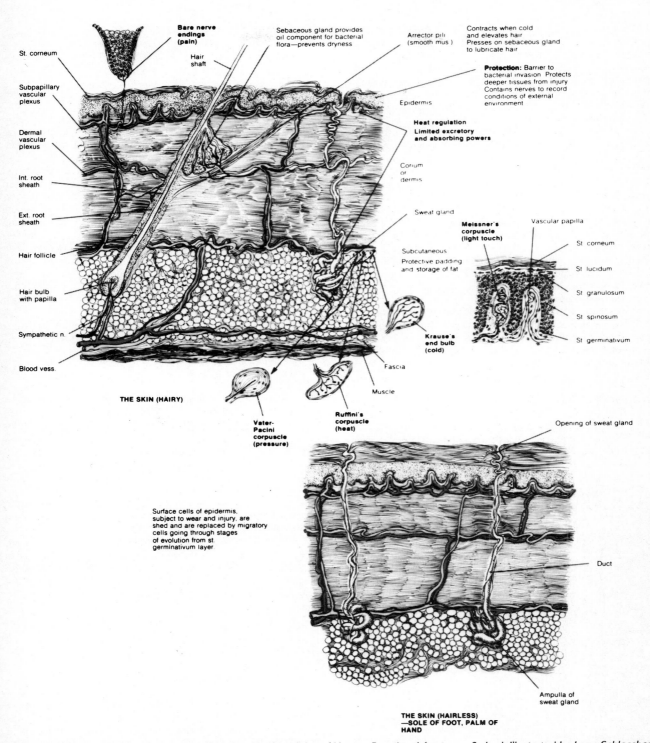

St. corneum

Subpapillary vascular plexus

Dermal vascular plexus

Int. root sheath

Ext. root sheath

Hair follicle

Hair bulb with papilla

Sympathetic n.

Blood vess.

Bare nerve endings (pain)

Hair shaft

Sebaceous gland provides oil component for bacterial flora—prevents dryness

Arrector pili (smooth mus.)

Contracts when cold and elevates hair Presses on sebaceous gland to lubricate hair

Protection: Barrier to bacterial invasion. Protects deeper tissues from injury. Contains nerves to record conditions of external environment

Epidermis

Heat regulation Limited excretory and absorbing powers

Corium or dermis

Sweat gland

Meissner's corpuscle (light touch)

Vascular papilla

St corneum

St lucidum

St granulosum

St spinosum

St germinativum

Subcutaneous Protective padding and storage of fat

Krause's end bulb (cold)

Fascia

Muscle

THE SKIN (HAIRY)

Vater-Pacini corpuscle (pressure)

Ruffini's corpuscle (heat)

Surface cells of epidermis, subject to wear and injury, are shed and are replaced by migratory cells going through stages of evolution from st. germinativum layer.

Opening of sweat gland

Duct

Ampulla of sweat gland

THE SKIN (HAIRLESS) —SOLE OF FOOT, PALM OF HAND

Figure 1. The skin. (From Zuidema, G. D.: The Johns Hopkins Atlas of Human Functional Anatomy, 3rd ed. Illustrated by Leon Schlossberg. Baltimore, The Johns Hopkins University Press, 1986.)

BENIGN EPIDERMAL TUMORS

Seborrheic Keratosis

The lesions of seborrheic keratosis are very common, especially in older individuals. They may be single or multiple, and occur mainly on the trunk and face. They have distinct, sharp margins and a "stuck-on" appearance. Brown in color, they are of a greasy and warty character (Fig. 2). Histologically, they are composed of benign basaloid cells that proliferate in an exophytic manner. These lesions almost never show malignant change and are easily removed by excision, shaving, or curettage. The differential diagnosis includes actinic keratosis, squamous cell carcinoma, and malignant melanoma.

Leukoplakia

Leukoplakia (Gr. *leukos*, white) is a clinical term applying to white patches that develop on the mucous membranes of the mouth, lips, or vagina. These lesions are often associated with chronic irritation, such as ill-fitting dentures, tobacco, and alcohol abuse. If the lesion does not regress with removal of the possible offending agent, a biopsy should be performed to exclude a malignant process. Development of malignancy in leukoplakia is unusual, but both malignancy and leukoplakia are associated with the same types of irritative phenomena. Histologically, leukoplakia is associated with epithelial hyperplasia and chronic inflammation.

Trichoepithelioma

Usually, trichoepitheliomas occur as multiple lesions and are often inherited as a dominant trait. They present as round, firm, skin-colored nodules up to 1 cm. in diam-

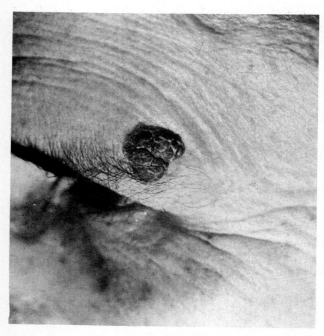

Figure 2. Seborrheic keratosis.

eter, primarily on the face. Histologically, the lesion is well circumscribed with a keratinized center surrounded by a lining of flattened basophilic ("basalioma") cells. Additional characteristics are tumor islands with peripheral palisading, not unlike that seen in basal cell carcinoma. These lesions can be difficult to differentiate histologically from basal cell carcinoma. Therefore, the clinical history is extremely helpful to the pathologist.

Warts

Warts are benign epidermal tumors caused by papilloma viruses (papovaviruses). The clinical appearance of the lesion depends on the virus subtype and the location. Verruca vulgaris is the most common type, occurring in childhood and adolescence and involving the hands and fingers. The warts may occur in groups and singly, often being spread by *autoinoculation*. Other types are the *plantar wart* and the *plane wart* (verruca plana). Helpful clinical observations are the presence of black dots of degenerating hemoglobin and a honeycomb appearance within the hyperkeratotic areas. Histologically, epidermal hyperplasia with perinuclear vacuolization and intranuclear inclusions are seen. The lesions may regress with time, but treatment is often necessary because of the size of the wart or for psychological reasons. Electrodessication or freezing with liquid nitrogen is frequently helpful. Recurrence is frequent, and new local lesions can develop following treatment, especially when excision and suture are done.

Cysts of the Epidermis

Epidermal cysts (wen, sebaceous cysts) are some of the most common lesions with which the surgeon deals. They develop when there is obstruction of the follicular infundibulum of the hair follicle by inflammation or sebum and desquamated keratinocytes (especially in acne). The cyst presents as a swelling, usually on the face, neck, or back. These cysts can remain stable for years, but occasionally will rupture in the surrounding dermis and produce a marked inflammatory reaction. Histologically, epidermal cysts are lined by stratified squamous epithelium and filled with laminated keratin debris.

"Sebaceous cyst" is a misnomer because there are no sebaceous glands or sebum in an epidermal cyst. These can be treated by simple excision, but it is necessary to excise the cyst wall entirely to prevent recurrence or inflammation secondary to the keratin remaining in the dermis.

PREMALIGNANT AND MALIGNANT EPIDERMAL TUMORS

Solar (Actinic, Senile) Keratosis

Actinic keratosis is a premalignant lesion developing on sun-exposed skin of the face, neck, and hands. This lesion is very common and is seen in persons with fair skin and those with occupations that require outdoor activity. The lesion is also now seen with increased frequency in persons who sunbathe frequently or experience a large sun exposure over a short period. Histologically, actinic keratosis shows dysplasia of the squamous epithelium. It is not unusual for these lesions to progress to squamous cell carcinoma. However, it is rare for a squamous cell carcinoma arising in an actinic keratosis to metastasize. Actinic keratosis is treated by excision and close follow-up for development of other actinic keratoses and squamous cell carcinoma.

Squamous Cell Carcinoma (Epidermoid Carcinoma)

Squamous cell carcinoma is the most common malignant tumor of the skin that has a potential for metastasis. Most of these tumors occur in older patients with a long history of sun exposure. However, one type of squamous cell carcinoma (Bowen's disease) can arise in mucous membranes or on non–sun-exposed skin. Other predisposing factors include arsenic ingestion; chronic ulcers (e.g., stasis ulcers); chronic sinuses (osteomyelitis); prolonged contact with organic hydrocarbons, tobacco and betel; radiation or thermal injury; and xeroderma pigmentosum. Carcinoma in sun-exposed skin clinically presents as a sharply defined plaque or as a single, painless, firm, red nodule with keratotic scales (Fig. 3) or a cutaneous horn. When the tumor becomes invasive, a shallow ulcer with wide, raised borders usually appears. Squamous cell carcinomas developing on mucous membranes often present as white patches (see the earlier discussion in leukoplakia).

Histologically, *in situ* squamous cell carcinoma (*Bowen's disease*) is composed of atypical squamous cells that replace the entire normal epidermis but do not invade the dermis. When there is breakthrough of the basement membrane, the carcinoma becomes invasive. The tumor cells show variation in size and shape, in nuclear hyperchromatism, and in high nuclear-to-cytoplasmic ratio. Most squamous cell carcinomas developing in sun-exposed skin are well differentiated and produce keratin with the formation of horn pearls (concentric layers of squamous cells with increasing keratinization centrally). Characteristic of squamous cell carcinoma is a heavy infiltrate of lymphocytes and plasma cells in the dermis beneath the tumor.

Biopsy should be done for all lesions suggestive of carcinoma. Excisional biopsy is preferable in small lesions.

Keratoacanthoma

Keratoacanthoma is a common lesion that occurs in elderly persons, usually solitary with a rapid onset. The lesion consists of a firm, dome-shaped nodule up to 2.5 cm. in diameter with a horn-filled crater in its center (Fig. 4). Most keratoacanthomas occur on the exposed surfaces of the body. Histologically, keratoacanthoma shows a crater-

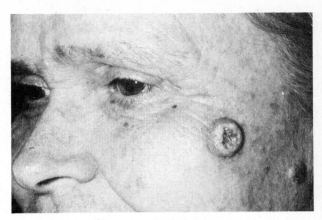

Figure 4. Keratoacanthoma.

form proliferation of squamous epithelium having glassy cytoplasm, dyskeratosis, and varying amounts of atypia. Some are difficult to differentiate from squamous cell carcinoma. Keratoacanthoma is a benign lesion and will regress if not treated. Most lesions are excised because of the clinical similarity to sqamous cell carcinoma.

Basal Cell Carcinoma

Basal cell carcinoma is a common, locally aggressive tumor of the skin that rarely metastasizes. It usually presents on the face and hair, bearing areas as a pearly-gray, semitranslucent papule with telangiectasia (Fig. 5). The

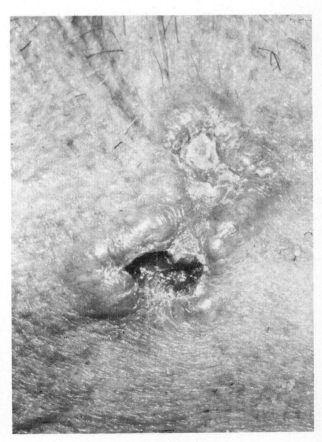

Figure 5. Basal cell carcinoma.

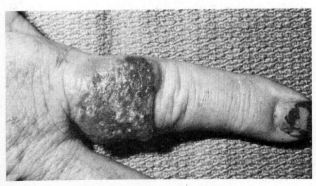

Figure 3. Squamous cell carcinoma.

lesions can present as black or brown nodules, plaques, or indurated areas with ulceration. Basal cell carcinoma is uncommon on the dorsum of hands and forearms, which are areas exposed to the sun. The lesions are common on the eyelids and the inner canthus, areas more protected from sunlight by dense pilosebaceous follicles. The rare *basal cell nevus syndrome* is a dominantly inherited disorder associated with the development, in early life, of numerous basal cell carcinomas and abnormalities of bone, skin, nervous system, eyes, and reproductive systems. In patients with xeroderma pigmentosum, there is also an increased risk of basal cell carcinoma developing.

There are several types of clinical presentations, but two are of special importance. *Superficial basal cell carcinoma* consists of nests of tumor cells budding from the lower epidermis and associated with an inflammatory fibrous stroma. This tumor does not invade beyond the papillary dermis. *Morphea-like basal cell carcinoma* consists of nests of tumor associated with a dense, sclerotic, fibrous stroma. The nests are so small that they can be overlooked on superficial examination.

Histologically, the tumor cells form nests, cords, and islands in the dermis. The cells are small and resemble normal basal cells of the epidermis. At the periphery of the nests, the basaloid cells tend to palisade, a characteristic and diagnostic feature. Mitotic figures are infrequent. Mucinous degeneration and differentiation toward appendiceal structures can occur. The relationship of basal cell carcinoma to its surrounding stroma appears to be important because there is a characteristic fibrovascular mucinous tissue surrounding the tumor nests.

In the past, basal cell carcinomas were considered to be slow-growing tumors of questionable malignancy. However, every clinician who has treated and followed such patients for a few years can attest that basal cell carcinoma is a malignant neoplasm. Early treatment directed toward eradicating the lesion is the best therapy. When basal cell carcinoma recurs several times, it becomes more and more difficult to treat. Excisional biopsy with a good margin is the treatment of choice. Basal cell carcinomas arising in the central triangle mid-third of the face (margins of nose to upper lip) tend to recur often after excision. They may become quite virulent and extremely invasive. Small basal cell carcinomas can be excised and curetted at the base. Often, large lesions need to be removed under microscopically controlled procedures in which the pathologist does multiple frozen sections of margins that have been mapped by the surgeon.

Patients with actinic changes in the skin and proven carcinomas are strongly advised to use sun screens for protection from further sun damage.

PIGMENTED LESIONS

Nevocellular Nevus (Pigmented Nevus, Mole)

Pigmented nevi are benign tumors of melanocytes and/or nevus cells. These moles are present in all individuals in varying numbers. They may be present at birth (congenital) (Fig. 6), but usually they appear in adolescence and increase in number through middle age (Fig. 7). They begin as small brown macules and then "mature," becoming dome-shaped and sometimes polypoid. Most become less pigmented after age 60.

Histologically, pigmented nevi show three different patterns. Lesions from young patients usually show nests

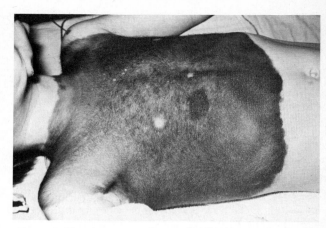

Figure 6. Giant hairy nevus (congenital "bathing trunk nevus").

of nevus cells at the dermal epidermal junction (*junctional nevus*). In older patients, nests will appear at the dermal epidermal junction and in the dermis (*compound nevi*). Nevi that have become less pigmented lose all junctional activity and have nests of nevus cells totally in the dermis (*intradermal nevus*). Sometimes it is difficult to differentiate these from neurofibromas (*neural nevus*).

UNCOMMON LESIONS

The *blue nevus* is an uncommon pigmented tumor composed of intradermal spindle and dendritic cells filled with coarse melanin pigment. As a result of the Tyndall effect of light scattering, reds are absorbed and deep blues are reflected back through the skin. Consequently, these lesions appear a deep blue-black, similar to the Mongolian spot of early childhood. They rarely become malignant.

The *spindle cell–epithelioid cell nevus* (Spitz tumor, benign juvenile melanoma) is an unusual lesion of children and, occasionally, adults. The lesion appears suddenly and grows rapidly over a few months' duration. The nevus is usually red, and the clinical diagnosis is pyogenic granuloma

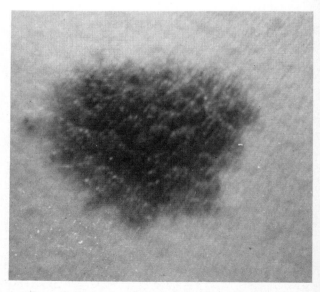

Figure 7. Common acquired pigmented nevus (mole).

or hemangioma. The histologic pattern can sometimes be difficult to interpret.

REMOVAL OF NEVI

Nevi are removed, usually for cosmetic reasons or when there is a clinical indication of malignant melanoma. If a patient is concerned that a nevus has changed, an excisional biopsy is recommended. For larger lesions, such as giant hairy nevi, incisional biopsies can be done when malignancy is suspected. Nevi should not be removed by shaving from the surface of the skin; such removal limits the pathologist's ability to determine the depth of invasion accurately if the lesion proves to be a melanoma.

RELATIONSHIP BETWEEN MOLES AND MELANOMA

Pigmented nevi are common, and malignant melanoma is relatively rare; therefore, malignant transformation of moles can be unusual. However, it is now known that between 20 and 40 per cent of patients with malignant melanoma have histologic evidence of an associated pre-existing benign nevus at the site of the melanoma. There is definitely an increased incidence of malignant melanoma in giant congenital pigmented nevi; in 5 to 40 per cent of these, melanoma develops.

Dysplastic Nevus Syndrome

An unusual type of nevus occurring in patients with melanoma and in many of their relatives has been designated the *B-K mole syndrome*, or dysplastic nevus syndrome.[1] Dysplastic nevi can also appear spontaneously in patients without the syndrome. Usually larger than ordinary melanocytic nevi, they measure 5 to 15 mm. in size. They have an irregular border and show a mixture of tan, brown, black, and pink colors. Because many of these patients with dysplastic nevus syndrome are at increased risk for malignant melanoma to develop, they should be thoroughly examined and closely followed, and family members should be examined for dysplastic nevi and malignant melanoma.

Histologically, the dysplastic nevus has a characteristic pattern. There are nests and cords of nevus cells at the rete ridge tips with slight to severe nuclear atypia associated with lamellar fibrosis and a variable chronic inflammatory infiltrate in the papillary dermis.

Malignant Melanoma

Malignant melanoma (Fig. 8) is still an uncommon neoplasm of the skin for which early diagnosis is of extreme importance. The incidence of melanoma has been increasing dramatically over the past two decades. The exact reason for this increase is not known, but speculations include changing dress codes and increased exposure to sunlight.

Malignant melanoma can arise *de novo* or in a pre-existing pigmented nevus. Four basic histologic types of melanoma are recognized: (1) superficial spreading, (2) lentigo maligna, (3) acra lentiginous, and (4) nodular. Superficial spreading malignant melanoma is the most common type in the United States. Lentigo maligna melanoma usually arises from a premalignant lesion lentigo maligna (Hutchinson's melanotic freckle).

Any pigmented lesion that has changed with variation in colors and with development of nodules or ulceration

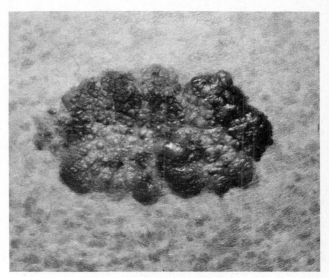

Figure 8. Malignant melanoma.

should be excised. After the diagnosis of melanoma has been confirmed, a wider excision is usually necessary. Regional lymph node dissection is performed if there is lymphadenopathy or if the lesion exceeds 0.85 mm. in thickness. Surgery remains the only successful therapy for melanoma.

SOFT TISSUE TUMORS

Keloids

Keloids are red, raised, firm nodules with a smooth, shiny surface (Fig. 9) that extends mushroom-like beyond

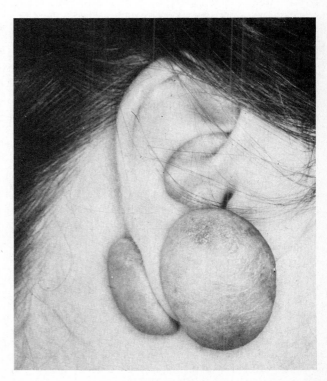

Figure 9. Keloid.

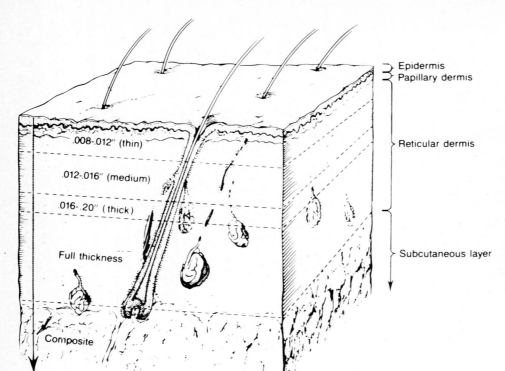

.008-.012" (thin)

.012-.016" (medium)

.016-.20" (thick)

Full thickness

Composite

Epidermis
Papillary dermis

Reticular dermis

Subcutaneous layer

Figure 10. Illustration depicting a cross section of skin indicating the varying thicknesses of skin grafts. Note that a full-thickness graft removes all of the epidermal appendages. Regeneration of the surface epithelium following a full-thickness skin graft is possible only from the periphery of the wound. The donor site for a full-thickness skin graft is usually closed primarily. (From Serafin, D.: The skin: Functional, metabolic and surgical considerations. In Sabiston, D. C., Jr. (Ed.): Textbook of Surgery, 13th ed. Philadelphia, W. B. Saunders Company, 1986, p. 1576.)

the borders of the original wound, thus being distinguished from *hypertrophic scars*. Hypertrophic scars have a similar clinical appearance, but they do not extend beyond the borders of the initial wound. Keloids are usually associated with antecedent trauma and are more common in blacks. There is an occasional familial predilection for keloid formation.

Treatment of keloids can be difficult because recurrence following excision is very frequent. Various therapies, such as intralesional steroids, cryotherapy, and irradiation, have been tried with variable results reported. When keloids are very large, excision with grafting becomes necessary (Fig. 10). In such circumstances, the excision is done intralesionally, leaving the borders intact. This appears to diminish the chance for recurrence. External elastic pressure for a protracted period can be used to treat hypertrophic scars and also to help reduce the recurrence of keloids.

Keloids, hypertrophic scars, and "normal" scars represent the spectrum of wound healing. All wounds become indurated and firm during the healing process. However, hypertrophic scarring and keloids, especially, are evidence of too much collagen production. In the case of the hypertrophic scar, the central enlargement of the scar does not overlap the original borders of the wound. These wounds are red and itchy. The reactivity in the wound is self-limited, and with time spontaneous resolution occurs. If the symptoms are annoying, the intralesional instillation of steroids (triamcinolone) will often hasten resolution and relieve the itching. For large wounds such as burns, fitted elastic garments apply a definite external pressure that tends to ameliorate the tendency to hypertrophic scarring.

Fibroma

Pure fibromas of the skin exist rarely, if at all. Soft fibromas (acrochordon, fibroepithelial papilloma, skin tags)

are common lesions that occur with increasing age in the neck and axillary areas. Histologically, these lesions show a fibrovascular stalk covered with stratified squamous epithelium. They can be treated easily by a shave biopsy flush with the skin.

Dermatofibromas (fibrous histiocytoma, sclerosing hemangioma) occur in the skin as firm, indolent, gray-brown nodules (Fig. 11). They usually present on the extremities and may or may not be related to a history of trauma. Histologically, these lesions show varying mixtures of fibroblasts, collagen, histiocytes, and blood vessels. Treatment is simple excision.

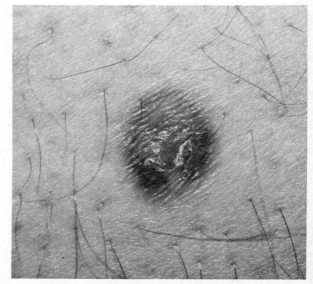

Figure 11. Dermatofibroma.

Lipoma

Lipomas are common skin tumors composed of mature fat cells. These tumors are soft, painless masses that occur singly and, rarely, multiply, and they usually are excised for cosmetic reasons. Occasionally, they produce symptoms of local discomfort possibly because of pressure on cutaneous nerves.

Hibernomas are a variety of lipoma in which the cells resemble the brown fat of hibernating animals. These multivacuolated mulberry-like cells are in fact immature fat cells that probably evolve by failure of an enzyme system that leads to maturation.

Neurofibroma

Neurofibroma is a benign tumor composed histologically of a mixture of fibrous tissue, nerves, and Schwann cells. The tumor may occur singly or in multiples in association with café au lait spots, the *sine qua non* of neurofibromatosis (von Recklinghausen's disease). Clinically, these lesions have a soft consistency and are skin-colored (Fig. 12). In some cases, neurofibroma presents as a subcutaneous nodule in peripheral nerves. Rarely, there are large flabby masses in which thickened, tortuous nerves are palpable. These plexiform neurofibromas are considered diagnostic of neurofibromatosis. In the solitary cutaneous neurofibroma, simple excision is curative. In patients with neurofibromatosis, close follow-up is necessary to observe malignant degeneration of the tumors. Plastic reconstruction is sometimes necessary because of the disfigurement produced.

Malignant Tumors of Soft Tissue

Dermatofibrosarcoma protuberans is a soft tissue tumor that arises in the dermis and subcutaneous tissue. It is of low-grade malignancy and expands the epidermis and underlying soft tissue. Histologically, there is a dense collection of fibrous tissue with a whorling pattern (storiform) that encroaches on the overlying epidermis and invades the subcutis. Mitotic figures are variable, but the anaplasia seen in more malignant tumors is absent. These should be treated with a wide local excision because they tend to recur locally and have been known to metastasize after several recurrences. Some pathologists believe that this tumor is malignant fibrous histiocytoma of the skin.

Malignant fibrous histiocytoma is the most common malignant tumor of soft tissue. This fact has become recognized only in the past 10 years. These pleomorphic tumors were previously diagnosed as variants of liposarcoma, fibrosarcoma, or rhabdomyosarcoma. They arise in the deep soft tissue, most commonly the thigh, and form a large mass that eventually may ulcerate the overlying skin. Initial treatment should be wide local excision, since more than half of the lesions recur locally and eventually metastasize.

VASCULAR TUMORS

Hemangioma

Hemangiomas are the most common benign vascular tumor of infants and children. There are two major types. The *capillary hemangioma* is very common in infancy and

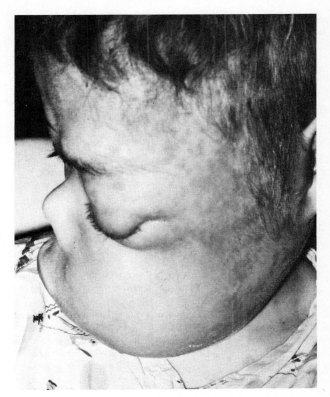

Figure 12. Neurofibroma.

childhood, usually presenting at birth as a bright-red, raised, circumscribed nodule or plaque (Fig. 13). It can grow rapidly and can be of concern to the parents and physician. Histologically, these lesions are composed of numerous small capillaries.

The *port wine stain* is a congenital, flat, dark lesion that is present at birth and is composed of small endothelium-lined channels. Pressure on the lesion will cause blanching. These tumors tend to appear more prominent

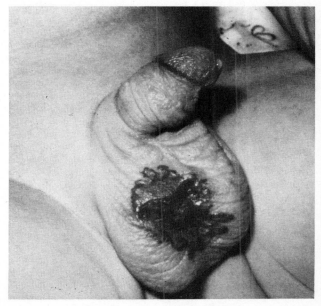

Figure 13. Capillary hemangioma.

with aging, in contrast to the capillary hemangiomas, which usually regress by the age of 5.

Cavernous hemangiomas are soft, blue, compressible masses (Fig. 14) composed of large, thin-walled, endothelium-lined channels. They increase in size and may ulcerate and bleed; they rarely regress. Lymphangiomas are similar tumors composed of channels filled with lymph instead of blood.

Treatment of hemangiomas requires patience and individualization in each case. Most capillary hemangiomas, especially the smaller ones, will regress by age 5, frequently with central clearing and fibrosis. Lesions located on the face, neck, hands, or vulva that are rapidly growing may require local excision for control. Although radiation was used extensively in the past to treat hemangiomas, it is employed less often today because of the long-term complications of radiation therapy and the fact that most capillary hemangiomas will regress. Treatment with systemic corticosteroids in large doses will occasionally initiate regression in rapidly growing lesions. External elastic pressure with a fitted garment can help reduce capillary hemangiomas and often can prevent enlargement of the cavernous variety.

The port wine nevus is a difficult cosmetic problem. The use of lasers has contributed to the therapy of these lesions, and it is to be hoped that such treatment will prevent the need for extensive surgery and grafting. Cosmetics are useful in the case of small lesions.

Malignant Vascular Tumors

Malignant vascular tumors are very rare and previously have been subclassified, but for practical purposes only three types merit mention. *Angiosarcoma* is a malignant tumor of endothelial cells and most commonly occurs on the head and neck of elderly people. Treatment consists of wide excision.

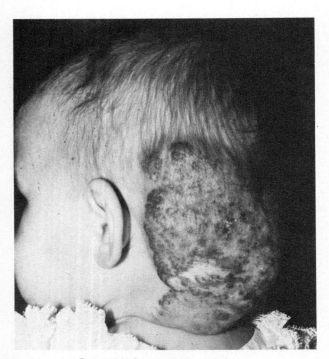

Figure 14. Cavernous hemangioma.

Kaposi's sarcoma, a clinicopathologic subtype of the malignant vascular tumor, is a slowly progressive lesion on the legs of men aged 40 to 70 years. The origin is probably a multipotential mesenchymal cell that can differentiate into the vascular and spindle components of the tumor. Kaposi's sarcoma is uncommon in the United States, but is endemic in certain parts of central Africa. This tumor has become more important within the past decade because of the recognition of the *acquired immune deficiency syndrome (AIDS)*. Many patients with AIDS present with an opportunistic organism infection and/or Kaposi's sarcoma. Kaposi's sarcoma usually begins on the lower extremities, but it can occur anywhere on the skin. The lesions enlarge, coalesce, and become nodular. Later, the lesions become disseminated through internal organs and lymph nodes. Treatment should be directed to local excision and any underlying disease.

The third type of angiosarcoma develops in an extremity with chronic edema. *Lymphangiosarcoma* may develop several years after a radical mastectomy in the edematous tissue of the ipsilateral arm. The cutaneous nodules have a bluish color, rapidly increase in size, and may ulcerate. Death usually occurs within 1 to 2 years after appearance of the angiosarcoma as a result of metastases, especially to the lungs.

MISCELLANEOUS LESIONS

Xanthomas

Xanthomas are tumors characterized histologically by collections of foamy (lipid-laden) histiocytes. They are ubiquitous, occurring in all races and in both sexes. Xanthomas are occasionally associated with familial or acquired disorders leading to hyperlipidemia, such as biliary cirrhosis, pancreatitis, and diabetes mellitus. However, in most individuals, xanthomas arise without an underlying cause. Xanthomas are classified according to their clinical appearance and location. The five types are eruptive, tuberous, tendon, plane, and xanthelasma. The eruptive xanthoma is the only type with consistent clinical correlation with the levels of plasma triglycerides and lipids. Xanthelasmas are soft yellow plaques that occur on the eyelids; these lesions can be treated by local excision.

Pilonidal Cysts

Pilonidal cysts and their accompanying sinuses are of congenital and ectodermal origin, although the exact etiology is unknown. Some theories suggest that they are produced by invaginations of ectoderm resulting from the traction by the caudal ligament, which attaches to the lower vertebrae; that they are the result of ectodermal invagination of the midline early in development; that they are abnormal rests on dormant dermoid cells; and that they occur because of persistence of a coccygeal vestige of the neural canal.

Pilonidal cysts and sinuses occur in the posterior midline near the tip of the coccyx; when obstructed, they may enlarge tremendously, leading to large abscesses. They may be difficult to eradicate surgically. Histologically, the sinuses are lined with stratified squamous epithelium with hair, hair follicles, and sweat glands. Usually, the cysts are lined with cuboidal epithelium plus rare hair follicles. With recurrences there may be innumerable tracts around the buttock and sacral region, making treatment difficult.

Hidradenitis Suppurativa

Hidradenitis suppurativa is a chronic, suppurative, and scarring disorder of apocrine gland–bearing areas. The etiology of this disease is not well understood, but it is probably due to a combination of factors, such as keratinous obstruction of the hair follicle followed by secondary bacterial infection. The patient presents with small red nodules or pustules that eventually drain. Eventually, sinus tract formation and scarring occur. The histopathology of early lesions, although only rarely are these examined, shows keratinous occlusion of the apocrine ducts and hair follicle. Neutrophil infiltration, intraglandularly and later in the surrounding dermis and subcutaneous tissue, is also seen. Later, the lesions show scarring, chronic and granulomatous inflammation, and sinus tracts lined by squamous epithelium.

Early therapy is of utmost importance. Systemic antibiotics and local drainage procedures are important in management. After scarring and sinus tract formation have become extensive, it is necessary to excise the involved areas.

SELECTED REFERENCES

Fitzpatrick, T. B., Eisen, A. Z., Wolf, K., Freedberg, I. W., and Austen, K. F.: Dermatology in General Medicine, 2nd ed. New York, McGraw-Hill, 1979.
Goldsmith, L. A.: Biochemistry and Physiology of the Skin. New York, Oxford Press, 1983.
Lever, W., and Schaumberg-Lever, G.: Histopathology of the Skin, 6th ed. Philadelphia, J. B. Lippincott Company, 1984.

REFERENCES

1. Green, M. H., Clark, W. H., Tucker, M. A., et al.: Acquired precursors of cutaneous malignant melanoma. N. Engl. J. Med., 312:91, 1985.

GYNECOLOGIC SURGERY

A. F. HANEY, M.D.

38

The evolution of gynecology as a specialty began in the 19th century with surgical specialization and has grown to include a broad range of topics, including embryology, endocrinology, genetics, infectious disease, and oncology. The clinical problems encountered by the gynecologist have many unique aspects corresponding to the role of the genital tract in reproduction. A high level of technical sophistication allows interruption of normal homeostasis, thus providing contraception, correction of reproductive failure, reduction of the morbidity and mortality from gynecologic disease, and stabilization of the effects of aging as they relate to the genital tract and reproductive hormones.

Although gynecologic diseases were certainly known to the ancients, the first successful abdominal operation on the pelvic organs was performed in 1809 by Ephraim McDowell, a rural practitioner in Kentucky. His removal of a large ovarian cyst heralded significant advances in gynecologic surgery paralleling those in other surgical specialties. A major advance is credited to J. Marion Sims in the mid-1800s for successful closure of vesicovaginal fistulas. By the turn of the century, Wertheim had performed a radical hysterectomy for cancer of the cervix with extensive node dissection, and the basic principles of that operation are utilized to this day. Those advances, as well as the general improvement in medical care, set the tone for the rest of the century, with a more scientifically oriented approach to women's health care.

In the 1920s, the modern era of gynecologic investigation began. Notable advances included Sampson's description of retrograde menstruation as the etiology of endometriosis, the synthesis of estrogen by Allen and Doisy, and the discovery of a fetal product in maternal urine, human chorionic gonadotropin (hCG), by Ascheim and Zondek. Cytologic evaluation of the genital tract for the detection of premalignant changes began in the 1940s with the major contribution of Papanicolaou and Traut. Recognition that choriocarcinoma had a high requirement for folic acid led Li, Hertz, and Spencer to use methotrexate to cure metastatic choriocarcinoma, dramatically demonstrating the potential of chemotherapy in selected malignancies.

The reproductive endocrinology of the female menstrual cycle began to be better understood in 1958 with Gemzell's induction of ovulation with human menopausal gonadotropins and was accelerated dramatically with the development of radioimmunoassay and the introduction of oral contraceptives addressing the most important problem facing mankind, overpopulation. This chapter is intended to give the medical student an overview of gynecology and to encourage further reading of research reports and reviews on individual aspects of this discipline.

GENITAL TRACT EMBRYOLOGY

Genital tract differentiation is a complex process that is dependent upon the genetic complement of the individual and the expression of gonadal hormones. Genital tract differentiation involves three separate genital tract compartments: the gonad, the internal duct structures, and the external genitalia. A wide variety of genital tract anomalies are encountered, and a knowledge of the mechanisms of embryogenesis will aid in understanding these problems and provide insights into appropriate therapy. Because of the parallel development and proximity of the genital and urinary tracts, simultaneous congenital defects are often present.

Ovarian Differentiation

Gonadal differentiation is dependent upon genetic sex, with a 46,XX genetic complement resulting in ovarian differentiation and a 46,XY testicular differentiation. The germ cells migrate from the yolk sac along the gut mesentery to an area of mesoderm on the posterior aspect of the abdominal cavity called the *gonadal ridge*. The oocytes initially undergo *mitosis*, reaching a maximal number of between 5 and 20 million by 20 weeks of gestation. The oocytes are invested by precursor follicular cells of uncertain origin. The oocytes then begin the process of *meiosis*, which is designed to reduce the chromosome number to a haploid complement. Meiosis is arrested in prophase of the first division and remains at that point until immediately prior to ovulation. The majority of follicular units undergo atresia *in utero*, leaving approximately 1 to 2 million present at birth. This loss continues in childhood, with approximately 100,000 to 200,000 oocytes present at the time of puberty, and virtually no oocytes at the climacteric, with only 300 to 400 being ovulated during a reproductive lifetime, indicating that the vast majority are lost through atresia. The rate of oocyte loss is unaffected by the use of agents such as oral contraceptives, which suppress pituitary gonadotropins and prevent ovulation, suggesting that the majority of follicular differentiation is gonadotropin-independent.

Recently, the understanding of the genetics of gonadal differentiation has been expanded by the demonstration of a specific genetic code for testicular differentiation. A surface protein, the Y-antigen, appears on cells of 46,XY individuals, and the genetic template resides on the Y chromosome. This gene can be translocated to another chromosome; hence, in some individuals with 46,XX karyotypes there can be testicular differentiation if the Y-antigen is present. Similarly, ovaries can develop in an individual with 46,XY complement in the absence of the Y-antigen. An understanding of the mechanism of abnormal gonadal differentiation should improve after more experience with this technique.

The Internal Genitalia

The vagina, cervix, uterus, and fallopian tubes are formed from the interaction of the mesonephric (wolffian) and paramesonephric (müllerian) ducts. Controversy still surrounds the specific contributions of each of these primordial structures to the developing genital tract, but there is no doubt that the urogenital sinus makes contact with the caudal portion of the paired müllerian ducts linking the female genital tract with the perineum. The lower portions of the two müllerian ducts fuse and form the upper portion of the vagina, cervix, and uterus (Fig. 1). The more cephalad portions remain separated and form the fallopian tubes. The genital tract is canalized, and the patency is established. The role of the mesonephric ducts in female differentiation is uncertain; while they undergo regression, they do appear necessary, probably by interaction with the adjacent müllerian structures. Mesonephric remnants are frequently observed lateral to the müllerian ducts, and it now appears that cells of mesonephric origin enter the developing ovarian stromal compartment as well, termed the *intraovarian rete*.

In the absence of testicular differentiation, the mesonephric ducts regress and the müllerian ducts persist, forming typical female internal genitalia. When testes are present, testosterone is produced by the Leydig cells in response to the hCG elaborated by the placenta. The high local concentration of testosterone is responsible for maintenance of the mesonephric ducts. The Sertoli cells produce a protein that causes regression of the müllerian ducts termed *müllerian-inhibiting substance* (MIS). In the absence of a normally functioning testis, these events do not occur and development proceeds along female lines despite the presence of a male gonad.

Development of the External Genitalia

Despite the obvious anatomic dissimilarity, male and female external genitalia are derived from the same embryonic structures. Analogous to the internal structures, in the absence of high levels of testosterone, the development will occur along female lines. The process of male differentiation is complicated by the presence of the nuclear enzyme 5-alpha-reductase in genital skin, converting testosterone to its more potent metabolite, dihydrotestosterone (DHT). Men genetically deficient in 5-alpha-reductase incompletely virilize their external genitalia, despite normal development of the mesonephric ducts, demonstrating the organ specificity of the virilization caused by DHT. Similarly, women exposed to androgens *in utero* may have virilized external genitalia, but because very high local concentrations of androgens are required for maintenance of the mesonephric ducts, the internal genitalia remain unchanged.

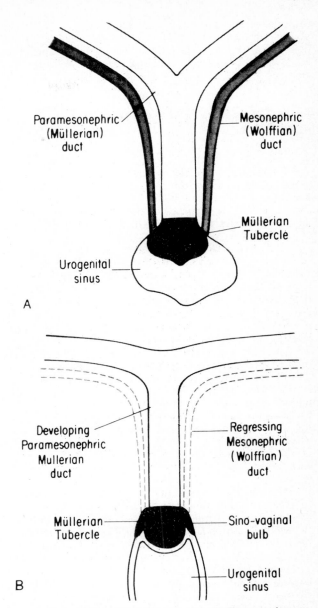

Figure 1. Embryology of the internal genitalia. The paired mesonephric (wolffian) and paramesonephric (müllerian) ducts are depicted in their proper anatomic relationship as they contact the urogenital sinus. In the absence of a testis, the mesonephric duct regresses and the urogenital sinus further differentiates (right). Beyond this point, the müllerian structures undergo canalization, yielding a patent reproductive tract.

PELVIC ANATOMY

The genital tract undergoes a series of dramatic transformations throughout a woman's lifetime, paralleling her reproductive status. At birth, the genital tract is minimally stimulated as a result of the high maternal estrogen levels during pregnancy. This estrogenization is rapidly lost post partum, and the genital structures remain in an immature state until puberty. Circulating sex steroids increase substantially at puberty, maturing and enlarging the pelvic organs in preparation for reproduction. The high levels of gonadal hormones remain throughout the menstrual years and are linked to the process of ovulation. During the climacteric, estrogen production declines, leading to atrophy of the genital tract. This portion of the chapter will not attempt to be a definitive anatomy text; rather, the focus will be on clinically important aspects of genital tract anatomy.

Vascular, Lymphatic, and Nerve Supply of the Pelvis

VASCULAR SUPPLY

There are three main vascular pathways supplying the pelvis: (1) the *ovarian arteries* originating from the aorta near the renal arteries, (2) the *hypogastric* or *internal iliac arteries* arising as branches of the common iliac arteries, and (3) branches from the *femoral arteries* supplying the vulva (Fig. 2).

The ovarian arteries descend to the pelvis by coursing over the psoas muscle, crossing over the external iliac vessels, and entering the ovary via its superior pole. The right ovarian vein empties directly into the vena cava, but the left ovarian vein empties into the left renal vein opposite the adrenal vein. The ovarian arteries send branches to the oviducts as well as to the ascending branches of the uterine arteries at the medial pole of the ovary.

The hypogastric arteries course posteriorly along the sciatic notch, yielding anterior branches supplying arteries to the uterus, bladder, vagina, rectum, and vulva. The *uterine artery* is the most important surgically. It is the major vessel to the uterus and courses just anterior to the ureter, reaching the uterus at the junction of the cervix and the uterine fundus, sending main branches to each. The ascending branches are tortuous and follow the lateral border of the uterus to join branches of the ovarian arteries. The descending branch supplies the cervix and upper vagina.

Separate *vaginal* and *anterior vesicle arteries* supply the remainder of the vagina and bladder, respectively. The vascular supply of the vulva is derived from branches of the *femoral* and *pudendal arteries*. The pudendal artery is the most caudal branch of the hypogastric artery and passes near the ischial spine, through the lesser sciatic foramen in its course to the vulva. As with most organ systems, collateral circulation is the rule with vascular connections to the femoral, hemorrhoidal, and contralateral ovarian and uterine arteries.

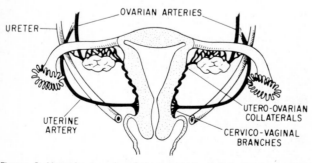

Figure 2. Vascular supply of the internal genital structures. Two pairs of arteries represent the main vascular supply of the internal genital structures, the uterine and ovarian arteries. This vascular pattern is important to the gynecologic surgeon because the two principal arteries have large collaterals. When gynecologic operations are performed, the proximity of the ureter to the uterine artery must be borne in mind to avoid ureteral injuries.

LYMPHATIC SUPPLY

The lymphatic channels parallel the vascular supply with the internal genitalia draining via the obturator and hypogastric nodes to the common iliac chain and on to the para-aortic nodes. Lymphatics, like blood vessels, have collaterals, and some lymphatic drainage of genital structures can occur through the external iliac and sacral nodes. Lymphatic drainage of the vulva is via subcutaneous vessels to the superficial and deep inguinal nodes and subsequently the femoral chain. The lower portions of the vagina and urethra may also drain by this pathway. A femoral canal lymph node, *Cloquet's node*, is often the first node involved in lymphatic spread of malignancies from the vulva and as such has great prognostic significance. Ovarian lymphatics course along with the ovarian vessels, bypassing the pelvic nodes, and communicate directly with the para-aortic lymphatics.

NERVE SUPPLY

The nerve supply to the pelvis comes from the fourth and fifth lumbar and first four sacral nerve roots. They form the *sacral plexus*, which gives rise to the pudendal nerve accompanying the pudendal artery to become the primary sensory and motor nerve to the vulva and perineal muscles. Both the preganglionic parasympathetic fibers to the viscera and the postganglionic sympathetic fibers from the hypogastric plexus are present.

External Genitalia

The *vulva* is the term generally applied to the external genitalia of the female (Fig. 3). Although the vulvar skin is histologically similar to the adjacent nongenital skin, including the presence of skin appendages (e.g., hair follicles, sweat glands), it is unique in its trophic response to gonadal hormones, the presence of apocrine glands similar to the axilla, and hair follicles responsive to androgens. Pubic hair develops during puberty in response to both ovarian and adrenal androgens. The total amount of pubic hair varies according to the genetic predisposition of the individual; in the absence of puberty, however, virtually none develops. The characteristic female hair pattern, or *escutcheon*, is that of an inverted equilateral triangle with the base parallel to the pubic bone covering the mons veneris and hair extending over the remainder of the vulva and laterally to the inner aspect of the thighs.

The *labia majora* are vulvar skin folds beginning lateral to the base of the clitoris in the mons and extending posteriorly to the perineal body surrounding the remainder of the genital structures. The perineal body is that midline coalescence of skin, subcutaneous tissue, and underlying connective tissue that separates the vaginal entrance anteriorly from the rectum posteriorly. The *labia minora* are parallel skin folds without hair follicles medial to the labia majora that enclose the *urethral meatus* and vaginal entrance, collectively known as the *introitus*. The labia minora begin anteriorly, forming the prepuce of the clitoris, and end at the top of the perineal body, forming the posterior fourchette.

The *clitoris* is the phallic structure analogous to the male penis and is sensitive to androgen action and tactile stimulation. Just posterior to the clitoris in the midline is the urethral meatus, which is surrounded laterally by periurethral glands exiting through Skene's ducts. Immediately posterior to the urethral meatus is the entrance to the

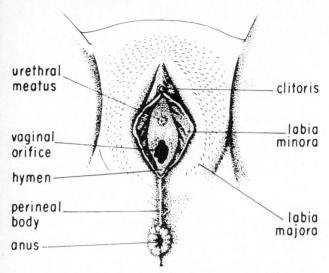

Figure 3. The vulva. A schematic diagram of the vulva is shown. Note the anatomic relationships between the introitus, perineal body, and anus.

vagina, which is initially covered by a thin fibrous membrane, the *hymen*, which is resorbed in the adult and manifested by only a fringe of irregular tissue. Occasionally, this membrane may remain intact, forming an imperforate hymen. Ducts draining two compound racemose glands—*Bartholin's glands*—enter the introitus laterally at the posterior aspect of the vaginal orifice. Their function is unknown, and they can be appreciated only when the ducts are obstructed and the glands are enlarged.

The Perineum

The perineum consists of several layers of fascia and muscle through which pass the urethra, anus, and vagina. The function of these layers is often overlooked when one details their complicated anatomy. They provide structural support for the three traversing canals, allowing continence of feces and urine yet retaining enough flexibility to allow coitus and the expulsion of the fetus during childbirth. Knowledge of this complex anatomy facilitates repair of these structures when they are weakened by childbirth or to provide adequate drainage of superficial infections that progress along the natural tissue planes.

Two superficial fascial layers present in the perineum, *Cruveilhier's* and *Colles' fascia*, are continuous with the fascial planes of the abdominal wall, Camper's and Scarpa's, respectively. The deep perineal fascia is also present in two layers. The first is composed of the fascial investments of the superficial perineal muscles, the bulbocavernosus, ischiocavernosus, superficial transverse perineal, sphincter urethrae, and sphincter ani muscles. The second layer is formed by the fascia covering the deep layer of muscles of the pelvic floor, the levator ani, the coccygeus, and the deep transverse perineal muscles, collectively known as the *urogenital diaphragm*.

The levator ani and external anal sphincter muscles provide continence of feces, and the act of defecation involves both relaxation of these muscles and a Valsalva maneuver to increase intra-abdominal pressure to expel stool. The urethra has its own muscular sphincter attached to periurethral connective tissue and the pelvic rami. Similar to the rectum, both the Valsalva maneuver and relaxation of the sphincter contribute to controlled micturition. The vaginal orifice is surrounded by the bulbocavernosus muscles, which blend superiorly with the ischiocavernosus muscle under the clitoris and posteriorly with the anal sphincter and transverse perineal muscles. Loss of integrity of these muscle groups, usually by childbirth trauma, may result in incontinence of urine or feces or in sexual dysfunction.

The Vagina

The vaginal entrance represents the junction between the müllerian ducts and the urogenital sinus. In contrast to the skin of the vulva, the rugated vaginal mucosa is non-keratinized, stratified squamous epithelium devoid of skin appendages. The thickness of the epithelium is increased by estrogen, making it well adapted to withstand the rigors of coitus and childbirth. The vagina contains no glands, and lubrication during coitus is secondary to a transudate of plasma induced by sexual arousal. A mucoepithelial discharge is normally present in the vagina along with both aerobic and anaerobic bacteria. The pH is usually acidic because of the production of lactic acid by the vaginal flora. The vagina is supported by an investment of connective tissue called the paravaginal fascia.

Several misconceptions are prevalent about the vagina. First, the vagina is usually described as a cylinder or tube; in actuality, it represents only a potential space because the walls are coapted. Second, the vagina is usually thought of as projecting directly cephalad into the abdominal cavity; actually, it is directed posteriorly toward the sacral promontory so as to be virtually horizontal when one is standing. Lastly, the vagina is not uniform in size; it has a large caliber and is distensible, and the apex is significantly larger than the introitus.

The Cervix

The uterus is divided into two distinct segments. The lower portion, or *cervix*, is lined by mucus-secreting columnar epithelium in direct continuity with the epithelium of the vagina. The *ectocervix* has stratified squamous epithelium similar to that of the vagina with a rather abrupt transition between the two, the squamocolumnar junction. The racemose glands of the *endocervix* are responsive to estrogen and progesterone, producing a unique hydrogel—*cervical mucus*—which varies dramatically in character through the menstrual cycle. The mucus provides a bacterial barrier between the sterile upper genital tract and the bacteria-containing vagina while facilitating sperm access around ovulation. The endocervical architecture is that of multiple crypts providing a reservoir for sperm in which they survive for up to several days after coitus.

After childbirth, the columnar epithelium is typically everted on the ectocervix and thus exposed to the vaginal environment. This environmental change initiates a process of squamous metaplasia, replacing or covering the columnar epithelium with metaplastic squamous epithelium. Entrapped mucus-secreting columnar epithelium continues to function, resulting in mucus-filled "Nabothian cysts" on the cervix. The diameter of the endocervical canal varies during the menstrual cycle, reaching its largest size (>1 cm.) at midcycle.

The Uterine Fundus

The upper segment, or *uterine corpus*, is a muscular, pear-shaped organ approximately 8 cm. in length with walls composed of smooth muscle, 1 to 2 cm. thick. The endometrial cavity is only a potential space because the walls are coapted. The oviductal ostia are located laterally high in the uterine fundus with a gradual transition from endometrium to the oviductal epithelium. The uterus protrudes into the abdominal-pelvic cavity between the bladder anteriorly and the rectum posteriorly. The peritoneum is continuous over all the pelvic structures, yielding indentations anteriorly, the uterovesical fold, and, posteriorly, the cul-de-sac, which is the most dependent portion of the abdomen.

The epithelium of the uterine cavity is truly unique, undergoing cyclic proliferation, secretory activity, and menstrual shedding (Fig. 4). The endometrium has both a cycling layer and a basal regenerative layer composed of glands and specialized stroma responsive to ovarian hormones. Unopposed estrogen stimulates proliferation of both the glandular and stromal elements; after ovulation, under the influence of both estrogen and progesterone, secretory activity occurs with decidualization of the stroma. In the absence of pregnancy, the steroid support is withdrawn and the complex event of menstruation occurs. The basic process is one of collapse with a decline in endometrial height; reversion to a proliferative pattern; and the loss of extracellular fluid, blood, and a relatively small number of glandular and stromal cells. Prostaglandins are mediators of the process, causing tissue hypoxia in the superficial layer of epithelium as well as uterine contractions to aid in expulsion of the menstrual debris.

The uterine wall is composed of estrogen-responsive smooth muscle; hence, the uterus enlarges at puberty and atrophies during the climacteric. The uterus is typically anteflexed toward the abdominal wall with flexion at the junction of the cervix and uterine fundus. A prominent but elastic structure, the *round ligament*, exits laterally from the uterine fundus anterior to the oviduct and courses retroperitoneally through the inguinal ring to insert in the mons veneris.

The Fallopian Tubes

The *oviducts*, or fallopian tubes, have three basic functions:

1. To act as a conduit for ascent of the mobile male gamete, i.e., sperm.

2. To provide an environment conducive to fertilization and early embryonic growth.

3. To pick up the immobile female gamete, i.e., the oocyte, and transport it, after fertilization, into the uterus in a timely fashion.

The oviducts enter the uterus laterally in the fundus and course along the broad ligament, curving around the ovaries with a vascular pedicle, the mesosalpinx, affording a great deal of mobility. The tubes are approximately 12 cm. long and separable into three distinct segments: (1) the isthmus, (2) the ampulla, and (3) the fimbria. The nearest to the uterus is the isthmic segment, characterized by a thick muscular wall and a relatively simple round lumen lined by columnar cells with relatively few cilia. There is a rather gradual transition into a much larger caliber segment, the *ampulla*. The muscular layer is attenuated, and the epithelium markedly enfolded with a large proportion of ciliated cells. This produces longitudinally oriented furrows extending to the fimbrial ostia. This is histologically similar to the ampulla, with the folds projecting through the ostia, increasing the surface area of epithelium. A specialized segment of this epithelium extends down to the surface of

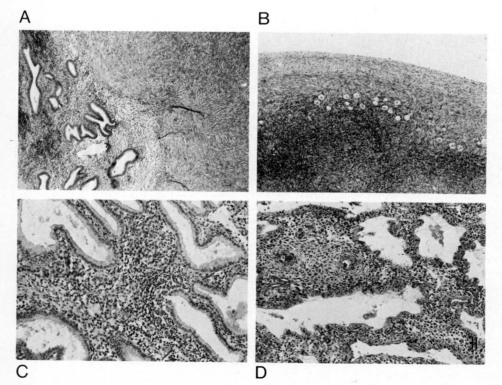

Figure 4. Histology of the genital tract.

A, Ovarian endometriosis is illustrated with typical endometrial glands and stroma adjacent to ovarian stroma (52×).

B, The primordial ovarian follicles are demonstrated near the ovarian capsule. Note that the oocytes have only a single layer of follicular cells and are surrounded by typical ovarian stroma (68×).

C, Typical late luteal endometrium is shown. The glands have a single layer of vacuolated columnar cells, there is secretory material within the glands, and the stroma is undergoing decidualization (170×).

D, The endometrium of early pregnancy is shown with intensely decidualized stroma, prominent vasculature, and hypersecretory glands with a serrated border (130×).

the ovary, termed the fimbria ovarica, contacting the ovarian capsule and enhancing the likelihood of oocyte retrieval. Peritoneum covers the external surface of the oviducts enclosing the vascular supply of the oviduct in the mesosalpinx. The fallopian tubes have great mobility and under physiologic conditions are found curled around the ovaries deep in the cul-de-sac. The aqueous environment allows exposure of the maximal fimbrial surface area, enhancing the likelihood of epithelium-oocyte contact.

The Ovary

The human ovary is an oblong structure with a glistening white convoluted surface approximately 2 × 3 × 3 cm. in size. The ovaries are located on the posterior aspect of the broad ligament inferior to the oviduct and lateral to the uterus with a vascular pedicle called the *mesovarium*. Structural support for the ovary comes not only from the mesovarium but also from a dense fibrous band attached medially to the uterus, the *utero-ovarian ligament*, and laterally by a condensation of connective tissue surrounding the ovarian vasculature, the *infundibulopelvic ligament*.

Histologically, the ovary is separable into the *cortex*, containing the follicular units (Fig. 4), and the *medulla*, composed primarily of steroidally active gonadal stromal cells. A single layer of cuboidal cells, the coelomic or germinal epithelium, covers the entire ovary. Primordial follicles contain an oocyte surrounded by a layer of follicular cells and an outer layer of specialized stromal cells called the *theca*. Under the influence of pituitary gonadotropins, the follicles enlarge, dramatically increasing the number of granulosa and thecal cells that produce both estrogens and androgens (Fig. 5). Follicular fluid accumulates, and as the follicle approaches 2 cm. in size, enzymatic digestion of the follicle wall and enclosing ovarian capsule results in the escape of the oocyte and follicular fluid, i.e., ovulation.

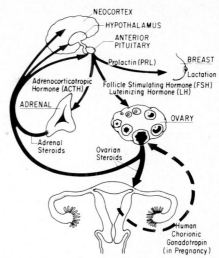

Figure 6. This schematic diagram depicts the major components of the female reproductive system. This is an interactive system involving the central nervous system, pituitary, ovary, and uterus. Both positive and negative feedback actions of gonadal and adrenal steroids are operative. When pregnancy is established, the chorionic gonadotropin elaborated by the fetus maintains luteal function.

Intraperitoneal bleeding may result from this process, and blood fills the ruptured follicle. The process of luteinization converts the follicle into a *corpus luteum*, which produces large amounts of progesterone (Fig. 5). In the absence of pregnancy, the corpus luteum regresses to form a hyalinized scar within the ovary, the *corpus albicans*. These dramatic events give the surface of a functional ovary an irregular, convoluted appearance.

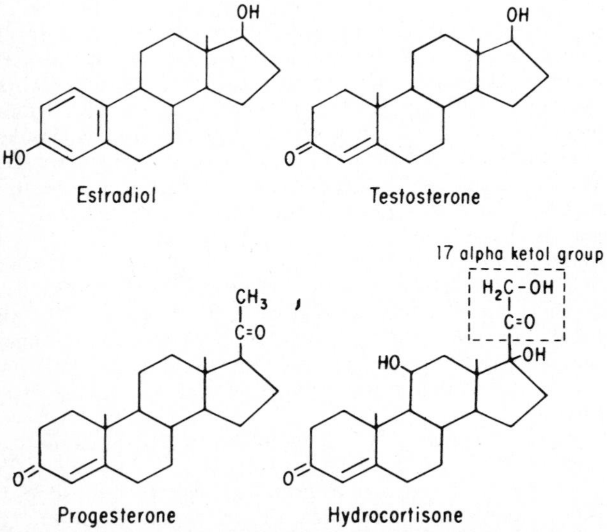

REPRODUCTIVE PHYSIOLOGY

Reproduction is a complex process involving behavior, gametogenesis, endocrine signaling, gamete and embryo transport, and pregnancy. In contrast to men, women have cyclic fluctuations in pituitary and gonadal hormones that prepare the genital tract for conception (Fig. 6). Recent discoveries and technological advances have increased our understanding of this unique physiology, thus enhancing our ability to treat reproductive endocrine disorders and infertility and to provide effective, safe contraception.

Puberty

The transition from childhood to sexual maturity begins typically between 8 to 10 years of age and takes 3 to 5 years to complete. This is a gradual process that involves accelerated growth velocity, *pubarche* (pubic and axillary hair development), *thelarche* (breast development), and *menarche* (vaginal bleeding) and that terminates in ovulatory menstrual cycles. The "trigger" for the initiation of puberty is unknown, but chronologic age, genetic factors, statural height, and body composition are undoubtedly involved. The mechanism appears to be a decrease in

Estradiol

Testosterone

17 alpha ketol group

H_2C-OH
$C=O$
$-OH$

Progesterone

Hydrocortisone

Figure 5. The gonadal hormones. The three main ovarian steroids important in reproduction are depicted and compared with the potent glucocorticoid hydrocortisone. Subtle differences in tertiary structure result in the ability to bind specific cellular receptors, conferring organ specificity.

sensitivity of the hypothalamus to the suppressive effects of gonadal steroids, requiring greater levels of circulating steroids to maintain low gonadotropins and prevent follicular development. The adrenal gland is also involved because an increase in adrenal androgens occurs simultaneously (*adrenarche*).

Precocious puberty is a relatively common clinical problem in girls, either as isolated thelarche or true isosexual puberty. Rarely, tumors in the hypothalamic-pituitary region or steroid-secreting ovarian neoplasms are encountered. In the large majority of cases, however, no underlying pathology is uncovered and they are simply termed "idiopathic" or "constitutional." Suppression of the hypothalamic-pituitary axis by progestogens, usually in the depo form, is most effective in delaying pubertal progression until close to the chronologically appropriate time.

Delayed menses is also a relatively common complaint, and the presence of some evidence of pubertal development, i.e., statural height, breast and pubic hair development, is useful in predicting which women require more detailed investigation. In the absence of any secondary sex characteristics, evaluation should begin by age 14 and proportionally later if some evidence of gonadal steroid production is present. With the exception of pregnancy, the same diseases that cause amenorrhea in the adult should be considered in the child with delayed puberty. An exception is one of the syndromes of gonadal dysgenesis. This may be the classic *Turner's syndrome*, with a 45,XO chromosomal complement, gonadal failure with a normal 46,XX karyotype, a mosaic of the two, or a structural aberration of the X chromosome. All these syndromes share in common the absence of oocytes in the ovary, and steroid production remains at prepubertal levels, resulting in the absence of puberty. Even more uncommon are central nervous system tumors that disrupt hypothalamic function. Again, the largest group of patients have no demonstrable pathology and, eventually, ovulatory function can be anticipated.

The Menstrual Cycle

A dynamic interactive feedback system between the ovary and the hypothalamic-pituitary axis results in timely follicular maturation, ovulatory corpus luteum formation, and, in the absence of pregnancy, menses (Fig. 7). The details of this system are still being evaluated, and this serves as a model for similar relationships between the hypothalamus and pituitary and the thyroid and adrenal. What follows is a practical outline of the menstrual cycle as it is currently understood.

The hypothalamus, with input from the cortex, releases pulses of a small peptide, gonadotropin-releasing hormone (GnRH), into the hypophyseal-portal system with its unique property of draining venous blood from the hypothalamus to the anterior pituitary. In response to pulses of GnRH, the pituitary releases both follicle-stimulating hormone (FSH) and luteinizing hormone (LH), collectively known as the *gonadotropins*, into the systemic circulation. Circulating gonadal steroids (estrogens, androgens, and progestogens) suppress LH and FSH release by classic negative feedback system.

In the ovary, small cohorts of follicles are continually initiating gonadotropin-independent maturation and after approximately 50 days reach a point of gonadotropin sensitivity. At this critical time, relatively high circulating levels of FSH continue this developmental process in selected

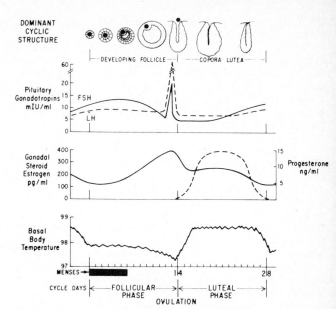

Figure 7. The female reproductive cycle. The dominant cyclic structure, pituitary gonadotropins, gonadal steroids, and basal body temperature are plotted over a single menstrual cycle. Note the lower temperature, low estrogen, and rising follicle-stimulating hormone (FSH) associated with a developing follicle early in the follicular phase. As the follicle matures and enlarges, the estrogen levels rise and have a positive feedback effect on the pituitary. The resultant surge in gonadotropins causes rupture of the follicle and release of the oocyte. After ovulation, the estrogen levels decline and the thermogenic steroid progesterone dominates the luteal phase. In the absence of conception, the luteal phase lasts 14 days, with the FSH levels beginning to rise late in the luteal phase, initiating follicle development for the ensuing cycle.

follicles in the cohort that have gained sufficient numbers of FSH receptors on the granulosa cells (Fig. 8). Typically, one follicle becomes dominant and the remainder undergo atresia by an as yet unrecognized mechanism. Luteinizing hormone stimulates androgen production by the thecal compartment, providing an estrogen substrate for the FSH-induced aromatase activity in the granulosa cells, which lack the ability to synthesize estrogen *de novo*. Estrogen production mirrors follicular development, and as circulating estrogen levels rise, the gonadotropins are suppressed. Paradoxically, with sustained estrogen levels, a positive feedback action is initiated in the pituitary, abruptly releasing large amounts of both FSH and LH, i.e., the midcycle surge. This precipitates the final maturation of the oocyte, enzymatic digestion of the follicle wall, and release of the oocyte. Other regulatory factors produced by the follicle (inhibin, oocyte maturation inhibitor, and luteinization inhibitor) are currently being investigated, but their role in the control of the menstrual cycle is unclear at this time.

After ovulation, the gonadotropins remain suppressed and the follicle undergoes conversion to a corpus luteum. The previously avascular granulosa layer is invaded by blood vessels from the theca, i.e., neovascularization. The granulosa cells undergo hypertrophy (morphologic luteinization), and the predominant steroid produced is progesterone. LH receptors are present on luteal cells awaiting the fetal signal, hCG, which stimulates these receptors, maintains progesterone production, and prolongs the life span of the corpus luteum.

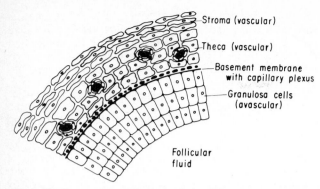

Figure 8. Compartmentalization of the follicle wall. The three follicular compartments are presented schematically, illustrating their anatomic relationship. The vascular ovarian stroma produces small amounts of steroids, predominantly androgens. The theca is well vascularized and produces large amounts of both androgens and estrogens. A capillary plexus is present under the basement membrane surrounding the avascular granulosa layer and enclosed follicular fluid. Thecal androgens are aromatized by the granulosa cells, resulting in extremely high estrogen concentrations in the follicular fluid.

The endometrium, initially in a proliferative pattern under the influence of follicular estrogen, undergoes a programmed pattern of secretory changes (see Fig. 4), presumably producing uterine proteins required for implantation and early embryonic development. These secretory proteins are relatively uncharacterized, and only prolactin (PRL) has been identified. The endometrial stromal cells undergo a decidual change and late in a nonconceptive cycle gain the ability to synthesize prostaglandins, important in the mechanism of menstruation.

In the absence of an hCG "rescue," the corpus luteum undergoes a programmed demise in 14 days by an obscure mechanism and menses ensues. Prior to menses, the FSH levels rise and another cohort of developing follicles at the gonadotropin-sensitive stage is recruited, with the process being repeated. As the number of oocytes declines, follicular maturation becomes erratic and vaginal bleeding ceases to be regular. Eventually, insufficient estrogen is produced to support endometrial growth and menopause occurs. In contrast to gonadal hormone production in men, gonadal hormone production in women is inexorably linked to the presence of gametes (oocytes); and because there is a fixed number of oocytes at birth, significant gonadal steroid output stops when no follicles remain. The negative feedback relationship of gonadal steroids to the hypothalamus continues to function after the *climacteric* (the decline in ovarian function) so that the circulating levels of FSH and LH rise dramatically. A similar rise in the gonadotropins is noted after surgical castration or in women with gonadal dysgenesis.

The climacteric gradually occurs over a period of several years, whereas the last vaginal bleeding episode is a point in time, i.e., *menopause*. Estrogen production not only is critical to the function of the reproductive tract but also maintains bone matrix and a normal cardiovascular system. Although it is not the only factor, loss of ovarian estrogen appears to be a significant contributor to osteoporosis, particularly in thin, light-skinned women with increased rates of pathologic fractures. The cardiovascular effects are less clearly defined. As our life expectancy is prolonged by more sophisticated biomedical science, this is an increasingly important issue.

In addition to atrophy of the genital structures, many women suffer from severe vasomotor "hot flushes." Not only are they annoying; they also alter normal sleep patterns and can alter the personality of severely affected women by the effects of chronic sleep deprivation. It is now apparent that an estrogen-sensitive nucleus in the brain is responsible for the episodic sympathetic discharges causing peripheral vasodilation and the subjective hot flush. Estrogen replacement therapy is extremely effective in the treatment of women symptomatic of estrogen deficiency (genital tract atrophy and vasomotor symptoms) and appears to be efficacious in reducing the incidence of symptomatic osteoporosis in selected high-risk populations of postmenopausal women. Whether estrogen replacement therapy should be universally given to postmenopausal women to forestall osteoporosis is a controversial issue because there are significant liabilities, such as estrogen-associated endometrial cancer.

THE CLINICAL EXAMINATION

The genital structures are unique, in that virtually the entire reproductive tract is accessible to direct examination and the majority of gynecologic disease can be readily detected. Who should be examined and how often are hotly debated issues currently. There is little question that women should begin having regular pelvic examinations by age 20, earlier if they are sexually active, have an aberration of puberty, or experience symptoms of gynecologic disease, such as irregular or heavy vaginal bleeding, severe dysmenorrhea, or pelvic pain. The main reason for regular pelvic examinations is health maintenance, and the optimal interval between examinations in asymptomatic women is unknown. Most gynecologists, however, suggest annual examinations, particularly if the patient does not see another physician and utilizes her gynecologist as her primary care physician. This annual visit should include examination of the abdomen, breasts, neck, and axilla as well as the pelvic area. It should be more extensive if warranted, based on additional symptoms or medical history.

Patient History

A thorough gynecologic history is paramount, beginning with a chronologic history of the present illness. Next, the patient's age, parity (number of previous pregnancies and the outcome of each), and menstrual pattern should be established. Specific note should be made of her preceding several menstrual periods and, specifically, of any irregular or heavy vaginal bleeding or dysmenorrhea. A chronologic history of contraceptive use is important, as well as any previous gynecologic problems, treatment, and their current status (i.e., previous abnormal Papanicolaou smear, ectopic pregnancy, or pelvic operations). Specific questioning as to other pelvic symptoms should be included, such as vaginal discharge, pelvic discomfort, urinary incontinence, and bladder or bowel dysfunction. Finally, a general medical history should be obtained, particularly with regard to nongynecologic abdominal or pelvic operations and systemic diseases undergoing treatment. Often patients will neglect to mention nongynecologic symptoms, feeling they are not related to the specific indication for the visit.

Pelvic Examination

Most women acknowledge the necessity for routine pelvic examinations, but present themselves for it only reluctantly. Evaluation of the genital structures should be treated like other aspects of the physical examination, with special attention to the sensitive nature of the examination. Privacy and dignity are greatly appreciated, and the use of drapes and a female chaperone afford the confidence necessary to gain the cooperation necessary for an adequate examination. Tell the patient exactly what each step will entail to minimize the element of surprise.

The examination should be performed with the patient in the dorsal lithotomy position and should begin with abdominal palpation, since many gynecologic problems (infections and large pelvic masses) can be appreciated through the abdominal wall. Inspection of the vulva is important, with attention to the pelvic hair distribution, clitoral size, vulvar and periurethral glands, and hormonal influence. Palpate the inguinal areas for lymphadenopathy or hernias. Prior to inserting the speculum, place a finger in the vaginal entrance to be sure the size of the speculum is appropriate. A variety of sizes and shapes are available, and a warmed instrument will minimize any discomfort. The speculum should be directed posteriorly toward the sacral promontory in the natural axis of the vagina and opened gently to visualize the cervix. Attention to any discharge present, the hormonal state of the vaginal wall, and the appearance of the cervix, including the nature of the cervical mucus, are important. Exfoliative cytology is usually obtained at this point by gentle scraping of the ectocervix and aspiration of the endocervical canal. Upon removal of the speculum, the patient should be asked to do a Valsalva maneuver so that the structural support of the uterus, bladder, and rectum can be evaluated.

With use of a lubricant, the index and middle finger of the examining hand should be placed in the vagina and the cervix, uterus, and adnexal structures should be palpated. Elevation of the uterus toward the abdominal wall, or at least fixation, aids in abdominal palpation by the other hand. Careful attention should be paid to the size, shape, and contour of the uterus; to the delineation of the ovaries to exclude enlargement; and to tenderness of any structure. A rectovaginal examination should be performed to study the rectal mucosa, the rectovaginal septum, and the posterior aspect of the uterus and cul-de-sac, which often are easier to examine through the rectum. In young girls, a rectal examination is usually well tolerated and can be a useful alternative to vaginal entry in excluding significant pathology.

Ancillary Clinical Evaluation

VAGINAL WET PREPARATION

When women complain of a vaginal discharge, an accurate diagnosis can usually be made by microscopic study of a vaginal wet preparation. Vaginal material, obtained with a clean cotton swab, is suspended in saline and transferred to a microscopic slide for inspection. *Trichomonas vaginalis* and *Candida albicans* are easily identified, the latter requiring the addition of potassium hydroxide for easy discrimination.

EXFOLIATIVE CYTOLOGY

No single contribution to the health care of women exceeds the pioneering work of Papanicolaou and col-

leagues, who identified premalignant cervical changes as well as occult cancer by simple, inexpensive exfoliative cytology. The genital tract is ideally suited for application of this technique, since a common site of genital malignancy—the cervix—is readily accessible on an outpatient basis. Other cancers higher in the genital tract, i.e., endometrial, tubal, and ovarian, occasionally are identified as they shed cells in the vaginal pool. Primary lesions of the vagina and vulva can also be readily identified, with scraping of the vulva required for adequate sampling. Similarly, a small brush can be inserted into the endometrial cavity to increase the collection of cells for cytologic evaluation.

It is important that the samples be collected properly, fixed immediately, adequately stained, and interpreted by an experienced cytologist. Air-drying prior to fixation presents a significant problem to the cytologist, and this should be borne in mind when the samples are collected. The cytologic impression should never be used as the sole basis for cancer treatment, but, rather, viewed as a screening test that requires histologic confirmation. Recently, a technique of cytologic evaluation of aspirated tissue fragments from inaccessible lesions has been developed, called *fine-* or *thin-needle aspiration*. With this technique, a fine needle (usually 22 gauge) is guided into masses that are not accessible and aspiration is applied as the needle is withdrawn. The intact tissue fragments aspirated are then smeared on a slide and prepared and evaluated by cytologic methods. This is a reliable technique, and malignancies can frequently be identified, sparing the patient a more serious surgical procedure. A negative aspirate cannot exclude a malignant process, since the aspiration technique may randomly remove only surrounding connective tissue.

Cytologic studies can be used in many other ways as well, such as for the detection of viruses (e.g., *herpes progenitalis*), identification of organisms responsible for vaginal infections (*Trichomonas vaginalis*, *Candida albicans*, and *Chlamydia trachomatis*), and the presence of sperm, useful in the medicolegal evaluation of alleged sexual assault. The hormonal status of the vagina can easily be determined; with estrogen exposure, cornified cells predominate, whereas in hypoestrogenic states, parabasal cells are observed. The sex chromosomal complement can be evaluated cytologically by means of buccal smears. The presence of an X-chromatin mass or *Barr body* indicates the presence of two X chromosomes, implying a 46,XX chromosomal complement. In the absence of a Barr body, only one X chromosome is present, implying either a 46,XY or 45,XO chromosome complement. The Y chromosome can readily be detected, since the distal two thirds of the long arm is highly fluorescent.

CERVICAL EVALUATION

The volume of cervical mucus and its quality reflect the hormonal status of women throughout the menstrual cycle. Clear, acellular mucus, demonstrating marked viscoelastic properties (spinnbarkeit), indicates high unopposed estrogen, typical immediately prior to ovulation. Cellular opaque mucus with poor spinnbarkeit is present after ovulation. An assessment of the fertility potential of a couple can be made by aspirating the mucus at midcycle after coitus and observing the number of motile sperm, i.e., the postcoital or *Huhner test*. *Neisseria gonorrhoeae* is harbored in the cervix, and Gram's stains of cervical swabs may demonstrate the typical gram-negative intracellular diplococci. Cervical cultures using selective media incubated in carbon dioxide readily enable growth of the gonococcus and are the standard for diagnosis.

Viewing the cervix through an operative microscope (the *colposcope*) is extremely helpful in evaluating abnormal Papanicolaou smears. After the cervix is washed with dilute acetic acid, the surface appearance of dysplastic areas is highlighted, allowing directed biopsy on an outpatient basis without anesthesia. This procedure has virtually eliminated the excisional biopsy of the cervix by cold-knife conization, now reserved only for occasional dysplasias not visible on colposcopy.

THE ENDOMETRIUM

The endometrium can be evaluated histologically by several techniques. Random endometrial biopsies can be obtained with the use of a small curette without anesthesia as an office procedure. These biopsies are useful in evaluation of the ovulatory status of infertile women or in detection of endometrial malignancies in women with abnormal uterine bleeding. The overall architecture of the endometrial cavity is readily outlined by hysterosalpingography. The presence of intrauterine polyps, myomas, or adhesions is easily detected. Recently, operative hysteroscopy, using a small fiberoptic instrument and a distending medium of high-molecular-weight dextran, has greatly improved diagnostic ability but has the drawback of requiring general anesthesia.

ULTRASOUND

Application of real-time diagnostic ultrasound scanning in gynecology has proved a useful adjunct to pelvic examination. Masses can be acoustically categorized as solid, cystic, or complex, and their location relative to other pelvic structures can be clarified. The acoustic appearance may be helpful for diagnosis; undoubtedly, however, the most useful aspect of ultrasound is the detection of a pregnancy within the uterus. The lack of potentially harmful ionizing radiation and the noninvasive nature of the technique are significant advantages.

DIRECT PELVIC INSPECTION

The widespread use of *laparoscopy* attests to its utility in gynecology. This has been made possible by advances in fiberoptic technology that allow direct pelvic inspection without committing the patient to a major abdominal procedure. This is particularly applicable to voluntary sterilization. The operative technique is simple; by placement of a blunt needle through the abdominal wall, the peritoneal cavity can be distended with carbon dioxide. A fiberoptic instrument can then be placed, usually in a periumbilical location, to visualize the pelvic structures. The pelvic viscera can virtually always be visualized because of their fixed position in the pelvis; however, other abdominal organs, such as the appendix, may be more difficult to visualize because of their variable anatomic location. Thus, laparoscopy seems better suited to gynecology than to any other surgical discipline.

DETECTION OF PREGNANCY

The early detection of pregnancy is of vital importance to the gynecologist. Crude urinary assays of hCG have been replaced by rapid, sensitive, qualitative, and quantitative serum assays of hCG, which can detect the presence of hCG at the time of the expected menses, day 29 of a conceptive cycle. These assays can be performed in as little as 2 hours, and by use of an antibody directed against the unique beta subunit of hCG, cross-reactivity with the other gonadotropins is eliminated. The availability of these assays has been a major advance in the diagnosis of pregnancy and has proved especially helpful in evaluation of women in emergency situations.

CONGENITAL ABNORMALITIES OF THE GENITAL TRACT

Müllerian and Urogenital Sinus Anomalies

Several types of müllerian defects are observed; the most common is incomplete fusion of the ducts, yielding an apparent "duplication" of the structures. When completely separate, the ducts form parallel normal-appearing vaginas and cervices with somewhat smaller separated uterine horns, each with a single fallopian tube. A general, but not inviolate, rule is that from the most caudal level of separation the further cephalad portions of the ducts remain apart. This results in a variety of anomalies dependent upon the degree of malfusion (Fig. 9). Occasionally, a portion of the fused duct structure does not fully develop, yielding anything from virtually complete agenesis of the entire reproductive tract to atretic segments (Fig. 9). A combination of incomplete fusion and partial agenesis is frequently present, leading to a variety of configurations with blindly ending portions of the ducts (Fig. 8). When endometrium is present in a blind horn, the menstrual debris has no route of drainage and retrograde menstruation may develop. This results in *endometriosis* and necessitates establishment of adequate drainage or excision of the remnant. Another anomaly results from normal fusion without resorption of the midline septum. The external surface of the uterus appears normal, but an internal longitudinal septum is present within the uterus (Fig. 10). Women with separated uterine horns generally have normal fertility, albeit with a higher rate of premature labor, and no surgical intervention is necessary. A uterine septum may be associated with habitual abortion, requiring excision of the septum to enable establishment of a viable pregnancy.

Anomalies involving the lower vagina may also occur, near the junction of the urogenital sinus and the müllerian ducts. A transverse vaginal septum or, rarely, an atretic lower vagina may be encountered (Fig. 10). Depending on the degree of vaginal development, the urogenital sinus portion and the remaining vaginal pouch may be surgically united. If this is not technically possible, the entire upper portion of the müllerian structures will have to be excised to prevent the development of severe endometriosis.

It should be emphasized that in all these anomalies the ovaries are normal and puberty progresses normally. Even when the entire upper genital tract is absent, the introitus invariably looks normal and no hint of a problem occurs until absence of menses or cyclic abdominal pain from retrograde menses brings the patient to the physician for evaluation. If a blind vaginal pouch of significant size is present, progressive dilatation with graduated dilators may enlarge the vaginal canal sufficiently for satisfactory coitus. When this is unsuccessful, a McIndoe vaginal creation can be performed using a split-thickness skin graft around a mold to create an artificial vaginal tube that functions normally for coitus.

The most common anomaly of all is a simple, imperforate hymen. Typically, young women will present to the

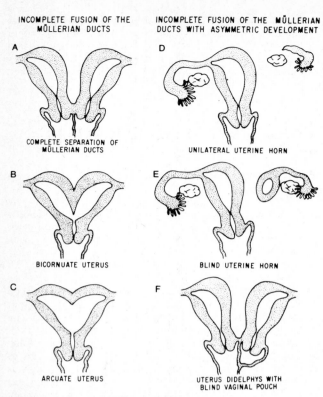

Figure 9. Defects of müllerian duct fusion.

A, Malfusion of the müllerian ducts is relatively common, and with complete separation "duplication" of the entire genital tract can occur.

B, C, Fusion of the caudal portion may result in variable degrees of uterine fundal separation. Occasionally, malfusion and asymmetric development occur simultaneously.

D, When an entire cephalad portion of a single duct is absent, the contralateral uterine horn functions relatively normally and the anomaly may go undetected.

E, F, When an incompletely developed müllerian duct contains endometrium without a route of vaginal drainage, either a hematometria (a blood-filled uterine cavity) or a hematocolpos (a distended blood-filled vagina) may result. This presents clinically with cyclic abdominal pain and endometriosis at the time of puberty.

gynecologist with normal pubertal status but with the absence of vaginal bleeding. A blood-filled, distended vagina (hematocolpos) with a bulging membrane over the vaginal entrance is appreciated. Simple incision and removal of the membrane are all that are required for excellent anatomic results.

Because the urinary tract is in intimate contact with the genital tract and develops at the same time *in utero*, it should come as no surprise that there is a high incidence of urinary tract abnormalities when a genital tract anomaly is present. This is particularly true when the defect is asymmetrical, and it suggests that radiographic investigation of the urinary tract is worthwhile whenever a genital tract anomaly is present.

Wolffian Remnants

Incomplete regression of the mesonephric (wolffian) ducts can result in cystic remnants anywhere along the course of this duct. These are retroperineal structures

adjacent to the vagina, uterus, and oviducts. Examples include Gartner's duct cysts in the vagina, paraovarian cysts within the broad ligament that may reach large size, and pedunculated fimbrial hydatid cysts of Morgagni. These are extremely common and need not be removed unless they undergo torsion or cause symptoms. These mesonephric remnants most likely represent the site of origin of the rare clear cell adenocarcinoma and other bizarre neoplasms in this region.

Intersex Problems

There are rare clinical situations in which the gonadal sex, internal genitalia, and external genitalia are not consistent. *Hermaphroditism* is the general term describing this situation, which has been known since antiquity.

CLASSIFICATION

With our current understanding, we can separate persons with an intersex problem into three basic categories: (1) true hermaphrodites, (2) virilized females (female pseudohermaphrodites), and (3) incompletely virilized males (male pseudohermaphrodites).

True Hermaphrodites. True hermaphroditism is the rarest entity and describes an individual with both ovarian and testicular tissue present. Because the internal and external genitalia are dependent upon gonadal hormone action, the degree to which each gonad functions will determine the anatomic appearance of the genitalia. True hermaphrodites may have a normal-appearing ovary and contralateral testicle or, more classically, an ovotestis, i.e., a single gonad with ovarian tissue at one pole and testicular tissue on the other.

Female Pseudohermaphrodites. The most common of the intersex problems is that of a virilized female or a

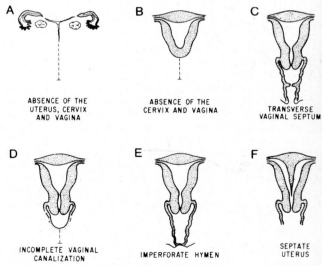

Figure 10. Abnormal müllerian development. A variety of unusual anomalies not related to malfusion can occur, varying from virtually complete absence of the internal structures (A), a simple imperforate hymen (E), to anything in between (B, D). A transverse vaginal septum (C) is thought to represent an error in the contact of the urogenital sinus and the caudal portion of the müllerian ducts. Failure to canalize the fused ducts properly results in a midline septum within the uterus, which has a normal exterior appearance (F).

female pseudohermaphrodite. This can be secondary to maternal ingestion of androgenic compounds, the presence of an androgen-secreting tumor in the mother, or congenital adrenal hyperplasia with excessive production of fetal adrenal androgens because of enzyme deficiencies in the pathway to production of cortisol. Oral contraceptives containing synthetic progestogens with androgenic properties are the most commonly ingested agents. Gonadal-stromal tumors or luteomas of pregnancy represent maternal sources of androgens during pregnancy. The two most common types of congenital adrenal hyperplasia are the 21- and 11-hydroxylase deficiencies inherited in an autosomal recessive pattern. The most severe form of the disease must be present to alter the development of the genital structures *in utero*. It is important to identify these patients and rear them as females because they are potentially fertile women.

Male Pseudohermaphrodites. The last group is that of incompletely virilized males, male pseudohermaphrodites, and it includes a diversity of syndromes. At one end of the spectrum is the woman with complete androgen insensitivity who has absent or nonfunctional androgen receptors inherited as an X-linked trait. These are phenotypically normal-appearing women with scant pubic hair, and the absence of müllerian structures (vagina, cervix, uterus, and tubes), as testicular production of MIS is normal. The testes should be left *in situ* until after puberty to ensure normal pubescence, attributed to aromatization of testosterone to estradiol. The testes should then be excised, since the potential for neoplasia is significant with an intra-abdominal gonad bearing a Y chromosome. A neo-vagina can be created at the same time if required. Incomplete forms of this syndrome are observed with a reduction rather than absence of androgen action, typically presenting as a phenotypic male with gynecomastia, oligospermia, and incomplete virilization of the external genitalia. Another unique syndrome in this category is the absence of the nuclear enzyme 5-alpha-reductase responsible for the conversion of testosterone to the more potent metabolite DHT. This is inherited in an autosomal recessive fashion, with the men having normal internal genitalia (the testosterone-responsive structures) and incompletely virilized external genitalia, which require DHT for complete virilization. Some further masculinization occurs at puberty with the marked increase in testosterone at that time.

EVALUATION AND MANAGEMENT

A thorough knowledge of all these syndromes is necessary to adequately evaluate and manage these rare clinical problems. The psychologic effects on the parents, the anatomic possibilities of corrective surgery, the sex of rearing, the anticipated effects of puberty, and the gender identity of the child must all be considered before irrevocable decisions are made. This is obviously an extremely stressful time for parents, requiring great skill by the physician to obtain their full cooperation for these difficult clinical decisions.

THE EXTERNAL GENITALIA

A variety of systemic or unique genital problems can be encountered on the vulva, ranging from infectious diseases to neoplasia. Because vulvular tissues are hormonally responsive, the effects of the systemic hormonal milieu can influence their appearance and must be borne in mind.

Although many of the clinical problems are symptomatic, the most serious—carcinoma of the vulva—produce no symptoms, making careful inspection of the vulva on routine pelvic examination mandatory.

Vulvitis

Symptomatic vulvar irritation can be present at any age, and a careful, skilled examination is required. Currently, a common etiology is *herpes progenitalis* (*herpes simplex*, Type 2) which is venereally transmitted and presents with painful vesicles on the vulva. The diagnosis can be confirmed by culture of the virus from the lesions. The vesicles tend to recur cyclically, but chronic use of acyclovir, an antiviral agent, may reduce the severity and frequency of the recurrences. Unfortunately, no *cure* for this unique viral infection is currently available. Another venereally transmitted virus causes venereal warts, or *condylomata acuminata*, which are papillary excrescences ranging in size from barely visible lesions to large masses. Excision or local destruction (cryotherapy and laser vaporization) is usually curative, but the warts may require repeated treatments. The most useful therapy has been topical application of the chemically destructive agents podophyllin and trichloroacetic acid. Both herpes and venereal warts can involve the vagina and cervix as well. Other venereally transmitted infections, such as syphilis, granuloma inguinale, lymphogranuloma venereum, and chancroid, can cause vulvar lesions, but these are rarely observed today.

Generalized vulvovaginitis can be a chronic and particularly annoying problem. Frequently, the excoriation caused by scratching leads to secondary bacterial infection of the subcutaneous tissue. This is a serious problem in the elderly diabetic patient with mycotic vulvitis, since necrotizing fasciitis secondary to gas-forming anaerobes can rapidly become a life-threatening infection. Treatment is rapid, wide, local excision of infected areas; control of diabetes; and, when available, hyperbaric oxygen therapy. In young women, candidal vaginitis is extremely common. Although irritating, it rarely produces serious sequelae and is amenable to topical antifungal agents.

The glands present on the vulva can become infected and present as localized abscesses. The Bartholin's glands in the lateral aspects of the posterior fourchette are often involved, causing a painful, unilateral vulvar abscess. Simple incision and drainage relieve the acute problem, but recurrences are common and require marsupialization of the abscess wall. Noninfected Bartholin's gland cysts also require either marsupialization or excision. The apocrine sweat glands on the vulva can be involved in a chronic inflammatory process, *hidradenitis suppurativa*, with intermittent draining purulent abscesses. This is often present also in the axilla and can be treated only by recurrent incision and drainage or excision of the vulvar skin, a skinning vulvectomy, with split-thickness grafting. Antibiotics are of little use, and the chronicity of the disease is particularly frustrating.

Vulvar Atrophy

Symptomatic degenerative changes of the vulva are common and typically occur after the spontaneous cessation of ovarian function. In addition to the distressing problems of dyspareunia, itching, and pain, these areas are often the site of vulvar carcinomas. Several histologic patterns have been described, including kraurosis vulvae (shrunken), leukoplakia (hypertrophic), and lichen sclerosus et atrophicus (atrophy). Topical treatment with hormone creams (estrogens and androgens) is helpful, but in some cases localized excision is required, including a skinning vulvectomy and skin grafting when the process involves a large area of the vulva.

Vulvar Neoplasia

Carcinoma *in situ* of the vulva can be a localized or generalized vulvar process. Scraping suspicious lesions for cytologic examination is useful. Colposcopy using 2 per cent acetic acid or a nuclear stain of 1 per cent toluidine blue is helpful in directing biopsy. A Keyes dermatologic punch is the best biopsy instrument. Histologic diagnosis is essential, and up to a third of women with preinvasive lesions of the vulva have or will later show similar findings in squamous epithelium higher in the genital tract, i.e., the vagina and cervix. Histologically, these areas appear similar to epidermoid cancers elsewhere but without evidence of invasion. Excision is the treatment of choice, and, as with degenerative changes, skin grafting is employed for multifocal or extensive lesions.

Invasive cancer of the vulva is clinically detected by presence of a vulvar mass, bleeding, ulcer, or localized irritation occurring in the postmenopausal years and is rare before the fourth decade of life (Fig. 11). Well-differentiated squamous carcinoma is the rule, with occasional adenocarcinomas arising in the Bartholin's glands and melanocarcinomas from pigmented cells. Paget's disease is a slowly progressive, acanthotic epidermal cancer characterized by well-circumscribed, hyperemic, indurated areas, with intradermal cells demonstrating distinctive, clear, granular cytoplasm. This may represent an unusual adenocarcinoma of sweat glands, and a similar process is encountered in the breast. Wide local excision is usually adequate therapy.

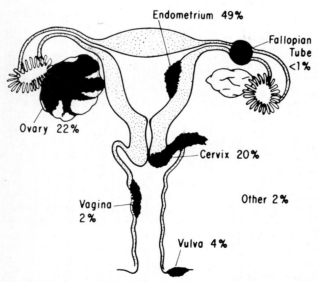

Figure 11. Sites of gynecologic cancer. The distribution of primary gynecologic cancers is illustrated. Cancers of the vulva, vagina, and cervix are of the squamous variety, whereas endometrial, ovarian, and tubal cancers are usually adenocarcinomas. Any tissues within the genital tract, such as oocytes, ovarian stroma, smooth muscle, blood vessels, and pigmented cells, can become malignant and comprise the other malignancies.

The main prognostic feature of vulvar carcinoma is the size of the primary lesion. When the primary tumor is 1 cm. or less, the probability of lymphatic spread is markedly reduced. Unfortunately, long delays in diagnosis are common; thus close scrutiny of any vulvar abnormality is urged. The lymphatic drainage of the vulva is via lymphatics to the superficial inguinal lymph nodes, then to the deep femoral chain, to the external iliac, and then to the internal iliac nodes. Infrequently, this pathway is bypassed with deep nodal metastases prior to spread to the inguinal nodes. Contralateral lymphatic drainage, however, is relatively common. The treatment is primarily surgical with radical vulvectomy and inguinal node dissection, careful attention being paid to Cloquet's node in the femoral canal. As with epidermoid carcinomas of other sites, chemotherapy and radiation therapy are of limited value and are usually reserved for palliation. This is a disease of elderly women, and preoperative evaluation as to the suitability of radical surgery is important. The 5-year survival rate approaches 80 per cent without nodal spread, but declines substantially with tumor present in lymph nodes. Direct extension to the urethra or rectum necessitates a pelvic exenteration.

THE VAGINA

The vagina represents the conduit through which male gametes enter the female reproductive tract as well as the route of expulsion of the fetus. With thick squamous epithelium, it is well designed to withstand the traumas of coitus and childbirth as well as to minimize the opportunity for pathogenic bacteria to enter the genital tract and gain access to the abdominal cavity. Under the influence of estrogen after puberty, the vaginal epithelium is thickened and contains glycogen, which the vaginal flora (diphtheroids, lactobacilli, and a variety of anaerobic bacteria) convert to lactic acid, maintaining a low pH and an inhospitable environment for bacterial growth.

Vaginitis

Infections of the vagina, although not of major clinical significance, may nonetheless be extremely uncomfortable. There are three major etiologies: (1) the protozoan *Trichomonas vaginalis*, (2) the fungus *Candida albicans*, and (3) the bacterium *Haemophilus vaginalis*.

Trichomonas is venereally transmitted and causes a foamy, greenish-yellow, malodorous discharge. A wet preparation reveals the typical flagellated organisms, which are actively mobile. Treatment is with metronidazole for both the patient and her sexual partner.

Fungal (yeast) vaginitis is characterized by an irritating, thick, white vaginal discharge and uncomfortable vulvar itching. Excoriation by scratching may provide an opportunity for bacterial infection, which is a serious problem in the diabetic with microvascular disease. With yeast vaginitis, the pH is more alkaline, and circumstances that reduce the glycogen (such as pregnancy and use of oral contraceptives) predispose to these infections. Many efficacious topical antifungal agents are available.

Haemophilus vaginitis causes a watery discharge and is treatable with sulfonamides and tetracyclines. Vulvar infections such as herpes and venereal warts may be present in the vagina as well.

Vaginal irritation is very common after cessation of ovarian function with the attendant genital tract atrophy.

This process can be reversed easily by the use of oral or topical estrogen. In children, foreign bodies in the vagina are the most common cause of vaginal discharge, with a rare cervical cancer—sarcoma botryoides—associated with vaginal bleeding.

Vaginal Neoplasia

Intraepithelial neoplasia may occur anywhere in the vagina in the squamous epithelium. It may develop in the vaginal fornices after treatment for cervical neoplasia, or it may be associated with multifocal dysplasias throughout the genital tract. It is typically detected by genital tract cytologic studies and can be localized for biopsy by colposcopy. Treatment consists of localized excision of the involved areas, including an upper vaginectomy if necessary.

Invasive vaginal cancer is usually of the squamous variety and is a rare lesion (Fig. 11). Vaginal melanomas may also occur as well as clear cell adenocarcinomas, associated with prenatal diethylstilbestrol (DES) exposure. The age range is from the late reproductive years and beyond; the patient most commonly presents with vaginal discharge and bleeding. Vaginal cancer is staged as follows:

Stage I—cancer limited to the vaginal wall.
Stage II—cancer involving the subvaginal tissue.
Stage III—the tumor extends laterally but is not fixed to the adjacent pelvic wall (side wall).
Stage IV—Tumor involves the symphysis or adjacent viscera.

Lymphatic spread is similar to that of cervical cancer when the lesion is in the upper vagina involving the obturator nodes and iliac system. In the lower vagina, lymphatic drainage may occur via the vulvar lymphatics to the inguinal nodes. Treatment is primarily radiation, with several delivery systems designed to deliver the therapeutic dose to the lesion within the vagina. Including nodal areas in the radiation fields is worthwhile when more advanced disease is present. Exenterative surgery may be helpful when the bladder or rectum is involved.

THE CERVIX

The cervix undergoes dramatic changes throughout the reproductive lifetime as well as within the menstrual cycle. The squamocolumnar junction normally is located in the endocervical canal, but it can be present well out on the ectocervix, either post partum or on a congenital basis. Cervical mucus is produced in response to estrogen, and with eversion of the mucus-secreting columnar cells on the ectocervix, a mucoid and sometimes purulent discharge may be experienced. Although this may cause a foulsmelling discharge, it is of no pathologic significance and appears not to alter reproductive capacity. Occasionally, condylomata acuminata or *herpes progenitalis* involves the cervix and can present with proliferative or ulcerative cervical lesions. Localized treatment with cryotherapy, cauterization, or laser vaporization can be effective in destroying the mucus-secreting epithelium and reducing the production of mucus. It is mandatory that cytologic or colposcopic screening be performed prior to therapy so that an occult cervical malignancy will not be overlooked.

Cervical Neoplasia

The main importance of routine cervical evaluation is to screen for cervical cancer, which accounts for approximately 20 per cent of gynecologic malignancies (Fig. 11). The unique aspect of this malignancy is its accessibility to cytologic screening and outpatient biopsy. Additionally, premalignant dysplasias can readily be identified and conservatively treated without removal of the uterus, preventing progression to invasive cancer. Because of the ability to visualize the cervix, the development of cervical cancer has been well studied. Everted endocervical epithelium undergoes a process of squamous metaplasia, replacing the columnar cells. The greater the area of the eversion, the larger the "transition zone" of squamous metaplasia. It is thought that in the presence of a carcinogen, abnormal maturation of squamous epithelium results, i.e., cervical intraepithelial neoplasia (CIN) or dysplasia. This can be graded, depending on the extent of the histologic change up to the point of a full-thickness epithelial change, carcinoma *in situ*.

In most instances, CIN precedes invasive cervical cancer by at least a decade and, although asymptomatic, it is easily detectable by cervical cytologic methods. The optimal interval between Papanicoloau smears is not clear, but most gynecologists recommend annual smears, particularly in young sexually active women at greater risk. CIN appears to be "venereal" in origin because it is associated with the early onset of sexual activity, high parity, and multiple sexual partners. The presence of a carcinogen appears necessary, and herpes simplex virus Type 2, human papilloma virus, and sperm proteins have been suggested, but no definitive carcinogen has been identified to date.

The abnormal Papanicolaou smear is a screening test rather than a definitive histologic characterization of the disease process. After an abnormal smear is obtained, colposcopic examination is performed to identify the abnormal area(s) for biopsy. Application of a 3 per cent acetic acid solution makes visualization easier, and several abnormal patterns are observed, including white epithelium, mosaicism, punctation, leukoplakia, and atypical vessels. An endocervical curettage (ECC) is required, since CIN may be present in the endocervical canal and may not be visualizable by colposcopy. In the presence of a negative ECC, if biopsies of the abnormal areas and the cytologic results are compatible, localized destructive therapy (i.e., cryosurgery, cauterization, laser vaporization) is appropriate and usually curative. Careful follow-up cytologic evaluation is required. An alternative, if pregnancy is not a factor, is simple hysterectomy. If the cytologic abnormality is not detected by biopsy, the colposcopic examination is technically unsatisfactory; or if the ECC result is positive, a cold-knife conization of the cervix is necessary to exclude the possibility of an invasive cervical cancer. Simple hysterectomy is acceptable treatment of CIN only after exclusion of invasive cervical cancer.

Cervical cancer is usually an epidermoid cancer arising from an area of CIN. Approximately 5 per cent of cervical cancers are adenocarcinomas, presumably arising from the columnar endocervical cells. Cervical cancer is staged as follows:

Stage 0—carcinoma *in situ*.
Stage I—carcinoma confined entirely to the cervix (I-A, early stromal invasion; I-B, all other Stage I lesions).
Stage II—carcinoma involving the upper two thirds of the vagina or the parametrial areas, but not extending to the pelvic side wall (II-A, only vaginal involvement; II-B, infiltration of the parametria).
Stage III—carcinoma involving the lower third of the vagina or extending to the pelvic side wall (III-A, involving the lower third of the vagina and the parametrium, but not the side wall; III-B, extension to the side wall; III-urinary, obstruction of one or both ureters regardless of other disease).

Stage IV—carcinoma outside the reproductive tract (IV-A, involving the mucosa of the bladder or bowel; IV-B, outside the pelvis).

This staging system is well correlated with the likelihood of nodal metastases with Stage I, 17 per cent; Stage II, 32 per cent; Stage III, 47 per cent; and Stage IV, 81 per cent. Independent of stage, the rate of nodal metastases increases with increasing size of the cervical lesion, being rare with primary lesions less than 1 cm. in size, 17 per cent for 1- to 3-cm. lesions, and 52 per cent at greater than 3 cm. Common sites for distant metastases are liver, lung, and bones.

Treatment of invasive cervical cancer is by a radical surgical procedure or radiation. Chemotherapy, as with most epidermoid cancers, is of little other than palliative benefit. Therapy should be individualized for every patient, the majority of gynecologic oncologists today favoring radiotherapy. This yields 5-year cure rates that are slightly higher than with the extended hysterectomy approach. With the high level of expertise available for radiation therapy, the complications of radiation sickness, radiation proctitis and cystitis, or necrosis of the vagina and cervix are rare. The surgical approach is limited to Stage I or II-A lesions and involves an extended hysterectomy, with removal of the uterus, the upper third of the vagina, the entire uterosacral and uterovesical ligaments, the entire parametrium, and a pelvic lymphadenectomy (ureteral, obturator, hypogastric, and iliac chains). The surgical approach requires a skilled operator, a favorable medical condition of the patient, and acceptance of serious morbidity such as ureterovaginal fistula in 1 to 5 per cent of the patients. For more advanced stages of cervical cancer, radiotherapy is the only reasonable therapeutic option.

THE UTERUS

The uterus is a muscular organ with a unique epithelium-lined cavity, and both uterine compartments are sensitive to the effects of ovarian steroids. The uterine smooth muscle cells undergo hypertrophy in response to estrogens, enlarging the overall uterine size. The endometrium proliferates in response to unopposed estrogen, changing to a secretory pattern under the influence of luteal progesterone. When pregnancy occurs, hCG maintains luteal progesterone production, causing a hypersecretory change in the endometrium. These physiologic growth characteristics herald the patterns of neoplasms observed in the uterus and suggest the etiology of some of these lesions as well as provide intriguing opportunities for therapy.

The Endometrium

Several diseases originating in the endometrium are prevalent in women, including adenomyosis, endometriosis, polyps, and hyperplasias.

ADENOMYOSIS

Normally, the endometrium is confined to the uterine cavity. Invasion of the myometrium by benign endometrium is called adenomyosis, resulting in a boggy, enlarged tender uterus, dysmenorrhea, and heavy menses. Typically, this problem affects parous women in their 30s and 40s and requires hysterectomy when symptoms are severe.

ENDOMETRIOSIS

Retrograde menstruation occurs in all women to some extent, but viable endometrial cells can be transplanted to the pelvic peritoneal surfaces, i.e., endometriosis. The implants are frequent on fixed pelvic structures that have good vascularity and·are in the dependent areas of the pelvis (see Fig. 4). Significant scarring is present surrounding the implants, giving them a nodular character. Endometriosis is associated with infertility, dyspareunia, and dysmenorrhea, and it occasionally involves other pelvic viscera. Prolonged suppression of ovarian function by synthetic steroids causes atrophy of the uterine endometrium as well as the ectopic implants. These agents include continuous birth control pills, danazol, and medroxyprogesterone acetate. The uterine endometrium has a stable regenerative layer and, with resumption of ovulation after the suppressive course, normal endometrium redevelops. The ectopic implants, however, do not have a regenerative layer and are resorbed. Unfortunately, the conditions leading to retrograde menstruation are not altered; therefore, prevention of ovulation or surgical removal of implants fails to prevent recurrence of the process.

POLYPS

Endometrial polyps represent localized polypoid areas of endometrium with underlying connective tissue. The epithelium on polyps may not be hormonally responsive and therefore may be out of phase with the remainder of the endometrium.

HYPERPLASIA

Adenomatous hyperplasia of the endometrium is commonly associated with the unopposed estrogen observed with chronic anovulation. Without the progesterone dominance of the luteal phase, continuous—albeit aberrant—proliferation is the histologic pattern and irregular heavy vaginal bleeding is common. If this continues over a long interval of time, adenomatous hyperplasia may develop, which is felt to represent a precursor of adenocarcinoma of the endometrium.

A variant seen in perimenopausal women is *benign cystic hyperplasia*. In this situation, the endometrium is in a proliferative pattern and the glands are large and cystic. Although the risk of neoplastic change is less with this lesion, the bleeding may still be heavy. Curettage removes the hyperplastic endometrium, but it does nothing to change the underlying problem. Recently, use of continuous oral progestogens to block gonadotropin stimulation of the ovaries and create decidual atrophy of the endometrium has been found to be therapeutically useful. At the minimum, frequent histologic sampling of the endometrium and cyclic intermittent progestogen administration are required.

ADENOCARCINOMA OF THE ENDOMETRIUM

The vast majority of cancers of the endometrium are adenocarcinomas and occur in the 50- to 70-year age group (Fig. 11). This represents the most common genital cancer, but the death rate for this disease is substantially less than with cervical and ovarian cancer. The reason for this optimistic therapeutic outlook is the early marker of neoplastic endometrial growth, postmenopausal bleeding. Heavy irregular bleeding in premenopausal women similarly can herald neoplastic changes as well and bears close evaluation. Fractional curettage is the principal diagnostic test, with cytologic sampling and endometrial biopsy occasionally identifying the cancer. There appears to be a histologic continuity from adenomatous hyperplasia to hyperplasia with cellular atypia and then to frank adenocarcinoma. This suggests that prolonged unopposed estrogen is etiologic in the development of this neoplasm and correlates with the observations that women with low parity, late menopause, and obesity (higher or more prolonged unopposed endogenous estrogen production) are at greater risk for the development of the disease. Aromatization of adrenal androstenedione to estrone occurs in many peripheral tissues, particularly fat, and probably accounts for the correlation with obesity. Likewise, estrogen replacement therapy in postmenopausal women carries with it a higher risk of adenocarcinoma of the endometrium. Fortunately, the benefits of estrogen replacement therapy on vasomotor symptoms, genital atrophy, and osteoporosis appear to be safely obtainable with the use of combined estrogen and progestogen replacement. The progestogen creates a secretory change in the endometrium that alters the continuous proliferative effects of unopposed estrogen.

Several histologic types of endometrial cancer are observed and have prognostic significance. These include, in order of worsening prognosis, (1) adenoacanthoma, (2) adenocarcinoma, (3) papillary, (4) adenosquamous, and (5) clear cell, with adenocarcinoma being by far the largest single group. Prognostic features for endometrial adenocarcinoma include the degree of histologic differentiation (grade), uterine size, stage of the disease, myometrial invasion, peritoneal cytology, lymph node metastasis, and involvement of the adnexal structures. Endometrial cancer is staged as follows:

Stage I—Carcinoma confined to the uterine corpus (Stage I-A, the uterine cavity is less than 8 cm.; Stage I-B, the uterine cavity is greater than 8 cm.). These cancers should further be classified as to histologic appearance: *Grade 1*—highly differentiated adenocarcinoma; *Grade 2*—differentiated adenocarcinoma with partly solid areas; and *Grade 3*—predominantly solid areas or undifferentiated carcinoma.

Stage II—Involvement of the uterine corpus and cervix.

Stage III—Involvement of the other genital structures or adjacent tissues but not the bladder or rectum.

Stage IV—Bladder or rectal involvement or disease outside the pelvis.

Current recommended treatment for endometrial cancer is controversial, involving primary surgery versus surgery plus adjunctive radiation. Both approaches yield excellent cure rates with Stage I disease. The main goal of radiation is to reduce the incidence of vaginal vault recurrences. This is accomplished with local vault radiation using vaginal and uterine applicators. Endometrial cancer spreads commonly to the adnexal structures (tubes and ovaries) and the vaginal vault. Nodal metastasis occurs via the pelvic nodal chains (obturator, external iliac, and common iliac nodes) with occasional isolated para-aortic nodal metastasis. Intraabdominal spread can occur and is usually detectable by peritoneal cytologic evaluation. The use of intraperitoneal P-32, a colloidal solution that gives peritoneal surface radiation, may be of benefit in these circumstances. Individualized therapy, including assessment of all the prognostic indicators, appears to be the current recommendation, with increasing use of adjunctive radiation with worsening prognosis.

As endometrial cells are converted from proliferative to secretory activity by progesterone, synthetic progestogens have been evaluated as to their effects in ameliorating the course of endometrial adenocarcinoma. They appear to be of no benefit prophylactically, but are of benefit for recurrent disease palliation in approximately a third of patients. The response to progestogens is positively correlated with earlier tumor grade and the presence of progesterone receptors in the tumor. The most frequently used agents are medroxyprogesterone acetate and megestrol acetate. Chemotherapy is of limited use in this neoplasm.

The Myometrium

Probably the most common benign neoplasms of the genital tract are uterine leiomyomas, also called myomas, fibroids, and fibromyomas (Fig. 12). These can occur at any age, but are more common in the latter reproductive years. Leiomyomas are more common in black women and can frequently attain extremely large size. They may be present anywhere in the uterus and occasionally become parasitic, draining their blood supply from adjacent pelvic structures. As they are rarely malignant, the main indications for removal are pain, pressure, large size, abnormal uterine bleeding, and infertility when the leiomyomas impinge on the uterine cavity.

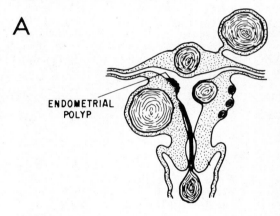

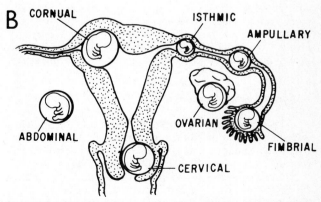

Figure 12. A, *Uterine leiomyomata. Leiomyomas of the uterus are composed of whorls of smooth muscle cells that can attain large size. They may occur anywhere in the uterus, but usually originate in the uterine fundus. Pedunculated, subserosal, transmural, submucosal, and intrauterine leiomyomas are observed. Pedunculated intrauterine leiomyomas are often extruded through the cervix. B, The sites of ectopic pregnancies are illustrated, tubal sites being the most common. The most dangerous sites are the abdominal cavity, the cervix, and the cornua, as the possibility of rapid massive bleeding is significant.*

Grossly, leiomyomas are usually ovoid, firm, multinodular masses arising from the uterus. On cut section, they are white and solid, with occasional degenerative areas of necrosis. Histologically, they are composed of whorls of interlacing smooth muscle and connective tissue. Hyalinization is observed after degeneration, and calcium deposition is common.

Treatment of uterine leiomyomas is excision, either by hysterectomy if childbearing is completed or by myomectomy if childbearing potential is desired. In the absence of pain, bleeding, or rapid growth, small leiomyomas need not be removed unless uncertainty exists as to the origin of the pelvic mass. Infertility can reliably be attributed to leiomyomas only when they impinge on the uterine cavity. Selective hysteroscopic removal of intrauterine or submucosal tumors is possible and reduces the need for laparotomy. Abdominal myomectomy is necessary for larger leiomyomas, and when the uterine wall has been incised, most gynecologists recommend abdominal delivery because the weakened uterine fundal incision may rupture during labor.

Sarcomas can originate from uterine smooth muscle cells, endometrial cells, or the underlying connective tissue and vascular elements. Other than the low-grade leiomyosarcomas, these cancers are associated with a poor prognosis with early metastasis, notably when the lungs are involved. Extirpative surgery is the mainstay of treatment, with neither chemotherapy nor radiation offering significant benefit.

THE OVARY

The ovary is composed of several specialized tissues, including germinal epithelium, oocytes, and gonadal stroma as well as the usual connective tissue and vascular components (see Fig. 4). Benign and malignant ovarian tumors can be present at any age, but the proportion that are malignant increases from 10 per cent in women under 30 years old to 20 per cent between 30 and 50, to 50 per cent in women over 50. Unfortunately, ovarian tumors are usually asymptomatic unless torsion or internal bleeding with rapid enlargement occurs. The symptom that brings most ovarian tumors to medical attention is abdominal enlargement, a late sign. For this reason, it is important to evaluate all adnexal masses carefully, using the clinical presentation to determine the urgency of surgical excision.

Benign Ovarian Neoplasms

The most common etiology of ovarian enlargement in women of reproductive age is a functional change, such as a hemorrhagic follicular or luteal cyst. Chronic anovulation is often associated with bilaterally large "polycystic" ovaries containing a large stromal compartment and multiple subcapsular follicles. For these reasons, adnexal masses in young women should be observed over a several-month interval, since most functional cysts will resolve, particularly if the gonadotropins are suppressed with oral contraceptives. Pelvic sonograms may be helpful in confirming the cystic natures of masses, since the probability of a true neoplasm is increased when the mass is solid.

Endometrial cysts, or *endometriomas*, are the most common benign ovarian tumors (see Fig. 4). These appear as "chocolate cysts" with a well-defined capsule surrounding a thick, brownish liquid felt to represent menstrual debris.

Simple cystic ovarian masses as well as serous and mucinous cystadenomas are common. The next most frequent is the *benign cystic teratoma*, or *dermoid cyst*, representing parthenogenetic cleavage of an oocyte. Skin, hair, bone, and teeth are common, but any tissue may be included. Approximately 25 per cent of dermoids are bilateral, and if immature elements are present, malignancy should be suspected (approximately 1 per cent).

Rarer benign neoplasms can also occur, including fibromas, adenofibromas, and Brenner tumors (Walthard's inclusion rests). The most dramatic presentation of an ovarian fibroma is that associated with massive ascites and occasionally a sympathetic hydrothorax (*Meig's syndrome*). Hormone-secreting gonadal stromal tumors (Leydig cell, hilus cell, granulosa cell, or thecal cell types) can produce both estrogens and androgens. Clinically, they may come to the physician's attention because of inappropriate estrogenization (postmenopausal bleeding) or virilization. This latter group makes up less than 3 per cent of the total. Non-ovarian pelvic tumors such as a leiomyoma, a hydrosalpinx, or a mesonephric duct remnant may be clinically indistinguishable from a true ovarian neoplasm and may require surgical exploration for diagnosis.

Surgical removal of ovarian tumors can usually be accomplished by excising the neoplasm and leaving the remainder of the ovary. If a benign neoplasm has completely replaced the ovary, an oophorectomy may be necessary, but all efforts should be made to preserve ovarian function in the young woman, for both childbearing and preservation of gonadal hormone production.

Ovarian Cancer

Although ovarian cancer represents 22 per cent of all reproductive tract neoplasms, it is responsible for 47 per cent of the deaths from gynecologic cancer (Fig. 11). This disparity is due to the fact it is an asymptomatic malignancy, leading to delays in diagnosis until the disease is advanced. The most common type of ovarian cancer is thought to originate from the *coelomic* or *germinal epithelium*, covering the ovary with four main histologic types: serous, mucinous, endometroid, and mesonephroid (clear cell) tumors. The next most common type is of *germ cell origin* (teratoma, dysgerminoma, embryonal cell, endodermal sinus, choriocarcinoma, and gonadoblastoma), followed by gonadal stromal tumors and neoplasms derived from the mesenchymal elements (sarcomas). The ovary is a common metastatic site for primary tumors of the gastrointestinal tract (Krukenberg tumor), breast, endometrium, and lymphatic system. Ovarian cancer is staged as follows:

Stage I—Cancer limited to the ovaries (I-A, one ovary; I-B, both ovaries; I-C, one or both ovaries with ascites or positive peritoneal cytology).

Stage II—Cancer involving one or both ovaries with pelvic extension (II-A, to the uterus and/or tubes; II-B, to other pelvic structures; II-C, either II-A or II-B with ascites or positive peritoneal cytologic results).

Stage III—Cancer involving one or both ovaries with widespread intraperitoneal metastasis.

Stage IV—Cancer involving one or both ovaries and spread outside the peritoneal cavity.

Clinically, ovarian cancer presents with abdominal swelling and pain, signs of widespread intra-abdominal metastasis (Stage III). Because the operability and survival are greater with detection at earlier stages, women should be urged to have pelvic examinations at least annually. In postmenopausal women, a palpable ovary should arouse suspicion, since the ovary should not be palpable after cessation of ovarian function.

Treatment of ovarian cancer is primarily surgical, involving removal of the uterus, tubes, ovaries, and omentum (a common site of spread) as well as obtaining a peritoneal cytologic evaluation. As much tumor as possible should be removed from other sites in the more advanced stages of the disease. Most gynecologic oncologists believe that additional therapy is mandatory for all patients in the form of chemotherapy, intraperitoneal radiotherapy (P-32), and pelvic and abdominal external radiation. Alkylating agents have been the most useful, with combination chemotherapy being occasionally of benefit. Many authorities also suggest a "second look" either by laparoscopy or laparotomy after adjunctive therapy to evaluate the disease status and further individualize the therapeutic efforts. Clearly, to improve the prognosis with this disease, major efforts will be required in earlier diagnosis, complete initial surgical extirpation of the disease, and enhanced effectiveness of adjunctive therapy.

THE FALLOPIAN TUBE

The human oviducts (fallopian tubes) are frequently the site of pelvic infections. *Salpingitis* often results in agglutination of the epithelial folds, which may lead to tubal obstruction at the fimbria. The endosalpinx continues to produce a watery secretion that distends the tube, creating a "hydrosalpinx." The increased intratubal pressure compromises the vascular supply of the epithelial folds, causing a loss of endothelium. A neosalpingostomy can be performed to reestablish patency of the tube, but the ability to transport oocytes and embryos is reduced, leaving higher rates of infertility and ectopic pregnancies. Uterotubal junction obstruction is also observed, but with a lower frequency than distal obstruction. Several distinct histologic patterns are observed, including endometriosis, fibrosis, and chronic inflammation. A nodular sclerotic process, salpingitis isthmica nodosa, creates diverticula lined by tubal epithelium and is associated with a high rate of tubal pregnancy. Tubal obstruction secondary to pelvic tuberculosis is rare in the United States today, but is still prevalent in underdeveloped countries. The diagnosis is established by culture of the endometrium, and virtually no surgical improvement in terms of fertility can be anticipated.

Cancer of the fallopian tube is a rare genital tract malignancy; the patient presents with a watery and often bloody vaginal discharge, pain, and a pelvic mass (Fig. 11). The histologic picture is that of a papillary adenocarcinoma almost indistinguishable from the papillary serous cystadenocarcinoma of the ovary. Treatment is essentially the same as for ovarian cancer; however, because of the rarity of tubal carcinoma, prognostic information is not available.

LOSS OF PELVIC SUPPORT

Support for the pelvic structures is provided by a variety of ligaments and fascial connections, both investing the vagina and cervix and fixing the uterine fundus to the pelvic side walls. The primary structural support for the uterus comes from the so-called cardinal ligaments, which are dense condensations of the endopelvic fascia extending laterally from the cervix and inserting into the pelvic side.

wall. The uterosacral and round ligaments add further support, as does the condensation of connective tissue between the bladder and anterior lower uterine segment. The vagina is invested by the connective tissue from the rectovaginal and vesicovaginal septae, called the pubocervical fascia. Childbirth requires significant distention of the reproductive tract, stretching the connective tissues that provide support. These changes, coupled with the general effects of aging on the connective tissues throughout the body, may result in loss of support for the genital structures as well as the adjacent pelvic viscera, i.e., bladder and rectum. The role of the hormonal changes occurring at menopause is uncertain.

Several structural defects can result from the loss of pelvic support with distressing effects on the lifestyle of the patient. A *cystocele* is a hernia of the bladder into the vagina (Fig. 13). On pelvic examination, a protrusion of the anterior vaginal wall is easily visible with the Valsalva maneuver, usually with an accompanying *urethrocele*. The size of the cystocele can vary dramatically and often is associated with a loss of the urethrovesical angle and urinary *stress incontinence*. Stress incontinence is defined as that which occurs with increases in intra-abdominal pressure, such as coughing and sneezing or assuming upright posture.

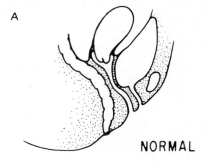

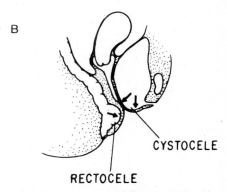

Figure 13. Pelvic relaxation: incontinence. With normal pelvic support, the urethra enters the bladder at approximately a right angle (A). Symptomatic pelvic relaxation may be manifested primarily by urinary incontinence. With weakening of the paravaginal fascia during childbirth, a cystocele or cystourethrocele (B) may distort the normal relationship between the bladder and the urethra to the extent that it does not function as part of the urethral sphincter. With the increases in intra-abdominal pressure associated with coughing and sneezing, urine escapes. Similarly, thinning of the fascia on the posterior vaginal wall may result in herniation by rectum, i.e., a rectocele (B).

This is specifically different from *overflow incontinence* and *enuresis*, which imply neurologic problems in the bladder itself, not weakness in the supporting connective tissue investments. Surgical closure of this anterior vaginal wall hernia, *anterior colporrhaphy*, or elevation of the bladder neck by a retropubic cystourethropexy or suburethral sling, recreates the normal urethrovesical relationship and restores continence. Often a *rectocele*, which is the analogous hernia of the posterior vaginal wall, the rectovaginal septum, may also be present (Fig. 13). A similar surgical repair, *posterior colporrhaphy*, is used to reduce this hernia and recreate an intact rectovaginal septum. These procedures should be delayed until childbearing is completed, since a subsequent delivery may recreate the defect, jeopardizing the surgical repair.

Mobility of the uterus is increased with the relaxation of the supporting structures after childbearing. When these changes are marked, the uterus can descend to the reproductive tract with the Valsalva maneuver to the point of presenting at the vaginal entrance (Fig. 14). This is uncomfortable and is often associated with a cystocele and stress incontinence. A hernia of the peritoneal cavity between the rectum and the uterus, an *enterocele*, is also common with uterine prolapse, complicating the surgical repair. Removal of the uterus, repair of the anterior and posterior vaginal septa, removal of the peritoneal hernia sac, plication of the uterosacral ligaments, and obliteration of the cul-de-sac can reduce this hernia. Occasionally, after hysterectomy the vagina itself will invert and prolapse, creating a hernia sac containing bowel. This requires fixation to a solid structure such as the sacrospinous ligament or sacral promontory because the pelvic connective tissues are unable to provide the necessary support.

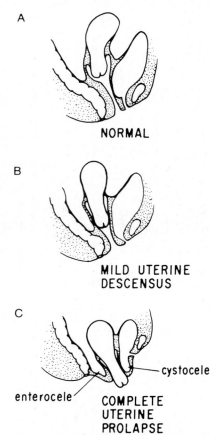

Figure 14. Pelvic relaxation: uterine descensus. Weakening of the supporting ligaments may allow the uterus to descend from its normal position (A) by inverting the vagina (B). Progressive descent may continue until the uterus is present at the vaginal entrance (C). Frequently, a cystocele and an enterocele (a peritoneal hernia posterior to the uterus) may also be present.

PELVIC INFLAMMATORY DISEASE

The genital tract is susceptible to infections because of (1) a surgical injury to the genital tract, i.e., hysterectomy, (2) it being optimal environment in which bacteria can gain access to the genitals, i.e., retained products of conception, and (3) the presence of an organism with a selective advantage for survival in the genital tract.

The most common organism in the latter category is *N. gonorrhoeae*. It is venereally transmitted and may be harbored in the cervix asymptomatically for substantial intervals of time. This accounts for the communicable spread of the disease through sexual contact, and cervical culture for gonococcus in high-risk patients (a history of gonorrhea, sexual contact with a known carrier) is urged. When cervical cultures are positive, aqueous procaine penicillin G, 4.8 million units intramuscularly (IM), preceded by 1 gm. of probenecid orally, should be administered. Alternatives include 3.5 gm. of ampicillin and 1 gm. probenecid orally or 500 mg. tetracycline orally four times a day for 5 days. A parenteral alternative for women allergic to penicillin is 2 gm. of spectinomycin IM. Reculture in 5 to 7 days is mandatory for a "test of cure," particularly with the emergence of penicillin-resistant strains. The community Public Health Department should be consulted because the recommendations may change with the local experience.

Clinically, symptomatic pelvic inflammatory disease usually presents as an acute febrile illness (temperature > 38°C.) with bilateral lower abdominal tenderness and a paucity of gastrointestinal symptoms. On examination, severe pelvic peritonitis is almost always present with exquisite tenderness on manipulation of pelvic structures. Adnexal masses may be present, but are far more common with recurrent infection. With a cervical Gram's stain, the presence of the intracellular gram-negative diplococci, characteristic of the gonococcus, can frequently be detected. Culture of the peritoneal cavity, however, yields a more diverse group of organisms and illustrates the polymicrobial nature of the disease when the gonococcus has colonized the genital tract. The reasons for this are not clear, but a breakdown in the cervical barrier to other bacteria, attributed to the gonococcus, is suspected.

Patients with clinically apparent pelvic infections should be hospitalized and aggressively treated with intravenous antibiotics. Current recommended regimens include 100 mg. doxycycline every 12 hours, with 2 gm. cefoxitin every 6 hours; 600 mg. clindamycin every 6 hours and an initial dose of 2 mg. of gentamicin or tobramycin, followed by 1.5 mg. every 8 hours in patients with normal renal function; and 100 mg. doxycycline and 1 gm. metronidazole every 12 hours.

Patients should be monitored closely for a clinical response, including pelvic examinations every 2 to 3 days to ensure resolution of the pelvic peritonitis. In the absence of significant clinical improvement in 24 to 48 hours, resistant organisms, a developing pelvic abscess, or an error in diagnosis with another cause of the peritonitis should be suspected.

Pelvic abscess formation can occur at any time and is

manifested by a tender, "doughy" mass in the pelvis. This can occur anywhere in the pelvis, but is most frequently lateral to the uterus, forming a tubo-ovarian abscess, or posterior to the uterus in the cul-de-sac. The latter typically dissects down the rectovaginal septum presenting as a mass in the posterior vaginal fornix. Colpotomy drainage of a cul-de-sac abscess usually results in a dramatic clinical improvement, but requires careful selection of patients so as not to rupture an abscess in the peritoneal cavity. Anaerobic bacteria such as *Bacteroides* and enteric bacilli are uniformly present in abscess cavities. Intravenous antibiotics are of little value because of the lack of vascularity of the abscess. This is a potentially life-threatening clinical problem, and if prompt regression of the signs and symptoms of the abscess does not occur, surgical intervention is mandatory. This most often requires removal of the uterus, tubes, and ovaries. Rarely, a unilateral tubo-ovarian abscess is amenable to adnexectomy, with preservation of the remainder of the genital tract. This approach demands careful selection of patients with optimal anatomic circumstances in a young, nulliparous woman strongly desirous of future childbearing. At the earliest sign of recurrent pelvic infection, removal of the remaining pelvic organs should be completed.

If a pattern of recurrent acute infections develops, these are likely due to nongonococcal anaerobic and enteric organisms. Chronic salpingo-oophoritis may cause intermittent pain with few other signs of acute infection. Under these circumstances, a white blood cell count and erythrocyte sedimentation rate (ESR) may be helpful in detecting the presence of a smoldering active infection. The pelvic structures typically are involved in extensive adhesions isolating the adnexal pedicle and obstructing the fallopian tube, thus preventing bacteria from gaining access to the peritoneal cavity. This may be life-saving in the acute illness, but it renders the patient infertile. Surgical attempts at repair of the oviduct and removal of peritubal adhesions are necessary to enhance the probability of conception. When the pain is debilitating, removal of the uterus, tubes, and ovaries may be the only alternative.

INFERTILITY

In American society today, the inability to conceive is an increasing problem that has been made all the more acute by easily available abortions and the fewer numbers of unmarried mothers placing babies for adoption. This is a devastating problem for most couples and should be approached just as seriously as any other medical problem. When to initiate the investigation should be a clinical judgment based on the couple's age, previous reproductive history, length of infertility, and any clinical history suggesting a specific fertility problem. The initial discussion should involve both the husband and wife, and the steps in the investigation should be outlined.

Fertility problems can be categorized into six basic types: (1) male factor, (2) cervical mucus, (3) uterine abnormalities, (4) tubal obstruction or adhesions, (5) ovulatory function, and (6) peritoneal factor, particularly endometriosis. Coital frequency and technique are rarely clinical problems.

Male factor can be evaluated by performing several semen analyses. Normally, fertile men have a sperm concentration greater than 20 million per milliliter and at least 60 per cent normal sperm motility and morphology. The value of the postcoital (Huhner) test remains controversial, but the presence of more than 3 to 5 motile sperm in well-

estrogenized cervical mucus several hours after coitus is reassuring. The uterine cavity can be assessed by hysterosalpingography (HSG) or hysteroscopy. The presence of a uterine septum, intrauterine polyp, or leiomyoma can have an adverse effect on fertility. Fallopian tube patency can be tested by HSG or at the time of laparoscopy. Direct visualization of the pelvis is indispensable for evaluation of peritubal or ovarian adhesions as well as the presence of endometriotic implants, which may be totally asymptomatic.

The most dramatic improvements in infertility care in the past decade have come with improved ovulation induction, the application of microsurgical techniques for repair of the oviducts, and, most recently, extracorporeal fertilization and embryo transfer.

AMENORRHEA

The absence of menses is a common complaint and may have a variety of etiologies, ranging from simple pregnancy to rare central nervous system tumors. A logical stepwise approach to evaluation requires a thorough understanding of the reproductive system (see Fig. 5) coupled with a complete history and physical examination. Without a doubt, the most common cause of amenorrhea in women of reproductive age is pregnancy, and this should always be considered. Localizing the etiologic site is the next step, considering the uterus, ovaries, pituitary, and hypothalamus.

A history of previous vaginal bleeding suggests the presence of a normal uterus, and except for intrauterine synechiae or cervical stenosis following a surgical procedure, this eliminates the uterus as a cause. These surgically induced uterine abnormalities can be confirmed by progestogen withdrawal, alone or after estrogen priming.

Ovarian dysfunction can occur at any age, varying from chronic anovulation to premature ovarian failure. Anovulation can clinically be divided into estrogenic or hypoestrogenic groups, with a positive progestogen withdrawal separating the former from the latter. Measurement of the gonadotropins is useful because these will be low or in the normal range, particularly FSH, since the levels will rise into the castrate range with ovarian failure. Higher centers are implicated if the lower genital tract is normal and the gonadotropins are low and hypoestrogenism is present.

The most common pituitary tumor in women secretes prolactin, and measurement of a serum prolactin level is mandatory. Radiographic assessment of the sella turcica and hypothalamus is helpful with other problems such as craniopharyngiomas, hypothalamic tumors, and arachnoid herniation through an incompetent diaphragma sellae, the "empty sella syndrome." Commonly, no pathologic etiology can be determined in women with low gonadotropins and hypoestrogenism; the process is thought to be secondary to intrinsic malfunction of the hypothalamus, termed "hypothalamic amenorrhea." Severe metabolic or psychologic stress can also induce amenorrhea. Examples include anorexia nervosa and excessive exercise.

PRENATAL EXPOSURE TO DIETHYLSTILBESTROL

Diethylstilbestrol is a nonsteroidal estrogen that was given to pregnant women from the late 1940s to the 1960s in an attempt to prevent spontaneous abortion. It did not prove efficacious, but acted as a teratogen, altering structures derived from the müllerian ducts. Prenatal DES exposure has also been associated with a previously rare clear cell adenocarcinoma of the vagina. These effects are consistent with either an unanticipated estrogen action *in utero* attributable to the unusual metabolism and transport of this xenobiotic or a unique teratogenic effect of the compound.

Prenatal DES exposure results in the presence of islands of mucus-secreting columnar epithelium in the vagina, i.e., vaginal adenosis. Usually, squamous metaplasia obliterates or covers these areas, and rarely (1 in 2 to 10,000 exposed women), a clear cell adenocarcinoma develops, presumably originating in areas of adenosis. The cancer develops after puberty and before the mid-20s, making frequent pelvic examination during this interval useful. Whether DES is carcinogenic or is simply a teratogen requiring the presence of a co-carcinogen to induce the neoplasm is unknown. Treatment of the vaginal cancer requires removal of the uterus and the involved segment of the vagina with wide margins and pelvic lymphadenectomy. The role of adjunctive therapy, chemotherapy, progestogens, and radiation is not clear because of the small number of cases.

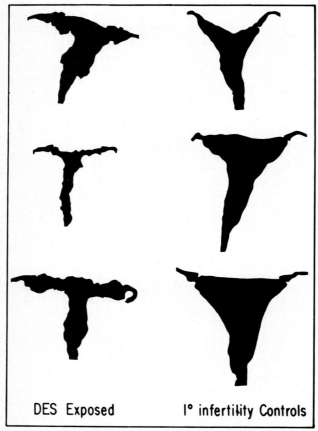

DES Exposed   **1° infertility Controls**

Figure 15. Upper genital tract effects of prenatal diethylstilbestrol (DES) exposure. Outlines of the hysterosalpingograms of infertile women with prenatal DES exposure are contrasted with those of infertile women without known exposure to DES. Note the smaller size, irregular contours, and typical T-shaped endometrial cavity. This is a unique effect and is present in over 75 per cent of women with the cervicovaginal changes associated with prenatal DES exposure. (From Haney, A. F., Hammond, C. B., Soules, M. R., and Creasman, W. T.: Fertil. Steril. 31:142, 1979.)

The cervix is also affected by prenatal DES with several anatomic deformities described. These include transverse cervical ridges, a cervical hood or collar, a cockscomb cervix, and pseudopolyp formation. The endocervical canal is narrow, and mucus production reduced. It is not clear whether the rate of cervical dysplasia in DES-exposed women is increased. The cervical cryotherapy utilized therapeutically to treat CIN results in a high rate of cervical stenosis in DES-exposed women because of the smaller dimensions of the endocervical canal.

The upper genital tract is also a müllerian duct structure and likewise affected, with the uterus typically being smaller and having an irregularly shaped endometrial cavity (Fig. 15). The fallopian tubes are rarely noted to be atretic. To date, there is no suggestion of a clinical significant effect on the ovary. Although these teratogenic effects have been associated with higher rates of spontaneous abortion, premature delivery, and ectopic pregnancy, the vast majority of DES-exposed women can successfully reproduce.

Male offspring are analogously affected in structures derived from the mesonephric ducts. Higher rates of retained testes, epididymal cysts, and oligospermia have been noted. The reduced sperm production, while measurable, probably does not reduce the fertility potential, since it is not below the level necessary for reproduction. Further time will be required to determine whether any neoplasia develops in the genital tract of these men.

ANDROGEN EXCESS

There are two sites of androgen synthesis, the ovary and the adrenal cortex. The symptoms of androgen excess in women vary, depending on the magnitude of the problem. With minor elevations, mild acne, facial and abdominal hirsutism, and irregular menses are common. When high levels of androgens are present, true virilization may occur with clitoromegaly, temporal hair recession, heightened libido, deepening of the voice, atrophy of the breasts, and increased muscle mass. When the androgens are produced by aberrant function, the process is typically mild and gradual, whereas with androgen-secreting tumors of the ovary and adrenal the virilization has an abrupt onset and is rapidly progressive.

Chronic anovulation represents almost 95 per cent of the clinically significant cases of androgen excess. This usually presents as cosmetically troublesome hirsutism and irregular menses in women in their late teens and early 20s. If cyclic ovulation is present, the hirsutism is more likely genetic because the degree of normal facial hair varies markedly on a familial basis. Women from around the Mediterranean, for example, can anticipate more "genetic" hirsutism than Asiatic or northern European women. Gonadal-stromal tumors of the ovary, such as an arrhenoblastoma or Leydig cell tumor, can produce either estrogens or androgens and tend to have a more abrupt and clinically progressive course. These tumors originate from the hormonally active stromal compartment and histologically may appear as any combination of Leydig cells, Sertoli cells, granulosa cells, or thecal cells, representing both male and female differentiation. Gonadal-stromal tumors are associated with marked elevations in serum testosterone when compared with the much more modest elevations of testosterone observed in women with chronic anovulation. When ovarian tumors are identified, they should be excised; occasionally, they may be so small as to be identifiable only by selective venous catheterization of the ovarian veins.

Women with chronic anovulation are best managed by suppression of gonadotropins, usually by oral contraceptives, in combination with one of the available anti-androgens, spironolactone or cimetidine.

An adrenal source of excess androgen is indicated by a marked elevation in the weak adrenal androgen dehydroepiandrosterone (DHEA), usually by measurement of its sulfated form. Adrenal tumors are rare and occasionally malignant, and they therefore should be removed. "Adult-onset" or "late" congenital adrenal hyperplasia secondary to mild deficiencies in 21- or 11-hydroxylase enzymes have been reported with an autosomal recessive inheritance pattern. These are not clinically apparent prior to puberty, probably because of the increase in adrenal steroid output beginning at that time. The steroids that immediately precede these hydroxylation steps, 17-hydroxyprogesterone and progesterone, are usually elevated and helpful in making the diagnosis. The lower cortisol output results in increased adrenocorticotropic hormone (ACTH) production and increased adrenal androgens. Physiologic replacement doses of glucocorticoids lower the ACTH drive and reduce the androgen burden.

ECTOPIC PREGNANCY

Spontaneously occurring extrauterine pregnancy is unique to humans and is frequently a life-threatening clinical problem (Fig. 12). Whether this is attributable to unique human diseases predisposing to ectopic pregnancy or less stringent requirements for embryo survival, allowing for implantation outside the uterus, is not known. Both factors may be involved, but regardless of the etiology the human embryo has aggressive growth characteristics and can establish an adequate blood supply by invading non-uterine tissues. This is undoubtedly suboptimal placentation, and the key to understanding the development of ectopic pregnancies is an appreciation of factors that prevent or retard embryo transport.

Sperm are small mobile gametes able to traverse the entire female reproductive tract even through a compromised tubal lumen. By contrast, the oocyte and embryo have no intrinsic mobility and require the oviducts to transport them. Approximately 4 to 6 days after fertilization, the embryo is ready for implantation; consequently, an alteration in the normal transport mechanism may result in implantation of an embryo outside the uterus. Embryo transport in the fimbrial and ampullary portions of the fallopian tube is by ciliary action along the longitudinal furrows created by the enfolded epithelium. When salpingitis causes intraluminal adhesions, obstruction of these furrows may block embryo transport and may result in implantation in the tube. Early in an ectopic gestation, the blood supply appears sufficient for normal embryonic development; consequently, the endocrine changes of early pregnancy may be indistinguishable from normal. As the gestation progresses, however, insufficient vascularity typically leads to falling hCG levels and lower gonadal steroid levels. Irregular vaginal bleeding results as well as loss of the subjective symptoms of early pregnancy, i.e., breast tenderness, nausea, and so on. Occasionally, the vascularity is adequate to sustain hCG levels for longer intervals of time and the hormonal milieu of early pregnancy is maintained.

By far the most common site of ectopic pregnancy is the oviduct, and the clinical circumstances in which pregnancy occurs can suggest increased awareness of this possibility by the physician (Fig. 12). A history of previous tubal infection, reconstructive tubal surgery, a previous ectopic pregnancy, or prenatal DES exposure should alert the clinician to consider the possibility of an ectopic gestation. An ultrasound scan at approximately 6 to 7 weeks from the last normal menstrual period can identify a normal intrauterine gestation. When this is not observed, an ectopic pregnancy should be considered. With this approach, more ectopic pregnancies will be identified prior to rupture and enhance the opportunities for conservative management.

Unsuspected ectopic gestations usually present with an aberration of menses, irregular vaginal bleeding, and abdominal pain. This can easily be confused with salpingitis, but the increased white blood cell count and fever are absent. Unfortunately, the classic presentation is not particularly common, and the symptoms overlap with normal pregnancy, dysfunctional uterine bleeding, and other gynecologic problems, making the diagnosis difficult and often delayed. When an ectopic pregnancy is suspected, the patient must be rapidly evaluated to exclude this possibility because of the life-threatening nature of the problem.

Diagnostic techniques today include (1) rapid, sensitive serum assays for hCG, which can detect low levels of this hormone, (2) ultrasound scanning of the uterus, which can detect an intrauterine pregnancy, (3) a *culdocentesis* to ascertain the presence of intraabdominal bleeding, and (4) laparoscopy to visualize the pelvic structures. When an ectopic pregnancy is identified, a *celiotomy* is performed for excision of the gestation to prevent further intra-abdominal hemorrhage. If the patient does not desire maintenance of reproductive potential, a salpingectomy is the procedure of choice. If preservation of reproductive potential is desired, a linear salpingostomy on the antimesenteric surface of the oviduct can frequently enable removal of the trophoblast and preservation of the tube. If rupture has already occurred, a segmental resection of the ectopic gestation can be performed, preserving as much tube as possible for later reconstruction. Whether to repair the tube at the time of ectopic removal is controversial since there is considerable distortion of the anatomy because of the bleeding. A higher rate of repeat tubal pregnancy can be anticipated in these oviducts, but this is in the range of 15 to 20 per cent, leaving the substantial majority of women who achieve pregnancy with normal intrauterine gestations. A significant number of these women will encounter infertility as a result of the inflammatory changes that led to the first ectopic pregnancy.

SURGICAL PROCEDURES DURING PREGNANCY

Although pregnant women occasionally require surgical procedures, whenever possible, operations should be delayed until after pregnancy or at least beyond the first trimester. The status of the fetus must be borne in mind, since there are now two interdependent patients—the mother and the fetus. Emergency considerations may demand immediate operative intervention, and under these circumstances good maternal health will undoubtedly be in the best interest of the fetus. The stress of a surgical procedure and anesthesia can induce abortion in the first trimester and can precipitate premature labor at later stages of pregnancy. The early losses appear to be hormonally related, since luteal function is adversely affected by surgical procedures. Unfortunately, there is nothing therapeutically available to prevent these endocrine changes and the clinical circumstances may leave no alternative. Premature labor, by contrast, has been successfully treated by beta-adrenergic receptor agonists. Consideration for such treatment should be given when the operative procedure is performed prior to 34 weeks' gestation. After that time, the probability for fetal survival with good neonatal care is virtually identical to that at term delivery.

Pelvic and abdominal anatomy is significantly distorted by the gravid uterus arising out of the pelvis. Both the anatomic and functional changes accompanying pregnancy may obscure the usual signs and symptoms of illness. Common clinical problems, such as appendicitis, cholecystitis, pancreatitis, and nephrolithiasis, may tax even the most skilled and experienced clinician during pregnancy.

Evaluating trauma during pregnancy requires knowledge of growth characteristics and susceptibility of the gravid uterus as well as an appreciation of the condition of the fetus. Early in pregnancy (less than 10 weeks), the uterus is well protected from abdominal trauma because it has not yet become an abdominal organ. It is shielded from abdominal trauma by the bony pelvis and cushioned by the urinary bladder, psoas muscles, and bowel. By contrast, later in pregnancy the uterus and fetus are more susceptible to abdominal trauma because of the protrusion of the uterus into the abdominal cavity. The fetus is not often injured despite significant trauma because it is within the aquatic environment, the *amnionic sac*, which cushions any trauma. The most frequent consequence of severe injury is premature separation of the placenta. Large amounts of retroplacental bleeding can occur with death of the fetus and massive hemorrhage, which usually initiates labor. Careful evaluation of uterine tone and vaginal bleeding is mandatory to detect a placental abruption, and rapid atraumatic delivery offers the best chance of survival for both mother and fetus. The vulva and vagina have a marked increase in their blood supply during pregnancy, and injuries can be anticipated to produce proportionally greater blood loss.

TROPHOBLASTIC NEOPLASIA

Gestational trophoblastic cancer can follow any type of pregnancy, but over 50 per cent follows a hydatidiform mole. Occasionally, no antecedent pregnancy can be identified. The several histologic types (invasive mole, choriocarcinoma, and anaplastic trophoblastic tumor) share in common hCG production, which is useful as a tumor marker. With a high proclivity to metastasize, malignant trophoblast is frequently detected only upon histologic evaluation of excised metastatic nodules. The most common sites are the vagina, lung, liver, brain, and bowel.

The hydatidiform mole is a benign trophoblastic process and the most common overall. Grossly, multiple grape-like clusters of vesicles are present in the uterus; histologically, these are large, hydropic, chorionic villi with trophoblastic proliferation. The incidence of moles varies geographically, with an incidence in the United States of approximately one in two thousand (1:2000) deliveries; it is more common in the Far East, occurring as often as one in 125 pregnancies. The clinical presentation is usually heavy vaginal bleeding early in the second trimester of pregnancy with no fetal heart tones in a large-for-dates uterus. Sonographically, multiple disorganized intrauterine echoes, rarely with a coexisting fetus, are diagnostic. A careful suction dilatation and curettage is required to evacuate the molar tissue, since perforation of the enlarged uterus can result in massive bleeding.

Choriocarcinoma has been an excellent example of the effectiveness of specifically targeted chemotherapy. Trophoblast has a high requirement for folic acid, making the tumor highly susceptible to the folic acid antagonist methotrexate. Multiagent chemotherapy with selective surgical excision and radiation therapy permanently cures the majority of patients even when distant metastases are present. Among patients with a good prognosis, this can usually be accomplished with chemotherapy alone, retaining reproductive function. Treatment should be conducted in one of the specialized trophoblastic disease centers, located around the United States, in which there has been extensive experience with this otherwise uniformly fatal malignancy.

SELECTED REFERENCES

General Gynecology

Bongiovanni, A. M. (Ed.): Adolescent Gynecology. New York, Plenum Press, 1981.
Children and adolescents often have gynecologic problems, but the spectrum of diseases is different from that encountered in the general practice of adult gynecology. This text provides a useful reference for the practicing physician dealing with the unique aspects of these patients, particularly infrequently encountered congenital anomalies and inborn errors of metabolism.

Buchsbaum, H. J. (Ed.): The Menopause. New York, Springer-Verlag, 1983.
Aging is undergoing intensive study, and this reference provides a current review of the consequences of the climacteric. It covers all the important aspects of this complicated process with special emphasis on the clinical management.

Duenhoelter, J. H.: Greenhill's Office Gynecology, 10th ed. Chicago, Year Book Publishers, 1983.
The primary strength of this book is its focus on the outpatient management of gynecologic problems. There are excellent sections devoted to the physical examination and outpatient surgical procedures. It is helpful to those practicing office gynecology, whether in specialty or in general practice.

Kase, N. G., and Weingold, A. B. (Eds.): Principles and Practice of Clinical Gynecology. New York, Wiley Publishing Company, 1983.
This is a comprehensive text on nearly every aspect of gynecology. It covers the physiologic principles of the discipline as well as a comprehensive clinical approach to women's health care.

Monif, G. R. G. (Ed.): Infectious Disease in Obstetrics and Gynecology. Philadelphia, Harper & Row, 1982.
This is an excellent reference source, a thorough review of infectious diseases in gynecology. The unique microbiologic and clinical aspects of pelvic infections are summarized, and this text is useful for both students and practitioners.

Nichols, D. H., and Randall, C. L.: Vaginal Surgery. Baltimore, Williams & Wilkins, 1983.
This is a well-illustrated guide for the gynecologic surgeon addressing a technically difficult aspect of the specialty. The basic principles and practical approaches to complicated vaginal operations are described and are of particular value to those interested in problems of pelvic support and gynecologic urology.

Novak, E. R., and Woodruff, J. D.: Novak's Gynecologic and Obstetric Pathology. Philadelphia, W. B. Saunders Company, 1979.
This book continues to be the definitive text devoted to gynecologic pathology. It serves as a guide for understanding gynecologic disease and those unique aspects of genital tract neoplasms. It is written with a clinical perspective and, consequently, is as useful to the student as the experienced practitioner.

Porter, C. W., Waife, R. S., and Holrop, H. R.: Contraception. New York, Grune & Stratton, Inc., 1983.
Contraceptive technology continues to undergo rapid changes, and this text is a practical guide to clinical contraception. While directed toward the practitioner, it includes ample reviews on the various methods, updating the current status of each.

Sciarra, J. J. (Ed.): Gynecology and Obstetrics. Philadelphia, Harper & Row, 1984.
This is a very comprehensive text, covering nearly every aspect of the discipline. There are numerous authoritative essays by recognized experts

designed to be updated in future editions. It is divided into several sections corresponding to the subspecialties of obstetrics and gynecology, and includes many related topics such as genetics, human sexuality, and fertility regulation.

Semm, K.: Atlas of Gynecologic Laparoscopy and Hysteroscopy. Philadelphia, W. B. Saunders Company, 1977.
Endoscopy has become an indispensable surgical technique for the gynecologist. This text provides the surgical principles of the techniques as well as many excellent color photographs of pelvic pathology. The student interested in these procedures will find this book invaluable.

Reproductive Endocrinology and Infertility

Aiman, E. J. (Ed.): Infertility: Diagnosis and Treatment. New York, Springer-Verlag, 1984.
All aspects of infertility are covered in this book, with many experts in the field contributing chapters on the various topics. It is comprehensive and well written and serves as an excellent reference for clinicians dealing with infertile couples.

Garcia, C-R., Mastroianni, L., Jr., Amelar, R. D., and Dublin, L. (Eds.): Current Therapy of Infertility: 1984–1985. Philadelphia, B. C. Decker, Inc., 1984.
Many expert contributors provide current therapeutic recommendations for treatment of infertility. This book is clinically focused and covers the entire subject, both for male and female factors. The emphasis is on the recent changes in the subspeciality.

Gomel, V.: Microsurgery in Female Infertility. Boston, Little, Brown and Company, 1983.
The advances in the surgical treatment of infertility are well demonstrated in this book. Of particular value are the large number of color plates graphically illustrating the advantages of the microsurgical approach to reconstruction of the pelvic viscera.

Siegler, A. M., and Lindemann, H. J.: Hysteroscopy: Principles and Practice. Philadelphia, J. B. Lippincott Company, 1984.
Hysteroscopy is a relatively new approach to sterilization, the diagnosis of uterine bleeding, and the evaluation of the uterine factor in infertility. This monograph provides an excellent place to begin familiarization with this technique. It gives practical instruction as well as providing a large number of color plates to illustrate the capability of the technique.

Speroff, L., Glass, R. H., and Kase, N. G.: Clinical Gynecologic Endocrinology and Infertility, 3rd ed. Baltimore, Williams & Wilkins, 1983.
This is an excellent guide to the principles and practice of reproductive endocrinology. The authors include the newer concepts of this rapidly changing field and incorporate them into the framework of their previous texts. It is particularly strong in providing insights into the physiologic basis of clinical practice.

Gynecologic Oncology

Coppleson, M. (Ed.): Gynecologic Oncology: Fundamental Principles and Clinical Practice. New York, Churchill Livingstone, 1981.
An excellent starting point for the student interested in gynecologic oncology is this comprehensive two-volume text. It covers the clinical aspects of genital cancer as well as the basic principles of chemotherapy and radiation.

DiSaia, P. J., and Creasman, W. T.: Clinical Gynecologic Oncology, 2nd ed. St. Louis, C. V. Mosby Company, 1984.
This is a well-written text covering the entire field of gynecologic oncology. It is easily readable and provides practical guidelines for the management of clinical problems. It integrates recent therapeutic recommendations with the basic principles of cancer therapy.

THE UROGENITAL SYSTEM

W. MARSTON LINEHAN, M.D.

39

Urologic surgery involves management of diseases of the urogenital tract in males and the urinary tract in females. The urinary system comprises the kidneys, ureters, bladder, and urethra and performs the functions of production, transportation, storage, and elimination of urine. The male genital system includes the testes, epididymides, vas deferens, seminal vesicles, prostate, and penis, and its primary function is reproduction.

ANATOMY AND PHYSIOLOGY[12, 17, 18, 20, 23]

Kidney

The primitive nephric system begins as the *pronephros*, which provides the earliest nephric function and disappears by the fourth week of gestation. Following the degeneration of the pronephros, the *mesonephric* tubules develop and provide nephric function. At the eighth week, a ureteral bud grows cephalad off the mesonephric duct and stimulates the development of the metanephrogenic cap and its subsequent cranial migration. From this ascending and developing metanephrogenic tissue and ureteral bud, the kidney, collecting system, and ureter develop.

The kidneys are paired retroperitoneal organs that lie along the border of the psoas muscle below the diaphragm and in proximity to the spinal column. The average kidney measures 11.5 cm. in length, is 150 gm. in weight, and is lined by a fibrous capsule. Outside the renal capsule there is a variable amount of perirenal fat. Surrounding the kidney and perirenal fat and extending from the diaphragm down to the ureter is a fascial tissue known as *Gerota's fascia*. The kidney comprises an outer cortex, a central medulla, calyces, and pelvis. In the cortex are the glomeruli and the proximal renal tubules. The medulla of the kidney is the site of the renal pyramids, which contain collecting ducts that drain into the calyces.

The primary function of the kidney is accomplished by the nephron, which consists of the glomerulus, tubules, and collecting duct. Blood is filtered across the glomerulus into Bowman's space and thence into the proximal tubule, where 70 per cent of filtrate resorption takes place. As the filtrate progresses through the loop of Henle, sodium and accompanying ions are resorbed. In the distal tubule, adjustments take place in pH and osmolality and there is a passive mechanism for resorption of calcium, phosphate, inorganic sulfate, and protein. The kidney plays an important role in acid-base regulation, particularly in hydrogen ion excretion

and production of bicarbonate. After the collecting duct empties its contents into the calyx, the urine passes through the renal pelvis and ureter into the bladder. The renal artery arises from the aorta and enters the kidney at the hilum, between the pelvis of the kidney and the renal vein. The first branch of the renal artery, which is posterior, supplies the upper and middle half of the dorsal aspect of the kidney. The anterior portion of the renal artery is divided into a superior, upper, middle, and lower segment. The renal veins are anterior to the arteries and may be multiple. Accessory renal veins are of clinical importance, since they may cross the ureter and cause hydronephrosis or may complicate renal surgical procedures. On the left side, the gonadal, vertebral, and adrenal veins empty into the renal vein; on the right side the gonadal and vertebral veins empty directly into the vena cava. The kidneys are drained by lymphatics that follow the vascular supply. The neural supply to the kidney is contained in a plexus located anterior to the aorta, which supplies the kidneys and upper ureters (Fig. 1)

The kidneys lie between the twelfth thoracic and second lumbar vertebrae, and are bounded medially by the psoas, posteriorly by the quadratus lumborum, laterally by the abdominal muscles, and superiorly by the diaphragm. The right kidney is generally 1 to 2 cm. lower than the left. The right kidney is bounded above by the right lobe of the liver, medially by the duodenum and inferior vena cava, and anteriorly by the hepatic flexure of the colon. The left kidney is bounded superiorly by the spleen and tail of the pancreas, anteriorly by the splenic flexure of the colon and the jejunum, and medially by the descending aorta. Superior and medial to each kidney is the adrenal gland.

The most common surgical approaches to the kidney are the flank approach, the transperitoneal abdominal approach, and the thoracoabdominal approach.

The *flank incision* is an extraperitoneal approach and provides excellent access to the renal parenchyma and collecting system. With the patient in the lateral position, this procedure is performed through the bed of the tenth, eleventh, or twelfth rib. The choice of rib is dependent upon the position of the kidney and the site of the lesion. This approach is commonly used to remove small renal tumors and kidney stones or to repair abnormalities in the kidney or collecting system.

The *abdominal approach* is used when early access to the renal pedicle is important, such as with trauma or a renal tumor. A vertical midline or an anterior subcostal incision may be used. The subcostal incision is made from the midaxillary line anteriorly across the rectus muscle and

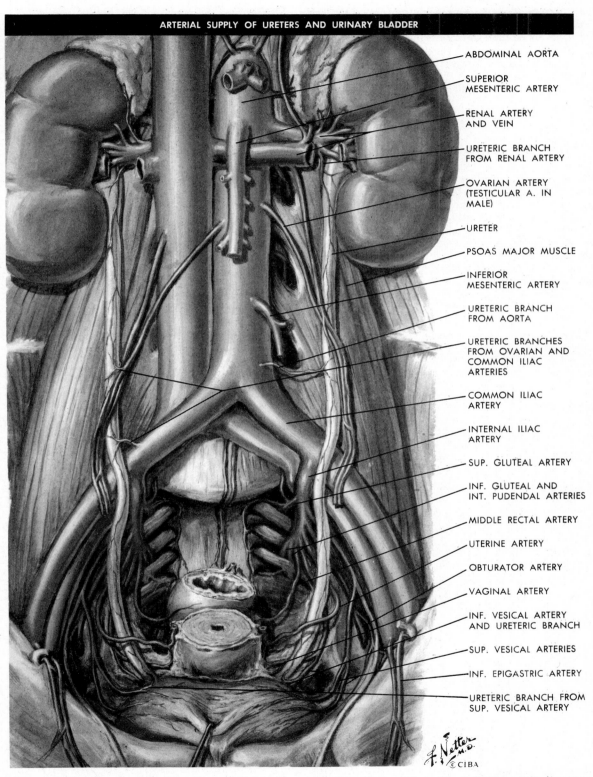

ARTERIAL SUPPLY OF URETERS AND URINARY BLADDER

- ABDOMINAL AORTA
- SUPERIOR MESENTERIC ARTERY
- RENAL ARTERY AND VEIN
- URETERIC BRANCH FROM RENAL ARTERY
- OVARIAN ARTERY (TESTICULAR A. IN MALE)
- URETER
- PSOAS MAJOR MUSCLE
- INFERIOR MESENTERIC ARTERY
- URETERIC BRANCH FROM AORTA
- URETERIC BRANCHES FROM OVARIAN AND COMMON ILIAC ARTERIES
- COMMON ILIAC ARTERY
- INTERNAL ILIAC ARTERY
- SUP. GLUTEAL ARTERY
- INF. GLUTEAL AND INT. PUDENDAL ARTERIES
- MIDDLE RECTAL ARTERY
- UTERINE ARTERY
- OBTURATOR ARTERY
- VAGINAL ARTERY
- INF. VESICAL ARTERY AND URETERIC BRANCH
- SUP. VESICAL ARTERIES
- INF. EPIGASTRIC ARTERY
- URETERIC BRANCH FROM SUP. VESICAL ARTERY

Figure 1. The arterial supply and relationship of organs of the urinary tract. (From Netter, F.H., in Ciba Collection of Medical Illustrations, Volume 6, Summit, N.J., 1953.)

may be performed bilaterally. The bilateral subcostal *incision* provides excellent exposure of both kidneys and their vascular supply and of both adrenal glands.

The *thoracoabdominal approach* is performed through the bed of the ninth, tenth, or eleventh rib and extends downward to divide the external oblique, internal oblique, and transversus muscles. The diaphragm is incised, and there is excellent access to the kidney, renal vessels, abdominal aorta, and vena cava. This incision is used when there is a large renal, adrenal, or other retroperitoneal lesion.

Ureter

The ureters are retroperitoneal conduits connecting the kidney with the bladder. Initially, the ureters pass through Gerota's fascia and then cross the psoas muscle and common iliac vessels. They course along the posterior aspect of the pelvis, under the vas deferens, and enter the base of the bladder at the trigone. The blood supply to the ureter is from the renal, gonadal, aortic, common iliac, and internal iliac vessels. The lymphatics accompany the arteries and drain into the hypogastric, iliac, and para-aortic nodes. Autonomic innervation of the wall of the ureter confers peristaltic activity in which rhythmic contractions emanating from a proximal pacemaker control the smooth and efficient transportation of urine from the renal pelvis to the bladder. The mucosa of the ureter is composed of transitional epithelium, which rests on a fibrous lamina propria. Under the lamina propria are the well-developed circular and longitudinal muscle layers and the adventitia.

Bladder

The bladder is a muscular organ that functions as the main reservoir of the urinary tract and has a capacity of 350 to 450 ml. The ureters enter the posteroinferior portion of the bladder at the trigone. The trigone forms the base of the bladder from the ureteral orifices to the bladder neck. Anterior to the bladder are the space of Retzius, which contains fatty tissue and a plexus of veins, and the pubic bone of the pelvis. Posterior to the bladder in the male are the seminal vesicles, vas deferens, ureters, and the rectum. In the female, the vagina and uterus are located between the bladder and the rectum.

The arterial supply to the bladder is derived from branches of the internal iliac artery—the superior, middle, and inferior vesical arteries. The veins from the bladder drain into the plexus of Santorini anteriorly and the pudendal plexus posteriorly. The lymphatic drainage of the ventral portion of the bladder drains into the external iliac nodes; the lymphatic drainage of the dorsal half of the bladder drains into the internal, external, and common iliac node chains. Histologically, the bladder is composed of a mucosal layer of transitional epithelium, a submucosa of connective and elastic tissue, and a detrusor muscle layer composed of longitudinal, spiral, and circular muscles. Pain, temperature, proprioception, and motor innervation to the bladder are provided by sacral nerve roots 2, 3, and 4 via the pelvic nerve. The sympathetic innervation to the bladder is derived from T11, T12, L1, and L2 through the hypogastric nerve. There is an involuntary physiologic internal sphincter at the bladder neck composed of smooth muscle, and a voluntary, external sphincter mechanism composed of striated muscle.

The control of voiding is a complex process that is coordinated by the micturition center in the cerebral cortex, which is connected to a pelvic reflex arch from the sacral spinal cord to the bladder. Normal voiding involves the simultaneous contraction of the detrusor muscle and the relaxation of the internal and external sphincters. Any disease process that affects the cortical micturition center, the motor or sensory spinal tracts, the peripheral nerves to the bladder, the bladder itself, or the sphincter mechanism may have an effect on bladder function or continence (Fig. 2).

Urethra

The urethra is the conduit for both urine and the products of the male genital system. The male urethra extends approximately 23 cm. from the bladder neck to the meatus and is divided into anterior and posterior portions.

The *anterior urethra* is divided into the bulbar, the penile, and the glandular urethra. The fossa navicularis is a small distal dilation in the glandular urethra. The anterior urethra is surrounded by an erectile body, the corpus spongiosum. The bulbourethral glands, also known as *Cowper's glands,* are located in the urogenital diaphragm and empty into the bulbar urethra. The penile urethra is lined by numerous small glands, the glands of Littre.

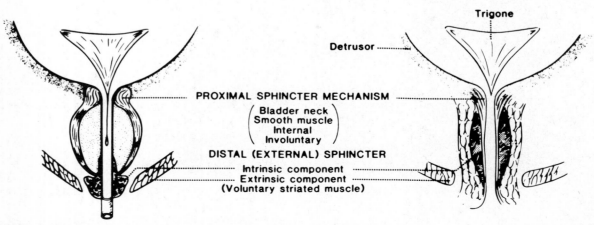

Figure 2. The sphincter mechanism in the male and female urethra. (From Webster, G. D.: In Paulson, D. F. (Ed.): Genitourinary Surgery. New York, Churchill Livingstone, 1984.)

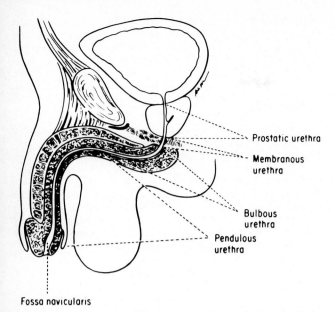

Prostatic urethra

Membranous urethra

Bulbous urethra

Pendulous urethra

Fossa navicularis

Figure 3. The divisions of the male urethra. (From Webster, G. D.: In Paulson, D. F. (Ed.): Genitourinary Surgery. *New York, Churchill Livingstone, 1984.)*

The *posterior urethra* is composed of the membranous and prostatic urethra. The prostatic urethra extends from the bladder to the membranous urethra and contains the verumontanum, a raised area at the distal portion of the base of the prostatic urethra that is formed by the entrance of the ejaculatory ducts and the utricle, which is a müllerian duct remnant (Fig. 3).

Prostate

The prostate gland is a fibromuscular organ that surrounds the vesical neck and proximal portion of the urethra in the male. It is approximately 20 gm. in weight in the adult male and is composed of an anterior and a posterior portion. Embryologically, the prostate gland is derived from five epithelial evaginations of the posterior urethra. The blood supply of the prostate is provided by the inferior vesical artery and enters at the posterolateral aspect of the vesical neck. The venous drainage of the prostate is diffuse and empties into the plexus of Santorini. The nerve supply of the prostate is predominantly of sympathetic origin from the hypogastric plexus and from fibers arriving from the third and fourth sacral nerves through the sacral plexus. The lymphatic drainage of the prostate is to the obturator, internal iliac, external iliac, and presacral nodes and is of considerable importance in evaluating the extent of spread of disease from the prostate.

Normal prostatic function is dependent on testosterone, produced by the Leydig cell of the testis in response to stimulation by luteinizing hormone (LH) from the pituitary gland. Testosterone is metabolized to dihydrotestosterone by 5α-reductase within the prostate and seminal vesicles.

Although the prostate is divided into five lobes (posterior, middle, anterior, and two lateral lobes), it is separated functionally into two independent structures. The interior periurethral glandular tissue gives rise to hyperplasia and is responsible for benign enlargement of the prostate seen in men of advancing age. The outer segment is a musculoglandular structure from which prostatic malignancies arise. Histologically the prostate is composed of connective tissue, smooth muscle fibers, and epithelial glands lined by tall columnar cells and a layer of flattened basilar cells.

Seminal Vesicle

The seminal vesicles are paired structures located beneath the trigone at the base of the bladder and are invested posteriorly by Denonvilliers' fascia, which separates them from the rectum. They enter the ampullae of the vas and form the ejaculatory ducts, which enter the prostatic urethra at the verumontanum. The seminal vesicles secrete a viscous, mucoid fluid that is the source of fructose in the ejaculate. Absence of fructose in the ejaculate indicates blockage or absence of the seminal vesicles.

Histologically, the mucous membrane of the seminal vesicles is pseudostratified and contains a submucosa of dense connective tissue that is covered by a thin layer of muscle that is contractile during ejaculation. The volume of the normal human ejaculate ranges from 2 to 6 ml. and is composed of two components, spermatozoa and seminal fluid. The seminal fluid is formed predominantly by the secretions of sexual accessory tissues, including the epididymides, vasa deferentia, ampullae, seminal vesicles, prostate, Cowper's glands, and the glands of Littre. Seminal fluid contains a high level of potassium, zinc, citric acid, fructose, spermine, and acid phosphatase.

Penis

The main body of the penis is composed of three erectile bodies. The *corpus spongiosum* is a ventromedial structure that surrounds the urethra. Dorsal and lateral to the midline corpus spongiosum, there are two other erectile structures, each known as the *corpus cavernosum* (plural, corpora cavernosa). Each of these erectile bodies is separately invested with fibrous tissue known as the *tunica albuginea*. These structures are collectively surrounded by fibrous tissue, known as *Buck's fascia*. Underneath the skin of the penis and scrotum is *Colles' fascia*, a fibrous tissue that extends from the base of the glans to the urogenital diaphragm and is contiguous with Scarpa's fascia of the abdominal wall. The penis and urethra are supplied by the internal pudendal artery, which divides into a profunda artery of the penis, a dorsal artery of the penis, and the bulbourethral artery. The deep dorsal vein of the penis courses beneath Buck's fascia adjacent to the dorsal arteries and drains into the internal pudendal vein via the pudendal plexus. The lymphatic drainage of the skin of the penis drains to the superficial and deep inguinal lymph nodes, while the lymphatic drainage from the glans penis and urethra is to the deep inguinal and external and internal iliac nodes. Embryologically, the penile urethra is formed by the fusion of the urethral folds of the ventral surface of the genital tubercle, which then becomes elongated to form the penis in the developing male.

Scrotum

The scrotum is dual-chambered and contains the testes, epididymides, and terminal portion of the spermatic cord. Beneath the scrotal skin is Darto's fascia, which contains elastic fibers, connective tissue, and smooth muscle. The blood supply to the scrotum is provided by the internal pudendal artery and by the deep pudendal branch of the femoral artery. The scrotal veins course with the internal pudendal and deep pudendal arteries and empty into the internal pudendal and saphenous veins. Cutaneous innervation to the scrotum is from branches of the ilioinguinal and external spermatic nerves, and lymphatic drainage is to the superficial and deep inguinal nodes. The scrotum is formed in the male by the fusion of the genital swellings that form the labia majora in the female.

Spermatic Cord

The spermatic cord, which suspends the testicle, is a fascial-covered structure that contains spermatic arteries and veins, the pampiniform plexus, lymph channels, the autonomic supply to the testicle, and the cremasteric muscle. The contractions of the cremasteric muscle change the position of the testis for temperature regulation. It is important that the temperature of the testis be maintained lower than that of the rest of the body for optimal spermatogenesis.

Testis

The testes are paired glands located in the scrotum and covered by the tunica albuginea. At the upper pole of the testis is a small pedunculated body, the appendix testis. The tunica vaginalis is a sheath that invests the testes and epididymis. The arterial supply to the testis is provided by the internal spermatic, deferential, and external spermatic arteries. The veins from the testis and epididymis form the pampiniform plexus in the spermatic cord, which then becomes the internal spermatic vein. The right spermatic vein empties into the vena cava; the left spermatic vein empties into the left renal vein. The lymph node drainage from the testes is to the retroperitoneum and to mediastinal and supraclavicular lymph nodes. The testis is composed histologically of a number of seminiferous tubules containing spermatogenic and Sertoli cells with a surrounding connective tissue stroma containing Leydig cells. The undifferentiated gonad starts to develop into a testis at about the seventh week of gestation. As the mesonephric duct develops, the müllerian duct regresses under the influence of müllerian inhibitory factor. The mesonephric duct differentiates into the male ductal system forming the epididymis, vas deferens, seminal vesicles, and ejaculatory duct. The testis progressively descends until it is in the scrotum at birth.

Epididymis

The epididymis is a coiled duct that lies posterolateral to the testis and consists of an upper portion, the globus major, and a lower portion, the globus minor. The globus major is connected with the testis by efferent ducts from the testis and is the site of the appendix epididymis. The arterial supply to the epididymis is provided by the internal spermatic artery and the deferential artery. The epididymal veins drain into the pampiniform plexus. The lymphatic drainage of the epididymis is to the external iliac and hypogastric nodes. Sperm passes into the epididymis through the efferent ducts from the rete testis and then through the vas deferens into the ampulla. In addition to providing a pathway for the spermatozoa, the epididymis also contributes to the maturation of the spermatozoa during transit. Damage to the epididymis from inflammation or trauma can lead to fertility problems.

EVALUATION

In the genitourinary evaluation,[17, 20, 23] it is important to ascertain whether the patient has had previous genitourinary surgery or has any history of congenital abnormalities. General features in the history such as weight loss, malaise, and fever should be sought, as an occult genitourinary malignancy can initially manifest itself as weight loss or malaise. Disorders such as prostatitis, pyelonephritis, or hydronephrosis secondary to a kidney stone or tumor may present with fever or pain. Since many genitourinary abnormalities manifest themselves as abnormalities in voiding, careful questioning about patterns, frequency, and character and control of voiding is essential.

Pain

Pain from the kidney is usually noted as a dull ache in the flank or lumbar area and is usually a late finding in a neoplasm involving the kidney. If a renal tumor or infection is extensive and involves the diaphragm, pain can be referred to the shoulder. Pain from the ureter is most commonly secondary to acute obstruction such as from a stone or blood clot; chronic obstruction and hydronephrosis may be totally asymptomatic. An acutely obstructing stone in the upper ureter is likely to cause pain in the flank or abdomen, and as the stone moves down the ureter, the pain moves progressively toward the groin. Pain from the bladder is most commonly due to either cystitis or acute outlet obstruction. When the bladder outflow tract is acutely obstructed, the bladder contracts in an attempt to empty itself and this may cause pain. A neoplasm in the bladder rarely causes pain until it is in a far advanced stage.

Pain in the scrotum may represent referred pain from the ureter, or it may be due to an abnormality of the epididymis or testis. Primary scrotal pain may be due to epididymitis, orchitis, or testicular torsion. A rapidly growing or necrotic testicular tumor may be painful; however, most testicular tumors do not present with pain. Chronic prostatitis can cause a dull ache in the perineum or lower back; acute prostatitis generally presents as pain in the perineum associated with fever. Prostatic carcinoma rarely presents with pain until it is quite advanced.

Abnormalities in Voiding

Hesitancy. Hesitancy refers to difficulty starting the urinary stream. This most commonly is due to outlet obstruction from an abnormality such as prostatic enlargement or urethral stricture. However, it can also be secondary to neurogenic bladder dysfunction.

Decreased Caliber. Decreased caliber and force of urinary stream are symptoms commonly associated with bladder outlet obstruction. This may be secondary to a benign or malignant enlargement of the prostate gland, a urethral stricture, or a neoplastic process involving the urethra.

Frequency. Frequency means that the patient voids more often than usual. This may be due to bladder irritation secondary to an infection or other inflammatory process, or it may be due to an unstable or chronically distended, poorly emptying bladder.

Urgency. Urgency signifies an abnormal urge to void and is generally associated with a bladder that is contracting inappropriately. Urgency may be secondary to inflammation or to another pathologic condition that results in bladder instability.

Nocturia. Nocturia indicates that the patient voids an unusual number of times during the night and may be a sign of an unstable bladder in which the normal nocturnal inhibition of the voiding sensation is no longer present. Nocturia, frequency, and urgency are symptoms of bladder instability.

Dysuria. Dysuria refers to painful voiding and is commonly secondary to a urinary tract infection. A nonbacterial inflammation, a stone, or a tumor can also cause dysuria.

Enuresis. Enuresis is the involuntary passage of urine at night or while asleep. Enuresis is normal up to a certain age, although if it is persistent it can be secondary to a congenital anatomic abnormality or neurologic dysfunction.

Polyuria. Polyuria is the voiding of an excessively large volume of urine. This is most commonly secondary to a primary renal disorder such as an abnormality in the urinary concentrating mechanism.

Incontinence. An incontinent patient is one who has an inability to prevent involuntary passage of urine. *Stress incontinence* refers to exertional leaking of urine as a result of coughing, sneezing, or other straining. *Urge incontinence* refers to leaking of urine associated with an uncontrollable urge to void and is usually a sign of an unstable bladder.

Pyuria. Pyuria signifies the presence of white blood cells in urine and often is associated with a urinary tract infection.

Pneumaturia. Pneumaturia means the passage of gas in the urine. This can be secondary to an infection by a gas-forming organism in the genitourinary system, although it most commonly indicates the presence of a urinary-enteric fistula.

Hematuria. Hematuria is a term used to signify the presence of blood in the urine. With gross hematuria, blood present in the urine is plainly visible; with microscopic hematuria, the presence of blood cells is detected by use of a microscope. In unexplained cases of either microscopic or gross hematuria, a thorough examination is required. A patient who is receiving chemotherapeutic agents or anticoagulants can also still have a bladder tumor, kidney tumor, or other abnormality as a cause of the hematuria, and these possibilities need to be ruled out.

Physical Examination

A thorough physical examination is an integral part of the evaluation of a patient with a genitourinary abnormality. Palpation in the right or left upper quadrants and flank may elicit tenderness in the renal fossa. An abdominal examination may reveal a retroperitoneal mass or distended bladder. Palpation of the scrotum is performed to detect abnormalities of the spermatic cord, epididymis, or testis. A thorough examination of each testis and epididymis should be performed for detection of a mass lesion or abnormalities in testicular size or location. In the penile examination, the foreskin should be retracted and the meatus inspected for position and for the presence of discharge or inflammation. The prostatic examination includes palpation of the prostate as well as examination of

the periprostatic tissue and rectal sphincter. Any abnormal prostate nodule found on examination should be evaluated further. Seminal vesicles are normally not palpable. However, seminal vesicles that are invaded by prostatic carcinoma may be hard, whereas seminal vesicles that are inflamed are usually nodular.

Radiographic Evaluation

PLAIN FILM

The plain film demonstrates bony abnormalities, calcifications, and abnormal fat or gas densities. A calcification on the plain film may indicate the presence of a urinary tract stone, or it may represent a calcification in the substance of the adrenal gland, kidney, collecting system, bladder, or an adjacent lymph node. Gallbladder stones can also mimic kidney stones on a plain film, and an intravenous pyelogram is often required to delineate the exact location of the opacity.

INTRAVENOUS PYELOGRAM

The intravenous pyelogram is a radiologic study in which sequential films are taken as the kidneys concentrate and excrete an intravenously injected contrast dye. This study provides anatomic information about the renal parenchyma, pelvis, ureter, and bladder and can provide information about renal function (Fig. 4). The initial phase, in which dye circulates into the kidney, is known as the *nephrogram phase*. Renal parenchymal abnormalities such as glomerulonephritis and pyelonephritis often produce an abnormal nephrogram phase on the intravenous pyelogram, and renovascular abnormalities, such as renal artery stenosis, may also be detected.

Following the nephrogram phase of the intravenous pyelogram, the collecting system is visualized as dye is excreted. This portion of the study may reveal filling defects, such as might be caused by a stone or tumor in the renal pelvis. Congenital abnormalities, such as ureteropelvic junction stenosis or a duplicated collecting system, may be identified. Finally, the cystogram phase should be examined for the presence of bladder trabeculation (hypertrophy of the muscular wall of the bladder) or diverticula (abnormal outpouchings of the bladder wall). Intravenous contrast dye can be toxic to the kidney, particularly when the kidney is involved with a disease process such as diabetes or multiple myeloma. Therefore, the indications for performing the study should always be clear, and good hydration prior to the study should be ensured in patients who are at particular risk.

CYSTOGRAM

A cystogram is performed by placing a catheter in the bladder and filling the bladder with contrast media. The cystogram provides information about bladder anatomy and the absence or presence of vesical masses, diverticula, or ureterovesical reflux.

RETROGRADE PYELOGRAM

Dye is injected into a catheter that is placed endoscopically in the ureter. This procedure is very useful in delineating upper tract anatomy when the intravenous pyelogram does not provide sufficient anatomic information, when there is a nonfunctioning kidney, or when it is not possible

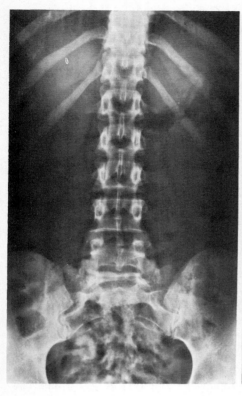
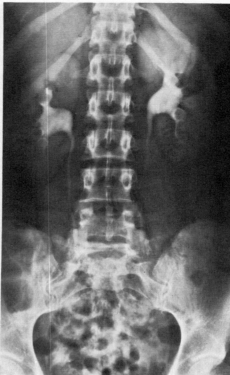

Figure 4. The plain film from the intravenous pyelogram (left) shows the renal outlines, psoas shadows, and bony structures. The film taken 5 minutes after contrast injection (right) shows the renal outline, collecting system, and upper ureters.

to perform intravenous pyelogram because of renal insufficiency, obstruction, or dye allergy.

RETROGRADE URETHROGRAM

Retrograde urethrography is performed by injecting contrast media into the urethra and obtaining a lateral x-ray of the urethra. This test provides information about the extent and location of strictures, diverticula, stones, or neoplastic disease (Fig. 5).

ULTRASOUND

Ultrasound, a noninvasive procedure that depends on differences in tissue echogenicity, has gained widespread use in the evaluation of genitourinary abnormalities. Renal ultrasound is particularly helpful in differentiating cystic from neoplastic lesions, and it may also be useful in the detection of hydronephrosis. Scrotal ultrasound is very accurate in differentiating lesions of the epididymis from those in the testis, and in detecting masses within the testis. Recently, transrectal ultrasound has been used for detection of prostatic tumors, and both transabdominal and transurethral ultrasound are currently being evaluated for staging bladder tumors.

COMPUTED TOMOGRAPHY

Computed tomography (CT) scans have become an integral part of the urologic evaluation of many genitourinary abnormalities. The CT scan is very accurate in the differentiation of cystic from solid renal masses and in some

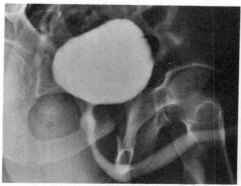
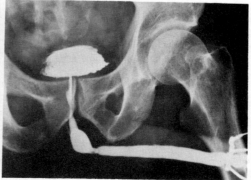

Figure 5. The voiding cystourethrogram on the left shows an oblique view of a normal urethra and bladder contrast study. The retrograde urethrogram on the right was performed on a patient with a bulbar stricture and demonstrates both the stricture and reflux in Cowper's glands.

instances has replaced the arteriogram. The CT scan is commonly used for preoperative evaluation and staging of patients with testicular and renal carcinoma and for surveillance after treatment. The CT scan has also been used in the evaluation of prostate and bladder lesions, but this technique has not yet gained widespread use.

ARTERIOGRAPHY

The renal arteriogram is the standard means of evaluating renal parenchymal mass lesions; it accurately defines the arterial supply of the renal lesion and that of the rest of the kidney. It is also used to obtain precise anatomic characterization of renal arterial lesions.

THE KIDNEY [2, 16, 17, 17a, 22, 24, 25]

Anomalies

Renal agenesis, the total absence of a kidney, can be unilateral or bilateral. Unilateral agenesis is usually accompanied by compensatory hypertrophy of the contralateral kidney.

In *renal aplasia*, nephrogenic tissue is present but fails to develop. This is generally due to either inadequate stimulation of the metanephros, a ureteral bud of poor quality, or inadequate vascularity of the metanephrogenic blastema.

In *renal hypoplasia*. the kidney is normal but small, and there is usually a poorly developed ureter and trigone. A hypoplastic kidney is generally not able to undergo hypertrophy if the opposite kidney is damaged or removed.

A kidney that is not in its normal position is termed an *ectopic kidney*. The ectopic kidney is usually malrotated and may even be on the side with the other kidney, in which case it is termed *crossed renal ectopia*. An ectopic kidney results from persistence of early embryonic vasculature, which prevents normal ascent of the kidney during development. Simple ectopia is found to be present in 1 of 800 patients and is three times more common on the left. Eight-five per cent of the time when there is crossed renal ectopia, there will also be fusion with the other kidney. The most common type of fusion anomaly is the *horseshoe kidney*, in which the lower poles of the kidneys are fused. A horseshoe kidney may be asymptomatic, or there may be renal pelvic obstruction and stone formation.

Renal Abnormalities

A wide range of renal abnormalities can be detected with currently available diagnostic techniques such as intravenous pyelogram, ultrasound, or CT scan. It is often difficult to differentiate initially a benign from a malignant lesion. A partial list of abnormalities that may be encountered includes renal cyst, polycystic kidney, renal dysgenesis, medullary cystic disease, renal adenoma, angiomyolipoma, xanthogranulomatous pyelonephritis, renal or perinephric abscess, and hypernephroma. In children, the differential of renal mass lesions include multicystic kidney, hydronephrosis, renal vein thrombosis, Wilms' tumor, and multilocular cystic nephroma.

SIMPLE RENAL CYST

Renal cysts are lesions predominantly seen in adults; they may vary in size and may be multiple or bilateral. Use of a renal ultrasound study or abdominal CT scan can often differentiate a benign renal cyst from a neoplastic lesion, although an arteriogram may be required. If it is not certain that an abnormality is benign, a cyst puncture plus a renal cystogram (an x-ray of the dye-filled cyst) may be performed. The cyst fluid is examined for presence of blood and/or abnormal cytology. In equivocal cases, exploration of the kidney with visual inspection of the lesion and removal of the cyst wall for histologic analysis may be the only way to make the definitive diagnosis.

POLYCYSTIC KIDNEY DISEASE

Adult polycystic kidney disease is an autosomal dominant disease in which there are multiple cysts of varying sizes in both the renal medulla and cortex. It generally manifests itself in the third or fourth decade, but there is usually normal renal function until late in life, at which time dialysis or renal transplantation may be required. These patients commonly have cysts in other areas such as the liver, and up to 15 per cent have cerebral aneurysms. *Infantile polycystic renal disease* is an autosomal recessive disease that presents typically as bilateral flank masses with multiple renal cortical and medullary cysts. The diagnosis can be established by ultrasound or by intravenous pyelogram.

ANGIOMYOLIPOMA

Angiomyolipoma is a benign renal tumor that is often mistaken for a malignant lesion. Histologically, this tumor contains vascular and muscle elements and fat cells. This tumor is generally considered benign, though metastases to regional lymph nodes have been documented. The standard treatment for an angiomyolipoma is nephrectomy.

MEDULLARY CYSTIC DISEASE

Medullary cystic disease can be an isolated occurrence or part of an autosomal dominant disorder. Medullary cystic disease does not often necessitate surgical management and, although small renal stones may form, this disorder is consistent with a normal life span.

MULTICYSTIC KIDNEY

Multicystic kidney is a nonhereditary, developmental anomaly in which there are ten to 20 variable-sized renal cysts that do not communicate with the collecting system. A small renal pelvis is usually present. This disorder typically presents as a unilateral mass in a neonate and is diagnosed by ultrasound.

URETEROPELVIC JUNCTION OBSTRUCTION

Idiopathic ureteropelvic junction obstruction is the most common cause of congenital hydronephrosis. Intravenous pyelography typically shows delayed function and a dilated collecting system. Retrograde pyelography will often show an abnormally high insertion of the ureter on the renal pelvis. A pyeloplasty is performed to repair the stenotic ureteropelvic junction and to resect a portion of the redundant pelvis.

XANTHOGRANULOMATOUS PYELONEPHRITIS

Xanthogranulomatous pyelonephritis is an uncommon lesion of the kidney that is generally seen in association with diabetes mellitus, chronic renal stones, or obstruction.

Pyelography often reveals a nonfunctioning kidney with stones, pyonephrosis, or renal abscess. The standard treatment for this lesion is nephrectomy.

Perinephric Abscess

A perinephric abscess may result from pyelonephritis or from the rupture of a renal abscess, or it can be secondary to hematogenous spread of infection from another part of the body. Perinephric abscess is often seen in patients with chronic urinary tract infection or diabetes mellitus. Patients commonly present with fever, abdominal or flank pain, and tenderness in the flank. The arteriogram is not usually of benefit, but ultrasound can be very helpful in leading to a diagnosis. Treatment often consists simply of an incision and drainage, although at times a nephrectomy is required.

Malignant Lesions

Since the first planned nephrectomy for renal carcinoma was performed by Grawitz in 1883, *renal carcinoma* has continued to be a difficult problem for the clinician. This tumor, which is thought to originate in the proximal renal tubule, occurs in 15,000 patients in the United States each year and accounts for 6000 deaths annually. Renal carcinoma is predominantly a disease of adults, although it has been reported in patients as young as 6 months of age. This disease often presents in an advanced stage as a result of the fact that the kidneys are located in the retroperitoneum and the malignancy can progress undetected. There is a male:female ratio of 2:1, which is thought to be due to greater exposure to environmental toxins among men. Although the etiology of kidney carcinoma in humans is not clearly defined, there is an association with cigarette and pipe smoking. In adult hamsters treated with diethylstilbestrol (DES), renal tumors have been found to develop but no hormonal mechanism for tumorigenesis has been identified in man. Renal carcinoma has been found in association with von Hippel–Lindau disease and polycystic kidney disease. Histologically, the tumor is most often composed of clear or granular cells arranged in a tubular, papillary, or solid pattern. Hemorrhage, necrosis, and calcification are common, particularly in large tumors.

The most common symptom associated with hypernephroma is hematuria, which occurs in two thirds of patients and is often painless. The classic triad of pain, hematuria, and flank mass is usually encountered only in advanced cases. The patient may complain only of a dull ache or fever. The presence of a nonfunctional kidney on intravenous pyelogram in a patient with flank pain and fever should be considered carcinoma until proven otherwise. Four per cent of hypernephromas are associated with erythrocytosis, although the patient may present with anemia if the disease is advanced. Hypercalcemia has been found in patients with metastatic hypernephroma and is thought to be secondary to the production of a parathyroid hormone–like factor that stimulates bone resorption. Hepatic dysfunction in the absence of liver metastasis can be associated with hypernephroma and resolves once the tumor is removed.

The clinical course of patients with kidney carcinoma can be extremely variable. The disease may not progress for years, and there have been a few cases of spontaneous regression reported. Most patients with metastatic disease, however, experience a progressive downhill course. Survival is generally dependent on extent of disease at time of presentation. The 5-year survival for patients who present with Stage I renal carcinoma (tumor confined within the kidney capsule) is 70 per cent, with Stage II (invasion of perirenal fat) 50 to 60 per cent, with Stage III (local spread to renal vein, vena cava or lymph nodes) 30 to 50 per cent, and with Stage IV (metastatic tumor) 0 to 10 per cent. Renal vein involvement does not have a significant negative impact on survival, but lymph node or other adjacent organ involvement is associated with markedly decreased survival.

The intravenous pyelogram of a patient with hypernephroma usually shows a mass lesion, and there may be splaying of the calyces or displacement of the kidney. Computed tomography of the kidney will often reveal a mass lesion (Fig. 6) with density similar to that of renal parenchyma but that only takes up a small amount of renal contrast media. Arteriography typically demonstrates neovascularity and pooling of contrast dye within the tumor. An inferior vena cavagram is usually performed with the arteriogram and provides information about involvement of the vena cava.

The standard treatment for localized renal carcinoma is radical nephrectomy, which is the removal of the kidney plus Gerota's fascia. There is no convincing evidence favoring the routine use of a regional lymphadenectomy with radical nephrectomy, although most surgeons remove suspicious nodes at the time of nephrectomy. For patients in whom a tumor occurs in a solitary kidney, partial nephrectomy may be used in selected cases. A transabdominal, flank, or thoracoabdominal incision can be used for the removal of renal tumor, depending on the size and location of the tumor. It is important that the surgeon choose the approach that will enable safe removal of the tumor while maintaining control of the vascular supply. A tumor thrombus in the vena cava can most often be successfully removed with resulting low morbidity. If the vena cava is invaded by tumor, resection of a portion of the vena cava may be required.

Systemic chemotherapy for the treatment of metastatic renal carcinoma has met with only limited success. The response rate to different chemotherapeutic regimens is 15 to 35 per cent, and long-term survival is uncommon. This tumor is most often radioresistant, and at the present time most reserve radiotherapy for persistent disease after nephrectomy or for symptomatic osseous metastases.

A new approach to the therapy of cancer has been developed that is based on the adoptive transfer of autologous lymphokine-activated killer cells and recombinant interleukin-2. This therapy has been shown to be associated with objective regression of a number of different types of cancer, including renal carcinoma, and clinical trials are currently under way to evaluate its effectiveness.

Metastatic tumors to the kidney are twice as common as primary renal neoplasms; they tend to be bilateral and are infrequently removed surgically. The most common tumors to metastasize to the kidney are lung, breast, and stomach carcinoma. It is also not uncommon for a tumor to metastasize from one kidney to another.

Wilms' Tumor

Wilms' tumor, or *nephroblastoma*, is the most common solid mass seen in children. The peak incidence is during the second year of life and 75 per cent present before the age of 5. These patients present with hypertension, abdominal pain, or gross hematuria, and in 60 per cent there are palpable masses. The histologic characteristics include spindle cell elements and poorly differentiated skeletal, smooth muscle, and epithelial components. The combined use of

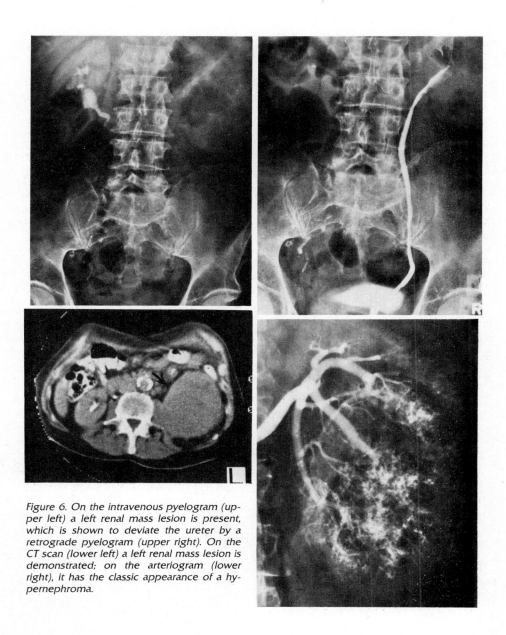

Figure 6. On the intravenous pyelogram (upper left) a left renal mass lesion is present, which is shown to deviate the ureter by a retrograde pyelogram (upper right). On the CT scan (lower left) a left renal mass lesion is demonstrated; on the arteriogram (lower right), it has the classic appearance of a hypernephroma.

surgery, radiation therapy, and chemotherapy has greatly increased the survival rate in children with Wilms' tumor.

Renovascular Disorders[8, 10, 23]

Five to 15 per cent of the hypertensive population in the United States has renovascular disease. With an increased understanding of the renin-angiotensin axis and improved medical, surgical, and radiographic techniques, there have been great advances in the diagnosis and treatment of this disease.

Atherosclerosis and *fibrous dysplasia* account for approximately 90 per cent of renal artery lesions. Atherosclerotic lesions tend to occur in the proximal third of the renal artery, are bilateral in approximately a third of patients, and affect men more often than women. Fibrous dysplasia produces lesions of greater length that are often multiple and bilateral. It affects females more often than males by a ratio of 4:1. Renin, which plays a role in the initiation of renovascular hypertension, is a proteolytic enzyme secreted by the kidney from the juxtaglomerular apparatus. Renin acts on renin substrate to form angiotensin I. Angiotensin I is metabolized by converting enzyme in the lung and kidney to angiotensin II, a potent vasoconstrictor that stimulates aldosterone secretion.

A number of diagnostic tests and anatomic studies are used in the assessment of a patient with suspected renovascular hypertension. The rapid-sequence intravenous pyelogram provides information about perfusion, renal function, and relative kidney size, but alone it cannot reliably exclude the diagnosis of renovascular hypertension. The radioactive renogram is a useful noninvasive test that, along with the intravenous pyelogram, may identify patients who would benefit from more sophisticated evaluation. Renal arteriography is the most accurate method for anatomic localization of renal artery lesions. Peripheral and selective renal vein renin determinations, renal function tests, and pharmacologic angiotensin blocking tests are used to determine whether the hypertension is due to a specific renal lesion.

When it has been established that the hypertension is due to a renal artery lesion, a number of surgical options are available. Renal artery endarterectomy, bypass with a synthetic graft or portion of saphenous vein, splenorenal shunt, and patch angioplasty are among the surgical procedures employed. The recently developed technique of percutaneous transluminal balloon angioplasty has gained widespread use and may become the treatment of choice for uncomplicated cases of renal artery stenosis. The choice of surgical procedure depends on the extent and location of the lesion and the preference of the surgeon.

Urinary Tract Calculi[7, 20]

A stone within the genitourinary tract can be due to a number of causes. Stone formation may be secondary to a primary metabolic disorder or to an obstruction causing urinary stasis and infection, or it can be idiopathic. Urinary tract calculi are most commonly composed of calcium oxalate, calcium oxalate plus hydroxyapatite, or magnesium ammonium phosphate (struvite). Uric acid or cystine stones are encountered less frequently. When recurrent urinary tract stones form, a metabolic evaluation is indicated. It is also important to identify whether there is a predisposing condition that might lead to stone formation, such as a history of gout, urinary tract infection, immobilization,

recent trauma, bowel or bone disease, hyperthyroidism, hyperparathyroidism, or malignancy. Initial laboratory assessment includes a determination of serum electrolytes, calcium, uric acid, and phosphorus as well as 24-hour urine calcium, uric acid, and oxalate excretion. If the patient is found to have hypercalciuria, a calcium load test may be used to differentiate absorptive, resorptive, or primary renal-leak hypercalciuria.

Urinary tract stones can occur in the pelvis of the kidney, in the ureter, in the bladder, or in the urethra. With the introduction of percutaneous ultrasonic lithotripsy, ureteroscopy, ureteroscopic ultrasonic lithotripsy, and extracorporeal shock wave lithotripsy, the indications for open surgical removal of calculi are changing. Stones that present in the pelvis of the kidney may be removed by pyelolithotomy. If the stone in the pelvis fills the entire collecting system, it is known as a *staghorn calculus* (Fig. 7); the standard method of removal has been an anatrophic nephrolithotomy, performed through an extended incision through the lateral aspect of the parenchyma of the kidney. Stones that originate in the kidney and travel down the ureter are most likely to lodge at one of three locations: at the ureteropelvic junction, at the point where the ureter crosses the iliac vessels, or at the ureterovesical junction. Eighty per cent of the stones that reach the ureter pass spontaneously. A small stone that lodges in the lower third of the ureter may often be removed endoscopically. Stones that are greater than 1 cm. in size usually will have lodged higher and need to be removed surgically. Ureteral stones that are too large or too high to be removed by basket extraction may be removed with a flank or lower abdominal incision. Primary vesical stones are rare in the United States, but are not uncommon in the Middle East and Africa. In the United States, vesical stones are usually secondary to bladder outlet obstruction with infection of residual urine. Small vesical stones can often be removed transurethrally, but larger stones necessitate a transvesical approach.

Recently, a number of techniques have been introduced that have revolutionized the surgical management of

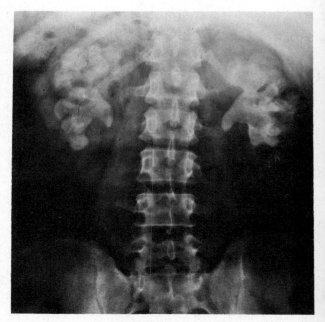

Figure 7. Large bilateral staghorn calculi completely outline the calyceal system and the pelvis of each kidney.

urolithiasis. In one technique, a small *nephrostomy catheter* is placed in the kidney percutaneously with the aid of fluoroscopic guidance. This percutaneous nephrostomy allows the endourologic removal of small stones with grasping forceps without the need for the standard surgical approach. Percutaneous or endoscopic ultrasonic *lithotripsy* causes the renal or ureteral stones to break into fine granules, which are then evacuated by suction. Therefore, urinary tract calculi may be extracted percutaneously or endoscopically with the aid of the ultrasonic lithotriptor without the need for an open surgical procedure. Another recent innovation has been the introduction of nonsurgical treatment of renal calculi by extracorporeal *shock wave* lithotripsy. By this method a patient under anesthesia is placed in a tub of water and under radiographic control a low-energy shock wave is applied that breaks the stone into small fragments, which are passed spontaneously. At present, the indications for extracorporeal shock wave lithotripsy are being greatly expanded, and this technology will probably almost completely replace the surgical removal of urinary tract calculi.

Tumors of the Renal Pelvis and Ureter

Tumors can occur in the renal collecting system, pelvis, or ureter either in association with tumors of the bladder or as isolated events.[13, 23, 25] There are a number of categories of patients who are at high risk for upper tract neoplasms. *Balkan nephropathy* is a disease of obscure etiology associated with a high rate of tumors of the renal pelvis and ureter. The abuse of phenacetin, an aniline derivative, has been reported to be associated with papillary necrosis, obstruction, and infection, and there is a very high rate of both bladder and renal pelvic cancer in these persons.

In 75 per cent of patients with renal pelvic tumors, hematuria develops. The tumors usually appear late in life, tend to be painless, and are most often transitional cell carcinomas. Physical examination is usually normal until late in the course of the disease. These tumors may invade locally into nodes or adjacent organs or metastasize to liver, lungs, or brain. The intravenous pyelogram may outline a filling defect in the collecting system, although a radiolucent stone or blood clot can be mistaken for a tumor. A tumor in the ureter classically causes a dilation of the ureter below the expanding lesion. There may also be a hydroureter above the tumor if the obstruction is complete. A retrograde pyelogram is often helpful in delineating the abnormality, and urinary cytology and a brush biopsy should be obtained. It is important, when a renal mass lesion is being evaluated, to consider the possibility of a neoplasm originating in the collecting system.

The standard treatment for a high-grade tumor in the renal pelvis or ureter is total nephroureterectomy with the removal of a small cuff of bladder. The distal ureter and bladder cuff are removed because there is a high rate of occurrence in the ureteral stump when it is not removed. In well-selected patients with a localized, low-grade tumor of the ureter or renal pelvis, a segmental resection may be performed.

THE BLADDER

Anomalies of the Bladder and Ureter[17, 20]

A ureter that enters the bladder in an area other than the trigone is termed *ectopic*. The ureter may enter anywhere in the bladder, vesical neck, prostatic urethra, sem-

inal vesicle, or vas deferens. In the female, the ureter may enter the vagina, cervix, uterus, or rectum. Eighty per cent of ectopic ureters are associated with a duplicated collecting system. In this case, the ureter from the upper collecting system is most often associated with an ectopic insertion of the ureter. A *ureterocele* is a cystic dilation of the distal portion of the ureter and may be diagnosed by intravenous pyelogram or cystogram. Ureteroceles are commonly associated with duplicated collecting systems and often become obstructed.

Vesicoureteral reflux is a congenital condition caused by a malformation of the ureterovesical junction in which there is lack of a sufficient intramural tunnel to provide the normal antireflux mechanism. Reflux may be mild or severe, and is commonly associated with ureteral ectopia. The diagnosis of reflux is made on cystogram. The treatment is reimplantation of the ureter into the bladder, for which there are a number of techniques available.

Persistence of the *urachus*, which is the canal in the fetus connecting the bladder with the umbilical cord, is one of the more common abnormalities of bladder development. This abnormality can manifest itself as a small diverticulum in the dome of the bladder or as a completely patent urachus.

Bladder abnormalities such as agenesis, hypoplasia, duplication, and *exstrophy* are rare. Exstrophy is a severe congenital malformation that occurs in 1 of 40,000 births and results from a failure of the mesoderm structures of the abdominal wall to develop. Exstrophy can present as *epispadias*, the failure of closure of the dorsal aspect of the urethra, to complete exstrophy with pubic separation and a persistent cloaca. Surgery to correct the exstrophy and achieve urinary continence has recently achieved marked success.

Bladder Neoplasms[9, 14, 15, 17, 20, 23]

There are 22,000 new cases of bladder carcinoma with 9800 deaths per year in the United States. The incidence of bladder carcinoma in males is five times greater than it is in females. Bladder carcinoma tends to be a disease seen in older age groups and is the fifth leading cause of deaths in males 75 years of age and older. There is an increased incidence of this disease among dye workers, nurses, tailors, hairdressers, leather workers, tire workers, and cigarette smokers. The risk of carcinoma of the bladder increases in highly industrialized areas; men who live in urban communities have a 50 to 75 per cent greater risk of developing bladder carcinoma than do men in rural areas. There have been some studies suggestive of an association between sugar substitutes and bladder cancer, but a definite relationship has not been convincingly demonstrated. With exposure to medications such as phenacetin and cyclophosphamide, there is an increased incidence of bladder carcinoma, as there is in patients who have bladder outlet obstruction, neurogenic bladder, and chronic urinary tract infections.

GRADE AND STAGE OF TUMOR

Both the grade and stage of the bladder tumor are important for planning appropriate treatment (Fig. 8). Bladder tumors are graded from 1 to 3, with *Grade 1* tumors having a well-differentiated, a five- to seven-cell mucosal layer with minimal variation in size and shape of the nuclei. *Grade 2* tumors show less differentiation with nuclei that are hyperchromatic and variable in size and shape. *Grade 3* tumors are characterized by marked ana-

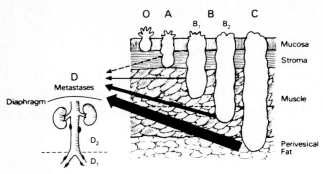

Figure 8. The staging of bladder cancer. (From Skinner, D. G.: Cancer Res., 37:2838, 1977.)

plasia, extreme variation in size and staining of the cells, and numerous mitotic figures.

The importance of the stage of bladder cancer on treatment and prognosis was first recognized by Jewitt and Strong. The currently used Jewitt-Marshall classification divides bladder tumors into five categories:

(1) *Stage 0* represents a mucosal papillary tumor; (2) *Stage A* tumor has invaded the lamina propria; (3) *Stage B* signifies that the tumor has invaded either the superficial (*B1*) or deep (*B2*) muscle; (4) a *Stage C* tumor has extended beyond the muscle into the perivesical fat; and (5) a *Stage D* tumor is metastatic.

CELL TYPE

Ninety per cent of bladder tumors are transitional cell carcinomas, 7 per cent are squamous cell type, 2 per cent are adenocarcinoma, and 1 per cent are undifferentiated. Squamous cell carcinoma of the bladder is often related to long-standing infection or inflammation. The patient may have a history of urinary tract infection, bladder calculi, or an indwelling catheter. These radioresistant tumors are associated with a very poor prognosis, and there is only a 20 to 30 per cent 1-year survival rate. Squamous cell carcinoma is very common among patients with *Schistosoma haematobium.* In Africa and the Middle East, where schistosomiasis is prevalent, squamous cell carcinoma accounts for 90 per cent of bladder tumors. The squamous cell carcinoma associated with schistosomiasis is a relatively unaggressive tumor with a much better prognosis. Adenocarcinoma may be urachal or non-urachal in origin and is seen in a high percentage of patients with exstrophy. Chronic infection may lead to the development of cystitis glandularis followed by overt adenocarcinoma. Adenocarcinoma is an aggressive lesion in which early invasion and metastases are common.

CLINICAL FINDINGS

The most common clinical symptom associated with bladder carcinoma is hematuria. The hematuria may be profuse or mild, continuous, or intermittent. The patient can present with flank pain from hydronephrosis if a ureter is obstructed or with weight loss and malaise with metastatic disease. Physical examination findings are most often normal when the tumor is small or confined to the bladder. Laboratory evaluation includes urinalysis and urine cytology, blood count, blood urea nitrogen, and creatinine. The blood count may reveal anemia in a patient with chronic blood loss; renal function studies usually are normal unless the tumor has caused significant renal obstruction.

STAGING

The clinical staging of a patient with a known or suspected bladder carcinoma includes an intravenous pyelogram, cystourethroscopy, and an examination under anesthesia. Cystourethroscopy provides information about the position of the tumor and helps determine whether it is localized or multicentric. A biopsy is performed of the tumor and its base in order to assess the extent of muscle invasion. Biopsies are also performed in other areas of the bladder in order to identify unsuspected tumor or carcinoma *in situ.*

TREATMENT

A low-grade and superficial tumor is treated by endoscopic resection (Fig. 9) followed by instillation of intravesical chemotherapy such as thiotepa, mitomycin, or Adriamycin up to 1 year. Intravesical chemotherapeutic agents have a response rate of 45 to 85 per cent and have been shown to decrease the rate of tumor recurrence and progression. Bacillus Calmette-Guérin (BCG) has been used as an intravesical agent in the treatment of superficial tumors. The early results suggest that BCG may be an effective agent for preventing tumor recurrence, but its effectiveness relative to the more commonly used chemotherapeutic agents will not be completely defined until larger comparative trials are completed. Patients treated for superficial bladder carcinoma are followed closely for recurrence or progression. This involves cystourethroscopy and urine cytologic studies every 3 months for up to 2 years followed by repeat examinations at less frequent intervals.

Radical cystectomy is the standard treatment of invasive bladder carcinoma. This procedure includes removal of the pelvic lymph nodes, and, in the male, the prostate and seminal vesicles. In the female, the ovaries and uterus are generally removed along with a small anterior cuff of vagina. Many surgeons routinely remove the urethra in the male, while others perform a urethrectomy only if there is carcinoma *in situ* present or tumor involvement of the bladder neck or prostatic urethra. The most common type

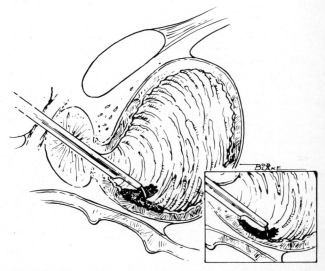

Figure 9. In the transurethral removal of a bladder tumor, the initial superficial resection is followed by a deeper cut to make certain that a portion of the bladder wall is removed so that the depth of invasion by tumor can be properly assessed. (From Benson, M., and Olsson, C. A.: In Paulson, D. F. (Ed.): Genitourinary Surgery. New York, Churchill Livingstone, 1984.).

of urinary diversion following cystectomy is the *Bricker ileal conduit*. In this procedure, the ureters are attached to a segment of distal ileum that is isolated from the intestinal tract and brought out through the abdominal wall. This isolated segment of ileum forms a reservoir for urine and a conduit for its elimination. A reanastomosis is performed in the intestinal tract so that intestinal function remains essentially normal. Perioperative complications of this procedure include anastomotic leak and anuria; later complications include reflux, renal insufficiency, and ureteroileal anastomotic stenosis. Ureterojejunal cutaneous diversion may be considered for those patients in whom the ileum is not suitable because of disease or radiation damage. The technique for constructing a jejunal conduit is essentially the same as for an ileal conduit. In these patients there is a tendency to develop hypochloremic acidosis and azotemia, and this procedure is contraindicated in patients with renal insufficiency or hypertension. In a ureterosigmoidostomy, the most common type of urinary diversion prior to 1950, the ureters are anastomosed to the lower sigmoid colon. This procedure is less satisfactory than the standard ileal conduit because of problems with incontinence and the fact that pyelonephritis, ureteral obstruction, calculi, or electrolyte imbalance often develops in these patients. Some degree of hypokalemic, hyperchloremic metabolic acidosis occurs in about half of the patients undergoing this procedure.

A recent innovation in urinary diversion has been the introduction of the *Kock pouch*, in which a pouch of approximately 80 cm. of ileum is made into a continent, nonrefluxing reservoir. This procedure has the advantage of allowing patients to empty the reservoir with a catheter four to six times per day. An abdominal urinary collection device is not required and the abdominal stoma is small and necessitates only a bandage for cover. Although experience with this innovative procedure is limited at the present time, it holds promise for providing patients greater convenience and an improved self-image.

Many surgeons use external beam radiotherapy in the preoperative period before cystectomy. Radiotherapy may prevent seeding from tumor spillage during a radical cystectomy, or it may prevent the progression of disease locally from undetected micrometastases. However, it has not been clearly demonstrated that preoperative radiotherapy has a significant impact on survival. The 5-year survival rates for patients with Stage B bladder carcinoma, with or without preoperative radiotherapy, are in the 40 to 50 per cent range. Patients who have Stage C bladder carcinoma have a 25 to 35 per cent 5-year survival.

Partial or segmental cystectomy may be appropriate for invasive transitional cell carcinoma or adenocarcinoma in very specific circumstances. Random bladder biopsies should reveal neither papillary tumor nor carcinoma *in situ* in other areas of the bladder. The tumor should be solitary and in a location of the bladder where it can be removed with a 2-cm. margin. Multifocal or recurrent disease offers little chance for cure with segmental resection.

CARCINOMA IN SITU

Carcinoma *in situ* is a bladder lesion in which there is cellular anaplasia with no papillary component or lamina propria invasion. Histologically, carcinoma *in situ* is characterized by severe cellular anaplasia with marked variety in size, shape, and staining intensity of nuclei. The appropriate management of carcinoma *in situ* depends on a number of factors such as chronicity of the disease, symp-

toms, and extent of bladder involvement. Carcinoma *in situ* is an insidious disease, in that invasion or progression can occur in an unpredictable fashion. If the lesion is confined to a small area in the bladder and if biopsy specimens of the urethra, trigone, and vesical neck are negative, intravesical chemotherapy may be used and achieves a 40 to 55 per cent response rate. If this disease is widespread, if the patient is symptomatic, or if there is disease in the urethra, prostatic ducts, or lower ureters, a radical cystectomy is generally recommended.

Neurogenic Bladder, Incontinence[3, 12, 17]

Normal control of micturition is maintained by a complex mechanism involving interaction of the cerebral cortex, spinal cord, bladder, and the vesical sphincter mechanism. The control of micturition is dependent on a number of nuclei in various portions of the nervous system which are connected by axonal pathways.

Bradley has divided these pathways into four loops or reflex arches. Loops I and II involve the innervation of the detrusor muscle; loops III and IV, the innervation of periurethral striated muscle. Loop I consists of connections from the cortical micturition center in the cerebral cortex to the brain stem detrusor nucleus. Loop II connects the brain stem detrusor nucleus with the detrusor muscle nuclei in the sacral gray matter. Loop III consists of fibers from the detrusor muscle to the motor neurons of the conus medullaris, which connect with the periurethral striated muscle through the pudendal nerve. Loop IV connects the conus medullaris motor neurons through the spinal pyramidal tract with the motor cortex in the frontal lobe.

In the evaluation of patients with disorders of micturition, it is important to bear in mind that any physiologic or anatomic abnormality along this pathway can cause a neurogenic bladder dysfunction. Neurogenic bladder disorders are not uncommon in patients with multiple sclerosis, myelodysplasia, spinal cord injury, or diabetes mellitus or after pelvic surgery or injury. The goals of management in patients with neurogenic bladder dysfunction are (1) preservation of renal function, (2) achievement of continence, (3) prevention of upper and lower urinary tract deterioration, and (4) prevention of urinary infection. The evaluation of a patient with neurogenic bladder should include a thorough neurologic examination, since bladder dysfunction may be the primary manifestation of a more widespread neurologic disorder. In patients with myelodysplasia, a multidisciplinary approach including orthopedic and neurologic surgeons, physical therapists, and psychologists has greatly improved management.

The initial evaluation of a patient with neurogenic bladder includes an intravenous pyelogram, a voiding cystourethrogram, and a urodynamic evaluation. A urodynamic study includes cystometry, measurement of the urinary flow rate, sphincter electromyography, and a urethral pressure profile. Cystometry is the representation on a graph of bladder pressure as a function of time and provides data about bladder sensation, compliance, and capacity. During this test, voluntary and involuntary contractions can be objectively measured and provocative tests performed to stimulate involuntary contractions. The effect of pharmacologic agents on bladder function can also be assessed. Urinary flow rate provides information about detrusor function and the sphincter mechanism. The voiding cystourethrogram is a radiographic visualization of the lower urinary tract during filling, storage, and voiding. This test provides objective, visual evidence about sphincter competence and serves to pinpoint the anatomic site of outflow obstruction or reflux. Information about the striated muscles of the external sphincter is gained from the sphincter electromyogram. The patient's ability to relax and contract the external sphincter and the sphincter's activity during voiding provide valuable information about the sphincter's role in voiding abnormalities. The urethral pressure profile records intraurethral pressure at successive points in the urethra and helps identify sites of obstruction.

Objective data generated by urodynamic testing have led to great advances in the treatment of neurogenic bladder dysfunction and have provided a more objective basis for the use of pharmacologic agents in the management of this disorder. Cholinergic agents such as bethanacol stimulate muscarinic receptors, increase detrusor tone, decrease bladder capacity, and may be used in association with an alpha blocking agent, such as dibenzylene, for treatment of urinary retention or vesical areflexia. The anticholinergic agent propantheline may be of use with an unstable or hyperreflexic bladder. Adrenergic agents such as phenylephrine or phenylpropanolamine increase sphincter tone and may be useful in the treatment of sphincter incompetence or enuresis. Phenoxybenzamine, an alpha-adrenergic blocking agent, provides a prolonged lowering of the urethral pressure and is sometimes useful for neurogenic sphincter dyssynergia. The goal of pharmacologic manipulation is to enable the patient with neurogenic bladder dysfunction to void normally while maintaining continence. If a patient is continent but cannot void adequately, self-intermittent catheterization may be recommended.

Stress Urinary Incontinence

Stress urinary incontinence is an abnormality that involves the involuntary loss of urine associated with an increase in intra-abdominal pressure caused by coughing, sneezing, or straining.[12, 17, 20, 23] On physical examination of a patient with stress incontinence, an assessment of the pelvic floor support and urethral hypermobility is made. Then, with the bladder filled with fluid, the patient is observed for leakage while coughing or straining. When this procedure is repeated, with the examiner providing urethral and bladder support, there should be no leakage. It is important to obtain a careful history to ascertain whether there is bladder instability, which is suggested by urgency, urge incontinence, or leakage when the patient is supine. If instability is suspected, a urodynamic evaluation is indicated, since patients who have only bladder instability will not benefit from a surgical procedure.

The Marshall-Marchetti-Kranz method is the standard surgical procedure for stress incontinence and consists of urethrovesical suspension. The Burch modification incorporates a colposuspension, which gives broad support to the urethra and bladder base by the suture fixation of the lateral vaginal fornix to Cooper's ligament. In procedures described by Stamey and Peyera, a retropubic urethral suspension is performed by passing a special needle and suture through a small suprapubic incision down through the vaginally exposed periurethral tissue. This permits the relocation of the proximal urethra and vesical neck to its normal anatomic position without extensive retropubic dissection. Successful results are achieved in 85 to 95 per cent of patients with these procedures. Failure may be due to unsuspected bladder instability or unsuccessful retropubic urethropexy.

For incontinent males who fail to respond to conservative measures, a number of surgical procedures have been developed to provide continence. One technique that has recently gained widespread acceptance is the surgical implantation of an artificial sphincter. An inflatable cuff is placed around the bulbar urethra or bladder neck. When the cuff is deflated, the bladder empties, after which the cuff is gradually reinflated to prevent urine leakage.

Cystitis

Cystitis[15, 17, 20] is more frequent in females than in males and is often accompanied by dysuria, urgency, or a low-grade fever. In females, cystitis is caused by organisms that have colonized the urethra or vagina and it may often follow sexual intercourse. Recurrent bacterial cystitis is often encountered in women with diabetes, pregnancy, or congenital anomalies that result in secondary infection. Recurrent or persistent infection may require prophylactic, low-dose antibiotic treatment. In the male, cystitis is usually secondary to a prostate or kidney infection or to retention of residual urine. Tuberculous cystitis may be due to a descending infection or to genital tuberculosis. Chronic tuberculous involvement can lead to a severely contracted, poorly functioning bladder and should be suspected when chronic cystitis fails to respond to antibiotic therapy. External beam radiotherapy can also cause acute cystitis. Radiation-induced changes include ulceration and necrosis of the wall and may produce a contracted bladder. Radiation-induced cystitis usually responds to symptomatic management.

Interstitial cystitis is a lesion that can occur in either sex, but it is more commonly seen in females. The exact etiology of this disorder is unclear, although it is thought to be an autoimmune phenomenon. Patients with interstitial cystitis present with dysuria, frequency, and painful voiding. Endoscopically there are small, discrete hemorrhages of patchy distribution. Histologic examination of these lesions reveals hemorrhage, edema, and lymphocytic infiltrates. Steroids, anti-inflammatory medications, and antihistamines have all been used for treatment with variable success. Patients with persistent symptoms may be treated with fulguration or with bladder distention under anesthesia. In severe, refractory cases, bladder denervation or even replacement by cecocystoplasty may be employed.

THE PROSTATE[4, 10, 14, 15, 20]

Congenital Anomalies

A small or absent prostate gland is a rare congenital abnormality that may be associated with malformations of the cloaca, urethra, and testes. Asymmetric development of the prostate is often associated with ductus deferens and seminal vesicle abnormalities and the presence of a malformed or absent kidney. Congenital fistulas may develop between the prostatic urethra and the rectum.

Prostatitis

ACUTE PROSTATITIS

Patients with acute prostatitis present with fever, chills, dysuria, and perineal pain. The patient may have bladder irritability, hematuria, bladder outlet obstruction, or prostatic abscess formation. Histologically, acute prostatitis is marked by the presence of polymorphonuclear leukocytes and a variable number of lymphocytes, plasma cells, and macrophages.

Patients with acute prostatitis usually respond dramatically to intravenous antibiotics and hydration. Following the inital treatment, antibiotic treatment for 6 weeks to 6 months is often required to prevent the development of chronic prostatitis. Anatomic abnormalities such as stricture, benign prostatic hypertrophy, prostatic carcinoma, and neurogenic bladder can predispose to acute prostatitis and should be considered when the acute condition has improved.

CHRONIC PROSTATITIS

Chronic prostatitis is usually secondary to invasion of bacteria from the urethra, but it may arise from a hematogenous source or may be secondary to inadequate treatment of acute prostatitis. Chronic prostatitis can be caused by a gram-negative organism such as *Escherichia coli* or an agent such as *Chlamydia trachomatis* or *Trichomonas*. These patients may present with aching in the perineum and low back pain or a low-grade fever; they may also complain of burning with ejaculation, bladder irritability, frequency, or urgency. Histologically, there is infiltration by inflammatory cells and destruction of glandular epithelium. Physical examination will reveal a tender prostate that often has crepitus. Cultures of the expressed prostatic secretions from the prostatic massage should be made and examined under the microscope. If the cultures are positive for a pathologic organism, specific therapy is initiated. If the culture results are negative, as is most common, the patient may be treated with nonspecific antimicrobial agents. Trimethroprim-sulfamethoxazole or minocycline may be given for 2 to 6 weeks. If *Chlamydia* or *Trichomonas* is found, treatment by erythromycin or metronidazole is indicated. Nonspecific measures such as daily sitz baths or enhanced sexual activity may also help alleviate the symptoms. This disease is often very difficult to treat successfully, and chronic antibiotic suppression may be the only acceptable solution.

GRANULOMATOUS PROSTATITIS

Granulomatous prostatitis, which occurs in the fifth and sixth decades of life, is commonly mistaken for prostatic carcinoma. The patients present with terminal hematuria, perineal pain, and discomfort, and on physical examination there is likely to be a firm, hard nodular texture to the prostate. The diagnosis is made by biopsy, which will show noncaseating granuloma, multinucleated giant cells, and foamy histiocytes. The symptoms may totally resolve after a few days of catheter drainage, but many patients will require some form of prostatectomy to obtain total relief. Postoperatively, these patients tend to do very well and will often have a normal prostate when examined in 3 to 6 months.

TUBERCULOUS PROSTATITIS

Another lesion that can mimic prostatic carcinoma on physical examination is tuberculous prostatitis. This uncommon lesion should be suspected in a patient who has firm nodules in the prostate and evidence of upper tract or bladder involvement with tuberculosis. If the infection in the prostate progresses untreated, the prostate will become small and fibrotic and the seminal vesicles and epididymis can become involved.

Benign Prostatic Hypertrophy

Benign prostatic hypertrophy is a disease of older males and is rarely encountered before the age of 40. The normal prostate in man undergoes a slow increase in size from birth to puberty; at that time there is a rapid increase in size, which continues until the late 30s. Midway through the fifth decade, the prostate may undergo hypertrophic changes. The exact etiology of benign prostatic hypertrophy is not clear, although it is not seen in men castrated prior to puberty and it does not progress after castration. This abnormality may be associated with an increase in tissue dihydrotestosterone content or with a change in the ratio of androgen to estrogen, which is known to change with aging. Approximately 1 in 100 men will require surgery for this condition.

Benign prostatic hypertrophy occurs in the periurethral glandular tissue, which is involved with neither essential functions of the prostate nor the origin of malignancy. The periurethral glandular tissue expands, and the portion of the prostate that is compressed is termed the "surgical capsule." The hyperplastic tissue may be composed of one of five histologic patterns: (1) stromal, (2) fibromuscular, (3) muscular, (4) fibroadenomatous, or (5) fibromyoadenomatous. Histologically, there are increases in fibromuscular stroma and in the number and size of acini.

CLINICAL PRESENTATION AND EVALUATION

Patients with bladder outlet obstruction secondary to benign prostatic hypertrophy may present with difficulty in initiating voiding, incomplete emptying, dribbling, frequency, or total urinary retention with complete inability to void. With development of a slow, progressive obstruction, the patient may be unaware of the abnormality. With chronic borderline inability to void, acute urinary retention may be precipitated by alcohol ingestion, a prolonged delay in voiding, anticholinergic medication, tranquilizers, or antidepressants. The enlarging prostate produces urinary obstruction and persistently increased intravesical pressure, which will result in detrusor hypertrophy, bladder trabeculation, and formation of diverticuli. This process can progress to hydronephrosis and upper tract deterioration.

Neither prostatic size nor degree of outlet obstruction can be accurately determined on physical examination. Urinary retention may occur with a gland that feels normal on rectal examination; conversely, a gland that seems significantly enlarged may produce no bladder outlet obstructive symptoms. A post-void catheter residual urine volume aids in determination of inadequate bladder emptying; the normal post-void residual urine volume in an adult male is approximately 35 ml. Measurement of urinary flow rate is an accurate screening tool for evaluation of bladder outlet obstruction. The average urinary flow rate in a male is 16 ml. per second; patients with prostatic hypertrophy usually have flow rates less than 10 ml. per second. An acid phosphatase determination is routinely performed to detect the presence of occult malignancy, but is best obtained prior to rectal examination because of the potential for producing false elevations of acid phosphatase with prostatic examination. An intravenous pyelogram may be obtained in order to identify the location and caliber of the ureters. Cystourethroscopy, a procedure in which a cystoscope with fiberoptic illumination is introduced through the urethra to the bladder, forms an important part of the preoperative evaluation. This procedure allows the surgeon to make an estimation of the size and anatomic configuration of the prostate as well as the length of the prostatic urethra. The bladder is also examined for the presence of trabeculation, diverticula, intravesical stones, or malignant disease, and location of the ureteral orifices.

TREATMENT

At present there is no acceptable medical treatment for benign prostatic hypertrophy; the only effective treatment is surgery. Indications for surgery include (1) acute urinary retention, (2) hydronephrosis, (3) recurrent urinary tract infection, (4) hematuria, or (5) symptoms that are of significant magnitude for the patient to desire surgical treatment. The goal of surgery is to relieve symptoms while preserving anatomic integrity and function.

There are four standard surgical approaches to the removal of prostate for benign prostatic hypertrophy (Fig. 10): (1) transurethral, (2) transvesical, (3) retropubic, or (4) perineal. Regardless of the surgical approach chosen, the operation is performed to remove the adenomatous portion of the prostate which is located within the surgical capsule. Total removal of both the prostate and seminal vesicles is reserved for malignant disease.

Transurethral Resection

Transurethral resection of the prostate enables the surgeon to relieve the obstruction with a minimum of morbidity and a relatively short postoperative course. By use of a resectoscope employing current from an electrosurgical unit, the surgeon resects prostatic tissue with a wire

loop. Following resection, subsequent healing takes place by granulation and re-epithelialization of the prostatic urethra. Irrigation fluid, such as isotonic glycine, is used during transurethral resection to clear the operative field. Fluid is often absorbed into the bloodstream through open venous channels of the prostatic capsule during resection, and therefore the fluid must be isotonic. If hypotonic fluid is used, hemolysis and renal damage could occur. If a high conductivity solution such as saline were used, cutting and coagulation would not be possible because the electrocautery would be ineffective. The absorption of large amounts of the irrigation fluid during the procedure can cause hyponatremia and result in agitation, restlessness, nausea, vomiting, and confusion. If symptoms develop in a patient undergoing a transurethral resection, an immediate serum sodium and electrocardiogram should be obtained. The standard treatment of this syndrome consists of administration of diuretics and the judicious use of intravenous hypertonic saline. The incidence of pulmonary emboli after transurethral prostatectomy is 0.3 to 2.2 per cent and is highest in patients who have been hospitalized for a number of days prior to operation. The incidence of urethral stricture following transurethral resection is approximately 6 per cent. Transurethral prostate resection should have no adverse effect on potency.

Suprapubic Prostatectomy

The first planned suprapubic prostatectomies were performed in the 1880s by Dittel and Belfield. The suprapubic, transvesical approach is used when there is a large gland with a significant intravesical component. This approach allows the surgeon to visualize the ureteral orifices, to protect them during the procedure, and to simultaneously treat other intravesical lesions, such as diverticula or calculi. The suprapubic prostatectomy is performed through a low midline abdominal incision, through which the bladder is opened, and the prostatic adenoma is digitally enucleated along the plane of the surgical capsule. Postoperatively, a urethral catheter and suprapubic catheter are employed for drainage.

Retropubic Prostatectomy

The first report of retropubic prostatectomy was in 1909 by Van Stockum. This operation was performed sporadically until it was popularized in the 1940s by Millen. This procedure is performed through a low abdominal approach, and a transverse incision is made through the prostatic capsule. After the prostate is enucleated, hemostatic sutures are placed and a wedge of bladder neck is removed to prevent stenosis. After a urethral catheter is placed in the bladder, the prostatic capsule is closed. This procedure can be performed very rapidly, and there are few postoperative complications. It is best suited to patients who do not have a small, fibrotic gland or who are not significantly obese.

Perineal Prostatectomy

Ferguson performed perineal prostectomies along with lithotomy in the 1850s, but Young in 1903 described the perineal prostatectomy that is performed today. With the patient in an exaggerated lithotomy position, a perineal incision is made and the dissection proceeds through the central tendon and rectourethralis muscle to expose the prostate. An incision is made through the prostatic capsule,

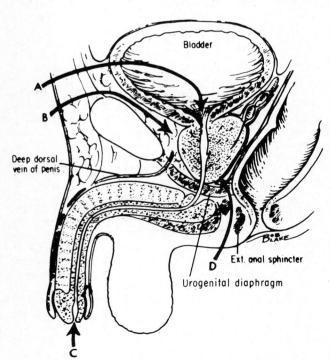

Figure 10. Four approaches to the surgical removal of benign prostatic adenoma: A, Transvesical. B, Retropubic transcapsular. C, Transurethral. D, Perineal. (From Paulson, D. F. (Ed.): Genitourinary Surgery. New York, Churchill Livingstone, 1984.)

and the adenoma is enucleated from below. Postoperatively, up to 50 per cent of patients who undergo this procedure are impotent. The high impotence rate and the technical difficulties of the operation are the reasons that this procedure is used infrequently.

Prostatic Carcinoma

Prostatic carcinoma accounts for 17 per cent of tumors in men and is the second most common malignancy in males. It is the third most common cause of cancer death in men over 55 and the most common cause of cancer death in men over 75. There are presently 65,000 new cases of prostatic carcinoma per year, and it causes 21,000 deaths annually. Prostatic carcinoma is predominantly a disease of elderly males, with the peak incidence in the late 60s and early 70s; fewer than 1 per cent are younger than 50 years old. The incidence of prostatic carcinoma found at autopsy is the same worldwide; however, the clinical incidence of this disease is relatively higher in the United States and Western Europe and lower in the Orient. The incidence in the American black population is 50 per cent higher than that of the population as a whole.

The etiology of prostatic carcinoma is unknown, but a number of observations suggest a hormonal role. The disease is not found in eunuchs, and there is often marked tumor regression seen after orchiectomy. High prostatic carcinoma rates have been found in men exposed to cadmium, in tire workers, in painters, and in farmers. The fact that vegetarians and Japanese show low rates of prostatic carcinoma has led some investigators to suggest a dietary etiology.

Prostatic carcinoma may be divided into four stages:

1. Stage A carcinoma is diagnosed by endoscopic resection of the prostate. In Stage A1 disease, there is a microscopic focus of well-differentiated adenocarcinoma present in fewer than three microscopic foci; in Stage A2, there is diffuse involvement of the gland.

2. Stage B1 carcinoma is confined to the prostate in a discrete nodule detected by rectal examination; Stage B2 indicates large or multiple nodules.

3. In Stage C the carcinoma has grown outside the prostatic capsule to the periprostatic area.

4. Stage D is metastatic prostatic carcinoma; Stage D1 indicates metastases to pelvic lymph nodes, and Stage D2 is defined as metastatic disease in bone, distant lymph nodes, or soft tissue.

Histologically, prostatic carcinoma may be well, moderately, or poorly differentiated. In well-differentiated carcinoma, the glands are proximal and smaller than normal and lack the typical papillary configuration of benign hyperplasia. In moderately differentiated carcinoma, the glands are more haphazardly distributed and there is mild cellular anaplasia. In poorly differentiated carcinoma, the tumor may occur as solid sheets of anaplastic cells with dense nuclei and no glandular formation. Gleason developed a pathologic classification in which histologic characteristics of the tumor are combined to produce a prognostic score of 2 to 10, which may be of use in predicting the course of the disease.

The evaluation and staging of patients with prostatic carcinoma include a serum acid phosphatase determination, bone scan, and intravenous pyelogram. Acid phosphatase elevation in prostatic carcinoma was first described in 1938 by Gutman and Gutman, and, in 1953, the tartrate inhibitable prostatic fraction was identified by Fishman and Lerner. Bone is the most frequent site of hematogenous metastases of prostate carcinoma, and the bone scan is a very sensitive test for detecting metastases. The most common bony sites involved are the pelvis, lumbar spine, and femur. The intravenous pyelogram provides information about possible upper tract involvement; it is not uncommon for metastatic prostatic carcinoma to obstruct a ureter because of disease in the pelvic lymph nodes. When a suspected prostatic nodule is palpated, histologic confirmation of the presence of malignant disease is obtained by transrectal biopsy with a closed needle. If the acid phosphatase, bone scan, and intravenous pyelogram results are normal, the next step in staging is a pelvic lymphadenectomy, which involves the bilateral removal of the obturator and hypogastric lymph nodes. The pelvic lymphadenectomy is important because 14 to 40 per cent of patients thought to have disease confined to the prostate will have pelvic nodal metastases.

TREATMENT

There are a number of therapeutic options available for the treatment of prostatic carcinoma, depending on the stage of the disease.[17, 19, 21, 23] The available treatment modalities include (1) radical prostatectomy (Fig. 11), (2) external beam radiotherapy, (3) interstitial irradiation, (4) hormone manipulation, and (5) chemotherapy.

Stage A1

Stage A1 prostatic carcinoma is managed conservatively, and a repeat resection of the prostate is performed in 6 months. This type of carcinoma has very little propensity to progress or metastasize, and the prognosis is excellent.

Stage A2, B1, and B2

Stage A2, B1, and B2 carcinoma may be treated by *radical prostatectomy*. Radical prostatectomy involves the total removal of the prostate gland, the prostatic capsule, the ampullae, and the seminal vesicles. The two surgical approaches used are the radical *perineal* prostatectomy and the radical *retropubic* prostatectomy.

The *perineal approach* provides good exposure for reconstruction of the vesicourethral anastomosis and is well tolerated in elderly patients who might otherwise have difficulty with an abdominal operation. The operation does

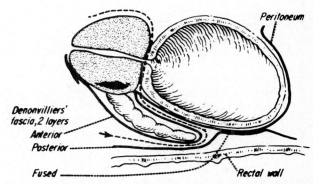

Figure 11. In a radical prostatectomy the entire prostate and seminal vesicles are removed. (From Paulson, D. F. (Ed.): Genitourinary Surgery. New York, Churchill Livingstone, 1984.)

not allow for simultaneous pelvic lymphadenectomy, and therefore two operations are required. This procedure is contraindicated in patients with ankylosis of the hips or in patients who have had previous prostatic surgery with subsequent fibrosis in the region of the prostate.

With the *radical retropubic prostatectomy,* there is the significant advantage of allowing the surgeon simultaneously to perform a pelvic lymphadenectomy and inspection for and repair of ureteral damage or involvement. A recent innovation by Walsh has been the development of a nerve-sparing radical retropubic prostatectomy in which postoperative potency is maintained in a high percentage of patients.

Stage C

Stage C carcinoma has been treated in the past by radical prostatectomy, cystoprostatectomy, radical prostatectomy plus hormone therapy, interstitial irradiation, and external beam radiotherapy. However, it has not been clearly demonstrated that any of these treatments increase survival and most clinicians today treat an asymptomatic patient with Stage C carcinoma conservatively.

Stage D

Huggins and Hodges opened a new era in the treatment of prostatic carcinoma when they reported the use of orchiectomy and DES for the treatment of metastatic disease. Since that time, the use of orchiectomy and/or estrogen treatment for metastatic prostate carcinoma has become widespread. Other types of endocrine manipulation have also been used, including adrenalectomy, hypophysectomy, luteinizing hormone–releasing hormone (LHRH) analogs, and androgen-blocking agents.

Orchiectomy and Estrogen. Bilateral orchiectomy, the most direct method of removal of testosterone, causes a prompt decline in plasma testosterone from approximately 700 to 50 ng. per 100 ml. The patient is rendered impotent after orchiectomy, and some patients may undergo a change in self-image. Diethylstilbestrol functions by inhibiting the release of LH from the pituitary gland and thereby decreasing the release of testosterone from the testis; it may also have a direct effect on the Leydig cell as well as on the metabolism of prostatic cells.

Adrenalectomy. The adrenal gland produces circulating androgens, and adrenalectomy has been performed to remove this additional androgen source. Adrenalectomy has been found to produce only a short-lived partial response in patients for whom conventional hormone manipulation has failed, and prolonged survival is unusual.

Hypophysectomy. Hypophysectomy, which results in removal of the source of LH, has also been used to treat patients with hormone-unresponsive metastatic prostate carcinoma. These patients show generally only limited subjective and objective improvement, and this procedure has not gained widespread use.

Androgen Blocking Agents and LHRH. Antiandrogens are used to block the effect of testosterone on the target tissue. These agents prevent dihydrotestosterone binding to the nuclear chromatin and inhibit mRNA formation and protein synthesis. Antiandrogens have not been found to be useful in cases of conventional treatment failure, but they may have a role in the treatment of patients who have not received hormone treatment. Some investigators have advocated the use of both an antiandrogen plus hormone manipulation with either LHRH analogs or orchiectomy as primary therapy in patients who have not received prior hormonal treatment. The early results

with this approach were encouraging; however, longer-term studies so far have failed to demonstrate an advantage of this form of treatment over standard hormone manipulation by DES or orchiectomy alone.

Chemotherapy. Chemotherapy for metastatic prostatic carcinoma that has failed to respond to endocrine manipulation has not been effective. As a single agent, hydroxyurea or *cis*-platin has been found to have a 40 to 45 per cent response rate, nitrogen mustard 39 per cent, Adriamycin 29 per cent, and 5-fluorouracil (FU) 23 per cent. The combination of cytoxan, 5-FU, and Adriamycin has been reported to have an initial response rate as high as 50 per cent, but long-term survival benefits have yet to be demonstrated.

Radiation Therapy. Radiation therapy is advocated by some for primary treatment of localized prostatic carcinoma. With this treatment, which usually consists of 6500 to 7500 rads, patients with Stage B carcinoma achieve 80 to 90 per cent tumor control in the prostate. In patients with Stage C disease, 7000 rads has been reported to control the tumor in 80 per cent. Patients may suffer bladder or rectal irritation as a result of radiation, but symptoms tend to be transient and major complications (such as small bowel obstruction, severe hemorrhagic cystitis, or proctitis with stricture) occur in only 3 per cent. Chronic cystitis or proctitis occurs in approximately 15 per cent of the patients, erectile impotence in 30 per cent. There have been large series of patients with long-term follow-up treated with radical surgery or external beam radiotherapy, but there have been few prospective randomized studies from which to compare radiation with surgery. External beam radiotherapy is very useful in the treatment of symptomatic osseous metastases.

Interstitial Irradiation. Another addition to the therapeutic armamentarium for localized prostatic carcinoma is interstitial irradiation. A staging pelvic lymphadenectomy is done, followed by the implantation of ^{125}iodine seeds into the prostate. This procedure is associated with less morbidity than radical surgery, and disease control is achieved in a significant number of patients. Postoperative complications may include transient voiding symptoms, genital edema, and lymphocele (a localized collection of lymph fluid). Late complications include rectal discomfort, urinary irritability, impotence, and proctitis.

THE SEMINAL VESICLES

Seminal vesicle cysts, which are rare, are usually congenital in origin, although ejaculatory duct obstruction can also cause them.[10, 17] The cysts can be removed transvesically or perineally (Fig. 12). Inflammatory disease may affect the seminal vesicles and can cause hematospermia and painful ejaculation. Rectal examination often reveals tenderness and induration in one or both seminal vesicles. Seminal vesicle abnormalities may be detected by retrograde seminal vesiculogram, needle aspiration, or ultrasound. Inflammatory seminal vesiculitis is almost uniformly responsive to broad-spectrum antibiotics. In the rare instance in which pain and discomfort persist despite conservative management, transvesical seminal vesiculectomy is performed.

THE PENIS[5, 17, 18a, 20, 23, 26]

Phimosis

Phimosis is a condition in which it is not possible to retract the foreskin on the penis. This may be a complica-

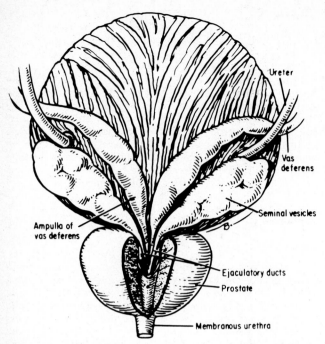

Figure 12. The anatomic relationship of the posterior aspect of the prostate, seminal vesicles, vas deferens, and bladder. (From Paulson, D. F. (Ed.): Genitourinary Surgery. New York, Churchill Livingstone, 1984.)

tion of circumcision in which too much foreskin is left, or it may be secondary to an infection that occurs under redundant foreskin. In the latter, the prepuce becomes chronically fibrotic and adhesions form beneath the prepuce and prevent retraction. This condition is commonly a result of poor hygiene, and treatment involves local measures to eradicate the infection. A dorsal slit of the prepuce may be necessary. When the acute infection and inflammation resolve, the definitive treatment is circumcision.

Paraphimosis

Paraphimosis is a condition in which the foreskin, once retracted behind the glans, cannot be returned to its original position. The foreskin becomes entrapped behind the coronal sulcus by secondary swelling of the glans. This can usually be resolved by gentle pressure. If the glans is left unreduced, continued swelling may render reduction impossible. To treat the acute condition, an incision may be made to incise the constricting lesion. Circumcision may be required at a later date to prevent recurrence.

Balanitis

Balanitis is an inflammation of the glans penis; balanoposthitis is an inflammation of both the glans and the foreskin. Balanitis is most commonly due to redundant foreskin and poor hygiene. However, a more ominous disease such as squamous cell carcinoma can cause balanoposthitis, and if the inflammation does not clear with good hygiene, further evaluation is necessary. Erosive balanitis may be due to an infection of *Borrelia refringens* and *Vibrio*.

Circumcision

Circumcision is performed in most countries and prevents phimosis, paraphimosis, and balanitis. There are a number of techniques available for circumcision. In the sleeve resection technique, after the skin is incised circumferentially at the base of the foreskin, the foreskin is retracted and another incision is made proximal to the coronal sulcus. The foreskin is removed, hemostasis is achieved and the two skin edges are reapproximated. In the neonate and young infant, circumcision is often performed with the use of a Gomco clamp.

Priapism

Priapism is a rare disorder in which a male experiences a prolonged erection that is unassociated with sexual stimulation and that may be painful. In this condition, which may persist for days if left untreated, the corpus cavernosum fills with viscous blood. In 60 per cent of patients, priapism is idiopathic. It also may be associated with leukemia, metastatic carcinoma, local trauma, and sickle cell anemia. Numerous types of nonsurgical management have been attempted with varying amounts of success. Ganglionic blocking agents, spinal anesthesia, hypotensive anesthesia, DES, and anticoagulants have all been employed with mixed results. The child with sickle cell anemia usually responds to exchange transfusions. In a patient with leukemia, the priapism will often resolve as the leukemia is successfully treated. If conservative management fails, surgical intervention is indicated. Surgical procedures have been devised to shunt the blood from the corpora cavernosa, to create a flaccid penis, and to prevent long-term complications such as impotence. In the Winter's shunt procedure, several fistulas are created with a biopsy needle from the glans corpus spongiosum to the corpora cavernosa. Another shunting procedure that has been widely used is the corpus cavernosum–spongiosum shunt. In this operation, an incision is made at the base of the penis and a window of tunica albuginea is removed from the corpus cavernosum and corpus spongiosum, which are then sutured together. This allows blood from the engorged corpus cavernosum to flow through the corpus spongiosum. The anastomosis of saphenous vein to corpus cavernosum has also been used to shunt blood from the corpora cavernosa. In the management of a patient with priapism, it is important to remember that impotence is often a sequela of priapism itself. Despite appropriate and timely surgical intervention, the patient may still become permanently impotent.

Peyronie's Disease

Peyronie's disease is a fibrotic process of the sheath of the corpus cavernosum that usually begins with pain followed by development of plaque in the sheath. This area then becomes fibrotic and causes curvature during erection. In most patients, symptoms resolve spontaneously with conservative management. However, in a small percentage of patients, painful erections persist and the penile curvature may be of such severity that sexual intercourse is not possible. Medical treatment has been unsatisfactory in the treatment of this disorder, and a number of surgical procedures have been developed. One approach is to resect the plaque and replace it with a dermal graft. The curvature may also be corrected by the surgical removal of a wedge of corpus cavernosum on the contralateral side of the penis. If impotence is associated with this disease, a penile prosthesis can be placed at the time of surgery.

Lymphogranuloma Venereum

Lymphogranuloma venereum is an infectious venereal disease caused by *Chlamydia trachomatis.* A penile lesion typically develops 30 to 60 days after exposure, heals spontaneously, and may be overlooked by the patient. This genital lesion is followed by lymphadenitis and, in the female, rectal stricture. The involved inguinal nodes suppurate and form multiple sinuses. The diagnosis is made by a positive complement fixation test. Tetracycline is effective treatment for the primary disease, although sulfonamides may be needed to control secondary infection. The draining sinuses may have to be resected, and the rectal strictures can necessitate surgical correction.

Granuloma Inguinale

Granuloma inguinale is a chronic venereal infection of the skin and subcutaneous tissues involving the genital areas, perineum, and inguinal regions. The infectious agent is a bacterium related to *Klebsiella pneumoniae.* The initial genital lesion forms a nodule that fragments and ulcerates. This ulcer is painful, may bleed, and can spread extensively. The diagnosis is made by the identification of Donovan bodies, which are organisms located inside monocytes. Secondary infection, ulceration, and sinus formation are common. Therapeutic agents include tetracycline, chloramphenicol, or streptomycin.

Condyloma Acuminatum

Condylomata acuminata, or *venereal warts,* are caused by a virus that has a propensity for residing in moist areas in the genital region. Histologically, they are keratin-covered papillary projections from the surface of the penis. The growth down into the stroma is characterized by normal maturation without anaplasia, although there may be some abnormal mitotic activity. When the lesions are on the penis, they are treated with podophyllin. When condylomata acuminata involve the urethra or bladder, they can be very difficult to treat. If there are only a few small urethral lesions, they may be treated by endoscopic resection. When the lesions are large or multiple, 5-FU or thiotepa instillations may be required.

Giant condylomata acuminata of the Buschke-Lowenstein type are characterized by deep tissue penetration. Treatment consists of surgical removal because this entity may represent a type of verrucous carcinoma.

Herpes Progenitalis

Genital herpes, usually caused by herpesvirus type II, is characterized by vesiculopustular lesions and may include adenopathy. These lesions, which can be painful and recurrent, often appear on the foreskin or glans penis and coalesce to form a superficial, spontaneously healing ulcer.

Syphilis

Syphilis, caused by the spirochete *Treponema pallidum,* typically produces a painless ulcer 2 to 4 weeks after sexual exposure. The lesions may appear on the glans, corona, foreskin, or shaft of the penis. Histologically, the lesion contains small round cells plus plasma cells and contains neutrophils if there is a secondary infection. The diagnosis is made by finding spirochetes on darkfield examination of serous exudate from the lesion. Serologic testing is useful, but there may be negative results for up to 3 weeks after appearance of the penile lesion. All penile ulcers should be considered syphilitic until proven otherwise. The recommended treatment is penicillin.

Neoplasms

PREMALIGNANT LESIONS

Erythroplasia in Queyrat's and Bowen's disease is a histologically similar lesion which may represent carcinoma in situ. Bowen's disease is associated with a high incidence of internal malignancy and can occur anywhere on the body. When Bowen's disease occurs on the penis, it occurs on the penile shaft; Queyrat's erythroplasia occurs on the glans or coronal sulcus. Histologically, both diseases show marked anaplasia of cells and variation in size and shape of the nuclei.

If the lesion is on the prepuce, a circumcision will be sufficient treatment. A small lesion may be treated by a total excision; however, if the lesion is too large to be removed with local excision, topical 5-FU is applied. Follow-up examination and re-biopsy are important to identify persistent or progressive disease, which may necessitate amputation.

MALIGNANT LESIONS

Most tumors of the penis are epithelial and are related to chronic infection and inflammation of the foreskin or glans. Carcinoma of the penis is unusual in countries where neonatal circumcision is practiced, but it is prevalent in areas such as Africa and Southeast Asia, where circumcision is not routinely performed. In the United States, carcinoma of the penis accounts for fewer than 1 per cent of malignancies, whereas in Southeast Asia it accounts for 10 to 15 per cent. Carcinoma of the penis usually arises on the glans or inner surface of the foreskin and may appear as an erythematous plaque or an ulcer. Histologically, this disease, which is squamous cell carcinoma, presents as dark-staining basal cells that are anaplastic, form keratin pearls, and lose their normal polarity. If the lesion has grown into the corpus cavernosum, the incidence of metastatic disease is increased and survival is significantly decreased. The tumor normally metastasizes initially to the femoral and iliac lymph nodes. Stage A penile carcinoma is restricted to the glans or foreskin; Stage B involves the shaft of the penis and/or the corpus cavernosum. Stage C involves the inguinal lymph nodes, and Stage D involves metastasis beyond the inguinal pelvic nodes. There is an increased incidence of hypercalcemia of malignancy with penile carcinoma that resolves when the tumor is removed.

Surgical removal of the primary lesion is effective for local control of the tumor if a 2-cm. margin of normal tissue can be obtained. Sexual function and a normal voiding pattern may be preserved if partial penectomy is performed. Total penectomy with perineal urethrostomy is indicated when the tumor is present on the proximal aspect of the penis. In a young, sexually active patient with a small noninvasive tumor, radiation therapy may be an alternative to penile amputation. In carefully selected patients, the results of this form of treatment are acceptable. These patients must be followed closely, and a re-biopsy of the lesion is necessary to confirm disease control. The most common complication of radiation is urethral stricture.

Approximately 50 per cent of patients who present with penile carcinoma will have palpable inguinal adenopathy, but only half of these patients will have positive nodal disease. Although there is not total agreement about the best method for dealing with inguinal nodes, most clinicians recommend an inguinal lymphadenectomy if the adenopathy is still palpable 6 weeks after surgical removal of the primary tumor. Without treatment, 5-year survival is rare if the inguinal nodes are positive, but with lymphadenectomy the 5-year survival is in the 50 per cent range. In the treatment of metastatic carcinoma of the penis, bleomycin, cis-platin, and methotrexate have been used with reasonable success.

Sexual Dysfunction

The exact mechanism of penile erection is incompletely understood. The stimulus for erection is complex and of both somatic and psychogenic origin. The psychogenic stimuli are mediated via a cerebral erotic center, and local stimulatory input is mediated through the sacral spinal cord. Penile parasympathetic innervation is via the pudendal nerves and S2, S3, S4. During erection, which is under parasympathetic control, the vascular spaces in the corpora cavernosa and corpus spongiosum fill with blood. At the time of ejaculation, which is controlled by the sympathetic system, the bladder neck closes and the ejaculate is propelled out through the urethra.

Male sexual dysfunction is a complex phenomenon that can be associated with a number of disorders. Impotence is defined as erectile dysfunction that is characterized by the persistent inability to obtain or sustain an erection that is adequate for intercourse. In an impotent patient, a psychogenic component should always be considered. An assessment of male sexual dysfunction should also include both partners. There is a wide range of causes of male sexual dysfunction including vascular, metabolic, and medication-related problems. Vasculogenic causes for impotence can be arterial or venous in origin. Atherosclerotic lesions involving the internal pudendal or penile arteries are a common cause of impotence. The incidence of impotence associated with atheromatous aortoiliac disease approaches 60 per cent and venous abnormalities of the corpus cavernosum have also been reported to be associated with this disorder. There is a long list of pharmacologic agents that have an adverse effect on sexual function in the male. Anticholinergic medications, antidepressants, psychotropic agents, and antihypertensive medications such as methyldopa, clonidine, and propranolol are associated with erectile dysfunction. Diabetes is one of the more common causes of impotence in men and is seen in up to 59 per cent of impotent patients. Surgical procedures, such as aortoiliac bypass, radical prostatectomy, cystectomy, and abdominoperineal resection, may all cause impotence. Neurogenic causes can include spinal cord injury, multiple sclerosis, myelodysplasia, and peripheral neuropathy. En-

docrine disorders, such as abnormalities of the pituitary-testis axis and thyroid dysfunction, account for 10 per cent of cases. Penile injury, pelvic fracture, Peyronie's disease, and priapism can also cause sexual dysfunction.

The evaluation of a patient with sexual dysfunction includes a total medical and sexual history and a complete physical examination. Initial laboratory tests include blood count, urinalysis, examination of the expressed prostatic secretion, and measurement of blood sugar and serum creatinine. Endocrine tests include determinations of testosterone, prolactin, FSH, and LH. A nocturnal penile tumescence test is often of value. This test measures occurrence of erection while the patient is asleep and may help distinguish psychogenic from organic impotence. The measurement of penile blood pressure gives an indication of a possible vascular etiology and measurement of the bulbocavernosus reflex provides objective information about neurologic abnormalities.

Few forms of medical treatment for impotence have been successful. If an endocrinologic abnormality exists that results in impotence, its correction should allow normal sexual function to return. A patient in whom diabetes is under poor control will often regain potency when the diabetes is brought under better control. Neurogenic impotence secondary to a vitamin deficiency or pernicious anemia may also be reversible.

There are a number of surgical procedures available for the treatment of impotence. The Small-Carion semirigid penile prosthesis is a silicon rod that is placed inside the corpora cavernosa through a penile, scrotal, or perineal incision. This prosthesis provides permanent semirigidity to the penis and is associated with a 90 to 95 per cent success rate. The Jonas prosthesis has a silver wire center that enables the penis to be directed and stabilized in a certain position. An inflatable penile prosthesis developed by Scott consists of inflatable cylinders connected to a small pump and fluid reservoir by Silastic tubing. The cylinders placed in the corpora are inflated by compression of the pump and are deflated after intercourse. Primary corpus cavernosum revascularization has been performed with mixed results, although recent attempts in microvascular repair have been encouraging.

Recently, a new pharmacologic strategy has been developed for the management of impotence. This therapy involves the injection of papaverine hydrochloride with phentolamine mesylate directly into the corpus cavernosum of the penis. Both of these agents cause vasodilation. Papaverine is a smooth muscle relaxant, and phentolamine is an alpha-adrenergic blocking agent. Intracavernous injection of the combination of papaverine and phentolamine results in an erection in responding men usually within 10 minutes. Following self-injection of the medications, the patient will have an erection for approximately 2 hours, during which time intercourse may be performed, often with ejaculation. Current recommendations are that the patient perform self-injection no more than once every 3 days. Patients are followed monthly with detailed history, physical examinations, and liver function tests as well as careful monitoring for side effects. Reported complications to date have been few; however, they include priapism, corpus cavernosum scarring, and potential hepatotoxicity. Although there is as yet a relatively limited experience with papaverine-phentolamine intracavernous injection, more widespread use will provide important information about safety and long-term efficacy. Intracavernous injection expands the surgeon's therapeutic options and, in selected patients, provides an alternative to prosthesis implantation, which will most likely play a major role in the management of impotence in the future.

Surgical interference with the sympathetic nerves may result in ejaculatory dysfunction. A certain percentage of patients who undergo retroperitoneal node dissection for metastatic testicular carcinoma, sympathectomy for peripheral vascular disease, abdominoperineal resection of the rectum, and aortoiliac surgical procedures will have ejaculatory dysfunction. Patients may experience retrograde ejaculation after a transurethral resection of the prostate when the bladder neck internal sphincter has been resected. Retrograde ejaculation as a result of damage to the sympathetic chain may sometimes be successfully treated by pharmacologic manipulation to increase the tone of the internal sphincter.

THE URETHRA[17, 23, 25]

Urethral Valves

Urethral valves are folds of the mucosa that arise from the floor of the prostatic urethra. Patients with urethral valves may present with mild or moderate obstruction with mild voiding problems, or they may present with severe obstruction and upper tract deterioration. Obstruction from urethral valves can result in dilation of the prostatic urethra and hypertrophy of the detrusor muscle with concomitant trabeculation and formation of vesical diverticula. In neonates with severe obstruction, a kidney can rupture and urinary ascites and pulmonary compromise can be present. These infants typically have a palpable, hypertrophied bladder with poor urinary stream. Excretory urogram will demonstrate the hydroureter and hydronephrosis and will show residual contrast medium on a post-void film. The voiding cystourethrogram demonstrates the wide dilation of the prostatic urethra, and shadows representing the valves may be visible. Cystourethroscopy is performed to identify the mucosal diaphragms in the prostatic urethra. The treatment depends upon the extent of disease. In children with only moderate anatomic changes, simple destruction of the valves is adequate; in children with more advanced disease, a temporary urinary diversion may be necessary.

Hypospadias

In hypospadias, which occurs in 8 per 1000 male infants, the urethral meatus is situated in a more proximal position than normal on the ventral aspect of the penis. The meatus can be located as far back as the perineum, but the more distal hypospadias is more common. Hypospadias tends to be familial and is often associated with chordee, a ventral curvature of the penis. It may also be associated with undescended testes or other genitourinary abnormalities. Severe hypospadias is more likely to be associated with other genitourinary anomalies. A variety of surgical repairs have been devised for the repair of hypospadias. The success rate for hypospadias repair has increased substantially owing to an understanding of the importance of meticulous handling of tissues and also to improved surgical techniques. Complications such as fistula formation and postoperative stricture occur in approximately 15 to 20 per cent of patients. These problems are kept to a minimum when reconstructions are performed by

surgeons who are experienced in dealing with this abnormality and who are familiar with the many surgical options available.

Epispadias

In epispadias, an uncommon disorder that occurs in 1 per 120,000 males, the urethral meatus opens on the dorsal aspect of the penis. Epispadias is often associated with exstrophy and the combination of epispadias and exstrophy occurs in 1 of 30,000 births. Epispadias can be glandular, penile, or penopubic. Incontinence is often associated with exstrophy and is seen with proximal involvement of the penis or pubis. Surgical repair is most often a multistage procedure, the objective of which is to achieve continence, normal sexual function, and a satisfactory cosmetic result.

Urethral Stricture Disease

Urethral stricture disease is usually secondary to trauma or inflammation. Gonococcal disease is a leading cause of inflammation, and frequent traumatic causes may include pelvic fracture, instrumentation, or long-term urinary catheter drainage. When the mucosa is traumatized, urine tends to extravasate and the resulting scarring causes a stricture. The patient with stricture may present with a urinary tract infection or a decrease in size and force of urinary stream. The symptoms may be identical to those seen in benign prostatic hypertrophy in an elderly male.

In the evaluation of a patient with stricture disease, a urinalysis, urine culture, intravenous pyelogram, and retrograde urethrogram should be obtained. The excretory urogram will identify bladder or upper tract problems that may be associated with the stricture. The retrograde urethrogram is the mainstay of diagnosis and will identify the caliber, location, and extent of stricture involvement.

In many cases, urethral strictures can be managed by dilation or direct vision internal urethrotomy. In selected patients with short strictures, internal urethrotomy, performed endoscopically with a small cutting instrument, has produced excellent results. When frequent dilation is required, when there are multiple or long strictures, when the dilation is too difficult, or when the stricture presents in a child, open surgical intervention is indicated. There are many one-stage and two-stage surgical procedures that may be used. The choice of procedure depends on the location and extent of the stricture and the preference of the surgeon (Fig. 13).

Inflammatory Disease

Neisseria gonorrhoeae is a gram-negative organism that is transmitted by sexual contact. The patient typically presents with a discharge, dysuria, and pyuria 2 to 10 days after sexual exposure. The diagnosis is made by culture or the urethral discharge and by identification of gram-negative intracellular diplococci on Gram stain or culture. The gonococcus invades the periurethral glands, and during the healing process there are inflammation and fibrosis, which cause scarring and stricture formation. Urethral stricture disease secondary to gonococcus tends to be more extensive than that due to simple trauma and often occurs in multiple areas of the urethra. Gonococcal infection can cause prostatitis and epididymitis, and it can result in infertility. The

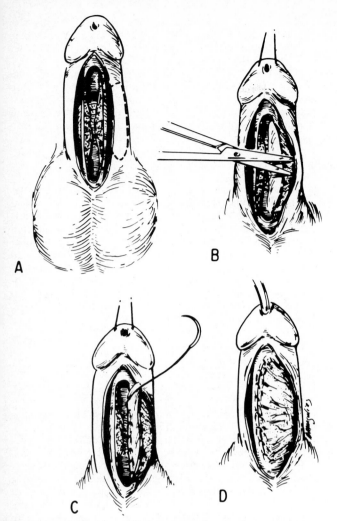

Figure 13. Repair of the penile urethral stricture by the Orandi-penile skin island flap urethroplasty method. (From Webster, G. D.: In Paulson, D. F. (Ed.): Genitourinary Surgery. New York, Churchill Livingstone, 1984.)

present recommendation for treatment of gonococcal infection is penicillin. The diagnosis of nongonococcal urethritis is made when urethritis and discharge are present but gonococcus is not identified. The two most common causes for nongonococcal urethritis are *Chlamydia trachomatis* and *Ureaplasma urealyticum*.

The treatment of nongonococcal urethritis consists of tetracycline or erythromycin. *Chlamydia* and *Ureaplasma* are found in a high percentage of patients who continue to have urethritis after treatment with penicillin for gonococcal urethritis, and frequently patients will have both gonococcal and nongonococcal urethritis.

Urethral Carcinoma

Urethral carcinoma is rare; there have been fewer than 500 cases reported in males. The etiology of urethral carcinoma is unclear, although it is associated with chronic irritation and tissue injury. The majority of males with urethral carcinoma present with a history of venereal dis-

ease or urethral stricture with chronic infection. Seventy-five per cent of the cases in males are squamous cell carcinoma, although transitional cell carcinoma and adenocarcinoma may also occur. Patients commonly present with obstructive symptoms, and the disease is often initially assumed to be a stricture. The treatment depends on the location of the tumor. If the tumor is present in the distal urethra, a partial urethrectomy may be adequate. When the tumor occurs in the bulbar urethra, the treatment is total penectomy and cystoprostatectomy. The 5-year survival rate for patients with urethral carcinoma in the penile urethra is approximately 40 per cent; when the disease occurs in the bulbar urethra, it is 10 per cent. The 5-year survival rate for urethral carcinoma in the female is from 10 to 40 per cent, depending on the location of the tumor.

THE SCROTUM[17, 20, 23]

Neoplasms

Scrotal tumors are uncommon and appear to be secondary to an occupational exposure to carcinogens such as soot, tar, creosote, or various petroleum products. There is a high incidence of scrotal carcinoma, for example, among chimney sweeps. In the management of a tumor localized to the scrotum, a partial scrotectomy is often sufficient; when inguinal nodes are involved, a bilateral inguinal lymph node dissection is indicated. Most scrotal tumors are of squamous cell origin, but other tumors such as rhabdomyosarcoma, leiomyosarcoma, and liposarcoma may also occur.

Gangrene

Scrotal gangrene is encountered in a number of different clinical situations. Gangrene of the scrotum can be a sequela of urinary tract extravasation, epididymitis, or prostatoseminovesiculitis. Fournier's gangrene is a particularly ominous variant of inflammatory disease of the scrotum usually seen in middle-aged or older men. This disease undergoes an explosive, fulminant course that presents in the scrotum and may involve the abdominal wall to the axillae within a short period of time. Fournier's gangrene is thought to be secondary to either a streptococcal or an anaerobic infection.

The initial treatment is directed to the underlying abnormality, such as the urinary extravasation, and the patient should immediately be placed on antibiotic therapy. Prompt surgical drainage of the edematous tissues or abscess is of benefit, and early extensive resection of involved tissues is essential. The mortality rate with Fournier's gangrene is high and optimal successful management lies in early diagnosis and prompt, aggressive treatment.

Hydrocele

A hydrocele is a serous collection of fluid that develops between the visceral and parietal layers of the tunica vaginalis. Primary hydroceles are seen in children and result from failure of closure of the processus vaginalis, an embryonic peritoneal diverticulum that traverses the inguinal canal and forms the tunica vaginalis. In a hydrocele that presents in a neonate, surgery is delayed up to 2 years because the patent processus vaginalis will usually close. In adults, secondary hydroceles tend to develop slowly over a period of time and are thought to be secondary to lymphatic outflow obstruction. The diagnosis of hydrocele can be made by transillumination of the scrotum. A hydrocele will transilluminate, whereas a hernia, tumor, or enlarged testis from orchitis will not. In the surgical repair of a hydrocele, the redundant portion of the hydrocele sac is resected and the remaining portion is everted and sutured behind the testis.

THE SPERMATIC CORD[17, 20, 23]

Varicocele

A varicocele is a dilation of the pampiniform plexus of veins above the testis. It is a common finding in young males and is most often seen on the left. The pampiniform plexus empties into the internal spermatic vein, which drains into the renal vein on the left and the vena cava on the right. The frequent occurrence of this abnormality on the left side is thought to be related to the fact that the left spermatic vein empties into the renal vein and the combination of upright position and incompetent valves may increase pressure and result in varicocele formation. A varicocele may also be associated with a renal tumor or other retroperitoneal neoplasm. The examination of a patient with a varicocele should be performed with the patient in the upright position. A palpable mass of veins will be present in the scrotum, and the testis may be atrophic. If the lesion becomes painful or is associated with infertility, repair is indicated. The repair involves the ligation of the internal spermatic vein in the inguinal canal or just above the internal ring.

Neoplasms

Most spermatic cord tumors are benign. Lipoma, fibroma, leiomyoma, and myxofibroma may occur in the spermatic cord and are treated by simple excision. Malignant tumors are usually sarcomas, such as leiomyosarcoma, liposarcoma, or rhabdomyosarcoma, that present in middle age and may initially be mistaken for an inguinal hernia. These tumors tend to metastasize early.

THE EPIDIDYMIS[17, 20, 23]

Epididymitis

Epididymitis may be caused by a number of organisms. In the male over the age of 35, *Escherichia coli* is the most common cause of epididymitis; in men under 35, *Chlamydia trachomatis* is the most common organism. Epididymitis may occur spontaneously, or it may follow a surgical procedure such as prostatectomy. If the patient has a urethral stricture or prostatic hypertrophy, bacteria can also pass back down the vas deferens to infect the epididymis. In the acute stage of epididymitis, there may be pain, swelling, and low-grade fever. Cystitis and prostatitis are commonly encountered, and the patient may present with a mild urethral discharge, leukocytosis, or a urinary tract infection. On physical examination, the scrotum is enlarged, spermatic cord tenderness may be present, and palpation reveals a thickened, painful epididymis. It can be difficult to differentiate epididymitis from testicular torsion. Slight elevation of the scrotum tends to make epididymitis less painful, but this maneuver exacerbates pain from testicular torsion. Epididymitis usually occurs in older men, although it is sometimes seen in younger males.

Treatment involves scrotal elevation and antibiotic therapy. Treatment should be initiated as soon as the diagnosis is made and should continue until symptoms are totally resolved. If acute epididymitis is allowed to become chronic, the epididymis can scar and infertility may result.

Neoplasms

Three fourths of epididymal tumors are benign. Adenomatoid tumor, the most common benign epididymal tumor, appears between the third and sixth decade and is thought to take its origin from müllerian mesenchymal elements. Leiomyoma can also appear in the epididymis. This benign tumor is multicentric, sometimes bilateral, and is associated with von Hippel–Lindau disease. Malignant fibrosarcoma and rhabdomyosarcoma occur in the epididymis of younger patients and are treated by radical removal of the cord, epididymis, and testis. Radiation therapy, chemotherapy, or both may also be used.

THE TESTIS[17, 20, 23]

Anorchia

Gonadal abnormalities may be divided into anomalies of development and anomalies of position. Testicular absence, termed anorchia, is an uncommon finding that occurs in approximately 1 in 5000 births. The fetal testis is essential to the development of the wolffian duct system and for the degeneration of the female müllerian duct system. For a male phenotype to develop, the testis must be present until at least the 16th week of gestation. Therefore, in a normal phenotypic male with an XY karyotype and anorchia, some type of injury must have occurred to the developing gonad after the 16th week such as torsion of the vessels, infection, or trauma. It must be established whether or not a testis is actually absent or only incompletely descended, since a testis that remains intra-abdominal has a 40-fold greater chance of developing a testicular tumor than a normal testis. In the evaluation of a patient with bilateral nonpalpable testes, human chorionic gonadotropin (hCG) is administered. If there is no rise in serum testosterone after hCG is given, it is assumed that there is no testicular tissue present and no further investigation is needed. A spermatic arteriogram or venogram can be useful in locating a nonpalpable testis, as can a pelvic CT scan. If the presence or absence of a nonpalpable testis is unresolved, surgical exploration is indicated. The finding of a blind ending vas deferens and spermatic vessels is considered diagnostic of anorchia. In either anorchia or monorchia, a Silastic testicular prosthesis can be placed in the scrotum. A man with bilateral anorchia managed with testosterone supplementation may have normal sexual function, although he will be infertile.

Undescended Testes

There are two types of undescended testes: an *ectopic* testis lies outside the normal path of descent, and a *cryp-*

torchid testis is one in which descent has been arrested along the correct pathway before reaching the scrotum.

Ectopic testes are thought to be due to an abnormality of the gubernaculum, which normally guides the descent of the testis. Ectopic testes may be found in the superficial inguinal region, over the pubis, in the perineum, or, rarely, under the skin at the base of the penis. *Cryptorchidism* occurs in 3.4 per cent in full-term infants. Fifty per cent of the time, these testes will descend during the first month of life. Cryptorchidism is thought to be due to an intrinsic testicular defect, deficient hormonal stimulation, or an abnormality of the gubernaculum. A cryptorchid testis may be found in the abdomen, upper or lower inguinal canal, or high scrotum. The majority of these testes lie in the inguinal canal, although 15 per cent will be abdominal.

Some clinicians administer a trial of gonadotropins in order to induce an undescended testis to descend properly, and success has been reported with this therapy in up to 20 per cent of patients. If hormone therapy fails or if an inguinal hernia is present, surgery is indicated. The surgical goal of placing a viable testis in the scrotum is sometimes not possible because of insufficient length of the vascular pedicle. A number of alternate approaches have been developed to deal with this problem. The surgeon may place the testis in the scrotum after dividing the spermatic vessels, taking care to preserve the collateral circulation to the vas deferens, cremasteric muscle, and scrotum. Another approach involves a two-stage procedure in which the testis is brought down to the inguinal canal in the first stage and at a later time the testis is placed in the scrotum. A third approach involves the microvascular anastomosis of the spermatic vessels to the inferior epigastric artery and vein. Surgery is usually performed before the child reaches the age of 2; there is permanent damage to a testis left in place past 5 years of age.

Torsion[17, 23]

In testicular torsion, a disease of prepubertal and pubertal males, there is incomplete reflection of the tunica vaginalis on the testis and epididymis. This deformity permits the testis to rotate within the tunica vaginalis and causes strangulation of the blood supply. The testis will undergo permanent damage unless the abnormality is promptly corrected. Young males with testicular torsion are typically awakened from sleep with scrotal pain and may present with nausea, vomiting, and scrotal edema. On physical examination, the testis on the affected side is often higher than the opposite side and it may have a transverse position. The testis is generally very tender, and elevation does not relieve the pain as it often does with epididymitis. Radionuclide testicular scan and Doppler stethoscopic examination may be helpful to determine vascularity in an equivocal case. However, any young male with a normal urinalysis who presents with a painful scrotum should be strongly considered for exploration.

Once the decision to operate has been made, the procedure should be performed as soon as possible because the greater the amount of time that elapses between the onset of symptoms and surgical repair, the greater the chance for testicular loss. In the surgical procedure, performed through a transcrotal incision, the testis is uncoiled and an absorbable suture is placed to secure the testis from rotating again (Fig. 14). The contralateral side is also secured by a suture because the deformity tends to be bilateral and the contralateral side is at increased risk for torsion at a later date.

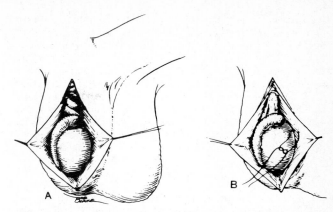

Figure 14. In a testicular torsion repair, the cord is straightened and a suture is placed through the testis and sac. (From Donohue, J. P.: In Paulson, D. F. (Ed.): Genitourinary Surgery. New York, Churchill Livingstone, 1984.)

Orchitis[10, 20, 23]

Acute infection may reach the testis by a hematogenous route, by lymph channels, or down through the vas deferens. Any agent causing bacteremia can infect the testis, and *Escherichia coli, Klebsiella*, streptococcus, and staphylococcus are not uncommonly encountered. The most common causes of bacterial orchitis are epididymitis, prostatitis, or urinary tract infection. Treatment depends on the extent to which the testis is involved, and in most cases specific antibiotic therapy is sufficient. Rarely, the testis is suppurative to the extent that orchiectomy is the only alternative. Orchitis can occur with a number of mycotic or viral illnesses, but mumps is the most common cause of testicular inflammatory disease. Mumps orchitis is rare before puberty, but it occurs in 18 per cent of adult males who contract the disease. Seventy per cent of the time, patients will have only unilateral involvement and 50 per cent of involved testes will later show testicular atrophy. The seminiferous tubules in the testis are particularly sensitive to infection and inflammation. Often the germ cells are damaged in an atrophied testis, but the interstitial cells continue to function and produce testosterone.

Testicular Neoplasms[10, 20, 23]

Carcinoma of the testis has an incidence of 2.8 per 100,000 and is the most common solid neoplasm occurring in males between the ages of 15 and 45. Testicular carcinoma is rare in the black population and only 3 per cent occurs in children. The germ cell tumors that account for 95 per cent of testicular neoplasms include classic seminoma, spermatocytic seminoma, embryonal carcinoma, yolk sac tumor, teratoma, and choriocarcinoma. Testicular tumors tend to spread early to the retroperitoneal lymph nodes. The initial embryologic development of the gonads originates in the area adjacent to the developing nephrogenic tissue, and even though the testis descends to the scrotum, the primary lymph drainage remains retroperitoneal. Testicular carcinoma is divided into three stages: *Stage I* is confined to the testis; *Stage II* has spread to the retroperitoneum; and *Stage III* has metastasized outside the retroperitoneum.

A patient with a suspected testicular tumor should always undergo an inguinal exploration because a transcrotal approach may spread tumor and complicate future management. In staging of a testicular mass suspected of being malignant, the serum tumor markers, alpha-fetoprotein (AFP) and hCG, are measured. These tumor markers are important in the initial evaluation of a patient with a suspected testicular tumor and in the surveillance period after removal of the tumor. Elevated tumor markers may be the earliest indication that the tumor has recurred and are helpful in following response to chemotherapy. An abdominal CT scan or lymphangiogram provides information about the presence of retroperitoneal metastases.

The role of surgical procedures in the management of testicular carcinoma is evolving. Retroperitoneal node dissection (Fig. 15) is used to assess the extent of spread of testicular carcinoma to the retroperitoneum and is commonly performed after orchiectomy in Stage I nonseminomatous carcinoma and in Stage II disease either before or after chemotherapy. A retroperitoneal node dissection may also be performed in Stage III nonseminomatous testicular carcinoma after chemotherapy in order to identify the presence of persistent malignant disease or to remove teratoma. Metastatic nonseminomatous testicular carcinoma may undergo degeneration to teratoma during chemotherapy. This teratomatous tissue needs to be removed because it may invade local structures, although it is not considered malignant tissue. The use of combination chemotherapy has revolutionized the treatment of nonseminomatous testicular carcinoma and has significantly improved survival. Disease-free survival for Stage I nonseminomatous testicular carcinoma is 99 per cent, 87

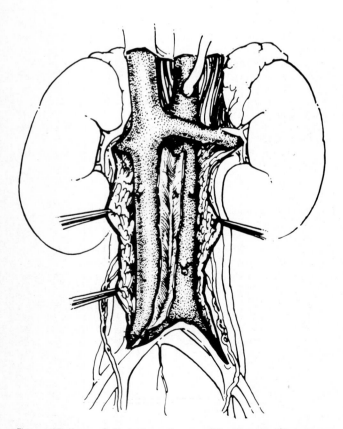

Figure 15. Area of dissection of a suprahilar and infrahilar retroperitoneal node dissection for testicular carcinoma. (From Donohue, J. P.: In Paulson, D. F. (Ed.): Genitourinary Surgery. New York, Churchill Livingstone, 1984.)

per cent for Stage II, and 57 per cent for Stage III testicular carcinoma.

SEMINOMA

Seminomas tend to occur in the fifth and sixth decade of life and represent about 40 per cent of testicular tumors seen in adults. Histologically, these have a uniform appearance with distinct cell borders, round nuclei, and aggregates of lymphocytes. The hCG may be elevated in a patient with seminoma, but an elevated AFP indicates the presence of nonseminomatous elements. The prognosis for early stage seminoma is very good.

The standard treatment for Stage I, II, and III seminoma involves radiation therapy. Recently, it has been observed that seminoma responds to combination chemotherapy, and trials are in progress to evaluate the use of chemotherapy with or without radiation therapy for Stage II or Stage III disease. Some advocate the use of retroperitoneal lymphadenectomy in a patient with seminoma to exclude a microscopic focus of a nonseminomatous tumor, but this is not a uniformly held view and most physicians initiate treatment without lymphadenectomy.

SPERMATOCYTIC SEMINOMA

Spermatocytic seminoma occurs in men over 65 and is considered a benign tumor. Histologically, these tumors form solid sheets of cells of varying sizes without a lymphocytic infiltrate. Patients with this tumor are treated conservatively with orchiectomy. Only three deaths from spermatocytic seminoma have been reported.

EMBRYONAL CARCINOMA

A highly malignant tumor, embryonal carcinoma represents 20 per cent of testicular tumors in adults. This tumor forms glandular and papillary structures with irregular nuclei, hemorrhage, and necrosis. Serum AFP may be elevated, but hCG is not elevated in pure embryonal carcinoma. This tumor characteristically metastasizes rapidly to the retroperitoneum or lungs.

YOLK SAC TUMOR

The yolk sac tumor accounts for 60 per cent of testicular tumors in children. This is a particularly malignant tumor that rarely presents in adults in its pure form but commonly accompanies embryonal carcinoma or teratocarcinoma. Histologically, this tumor consists of anastomosing tubular and acinar structures. Serum AFP elevations are seen commonly, and yolk sac tumor is thought to be related to embryonal carcinoma.

TERATOMA

Teratomas account for 7 per cent of testicular tumors in adults and 40 per cent in children. Histologically, this tumor combines elements of fetal and adult structures originating from three germ cell layers: endoderm, ectoderm, and mesoderm. This tumor is considered benign in children, but in adults a significant number of teratomas metastasize.

CHORIOCARCINOMA

In its pure form choriocarcinoma is a rare, aggressive tumor. Choriocarcinoma often occurs mixed with other germ cell elements and consists of two cell types, syncytio-trophoblasts and cytotrophoblasts. Serum hCG levels are typically very high with choriocarcinoma. The primary tumor in the testis can often go unnoticed, and the patient may present with symptoms of advanced metastatic disease.

NON–GERM CELL TUMORS

Although non–germ cell tumors of stromal origin tend to be benign, 10 per cent are malignant. Leydig cell tumors and Sertoli cell tumors are the most common stromal tumors. Evaluation includes tumor marker determination, CT scan or lymphangiogram as well as complete endocrine evaluation. If the CT scan and lymphangiogram are normal, these patients do not generally require a retroperitoneal lymphadenectomy and may be managed conservatively with orchiectomy alone.

INFERTILITY[17, 20, 23]

Infertility has become an increasingly common problem that affects approximately 14 per cent of couples. A couple is not considered to have an infertility problem until there has been unprotected intercourse without conception for a period of no less than 12 months. The evaluation of an infertile couple includes an examination of both partners, and in approximately 50 per cent of the cases the cause of infertility has been found in the male.

A wide range of abnormalities can have an adverse effect on male fertility. There may be germ cell aplasia, a congenital defect in development of the seminal cells, or spermatogenic arrest, a developmental abnormality of maturation. Cryptorchidism is associated with an increased infertility rate. The cryptorchid testis is subjected to a higher temperature than the normal testis and is also likely to have other associated developmental abnormalities besides failure of descent. Mumps orchitis or radiation orchitis can cause damage to the spermatogenic cells. The ductal system can become obstructed by inflammation caused by epididymitis or vasitis, or there can be a congenital absence of the vas deferens. Pituitary abnormalities can also lead to abnormalities in testicular function. In hypopituitarism a lack of FSH can cause maturation delay of the spermatogenic cells. Pituitary hyperfunction can have an adverse effect on the testis through LH or indirectly through the effect of hyperadrenalism. In hypogonadism from primary testicular failure, an example of which is *Klinefelter's syndrome,* poorly formed seminiferous tubules show only marginal function. A varicocele may be associated with a decreased sperm count, an increase in immature forms, and a decrease in motility.

In the evaluation of a couple with infertility, it is important to obtain information about the duration of sexual relations without preventative measures, the method of birth control, and the frequency and timing of coitus. Any problem relating to testicular descent, the onset of puberty, or a history of prior surgical procedures should be identified. Information should be sought about urinary tract infections, venereal disease, mumps, renal disease, diabetes, tuberculosis, or other febrile or viral illnesses. Medication history is informative, since drugs can interfere with spermatogenesis, erection, or ejaculation. An occupational history should elicit information about exposure to prolonged heat or chemicals. Information about previous pregnancies or offspring or a family history of testicular atrophy, hypogonadism, or cryptorchidism should also be identified.

On physical examination, general habitus, hair distribution, and secondary sexual characteristics are noted. The neurologic examination will identify visual field defects, anosmia, or defects in rectal sphincter tone or perineal sensation. In the genitourinary examination, particular attention is given to evaluation of testicular size and consistency, inspection of the epididymis and vas deferens, and examination of the penis and corpora cavernosa. Laboratory evaluation includes urinalysis, semen analysis, serum testosterone, FSH, and LH. A buccal smear is performed if Klinefelter's syndrome or other chromosomal abnormality is suspected. A semen specimen should be obtained after 3 days' abstinence. The semen is examined for volume, motility, count, maturation, and presence of cell clumping. If the volume is low, below 3 to 5 ml., artificial insemination with the husband's semen may be successful. If the volume is high, a split-ejaculate technique is recommended. Normal motility should be seen in at least 50 per cent of the sperm cells. Treatment of patients with low motility is rarely successful. If clumps of white blood cells are seen, the patient may be treated with erythromycin or doxycycline (Vibramycin). Sperm counts of less than 20,000,000 per ml. on three semen analyses at least 1 week apart are considered low, and these patients are generally at least subfertile. Azospermia may be due to spermatogenic maturation arrest, Sertoli-only syndrome, Klinefelter's syndrome, or ductal obstruction. A serum fructose level will indicate whether the seminal vesicles are present. A testicular biopsy is indicated in certain instances, such as azospermia, and can provide information about the etiology of infertility and prognosis for treatment.

INTERSEX[5, 20, 23]

A newborn infant who presents with ambiguous genitalia has an urgent problem that needs immediate evaluation. An early decision should be made about the gender status. The choice of gender often depends upon the infant's anatomic characteristics. If there is inadequate phallus, the child should be reared as a female regardless of genetic sex. There are four major intersex abnormalities in newborns: (1) female pseudohermaphroditism, (2) male pseudohermaphroditism, (3) mixed gonadal dysgenesis, and (4) true hermaphroditism.

Female Pseudohermaphroditism

Female pseudohermaphrodites are generally genetic females who have been exposed to endogenous or exogenous androgens during development. In congenital adrenal hyperplasia, the most common type of female pseudohermaphroditism, there is an overproduction of adrenal androgen that virilizes the female fetus. These patients have normal female internal structures with partially masculinized external genitalia. With adrenal hyperplasia, there is often excess mineralocorticoid; this leads to sodium retention and hypertension, although there may be a deficit in mineralocorticoid production resulting in salt loss. The enzyme abnormality in adrenogenital syndrome is a deficiency in either 21-hydroxylase, 11-hydroxylase, or 3 β-dehydrogenase. The diagnosis is made by the determination of elevated urinary ketosteroids. Female pseudohermaphrodites are reared as females and may require clitoral reduction, labial-scrotal reduction, and vaginoplasty.

Male Pseudohermaphroditism

Male pseudohermaphrodites are genetic males who have gonads but incompletely masculinized genital ducts and external genitalia. This syndrome can result from (1) failure of testicular differentiation, (2) failure of secretion of müllerian inhibitory factor, (3) failure to target tissue to respond to testosterone, or (4) failure of conversion of testosterone to dihydrotestosterone owing to deficiency of 5α-reductase. There is a broad variation in presentation, and these patients may present with only mild hypospadius or complete testicular feminization. Patients with testicular feminization typically present as fully developed females who do not experience menarche. These patients are supported as females and undergo bilateral orchiectomy of the undescended testes to lessen the chance of developing testicular malignancies.

Mixed Gonadal Dysgenesis

Mixed gonadal dysgenesis is the second most common cause of ambiguous genitalia in the newborn. These children often have karyotypic mosaicism, the etiology of which is unknown. They present with asymmetry of ambiguous external genitalia, a dysgenetic testis on one side and a streak gonad on the other side. A uterus, vagina, and at least one fallopian tube are commonly present, and these children are most often reared as females. If they are assigned to male gender, they require multiple surgical procedures for reconstruction of the external genitalia. There is an increased risk of neoplasm in the dysgenetic gonads, and the current recommendation is for early removal.

True Hermaphroditism

True hermaphroditism is a rare disorder in which both ovarian and testicular tissue is present. There is a variable differentiation of both the internal and external genitalia, and the external genitalia are ambiguous. Cryptorchidism and hypospadias are common, and a uterus is present. The management of true hermaphroditism is dependent on the age of diagnosis, functional capacity of the gonads, and degree of development of the phallus.

Transsexualism

Transsexualism[8] is a psychiatric condition in which a person feels that he or she has the wrong physical sex. These patients, who are normal anatomically, seek to change their physical appearance to conform to the image that they have of themselves as a member of the opposite sex. Psychotherapy may be unsuccessful in reorienting these patients to their true anatomic sex, and after intensive evaluation by a multidisciplinary group transsexual surgery may be elected.

In this procedure, a bilateral orchiectomy and partial urethrectomy are performed, a perineal urethrostomy is created and a neovagina is constructed between the bladder and rectum. Surgery for female transsexuals to male is technically feasible but less satisfactory than surgery for male transsexuals. The early enthusiasm for this procedure has abated, and the long-term role of surgery in the treatment of this condition is as yet incompletely defined.

SELECTED REFERENCES

Glenn, J. F. (Ed.): Urologic Surgery, 3rd ed. Philadelphia, J. B. Lippincott Co., 1983.

This text, with over 100 contributors, provides descriptions and artistic presentations of the vast array of operations performed in urologic surgery. These are descriptions of preoperative and postoperative management as well as detailed explanations of indications for surgery and specifics of surgical techniques.

Paulson, D. F. (Ed.): Genitourinary Surgery. New York, Churchill Livingstone, 1984.

This two-volume work comprises contributions from 15 recognized authorities in the field. It details clearly the embryology, anatomy, and physiology of each organ in the genitourinary system and provides an excellent series of illustrations that clearly depict both basic and complex urologic surgical procedures.

Walsh, P. C., Gittes, R. F., Perlmutter, A. D., and Stamey, T. A. (Eds.): Campbell's Urology, 5th ed. Philadelphia, W. B. Saunders Company, 1986.

This is a highly regarded and recently updated textbook which has long been a standard in the field. It is highly recommended.

Witten, D. M., Utz, D., and Myers, G. (Eds.): Emmett's Clinical Urography, 4th ed. Philadelphia, W. B. Saunders Company, 1977.

This three-volume work provides complete consideration of the entire spectrum of radiographic techniques used in the diagnosis of genitourinary disease. The reference provides a detailed explanation of the rationale behind each test and a description of how each test is performed. It contains excellent illustrations of radiographs demonstrating the entire scope of uroradiographic diagnosis.

REFERENCES

1. Bergman, H. (Ed.): The Ureter. New York, Springer-Verlag, 1981.
2. Bennington, J. L., and Beckwith, J. B.: Tumors of the Kidney, Renal Pelvis, and Ureter. Washington, D.C., Armed Forces Institute of Pathology, 1975.
3. Bradley, W. E.: Innervation of the male urinary bladder. *In* Kaufman, J. J., and Raz, S. (Eds.): Urol. Clin. North Am., 5:279, 1978.
4. DeVita, V. T., Hellman, S., and Rosenberg, S. A. (Eds.): Cancer, Principles and Practices of Oncology, 2nd ed. Philadelphia, J. B. Lippincott Co., 1985.
5. Donahoe, P. K., and Crawford, J. D.: Management of neonates and children with male pseudohermaphroditism. J. Pediatr. Surg., 12:1045, 1977.
6. Eckstein, H. B., Hohenfellener, R., and Williams, D. I.: Surgical Pediatric Urology. Philadelphia, W. B. Saunders Company, 1977.
7. Finlayson, B., and Roth, R. A.: Stones, Clinical Management of Urolithiasis. *In* Lippertino, J. A. (Ed.): International Prospectives in Urology. Baltimore, Williams & Wilkins, 1983.
8. Glenn, J. F. (Ed.): Urologic Surgery, 3rd ed. Philadelphia, J. B. Lippincott Co., 1983.
9. Javadpour, N. (Ed.): Principles and Management of Urologic Cancer. Baltimore, Williams & Wilkins, 1983.
10. Kaufman, J. J. (Ed.): Current Urologic Therapy, 2nd ed. Philadelphia, W. B. Saunders Company, 1986.
11. Kelalis, P. P., King, L. R., and Belman, A. B. (Eds.): Clinical Pediatric Urology, 2nd ed. Philadelphia, W. B. Saunders Company, 1985.
12. Krane, R. J., and Siroky, M. B. (Eds.): Clinical Neuro-urology. Boston, Little, Brown and Co., 1979.
13. Matonoski, G. M., and Elliott, E. A.: Bladder cancer epidemiology. Epidemiol. Rev., 3:203, 1981.
14. Mostofi, F. K.: Testis, Scrotum, and Penis. *In* Anderson, W. A. D., and Kissane, J. M. (Eds.): Pathology. St. Louis, C. V. Mosby Co., 1977, p. 1013.
15. Mostofi, F. K., and Davis, C. J.: Genitourinary pathology course proceedings. Washington, D.C., Armed Forces Institute of Pathology, 1984.
16. Munday, G. R., Ibbotson, K. J., D'Souza, S. M., Simpson, E. L., Jacobs, J. W., and Martin, T. J.: The hypercalcemia of cancer: Clinical implications and pathogenic mechanisms. N. Engl. J. Med., 310:1718, 1984.
17. Paulson, D. F. (Ed.): Genitourinary Surgery. New York, Churchill Livingstone, 1984.
17a. Rosenberg, S. A.: Adoptive immunotherapy of cancer using lymphokine activated killer cells and recombinant interleukin-2. *In* DeVita, V. T., Hellman, S., and Rosenberg, S. A. (Eds.): Important Advances in Oncology 1986. Philadelphia, J. B. Lippincott Company, 1986.
18. Sabiston, D. C., Jr. (Ed.): Davis-Christopher Textbook of Surgery. Philadelphia, W. B. Saunders Company, 1981.

18a. Sidi, A. A., Cameron, J. S., Duffy, L. M., and Lange, P. H.: Intravenous drug-induced erections in the management of male erectile dysfunction: Experience with 100 patients. J. Urol., *135*:704, 1986.

19. Skinner, D. G., and deKernion, J. B. (Eds.): Genitourinary Cancer. Philadelphia, W. B. Saunders Company, 1978.

20. Smith, D. R. (Ed.): General Urology, 10th ed. Los Altos, Calif., Lang Medical Publications, 1981.

21. Smith, R. B., and Skinner, D. G. (Eds.): Complications of Urologic Surgery. Philadelphia, W. B. Saunders Company, 1976.

22. Strewler, G. J., Williams, R. D., and Nissenson, R. A.: Human renal carcinoma cells produce hypercalcemia in the nude mouse and a novel protein recognized by parathyroid hormone receptors. J. Clin. Invest., *71*:769, 1983.

23. Walsh, P. C., Gittes, R. F., Perlmutter, A. D., and Stamey, T. A. (Eds.): Campbell's Urology, 5th ed. Philadelphia, W. B. Saunders Company, 1986.

24. Williams, D. I., and Johnson, T. H. (Eds.): Paediatric Urology, 2nd ed., London, Butterworth Scientific, 1982.

25. Witten, D. M., Myer, G. H., and Utz, D. C. (Eds.): Emmett's Clinical Urography, 4th ed. Philadelphia, W. B. Saunders Company, 1977.

26. Zorgniotti, A. W., and Lefleur, R. S.: Auto-injections of the corpus cavernosum with a vasoactive drug combination for vasculogenic impotence. J. Urol., *133*:39, 1985.

NEUROSURGERY

DENNIS E. BULLARD, M.D.

> Perhaps if one were to cut out a ... single convolution of the brain, and paste it to a page, it would speak with more eloquence than all the words of Balzac.
>
> *Richard Selzer*, Mortal Lessons: Notes on the Art of Surgery[23]

40

The neurosurgeon has the privilege of dealing intimately with the human nervous system, and to do it well requires a basic knowledge of the function of the nervous system, a standard of technical competence, and a committed concern for the patient.

HISTORIC ASPECTS

From skeletons dating back to the neolithic period, there is strong archaeologic evidence that trepanation (creation of holes in the skull) was performed in widely separated parts of the world at the beginning of human civilization.[27] Trepanated skulls have been found among pre-Columbian civilizations, the later Inca culture in South America, and neolithic peoples in nearly all countries of Europe. This practice, described in great detail in the Greco-Roman literature, continued to be utilized into the 19th century by primitive African, Micronesian, and South American cultures. The context for these procedures is open to intriguing speculation; during the renaissance of medicine in the Salerno school in the ninth century A.D., trepanation was proscribed to treat mania or melancholy and to allow the escape of noxious humors. Later it was used for similar reasons, including treatment of headaches and trauma.

The concept of the nervous system held by earlier cultures is equally fascinating. As early as during the Babylonian civilization, an association between headache and fever was made. In the Edwin Smith papyrus, which dates to the second millennium B.C., are descriptions of the external surface of the brain and cerebrospinal fluid (CSF). Hippocrates covered several neurologic topics, including epilepsy, compression of the spinal cord, and open head injuries. However, over the next 2000 years, progress was limited, although increased knowledge of the anatomy and physiology of the central nervous system (CNS) was made by such pioneers as Willis, Vesalius, Morgagni, Eustachius, and Fallopius. It was not until the late nineteenth century that significant advances in clinical neurosurgery were made. Then, as now, progress in neurosurgery was made possible by developments in other areas, specifically the development of anesthesia and asepsis. In Britain, Macewen, Professor of Surgery at the University of Glasgow, developed an interest in neurosurgery and, utilizing many of the principles learned from his mentor Lister, applied aseptic surgical techniques successfully to the treatment of intracranial abscesses. With these techniques and the con-

cept of cerebral localization, which had been developed through the German, French, and British schools of neurology, Godlee in 1884 became the first surgeon to correctly localize and operate upon an intracranial tumor. However, it is Horsley who is remembered as the neurosurgical figure of that period. In 1887, taking advantage of the clinical acumen of the neurologist Gowers, Horsley successfully removed a neoplasm from the spinal canal. Over the next 20 years, his contributions to neurosurgery were numerous, including pioneering work with Clarke in stereotactic neurosurgery and initial efforts in the treatment of trigeminal neuralgia by retrogasserian neurotomy.

This close working relationship between neurologists and surgeons provided the early foundation for surgical exploration of the nervous system. It was at this time that Cushing, a brilliant neurosurgeon, applied formidable talents solely to the development of the field. Using the principles learned from Halsted, Cushing developed the surgical techniques necessary to operate successfully upon the human brain. His contributions to neurosurgery are encyclopedic and include the development of the blood pressure cuff, the classification of brain tumors, the development of the electrocautery, and the establishment of a formal neurosurgical residency training regimen. It is upon this pioneering work that the modern discipline of neurosurgery is based.

ANATOMY

The nervous system is composed of nerve cells (neurons), which have a body, axon, and several dendrites. The neuron generates and propagates an electrical signal from the body down the axon and is transmitted via a synapse with other cells. The neurotransmitters released at the synapse vary and are currently known to include acetylcholine, dopamine, norepinephrine, serotonin, gamma aminobutyric acid (GABA), and glycine. The supporting cells of the nervous system include the glia and the oligodendrocytes; the latter provide myelination for the CNS, compared with the Schwann cells, which provide myelination for the peripheral nervous system (PNS). This division between central and peripheral nervous system is based primarily on whether the components are inside or outside the skull and vertebral column. The CNS is composed of the brain, which lies within the skull, and the spinal cord, which lies within the vertebral column. The brain is composed of the cerebrum, the brainstem, and the cerebellum. In general, higher cortical functions reside in the cerebrum, whereas the brainstem serves as both a connection between the higher and lower centers and the center for most visceral and autonomic functions such as heart rate and respiration. The cerebellum provides coordination between the cerebrum and the spinal cord and appears to act primarily as a modulator.[6]

During the embryologic formation of the nervous system, a cavity is formed within the cerebral vesicle, which becomes the *lateral ventricle*.[11] Within the diencephalic portion of the midbrain, a narrow chamber called the *third ventricle* forms; this communicates with the paired lateral ventricles via the foramen of Monro. Inferiorly, the third ventricle becomes a small passage within the midbrain, which opens into the *fourth ventricle* situated in the metencephalon (*cerebellum* and *pons*) and myelencephalon (*medulla*). The fourth ventricle opens into the *subarachnoid space*, which in turn communicates over the entire CNS. Within the spinal cord, a residual small spinal canal, lined by the same ependymal cells that line the other ventricular chambers, exists. Cerebral spinal fluid is formed primarily from the *choroid plexus*, which is present in the lateral, third, and fourth ventricles. This fluid exits from the fourth ventricle, surrounds the brain and spinal cord, and eventually is absorbed into the venous system by way of the arachnoid granulations that surround the superior sagittal sinus, which is formed by the dural covering layers between the two cerebral hemispheres. Normally, CSF is produced at a constant rate of 0.35 ml. per minute in adults and 0.15 ml. per minute in infants. In adults, the total volume is in the range of 150 ml. The *dura*, one of the three meningeal layers that surround the nervous system, is the outer, tough, connective tissue layer that lies immediately adjacent to the bone of the skull and vertebral column. Within the dura is the *arachnoid*, a delicate membrane that attaches the dura to the pia mater and lies immediately adjacent to the brain. The space within the arachnoid is filled with CSF and is known as the subarachnoid space. The *pia mater* is closely attached to the external surface of the brain and extends into the sulci and fissures of the cerebrum and cerebellum, fusing with the dura and perineurium of the cranial and peripheral nerves as they exit the CNS. The blood vessels supplying the CNS are surrounded by the pia as they penetrate the nervous system.

Although the adult brain represents only 2 per cent of the total body mass, it utilizes 20 per cent of the total body oxygen consumption, 25 per cent of the entire body's glucose consumption, and 20 per cent of the total cardiac output each minute. It is extremely sensitive to reduction in any of these basic components, with prolonged deprivation resulting in irreversible brain damage. These components are all provided to the brain by the cerebral circulation. This is formed by the paired internal carotid and vertebral arteries, which join around the brainstem to form the circle of Willis (Fig. 1). This anastomosing circuit allows collateral flow for the 800 ml. of blood per minute, which is normally provided the adult brain. The average regional blood flow is approximately 50 ml. per 100 gm. per minute, varying between 15 to 20 ml. per 100 gm. per minute in the cerebral white matter to 65 to 75 ml. per 100 gm. per minute in the gray matter. At blood flow less than 12 ml. per 100 gm. per minute, cell death occurs. The rate of cerebral blood flow is a function of the cerebral perfusion pressure (CPP) and the cerebral vascular resistance (CVR). In turn, the CPP is a function of the systemic mean arterial pressure (SAP) and the intracranial pressure (ICP).

$$\frac{CBF\ =\ CPP/CVR}{CPP\ =\ SAP\ -\ ICP}$$

In adults, the ICP can be measured either by insertion of a catheter into the lateral ventricle or by the more standard lumbar puncture into the lumbar subarachnoid space. In adults, normal values for ICP are 40 to 210 mm. of CSF. Normally, the brain is protected from systemic blood by the blood-brain barrier (BBB). Anatomically and physiologically, this barrier prevents the movement of ionic compounds, molecules of large molecular weight, and polar

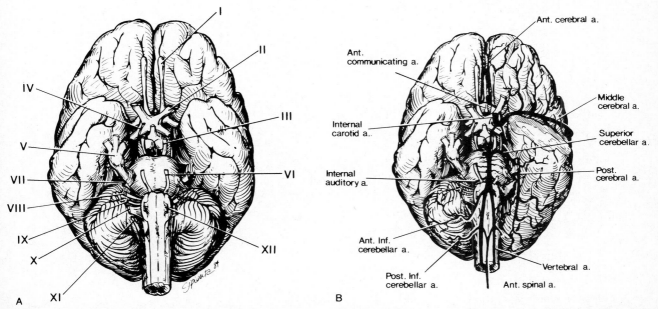

Figure 1. The brain. A, A basal view of the brain and upper spinal cord demonstrating the cranial nerves. B, A basal view of the brain demonstrating in a schematic fashion the vascular supply. (Modified from DeJong, R. N.: The Neurologic Examination, 4th Ed. Hagerstown, Md., Harper & Row, 1979.)

nonelectrolytes from the blood into the brain. Although the structure of this barrier is not precisely known, anatomically the tight junction of the cerebral capillary endothelia appears to form an important role. The BBB is extremely important because it may preclude the passage of therapeutic agents from the systemic circulation into the brain.

CLINICAL DIAGNOSIS AND MANAGEMENT

Patient History

It has been often stated that the diagnosis in most neurosurgical patients can be made by a carefully elicited, pertinent history from the patient and family.[6] This provides not only an assessment of the neurologic dysfunction but also insight into the patient and the environment. Because neurologic diseases often impair the ability of the patient to relate the history accurately, it is crucial that family and friends be consulted for confirmation and additional data. Inconsistencies in the history must be rigorously pursued to obtain an exact understanding of the patient's problem. With the exception of certain emergent situations, a detailed and complete history should be obtained *before* the neurologic examination. Routinely, a general physical ex-

amination is performed, followed by evaluation of higher cortical functioning and mental status, detailed evaluation of the cranial nerves, motor, sensory and reflex testing, and finally evaluation of coordination to include gait and station. A thorough examination of the nervous system is an endeavor requiring much practice and study. Examination of comatose patients, psychiatric patients, infants, or small children, and those in emergent situations requires special talent.

Localizing Concepts

With increasing reliability of imaging techniques for the CNS, it has become apparent that the rigidly held localizing principles previously taught do not always exist. Nevertheless, certain localizing concepts should be learned by all interested in the CNS.[6]

In general, the *cerebral functions* of the left hemisphere control the motor and sensory functioning of the contralateral face and body. In right-handed individuals, the left frontal, temporal, and parietal regions generally control expressive and receptive speech (Fig. 2). The hemisphere controlling these language functions is termed the *dominant* hemisphere. Other localizing hemispheric regions include the frontal eye fields. With irritative lesions, such as an

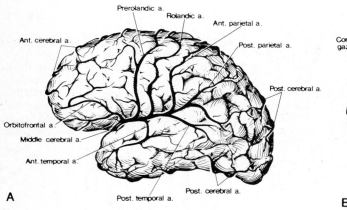

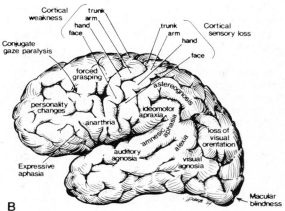

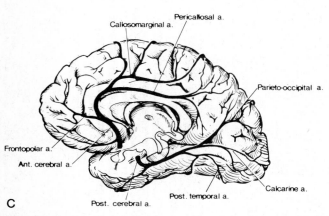

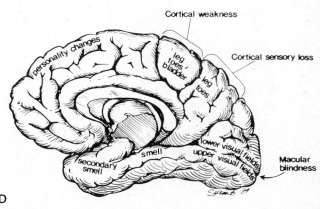

Figure 2. Cerebral hemisphere. A, Lateral view, showing the generalized arterial distribution. B, Lateral view (dominant hemisphere), showing a schematic picture of the deficits associated with lesions in certain areas of the brain. C, Medial view, showing an idealized arterial vascular pattern. D, Medial view, demonstrating functional areas and the resultant deficits associated with lesions. (Modified from DeJong, R. N.: The Neurologic Examination, 4th Ed. Hagerstown, Md., Harper & Row, 1979.)

epileptic focus, stimulation in this region results in the head and eyes turning toward the opposite side. In a destructive lesion, such as a stroke, the converse is true, and the eyes turn to the affected side. The motor control previously mentioned is localized in the precentral gyrus or motor strip. This region is topographically oriented so that the body control is organized with the face, tongue, hand, arm, and trunk along the lateral hemisphere with the leg and foot along the medial portion of the hemisphere. The postcentral gyrus is involved with cortical sensation, and lesions in this region cause a loss of discriminative sensation. Primary sensory modality, such as light touch and pain, appears to be subserved in more caudal structures, primarily the sensory thalamus. The sensory-association areas are located in the posterior parietal region. In the dominant hemisphere, these involve interpretation and analysis of both written and verbal language. In the nondominant hemisphere, lesions generally cause defects in spatial orientation and body awareness. Lesions in either side, however, may result in sensory inattention in the contralateral body. The occipital lobes are concerned primarily with vision. The visual receptive area is located medially along the lips of the calcarine fissure. A lesion in one hemisphere produces a loss of vision in the contralateral homonymous visual field. Lesions in the medial temporal region, or the group of structures termed the limbic system, may cause resultant personality changes, olfactory or gustatory hallucinations, or alterations in memory. Subcortically, the posterior internal capsule transmits the motor fibers from the motor cortex to the spinal cord, with resulting lesions causing a contralateral hemiparesis. The internal capsule is surrounded by the basal ganglia, where lesions can produce a variety of involuntary movements. Lesions of the brainstem can be quite complex. Often, however, because of the arrangement of the cranial nerve nuclei and the descending pyramidal motor tract, a lesion on one side produces an alternating hemiplegia, an ipsilateral cranial nerve deficit in association with a contralateral body hemiplegia. Lesions in the anterior part of the third ventricle or sellar region can produce both endocrine dysfunction and/or lesions of the third through sixth cranial nerves, which emerge from the brainstem and enter the orbit by way of the cavernous sinus. Lesions of the cerebellum, which is the chief component of the posterior fossa, often produce either lateralizing or truncal incoordination. This may present as an ataxia of the arms and legs or as a dysarthria of speech or vertical nystagmus. In left-handed patients, either the right or left hemisphere, or a combination of both, may subserve this dominant status.

The *spinal cord*, which extends within the vertebral column, has a central gray matter with surrounding white matter tracts in the reverse of the organization found at the cerebral level. Within the anterior gray column are the anterior horn cells that serve as the final common pathway for movement. Interspersed among these large motor cells are smaller neurons, the *gamma neurons*, which supply the contractile elements of the muscle spindle providing maintenance of muscle tone and serve as a mechanism for supraspinal modulation. Afferent impulses are brought into the CNS by way of the posterior dorsal root ganglion and dorsal root entry zone. The ascending and descending fiber tracts, which surround the spinal gray matter, allow transmission of impulses and thereby exchange of information both rostrally and caudally. This allows the spinal cord to be organized to allow segmental or localized control of movement while motor and sensory information is simultaneously being integrated via the ascending and descending tracts on a suprasegmental basis.

Perioperative Management

Preoperatively, the neurosurgeon must be thoroughly aware of systemic problems that may compromise the patient during an intracranial or intraspinal operation. An example would be a prior history of hypertension, which would be associated with the decreased ability of the patient to maintain adequate cerebral perfusion at lower blood pressures; another example is the susceptibility of patients with marked baseline increases in ICP to further increase with the induction of anesthesia.

Intraoperatively, attention must be given not only to direct trauma to the intracranial or intraspinal structures but also to the influence that factors such as operative positioning of the patient and alterations in blood pressure or oxygenation may play.[10] Specifically, the sitting position may be associated with intraoperative venous air embolism and a decreased ability for autoregulation of vascular perfusion to the brain and spinal cord, while the prone position may provide decreased visualization secondary to the pooling of blood in the operative field.

Postoperatively, patients are susceptible not only to intracranial bleeding, increased ICP from edema, and alterations in functioning secondary to infection but also to problems with the hypothalamic-pituitary system, such as the syndrome of inappropriate antidiuretic hormone release (SIADH) or central salt loss. Postoperatively, frequent evaluation of the vital signs and the neurologic status is crucial. Early signs of increased intracranial pressure and brain herniation, such as alteration in level of mentation or abnormalities in the blood pressure or pulse rate, must be detected early and treated aggressively. Following intracranial procedures, cerebral edema in particular is prone to develop and fluid overload must be avoided in this critical period. This may necessitate not only relative fluid restriction, approximately 75 to 100 ml. per hour in adults, but also use of steroids or hyperosmolar agents. When the potential for seizure activity is present, the patient must be maintained on therapeutic anticonvulsant levels in both the preoperative and postoperative periods. If the patient is unable to eat, it is necessary to provide early and adequate caloric intake to prevent the catabolic state with increased potential for infections and skin problems. In patients with spinal cord lesions, particular care must be given to protection of the skin and prevention of urine or fecal retention.

Diagnostic Studies

RADIOGRAPHS OF THE SKULL AND SPINE

Plain films of the skull and spine are important in the screening of trauma, bony infections, neoplasms, congenital abnormalities, and degenerative disease.[5, 7] Changes from a normal configuration, such as enlargement of the pituitary fossa, the presence of abnormal vascular grooves or aberrant calcification can be seen in the skull films of adults. In children, the status of the cranial sutures can be seen with specific attention to separation associated with increased intracranial pressure or premature closure (craniosynostosis). Similarly, spine films have an important role in evaluation of degenerative, traumatic, congenital, and neoplastic diseases of the spine by demonstrating variance from the normal anatomy and normal structural relationships.

When added detail of the bony structure is needed, hypocycloidal polytomography consisting of moving the x-ray source and film in relationship to each other to focus on only one anatomic plane is useful. Increased specificity and degree of spatial resolution can thus be obtained.

Myelography

Because plain films do not allow visualization of the intraspinal soft tissue, it is frequently necessary in the evaluation of spinal disease to utilize a contrast agent. By injection of air, oil-based contrast, or water-soluble dyes into the subarachnoid space, the base of the brain, spinal cord, and nerve roots can be well visualized. Currently, the water-soluble dyes are utilized in most medical centers, since they provide greater anatomic definition, a lower incidence of arachnoiditis, more versatility, and the potential for additional contrast imaging with CT scans (Fig. 3). When used in combination with CT scanning, an extremely high degree of sensitivity can be obtained with excellent visualization of lesions of the brainstem and spine, including a ruptured disc, small tumors, congenital anomalies, and vascular lesions.[5]

Computed Tomography

The impact of computed tomography (CT) scanning upon neurosurgery cannot be overestimated. This modality utilizes the same principle as tomography but, in addition, employs multiple radiation detectors and a computer to digitize and reconstruct the data, permitting the head or spine to be visualized as a series of thin, well-defined images. The differing tissues are visualized on a white-black scale, varying according to their biologic attenuation coefficient (Fig. 4). By combining intravenous (IV) or intrathecal (IT) iodinated contrast material, an extremely high degree of resolution can be obtained (Fig. 5). For these reasons, CT has largely supplemented pneumoencephalography, angiography, and standard myelography as the initial study for neurologic disease. Uses of this technique have steadily multiplied, and today previously occult lesions can be visualized by the use of delayed scanning or higher contrast doses.

Emission Tomography

Computed tomography has largely replaced radionuclide scanning because of its higher degree of specificity and spatial resolution. However, a recently developed technique called *emission computed tomography* (ET), which allows radionuclide data to be reconstructed in a manner similar to CT, shows promise. Currently, there are two general types of ET: single-photon emission (SPECT), and positron emission tomography (PET). The latter is the more widely used and employs biologic compounds labeled with a radioactive isotope that decays by emitting a positron. After administration, the radionuclide compound localizes within the body and is imaged by an array of gamma detectors. The computerized reconstruction of the anatomic distribution of the positron emission allows biochemical and metabolic localization to be determined. Currently, the short half-lives of the isotopes employed and the necessity for having a cyclotron immediately available have resulted in limitations in the use of this technique. In contrast, SPECT scanning is much less expensive but has less spatial resolution. Both of these techniques are under active investigation at this time to determine their potential uses in neuroimaging.

Magnetic Resonance

Magnetic resonance (MR) is a tomographic method of imaging the body based upon the response of tissue protons to radiofrequency (RF) while in a magnetic field. This innovative form of imaging is currently in its infancy but already has shown tremendous potential for studying the brain and spinal cord. In contrast to the other tomographic techniques, MR has multiple advantages: There is no radiation exposure to the patient, bone artefact is minimal, images may be made in multiple planes simultaneously, and results appear to be more sensitive in the detection of

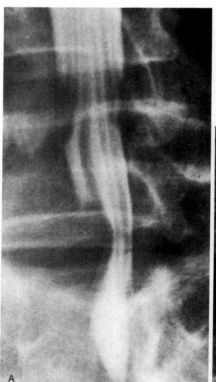

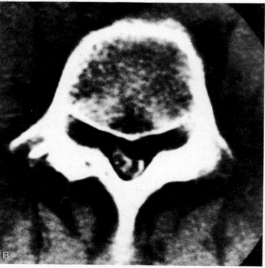

Figure 3. A, A metrizamide myelogram demonstrating in the oblique projection effacement of the nerve root secondary to a ruptured lumbar disc. B, CT scan of the same area demonstrating the ruptured disc as a soft tissue mass compressing the thecal sac.

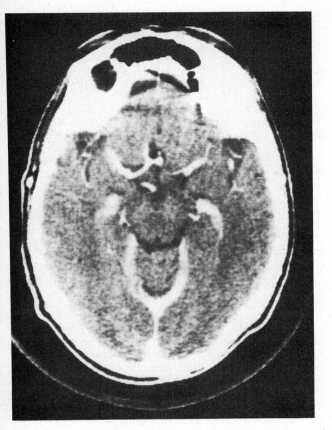

Figure 4. An enhanced CT scan of the brain demonstrating normal anatomy, including portions of the anterior circle of Willis, the choroid plexus in the choroidal fissure, the brainstem, and a portion of the cerebellum at the tentorial notch.

early infarction and demyelinating disease. Although the high cost of these units now limits their widespread use, their tremendous potential makes it likely that MR will become a dominant form of neuroimaging within the near future.

ELECTRICAL DIAGNOSTIC STUDIES

Among the electrical techniques for evaluating the nervous system, three are most frequently used: electroencephalography (EEG), evoked potentials (EP), and electromyography (EMG) with nerve conduction velocities (NCV).[8]

Electroencephalography. This technique involves the measurement of amplified electrical signals from the scalp. Electroencephalography has proved to be the most reliable method for evaluation of seizure disorders but has also proved applicable in the study of sleep apnea and certain progressive neurologic diseases.

Evoked Potentials. In contrast, EP consists of the recording of the electrical activity from the scalp following specific stimulation of the visual, auditory, or somatosensory receptors. The recorded EP is the computed average of multiple stimuli and responses and provides documentation of the functional integrity of a given afferent pathway. Depending upon the pathway stimulated, varying degrees of localizing potential are available. Clinically, EP has proved valuable in the evaluation of multiple sclerosis, optic nerve functioning, and brainstem integrity and, most recently, it has been utilized intraoperatively for both posterior fossa and spinal procedures.

Electromyography with Nerve Conduction Velocities. The last of the electrical studies to be covered are those designed to evaluate the motor unit, which includes the anterior horn cell, ventral root, nerve plexus, peripheral nerve, myoneural junction, and the muscle fiber. The two general types of studies are EMG, which records the electrical activity induced within the muscle with varying degrees of activity, and NCV, which are recordings of the rate at which a stimulated nerve can conduct electrical activity. When used in combination, these techniques are valuable for the evaluation of myopathies, peripheral nerve injuries, and radicular lesions. As with all of the electrical studies, interpretation is highly dependent upon the clinical history and examination.

DIGITAL SUBTRACTION ANGIOGRAPHY

In the past, the standard technique for evaluating intracranial and spinal vessels was the *arteriogram* (Fig. 6).

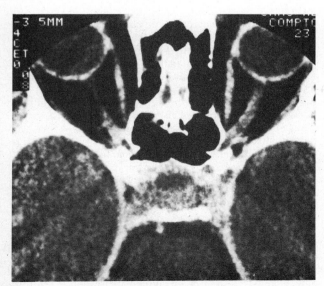

Figure 5. CT scan demonstrating a pituitary adenoma (low density) within the pituitary fossa.

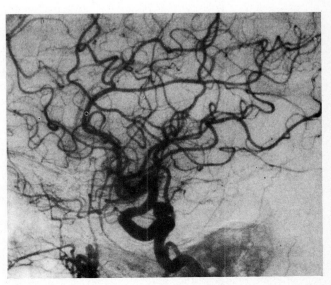

Figure 6. Lateral carotid arteriogram demonstrating a posterior communicating artery aneurysm.

In this technique, a radiopaque dye is injected into the vascular system and rapid-sequence films are obtained subsequently. Such films demonstrate the intracranial vascular anatomy, and the displacement of normal vessels or abnormal vascularity can be quite helpful in the diagnosis of specific CNS pathology. Recently, the use of computers to interpret the x-ray data digitally has created a new technique called intravenous digital subtraction angiography (DSA). This method is far less invasive and requires less contrast medium than standard angiography. It has limitations with spatial resolution, which is most notable in attempts to use it intracranially, but it does appear to be a useful technique for the evaluation of extracranial vessels and may have a more widespread applicability as its technology improves.

INTRACRANIAL TUMORS

Tumors involving the CNS are among the most devastating of neoplasms. They are estimated to account for approximately 2.5 per cent of all mass lesions, resulting in approximately 3.9 to 4.4 deaths per 100,000 population per annum in the United States. The age incidence of brain tumors peaks in childhood and middle-to-late adult life for primary tumors and in later adult life for metastatic tumors (Fig. 7). The age incidence for primary tumors makes the economic and personal impact of these tumors far greater than sheer numbers alone would indicate. Second to leukemia, brain tumors are the leading cause of cancer death in children, while malignant gliomas in adults have an enormous economic impact, ranking fourth among males and eighth among females in order of neoplastic causes for lost work years. The biologic behavior and prognosis of primary intracranial tumors are as heterogeneous as their histopathologic features, ranging from the cystic cerebellar astrocytoma of childhood, which is cured by removal alone, to the malignant glioblastoma multiforme, which is uniformly fatal despite all known therapy.[3, 4]

Presentation

The location of the tumor within the CNS and its biologic behavior determine the neurologic presentation of the patient. When a tumor grows slowly in a neurophysiologically silent area of the brain or within the intraventricular cavity, it may first present in a nonfocal manner with headache, nausea, vomiting, alteration in personality, or changes in level of consciousness on the basis of increased intracranial pressure. This is especially true in childhood because of the increased occurrence of infratentorial neoplasms rather than tumors in the cerebrum, which tend to obstruct the ventricular system with resultant hydrocephalus, irritability, or lethargy.[14] In contrast, tumors involving the speech areas or cortical motor strip may present with unilateral weakness or dysphasia long before there is a generalized increase in intracranial pressure. Depending upon the location of the tumor, other clinical abnormalities may be present, and these include endocrine abnormalities in association with pituitary and hypothalamic tumors, hearing loss in association with cerebellopontine angle tumors, ataxia in association with cerebellar tumors, and visual deficits in association with tumors involving the optic nerve or chiasm. Frequently, the history and clinical findings in association with the age of the patient may provide the clinician with a reasonably circumscribed differential diagnosis.

Diagnosis

With the development of CT scanning, the ability to visualize the CNS in a relatively noninvasive manner has resulted in the early diagnosis of many tumors. Although it has not obviated the need for tissue diagnosis of intracranial lesions, a cumulative experience with CT patterns has allowed better guidance for the early management of these patients. The addition of IV or IT contrast material has increased the detection of occult lesions by accentuating the absorption contrast between normal and abnormal brain. The versatility of CT scanning has resulted in marked reduction in the use of such studies as pneumoencephalography, radionuclide scanning, and polytomography. Angiography still has a role, both diagnostically and in the preoperative planning, in certain patients. In the majority, a *tissue diagnosis* is mandatory prior to commitment to therapy. Despite the increased sensitivity of current imaging techniques, differing diseases continue to mimic one another and defy best efforts of noninvasive diagnosis.

Treatment

The goal of therapy for intracranial tumors is to maximize the quality of life for the patient and to increase the time of functional survival. This often requires the physician to make difficult decisions that must be based upon a thorough understanding of the underlying disease and the therapeutic alternatives.

For most tumors, the first and primary goal is to optimally reduce the tumor burden. In most cases, this necessitates *operative intervention*, which provides a definite histologic diagnosis, effectively removes viable and nonviable tumor burden, and can result in marked symptomatic improvement. With certain tumors, such as cerebellar astrocytomas in children and acoustic neuromas in adults, this alone is the treatment of choice. In other tumors, especially the malignant primary and metastatic tumors, *additional radiation therapy* is required for maximal palliation. Radiation causes ionization in dividing cells. Since most CNS cells are either nondividing or slowly dividing, this generally allows a therapeutic index for treatment. However, radiation is associated with multiple side effects, including, among others, increased edema and long-term demyelination and necrosis. The complications of radiation are most pronounced in early childhood, and for these reasons it must be used judiciously. In addition, many primary and metastatic tumors are relatively radiation-resistant.[3, 4] In certain brain tumors, most notably the more malignant ones, *chemotherapy* has been of benefit; in most instances, however, the role of chemotherapy has yet to be unequivocally demonstrated. This relative resistance of malignant tumors, specifically the malignant gliomas, appears to be due primarily to the heterogeneity of the tumors and to certain unique problems, including delivery of the agent across the blood-brain barrier.

Intracranial tumors often cause unique problems. Among these are those directly associated with the sensitivity of the CNS to increased intracranial pressure. Increased ICP may be the result of enlarging tumor mass, cerebral edema, or obstruction of the CSF pathways with subsequent hydrocephalus. For increasing tumor mass, the only effective therapy is *direct reduction* in the neoplastic burden. Of the methods available, *surgical excision* is the only one that results in an immediate response. Steroids have proved extremely effective in the reduction of the vasogenic component of cerebral edema. When used in

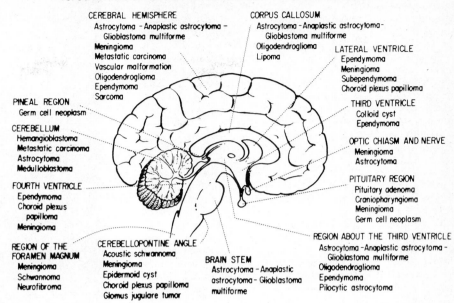

TOPOGRAPHIC DISTRIBUTION OF INTRACRANIAL TUMORS IN ADULTHOOD

CEREBRAL HEMISPHERE
Astrocytoma - Anaplastic astrocytoma -
Glioblastoma multiforme
Meningioma
Metastatic carcinoma
Vascular malformation
Oligodendroglioma
Ependymoma
Sarcoma

CORPUS CALLOSUM
Astrocytoma - Anaplastic astrocytoma-
Glioblastoma multiforme
Oligodendroglioma
Lipoma

LATERAL VENTRICLE
Ependymoma
Meningioma
Subependymoma
Choroid plexus papilloma

PINEAL REGION
Germ cell neoplasm

THIRD VENTRICLE
Colloid cyst
Ependymoma

CEREBELLUM
Hemangioblastoma
Metastatic carcinoma
Astrocytoma
Medulloblastoma

OPTIC CHIASM AND NERVE
Meningioma
Astrocytoma

FOURTH VENTRICLE
Ependymoma
Choroid plexus
papilloma
Meningioma

PITUITARY REGION
Pituitary adenoma
Craniopharyngioma
Meningioma
Germ cell neoplasm

REGION OF THE
FORAMEN MAGNUM
Meningioma
Schwannoma
Neurofibroma

CEREBELLOPONTINE ANGLE
Acoustic schwannoma
Meningioma
Epidermoid cyst
Choroid plexus papilloma
Glomus jugulare tumor

BRAIN STEM
Astrocytoma - Anaplastic
astrocytoma - Glioblastoma
multiforme

REGION ABOUT THE THIRD VENTRICLE
Astrocytoma - Anaplastic astrocytoma -
Glioblastoma multiforme
Oligodendroglioma
Ependymoma
Pilocytic astrocytoma

A

Figure 7. Topographic distribution of intracranial tumors in adulthood (A) and childhood (B). (From Burger, P. C., and Vogel, F. S.: Surgical Pathology of the Nervous System and Its Coverings. New York, John Wiley & Sons, 1982.)

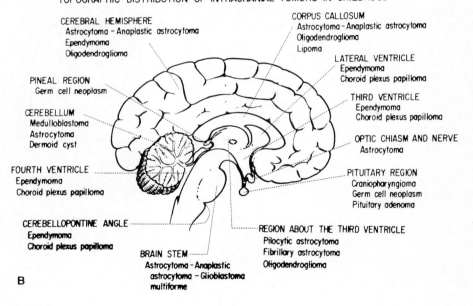

TOPOGRAPHIC DISTRIBUTION OF INTRACRANIAL TUMORS IN CHILDHOOD

CEREBRAL HEMISPHERE
Astrocytoma - Anaplastic astrocytoma
Ependymoma
Oligodendroglioma

CORPUS CALLOSUM
Astrocytoma - Anaplastic astrocytoma
Oligodendroglioma
Lipoma

LATERAL VENTRICLE
Ependymoma
Choroid plexus papilloma

PINEAL REGION
Germ cell neoplasm

THIRD VENTRICLE
Ependymoma
Choroid plexus papilloma

CEREBELLUM
Medulloblastoma
Astrocytoma
Dermoid cyst

OPTIC CHIASM AND NERVE
Astrocytoma

FOURTH VENTRICLE
Ependymoma
Choroid plexus papilloma

PITUITARY REGION
Craniopharyngioma
Germ cell neoplasm
Pituitary adenoma

CEREBELLOPONTINE ANGLE
Ependymoma
Choroid plexus papilloma

BRAIN STEM
Astrocytoma - Anaplastic
astrocytoma - Glioblastoma
multiforme

REGION ABOUT THE THIRD VENTRICLE
Pilocytic astrocytoma
Fibrillary astrocytoma
Oligodendroglioma

B

effective dosages, ranging from 4 to 120 mg. per day of dexamethasone, rapid improvement in clinical status can often be achieved. This improvement, however, is based only on reduction in edema, and steroids have no direct tumoricidal effect. In certain circumstances, generally in the postoperative period or at the time of acute deterioration associated with increased edema or intratumoral hemorrhage, the short-term use of hyperosmolar agents, such as mannitol, may be necessary to provide an immediate but transient reduction in intracranial pressure. Hydrocephalus, which results from obstruction of normal CSF pathways, may be treated temporarily by external drainage, when it is a transient problem, or by the insertion of an internal shunt when the hydrocephalus is likely to be a permanent

problem. This is generally very effective, but in certain circumstances, such as medulloblastomas in children, shunting has been reported to result in an increase in systemic metastasis.

SPINAL TUMORS

Classification

Tumors involving the spine are generally classified into three groups: (1) intramedullary, (2) intradural-extramedullary, and (3) extradural.[4]

Intramedullary. The majority of intramedullary tumors encountered are glial in origin and include astrocytomas, ependymomas, and oligodendrogliomas. The *astrocytomas*, unlike their intracranial counterparts, tend more often to be well differentiated histologically. These tumors can infiltrate widely without well-defined margins, making surgical excision extremely difficult. In contrast, *ependymomas* and *oligodendrogliomas* tend to be better defined. The myxopapillary ependymoma is a variant that occurs almost exclusively in the area of the cauda equina. These tumors are histologically distinctive with the presence of fibrillated or epithelial glia in association with a mucoid-type material. *Hemangioblastomas* may also occur as intramedullary tumors, although in a somewhat lesser frequency than as cerebellar lesions, and they may be seen in the context of the von Hippel–Lindau syndrome. These tumors are generally discrete and highly vascular with large leptomeningeal feeding vessels present on the surface of the spinal cord. This appearance may mimic that of a vascular malformation. *Metastatic* intramedullary tumors may also occur, but are extremely rare. All of the primary intramedullary tumors may be associated with cysts or syrinx formation.

Intradural-Extramedullary. Among the intradural-extramedullary tumors, *meningiomas* and *schwannomas* are the most common. Meningiomas represent 25 to 33 per cent of all primary intraspinal tumors and generally occur in females in the thoracic region. These tumors arise from meningothelial cells in the region of the dorsal root ganglia and are usually amenable to total excision. The schwannomas arise from the Schwann cells, which invest the more distal spinal roots, constitute approximately 30 per cent of intraspinal tumors, and are evenly distributed within the vertebral column. Although tumors tend to occur laterally, the meningioma is more likely to involve the overlying dura. Plexiform neurofibromas may also occur in the spinal cord and are strongly indicative of von Recklinghausen's disease. Other congenital tumors, such as *dermoids* and *epidermoids*, may also occur in the intradural-extramedullary location, as can metastatic lesions from both systemic and primary tumors (Fig. 8).

Extradural. Extradural tumors are most frequently metastatic lesions, *lymphomas* or *multiple myeloma/plasmocytomas* and are relatively frequent complications of systemic disease, which may present solely as painful vertebral lesions or as space-occupying epidural masses compressing the spinal cord. Metastatic lesions from the lung, breast, unknown primary sites, and lymphomas constitute approximately half of all spinal metastases. Other less commonly occurring metastatic primary sites are the prostate, kidney, and gastrointestinal tumors. Metastases can involve any part of the spinal cord, but the thoracic region appears to be the most commonly involved.

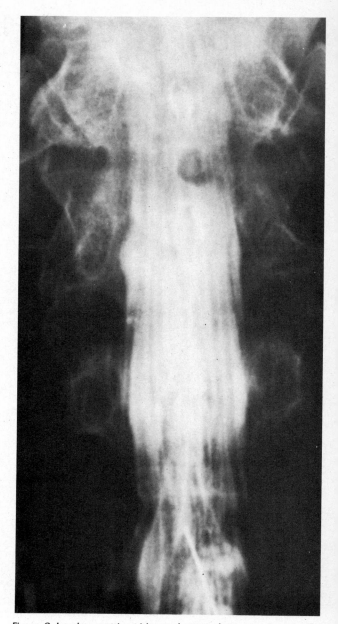

Figure 8. Lumbar metrizamide myelogram demonstrating an adenocarcinoma from the lung that has metastasized to the region of the cauda equina. Earlier, this patient had been found to have an intracranial metastasis. It is from this lesion rather than the lung itself that the subarachnoid metastasis most likely derived.

Symptoms and Signs

Back pain is the most common presenting symptom of most spinal tumors, especially *extradural* tumors. With extrinsic lesions, long tract dysfunction is usually more pronounced and focal pain to external percussion evident. The intrinsic lesions, in contrast, more frequently present with dysfunction in either the upper or lower extremities with an ill-defined nocturnal pain syndrome. On examination, the decussating pain fibers are more often involved with less compromise of the long tracts until the later stages of the disease. The rate of growth of the tumor strongly influences the degree of disability because of the poor compensatory potential for acute compression of the spinal cord.

Diagnosis and Treatment

Plain film findings of the spine are frequently positive for metastatic diseases. This is usually seen as early loss of a pedicle or with osteoblastic or osteolytic lesions in the involved vertebral bodies. *Isotope bone scans* may also be helpful in assessing the extent of disease within the vertebral column. With intrinsic or intramedullary-extradural tumors, plain films may show widening of the internal diameter of the canal with sclerotic changes in the pedicles. To determine the true extent of spinal involvement, however, high-resolution myelography, often in conjunction with CT scanning, is mandatory.

Surgical exploration is necessary to establish a diagnosis of intradural tumors. With the infiltrative, poorly defined astrocytomas, limited biopsy, however, may be all that is achievable. The ependymomas and hemangioblastomas may be better defined and more amenable to surgical resection. The role of radiation therapy is still debatable for these tumors, but appears to have a place in the treatment of the more malignant and less well defined tumors. For benign intradural-extramedullary tumors, surgical resection is the treatment of choice and, in most cases, radiation has no role. For metastatic tumors, conflict still exists as to the best form of treatment. In the short term, surgical excision, radiation, and/or combination of both appear to be equally effective in treating the spinal cord compression. For patients ambulating prior to treatment, the prognosis for short-term continued function is relatively good. For those patients who are unable to walk, the potential for further ambulation is poor, regardless of the type of treatment. For ambulatory patients, limited data have suggested that surgery may prolong the interval of functional ambulation. For hematogenous tumors, radiation and appropriate medical management of the underlying disease are crucial factors in the treatment of the patient.

CEREBROVASCULAR DISEASE

Cerebrovascular diseases are among the most common neurologic disorders of adults.[18] *Stroke* is the most common and is the third most frequent cause of death in the United States. Cerebrovascular disease (CVD) is manifest in two general ways, by *hemorrhage* or *ischemia*. In the former, the leakage of blood occurs into the subarachnoid space, the ventricular system, or directly into the parenchyma of the brain. In the latter, the blood supply to a region of the brain is reduced by hypotension or by thrombotic or embolic obstruction of an artery. If the ischemia is sufficiently severe, irreversible brain damage, infarction, occurs. The vast majority of patients with CVD present with stroke, which is a nonconvulsive, acute, focal neurologic deficit. The extent of neurologic deficit reflects the nature and severity of the insult, as well as the location in which it occurs.

Subarachnoid Hemorrhage

Classically, adults with a subarachnoid hemorrhage (SAH) have the acute onset of an excruciating headache in association with nausea and vomiting, with or without loss of consciousness or a seizure. This presentation is the result of the acute exposure of the intracranial subarachnoid space and brain to arterial blood at its significantly higher pressure. Not all patients appear with the classical history, however, and the physician must be aware that an SAH presentation can range from a mild headache to instantaneous death.

On examination, the majority of patients are found to be hypertensive and to have meningismus secondary to blood in the CSF. Neurologically, they range from normal to comatose. A clinical grading system for patients with SAH was originally proposed by Botterell and has subsequently been amended by others (Table 1). Certain focal

TABLE 1. Neurologic Grading following Subarachnoid Hemorrhage*

Grade	Definition
I	Symptom-free
II	Minor symptoms (headache, meningeal irritation, diplopia)
III	Major neurologic deficit but fully responsive
IV	Impaired state of alertness but capable of protective or other adaptive responses to noxious stimuli
V	Poorly responsive but with stable vital signs
VI	No response to address or shaking, nonadaptive response to noxious stimuli, and progressive instability of vital signs

*From Nebbelink, D. W., Forner, J. C., and Henderson, W. B.: et al: Stroke, 8:202, 1977.

neurologic signs are suggestive of the location of an intracranial aneurysm as the source for the SAH, such as an ipsilateral third nerve palsy in association with a posterior communicating aneurysm. Retinal hemorrhages may also be seen and are thought to be secondary to compression of the central retinal vein with secondary retrograde venous distention.

Following initial evaluation and stabilization, CT scanning is the procedure of choice. Previously, the diagnosis of SAH was based upon the presence of blood in the CSF on lumbar puncture (LP). With the recent generation CT scanners, however, an LP is often not required. In addition, the presence of intracerebral hematomas in association with the SAH can be assessed. The presence of a hematoma may necessitate emergency evacuation because of the mass effect or, in the case of accumulations of blood in the basilar cisterns, may be an important prognostic sign for the future development of cerebral vasospasm. Following confirmation of the SAH, arteriography should be performed in order to diagnose the site of bleeding and the vascular anatomy. Generally, in adults, one half to two thirds of SAHs cases will be due to the rupture of an intracranial aneurysm, 5 to 6 per cent will be due to bleeding from an arteriovenous malformation (AVM), and the remainder may never have a site of bleeding established or they may be secondary to relatively rare causes, such as primary or metastatic brain tumors, blood dyscrasias, eclampsia, hypertensive hemorrhage, or spinal AVM. In children, the incidence of AVMs is ten times that of aneurysms, although specifically for the presence of SAHs approximately 50 per cent are caused by aneurysms, 25 per cent by AVMs, 20 per cent by unknown causes, and less than 5 per cent by other factors, such as moyamoya disease, neoplasm, and hypertension.

Intracranial aneurysms classically originate at the bifurcation of major intracranial vessels (see Fig. 6). Although it appears that these are congenital lesions and may be associated with other congenital anomalies, such as coarctation of the aorta or polycystic kidney disease, the low incidence of SAH from an aneurysm in infancy and childhood supports an additional degenerative component. The presence of these aneurysms may also be rarely associated with prior trauma, infection, or brain tumors. Two types of aneurysm that occur less frequently are *arteriosclerotic* and *mycotic*. The former are ectatic dilations of severely involved arteriosclerotic intracranial vessels. Generally, these occur on the vertebral-basilar system and present by compression of the adjacent structures. They rarely bleed, but may clinically be quite serious because of their mass effect and relative inaccessibility or tendency to thrombose with subsequent infarction. Mycotic aneurysms result from weakening of the wall of the distal intracranial arterial tree from sepsis or meningitis. Because of their difference in location from that of congenital aneurysms and their tendency to be multiple, they can often be clinically suspected by the arteriographic picture. As with congenital aneurysms, they are best treated by surgical clip ligation. Approximately 85 per cent of the congenital aneurysms occur on the anterior component of the circle of Willis. They may occur at almost any bifurcation, but certain locations are most frequent, e.g., the junction of the posterior communicating artery with the internal carotid artery, the junction of the anterior communicating artery with an anterior cerebral artery, and the first branching of the middle cerebral artery. When they occur on the posterior circulation, the terminal bifurcation of the basilar artery is the most frequent site. In approximately 20 per cent of patients, more than one aneurysm will be seen.

Following initial presentation and diagnosis of SAH secondary to an intracranial aneurysm, three major problems confront the neurosurgeon: the risk of recurrent SAH, delayed vasospasm with resultant ischemia or infarction, and the development of communicating hydrocephalus. Following SAH, the highest incidence of rebleeding occurs within the first 2 weeks with gradual decrease over the next 4 weeks to a plateau with an annual rebleed incidence of 3 to 4 per cent per year. The morbidity associated with rebleeding is much higher than that seen initially and the mortality from rebleeding is approximately 45 per cent. It is estimated that 50 per cent of ruptured aneurysms will bleed again within 6 months if not treated. Clinically significant vasospasm occurs in approximately 20 to 36 per cent of patients and usually occurs between 4 and 16 days after initial hemorrhage. This is a major problem associated with a high incidence of clinical morbidity, infarction, and even death. The cause for vasospasm is unknown, although the increased incidence in patients with larger amounts of subarachnoid blood suggests a blood component or byproduct plays a role. Communicating hydrocephalus occurs in 15 to 25 per cent of patients.

The definitive treatment of an intracranial aneurysm is surgical clip ligation.[18] Aneurysms of the internal carotid artery may be treated by progressive compression of the cevical carotid artery. In most modern medical centers, the overall operative mortality of this procedure is less than 5 per cent. The range in mortality, however, varies drastically with the neurologic status of the patient, ranging from less than 1 per cent in Grade I patients to 20 to 30 percent in Grade III patients, and with the skill of the surgeon. Initially, ruptured aneurysms were treated as acute emergencies and surgical ligation was performed on an emergent basis. However, the poor results obtained with early intervention during the 1950s led most neurosurgeons to postpone operation for 2 to 3 weeks following the acute episode. From early data, it appeared that the marked improvement in the surgical outcome obtained by delaying operation was based upon fewer technical problems and a reduced incidence of postoperative vasospasm. As this became the standard method of treatment, medical management was directed toward reduction in the incidence of rebleeding and the control of vasospasm. In the hope of preventing a sudden increase in blood pressure, which may result in rupture of the aneurysm, patients are kept at bed rest in a quiet room, they are given stool softeners, and indwelling urinary catheters are used. Antifibrinolytic therapy to prevent dissolution of the perianeurysmal clot decreases the incidence of rebleeding during the first 2 weeks following

initial SAH, although recent studies have suggested no long-term reduction in morbidity or mortality because of an associated increase in the incidence of vasospasm. Data have also been generated to suggest that vasospasm may be reduced by increasing the intravascular volume of the patient. This is best accomplished by increasing the patient's blood volume with blood products or colloid solutions. The optimal hematocrit appears to be approximately 35. Because the goal is increased blood volume and cardiac output rather than increased blood pressure, a Swan-Ganz catheter may be required for optimal monitoring. Multiple drug regimens have been employed in an attempt to reduce spasm, but none has consistently shown any benefit. Currently, calcium channel antagonists, such as nifedipine, are being evaluated for this purpose.

With advances in both medical and technical areas, attempts to reintroduce early operation for aneurysms have reappeared and currently the timing of operation for ruptured aneurysms is a major neurosurgical controversy. For Grade I or II patients, early operation within the first 3 days or delayed surgery appears to be reasonable. For Grades III through V, medical management with bed rest, controlled hypotension, concomitant vascular loading, and treatment with antifibrinolytic agents appears to be the optimal initial form of therapy during the first 2 to 3 weeks. With these, it is often possible to delay operation until the patient has clinically improved and conditions are more favorable for an improved result.

Surgical therapy of an aneurysm is based upon obliterating the neck of the aneurysm, strengthening the wall of the aneurysm with reinforcing materials, or reducing the arterial pressure within the aneurysm. The first of these is the most commonly used and consists of surgically exposing the aneurysm and placing a metal clip or ligature across the neck (Fig. 9). Although this is the optimal form of therapy, at times it may be anatomically impossible because the aneurysmal neck may be surgically inaccessible or is so broad-based that it cannot be isolated. Under these circumstances, the wall of the aneurysm can be reinforced with strips of muscle, fascia, or plastic. A final option is ligation, either proximally or both distally and proximally, of the vessels supplying the aneurysm. This may be utilized with proximal internal carotid artery aneurysms. The overall results from the latter two types of treatment have not been as satisfactory, but under certain circumstances they may be the only reasonable alternatives. For aneurysms of the posterior circulation, specal problems and hazards exist and certain of these lesions are considered inoperable by most neurosurgeons. When the aneurysm has been surgically treated, the primary goal is to reduce the incidence of delayed vasospasm and/or the development of hydrocephalus. The first of these is approached by volume expansion and the second by placement of either a temporary ventriculostomy or a permanent indwelling shunt.

Arteriovenous Malformation

Arteriovenous malformations of the brain are congenital lesions in which arteries and veins are in direct communication without the normal intervening smaller vessels. Although the categorization of the different types of AVM is debatable, for practical purposes these can be divided into four categories:

1. *Telangiectasias*, which are capillary cuffs separated by normal brain.

2. *Cavernous angiomas*, which are small, solitary le-

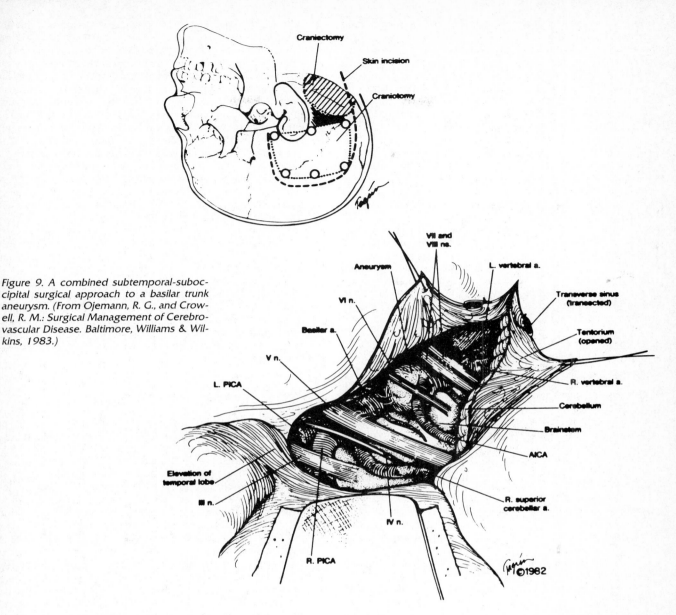

Figure 9. A combined subtemporal-suboc-cipital surgical approach to a basilar trunk aneurysm. (From Ojemann, R. G., and Crowell, R. M.: Surgical Management of Cerebrovascular Disease. Baltimore, Williams & Wilkins, 1983.)

sions composed of sinusoidal vessels with no interposed normal brain tissue.

3. *Venous angiomas*, which are composed of enlarged, normal veins with normal tissue interposed.

4. *True* AVMs, which are generally large lesions with both arterial and venous components with no intervening capillaries.

In childhood, the most frequently occurring AVM is in the region of the great vein of Galen. This malformation may present as cardiac failure, hydrocephalus, or craniomegaly, depending upon the time of presentation.[14]

In adult life, AVMs may present with headaches, seizure activity, or bleeding into the subarachnoid space or, more commonly, into the parenchyma of the brain or ventricular system. Telangiectasias and cavernous angiomas are generally small and may be detected only by biopsy of the walls of the hematoma. The prognosis for patients with these AVMs is generally good, depending upon the initial neurologic damage sustained. The larger AVM can usually be seen angiographically. These lesions are often quite large and have a conical shape, with the superficial portion covering larger areas of the cerebral surface with extension of the lesion deep to the ventricular surface. When large or critically situated, the AVM may "steal" blood from surrounding brain, resulting in progressive neurologic deterioration secondary to ischemia and infarction. Generally, AVMs have a much slower incidence of bleeding than do intracranial aneurysms. The mortality associated with bleeding also appears to be less, being approximately 10 per cent at the initial episode, increasing to approximately 20 per cent by the third episode. From retrospective analysis, it appears that AVMs presenting with hemorrhage have a fourfold higher annual incidence of rebleeding than those presenting with seizures. If an AVM has bled twice, the rebleed incidence markedly increases from approximately 4 per cent per year to 25 per cent. With both types of presentation, however, a significant chance of later bleeding or progressive neurologic dysfunction exists. When accessible, the treatment of choice for these lesions is surgical resection. These lesions can be extremely difficult to resect without neurologic damage to the patient, and treatment must be individualized. Radiation therapy or artificial embolization appears to have a role in otherwise unresectable lesions and may be of benefit as adjunctive forms of therapy for potential surgical candidates. Limited ligation of the dominant feeding vessels is of virtually no value in the treatment of AVMs because of the rapid development of collateral flow through the lower resistance offered by the vascular bed of the AVM.

A variant of the intracranial AVM is the dural AVM, which is formed by abnormal communication between branches of the external carotid, internal carotid, vertebral arteries, and dural venous sinuses. These lesions are also probably congenital in origin, although in some there is a definite prior history of trauma. These lesions usually present with a pulsatile tinnitus, but may also be associated with focal neurologic deficits, increased intracranial pressure, or intracranial hemorrhage into the subarachnoid space or parenchyma.

The treatment of choice is surgical resection. Embolization appears to be of benefit in some patients and because of the intermittent clinical association with hydrocephalus shunting may be required. The overall prognosis for these patients is quite good.

Intracerebral Hemorrhage

All of the previously mentioned entities may present with intracerebral rather than subarachnoid hemorrhage, or with combinations of the two. Of these, the vascular malformation is the most common intracerebral hemorrhage. In addition, several disease entities most frequently present as intracerebral rather than subarachnoid hemorrhages. The most common of these is the *hypertensive intracranial hemorrhage*. With prolonged hypertension, there is a fibrinoid necrosis of the walls of small arteries and arterioles with frequent formation of multiple small vessel dilations known as *Charcot-Bouchard aneurysms*. These form on the small, deep penetrating arteries in a distribution similar to that noted with hypertensive hemorrhage, although a direct cause-and-effect situation has not been established. Hemorrhage associated with hypertension occurs most frequently within the basal ganglia, pons, and cerebellum, although it may occur in other intracranial sites. Depending upon the location of the hemorrhage, the clinical presentation tends to be uniform with the acute onset of headache and neurologic deficit. When a prior history of hypertension is known and the CT scan is compatible with the known patterns for hypertensive hemorrhage, no further diagnostic studies are usually indicated. However, when the clinical history or CT pattern is abnormal, a cerebral arteriogram should be obtained to exclude an underlying structural lesion, such as an AVM or tumor. Because of the acute mass effect associated with the hemorrhage, a small lesion may not be demonstrated at this time. When a high index of suspicion is present, the patient should be re-evaluated with an enhanced CT scan 2 to 4 months following the acute episode.

The treatment of these cerebral hematomas is currently being re-examined. The acute neurologic deficit produced by the tissue destruction associated with the hematoma obviously will not be reversed by surgical resection. However, the mass effect of the hematoma and the subsequent development of edema with increasing pressure effect may be prevented or improved by evacuation. In general, with or without operation, patients in good neurologic condition following hemorrhage do well whereas comatose patients do poorly. Operation appears to be of benefit primarily in those patients who are stuporous or who are originally alert with subsequent neurologic deterioration in association with progressive mass effect. Hematomas closer to the cortical surface generally are better managed surgically than those situated in the basal ganglia. When the hematoma is in the cerebellum, the circumstances are altered. In this group of patients, who constitute between 5 and 6 per cent of all those with intracranial hematomas, the problem of brainstem compression and hydrocephalus becomes extremely important and may produce rapid neurologic deterioration. Moreover, in this group of patients, the subsequent long-term disability is not directly related to preoperative neurologic deficit in the same manner as cerebral lesions. Because of this, most patients with posterior fossa hematomas should undergo surgical evacuation. The two exceptions are patients who are in good clinical condition with small clots following hemorrhage and those who present essentially brain dead.

Intracranial hemorrhage is also associated with hematologic disorders, such as leukemia, aplastic anemia and thrombocytopenic purpura, liver disease, anticoagulant therapy, occult neoplasms, and congophilic angiopathy. Treatment must be individualized to the type and stage of the underlying disease and the neurologic state as well as the location of the hemorrhage.

Cerebral Ischemia

The surgical management of extravascular cerebral disease is discussed in Chapter 41, and recent developments in neurosurgical technology are pertinent to this problem. The first extracranial-to-intracranial (EC-IC) anastomoses of the superficial temporal artery to a cortical branch of the middle cerebral artery for the treatment of extracranial vascular disease were performed in 1968. Technically successful EC-IC bypasses have been performed to most major vessels on the intracranial carotid, vertebral, or basilar systems utilizing direct anastomosis of venous grafts. This rapid technological development has resulted in varying criteria for operation and a lack of clarity for the therapeutic value of these prodecures. Currently, a large cooperative study is under way to evaluate the exact role of EC-IC bypasses in the treatment of extracranial carotid disease. When stenosis or occlusion of the extracranial or proximal intracranial arteries is present and is anatomically consistent with the patient's clinical ischemic events, EC-IC revascularization may be of benefit. With posterior circulation lesions and symptoms of brainstem ischemia, revascularization of the distal vertebral or basilar circulation may be considered. Additional uses for this technique are *prophylactic* vascularization prior to attempted ligation of giant intracranial aneurysms or attempted resection of benign tumors involving the major intracranial vessels.

Spinal Vascular Disease

Vascular diseases of the spinal cord include the same general categories as intracranial vascular diseases. Spontaneous intraspinal hemorrhages may occur secondary to angiomatous malformations, neoplasms, or vascular diseases. The angiomatous malformations of the spinal cord are anatomically divided into those that are primarily intramedullary or extramedullary. In the former, hemorrhage or infarction of the lesion will result in primary cord damage with a secondary myelopathy. In contrast, hemorrhage from a largely extramedullary lesion produces subarachnoid blood, which may present by acute cord compression or which may, in fact, present as a suspected intracranial subarachnoid hemorrhage. Clinically, the malformations usually present with a progressive dysfunction associated with acute exacerbations. Most lesions are present on myelography with water-soluble dyes. However, the anatomy and distribution of these lesions require detailed visualization utilizing selective arteriography. Because these lesions may feed from multiple intracostal arteries in addition to branches of the vertebral-basilar system, this may be quite an extensive diagnostic undertaking.

Operative intervention requires a high degree of neurosurgical sophistication to prevent further damage to the spinal cord. Numerous tumors, most frequently the angioblastomas, also present with spontaneous intramedullary or extramedullary hemorrhages. These lesions require resection for decompression of the hemorrhage as well as surgical diagnosis and treatment.

CRANIOCEREBRAL INJURIES

Head injury is a frequent cause of morbidity and mortality worldwide.[1] Despite a progressive decline in the number of fatal and severe head injuries since the nationwide reduction in the highway speed limit, more stringent prosecution of drunken drivers, and the increased use of seat belts, road accidents still are responsible for more than half of these injuries and are the leading cause of death in patients below the age of 45. More than 70 per cent of patients involved in such accidents sustain trauma to the head. The type of damage following trauma can be classified as a *primary injury*, one that occurs at the time of the accident, or as a secondary injury, one that results from subsequent increased intracranial pressure, anoxia, ischemia, infarction, and metabolic alteration. The primary goal of the neurosurgeon is to minimize the extent of secondary injuries by appropriate diagnosis and treatment of the primary injuries.

Primary Assessment and Treatment

Patients who present with significant cranial trauma frequently also have associated injuries to the spine and other organs. Evaluation of these patients requires judicious triage with the establishment of an adequate airway and control of shock as the first orders of importance.

Following stabilization, a precise history and physical examination must be performed. Knowledge of the details of the accident or of prior medical problems may be of critical importance. The general examination, including signs of external trauma and the presence of other organ involvement, must be performed carefully, yet expeditiously. Vascular instability should alert the physician to the presence of non-CNS injury, including rupture of an abdominal organ, long bone fracture, or vascular injury. The structure of the neurologic examination in an emergency is basically as in the standard examination, but by necessity may be more abbreviated. The mental status of the patient is established by the level of consciousness and response to verbal and painful stimuli. Examination of the cranial nerves begins with pupillary status and response, the presence of extraocular eye movement, facial symmetry

TABLE 2. Glasgow Coma Scale*

Eye Opening (E)	
Spontaneous	4
To speech	3
To pain	2
Nil	1
Best Motor Response (M)	
Obeys	6
Localizes	5
Withdraws	4
Abnormal flexion	3
Extensor response	2
Nil	1
Verbal Response (V)	
Oriented	5
Confused conversation	4
Inappropriate words	3
Incomprehensible sounds	2
Nil	1

*Coma score = E + M + V.

and sensation, the presence of a gag response, and movement of the tongue. During this time, the neck must be stabilized until spinal instability can be excluded. In a comatose patient, extraocular eye movement may be tested by oculocaloric testing in order to establish brainstem integrity. Movement of the arms and legs is tested according to power, symmetry, and the stimulus required to obtain optimal response (Table 2). In the comatose patient, the sensory examination is by necessity integrated with the motor examination. In a more alert individual, detailed testing of response to pinprick, vibration, and joint position sense can be performed. The symmetry and presence of deep tendon responses are then evaluated. Finally, the presence of abnormal responses, such as extensor plantars, is noted.

It is obvious that the emergent situation may necessitate altering the sequence and extent of testing. During initial stabilization and evaluation, appropriate blood studies should be obtained, including a complete blood count, samples for type and cross-matching, electrolytes, arterial blood gases, and, when pertinent, blood screens. Urine is examined to evaluate the presence of blood and/or toxins. Next, radiographic evaluation should be performed; in the comatose and potentially unstable patient, a single crosstable cervical spine x-ray followed by CT scan of the head is the first priority.[7] When cervical injury cannot be excluded, the patient's neck should be stabilized with a cervical collar and the patient should be moved with great care. Excluding emergent situations, skull films may be of value prior to CT scanning and in a patient with minor head trauma may preclude the need for CT scan. In the pediatric age group, however, skull films are generally less revealing.

On a neurosurgical basis, immediate attention is given to the exclusion of a life-threatening intracranial hemorrhage or the presence of an unstable spinal injury. In all patients with suspected head injury, it is critical that cervical spine injury be excluded. During this initial evaluation and treatment, a judicious set of priorities must be established by those managing the patient. When the patient is stabilized, specific attention can then be given to the further clarification of the nature and extent of the intracranial injury. In patients with less severe injury, the question of admission to the hospital for further observation often arises. All patients with altered levels of consciousness, persistent nausea or vomiting, focal neurologic deficits, fever, or skull fractures should be observed in the hospital over the next 24 hours. This is especially true in elderly patients, alcoholics, persons who live alone, and children. In children, any head injury that results in even a transient loss of consciousness should not be underestimated. Children appear to have the potential for a unique response of rapid vascular congestion intracranially secondary to marked increase in CBF with hyperemia and congestion.

With the development of CT scanning, it has become apparent that the spectrum of intracranial injury can be very complex. Because of this, it is rare that the neurosurgeon is faced with the situation of performing an emergency decompressive procedure without a prior CT scan. The CT scan allows visualization of the intracranial contents with subsequent diagnosis of extradural, subdural, and intracerebral mass lesions, specifically hematomas, the presence of hydrocephalus, or extensive edema. With the development of recent generation CT scanners, better definition of bony trauma is now available.

When the extent of the intracranial injury can be assessed, the decision of medical versus operative therapy can be made. When operation is not warranted, close observation of the patient both neurologically and systemically is mandatory. In many centers, the *Glasgow coma scale* (Table 2) is used to objectively follow the neurologic status of the patient. Medical management of the patient with severe trauma is directed toward stabilizing vascular volume, reducing intracranial pressure when elevated, and preventing the multitude of complications associated with systemic trauma and loss of consciousness. Generally, the foundation for reducing increased intracranial pressure involves controlled hyperventilation to maintain carbon dioxide between 20 and 25 mm. Hg and the administration of hyperosmolar agents (such as mannitol) or diuretic agents (such as furosemide) to reduce the intracranial pressure. When these agents are used, it is important that the intracranial pressure of the patient be monitored; generally, a catheter is inserted into the ventricular system or a solid-state transducer is inserted into the subarachnoid or epidural space. The former technique has the advantage of also providing the therapeutic option of directly releasing CSF. In normal patients, ICP pressures greater than 10 mm. Hg are noted only with Valsalva maneuver or straining and prolonged pressures above 20 mm. Hg do not occur. Although this practice is somewhat arbitrary, most physicians attempt to maintain the ICP below 15 to 20 mm. Hg in patients with head injuries. The use of intravenous mannitol administered in doses of 0.5 to 1 gm. per kg. on an empiric or 3- to 6-hour basis can be beneficial. When mannitol is used, the serum osmolarity should not be allowed to rise above 320, since beyond this point no increase in effect is noted and renal toxicity can be encountered. When intracranial pressure cannot be controlled by these methods, some advocate administering short-acting barbiturates until reduction in ICP or vasomotor instability occurs. Successful results in association with barbiturate doses that produce burst suppression on the EEG have been reported. Improved results, however, have not been consistently noted; the use of barbiturates is associated with the potential risk of cardiovascular instability, and the exact role of these agents in the treatment of severe head injury has yet to be determined. Similarly, many advocate the use of corticosteroids for the treatment of severe head injury. However, in *controlled* trials, no benefit has been demonstrated and the author does not recommend their routine use. In these extremely fragile patients, careful observation is required for the development of additional medical problems, such as infection, SIADH release, stress ulcers, and others.

Traumatic Neurosurgical Syndromes

Although the spectrum of injury associated with trauma is wide, certain reasonably well defined entities occur. These range from simple scalp lacerations to acute epidural hematomas.

SCALP LACERATIONS

Scalp lacerations may be the cause of profound blood loss and in a child may produce shock, although such is unlikely in the adult, despite significant blood loss. Following initial stabilization and treatment, scalp wounds should be closed primarily. Cleansing of the wound with extensive irrigation and débridement of all nonviable tissue is of maximal importance in view of the high incidence of infection resulting from inadequate débridement. The scalp edges should be closed without tension, and if this is impossible, a rotation flap, local pedical flap, or free flap may be necessary, with or without additional split-thickness skin grafting.

SKULL FRACTURES

Four general types of skull fractures occur: (1), linear, (2) depressed, (3) diastatic, and (4) basilar. These can be further classified as *open* or *closed*, depending upon whether the scalp is intact.

Linear Fractures. The linear skull fracture is often not of major importance and requires only close observation during the post-traumatic period. When a linear fracture involves the perinasal air cavities, the potential for the development of CSF *rhinorrhea* or *otorrhea* exists. Open linear skull fractures cannot be viewed as a static phenomenon. Almost invariably at the time of injury, the bony edges are widely separated with resultant closure and trapping of foreign material. In this situation, débridement of the wound and evaluation of the dural integrity are mandatory. In children, closed linear fractures may later develop into progressively enlarging leptomeningeal cysts with secondary herniation of intracranial contents. When the linear skull fracture extends across major vascular channels, such as the middle meningeal groove, the most frequent side of epidural hematomas or the major draining venous channels, the superior sagittal sinus and transverse sinus, it becomes potentially more critical.

Depressed Fractures. In a depressed skull fracture, the outer table of one or more of the segments is displaced below the level of the inner table of the surrounding intact skull. Depressed fractures may be treated in the same way as linear skull fractures unless the degree of depression of the inner table is greater than 3 to 10 mm. In this circumstance, as in open linear fractures, the extent of intracranial damage may be greater than is apparent on plain skull films, particularly in children. If a depressed fracture is associated with the major vascular channels, arteriography and operative intervention are also generally necessary. Compound depressed skull fractures must be satisfactorily débrided and a water-tight drill integrity established. Devitalized brain should be removed. In the case of children, it has been reported that the bone fragments may be replaced if they are thoroughly cleansed. The risk of infection must be weighed carefully, however, with the cosmetic result and the advantages and disadvantages of a delayed cranioplasty.

Diastatic Fractures. A diastatic skull fracture is one that follows the diastases of the skull. Leptomeningeal cysts usually occur in children under the age of 3, often in association with a long diastatic fracture. The subsequent development of an enlarging, pulsatile mass occurs because the initial injury causes a tear in both the dura and arachnoid, followed by pulsatile enlargement of the fracture by the CSF pulsations. These should be treated by surgical repair.

Basilar Fractures. Basilar skull fractures are those occurring at the base of the skull. Sometimes these cannot be directly visualized on plain films and are clinically diagnosed by the presence of such associated clinical features as a hemotympanum (Battle's sign) or radiographically by an air-fluid level in the sphenoid sinus on supine skull films. These fractures are frequently associated with CSF rhinorrhea or otorrhea. When this occurs, close observation for 7 to 14 days with bed rest and antibiotic coverage may be adequate for a spontaneous cessation of the leak. This is especially true with otorrhea. However, if the spontaneous cessation of the CSF leak does not occur by this time, intracranial repair of the dural leak is required. The specific site of the leakage may require extensive radiographic evaluation, including either radioisotope scanning or CT scanning with the contrast agent injected intrathecally and monitoring pledgets placed within the nasal cavity. If displaced fractures join the subarachnoid space with the air-containing cavities, immediate surgical *replacement* is the treatment of choice. In this circumstance, dural repair, exenteration of the sinus, and débridement of the wound are required. Postoperatively, the patient requires a lumbar drain for 3 to 5 days with bed rest and antibiotic coverage.

Subdural Hematomas

Classically, subdural hematomas can be (1) acute, (2) subacute, or (3) chronic. With the development of the CT scan, however, the division between these has become somewhat obscured, although in general the three entities continue.

Acute. Acute subdural hematomas have their clinical onset within 24 hours after injury and may be extremely difficult to differentiate clinically from an acute epidural hematoma. The compression is usually secondary to a solid blood clot formed by a torn subdural vein. It is difficult to evacuate this type of lesion through a burr hole alone, and multiple trepanations or a craniotomy may be required. These lesions are usually associated with a significant degree of head injury and may be bilateral. Despite the development of CT scanning and better medical management, operative mortality remains 75 per cent or more.

Subacute. The subacute subdural hematoma generally presents 2 to 14 days after the injury and is seen in less severe injuries. The consistency of the lesion varies from solid clot to liquefied material and can often be evacuated through one or two well-placed trepanations.

Chronic. In contrast, the chronic subdural hematoma is often seen in elderly patients, in patients with bleeding disorders, or in chronic alcoholics following minor head injury. In some instances, a prior history of trauma cannot be elicited. These patients often present with headaches and progressive alterations in mentation or level of consciousness. Focal neurologic deficits are less likely, although they may be present. The CT scan shows these lesions to often be of low density, and they may be extremely large in a relatively asymptomatic patient.

Skull fractures are infrequent, as are overt signs of external trauma, and these can generally be evacuated through a single burr hole. Multiple adjunctive forms of operative management have been advocated, varying from external drainage to perfusion of the subarachnoid space via a lumbar puncture. The purpose of all of these procedures is prevention of recurrence of the hematoma which, unfortunately, is an all too common phenomenon. The mechanism for this is unknown, but it appears to be related to the often underlying cerebral atrophy. In the past, the presence of a thickened membrane was thought to necessitate a craniotomy. This no longer is regarded as necessary, although communication and thorough irrigation of the hematoma cavity is still essential for successful results. Following evacuation, most patients are maintained with the head at 0 degrees for 2 to 5 days, then progressively mobilized. The presence of persistent shift and fluid on CT scan is not infrequent, and repeat operative intervention should be determined only on clinical grounds or by the presence of a persistent lesion 3 months following operation.

Epidural Hematoma

As previously mentioned, the most acute and devastating of the intracranial traumatic injuries is the epidural hematoma. Most frequently, this is associated with a fracture across the middle meningeal artery groove with resultant tear. Classically, it has been taught that patients present with trauma and loss of consciousness, followed by a lucid interval with subsequent acute progressive deterioration. Unfortunately, significant variations occur in presentation, and when time permits, the CT scan is of great benefit. However, the neurosurgeon can be confronted with a patient with acute deterioration to the extent that brainstem compression is obvious. In this circumstance, endotracheal intubation with hyperventilation and the emergent administration of hyperosmolar agents are indicated. When a CT scan cannot be performed emergently, an exploratory burr hole should be considered as the primary diagnostic and therapeutic procedure. In this situation, the side of the head to be explored should be based upon the following criteria in descending order of importance: (1) an ipsilateral dilated pupil, (2) the presence of an ipsilateral skull fracture, or (3) the side contralateral to progressive motor weakness or posturing. The incision should involve the temporal region, specifically the area overlying the middle meningeal artery in order to exclude an acute epidural hematoma; however, the side of the head should be prepared in such a way that if an epidural hematoma is not found, a large craniotomy flap can be rotated in order to allow the evaluation of the presence of a subdural or intracerebral hematoma and/or contusion (Fig. 10). It is to be emphasized, however, that this situation is extremely rare and, whenever possible, a CT scan should precede operative treatment of cerebral trauma.

Spinal Trauma

Although approximately 10 per cent of head injuries are associated with spinal injury and although spinal injuries can occur frequently without head injury, the majority of closed spinal injuries do not produce significant spinal cord

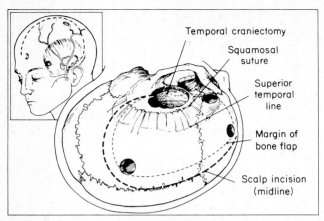

Temporal craniectomy

Squamosal suture

Superior temporal line

Margin of bone flap

Scalp incision (midline)

Figure 10. A craniotomy flap can be utilized for evacuation of acute epidural, subdural, and intracerebral hematomas. The surgical exposure allows relatively rapid access to the frontal, temporal, and parietal regions of the brain, which are most likely to be involved with these traumatic injuries. (From Becker, D. P., Miller, J. D., Young, H. F., et al.: Diagnosis and treatment of head injuries in adults. In Youmans, J. R. (Ed.): Neurological Surgery. Philadelphia, W. B. Saunders Company, 1982.)

or nerve root injury. When present, however, they are often devastating. As with head injuries, these are primary and secondary injuries associated with trauma to the spine. Surgery cannot reverse the damage done by primary injuries occurring at the time of injury, but it can be of significant benefit to the patient by minimizing the secondary injuries resulting from ischemia, continued cord compression, or a host of other problems occurring in these patients.

SPINAL FRACTURES

Spinal fractures with subsequent neurologic damage are the result of direct or indirect trauma applied to the spine.[7] Trauma of the cervical spine is most often the result of indirect trauma following excessive movement of the head in relationship to the body. This is caused by sudden acceleration/deceleration, as is frequently seen in motor vehicle accidents. The vast majority of fractures occur at two levels within the vertebral column: in the lower cervical region or at the thoracolumbar junction. These areas have in common the junction between the relatively fixed thoracic spine and the more mobile lumbar or cervical region. The fractures of the vertebrae involve the vertebral body and/or the vertebral arch.

The classification of spinal fractures varies, although certain ones, such as Jefferson's fracture of the atlas or the pedicle fracture of the atlas (which is often referred to as the "hangman's fracture)," are well-described clinical entities. Cervical fractures can generally be categorized as the result of hyperflexion, hyperextension, hyperrotation, or lateral hyperflexion. In these descriptions, it is also important to categorize whether dislocation exists. A similar scheme exists in the thoracolumbar region, where the fractures can be categorized as the result of flexion, extension, vertical compression, or lateral bending. For all regions of the spine, the crucial question for the physician and patient is whether the injury is stable or unstable in terms of the supporting elements surrounding the spinal cord.

When a patient who has sustained trauma is initially evaluated, a high index of suspicion must always be held

for the existence of a spinal fracture. It is mandatory that the patient undergo adequate neurologic evaluation, followed by appropriate diagnostic x-ray studies. In the cervical region, five types of film constitute the baseline evaluation: (1) the lateral cross-table x-ray, (2) bilateral 30-degree oblique studies, (3) anteroposterior (AP) x-rays of the lower cervical spine, (4) AP views of the atlas-axis, and (5) the vertebral arch field. These studies can be done with the patient supine without any necessity of moving the head, and similar sets are also performed when thoracic or lumbar injuries are suspected. Following these baseline studies and stabilization of the patient, it is often necessary to obtain more detailed anatomic information, which can be generally given by polytomography, CT scanning, and, in certain instances, myelography.

For dislocated *cervical injuries*, reduction of the fracture is the first order of management following initial stabilization. This is usually achieved by the application of a halo skull fixation and continuous traction with varying amounts of weight. Maintenance of the neck in a neutral position is usually maintained with 5 pounds of traction, whereas reduction may require significantly more. If reduction is not achieved over a 12- to 24-hour period by this technique, manipulation of the spine under general anesthesia or muscle relaxant control may become necessary. When this does not produce adequate reduction of the fracture, an open operative procedure with fusion is generally required. The timing must be balanced between optimal stabilization of the patient and institution of scarring of the fracture out of alignment. Following reduction, fixation of alignment can be maintained externally utilizing the halo skull traction in association with a chest brace.

For *thoracolumbar fracture-dislocations*, there is a greater degree of associated stability. The options of treatment for an assumed unstable fracture are prolonged bed rest with subsequent external support or internal compression and stabilization.

Following the early management of the acute injury, patients with neurologic deficits should almost immediately begin a program to minimize secondary lesions and begin rehabilitation. The problems confronting these patients are multitudinous and include pressure sores, chronic bladder infections, contractures, and poor wound healing because of catabolic state. Appropriate management requires close cooperation between the neurosurgical, orthopedic, and rehabilitation services.

CLINICAL SYNDROMES

Superimposed on virtually all major spinal cord injuries is a state of *spinal shock* with loss of transmission of impulses below the level of injury with resultant flaccid paralysis and dysfunction of the bladder. Recovery may be sudden or may take up to several weeks. In all patients with spinal cord syndromes, careful clinical observation to identify clinical progression is critical.

However, the clinical syndromes associated with spinal cord injury often conform to certain general patterns. With cervical lesions, the anterior cord, central cord, and Brown-Séquard syndromes are the most common and well described.

Anterior Cord Syndrome. The anterior cord syndrome produces dysfunction of the anterior portion of the spinal cord, most often from primary or secondary occlusion of the anterior spinal artery or a dominant radicular branch feeding into this artery. The clinical syndrome is best understood by viewing the damage that would result from loss of the regions in this portion of the cord. Such patients generally experience complete paralysis below the level of trauma with decreased light touch and sensation in the same distribution, although, because of the presence of higher level crossing fibers within the spinal thalamic system, the sensory and motor areas may not be identical. Finally, there is relative preservation of the posterior column function.

Central Cord Syndrome. In contrast, the central cord syndrome involves the center of the cord, primarily the gray matter. This syndrome is characteristically seen in elderly patients with prior compromise of the cervical canal following relatively minor hyperextension injuries. The basis of this injury appears to be infarction in the watershed central distribution. Because of this distribution, characteristically the patients have much greater deficits in the upper extremities than in the lower. The sensory loss can be variable. In the past, because initial recovery often resulted in significant functional improvement in the lower extremities and proximal arms, there was thought to be relatively good prognosis with this syndrome. However, follow-up studies appear to indicate that late progressive spasticity in the lower extremities often results in relatively poor long-term prognosis.

Brown-Séquard Syndrome. The Brown-Séquard syndrome is anatomically based on dysfunction of one half of the symmetrical spinal cord. Clinically, patients have ipsilateral spastic paralysis and loss of dorsal column function in association with contralateral loss of spinal thalamic function, pain and temperature, usually one to two dermatomes below the level of injury.

Peripheral Nerve Injuries

CLASSIFICATION

Peripheral nerve injuries include trauma to the proximal plexuses as well as injury to the more peripheral nerves on the basis of acute trauma or entrapment syndromes. Classification of nerve injuries can be quite complex, but the simplified categories used by Seddon appear to be quite adequate for most injuries.[22] In this system, there are three degrees of injury: (1) neurapraxia, (2) axonotmesis, and (3) neurotmesis.

Neurapraxia. Neurapraxia is the result of selective demyelination of large nerve fibers with a resultant motor weakness and general sparing of sensory and autonomic fibers. Because electrical conduction distal to the lesion is preserved, very little muscle atrophy ensues. This type of injury usually heals spontaneously within days to weeks, and the prognosis is excellent without surgical intervention. This injury is essentially a physiologic one rather than an anatomic one.

Axonotmesis. Axonotmesis involves loss of continuity of the axons without interruption of the supporting structures. Because the Schwann sheath is intact, anatomic continuity of the nerve continues to exist and recovery can occur on the basis of axonal regeneration. Clinically, complete dysfunction of the nerve generally exists and a degree of muscle atrophy will ensue. Classically, recovery occurs on the basis of axonal regeneration at a rate of approximately 1 mm. per day (1 inch per month). The patients have a good prognosis without operative intervention.

Neurotmesis. The most severe of the injuries, neurotmesis, involves complete disruption of the nerve and supporting structures. Distal wallerian degeneration occurs with complete dysfunction distally and progressive atrophy.

Although axonal regeneration follows, the loss of continuity of the supporting structures precludes successful distal regeneration without surgical intervention.

NERVE REGENERATION

When axonal damage occurs, the basis of regeneration is axonal sprouting, which occurs 10 to 20 days following injury and subsequent regrowth of the axons distally with reinnervation. Functional recovery depends upon the reinnervation. The regeneration of a nerve is dependent upon multiple factors. These include the age of the patient, type of nerve, extent of injury, and distance between the level of injury and the muscles to be reinnervated. Older patients, mixed sensory and motor nerves, severely disruptive injuries, and proximal injuries respond poorly. Clinically, this often influences the decision of which nerves to repair surgically. The poor prognosis associated with proximal ulnar and peroneal nerves makes repair generally unsatisfactory. In contrast, distal radial or tibial nerve injuries may result in satisfactory motor recovery. Unfortunately, because of the nature of the complexity of reinnervation, recovery is seldom, if ever, 100 per cent.

NEUROLOGIC EXAMINATION

The choice of therapy for peripheral nerve injuries is based upon a detailed and cognizant neurologic examination. Because of the complexity of movement in the upper extremity, the physician must be careful to isolate and correctly evaluate motor activity so that secondary or compensatory movements will not be misunderstood. The sensory examination, while beneficial, has such variation that it can provide only supportive evidence of dysfunction or recovery in most patients. *Tinel's sign*, consisting of the elicitation of a tingling paresthesia with gentle percussion over the nerve trunk, is often used to assess the site of subacute entrapment or distal progression of recovery. Also important in assessment of injury and regeneration is a carefully performed electrical study, and the EMG and NCV have been previously discussed. When performed carefully in an appropriate clinical setting, such studies can be of much value in determining the presence of denervation or reinnervation.

CLINICAL SYNDROMES

Certain clinical syndromes are frequently seen. *Brachial plexus injuries* may result from excessive stretch during traumatic injuries to the arm, shoulder, or neck or from direct penetrating injuries. Careful examination at the time of injury may give important information concerning both the distribution and nature of the injury. The presence of winging of the scapula, weakness of the rhomboids, paralysis of the ipsilateral diaphragm, or a *Horner's syndrome* each suggests avulsion of the nerve root supplying the brachial plexus from the spinal cord. Because of the proximity of the subclavian and axillary arteries and veins, assessment of integrity is also required. More distal acute injuries and chronic or subacute entrapment syndromes include the supravascular nerve at the scapular notch, the axillary nerve in association with proximal humeral or shoulder injuries, the median nerve in the forearm or at the wrist, the ulnar nerve at the elbow or wrist, and the radial nerve in the axilla, distal arm, or proximal forearm. In the lower extremity, peripheral nerve injury must be carefully differentiated from cauda equina or root injuries.

This involves careful physical examination and frequently specific electrical studies. The most frequent sites for lower extremity peripheral nerve injuries or entrapment include the lateral femoral-cutaneous nerve at the inguinal ligament, the obturator nerve at the obturator canal, the femoral nerve proximally within the psoas muscle or at the level of the inguinal ligament, and the sciatic nerve at the sciatic notch or either of its two components—the peroneal nerve at the fibular head or the tibial nerve distally at the tarsal tunnel.

TREATMENT

Surgical therapy is designed to provide maximal opportunity for reinnervation. In association with disruption of the nerve, neurotmesis, intervention may occur primarily at the time of injury or secondarily. In the past, primary intervention was generally limited to sharp lacerations of the nerve with virtually all intervention occurring secondarily. Some authors now favor primary repair because of the ease of identifying the pertinent structures in the absence of scar tissue. However, it is often difficult, even when utilizing microsurgical techniques, to identify the true extent of injury at this time. In general, it is probably preferable to limit the primary intervention to repair of sharply lacerated nerves and to débridement of other wounds with identification and débridement of the pertinent tissue in order to prevent infection and to allow later identification of the nerves at the time of secondary repair. With secondary repair, when primary anastomosis cannot be achieved without excessive tension, the use of nerve grafts from cutaneous nerves, such as the sural or intracostal, may be necessary. Although necessary, the regeneration of injuries requiring nerve grafts is usually not as satisfactory as that obtained from direct reanastomosis. The use of nerve grafts becomes a complex issue when the injured nerve is still in anatomic continuity. If electrical stimulation of the nerve proximally does not indicate transmission across the traumatic regions at a clinically appropriate time following injury, excision of the region of injury with use of nerve grafts is indicated. In contrast, if transmission occurs, external decompression of the nerve is the treatment of choice.

Following partial nerve injuries, peripheral and eventually central pain syndromes may occur. Causalgia is an intense burning pain usually seen in association with partial injury of a mixed peripheral nerve. Clinically, autonomic and atrophic changes are frequently found. The treatment of choice is usually sympathectomy, often in association with intensive medical management.

CONGENITAL ABNORMALITIES

Embryologic Defects

During the second week following conception, the neural plate appears as a midline proliferation of ectodermal cells in the dorsal portion of the embryo.[11] Subsequently, the neural plate invaginates, forming first a groove and then a tube during the third through fifth weeks of gestation. The neural tube then separates from the ectodermal layer and becomes encircled by mesodermal tissue, which later forms the vertebral column, skull, and supporting connective tissue. From the relatively high rate of midline fusion defects that are seen clinically, the embryo must be particularly prone to insults during this phase of development.

While the majority of these are recognized at birth, or shortly thereafter, many do not become clinically obvious until adult life, and, in certain circumstances, may never present as a clinical problem. The spectrum of diseases is extensive and may involve all embryologic components or merely the supporting structures, depending upon the severity of the error and when in the course of embryologic development it occurs. Many theories have been developed to explain the etiology of these lesions, although none clearly describes the spectrum of entities seen.[14]

Spinal and *cranial dysraphism* encompasses a wide variety of lesions. In its most severe form, *craniospinal rachischisis*, there is a failure of dorsal closure of both the ectodermal and mesodermal layers with subsequent lack of development of the brain and spinal cord. At the opposite end of the spectrum, both the neural development and overlying mesodermal and ectodermal components may be intact with the exception of midline failures of fusion of the bone: *spina bifida*, when it occurs in the spine, and *cranium bifidum*, when it involves the skull. Between these extremes, there are many variations.

Myelomeningoceles

The myelomeningoceles (*spina bifida cystica*) are probably the most important of the midline fusion defects (Fig. 11). These lesions most often occur in the caudal aspect of the spine and involve the lower thoracic, lumbar, and sacral regions. By definition, myelomeningoceles, in contrast to *meningoceles*, involve neural tissue in addition to the skin and meningeal covering. They can vary in this superficial covering from full-thickness skin to virtually no tissue

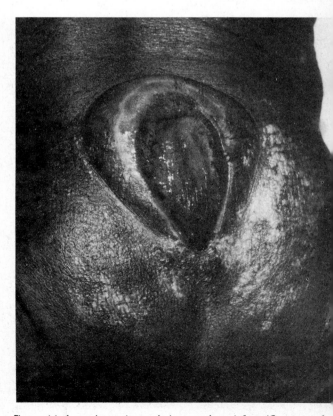

Figure 11. A myelomeningocele in a newborn infant. (Courtesy of Dr. W. Jerry Oakes.)

overlying the neural elements. Commonly, myelomeningoceles are associated with a group of cranial and cervical anomalies, which include the Chiari malformations, aqueductal forking, and hydromyelia. The complexity of associated lesions clearly demonstrates the interaction among the different levels of the CNS at the earlier stages of development. Specifically, the Type II Chiari malformation, which involves a complex hindbrain deformity, is almost never seen without an associated myelomeningocele. Conversely, except in the case of small or sacral myelomeningoceles, a Chiari Type II malformation is always present. This lesion consists of a small posterior fossa with caudal displacement of the cerebellar vermis and the fourth ventricle. There is associated beaking of the fused quadrigeminal plate, kinking of the cervicomedullary junction, and a forking of the aqueduct of Sylvius. The reason for the association between the Type II Chiari malformations and myelomeningoceles has been ascribed to a multitude of etiologies, including tethering of the spinal cord secondary to the myelomeningocele, a displacement of the hindbrain secondary to hydrocephalus, and to a common insult occurring to the fetus prior to the fusion of the dorsal and caudal neuropores. A multitude of additional congenital anomalies may also be seen in association with myelomeningoceles, including craniolacunia, basilar impression, platybasia, Klippel-Feil deformity, congenital heart disease, and anomalies of the gastrointestinal system.

Clinically, patients with myelomeningoceles can be complex and each must be evaluated on an individual basis. The physician is responsible for carefully describing and documenting these prior to consideration of therapeutic intervention. During this time, it is important to protect the lesion by keeping it moist and uncontaminated. Neurologically, deficits may be quite variable and require careful evaluation. With less severe sacral lesions, the neurologic examination may be intact while paraplegia is frequently seen with the lumbar lesions and quadriplegia with the cervical lesions. Often it is difficult to truly evaluate motor response because of the presence of either spinal shock or reflex motor withdrawal. It is important, therefore, to assess which motor function is normal or spontaneous and which is the result of segmental reflex activity. A complete assessment of the degree of physical disability cannot necessarily be made at this time; therefore, because of the need for an early decision regarding therapy, there are few easy answers for the family or the physician in most circumstances. Attempts to predict future intellectual function or impairment based upon clinical criteria at birth have been conflicting, and attempts to predict which criteria obviate operation have been nearly impossible because of the overlying social and moral factors.

When operative treatment is elected, the goals are to prevent infection and further loss of neurologic function by replacing the neural elements within the spinal canal, maximizing the dorsal covering elements to minimize trauma, and closure of the dura and skin to prevent drying and infection. During closure of the defect, careful handling of both the neural structures and the skin is mandatory. Following closure of the defect, the patient must be carefully followed for the subsequent development of hydrocephalus. With larger or more rostral lesions, the incidence of subsequent hydrocephalus becomes quite high. During this initial period, serial ultrasound or CT scans in addition to daily measurement of head circumference may be necessary. Because of the multitude of problems, both physical and social, which face these patients and their families, their subsequent care is generally best managed by a multispecialty approach.

Meningoceles, in contrast, contain no nervous tissue. The neurologic examination in these patients is usually normal. These lesions are generally found in the lower fourth of the spine, although they may occur at any point, and in approximately 10 per cent of patients may actually present anteriorly as a pelvic or mediastinal mass. Small lesions may be treated conservatively, but larger lesions, or those without a full thickness of skin, require operative repair. The prognosis for these patients is generally good, and additional congenital anomalies are only rarely associated.

Occult Spinal Dysraphism

With increasing sophistication, both among patients and in diagnostic studies, the occurrence of clinically occult closure defects in the posterior neural arches is being noted more frequently and is currently estimated to occur in approximately 5 to 10 per cent of the population. The majority of these occur in the lumbar spine and may be associated with a cutaneous abnormality, such as a vascular or hairy patch or a sinus tract. Although the majority of the simple cases of spina bifida occulta are not clinically important, when associated with cutaneous manifestations a higher incidence of intraspinal lesions is noted. These lesions include intraspinal lipomas, dermoid tumors, and diastematomyelia and may present in adolescence or early adult life as slowly progressive foot deformities, muscle atrophy, and problems with gait or sphincter control. Such lesions may be seen in conjunction with a caudal displacement of the spinal cord. Originally, this syndrome was described in association with a thickened filum terminale and the presence of the conus medullaris below the normal L1-L2 level. However, more recently, evidence for tethering of the spinal cord, thereby making it more susceptible to repeated trauma with flexion and extension of the lumbar spine, has been reported with other entities. When treated early, this condition can often be successfully resolved by either section of the thickened filum or release of the constricting lesions. Unfortunately, however, this may result in only cessation of neurologic deterioration rather than reversal of existent neurologic deficits.

Dermal Sinus Tracts

Embryologically, when the normal separation of the neuroectoderm from the epithelial ectoderm does not occur, a stratified squamous epithelial tract may extend between the two layers. With development and migration of the two layers, a tract or deposit of epithelial tissue is brought into a final ectopic location. These lesions occur most frequently in either the lumbosacral or occipital regions, as would be expected if an association with either posterior or anterior neuropore closure existed. While most are quite superficial, some may extend for long distances and end intradurally. In this event, they are often associated with intracranial or intraspinal dermoid tumors. In the fortunate patient, the dermal sinus is recognized as a midline lesion and is treated appropriately by complete operative resection. Unfortunately, this is often not the situation and the patient presents with multiple episodes of meningitis, usually secondary to *Staphylococcus aureus* or *Escherichia coli*, or, more rarely, meningitis may occur following excision of what was mistakenly thought to be a superficial lesion. When an infection has occurred, resection of these lesions becomes more difficult because of surrounding tissue reaction. In some patients, the dermoid tumor rather than the tract will be the primary problem and neurologic dysfunction will be present secondary to a mass lesion. The treatment of choice for these lesions is complete excision. Preoperatively, the anatomic features should be defined by myelography rather than by an attempt to inject contrast through the dermal opening itself.

Lipomeningocele

Lipomeningoceles are abnormal accumulations of fatty tissue usually found in the lumbar region and may reach large size. Fortunately, lipomeningoceles are only very rarely associated with other congenital anomalies, including hydrocephalus, and in almost all patients the neurologic examination is normal at birth. However, it appears that if not treated soon after birth, a progressive neurologic deficit occurs in most patients secondary to tethering of the spinal cord. Clinically, the syndromes are similar to those seen with cord tethering from other causes. The two goals of operation are the relief of tethering of the spinal cord and assurance of a satisfactory cosmetic result.

Neuroenteric Cysts

When the primitive endoderm is not correctly separated from the notochordal plate, endodermal tissue may be retained within the vertebral canal. This produces an anterior bony defect and an intraspinal cyst. The cyst may be lined by a spectrum of tissue types ranging from a single layer of epithelium to a multilayered, mucus-secreting tissue. These tissues may resemble elements of the respiratory or gastrointestinal tract and occur at any point within the vertebral column, but most frequently arise between C5 and T2 where the primitive lung bud evolves from the primitive gastrointestinal system. The cyst may be intramedullary or, more rarely, intraneural-extramedullary, or extradural. The lesions usually present as a slowly progressive mass lesion and are best treated by resection.

Diastematomyelia

The term diastematomyelia is almost self-explanatory, meaning two spinal cords. In actuality, the spinal cord is separated by a longitudinal cleft that contains bone, cartilage, or fibrous tissue. These are usually seen at or below the T10 level. Frequently, there is an occult bony defect or an overlying cutaneous lesion within one to two levels of the septum. Only rarely is hydrocephalus or a Chiari malformation associated, and the patient usually presents in childhood with a progressive spastic paraparesis with thoracic lesions or a spinal tethering syndrome from lesions in the lumbar region. In addition, the patient may present solely with bony abnormalities of the back or legs, such as scoliosis, kyphosis, or clubfoot. Clinically, the course is almost invariably progressive and operative intervention is warranted even in neurologically intact patients.

Preoperatively, the anatomy of the lesion should be defined both by plain films and by metrizamide myelography with CT scanning. The goal of operation is removal of the tethering effect of the lesion, whether it be bony or fibrous. Subsequent spinal fusion may be required when multiple levels are involved by laminectomies.

Sacrococcygeal Teratoma

Although sacrococcygeal teratoma occurs only rarely, it may be confused with a myelomeningocele because of its location. It occurs in the dorsal midline, although the mass of the lesion may be within the abdominal cavity. The correct diagnosis is of importance because with increasing age a progressive increase in the incidence of malignant tissue occurs in these lesions, ranging from 10 per cent or less at birth to greater than 50 per cent by 2 months of age. These tumors are treated by complete removal of the mass, including its presacral portion, because they may metastasize, most frequently to the lungs. Neither radiation nor chemotherapy has been shown to be effective in treating primary or metastatic lesions.

Syringomyelia

In adults, Type I Chiari malformation may be associated with the downward displacement of the cerebellar tonsils and a cystic dilation of the spinal cord, syringomyelia. Syringomyelia may also be associated with a multitude of other lesions, including spinal tumors or trauma. Classically, patients with syringomyelia present with a suspended loss of pinprick and a lower motor neuron syndrome in the upper extremities with spastic paraparesis in the lower extremities. However, the presenting manifestations of this syndrome can be protean. The diagnosis is established by metrizamide myelography and CT scanning through the cervicomedullary junction with demonstration of displacement of the tonsils and/or a delayed intramedullary uptake of dye. Multiple types of operative intervention have been advocated, including posterior fossa decompression, shunting of the syrinx, and even drainage of the cystic cavity through an opening in the lower spinal cord. Currently, bony decompression of the posterior fossa with dural grafting or the insertion of a catheter to allow communication between the intraventricular and the subarachnoid space is the most commonly utilized procedure. Although controversial, the goal of therapy is to alter a pressure gradient that is generated between the intraventricular and subarachnoid spaces. From simultaneous recordings of pressure within the ventricle and within the lumbar space, it appears that a sustained increase in an intravenous pressure gradient causes the formation and continuation of the intramedullary cyst. In clinical terms, the goal of therapy is to prevent further deterioration; however, improvement occurs in only a small percentage of patients. In the past, a distinction has been made between hydromyelia and syringomyelia. Currently, most authors do not believe that this is clinically beneficial.

Cranium Bifidum

Defects in the closure of the cephalic end of the neural tube may also occur and are manifest by lesions in the cranium (Fig. 12). These range from near absence of the brain, *anencephaly*, to occult midline defects in the vertex of the skull, *cranium bifidum occulta*. When brain tissue is involved in the midline brain defect, the term *encephalocele* is applied. In Western cultures, the posterior encephalocele, which is usually centered over the inion, is more common than the frontal encephalocele. These dilated soft tissue masses usually enclose abnormal neural tissue and are associated with other intracranial anomalies such as agenesis of the corpus callosum or holoprosencephaly. Frontal encephaloceles, in contrast, are more often noted among Asians. These occur in the midline above the nasion and are often associated with hypertelorism or other midline facial anomalies. The extent of cranial dysfunction with frontal encephaloceles is generally less severe than that seen with posterior encephaloceles. As with myelomeningoceles, the decision to operate on children with moderate-to-severe posterior encephaloceles is a complex one with multiple social and moral implications. When operation is to be performed, the goal is salvation of normal tissue, a watertight dural closure, and a satisfactory cosmetic result. Later, procedures such as shunting or cranioplasties may be required. Almost invariably a degree of cerebral dysfunction is present.

Craniosynostosis

In the normal infant, there is sequential closure of the cranial sutures. When a premature closure of any of these occurs, a cosmetic defect results. If only one suture is involved, no neurologic involvement may be noted. However, if multiple sutures prematurely fuse, a significant neurologic impairment may result. The cosmetic impairment associated with craniosynostosis can be visualized by the resultant accentuated growth along the vectors of the unfused sutures. Therefore, an abnormally elongated head in the sagittal plane, *scaphocephaly*, is the result of a premature closure of the sagittal suture with expansion of the head frontally and occipitally. This is the most common of the craniosynostoses. Others include *brachycephaly*, which is a shortening of the anteroposterior diameter of the head secondary to the premature closure of both coronal sutures. When the coronal suture is fused unilaterally, often in association with the ipsilateral frontosphenoidal or frontoethmoidal sutures, the condition is termed *plagiocephaly*.

These syndromes may be inherited on a dominant basis in association with facial (*Crouzon's syndrome*) and/or extremity involvement (*Alpert's syndrome*). To obtain maximal cosmetic benefit, patients should be operated upon as soon as possible. If operation is delayed beyond 1 year of age, major reconstruction is required, which may best be postponed until later childhood.

Hydrocephalus

Hydrocephalus is a broad complex of syndromes resulting from an imbalance between the production, absorption, or flow of CSF. Clinically, two general categories are recognized: communicating and noncommunicating. With communicating hydrocephalus, the obstruction to flow occurs external to the ventricular system, most often at the basilar cisterns or at the pacchionian granulations. Noncommunicating hydrocephalus, in contrast, occurs when the obstruction is within the ventricular system. This most often occurs at the aqueduct of Sylvius, the foramina of Monro, or the outlets of the fourth ventricle. In the vast majority, hydrocephalus is the result of decreased absorption or impairment to flow rather than increased production. In childhood, hydrocephalus occurs alone on a congenital basis or may be associated with other congenital or acquired entities, such as meningomyeloceles, after meningitis, SAH, or other etiologies.

In the past, the diagnosis of hydrocephalus was made by a rapidly enlarging head out of proportion to body growth. In older references, one may see illustrations of children with enormous heads, but with increasing levels of parental awareness and the availability of ultrasound and CT for diagnostic evaluation, this has become less frequent. In the neonate, ultrasonography can be quite helpful; in older children, CT scanning is generally required. At times, the addition of positive contrast, through either the lumbar subarachnoid space or ventricular system, may be required

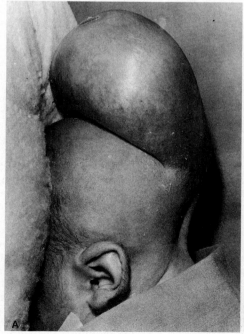 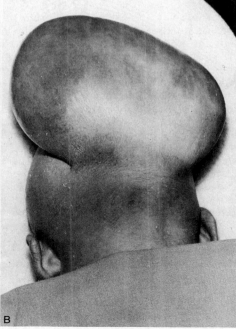

Figure 12. An occipital encephalocele (A, B) in a newborn infant. (Courtesy of Dr. W. Jerry Oakes.)

to define the anatomy of the lesion. Currently, the standard treatment is insertion of a ventriculoperitoneal (VP) shunt. This procedure appears to be associated with the lowest incidence of serious complication and requires fewer later revisions. Alternative procedures include ventriculoatrial shunting or ventriculopleural shunting. Potential complications associated with any form of shunt insertion are multiple, but with careful insertion the complication rate should be less than 10 per cent.

DEGENERATIVE SPINAL DISEASE

Degenerative disease of the spine is a frequent clinical problem. In the lumbar region, it has been estimated that in greater than 70 per cent of the adult population, low back pain and/or sciatica has developed or will develop at some time during life.[20] In the thoracic spine, clinical syndromes are relatively rare because of the stabilization of the spine by the rib cage; in the cervical region, degenerative disease is more frequent and may present as compression of a nerve root with radicular arm pain or as generalized dorsal encroachment of the spinal canal with a resultant myelopathy. These disease problems are among the most common challenges seen by neurosurgeons in the United States today.

Anatomy

The spine generally comprises 33 vertebrae (seven cervical, twelve thoracic, five lumbar, five sacral bodies, the last composed of five fused bodies and four or five inferior ossicles which form the coccyx). Although continuous variation occurs in structure within this segmental column of bones that form the axial skeleton, the typical vertebra generally is composed of a ventral body and a dorsal vertebral arch. The arch is connected to the body dorsilaterally by the two pedicles and is fused dorsally into the paired, flattened laminae that fuse into a single dorsal spinous process. The spinal cord is contained within the circular cavity formed by the dorsum of the body, the pedicles, and the laminae. Dorsilaterally the superior and inferior articular processes form diarthroidal articulations between the vertebral arches. The opposing superior and inferior notches form the intervertebral foramen through which the nerve roots and radicular arteries pass. Variations in structure are related to variations in function. In the cervical spine, which bears the least weight, the bodies are relatively smaller proportionately than the lumbar bodies.

Between the bodies is the intervertebral disc. This consists of the nucleus pulposus, the residual of the notochord, which is encircled by the fibrous anulus fibrosus. Anteriorly, the anulus fibrosus is bordered by the anterior longitudinal ligament; posteriorly, it is bordered by the posterior longitudinal ligament. Further posteriorly, the laminae are connected by the elastic ligamentum flavum.

In the cervical spine, the upper two cervical vertebrae differ significantly in their anatomic structure from the remaining cervical vertebrae. The *atlas*, or first cervical vertebra, has a circular shape and is lacking either a true spinous process or body. The axis, or second cervical vertebra, has an enlarged body secondary to the fusion of the body of the atlas. The first cervical nerve root emerges laterally through a hole in the atlanto-occipital ligament above the first vertebra. This sequence of the nerve root exiting above the concomitant vertebral body continues until the space between the seventh cervical and first

thoracic vertebral bodies where an eighth cervical nerve is arbitrarily designated. Subsequently, the equivalent nerve root exits below the designated vertebral body. Clinically, however, in both the cervical and lumbar spine, a ruptured disc at a given interspace usually involves the lower nerve root (Table 3). This is due to the altered relationships of the nerve roots and spinal cord to the vertebral body that occur following the disproportionate growth of the axial skeleton in early life.[11] The spinal cord generally ends at the upper L1 vertebral body level in all patients above the age of 2 months. Below this termination of the spinal cord, the conus medullaris, the lumbar and sacral roots form the cauda equina. Both cord and roots lie within the subarachnoid and dura. The epidural space, which lies within the spinal canal, contains varying amounts of fat as well as the exiting nerve roots and epidural veins.

Clinical Syndromes

In both the cervical and lumbar regions, clinical radiculopathies can result from herniation of the nucleus pulposus dorsilaterally to compress the adjacent nerve root or from the formation of osteophytes that extend dorsilaterally from the adjacent vertebral bodies and/or oncovertebral joints to encroach upon the neural foramina. In the cervical and thoracic regions, the additional syndrome of spinal cord compression or myelopathy can result from the dorsal rupture of disc material or the dorsal projection of osteophytic material to compress the spinal cord. There is a significant amount of overlap between these disease entities, but dominant clinical patterns generally occur.

CERVICAL RADICULOPATHY

Although cervical radiculopathy secondary to a lateral cervical disc had been previously described, not until 1943 was it clearly and concisely described in such a way that it became widely accepted as a clinical syndrome.[24] Statistically, cervical radiculopathy is most frequently due to a soft disc, the rupture of actual disc material. However, radiculopathy due to osteophytic compression (*spondylosis*) is also a common problem and there is a significant degree of overlap between the two entities. Most frequently patients will present with involvement of the sixth cervical root secondary to compression between the fifth and sixth vertebral bodies or by compression of the seventh cervical root at the interspace below. Patients may present either acutely with the sudden onset of pain radiating into the neck and down the arm or subacutely with chronic neck pain and the insidious onset of arm pain. The clinical syndromes associated with specific nerve root encroachment are well characterized, although variable (Table 3). Pain secondary to a cervical disc is usually aggravated by movement of the neck and by any Valsalva maneuver, such as coughing, sneezing, or straining, which increases the intrathoracic pressure with a resulting increase in epidural venous pressure and compression of the involved nerve root. Although it would appear that, from the etiology of the two causes for cervical radiculopathy, the onset of a soft disc would be more acute than that of a hard disc, this is not an absolute finding.

Plain films of the cervical spine are routinely obtained to assess the degree of degenerative change and to exclude any congenital, neoplastic, or traumatic lesions. In most patients, however, the use of a contrast study is required for absolute diagnosis. Currently, myelography with water-soluble dyes and/or CT scanning provides the optimal radiographic assessment (see Fig. 3).

For all patients with cervical radiculopathy, a trial of medical management should be initially employed unless marked motor weakness is present. Medical management usually involves restricted activity, analgesics, nonsteroidal anti-inflammatory agents (NSAIDs), and immobilization of the neck. This last feature may be accomplished either by a cervical collar or by halter traction utilizing 5 to 10 pounds. Physical therapy and deep heat may also be of symptomatic benefit. During the trial of conservative therapy, it is important that the patient be closely monitored for the development of motor weakness or signs of myelopathy, either of which is an indication for operative intervention. When used judiciously, operation has been quite effective in the treatment of patients with cervical radiculopathy.

Although many operative procedures have been employed, there are two general types: (1) the *anterior approach* and (2) the *posterior approach*. The anterior operative approach consists of exposing the vertebral body through the anterior neck with resection of the involved disc. In association with this, the ruptured disc or osteophytes may be removed and a bone graft may or may not be placed. The posterior approach, in contrast, consists of the decompression of the lamina and facets posteriorly, exposing the underlying nerve root at the foramen. Soft discs may be approached posteriorly, while osteophytes can be managed anteriorly with decompression and insertion of a bone graft. The basis for this is the view that the posterior approach does not deal effectively with the anteriorly placed osteophyte but allows easy removal of a ruptured soft disc with a lower overall incidence of associated morbidity than the anterior approach. However, review of the literature and the experience of others clearly show that when used judiciously both approaches are very successful with both soft and hard discs. The incidence of complications associated with the anterior approach is somewhat higher but not prohibitive. In certain circumstances, nearly all authors agree upon the posterior approach, including lesions above C3-4 or below C6-7, when the diagnosis is in question, when an associated spinal stenosis exists, when more than two to three levels are involved, or when there is a possibility of a neoplastic lesion.

CERVICAL MYELOPATHY

In 1952, Brain and co-workers described the association of cervical myelopathy with cervical spondylosis, providing both the classical description of the disease entity and clearly elucidating many of the associated factors.[2] Subsequently, other factors, including a congenitally shallow spinal canal, 10 mm. or less, have been defined. Clinically, cervical myelopathy generally presents insidiously, with the patient complaining of chronic gait difficulties, subjective sensations of weakness in the lower extremities, or, less frequently, neck pain. Patients may also present with bladder dysfunction, but this usually occurs late in the disease and is a poor prognostic sign. Neurologic examination generally reveals increased tone, which may range from mild to severe with bilateral spasticity. These are generally more marked in the lower extremities and may be associated with distal lower extremity weakness. The arms are usually less involved unless there is direct root compromise with a superimposed radicular component. As expected, the tendon reflexes are increased and pathologic reflexes such as a plantar extensor may be present. Sensory abnormalities usually consist of reduced vibratory and position sense in the lower extremities with varying degrees of alteration in superficial sensations, such as pain and temperature.

Cervical spine films are obtained, although the presence of cervical spondylosis in over 75 per cent of asymptomatic patients above the age of 50 reduces the diagnostic value of this finding. As with cervical radiculopathy, the diagnostic procedure of choice is water-soluble myelography and/or CT scanning.

The natural history of this disorder is quite variable and has made the influence of various therapeutic regimens difficult to ascertain. Medical management with a trial of bed rest and cervical immobilization with a soft collar may be of benefit, although in most cases this is unsuccessful in reversing any of the neurologic deficits. With progression, most recommend operative intervention. Unfortunately, the role of operation appears largely that of preventing further deterioration rather than producing improvement. Because of the uncertainty of the natural history, the question of when to intervene is difficult to establish clearly. The more minor the neurologic findings, the less prone one is to recommend operation, yet the more advanced the disease the less satisfactory the results. In most cases, it is best to determine the tempo of disease progression for each individual patient, although when the sagittal diameter of the spinal canal is reduced statically or dynamically to 10 mm. or less, preventive operation can be strongly recommended. Operative procedures, both anteriorly and posteriorly, have been used; in general, when multiple levels are involved, a posterior decompression is more appropriate. In contrast, when the spinal cord compression appears to be based upon an anterior bar at one or two levels alone, an anterior approach is a reasonable alternative.

THORACIC DISC DISORDERS

The incidence of thoracic disc disorders is quite low; nearly all occur below the fifth thoracic vertebra, and in a significant number, onset of symptoms occurs in relationship to an injury. Clinically, the distribution of pain is onto the chest wall or abdomen and may be easily mistaken for thoracic or abdominal disease. A prolapsed disc or degen-

TABLE 3. *Frequent Clinical Findings with Radicular Disease*

Involved Root	Clinical Findings		
	Motor Deficit	*Sensory Change*	*Reflex Loss*
C5	Deltoid	Proximal shoulder	None
C6	Biceps	Thumb	Biceps
C7	Triceps	Long finger	Triceps
C8	Intrinsic hand muscles	Ring and little fingers	None
T4	None	Nipple	None
T10	None	Umbilicus	None
L4	Quadriceps	Anterior thigh, medial calf	Knee jerk
L5	Foot dorsiflexion	Lateral calf, medial dorsum of foot	None
S1	Foot plantar flexion	Lateral calf and foot	Ankle jerk

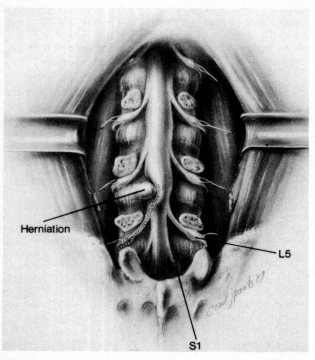

Figure 13. A posterior schematic view of the lumbar spine with the posterior elements removed, showing the relationship between the nerve roots, the disc, and the bony structures. Note that a ruptured disc at L4-5 would normally compress the L5 nerve root and would involve only the L4 nerve root were it to be superiorly or far laterally placed.

erative change can also present as a painless myelopathy. The clinical syndrome is confined generally to spastic paraparesis and decreased pinprick and light touch in the lower extremities. Dorsal column function is generally spared. Myelography best defines the level of involvement, and because of the anatomic locations of these lesions an anterolateral decompression is generally recommended. Extreme care must be utilized in manipulating a thoracic spinal cord that is already compromised. Often, cessation of progression rather than improvement is the result.

LUMBAR RADICULOPAHTY

As in the cervical spine, compression of the lumbar nerve roots may be on the basis of a ruptured disc or bony encroachment on the lateral foramen (Fig. 13). Pathologically, soft discs appear to result from the progressive development of a defect posterolaterally in the anulus fibrosus. Clinically, a history of progressive low back pain with subsequent referred pain into the buttock or proximal leg is obtained, which progresses to involve the entire leg in a radicular manner. It is thought that this is on the basis of progressive protrusion of the nucleus pulposus through the anulus with eventual rupture through the posterior longitudinal ligament, resulting in compression of the nerve root. A spectrum of disease appears to exist, ranging from mild asymmetry in the anulus to a freely ruptured disc fragment in the epidural space. The general clinical syndromes associated with specific root involvement are outlined in Table 3. Clinically, more than 90 per cent of lumbar disc herniations occur at either the L5-S1 or L4-5 levels. Rarely, a disc may herniate posteriorly with compression

of the cauda equina resulting in bowel and bladder dysfunction in addition to severe bilateral neurologic deficits.

Alternatively, lumbar radiculopathy may also be on the basis of bony disease with more lateral compression. With progressive degeneration in the lumbar spine, formation of posterior and posterolateral osteophytes, narrowing of the lateral recesses and foramen, and hypertrophy of the posterior elements (including the laminae, facet joints, and ligamentum flava) are present. The overall result is similar to that seen in the cervical spine with a narrowing of the spinal canal. However, because in the lumbar spine the cauda equina rather than spinal cord occupies this space, the clinical presentation is more radicular from the lateral root encroachment on the nerve roots than from the midline compression, which causes a myelopathy. In general, these clinical syndromes appear to be less acute historically than those seen with soft disc ruptures. With these lesions, the patient may present with standard low back pain and sciatica or with central or lateral claudication syndromes associated with walking, sitting, or standing for prolonged periods of time.

On physical examination, the patient with an active radiculopathy usually has evidence of nerve root irritation. These include mechanical signs, such as paravertebral muscle spasm, decreased range of motion of the lower back, lumbar scoliosis, radicular pain in association with flexion of the straight leg at the hip, or compression of the sciatic nerve at the sciatic notch or at the popliteal fossa. The specific neurologic deficits associated with radicular syndromes are shown in Table 3.

Baseline plain films are obtained to exclude neoplastic, infectious, or congenital malformations. With the exception of the acute onset of sphincter dysfunction or weakness in dorsiflexion of the foot, all patients should be treated medically in the initial period. Medical management consists of restricted activity, analgesics, NSAID, and muscle relaxants. Locally applied heat or ultrasonic deep heat may also be of benefit. When the patient again becomes ambulatory, a lumbosacral corset can be useful in reducing discomfort. In patients who respond to conservative management, a regimen of exercises to increase the abdominal muscle tone and rigid adherence to maintaining an optimal weight are strongly recommended. Following an acute episode of low back or radicular pain, avoidance of frequent bending at the waist and the lifting of heavy objects will be necessary. When conservative management fails, the patient should undergo diagnostic studies as a prelude to operative intervention. In the past, myelography, electromyography, or both were the diagnostic studies of choice. Recently, the development of high-resolution CT scanning has proved to be quite useful in the evaluation of low back and leg pain in individuals who have not had previous surgery. The value of the EMG is primarily in equivocal cases where confirmatory evidence for disease at a specific level is required.

For ruptured lumbar disc, the standard operative treatment is partial hemilaminectomy with exploration and decompression of the involved nerve root. This consists of a midline lumbar incision with anatomic dissection to expose the laminae and facets at the involved level. Partial removal of the laminae, medial facets, and ligamentum flavum is performed, exposing the dural sac and the nerve root. All freely ruptured disc material should be removed. Further removal of degenerative disc material within the interspace is then performed by most surgeons. Decompression of lateral bony encroachment is performed when necessary. It is important that the nerve root be explored as far laterally as necessary in order to ensure satisfactory decompression. When excessive spinal mobility appears to be a clinical problem, the addition of posterolateral lumbar fusion may be indicated. In the presence of severe canal compromise secondary to either disc herniation or degeneration of the bony and supporting structures, laminectomy rather than partial hemilaminectomy is the procedure of choice. In this instance, a midline approach is used to expose the spinous processes and laminae. The surgeon then removes both laminae, the ligamentum flavum, and, when indicated, portions of the facets in order to provide adequate posterior and/or posterolateral decompression.

Chymopapain is a proteolytic enzyme that produces rapid hydrolysis of the noncollagenous polypeptides or proteins forming the chondromucoproteins of the nucleus pulposus. When used judiciously, chymopapain appears to be a reasonable alternative to operation for patients with ruptured discs that remain in communication with the disc space. Severe anaphylactic reactions, postinjection acute transverse myelopathy, and other serious systemic and neurologic complications have occurred following the use of this drug. Careful patient selection and familiarity with the potential problems associated with chymopapain are mandatory for those selecting this type of therapy modality.

FUNCTIONAL NEUROSURGERY

Functional neurosurgery is the term applied to neurosurgical areas associated with the study and treatment of movement disorders, epilepsy, pain, and mental illness.[21] In general, functional neurosurgery is based upon the concept that altered functioning of the CNS involves an abnormal neurophysiologic equilibrium. With this premise, treatment is directed toward establishing a normal balance by *ablative* procedures of the relatively hyperactive component or *stimulation* of the relatively hypoactive component. Ablation may be performed by dividing a specific pathway or, more commonly, by the stereotactic radiofrequency-, chemical-, or temperature-controlled ablation of a specific structure or area. Stimulation procedures, although much less common, are performed by utilizing the implantation of indwelling electrodes or, most recently, by the intracranial transplantation of embryonic tissue.[12]

Stereotactic Neurosurgery

With the development of stereotactic procedures for humans in 1947 by Spiegel and Wycis, the field of functional neurosurgery began to expand dramatically. Stereotactic surgery utilizes the identification of intracranial structures by their anatomic relationship to defined external or internal landmarks.[21] This concept first evolved in 1908, when Horsley and Clarke devised an animal stereotactic instrument to produce localized lesions in cerebellar nuclei.[9] In 1947, Spiegel and Wycis applied this concept to man utilizing a fixed external frame and the ventricular system to provide internal landmarks.[25] With the discovery that lesions in the basal ganglia were of therapeutic benefit in the treatment of the tremor and rigidity of Parkinson's disease, stereotactic neurosurgery rapidly evolved to a frequently performed and generally successful endeavor. With the introduction of effective medical therapy for Parkinson's disease, a relatively frequent disorder, the use of stereotactic surgical procedures declined. Although the technique remained generally successful in the treatment of various other types of movement disorders and in the evaluation and treatment of certain types of pain and seizure disorders, its utilization became largely limited to specialized centers. More recently, renewed interest in this area has occurred with the interfacing of external visualization using the CT scanner with stereotactic technology (Fig. 14). A multitude of CT compatible frames have evolved, and the ability to safely and successfully utilize CT-guided stereotaxy for the biopsy of intracranial lesions has allowed its widespread use in neurosurgery.

The key concept in stereotactic neurosurgery is that the CNS with its various structures can be defined in three-dimensional space utilizing internal and/or external landmarks. In general, a patient's head is fixed with a stereotactic frame that allows absolute definition of coordinates on a three-dimensional scale. In the past, internal landmarks, usually the anterior commissure (AC) and posterior commissure (PC), as defined by ventricular contrast studies, were first visualized, and using a stereotactic atlas of the brain, which defines anatomic structures in relationship to the anterior and posterior commissures in either one human brain or statistically in relationship to multiple human brains, a given target, such as the ventrolateral (VL) thalamus, was approached by its spatial relationship to the AC-PC line. An electrode is inserted to the calculated

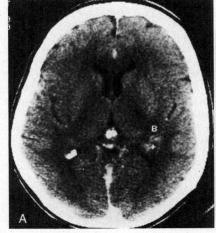

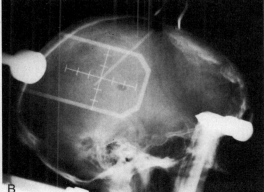

Figure 14. A, CT scan demonstrating a small contrast enhancing lesion in the parietal region. With the use of coordinates generated by the CT scanner, a target point for biopsy was selected (B). B, A lateral skull film obtained intraoperatively demonstrating insertion of a biopsy needle to the predetermined target point.

target point, and either stimulation or recording is performed. This neurophysiologic verification of the site of the electrode insertion is crucial because of the anatomic variability among individuals. The neurophysiologic techniques employed have ranged from relatively simple stimulation to define the internal capsule to exquisitely elaborate single unit recordings during operation. This interface between neuroanatomy and neurophysiology has allowed a much better understanding of the three-dimensional structure and functioning of the basal ganglia.

When lesions are made in the CNS, multiple techniques have been applied, the most frequent being insertion of an electrode for subsequent radiofrequency lesioning. When an alternating current of 50,000 to 2,000,000 Hz is used, heat is generated at the tip of the electrode, producing a well-circumscribed lesion. Most electrodes have thermistors in the tip that allow the temperature generated to be monitored with excellent control of the size of the lesion produced. By variation of the size of the electrode and the temperature generated, specifically shaped lesions in different areas can be produced. Alternatively, a cryoprobe cooled by liquefied nitrogen to produce a freezing artefact or the direct injection of a toxic chemical, such as absolute alcohol, may be employed. When chronic stimulation is to be performed, indwelling electrodes attached to implantable receivers are inserted. An external power supply and control unit then allow control of the stimulation via the internalized radioreceiver and electrode. These systems have been employed successfully to treat movement disorders and chronic pain. Most recently, work has begun in the transplantation of embryonic cellular tissue to predefined intracranial target points in an attempt to restore biochemical and physiologic homeostasis.[12] Although still in its earliest phase, this area of research has generated much enthusiasm in a short time.

Movement Disorders

The treatment of involuntary movement disorders (MDs) began in 1909, when Horsley advocated relief of a hemiathetosis by resection of the precentral gyrus. Subsequently, many investigators placed lesions in various points along the pyramidal tract to control aberrant movements. Subsequent development of improved instrumentation and the publication of human stereotactic atlases allowed the development of stereotactic procedures for the treatment of these disorders. Currently, most surgeons utilize a radiofrequency lesion in the region of the VL thalamus for the treatment of the vast majority of MDs. This procedure is generally effective in patients with parkinsonian tremors, MDs associated with dystonia musculorum deformans, choreoathetosis, cerebral palsy, and MDs that develop following stroke or trauma. Although parkinsonian tremor has responded well to the medical re-establishment of increased dopamine levels in the striatum, most other MDs have not responded favorably to pharmacologic management. Despite extensive investigation, relatively little is basically understood about MDs. Most of what is known is based upon data generated with Parkinson's disease, which may or may not be directly pertinent to the other types of MDs. Currently, the working hypothesis is that aberrant movements and resulting dyskinesias are a consequence of altered gamma and alpha equilibrium. The anatomic basis for this appears to be centered in the cerebellum and basal ganglia, although ascending and descending fiber tracts are also involved. Theoretically, lesions in the thalamus are of benefit because of interruption of the two major extrapyramidal systems in this region: a pallidofugal system that arises from the globus pallidus and enters the inferior thalamus before proceeding to the cortex, and a pathway that arises in the contralateral cerebellar nuclei and enters the thalamus more posteriorly. These two pathways appear to have a major role in the development of rigidity and tremor in association with Parkinson's disease and the other MDs. The placement of a lesion in the VL thalamus is then theoretically beneficial because it reduces gamma system inhibition and direct alpha drive. However, the complexity of the wide spectrum of MDs is such that a high degree of expertise and experience is required for physiologic recording and specific placement of the lesions. When the technique is used appropriately, improvement in tremor occurs in 80 to 85 per cent of patients with Parkinson's disease, in over 75 per cent of patients with posttraumatic movement disorders, and in approximately 50 per cent of patients with dystonia musculorum deformans and cerebral palsy.

Epilepsy

Epilepsy is a syndrome consisting of the sudden onset of altered neurologic function on the basis of sudden, excessive neuronal activity. Although epilepsy has been known as a clinical entity since Hippocrates, the basic mechanisms associated with this disorder are still relatively unknown. It appears that involved neurons have a degree of instability in their membrane with a resultant episodic abnormal depolarization. Although the syndrome was generally thought to originate from a specific focus in most patients, the widespread results and the probable progressive nature of seizures make them quite complex. Although epilepsy is estimated to affect 0.5 to 5 per cent of the population, the neurosurgeon generally sees this problem in two specific circumstances. In the first, it is seen in association with localized or generalized damage to the brain caused by trauma, stroke, or brain tumors. In this situation, the problem is making the appropriate diagnosis and beginning therapy with anticonvulsants. In the second circumstance, the neurosurgeon is confronted with those patients who have intractable epilepsy and have failed to respond to optimal medical management and therefore become candidates for neurosurgical treatment.[17]

As expected, the description in nomenclature for seizures is complex and variable. Recently, the International League Against Epilepsy established a complex classification system made up of partial and generalized seizures.[17]

Partial seizures are clinically focal with a localizing nature. These seizures may be elementary without loss of consciousness or complex and associated with alterations in consciousness. They may also become secondarily generalized but always with some evidence of an initial focal origin. The signs may include a turning of the head and eyes in association with a frontal location, tonic-clonic movements in the opposite body secondary to motor cortex involvement, focal paresthesias from parietal lobe involvement or the wide spectrum of behavioral alterations associated with complex partial seizures arising from the temporal lobe.

Generalized seizures, in contrast, begin without focal onset and are often associated with immediate alterations in consciousness or bilateral motor activity. Clinically, seizures most often seen in this category are:

1. The *petit mal* seizure seen in childhood with its characteristic 3 per second spiking wave pattern on EEG.

2. The akinetic seizures associated with the Lennox-Gastaut syndrome.

3. The tonic-clonic generalized seizures seen in adults, often in association with withdrawal from alcohol or drugs or caused by metabolic changes.

In regard to the approach for the patient with a suspected seizure disorder, the first goal is to establish the diagnosis for any underlying problems that have caused the seizure disorder. In the population seen by neurosurgeons, the most common problems for an adult onset of seizures are brain tumors and cerebrovascular disease for focal seizures, drug withdrawal, metabolic abnormalities, degenerative disease, or infection for generalized seizures. For most of these patients, the history and physical examination will provide the majority of the information needed with supplementation being provided by CT scan of the brain, EEG, metabolic laboratory evaluation, and, in some circumstances, a lumbar puncture. After establishment of the correct diagnosis and therapeutic intervention of the etiology of the seizures, further treatment is based upon institution of appropriate anticonvulsant therapy. In most instances, therapy should be initiated with a single drug, which is increased until either therapeutic control or toxicity is obtained. For most generalized and focal seizure disorders, carbamazepine, phenytoin, or phenobarbital is the preliminary drug of choice. For petit mal seizures, ethosuximide, clonazepam or valproic acid is utilized. During institution of therapy, frequent clinical and laboratory assessment of the patient should be obtained.

Rarely, the neurosurgeon is confronted with a patient in status epilepticus. This frightening and not infrequently fatal situation occurs when the repetitiveness of the seizure disorder does not allow the patient to regain consciousness between seizures. The significance and potential mortality associated with these cannot be overemphasized. The physician must treat this disorder aggressively, which requires the establishment of control of the vascular space and airway of the patient, followed by immediate institution of anticonvulsant therapy. The patient should be given diazepam for initial control of the seizures; in addition, a longer-acting anticonvulsant, such as phenytoin, should be initiated early to prevent the patient from immediately relapsing into status epilepticus following initial control. Because these agents are respiratory depressants, it is crucial that control of the airway be obtained. It is also important that any underlying metabolic abnormalities be corrected as soon as possible in order to allow efficacy of the drugs given. In a small percentage of patients, the use of general anesthesia will be required in order to obtain control of the seizures. In patients with continuous focal seizures, the same urgency is not present. However, the underlying cause of this must be determined. In the neurosurgical population, this is generally the result of infection or a vascular insult.

To treat epilepsy in a patient with intractable seizures, extensive facilities for monitoring are required. Although surgical intervention is frequently successful in these patients, it should be limited to those who have had an extensive trial of medical therapy, in those in whom the epilepsy constitutes a significant medical and social problem, and in those in whom satisfactory localization is present. The patients who meet these criteria are usually limited to individuals with temporal lobe or psychomotor seizures. These patients frequently exhibit complex emotional and behavioral manifestations of their underlying disease process. Because the resection of tissue is keyed to both successful operative treatment and minimization of neurologic deficit postoperatively, preoperative monitoring with depth electrodes and intraoperative cortical mapping are generally required. When these procedures are performed judiciously, unilateral temporal lobe epilepsy treated surgically yields improvement in almost 80 per cent of patients.

The second situation is intractable epilepsy caused by infantile hemiplegia. Both clinically and electrically, these are widespread epileptic foci originating from the damaged hemisphere with secondary spread to the opposite cerebral hemisphere. Excision of the hemisphere with additional resection of portions of the basal ganglia may be of significant benefit in the management of these patients. Postoperatively there may be additional hemispheric dysfunction, although this is unusual, or hydrocephalus may develop secondary to alterations in the absorption of CSF. Other surgical procedures, such as resection of corpus callosum, have been reported beneficial in certain patients, including adults with multifocal cortical epilepsies and children with atonic or akinetic seizures.

Pain

Chronic pain is one of the most complex problems in medicine. Fortunately, over the past decade, considerable progress has been made in the understanding of this problem with the discovery of the endorphins, substance P, and other peptides that appear to act as transmitters. There is also an improved understanding that pain appears to extend beyond the simple sensation conveyed in the lateral spinal thalamic pathway.[26] The key to understanding the current neurosurgical approaches to the relief of pain is to understand the anatomic pathways that subserve pain.

Pain-generated peripheral impulses appear to evolve from various types of receptors. In primates, three types of nociceptors have been described. Two are associated with small *myelinated primary afferents*, A, while the third is an *unmyelinated C fiber*. Each of the different nociceptive units appears to be responsive to different stimuli with the generation of potentially different transmitter substances. There is considerable evidence that these are peptides, most specifically substance P, but this has not been completely established. These fibers then transmit through the dorsal ganglia to the dorsal root entry zone (DREZ) of the spinal cord. The dorsal root fibers approach the cord, becoming organized into small fibers laterally, which represent the bulk of those subserving pain, and larger fibers medially. The more lateral fibers enter the substance of the spinal cord in the region of the DREZ with nearly all of the primary pain afferents terminating in the two most superficial laminae of the spinal gray matter. Some of these fibers, however, may ascend or descend for two to three segments in the tract of Lissauer before termination. There is also some evidence that some pain fibers will enter the spinal cord through the ventral root, although they may terminate in the same fashion as those that enter more dorsally. The area of termination of the C fibers in the DREZ and dorsal horn corresponds to the distribution of substance P and to the distribution of opiate-binding sites. There also appear to be collaterals from the more medially placed larger mechanoreceptors, which make axo-axonic contact with the small fibers in the posterior dorsal horn. It has been speculated that these collaterals may presynaptically block the liberation of transmitter substances, thereby explaining why some types of pain may be improved by *transcutaneous nerve stimulation* (TNS). The interaction between these receptors and the various types of stimuli and ascending and descending pathways has been formulated into the *gait control theory* of pain first proposed by Melzack and Wall in 1965.[13]

Multiple tracts convey pain cephalad, including the

neospinothalamic (lateral) tract, the paleospinothalamic tract, and the archeospinothalamic system. Of these, the *neospinothalamic tract* is the best described. After termination of the first-order neurons in the posterior horn, the second-order cells are found anterior to the substantia gelatinosa where they project fibers across the midline in the anterior white commissure to ascend in the contralateral anterolateral quadrant as a lateral spinothalamic tract. This tract then proceeds through the medial lemniscus to the ventral posterolateral nucleus of the thalamus. In contrast, the *paleospinothalamic tract* involves neurons that provide collaterals to the reticular formation at the level of the pons and midbrain with the formation of a multisynaptic pathway that appears to interact with the hypothalamus, the intralaminar nuclei of the thalamus, the centrum medianum, and the limbic lobe. This pathway, in contrast to the spinothalamic tract, is much less well topographically organized and appears to be more involved with the suffering component of pain. The *archeospinothalamic tract* is only poorly understood but also appears to involve the diencephalon and limbic system in a multisynaptic pain pathway. Following general organization of sensory input in the thalamus, projections from the thalamus extend to the sensory cortex. However, the perception and localization of pain appear to occur at the subcortical level. It is also likely that there is significant integration of the various afferent components at this level, with a balance being obtained between stimulatory and inhibitory influences. Recent evidence has strongly suggested that efferent axons from the periaqueductal gray matter (PAG) in the midbrain descend to nuclei in the reticular formation of the lower brainstem, which, in turn, send impulses caudad to terminate in the spinal cord. In this system, there appear to be opiate-binding synapses with active inhibitory and stimulatory interconnections.

Pain can then be conceived both as a primary and a secondary problem. In the primary sense, it is the perception of a noxious stimulus and with removal of the stimulus the perception of pain is resolved. As a secondary phenomenon, it appears that pain can become an ongoing central process that is relatively independent of the original pathologic event. This type of central pain syndrome is often seen after traumatic peripheral injuries or with cancer, or it may be seen with degenerative disease in the CNS, such as with multiple sclerosis. This type of pain is intense, chronic, and often associated with a marked emotional overlay. Frequently, these patients become addicted to drugs and will show marked alteration in their normal personality.

In confronting chronic pain, the neurosurgeon must first exhaust the medical modes of therapy with appreciation of the elements that are involved, such as anxiety, depression, and frustration. Often, this requires treatment with agents beyond simple analgesics, such as antidepressants, tranquilizers, anti-inflammatory agents, or anticonvulsants. When maximal response to these has been obtained, functional neurosurgical intervention may be necessary. Although the treatment of pain may be quite complex, several general principles do appear to hold. The surgical treatment of pain should be designed to provide the least alteration in sensory function and should be performed at the most peripheral level possible.

The most peripheral procedure is the *ablation of a peripheral nerve*. This can be done by surgical sectioning, avulsion, or the injection of alcohol or phenol. An example is the injection of alcohol into the mental division of the trigeminal nerve for trigeminal neuralgia involving just the chin. The advantage is the small area deafferented and the relative safety of this procedure. However, there is a tendency for the pain to later recur or to involve larger areas of the face, at which time a more proximal procedure is required.

The next most distal procedure is the *sensory rhizotomy* involving the section of several dorsal roots. Denervation of multiple segments is required because of the normally occurring overlap of sensory innervation. Dorsal rhizotomies may be applicable in treating cancer pain that originates from a specific nerve or plexus, and the potential for relief can be evaluated preoperatively by selective blocking of the nerves to be ablated. Unfortunately, this procedure produces a totally insensitive area, which may be of greater aggravation to the patient than the original pain.

A major improvement in the treatment of brachial plexus avulsion injuries, post-herpetic neuralgia, and central pain following traumatic spinal injuries has occurred with the development of the *DREZ lesion*.[15] This procedure consists of radiofrequency- or laser-controlled coagulation of the DREZ in the involved region of the spinal cord. With refinement in this technique, damage to the adjacent cortical spinal tract and dorsal columns has been virtually eliminated. The mode of action of this operative approach is still unsettled, although numerous theories have been proposed.

One of the most successful and frequently performed neurosurgical procedures for pain is the *percutaneous spinal chordotomy*. Originally performed as an open procedure involving laminectomy and sectioning of the lateral spinothalamic tract contralateral to the painful side, the percutaneous C1-2 chordotomy is now being used more frequently. With the patient under local anesthesia, a radiofrequency needle is inserted into the lateral spinothalamic tract contralateral to the painful side. Because of the ascending nature of pain fibers, it is necessary that the pain not extend above the shoulder if a successful result is to be obtained. The extent of lesioning and the specificity of the area of denervation are controlled by the experience of the surgeon and the variability of the anatomic distribution of the pain. When judiciously used, this procedure can result in marked improvement in patients severely incapacitated by cancer-related pain in the lower extremity, distal arm, or chest. A percutaneous chordotomy should be reserved for patients with a short life expectancy because of the potential for the development of severe deafferentation pain in long-term survivors. Although this procedure can be performed bilaterally, a significant risk of subsequent noctural respiratory failure is associated with bilateral high cervical chordotomies. This type of procedure is not indicated for midline pain.

An alternative is the *commissural myelotomy*, which involves sectioning of the spinal cord to interrupt the decussating spinothalamic tract in the anterior white commissure. This procedure can be of benefit to patients with bilateral or midline pain, most notably those with pelvic cancers. An *extralemniscal myelotomy* involves the insertion under stereotactic control of an electrode into the midline between the posterior arch of C1 and the foramen magnum with a lesion produced at the point where stimulation results in lower extremity response. This procedure appears to be of benefit in certain cancer patients, although it has not gained wide acceptance.

When pain involves the head, face, or neck in a distribution too high to be relieved by chordotomy, *medullary tractotomy* may be beneficial. In the more recently utilized stereotactic variation of this procedure, an electrode can be inserted into the mesencephalon in the region of the superior colliculus in patients with intractable facial pain from malignant etiology. By careful preoperative stimulation, a well-circumscribed lesion abutting on the PAG can be made with excellent relief of pain. Postoperatively, an associated loss of upgaze, double vision, or contralateral weakness has been reported in rare instances.

With widespread pain and a significant element of suffering, a stereotactic lesion in the thalamus may be considered. Although multiple types of thalamic lesions have been described, the more extensive *medial thalamotomy* with expansion of the lesion to involve the intralaminar nuclei and centrum medianum appears to be the most effective and does not seem to be associated with a significantly increased incidence of complications compared with the more circumscribed *basal thalamotomy*. Unfortunately, although satisfactory results have been reported with this procedure in some series, the pain relief may be short-lived and alterations in speech or memory may occur when performed in the dominant hemisphere. A relief in the suffering component of pain may also be achieved with a lesion of the cingulate gyrus. Although this procedure appears to be quite effective in certain circumstances and is much less destructive than the previously performed frontal leukotomy, current social situations generally preclude its use in many medical centers.

It appears that long-term electrical stimulation may produce significant relief of certain central pain syndromes. Insertion of electrodes into the PAG of the midbrain has been reported to be beneficial in both malignant and nonmalignant chronic pain. It is hypothesized that this is because an alteration in the paleospinothalamic tract and in the descending inhibitory circuits occurs. Preliminary reports concerning the implantation of catheters to allow selective infusion of morphine have also shown promise for the treatment of various types of pain, most notable cancer-related pain. Multiple types of systems have been utilized, including external catheter systems, implanted reservoirs, and constant-rate pumps. These systems have been implanted both intradurally and extradurally in the spinal canal and intraventricularly in the cranial region. The chronic epidural or subarachnoid infusion of morphine has allowed reduced levels of morphine to be employed and has improved the response rate in many situations. However, prior to insertion it must first be determined that the patient's pain is sensitive to morphine; following insertion of the system, most especially in the intraventricular region, careful monitoring for infection and for the potential of respiratory depression is essential.

Empirically, diffuse bone pain associated with hormone-responsive tumors, such as metastatic breast or prostate cancer, has shown significant improvement after pituitary ablation surgically or by the transphenoidal injection of alcohol stereotactic implantation of radioactive pellets or "lesioning" with thermal probes. These procedures appear to be most effective in hormone-sensitive tumors and in patients who have shown a response to prior hormone manipulation, such as oophorectomy in females or orchiectomy in males. However, successful results have also been achieved in patients with pulmonary neoplasms and melanoma, suggesting additional factors beyond hormonal manipulation involved in the result.

INFECTIONS OF THE CENTRAL NERVOUS SYSTEM

Both the CNS and its coverings may be involved with bacterial, viral, and fungal infections.[28] In the past, cranial infections, including osteomyelitis, epidural abscesses, and subdural empyema, were relatively common because of the high incidence of secondary infections from the perinasal air spaces. With improved treatment, the incidence of these complications has significantly decreased, but they continue to occur, often on an emergency basis. Other sources for intracranial abscesses or osteomyelitis include previous operations, penetrating cranial injuries, and, rarely, hematogenous spread of organisms.

The clinical presentation for these is largely based upon which intracranial cavity is involved. With osteomyelitis, only focal tenderness may be involved, whereas a subdural empyema in a child may present as acute deterioration with relatively little warning. Treatment of these is directed toward making the appropriate microbiologic diagnosis and instituting systemic antibiotics. When bone is involved, débridement generally precludes a continued nidus for reinfection. An epidural abscess generally responds to drainage and treatment of the underlying source of the infections. Subdural empyemas, especially in children, are complex problems that require extensive drainage and frequently recur despite prolonged therapy with appropriate antibiotics.

Any bacterial organism can cause meningitis, but 80 to 90 per cent of cases are caused by *Pneumococcus pneumoniae*, *Haemophilus influenzae*, and *Neisseria meningitidis*. In association with head trauma or operation, group A streptococcus or *Staphylococcus aureus* becomes more common, whereas in the newborn gram-negative enteric organisms are seen in over 50 per cent of patients. The involvement of the subarachnoid space with bacterial or fungal meningitis may necessitate neurosurgical intervention when the underlying etiology of the infection is a lesion such as a spinal dermal sinus tract (in which case resistance to systemic therapy necessitates the insertion of an indwelling reservoir for intrathecal drug therapy) or when the meningitis results in a secondary chronic effusion. Classically, this last problem occurs in children following meningitis with *H. influenzae*. The subdural effusions should initially be treated by repeated aspirations through the patent suture, but when resistance to this form of therapy occurs, a craniotomy for the insertion of internalized shunts may be necessary.

The brain may be involved by a multitude of infectious agents, including bacteria, fungi, and viruses. The extent of involvement may also be quite diverse, ranging from a superficial cerebritis to a deep-seated brain abscess. The origin of the infectious agent may be through the perinasal sinuses, through hematogenous spread, or via direct inoculation, such as in the postoperative or post-traumatic situation. In the past, the diagnosis was often quite difficult and required invasive studies to localize the lesion. With the development of CT scanning, the anatomic structures involved can be clearly defined preoperatively. In this regard, some controversy has evolved in the management of intracranial abscesses. Previously, the neurosurgeon awaited the development of a well-circumscribed abscess prior to operative intervention, which usually consisted of resection of the encapsulated abscess. With the development of CT scanning and the ability to directly aspirate and follow the intracranial lesions, the tendency is now toward initial bacteriologic diagnosis followed by long-term antibiotic therapy with serial CT scans. For most patients, this appears to be adequate and in only limited situations is total excision of the wall of an abscess now indicated. For suspected viral infections, tissue biopsy to establish definitive diagnosis may be required.

In neurosurgical patients, a foreign body is often present in such situations as a cranioplasty or a ventriculoperitoneal (VP) shunt and provides a potential nidus for infection. In the past, removal of nearly all foreign bodies were required. However, recent evidence suggests that with infected VP shunts some may be salvaged by long-term treatment with intraventricular and systemic antibiotics.

Tuberculosis has been a major factor historically, but today it is of much less significance. In the developing world, however, tuberculosis and cysticercosis as well as certain parasitic infections remain major causes of CNS infection.

Bacterial infections may also involve the spinal column, and spinal epidural empyema may be seen with hematogenous spread, following spinal operations, or adjacent to osteomyelitis involving the vertebral bodies. For the vast majority, surgical decompression is an absolute requirement when any evidence of spinal cord compression exists. In mild infections, medical therapy alone may be satisfactory. Subdural infections are much less common, and intramedullary viral or bacterial infections are extremely rare. Disc space infection following spinal procedures may occur and is best treated by immobilization and appropriate long-term antibiotic coverage. In the treatment of CNS infections, both the sensitivity of the organism to a given agent and the ability of the agent to cross the blood-brain barrier must be considered. In the past, penicillin and chloramphenicol were the most widely employed agents in treating most gram-positive bacterial infections. With the development of metronidazole and other synthetic agents, the armamentarium has been greatly improved. This is especially the situation in the use of third-generation cephalosporins and the newer aminoglycosides for the treatment of both gram-positive and gram-negative organisms.

SELECTED REFERENCES

Burger, P. C., and Vogel, S. F.: Surgical Pathology of the Nervous System and its Coverings, 2nd ed. New York, John Wiley & Sons, 1982.
A superbly written and illustrated monograph on surgical neuropathology. This text contains an extremely well written discussion on nearly all of the topics covered and provides enjoyable reading.

DeJong, R. N.: Neurologic Examination: Incorporating the Fundments of Neuroanatomy and Neurophysiology. Hagerstown, Md., Harper & Row, 1979.
This lucid text provides a superb introduction to the beginner as well as an excellent review for those already possessing knowledge of the functioning of the central nervous system.

Penfield, W., and Jasper, H.: Epilepsy and the Functional Anatomy of the Human Brain. Boston, Little, Brown and Co., 1954.
This book provides an excellent analytical analysis of the extensive experience of two pioneers in the field of epilepsy research. It remains one of the best references in this fascinating field.

Schaltenbrand, G., and Walker, A. E. (Eds.): Stereotaxy of the Human Brain. New York, Thieme-Stratton, Inc., 1982.
This multiauthored text provides a detailed introduction and extensive review of functional neurosurgery. The multiple sections are well orchestrated so that virtually all aspects of stereotactic procedures and the underlying basic science are covered without redundancy. Although many of the sections are beyond the introductory phase, the text is the best introduction to this intriguing field.

Walker, A. E.: History of Neurological Surgery. Baltimore, Williams & Wilkins Company, 1951.
A detailed and well-written history of neurosurgery. An extensive bibliography is provided, allowing the reader to pursue the history of neurological surgery in great detail.

Youmans, J. R. (Ed.): Neurological Surgery, 2nd ed. Philadelphia, W. B. Saunders Company, 1982.
This is an encyclopediac neurosurgical reference and remains the best standard resource for those interested in neurosurgery. Most aspects of the discipline are covered in great depth with extensive bibliographies for further reference.

REFERENCES

1. Becker, D. P., Miller, J. D., Young, H. F., et al.: Diagnosis and treatment of head injury in adults. *In* Youmans, J. R. (Ed.): Neurological Surgery, 2nd ed., Vol. 4. Philadelphia, W. B. Saunders Company, 1982.
2. Brain, W. R., Northfield, D., and Wilkinson, M.: The neurological manifestations of cervical spondylosis. Brain, 75:187, 1952.
3. Bullard, D. E.: Brain tumors, *In* Rakel, R. F. (Ed.): Conn's Current Therapy. Philadelphia, W. B. Saunders Company, 1985.
4. Burger, P. C., and Vogel, S. F.: Surgical Pathology of the Nervous System and Its Coverings, 2nd ed. New York, John Wiley & Sons, 1982.
5. Burrows, E. H., and Leeds, N. E.: Neuroradiology, Vols. 1 and 2. New York, Churchill Livingstone, 1981.
6. DeJong, R. N.: Neurologic Examination: Incorporating the Fundamentals of Neuroanatomy and Neurophysiology, 4th ed. Hagerstown, Md., Harper & Row, 1979.
7. Gehweiler, J. A., Osborne, R. L., and Becker, R. F.: The Radiology of Vertebral Column. Philadelphia, W. B. Saunders Company, 1980.
8. Goodgold, J., and Eberstein, A.: Electrodiagnosis of Neuromuscular Diseases, 3rd ed. Baltimore, Williams & Wilkins, 1983.
9. Horsley, V., and Clarke, R.: The structure and functions of the cerebellum examined by a new method. Brain, 31:45, 1908.
10. Horwitz, N. H., and Rizzoli, H. V.: Postoperative Complications of Intracranial Neurological Surgery. Baltimore, Williams & Wilkins, 1982.
11. Lemire, J., Loeser, D., Leech, R. W., et al: Normal and Abnormal Development of the Human Nervous System. Hagerstown, Md., Harper & Row, 1975.
12. Mark, V. H., Gildenberg, P. L., and Franklin, P. O.: Proceedings of the colloquium on the use of embryonic cell transplantation for correction of CNS disorders. Appl. Neurophysiol., 47:1, 1984.
13. Melzack, R., and Wall, P. D.: Pain mechanisms: A new theory. Science, 150:971, 1965.
14. Milhorat, T. H.: Pediatric Neurosurgery. Philadelphia, F. A. Davis, 1978.
15. Nashold, B. S., Jr., Ostdahl, R. H., Bullitt E., et al.: Dorsal root entry zone lesions: A new neurosurgical therapy for deafferentation pain. Adv. Pain Res. Ther., 5:739, 1983.
16. Nibbelink, D. W., Forner, J. C., and Henderson, W. B.: Intracranial aneurysms and subarachnoid hemorrhage: Report on a randomized treatment study. Stroke, 8:202, 1977.
17. Niedermeyer, E.: Epilepsy Guide: Diagnosis and Treatment of Epileptic Seizure Disorders. Baltimore, Urban and Schwarzenberg, 1983.
18. Ojemann, R. G., and Crowell, R. N.: Surgical Management of Cerebrovascular Disease. Baltimore, Williams & Wilkins, 1983.
19. Penfield, W., and Jasper, H.: Epilepsy and the Functional Anatomy of the Human Brain. Boston, Little, Brown and Co., 1954.
20. Rothman, R. H., and Simeone, F. A.: The Spine, 2nd ed., Vols. 1 and 2. Philadelphia, W. B. Saunders Company, 1982.
21. Schaltenbrand, G., and Walker, A. E. (Eds.): Stereotaxy of the Human Brain. New York, Thieme-Stratton, Inc., 1982.
22. Seddon, H.: Surgical Disorders of the Peripheral Nerves. Baltimore, Williams & Wilkins Co., 1972.
23. Selzer, R.: Mortal Lessons: Notes on the Art of Surgery. New York, Simon and Schuster, 1974.
24. Semmes, R. E., and Murphey, M. F.: The syndrome of unilateral rupture of the sixth cervical intervertebral disk with compression of the seventh cervical nerve root: A report of four cases with symptoms simulating coronary disease. J.A.M.A., 121:1209, 1943.
25. Spiegel, E. A., Wycis, H. T., Marks, M., et al.: Stereotactic apparatus for operations on the human brain. Science, 106:349, 1947.
26. Swerdlow, M.: Relief of Intractable Pain. New York, Elsevier, 1983.
27. Walker, A. E.: History of Neurological Surgery. Baltimore, Md., Williams & Wilkins, 1951.
28. Wilson, N.: Infections of the Nervous System. Philadelphia, F. A. Davis, 1979.

THE ARTERIAL SYSTEM

ROBERT W. BARNES, M.D.

41

This chapter has several objectives that will permit the reader to:

1. Recognize clinical features that differentiate peripheral arterial disease from other disorders.

2. Recognize the four basic morphologic disorders that lead to clinical manifestations of peripheral arterial disease.

3. Understand the pathophysiologic disturbances that lead to clinical symptoms of peripheral arterial disease.

4. Recognize the relative importance and salient features of the history, physical examination, noninvasive diagnostic techniques, and invasive angiographic methods used to evaluate peripheral arterial disease.

5. Understand the natural history of various peripheral arterial disorders.

6. Develop a systematic approach to diagnostic evaluation and therapy of peripheral arterial disease based upon risk priorities (life, limb or organ, functional disability or asymptomatic status), using algorithms as guidelines.

7. Become familiar with the ten most common peripheral arterial disorders, including their clinical hallmarks, prevalence, pathogenesis, pathophysiology, diagnostic approaches, differential diagnosis, natural history, therapeutic principles, complications, and prognosis.

The initial section of this chapter will review definitions and classifications and discuss the basic principles that are common to all peripheral arterial disorders, including pertinent anatomy and morphologic abnormalities, pathophysiology, diagnostic and therapeutic principles, natural history, and complications of peripheral arterial disease. The last section of the chapter will discuss in greater detail the ten common peripheral arterial diseases, including:

1. Acute arterial occlusion.
2. Arterial trauma.
3. Aneurysm.
4. Chronic arterial occlusion.
5. Arteritis.
6. Thoracic outlet compression syndrome.
7. Raynaud's syndrome.
8. Cerebrovascular disease.
9. Renovascular hypertension.
10. Mesenteric vascular insufficiency.

DEFINITIONS AND CLASSIFICATION

Peripheral vascular disease refers to disorders of arteries, veins, and lymphatics exclusive of the heart. By convention, diseases of the ascending aorta and aortic arch as well as of intracranial vessels are usually excluded from a discussion of peripheral vascular disease, because such disorders are in the special therapeutic provinces of cardiac and neurologic surgeons, respectively. This chapter will review the common disorders of peripheral arteries, exclusive of arteriovenous fistula.

Peripheral arterial disease may be classified in a variety of ways, many of which are of functional clinical importance. The following classification methods include examples of specific arterial disorders reflecting each category.

Anatomic Classification

Anatomic classification of peripheral arterial disease includes disorders of the extremities, the cerebral circulation, and the visceral arteries (Fig. 1). Peripheral arterial disease most commonly affects the vessels of the lower extremities and the extracranial cerebral circulation. Lower extremity arterial disease is often subclassified as *inflow* disease, including lesions of the aorta and the iliac and the common femoral arteries, *outflow* disease of the femoropopliteal system, and *runoff* disease of the tibial and peroneal arteries. *Small vessel disease* is, by definition, disease of unnamed arteries including arterioles and capillaries. Although such disease may occur in diabetes mellitus, particularly in the retina or kidney, true small vessel disease is rarely responsible for clinical symptoms in the extremities. Physicians should not attribute manifestations of peripheral arterial disease in diabetics, including claudication, ischemic rest pain, and gangrene, to small vessel disease. Such patients usually have atherosclerotic occlusive disease of named arteries, particularly in the femoropopliteal or tibial arterial system, although the lesions may be distributed more distally than in nondiabetic subjects.

Upper extremity arterial disease may involve the subclavian, axillary, brachial, radial, or ulnar arteries or the arteries of the palms and digits. Such disease is much less common than is disease of the lower extremities.

Extracranial cerebrovascular disease is usually subdivided into carotid and vertebrobasilar disease. Lesions of the subclavian artery may lead to cerebrovascular symptoms, particularly if collateral circulation develops via the vertebral arteries (subclavian steal).

Visceral arterial disease involves lesions of branches of the abdominal aorta, including the celiac, mesenteric, and renal arteries. Such lesions may lead to acute or chronic mesenteric ischemia or disturbances of renal function including renovascular hypertension and progressive renal failure.

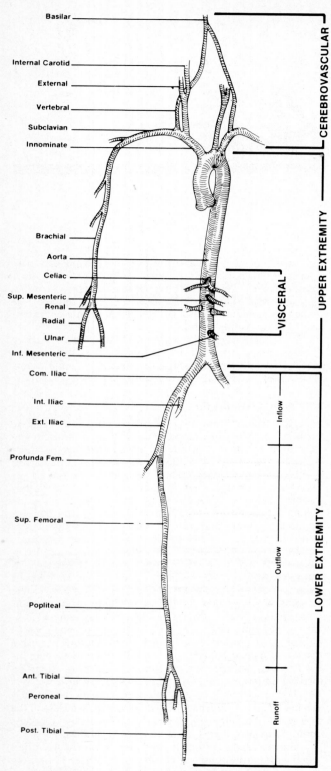

Figure 1. Pertinent anatomy of peripheral arterial disease.

Labels (top to bottom, left side): Basilar, Internal Carotid, External, Vertebral, Subclavian, Innominate, Brachial, Aorta, Celiac, Sup. Mesenteric, Renal, Radial, Ulnar, Inf. Mesenteric, Com. Iliac, Int. Iliac, Ext. Iliac, Profunda Fem., Sup. Femoral, Popliteal, Ant. Tibial, Peroneal, Post. Tibial

Brackets (right side): CEREBROVASCULAR, UPPER EXTREMITY, VISCERAL, LOWER EXTREMITY, Inflow, Outflow, Runoff

Etiologic Classification

Etiologic classification of peripheral arterial disease includes *congenital* and *acquired* disorders. Most arterial diseases are acquired, usually as the result of degenerative conditions, particularly atherosclerosis. *Congenital* lesions include coarctation of the aorta, possibly fibromuscular dysplasia, and cystic adventitial degeneration. The most common congenital vascular abnormality is arteriovenous fistula, which is discussed in another chapter.

Temporal Classification

Temporal classification of arterial disease includes acute and chronic disorders. *Acute* arterial occlusion refers to disorders of relatively rapid onset and often fairly severe symptoms, e.g., thrombosis, embolism, and trauma. Cerebrovascular symptoms are classified on a temporal basis, with transient ischemic attacks lasting less than 24 hours and stroke lasting for more than 24 hours. *Chronic* arterial disease includes most atherosclerotic occlusive disease and arterial aneurysms.

Mechanistic Classification

Mechanistic classification of arterial disease includes organic and functional disorders. *Organic* arterial disease refers to structural changes in arteries within either the lumen or the arterial wall or extravascular compression. *Functional* arterial disorders include states of reversible abnormal narrowing (vasoconstriction) or enlargement (vasodilatation), often called vasomotor disturbances. Raynaud's disease is an example of such a functional disorder.

Morphologic Classification

Morphologic classification of peripheral arterial disease categorizes lesions into one of four arterial disorders that may lead to clinical symptoms: (1) obstruction, (2) dilatation, (3) disruption, and (4) fistula (Fig. 2).

Most arterial disorders result from *obstruction* to blood flow and include acute or chronic arterial occlusive disease due to thrombosis, embolism, atherosclerosis, or trauma. Abnormal permanent *dilatation* of an artery is termed an aneurysm and, because of the absence of obstruction to flow, may be asymptomatic until complications (rupture or thrombosis) ensue. *Arterial disruption* is common in arterial trauma and may be partial or complete with resultant hemorrhage or arterial occlusion. Fistula formation between an artery and an adjacent vein is termed *arteriovenous fistula* and will be discussed in a separate chapter.

Arterial obstruction may be subclassified as intraluminal, including thrombosis or embolism; *mural*, typified by atherosclerosis or arterial dissection; and *extramural*, exemplified by neurovascular compression syndromes, compartment syndrome, or compression by adjacent tumor or other masses.

More specific morphologic subclassification of arterial disease may be based upon the underlying *pathology*. The most common pathologic causes of peripheral disease are atherosclerosis, trauma, and thromboemboli. Less common pathologic entities include fibromuscular dysplasia, arteritis, neurovascular compression syndromes, cystic medial or subadventitial degeneration, coarctation, and primary arterial tumors.

Hemodynamic Classification

Hemodynamic classification separates arterial disorders into those with reduced circulation (ischemia), normal

A. OBSTRUCTION

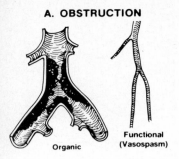

Organic

Functional
(Vasospasm)

B. DILATATION

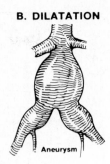

Aneurysm

C. DISRUPTION

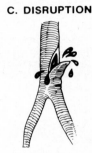

Trauma

D. FISTULA

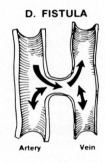

Artery   Vein

Figure 2. Principal morphologic lesions underlying peripheral arterial disorders.

circulation, or increased circulation (hyperemia). Most arterial occlusive disease results in reduced circulation either with exercise or, in more advanced disease, at rest. Arterial aneurysms usually do not affect the peripheral arterial circulation unless thromboembolic complications ensue. An arteriovenous fistula characteristically results in increased arterial circulation proximal to and at the site of the fistula with reduced circulation distal to the fistula, the magnitude of which depends on the size of the fistula.

Prognostic Classification

A *prognostic classification* of peripheral arterial disease reflects the four potential risks of arterial disorders: life-threatening disease, such as ruptured aneurysm; limb- (or organ-) threatening disease, such as acute arterial occlusion or advanced chronic arterial insufficiency; functionally disabling disease, as in chronic arterial occlusive disease, which may interfere with self-care or occupational or recreational activities; and nondisabling conditions such as mild arterial occlusive disease or asymptomatic aneurysm. This chapter emphasizes the importance of rapid recognition of the potential risk of arterial disorders to permit appropriate management to prevent loss of life, limb, or functional well-being. Protocols for managing specific arterial disorders will be illustrated by diagnostic and therapeutic algorithms.

PATHOPHYSIOLOGY

Excluding arteriovenous fistula, peripheral arterial disease produces clinical manifestations via one of three mechanisms: obstruction to arterial flow, aneurysmal dilatation,

or arterial disruption with hemorrhage. Because the pathophysiology of arterial hemorrhage is well reviewed in other sections of this text, this discussion will focus upon the pathophysiology of arterial obstruction and dilatation. To understand the pathophysiology of arterial disease, one must first have an appreciation of normal hemodynamics.[2,17]

Hemodynamics of Normal Circulation

Blood moves through the circulation as a result of differences in *total fluid energy*. Although pressure gradients are often considered to be the driving force for blood flow, other forms of fluid energy also affect the circulation. Total fluid energy includes potential energy and kinetic energy. *Potential energy* includes intravascular pressure and gravitational energy. *Intravascular pressure* is the result of the pumping action of the heart but is also influenced by *hydrostatic pressure* and, to a slight degree, *static pressure* (the residual pressure of the blood within the elastic vascular system in the absence of the circulation). Hydrostatic pressure (P) is the negative product of the specific gravity of blood (ρ), the acceleration of gravity (g), and the distance (h) above the phlebostatic axis (level of the right atrium):

$$P_{HYDROSTATIC} = -\rho gh$$

Gravitational potential energy ($+\rho Pgh$) expresses the ability of blood to perform work based on its position above a reference point and is equal to, but opposite in mathematical sign of, hydrostatic pressure. Because hydrostatic pressure and gravitational potential energy usually cancel each other out and static pressure is relatively low (5 to 10 mm. Hg), intravascular pressure produced by cardiac contraction represents the primary component of potential energy that propels the blood.

Kinetic energy (KE) reflects the ability of blood to perform work on the basis of its motion and is proportional to the square of the blood velocity (v):

$$KE + \frac{1}{2}(\rho v^2)$$

Under conditions of steady blood flow in a frictionless system, the total fluid energy (pressure and gravitational and kinetic energies) in a given streamline is the same at any point along the circulation, as expressed by the Bernoulli equation:

$$P_1 + \rho gh_1 + \frac{1}{2}\rho v^2 = P_2 + \rho gh_2 + \rho v_2^2$$

Because of friction in the human circulation, some energy is dissipated as heat, which must be added to the right side of the above equation.

There are two forms of energy loss due to blood flow: viscous and inertial losses. *Viscous losses* are the result of blood viscosity, which results in friction between adjacent layers of blood. *Inertial losses* result from alterations in blood flow velocity or new direction.

Viscous energy losses are expressed by Poiseuille's law, which states that the pressure gradient across a rigid tube (P_1-P_2) is proportional to fluid flow (Q) or mean velocity ($\bar{V}$), the tube length (L), and the fluid viscosity (η) and is inversely proportional to the fourth power (or second power if velocity is used) of the tube radius (r):

$$P_1 - P_2 = Q(8L\eta/\pi r^4)$$

or

$$P_1 - P_2 = \bar{V}(8L\eta/\pi r^2)$$

Poiseuille's equation forms the basis of the familiar relationship:

$$\text{pressure} = \text{flow} \times \text{resistance}$$

The factors contributing to hemodynamic resistance in Poiseuille's equation include fluid viscosity and tube length and radius, the latter being the most important variable. It is important to realize that Poiseuille's law applies only to the idealized conditions of steady (nonpulsatile), laminar (nonturbulent), irrotational flow of a Newtonian fluid (viscosity unaffected by velocity) in a straight, rigid, cylindrical tube. Because few of these conditions apply to the human circulation, Poiseuille's law can only serve as a guide to the minimal pressure gradient or resistance that may be expected in man.

Hemodynamics of Arterial Obstruction

In arterial occlusive disease, inertial energy losses may exceed viscous losses. Inertial losses are proportional (with a probability constant (k) to the density or specific gravity of blood (ρ) and the square of the blood velocity (v):

$$P = k \tfrac{1}{2} \rho v^2$$

The measured pressure drop across a given vascular segment at varying flow rates does not follow the linear relationship of Poiseuille's law. Rather, the observed pressure gradients fit a line with both linear and squared flow terms, corresponding to both viscous and inertial energy losses. Inertial losses account for much of the energy dissipation as blood flows through an arterial stenosis (Fig. 3). The energy losses occur at both the entrance (contraction effects) and exit (expansion effects) and are particularly prominent at the exit of the stenosis. As shown in Figure 3, most of the energy dissipation across a stenosis is due to kinetic energy loss, particularly at the exit.

The ratio of inertial forces to viscous forces acting on blood is reflected in the Reynold's number (Re):

$$Re = \rho v d$$

where d is the vessel diameter. At a Reynold's number of over 2000, inertial forces may disrupt normal laminar blood flow, resulting in turbulent flow in random directions and velocities. Such turbulent blood flow is uncommon in the peripheral circulation, where Reynold's numbers are usually below 2000. However, blood flow is frequently disturbed in human circulation. Steady laminar blood flow results in a parabolic blood velocity profile across the diameter of the vessel, whereas disturbed or turbulent flow results in a more blunt profile. In pulsatile blood flow in the human circulation, the velocity profile constantly changes throughout the cardiac cycle and may vary from flat to nearly parabolic (during peak systole) and may include periods of transient reverse blood flow in early diastole. This reverse blood flow is typical of major arteries and may be detected with simple directional Doppler ultrasonic velocity instruments. The arterial velocity patterns are disturbed distal to arterial obstruction, and there is loss of the normal reverse flow in diastole. Such abnormality may be readily detected by Doppler ultrasound.

The degree of narrowing of an artery required to produce a detectable pressure gradient or reduction in blood flow is called the critical stenosis. A stenosis in most

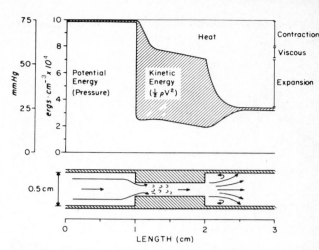

Figure 3. Schematic diagram of factors contributing to viscous and inertial energy losses associated with a stenosis. (After Sumner, D. S.: Hemodynamics and pathophysiology of arterial disease. In Rutherford, R. B. (Ed.): Vascular Surgery, 2nd ed. Philadelphia, W. B. Saunders Company, 1984, pp. 19–44.)

peripheral arteries does not become significant until the lumen cross-sectional area is reduced by at least 75 per cent, which corresponds to a diameter reduction of 50 per cent. The pressure drop across a given stenosis is proportional to the flow across the narrowing, which explains why relatively insignificant stenoses at rest may be associated with significant pressure gradients and, thus, symptoms, during the increased blood flow associated with exercise.

In order to understand the hemodynamics of peripheral arterial occlusive disease, one must understand the various components of the arterial circulation that result in altered hemodynamics in the presence of arterial occlusive disease (Fig. 4). When arterial stenosis develops, the resulting pressure gradients may lead to enlargement of adjacent blood vessels circumventing the obstruction, the so-called collateral arteries. In addition, the reduction in pressure more distally in the circulation may result in vasodilatation of the distal circulatory bed, the so-called peripheral vascular resistance. The combined resistance of the segmental arterial stenosis and the adjacent collateral vessels may be considered the segmental resistance. The resistances are parallel and are related by the following reciprocal formula:

$$1/R_{\text{SEGMENTAL}} = 1/R_{\text{STENOSIS}} + 1/R_{\text{COLLATERAL}}$$

The segmental resistance is in series with the peripheral vascular resistance of the distal arterioles and capillaries, the combined resistance of which is expressed by the following formula:

$$R_{\text{TOTAL}} = R_{\text{SEGMENTAL}} + R_{\text{PERIPHERAL}}$$

Normally the segmental vascular resistance of major arteries is low and the peripheral vascular resistance is relatively high. The resting blood flow through major arteries normally has a large pulsatile component and a low mean blood flow component, with little associated segmental pressure drop. With exercise, the peripheral resistance decreases and flow through segmental arteries increases as much as 10 or 20 times resting values, again with relatively little pressure drop.

With moderate arterial occlusive disease, the segmental

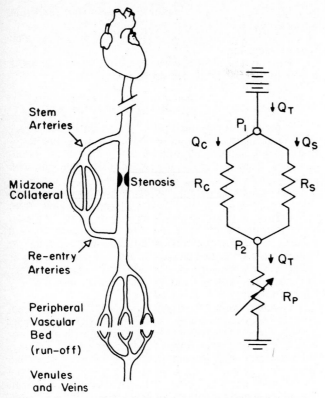

Stem
Arteries

Midzone
Collateral

Stenosis

Re-entry
Arteries

Peripheral
Vascular
Bed
(run-off)

Venules
and Veins

Figure 4. Schematic illustration and electrical analogue of factors contributing to segmental peripheral arterial resistance. (After Sumner, D. S.: Hemodynamics and pathophysiology of arterial disease. In Rutherford, R. B. (Ed.): Vascular Surgery, 2nd ed. Philadelphia, W. B. Saunders Company, 1984, pp. 19–44.)

resistance in the affected artery is increased, but resting blood flow may be normal as a result of compensatory decrease in the peripheral vascular resistance. The increased segmental resistance results in a reduction in the pulsatile component of blood flow through the affected area and is associated with an abnormal resting pressure gradient across the segment. With exercise, the peripheral vascular resistance further decreases, but its capacity to do so is limited by the compensatory decreased resistance at rest such that exercise blood flow is lower than normal. Exercise blood flow is further limited by the increased pressure drop across the segmental resistance at increased flow rates. As a result, muscle ischemia (claudication) results during exercise.

With advanced peripheral arterial occlusive disease, resting blood flow may be reduced despite maximal reduction in peripheral vascular resistance, and ischemic rest pain or tissue necrosis may develop. There is minimal pulsatile blood flow with predominant mean blood flow and a marked pressure drop across the segmental resistance. With exercise, little or no increase in blood flow can occur as a result of the maximal peripheral vasodilatation, and claudication occurs rapidly, usually with a marked reduction in pressure across the segmental resistance.

Despite the development of prominent collateral blood vessels, the resistance of the collateral circuits is always greater than that of the original unobstructed artery. If the collateral vessel was as large as one fourth the diameter of the main artery, 256 such vessels would be required to equal the resistance of the original artery. Usually collateral

vessels are much smaller than this. As a result, despite extensive collateral circulation, resting systolic pressure gradients are almost always recordable across segments of arteries involved by arterial occlusive disease.

These hemodynamic factors explain the common symptoms and signs of peripheral artery occlusive disease. Because of the reduction in pressure across diseased vascular segments, pulses become weaker or unpalpable. Patients with weak pulses at rest may have disappearance of pulses with exercise as a result of a further decrease in distal arterial pressure associated with the increased blood flow across the segmental vascular resistance. Recordings of systolic blood pressure in an extremity distal to an obstruction reveal abnormally low systolic pressures when related to a normal arm systolic pressure. The pulse amplitude of Doppler velocity tracings or plethysmographic recordings will become progressively attenuated as a result of the dampening of the peripheral arterial velocity and pulse waveform associated with the stenosis. Because of the progressive vasodilatation of the peripheral arterioles distal to an arterial obstruction, little therapeutic effect can be expected from oral vasodilators or lumbar sympathectomy for most patients with advanced peripheral arterial occlusive disease.

Hemodynamics of Arterial Aneurysm

Peripheral artery aneurysms rarely result in significant reduction in blood flow unless complications of thrombosis or embolism develop. Although an arterial dilatation may result in local flow disturbances including zones of flow separation and eddy currents, the body often adapts to such flow disturbances by developing layers of laminated thrombus that line the aneurysm, resulting in a flow channel of relatively normal dimensions. Such a laminated thrombus often results in a misleading arteriographic image of relatively normal vascular lumen, which belies the presence of a sizable arterial aneurysm. For this reason, other diagnostic methods should be relied upon to estimate the size of peripheral aneurysms.

The principal pathophysiology of arterial aneurysms relates to the altered mechanical properties of the vessel wall. Normal blood vessels are viscoelastic, with varying proportions of elastin, smooth muscle, and collagen contributing to the wall properties. Large arteries, particularly the aorta, have a relatively greater amount of elastin to provide the elasticity necessary to absorb the energy of the cyclic cardiac output. Such elasticity also aids in maintaining relatively steady peripheral blood flow. As the elastic elements deteriorate with age, atherosclerotic disease, or other degenerative or inflammatory disorders, the distensibility of the vessel wall decreases. Although atherosclerosis is the most common pathogenic lesion associated with aneurysm, the exact cause of aneurysm is unknown. The predilection of the infrarenal abdominal aorta to aneurysm formation has been considered the result of excessive forces at this location in the arterial system resulting from reflected pulse waves from the aortic bifurcation. An alternative explanation of the frequency of infrarenal aneurysmal disease is the paucity of fibromuscular lamellae, which are relatively avascular and under greater tension in this location of the aorta.

The increased tension in the wall of an aneurysm is usually considered a reflection of Laplace's law:

$$\text{tension} = \text{pressure} \times \text{radius}$$

However, this law applies only to infinitely thin-walled structures, such as soap bubbles. A more appropriate relationship of the wall stress (τ) in an aneurysm must include the contribution of the wall thickness (δ):

$$\tau = (P \times r_{INSIDE})/\delta$$

This formula suggests that the wall stress of a 6.0-cm. (diameter) aortic aneurysm, with a proportionate reduction in wall thickness, would be about 12 times the stress of a normal 2.0-cm. aorta, which is a much greater tension than that predicted by Laplace's law. Intraluminal thrombus may reduce the tension in the outer wall of the aneurysm, but this protective effect is lost if the thrombus is incomplete or has a fissure in it. This formula also illustrates the importance of hypertension in increasing wall stress and thus the risk of rupture of an arterial aneurysm.

DIAGNOSTIC PRINCIPLES

The evaluation of patients with suspected peripheral arterial disease may involve one or more of the following: history, physical examination, noninvasive diagnostic techniques, and invasive radiologic methods, particularly arteriography.[3] Although some patients may require all four steps of the evaluation, many individuals need only a careful history and physical examination, with or without some objective validation of the presence, location, and magnitude of arterial disease using noninvasive methods. Although physicians and patients are increasingly aware of the technologic advances in medicine, the physician should avoid unnecessary invasive diagnostic methods in a patient with suspected peripheral arterial disease unless major surgical intervention is contemplated. Some general principles of the diagnosis of patients with vascular disease will be reviewed in this section with more specific diagnostic techniques for each vascular condition described later in this chapter.

History

The history is the most important body of information in evaluating and managing a patient with peripheral arterial disease. An exception to this is the patient with arterial aneurysm, who may have no symptoms and may be correctly diagnosed only with a careful examination. Patients with arterial trauma usually have an evident history. Because arterial occlusive disease is the most common form of arterial disorder, the following section will review the important elements of the history in a patient with suspected arterial occlusive disease in the lower extremity. Many of these principles also apply to patients with arterial disease of the upper extremity as well as cerebrovascular or visceral artery disease. A more complete description of these specific conditions will be reviewed later in this chapter.

In a patient with suspected chronic arterial occlusive disease of the lower extremities, the history should endeavor to answer the following eight questions:

1. Are the patient's symptoms due to *arterial* disease?
2. What is the probable *etiology* of the arterial obstruction?
3. What is the anatomic *location* of the obstruction(s)?
4. What is the *functional impairment* of the patient?
5. Does the patient have *atherosclerotic risk factors*?
6. Will the patient benefit from *medical therapy*?

7. Is the patient a candidate for *operation* (and thus arteriography)?
8. What are the *operative risks* (and, therefore, what type of operation)?

The features of the history that permit answers to these questions will be elaborated upon in turn.

ARE THE PATIENT'S SYMPTOMS DUE TO ARTERIAL DISEASE?

Patients with peripheral arterial occlusive disease usually present with one or more of the following manifestations: asymptomatic, intermittent pain with exercise (claudication), persistent pain at rest, or tissue necrosis with either ulceration or gangrene.

Asymptomatic patients are discovered to have arterial occlusive disease incidentally upon physical examination, either with peripheral pulse deficits or the presence of an arterial bruit. A bruit in the neck may signify carotid stenosis, a bruit in the epigastrium may indicate celiac or mesenteric artery stenosis, and a bruit in either flank or either hypochrondrium may be indicative of renal artery stenosis. The latter condition may be accompanied by hypertension.

Claudication is, by definition, intermittent muscle pain brought on by *reproducible* exercise and relieved by a *brief* period of rest. The patient characteristically complains of muscle cramping after a well-defined distance of walking, although the muscle discomfort may be variously described as fatigue, weakness, or numbness of the extremity. The pain should be relieved by cessation of walking even though the patient continues to stand. It is important to differentiate these features from *pseudoclaudication* due to neurospinal or musculoskeletal conditions, which may result in lower extremity pain after *variable* periods of exercise with relief occurring only after a more *prolonged* period of rest or after sitting or lying down.

Ischemic *rest pain* involves sharp or burning pain or numbness in the most distal aspect of the affected extremity, including the toes, forefoot, or heel. Rest pain often occurs at night and interferes with sleep and may be characteristically relieved by hanging the extremity in a dependent position or by a brief period of walking about the room. Ischemic rest pain must be differentiated from night cramps, which are muscle cramps in the calf or foot that are usually relieved by massage or by medications such as quinine or chlorpheniramine. Ischemic rest pain must also be differentiated from peripheral neuropathy, which frequently affects patients with diabetes mellitus, resulting in a burning pain in a stocking distribution that is not relieved by positional changes.

Tissue necrosis represents the most severe expression of peripheral arterial occlusive disease. *Ischemic ulceration* usually occurs on the distal aspect of the extremity or foot in areas predisposed to trauma, including the toes, dorsum of the foot, and malleoli. Ischemic ulcers are characterized by poor granulation tissue in the base and lack of epithelialization of the margins. Such ulcers should be differentiated from venous stasis ulcers, which usually occur on the medial aspect of the lower leg with a surrounding area of hyperpigmentation and stasis dermatitis. Venous ulcers usually show good granulation tissue and epithelium at the margins if properly treated. Neurotrophic ulcers characteristically occur on the soles of the feet beneath the metatarsal heads, frequently in diabetic patients with peripheral neuropathy. Such ulcers are deeply punched out and may extend to, and infect, the metatarsal heads (mal perforans). However, such ulcers will usually heal if pressure is relieved with properly fitting shoes or a period of bed rest. Other less common forms of ulceration that must be differentiated from ischemic ulcers include ulceration associated with hypertension and arteritis.

Gangrene in peripheral arterial occlusive disease usually affects the toes, foot, or distal leg. Most gangrene is dry and noninfected, especially with severe ischemia of acute or chronic arterial occlusion. Wet or infected gangrene most often occurs in diabetics with less severe ischemia but with neglected superficial wounds associated with neuropathy, which may become secondarily infected. Gangrene due to arterial occlusive disease must be differentiated from other types of gangrene, including venous gangrene associated with massive deep vein thrombosis (phlegmasia cerulea dolens). Venous gangrene can be differentiated by the warmer cyanotic and markedly edematous extremity. Gangrene associated with frostbite is evident from a history of exposure to cold. Symmetrical gangrene of the toes, fingers, or distal portions of the extremities, despite the presence of peripheral pulses, should suggest serious underlying systemic disease such as disseminated intravascular coagulation (DIC) or the low cardiac output syndrome associated with severe cardiogenic shock, particularly in the presence of vasopressors or cardiotonic medications.

A pregangrenous condition that is being increasingly recognized is the so-called *blue toe* syndrome. This condition is manifested by painful mottling or cyanosis of one or more toes that may eventually result in epidermolysis or gangrene. This syndrome may develop despite the presence of palpable peripheral pulses. The etiology of the ischemic digit(s) is usually a microembolus from a proximal arterial lesion, often an aneurysm or an atherosclerotic plaque.

WHAT IS THE PROBABLE ETIOLOGY OF THE ARTERIAL OBSTRUCTION?

The history will often suggest the underlying cause of the arterial occlusive disease. Atherosclerosis is the most common disorder resulting in arterial obstruction. Atherosclerosis is suggested by other systemic manifestations of this disease, such as angina pectoris, a previous myocardial infarction or stroke, or a family history of atherosclerosis. The presence of atherosclerotic risk factors may be evident and will be discussed further in another section.

Diabetes mellitus is a common predisposing factor to peripheral atherosclerosis. However, as previously mentioned, diabetic patients with manifestations of arterial obstruction should not be considered to have "small vessel disease" as the explanation for their ischemic extremity. Claudication, ischemic rest pain, or gangrene in diabetic patients is almost always the result of atherosclerosis of named arteries, which are by definition not "small vessels." While it is true that the atherosclerosis of diabetic patients is often distributed in more distal vessels (popliteal and tibial arteries) than that of nondiabetic patients who have more proximal occlusive disease (aorta, common iliac, or femoral arteries), diabetic patients often have reparable peripheral atherosclerosis. Attributing diabetic vascular disease to "small vessel" disorders may result in a nonaggressive diagnostic and therapeutic approach, which may jeopardize a patient's extremity.

Thrombosis or embolism is suggested by a history of sudden onset of leg symptoms. A history of prior claudication suggests thrombosis, whereas embolism may be suggested by a history of rheumatic fever, valvular heart disease, atrial fibrillation, or the presence of a proximal arterial aneurysm.

Other causes of arterial obstruction may be evident from the history. Trauma is usually self-evident. However, iatrogenic trauma due to cardiac or peripheral arterial catheterization may be initially asymptomatic, and the patient will manifest symptoms only after activity increases after hospital discharge. Thromboangiitis obliterans (Buerger's disease) is suggested by *foot* claudication because of the distal tibioperoneal or plantar arterial disease associated with this condition. Foot claudication may occasionally occur in diabetic patients but is unusual because of associated peripheral neuropathy. Patients with Buerger's disease are usually younger than diabetic patients, most commonly males, and are addicted to cigarette smoking. They may have associated cold sensitivity and recurrent ischemic ulcerations and infections with autoamputations of the fingers and toes. Manifestations of peripheral arterial occlusive disease in patients without a history of cigarette smoking or diabetes mellitus may suggest unusual congenital or structural anomalies, such as muscular entrapment or cystic adventitial degeneration of the popliteal artery, most commonly in young men, or fibromuscular dyplasia, which occurs in young women. Abdominal aortic coarctation or hypoplasia also may occur in young women.

WHAT IS THE ANATOMIC LOCATION OF THE OBSTRUCTION(S)?

The history may suggest the anatomic location of the arterial obstruction. Aortoiliac (inflow) disease, so-called Leriche's syndrome, is suggested by claudication that involves the buttock as well as more distal parts of the extremity. Impotence may be present in male patients. Thigh claudication suggests occlusive disease of the common femoral or external iliac artery or *both* superficial femoral and perfunda femoris arteries. Calf claudication is the most common location of leg pain caused by peripheral arterial occlusive disease at any location in the extremity because of the marked metabolic requirements for this active muscle group associated with walking. Superficial femoral or popliteal artery occlusive disease (outflow disease) characteristically results in claudication of the calf, but calf claudication may also be the only manifestation of aortoiliac occlusive disease. Foot claudication, as mentioned previously, characteristically occurs in Buerger's disease, which has a predilection for tibial and peroneal arteries as well as more distal plantar and digital arteries of the foot.

WHAT IS THE FUNCTIONAL IMPAIRMENT OF THE PATIENT?

One of the most important features of the patient's history is the definition of functional impairment, which dictates the extent of diagnostic and therapeutic intervention. The history should accurately define the level of disability, which falls into one of four broad categories:

1. Life-threatening condition, such as ruptured abdominal aortic aneurysm, wet (infected) gangrene, arterial trauma with hemorrhage, acute mesenteric artery occlusion, or stroke.

2. Limb- or organ-threatening condition, such as acute arterial occlusion, chronic arterial obstruction with ischemic rest pain or gangrene, chronic mesenteric arterial occlusion (intestinal angina), renovascular hypertension, or cerebral transient ischemic attacks.

3. Functional disability, such as claudication that interferes with self-care, occupation, or recreation.

4. Asymptomatic disease, such as arterial aneurysm or asymptomatic carotid bruit.

Does the Patient Have Atherosclerotic Risk Factors?

The history may reveal risk factors that predispose to peripheral atherosclerosis. *Cigarette smoking* is the leading risk factor for peripheral arterial occlusive disease. Atherosclerosis is an unlikely cause of peripheral arterial obstruction in a patient who has never smoked cigarettes unless the patient has diabetes mellitus. *Diabetes mellitus* is a strong risk factor for peripheral atherosclerosis, particularly of more distal vessels of the extremity. *Hyperlipidemia* is not common in patients with peripheral arterial occlusive disease, although hypertriglyceridemia is the most frequent abnormality of such patients. *Hypertension* may contribute to peripheral atherosclerosis and is a leading risk factor for cerebrovascular disease and stroke. Obesity may aggravate claudication but, by itself, is a weak risk factor for peripheral atherosclerosis. Sedentary activity may predispose to atherosclerosis, but its relationship as a risk factor is not well documented.

Will the Patient Benefit from Medical Therapy?

The history remains the cornerstone for deciding whether a patient should have an initial trial of medical therapy or whether a more invasive procedure, such as interventional radiography or operation, is indicated. Patients who have a history of recent onset of claudication and who have not been given adequate medical therapy should initially be treated medically, particularly with an exercise program and a concerted effort to cease smoking. However, if a patient's occupation or daily activity has involved maximal exercise and the claudication has become progressively limiting to the patient, particularly if present for many months or years, surgical therapy may be indicated. Medical therapy is suggested for patients who are either asymptomatic or have mild functional disability, whereas surgical (or radiologic) intervention is indicated in a patient with life- or limb-threatening ischemia.

Is the Patient a Candidate for Operation?

The history usually indicates the need for operation; only after this decision is made should arteriography be considered. The operative indications fall into one of four broad categories, which are listed in their order of importance:

1. Life salvage, such as repair of a ruptured aortic aneurysm or arterial trauma or amputation for wet (infected) gangrene.
2. Limb salvage, with radiologic or surgical intervention to prevent limb loss secondary to gangrene, ischemic ulceration, or intolerable vascular rest pain.
3. Preservation of function such as radiologic or surgical intervention to treat *disabling* claudication that limits self-care, occupation, or desired recreation.
4. Prophylaxis, such as resection of an asymptomatic aortic aneurysm to prevent rupture, repair of a popliteal aneurysm to prevent thrombosis or embolism, or carotid endarterectomy of asymptomatic carotid stenosis to prevent stroke.

What Are the Operative Risks?

The final feature of the history that is of importance in planning therapy is the definition of operative risks, which, in turn, may influence the type of operation that may be performed. The history may reveal associated systemic disease such as coronary artery disease, pulmonary insufficiency, chronic renal failure, severe hypertension, cerebrovascular disease, or associated malignancy. Such patients may not be candidates for major vascular reconstructions that carry increased risks, such as procedures that involve entry into the thoracic or abdominal cavity. Such patients may require "extra-anatomic" reconstruction with bypass procedures that do not enter body cavities, such as femorofemoral bypass, axillofemoral bypass, or femoropopliteal or -tibial bypasses. These operations can generally be performed with no greater risk than that associated with amputation. If, however, the patient has few or no major operative risk factors, "anatomic" reconstruction, such as aortoiliac endarterectomy or aortofemoral bypass, may be feasible. The history may reveal a patient with advanced leg ischemia who has no future potential for walking because of severe fixed flexion contracture or disabling stroke. Such a patient may then be a candidate for amputation rather than arterial reconstruction.

The aforementioned features of the history reveal the importance of these data in planning further work-up and treatment of the patient. Although the physical examination, noninvasive diagnostic techniques, and arteriography all provide objective documentation of the presence, location, and extent of arterial occlusive disease, the patient's testimony remains the single most important body of information that dictates the extent of the diagnostic and therapeutic management to be pursued.

Physical Examination

The physical examination includes inspection, palpation, and auscultation of the vascular system and provides confirmation of the presence, location, and severity of peripheral arterial occlusive disease.

Inspection

Inspection usually reveals abnormalities only in patients with advanced arterial occlusive disease. Color changes are usually seen in the lower extremity only in patients with ischemic rest pain or tissue necrosis. Pallor of the foot with elevation of the lower extremity indicates severe arterial occlusive disease, with an ankle blood pressure usually less than 60 mm. Hg. Dependent rubor reflects maximal peripheral vasodilatation after ischemia of the foot with elevation. Delayed refilling of superficial veins is an additional sign of advanced ischemia. Signs of pregangrenous changes, such as "blue toe" syndrome, as well as ischemic ulceration and gangrene have been mentioned previously. These changes reflect advanced arterial occlusive disease.

Trophic changes also reflect ischemia of the extremity at rest, which alters the function of skin appendages with resultant thickening of the nails, hair loss, and dryness or atrophy of the skin. The thickened toenails must be differentiated from fungal infection of the nails, particularly in diabetic patients. The hair loss characteristically occurs on the toes. Hair loss on the lower legs is usually of no diagnostic significance.

Particular attention should be paid to inspection of the retina in patients with cerebrovascular disease. Evidence of microemboli may be identified in branches of the retinal arteries. With experience one may differentiate the character of the microembolus, be it platelet, thrombus, calcium, or cholesterol debris. The characteristics of retinal emboli will be discussed in a later section of this chapter.

PALPATION

Palpation should include assessment of skin temperature, grading of peripheral pulses, and palpation for thrills. Coolness of an extremity is of no particular diagnostic value unless there is asymmetry in temperature between two extremities. Symmetrical coolness of the acral portions of the body is commonplace, usually reflecting increased sympathetic vasomotor tone.

Palpation and grading of peripheral pulses is an important part of the physical examination of the arterial system. Although a number of different grading schemes have been suggested, the most practical method is to use a 2+, 1+, and 0 grading system to reflect normal, reduced, and absent pulses, respectively. Assessment of extracranial cerebrovascular pulses should include palpation of each common carotid, subclavian, and superficial temporal artery. The carotid bifurcation should not be manually compressed to avoid reflex bradycardia or dislodgement of emboli from a diseased carotid bifurcation.

The common carotid artery should be palpated low in the neck between the sternocleidomastoid muscle and trachea. The subclavian artery pulse may be felt in the supraclavicular fossa. In the upper extremity, the brachial, radial, and ulnar pulses should be elicited. In the abdomen, the abdominal aorta pulse should be palpated above the level of the umbilicus, and the aorta should be simultaneously assessed for the presence of aneurysm. Each common iliac artery may be palpated in a thin patient. In an obese patient, the external iliac artery may be palpated immediately above the inguinal ligament. In the lower extremity, the common femoral artery pulse may be palpated in the groin at the midpoint between the anterior superior iliac spine and the pubic tubercle. The superficial femoral artery pulse may be palpated in the proximal thigh just distal to the common femoral artery pulse. The popliteal artery pulse may be difficult to palpate but should be examined with the fingers of both hands in the popliteal fossa with the thumbs in front of the proximal tibia. The artery is usually 1 or 2 cm. lateral to the midline in the popliteal fossa and may be palpated by using the fingers to gently compress the vessel anteriorly against the posterior surface of the tibia. If a prominent popliteal pulse is readily palpated, one should suspect a popliteal artery aneurysm. At the ankle, the posterior tibial pulse is palpated just posterior to the medial malleolus. The dorsalis pedis pulse is palpated on the dorsum of the foot between the first and second metatarsal bones. More laterally on the dorsum of the foot, a pulse may be felt in the terminal branch of the peroneal artery after it perforates the interosseous membrane to join the dorsalis pedis artery on the dorsum of the foot.

The grading of pulses must be based upon the amplitude of the normal pulse for a given patient. Pulses are much more readily palpated in some patients compared with others. A normal pulse from an unaffected extremity, such as an upper extremity, for a given patient should be considered a 2+ pulse and the remaining pulses in that patient graded accordingly. A 2+ pulse implies no significant obstruction of the circulation proximal to the pulse so graded. A 1+ pulse may signify a stenosis or occlusion with good collateral circulation proximal to the affected pulse. Differentiation of stenosis from occlusion is based upon the presence or absence of a vascular bruit, as described hereafter. An absent pulse signifies occlusion (or severe stenosis) proximal to the reduced pulse. From such information, the examiner should be able to clearly delineate the anatomic level of arterial occlusive disease based on the presence and location of pulse deficits.

A palpable *thrill* suggests a severe stenosis or an arteriovenous fistula. A stenosis is suggested by a thrill only during systole, whereas an arteriovenous fistula may be accompanied by a thrill throughout the cardiac cycle.

The patient with suspected cerebrovascular disease should undergo a complete neurologic evaluation including assessment of sensory and motor deficits as well as of deep tendon and other reflexes.

AUSCULTATION

Auscultation should include measurement of blood pressure and assessment for vascular bruit. The blood pressure should be measured in both upper extremities to identify possible subclavian obstruction and concomitant subclavian steal syndrome. Normally, the systolic blood pressures in both arms should be within 20 mm. Hg of each other. An arm systolic pressure that is more than 20 mm. Hg below that of the contralateral arm suggests proximal arterial obstruction in the affected extremity.

Vascular *bruits* are the result of abnormal wall vibrations associated with an arterial stenosis or an arteriovenous fistula. Most peripheral vascular bruits occur only in the systolic portion of the cardiac cycle. Exceptions to this are continuous bruits throughout the cardiac cycle associated with an arteriovenous fistula. Severe stenosis of the internal carotid artery may also be associated with a systolic bruit that extends into diastole. This phenomenon is a reflection of the relatively low cerebrovascular resistance that permits high flow in the internal carotid artery during diastole as well as systole.

Extensive auscultation of the major peripheral arteries may reveal stenoses that might otherwise be overlooked by an incomplete vascular examination. A bruit over the common carotid artery low in the neck implies common carotid stenosis. A bruit in the supraclavicular fossa suggests subclavian artery stenosis. A bruit over the right subclavian and right common carotid arteries suggests innominate artery stenosis. A bruit over each subclavian and common carotid artery bilaterally suggests radiating bruits from the thorax associated with conditions such as aortic stenosis or aortic arch vessel disease. A bruit that is maximal over the distal carotid artery near the angle of the mandible suggests carotid bifurcation stenosis. Such a bruit may emanate from either the internal or external carotid artery. However, as mentioned previously, if the bruit extends into early diastole, severe internal carotid stenosis is suggested. A bruit posterolateral to the sternocleidomastoid muscle suggests vertebral artery stenosis. The bell of the stethoscope should be applied to the closed eyelid to elicit a bruit associated with carotid siphon stenosis.

In the abdomen, a bruit in the epigastrium that decreases with inspiration and increases with expiration suggests functional celiac artery stenosis associated with compression by extrinsic neural or diaphragmatic structures. A bruit in each hypochondrium or each flank suggests renal artery stenosis. If the bruit extends into early diastole, severe renal artery stenosis is suggested. A bruit immediately below the umbilicus on one side or the other suggests common iliac artery stenosis. If the bruit is maximal just above the inguinal ligament, external iliac artery stenosis is implied. If the bruit is maximal just distal to the inguinal ligament, common femoral artery stenosis exists. Superficial femoral artery stenosis may be documented by a bruit along the course of this vessel in the adductor canal. A bruit that is maximal in the popliteal fossa suggests popliteal artery stenosis.

From the aforementioned information, the examiner

	BP	R	U	Br	Sc	CC	CB	ST	Or	V	A	Re	Cl	El	CF	SF	P	PT	DP	Pe
Right	190/110	++	++	++	++B	++B	++	++	B	B	++	B	+B	+	+	0	0	0	0	0
Left	130/70	+	0	+	0	++	++B	+	−	−		−	++	++	++	+B	+	+	+	0

Figure 5. Record of peripheral pulses, bruits, and blood pressure. BP = Blood pressure; R = radial; U = ulnar; Br = brachial; Sc = subclavian; CC = common carotid; CB = carotid bifurcation; ST = superficial temporal; Or = orbit; V = vertebral; A = aorta; Re = renal; Cl = common iliac; El = external iliac; CF = common femoral; SF = superficial femoral; P = popliteal; PT = posterior tibial; DP = dorsalis pedis; Pe = peroneal; + + = normal pulse; + = reduced pulse; 0 = absent pulse, B = bruit; minus (−) infers no bruit (not used in all locations, only for orbital, vertebral, and renal arteries, which cannot be palpated and thus have no pulse record).

should be able to be explicit in the diagnostic impression regarding the presence, location, and severity of arterial disease. A typical record of peripheral pulses, bruits, and blood pressure is presented in Figure 5. Using this record, the examiner should be able to make an explicit anatomic diagnosis as follows:

1. Innominate artery stenosis, mild.
2. Left subclavian artery occlusion, ? subclavian steal.
3. Left external carotid stenosis, ? internal carotid stenosis.
4. Right internal carotid siphon stenosis.
5. Right vertebral artery stenosis.
6. Right renal artery stenosis.
7. Right common iliac artery stenosis.
8. Right superficial femoral artery occlusion.
9. Left superficial femoral artery stenosis.

Noninvasive Diagnostic Techniques

The noninvasive peripheral vascular laboratory provides objective physiologic information for the detection, localization, and quantification of peripheral arterial, cerebrovascular, and venous disease.[1] These studies do not substitute for a careful history and physical examination nor do they replace angiography in selected patients. However, noninvasive techniques do provide complementary functional data to confirm the diagnosis, predict therapeutic results, monitor medical or surgical therapy, and follow the natural history or efficacy of treatment for peripheral vascular disease. A detailed description of noninvasive techniques is out of the scope of this chapter. However, in this section the basic principles of some of the more practical methods used to evaluate peripheral arterial and cerebrovascular disease will be discussed.

The two most common instruments used for noninvasive vascular testing are Doppler ultrasound and plethysmography. The Doppler ultrasound velocity detector is sensitive to frequency shifts of ultrasound reflected from moving blood cells. Both simple portable devices and more complex laboratory instruments that permit interpretation of artery or venous flow signals by means of audible signals, recordable analogue waveforms, or sound spectral analysis are available. Some devices are also capable of generating images of vessels on a storage oscilloscope. Doppler devices may be used to detect velocity waveforms in arteries and veins, measure segmental limb blood pressures, or generate ultrasonic images of the lumen of blood vessels.

Plethysmography permits recording of dimensional changes of a digit, limb, eye, or other body part with each heartbeat or in response to temporary obstruction of venous return (venous occlusion plethysmography). A variety of plethysmographic transducers are available including strain-gauge, photoelectric, impedance, air, and water techniques. Plethysmography is useful in recording arterial pulsations in a digit, extremity, or eye; measuring segmental digit or limb blood pressures; recording pulse wave arrival times in each eye; or determining venous outflow or venous reflux in chronic venous disease.

An additional instrument used in noninvasive laboratory to record bruits is the so-called phonoangiograph. This instrument permits a graphic recording of the amplitude of a vascular bruit with respect to time. Some computerized devices are also capable of analyzing the spectrum of sound frequency in bruits to permit a more accurate assessment of the residual lumen diameter.

Doppler ultrasound is the simplest, most inexpensive, and versatile technique used to screen for peripheral arterial disease. The normal arterial velocity waveform is multiphasic with a prominent systolic component and one or more diastolic sounds. In the presence of arterial obstruction, the Doppler velocity signal is attenuated distal to the obstruction with a more monophasic signal and absence of the discrete diastolic sounds. The pitch of the Doppler signal is proportional to blood flow velocity. If the Doppler is used as a sensitive electronic stethoscope along the course of an artery, sites of stenosis may be identified as locations of increased pitch of the Doppler signal.

The most objective method for the screening of arterial occlusive disease is to measure distal limb blood pressure with Doppler ultrasound. In the lower extremity, the ankle systolic pressure may be recorded with a pneumatic cuff placed above the malleolus and the Doppler signal elicited from the posterior tibial or dorsalis pedis artery on the foot (Fig. 6). The cuff may be the same width as that used for the arm. The cuff is inflated until the Doppler signal disappears, and as the cuff is slowly deflated the ankle systolic pressure is noted at that point where the Doppler signal returns. The ankle systolic pressure may be divided by the arm systolic pressure to calculate the ankle/brachial pressure index (API). Normally the ankle pressure is equal to or greater than that of the arm. In the presence of arterial occlusive disease, the ankle pressure will be below that of the arm by an amount proportional to the severity

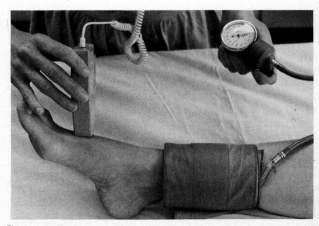

Figure 6. Technique of measurement of ankle systolic blood pressure using Doppler ultrasound.

of arterial obstruction. Patients with claudication normally have an ankle pressure index between 0.5 and 1.0. Patients with ischemic rest pain usually have an ankle pressure index less than 0.5 with an absolute ankle pressure usually less than 50 mm. Hg.

Using specially designed cuffs with longer inflatable bladders, segmental leg blood pressure can be obtained at the proximal thigh, above the knee, below the knee, and at the ankle. Such information permits objective documentation of the anatomic location of arterial occlusive disease in the limb. Digit blood pressures may be obtained with cuffs specially designed to fit on the proximal phalanx of the toe. A plethysmograph is usually necessary to record digit blood pressures. Normally the toe blood pressure is at least 60 per cent of the ankle pressure. Similar methods of segmental pressure measurements may be used on the upper extremity. The measurement of penile blood pressure permits assessment of vasculogenic impotence. Normally the penile systolic pressure is at least 70 per cent of the brachial systolic pressure. Reductions in penile pressure are suggestive of a vascular cause of impotence.

Ankle blood pressures may be recorded before and after treadmill exercise or after deflation of an arterial tourniquet on the leg during the ensuing reactive hyperemia. Normally, there is little drop in ankle pressure after a standard walking pace of about 1.5 to 2.0 mph. In patients with arterial occlusive disease, there will be an abnormal drop in ankle pressure, often to very low or unobtainable levels, with a prolonged recovery over the ensuing 10 or 20 minutes. The magnitude of this abnormal ankle pressure response to exercise is indicative of the severity of arterial occlusive disease.

Assessment of cerebrovascular disease may involve the use of Doppler ultrasound, ocular plethysmography, or real-time imaging of the carotid bifurcation using B-mode ultrasound. Indirect cerebrovascular screening techniques assess altered flow or pressure in branches of the ophthalmic artery, which is the first major intracranial branch of the internal carotid artery. Severe internal carotid artery obstruction may result in abnormal flow in ophthalmic artery branches, which may be detected by Doppler ultrasound. Alternatively, abnormal ocular pulse arrival time or retinal artery pressure may be recorded with ocular plethysmographs. Carotid artery bruits may be recorded with a carotid phonoangiograph. Direct assessment of the presence of internal carotid artery stenosis or occlusion is possible using Doppler ultrasound or Doppler or B-mode ultrasonic arteriography (Fig. 7).

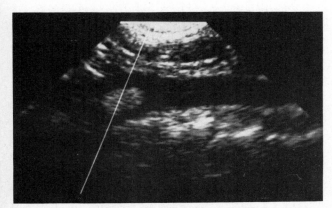

Figure 7. Combined echo-Doppler (duplex) ultrasonic scan of carotid bifurcation.

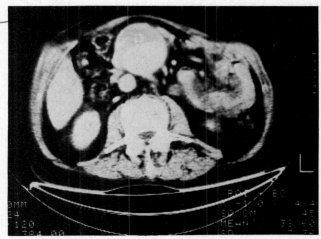

Figure 8. Computed tomogram of abdominal aortic aneurysm.

Real-time imaging with B-mode ultrasound is commonly used to screen for abdominal or peripheral artery aneurysms. Such ultrasonic sonograms provide the most accurate method of defining the true diameter of such aneurysms. Arteriograms may be misleading because of the presence of mural thrombus lining the aneurysm.

Computed tomography (CT) may also be used to assess the peripheral arterial system for true aneurysms or aortic dissection. Computed tomography is more expensive than ultrasonography, but it is particularly helpful in assessing suprarenal aortic aneurysms or aortic aneurysms or dissection in the thorax, which cannot be interrogated by ultrasound (Fig. 8). Computed tomography is also useful for assessing patients for complications after arterial reconstruction, such as false aneurysms or prosthetic infections, and is of great value in assessing patients with stroke for evidence of cerebral hemorrhage or infarction.

Arteriography

Arteriography involves the use of contrast medium to provide morphologic radiographic images of peripheral arterial disease (Fig. 9). The invasive studies constitute the diagnostic standard for the evaluation of peripheral artery disease but must be performed only for specific diagnostic indications. Although contrast arteriography has been conventionally performed by introduction of contrast medium into the arterial system, recent advances in digital subtraction angiography (DSA) permit imaging of major arteries using intravenous injections. The latter technique is somewhat less expensive and carries less risk and discomfort to the patient. However, intravenous DSA requires more contrast material and provides less imaging resolution than conventional intra-arterial angiography.

Peripheral arteriography is indicated only in patients for whom an operation or other major intervention is planned. Arteriography should not be considered routinely for diagnosis for peripheral arterial disease. The objective of arteriography is to provide anatomic information regarding the reconstructability of the arterial lesions. Arteriography may be performed percutaneously by introducing a catheter into the abdominal aorta via the translumbar route or via more peripheral arteries such as the femoral or axillary artery. Intravenous DSA is usually performed through a central venous injection using a catheter introduced into a brachial vein.

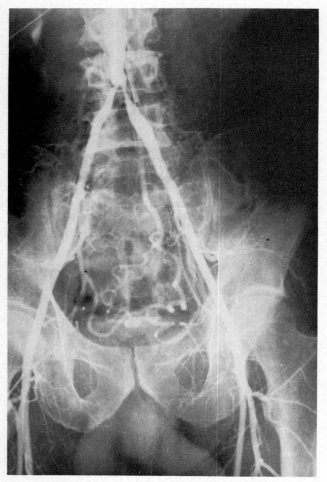

Figure 9. Transfemoral aortogram showing atherosclerotic stenosis of aortic bifurcation and common iliac arteries.

Cerebrovascular arteriography is indicated for patients with transient ischemic attack or patients who have had stroke with a significant recovery of function. Patients with atypical cerebrovascular symptoms and select patients with asymptomatic carotid bruits may also undergo arteriography if carotid endarterectomy is being considered. Intravenous DSA may be indicated in patients in whom a significant carotid lesion is suspected, particularly if identified by noninvasive screening techniques. Other patients are best evaluated by intra-arterial cerebral angiography, usually by transfemoral or transaxillary approach. Direct carotid puncture is occasionally performed to identify cerebrovascular lesions.

The risks of arteriography include thrombosis, embolism, hemorrhage, arteriovenous fistula, stroke, and allergy to contrast medium. Most allergic sequelae are readily controlled by medication, but occasionally cardiovascular collapse may occur. Because of the risk and expense of arteriography, these studies are considered only for patients in whom major therapeutic intervention is planned.

THERAPEUTIC PRINCIPLES

When faced with a patient with suspected arterial disease, the physician should develop a systematic method of evaluating the extent of the disease so that the diagnostic

and therapeutic decisions may be intelligently addressed. An example of a management algorithm for patients with suspected arterial disease is shown in Figure 10. This algorithm is based upon classification of the arterial disease into one of the following four levels of severity:

1. Life-threatening condition.
2. Limb- or organ-threatening condition.
3. Functionally disabling condition.
4. Asymptomatic status.

If the patient's life is threatened, as with arterial trauma and hemorrhage, a ruptured abdominal aneurysm, infected gangrene, or mesenteric artery occlusion, immediate emergency operation may be indicated. If a limb or organ is threatened, as with acute arterial occlusion, ischemic rest pain, gangrene, transient ischemic attack, (TIA) or recovery from stroke, an urgent arteriogram and operation (or, alternatively, fibrinolytic therapy and balloon dilatation) may be indicated. If the patient has a functional disability, the rapidity and extent of work-up and therapy may depend upon the extent of the disability. If the patient is unable to perform self-care activities, urgent angiography and radiologic or surgical intervention may be necessary. However, if the patient has disabling claudication and has not yet had an adequate trial of medical therapy, the latter should be initiated. Only if medical therapy fails should elective arteriography and interventional radiography or operation be considered. If the patient is asymptomatic, the clinican must determine whether or not a prophylactic intervention, such as resection of an abdominal aortic aneurysm, is necessary. Similarly, patients with asymptomatic carotid disease must be individually assessed for the relative risk of stroke without operation versus the risk of prophylactic carotid endarterectomy. For all other patients with asymptomatic peripheral arterial occlusive disease, observation is indicated and arteriography is not recommended. Medical therapy, particularly intervention for atherosclerotic risk factors, may be appropriate for such individuals.

Using the aforementioned systematic approach, the clinician should be able to appropriately select medical, radiologic, or surgical therapy based upon a careful history and physical examination. Noninvasive diagnostic techniques may be appropriate to quantify the presence and extent of arterial occlusive disease or the size of small abdominal aortic aneurysms. Such objective information is also useful in following the natural history and the influence of medical therapy on vascular disease. Arteriography and interventional therapy should be reserved for those patients who fulfill the aforementioned criteria for such invasive approaches.

ACUTE ARTERIAL OCCLUSION

Acute arterial occlusion represents sudden obstruction of a peripheral artery by one of two principal mechanisms: embolism or thrombosis.

Clinical Hallmarks

Acute arterial occlusion should be suspected in the presence of the "6 Ps," which include:

1. Pain.
2. Pallor.
3. Paresthesias.
4. Paralysis.
5. Pulselessness.
6. Polar (cold) sensation.

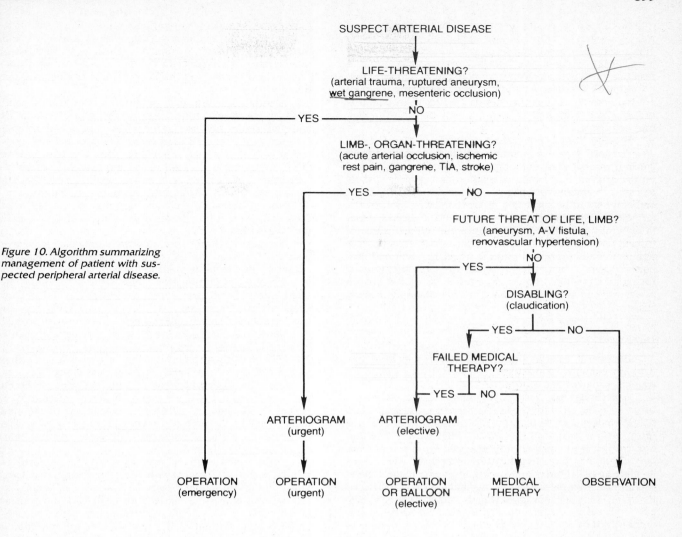

Figure 10. Algorithm summarizing management of patient with suspected peripheral arterial disease.

Pathology

Acute arterial occlusion results from either embolic or thrombotic obstruction of a peripheral artery.[17] Embolism consists of thrombotic, atheromatous, or other material that migrates from a proximal portion of the circulation to a more distal site where it obstructs arterial flow. Thrombotic material is the most common component of an embolus. The location and duration of development of the thrombotic mass may indicate the source of embolus. Embolus from a left atrial appendage may show alternating layers of red and white blood cells and platelet or fibrin debri; the embolus from a proximal ulcerated atheromatous plaque may consist of plaque constituents including cholesterol and calcium. Cholesterol clefts may be seen in sections taken from digits suffering small vessel microemboli ("blue toe" syndrome). Emboli from arterial aneurysms may contain fibrin and platelet debris, so-called white thrombi.

Thrombosis represents blood coagulum forming on an underlying arterial lesion, which eventually occludes the lumen. Most commonly, thrombosis occurs at sites of atherosclerotic plaques or in peripheral arterial aneurysms. Thrombosis may also occur with less common arterial disorders such as Buerger's disease, muscular entrapment, or cystic adventitial degeneration.

Etiology

EMBOLISM

There are four principal causes of arterial embolism: cardiac disease, arterial disease, venous disease, and foreign body.

Cardiac Disease. Cardiac disorders that may lead to peripheral arterial embolism include atrial fibrillation, myocardial infarct, ventricular aneurysm, mitral stenosis, prosthetic cardiac valve, bacterial endocarditis, and atrial myxoma. Currently the most common cardiac causes of peripheral arterial embolism are atrial fibrillation and mural thrombi associated with myocardial infarct, including ventricular aneurysm. Although atrial myxoma is a rare cause of peripheral arterial emboli, its detection requires routine histologic examination of all embolic material removed at operation, because a myxoma may appear similar to a thrombus.

Arterial Disease. Arterial causes of peripheral arterial embolism include thromboembolic debris from arterial aneurysm or ulcerated atheromatous plaque as well as atheromatous debris from atherosclerotic ulcers. Atheroembolism may result in the "blue toe" syndrome or may cause rather diffuse microinfarcts of the skin mimicking livedo reticularis. Visceral atheromatous emboli may lead to infarction or ulceration of the small or large intestine as well as progressive renal failure. Although the most common location of peripheral arterial aneurysms is the infrarenal aorta, popliteal artery aneurysms are most prone to result in thrombosis or distal emboli of the lower extremity.

Venous Disease. Although a rare cause of peripheral arterial emboli, venous thrombosis may result in *paradoxical embolism* through an atrial septal defect or patent foramen ovale.

Foreign Body. *Foreign bodies* are an occasional cause of peripheral arterial embolism. Bullets associated with gunshot wounds may either enter or erode through a vessel on the arterial side of the circulation and migrate distally to result in embolic peripheral arterial occlusion. A bullet embolus should be suspected in a patient who has a bullet entrance wound but no exit wound and in whom signs of peripheral arterial occlusion are present. Other causes of foreign body embolus include monitoring catheters that are unintentionally dislodged into the arterial system and misplaced or migrating foreign bodies inserted intentionally for radiologic obliteration of an arterial vascular bed, such as arteriovenous fistula or pelvic arterial traumatic hemorrhage.

THROMBOSIS

Peripheral arterial thrombosis may result from one of four common conditions: atherosclerosis, aneurysm, trauma, or iatrogenic injury.

Atherosclerosis. The most common cause of arterial thrombosis is an underlying *atherosclerotic plaque*. This plaque may cause severe stenosis, which results in eventual thrombotic occlusion of the lumen. Alternatively, the atherosclerotic lesion may not produce significant stenosis but may develop surface irregularity or ulceration, which leads to platelet and fibrin deposition and eventual thrombotic occlusion. Other pathologic lesions that may lead to arterial thrombosis include fibromuscular dysplasia, Buerger's disease, muscular entrapment, and cystic adventitial degeneration. Arterial dissection may lead to sufficient compromise of the lumen to result in eventual thrombosis of the artery.

Aneurysm. Peripheral arterial aneurysms are often lined by thrombotic material to maintain a relatively normal diameter of the arterial lumen. Excessive deposition of platelet and fibrin debris may eventually lead to thrombosis of the lumen, which is most common with popliteal artery aneurysms, less common in femoral artery aneurysms, and uncommon in infrarenal aortic aneurysms.

Trauma. Trauma may result in arterial thrombosis owing to contusion, intimal disruption, or laceration of the artery.

Iatrogenic Injury. Iatrogenic injury may cause arterial thrombosis from arterial catheterization for coronary or peripheral angiography, arterial monitoring of arterial blood pressure or blood gases, or blood gas sampling through repeated arterial needle puncture.

Clinical Manifestations

Acute arterial occlusion may occur in any part of the arterial system. Occlusion in the cerebrovascular, renal, and mesenteric circulations will be discussed in later sections of this chapter. Clinical manifestations of acute arterial occlusion of vessels to the extremities characteristically result in the "six Ps" of pain, pallor, paresthesias, paralysis,

pulselessness, and polar (cold) sensation. These manifestations may be similar for both arterial embolism and thrombosis. However, certain distinguishing characteristics may permit the examiner to differentiate these two conditions, which is important in planning further diagnosis and therapy.

Arterial embolism may be differentiated from thrombosis by the more abrupt and sudden onset of symptoms and signs of arterial insufficiency. The patient with arterial embolism often can relate the exact time or activity associated with the onset of extremity pain. The patient with arterial thrombosis may note more gradual onset of symptoms and often may notice numbness, pain, or weakness in the extremity after arising from sleep or a seated position. A history of antecedent claudication may be elicited from the patient with arterial thrombosis, whereas embolism may not be associated with symptoms or signs of chronic occlusive disease. However, the patient with embolism may have history of cardiac disease or arrhythmia, which may be absent in the patient with arterial thrombosis.

On physical examination, some signs may permit differentiation of embolism from thrombosis. The patient with acute arterial embolism may have a pale and waxy or cadaveric appearance to the extremity. Patients with arterial thrombosis may have less severe signs of ischemia because of chronic occlusive disease and collateral development. The patient with thrombosis may thus have a somewhat pale but mottled or slightly cyanotic extremity. In both conditions the superficial veins are collapsed. Edema should not be present unless the ischemia has been present for a period of time during which the patient has maintained dependency of the limb to relieve ischemic rest pain. The temperature of the affected extremity will be lower than that of the opposite limb.

Pulse deficits will be present distal to the level of arterial occlusion. Patients with arterial embolism may have pulses in the contralateral extremity, whereas patients with arterial thrombosis may have both ipsilateral and contralateral pulse deficits. Similarly, arterial bruits may be present in patients with arterial thrombosis but are uncommon in patients with embolism. In both conditions the patients develop increasing ischemic foot or leg pain with elevation of the extremity above the level of the heart.

The severity of the ischemia will be reflected in the extent of sensory or motor disturbance. With sufficient collateral circulation, paresthesias or motor weakness may not be present. With increasing ischemia, paresthesias and sensory deficits may be present. With extreme degrees of ischemia, anesthesia and motor paralysis develop, beginning in the foot and distal extremity. If muscle rigor is present, the ischemia may be irreversible and amputation may be necessary.

Differential Diagnosis

Neurospinal or musculoskeletal problems are usually readily distinguished by the absence of signs of limb ischemia. Acute *deep vein thrombosis* is the principal condition that must be distinguished from acute arterial occlusion. Patients with venous thrombosis usually experience more gradual onset of limb pain. Antecedent claudication and cardiac disease are usually absent. The affected extremity is more cyanotic, with distention of superficial veins and edema often being prominent. Extensive deep vein thrombosis (phlegmasia cerulea dolens) may result in gangrene of the distal extremity due to increased interstitial pressure and reduction in capillary perfusion (venous gangrene). Deep vein thrombosis may be further distinguished from acute arterial occlusion by increased warmth of the extremity and the presence of peripheral pulses, although the latter may be difficult to palpate if there is significant edema. Doppler assessment of ankle pressure may be necessary to assess the status of the arterial circulation. Patients with venous thrombosis are further distinguished from those with arterial occlusion by improvement in leg symptoms with leg elevation and worsening of symptoms with limb dependency.

Diagnostic Evaluation

Non-invasive diagnostic techniques permit rapid objective assessment of patients with suspected acute arterial occlusion. In the affected extremity, Doppler arterial signals may be abnormal or absent distal to the site of obstruction. Ankle systolic blood pressures are reduced or unobtainable, with an ankle/arm index usually below 0.5. Patients with suspected arterial thrombosis may have abnormal Doppler signals and ankle/arm pressure indices in the contralateral extremity.

Patients with suspected arterial embolism require cardiac evaluation. An electrocardiogram may reveal atrial fibrillation or evidence of an old myocardial infarct. Echocardiography may reveal atrial or mural ventricular thrombus. Holter monitoring may be necessary to exclude periodic dysrhythmias that may predispose to atrial thrombi.

Arteriography is the definitive invasive diagnostic technique used to evaluate patients with acute arterial occlusion. Whereas most patients may be candidates for arteriography, patients with severe limb-threatening ischemia may be candidates for immediate operative intervention, particularly those with suspected acute arterial embolus. Most other patients are candidates for arteriography to localize and characterize the occlusive process. Such radiologic intervention also permits possible thrombolytic therapy, particularly in patients with distal emboli or thrombosis, which may be difficult to manage surgically.

Medical Therapy

Medical therapy, although not a definitive treatment for acute arterial occlusion, may be helpful during the initial management of patients with acute arterial occlusion. Unless there are absolute contraindications to anticoagulation, heparin should be administered intravenously, usually with a 5000-unit bolus followed by approximately 1000 units per hour to maintain the partial thromboplastin time or the clotting time approximately twice the control value. The goal for heparin therapy is to prevent extension of the thrombus into areas of poor collateral circulation and to reduce the risk of recurrent embolus if the latter is responsible for the acute arterial occlusion. The affected limb should be maintained in a horizontal or slightly dependent position. The extremity should *not* be elevated above the atrial level, which would reduce peripheral perfusion. Although blankets may be used to cover the affected extremity, external application of heat must be *avoided* to prevent severe burns because of the inadequate cutaneous circulation.

Interventional Radiology

In select patients, thrombolytic agents may be infused by percutaneous catheter to lyse the offending thrombus or embolus. Direct infusion of streptokinase or urokinase into the thrombus or embolus provides the greatest possibility for dissolution of the obstruction. Such therapy is most effective if employed within 72 hours of the onset of arterial obstruction. Because of the risk of bleeding from fibrinolytic agents, such therapy must be considered before repeated vascular punctures or operative intervention has taken place. Thrombolytic therapy is recommended only for patients with distal arterial occlusive lesions (distal to the popliteal artery) or patients who are not good candidates for arterial reconstruction.

If thrombolytic therapy clears a thrombotic occlusion in a patient with underlying focal arterial stenosis, balloon dilatation or *percutaneous transluminal angioplasty* (PTA) may be employed to dilate the offending stenosis. Such radiologic intervention is particularly helpful in patients who develop thrombosis of bypass grafts owing to neointimal hyperplasia at the distal anastomosis. However, the long-term efficacy of interventional radiologic procedures remains to be established.

Operative Therapy

Patients with acute arterial embolism may undergo *embolectomy* using a Fogarty balloon catheter introduced by cutdown on the femoral artery (or brachial artery for upper extremity emboli). The catheter is passed both proximally and distally via an arteriotomy. The balloon is inflated and the catheter then gently withdrawn to retrieve all embolic debris. Care must be taken in the use of this catheter to avoid excessive denuding of intima, arterial dissection, perforation, or arteriovenous fistula.

Patients with thrombosis due to underlying arterial occlusive disease may require arterial *reconstruction* to restore normal circulation. Patients with focal atherosclerosis in accessible vessels may undergo endarterectomy. However, most patients have more extensive arterial occlusive disease requiring bypass using prosthetic materials (for aortoiliac occlusive disease) or autogenous saphenous vein (for femoropopliteal or tibial artery occlusive disease). Patients at increased operative risk may undergo extraanatomic bypass, particularly of aortoiliac disease, using techniques such as axillofemoral or femorofemoral bypass.

If arterial reconstruction or embolectomy has restored circulation after a prolonged period of limb ischemia, increased pressure may develop in muscular compartments of the extremity. Such increased pressure may compromise tissue perfusion to muscles and nerves in the affected compartment(s). Such neuromuscular compression may develop despite the presence of palpable distal pulses in the extremity. Early signs of compartmental compression include pain over the affected compartment and sensory deficit in the distribution of nerves running through the compartment. In the lower extremity, the anterior compartment is most commonly affected. An early sign of anterior compartment syndrome is elicited by anesthesia in the dorsal web space between the great and second toes, which is innervated by the deep peroneal nerve, which passes through the anterior tibial compartment. Additional early signs include pain upon passive movement of the great toe or the foot. Objective measurement of compartmental pressures is possible by intermittent needle puncture or by continuous pressure measurement using a wick catheter. If compartmental pressures exceed 30 to 40 mm. Hg, decompression of the compartment(s) by fasciotomies and extensive skin incisions may be necessary. Failure to treat developing compartmental syndromes early may result in severe and irreversible neuromuscular deficits.

Patients who undergo successful revascularization after a period of prolonged ischemia may develop serious systemic metabolic complications associated with hyperkalemia, renal failure, pulmonary insufficiency, or cardiac decompensation. Each of these metabolic insults will require specific supportive therapy.

Patients who show signs of irreversible extremity ischemia, including gangrene and extensive rhabdomyolysis, particularly in the presence of muscle rigor, may be candidates for amputation. Such advanced ischemia may result from either delay in appropriate treatment or failure of arterial revascularization attempts.

Postoperative Management

Patients who are successfully treated for peripheral arterial embolism should have appropriate therapy of the underlying cardiac or proximal vascular disorder. This may include chronic anticoagulation for patients with a cardiac source of embolus. Patients with proximal atherosclerosis or arterial aneurysm should be considered for elective surgical intervention.

Prognosis

The prognosis for limb salvage in patients with acute arterial occlusion ranges between 80 and 90 per cent, depending on the adequacy of the collateral circulation and the rapidity of therapeutic intervention. The patient survival also ranges between 80 and 90 per cent, with mortality usually reflecting underlying severe cardiac disease.

Algorithm

Figure 11 reviews in algorithmic format the principles of diagnosis and therapy of patients with suspected acute arterial occlusion. Unless contraindicated, intravenous heparin therapy is initiated. The physician must then attempt to differentiate embolism from thrombosis based upon symptoms, antecedent history, and clinical signs. After obtaining validating non-invasive studies, if available, further diagnostic or therapeutic intervention depends upon the severity of the ischemia. If embolism is suspected and the extremity is markedly ischemic, emergency operation with attempted embolectomy is indicated. If ischemia is less severe and the embolus is distal to the popliteal artery, fibrinolytic therapy should be considered, particularly in patients who are at high risk of operation. After fibrinolytic or surgical therapy, further cardiac evaluation or assessment of proximal arterial occlusive disease or aneurysm is indicated. If arterial reconstruction is successful, prolonged

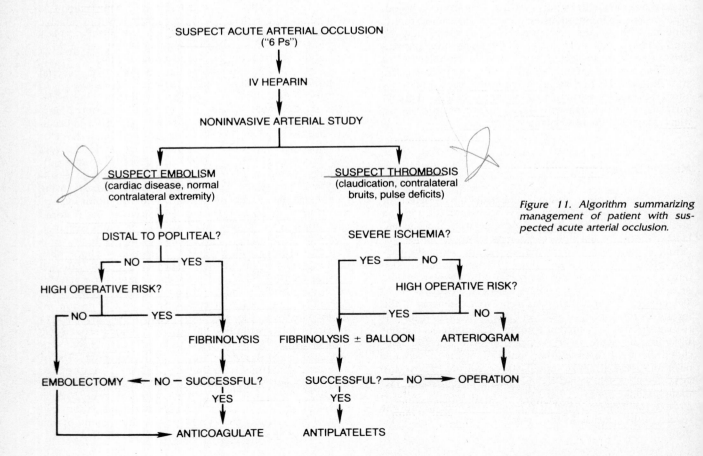

Figure 11. Algorithm summarizing management of patient with suspected acute arterial occlusion.

anticoagulation may be necessary for patients with cardiac causes of embolism.

In patients with suspected thrombosis, arteriography should be considered unless severe ischemia or prohibitive operative risk is present, in which case fibrinolytic therapy and possible balloon dilatation should be entertained.

ARTERIAL TRAUMA

Arterial trauma represents arterial injury due to blunt or penetrating forces that may result in hemorrhagic or thrombotic complication.

Clinical Hallmarks

Arterial trauma should be suspected if one or more of the following "nine Ps" are present:
1. Puddling (bleeding).
2. Protuberance (expanding hematoma).
3. Proximity of penetrating wound to neurovascular trunks and any other of the "six Ps" of acute arterial occlusion:
4. Pain.
5. Pallor.
6. Paresthesias.
7. Paralysis.
8. Pulselessness.
9. Polar (cold) sensation.
Other signs of possible arterial trauma include:
10. Hypotension.
11. Bruit.
12. Associated nerve or vein injury.

Etiology

Arterial trauma may result from one or more basic mechanisms of injury: penetrating injury, blunt injury, fracture or dislocation, or iatrogenic injury.[15] *Penetrating* injuries are usually classified as low- or high-velocity injuries. Low-velocity injuries include stab wounds and gunshot wounds from firearms with a muzzle velocity of less than 2000 feet per second. High-velocity missile injuries are frequently encountered with military weapons and firearms used for large game hunting. *Blunt injuries* are common in pedestrian and motor vehicle accidents and following falls. Arterial injuries may accompany fractures or dislocations, particularly those around the knee or elbow. Iatrogenic arterial injuries may result from complications of arterial catheterization or monitoring, including punctures associated with arterial blood gas sampling.

Pathology

Arterial injury usually results in hemorrhage and/or thrombosis of the affected artery. Incomplete arterial disruption or laceration may result in greater hemorrhage, owing to the inability of the vessel to retract, than may be the case with complete transection of the artery. Arterial contusion reflects varying degrees of mural damage without disruption of the full thickness of the arterial wall. Contusion may result in only subadventitial or subintimal hemorrhage, although more severe damage associated with contusion may result in intimal disruption or arterial dis-

section and spasm with resulting intraluminal thrombosis. Arterial laceration may lead to contained adjacent hematoma resulting in a pulsatile false aneurysm. Injury of both artery and adjacent vein may lead to traumatic arteriovenous fistula.

Clinical Manifestations

The aforementioned "nine Ps" may make acute arterial trauma self-evident on initial inspection. It is important to obtain a clear history of blood loss at the scene of the accident. Obvious arterial injury may be evident with penetrating trauma and brisk hemorrhage of bright red blood. Arterial injury may be more difficult to recognize in blunt injury, particularly if there is incomplete arterial disruption or intimal tears with persistent pulses. An expanding hematoma or a wound in proximity to a neurovascular bundle should always suggest the possibility of arterial trauma. A continuous bruit is pathognomonic of an arteriovenous fistula. An expanding hematoma and the signs of acute arterial occlusion should always lead the examiner to suspect arterial injury.

Diagnostic Evaluation

Noninvasive diagnostic studies may suggest arterial obstruction based on abnormal peripheral arterial signals or reduced segmental limb blood pressures. However, the presence of normal Doppler pressures and signals does not exclude an arterial injury, and the aforementioned clinical manifestations should always prompt arteriography in patients with possible minor arterial injury and sustained peripheral perfusion. Arteriography is necessary to exclude intimal disruption or continuing hemorrhage, which may not result in distal limb hypoperfusion. Arteriography is unnecessary in patients with obvious arterial injury, particularly localized penetrating trauma such as gunshot or stab wounds with external hemorrhage or peripheral pulse deficits. However, shotgun wounds and blunt trauma, both of which may lead to more extensive arterial injury, are best evaluated by preoperative arteriography.

Preoperative Management

Initial management of arterial trauma involves the general principles of trauma management, including the "ABCs" (airway, breathing, circulation). External bleeding is controlled by direct pressure with dressings and manual pressure or an elastic bandage. Large bore intravenous lines must be inserted in uninjured extremities and crystalloid solutions infused while blood is being typed and crossmatched. Fractures should be splinted and dislocations reduced if possible. Nasogastric and Foley catheters are inserted. The patient should receive tetanus prophylaxis and intravenous antibiotics. Appropriate x-ray films should be ordered, including arteriography if indicated. The resuscitation should be as prompt as feasible so that operative intervention need not be unnecessarily delayed.

Operative Therapy

Operative intervention is tailored to the site of arterial injury. The principle of arterial repair includes lateral arteriorrhaphy for closure of a clean arterial laceration.

More extensive arterial injury may require local resection with end-to-end anastomosis or interposition or bypass grafting, preferably with autogenous saphenous vein. Arterial injuries of vessels that may be sacrificed may be treated with ligation, such as injuries to one of the arteries of the forearm or one of the tibial vessels, providing normal circulation is present in the other distal vessels. External or internal fixation of fractures should be performed in concert with orthopedic surgeons. If severe arterial ischemia is present, initial repair of the artery may be necessary with subsequent fixation of fractures. However, where possible, stabilization of fractures and maintenance of appropriate limb length should be considered prior to completing definitive arterial reconstruction. If marked ischemia has been present for several hours, postoperative fasciotomy should be considered to relieve or prevent the compartment compression syndrome. Amputation is reserved for irreversible ischemia (muscle rigor), gangrene, or for arterial reconstruction failure with advanced limb ischemia.

Postoperative Management

In the postoperative period, peripheral pulses should be recorded; if available, objective measurement of distal limb systolic pressures using Doppler ultrasound is advisable. Reoperation may be necessary for thrombosis of operative repairs. Appropriate maintenance of blood volume with intravenous infusions and prophylactic antibiotics for 24 to 48 hours is an adjunct to postoperative care. Complications of thrombosis or hemorrhage may require reoperation. Infection may occur early or late in the postoperative period and usually responds to open wound care unless a prosthetic graft becomes infected. In the latter circumstance, the graft must be removed and revascularization attempted using autogenous materials through uninvolved tissue planes. If fasciotomy was not performed at the initial operation, monitoring of compartment pressures is advisable to detect the compartment compression syndrome. Late complications of arterial injury include false aneurysm and arteriovenous fistula which, if detected, require operative repair.

Algorithm

Figure 12 shows an algorithm summarizing the assessment and management of patients with suspected arterial

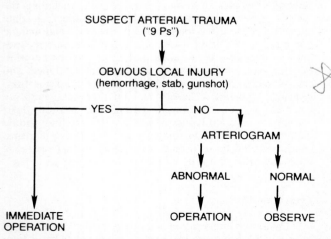

SUSPECT ARTERIAL TRAUMA
("9 Ps")
↓
OBVIOUS LOCAL INJURY
(hemorrhage, stab, gunshot)

YES — NO
ARTERIOGRAM
ABNORMAL — NORMAL
IMMEDIATE OPERATION — OPERATION — OBSERVE

Figure 12. Algorithm summarizing management of patient with suspected acute arterial trauma.

trauma. If local obvious injury is present, such as hemorrhage from a stab or gunshot wound, immediate operative intervention is advisable. If such injury is not evident or if more extensive arterial injury is suspected from blunt trauma or gunshot wounds, arteriography should be performed. Any abnormalities should be considered for operative repair. Patients with normal arteriograms may be observed.

ARTERIAL ANEURYSM

An aneurysm is an abnormal dilatation of a focal or diffuse segment of artery, involving either all layers of the arterial wall (true aneurysm) or only a portion of the vessel wall or surrounding tissue (false aneurysm).

Clinical Hallmarks

An aneurysm should be suspected in any patient with a pulsatile mass. A ruptured aneurysm is characterized by the "three Ps":
1. Pain.
2. Pulsatile mass.
3. Pressure drop (hypotension).

Etiology

Aneurysms are usually caused by one of four conditions: degenerative, inflammatory, mechanical, or congenital.

Degenerative Conditions. The most common degenerative cause of peripheral arterial aneurysm is atherosclerosis. Although atherosclerosis most commonly causes an infrarenal abdominal aortic aneurysm, other contributory factors may be present, such as abnormalities in vessel wall metabolism, increased wall stresses associated with reflected pressure waves, or inadequate aortic wall nutrition or insufficient numbers of musculoelastic lamellae. Fibromuscular dysplasia is a less common cause of aneurysms but may result in small multiple aneurysms of the renal or carotid arteries. Cystic medial necrosis is a common predisposing factor to dissecting aneurysms, especially in patients with hypertension or Marfan's syndrome.

Inflammatory Condition. Inflammation or infection may result in arterial aneurysms. In the past syphilis was the most common cause of aortic aneurysms, particularly in the ascending aorta. However, currently syphilis is much less common than atherosclerosis as a cause of aneurysms. Other infections may result in so-called mycotic arterial aneurysm, including a variety of gram-positive or gram-negative bacteria. *Salmonella aortitis* is a particularly frequent cause of mycotic aneurysm. Noninfectious arteritis, such as giant cell arteritis or polyarteritis nodosa, may result in arterial aneurysm.

Mechanical Condition. Mechanical causes of aneurysm include posttraumatic false aneurysm, poststenotic aneurysms (common distal to a coarctation), and anastomotic false aneurysms associated with breakdown of a suture line due to wall stress, infection, or degeneration of the adjacent host artery.

Congenital Disorders. Congenital aneurysms include the common cerebral (berry) aneurysm and aneurysms associated with inherited disorders of metabolism such as Ehlers-Danlos syndrome or Marfan's syndrome.

Pathology

Aneurysms may be characterized by the amount of involvement of the vessel wall, the shape, the location, and the histopathology, which reflects the underlying etiology.

VESSEL WALL INVOLVEMENT

True aneurysms involve all layers of the vessel wall and include most forms of degenerative and inflammatory types of aneurysms. *False aneurysms* involve only a portion of the vessel wall, e.g., berry aneurysms, in which there is deficiency of the arterial media, particularly at branch points of vessels at the base of the brain. Other forms of false aneurysm include posttraumatic or anastomotic aneurysms in which little or no vessel wall is present and the boundary of the aneurysm is adjacent tissue.

SHAPE

Aneurysms classified by their shape may be saccular, fusiform, and dissecting. *Saccular* aneurysms involve only a portion of the circumference of the vessel. Syphilitic aneurysms are characteristically saccular, but other mycotic infections and occasional atherosclerotic aneurysms may be saccular. *Fusiform* aneurysms involve uniform dilatation of the entire circumference of the vessel. Such aneurysms are common with atherosclerosis. *Dissecting* aneurysms involve separation of layers of the arterial wall (usually the media) for varying lengths of the vessel. Such aneurysms often result from cystic medial necrosis, particularly in patients with hypertension or Marfan's syndrome.

LOCATION

The most common location of arterial aneurysms is the infrarenal abdominal aorta, usually as the result of atherosclerosis. Aortic aneurysms may also involve the thoracic aorta, including the ascending, arch, or descending portion. Aortic aneurysms involving both the thoracic and abdominal portions are termed thoracoabdominal aneurysms. Peripheral arterial aneurysms may include iliac aneurysms, usually associated with infrarenal aortic aneurysms. Femoral and popliteal aneurysms may occur, often bilaterally, and are frequently associated with abdominal aortic aneurysm. These aneurysms are usually the result of atherosclerosis. Subclavian or axillary aneurysms may occur, due to either atherosclerosis or repeated trauma, such as that caused by prolonged use of crutches. Splanchnic artery aneurysms may involve the celiac and mesenteric arteries or their branches. These aneurysms may be due to atherosclerosis, fibromuscular dysplasia, or infection (mycotic). Renal artery aneurysms are commonly associated with hypertension and may be due to atherosclerosis (poststenotic) or fibromuscular dysplasia, frequently in women. Carotid aneurysms are uncommon but may be the result of atherosclerosis or fibromuscular dysplasia. Cerebral aneurysms are usually the result of congenital abnormality, particularly deficiency in the media at the point of arterial branching (berry aneurysm).

HISTOPATHOLOGY

The histopathology of arterial aneurysms depends upon the underlying etiology. Atherosclerosis results in deposition of lipid, initially in the arterial media, with subsequent evolution of the atheroma into more complex deposits of fibrous tissue, calcification, or hemorrhage. As the process extends into the media of the vessel, there is disruption of the normal elastic and smooth muscle fibers with progressive fibrosis, which does not withstand repeated arterial pulse pressure with the same viscoelastic properties as the normal arterial wall. Progressive dilatation results in increased arterial wall tension, which perpetuates the dilating process. The lumen of the aneurysmal portion of the arterial wall is often lined by platelet and fibrin debris to maintain a blood flow channel of relatively normal dimensions.

Syphilis results in characteristic gummata and destruction of the normal musculoelastic layers of the vessel wall. Fibrous tissue replacement undergoes progressive aneurysmal dilatation because of the abnormal viscoelastic properties of connective tissue. Other forms of inflammatory aneurysm may reveal varying stages of acute or chronic inflammatory cells and offending bacteria. Giant cell arteritis is characterized by a chronic mononuclear infiltrate with associated giant cells.

Fibromuscular dysplasia is characterized by areas of fibrous tissue proliferation that may involve the intima, media, or adventitia. An uncommon form of fibromuscular dysplasia involves hyperplasia of the smooth muscle of the media. Between areas of fibrosis, there is thinning of the arterial wall with aneurysmal dilatation.

False aneurysms are characterized by loss of the normal histologic layers of the vessel wall with the aneurysm wall lined by fibrous tissue, which usually represents adjacent tissue around the artery. Anastomotic false aneurysms may be the result of either fragmentation of the suture material, infection with dissolution of the adjacent artery, or true aneurysmal dilatation of the atherosclerotic host artery.

The Ehlers-Danlos syndrome is characterized by fragmentation of the elastic tissue in the media of the artery with multiple areas of aneurysmal dilatation. Marfan's syndrome is histologically characterized by areas of cystic medial destruction with aneurysmal dilatation or arterial wall dissection.

Manifestations

Aneurysms may become manifest in one of three ways: asymptomatic (incidental discovery on physical examination), rupture, or thromboembolic complication.

Asymptomatic Aneurysms. In most patients, an aneurysm is discovered on a routine physical examination. Occasionally, asymptomatic aneurysms are discovered incidentally on plain x-ray films or arteriograms.

Rupture. Patients in whom an aneurysm ruptures classically have the clinical triad of pain, an expanding pulsatile mass, and signs of hypotension. Rupture of an infrarenal abdominal aortic aneurysm may develop either contained retroperitoneal hematoma or exsanguinating free intraperitoneal rupture. A contained rupture usually presents with severe pain in the low back that may radiate to the genitalia. On abdominal examination a large pulsatile abdominal mass may be felt unless the patient is very obese. If the rupture is contained and the amount of hemorrhage is small, the blood pressure may be unaffected or the patient may become hypertensive because of the pain. However, with progressive hemorrhage signs of hemorrhagic shock develop.

Thromboembolic Complication. An aneurysm that develops thrombosis or distal embolization will present with clinical signs of acute arterial occlusion. Thromboembolic complications are much more common with peripheral aneurysms of the popliteal or femoral artery than with aortic aneurysms.

Diagnosis

Most aneurysms should be discovered on physical examination. The examiner should always attempt to determine the diameter of the abdominal aorta above the level of the umbilicus. Normally the abdominal aorta is less than 2.5 cm. in diameter. If a prominent aortic pulsation is felt, particularly in an obese individual, an abdominal aortic aneurysm should be suspected. Likewise, if the popliteal pulse is more readily felt than usual, a popliteal aneurysm must be considered.

Plain radiographs may reveal calcification of an aneurysmal wall, particularly of the infrarenal aorta. Such calcification may be more readily seen on a lateral (cross-table) view. However, many aneurysms do not contain calcium and may not be seen on routine films.

Abdominal or peripheral artery aneurysms may be visualized with real-time B-mode ultrasonic scans (sonograms).[6] The sonogram usually provides the most accurate method of determining the overall size and extent of abdominal aortic aneurysm. Sonograms are also useful to evaluate femoral or popliteal aneurysms. Occasionally sonograms may identify a contained rupture with extravasation of blood outside the aneurysmal wall. However, any patient with suspected ruptured aneurysm should not undergo ultrasonic or radiologic study but should be considered for immediate operation.

Computed tomography may be useful to evaluate aneurysms that are not readily evaluated by ultrasonography, such as suprarenal or thoracic aortic aneurysms, dissecting aneurysms, true pelvic aneurysms, postoperative (false) aneurysms, or suspected infected or inflammatory aneurysms.

Arteriography may be useful when planning operative intervention. However, routine arteriograms are not necessary for most infrarenal abdominal aortic aneurysms unless there is associated peripheral arterial occlusive disease, suspected renovascular disease in severely hypertensive patients, or anticipated suprarenal aneurysmal extension. An arteriogram is not useful to determine the size of an abdominal aortic aneurysm because the contained thrombus may result in a relatively normal lumen dimension. Arteriography may be indicated if associated visceral artery disease is suspected.

Therapy

There is no medical therapy of arterial aneurysm other than treatment of hypertension for patients who are being followed for small aneurysms or who have absolute contraindications to operation. Except for rare instances of treatment of aneurysms by interventional radiology (catheter-induced thrombosis of nonvital arteries, such as splanchnic or internal iliac aneurysms), operative intervention is usually the treatment of choice.

Operation is usually recommended for one of three reasons: prophylaxis against rupture, treatment of rupture, or treatment of thromboembolic or other complications.[18] The risk of rupture of an arterial aneurysm is proportional to the size of the aneurysm. This risk is a logarithmic relationship, and crude statistics of abdominal aortic aneurysm are presented in Table 1.

The risk of rupture also depends upon the location of the aneurysm and the tamponading effect of adjacent tissue. For an intraperitoneal rupture of an abdominal aorta, the immediate mortality rate is between 50 and 80 per cent. A 5 to 10 per cent initial mortality exists for retroperitoneal rupture of the abdominal aorta with a progressive increasing mortality depending upon the delay in instituting appropriate treatment. The risk of rupture of femoral or popliteal aneurysms is lower in terms of risk to life but higher in terms of risk to the viability of the affected limb.

The indications for operative intervention of a abdominal aortic aneurysm include the following:

1. All aneurysms greater than 6 cm. in diameter, providing there are no prohibitive risk factors.
2. A painful or tender aneurysm.
3. An aneurysm enlarging by more than 0.5 cm. per year as demonstrated by ultrasonography.
4. Signs of compression of adjacent tissue (intestine, ureter).
5. Signs of intestinal bleeding.
6. Signs of rupture.
7. Severe associated hypertension.
8. Signs of associated disabling peripheral arterial disease or embolization.
9. An aneurysm of less than 6 cm. in diameter in a good risk patient.

Operative repair usually involves an interposition Dacron prosthesis. For abdominal aortic aneurysms, the prosthesis is sutured end-to-end to the nondiseased portion of the abdominal aorta with distal anastomosis to the terminal aorta, the common iliac arteries, or the femoral arteries depending upon the extent of aneurysmal or occlusive disease.

Aneurysms of the common femoral artery are usually repaired by interposition of a Dacron prosthesis. Aneurysms of the popliteal artery are usually bypassed with autogenous saphenous vein. The aneurysm may be ligated proximally and distally, or the aneurysm may be opened with individual ligation of the branches of the artery to reduce the mass effect of a large popliteal aneurysm remaining in the popliteal fossa.

Postoperative Complications

Specific early postoperative complications after repair of aneurysms include hemorrhage and thrombosis or distal embolization. Abdominal aortic aneurysmectomy may be accompanied by renal failure, but this has been reduced with improved methods of anesthesia, hydration, and selective use of diuretic agents intraoperatively. Urologic complications, including obstruction of the ureter by inadvertent positioning of the aortofemoral bypass prosthesis anterior to the ureter, may occur. Large aneurysms of the iliac arteries may make dissection difficult, and the ureter may be injured or transected at the time of operation.

TABLE 1. *Risk of Rupture of Abdominal Aortic Aneurysm (in Five Years)*

Aortic Diameter (cm.)	Risk (%)
2.5 (normal)	0
4	15
5	20
6	30
7	50
8	75

Ischemia of the colon may occur as a result of sacrifice of the inferior mesenteric artery and exclusion of the internal iliac artery circulation from the vascular repair. Normally colon ischemia can be avoided if blood flow to one of the internal iliac arteries is preserved. Alternatively, the inferior mesenteric artery may be reanastomosed to the prosthetic graft. Colon ischemia is manifested by bloody diarrhea in the early postoperative period. Sigmoidoscopy should be performed, and if severe ischemia is present reoperation may be necessary with the creation of a colostomy and resection of gangrenous bowel. Milder degrees of colon ischemia may be treated nonoperatively, although stricture of the sigmoid colon may develop in the postoperative period.

Disturbances of sexual function are common after aortoiliac reconstructive operation. One of the most common disorders is retrograde ejaculation due to interruption of preaortic sympathetic innervation. Less commonly, impotence may develop after aortoiliac operative procedures. A rare neurologic complication is paraplegia due to interruption of blood supply to the lower spinal cord when the arteria radicularis magna (Adamkiewicz) rises from the infrarenal aorta.

Late complications after repair of arterial aneurysm include the development of false aneurysm, which may occur as the result of infection, fracture of the anastomotic suture, or degeneration of the wall of the artery adjacent to the prosthesis. Infection of an arterial prosthesis may occur at any time in the late postoperative period. Although indolent organisms such as *Staphylococcus epidermidis* may lead to late prosthetic infection from inoculation at the time of operation, infection may also result from transient bacteremia in the postoperative period. For this reason patients should be placed on prophylactic antibiotics if any dental or medical interventions are undertaken that could cause bacteremia. An infected arterial prosthesis usually requires removal with arterial reconstruction through clean, uninvolved extra-anatomic planes. Abdominal aortic aneurysmectomy and aortoenteric fistula may develop because of infection or mechanical erosion of the prosthesis into adjacent bowel, usually the fourth portion of the duodenum.

This complication can be minimized by covering the prosthesis and the proximal suture line with remnants of the aneurysm wall or with retroperitoneal tissue or omentum. Any patient who develops gastrointestinal hemorrhage after previous prosthetic aortic graft reconstruction should be considered to have an aortoenteric fistula until proven otherwise.

Thrombosis of an arterial prosthesis after aneurysm repair may develop at any time during the postoperative period, most commonly owing to progressive atherosclerotic peripheral arterial occlusive disease. However, subclinical graft infection may be first manifest as occlusion of limb of an aortofemoral prosthesis.

Algorithm

Figure 13 is an algorithm that summarizes the important principles in the diagnosis and management of a patient with a suspected abdominal aorta aneurysm. If rupture of the aneurysm is suspected, the patient should be considered for immediate emergency aneurysmectomy unless there is a prohibitive operative risk and the diagnosis is unclear. In such instances, a CT scan or sonogram may be considered if the patient is stable to establish unequivocally the diagnosis of rupture. If rupture is not suspected, an ultrasonogram may be advisable if there is uncertainty whether the aneurysm is of sufficient size to warrant operation. If the aneurysm is less than 5 cm. in diameter, observation may be recommended with repeated ultrasonograms at 3- to 6-month intervals to determine the rate of enlargement. Operative intervention would be considered if the aneurysm increases by more than 0.5 cm. during the course of one year or if signs of rupture develop. For aneurysms larger than 5.0 cm., operation should be considered unless there are prohibitive operative risks. If associated disease, such as hypertension, peripheral vascular disease, or renal failure, is present or if there is a question about suprarenal extension, arteriography would be advisable prior to operation. Otherwise, patients may be considered for aneurysmectomy without arteriography. However, some surgeons

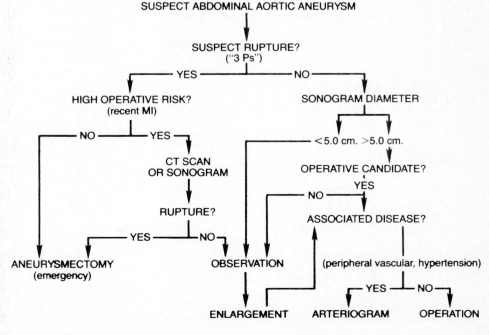

Figure 13. Algorithm summarizing management of patient with suspected abdominal aortic aneurysm.

routinely perform arteriography to identify any unsuspected vascular disease prior to operative intervention.

CHRONIC ARTERIAL OCCLUSIVE DISEASE

Chronic arterial occlusive disease refers to organic obstruction of a segment or multiple segments of the peripheral arterial system, usually due to atherosclerosis, which may lead to symptoms of peripheral arterial insufficiency with exercise or at rest. This section will be limited to chronic arterial occlusive lesions of the extremities, particularly the lower extremity. Chronic arterial occlusive disease of other vascular beds will be discussed in subsequent sections of this chapter.

Clinical Hallmarks

Chronic arterial occlusive disease should be suspected in a patient who manifests one or more of the following:
1. Reproducible muscle pain with exercise relieved by brief rest (claudication).
2. Pain in the distal extremity at rest (ischemic rest pain).
3. Ischemic nonhealing ulceration.
4. Gangrene.
5. Pulse deficits.

Etiology

Most chronic arterial occlusive disease is the result of atherosclerosis. Less common causes of chronic occlusive disease include fibromuscular dysplasia, thromboangiitis obliterans (Buerger's disease), muscular entrapment, and subadventitial cystic degeneration. The latter two conditions should be suspected in any young adult male who develops symptoms or signs of chronic occlusive disease, particularly if the patient has never smoked cigarettes. Muscular entrapment most commonly involves the popliteal artery, which may course anomalously around the medial aspect of the medial head of the gastrocnemius muscle. Alternatively, the artery may be compressed by an anomalous muscle or fascial band in the popliteal fossa. Cystic adventitial degeneration involves a subadventitial cyst that contains clear mucous fluid, which results in a characteristic "hour glass" deformity of the arterial lumen on arteriography. Both muscular entrapment and subadventitial cystic degeneration may progress to total thrombotic occlusion of the popliteal artery.

Pathology

Atherosclerosis is the most common underlying lesion in chronic arterial occlusive disease. The pathology of the atherosclerotic lesion has been described in earlier sections of this chapter and other chapters of this textbook. The location of the atherosclerosis will influence the clinical manifestations and functional extent of the arterial occlusive disease. Atherosclerosis is often segmental and may involve a single segment of the arterial system (such as the aorto-iliac, femoropopliteal, or tibioperoneal artery segments in the lower extremity). A single level of occlusive disease leads to less severe symptoms than does multisegmental

disease. Symptoms may result from either narrowing of the vessel (stenosis) or total obstruction of the lumen (occlusion). The atheromatous plaque may only partially obstruct the lumen, whereas superimposed thrombus results in total occlusion of the vessel. The atherosclerotic plaque may ulcerate and discharge athermomatous contents as distal emboli (cholesterol embolization). Alternatively, superimposed thrombotic debris may become dislodged and result in distal emboli.

The pathology of fibromuscular dysplasia and thromboangiitis obliterans (Buerger's disease) is discussed in separate sections of this chapter.

Clinical Manifestations

Patients with chronic arterial occlusive disease may present in one of four ways: asymptomatic, claudication, ischemic rest pain, or tissue necrosis.

ASYMPTOMATIC DISEASE

Asymptomatic patients may be identified on the basis of pulse deficits or vascular bruits during the course of routine physical examination. The remaining manifestations of symptomatic patients are usually diagnostic of chronic arterial occlusive disease, and a careful history and physical examination should lead to an accurate clinical diagnosis in most patients.

CLAUDICATION

Claudication is defined as *reproducible* muscle pain with exercise that is relieved by a *brief* period of rest, usually in the standing position. This definition is important because it permits the examiner to differentiate true claudication from "pseudoclaudication," which may mimic vascular disease but actually results from neurospinal or musculoskeletal disease.

Claudication due to chronic arterial occlusive disease characteristically causes intermittent pain after a reproducible amount of exercise, which is often graded into the number of city blocks that the patient can walk. There should be a little day-to-day variability in the walking distance that elicits extremity pain. The muscle pain should be relieved by a brief period of rest in the standing position (less than 5 minutes). Patients with pseudoclaudication have a history of lower extremity pain after walking variable distances. They may also complain of pain in the major muscle groups of the extremity while at rest. Furthermore, pseudoclaudication may require a specific position for relief, such as sitting or lying down.

Claudication most commonly occurs in the calf, although posterior thigh or buttock pain may occur with common femoral or aortoiliac occlusive disease, respectively. Patients with pseudoclaudication due to neurospinal or musculoskeletal disease often complain of pain in the anterior thigh or leg or in the low back. Patients with claudication characteristically complain of cramping or aching in the extremity, although occasionally weakness or numbness may be described. Patients with pseudoclaudication may complain of burning or lancinating pain or hyperesthesias of the extremity.

ISCHEMIC REST PAIN

Ischemic rest pain must be differentiated from common muscle cramps, which are unrelated to arterial occlusive disease. Patients with ischemic rest pain have advanced arterial insufficiency, which becomes manifest in the most distal parts of the extremity, including the toes, forefoot, and heel. Patients with the so-called night cramp syndrome usually complain of muscle cramps in the calf or the arch of the foot. Ischemic rest pain is characterized as burning, aching, or numbing, although severe, constant, deep pain may be noted. Patients with muscle cramps complain of actual cramping of muscle groups, and the toes or foot may become flexed as a result of the muscle contraction. Ischemic rest pain usually occurs at night but may become constant at all times of the day and night with advancing arterial occlusive disease. Muscle cramps usually occur soon after retiring.

Ischemic rest pain may be relieved by hanging the foot in the dependent position or by a brief walk about the room. Patients with night cramps may relieve their discomfort by massaging the affected muscle group or by walking. Ischemic rest pain may become severe and unremitting with little relief even from strong narcotic agents. Night muscle cramps are characteristically relieved with quinine or chlorpheniramine.

TISSUE NECROSIS

Advanced arterial occlusive disease may result in tissue necrosis, which may be manifest by either *ischemic ulceration* or *frank gangrene*.

Ischemic Ulceration

Ischemic ulcers must be differentiated from other causes of cutaneous ulceration. Ischemic ulcers characteristically occur on the toes, heel, foot, or malleoli. The most common leg ulcer that may be confused with ischemic ulcer is the chronic venous stasis ulcer due to deep venous insufficiency. Venous stasis ulcers usually occur above the medial malleolus on the lower leg. Ischemic ulcers are characterized by severe pain, except in patients with neuropathy, such as individuals with diabetes mellitus. Venous stasis ulcers are usually much less painful. The pain may be relieved in patients with ischemic ulceration by hanging the extremity in a dependent position. Patients with venous stasis ulcers obtain maximal relief by elevating the extremity.

The base of an ischemic ulcer may be necrotic and usually has poor or absent granulation tissue. With appropriate medical management, patients with venous stasis ulcer develop excellent granulation at the base of the ulcer. The margins of an ischemic ulcer have little or no healing epithelium, whereas venous stasis ulcers usually show a gray or bluish healing neoepithelium at the ulcer border. The skin surrounding an ischemic ulcer is usually atrophic, whereas the skin surrounding a stasis ulcer may show stasis hyperpigmentation.

Other chronic lower extremity ulcers must be differentiated from ulceration. Trophic ulcers characteristically appear as punched-out ulcers on the plantar aspect of the foot beneath the heads of the metatarsal bones. These characteristically occur in patients with diabetes mellitus and peripheral neuropathy. A surrounding callus is typically present, and the ulcer base may be granulating, although deep necrosis may develop with secondary infection of the metatarsal head. Arteritis may lead to punched-out ulcers on the lower leg, which may be slow to heal. Traumatic ulcers usually occur on the pretibial area of the lower leg and are often slow to heal, even in patients with normal

peripheral circulation. Hypertensive ulcers are characterized by severe pain, surrounding violaceous discoloration, and a history of severe hypertension. Patients with rheumatoid arthritis or other collagen vascular disease may develop chronic ulcers on the lower extremity, which are slow to heal.

Gangrene

Gangrene is ischemic necrosis of tissue that usually appears as dark blue or black mummification of a portion of the extremity. Gangrene due to arterial occlusive disease usually involves the toes, heel, or other portion of the foot or the malleolus. Progressive arterial occlusive disease may result in gangrene of the entire foot and lower leg. *Dry gangrene* is most common in patients with arterial occlusive disease and is noninfected necrosis of tissue. *Wet gangrene* indicates infected necrosis, which is more common in patients with diabetes mellitus.

Gangrene may also occur in other conditions that do not represent chronic arterial occlusive disease. Frostbite may lead to gangrene of digits or more proximal portions of the extremity. A history of exposure to cold should make the diagnosis obvious. Gangrene in patients with diabetes mellitus may involve the toes, the forefoot, or the entire foot. Although chronic arterial occlusive disease may contribute to diabetic gangrene, neuropathy, minor trauma, and uncontrolled invasive infection may lead to extensive gangrene despite intact major circulation. Unfortunately, many patients with diabetes mellitus develop extensive gangrene owing to unrecognized infection from wounds on the toes, interdigital clefts, or soles of the feet. Deep plantar space infection may be difficult to recognize clinically and may lead to secondary thrombosis of plantar or digital arteries, with resultant extensive tissue necrosis. For this reason, all patients with diabetes mellitus must be instructed on rigorous foot hygiene and must be rapidly treated for any breaks in the continuity of the skin.

Two conditions may lead to symmetrical digital or extremity gangrene in the absence of chronic arterial occlusive disease. *Disseminated intravascular coagulation* may lead to acute occlusions of the microcirculation in the digits or distal extremities with resultant symmetrical gangrene. It may be caused by a number of conditions, including septicemia, shock, and amniotic fluid embolism. Another cause of progressive symmetrical digital lower extremity gangrene is the *low cardiac output syndrome*. Such patients are characteristically in severe acute or chronic congestive heart failure and may be receiving sympathomimetic agents, which lead to a further reduction in distal extremity perfusion. Other causes of gangrene unrelated to chronic occlusive disease include venous gangrene associated with extensive deep vein thrombosis (phlegmasia cerulea dolens) and the crush syndrome due to prolonged compression of the extremity, particularly in patients suffering trauma coma, or drug overdose.

Physical Examination

Patients with suspected chronic arterial occlusive disease should be carefully evaluated by inspection, palpation, and auscultation. Patients who are asymptomatic or have mild or moderate claudication may have no abnormality on inspection of the affected extremity. *Trophic changes*, including hair loss on the toes, thickened nails, and dry atrophic skin, usually indicate advanced arterial occlusive disease. Similarly, elevation pallor and dependent rubor are seen only in patients with ischemic rest pain or tissue necrosis. The characteristics of ischemic ulcers and gangrene have been mentioned in the previous section.

Pulse deficits are important to elicit in patients with chronic arterial occlusive disease. The technique of pulse palpation and the method of grading peripheral pulses have been previously discussed. The examiner should attempt to define the anatomic levels of chronic arterial occlusion based on the pulse deficits and the location of vascular bruits. Absent femoral pulses indicate aortoiliac occlusive disease. Absence of a popliteal pulse should suggest superficial femoral or popliteal artery obstruction. Absent pedal pulses in the presence of more proximal pulses reflect tibioperoneal artery occlusive disease, which is particularly common in diabetic patients. The presence of bruit signifies arterial stenosis.

Diagnostic Evaluation

After a careful history and physical examination, the examiner should be able to develop an anatomic diagnosis and plan further diagnostic intervention or therapy. Noninvasive diagnostic studies provide an objective baseline of the presence and location of chronic arterial occlusive disease and any functional impairment. For chronic peripheral arterial occlusive disease, resting recordings of Doppler arterial velocity signals and measurement of segmental limb blood pressures are appropriate. Digit plethysmography should be performed, particularly if digit artery occlusive disease is present or if one must differentiate painful diabetic neuropathy from ischemic rest pain. Hyperemia testing with treadmill exercise or reactive hyperemia should be employed only for patients with claudication. Patients with suspected neurospinal or musculoskeletal disease are best evaluated with a treadmill test to differentiate pseudoclaudication from true claudication if there is associated arterial obstruction.

Arteriography should be considered only if the patient is a candidate for operation. The decision to intervene operatively should be based upon principles reviewed in the earlier sections of this chapter. If arteriography is to be undertaken, the radiologist should be consulted carefully to define the objectives of the diagnostic study as well as to consider possible interventional procedures such as balloon dilatation (percutaneous transluminal angioplasty). Most patients undergoing arteriography should have visualization of the entire arterial tree from the infrarenal abdominal aorta to the tibial arteries in the lower leg and, if possible, the plantar arterial arch in the foot. The arteriogram may be performed using translumbar or percutaneous femoral artery techniques.

Prognosis

Most patients with chronic arterial occlusive disease do not require operative intervention and will not be threatened by limb loss. Approximately 90 per cent of patients can be managed medically. Approximately 10 per cent of patients may eventually require surgical therapy, with the risk of limb loss during the patient's lifetime being approximately 5 per cent. The major risk to patients with chronic arterial occlusive disease is atherosclerosis involving the heart or brain. Approximately 25 to 50 per cent of patients with symptomatic peripheral arterial occlusive disease will die within 5 years of the initial diagnosis, usually from myocardial infarction or stroke.

Medical Therapy

Most patients are candidates for medical therapy. Physicians should make an aggressive effort to intervene with atherosclerotic risk factors. Unfortunately, most patients who do not require operation seldom are carefully instructed in the various nonoperative measures that improve the prognosis of peripheral arterial occlusive disease.

EXERCISE

The most important recommendation for patients with symptomatic claudication is an explicit *exercise* program. Regular exercise is the best stimulus for improving collateral circulation and muscle metabolism in patients with chronic arterial occlusive disease. The patient should be instructed to determine the maximal walking distance (MWD), which is that distance that brings about severe claudication, forcing the patient to stop walking. The patient should then begin a daily exercise program of walking three fourths of this MWD, which should be a distance that leads to definite but moderate and tolerable claudication. The patient should then stop and rest for 3 to 5 minutes and then repeat this amount of exercise at least 5 times daily, with brief periods of rest between each exercise period. This exercise program should involve approximately 1 hour of walking every day. After 4 to 6 weeks the patient should redefine the MWD and then adjust the daily repetitive exercise distance accordingly. With strict adherence to such an exercise program, many patients with disabling claudication may develop significant improvement in their walking tolerance, and a number of patients may actually have remission of claudication for an extended period of time.

SMOKING

The second most important recommendation for patients with symptomatic chronic occlusive arterial disease is an unequivocal commitment to cease smoking in any of its forms. Although many patients do not successfully give up smoking, there is no other accomplishment that can be of greater benefit to the patient than to eliminate this leading risk factor for peripheral arterial occlusive disease. The physician should encourage the patient to solicit adjuncts that may aid in breaking the smoking habit, including enrollment in group therapy, use of adjunctive medications including nicotine-containing chewing gum, participation in biofeedback or hypnotherapy, and other methods to eliminate this habit. Unfortunately, continuance of the smoking habit may result in significant disease progression with an increased risk of future limb loss or failure of surgical therapy.

OBESITY AND RELATED RISK FACTORS

Other interventions with risk factors should be recommended. Obese patients should be encouraged to lose weight, not only to reduce the risk of atherosclerotic disease progression but also to improve the walking distance because of decreased work load. Although hyperlipidemia is not common in patients with peripheral arterial occlusive disease, any derangement in serum lipids should be appropriately treated by diet or drug therapy.

Diabetes mellitus should be strictly controlled. Hypertension should be treated, even though significant reductions in blood pressure may lead to some increase in claudication. However, the incidence of atherosclerotic disease progression may be reduced by appropriate control of blood pressure, which is also necessary to reduce cardiac and cerebral complications.

FOOT HYGIENE

An important aspect of medical care is instructing patients in appropriate foot hygiene. Most patients in whom tissue necrosis develops will have skin lesions that could have been prevented with appropriate foot care. The patient should be instructed to trim toenails carefully; this may require podiatric consultation, particularly in diabetic subjects. The feet should be kept clean and dry. Fungal infection of the nails or interdigital areas should be carefully treated. The patient should be instructed to wear properly fitting shoes. Patients or family members should inspect the shoes daily for foreign bodies if neuropathy is present. Calluses or corns should be treated only by an experienced individual, preferably a podiatrist. The patient should be instructed to avoid hot water and heating pads, particularly in the presence of chronic arterial occlusive disease. A family member may be instructed to be responsible for regular inspection of the patient's feet as well as footwear.

VASODILATORS

Vasodilator drug therapy has little role in the treatment of chronic arterial occlusive disease. Although many patients are prescribed vasodilators and some claim benefit from these agents, few studies show objective improvement with such therapy. Many patients may increase their walking distance as a result of vasodilator therapy. The exercise program may be the primary stimulus for improved circulation, not the vasodilators themselves. Indeed, most vasodilators may cause a mild reduction in systemic blood pressure because of nonspecific generalized vasodilation. Such reduced systemic blood pressure may lead to an increase in claudication. The objective of any therapy should be regional vasodilation in the affected extremity. Exercise is the best method to accomplish this goal. Recently, some vasodilators with properties that reduce blood viscosity have been reported in randomized studies to improve claudication in patients with chronic arterial occlusive disease. The author feels that pharmacologic therapy has little use in a patient with chronic arterial occlusive disease.

Interventional Radiology

Patients who are candidates for operative therapy may be considered for interventional radiologic procedures, particularly those at high operative risk. Catheter infusion of streptokinase or urokinase may be considered in patients at high operative risk or with distal arterial occlusive disease, in a manner similar to that for acute arterial occlusion. However, thrombolytic therapy in patients with chronic arterial occlusive disease is not as successful as in patients with acute arterial occlusion.

Balloon dilatation (percutaneous transluminal angioplasty [PTA]) may be considered in patients with localized stenoses of major arteries, particularly the common iliac artery. Such therapy is particularly helpful in male patients with claudication and good arterial runoff. Balloon dilatation reduces the risk of sexual dysfunction in patients with localized common iliac artery stenosis. More distal arterial stenoses or more extensive atherosclerotic vascular disease is best treated by surgical therapy.

Operative Therapy

Patients with chronic arterial occlusive disease are candidates for operation for the purposes of limb salvage or preservation of function. Patients with gangrene, ischemic ulceration, or ischemic rest pain are at risk of limb loss and are appropriate candidates for operative intervention. Patients with disabling claudication of greater than 3 months duration who have failed medical therapy are candidates for operation if the claudication interferes with self-care, occupation, or recreation.

Patients for arterial reconstruction should be assessed for their operative risk factors. If there is no major contraindication to operation, anatomic reconstruction of the peripheral circulation is preferable, with endarterectomy or bypass of arterial occlusive segments, depending upon the location of the occlusive disease. An underlying principle of arterial reconstruction is to correct the most proximal occlusive lesions before considering more distal reconstruction. Often repair of the most proximal lesions of the segmental arterial occlusive disease will result in significant improvement in claudication or limb salvage, even though more distal occlusive lesions remain. Thus, aortoiliac reconstruction should be considered before treating femoropopliteal or more distal arterial occlusive disease.

Aortoiliac atherosclerosis may be treated by endarterectomy, particularly if localized to the terminal aorta or the common iliac arteries. More extensive disease involving the external iliac or femoral vessels usually requires prosthetic bypass using a Dacron bifurcation graft.[10] The bypass is usually carried to the common femoral or profunda femoris artery. Patients with residual superficial femoral artery occlusive disease are often significantly improved by the inflow reconstructive procedure.

Patients with isolated femoropopliteal artery occlusive disease may be candidates for a femoropopliteal bypass. Localized stenoses in the superficial femoral artery occasionally are amenable to local endarterectomy. However, more extensive disease usually requires bypass, preferably with an autogenous saphenous vein graft. Saphenous vein bypass grafts may be performed by reversing the vein to permit antegrade flow through the saphenous venous valves. More recently, so-called *in situ* vein bypass grafts have been performed by excision or incision of the venous valves while leaving the vein undisturbed in the subcutaneous position. The latter procedure may improve the preservation of venous endothelium and permit more appropriate tailoring of the ends of the saphenous vein to the proximal and distal arteries in the leg. Patients in whom the saphenous vein is of unsuitable caliber (less than 4 mm. in diameter) or in whom there is surgical absence of the vein may be candidates for bypass using prosthetic (polytetraflouroethylene) or other biologic substitutes (glutaraldehyde starch-preserved human umbilical vein).

In patients who are at high risk of intra-abdominal anatomic reconstruction for aortoiliac occlusive disease, extra-anatomic bypass using prosthetic grafts in the axillofemoral or femorofemoral position may be advisable.

Patients who are not candidates for arterial reconstruction are occasionally considered for lumbar sympathectomy.

This procedure may improve cutaneous circulation in the foot of patients with early ischemic rest pain or minor tissue necrosis. However, this procedure has little role in patients with more advanced arterial occlusive disease and does not improve claudication.

Patients with intolerable ischemic rest pain or gangrene who are not candidates for arterial reconstruction should be considered for amputation. Amputation should be performed at the most distal level compatible with healing. Although a digit or forefoot (transmetatarsal) amputation may be considered in some patients with diabetes mellitus, most patients with advanced arterial occlusive disease require major extremity amputation at the below-knee or above-knee level. Clinical and noninvasive diagnostic techniques may help predict the most appropriate level of amputation wound healing. The amputation technique must be meticulously performed. Pre- and postoperative physical therapy is important. The amputation wound may be dressed in elastic bandage or in a plaster cast to avoid trauma or excessive edema, which impedes wound healing. Rehabilitation requires vigorous physical therapy and appropriate protection of the amputation stump. With appropriate wound care, a temporary prosthesis may be prescribed 4 to 6 weeks after amputation. A permanent prosthesis is prescribed 3 or 4 months later after maximal stump shrinkage has occurred. Some patients who are markedly debilitated may not be candidates for prosthetic rehabilitation.

Complications

Postoperative complications are similar to those mentioned following operative therapy for arterial aneurysms. Myocardial infarction and stroke are more common in patients with arterial occlusive disease.

Prognosis

The operative mortality after vascular reconstruction depends upon the clinical status of the patient. Overall, there is approximately a 3 to 5 per cent risk of death, usually from myocardial infarction, after arterial reconstruction. Perioperative mortality following amputation may be higher because of the more advanced arterial occlusive disease of such patients. The late postoperative mortality varies between 25 and 50 per cent, usually the result of myocardial infarction or stroke.

The risk of arterial reconstruction in terms of limb loss is approximately 5 per cent in the perioperative period and 10 to 20 per cent in the late postoperative period.

Graft patency following aortofemoral bypass is approximately 90 per cent over a 5-year period. A similar patency rate has been noted following aortoiliac endarterectomy. The patency of femoropopliteal bypass grafts over 5 years varies between 60 and 75 per cent, depending upon the extent of peripheral arterial occlusive disease. The patency rate for prosthetic grafts is less than that, with fewer than 50 per cent patent grafts distal to the knee. Likewise, femorotibial bypass vein grafts have an overall patency rate of about 50 per cent in 5 years.

Algorithm

Figure 14 is an algorithm that summarizes the therapeutic principles in a patient with suspected chronic arterial occlusive disease. The clinician must first define whether or not the patient is threatened with limb loss. If ischemic rest pain or tissue necrosis is present, an arteriogram should be considered with subsequent radiologic or surgical intervention. If, however, limb salvage is not a consideration, the next concern should be whether or not the patient has truly disabling claudication. If not, the patient should be considered for medical therapy. If claudication is disabling but of relatively short duration, medical therapy should be considered in an attempt to improve collateral circulation. If disabling claudication has been present for more than 3 months but the patient has not had an adequate trial of medical therapy, nonoperative therapy should be instituted. If the patient has persistent disabling claudication despite adequate medical therapy, arteriography should then be considered unless the patient is not an operative candidate. If the arteriogram reveals a localized stenosis, particularly of the common iliac artery, balloon dilatation should be considered. If more extensive atherosclerotic disease is present, either anatomic or extra-anatomic arterial reconstruction should be considered, depending upon the patient's operative risk factors.

ARTERITIS

Arteritis refers to an inflammatory disorder of an artery, which may be caused by an infectious agent or noninfectious conditions such as autoimmune disease. The three most common arteritides that will be included in this section are thromboangiitis obliterans (Buerger's disease), Takayasu's arteritis, and giant cell or temporal arteritis.

Clinical Hallmarks

Buerger's disease should be suspected in a patient with one or more of the following:
1. Painful ischemic digits of the upper and lower extremities in a young adult male with a heavy smoking history.
2. Foot claudication.
3. Recurrent superficial thrombophlebitis.
4. Raynaud's syndrome (see subsequent section).

Takayasu's arteritis should be suspected in a patient with one or more of the following:
1. Initial fever, malaise, and arthralgia in a young adult female.
2. Bruits and pulse deficits of the brachiocephalic arteries.
3. Congestive heart failure, coronary artery disease, hypertension, or stroke in a young adult female.
4. Elevated erythrocyte sedimentation rate.

Temporal arteritis should be suspected in an elderly patient with one or more of the following:
1. Recurrent severe headache.
2. Polymyalgia rheumatica.
3. Temporal artery tenderness or nodularity.
4. Visual blurring or other visual disturbances.
5. Elevated erythrocyte sedimentation rate.

Pathology

Buerger's disease is characterized pathologically as a panangiitis of medium and small blood vessels including both arteries and adjacent veins.[13] The inflammatory arte-

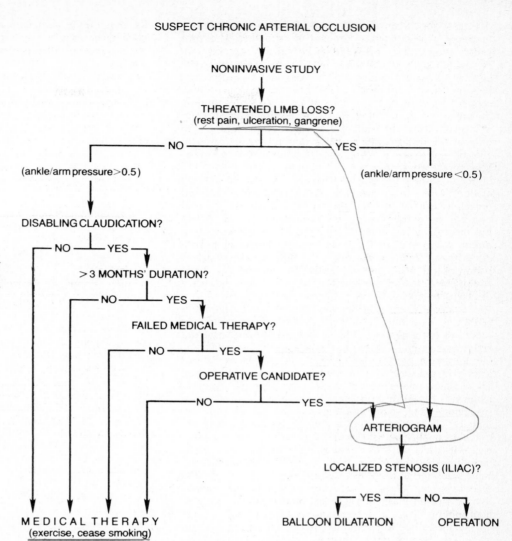

Figure 14. Algorithm summarizing management of patient with suspected chronic arterial occlusive disease.

ritis is accompanied by intravascular thrombosis, which likewise affects both arteries and veins. Recurrent migratory superficial thrombophlebitis may occur. The vascular involvement shows a predilection for distal extremity vessels including digital, palmar and plantar, and tibioperoneal arteries. Visceral vessels including mesenteric arteries may be involved.

Takayasu's arteritis is characterized by a nonspecific inflammation that progresses to fibrosis and thrombosis of arteries, particularly brachiocephalic arterial branches of the aortic arch.[16] Pulmonary arterial disease may also occur. In the abdomen, mesenteric artery, suprarenal and infrarenal aorta, and renal artery involvement may occur with resultant mesenteric vascular insufficiency or renovascular hypertension.

Giant cell arteritis, including temporal arteritis, is characterized by inflammation involving giant cells of the aortic arch and its branches, particularly the temporal arteries.

Other types of arteritis that will not be discussed in this section include such disorders as polyarteritis nodosa, mycotic (infectious) arteritis, rheumatoid vasculitis, and other types of collagen vascular disease.

Etiology

The etiology of Buerger's disease, Takayasu's arteritis, and giant cell arteritis is unknown. Autoimmune causes and allergy or hypersensitivity reactions have been implicated. In Buerger's disease, the association with cigarette smoking is a striking characteristic, with affected patients usually severely addicted to smoking. A possible allergy or hypersensitivity to a component of cigarette smoke may contribute to this disorder. Patients rarely are able to cease smoking despite progressive peripheral vascular disease, which may result in extensive digital and extremity amputations.

Clinical Manifestations

Buerger's disease usually affects young adult men between the ages of 20 and 40. About 10 per cent of the patients are women. Affected individuals have a history of heavy cigarette smoking, usually greater than 20 cigarettes daily. The earliest manifestation may be claudication of the arch of the foot, which is pathognomonic of Buerger's disease. Foot claudication rarely occurs in diabetic patients because of associated peripheral neuropathy. The foot claudication is a reflection of the distal arterial occlusive disease affecting the tibioperoneal or plantar arteries. Ischemic rest pain develops progressively and may affect not only the toes but also the fingers. Affected digits may show signs of cyanosis or dependent rubor. Frequently there is inflammation of the nail fold and resultant paronychia. Small infarcts of the skin may develop, particularly of the pulp of the distal phalanx, which may progress to painful chronic ulceration or gangrene. Superficial thrombophlebitis may be present as tender, painful cords of veins of the upper or lower extremities. Raynaud's syndrome may be evident with classic triphasic color changes of marked blanching and pallor of the affected digit followed by painful cyanosis and subsequent rubor. Pulse deficits usually affect the most distal portions of the extremity, including diminution or absence of the pedal, radial, and ulnar pulses. An Allen test may be positive, as manifested by persistent pallor of the hand after releasing a clenched fist while compressing the radial or ulnar artery. This test is indicative of occlusive disease of the palmar arterial arch.

Takayasu's arteritis may lead to varying clinical manifestations depending on the stage of the disease. Initially there are systemic signs of fever, malaise, pallor, anorexia, arthralgias, night sweats, and weight loss. There may be pain in the neck, shoulder, or chest. Subsequently, signs of arterial insufficiency develop, particularly in the distribution of brachiocephalic vessels. Transient ischemic attacks, amaurosis fugax, or stroke may occur, and the diagnosis is suspected when such symptoms occur in a young adult female. There may be pulse deficits and bruits over the brachiocephalic vessels. Occasionally, arterial occlusive disease will affect the lower extremities or the visceral vessels including the mesenteric or renal arteries. Subsequently, signs of arterial occlusive disease of the coronary and cerebrovascular beds may develop, with increasing congestive heart failure, angina pectoris, myocardial infarct, and hemispheric stroke or vertebrobasilar insufficiency.

Giant cell or temporal arteritis may be considered in an elderly patient who develops recurrent headache, arthralgias, particularly of the shoulder girdle muscles, and visual disturbances including blurring or decreased visual acuity. There may be tenderness and nodularity along the course of the affected temporal artery.

Differential Diagnosis

Buerger's disease must be differentiated from atherosclerotic chronic arterial occlusive disease. The latter condition rarely affects the upper extremities. Diabetic atherosclerotic occlusive disease occurs in the same distribution as thromboangiitis obliterans, but the accompanying neuropathy usually precludes the development of foot claudication. Idiopathic thrombosis or embolism may mimic Buerger's disease. Digital artery involvement on the basis of atheroembolism ("blue toe" syndrome) is usually associated with proximal arterial or cardiac disease, which is unusual in patients with Buerger's disease. Scleroderma or other collagen vascular diseases must be differentiated from Buerger's disease with associated Raynaud's phenomena. Raynaud's disease in the absence of underlying systemic disease does not result in ulcerations or gangrene of the digits.

Takayasu's arteritis must be differentiated from atherosclerotic aortic arch vessel disease and is more common in young adult women, particularly in individuals of Oriental extraction.

Giant cell or temporal arteritis must be differentiated from other causes of headache and other forms of arthritis. The visual blurring associated with temporal arteritis must be differentiated from amaurosis fugax associated with atheroembolic cerebrovascular disease. The arteritides are generally differentiated from atherosclerosis by signs of systemic inflammation including elevated erythrocyte sedimentation rate.

Diagnostic Evaluation

Buerger's disease is usually suspected based on the clinical manifestations. Arteriography is not pathognomonic but may show multiple segmental occlusions of distal arteries with variable degrees of collateral circulation, which may be of a fine "cork screw" configuration. Histologic section of amputated tissue reveals non-necrotizing segmental chronic panarteritis with thrombosis of small arteries and adjacent thrombophlebitis.

Takayasu's arteritis may lead to blood abnormalities, including anemia, leukocytosis, and elevated gamma and alpha-2 globulins and fibrinogen. There is an elevated erythrocyte sedimentation rate (ESR) during the active phase of the disease. Arteriography reveals "atypical coarctation" with long stenotic segments or occlusions of the brachiocephalic vessels and occasional similar lesions in the suprarenal or infrarenal abdominal aorta and its branches, including the mesenteric, renal, and iliac arteries. Long stenotic segments of the pulmonary arteries may also be seen on pulmonary arteriography.

Temporal arteritis is associated with an elevated ESR and segmental stenoses or occlusions on temporal arteriography. Biopsy of the temporal artery may reveal segmental areas of arteritis with the presence of giant cells.

Treatment

Medical treatment of patients with Buerger's disease must begin with an intensive effort to convince the patient to cease smoking. If the patient is successful in stopping smoking, the disease will arrest at the level of involvement at the time therapy is instituted. Unfortunately, most patients are unable to cease smoking and disease progression is the rule. Local wound care, including soaking affected digits and using proteolytic enzymes, may be helpful. Antibiotics are indicated for secondary infection. Calcium channel–blocking agents such as nifedipine are the best pharmacologic agents available for treating associated Raynaud's phenomenon. Vasodilators are of little value. Surgical therapy of Buerger's disease includes conservative débridement of necrotic or gangrenous tissue, conservative amputation with preservation of maximal length of digits or limbs, and occasional lumbar sympathectomy of palmar or digital sympathectomy. Sympathectomy, however, is rarely of lasting benefit for the patient.

The therapy of Takayasu's and giant cell or temporal arteritis includes corticosteroid therapy and occasional reconstructive vascular surgery for major vascular occlusive disease of the brachiocephalic or abdominal aorta and its branches. Bypass prosthetic grafts are preferred to endarterectomy, which is usually difficult and with which recurrent occlusive lesions are likely.

Prognosis

Patients with Buerger's disease who stop smoking will have arrest of their disease. Continued smoking results in progressive ischemia with autoamputation or surgical amputation of digits and progressive, more proximal, major limb amputations. Some patients have been noted to continue to smoke despite loss of all four extremities. The life expectancy is normal.

Patients with Takayasu's arteritis often suffer progressive occlusive disease and stroke or myocardial infarction. Patients with temporal arteritis may suffer progressive blindness unless corticosteroid therapy is promptly instituted.

THORACIC OUTLET COMPRESSION SYNDROME

Thoracic outlet compression syndrome refers to a constellation of symptoms produced by compression of the subclavian artery or vein of the brachial plexus due to congenital or acquired structural processes of the bony and muscular borders of the thoracic outlet.[12]

Clinical Hallmarks

Thoracic outlet compression syndrome should be suspected in a patient with one or more of the following:
1. Chronic pain of the neck, shoulder, and upper extremity, particularly with the extremity in a provocative position.
2. Signs of arterial insufficiency with the upper extremity in a provocative position, particularly when hyperabducted.
3. Signs of venous congestion with the arm in a provocative position.
4. Signs of distal arterial microemboli in the hand or Raynaud's syndrome.

Pathogenesis

Thoracic outlet compression of the subclavian artery or vein of the brachial plexus may occur from three principal mechanisms. A cervical rib or fibrous band, including a prominent scalenus anticus muscle, may compress the superior border of the subclavian artery as it courses over the first rib. This may be intensified by inspiration, extension of the neck, and turning of the patient's head to the side of, or away from, the affected extremity (Adson maneuver). The rib, band, or hypertrophic muscle may also compress the lower roots of the brachial plexus. A second mechanism of thoracic outlet compression may result in extrinsic neurovascular compression by the clavicle against the first rib as the patient braces the shoulders in an exaggerated military position of attention, with the shoulder thrown posteriorly and caudally (costoclavicular maneuver). A third mechanism is the extrinsic compression of the vessels or nerves by hyperabduction of the arm, with resultant compression as the neurovascular bundle passes beneath the coracoid process of the scapula (hyperabduction maneuver).

Differential Diagnosis

The thoracic outlet compression syndrome may be mimicked by two other neurologic compression syndromes,

that associated with the carpal tunnel and the syndrome resulting from extrusion of a cervical intervertebral disc upon the cervical nerve roots. The symptoms and signs as well as the diagnostic studies that differentiate these conditions will be discussed in the following section. Other disorders that occasionally mimic thoracic outlet compression include such musculoskeletal problems as sprain, rotator cuff injury, tendonitis, and subacromial bursitis of the shoulder. Cervical spondylosis, ulnar nerve compression at the elbow, multiple sclerosis, and spinal cord tumor are neurologic conditions that also require differentiation. Finally, shoulder or arm pain on the left side may be due to angina pectoris.

Clinical Manifestations

Clinical manifestations of thoracic outlet compression syndrome will be compared with those symptoms characteristic of carpal tunnel and cervical disc syndromes. The pain of thoracic outlet syndrome usually involves the neck, shoulder, and upper arm and is intermittent at the outset, particularly when exacerbated by provocative neck or arm positions. The pain associated with carpal tunnel syndrome is usually intermittent and affects the first, second, and third fingers, wrist, and volar aspect of the forearm. The pain associated with cervical disc syndrome is constant and affects the neck and shoulder. Numbness associated with thoracic outlet syndrome may involve the distribution of the ulnar nerve or the whole hand and arm. Numbness associated with carpal tunnel syndrome affects the distribution of the median nerve, including the second, third, and fourth fingers, and occasionally the first finger. The numbness associated with the cervical disc syndrome usually affects the radial nerve, involving the dorsal web space between the first and second fingers. Muscle weakness or awkwardness may be noted in the thoracic outlet syndrome and affects all fingers or the fourth and fifth fingers. In the carpal tunnel syndrome the motor deficit affects the first, second, and third fingers. In the cervical disc syndrome usually the thumb is most affected. Positions that aggravate symptoms in the thoracic outlet syndrome are neck hyperextension and turning of the head, posterior and caudal positioning of the shoulder (exaggerated military posture of attention), and hyperabduction of the arm above the head. Positions that aggravate symptoms in the carpal tunnel syndrome are a sustained hand grip and pinching movements of the fingers. Aggravating positions in the cervical disc syndrome are turning of the neck and stretching of the arm.

Physical Examination

The color of the skin of patients with thoracic outlet compression syndrome is usually normal, although occasionally pallor of the hand and upper extremity may be noted if arterial compression occurs with a particular thoracic outlet maneuver. If venous congestion is prominent, the extremity may be cyanotic or have a splotchy discoloration associated with increased sympathetic vasomotor tone. Patients with carpal tunnel or cervical disc syndrome usually have normal skin color, although occasional rubor or splotchy discoloration may be seen. Edema is occasionally noted in patients with the thoracic outlet compression syndrome if there is venous congestion. Edema of the hand may also occur in the carpal tunnel syndrome but is not present in patients with the cervical disc syndrome. Percussion tenderness and reproduction of neurologic symptoms may occur by compression of the affected portion of the brachial plexus in patients with thoracic outlet compression syndrome. In patients with the carpal tunnel syndrome, compression of the volar carpal ligament at the wrist may result in paresthesias or lancinating pain in the distribution of the median nerve (positive Tinel sign). Patients with cervical disc syndrome may have reproduction of symptoms by percussion over the affected cervical disc. Wrist flexion may result in reproduction of symptoms in patients with the carpal tunnel syndrome (positive Phelan sign). Compression of the neck and brachial plexus may aggravate symptoms in the cervical disc syndrome. Patients with thoracic outlet compression syndrome may have further reproduction of symptoms by hyperabduction of the arm, a costoclavicular maneuver, or an Adson maneuver. Cervical disc symptoms may be aggravated by turning or tilting the head or by axial compression of the head.

Diagnosis

Differentiation of the thoracic outlet compression syndrome from the carpal tunnel and cervical disc syndromes is usually based upon the aforementioned history and physical examination. Nerve conduction studies are usually unreliable if negative but may show slowing of conduction across the affected portion of the brachial plexus in the thoracic outlet compression syndrome. Delay of nerve conduction across the wrist suggests carpal tunnel syndrome.

Plain radiographs are frequently normal in the thoracic outlet compression syndrome. However, occasionally a cervical rib or a long process of the seventh cervical vertebra may be seen. Radiographs of the wrist may be normal in the carpal tunnel syndrome, although occasionally arthritis or old trauma may be suggestive of the diagnosis. In the cervical disc syndrome, degenerative arthritis and narrowed intervertebral disc space may be seen.

Contrast arteriography should be considered in patients with thoracic outlet compression symptoms suggestive of arterial or venous obstruction. The extremity should be placed in the position that provokes clinical symptoms. Occasionally, repeated extrinsic arterial compression may lead to intraluminal neointimal hyperplasia, with resultant stenosis, poststenotic dilatation, or aneurysm formation. In patients who show signs of microemboli to the hand or Raynaud's syndrome, microdigital artery occlusive disease may be seen on arteriography. Contrast studies are usually negative in the carpal tunnel syndrome. A myelogram is usually abnormal in approximately 80 per cent of patients with the cervical disc syndrome.

Treatment

Most patients with the thoracic outlet compression syndrome can be managed conservatively with physical therapy to strengthen the shoulder girdle muscles. This should include shoulder shrugging exercises and other specific exercises to prevent drooping of the shoulders. In the carpal tunnel syndrome, conservative therapy should include splinting of the wrist, avoidance of grasping maneuvers, and, occasionally, steroid injection. Conservative management of the cervical disc syndrome includes cervical traction, exercise, or a cervical collar to maintain neck immobility.

The indications for operation in thoracic outlet compression syndrome are failure of conservative treatment

and persistent severe pain or neurogenic deficits, including loss of hand function. In addition, signs of persistent venous obstruction or arterial insufficiency, including microembolization, indicate the need for surgical intervention. Carpal tunnel syndrome requires operation if recurrent symptoms develop despite conservative therapy and there is severe pain or loss of hand function. Similarly, severe pain or neurologic deficits are an indication for removal of an offending cervical disc.

Operative treatment of thoracic outlet compression syndrome should be directed toward the offending mechanical problem. This usually involves resection of the first rib along with any band or cervical rib. This is most commonly accomplished by a transaxillary approach, although a supraclavicular or posterior muscle splitting approach may be necessary in certain circumstances. Associated arterial disease may require endarterectomy of resection with bypass grafting. Rarely, venous thrombosis may be treated by venous thrombectomy, anticoagulants, or fibrinolytic therapy. If thrombectomy or fibrinolytic therapy is successful, subsequent operation to remove the mechanical compression is necessary to prevent recurrent venous thrombosis. Operative treatment of the carpal tunnel syndrome involves resection of the carpal ligament. The cervical disc syndrome is treated by discectomy with cervical fusion.

RAYNAUD'S SYNDROME

Raynaud's syndrome represents a constellation of disorders characterized by episodic attacks of digital vasoconstriction manifested by sequential color changes of pallor, cyanosis, and rubor, often triggered by cold or emotion. The syndrome may be a functional disorder of unknown cause (Raynaud's disease) or secondary to distal arterial occlusive lesions associated with local or systemic disorders (Raynaud's phenomenon).

Clinical Hallmarks

A patient should be considered to have Raynaud's syndrome if one or more of the following are present:
1. Episodic attacks of digital ischemia with triphasic color changes of pallor, cyanosis, and rubor.
2. Precipitation of digital ischemia by cold or emotion.
3. Digital ischemia with or without gangrene in patients with underlying systemic disease, such as scleroderma, Buerger's disease, frostbite, occupation trauma, or hematologic disorder.

Etiology

Classically, Raynaud's syndrome has been divided into two disorders: Raynaud's disease and Raynaud's phenomenon.[14] Although there are diagnostic criteria that differentiate these two conditions, with time many patients with Raynaud's disease eventually prove to have an underlying local or systemic disorder that results in reclassification to Raynaud's phenomenon.

Raynaud's disease is characterized by episodic attacks of digital vasoconstriction in response to cold or emotion, typically manifested by sequential triphasic color changes of pallor, cyanosis, and rubor, without discernible underlying disease. Patients with Raynaud's disease should satisfy the following diagnostic criteria as originally described by Allen and Brown of the Mayo Clinic:

1. Intermittent attacks of triphasic discoloration of the digits of the extremities.

2. Absence of organic arterial occlusion.

3. Symmetrical bilateral distribution.

4. Absence of gangrene or significant cutaneous trophic changes.

5. Predominant occurrence in young women.

6. History of symptoms for at least 2 years without development of manifestations of underlying conditions associated with Raynaud's phenomenon.

Raynaud's phenomenon represents manifestations of episodic digital ischemia similar to that of patients with Raynaud's disease but in the presence of an underlying systemic or local disease, which may include one or more of the following:

1. Collagen diseases, including scleroderma, lupus erythematosus, rheumatoid arthritis, or dermatomyositis. Scleroderma or its variant, the CRST syndrome (calcinosis cutis, Raynaud's phenomenon, sclerodactyly, telangiectasia), is the most common cause of secondary Raynaud's phenomenon.

2. Atherosclerosis, particularly with digital microembolism of thrombotic or cholesterol debris.

3. Buerger's disease.

4. Frostbite, particularly several years after the cold exposure.

5. Nerve injury, including carpal tunnel syndrome, thoracic outlet compression syndrome, ulnar nerve entrapment, and traumatic nerve injury. The latter condition may lead to classic causalgia, which is a disabling syndrome of increasing extremity pain, edema, increased vasomotor tone, and osteoporosis, which may respond to early sympathetic nerve blocks or sympathectomy.

6. Occupational trauma, including prolonged exposure to chain saws or pneumatic hammers or repetitive digital exercise (concert pianist).

7. Hematologic disorder, including cryoglobulinemia, macroglobulinemia, and cold agglutinins.

Pathophysiology

The hemodynamic alterations associated with Raynaud's syndrome include initial arterial and arteriolar spasm, producing the marked blanching or pallor of the affected digits. Subsequent capillary and venular dilatation results in the ensuing cyanosis. Arteriolar dilatation eventually produces the rubor in the third phase of the color changes.

The principal underlying cause of the altered vasoreactivity is unknown. Etiologic hypotheses have included intrinsic abnormal vasoreactivity of the arterial and anteriolar walls and sympathetic hyperactivity. Recently, autoimmune abnormalities have been implicated. It has been hypothesized that a cold-stimulated autoantibody forms an immune complex that binds complement in the peripheral circulation with resultant chemical stimulation of the arterial smooth muscle through the sympathetic neuromuscular end plate.

Clinical Manifestations

The episodic digital vasoconstriction classically involves three changes in the color of affected digits. The patient can usually describe the affected fingers as becoming completely colorless, often as white as a bed sheet. There is usually a clear line of demarcation between the affected portion of the digit and the normal adjacent tissue. During this phase the digit may become numb because of the marked ischemia. As color begins to return to the digit the initial reperfusion with slowed circulation results in cyanosis of the digit. During this phase the digit may become painful. The pain increases during the subsequent period of arteriolar dilatation, with resultant rubor and burning dysesthesias. Some patients do not experience all three of the classic triphasic color changes. Some will notice only cyanosis and subsequent rubor, whereas others will notice only a blanching of the digit with subsequent rubor.

Precipitating factors most commonly involve exposure to cold, such as a refrigerator or a glass of ice cold liquid. However, some patients may experience attacks of digit vasoconstriction with only minor reduction in temperature, as associated with a cool breeze or a cool room. Patients may also experience Raynaud's attacks in response to emotional stimuli when they become upset, angry, or frightened. Patients often learn to avoid the stimuli that produce the digital ischemia.

Patients with Raynaud's disease are usually young adult females. They may complain of symptoms in both hands, although the attacks may also affect the feet, where the ischemia is generally not as symptomatic.

Patients with secondary Raynaud's phenomenon may develop milder attacks of color change but may notice more severe symptoms associated with digital artery occlusive disease and secondary tissue necrosis with resultant ulceration or gangrene of the fingertips. The disease results in progressive loss in soft tissue with recurrent ulcers, which may heal and lead to contracted tissue of the distal digit pulp. Patients with thromboangiitis obliterans may also notice infections and paronychia in addition to the ischemic ulceration. Digital ulceration or gangrene does not occur in patients with pure vasospastic Raynaud's disease.

Other digital abnormalities may be noted in patients with secondary Raynaud's phenomenon, such as the sclerodactyly associated with scleroderma or cutaneous evidence of microemboli in patients with proximal atherosclerosis or thoracic outlet compression syndrome.

Diagnosis

Patients can usually be classified as having primary Raynaud's disease or secondary Raynaud's phenomenon based on a careful history and physical examination. Patients with Raynaud's disease should be thoroughly evaluated for underlying etiology, including a complete laboratory evaluation, non-invasive vascular diagnostic studies, and possible arteriography.

A platelet count should be obtained, inasmuch as thrombocytosis may create symptoms similar to those of Raynaud's syndrome. The ESR may be elevated in patients with underlying systemic disease such as collagen disease or thromboangiitis obliterans. Serum protein electrophoresis should be obtained along with serum cryoglobulins, macroglobulins, and cold agglutinins. Collagen diseases may be identified by the presence of antinuclear antibodies, rheumatoid factor, complement C-3, antinative DNA antibody, lupus erythematosus preparations, and a positive Coombs' test. Immunoglobulin electrophoresis should also be obtained. Patients with scleroderma may manifest abnormalities on an esophagogram with altered esophageal motility even before cutaneous signs of sclerodactyly become apparent. Skin and muscle biopsies may be helpful to diagnose other collagen disease. If nerve compression is suspected, appropriate nerve conduction tests should be ordered.

The noninvasive vascular diagnostic techniques should provide objective evidence about the presence of proximal and digital arterial occlusive disease. Digit plethysmography may reveal an abnormal "peaked" pulse contour, which consists of an anacrotic notch on the upslope, a sharp pointed peak, and a dicrotic wave high on the downslope of the digit pulse tracing. However, such pulse wave abnormalities are not always present in patients with Raynaud's syndrome. If an obstructive digit pulse contour is present after reflex body heating, digital artery occlusive disease or proximal arterial obstruction should be suspected. The presence of proximal or distal arterial occlusive lesions may be documented by segmental limb blood pressures and digit blood pressures. These studies should be performed after reflex body heating to exclude abnormally low digit blood pressures due to functional vasoconstriction. Digit pressures and temperatures should be recorded before and after cold stimuli, such as immersion of the hand in ice water. Patients with Raynaud's syndrome have a critical closing pressure of the digital arteries at an abnormally high digit temperature. Patients also have delayed recovery in digit temperature (greater than 15 minutes) after immersion of the hand in ice water for 20 seconds. Additional noninvasive studies should be performed including thoracic outlet compression maneuvers and measures to assess the continuity of the palmar arterial arch.

Arteriography is indicated if patients are suspected of having organic digit arterial occlusive disease or possible small arterial obstructions that may contribute to digit ischemia on an occlusive or microembolic basis. Arteriography should be of high quality and should include magnified views of digital circulation before and after exposure to ice water and after injection of vasodilators. The presence of organic occlusive lesions signifies secondary Raynaud's phenomenon. Patients with Raynaud's disease may show abnormal vasospasm in response to cold but should have normal digital arterial circulation with rewarming or vasodilatation.

Treatment

Patients with Raynaud's syndrome should be advised to avoid cold exposure and to dress warmly in cold weather. It is important that the patient be advised not only to protect the affected extremities but to dress with more total body protection from the cold than he or she might otherwise be inclined to do. The resultant increase in body temperature may lead to reflex vasodilatation, which may further minimize the occurrence of Raynaud's attacks. Patients who smoke cigarettes should be advised to stop.

Oral vasodilators may be of some benefit for patients who continue to have symptoms despite the previously mentioned measures. Recently, the most efficacious medication has been one of the calcium channel–blocking agents, such as nifedipine. Prazosin has also been effective in diminishing Raynaud's attacks. Other oral agents include guanethidine, phenoxybenzamine, alphamethyldopa, tolazoline, and reserpine. Patients with suspected hypothyroidism may develop significant improvement in Raynaud's attacks with thyroid replacement.

Intra-arterial injections of reserpine may lead to significant improvement over the subsequent 1 or 2 weeks. Injections may be repeated, but are of limited usefulness. The recent availability of calcium channel–blocking agents has reduced the need for intra-arterial drug injection.

Sympathectomy plays a limited role in patients with Raynaud's syndrome. Patients with primary Raynaud's disease may achieve long-term benefit in 50 to 60 per cent of cases. Lower extremity sympathectomy is usually more lasting than thoracodorsal sympathectomy. Patients with Raynaud's phenomenon secondary to underlying systemic disease only occasionally benefit from sympathectomy. There is little benefit for patients with scleroderma. Patients with progressive digital gangrene despite maximal medical therapy may occasionally benefit from digital sympathectomy; however, most patients with severe collagen disease may eventually lose digits despite medical or surgical intervention.

EXTRACRANIAL CEREBROVASCULAR DISEASE

Extracranial cerebrovascular disease includes occlusive lesions of the aortic arch vessels or carotid or vertebral arteries, which may be manifest as asymptomatic bruits, intermittent attacks of cerebral ischemia (TIA), atypical symptoms, or brain infarction (stroke).

Clinical Hallmarks

Patients should be suspected of having extracranial cerebrovascular disease if there is intermittent (TIA) or persistent (stroke) disturbance in neurologic function involving one of the four "Ss":
1. Sight.
2. Sensation.
3. Strength.
4. Speech.

Extracranial cerebrovascular disease may also be suspected if the patient has:
5. Asymptomatic cervical bruit.

Epidemiology

Stroke is the third leading cause of death in the United States. Over 300,000 new strokes occur each year. At any given time, there are approximately 1,500,000 patients who have suffered stroke. Approximately 70 per cent of individuals who have had a stroke will have a persistent neurologic defect. Thirty eight per cent of patients will die of their initial stroke, and 10 per cent will die of a subsequent stroke. Approximately 10 per cent of patients have recurrent stroke in the first year, and 20 per cent will suffer another stroke within 5 years.

There are several risk factors that contribute to stroke. Although not traditionally considered a risk factor, TIA is the leading predictor of a future stroke, inasmuch as approximately 30 per cent of patients suffering a TIA will eventually have a stroke. It thus becomes incumbent upon all physicians to recognize TIAs and to teach their patients who are at risk of stroke to recognize TIAs.

The presence of an asymptomatic cervical (carotid) bruit may be a risk factor of future stroke. Approximately 10 to 20 per cent of patients with known carotid bruits may eventually suffer stroke.

Hypertension is the leading traditional risk factor for stroke. Whereas many patients with hypertension have associated extracranial cerebrosvascular disease, many strokes in hypertensive patients are the result of intracranial vascular disease or hemorrhage. The improvement in detection and treatment of hypertension over the past 20 years may be a significant factor in the overall reduction in the incidence of stroke during this period. Other risk factors that may contribute to stroke include a strong family history of stroke, associated peripheral or coronary artery occlusive disease, diabetes mellitus, cigarette smoking, and hyperlipidemia. Advancing age correlates closely with stroke risk, with patients over 70 years of age having 8 times the risk of stroke of patients aged 50.

Classification

There are several methods of classifying cerebrovascular disease, including temporal, anatomic, pathologic, and symptomatic classifications.

TEMPORAL CATEGORIES

Symptoms of cerebrovascular disease may be classified into one of the following three temporal categories:
1. Transient ischemic attack.
2. Reversible ischemic neurologic deficit (RIND).
3. Stroke (cerebrovascular accident [CVA]).

A TIA consists of an acute, focal, encephalic deficit of vascular origin that results in a neurologic disability lasting usually only a few minutes, occasionally a few hours, but never more than 24 hours. A TIA does not leave a residual neurologic deficit. Thus, a TIA implies only transient nerve cell dysfunction without neuronal infarction.

A RIND is a acute, focal, encephalic deficit of vascular origin with a neurologic disability lasting more than 24 hours but less than 3 weeks. A RIND is accompanied by eventual complete recovery, implying a small area of neuronal infarction or neurapraxia with eventual "recruitment" of nerve cell formation. A RIND is sometimes called TIA with incomplete recovery, a protracted TIA, or a stroke with recovery.

A *stroke* is a focal, encephalic deficit of vascular origin, usually of abrupt or rapid onset, with a neurologic disability lasting more than 24 hours and a variable total duration depending upon the extent of recovery. A stroke may have a variable course, which may include complete recovery, incomplete recovery (so-called partial nonprogressive stroke [PNS]), or no recovery, a so-called *completed stroke.* A stroke may manifest increasing deficit over minutes, hours, or days, reflecting hemorrhage, edema, progressive thrombosis, or vasospasm. Such a stroke may be termed a *stroke in evolution* or a progressing stroke. Finally, a stroke may be accompanied by waxing and waning of symptoms, suggesting a critical flow-reducing lesion, incomplete thrombosis, or hemodynamic instability, in the so-called *fluctuating stroke.*

ANATOMIC CATEGORIES

Extracranial cerebrovascular disease may be classified anatomically into *carotid territory* and *vertebrobasilar disease. Carotid* territory disorders (hemispheric or anterior circulation disease) may include deficits in the ipsilateral eye or hemisphere. Ipsilateral monocular visual disturbances may be transient (amaurosis fugax) or permanent (retinal infarct). Ipsilateral hemispheric deficits, with contralateral symptoms and signs, include TIA, stroke, and lacunar infarction. *Vertebrobasilar insufficiency* (VBI) (or posterior circulation disorders) include TIAs, stroke, subclavian steal syndrome, and lateral medullary syndrome, which will be discussed hereafter. Finally, atypical symptoms that cannot be discretely classified as carotid territory or vertebrobasilar insufficiency may be classed as *nonspecific* symptoms (pseudo TIAs, nonlateralizing or global symptoms).

PATHOLOGIC CATEGORIES

Cerebrovascular disease may be classified pathologically into one of five categories:
1. Ischemic stroke (cerebral infarction), which accounts for approximately 80 per cent of all stroke syndromes.
2. Hemorrhagic stroke (cerebral hemorrhage), accounting for approximately 15 per cent of strokes.
3. Subarachnoid hemorrhage.
4. Subdural hematoma.
5. Epidural hematoma.

These pathologic disorders will be discussed further hereafter.

SYMPTOMATIC CATEGORIES

Finally, cerebrovascular disease may be classified *symptomatically* according to the following categories:
1. Symptomatic patient, with classic TIA, RIND, or stroke.
2. Atypical symptoms (nonspecific, nonlateralizing, or global symptoms).
3. Asymptomatic patient, with a cervical bruit or abnormal noninvasive cerebrovascular screening study.

Pathology

ATHEROSCLEROSIS

Atherosclerosis accounts for most instances of extracranial cerebrovascular disease. Sixty seven per cent of all lesions are extracranial and surgically accessible, whereas 33 per cent are intracranial or surgically inaccessible by conventional surgical techniques. However, the recent development of neurosurgical techniques has allowed greater access to the therapy of intracranial lesions. Thirty eight per cent of cerebrovascular lesions are at the carotid bifurcation, 20 per cent at the origin of the vertebral arteries, and 9 per cent are in the aortic arch branches.

FIBROMUSCULAR DYSPLASIA

Fibromuscular dysplasia is the second most common cause of extracranial cerebrovascular disease. This vascular abnormality usually occurs in young or middle-aged women and is often associated with hypertension due to concomitant fibromuscular dysplasia in the renal arteries.

EXTRINSIC COMPRESSION

Other types of extracranial cerebrovascular disease include extrinsic compression caused by osteophytes of the vertebral column. Such cervical spondylosis may result in stenosis of the midportion of the vertebral arteries, which may result in vertebrobasilar insufficiency with extension of the neck or turning of the head. Kinking and coils of the carotid artery are often found in children and constitute one of the more common causes of a bruit in childhood. Most of these lesions are asymptomatic, although kinking in the adult patient may be the result of concomitant atherosclerosis, which may cause symptoms. Neck irradiation may result in fibrosis of the carotid artery, and irradiation injury may also cause accelerated atherosclerosis. Trauma or dissection of the carotid artery should be suspected in any patient who develops neurologic symptoms after injury. Some carotid dissections may occur spontaneously and are manifested by a long, tapering stenosis of the internal carotid artery on arteriogram. Such lesions may regress and improve with nonoperative management. Finally, arteritis may result in symptoms of extracranial cerebrovascular disease, as mentioned previously under the Takayasu syndrome.

ISCHEMIC STROKE

Ischemic stroke may result from one of two pathogenic mechanisms: cerebral thrombosis or cerebral embolism.

Cerebral Thrombosis. This represents thrombotic occlusion of the carotid or vertebral artery or branches, usually due to underlying atherosclerosis. The process often occurs during sleep, and the onset may result in sudden and complete stroke. Alternatively, the deficit may develop progressively over hours or intermittently over several hours or days.

Cerebral Embolism. This results from occlusion of the carotid or vertebral artery or its branches by thrombus or other material embolizing from a proximal source, such as the carotid artery bifurcation or the heart. Emboli from the carotid bifurcation are usually the result of hemorrhage into a plaque or overlying ulceration with superimposed thrombus or discharge of atheromatous material from the plaque itself. Cardiac emboli may result from atrial fibrillation, mitral and/or aortic valvular stenosis, mitral valve prolapse, myocardial infarction, ventricular aneurysm, subacute bacterial endocarditis, or cardiac myxoma. Cerebral embolism is often of sudden onset, unheralded, and associated with throbbing headache.

HEMORRHAGIC STROKE

Hemorrhagic stroke results from hemorrhage of the brain, often associated with hypertension, with resultant focal, small vessel necrosis, particularly of arteries in the internal capsule. The onset is often gradual with progressive increasing neurologic deficit, which may occur during periods of activity. Progressive neurologic deficit may eventuate in deep coma, and the prognosis is poor, often with a fatal outcome.

SUBARACHNOID HEMORRHAGE

Subarachnoid hemorrhage results in bleeding into the cerebrospinal fluid, often from a ruptured berry aneurysm or arteriovenous malformation. The patient may manifest severe headache of rapid onset and progressive neck stiffness. The onset is usually during activity, especially in young, otherwise heathy patients. There may be no localizing signs.

HEMATOMA

A subdural hematoma may be acute or of chronic duration with a collection of blood in the subdural space. There is often a history of minor precipitating trauma. The patient develops a mass effect with sudden or insidious onset of increasing lethargy, throbbing headache, and ill-defined neurologic deficits with fluctuating or worsening signs.

An *epidural hematoma* may occur with acute or, rarely, a chronic collection of blood in the epidural space, usually the result of head trauma with fracture. Often there is laceration of the middle cerebral artery. The patient may initially lose consciousness and then awaken with a "lucid" interval, only to develop progressive loss of consciousness, deviation of the eyes away from the lesion, inequality of the pupils, and eventual development of other signs of brain stem compression from cerebral herniation through the tentorium. Rapid recognition is necessary to allow expeditious neurosurgical intervention to prevent death.

Pathophysiology

Cerebrovascular disease may result in symptoms on the basis of one of two principal mechanisms: embolism or reduction of blood flow.

EMBOLISM

Embolism probably accounts for most of the neurologic deficits associated with extracranial cerebrovascular disease. As previously mentioned, the embolus may originate from disease in one of the extracranial cerebrovascular arteries, most commonly the carotid bifurcation. Evidence of the embolic cause of cerebrovascular disease was given credence with the discovery of retinal artery emboli on fundoscopic examination. Platelet, thrombotic, or cholesterol emboli may be distinguished by their physical characteristics in the retinas of patients who develop monocular symptoms of transient or permanent visual deficit. Cardiac sources of cerebral emboli were already mentioned. Rarely, cerebral emboli may originate from the venous system as a result of paradoxical embolism through a cardiac septal defect.

BLOOD FLOW REDUCTION

Cerebrovascular symptoms may be the result of extracranial blood flow reduction due to high-grade arterial obstruction or systemic hypotension of any cause. Although advanced carotid atherosclerosis may lead to discrete cerebrovascular symptoms, many patients have severe (greater than 75 per cent) carotid stenosis or occlusion without cerebrovascular symptoms. The presence or absence of symptoms may depend upon the adequacy of collateral circulation, particularly via the circle of Willis. Many patients with focal transient ischemic attacks or stroke in the presence of severe carotid disease may suffer distal emboli from the diseased carotid bifurcation. Symptoms of more generalized cerebral ischemia, such as dizziness, syncope, or decreased mentation, may occasionally result from high-grade carotid occlusive disease that results in global reduction in cerebral perfusion. Cardiac arrhythmias or shock may similarly result in global cerebral hypoperfusion.

Manifestations of Carotid Territory Ischemia

Carotid artery disease may manifest itself with either *ocular* or *hemispheric symptoms*, which may be transient (TIA) or persistent (stroke).

OCULAR SYMPTOMS

Ipsilateral monocular visual disturbances are the most specific manifestations of carotid artery disease. *Amaurosis fugax* ("fleeting blindness" or retinal "TIA") is the most diagnostic symptom of ipsilateral carotid bifurcation athero-sclerosis. Amaurosis fugax is manifest as transient, mon-ocular, painless visual loss (obscuration of vision) where none existed previously, usually lasting 2 or 3 minutes and rarely 5 to 10 minutes. The visual disturbance may involve upper or lower altitudinal visual loss, often described as a film, "skim," curtain, or window shade being pulled over the eye. The visual disturbance clears, often in the reverse direction, and leaves no sequelae. Occasionally, amaurosis fugax may be manifest as a general peripheral loss of vision (gun-barrel vision mimicking the effect of closing down the diaphragm of a camera) or occasionally a total blackout or central blurring of vision. Attacks of amaurosis fugax are frequently abrupt and may occasionally be accompanied by photopsia or crude visual hallucinations. Occasionally, scin-tillating scotomata or bright, zig-zag, sparkling light effects may be described by the patient. Persistent monocular visual loss is termed *retinal infarction* and is associated with embolic occlusion of the central retinal artery or one or more of its branches.

HEMISPHERIC SYMPTOMS

Hemispheric ischemia from carotid artery occlusive disease may be transient (TIA) or persistent (stroke). Hemispheric symptoms include focal neurologic deficits involving one or more of the following:

1. A motor deficit involving weakness, paralysis, and poor use or clumsiness of one or both extremities on one side of the body contralateral to the affected hemisphere.

2. A sensory defect involving numbness, including loss of sensation, or paresthesias of one or both extremities on one side of the body contralateral to the affected hemi-sphere.

3. Speech or language disturbance, including aphasia or dysphasia, which may be only a minor defect or global, including difficulty in reading, writing, and performing calculations. This manifestation usually results from is-chemia of the dominant hemisphere.

4. A visual field deficit involving loss of the visual field on one side (homonymous hemianopia).

A hemispheric TIA or stroke is often more sympto-matic in the upper extremity. Hemiplegia with cortical signs of aphasia or neglect of contralateral space suggests a large cortical defect. Hemiplegia without cortical signs or sensory signs suggests a small (lacunar) infarct (internal capsule). Hemiplegia with obtundation or hemianopia suggests a large cortical and white matter infarct. Faciobrachial mono-plegia suggests a middle cerebral artery territory stroke, usually accompanied by cortical signs. Hemiparesis, contra-lateral spatial neglect, and weakness maximal in the shoul-der suggest a border zone infarction involving decreased flow between two major vascular territories of the anterior and middle cerebral arteries. Hemiplegia with maximal involvement of the leg and urinary incontinence with prim-itive reflexes suggest anterior cerebral artery thrombosis.

Lacunar infarction represents a small infarct in the territory of small perforating basal arteries, usually 1 to 5 mm. in diameter, in specific locations such as the internal capsule, basal ganglia, thalamus, pons, or cerebellum. Symptoms commonly involve pure motor hemiplegia of the face, arm, and leg without alteration of consciousness, vision, sensation, or intellect. Lacunar infarcts are often preceded by transient ischemic attacks and a history of hypertension. A pure sensory stroke suggests a lesion in the thalamus or cerebral cortex. A sensory deficit of the face, arm, and leg suggests a thalamic lesion. Selected

involvement of some, but not all, of the fingers suggests a cortical defect. Numbness involving the thorax and abdo-men suggests a thalamic lesion. Other syndromes include dysarthria and motor impairment of the hand (clumsy hand syndrome), crural monoparesis, and homolateral ataxia and weakness of the leg.

Manifestations of Vertebral Basilar Insufficiency

Vertebral basilar insufficiency involves transient insults or permanent deficits in the area of distribution of the vertebrobasilar system or its branches, including one or more of the following:

1. Motor deficits involving weakness, clumsiness, or paralysis in one or more limbs in any combination, often on varying sides of the body and with varying degrees of severity.

2. Sensory deficits involving numbness, including loss of sensation or paresthesias, in any combination of extrem-ities, including all four or involving both sides of the face or mouth. The deficit is frequently bilateral or may change from side to side in different attacks.

3. Loss of vision, partial or complete, in both homon-ymous fields (bilateral homonymous hemianopia).

4. Homonymous hemianopia.

5. Ataxia, imbalance, unsteadiness, or disequilibrium not associated with vertigo.

6. Vertigo, with or without vomiting, diplopia, dys-phasia, or dysarthria in any combination.

7. *Drop attack*, which is the sudden loss of motor power in the lower extremities, resulting in falling to the ground *without* loss of consciousness, which is usually pathognomonic of vertebrobasilar insufficiency but must be distinguished from syncope, which is not a transient is-chemic attack.

Transient ischemic attacks, which are indeterminant with respect to carotid or vertebrobasilar disease, include dysarthria and homonymous hemianopia if either of these symptoms occurs alone.

Manifestations of Subclavian Steal Syndrome

The subclavian steal syndrome is a surgically correct-able cause of vertebrobasilar insufficiency resulting from reverse flow in the ipsilateral vertebral artery distal to a proximal subclavian (or innominate) artery stenosis or occlusion (the subclavian artery "steals" blood from the vertebrobasilar system). Subclavian atherosclerosis is the most common cause of a cervical (supraclavicular) bruit. Subclavian artery obstruction occurs on the left side 70 per cent of the time. In 70 per cent of patients with subclavian steal physiology there are no symptoms because of sufficient collateral circulation to the brain and arm.

Subclavian steal symptoms usually fall into one of two mutually exclusive categories: vertebrobasilar insufficiency or arm claudication. Symptoms of vertebrobasilar insuffi-ciency are usually not precipitated by arm exercise, as is commonly believed, but occur as random events. Symptoms of arm claudication are usually the result of inadequate collateral circulation to the arm. Often the subclavian artery obstruction is not accompanied by reversed vertebral artery flow, thus accounting for the absence of cerebral symptoms in patients with arm claudication. Conversely, patients with subclavian steal physiology often are asymptomatic because the contralateral vertebral artery can supply sufficient blood flow to both the hindbrain and the affected arm. Patients who develop symptoms of vertebrobasilar insufficiency associated with subclavian steal often have concomitant advanced carotid occlusive disease, which, if corrected, may relieve the vertebrobasilar symptoms. Subclavian steal symptoms usually do not progress to stroke but may become sufficiently disabling to require surgical intervention.

Manifestations of Atypical Cerebrovascular Symptoms

Atypical (nonlateralizing or nonspecific) symptoms of cerebrovascular disease that occasionally result from advanced extracranial occlusive disease and may be relieved by cerebrovascular reconstruction include any of the following when occurring in isolation:

1. Unconsciousness, including syncope.
2. Tonic and/or clonic motor activity.
3. March of motor and/or sensory deficit.
4. Vertigo alone with or without nausea or vomiting, which is a definite rotational sensation or illusion of motion reflecting dysfunction of the vertebrobasilar system.
5. Dizziness, giddiness, wooziness, or lightheadedness alone, which is a nonspecific symptom, usually manifested by an unpleasant sensation of disturbed relationship with surrounding objects. Symptoms may also include feelings of faintness, lightheadedness, dizziness, and swaying due to vestibular, neurologic, cardiovascular, psychiatric, or other disorders.
6. Headache.
7. Migraine with focal neurologic symptoms.
8. Confusion alone.
9. Amnesia alone.
10. Forgetfulness or memory disturbance.
11. Senility or dementia.
12. Mental confusion alone.
13. Disorientation.
14. Impaired vision associated with alteration of consciousness.
15. Scintillating scotomata.
16. Dyplopia alone.
17. Dysarthria alone.
18. Dysphasia alone.
19. Incontinence of bladder or bowel alone.

Manifestation of Asymptomatic Carotid Disease

Asymptomatic carotid disease refers to patients with an incidentally discovered asymptomatic cervical bruit or an occlusive carotid lesion discovered by noninvasive testing or angiography. Carotid bruits must be differentiated from other causes of cervical bruit, including subclavian or innominate artery stenosis, radiating bruits from aortic valve disease, cervical venous hums, bruits over the thyroid (particularly in hyperthyroid individuals), and iatrogenic causes of bruit due to excessive pressure of the stethoscope. A carotid bruit is loudest over the carotid artery either low in the neck or, more commonly, at the carotid bifurcation near the angle of the mandible. Patients with asymptomatic carotid disease are usually discovered in one of the following three situations:

1. Isolated carotid bruit, discovered incidentally on physical examination.
2. Contralateral carotid disease, discovered on arteriogram on the side opposite symptomatic carotid disease.

3. In the preoperative patient discovered to have a carotid bruit or noninvasive evidence of significant carotid obstruction prior to major operation, such as coronary artery or peripheral artery reconstruction.

Asymptomatic carotid bruits are more prevalent in older patients, patients with hypertension and diabetes mellitus, and women. The risk of stroke in patients with asymptomatic carotid disease is unknown, although retrospective studies suggest a stroke risk over the course of 5 years of 15 to 20 per cent. Prospective studies suggest an increased stroke risk of approximately 15 per cent, but often the stroke is not on the side of the bruit. Asymptomatic carotid disease correlates with a future risk of myocardial infarction and death from coronary artery disease. An asymptomatic carotid bruit does not always correlate with the presence of significant internal carotid artery stenosis, inasmuch as approximately 20 to 50 per cent of patients will have normal noninvasive diagnostic studies. Furthermore, many patients with significant carotid disease by noninvasive diagnostic screening will have no audible cervical bruit. Nevertheless, the presence of significant internal carotid artery stenosis by noninvasive testing correlates with an increased risk of stroke of approximately 7 to 11 per cent over the course of 5 years when compared with a 1 to 2 per cent stroke risk in patients with normal noninvasive studies.

Patients with asymptomatic carotid artery disease contralateral to symptomatic lesions generally do not face a increased stroke risk without an antecedent transient ischemic attack. Several retrospective studies suggest that about 10 to 20 per cent of patients may develop a transient ischemic attack if the asymptomatic carotid lesion is carefully followed. However, the risk of future stroke without antecedent TIAs is under 5 per cent. It thus behooves the physician to emphasize the importance of recognizing the characteristic symptoms of transient ischemic attack so that appropriate surgical intervention may be instituted once the patient becomes symptomatic.

The risk of stroke from asymptomatic carotid disease in the preoperative patient is controversial. Retrospective studies suggest that patients with an asymptomatic carotid bruit have no greater risk of perioperative stroke than do patients without cervical bruits. Several prospective studies using noninvasive screening techniques confirm that patients with significant internal carotid artery stenosis may safely undergo coronary or peripheral vascular reconstruction without a significantly increased risk of perioperative stroke.[14] However, the author's follow-up data of such patients suggest that a significant number, perhaps 20 per cent, will eventually develop transient ischemic attacks in the postoperative period and require treatment of the carotid occlusive disease. However, these studies do not suggest the need for routine prophylactic carotid endarterectomy of asymptomatic carotid lesions prior to needed major cardiovascular operations. These studies, however, do suggest that patients with asymptomatic carotid disease are at increased risk of perioperative or late myocardial infarction or death from coronary artery disease.

Physical Examination

The physical examination will often provide valuable information in documenting the presence of extracranial cerebrovascular disease. One of the most specific indicators of extracranial carotid bifurcation atherosclerosis is the presence of *retinal emboli* visualized on fundoscopic examination. The causes of amaurosis fugax or retinal infarct may occasionally be documented by distinguishing the different types of emboli seen in the retinal artery or its branches. *Cholesterol* emboli appear as bright yellow, highly refractile (birefringent) bodies in the retinal artery branches, particularly at bifurcations. *Platelet* emboli appear gray white in color, whereas *calcium* emboli are chalky white in color. *Thrombi* may appear reddish-purple and may be difficult to distinguish from the blood in the retinal vessels. A retinal infarct may lead to pallor of the affected portion of the retina. Other abnormalities include hemorrhage and hypertensive arterial changes in the retina. If unilateral arcus senilis is present, significant carotid artery obstruction should be suspected on the side without the arcus. Xanthelasma are further indicators of hypercholesterolemia, which may predispose to carotid atherosclerosis.

Careful examination of upper extremity and cerebral vascular pulses may suggest extracranial cerebrovascular disease. Reduction in the right subclavian and common carotid pulses suggests innominate artery occlusive disease. Significant internal carotid artery obstruction normally does not alter the common carotid artery pulse. If the carotid pulse is unequivocally diminished, common carotid (or innominate artery) obstruction is suggested. Diminution in the temporal artery pulse suggests external carotid artery obstruction.

Examination of cervical bruits should be systematic to localize the site of arterial obstruction. Subclavian (or innominate) artery stenosis results in a bruit that is loudest in the supraclavicular fossa. Common carotid artery stenosis is suggested by a bruit low in the neck adjacent to the trachea. A bruit in the neck near the angle of the mandible suggests carotid bifurcation stenosis. Stenoses of the internal and external carotid arteries are indistinguishable unless the bruit extends into diastole, which is pathognomonic of severe internal carotid artery stenosis. A bruit over the orbit implies stenosis of the internal carotid siphon. A bruit posterolateral to the sternocleidomastoid muscle may occur with proximal vertebral artery stenosis.

Blood pressures should always be obtained in both arms. A reduction in blood pressure by more than 20 mm. Hg in one arm suggests possible subclavian artery obstruction in that extremity, which may be the first sign of the subclavian steal syndrome.

Finally, a careful cardiac and neurologic examination should be performed in patients with suspected cerebrovascular disease.

Noninvasive Diagnostic Studies

The role of noninvasive vascular testing for extracranial cerebrovascular disease varies depending on the symptomatic status of the patient. Patients who have classic hemispheric or vertebrobasilar TIAs are probably candidates for cerebrovascular angiography and, if an appropriate extracranial cerebrovascular lesion is found, surgical intervention. In such patients, noninvasive cerebrovascular studies should not dictate the decision to proceed with angiography. However, such patients may be screened by noninvasive techniques in order to document the presence of extracranial cerebrovascular disease, to aid in the decision about obtaining angiography by the intravenous versus the intra-arterial route, and to serve as a baseline for future intra-operative and postoperative diagnostic studies with noninvasive techniques. Nevertheless, patients with normal noninvasive studies who are symptomatic still require con-

trast angiography to define the presence of a correctable lesion. Patients without obstruction but with ulcerated plaques may not be detected by noninvasive study and require angiography for confirmation of the lesion.

Atypical symptoms, including dizziness, memory disturbance, bilateral visual disturbances, syncope, and so on, are ideal candidates for noninvasive cerebrovascular screening. Most patients with these nonspecific symptoms have normal noninvasive studies and require no further vascular work-up. However, patients with severe carotid occlusive disease detected by noninvasive techniques may be candidates for angiography and carotid endarterectomy, which may relieve the atypical symptoms.

Patients with an asymptomatic cervical bruit should be evaluated by noninvasive screening studies. Although the role of prophylactic carotid endarterectomy in such patients remains controversial, many patients with an asymptomatic cervical bruit have no evidence of significant internal carotid artery obstruction. Such patients are at low risk of future stroke and require no further diagnostic or therapeutic intervention. Patients with significant internal artery stenosis may be at increased risk of stroke and may be either carefully followed for the development of TIAs or undergo arteriography and prophylactic carotid endarterectomy, depending upon the philosophy of the patient's physician. In addition, noninvasive techniques permit assessment of the integrity of the circle of Willis, which may influence the advisability of intervening with prophylactic carotid endarterectomy, particularly in those patients whose cerebral perfusion may be dependent upon the patency of the diseased carotid artery.

The noninvasive techniques that are appropriate for screening patients with suspected cerebrovascular disease were discussed in the first portion of this chapter. Indirect (periorbital) screening techniques are commonly used but suffer the disadvantage of being insensitive to nonobstructive ulcerated carotid plaques. Furthermore, an abnormal study does not differentiate an operable carotid stenosis from an inoperable occlusion. Recently, increasing emphasis has been placed on the use of direct carotid screening techniques using Doppler flow analysis and real-time imaging of the carotid bifurcation. These techniques, although more sophisticated and expensive, permit more accurate assessment of carotid artery disease and also permit differentiation of carotid stenoses from occlusions.

Arteriography

Arteriography is indicated for any patient with carotid territory TIA or stroke with partial or complete recovery who is a potential candidate for operation. In addition, arteriography is indicated for patients with atypical cerebrovascular symptoms associated with noninvasive evidence of severe carotid occlusive disease. Finally, patients with an asymptomatic carotid bruit or noninvasive evidence of asymptomatic carotid occlusive disease, particularly in the absence of collateral circulation via the circle of Willis, may be candidates for arteriography and possible prophylactic carotid endarterectomy in selected instances. Conventional intra-arterial contrast arteriography, including views of the aortic arch and its branches as well as selective views of all four extracranial and intracranial cerebrovascular systems, should be considered in symptomatic patients with noninvasive evidence of minimal or no carotid artery disease (to exclude ulcerated plaques) and patients with suspected intracranial disease (ocular bruit or normal direct and abnormal indirect carotid screening studies). Intra-arterial angiography is also indicated for patients in whom significant extracranial carotid stenosis exists by noninvasive screening but in whom digital intravenous angiography is either inconclusive or technically unsatisfactory or unavailable. Digital subtraction intravenous angiography may be considered in patients with noninvasive evidence of significant extracranial internal carotid stenosis.

Other Diagnostic Studies

Computed tomography may be indicated in patients who have suffered stroke in order to differentiate cerebral hemorrhage from infarction. Computed tomograms aid in the timing of operation after acute stroke and the evaluation of patients with RIND. Computed tomography is also indicated to assess patients with fluctuating or worsening symptoms and those who develop postoperative neurologic deficit.

Electroencephalography is often used to evaluate patients with stroke, to provide a preoperative baseline, and to monitor patients intraoperatively during carotid endarterectomy. The electroencephalogram (EEG) may identify those patients who require a shunt during carotid clamping. Electroencephalograms are also useful to evaluate postoperative neurologic deficits.

Cardiac evaluation, including Holter monitoring, echocardiography, stress electrocardiography, and possible coronary angiography with ventriculography, may be useful in patients with suspected cardiac causes of cerebrovascular disease. Such studies may also be indicated in patients with carotid territory symptoms who have normal noninvasive and arteriographic studies.

Medical Therapy

Specific medical therapy for symptomatic cerebrovascular disease consists of antiplatelet or anticoagulant medication. Several prospective studies suggest that antiplatelet therapy may reduce the risk of cerebrovascular and other cardiovascular morbidity in patients with symptoms of transient ischemic attack.[11]

Aspirin has been widely used. Recent evidence suggests that relatively low doses of aspirin may suffice to suppress platelet function while minimizing the inhibition of prostacyclin production by the vascular endothelium. Daily doses of aspirin of between 60 and 300 mg. may give sufficient antiplatelet effect. The additive value of dipyridamole in daily doses of 75 to 200 mg. has been suggested by some investigators. Sulfinpyrazone and ibuprofen have also been recommended as alternative antiplatelet medications.

Anticoagulants have been shown to reduce the incidence of stroke after TIA in some prospective studies. Initial anticoagulation with intravenous heparin followed by oral anticoagulants (warfarin) has been recommended. Most neurologists suggest that anticoagulants be used only for 6 to 12 months and antiplatelet agents be considered thereafter. Anticoagulants may have the greatest efficacy in patients with vertebrobasilar insufficiency.

Other methods of medical therapy include treatment of hypertension, elimination of cigarette smoking, and control of hyperlipidemia. Vasodilators have been widely used but are of no proven value in patients with cerebrovascular insufficiency.

The use of antiplatelet therapy in asymptomatic patients is controversial. Although aspirin is widely prescribed for patients with an asymptomatic carotid bruit, there are no objective data to suggest that such therapy reduces the incidence of future TIAs or stroke in asymptomatic patients. Because symptomatic lesions are often found to contain hemorrhage at the time of carotid endarterectomy, some investigators have questioned the value of antiplatelet or anticoagulant therapy in asymptomatic patients.

Surgical Therapy

Surgical therapy may be indicated in patients with hemispheric symptoms, vertebrobasilar insufficiency, and select patients with asymptomatic carotid artery occlusive disease. The role of surgery in these separate conditions will be discussed in turn.

Carotid endarterectomy is the most common procedure employed for patients with angiographically proven lesions that are appropriate for ocular or hemispheric symptoms of cerebrovascular insufficiency. Carotid endarterectomy is most appropriate for patients who have suffered amaurosis fugax or hemispheric TIA. Patients with RIND or stroke with partial or complete recovery are also potential surgical candidates. Patients with severe carotid artery occlusive disease and symptoms of vertebrobasilar insufficiency may have relief of symptoms following carotid endarterectomy. Patients with atypical or nonlateralizing symptoms and proven severe carotid stenosis are also surgical candidates. The role of carotid endarterectomy in patients with asymptomatic carotid bruit or noninvasive evidence of asymptomatic carotid disease is controversial. Although some surgeons recommend routine prophylactic carotid endarterectomy for any patient with severe (greater than 50 per cent) carotid stenosis, the author recommends a more conservative approach. Candidates for prophylactic carotid endarterectomy include those with severe carotid stenosis and contralateral internal carotid occlusion, patients with a strong family history of stroke, and patients with noninvasive evidence of an incomplete circle of Willis without collateral circulation around the asymptomatic carotid lesion.

Contraindications to carotid endarterectomy include recent completed stroke without recovery, progressive stroke (stroke in evolution), and internal carotid artery occlusion. An exception to the latter is a patient who develops a recurrent TIA after angiographically proven internal carotid occlusion. Some patients may be candidates for external carotid endarterectomy if a significant external carotid stenosis is present. Some patients also have a "blind stump" of the internal carotid artery with a large cul-de-sac that may contain thrombotic debris that may embolize to the brain via branches of the external carotid and ophthalmic arteries. In such instances external carotid endarterectomy and elimination of the internal carotid artery stump may be indicated.

The technique of carotid endarterectomy should be meticulous and deliberate, because the risk of operation is inversely proportional to the skill of the surgeon.[19] Endarterectomy may be performed under general or regional anesthesia.

Many surgeons employ electroencephalographic monitoring in addition to routine monitoring by the electrocardiogram and arterial blood pressure. The carotid artery is carefully exposed through either a longitudinal or transverse cervical incision. Care must be taken to avoid unnecessary handling of the carotid bifurcation prior to clamping, to prevent cerebral emboli from the diseased carotid bifurcation. After systemic heparinization, the carotid artery and its branches are clamped and an arteriotomy opened along the common and internal carotid artery. Some surgeons routinely use an indwelling plastic shunt to provide cerebral blood flow during carotid clamping. However, few patients require such shunting, and many surgeons selectively shunt based upon slowing of the electroencephalogram or a low internal carotid back pressure (less than 25 to 50 mm. Hg, as determined prior to carotid clamping). The atheromatous plaque is then carefully removed in a cleavage plane that readily develops in the outer media. The artery is then gently cleared of all particulate debris and the arteriotomy is closed, usually without need for a patch. Flow is carefully restored to the branches of the external carotid artery prior to being restored to the internal carotid artery and the brain. The integrity of the carotid endarterectomy may be assessed intraoperatively by means of a sterile Doppler probe, real-time B-mode ultrasonogram, or operative arteriogram.

Operative therapy for vertebrobasilar insufficiency may also include procedures to increase flow in the affected vertebral system. Most commonly, the subclavian steal syndrome may be treated by procedures designed to improve flow and blood pressure in the distal subclavian artery. Although direct procedures on the proximal subclavian (or innominate) artery were originally recommended, such procedures as endarterectomy or bypass required transthoracic procedures. Extrathoracic approaches prove safer and initially involved ligation of the vertebral artery, which carried reverse flow to the arm. Subsequent reconstructive extrathoracic procedures proved efficacious, including bypass grafts from the ipsilateral common carotid to the subclavian artery distal to the vertebral takeoff. Alternative procedures include subclavian or axillary-axillary bypass grafts using prosthetic or autogenous vein grafts. Occasionally proximal vertebral artery stenosis may be treated by endarterectomy or bypass grafts. Alternatively, transposition of the vertebral artery to the side of the common carotid artery has been recommended for proximal vertebral artery stenosis. Rarely, patients with extensive aortic arch vessel disease require bypass procedures from the ascending aorta to the distal branch vessels using prosthetic grafts inserted via a median sternotomy.

Patients with inaccessible intracranial artery disease or occlusion of the internal carotid artery are occasional candidates for neurosurgical bypass procedures, commonly termed extracranial-intracranial (EC-IC) bypass. Usually a branch of the temporal or occipital artery is mobilized and attached end-to-side to a cortical branch of the middle cerebral or other cerebral artery. Although these procedures can be performed with 80 to 90 per cent technical success rates, the efficacy of the procedure in preventing future stroke in patients with asymptomatic internal carotid artery occlusion has not been established. Nevertheless, the procedures may be useful to relieve symptoms in patients with persistent transient ischemic attacks after internal carotid occlusion or with inaccessible intracranial artery disease.

Postoperative Complications

Surgical therapy for cerebrovascular disease should be performed in selected patients with a mortality rate of less than 2 per cent. Most perioperative deaths are the result of myocardial infarction. The incidence of stroke in extra-

cranial cerebrovascular reconstruction should be less than 5 per cent, preferably under 3 per cent. Most perioperative neurologic deficits are the result of emboli because of technical imprecision and are uncommonly the result of inadequate cerebral protection during carotid clamping.

Other postoperative complications after cerebrovascular operations include cranial nerve injury, particularly the superior laryngeal, hypoglossal, vagus, spinal accessory, glossopharyngeal, or greater auricular nerves. Postoperative hemorrhage may require evacuation to prevent respiratory embarrassment. Hypertension requires vigorous treatment to prevent stroke, cerebral hemorrhage, or myocardial infarction. Hypotension most commonly occurs if there has been disturbance of the carotid baroreceptors, particularly after staged bilateral carotid endarterectomy. Myocardial infarction is one of the most common postoperative complications following carotid endarterectomy and is more prevalent in patients with pre-existing coronary artery disease and intraoperative hypertension.

Prognosis

The prognosis of patients with untreated TIA is variable, but several studies suggest that about one third of patients will develop a stroke, one third will develop recurrent TIAs, and one third will become asymptomatic. The prognosis of a patient with *stroke* depends upon the pathologic type of stroke and the general clinical status of the patient. Overall about one third of patients will die of their initial stroke and approximately 10 per cent will subsequently die each year. About one third of stroke survivors will be disabled, one third will have minimal to moderate disability, and one third will recover complete neurologic function. One third of the patients will develop recurrent stroke or TIA, and two thirds of those suffering recurrent stroke will die.

The natural history of patients with untreated *asymptomatic bruit* is unknown. Several studies suggest that 10 to 20 per cent of such patients will develop a future stroke. Most strokes are probably preceded by TIAs, which are often unrecognized by the patient and physician alike. If patients with asymptomatic bruit are found to have noninvasive evidence of severe carotid stenosis, 10 to 15 per cent may develop future stroke, whereas patients with normal noninvasive studies have a future stroke risk of less than 5 per cent. Although many physicians claim a significant beneficial effect of prophylactic carotid endarterectomy in patients with asymptomatic carotid disease, the validity of this treatment remains to be established. The author recommends careful follow-up and education of the patient and the referring physician about the nature and significance of TIA, which should be the primary indication for subsequent angiography and prophylactic carotid endarterectomy.

Antiplatelet therapy may reduce cerebral and vascular ischemic events in patients with extracranial carotid occlusive disease by as much as 50 per cent, with reported event rates being reduced from 30 to about 15 per cent. Antiplatelet therapy has yet to be established to be of proven value in reducing the incidence of stroke or stroke-related deaths. Likewise, antiplatelet therapy has a less beneficial effect in women. Aspirin therapy is beneficial in reducing postoperative cerebral ischemic events in patients undergoing successful carotid endarterectomy, and such therapy may also reduce the incidence of postoperative recurrent carotid stenosis due to neointimal hyperplasia.

Anticoagulant therapy is of benefit in patients with

vertebrobasilar insufficiency, but its role in treating patients with symptomatic TIA or stroke remains to be established.

Surgical therapy in experienced hands may reduce the risk of future stroke in the territory of the operated carotid artery to about 5 per cent over a 5- to 10-year follow-up period. Recurrent carotid stenosis, which is usually asymptomatic, varies in incidence depending upon the technique of detection. Clinical symptoms recur in less than 2 per cent of patients, but noninvasive evidence of recurrent stenosis may be identified in 5 to 40 per cent of patients, depending upon the operative technique, the use of intraoperative monitoring, and postoperative antiplatelet therapy.

Algorithms

Figure 15 presents a diagnostic and management algorithm that the author employs for patients with symptomatic carotid artery disease. Such patients initially undergo noninvasive carotid evaluation to define the presence or absence of significant stenosis or occlusion of the internal carotid artery. If advanced carotid disease is identified, intravenous digital subtraction angiography permits morphologic validation of such lesions. If an occlusion is present, the patient is observed and extracranial-intracranial bypass considered only for patients with recurrent TIAs. If significant internal carotid stenosis is documented, prophylactic endarterectomy is performed. If noninvasive studies identify insignificant carotid disease or a normal carotid artery, intra-arterial angiography is recommended. If an ulcerated carotid plaque is found, endarterectomy is performed. If a normal arteriogram is demonstrated, medical therapy (antiplatelet agents) is recommended.

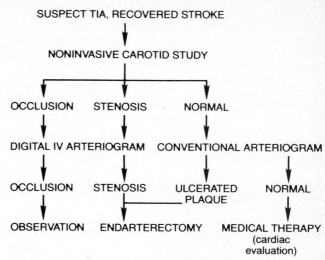

Figure 15. Algorithm summarizing management of patient with suspected hemispheric transient ischemic attack (TIA) or recovered stroke.

Figure 16 illustrates an algorithm for the evaluation of patients with suspected vertebrobasilar insufficiency or atypical (nonlateralizing) cerebral symptoms. Noninvasive studies are recommended to define the presence or absence of significant associated carotid disease. If such disease is present, intra-arterial angiography is recommended to confirm the carotid disease and also to evaluate associated vertebral artery disease. If carotid stenosis is present endarterectomy is recommended. If the noninvasive study shows no evidence of carotid disease and the symptoms are

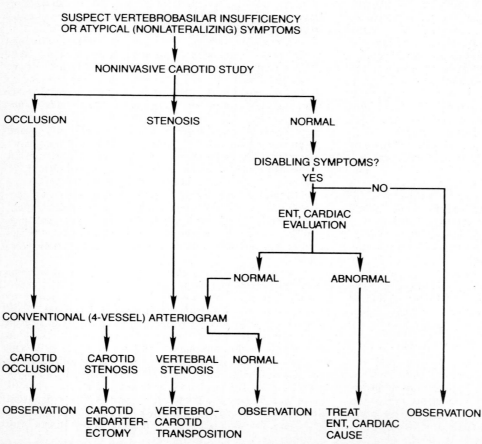

Figure 16. Algorithm summarizing management of patient with suspected vertebrobasilar insufficiency or atypical (non-lateralizing) symptoms.

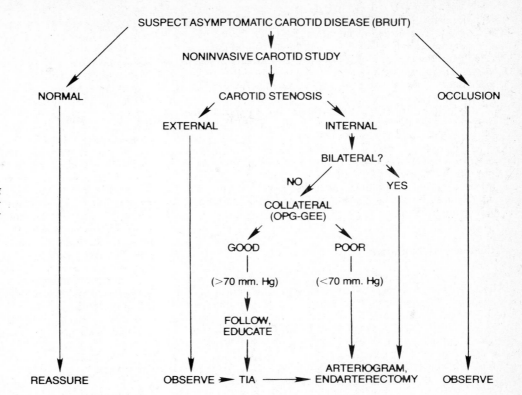

SUSPECT ASYMPTOMATIC CAROTID DISEASE (BRUIT)

NONINVASIVE CAROTID STUDY

NORMAL   CAROTID STENOSIS   OCCLUSION

EXTERNAL   INTERNAL

BILATERAL?

NO   YES

COLLATERAL
(OPG-GEE)

GOOD   POOR

(>70 mm. Hg)   (<70 mm. Hg)

FOLLOW,
EDUCATE

REASSURE   OBSERVE → TIA ——→ ARTERIOGRAM,
ENDARTERECTOMY   OBSERVE

Figure 17. Algorithm summarizing management of patient with suspected asymptomatic carotid disease or bruit.

disabling, specialty consultation, including otolaryngology and cardiology examinations, is recommended. If specific abnormalities are found, these should be treated. If such evaluation fails to define a cause for the disabling cerebrovascular symptoms, intra-arterial angiography is recommended to define operable extracranial vertebral artery disease.

Figure 17 depicts an algorithm for evaluating patients with asymptomatic carotid disease. Noninvasive studies are performed to define the presence or absence of significant internal carotid artery obstruction. If the study is normal or external carotid stenosis is found, the patient may be reassured and observed. If internal carotid artery stenosis is present, the management depends upon the status of the contralateral carotid artery. If unilateral disease is present and the collateral circulation is adequate, the patient is followed with medical management and educated to recognize the significance and presence of symptoms of TIAs. If subsequent TIAs develop, intravenous angiography and prophylactic endarterectomy are recommended. If the carotid artery disease is bilateral or if poor collateral circulation is present with unilateral carotid disease, prophylactic endarterectomy is advisable. If the noninvasive studies suggest internal artery occlusion, the patient is observed, and intervention is undertaken only if symptoms of recurrent TIA develop.

RENOVASCULAR HYPERTENSION

Renovascular hypertension refers to a potentially curable form of hypertension caused by significant obstruction of one or both renal arteries.

Clinical Hallmarks

A patient should be considered to have renovascular hypertension if one or more of the following are present:

1. Severe, uncontrollable hypertension.
2. Severe hypertension of recent onset.
3. Rapid progression of previously mild hypertension.
4. Hypertension in childhood or young adults.
5. A bruit in the hypogastrium or flank.

Etiology

Hypertension is of unknown cause (essential) in 90 per cent of patients. However, the most common curable form of hypertension is renal artery stenosis or occlusion, which may account for 5 to 10 per cent of patients with hypertension.[9] Less common causes of surgically curable hypertension include primary hyperaldosteronism (0.5 to 3 per cent of patients), unilateral parenchymal disease (1 per cent of patients), coarctation of the aorta (0.1 to 0.2 per cent of patients), pheochromocytoma (0.1 to 0.2 per cent of patients), and Cushing's disease (0.1 to 0.2 per cent of patients).

Most patients with renovascular hypertension have renal artery atherosclerosis. Fibromuscular dysplasia is the second most common cause of renovascular hypertension, particularly in young adult women. Less common causes of renovascular hypertension include embolism, trauma, unilateral hydronephrosis, renal cysts, and renin-secreting tumor.

Pathophysiology

Renovascular hypertension may be caused by unilateral renal artery stenosis (with a normal contralateral kidney) or bilateral renal artery stenosis or parenchymal disease. The physiology of these conditions differs. Patients with unilateral renal artery stenosis and a normal contralateral kidney develop decreased renal blood flow and glomerular filtration, with subsequent release of renin from the kidney.

Renin results in the formation of angiotensin-II, which results in vasoconstriction and secretion of aldosterone from the adrenal glands. There is consequent suppression of renin from the contralateral kidney and contralateral natriuresis. There is sustained release of renin from the ipsilateral affected kidney with resultant increased peripheral vein renin activity.

Patients with unilateral renal stenosis (or parenchymal disease) and contralateral disease develop decreased ipsilateral renal blood flow and glomerular filtration. Release of renin from the affected kidney results in the formation of angiotensin-II. Vasoconstriction and aldosterone secretion ensue. The contralateral renal disease prevents natriuresis. Consequent volume expansion develops with ipsilateral renin suppression, with resultant normal peripheral vein renin activity.

Clinical Manifestations

There are several features that distinguish renovascular hypertension from essential hypertension. The clinical characteristics of patients with atherosclerotic or fibromuscular causes of renovascular hypertension have been distinguished from those of patients with essential hypertension. The latter condition is more prevalent in patients with a longer history of hypertension and in black subjects. Essential hypertension is more common in obese patients. Atherosclerotic renovascular hypertension occurs more commonly in older individuals and in patients with severe hypertensive retinopathy and abdominal or flank bruits. Fibromuscular hypertension occurs more frequently in young adult females and is frequently accompanied by an abdominal or flank bruit.

Diagnostic Evaluation

Patients with hypertension should have routine serum chemistries to include electrolytes, blood urea nitrogen, creatinine, cholesterol, and blood sugar. Urinalysis, electrocardiogram, and plain chest film are also advisable.

The role of rapid-sequence (hypertensive) excretory urography is controversial. The sensitivity of this study in identifying abnormalities suggestive of an ischemic kidney is about 83 per cent. The cost-effectiveness of this study has been questioned.

Plasma renin activity in relation to 24-hour urine sodium excretion has a sensitivity and specificity of about 85 per cent. The test requires that the patient be off antihypertensives and diuretic medications for about 3 weeks. Differential renal vein renin studies have been widely used to assess the functional significance of renal artery stenoses. Blood samples from each renal vein are compared and related to the renin concentration in peripheral arterial blood or samples from the low inferior vena cava. Renovascular hypertension is suggested by a renal vein renin concentration of 1.5 to 2 times higher on the affected side. Alternatively, a ratio of renal vein renin minus peripheral renin divided by the peripheral renin of more than 0.48 on the diseased side with contralateral suppression of renin in the uninvolved kidney (renal vein renin equal to peripheral renin activity) is indicative of renovascular hypertension.

Recently the blood pressure response to various blocking agents, such as angiotensin-II blockade with saralasin or significant blood pressure drop with converting enzyme inhibitor (captopril), has been recommended as a screening test for renin-dependent hypertension.

Differential renal function studies (Howard or Stamey tests) have been developed to document the increased fractional reabsorption of sodium and water in the affected kidney as a result of reduced blood flow and glomerular filtration. The sensitivity of these tests has been about 85 per cent, but the specificity is only about 65 per cent. The tests are difficult to perform in the absence of an experienced urologic team.

Renal angiography remains the definitive anatomic method for detecting significant renal artery occlusive disease. Digital intravenous angiography has been suggested for screening, but intra-arterial angiography with multiple projections to identify the orifices of the renal arteries remains the diagnostic standard. Arteriography, however, has generally been recommended only for patients who are at high likelihood of harboring renal artery disease. The cost and risk of routine angiography preclude its use as a screening procedure.

Initial reports of noninvasive interrogation of renal artery morphology and velocity using combined echo-Doppler ultrasound (duplex scanning) suggest a possible role of this modality for screening patients with suspected renovascular disease.

Treatment

Most patients with hypertension are initially given a trial of medical management. Recent development of potent antihypertensive agents has made the medical control of hypertension the rule rather than the exception. A major objective in health care delivery is to identify patients with hypertension who may not be aware of their disorder. The best method of medically managing hypertension of varying degrees of severity remains to be established. Recent emphasis has suggested that restriction of dietary salt intake and the use of thiazide diuretics will control most hypertension. More severe hypertension may respond to alpha methyldopa, beta blockade, or converting enzyme inhibitors.

Patients who are poorly controlled on medical management or who develop signs of progressive renal impairment should be considered for angiography and possible radiologic or surgical intervention. If an offending renal artery stenosis is identified, some physicians would treat the patient based upon the history and the established presence of renal artery stenosis. The role of functional assessment by renin studies remains to be established.

Recent advances in interventional radiology suggest that some patients with renal artery stenosis are amenable to balloon dilatation (percutaneous transluminal angioplasty [PTA]). This procedure is most successful for unilateral localized stenosis in the main renal artery and particularly in patients with fibromuscular dyplasia of the main renal artery. The procedure is least successful in patients with bilateral renal artery stenosis, which involves ostial lesions in conjunction with a calcified aortic plaque. The procedure carries a small risk of renal artery dissection, renal artery rupture or thrombosis, and consequent loss of renal function. Preliminary reports suggest that 80 to 90 per cent of patients may develop a salutary result following balloon dilatation of unilateral renal artery stenosis. The long-term success of this procedure remains to be established.

Surgical intervention should be considered for patients

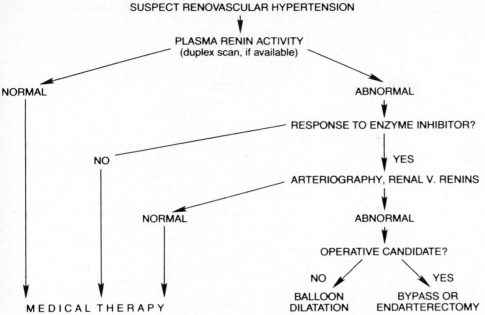

Figure 18. Algorithm summarizing management of patient with suspected renovascular hypertension.

with severe uncontrolled hypertension or who are young or are losing renal function. Renal artery bypass is most commonly employed from the aorta to the distal renal artery using autogenous saphenous vein, autogenous artery (hypogastric or splenic artery), or prosthesis (Dacron or polytetrafluoroethylene). Occasionally renal artery stenoses are amenable to transaortic endarterectomy, particularly if bilateral disease is present near the renal artery orifices.

Algorithm

Figure 18 depicts a diagnostic and management algorithm for patients with suspected renovascular hypertension. If patients have clinical features suggesting a likely vascular cause, initial screening for plasma renin activity may be performed; if the technology is available, duplex scanning could also be used to identify possible high-grade renal artery stenoses. If the screening study is normal, medical therapy is advised; if there is increased plasma renin activity, the patient may be evaluated for blood pressure response to converting enzyme inhibitor. If the study is negative, medical therapy is recommended. If a significant drop in blood pressure occurs, intravenous digital subtraction angiography may be performed, with or without concomitant determination of renal vein renin activity. If the study is normal, medical therapy is advisable. If renal artery stenoses are documented, surgical intervention should be considered unless lesions favorable for balloon dilatation are found or if the patient is at high risk for operation. Any patient undergoing balloon dilatation should be advised that emergency surgical intervention may be required if significant complications develop following angioplasty.

MESENTERIC VASCULAR INSUFFICIENCY

Mesenteric vascular insufficiency refers to acute or chronic ischemia of the intestine due to organic arterial occlusive disease, nonocclusive (vasospastic) obstruction, or mesenteric venous thrombosis.[5]

Clinical Hallmarks

Acute mesenteric arterial ischemia should be suspected in patients with one of the following:
1. Sudden severe abdominal pain.
2. Bowel evacuation (vomiting and diarrhea).
3. Signs of acute abdomen.

Patients should be suspected of having chronic mesenteric ischemia if one or more of the following are present:
1. Postprandial abdominal pain ("food fear" or "small meal" syndrome).
2. Weight loss.
3. Epigastric bruit.

Etiology

Acute mesenteric arterial ischemia may be classified as occlusive or nonocclusive. Occlusive arterial disease includes embolism, thrombosis, dissection, and trauma. Nonocclusive mesenteric arterial insufficiency may occur as a result of low cardiac output syndrome from advanced cardiac disease, shock of any etiology, or medications that result in mesenteric vasoconstriction, including digitalis and other catecholamines used to increase cardiac output.

Chronic mesenteric artery insufficiency is most commonly caused by atherosclerosis. Less common causes include celiac axis compression syndrome from extrinsic neural compression or compression from fibrous tissue at the aortic hiatus through the diaphragm. Less commonly, chronic mesenteric arterial ischemia may occur from Buerger's disease, collagen disease, radiation, or Crohn's disease.

Mesenteric venous thrombosis is a rare cause of mesenteric vascular insufficiency. Its etiology is unknown but may occur in conditions that may predispose to venous thrombosis, such as chronic congestive heart failure, malignancy, chronic liver failure, and so on.

Clinical Manifestations

Acute mesenteric arterial ischemia should be suspected in any patient who develops sudden severe abdominal pain, vomiting, and diarrhea. Late in the course of the disease the diarrhea may become bloody and the abdomen may be distended. In elderly patients the abdominal signs may be minimal. A striking feature of acute mesenteric arterial insufficiency is the discrepancy between the severity of abdominal pain and the findings upon palpating the abdomen. Bowel sounds may be hyperactive, hypoactive, or absent depending upon the stage of the disease.

Patients with chronic mesenteric arterial insufficiency present with recurrent postprandial abdominal pain, which may lead to significant weight loss. The pain, so-called intestinal angina, characteristically occurs from one half to 1 hour after eating and may be severe and cramping or sharp and boring in character. Pain is severe enough in many circumstances to result in a fear of eating. Some patients may obtain relief only by taking frequent, small meals. Malabsorption is uncommon but may occur in some patients and lead to steatorrhea or signs of vitamin deficiency. On physical examination, the abdomen may be normal except for the presence of an epigastric systolic bruit. If the bruit diminishes with inspiration, celiac axis compression syndrome is suggested. Signs of associated coronary, peripheral, or cerebrovascular atherosclerotic disease may suggest an atherosclerotic etiology, which is the most common cause of chronic mesenteric insufficiency.

Mesenteric venous thrombosis presents with signs of an acute abdomen with pain, nausea, or vomiting and occasional diarrhea. If the ischemia progresses to infarction, the patient may develop signs of intestinal perforation and peritonitis. Often mesenteric venous thrombosis is discovered only at operative exploration for an acute abdomen.

Diagnosis

Patients with acute mesenteric arterial ischemia may show a leukocytosis with a shift to the left. Hemoconcentration may be the result of fluid sequestration in the gut. A pronounced metabolic acidosis develops as the disease progresses and may be resistant to medical therapy. Hyperamylasemia and elevation in other serum enzymes (LDH, SGOT, SGPT, and CPK) occur late in the disease.

Plain radiographs of the abdomen may reveal nonspecific findings of dilated small and large bowel loops. There may be thickened muscosal folds and interloop edema. Late in the course of the disease free air may occur with perforation of the intestine.

Arteriography should be considered early in any patient with suspected acute mesenteric artery insufficiency. Both anteroposterior and lateral views of the abdomen should be obtained to clarify the mesenteric arterial anatomy. Arteriography also may delineate conditions that may be treated by interventional radiography at the time of the diagnostic procedure (see hereafter).

Patients with chronic mesenteric ischemia are best evaluated by arteriography if the diagnosis is suspected. Patients who manifest symtoms of malabsorption may be evaluated by the D-xylose test of intestinal absorption, but this test is unreliable in establishing the presence of chronic mesenteric ischemia. Barium contrast studies are usually normal. Arteriography provides a definitive diagnosis, especially with lateral views of the mesenteric arteries. In addition to obstruction of the main trunks, evidence of large collaterals ("meandering mesenteric artery") may document the diagnosis. In general, at least two of the three main arterial sources of mesenteric circulation must be obstructed to account for symptoms of chronic mesenteric ischemia.

Treatment

Patients with acute mesenteric arterial insufficiency should receive aggressive resuscitation with fluids and electrolytes. Antibiotics are administered intravenously. Cardiac support should be monitored with a Swan-Ganz catheter with appropriate use of cardiotonic agents. If there are signs of peritonitis, immediate operative exploration is indicated; otherwise, the patient should be considered for emergency mesenteric angiography.[8] If nonocclusive mesenteric artery insufficiency is documented, vasodilators such as tolazoline should be infused in the indwelling mesenteric catheter. If an embolus is visualized, emergency operation and thrombectomy are indicated. Alternatively, fibrinolytic therapy may be considered. If thrombosis is suspected, emergency revascularization should be considered. The use of fibrinolytic therapy and balloon dilatation of atherosclerotic mesenteric artery stenoses has been reported, but long-term experience with this approach has not been established.

At operation gangrenous bowel may require resection. Often a bowel with marginal circulation is found, which may be left behind and then re-examined at a "second look" reoperation, in 24 hours, to identify progression of ischemia.

Patients with chronic mesenteric ischemia are candidates for bypass or endarterectomy of the offending lesion. Patients with celiac axis compression syndrome may be helped by excision of the extrinsic compression of the celiac axis. Occasionally secondary intraluminal lesions of the celiac artery require endarterectomy or bypass for relief of symptoms.

Patients with mesenteric venous thrombosis may require segmental intestinal resection and reanastomosis. Postoperatively such patients may benefit from cautious anticoagulation therapy to prevent recurrent disease.

Prognosis

Patients with acute mesenteric ischemia have traditionally suffered a mortality rate exceeding 50 per cent. Most patients are not identified early enough in the course of the disease to prevent extensive intestinal infarction. After massive bowel resection, the short gut syndrome may develop. Progressive bowel necrosis, anastomotic leaks, and sepsis are common.

Patients with chronic mesenteric ischemia may be improved dramatically with revascularization of the ischemic intestines. Some patients develop thrombosis of reconstructed arterial segments and may suffer consequent intestinal angina or necrosis after successful vascular reconstruction.

Algorithm

Figure 19 illustrates an algorithm for patients with suspected acute mesenteric ischemia. If patients show signs of acute intestinal perforation, such as peritonitis or free

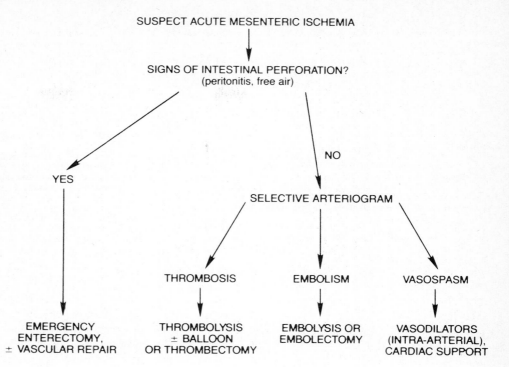

SUSPECT ACUTE MESENTERIC ISCHEMIA

SIGNS OF INTESTINAL PERFORATION?
(peritonitis, free air)

YES

NO

SELECTIVE ARTERIOGRAM

THROMBOSIS   EMBOLISM   VASOSPASM

EMERGENCY
ENTERECTOMY,
± VASCULAR REPAIR

THROMBOLYSIS
± BALLOON
OR THROMBECTOMY

EMBOLYSIS OR
EMBOLECTOMY

VASODILATORS
(INTRA-ARTERIAL),
CARDIAC SUPPORT

Figure 19. Algorithm summarizing management of patient with suspected acute mesenteric arterial insufficiency.

intra-abdominal air, emergency operation and resection of the involved intestine are indicated. If signs of intestinal perforation are absent, immediate arteriography should be performed. If thrombosis is documented, operative arterial reconstruction is indicated unless thrombolysis and balloon dilatation are feasible. If an embolism is documented, emergency operation with embolectomy is recommended, although thrombolysis may be considered. If nonocclusive mesenteric vasoconstriction is documented, administration of vasodilators by an indwelling arterial selective catheter is recommended along with medical management to support cardiac output.

SELECTED REFERENCES

Bernstein, E. F. (Ed.): Noninvasive Diagnostic Techniques in Vascular Disease, 3rd ed. St. Louis, C. V. Mosby Co., 1985.
This book represents the third edition of a work encompassing an exhaustive review of the principles and techniques of noninvasive vascular diagnostic technology. The book is organized into three parts. The first part represents fundamental measurement and current instrumentation, including velocity measurement, pressure measurement, volume measurement, radionuclide techniques, vascular imaging, and data base methodology. The second part describes areas of application including detection, quantitation, and prediction of outcome of vascular disease in the areas of extracranial cerebrovascular disease, peripheral arterial disease, and venous disorders. The third part reviews practical aspects of organization of a vascular laboratory and data analysis and interpretation. This book represents the most complete review of current state-of-the-art techniques in noninvasive methods to diagnose peripheral vascular diseases.

Juergens, J. L., Spittell, J. A., Jr., and Fairbairn, J. F., II: Peripheral Vascular Disease, 5th ed. Philadelphia, W. B. Saunders Company, 1980.
This book represents the fifth edition of the classic textbook on peripheral vascular diseases originally published by Allen, Barker, and Hines of the Mayo Clinic. The three editors are all currently members of the Division of Cardiovascular Diseases and Internal Medicine at the Mayo Clinic. The book reviews basic considerations of peripheral vascular disease, vascular pathology, hemodynamic physiology, coagulation and hemostasis, and vascular imaging. Subsequent sections are devoted to

degenerative arteriopathies, vascular diseases of diverse origin, venous and lymphatic diseases, and principles of management. This textbook is particularly excellent for review of medical aspects of vascular disease and unusual vascular conditions such as vasculitis, vascular diseases related to environmental temperature, and vascular disorders of the skin.

Rutherford, R. B. (Ed.): Vascular Surgery, 2nd ed. Philadelphia, W. B. Saunders Company, 1984.
This textbook represents the second edition of a work devoted to the current state-of-the-art principles of vascular diseases and vascular surgery. The editor calls upon numerous authorities to review problems of hemodynamics of the peripheral circulation, principles of angiography, fundamental methods of vascular surgery, and management of peripheral arterial, cerebrovascular, and venous diseases including acute arterial insufficiency, chronic ischemia of the lower extremities, neurovascular diseases of the upper extremity, arterial aneurysms, arteriovenous fistulae, visceral ischemic syndromes, portal hypertension, renovascular disorders, extracranial cerebrovascular disease, venous and lymphatic disease, and amputation principles and techniques.

Strandness, D. E., Jr., and Sumner, D. S.: Hemodynamics for Surgeons. New York, Grune & Stratton, New York, 1975.
This compendium is the largest single collection of hemodynamic principles in vascular disease. The title is somewhat of a misnomer, inasmuch as the hemodynamic principles described in this book apply to all medical disciplines that relate to vascular disorders. However, the authors, who are leaders in the field of peripheral hemodynamics, relate basic engineering and hydraulic principles to clinical surgery. The book is in three parts. The first section covers basic principles of arterial and venous pressure and blood flow measurements, cardiac hemodynamics, and mechanical properties of blood vessel walls. The second section on regional hemodynamics covers principles of the blood flow to the limbs and the therapy of arterial occlusive disease, venous valvular physiology, extracranial cerebrovascular disease, portal hypertension, and renovascular hypertension. The final section on specific problems includes chapters on Raynaud's syndrome, cold injury, and arteriovenous fistula.

References

1. Barnes, R. W.: Noninvasive diagnostic techniques in peripheral vascular disease. Am. Heart J., 97:241, 1979.
2. Barnes, R. W.: Hemodynamics for the vascular surgeon. Arch. Surg., 115:216, 1980.
3. Barnes, R. W.: Managing peripheral vascular disease. J. Cardiovasc. Med., 6:33, 1981.

4. Barnes, R. W., Leibman, P. R., Marsalek, P. B., Kirk, C. L., and Goldman, M. H.: The natural history of asymptomatic carotid disease in patients undergoing cardiovascular surgery. Surgery, *90*:1075, 1981.

5. Bergan, J. J., Dry, L., Conn, J., Jr., and Trippel, O. H.: Intestinal ischemic syndromes. Ann. Surg., *169*:120, 1969.

6. Bernstein, E. F., Dilley, R. B., Goldbeyer, L. E., Gosink, B. B., and Leopold, G. R.: Growth rates of small abdominal aortic aneurysms. Surgery, *80*:765, 1976.

7. Blaisdell, F. W., Steele, M., and Allen, R. E.: Management of acute lower extremity arterial ischemia due to embolism and thrombosis. Surgery, *84*:822, 1978.

8. Boley, S. J., Sprayregen, S., Siegelman, S. S., and Vieth, F. J.: Initial results from an aggressive roentgenological and surgical approach to acute mesenteric ischemia. Surgery, *82*:848, 1977.

9. Dean, R. H., Kieffer, R. W., Smith, B. M., Oates, J. A., Nadeau, J. H. J., Hollifield, J. W., and DuPont, W. D.: Renovascular hypertension. Arch. Surg., *116*:1408, 1981.

10. Edwards, W. S.: Arterial grafts: past, present and future. Arch. Surg., *113*:1225, 1978.

11. Fields, W. S., Lemak, N. A., Frankowski, R. F., and Hardy, R. J.: Controlled trial of aspirin in cerebral ischemia. Stroke, *8*:301, 1977.

12. Kelly, T. R.: Thoracic outlet syndrome—current concepts of treatment. Ann. Surg., *190*:657, 1979.

13. McPherson, J. R., Juergens, J. L., and Gifford, R. W.: Thromboangiitis obliterans and arteriosclerosis obliterans: Clinical and prognostic differences. Ann. Intern. Med., *59*:288, 1963.

14. Porter, J. M.: Raynaud's syndrome and associated vasospastic conditions of the extremities. *In* Rutherford, R. B. (Ed.): Vascular Surgery, 2nd ed. Philadelphia, W. B. Saunders Company, 1984, pp. 697–707.

15. Snyder, W. H., Thal, E. R., and Perry, M. O.: Peripheral and abdominal vascular injuries. *In* Rutherford, R. B. (Ed.): Vascular Surgery, 2nd ed. Philadelphia, W. B. Saunders Company, 1984, pp. 460–500.

16. Strachan, R. W.: The natural history of Takayasu's arteriopathy. Quart. J. Med., *33*:57, 1964.

17. Sumner, D. S.: Hemodynamics and pathophysiology of arterial disease. *In* Rutherford, R. B. (Ed.): Vascular Surgery, 2nd ed. Philadelphia, W. B. Saunders Company, 1984, pp. 19–44.

18. Szilagyi, D. F., Smith, R. F., De Russo, F. J., Elliott, J. P., and Sherrin, F. W.: Contribution of abdominal aortic aneurysmectomy to prolongation of life. Ann. Surg., *164*:678, 1966.

19. Thompson, J. E., Patman, R. D., and Talkington, C. M.: Carotid endarterectomy: Long-term outcome of patients having endarterectomy compared with unoperated controls. Ann. Surg., *188*:308, 1978.

SURGICAL DISORDERS OF THE VEINS

WORTHINGTON G. SCHENK III, M.D.

42

ANATOMY AND PHYSIOLOGY

The lower extremities are prone to disorders of the veins primarily because of the increased hydrostatic pressure secondary to gravitational effects on the upright posture. Although occlusion, obstruction, thrombosis, and inflammation occur in venous beds elsewhere, these phenomena are much more common in the lower extremities.

The primary function of veins is to serve as a conduit for the return of blood to the right heart; secondary functions include blood volume capacitance and thermal regulation. Venous blood flow occurs actively as well as passively; passive flow is governed by the hydrostatic pressure gradient between the postcapillary venules and the right atrium, and active flow is affected by the musculovenous pump mechanism. Passive venous return from the lower extremities is satisfactory in the supine position, but may be inadequate in the erect posture. Hydrostatic pressure of 10 to 15 mm. Hg in the postcapillary venules represents the residual energy from cardiac work, the rest having been dissipated in the small arteries, arterioles, and capillaries. The upright position imposes the additional hydraulic pressure resulting from the vertical column of blood extending from the ankle to the right atrium, which can add 100 mm. Hg to the total pressure within the veins of the lower extremity. This may result in stasis and distention of the thin-walled, high-compliance deep veins of the lower extremity, but is counteracted by the musculovenous pump. Rhythmic contraction/relaxation of the muscles of the lower extremity (such as during walking) causes intermittent compression of the deep venous channels of the lower extremity with retrograde flow prevented by the presence of valves. As a result, muscle contraction produces augmentation of blood flow in an antegrade direction whereas relaxation encourages emptying of the superficial veins into the deep venous system.

The thermoregulatory functions of veins include both heat conservation and dissipation. Heat conservation occurs passively through a countercurrent exchange mechanism made possible by the close apposition of deep arteries and veins. Cooler blood returning from the periphery absorbs heat from the adjacent arteries, thus cooling distal arterial blood leading to diminished heat loss in the extremities. Heat dissipation occurs in the relatively large subcutaneous veins of the extremities. Relaxation of smooth muscle tone in precapillary arterioles, under sympathetic control, results in a relatively high flow of blood into these channels where heat is easily dissipated.

The capacitance function of veins, particularly the veins of the pelvis and lower extremities, effectively buffers changes in circulating blood volume. Venous return to the right heart can be maintained despite blood loss by reducing the capacity of these channels through their sympathetic innervation. This phenomenon can be simulated therapeutically to treat hypovolemic shock: elevation of the lower extremities reduces the capacity of this compartment, resulting in a central shift of the total blood volume, as does external compression of the pelvis and lower extremities with a MAST (Military Anti-Shock Trousers) garment.

The extremities have three anatomically and functionally distinct sets of veins: deep, superficial, and perforating.

The *deep veins* accompany the named arteries of the extremities and tend to be closely apposed to them.[27] One to three veins accompany each artery with interconnected sinus-like channels and have a total cross-sectional area several times that of the accompanying artery at each level.

The *superficial veins* are thick-walled and muscular, and are located in the subcutaneous space. Many of the multiple subcutaneous veins and branches are quite variable in occurrence, size, and location. However, the two primary systems in the lower extremity, the long and short saphenous systems, have primary channels that are quite constant.

The *long saphenous vein* arises from the confluence of tributaries of the dorsum of the foot and can be found on the medial aspect of the ankle passing midway between the medial malleolus and the tibialis anterior tendon. It ascends on the medial aspect of the calf and thigh, passing 5 cm. posterior to the medial aspect of the patella, and terminates at its junction with the common femoral vein at the fossa ovalis. This landmark is found just medial to the femoral pulse and distal to the inguinal ligament, located 3 cm. lateral to and 1 cm. inferior to the pubic tubercle.

The *short saphenous vein* arises from tributaries on the lateral and plantar aspect of the foot, passes midway between the lateral malleolus and Achilles tendon, ascends vertically in the subcutaneous space, and passes through the superficial fascia to join the popliteal vein between the medial and lateral heads of the gastrocnemius muscle.

The *perforating veins* connect the superficial with the deep venous system, and normally functioning valves in those perforators plus physiologic changes in the pressure gradient result in blood flow from superficial to deep. Pathologic conditions can result in reversal of that flow.

A unique anatomic feature of all three groups of veins in the extremities is the presence of thin-walled, bicuspid valves. The renal, portal, and mesenteric veins as well as

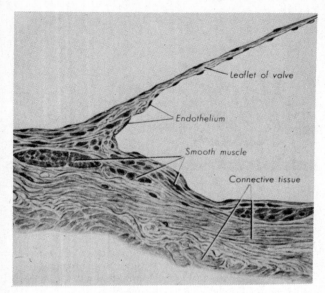

Figure 1. Microscopic features of a medium-sized vein. The adventitia merges with surrounding connective tissue. The thin wall has a few smooth muscle fibers and no elastic tissue. The valve leaflet is thin and delicate, endothelium-lined on both sides, with the free edge pointing in the direction of blood flow.

the superior and inferior venae cavae do not have valves. The two valve cusps are attached to a ring of slight thickening in the valve wall; the valve sinus, an area of slight dilatation around and just proximal to the valve leaflets, is visible on careful observation. Valves tend to be located just distal to major tributaries. They prevent retrograde flow and are critical to the musculovenous pump function. The orientation of the valves in the perforating veins of the extremities directs flow from superficial to deep, except in the veins of the hands, feet, and distal forearm, where the venous return is preferentially through the superficial veins.

The important histologic features of veins are illustrated in Figure 1. Veins possess varying amounts of smooth muscle in their media, and the wall thickness increases in the more dependent veins, being greater in the superficial than in the deep veins. There is no true elastic tissue in veins, and the intima consists of a monolayer of endothelium. The valve cusps consist of an extremely thin connective tissue superstructure covered on each side with endothelium virtually apposed back to back. The vasa vasorum of veins, where present, do not communicate with the lumen.

DIAGNOSTIC TECHNIQUES FOR THE EVALUATION OF VENOUS DISORDERS

The diagnostic techniques available are listed in Table 1. It is generally advisable to begin with the less invasive tests and to proceed to the more complex, when necessary, to answer specific questions or to select appropriate therapy.

Physical Examination

The lower extremities should be inspected for the presence, distribution, and pattern of visible varicose veins.

The presence of subcutaneous veins that are tender to direct palpation, including thrombosed veins or subcutaneous cords that may be associated with overlying erythema, is usually diagnostic of superficial thrombophlebitis. Associated trauma, nearby intravenous catheter sites, and associated lymphadenopathy or lymphangitis should also be sought.

The presence of *Homans' sign* is sometimes elicited in deep vein thrombophlebitis. The sign is positive when there is exquisite tenderness in the popliteal fossa and upper posterior calf on passive dorsiflexion of the foot. Unfortunately, this sign is neither sensitive nor specific for deep venous thrombosis. The extremity should be inspected for edema and the presence, location, and extent of pitting should be noted. Objective measurements should be obtained, including circumferential measurements at carefully specified locations at the ankle, upper calf, and lower and upper thigh, and compared with those of the contralateral extremity. The presence of abnormal coloration as well as positional changes in color should be noted. Severe venous outflow obstruction, such as is seen with extensive deep vein thrombosis, can result in a cyanotic plethora, whereas dependent rubor that is alleviated by elevation is more characteristic of chronic arterial insufficiency.

The presence, character, and location of peripheral pulses should be carefully recorded. Arterial insufficiency should not be confused with venous disease as the cause of skin changes and ulceration, but the two are occasionally present concurrently. The skin changes of arterial insufficiency characteristically include loss of hair growth, pallor, and a translucent, waxy, atrophic character of the skin. In contrast, long-standing venous disease produces a brawny and thickened character of the skin, associated with reddish-brown pigment deposition, and ulceration. The characteristic skin appearance and ulceration of venous disease is illustrated in Figure 2. Classically, the ulcers of venous insufficiency are located at or above the malleolus, whereas ulcerations secondary to arterial insufficiency are below the malleolus. When ulceration is noted, concurrent infection, cellulitis, drainage, and lymphadenopathy should be sought during examination.

The *Trendelenburg test* is a reliable maneuver for distinguishing deep venous from superficial or communicating venous valvular incompetence. It is vital to assess the condition of the deep venous system, particularly for patients with extensive superficial varicose veins. While the patient is standing in the upright position, one or more easily visible and palpable subcutaneous veins on each lower

TABLE 1. Diagnostic Modalities for the Evaluation of Venous Disorders

Physical Examination
 Inspection
 Homans' sign
 Trendelenburg test
 Ochsner-Mahorner test

Noninvasive Testing
 Doppler ultrasound
 B-Mode ultrasound imaging
 Impedance plethysmography

Nuclear Medicine
 Fibrinogen I-125 uptake test
 Radionuclide angiography

Radiologic
 Conventional contrast venography
 Descending venography

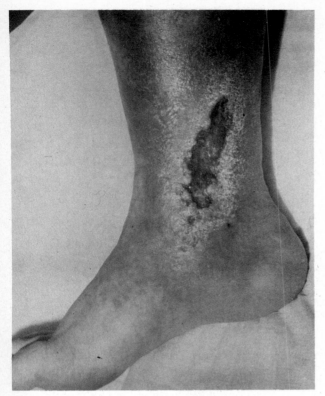

Figure 2. Appearance of a typical venous stasis ulcer. There is brawny edema, thickening of the skin, and pigment deposition. The ulcer is located at and slightly above the lateral malleolus, with hypertrophic edges.

extremity are marked. With the patient lying on the examining table with the leg in question raised passively to a 45-degree angle for several seconds, the leg is quickly lowered and the patient brought to an upright position while the time required for the marked vein to fill with blood is noted. The end point of venous filling may be best judged by a combination of observation and palpation. The venous filling time is recorded as the time in seconds from the moment the leg is lowered until the moment the vein becomes full. With no tourniquet used, a venous filling time of 30 seconds or more is normal, i.e., blood coming from the capillaries and filling the veins from below upward should take at least 30 seconds. Substantial arterial insufficiency will prolong venous filling time. However, when the venous filling time is 30 or more seconds without the use of a tourniquet, the valves of the lower extremity veins are considered competent and no further Trendelenburg testing is indicated. If the filling time is abnormally rapid, further testing as described next is indicated.

A good *venous tourniquet* is required for further testing. With the patient again lying supine and with the leg elevated at 45 degrees for 15 seconds or longer, the tourniquet is applied high on the thigh tightly enough to occlude the superficial veins. If the previously abnormal filling time now increases to 30 or more seconds when the patient stands with the tourniquet in place, only the superficial veins are incompetent and no further testing needs to be conducted. If, however, the filling time remains short as when no tourniquet was used, some veins in addition to the superficial veins are incompetent, filling in a retrograde manner by some other route than the superficial veins, and further testing is necessary. In that case, the tourniquet is removed and reapplied just above the knee, again with the patient's leg elevated to empty the lower extremity veins. If this results in prolongation of the venous filling time to normal, the observer concludes that in addition to superficial veins, the communicating veins in the thigh are also incompetent, that is, the blood from deep veins is able to pass into the superficial veins in a retrograde manner through communicating veins above but not below the knee. If the filling time is not appreciably lengthened by a tourniquet just above the knee, the incompetence must be of perforators at or below the knee, of the deep veins, of the short saphenous veins entering the deep system at or near the knee, or some combination of these. If the filling time is still abnormally short, the test is repeated with a tourniquet on the high calf. If use of the high calf tourniquet fails to lengthen an abnormally short filling time, the deep veins above or below the knee, or both, are incompetent.

A refinement of the tourniquet test to isolate the location of incompetent perforating veins is the *Ochsner-Mahorner test*. This test is performed in a manner similar to that of the Trendelenburg test, but with multiple venous tourniquets. With the patient supine and the leg elevated in a similar manner to empty the veins of the lower extremity, three tourniquets, high thigh, just above the knee, and high calf, are applied simultaneously. With the patient brought to a standing position, the veins in each of the three segments of the lower leg are then observed. The segment that exhibits an abnormally shortened filling time contains an incompetent venous perforator. The visualization of the incompetent segment can be enhanced by having the patient exercise by walking with the tourniquets in place.

Deep venous obstruction, in contrast to incompetence, may be excluded with some reliability by occlusion of the superficial veins. With this test, the limb in question is elevated as in the Trendelenburg test and firm pressure is provided with a snug elastic bandage applied from the foot to the high thigh, compressing the superficial veins only. The patient is then allowed to walk for 5 to 10 minutes. Incompetence of the superficial veins only should produce no pain and may actually be associated with improvement of symptoms. In the presence of significant obstruction to deep vein outflow, walking for 5 minutes or more will cause severe pain.

Noninvasive Testing

DOPPLER ULTRASOUND

The Doppler ultrasound blood flow detector instrument has proved to be valuable for noninvasive evaluation of the arterial system as described elsewhere. This instrument is also useful in demonstrating functional obstruction or incompetence in the deep venous system. Its only disadvantage is that its findings are somewhat more subjective and user-dependent than the objective pressure recordings and pulse volume recordings obtainable in evaluation of the arterial system.

The examination is ordinarily conducted with the patient supine and the legs level. The ultrasound probe is applied first at the palpable femoral pulse at the groin. When the audible phasic arterial signal is identified, the typical venous signal is identified just medial to the artery. This audible signal can be easily detected with some practice and is variously described as the sound of ocean waves or wind blowing through trees. The signal is ordinarily continuous rather than pulsatile, except for the frequent overlap of the signal from the adjacent artery.

The ability to compare findings to the opposite extremity is of valuable help in a unilaterally symptomatic extremity. The first notation is of the presence or absence of a spontaneous venous signal. Second, the patient is asked to take several slow deep breaths, to hold a Valsalva maneuver, and then release it. This should result in an easily discernible respiratory variation in the intensity of the venous signal. The venous blood flow may be either augmented or suppressed with inspiration, depending on whether the patient is primarily a thoracic or abdominal breather. The Valsalva maneuver should abruptly and totally occlude the venous flow, which should promptly return with an augmented flow when the Valsalva is released. If these findings are normal, it suggests that there is normal patency of venous channels between the common femoral vein and the inferior vena cava. It is a highly reliable test for acute iliofemoral thrombosis, with a sensitivity of approximately 95 per cent. There may be a 15 per cent false-negative rate with chronic iliofemoral thrombosis because the test findings may return to normal with recanalization or formation of collaterals.

The next part of the examination is to assess the augmentation of flow, or "A-waves." With the examiner still listening to the venous signal at the groin, A-waves are elicited by sequentially squeezing the midthigh, compressing the midcalf, and dorsiflexing the foot. Each of these maneuvers should result in a characteristic "pistol-shot" augmentation A-wave from the transmission of a wave of augmented flow through the deep veins. A progressively increasing delay between the compression and the audible signal as the examiner proceeds distally is normal. Absence of A-waves indicates venous occlusion between the compression and the common femoral vein. The examination may show deep vein valvular incompetence. The compression at a given location is held several seconds until the passage of the augmentation wave, then abruptly released. The presence of an A-wave upon release of the compression suggests retrograde flow indicative of valvular incompetence. If normal A-waves from the ankle to the groin are detected, no further Doppler examination is necessary. If they are not detected, the test can be further refined by applying the instrument to the popliteal area. With the patient in the prone position, a popliteal venous signal is detected in a manner similar to that described for the common femoral vein signal. Unfortunately, there is greater variability in the anatomy of the popliteal vein, which may be single or multiple. If a popliteal venous signal cannot be clearly distinguished, it may be due to an anatomic variation, and it should not be concluded that the popliteal vein is thrombosed. If a popliteal venous signal can be identified and an A-wave can be produced with foot dorsiflexion, there is physiologically unimpeded flow in the deep veins from the ankle to the knee.

The sensitivity of the Doppler examination for venous thrombosis in the tibial, soleal, popliteal, and superficial femoral veins is considerably less than that for iliofemoral thrombosis, primarily because there are frequently multiple channels in these deep veins and the Doppler testing for physiologic obstruction to venous flow is abnormal only in complete or near complete obstruction. Although the test is useful when results are unequivocally abnormal, a normal Doppler examination of the more distal lower extremity does not exclude the presence of significant deep vein thrombosis.

B-MODE ULTRASOUND IMAGING

A more recent development in noninvasive vascular investigation is B-mode ultrasound imaging. The fluid filled

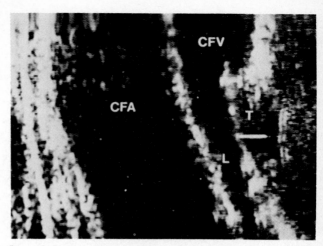

Figure 3. B-mode ultrasound appearance of the common femoral vein at the inguinal ligament. The vein is identified just medial to the common femoral artery. Thrombus adherence to the wall and residual or recannalized lumen is evident. CFA = Common femoral artery; CFV = common femoral vein; T = thrombus; L = lumen. (From Sullivan, E. D., Peter, D. J., and Cranley, J. J.: J. Vasc. Surg., 1:465, 1984.)

vein, surrounded by tissues of different acoustical density, can be imaged with high-resolution B-mode ultrasound scanning. This technique is capable of imaging patency and/or thrombosis of the lumen of large veins of the pelvis and lower extremities. A B-mode ultrasound image of the common femoral artery and vein at the groin is depicted in Figure 3. A recanalized lumen and the presence of adherent chronic thrombosis is demonstrated. This noninvasive imaging of anatomic detail of the venous system is proving to be a useful adjunct when combined with noninvasive physiologic testing.

IMPEDANCE PLETHYSMOGRAPHY

A noninvasive assessment of obstruction to venous outflow can be obtained with impedance plethysmography, which quantitates the rate of venous emptying in the calf after release of a temporary venous tourniquet on the thigh. This device records changes in blood volume in the extremity as reflected by changes in electrical resistance and is conducted by temporarily inflating a pneumatic venous tourniquet on the thigh while measuring the increase in venous capacity on the calf. The blood volume tracing reaches a plateau, after which the occluding cuff is deflated and the rate of venous outflow is recorded.

Typical venous plethysmography tracings in a patient with deep vein thrombosis in the right leg are shown in Figure 4. The technique is rapid and safe, with an overall sensitivity of approximately 94 per cent. A normal venous plethysmographic study has great value in excluding significant deep vein thrombosis. Small hemodynamically insignificant thrombi in calf veins may go undetected by this technique because the reduction in total venous outflow may be trivial. However, thrombi in small calf veins appear to be rarely associated with clinically significant pulmonary emboli. Because the risk of pulmonary embolism in patients with negative results appears to be significantly less than the risk associated with anticoagulation, the study has great value in enabling one to make a clinical decision. A patient being evaluated for suspected deep vein thrombosis who is found to be normal by an impedance plethysmographic study need not undergo treatment or further investigation.[14]

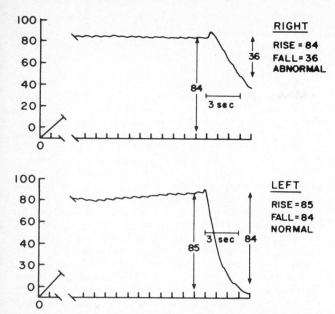

Figure 4. Lower extremity venous plethsymography in a patient with acute onset of pain and swelling in the right lower extremity. The abnormal right side is compared with the normal left side. The plethsymography is normal if the fall in 3 seconds exceeds 50 per cent of the rise to a plateau. The units on the ordinate are arbitrary.

However, a number of technical factors contribute to the false-positive rate, which is approximately 6 to 8 per cent. Vasoconstriction, pain, anxiety, hypotension, cold, and tight clothing can produce physiologic extrinsic compression of the venous system and yield false-positive results.[1] Thus, a patient with positive venous impedance plethysmographic findings is frequently further evaluated by *contrast venography* prior to the institution of anticoagulation.

Nuclear Medicine

FIBRINOGEN UPTAKE TEST

The fibrinogen I-125 uptake test has been used to detect the presence of thrombi in lower extremity veins and the incorporation of tagged fibrinogen in new or developing intravascular thrombi. Counts are taken at measured intervals on each lower extremity, typically on several sequential days. A 20 per cent increase in counts in an area, when compared with adjacent areas, contralateral extremity, or previous day, is ordinarily accepted as a positive result. This test has proved to be very valuable in quantitating thrombus formation in clinical studies directed toward evaluating methods for prophylaxis of deep vein thrombosis. Unfortunately, use of this test consistently leads to the overestimation of deep vein thrombosis. The clinical relevance of radionuclide-detectable fibrinogen deposition in deep veins in the lower extremities is uncertain and has limited the practical utility of this test. The prevalence of a positive result in patients undergoing abdominal operations with general anesthesia is estimated at 24 to 40 per cent.[8, 21]

RADIONUCLIDE ANGIOGRAPHY

Technetium radionuclide angiography is capable of producing images of the flow of the tracer through the vascular channels. Although it has proved useful as an investigational study and in certain specific clinical conditions, its sensitivity and resolution are such that it is a poor screening test for anatomically or physiologically important disorders of the veins. It is capable of noninvasively and repeatedly demonstrating flow through arteriovenous fistulas, previously thrombosed venous channels, and operative reconstructions of occluded or incompetent veins.

Radiologic Testing

CONTRAST VENOGRAPHY

The standard for anatomic imaging of the venous system is contrast venography. As the contrast mixes with and displaces blood in the veins of the extremity, obliterated veins, abnormal venous flow patterns, and partially occluding intravascular thrombi can be detected. The resolution of this test diminishes proximally as the contrast becomes progressively more dilute, and adequate imaging of iliac veins may require a very large volume injection.

Risks associated with the study include nephrotoxicity and allergic reactions to iodinated contrast, and the contrast agent itself is harmful to the vascular endothelium and may increase the risk of venous thrombosis. However, because of the risks inherent to full anticoagulation in a patient with suspected deep vein thrombosis, verification of the diagnosis by contrast venography is often recommended unless the clinical and noninvasive diagnosis is unequivocal. Unlike arteriography, with its large-bore puncture of major arteries, conventional venography can be safely performed on an outpatient basis.

DESCENDING VENOGRAPHY

Anatomic imaging of incompetent venous valves requires a modification of the technique referred to as descending venography. In this test, a catheter is passed from above into the inferior vena cava, typically by threading a long catheter fluoroscopically from an antecubital vein through the superior vena cava and right atrium. With the patient on a tilting fluoroscopic table, iodinated contrast is injected into the superior vena cava and an attempt made to visualize retrograde flow through the iliac and femoral veins. It is only by this technique that precise localization of incompetent vein valves in the iliofemoral system can be identified. However, the use of this test is reserved for patients in whom direct reconstruction or repair of valvular incompetence is anticipated. Examples of conventional antegrade and descending venograms are shown in Figures 5 and 6.

VARICOSE VEINS

Etiology, Signs, and Symptoms

Varicose veins of the lower extremities are an extremely common affliction, affecting 15 to 20 per cent of the adult population. A familial history may be obtained in about 15 per cent of patients. The affliction is more prevalent among females (the female-to-male ratio is 5:1), with many women dating the onset of visible and symptomatic varices to the time of pregnancy. Varicose veins are classified as primary and secondary. *Primary varicose veins* are an isolated disorder of the superficial veins of the lower extremities and are not a sequel of deep venous thrombosis.

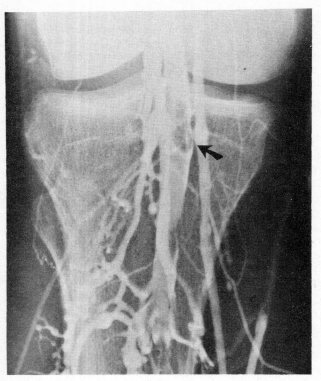

Figure 5. Conventional contrast venography. Iodinated contrast has been injected into a vein of the foot, and an image of opacification of the veins of the popliteal area has been obtained. A partially occluding thrombus in the popliteal vein appears as a lucent filling defect and is indicated by the arrow.

Secondary varicosities are a manifestation of deep venous insufficiency and are associated with multiple stigmata of chronic venous insufficiency, including edema, skin changes, stasis dermatitis, and ulceration. This condition has a distinctly different pathophysiology from primary varicose veins and should be carefully distinguished because its prognosis and treatment should be approached differently. (See "Chronic Venous Insufficiency and Postphlebitic Syndrome" later in this chapter.)

Continuous and prolonged overdistention of the relatively thin-walled veins of the lower extremity produces enlargement in both the transverse and longitudinal dimensions. The longitudinal enlargement produces the characteristic tortuosity of the subcutaneous veins, and the transverse distention results in the visible and palpable engorgement responsible for the symptomatic and cosmetic features. The common denominator in the pathophysiology of the production of varicose veins is loss of valvular competence; operative therapy, when indicated, is ablative and consists of destruction or removal of the veins, rather than correction of the valvular incompetence.

Factors contributing to the development of varicose veins include congenital weakness or absence of valve leaflets, incompetent perforating veins with reversal of venous blood flow from deep to superficial, volume expansion and hormonal influences of pregnancy, the effects of gravity on hydrostatic pressure, most notably in individuals whose occupations result in standing or sitting for prolonged periods without intermittent calf muscle contraction, and occasionally direct trauma to the valves of perforating veins. It is postulated that varicose veins propagate from proximal to distal. The combined effects of gravity and volume expansion may first render the valve at the saphenofemoral junction incompetent, resulting in a longer column of blood acting on the next lower valves, which would become similarly overdistended to the point of incompetence, and so forth.

The majority of patients complain primarily of the cosmetic aspect of multiple visibly distended veins of the lower extremities. Other complaints include a fatigued and heavy sensation particularly upon standing for a long period, characteristically relieved by elevation of the leg. A more disabling pain may occasionally be noted, and hem-

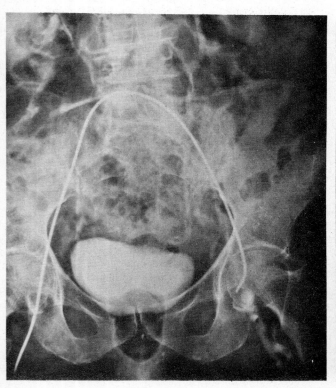

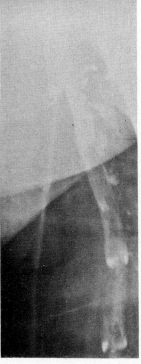

Figure 6. Descending venogram. A left descending venogram has been obtained by advancing a catheter percutaneously through the right common femoral vein, across the confluence at the inferior vena cava, and the tip is positioned in the left common femoral vein. The x-ray table has been tilted into a semi-upright position as a bolus of iodinated contrast has been injected. The contrast can be seen to reflux down the femoral vein instead of flowing cephalad to the common iliac vein. The inset demonstrates reflux in both the deep and superficial (great saphenous) veins, and several incompetent valves are identified.

orrhage, either spontaneous or from minor trauma, has been reported but is unusual.

The history should include a careful search for previous injury or previous deep venous thrombophlebitis. Previous treatment of varicose veins should also be noted in view of their recurrent nature. The physical examination should include a search for stasis dermatitis, pigmentation, edema, and ulceration, since these may all be evidence of more significant deep venous insufficiency.

Whenever any form of therapy is planned, it is important to confirm the patency and competency of the deep venous system. If the patient improves with the application of a well-fitted elastic stocking, normal function of the deep venous system is suggested, since obliteration of the superficial veins in the presence of inadequacy of the deep veins would be expected to make the patient worse. Noninvasive confirmation of deep venous function should be performed with the Trendelenburg test and venous plethysmography confirming normal venous outflow. Contrast venography is not necessary prior to the institution of treatment for primary varicose veins if the other noninvasive tests described previously are normal.

Indications for Treatment

Minor involvement should be treated conservatively, symptomatically, and nonoperatively. The first therapeutic approach is avoidance of prolonged standing, encouragement of weight loss and muscular activity such as walking, and reassurance that minor cosmetic concerns are not a health hazard. The use of light comfortable support hose may be quite helpful. Knee-length stockings with a tight elastic top are particularly to be avoided because of their tourniquet effect on superficial veins. For more symptomatic patients with significant discomfort and those whose occupation requires them to endure the deleterious effects of gravity, a graded-pressure, custom-fitted elastic garment should be prescribed.

The treatment options for more severe symptomatic and refractory involvement include *excision* and *injection sclerotherapy*. The patient's expectations and anticipated outcome should be carefully considered when the indications for treatment are solely for cosmetic reasons. Many patients with uncomplicated varicose veins can be treated equally well with ligation and stripping or injection sclerotherapy. Sclerotherapy has been shown to be an alternative to operative therapy in a randomized trial,[13] and for isolated enlarged veins, particularly those that may recur following surgical excision, sclerotherapy may be the treatment of choice. It is clearly an alternative for patients who are poor operative candidates. However, patients with demonstrable saphenofemoral regurgitation appear to have a significant recurrence rate following sclerotherapy[24] and should probably be treated with ligation and stripping. Saphenofemoral reflux can usually be demonstrated on physical examination. With the leg elevated, the saphenous bulb is occluded with localized digital pressure and the patient is then allowed to stand while this pressure is maintained. If the veins of the long saphenous system are seen to fill promptly on release of this digital pressure, saphenofemoral incompetence is present and injection sclerotherapy alone is less likely to be satisfactory because of the venous collaterals in this area.

Vein Stripping

Ligation plus excision, or "vein stripping," constitutes the operative method of removing varicose subcutaneous veins. Preoperatively, the visible and palpable engorged subcutaneous veins should be marked with indelible ink, with the patient standing in an upright position. Ink that is not removed by bathing, alcohol, or surgical scrub must be used. General or spinal anesthesia is appropriate, and a time-consuming procedure should be anticipated.

The goal of the operation is ligation and removal of the involved subcutaneous veins with ligation of the deep communicating perforators. The entire lower extremity, including the lower abdomen to the waist, is prepared circumferentially. The procedure is frequently done bilaterally. Isolated varices are excised prior to the stripping of the long and short saphenous veins for reasons described later. These individual veins are meticulously excised through separate small transverse incisions directly over the marked skin. Incisions are closed in layers, and a subcuticular technique is frequently employed.

The entire long saphenous system can be removed by use of the internal vein stripper. This is done last so that a compressive dressing can be applied immediately, thus reducing the risk of subcutaneous bleeding and hematoma formation. Separate incisions following the skin creases are made two finger breadths below the inguinal ligament and just medial to the femoral pulse, and just anterior to the medial malleolus. The saphenous vein is isolated at the ankle, and available branches are ligated and divided so that the intraluminal stripper can be passed upward from below. Through the groin incision, the entrance of the long saphenous vein into the common femoral vein at the fossa ovalis is identified and all tributary veins to the saphenofemoral junction are carefully identified, doubly ligated, and divided.

Finally, the saphenous bulb is suture ligated and the long saphenous vein divided so that the internal stripper can be passed up the entire length of the vein with exit through the opening in the groin incision. The handle to the stripper is then attached at this end so that the vein can be stripped distal to proximal. The olive tip is then applied to the lower end of the stripper, and the stripping process is begun for several centimeters cephalad to the ankle incision so that this incision can be closed. The groin incision can also be closed at this time, except for a 1-cm. opening to allow withdrawal of the instrument and the excised vein. The instrument is then slowly but forcibly extracted from the upper incision while simultaneously a compressive dressing is applied from the ankle upwards. The remaining opening of the groin incision is closed as the instrument is withdrawn with the entire long saphenous vein captured on its shaft. The details of this procedure are depicted in Figure 7.

The importance of the immediate application of the compressive dressing from below must be emphasized, since many branches of the long saphenous vein are avulsed by the stripping process. Some advocate stripping only from the knee to the groin if the vein in the lower leg is not involved, but most agree that the long saphenous system should be removed in apparent cases of varices isolated to the short saphenous system.

Complications include trauma to the saphenous and sural nerves with accompanying cutaneous hypesthesia, subcutaneous hematoma formation, and rare inadvertent arterial stripping. Removal of the superficial veins when they are dilated secondary to occlusion of the deep venous system is catastrophic, and thus the importance of proper preoperative evaluation is emphasized. Patient dissatisfaction should be expected if the patient seeking cosmetic improvement does not fully understand that the procedure is exchanging unsightly veins for multiple incisions. Some degree of recurrence of remaining and collateral veins is

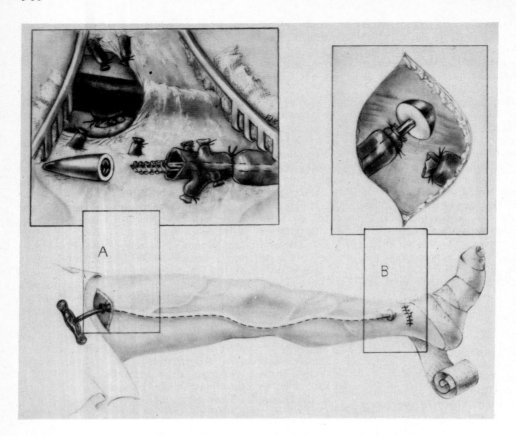

Figure 7. Stripping of the long saphenous vein. The long saphenous vein is isolated proximally at the fossa ovalis and distally at the medial malleolus. Inset A shows ligation and division of all tributaries to the saphenous bulb. The saphenous bulb has been divided and suture ligated flush with the common femoral vein. Inset B illustrates passage of the flexible intraluminal stripper from distal to proximal and ligation of the vein onto the shaft of the stripper just beneath the olive tip. After the stripper emerges at the groin, the interchangeable tip can be replaced by a handle. The stripping procedure is begun for a centimeter or two, and the distal incision at the ankle can be closed. A compressive dressing is then applied from distal to proximal as the stripper is withdrawn from the groin incision, capturing the vein on its shaft. See text for details.

not uncommon, and patients should also be counseled in this regard.

Postoperatively, the extremity should be elevated for 4 to 6 hours and the compressive dressing applied in the operating room should remain in place for 4 to 6 days. Twenty-four to 48 hours postoperatively, a program of progressive ambulation should begin. The patient is allowed to walk several minutes per hour, gradually increasing daily, and remains supine with the extremities elevated when not walking. Standing (without walking) and sitting are carefully avoided, and custom-fitted elastic stockings should be worn for several months.

Sclerotherapy

Nonoperative obliteration of dilated subcutaneous veins has waxed and waned in popularity since the time of Hippocrates. The method of sclerosis/compression therapy as described by Fegan and others appears to be successful in properly chosen cases.[6] The method has been used by Sigg and Zelikovski in more than 58,000 cases in Switzerland.[23] A detailed description of the preparation and technique is given by Sladen.[24]

With the patient in the upright position, the veins are marked and then individually injected through fine-bore needles with 3 per cent sodium dodecylsulfate in benzyl alcohol (Sotradecol). Particular attention is paid to the identification of the location of "blowouts," i.e., points of incompetent deep venous perforators, so that injections can be made at or close to these sites. The injection of no more than 0.5 ml. of sclerosant is made at each site with the leg elevated, although the actual needle insertion may be aided by temporarily allowing the extremity to hang over the side of the examining table. The most distal veins

are injected first, and a compressive dressing is applied from below upwards as the injections are made. As many as 10 to 20 sites can be injected at a single visit, and residual sites can be injected at the follow-up visit 7 days later. It is important that the compressive dressing consisting of elastic bandage reinforced with elastic tape remain in place for 7 days. This immediate compression encourages apposition of the walls of the superficial veins to obliterate them by direct fibrosis rather than thrombosis, and recanalization will not occur. It is also important for the patient to walk for 1 hour immediately following the treatment and for at least 1 hour each day throughout the treatment period. Compressive hose are prescribed for at least 2 months following the treatment, except for "touch-up" injections of isolated veins. Symptomatic relief and patient satisfaction with the cosmetic result are expected in 90 per cent of cases.

Serious allergic reactions and unsightly skin discoloration or necrosis are much less likely with Sotradecol than with the previously used sclerosing agent sodium morrhuate. Mild allergic reaction is seen in 0.05 per cent; 10 to 20 per cent of patients will have recurrence via persistent or collateral veins. However, the technique is well suited to isolated recurrences, whether following medical or surgical therapy. Efforts at prospective random trials comparing surgery and sclerotherapy have shown similar results with both techniques.[13]

PROPHYLAXIS OF POSTOPERATIVE DEEP VENOUS THROMBOSIS

Several characteristics of the surgical patient population tend to result in the development of acute deep venous thrombosis of the lower extremities. Factors that increase this risk include advanced age, malignancy, immobilization, orthopedic procedures, prolonged enforced bed rest, inhibition of the musculovenous pump by prolonged anesthesia, and, possibly, the induction of a hypercoagulable state by surgical trauma. The most serious sequela of acute deep venous thrombosis in the hospitalized patient is fatal pulmonary embolism,[22] and both of these subjects are discussed in Chapter 43.

ACUTE THROMBOPHLEBITIS

Acute thrombophlebitis may be *superficial* or *deep*. Superficial thrombophlebitis is generally a benign condition, but deep thrombophlebitis can be a morbid condition. The most severe form is *acute iliofemoral thrombosis*, and there are a number of chronic sequelae that are of considerable consequence.

Superficial Thrombophlebitis

Superficial thrombophlebitis is an intensely painful condition involving intravascular thrombosis and an intense inflammatory reaction in the superficial veins. It is frequently associated with intravenous cannulation sites. The diagnosis is confirmed by the presence of linear erythema visible in the overlying skin, exquisite tenderness to palpation, and, occasionally, a palpable cord. The condition is frequently seen in the upper extremities of hospitalized patients as a complication of intravenous fluid therapy. Careful nursing care of intravenous cannula sites and routine 72-hour cannula site rotation are important prophylactic measures. This condition is *not* associated with long-term disabling sequelae, nor is it a significant risk for pulmonary embolism. The treatment is symptomatic; the indwelling catheter is removed, and patients should be treated with adequate analgesia, elevation of the affected extremity, application of moist heat, and salicylates. Heparin anticoagulation is unnecessary, but long-term, low-dose salicylate treatment may be employed in persistent or recurrent cases. Because this condition involves a serious risk if it extends into the deep venous system, screening with noninvasive studies to exclude deep vein involvement may be employed when the lower extremities are involved.

Deep Venous Thrombophlebitis

Involvement of the deep venous system produces much less pain and tenderness, and objective signs and symptoms may be subtle. The diagnosis and treatment of deep venous thrombophlebitis of the lower extremities are described under the next section, "Acute Iliofemoral Thrombosis." Extensive deep vein thrombosis of the upper extremity can result in chronic edema, pain, disability, and, infrequently, pulmonary embolization. It can occur secondary to trauma, subclavian vein cannulation for central venous access, or occasionally "effort thrombosis," which can be related to very strenuous physical activity, such as wrestling or weight-lifting. The diagnosis is usually confirmed by venography; treatment consists of intravenous heparin administration, frequently given through a peripheral vein in the affected extremity, in a manner similar to that used for lower extremity deep vein thrombosis.

ACUTE ILIOFEMORAL THROMBOSIS

Diagnosis

The recognition of florid acute iliofemoral venous thrombosis is usually straightforward. Edema involves the entire extremity up to the groin, pain may be intense in ambulatory patients, there may be tenderness to palpation because of edema in deep muscle compartments, and the color is likely to be deeper than normal. Subcutaneous collateral veins may appear visibly distended, and mild inflammation and low-grade fever are not unusual. Signs and symptoms will be bilateral if both iliofemoral systems or the inferior vena cava is involved. The diagnosis is easily suspected clinically in these florid cases, although in as many as half of the cases iliofemoral thrombosis is asymptomatic and unsuspected, accompanied only by edema of gradual onset frequently in bedridden patients, and suspected only on the basis of pulmonary embolization or lower extremity edema. A secure diagnosis must be established before undertaking medical or surgical therapy. Noninvasive studies, including Doppler flow analysis and venous plethysmography, are useful. If the Doppler study is unequivocally abnormal, this is sufficient for initiating therapy. If plethysmographic studies are unequivocally normal, no further evaluation is necessary.[28] In other cases, contrast venography remains the standard for diagnosis.

In its most severe form, iliofemoral venous thrombosis can lead to impending or actual gangrene and tissue loss. The venous thrombosis may be accompanied by arterial spasm resulting in swelling, pain, and pallor of the leg, referred to as *phlegmasia alba dolens*. This condition, sometimes called "milk leg," was attributed to deposition of milk in the extremity in postpartum women in the 1700s.[3] Iliofemoral thrombosis with accompanying arterial spasm is now known to be the etiology.[4] Prompt recognition and treatment of this condition are vital to avoid progression to *phlegmasia cerulea dolens*, which is a more virulent form with a mortality as high as 50 per cent.[12] In this rare but severe form, the leg is not only swollen to the inguinal ligament but it is also cold and frankly cyanotic and progresses to bullae formation and tissue necrosis. The venous thrombosis is probably more extensive, occluding all venous collaterals, and is associated with arterial spasm.

Treatment

The treatment of iliofemoral thrombosis consists of anticoagulation and, more recently, thrombolytic therapy. Enthusiasm for operative intervention has varied in the past. Thrombectomy is generally reserved for patients with actual or impending tissue loss caused by an associated arterial insufficiency as with phlegmasia cerulea dolens.

The usual treatment of acute iliofemoral thrombosis is full therapeutic anticoagulation with heparin, bed rest, and elevation of the affected extremity. Anticoagulation with heparin is initiated promptly usually as a continuous intravenous infusion, which is the safest mode of administration.[10] A loading dose of 75 to 100 units per kg. is given, followed by continuous infusion of 800 to 1200 units per hour, depending upon the patient's weight, and monitored by blood coagulation studies. Maintaining the activated partial thromboplastin time (aPTT) at twice normal is an accepted therapeutic goal. A decrease in pain and edema should be noted within 24 hours, and full therapeutic heparinization is usually continued for 5 to 7 days before conversion to an oral warfarin anticoagulant. Heparin anticoagulation is allowed to overlap with sodium warfarin (Coumadin) anticoagulation and tapered off over 48 hours. Warfarin anticoagulation to a prothrombin time (PT) of one and one-half to two times control is sought. Coumadin anticoagulation is continued along with the use of custom-made, graded-pressure stockings for 4 to 6 months. Following this, there is no agreement on long-term therapy, although some surgeons recommend aspirin in a dose of one-half to one tablet once or twice daily.

The use of thrombolytic therapy with streptokinase has theoretical advantages over heparin anticoagulation alone in that it may produce more rapid resolution of intravascular thrombosis.[15] There is some evidence that long-term preservation of venous valvular function may be improved with streptokinase over heparin therapy alone.[2, 11] Streptokinase is most commonly administered as a continuous peripheral infusion. This consists of an infusion of 250,000 units over the first hour and 100,000 units per hour for approximately 72 hours, followed by conversion to heparin anticoagulation and subsequently to warfarin in the manner described earlier. The duration of fibrinolytic therapy may be determined by the use of noninvasive venous studies to confirm re-establishment of deep venous patency. The course of fibrinolytic therapy is rarely less than 48 hours, is usually continued for 72 to 96 hours, but is seldom beneficial if continued beyond 6 days. There is some enthusiasm for direct infusion of a lower dose of streptokinase directly into thrombosed vessels, such as coronary arteries, thrombosed mesenteric arteries, and thrombosed vascular grafts. A direct infusion of 5000 to 10,000 units per hour directly into the thrombosed vessel produces a higher local concentration of the agent, but this mode of therapy has rarely been employed for extensive venous thrombosis.

Full pharmacologic anticoagulation with either heparin or warfarin is associated with a significant risk of complication, which increases with the duration of treatment. Complications such as gastrointestinal bleeding, hematuria, external hemorrhage from minor trauma, and cerebrovascular stroke underscore the need for careful monitoring. The PT is assessed at least daily while warfarin dosage is being adjusted, weekly when a stable dose is established and at least biweekly for the duration of treatment. The list of medications that interfere with the actions of warfarin is extensive, and careful patient education is necessary for chronic anticoagulation to be safely maintained.

Surgical treatment of acute iliofemoral venous thrombosis remains controversial. Acute results are often dramatic, but long-term function is frequently disappointing.[12, 19] For these reasons, direct thrombectomy is rarely if ever considered except for impending loss of tissue.[9] Another adjunct to medical therapy in phlegmasia cerulea dolens is *sympathectomy*, either pharmacologic or surgical, to alleviate the vascular spasm component of this disorder. This is perhaps best accomplished by the placement of an epidural catheter (more safely accomplished prior to the initiation of anticoagulation) for the continuous or intermittent infusion of anesthetic agents to produce sympathetic blockage.

CHRONIC VENOUS INSUFFICIENCY AND POSTPHLEBITIC SYNDROME

Pathophysiology

Chronic venous insufficiency results from a mechanical or physiologic interference with venous outflow from the lower extremities. This syndrome requires obstruction or incompetence of the deep venous system; obliteration of the superficial venous system alone will not result in gross venous insufficiency. Congenitally absent or insufficient veins of the lower extremity is extremely uncommon. Iatrogenic or traumatic interruption of main venous channels from the infrarenal inferior vena cava to the common femoral vein can result in disability, although the establishment of adequate venous return through collaterals is the rule. The syndrome arises most commonly as a consequence of deep venous thrombosis. An episode of symptomatic deep thrombophlebitis can frequently be elicited (as described earlier under "Acute Iliofemoral Thrombosis"). Alternatively, a past episode of silent thrombophlebitis is frequently implied; a history of trauma, fracture, or transient lower extremity edema may be elicited despite the absence of a recognized diagnosis of thrombophlebitis.

Although a properly treated episode of deep vein thrombosis may resolve with normal vein function,[16] the episode may resolve with permanent obliteration of major venous channels, or these channels may recanalize with destroyed or defective valves, subjecting the deep venous system to the gravitational effects of hydrostatic pressure, especially in the upright position. Valvular incompetence must be distinguished from insufficient venous outflow when operative therapy is being considered. Either situation can result in a series of changes ultimately leading to the disability associated with the *postphlebitic syndrome*, in which the deep veins of the lower extremity become overdistended and reversal of flow in the perforating veins occurs and may lead to secondary varicose veins. Dependent edema results from elevation of capillary and postcapillary pressure. Inflammation, fat necrosis, and, eventually, calcification occur in the subdermal soft tissues, a result of pressure necrosis arising from increased pressure from within. Microextravasation of red cells in the dermal and subdermal tissues results in pigment accumulation in the typical reddish-brown hyperpigmented appearance of the postphlebitic limb, especially in the supramalleolar area. Full-thickness dermal necrosis produces skin ulceration, which in this condition can heal only by epithelialization over the granulation tissue bed. Because of the poor mechanical characteristics of this unsupported epidermis and because the underlying disorder persists, poor wound healing, repeated breakdown and reulceration, chronic recurrent soft tissue infection, and an alarming degree of disability are the end result. The typical appearance of a chronic postphlebitic lower extremity is shown in Figure 2.

Diagnosis and Treatment

The history may reveal a clear episode of acute thrombophlebitis. The absence of such a history does not preclude the diagnosis, however, because an episode of silent thrombophlebitis is much more likely than the primary occurrence of symptoms. Physical examination of the lower extremities may reveal edema, ulceration, hyperpigmentation, and the typical inflexible, scarred, woody characteristic of the subcutaneous tissue. Accompanying infection, drainage, or cellulitis should be noted. The presence of inframalleolar ulceration, pulse deficit, shiny atrophic skin without pigment deposition, or a history of claudication should alert the physician to the possibility of ulceration caused by arterial rather than venous insufficiency. The possibility of concomitant arterial and venous disease should not be overlooked; the noninvasive laboratory tests can be most helpful in this regard with Doppler analysis, sequential pressure measurements, pulse volume recording, and exercise tolerance testing to aid in excluding concomitant arterial insufficiency.

Treatment of the Postphlebitic Syndrome

Treatment for the postphlebitic extremity may be begun without contrast venography confirmation of the anatomic extent of pathology, the latter being reserved to answer specific questions when surgical therapy is considered.

Treatment of the postphlebitic lower extremity should be initially conservative and nonoperative. The patient with classic stigmata of chronic venous insufficiency of the lower extremity, including edema, pigment deposition, and ulceration, should be advised of the chronic relapsing and usually incurable nature of this condition. Meticulous skin care, avoidance of local trauma, and the use of compressive stockings should be emphasized. For the atrophic skin of the postphlebitic extremity which progresses to frank ulceration, the use of the "Unna boot" is frequently employed for outpatient management. This compressive/supportive dressing consists of an absorbent dressing applied directly over the ulcer, followed by wrapping the leg from the metatarsal heads to the upper calf with gauze impregnated with a gelatin/calamine compound. This semirigid compressive dressing typically remains in place for 5 to 7 days and is reapplied as necessary until the ulcer heals. In refractory cases, hospitalization with continuous elevation of the leg, aggressive wound care, daily whirlpool treatment, and antibiotic therapy when needed nearly always results in healing the acute ulcers.

Patients in whom healing fails or those who experience multiple recurrences and incapacitation may become candidates for more aggressive surgical therapy. If incompetence of the superficial venous system can be documented in conjunction with a patent deep venous system, ligation and stripping of the greater and lesser saphenous systems may be beneficial. Simple split-thickness skin grafting alone for venous stasis ulcers has a relatively high rate of recurrence because covering the granulating ulcer with epidermis alone has the same recurrence tendency as a spontaneously epithelialized ulcer: the thin epidermis is unsupported by normal underlying dermis and the basic venous insufficiency disorder remains. Therefore, incompetent veins should be treated appropriately. Rotation flaps, myocutaneous flaps, and composite microvascular free flaps have not been widely used because the creation of a large wound in an extremity in which the primary venous problem remains uncorrected may lead to an even larger nonhealing wound. Therefore, the next step in the surgical management of the postphlebitic syndrome is isolation of the dermis from the deep venous system by ligation of all perforating veins, a concept first proposed by Linton.[20] In this procedure, longitudinal incisions are made on the medial and lateral aspects of the leg with complete separation of the superficial tissues at the fascial level and identification and ligation of all venous perforators emerging from the muscle fascial level. The procedure must frequently be accompanied by a skin graft over large ulcerated areas. This more aggressive procedure is reserved for disabling and recurrent postphlebitic syndrome despite efforts at good nonoperative care, although the long-term results are quite good when it is employed. The fundamental aspects of the Linton operation are illustrated in Figure 8.

Since 1975, direct correction of the venous pathophysiology has been approached operatively. These corrective operations involve venous bypass, venous valvular repair,

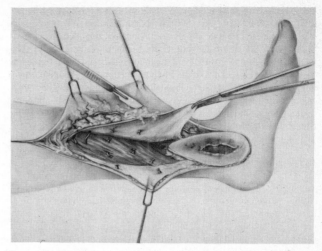

Figure 8. The Linton procedure for postphlebitic ulceration. Through a longitudinal incision, the incompetent perforating veins are ligated as they emerge from the muscle compartment. Elevating the muscle fascia facilitates the identification of these veins. The abnormal tissue between the skin and muscle is dissected and removed. The ulcer is excised and often requires skin grafting. The complete procedure includes a similar dissection laterally.

or the interposition of autologous venous valves.[7, 18] Direct repair of the abnormal venous system is intellectually appealing, but because the immediate results are quite variable and the long-term recurrence rate remains high, the use of these corrective operations remains somewhat controversial. These operations are best employed at centers with a specific interest in corrective venous procedures. To be considered for such an operation, precise anatomic definition of the venous pathology is critical. Chronic venous outflow obstruction must be distinguished from venous valvular incompetence. This is ordinarily performed with a series of noninvasive examinations supplemented by venography to assess incompetence of the venous valves in the deep venous system. If chronic venous outflow obstruction is documented by venography and impedance plethysmography, the patient may be a candidate for venous bypass surgery. Depending upon the anatomy, the contralateral saphenous vein may be used as a venous shunt. The vein is dissected from the saphenous bulb to below the knee, left attached at the saphenofemoral junction, and tunneled subcutaneously anterior to the pubis to be connected to the deep venous system in the contralateral leg distal to the area of occlusion. In the rare circumstance when it can be documented that the deep venous system is occluded proximally but the ipsilateral superficial (great saphenous) system is patent, a saphenous to popliteal vein anastomosis may be performed to shunt venous blood from the popliteal vein into the superficial system. The most commonly found pathophysiology in the chronic postphlebitic limb is that of deep venous valvular incompetence without venous outflow obstruction, which can be confirmed by appropriate noninvasive studies. Bypass or shunting procedures would obviously be ineffective in this circumstance, but two approaches which have been attempted for direct correction of this condition are *venous valvular repair* and *autologous valve interposition*. For venous valvular repair to be considered, descending venography is first employed to identify the sites of deep vein valves that are present but incompetent. This operation consists of meticulous resuspension of the individual incompetent valve leaflets using microvascular techniques. The details are illustrated by Kistner,[17] who reported 90 per cent symptomatic relief up to 7 years in selected patients. Alternatively, a segment of normal vein containing a competent valve, typically a segment of brachial vein taken from the arm, can be interposed into the femoral vein to restore venous valvular competence.[26] Taheri and co-workers reported corrected venous flow physiology in 13 of 30 patients undergoing this procedure; 14 retained venous reflux and three developed thrombosis of the femoral vein.[25]

SELECTED REFERENCES

Kistner, R. L.: Surgical repair of the incompetent femoral vein valve. Arch. Surg., *110*:1336, 1975.
Dr. Kistner has an extensive experience with the direct microvascular repair of incompetent vein valve leaflets in the deep venous system of the lower extremity. This report details the operative technique, summarizes his results, and emphasizes the importance of concomitant conventional medical and surgical therapy for optimal results in these patients.

Sigg, K., and Zelikovski, A.: "Quick treatment"—a modified method of sclerotherapy of varicose veins. Vasa, *4*:73, 1975.
The technique of compression sclerotherapy is emerging as a cost-effective option to surgical treatment of simple varicose veins. This article summarizes the results of 58,000 cases treated in Switzerland.

Thomson, H.: The surgical anatomy of the superficial and perforating veins of the lower limb. Ann. R. Coll. Surg. Engl., *61*:198, 1979.
This is an excellent review of the relevant surgical anatomy of the venous system of the lower extremities.

REFERENCES

1. Anderson, F. A., Jr., and Cardullo, P. C.: Problems commonly encountered in IPG testing and their solution. Bruit, *4*:21, 1980.
2. Arnesen, H., Holseth, A., and Lyle, B.: Streptokinase or heparin in the treatment of deep vein thrombosis: Follow-up results of a prospective study. Acta Med. Scand., *211*:65, 1982.
3. Davis, D. D.: An essay on the proximate cause of the disease called phlegmasia dolens. Trans. R. Med. Surg. S.D.C. London, *12*:419, 1923.
4. DeBakey, M. E., and Ochsner, A.: Phlegmasia cerulea dolens and gangrene associated with thrombophlebitis: Case reports and review of the literature. Surgery, *26*:16, 1949.
5. Diserio, F. J., Sasahara, A. A.: United States trial of dihydroergotamine and heparin prophylaxis of deep vein thrombosis. Am. J. Surg., *150* (Suppl. 4A):35, 1985.
6. Fegan, G.: Varicose Veins: Compression Sclerotherapy. Springfield, Ill., Charles C Thomas, 1967.
7. Ferris, E. B., and Kistner, R. L.: Femoral vein reconstruction: The management of chronic venous insufficiency. A fourteen-year experience. Arch. Surg., *117*:1571, 1982.
8. Flanc, D., Kakkar, V. V., and Clarke, M. B.: The detection of venous thrombosis of the legs using 125-I-labelled fibrinogen. Br. J. Surg., *55*:742, 1968.
9. Fogarty, T. J., Dennis, D., and Krippaehne, W. W.: Surgical management of iliofemoral thrombosis. Ann. Surg., *112*:211, 1966.
10. Glazier, R. L., and Crowell, E. G.: Randomized prospective trial of continuous versus intermittent heparin therapy. J.A.M.A., *236*:1365, 1976.
11. Goldhaber, S. Z., Buring, J. E., Ipnick, R. J., and Hennekens, C. H.: Pooled analysis of randomized trials of streptokinase and heparin in phlebographically documented acute deep venous thrombosis. Am. J. Med., *76*:393, 1984.
12. Haller, J. A., Jr., and Abrams, B. L.: Use of thrombectomy in the treatment of acute iliofemoral thrombosis in forty-five patients. Ann. Surg., *158*:561, 1963.
13. Hobbs, J. T.: Surgery and sclerotherapy in the treatment of varicose veins: A random trial. Arch. Surg., *109*:793, 1974.
14. Hull, R., Hirsh, J., Sackett, D. L., and Stoddart, G.: Cost-effectiveness of clinical diagnosis, venography, and non-invasive testing in patients with symptomatic deep vein thrombosis. N. Engl. J. Med., *304*:1561, 1981.
15. Hull, R., Raskob, G., and Hirsh, J.: A cost-effectiveness analysis of alternative approaches for long-term treatment of proximal venous thrombosis. J.A.M.A., *252*:235, 1984.
16. Kakkar, V. V., Howe, C. T., Flanc, C., et al.: Natural history of postoperative deep vein thrombosis. Lancet, *2*:230, 1969.
17. Kistner, R. L.: Surgical repair of the incompetent femoral vein valve. Arch Surg., *110*:1336, 1975.
18. Kistner, R. L., and Sparkuhl, M. D.: Surgery in acute and chronic venous disease. Surgery, *85*:31, 1979.
19. Lansing, A. M., and Davis, W. M.: Five year follow-up study of iliofemoral venous thrombectomy. Ann. Surg., *168*:620, 1968.
20. Linton, R. R.: The communicating veins of the lower leg and the operative technique for their ligation. Ann. Surg., *107*:582, 1938.
21. Multicenter Trial Committee: Dihydroergotamine-heparin prophylaxis of postoperative deep vein thrombosis. J.A.M.A., *251*:2960, 1984.
22. Sasahara, A. A.: International Multi-Center Trial: Prevention of fatal postoperative pulmonary embolism by low doses of heparin. Lancet, *2*:45, 1975.
23. Sigg, K., and Zelikovski, A.: "Quick treatment": A modified method of sclerotherapy of varicose veins. Vasa, *4*:73, 1975.
24. Sladen, J. G.: Compression sclerotherapy: Preparation, technique, complications, and results. Am. J. Surg., *146*:228, 1983.
25. Taheri, S. A., Heffner, R., Elias, S. M., Lazar, L., and Marchand, P.: Vein valve transplant. Contemp. Surg., *22*:17, 1983.
26. Taheri, S. A., Lazar, L., Elias, S. M., and Marchand, P.: Vein valve transplantation. Surgery, *91*:28, 1982.
27. Thomson, H.: The surgical anatomy of the superficial and perforating veins of the lower limb. Ann. R. Coll. Surg. Engl., *61*:198, 1979.
28. Wheeler, H. B., Anderson, F. A., Jr., Cardullo, P. A., Patwardhan, N. A., Jiang-Ming, L., and Cutler, B. S.: Suspected deep vein thrombosis: Management by impedance plethysmography. Arch. Surg., *117*:1206, 1982.

PULMONARY EMBOLISM

H. KIM LYERLY, M.D. • DAVID C. SABISTON, JR., M.D.

43

I

Overview

Pulmonary embolism continues as a serious complication of a variety of primary medical and surgical disorders. There is current evidence that more than 600,000 patients develop this complication annually in the United States, with some 200,000 deaths attributed to pulmonary embolism each year.[13] It is an interesting fact that the majority of patients with acute pulmonary embolism have this complication as a result of a serious *medical* disorder. However, the incidence of pulmonary embolism in *postoperative* patients remains significant and often presents as an acute emergency. The seriousness of this problem is illustrated by the fact that, in routine autopsies in patients over the age of 40, two thirds have evidence of either microscopic or gross pulmonary embolism. It should be emphasized that in most of these patients this finding is incidental, but in others it contributes to death and in a small number is the *principal cause of death*.

HISTORIC ASPECTS

In 1819, Laennec described "pulmonary apoplexy,"[28] which, in retrospect, was probably pulmonary embolism. In describing infarcts of the lung, Cruveilhier, in 1829,[12] made the observation that "all arterial branches which lead to those lesions were filled with clots that branched according to the vascular tree." However, it is to Rudolph Virchow, the father of modern pathology, to whom primary credit is due for introducing the embolic concept of pulmonary embolism. Prior to his observations, it was felt that thrombi in the pulmonary arteries arose *in situ* in the vessel and had no connection with distant venous thrombosis. Virchow studied a series of patients at autopsy, each of whom had sudden onset of severe respiratory insufficiency while in the hospital for an entirely different reason; he found emboli in the pulmonary arteries in every patient. When a careful search was conducted to identify the *origin* of these emboli, evidence of thrombi was found in the iliofemoral or pelvic veins in each of these patients. With these data Virchow conclusively demonstrated for the first time the *embolic* basis of this condition.[56]

PATHOGENESIS OF VENOUS THROMBOSIS

Virchow is known for his *triad* of causes of venous thrombosis:
1. Stasis of the blood in the veins.
2. Injury to the intimal surface of the veins, predisposing them to thrombosis
3. A generalized state of hypercoagulability.

Stasis

In postoperative patients, *stasis* is often important since they do not move nearly as much as they would normally, particularly if the incision is painful on motion of any part of the body. In this connection, adequate analgesia for relief of pain is important in maintaining the patient's normal mobility in the postoperative period. The histologic development of a thrombus is interesting, in that platelets usually become adherent to the recesses of the venous valves because they are located in a site of reduced velocity of blood flow. As the platelets, together with leukocytes and fibrin, accumulate on the endothelium along with erythrocytes, a thrombus develops. Ultimately the thrombus involves the entire vessel wall, thus totally occluding the venous lumen (Fig. 1).[11]

Injury

Venous emboli also form as the result of *injury* to the venous wall, either by blunt trauma or as the result of operative procedures in the region, particularly the thigh and leg.

Hypercoagulability

Although *hypercoagulability* is not well understood, it is generally defined as "the existence of an excessive amount

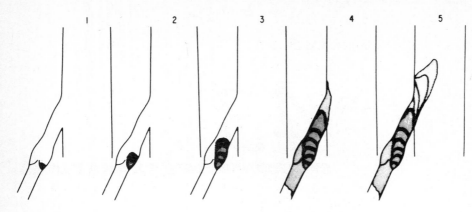

Figure 1. Illustration showing propagation of deep thrombus arising in a valvular pocket with deposition of successive layers and ultimate extension of the nonadherent red thrombus into the lumen of a larger parent vein. (From Cox, J. L., and Sabiston, D. C., Jr.: Phlebitis, thrombosis, and pulmonary embolism. In Condon, R. E., and DeCosse, J. J. (Eds.): Surgical Care: A Physiologic Approach to Problems in the First Fifteen Postoperative Days. Philadelphia, Lea & Febiger, 1980.)

of activity of one or more procoagulant substances or a decrease in anticoagulant factors."[2, 3] There are a large number of hypercoagulable disorders (Table 1).[52] These include antithrombin III, protein C, fibrinogen, and plasminogen activator deficiencies. Elements of the hemostatic system associated with primary hypercoagulability disorders are depicted in Figure 2. There are also *secondary* states, including the postoperative period, presence of malignant (particularly metastatic) disease, all oral contraceptives and estrogens, and pregnancy. In addition, a number of platelet disorders have, at times, been incriminated. Also, there are specific defects in the hemostatic system that occur in the presence of a state of hypercoagulability (Table 2).

When patients with a suspected hypercoagulable state are examined, several features should be carefully sought, beginning with a detailed family history of possible thromboembolism. Other features are listed in Table 3. The *laboratory tests* are important in determining the presence of hypercoagulability, and these are listed in Table 4. The specific coagulable states are listed in Table 5, together with the appropriate assay employed in the laboratory to

assess the problem as well as comments about each. Many of the aspects relating to the hypercoagulable state have specific relevance to the pathogenesis, clinical manifestations, and management of patients with *chronic and recurrent* pulmonary embolism, which are discussed later in this chapter. This condition is quite serious since it is generally associated with a progressive course of pulmonary insufficiency, pulmonary hypertension, right ventricular failure, and, ultimately, death.

PATHOLOGIC ASPECTS

Autopsy Findings

Evidence of pulmonary embolism at autopsy is quite common, and fresh or old pulmonary emboli are present in 64 per cent of autopsies of individuals over the age of 40.[16] Although *reflex* responses are of importance in the physiologic changes that follow pulmonary embolism, these responses are often of short duration and disappear in a matter of minutes or several hours. The *mechanical* factors are of primary significance, and the seriousness of clinical pulmonary embolism is most frequently due to the magnitude of pulmonary embolism or, more precisely stated, the percentage of occlusion of the pulmonary arterial tree. In most autopsy series, it has been shown that more than half of the total pulmonary arterial circulation must be occluded to produce serious physiologic changes in *otherwise normal patients*. However, if a patient has underlying cardiac or pulmonary insufficiency, smaller amounts of pulmonary embolism can be associated with serious clinical manifestations. It is an interesting fact that both experimental and clinical pulmonary emboli undergo spontaneous thrombolysis within the pulmonary arterial system with the passage of time.[15, 29, 46] This resolution is due to naturally circulating *thrombolysins* in both the experimental animal and man. A patient with total acute occlusion of the left pulmonary artery by pulmonary emboli with complete resolution by the fifteenth day is presented in Figure 3.[44]

In patients dying of pulmonary embolism, autopsy findings usually show the emboli to range from 1 to 1.5 cm. in diameter, obviously having arisen in veins of sizable diameter. Some thrombi are as long 50 cm., but most are smaller. Moreover, it is evident that thrombi passing through the heart fragment in their course to the lungs. The vast majority of pulmonary emboli arise in the systemic circulation, primarily from the iliac, femoral, and pelvic veins.[17, 31, 43] It is noteworthy that thrombophlebitis generally develops in the veins below the knee in the calf vessels,

---

TABLE 1. Hypercoagulable Disorders*

Primary
1. Antithrombin III deficiencies (congenital or acquired)
2. Protein C deficiency
3. Abnormal fibrinogen
4. Decreased or abnormal plasminogen
5. Vascular plasminogen activator deficiency
6. Plasminogen activator inhibitor
7. ? Factor XII deficiency
8. Homocystinuria

Secondary
1. Immobilization
2. Postoperative state
3. Malignancy
4. Pregnancy
5. Oral contraceptives and estrogens
6. Nephrotic syndrome
7. Other drugs: heparin, EACA, prothrombin complex concentrates (Proplex, Konyne)
8. "Lupus-like anticoagulant"
9. Platelet disorders: e.g., myeloproliferative disorders, paroxysmal nocturnal hemoglobinuria, diabetes mellitus, hypercholesterolemia (?)
10. "Hyperviscosity": e.g., Waldenström's macroglobulinemia, polycythemia
11. Prosthetic surfaces

*From Stead, R. B.: The hypercoagulable state. In Goldhaber, S. Z. (Ed.): Pulmonary Embolism and Deep Venous Thrombosis. Philadelphia, W. B. Saunders Company, 1985.

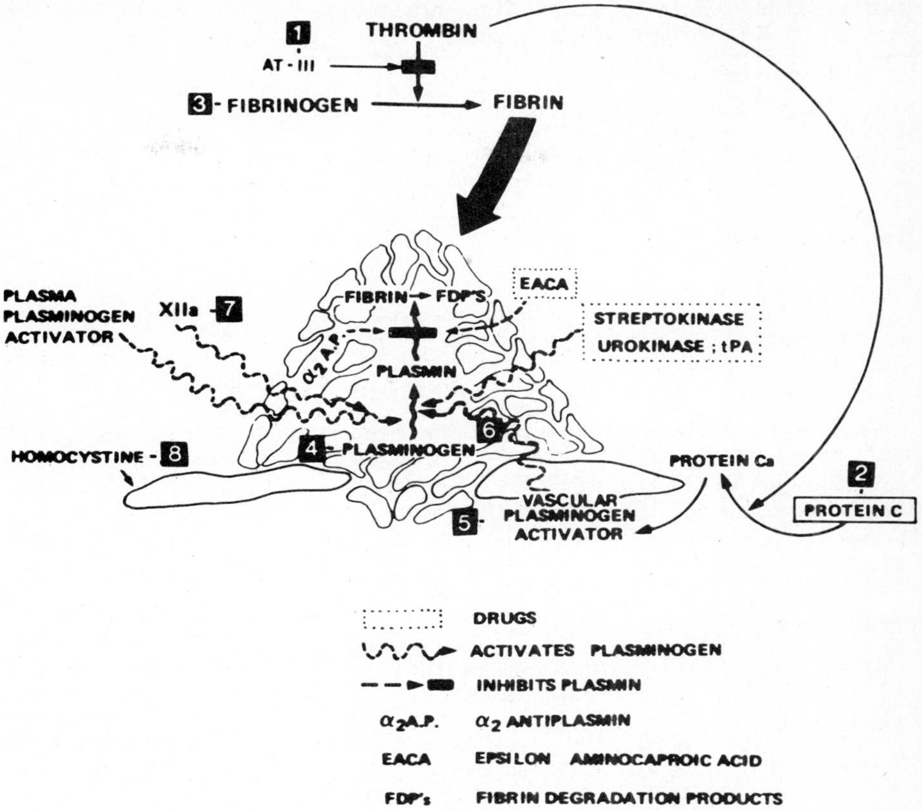

Figure 2. Elements of the hemostatic system that have been associated with primary hypercoagulable disorders. (From Stead, R. B.: The hypercoagulable state. In Goldhaber, S. Z.: Pulmonary Embolism and Deep Venous Thrombosis. Philadelphia, W. B. Saunders Company, 1985.)

but these are veins of small diameter, and if the venous thrombosis is localized solely to these veins, few, if any, serious complications are apt to occur even if the thrombi embolize to the lungs. It is the *larger* veins, such as the femoral and iliac vessels, that cause most of the serious clinical problems, since by virtue of their size they cause greater occlusion.

Material Other Than Thrombi

It should be remembered that material other than thrombi can embolize to the lung, including tumor embolization (especially renal cell carcinoma) and missiles (such as bullet embolization). When missiles are present in the pulmonary arteries, it is generally wise to remove them since they cause complications, including death.[53] Primary pulmonary neoplasms can mimic pulmonary embolism.[37] Pulmonary embolism should be carefully differentiated from pulmonary infarction, since only 10 per cent of patients with embolism develop pulmonary infarcts and such patients usually have hemoptysis, which can also occur *without* infarction.

Predisposing Factors

There are a number of *predisposing factors* in addition to stasis, injury, and hypercoagulability. Among these is *age* (emboli are rare in the young). Only about 1 per cent of all pulmonary emboli occur in children.[23] Heart disease (particularly congestive heart failure and atrial fibrillation), carcinomatosis, serious infections, and cerebrovascular accidents are often found to be predisposing causes of pulmonary embolism. Patients with various traumatic lesions,

particularly fractures of the hip and extensive soft tissue damage to the lower extremities, have a higher incidence of pulmonary embolism. It has long been known that surgical procedures, particularly prostatectomy, hip fracture repairs, and operations on the lower extremities, are also associated with a higher risk of pulmonary embolism. Oral contraceptives are also known to increase the incidence of both thrombophlebitis and pulmonary embolism.[32, 55]

PHYSIOLOGIC RESPONSES TO PULMONARY EMBOLISM

Patients with a pneumonectomy but an otherwise normal remaining lung have little difficulty with respiratory insufficiency, particularly at rest. Therefore, 50 per cent of the pulmonary arterial circulation can be occluded with few serious clinical symptoms. Moreover, in normal experimental animals and man, occlusion of a pulmonary artery by a balloon or clinical emboli causes few symptoms until more than 50 per cent of the arterial bed is occluded. These data correlate well with the postmortem studies demonstrating few serious physiologic changes in otherwise normal patients unless more than 50 per cent of the pulmonary arterial circulation is occluded. However, as the percentage of occlusion increases, respiratory insufficiency ensues, particularly if there is any pre-existing cardiac or respiratory disease.

DIAGNOSIS OF PULMONARY EMBOLISM

The *clinical manifestations* of pulmonary embolism are primarily dyspnea, chest pain, and hemoptysis (Table 6).

TABLE 2. Defects in the Hemostatic System Associated with the Hypercoagulable State*

Defective Hemostatic Component	Example
Abnormalities in blood flow	Sickle cell anemia Waldenström's macroglobulinemia Venous stasis
Abnormal vessel wall	Prosthetic heart valves; shunts Homocystinuria (?)
Platelet abnormalities Elevated platelet count (>10⁶/mm³)	Usually not, but may be in patients with myeloproliferative disorders, especially after splenectomy
Qualitative platelet defects	Myeloproliferative disorders Diabetes mellitus Hypercholesterolemia
Abnormal clotting factors	Factor XII deficiency
Abnormal or deficient inhibitors	Antithrombin III deficiency (qualitative or quantitative) Protein C deficiency
Circulating, activated clotting factors	Malignancy Disseminated intravascular coagulation (DIC) Liver disease
Abnormal fibrinolysis	Dysfibrinogenemia (usually more susceptible to bleeding but some examples of resistance to fibrinolysis) Diminished release of vascular plasminogen activator Qualitative or quantitative decrease in plasminogen

*From Stead, R. B.: The hypercoagulable state. *In* Goldhaber, S. Z. (Ed.): Pulmonary Embolism and Deep Venous Thrombosis. Philadelphia, W. B. Saunders Company, 1985.

Clinical signs, in order of incidence, include tachycardia, fever, rales, tachypnea, and evidence of thrombophlebitis in the lower extremities.

Asymptomatic pulmonary embolism is very common, and in one series of 158 postoperative patients following either hip reconstruction or major amputation, pulmonary scans showed that 33 had strong evidence of pulmonary embolism. Twenty-one underwent pulmonary arteriography, with 19 being positive. It is to be emphasized that

TABLE 3. When to Suspect Primary Hypercoagulable Disorders: Clinical Features*

Strong family history of "idiopathic" thromboembolism

Onset at an early age (less than age 35)

Two or more *well-documented* recurrences

Refractory to conventional therapy or early recurrence following discontinuation of prolonged therapy

Absence of other predisposing systemic disease, e.g., malignancy

Unusual location or presentation, e.g., mesenteric or axillary vein thrombosis; DVT *early* in pregnancy

*From Stead, R. B.: The hypercoagulable state. *In* Goldhaber, S. Z. (Ed.): Pulmonary Embolism and Deep Venous Thrombosis. Philadelphia, W. B. Saunders Company, 1985.

in each of these patients there were no *clinical symptoms* of pulmonary embolism. Moreover, autopsy data have confirmed similar findings in many reports.

LABORATORY FINDINGS

The plain chest film may show evidence of *diminished vascular markings* in the area of pulmonary emboli (Westermark's sign). Later, signs of congestion or atelectasis may appear in areas of embolism. A slight elevation in bilirubin, due to resolution of the emboli in the lungs, is sometimes present, and lactate dehydrogenase (LDH) activity may be increased. The electrocardiogram (ECG) is seldom specific for pulmonary embolism, and not more than 20 per cent of patients with proven pulmonary emboli demonstrate any ECG changes of significance. Electrocardiographic alterations include disturbances of rhythm, such as atrial fibrillation, ectopic beats, or heart block, and enlargement of the P waves, ST-segment depression, and T wave inversion may be seen.

Levels of Po_2 in the arterial and venous blood, together with the pH, are of importance. In patients who are otherwise normal, reduced arterial Po_2 (particularly in the range of 50 to 70 mm. Hg) is strong evidence of pulmonary embolism. Moreover, carbon dioxide retention is common, with an increase in the Pco_2 level. The echocardiogram, especially a two-dimensional study, can be helpful in the diagnosis of massive pulmonary embolism by demonstrating an enlarged, volume-overloaded right ventricle. This is

TABLE 4. Nonspecific Tests Available for the Laboratory Evaluation of the Suspected Hypercoagulable Patient*

A. Tests that detect transient responses to trauma and inflammation

  Elevated levels of "unactivated" clotting factors: fibrinogen, factors V, VII, VIII

  Elevated platelet count

  Reduced levels of antithrombin III

  Reduced fibrinolytic activity
    Prolonged euglobulin lysis time
    Elevated antiplasmin time

B. Tests that detect clinical or subclinical thrombosis

  Platelet activation or release
    Shortened platelet survival
    Elevated thromboxane B_2 (TxB_2)
    Elevated platelet factor 4 (PF4)
    Elevated beta thromboglobulin (βTG)
    Elevated circulating platelet aggregates
    Spontaneous or hyperreactive platelet aggregation

  Activation of coagulation enzymes
    Fibrin formation
    Elevated fibrin split products (FSPs)
    Elevated fibrin monomer complexes
    Increased fibrinogen turnover
    Elevate fibrinopeptide A (FPA)
    Elevated fibrin (fibrinogen fragment E)

  Thrombin generation
    Elevated F_{1+2} fragment
    Elevated thrombin:antithrombin complexes

  Plasmin:antiplasmin complexes

*From Stead, R. B.: The hypercoagulable state. *In* Goldhaber, S. Z. (Ed.): Pulmonary Embolism and Deep Venous Thrombosis. Philadelphia, W. B. Saunders Company, 1985.

TABLE 5. *Specific Tests Available for Laboratory Evaluation of the Suspected Hypercoagulable Patient**

Condition	Assay	Comments
Abnormal or deficient inhibitors of coagulation		
1. AT III deficiency	Immunologic Functional	Assay widely (commercially) available; warfarin may elevate levels and heparin may decrease levels. Depressed levels may be associated with secondary hypercoagulable state
2. Protein C deficiency	Immunologic Functional	Assay not readily available; must be measured for anticoagulants or normalized for anticoagulant effect
Defective fibrinolysis		
1. Defective release of plasminogen activator	Functional	Assay not widely available
2. Factor XII deficiency	Functional	PTT prolonged; assay widely available
3. Plasminogen activator inhibitor	Functional	Impaired fibrinolysis
4. Abnormal fibrinogen (dysfibrinogenemia)	Functional	Usually associated with bleeding but may be associated with thrombosis
5. Abnormal plasminogen	Immunologic Functional	Assay not widely available
Other		
1. Homocystinuria	Biochemical	Arterial and venous events commonly associated with endothelial damage
2. Myeloproliferative disease		Usually associated with bleeding, but may be associated with thrombosis. No assay available, clinical features of myeloproliferative disease apparent (e.g., splenomegaly, abnormal CBC, platelet count, karyotype, LAP score)
3. "Lupus-like anticoagulant"	Functional	PTT prolonged; assay widely available. May be associated with a secondary hypercoagulable state

*From Stead, R. B.: The hypercoagulable state. In Goldhaber, S. Z. (Ed.): Pulmonary Embolism and Deep Venous Thrombosis. Philadelphia, W. B. Saunders Company, 1985.

particularly apt to occur in a patient with severe, massive embolism with hypoxemia and shock (Fig. 4).[22]

Pulmonary scanning is a helpful screening device, particularly if the plain chest film is otherwise *completely normal*. It should be emphasized that if there are any radiopacities in the lung, which may be caused by atelectasis, pneumonitis, neoplasm, fluid, or hemothorax, these areas are not amenable to interpretation on the scan, since each of these conditions reduce pulmonary arterial blood flow in the area involved, producing a *positive* perfusion defect. Thus, if the plain film is abnormal, one should not generally proceed with a radioactive pulmonary scan but move directly to pulmonary arteriography, which is the most objective test that can be employed. If significant pulmonary embolism is present, it will almost always be demonstrable by pulmonary arteriography.

MEDICAL MANAGEMENT

Heparin

It is essential to establish a *firm* diagnosis of pulmonary embolism, either by radioactive scan (technetium-99m or iodine-131) or pulmonary arteriogram, prior to beginning definitive therapy, since this therapy may be associated with complications.[37] The standard management regimen of proven pulmonary embolism includes intravenous heparin. Generally, 15,000 units should be administered intravenously as the initial dose, with 5000 to 10,000 units administered every 4 to 6 hours thereafter. It is preferable to deliver the heparin by continuous intravenous drip with a motor-driven pump. The amount of heparin administered depends upon the prolongation of the activated partial thromboplastin time (APTT) to approximately twice the patient's pre-heparin time. The duration of heparin therapy

is individualized depending upon the clinical course. In general, 8 to 10 days of heparin therapy are recommended; therapy may be discontinued after this time provided there has been no evidence of further emboli.

Coumarin

Oral coumarin administration is begun several days prior to cessation of heparin therapy to allow the required period for adequate prolongation of the prothrombin time (PT). Although there is a difference of opinion concerning the length of time that coumarin should be given, varying from not at all to an indefinite period of anticoagulation, most believe that a period of 3 to 6 months is adequate. If there are no further clinical manifestations of thrombophlebitis or pulmonary embolism at that time, coumarin can be safely discontinued.

Thrombolytics

In the recent past, *thrombolytic agents* have been used effectively in patients, particularly those with *acute* and *early subacute* pulmonary emboli. Under normal circumstances, plasminogen is present in the blood and tissues, and two thrombolysins, streptokinase and urokinase, have been studied extensively. Both of these act by transforming plasminogen to plasmin. In the recent past the introduction of human plasminogen activator has lessened the likelihood of toxic reactions to these lytic agents; it has also been found quite useful in resolution of emboli.[6, 10]

Recombinant tissue type plasminogen activator has also been utilized for thrombolytic therapy in patients with massive pulmonary embolism.[8] It has been shown that defective release of tissue plasminogen activator (t-PA), as stimulated by venous occlusion, correlates quite well with

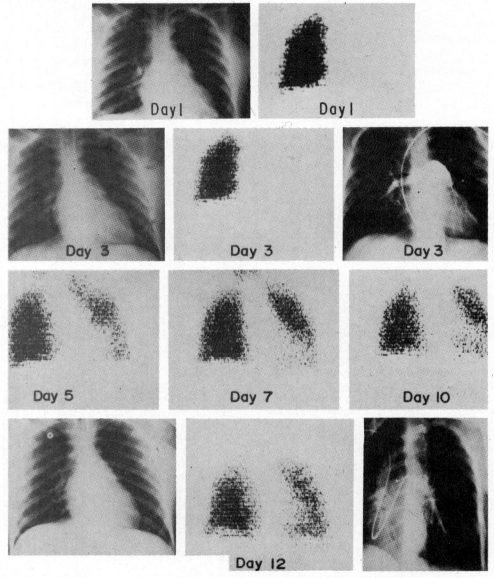

Figure 3. Serial chest films and scans following a massive pulmonary embolus to the left pulmonary artery in a 25-year-old woman after a pelvic operation. On the fifth postoperative day, discomfort was noted in the left chest with dyspnea. A plain chest film taken on this day (day 1) showed diminished vascular markings (Westermark's sign). A radioactive pulmonary scan showed no evidence of pulmonary flow to the entire left lobe. Beginning on the third day after the embolus, the scan and arteriogram both showed evidence of flow to the left lung. In subsequent scans and pulmonary arteriograms, resolution of the thrombus occurred with progressively increasing amounts of flow by the twelfth day. (From Sabiston, D. C., Jr.: Pulmonary embolism. In Sabiston, D. C., Jr. (Ed.): Textbook of Surgery, 13th ed. Philadelphia, W. B. Saunders Company, 1986.)

TABLE 6. Clinical Manifestations in 1000 Patients with Pulmonary Embolism at the Duke University Medical Center*

Symptoms	Per Cent
Dyspnea	77
Chest pain	63
Hemoptysis	26
Altered mental status	23
Dyspnea, chest pain, hemoptysis	14

Signs	Per Cent
Tachycardia	59
Recent fever	43
Rales	42
Tachypnea	38
Leg edema and tenderness	23
Elevated venous pressure	18
Shock	11
Accentuated P_2	11
Cyanosis	9
Pleural friction rub	8

*From Sabiston, D. C., Jr.: Pulmonary embolism. *In* Sabiston, D. C., Jr. (Ed.): Textbook of Surgery, 13th ed. Philadelphia, W. B. Saunders Company, 1986.

venous thromboembolic disease.[41] A fast-acting inhibitor of t-PA has also been identified and measured in human plasma.[9, 25] Recently it has shown that patients reported to have certain forms of venous thrombosis have an imbalance between activator and inhibitor levels rather than an actual deficiency of t-PA.[42]

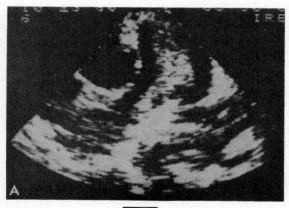

Figure 4. Thrombus in pulmonary artery. A, Two-dimensional echocardiogram in the short-axis parasternal view. B, Schematic drawing in the pulmonary artery. (From Hoagland, P. M.: Massive pulmonary embolism. In Goldhaber, S. Z.: Pulmonary Embolism and Deep Venous Thrombosis. Philadelphia, W. B. Saunders Company, 1985.)

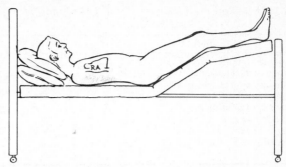

Figure 5. Correct positioning of lower extremities in prophylaxis of pulmonary embolism. Note the additional break at the knee. It is important that the level of the veins in the lower extremities be above the mean level of the right atrium (RA). (From Sabiston, D. C., Jr.: Pulmonary embolism. In Sabiston, D. C., Jr. (Ed.): Textbook of Surgery, 13th ed. Philadelphia, W. B. Saunders Company, 1986.)

PROPHYLAXIS OF PULMONARY EMBOLISM

Much has been written concerning the various approaches to the prophylaxis of venous thrombosis and pulmonary embolism. For example, increased physical activity, elevation of the lower extremities while in bed, stocking compression of the legs, and prophylactic anticoagulation have each been recommended. Clearly, stasis is eliminated if the thighs and legs are elevated above the level of the right atrium (Fig. 5).[44] Gravity can always be relied upon to drain venous blood from the legs rapidly and thus greatly reduce the likelihood of stasis emboli. Although there have been many advocates of low-dose heparin therapy,[26] considerable doubt exists as to whether this form of therapy is actually beneficial.[34] Postoperatively, bleeding can be a problem in patients receiving low-dose heparin therapy.

SURGICAL MANAGEMENT

Although anticoagulant therapy is usually successful in preventing further pulmonary emboli, occasionally recurrent emboli persist. At this point surgical therapy may be indicated. Whereas in the past there had been considerable support for interruption of the inferior vena cava, support has decreased during the past decade due, in large part, to the complications that have been reported following this procedure.[14] Interruption of the inferior vena cava can be considered for several special situations (Table 7).[7] Complications of caval interruption include persistent leg edema and ulceration; in addition, recurrent emboli and death may occur following caval interruption.[5, 38] The results of vena caval ligation in a large collected series are shown in Table 8.[1, 4, 5, 27, 33, 35, 36, 38, 40, 48, 57]

In an attempt to reduce the complications of inferior vena caval interruption, whether by ligation, plication, filters, or clips (Fig. 6),[44] a cone umbrella-like filter was designed to interrupt *large* emboli passing into the inferior vena cava (Fig. 7). This has been reported to be quite effective[18-20] and can be placed with the patient under local anesthesia. However, these filters can migrate and have been found in the right atrium and the pulmonary artery and have eroded through the vein into the retroperitoneum

TABLE 7. Reported Indications for Interruption of the Inferior Vena Cava

Indication	N	%
Complication or failure of AC	502	44
Heparin contraindicated	257	23
Caval/iliofemoral vein thrombosis	152	13
Prophylactic	92	8
Severe PE initial therapy	87	8
PE requiring embolectomy	25	2
Recurrent PE	24	2
Septic thrombophlebitis or PE	19	2
Total	1133	102

From Bomalaski, J. S., et al.: Chest, *82*:767, 1982.

Abbreviations: AC = Anticoagulants; N = number of patients; PE = pulmonary embolism; % = percentage of total patients reported receiving vena caval interruption. Total percentage is greater than 100 per cent owing to multiple indications in some patients.

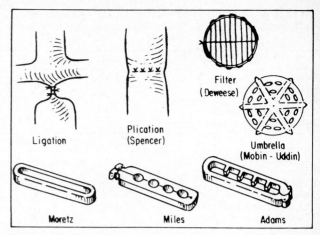

Figure 6. Diagrammatic representation of surgical approaches for interruption of the inferior vena cava in prevention of pulmonary embolism. The umbrella and the clips are constructed of plastic material. (From Sabiston, D. C., Jr.: Pulmonary embolism. In Sabiston, D. C., Jr. (Ed.): Textbook of Surgery, 13th ed. Philadelphia, W. B. Saunders Company, 1986.)

(Table 9).[22] Some have also passed into both of the right common iliac vessels, and others have been found in the renal pelvis.[58] For these reasons, some favor the continuation of heparin anticoagulation therapy despite recurrent emboli in the hope of avoiding problems that various caval procedures produce.[21, 51]

PULMONARY EMBOLECTOMY

First performed in 1908 by Trendelenburg, pulmonary embolectomy was originally a hazardous procedure. However, with the advent of extracorporeal circulation, it now has very definite indications in patients with massive embolism and profound circulatory collapse. Although most patients with pulmonary embolism, even though quite extensive, can be resuscitated with inotropic agents and respiratory support with endotracheal intubation and mechanical respiration, some remain in refractory shock. In this event, they become candidates for direct pulmonary embolectomy employing extracorporeal circulation. In general, such patients have a low arterial Po_2, an elevated Pco_2, and an accompanying acidosis. Recent results with

pulmonary embolectomy have demonstrated survival rates as high as 70 per cent, whereas in most patients with pulmonary embolism it is 40 to 50 per cent.[30] The chest film of a 72-year-old patient with massive pulmonary embolism following extraction of cataracts is shown in Figure 8.[47] In this patient, pulmonary embolic occlusion of only the left lower lobe pulmonary artery resulted in refractory shock not responsive to any medical management. Pulmonary embolectomy was performed, and emboli were removed from the left lower lobe pulmonary artery. The patient made an uneventful recovery. This illustrates the fact that a small amount of pulmonary embolism can produce severe clinical manifestations if the patient has pre-existing respiratory and cardiac insufficiency, as was present in this 72-year-old male. Prior to placing a patient on cardiopulmonary bypass, it is essential that a firm, objective diagnosis of pulmonary embolism be made either by pulmonary radioactive scanning or by pulmonary arteriography (Figs. 9 and 10).[24]

TABLE 8. Effectiveness of Inferior Vena Caval Ligation*

Reference	Number of Cases	Operative Mortality (Per Cent)	Recurrent Emboli (Per Cent)	Fatal Emboli (Per Cent)	Postphlebitic Sequelae (Per Cent)
Krause et al. (1963)[27]	55	5	0	0	—
Miles et al. (1964)[33]	40	15	3	0	32
Nabseth and Moran (1965)[38]	75	19	3	1	14
Bergan et al. (1965)[5]	11	9	9	0	18
Mozes et al. (1966)[36]	118	12	4	1	13
Wheeler et al. (1966)[57]	35	6	0	0	32
Amador et al. (1968)[4]	119	39	—	—	—
Moran et al. (1969)[35]	25	20	0	0	6
Ochsner et al. (1970)[39]	286	8	0	0	4
Piccone et al. (1970)[40]	72	13	36	22	33
Adams et al. (1971)[1]	38	13	8	3	43
Schowengerdt and Schreiber (1971)[48]	48	11	6	0	21
TOTAL	922	—	—	—	—
MEAN	—	14.2	6.3	2.1	—

*Adapted from Bernstein, E. F.: *In* Moser, K. M., and Stein, M. (Eds.): Pulmonary Thromboembolism. Chicago, Year Book Medical Publishers, Inc., 1973. Used by permission.

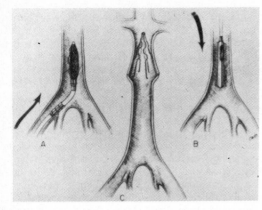

Figure 7. Insertion of the cone filter is accomplished by a carrier catheter inserted from the femoral vein (A) or retrograde from the jugular vein (B). To avoid misplacement into the right renal vein, the jugular inserter should be passed down to the level of the pelvis and then withdrawn to the level of L3 for discharge (C). Fixation is automatic, as the limbs spring open and the recurved hooks engage the wall of the inferior vena cava. (From Greenfield, L. J.: Curr. Probl. Surg., 13(4):1, 1976.)

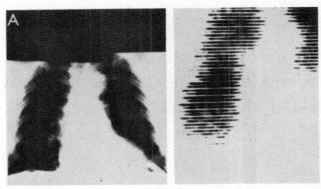

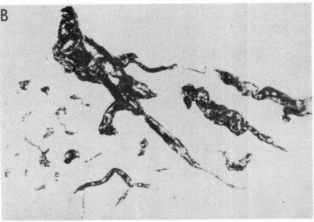

Pulmonary embolectomy for acute embolism is best performed through a median sternotomy. The pericardium is opened, and the patient is attached to cardiopulmonary bypass. The pulmonary artery is opened and the emboli are extracted. Both pulmonary arteries are copiously irrigated with saline to remove any small emboli. Passage of a Fogarty balloon catheter into the distal pulmonary arterial tree is effective in removing smaller emboli. Following closure of the pulmonary arteriotomy, the patient can be removed from cardiopulmonary bypass with resumption of acceptable cardiorespiratory function. If appropriate, interruption of the vena cava can be performed. The pulmonary scan of a patient with acute *massive* pulmonary embolism and intractable shock refractory to maximal resuscitation is shown in Figure 9.[45] The large emboli removed from the right and left pulmonary arteries are also shown.

Figure 8. A, Chest film from a postoperative patient with pre-existing cardiac and respiratory insufficiency. Pulmonary emboli are present in the left lower lobe. The patient was in severe and refractory shock. B, Emboli removed from the left lower lobe pulmonary artery at embolectomy. This resulted in improvement in the patient's signs and symptoms, and he made an uneventful recovery. (From Sabiston, D. C., Jr., and Wolfe, W. G.: Pulmonary embolectomy. In Moser, K. M., and Stein, M. (Eds.): Pulmonary Thromboembolism. Chicago, Year Book Medical Publishers, 1973.)

TABLE 9. Comparison of Transvenous Devices*

Reference	Number of Patients	Mortality	Venous Problems	Recurrent Emboli	Patency Rate
Mobin-Uddin Device					
MGH	41	5%	56%	10%	—
Wingerd	38	0%	75%	3 fatal	45%
Bomalaski	2,966	0.6%	9%	3.4%	40%
Cimochowski	65	4%	—	—	27%
Edwards Labs.	4,700	—	5%	2.2%	—
Mobin-Uddin	100	15%	—	45	—
Fullen	80	15%	—	2%	—
Lawrence	28	1%	—	11%	—
Senties	51	0%	—	0%	—
Menzoian	128	7%	—	0%	—
Schlosser	125	—	—	2%	—
Kimray-Greenfield Device					
MGH	56	5%	13%	3.6%	—
Wingerd	33	0%	38%	none fatal	95%
Bomalaski	141	3.5%	15%	—	—
Cimochowski	32	4%	—	—	95%
Greenfield	152	0%	17%	2% (none fatal)	95%

*Adapted From Hoagland, P. M.: *In* Goldhaber, S. Z. (Ed.): Pulmonary Embolism and Deep Venous Thrombosis. Philadelphia, W. B. Saunders Company, 1985.

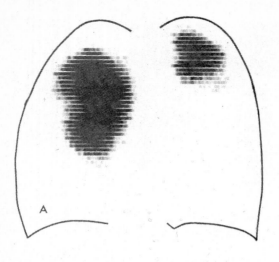

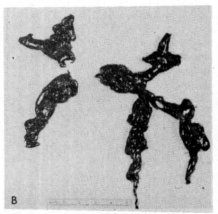

Figure 9. *Illustrations from a patient with massive pulmonary embolism on the twelfth postoperative day following an orthopedic operation and accompanied by intractable shock. A, The pulmonary scan shows massive occlusion of the right lower and middle lobar pulmonary arteries as well as nearly all of the pulmonary arterial circulation to the left lung. B, Emboli removed from both pulmonary arteries at the time of embolectomy. (From Sabiston, D. C., Jr.: Adv. Surg., 3:351, 1968.)*

Transvenous catheter embolectomy has also been recommended,[18] although this technique has not yet been widely accepted.

FAT EMBOLISM

In 1862, the famous German pathologist Zenker first described fat embolism in the pulmonary tissues of patients dying of a variety of injuries.[59] Fat embolism develops when fat emboli are mobilized from traumatized bone marrow at fracture sites and pass into the bloodstream. It has also been suggested that chylomicrons are formed from the release of neutral fats, which act as pulmonary emboli in the lung following injury. The latter are primarily fat droplets that have toxic effects on tissues. Clinical manifestations of fat embolism generally appear on around the third day following injury and are a contributing cause to the respiratory distress syndrome.

A diagnosis of *fat embolism syndrome* (FES) is primarily made by manifestations of hypoxia, confusion, pe-

techia, tachypnea, cyanosis, and the appearance of fluffy densities on the chest film. Fat globules may appear in the urine, but this is not necessarily of diagnostic significance. Although serum lipase levels may be elevated, this is not a consistent finding. If FES is of clinical significance, the arterial PO_2 is low, generally less than 60 mm. Hg on room air. This is associated with an increase in pH and a decrease in PCO_2 secondary to hyperventilation. On further deterioration, the PO_2 falls further with an increasing PCO_2 and the development of acidosis.

The treatment of FES is controversial. Clearly, fractures should be stabilized to prevent fat embolism into the venous system. Some have advocated the use of colloids, particularly albumin as a volume expander, which may be effective. Large doses of steroids (30 mg. per kg. for 24 hours in divided doses) have been recommended on both therapeutic and prophylactic bases.[49, 50, 54] Ventilatory sup-

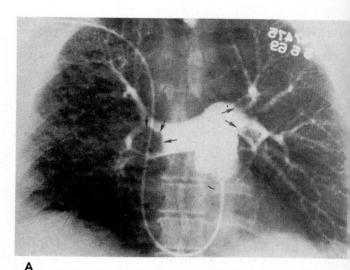

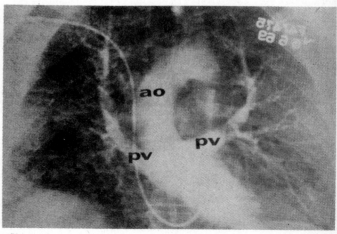

Figure 10. A, *Pulmonary arteriogram from patient with pulmonary embolism, indicating intraluminal defects and anatomic areas of occlusion by pulmonary emboli in both the right and left pulmonary arteries. B, Venous phase of pulmonary arteriogram showing return of contrast medium into pulmonary veins, left ventricle, and ascending aorta. Note that the most severe obstruction is in the pulmonary artery to the right lower lobe. Similarly, the venous drainage from the right inferior pulmonary vein is the least prominent. (From Jones, R. H., and Sabiston, D. C., Jr.: Surg. Clin. North Am., 56:891, 1976.)*

port is of definite value with the addition of positive end-expiratory pressure (PEEP). Therefore, this form of respiratory distress is similar to that of many other etiologic causes and generally should be managed similarly.

SELECTED REFERENCES

Bergqvist, D.: Postoperative Thromboembolism. Frequency, Etiology, Prophylaxis. New York, Springer-Verlag, 1983.
> *In this monograph, the author reviews the frequency, etiology, and prophylaxis of pulmonary embolism in postoperative patients. It also has one of the most extensive bibliographies available in the field (69 pages of references).*

Fishman, A. P.: Hypoxia on the pulmonary circulation: How and where it acts. Circ. Res., *38*:221, 1976.
> *This is an excellent review of the effects of hypoxia on the pulmonary circulation written by an outstanding investigator. The various potential mechanisms of hypoxia and its effect are reviewed in a highly recommendable manner.*

Goldhaber, S. Z. (Ed.): Pulmonary Embolism and Deep Venous Thrombosis. Philadelphia, W. B. Saunders Company, 1985.
> *This is an updated monograph that is quite complete and highly recommended to students wishing to consult an authoritative and considerably detailed series of presentations on all aspects of this subject.*

Gorham, I. W.: A study of pulmonary embolism. Parts I and II. Arch. Intern. Med., *108*:8, 189, 1961.
> *These companion papers emphasize the gross pathology of pulmonary embolism. Special emphasis is given the fact that in most patients with fatal embolism a substantial amount of the pulmonary arterial bed is occluded, generally more than half. This is one of the best pathologic studies in the literature.*

Moylan, J. A., and Evenson, M.: Diagnosis and treatment of fat embolism. Ann. Rev. Med., *28*:85, 1977.
> *These authors review the subject quite commendably, and they emphasize both management and prognosis.*

Sabiston, D. C., Jr., and Wolfe, W. G.: Experimental and clinical observations on the natural history of pulmonary embolism. Ann. Surg., *168*:1, 1968.
> *The natural history of pulmonary emboli in the experimental animal and man is presented. The gross and microscopic features and their changes with the passage of time are illustrated. The gradual resolution of the emboli and final disappearance in most instances are confirmed by serial scans and pulmonary arteriograms.*

Wagner, H. N., Jr., Sabiston, D. C., Jr., Ilio, M., McFee, J. G., Meyer, J. K., and Langan, J. K.: Regional pulmonary blood flow in man by radioisotope scanning. J.A.M.A., *187*:601, 1964.
> *The original experimental and clinical studies introducing the technique of radioactive pulmonary scanning are described.*

Wolfe, W. G., and Sabiston, D. C., Jr.: Pulmonary embolism. *In* Ebert, P. A. (Ed.): Major Problems in Clinical Surgery, Vol. 25. Philadelphia, W. B. Saunders Company, 1980.
> *This is a monograph with detailed consideration of the physiology, pathology, natural history, diagnosis, and management of all forms of pulmonary embolism.*

REFERENCES

1. Adams, J. T., Feingold, B. E., and DeWeese, J. A.: Comparative evaluation of ligation and partial interruption of the inferior vena cava. Arch. Surg., *172*:795, 1970.
2. Alexander, B.: Blood coagulation and thrombotic disease. Circulation, *25*:872, 1962.
3. Alexander, B., Meyers, L., Kenny, J., Goldstein, R., Gurewich, V., and Grinspoon, L.: Blood coagulation in pregnancy. Proconvertin and prothrombin, and the hypercoagulable state. N. Engl. J. Med., *254*:358, 1956.
4. Amador, E., Li, T. K., and Crane, C.: Ligation of inferior vena cava for thromboembolism. J.A.M.A., *206*:1758, 1968.
5. Bergan, J. J., Kinnaird, D. W., Koons, K., and Trippel, O. H.: Prevention of pulmonary embolism: Comparison of vena caval ligation, plication and filter operations in prevention of pulmonary emboli. Arch. Surg., *92*:605, 1966.
6. Bergman, S. R., Keith, A. A., Fox, M. B., et al.: Coronary thrombolysis achieved with human extrinsic plasminogen activator, a clot selective activator, administered intravenously. J. Am. Coll. Cardiol. *1*:615, 1983 (abstract).
7. Bomalaski, J. S., Martin, G. J., Jughes, R. L., and Yao, J. S. T.: Inferior vena cava interruption in the management of pulmonary embolism. Chest, *82*:767, 1982.
8. Bounameaux, H., Vermylan, J., and Collen, D.: Brief reports: Thrombolytic treatment with recombinant tissue-type plasminogen activator in a patient with massive pulmonary embolism. Ann. Intern. Med., *103*:64, 1985.
9. Chmielewska, J., Ranby, M., and Wiman, B.: Evidence for a rapid inhibitor to tissue plasminogen activator in plasma. Thromb. Res. 31:427, 1983.
10. Collen, D.: Tissue-type plasminogen activator: Therapeutic potential in thrombotic disease states. Drugs, *31*:1, 1986.
11. Cox, J. L., and Sabiston, D. C., Jr.: Phlebitis, thrombosis and pulmonary embolism. *In* Condon, R. E., and DeCosse, J. J. (Eds.): Surgical Care: A Physiologic Approach to Problems in the First Fifteen Postoperative Days. Philadelphia, Lea & Febiger, 1980.
12. Cruveilhier, J.: Anatomie Pathologique du Corps Humain. Paris, J. B. Bailliere, 1829–42.
13. Dalen, J. E., and Alpert, J. S.: Natural history of pulmonary embolism. Prog. Cardiovasc. Dis., *17*:259, 1975.
14. Donaldson, M. C., Wirthlin, L. S., and Donaldson, G. A.: Thirty-year experience with surgical interruption of the inferior vena cava for prevention of pulmonary embolism. Ann. Surg., *191*:367, 1980.
15. Fred, H. L., Axelrad, M. A., Lewis, J. M., and Alexander, J. K.: Rapid resolution of pulmonary thromboemboli in man. J.A.M.A., *196*:1137, 1966.
16. Freiman, D. G.: Pathologic observations on experimental and human thromboembolism. *In* Sasahara, A. A., and Stein, M. (Eds.): Pulmonary Embolic Disease. New York, Grune & Stratton, 1965.
17. Gibbs, N. M.: Venous thrombosis of the lower limbs with particular reference to bed rest. Br. J. Surg., *45*:209, 1957.
18. Greenfield, L. J.: Pulmonary Embolism: Diagnosis and Management. Current Problems in Surgery. Chicago, Year Book Medical Publishers, Inc., 1976.
19. Greenfield, L. J., McCurdy, J. R., Brown, P. P., and Elkins, R. C.: A new intracaval filter permitting continued flow and resolution of emboli. Surgery, *73*:599, 1973.
20. Greenfield, L. J., Zocco, J., Wilk, J., Schroeder, T. M., and Elkins, R. C.: Clinical experience with the Kim-Ray Greenfield vena caval filter. Ann. Surg., *185*:692, 1977.
21. Hirsh, J.: Venous thromboembolism: Diagnosis, treatment, prevention. Hosp. Prac., *10*:53, 1975.
22. Hoagland, P. M.: Massive pulmonary embolism. *In* Goldhaber, S. Z. (Ed.): Pulmonary Embolism and Deep Venous Thrombosis. Philadelphia, W. B. Saunders Company, 1985.
23. Jones, R. H., and Sabiston, D. C., Jr.: Pulmonary embolism in childhood. Monogr. Surg. Sci., *3*:35, 1966.
24. Jones, R. H., and Sabiston, D. C., Jr.: Pulmonary embolism. Surg. Clin. North Am., *56*:891, 1976.
25. Juhan-Vague, I., Moerman, B., DeCock, F., et al.: Plasma levels of a specific inhibitor of tissue-type plasminogen activator (and urokinase) in normal and pathological conditions. Thromb. Res., *33*:523, 1984.
26. Kakkar, V. V., et al.: Prevention of fatal postoperative pulmonary embolism by low doses of heparin: An international multicentre trial. Lancet, *2*:45, 1975.
27. Krause, R. J., Cranley, J. J., Hallaba, M. A. S., Strasser, E. S., and Hafner, D. D.: Caval ligation in thromboembolic disease. Arch. Surg., *87*:184, 1963.
28. Laennec, R. T. H.: De l'Auscultation Mediate. Paris, Brossen et Chaude, 1819.
29. Marshall, R., Sabiston, D. C., Jr., Allison, P. R., Bosman, A. R., and Dunnill, M. S.: Immediate and late effects of pulmonary embolism by large thrombi in dogs. Thorax, *18*:1, 1963.
30. Mattox, K. L., Feldtman, R. W., Beall, A. C., Jr., and DeBakey, M. E.: Pulmonary embolectomy for acute massive pulmonary embolism. Ann. Surg., *195*:726, 1982.
31. McLachlin, J., and Paterson, J. C.: Some basic observations on venous thrombosis and pulmonary embolism. Surg. Gynecol. Obstet., *93*:1, 1951.
32. Medical Research Council Subcommittee: Risk of thromboembolic disease in women taking oral contraceptives. Br. Med. J., *2*:355, 1967.
33. Miles, R. M., Chappell, F., and Renner, O.: Partially occluding vena caval clip for prevention of pulmonary emboli. Am. Surg., *30*:40, 1964.
34. Mitchell, J. R. A.: Can we really prevent postoperative pulmonary emboli? Br. Med. J., *1*:1523, 1979.
35. Moran, J. M., Kahr, P. C., and Callow, A. D.: Partial versus complete interruption for venous thromboembolism. Am. J. Surg., *117*:471, 1969.
36. Mozes, M., Bogolowsky, H., Antebi, E., Tzur, N., and Penchas, S.:

Inferior vena cava ligation for pulmonary embolism: Review of 118 cases. Surgery, *60*:790, 1966.

37. Myerson, P. J., Myerson, D. A., Katz, R., and Lawson, J. P.: Gallium imaging in pulmonary artery sarcoma mimicking pulmonary embolism: Case report. J. Nucl. Med., *17*:893, 1976.

38. Nabseth, D. C., and Moran, J. M.: Reassessment of the role of inferior vena cava ligation in venous thromboembolism. N. Engl. J. Med., *273*:1250, 1965.

39. Ochsner, A., Ochsner, J. L., and Sanders, H. S.: Prevention of pulmonary embolism by caval ligation. Ann. Surg., *171*:923, 1970.

40. Piccone, V. A., Jr., Vidal, E., Yarnoz, M., Glass, P., and LeVeen, H. H.: The late results of caval ligation. Surgery, *68*:980, 1970.

41. Pizzo, S. V.: Venous thrombosis. *In* Koepke, J. A. (Ed.): Laboratory Hematology, Vol. 2. New York, Churchill Livingstone, Inc., 1984, pp. 681–697.

42. Pizzo, S. V., Fuchs, H. E., Doman, K. A., Petruska, D. B., and Berger, H., Jr.: Release of tissue plasminogen activator and its fast-acting inhibitor in defective fibrinolysis. Arch. Intern. Med., *146*:188, 1986.

43. Rossle, R.: Uber die Bedeutung und die Entstehung der Wadenvenen-thrombosen. Virchows Arch. Pathol. Anat., *30*:180, 1937.

44. Sabiston, D. C., Jr.,: Pulmonary embolism. *In* Sabiston, D. C., Jr. (Ed.): Textbook of Surgery, 13th ed. Philadelphia, W. B. Saunders Company, 1986.

45. Sabiston, D. C., Jr.: Pathophysiology, diagnosis and management of pulmonary embolism. Adv. Surg., *3*:351, 1968.

46. Sabiston, D. C., Jr., and Wolfe, W. G.: Experimental and clinical observations on the natural history of pulmonary embolism. Ann. Surg., *168*:1, 1968.

47. Sabiston, D. C., Jr., and Wolfe, W. G.: Pulmonary embolectomy. *In* Moser, K. M., and Stein, J. (Eds.): Pulmonary Thromboembolism. Chicago, Year Book Medical Publishers, 1973.

48. Schowengerdt, C. G., and Schreiber, J. T.: Interruption of the vena cava in the treatment of pulmonary embolism. Surg. Gynecol. Obstet., *132*:645, 1971.

49. Shier, M. R., and Wilson, R. F.: Fat embolism syndrome: Traumatic coagulopathy with respiratory distress. Surg. Annu., *12*:139, 1980.

50. Shier, M. R., Wilson, R. F., James, R. E., et al.: Fat embolism prophylaxis: A study of four treatment modalities. J. Trauma, *17*:621, 1977.

51. Silver, D., and Gleysteen, J. J.: Paradoxical arterial embolism. Am. Surg., *36*:47, 1970.

52. Stead, R. B.: The hypercoagulable state. *In* Goldhaber, S. Z. (Ed.): Pulmonary Embolism and Deep Venous Thrombosis. Philadelphia, W. B. Saunders Company, 1985.

53. Stephenson, L. W., Workman, R. B., Aldrete, J. S., and Karp, R. B.: Bullett emboli to the pulmonary artery: A report of 2 patients and review of the literature. Ann. Thorac. Surg., *21*:333, 1976.

54. Stitt, R. W., and Adler, F.: The effects of corticosteroids on lung surfactant activity in experimentally produced fat embolism in rats. Surg. Forum, *28*:491, 1977.

55. Vessey, M. P., and Doll, R.: Investigation of relation between the use of oral contraceptives and thromboembolic disease. Br. Med. J., *2*:199, 1968.

56. Virchow, R.: Die Cellularpathologie in ihrer Begrundung auf physiologische and pathologische Gewebelehre. Berlin, A. Hirschwald, 1858.

57. Wheeler, C. G., Thompson, J. E., Austin, D. J., Patman, R. D., and Stockton, R. L.: Interruption of the inferior vena cava for thromboembolism: Comparison of ligation and plication. Ann. Surg., *163*:199, 1966.

58. Wolfe, W. G., and Sabiston, D. C., Jr.: Pulmonary embolism. *In* Ebert, P. A. (Ed.): Major Problems in Clinical Surgery, Vol. 25. Philadelphia, W. B. Saunders Company, 1980.

59. Zenker, F. A.: Bertrage zur normalen und pathologischen. Anatomie der Lunger. Dresden, Braunsdorf, 1862.

II

Chronic Pulmonary Embolism

Although pulmonary embolism usually presents as an acute clinical problem, it can also be manifested as a chronic disorder. In 1928, Ljungdahl[15] described chronic obstruction of the pulmonary arteries associated with progressive respiratory insufficiency ultimately leading to death. Although most patients with pulmonary embolism have a gradual resolution of the emboli *in situ* through mechanisms of the naturally occurring fibrinolytic systems in the body,[7, 8] in some instances, owing to inadequate fibrinolysis, the emboli fail to resolve and gradually accumulate in the pulmonary arterial system. The *hypercoagulable state* may be present in some patients with this disorder, and a detailed family history is very important in arousing clinical suspicion of this problem. The details concerning the causes and diagnosis of hypercoagulability have been presented earlier in this chapter, and they have a special relationship to some patients with *chronic, recurrent* pulmonary embolism with reduced natural thrombolysis. Such emboli may produce severe pulmonary arterial occlusion with resulting pulmonary hypertension, leading to symptoms of severe hypoxemia and right ventricular failure.[16, 18] It has been recently demonstrated that surgical removal of these emboli may reduce pulmonary hypertension and improve right heart failure with relief of respiratory insufficiency and clinical improvement for prolonged periods.

CLINICAL PRESENTATION

Patients with the syndrome of chronic pulmonary emboli usually have a history of exertional dyspnea that has progressed to severe respiratory insufficiency over a period of several months to years. They may also complain of recurrent episodes of thrombophlebitis, hemoptysis due to the dilated bronchial collateral circulation, and chest pain (Table 1). Physical findings include signs of severe pulmo-

TABLE 1. *Symptoms of Operable Patients in the Present Series with Chronic Unresolved Pulmonary Emboli (N = 14)**

Symptom	No. of Patients (%)
Dyspnea—exertion	12 (86)
Thrombophlebitis	11 (79)
Dyspnea—progressive	9 (64)
Hemoptysis	7 (50)
Chest pain	4 (26)
Fatigue	3 (21)

*From Chitwood, W. R., Jr., Lyerly, H. K., and Sabiston, D. C., Jr.: Ann. Surg., *201*:11, 1985.

TABLE 2. Initial Physical Findings in Operable Patients in This Series with Chronic Pulmonary Emboli (N = 14)*

Finding	No. of Patients (%)
Increased P$_2$	11 (78)
Cardiac murmur	8 (57)
Hepatomegaly	7 (50)
S$_3$ or S$_4$ gallop	6 (42)
Pulmonary rales	6 (42)
Jugular venous distention	4 (29)
Cyanosis	2 (14)
Clubbing	1 (7)

*From Chitwood, W. R., Jr., Lyerly, H. K., and Sabiston, D. C., Jr.: Ann. Surg., 201:11, 1985.

nary hypertension, often in conjunction with evidence of right ventricular failure, and may be manifested as an increased pulmonary second sound, a systolic murmur, hepatomegaly, and an S$_3$ or S$_4$ gallop. Other physical findings may include pulmonary rales, jugular venous distention, cyanosis, and clubbing (Table 2).

RADIOGRAPHIC STUDIES

Chest films usually demonstrate a dilated pulmonary artery and oligemic lung fields as well as right ventricular enlargement and pleural effusions (Fig. 1).[31] Arterial blood gases at room air reveal evidence of severe respiratory insufficiency with hypoxemia and mild respiratory alkalosis. Electrographic findings include right axis deviation and right ventricular hypertrophy suggestive of chronic cor pulmonale.

Ventilation and perfusion radionuclide scans performed during the evaluation are consistent with pulmonary embolism, with perfusion defects corresponding to oligemic regions on the plain film and arteriogram (Fig. 2). Pulmonary arteriography usually shows emboli in both lungs with between 55 and 75 per cent of the total pulmonary blood flow obstructed (Fig. 3). Pulmonary hypertension was present in all of 25 patients with chronic pulmonary emboli evaluated at Duke University Medical Center with a systolic pressure of 75.0 ± 8.0 mm. Hg, a diastolic pressure of 26.0 ± 3.0 mm. Hg, and a mean pressure of 42.0 ± 5.0 mm. Hg (Table 3).

Further preoperative studies include a thoracic aortogram, which usually shows dilated and tortuous bronchial vessels. The bronchial circulation is often considerably augmented and communicates through the pulmonary arteries, and in patients in which selective bronchial arteriograms were performed, patency of the distal pulmonary arteries was demonstrated in all but one (Fig. 4). When these are present, the prognosis following embolectomy is very favorable, since it can be established preoperatively that the distal pulmonary arterial bed is patent and removal of the proximal thrombus results in increased pulmonary arterial blood flow.

Right ventricular function may be assessed by first-pass radionuclide angiocardiography, which demonstrates severe chronic pulmonary arterial obstruction with a significant delay in arrival of the tracer. The mean resting ejection fraction for patients in our series was 23.5 ± 2.2 at rest and 28.0 ± 4.0 with exercise.

A thorough preoperative evaluation is necessary before suitability for operation in each patient can be determined. The most appropriate candidates for pulmonary embolectomy are those with severe respiratory insufficiency and a low arterial Po$_2$ and those who demonstrate enlarged bronchial vessels on thoracic aortography. A number of patients with this syndrome are found to be unsuitable candidates for embolectomy. The most common contraindication is distal pulmonary emboli that are diffusely spread throughout the small pulmonary arteries and are not amenable to surgical removal (Fig. 5). Other contraindications include severe cardiac failure and massive obesity. The majority of these patients are disabled with a New York Heart Association Class of IV (Table 4).

SURGICAL MANAGEMENT

Pulmonary embolectomy may be performed on one or both pulmonary arteries. In patients with bilateral pulmonary emboli or in those with involvement of the main pulmonary artery, extracorporeal circulation is generally indicated. In patients who have primarily unilateral involvement, either a right or left anterior thoracotomy can be performed with proximal occlusion of the vessel with distal embolectomy (Fig. 6). These emboli are densely adherent to the wall of the pulmonary artery, and considerable care must be taken in dissecting them. All distal emboli should

Text continued on page 963

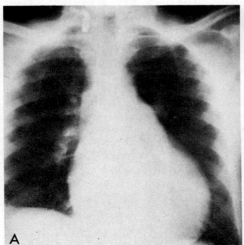
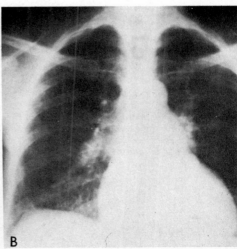

Figure 1. The anteroposterior chest film is shown before (A) and after (B) embolectomy of the right lower lobe pulmonary artery for chronic pulmonary emboli. Following operation, an increase in parenchymal flow to the right lower lobe was noted. Also note the decrease in the size of both the right main pulmonary artery and cardiac silhouette following embolectomy. (From Chitwood, W. R., Jr., Lyerly, H. K., and Sabiston, D. C., Jr.: Ann. Surg., 201:11, 1985.)

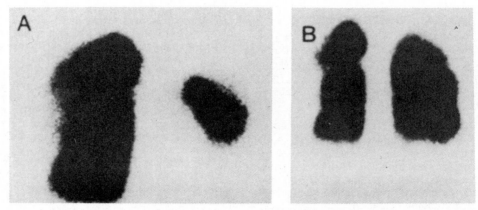

Figure 2. The posterior view of a pulmonary perfusion scan before (A) and 3 months after (B) embolectomy for a right lower lobe chronic pulmonary embolism. Note the re-establishment of flow to the right lower lobe. (From Chitwood, W. R., Jr., Lyerly, H. K., and Sabiston, D. C., Jr.: Ann. Surg., 201:11, 1985.)

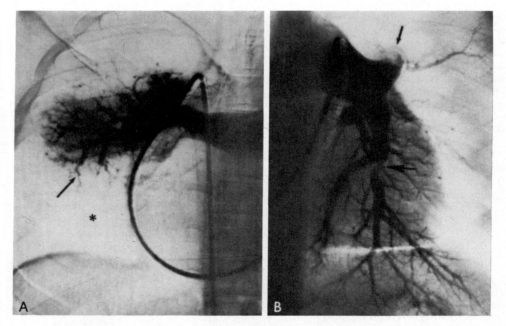

Figure 3. The preoperative angiogram of the same patient depicted in Figure 2 is shown. These represent the classic arteriographic findings of chronic pulmonary embolism. A, Tapered arterial defects are seen in distal pulmonary arteries (arrow) indicating chronic pulmonary emboli. Note total obstruction of the right lower lobe pulmonary artery leading to oligemia (asterisk). Moreover, segmental occlusion to the right upper lobe is also present. B, Proximal dilation of the main pulmonary artery is noted. A plaque is seen in the left upper lobe pulmonary artery (small arrow). In the left lower lobe pulmonary artery a residual web is evident (large arrow). This represents a partially resolved chronic pulmonary embolism. (From Chitwood, W. R., Jr., Lyerly, H. K., and Sabiston, D. C., Jr.: Ann. Surg., 201:11, 1985.)

TABLE 3. *Angiographic and Hemodynamic Data from Patients Undergoing Embolectomy for Chronic Pulmonary Emboli (N = 14)**

Patient	Leg Venogram	Vena Cavagram	Bronchial Angiogram	Pulmonary Angiogram		Pulmonary Artery Pressures					
				Major Occlusions	% P.A. Occlusions	Pre-Op			Post-Op		
						PAS	PAD	P̄A	PAS	PAD	P̄A
1	+	—	None	RLL / Left main (total)	65	75	20	32	35	14	20
2	+	+	None	RUL, RML, RLL / LLL (total)	60	48	18	30	37	14	21
3	+	—	Large bronchials—T7 / Large intercostal—T7 / Left lung only	RLL / Left main (total)	55	43	23	27	36	17	21
4	+	None	None	RUL, RLL / Ling, LLL (total)	55	44	18	28	38	12	21
5	—	—	None	RUL, RLL (total) / Ling, LLL	55	85	22	40	53	18	30
6	None	None	None	RLL / Left main (total)	65	100	30	45	100	20	46
7	+	—	Large bronchial—T7 / Both lungs; R > L	RLL (total), RML / LLL	60	65	30	42	None	None	
8	—	—	Large brnchial—T6 / Both lungs: L > R	RLL (diffuse) / Ling, LLL (total)	65	50	20	30	50	14	24
9	+	None	Large bronchials—T5 / Both lungs: R > L	RUL, RML, RLL / Ling	65	75	25	45	None	10†	None
10	+	None	Moderately dilated bronchials / No obvious flow	RUL, RML, RLL / (diffuse) / LLL (total)	60	95	30	54	54	14	27
11	+	None	Large bronchials: T6 and T7 / Both lungs: R > L	RUL (total), RLL (total) / LLL	70	130	55	82	65	15	32
12	—	None	Large bronchials—T7 / Left supplying right lung	RLL (total), RML / LLL (total), LUL	70	78	20	45	80	24	46
13	+	None	Large bronchials / Left lung only	RUL, RML (total) / LUL (total), LLL	60	58	17	32	None	10†	None
14	None	None	Large bronchials: T7 and T11 / Right lung only	Right main (total) / LUL (diffuse)	65	80	36	50	74	12	32

*From Lyerly, H. K., and Sabiston, D. C., Jr.: *In* Sabiston, D. C., Jr. (Ed.): Textbook of Surgery, 13th ed. Philadelphia, W. B. Saunders Company, 1986, p. 1751.
†Daggers indicate data obtained using Swan-Ganz pulmonary arterial catheters. Other postoperative hemodynamic data were obtained from cardiac catheterizations.
Abbreviations: R = Right, L = left, UL = upper lobe, ML = middle lobe, LL = lower lobe, and Ling = lingular.

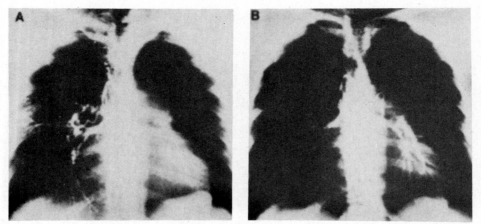

Figure 4. A, A selective bronchial arterial injection showing dilated bronchial collaterals on the right supplying the distal pulmonary parenchyma. B, A later phase of the same injection in which collaterals from the right side supply the distal pulmonary parenchyma in the left lower lobe. The left lower lobe pulmonary artery was noted to have a total proximal obstruction on the pulmonary arteriogram. (From Chitwood, W. R., Jr., Lyerly, H. K., and Sabiston, D. C., Jr.: Ann. Surg., 201:11, 1985.)

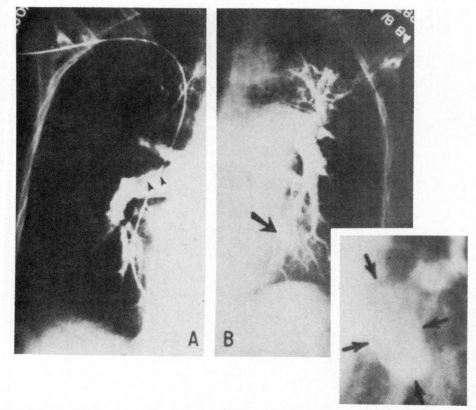

Figure 5. A pulmonary arteriogram from a patient demonstrates multiple peripheral filling defects. A, Organized emboli can be seen within the proximal right pulmonary arteries (arrows). B and Inset, In the left lower lobe a calcified embolus is present (arrows). (From Chitwood, W. R., Jr., Lyerly, H. K., and Sabiston, D. C., Jr.: Ann. Surg., 201:11, 1985.)

TABLE 4. *Arteriographic, Hemodynamic, and Functional Evaluation of 11 Patients Unsuitable for Pulmonary Embolectomy**

Patient	Age	Presenting NYHA Class	PA Systolic	PA Diastolic	PA Mean	% PA Occlusion	Contraindication to Surgery	Follow-Up Duration	Follow-Up NYHA Class
1	65	IV	80	33	50	80	Distal emboli	0	Expired, acute PE
2	40	III	95	30	50	45	Distal emboli	5 years	IV
							Massive obesity		
3	50	III	58	20	30	35	Distal emboli	1 week	Expired, respiratory distress
4	39	IV	107	45	70	85	Distal emboli	6 months	IV
5	69	III	85	25	45	75	Distal emboli	3 months	III
6	31	IV	145	45	80	(100% partial)	RV failure	2 months	IV
7	64	IV	90	20	45	35	Distal emboli	6 months	IV
8	39	II	60	25	35	55	Distal emboli	6 years	III
9	21	II	95	50	60	40	Massive obesity	3 months	Expired, RV failure
10	66	IV	70	32	45	(90% partial)	Distal emboli	2 months	IV
11	42	II	95	18	64	(100% partial)	Distal emboli	1 month	III

*From Chitwood, W. R., Jr., Lyerly, H. K., and Sabiston, D. C., Jr.: Ann. Surg., *201*:11, 1985.
Abbreviations: NYHA = New York Heart Association Classification, PE = pulmonary embolism, RV = right ventricular.

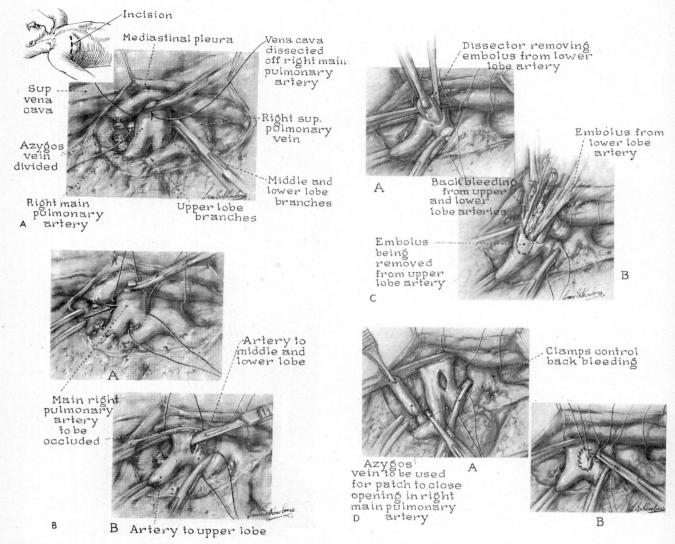

Figure 6. Technique of unilateral pulmonary embolectomy (without the necessity for extracorporeal circulation).

A, The incision is made in the right anterior chest with division of the pectoral muscles and entry into the pleural cavity in the third intercostal space. The lung is retracted and the anterior mediastinum opened posterior to the phrenic nerve. The azygos vein is ligated and divided for ideal exposure of the right pulmonary artery.

B, (A), A ligature is passed loosely around the right main pulmonary artery as well as its distal branches. The proximal right pulmonary artery is occluded with a vascular clamp, as are the distal branches. (B), An arteriotomy is made on the anterior surface of the right pulmonary artery for exposure of the embolus.

C, (A), The embolus is removed with forceps. (B), In patients with chronic pulmonary embolism, it may be necessary to dissect the embolus away from the arterial wall. If the embolism is chronic, prominent arterial back bleeding of bright red arterial blood should ensue when the embolectomy is complete.

D, (A and B), The arteriotomy in the right main pulmonary artery may be closed directly with a continuous suture, or a vein patch may be employed if it is thought that the primary closure would significantly reduce the lumen of the pulmonary artery. The venous graft may be easily obtained from the nearby azygos vein.

(From Sabiston, D. C., Jr., and Wolfe, W. G.: Pulmonary embolism. In Sabiston, D. C., Jr., and Spencer, F. C. [Eds.]: Gibbon's Surgery of the Chest, 4th ed. Phiadelphia, W. B. Saunders Company, 1983.)

Figure 7. A left anterolateral thoracotomy is made with entry into the pleural cavity through the third intercostal space. This is the approach for the main pulmonary artery and the left pulmonary artery. The venous outflow cannula may be placed in the outflow tract of the right ventricle through a purse-string suture as shown, and the arterial cannula is placed in the femoral artery. The main pulmonary artery is massively enlarged, with significant pulmonary hypertension. A tape is passed around the proximal pulmonary artery for control. If the right pulmonary artery requires exposure for embolectomy, the sternum can be transected and the incision extended into the right third intercostal space with entry into the right chest. In that instance, the venous return cannula may be placed in the right atrium, and the aorta can be used as the side for arterial inflow cannula. (From Wolfe, W. G., and Sabiston, D. C., Jr.: In Ebert, P. A. (Ed.): Major Problems in Clinical Surgery, Vol. 25. Philadelphia, W. B. Saunders Company, 1980.)

be removed until there is adequate back bleeding of bright red blood. It is usually preferable to close the arteriotomy with a pericardial patch to prevent constriction of the lumen.

When extracorporeal circulation is employed, the venous cannulation can be in either the right atrium or the outflow tract of the right ventricle. Involvement of the main pulmonary artery as well as the entire left pulmonary artery and its branches is depicted in Figure 7. Meticulous dissection is necessary, with removal of all distal emboli, in order to achieve an optimal postoperative result (Fig. 8). It is usually necessary to make a counterincision in the distal pulmonary artery to completely remove the adherent emboli in the secondary and tertiary branches of the pulmonary arteries (Fig. 9). Typical specimens removed at operation are shown in Figure 10.

Good distal back bleeding can usually be predicted in advance from the information gained by the thoracic arteriogram with selective injection of the bronchial arteries. These arteries are often dilated and tortuous and fill the distal pulmonary arterial circuit in a retrograde manner.

Postoperative Complications

Postoperatively, complications include severe right ventricular failure in those patients with long-standing cor pulmonale and pulmonary hypertension. One patient in our series died 3 days after operation of this complication despite removal of the chronic pulmonary emboli. Another complication that has been previously described is the hemorrhagic lung syndrome.

Following embolectomy and after re-establishment of pulmonary blood flow, massive parenchymal and intrabron-

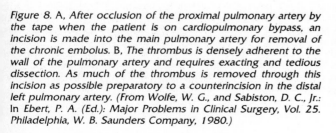

Figure 8. A, After occlusion of the proximal pulmonary artery by the tape when the patient is on cardiopulmonary bypass, an incision is made into the main pulmonary artery for removal of the chronic embolus. B, The thrombus is densely adherent to the wall of the pulmonary artery and requires exacting and tedious dissection. As much of the thrombus is removed through this incision as possible preparatory to a counterincision in the distal left pulmonary artery. (From Wolfe, W. G., and Sabiston, D. C., Jr.: In Ebert, P. A. (Ed.): Major Problems in Clinical Surgery, Vol. 25. Philadelphia, W. B. Saunders Company, 1980.)

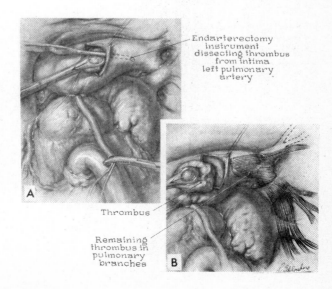

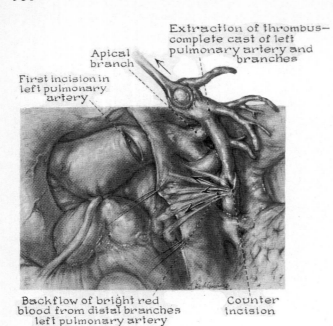

First incision in
left pulmonary
artery

Apical
branch

Extraction of thrombus—
complete cast of left
pulmonary artery and
branches

Backflow of bright red
blood from distal branches
left pulmonary artery

Counter
incision

Figure 9. Through a counterincision in the distal left pulmonary artery, the branches of the chronic embolus are removed as shown. Actually, the chronic embolus has formed a cast of the pulmonary arterial tree. After removal of this cast, a large amount of back bleeding occurs. The retrograde blood flow is bright red, indicating its source from the bronchial circulation being supplied by the aorta. The arteriotomies are closed. (From Wolfe, W. G., and Sabiston, D. C., Jr.: Pulmonary embolism. In Ebert, P. A. (Ed.): Major Problems in Clinical Surgery, Vol 25. Philadelphia, W. B. Saunders Company, 1980.)

chial hemorrhage during or following cardiopulmonary bypass may occur. Successful management of this complication can be achieved by use of a Carlens (Broncho-Cath) catheter for tracheal intubation. A Fogarty catheter is inserted to occlude the right or left mainstem bronchus and tamponade the blood within the lumen until appropriate blood coagulation can be achieved (Fig. 11). Usually the bleeding ceases when protamine is injected to counteract the heparin used for cardiopulmonary bypass.

Postoperative Results

Following embolectomy for chronic pulmonary embolism, an increase in PaO_2 is expected along with a rise in

the arterial $PaCO_2$ toward normal (Fig. 12). In our series 14 patients underwent embolectomy. Long-term follow-up data have demonstrated that the NYHA functional class of most patients changed quite significantly, moving from Class III or IV to Class I in most instances and in others to Class II, with only one patient showing a change from Class IV to Class III postoperatively (Fig. 13). These data, together with other similar series in the literature, indicate favorable results. A long-term follow-up arteriogram is demonstrated in Figure 14.

In contradistinction, those patients found unsuitable for embolectomy have a poor prognosis. In this group, three of 11 patients died, and the majority of the survivors are currently disabled at rest.

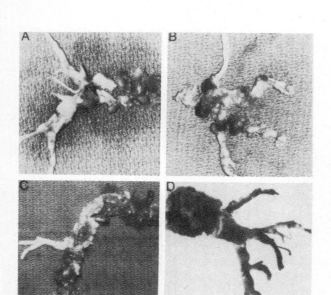

Figure 10. Chronic emboli removed from four patients undergoing pulmonary embolectomy. A to C, Patients underwent embolectomy via thoractomy and localized lobar pulmonary artery occlusion. D, This patient required cardiopulmonary bypass because of very proximal pulmonary artery involvement. Note the tenacious fibrotic material extended into the segmental vessels. In the majority of patients, distal branches could be embolectomized. (From Chitwood, W. R., Jr., Lyerly, H. K., and Sabiston, D. C., Jr.: Ann. Surg., 201:11, 1985.)

Figure 11. Method to control re-perfusion intrabronchial hemor-rhage.

A, The Broncho-Cath endo-bronchial tube in place with re-perfusion intrabronchial hemor-rhage from the left lung resulting in massive blood loss to the right lung and out the Broncho-Cath tube.

B, Inflation of the bronchial bal-loon and aspiration of blood from the right main bronchus.

C, Insertion of a Fogarty cath-eter into the endobronchial tube and inflation of the balloon to provide bronchial tamponade of the left main bronchus. Tampon-ade will be provided until coag-ulation factors are returned to normal, at which time the intra-bronchial reperfusion hemor-rhage should cease.

(From Lyerly, H. K., and Sabis-ton, D. C., Jr.: Diagnosis and man-agement of chronic pulmonary embolism. In Sabiston, D. C., Jr. (Ed.): Textbook of Surgery, 13th ed. Philadelphia, W. B. Saunders Company, 1986.)

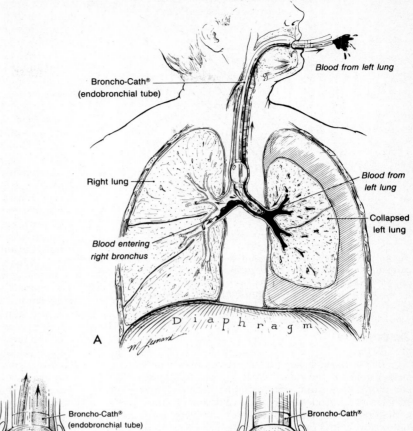

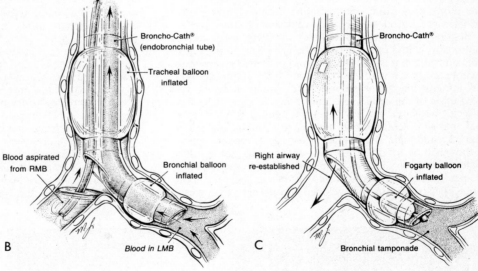

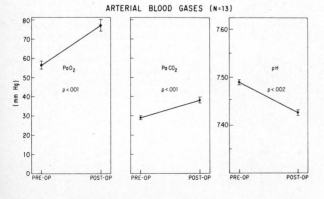

Figure 12. In the present series, arterial blood gases are shown before and following embolectomy. All values were statistically significant (P < 0.05). (From Chitwood, W. R., Jr., Lyerly, H. K., and Sabiston, D. C., Jr.: Ann. Surg., 201:11, 1985.)

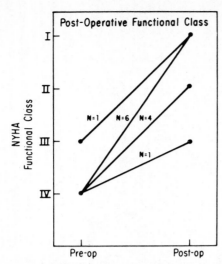

Figure 13. Preoperative and postoperative functional class of 12 patients undergoing successful pulmonary embolectomy. NYHA = New York Heart Association. (From Chitwood, W. R., Jr., Lyerly, H. K., and Sabiston, D. C., Jr.: Ann. Surg., 201:11, 1985.)

DISCUSSION

In the normal patient, an active fibrinolytic system is responsible for the rapid resolution of pulmonary emboli; therefore, most pulmonary emboli present as acute clinical problems. Clinical studies using pulmonary scans and arteriograms have demonstrated that complete dissolution of pulmonary emboli may occur as early as 8 to 14 days after the clinical event, although in some patients this response may be delayed for several months.[8, 23, 27, 30] In the majority of patients, the natural fibrinolytic sequences occur with resolution of the emboli and few, if any, long-term residual effects or symptoms. However, a significant number of patients with acute emboli have been shown to have continued pathologic stigmata as a long-term phenomenon,[8] although most of these chronic changes do not produce pulmonary hypertension. It was found in one series that of 22 per cent of patients with findings of unresolved emboli, only 2 per cent actually developed chronic cor pulmonale.[28]

Nevertheless, in a small but definite cohort, recurrent attacks of pulmonary emboli without resolution lead to a syndrome of chronic pulmonary hypertension and ensuing complications.

The failure of these emboli to resolve is thought to be due to inadequate fibrinolysis. Deficiencies of coagulant inhibitors lead to an inability to regulate intravascular clot formation. Antithrombin III (ATT III) is a protein essential for coagulation hemostasis. It is released during coagulation and inactivates thrombin and other serine proteases. Patients with deficiencies of ATT III have a hypercoagulable state clinically manifested by recurrent thrombosis and pulmonary embolism.[19] Deficiencies of activated protein C, which inhibits factors V and IV, and protein S, which serves as a cofactor for activated protein C, have also been reported to lead to an increased incidence of thromboembolism.[4, 6, 13] Besides inadequate fibrinolysis, embolization of previously organized thrombi that are resistant to dissolution may be another cause of chronic pulmonary emboli, but this is unproven.

Adequate anticoagulant therapy in patients with chronic emboli decreases the number of recurrent episodes of emboli to the pulmonary circulation. Despite anticoagulation, a small number of patients continue to have showers in the absence of significant resolution,[25] which may proceed to major pulmonary arterial obstruction, and pulmonary hypertension is present in 0.5 to 0.4 per cent of these patients.[5, 7, 11, 16] These emboli become infiltrated with fibroblasts and are refractory to fibrinolysis and may permanently occlude the lumen (Fig. 15).

In acute pulmonary embolism, the mean pulmonary arterial pressure rarely exceeds 40 mm. Hg.[16] Thus, higher pressures suggest a diagnosis of chronic obstruction with right ventricular enlargement. The presence of these elevated pressures is important, as it has been demonstrated that the natural history of this syndrome is related to the magnitude of the pulmonary arterial hypertension.[26] If the mean pulmonary artery pressure was greater than 30 mm. Hg, 5-year survival was only 30 per cent. In those patients with mean pressures greater than 50 mm. Hg, only 10 per cent were alive at 5 years (Fig. 16).

Medical management of chronic pulmonary emboli has included a number of fibrinolytic and vasodilator agents; however, these have been largely ineffective.[1, 9, 10, 14, 17, 21, 22] Recently, plasminogen activation has been shown to pro-

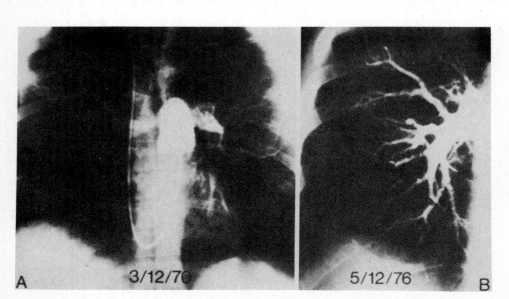

Figure 14. A, Pulmonary arteriogram in a patient prior to embolectomy. B, Six years following right lower lobe embolectomy. Note continued perfusion of the right lower lobe following embolectomy. (From Chitwood, W. R., Jr., Lyerly, H. K., and Sabiston, D. C., Jr.: Ann. Surg., 201:11, 1985.)

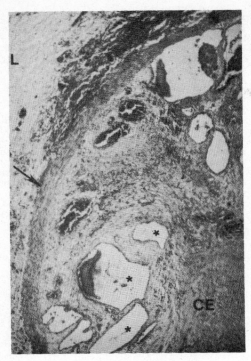

Figure 15. Photomicrograph of an organized chronic embolus within a large pulmonary artery. CE = Chronic embolus with fibrous ingrowth; L = lung parenchyma; arrow = medial elements of pulmonary artery; and asterisk = endothelium-lined channels indicating recanalization. Note pulmonary artery close adherence to the fibrotic embolic material (CE). (From Chitwood, W. R., Jr., Lyerly, H. K., and Sabiston, D. C., Jr.: Ann. Surg., 201:11, 1985.)

paired right ventricular function are appropriate candidates for surgical embolectomy.[2, 3, 24] In contrast, patients with this syndrome who have distal pulmonary emboli in the small arterial branches with patent proximal vessels, as well as those with severe right ventricular failure and massive obesity, are generally unsuitable for surgical management. Long-term follow-up of patients with operable pulmonary emboli shows quite favorable respiratory and cardiodynamic changes. Such patients experience relief of their incapacitating symptoms and maintain clinical improvement for prolonged periods.

SELECTED REFERENCES

Cabrol, C., Cabrol, A., Acar, J., Gandjbakhch, I., Guiraudon, G., Laughlin, L., Mattei, M.-F, and Godeau, P.: Surgical correction of chronic postembolic obstructions of the pulmonary arteries. J. Thorac. Cardiovasc. Surg., 76:620, 1978.
This article reports a series of patients with chronic pulmonary embolism managed by embolectomy. It is a relatively large series, and discussion is directed toward diagnosis, details of surgical management, and the results.

Chitwood, W. R., Jr., Lyerly, H. K., and Sabiston, D. C., Jr.: Surgical management of chronic pulmonary embolism. Ann. Surg., 201:11, 1985.
This is a report of the experience of a large series in the United States on surgical management of chronic pulmonary embolism. The clinical manifestations, management, and results are each evaluated in detail.

Goldhaber, S. Z. (Ed.): Pulmonary Embolism and Deep Venous Thrombosis. Philadelphia, W. B. Saunders Company, 1985.
This is a multiauthored monograph by a number of experts in the field. It is a valuable updated resource for all forms of pulmonary embolism, and, in addition, there is an excellent discussion of the hypercoagulable state in the management of massive pulmonary embolism and pulmonary thromboendarterectomy. It is a current resource for details of all aspects of pulmonary embolism.

REFERENCES

1. Benaim, R., Calvo, G., Fischler, M., and Chiche, P.: Les thromboembolies subaigues ou chroniques de l'artere pulmonaire las place du traitement fibrinolytique. Ann. Med. Intern., 127:767, 1976.
2. Bengtsson, L., Henze, A., Holmgren, A., and Bjork, V. O.: Thrombendarterectomy in chronic pulmonary embolism: Reports of 3 cases. Scand. J. Thorac. Cardiovasc. Surg., 20:67, 1986.
3. Chitwood, W. R., Jr., Lyerly, H. K., and Sabiston, D. C., Jr.: Surgical management of chronic pulmonary embolism. Ann. Surg., 201:11, 1985.
4. Clouse, L. H., and Comp, P. C.: The regulation of hemostasis: The protein C system. N. Engl. J. Med., 314:1298, 1986.
5. Comp, P. C., and Esmon, C. T.: Recurrent venous thromboembolism in patients with a partial deficiency of protein S. N. Engl. J. Med., 311:1525, 1984.
6. Cosgriff, T. M., Bishop, D. T., Hershgold, E. J., Skolnick, M. H., Martin, B. A., Baty, B. J., and Carlson, K. S.: Familial antithrombin III deficiency: Its natural history, genetics, diagnosis and treatment. Medicine, 62:209, 1983.
7. Dalen, J. E., and Alpert, J. S.: Natural history of pulmonary embolism. Prog. Cardiovasc. Dis., 17:259, 1975.
8. Dalen, J. E., Banas, J. S., Jr., Brooks, H. L., et al.: Resolution rate of acute pulmonary embolism in man. N. Engl. J. Med., 280:1194, 1969.
9. Dantzker, D. R., and Bower, J. S.: Partial reversibility of chronic pulmonary hypertension caused by pulmonary thromboembolic disease. Am. Rev. Respir. Dis., 124:129, 1981.
10. Dash, H., Ballentine, N., and Zelis, R.: Vasodilators ineffective in secondary pulmonary hypertension. N. Engl. J. Med., 303:1062, 1980.
11. deSoyza, W. D., and Murphy, M. L.: Persistent post-embolic pulmonary hypertension. Chest, 62:665, 1972.
12. Freiman, D. G., Suyemoto, J., and Wessler, S.: Frequency of pulmonary thromboembolism in man. N. Engl. J. Med., 272:1278, 1965.
13. Griffin, J. H., Bezeaud, A., Evatt, B., and Mosher, D.: Functional and immunologic studies of protein C in thromboembolic disease. Blood, 62:(Suppl. 1):301a, 1983.
14. Hollister, L. E., and Cull, V. L.: The syndrome of chronic thrombosis of the major pulmonary arteries. Am. J. Med., 21:312, 1956.
15. Ljungdahl, M.: Gibt es eine chronische Embolisierung der Lungenarterie? Deutsch Arch. Klin. Med., 160:1, 1928.

vide local thrombinolysis of relatively old thrombi in peripheral veins; this may lead to future resolution of chronic pulmonary embolism.[29] However, organized emboli with ingrowth of fibroblasts may be resistant to any form of thrombolytic therapy.

In summary, selected patients with symptoms of severe respiratory insufficiency, hypoxemia, and pulmonary hypertension with proximal pulmonary arterial occlusion and good bronchial collateral circulation with minimally im-

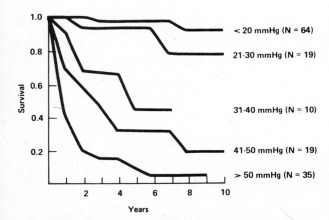

Figure 16. Survival in patients with pulmonary hypertension resulting from chronic recurrent emboli. Patient groups are compared at different mean pulmonary artery pressures. (From Chitwood, W. R., Jr., Sabiston, D. C., Jr., and Wechsler, A. S.: Clin. Chest Med., 5:507, 1984. Modified from Reidel, M., Stanel, V., Widimsky, J., et al.: Chest, 81:151, 1982.)

16. McIntyre, K. M., and Sasahara, A. A.: The hemodynamic response to pulmonary embolism in patients without prior cardiopulmonary disease. Am. J. Cardiol., *28*:288, 1971.

17. Olukotun, A. Y.: Vasodilator therapy for pulmonary hypertension. N. Engl. J. Med., *302*:1261, 1980.

18. Owen, W. R., Thomas, W. A., Castleman, B., and Bland, E. F.: Unrecognized emboli to the lungs with subsequent cor pulmonale. N. Engl. J. Med., *249*:919, 1953.

19. Paraskos, J. A., Adelstein, S. J., Smith, R. E., et al.: Late prognosis of acute pulmonary embolism. N. Engl. J. Med., *289*:55, 1973.

20. Riedel, M., Stanek, V., Widimsky, J., and Prerovsky, I.: Longterm follow-up of patients with pulmonary thromboembolism: Late prognosis and evaluation of hemodynamic and respiratory data. Chest, *81*:151, 1982.

21. Rubin, L. J., and Peter, A. M.: Primary pulmonary hypertension treated with oral phentolamine. Ann. Intern. Med., *302*:69, 1980.

22. Ruskin, J. N., and Hutter, A. M.: Primary pulmonary hypertension treated with oral phentolamine. Ann. Intern. Med., *90*:772, 1979.

23. Sasahara, A. A., and Hyers, T. M.: Urokinase pulmonary embolism trial: A national cooperative study. Circulation *47*:38, 1973.

24. Shuck, J. W., Walder, J. S., Kam, T. H., and Thomas H.: Chronic persistent pulmonary embolism: Report of three cases. Am. J. Med., *69*:790, 1980.

25. Sutton, G. C., Hall, R. J. C., and Kerr, I. H.: Clinical course and late prognosis of subacute massive, acute minor, and chronic pulmonary thromboembolism. Br. Heart. J., *39*:1135, 1977.

26. Tilkian, A. G., Schroeder, J. S., and Robin, E. D.: Chronic thromboembolic occlusion of main pulmonary artery or primary branches: Case report and review of the literature. Am. J. Med., *60*:563, 1976.

27. Tow, D. E., and Wagner, H. N., Jr.: Recovery of pulmonary arterial blood flow in patients with pulmonary embolism. N. Engl. J. Med., *276*:1053, 1967.

28. Wagenvoort, C. A., and Wagenvoort, N.: Pathology of Pulmonary Hypertension. New York, John Wiley & Sons, 1977, pp. 143–176.

29. Weimar, W., Stibbe, J., Van Seyen, A. J., et al.: Specific lysis of an iliofemoral thrombus by administration of extrinsic (tissue-type) plasminogen activator. Lancet, *2*:1018, 1981.

30. Wilhelmsen, L., Hagman, M., and Werko, L.: Recurrent pulmonary embolism: Incidence, predisposing factors and prognosis. Acta Med. Scand., *192*:565, 1972.

31. Woodruff, W. W., III, Hoeck, B. E., Chitwood, W. R., Jr., and Lyerly, H. K., Sabiston, D. C., Jr., and Chen, T. T.: Radiographic findings in pulmonary hypertension from unresolved embolism. AJR, *144*:681, 1985.

THE LUNGS AND CHEST WALL

44

I

Physiologic Aspects of Respiratory Function and Management of Respiratory Insufficiency in Surgical Patients

PETER K. SMITH, M.D.
DAVID C. SABISTON, JR., M.D.

Respiratory function is significantly altered by the performance of nearly all major surgical procedures. In the presence of pre-existing pulmonary disease, these alterations may lead to increased morbidity, respiratory failure, and even death. Although mortality is rare with modern anesthetic techniques and postoperative care, these advances have followed an improved understanding of the basic function of the respiratory system.[51] This allows appropriate preoperative and postoperative management and usually permits the accurate selection of patients who can be operated upon safely.[49]

CLINICAL EVALUATION OF PULMONARY FUNCTION

To integrate basic and clinical physiology and introduce commonly used terms, those parameters used to assess preoperative pulmonary function will be defined. The initial evaluation of the preoperative patient includes a complete history and physical examination. Disorders that place the patient at high risk include emphysema, bronchitis, asthma, and allergy. Exposure to environmental pollution, particularly smoking, should be documented. A history of dyspnea or shortness of breath, particularly with minimal exercise, should alert the physician to potential respiratory failure in the patient who has not yet been categorized by a physician. An insidious reduction of physical activity can mask respiratory dysfunction, and a history of such changes in lifestyle should be actively sought. The chronic production of sputum and any recent change in its degree or character mandate active evaluation. Physical examination will reveal

the overall configuration of the chest wall and can immediately reveal patients with obstructive lung disease. Peripheral or central cyanosis, a rapid respiratory pattern with the use of the accessory muscles of respiration, and the general demeanor of the patient can be revealing. The localized diminution of breath sounds, their character, and the presence of localized or generalized wheezing may indicate potentially reversible causes of respiratory dysfunction.

A chest film completes the routine preoperative evaluation. If conditions permit, the pursuit of more detailed information is usually obtained in patients with evidence of significant pulmonary disease or in patients undergoing thoracic or major upper abdominal procedures.

ASSESSMENT OF PULMONARY FUNCTION

Spirometric evaluation allows the estimation of the overall ability to ventilate. Variations from normal may be due to generalized pulmonary disease or to localized abnormalities. These tests are simple to obtain, but they must be carefully interpreted because there are wide variations in the normal population. The results obtained are highly dependent upon patient understanding and cooperation.[2]

Static Mechanics

The spirometric measurements of lung volumes and capacities are obtained initially.[16] These subdivisions of the

1. Total lung capacity (TLC)
2. Vital capacity (VC)
3. Inspiratory capacity (IC)
4. Functional residual capacity (FRC).

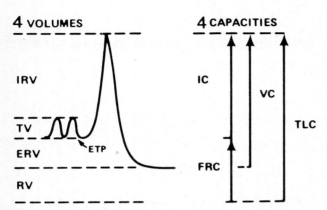

Figure 1. Four volumes and four capacities that subdivide the total lung capacity. For abbreviations and definitions, see text. (Reproduced from Tisi, G. M.: Pulmonary Physiology in Clinical Medicine, 2nd ed., Copyright 1983, by Williams & Wilkins, Baltimore.)

total lung capacity (TLC, liters) are illustrated in Figure 1. The TLC is divided into four lung volumes:

Tidal Volume (TV, L.). The volume of air inspired during a quiet normal respiration, begun at the end of a normal expiration from the end tidal point (ETP).

Inspiratory Reserve Volume (IRV, L.). The lung volume between the peak tidal point and the maximal inspiratory point.

Expiratory Reserve Volume (ERV, L.). The lung volume between the ETP and the maximal expiratory point.

Residual Volume (RV, L). The volume of air remaining in the lung at the maximal expiratory point.

Four lung capacities are defined by spirometry:

Total Lung Capacity (TLC, L.). The amount of air in the lungs following maximal inspiration.

Vital Capacity (VC, L.). The amount of air that can be expired following a maximal inspiration.

Inspiratory Capacity (IC, L.). The amount of air expired from the point of maximal inspiration to the ETP.

Functional Residual Capacity (FRC, L.). The amount of air within the lungs at the end tidal point.

It is apparent that RV is the only volume that cannot be determined from the spirometric tracing. Without a value for RV, TLC and FRC cannot be determined. In practice, RV can be determined by body plethysmography or by gas dilution techniques.[52] The values of lung volume and capacity are useful in the general categorization of patients into typical clinical patterns of pulmonary disease. They can be used to follow the progress of therapy perioperatively. Tidal volume and vital capacity can be determined quickly at the bedside with a minimum of equipment, and these measurements are particularly useful.

Dynamic Mechanics

The measurement of the ability to move air, through dynamic testing, has proved to be more sensitive in the prediction of postoperative pulmonary dysfunction.[51] *Airway obstruction*, a primary component of most lung diseases, is measured by recording air flow over time during spirometric testing. Those determinations most often used clinically are as follows:

Forced Vital Capacity (FVC, L.). The volume of air that can be forcibly expired with maximal expiratory effort.

Forced Expiratory Volume—One Second (FEV$_1$, L.). The amount of air that can be forcibly expired in first second of the FVC.

Maximal Voluntary Ventilation (MVV, L.). The amount of air that can be breathed in 1 minute during maximal effort, calculated from 15 seconds of actual ventilation.

FEV$_1$/FVC%. The fraction of the FVC maximally expired in 1 second.

Other values obtained include the maximal mid-expiratory flow rate or the forced expiratory flow rate from 200 to 1200 ml. below TLC (FEF 200–1200), which is less dependent on patient effort.[52]

Arterial Blood Gases

The measurement of the partial pressure of oxygen (Pao$_2$) and carbon dioxide (Paco$_2$) in arterial blood, as well as the pH, has become an integral part of the evaluation of the pulmonary patient. These values provide direct measures of the patient's ability to support oxidative metabolism.

Oxygen combines reversibly with hemoglobin according to the *oxyhemoglobin dissociation curve* (Fig. 2). The unusual shape of the curve allows the oxygen content of the blood to remain high over a wide range of Pao$_2$, a

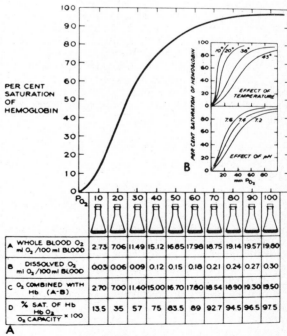

Figure 2. Hemoglobin dissociation curve for hemoglobin. A, The pH is 7.40 at 37°C. B, Effect of changing temperature and pH on the dissociation curve. Hb = Hemoglobin; HbO$_2$ = oxyhemoglobin. (Data of J. W. Severinghaus: J. Appl. Physiol., 21:1108, 1966. Reproduced with permission from Comroe, J. H., Jr.: Physiology of Respiration, 2nd ed., Copyright 1974, by Year Book Medical Publishers, Inc., Chicago.)

range usually easily achieved in the arterial blood. Additionally, the steep slope of the curve allows rapid release of oxygen in the tissues at a Pao_2 compatible with oxidative metabolism. Another feature of the curve is the rapid decline in Pao_2 that occurs when the oxygen content is lowered from full saturation. The mixture of desaturated blood with saturated blood, as occurs with a central right to left shunt, results in a stoichiometric alteration of oxygen content. The change in Pao_2 is much more dramatic, following the relatively flat portion of the dissociation curve. The importance of this phenomenon will be elaborated upon in a later section. The $Paco_2$ is a direct measure of alveolar ventilation. The normal range is 38 to 42 mm. Hg, with values greater than 46 mm. Hg indicating significant pulmonary insufficiency.

The arterial pH normally ranges from 7.37 to 7.43. The pH is maintained by the complex interactions of the blood buffer system, renal compensation, and ventilatory compensation. Acute deviations may be due to hyperventilation, causing a respiratory alkalosis (low $Paco_2$ and high pH). This is a common clinical finding, resulting from the anxiety of arterial puncture. Acidosis that is partially compensated for by hyperventilation (low $Paco_2$) usually indicates a metabolic abnormality or, more ominously, tissue hypoperfusion. Acidosis accompanied by an elevated $Paco_2$, perhaps partially compensated by renal retention of bicarbonate, is found in severe respiratory insufficiency.

DISTRIBUTION OF VENTILATION AND PERFUSION

Spirometric evaluation allows the estimation of the overall ability of a patient to ventilate. Of equal importance is the appropriate regional delivery to the inspired gases, coupled with a matching of regional perfusion to ventilation.

The distribution of ventilation is determined by many factors. The production of surfactant by terminal airways is important in maintaining small airway and alveolar expansion. Localized infections or secretions, as well as diffuse damage by chronic lung disease, can overwhelm this defense mechanism and cause regional airway collapse at the lobar, segmental, or even respiratory bronchiole level. Perfusion of nonventilated units leads to venous admixture, which can be viewed as the contamination of arterial blood with venous blood. Ventilation of nonperfused units is wasted ventilation, termed the *physiologic dead space*.

Ventilation

The interaction of the lung and chest wall generates negative intrapleural pressure during all phases of respiration with the exception of forced expiration. The pleural pressure so created varies from -10 cm. water (H_2O) at the apex to -2.5 cm. H_2O at the base, on average in the upright human. This gradient in pleural pressure depends on the recoil of both chest wall and lung, the phase of respiration, and body position. The intra-alveolar pressure is zero with the glottis open, and thus alveolar radius is related to the transmural (pleural–intra-alveolar) alveolar pressure and alveolar compliance. Thus, the pleural pressure gradient creates a gradient in alveolar size (given uniform alveolar compliance) wherein the apical alveoli are larger than basal alveoli.[6]

The effect of regional differences in alveolar (and by the same physical principles, airway) size is twofold. The low transmural basal pressure can result in alveolar and airway collapse, and the high apical transmural pressure places the alveoli near the limits of expansion. Studies using radioactive xenon gas have shown that both situations may occur in patients, as illustrated in Figure 3. The volume of the lung at which basilar alveolar and airway closure occurs is termed the *closing volume*. The relation of this volume to the FRC and age is illustrated in Figure 4.

Perfusion

The distribution of perfusion is largely affected by gravitational influences. The systolic pulmonary artery pressure rarely exceeds 30 mm. Hg in healthy individuals, and this can be insufficient to raise the fluid column (blood) to the apex of the upright lung.

Three zones of regional blood flow have been described

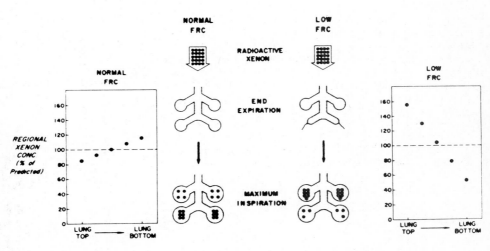

Figure 3. Effect of end-expiratory regional lung volume on the distribution of ventilation. Radioactive xenon was injected at the beginning of inspiration and measured with external counters. An inspiration from normal functional residual capacity (FRC) is distributed preferentially to the lung bottom, as the dependent alveoli are at minimal radius and capable of full expansion while apical alveoli are nearer full expansion. An inspiration from low FRC, where dependent air space is collapsed, results in a reversal of distribution, with the majority of ventilation occurring at the apex. (Reproduced with permission from Pontoppidan, H., Laver, M. B., and Geffin, B.: Acute respiratory failure in the surgical patient. Adv. Surg., 4:163, 1970. Copyright 1970, by Year Book Medical Publishers, Inc., Chicago. Redrawn from data of Milic-Emili, J., et al.: J. Appl. Physiol., 21:749, 1966.)

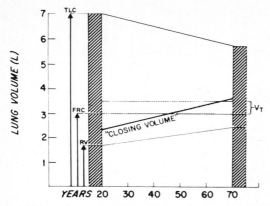

Figure 4. Effect of age on total lung capacity, functional residual capacity (FRC), residual volume, and closing volume. Values are for the normal, supine adult. In the fifth decade, closing volume exceeds the RFC during tidal ventilation, implying airway closure. The resulting ventilation-perfusion abnormality accounts for the hypoxemia seen with increasing age. A decrease in FRC, as seen with surgical incisions, anesthesia, and obesity, would have the effect of moving the tidal volume into the closing volume at a younger age and during a larger proportion of the tidal volume. The resulting ventilation-perfusion abnormality accounts for the hypoxemia seen with age and following surgical procedures.

(Reproduced with permission from Lumb, P. D.: Perioperative pulmonary physiology. In Sabiston, D. C., Jr., and Spencer, F. C. [Eds.]: Gibbon's Surgery of the Chest, 4th ed. Philadephia, W. B. Saunders Company, 1983. Modified from Pontoppidan, H., et al.: Acute Respiratory Failure in the Adult. Boston, Little, Brown and Company, 1973, using original data from Bates, D. V., et al: Respiratory Function in Disease. An Introduction to the Integrated Study of the Lung, 2nd ed. Philadelphia, W. B. Saunders Co., 1971; Sorbine, et al., Respiration, 25:3, 1968, and Leblanc, et al., J. Appl. Phyiol., 28:448, 1970.)

by West.[54] In the upright individual, *Zone 1* resides in the apex of the lung. Alveolar pressure is greater than both pulmonary artery pressure and pulmonary venous pressure. The alveolar pressure is directly transmitted to the pulmonary capillary resistance vessels, closing them and preventing perfusion altogether. Thus, Zone 1 is ventilated but not perfused, and constitutes a physiologic dead space.

Zone 2, in the midlung, occurs when the pulmonary artery pressure exceeds alveolar pressure, which in turn exceeds pulmonary venous pressure. The capillaries behave like flutter valves (Starling resistors) and flow is intermittent throughout the respiratory cycle. Pulmonary venous pressure has no effect on blood flow in this zone, the "vascular waterfall."

In *Zone 3*, the lung base, both pulmonary arterial and venous pressures exceed alveolar pressure, and flow thus occurs throughout the respiratory cycle. The magnitude of flow is dependent upon the pressure difference between pulmonary artery and pulmonary vein and upon the inherent resistance of the pulmonary capillaries modified by the distending pressure of the intraluminal blood. Regional flow is also controlled by the hypoxic vasoconstrictor reflex, which can reduce blood flow to nonventilated lung regions.[34]

REGIONAL MATCHING OF VENTILATION AND PERFUSION

It is apparent that the physical forces controlling regional ventilation and perfusion interact only in the broad-

est sense and are not generally self-corrective. Pleural pressure changes that would influence ventilation would not necessarily cause a corresponding change in perfusion. Likewise, diminution of pulmonary artery pressure increases the total Zone 1 volume but would not diminish wasted ventilation by the same mechanism. The hypoxic pulmonary vasoconstrictive response is physiologic and compensating, but it is not powerful enough to eliminate the adverse effects of ventilation-perfusion mismatch.

In the normal lung, ventilation and perfusion are closely matched, with the preponderance of both ventilation and perfusion distributed to the bases. Commensurate diminution of both ventilation and perfusion occurs in the midlung and apex. Basilar hypoventilation caused by changes in FRC or an elevated closing volume can cause a severe ventilation-perfusion abnormality. The consequences of this abnormality can be striking and are reflected in arterial oxygenation as well as in carbon dioxide metabolism. Ideal matching of ventilation and perfusion allows normal oxygen uptake and carbon dioxide elimination (Fig. 5, Panel I).

Oxygenation

If matching of ventilation and perfusion were ideal, the Pa_{O_2} would be equal to the partial alveolar pressure of oxygen (PA_{O_2}). While one is breathing 100 per cent oxygen, this can be calculated as follows[34]:

$$PA_{O_2} = PB - (PA_{CO_2} + PH_2O)$$

where PB = barometric pressure, PH_2O = water vapor pressure (corrected for temperature), and PA_{CO_2} = alveolar partial pressure of carbon dioxide (in practice, approximately equal to Pa_{CO_2}).

The degree to which there is a difference between PA_{O_2} and Pa_{O_2} (termed the $P(A-aD_{O_2})$) reflects the contamination of pulmonary venous blood with mixed venous blood, the result of perfusion of underventilated alveoli (Fig. 5, Panel II). This can be estimated while one is breathing 100 per cent oxygen, allowing easy calculation of PA_{O_2}. The actual magnitude of such mixed venous shunt flow can be calculated.

The product of the cardiac output (QT) and the arterial oxygen content (Ca_{O_2}) yields the amount of oxygen carried in the blood per unit of time. This blood can be viewed as a mixture of blood "shunted" through nonventilated alveoli (QS) and blood ideally perfused through ventilated alveoli (QC). The amount of oxygen carried in each is equal to the product of QS and the oxygen content of mixed venous blood (Cv_{O_2}) and the product of QC and the oxygen content of pulmonary end-capillary blood (Cc_{O_2}).

It follows that:

$$QT*Ca_{O_2} = (QC*Cc_{O_2}) + (QS*Cv_{O_2})$$

and that

$$QT = QC + QS$$

Solving these two questions yields the "shunt equation," which reflects the fraction of pulmonary flow that is "shunted" past nonventilated alveoli:

$$QS/QT = (Cc_{O_2} - Ca_{O_2})/(Cc_{O_2} - Cv_{O_2})$$

Cc_{O_2} can be calculated from nomograms describing the saturation of hemoglobin at the arterial pH and temperature of the patient, with 100 per cent saturation assumed. Similarly, Ca_{O_2} is calculated from the measured Pa_{O_2} and

Figure 5. Effect of changes in ventilation and perfusion on Pao$_2$ and Paco$_2$. Tidal volume is represented by black arrows, the thickness of the arrows representing changes in magnitude of the tidal volume.

Panel I, The normal lung is represented by two alveoli, each perfused by one half of the cardiac output.

Panel II, A and B, Acute collapse of an alveolus is associated with continued perfusion. Venous admixture results in arterial hypoxemia. An increase in the tidal volume to ventilated-perfused unit is unable to overcome the effect of venous admixture.

Panel II, C, Marked ventilation-perfusion abnormality is present. The left alveolus receives most of the perfusion and little ventilation, the blood remaining poorly oxygenated and with a high Pco$_2$. The reverse is the case for the right alveolus. The result is a decreased Pao$_2$ and an elevated Paco$_2$.

Panel III, A and B, Continued ventilation to a non-perfused alveolus results in dead space ventilation. Hyperventilation of the perfused alveolus can return Paco$_2$ to normal, usually requiring an increase in overall respiratory work. Hypotension can increase the amount of Zone 1 lung, increasing this "physiologic" dead space. Pulmonary embolism has a similar effect.

Panel III, C, A marked ventilation-perfusion imbalance induces a smaller dead space volume.

(Reproduced with permission from Laver, M. B., Austen, W. G. and Wilson, R. S.: Blood-gas exchange and hemodynamic performance. In Sabiston, D. C., Jr., and Spencer, F. C. [Eds.]: Gibbon's Surgery of the Chest, 3rd ed. Philadelphia, W. B. Saunders Co., 1976.)

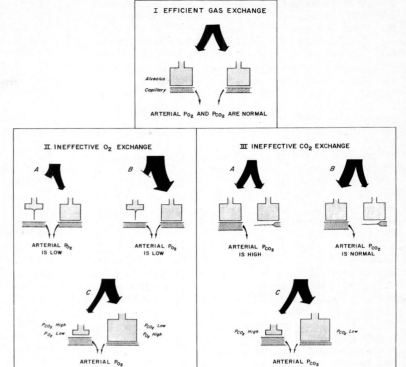

the hemoglobin content, and Cvo$_2$ from the measured partial pressure of oxygen in mixed venous blood.[34]

Carbon Dioxide

The Paco$_2$ is directly related to the magnitude of alveolar ventilation and the rate of carbon dioxide production by oxidative metabolism. The latter is relatively constant, although postoperative shivering may cause a significant increase in Paco$_2$. Ventilation of nonperfused air space results in wasted ventilation, and unless compensated for by increased tidal volume or increased respiratory rate, the Paco$_2$ will rise. The two sources of this "dead space" are anatomic and "physiologic."

The *anatomic dead space* is that portion of the upper airway that serves to transport respired air and has no intimate contact with the pulmonary capillaries. It is usually fixed in absolute volume (approximately equal in milliliters to the body weight in pounds) and is approximately one third of the tidal volume. The *physiologic dead space* is that portion of the lung where there is overventilation relative to perfusion. As physiologic dead space increases, minute ventilation must increase to compensate for what can be viewed as an encroachment on the tidal volume (Fig. 5, Panel III).

and the partial pressure difference across the tissue. Under normal conditions, the partial pressure difference is large (PAo$_2$ = 105 mm. Hg, mixed venous Po$_2$ = 40 mm. Hg). The rapid combination of oxygen with hemoglobin and the steep slope of the oxyhemoglobin dissociation curve tend to maintain this gradient. Thus, only approximately one third of the 0.75 second transit time of the red blood cell is required for near complete hemoglobin saturation. As a consequence, there is a large margin of safety in diffusion capacity of the normal lung. A large decrease in the pulmonary transit time, as in a septic hyperdynamic state, coupled with air space disease, can severely limit oxygen diffusion.[55]

Carbon dioxide is more than 20 times more soluble in tissue than is oxygen, allowing rapid transport. There is a lower partial pressure difference between the blood (mixed venous PCO$_2$ = 45 − 50 mm. Hg) and the inspired air (PCo$_2$ = O) than in the case of oxygen. Despite this, the higher molecular weight of CO$_2$ and the slower reaction rate in the dissolution of CO$_2$, diffusion impairment leading to hypercapnea is uncommon.[55] The measurement of diffusing capacity for O$_2$ and CO$_2$ is not possible clinically, but is approximated by the diffusion capacity of carbon monoxide (DLCO). DLCO can be determined rapidly and easily in the pulmonary function laboratory, and has become a routine part of pulmonary function testing.

IMPAIRED DIFFUSION CAPACITY

Oxygen must diffuse across the alveolar and capillary membranes and through the red blood cell membrane (a negligible amount of oxygen is dissolved in plasma). Gas diffusion depends upon distance (in this case, less than 0.5 micron), solubility of the gas, molecular weight of the gas,

SPECIFIC PULMONARY DISORDERS

Chronic obstructive pulmonary disease (COPD) is a general term describing a group of patients with respiratory disease. The common denominator is an element of expiratory obstruction.

Bronchitis is defined as chronic excessive mucous secretion in the bronchial tree and is usually accompanied by productive cough. Peribronchial inflammation and airway narrowing cause outflow obstruction. The FVC, FEV_1, and MVV are all decreased. Expiratory obstruction leads to air trapping, with an increase in the TLC and RV. Radioactive scanning techniques have demonstrated a predominant overperfusion of underventilated air spaces. As a consequence, hypoxia and hypercapnea are common features.[52]

Emphysema is characterized as the abnormal enlargement of air spaces distal to the terminal brochiole, associated with destruction of the alveolar architecture. There is loss of the normal elastic recoil of the lung as well as decreased elastic support of the peripheral airways. The TLC, FRC, and RV are increased. The FVC, FEV_1, and MVV are decreased. There is very little perfusion of nonventilated alveoli, but there is a large amount of physiologic dead space. Consequently, arterial oxygenation is often normal or only mildly depressed and the Pa_{CO_2} is usually normal.[6]

Restrictive lung disease can result from many diseases, including fibrothorax, kyphoscoliosis, sarcoidosis, interstitial pneumonitis, infiltrative neoplasms, myasthenia gravis, and cardiogenic pulmonary edema. Pulmonary compliance is decreased, and TLC, VC, and FRC are decreased. The airway size is increased, but the FEV_1 may be decreased, particularly in neuromuscular disorders. The $FEV_1/FVC\%$ is normal, however, when actual airway obstruction is not a component of the lung disease. Ventilation-perfusion abnormalities are common, resulting in hypoxemia. The development of hypercapnea is unusual and reflects the end stage of restrictive lung disease. The maintenance of normal arterial P_{CO_2} is the result of compensatory hyperventilation, which is achieved at a greatly increased work of breathing.[52]

THE EFFECT OF SURGICAL PROCEDURES ON PULMONARY FUNCTION

The degree of pulmonary dysfunction following operation is directly related to the type of procedure and the preoperative status of pulmonary function. For example, operations performed upon the extremities generally have little effect on pulmonary function.[52] Thoracic procedures, particularly those involving pulmonary resection, cause severe depression of respiratory function. Abdominal procedures can cause significant respiratory depression, especially with an upper midline incision.[32]

Total lung capacity and all the subdivisions of lung capacity are reduced following non-extremity procedures.[37, 47] This reduces the surface area available for gas exchange and promotes airway closure since the FRC is reduced below the closing volume. The resulting atelectasis, either macroscopic or microscopic, leads to arterial hypoxemia. Atelectasis can also be due to retained secretions, the quality of which may be altered by anesthetic agents. The elimination of these secretions is hampered by diminished cough, caused by pain or narcotic administration. There may be dysfunction of ciliary activity and clearance of microbial agents.

Airway closure is also due to postoperative splinting of the chest. The breathing pattern is characteristically altered to accomplish adequate minute ventilation with a lowered tidal volume at an increased respiratory rate. Sighing, a normal mechanism for opening the airways, is virtually eliminated in the early postoperative period.[27] Restriction of the patient to the bed, primarily in the supine position, is also deleterious.[53] Abnormal positioning of the

patient during operation can result in pulmonary dysfunction. This is particularly evident in the thoracic patient, for whom the lateral decubitus position can lead to dependent lung consolidation.[34]

PREOPERATIVE EVALUATION OF RISK

Increased age and a smoking history increase the closing volume.[27] Obesity diminishes the FRC and ERV, such that the end tidal point approaches the closing volume. Patients with obstructive pulmonary disease have a diminished ERV. The additive effect of a postoperative decrease in FRC and ERV results in airway closure and atelectasis in patients with these characteristics.

Obstructive pulmonary disease is the most important risk factor in surgical patients, the degree of expiratory obstruction being directly related to the risk of postoperative complications.[50] Restrictive lung disease is usually more easily tolerated, despite the fact that lung volumes are decreased postoperatively. This is due to better maintenance of expiratory flow and secretion clearing.

The use of preoperative pulmonary function testing has allowed an approximation of risk based on obstruction. An FEV_1 of greater than 2 liters is associated with minimal risk. Increased risk is associated with an FEV_1 of from 1 to 2 liters. When the FEV_1 is less than 0.8 liters, there is a moderate risk of severe complications, that risk becoming prohibitive with an FEV_1 less than 0.5 liters.[14] The 5-year survival of patients with an FEV_1 of less than 0.75 liters may be as little as 10 per cent, a factor that should be considered in elective surgical procedures.[13]

Thoracotomy and pulmonary resection are even less well tolerated.[14] The loss of functional pulmonary tissue and the more direct effects of thoracic incisions tend to depress postoperative pulmonary function more severely. The presence of pulmonary hypertension and hypercapnea probably contraindicate pulmonary resection. If the FEV_1 is less than 2 liters and the MVV less than 50 per cent of predicted, the patient is at increased risk for pulmonary resection and should probably not undergo a pneumonectomy. The quantitative lung scan can be helpful in borderline patients, in whom the removal of nonfunctioning lung tissue may be possible despite limited overall pulmonary function.[1]

PREOPERATIVE PREPARATION

Every effort should be made to convince the patient to cease smoking preoperatively. Ideally, this should be done at least 2 weeks before surgery, although there is marked benefit from cessation for as little as 1 week.

The identification of other treatable preoperative conditions is essential. In patients with a productive cough, sputum culture and the institution of appropriate antibiotics are imperative.

Patient education and training are very important parts of preoperative preparation. Breathing exercises strengthen the respiratory musculature. Instructions on coughing and deep breathing improve postoperative cooperation. Instruction in the use of p.r.n. (as needed) narcotics to allow coughing and deep breathing will give the physician a valuable ally in the titration of these drugs postoperatively. In patients with copious pulmonary secretions, chest percussion and postural drainage may be necessary.

POSTOPERATIVE MANAGEMENT

In general, if preoperative evaluation has been complete, this should be simply a continuation of preoperative therapy. Supplemental oxygen is administered to correct hypoxemia caused by central hypoventilation in the immediate postoperative period. Oxygen therapy is discontinued when its need is no longer required, as documented by arterial blood gas determinations. The patient is positioned with the head slightly elevated, if possible, and the position in bed changed at frequent intervals. It has been clearly demonstrated that inspiratory exercises, with the encouragement of deep breathing, are the most effective means of minimizing airway closure.[5] Narcotics are administered to minimize postoperative pain and to allow effective coughing. When the cough is ineffective, endotracheal suctioning may be necessary.

Early ambulation has proved to be an effective means to prevent postoperative pulmonary complications. Sitting upright and ambulation increase the FRC and lead to improvement in all lung volumes, counteracting the changes induced by surgery.[17] The risk of pulmonary embolism is also reduced.

MEDICAL MANAGEMENT OF BRONCHOSPASM

A larger variety of therapeutic agents are now available to optimize pulmonary function. An organized approach in the use of these agents is important, as there are many potential drug interactions and serious side effects that may limit therapy.

Theophylline

Theophylline is a member of the xanthine family and is currently the most popular bronchodilating agent. Its mechanism of action is unclear at this time, but it is known to inhibit phosphodiesterase and to specifically antagonize adenosine.

The specific effects of theophylline preparations are as follows:

1. Bronchodilatation.
2. Increase in respiratory drive.
3. Inhibition of mast cell mediator release.
4. Increase in mucociliary clearance.
5. Pulmonary arterial vasodilatation.
6. Increase in contractility and reduction in fatigability of the diaphragm.[4]

Bronchodilatation is dose-related over a relatively narrow therapeutic range (10 to 20 µg./ml.). The maintenance of appropriate serum theophylline levels has been made possible by the development of a clinically available radioimmunoassay. Adverse gastrointestinal effects can be seen with levels greater than 15 µg./ml. Cardiac effects are also seen at higher levels, but no studies have demonstrated adverse effects in the therapeutic range.

Intravenous loading with 5.6 mg. per kg. is indicated in acute bronchospasm, followed by a continuous infusion at a rate dependent upon age, smoking habits, and other medical conditions. Conversion to an oral preparation should be accomplished within 48 hours. Serum levels should be monitored throughout the initial period of use. The possibility that concomitant bronchodilatation and pulmonary arterial dilatation may be distributed in such a way

as to worsen ventilation-perfusion matching, and thus lead to hypoxia, should always be considered.[12, 18]

Adrenergic Agonists and Bronchodilator Aerosol Therapy

The effect of adrenergic agonists is primarily due to direct effects on bronchial smooth muscle, since there is no significant direct sympathetic innervation in the human. The beta-2 effects are bronchodilatory and anti-inflammatory by inhibition of mediator release. Mucociliary clearance is also improved.

The prototype sympathomimetic drug is epinephrine, but its use has been limited by adverse cardiac effects when given systemically and by poor bioavailability in oral forms. The development of metaproterenol and albuterol has allowed oral dosage and has minimized cardiac or beta-1 effects.

The effects of adrenergic agents are dose-related and show no response plateau. Therapy is limited by systemic side effects, which include tremor, nervousness, and cardiac arrhythmias. The use of an aerosol administration route allows greater effective dosing with fewer side effects. In acute bronchospasm, the aerosol route may not result in uniform airway distribution and effectiveness can be delayed. The bronchodilatory effects of the adrenergic agents are probably additive when used in combination with theophylline.[45]

Corticosteroids

The use of corticosteroids is usually avoided in the management of bronchospasm, if at all possible. If an acute bronchospastic episode cannot be broken with theophylline and beta-2 agents, systemic steroids are indicated. Patients already receiving chronic steroid therapy for obstructive lung disease should be given perioperative steroids because of adrenal suppression. In selected patients with severe bronchospasm, perioperative systemic corticosteroids can be beneficial.

The introduction of beclomethasone dipropionate has increased the therapeutic efficacy of steroid use, since it is administered by inhalation. Adrenal suppressive effects are not seen with normal prescription. Long-term studies have not shown any adverse histologic effects on the bronchial mucosa.[11]

Anticholinergic, Antimuscarinic Bronchodilators

The primary efferent innervation of the lung is parasympathetic, cholinergic, and excitatory, so that there is a predominant vagal tone resulting in bronchoconstriction and increased mucous secretion. Atropine has long been recognized as a potent bronchodilator, but its use has been limited by its side effects. Even with aerosol administration, systemic levels are high, resulting in bladder outlet obstruction, meiosis, and tachycardia. The dangers of inspissation of viscid secretions with chronic anticholinergic therapy may be only a theoretical adverse effect.

The introduction of the quaternary ammonium cogeners of atropine, atropine methonitrate, and ipratropium bromide, may result in the clinical revival of the anticholinergic agents. These drugs are poorly absorbed after aerosol administration and thus have few systemic effects. They are very potent bronchodilators, comparing favorably with the theophyllines and adrenergic agents. Additionally, they act to remove tonic stimulation and act synergistically with currently available agents. The most particular specific indication for these drugs is in the treatment of bronchospasm induced by beta blockage.[22] These agents are currently in use in Europe and are being considered for use in the United States.

Airway Management

The broad indications for intubation are upper airway obstruction, the need for ventilatory support, and the management of copious secretions. Ventilatory support may be required for hypoventilation, hypoxia, increased work of breathing, or combinations of these features in the clinical setting of *adult respiratory distress syndrome* (ARDS). Some specific indications for intubation and mechanical ventilation are outlined in Table 1, but these criteria should not be viewed as a substitute for clinical evaluation. The decision to intubate a patient in respiratory distress must be made prior to the development of an irreversible clinical state, and early intubation is preferable even if it may prove unnecessary.[42]

Intubation should be performed as an elective procedure, if at all possible. In this setting, nasotracheal intubation is preferred when prolonged support is anticipated because it allows a more mechanically secure airway and results in less tracheal mucosal damage than does orotracheal intubation.[20] In an emergency, orotracheal intubation is more rapid in experienced hands.

The safety of prolonged endotracheal intubation has

TABLE 1. Guidelines for Ventilatory Support in Adults with Acute Respiratory Failure*†

Datum	Normal Range	Indication for Tracheal Intubation and Ventilation
Mechanics		
Respiratory rate	12–20	>35
Vital capacity (ml./kg. of body weight‡)	65–75	<15
FEV₁# (ml./kg. of body weight‡)	50–60	<10
Inspiratory force (cm. H₂O)	75–100	<25
Oxygenation		
PaO₂ (mm. Hg)	100–75 (air)	<70 (on mask O₂)
P(A − aDO₂) (mm. Hg)§	25–65	>450
Ventilation		
PaCO₂ (mm.Hg)	35–45	>55¶
V_D/V_T	0.25–0.40	>0.60

*Reproduced with permission from Laver, M. B., and Austen, W. G.: Respiratory function: Physiologic considerations applicable to surgery. *In* Sabiston, D. C., Jr. (Ed.): Davis-Christopher Textbook of Surgery, 12th ed. Philadelphia, W. B. Saunders Co., 1981. Data from Wilson, R. S., and Pontoppidan, H.: Crit. Care Med., 2:293, 1974.

†The clinical evaluation of the patient should supersede intubation of a patient based on any single abnormal value. The clinical course of the patient will also modify the above values.

‡Ideal weight used if weight is grossly abnormal.

§Obtained after 10 minutes of 100 per cent oxygen.

¶Except in patients with chronic hypercapnea.

#First second forced expired volume.

been established for periods of up to 3 weeks.[33, 41] Advances in tube design, particularly the development of thin polyvinyl chloride, large-volume, high-compliance cuffs, has minimized the need for early conversion to tracheostomy. Skilled nursing care and the establishment of respiratory therapy departments have provided the constant surveillance of each patient that is required for successful longterm intubation. Meticulous attention to adequate humidification, sterile suctioning technique and frequent culturing of secretions have become routine intensive care practices.

Stauffer, in a prospective study, demonstrated that the complications of tracheostomy were more serious than those of intubation for airway control of less than 3 weeks' duration.[48] If more than 3 weeks of support become necessary, tracheostomy is required. If it is clear from the outset that prolonged intubation will be necessary, tracheostomy should probably be performed 7 to 10 days following intubation, before tracheal mucosal damage becomes severe.

Tracheostomy is currently most often performed as an elective procedure in the intubated patient. Operating room conditions should be duplicated if the procedure must be performed in the intensive care unit. Reliable lighting, sterile suctioning capability, sterile airway connectors, and expert anesthesia support are essential. Standard operative technique for tracheostomy is illustrated in Figure 6. Proper care in the aspiration of secretions, in avoidance of bacterial contamination, and in humidification of inspired gases is necessary to minimize complications. Special attention should be paid to proper support of ventilation attachments and to maintaining intracuff pressure in the 20 to 25 torr range to reduce tracheal trauma.[7]

Cricothyroidotomy has become recognized as a reasonable alternative to standard tracheostomy in recent years. Brantigan and Grow reported a series of 566 patients with excellent results.[10] Boyd and co-workers reported a 1 per cent incidence of glottic and subglottic stenosis in a more recent series, with these complications occurring only in patients operated upon after intubation for more than 7 days.[9] Cricothyroidotomy is preferred by some for longterm airway management of the postoperative cardiac patient because the incision is easily separable from the median sternotomy wound. Cricothyroidotomy is also preferable to emergency tracheostomy when endotracheal intubation cannot be performed, since it is faster and simpler and has a lower complication rate.

Ventilatory Support

Once airway control is established, mechanical ventilation is usually necessary. There is ample evidence that early aggressive respiratory support can minimize the morbidity of respiratory failure.[42] The goals of ventilatory support are to safely normalize minute volume and the distribution of ventilation and perfusion so as to provide for adequate oxygen delivery and carbon dioxide elimination.

Numerous mechanical ventilators are available, and more detailed descriptions are referenced.[36, 44] All ventilators deliver a mixture of humidified gases under positive pressure, with expiration being a passive process. The most popular ventilators volume cycle to the expiratory phase, good examples being the Bennet MA-1 and MA-2. This means that the inspiratory phase is accomplished with a controlled volume being administered in each cycle. The other major ventilator category, represented by the Bird

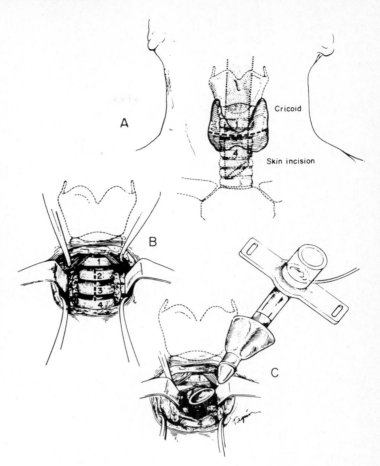

Figure 6. Technique of tracheostomy.

A, *The operation is performed in the intubated patient. The neck is slightly extended. A short horizontal incision is made to overlie the second or third tracheal ring, located by their relation to the palpated cricoid cartilage. The first and fourth rings are numbered.*

B, *The strap muscles are separated in the midline and retracted. The cricoid is identified as the primary landmark for counting the tracheal rings. The thyroid isthmus is usually divided between clamps and sutured to facilitate exposure, and the second and third tracheal rings are incised vertically. The first ring should never be incised.*

C, *Smooth thyroid pole retractors are illustrated as they expose the tracheal incision. The endotracheal tube has been retracted to a level just above the tracheal incision and should not be further removed until the tracheostomy tube has been demonstrated to be functional. A tracheostomy tube is then inserted and its flanges sutured to the skin. The tube is also secured with tapes placed around the neck. The incision may be closed with skin sutures, but this is not always required.*

(Reproduced with permission from Grillo, H. C.: Tracheostomy and its complications. In Sabiston, D. C., Jr. [Ed.]: Davis-Christopher Textbook of Surgery: The Biologic Basis of Modern Surgical Practice, 12th ed. Philadelphia, W. B. Saunders Company, 1981.)

ventilator, cycles to the expiratory phase based on system pressure during inspiration. With the pressure cycled ventilator, the tidal volume is not controlled per se but is dependent upon normal lung/chest wall compliance interacting with the tidal volume to cycle to the expiratory phase at a given achieved airway pressure. When compliance changes, the tidal volume also changes, making these respirators difficult to use properly in the postoperative period.

Ventilators can be used in a variety of ways to assist ventilation. Ventilation can be absolutely controlled only in the paralyzed or heavily sedated patient. Respiration is assisted by means of a variety of ventilatory modes, outlined as follows:

Assisted Ventilation (AV). The patient triggers a mechanical inspiration based on the generation of a small detected negative airway pressure.

Intermittent Mandatory Ventilation (IMV). The patient breathes on his own through the respirator circuit, but receives supplemental ventilation from the respirator at a controlled rate.

Pressure Support (PS) Ventilation. A constant inspiratory pressure is used to assist inspiration during IMV, a new technique that allows ventilator weaning by decreasing inspiratory support rather than by decreasing the IMV rate alone.

Continuous Positive Airway Pressure (CPAP). In adults, CPAP is used as pressure support to compensate for the resistive burden of the endotracheal tube during inspiration and to maintain FRC at end expiration.

Positive End Expiratory Pressure (PEEP). PEEP is used to maintain FRC in the patient supported for central

hypoventilation and therapeutically in respiratory distress syndromes to increase FRC and normalize the ventilation perfusion relationship.

High-Frequency Ventilation (HFV). Unusually high frequency ventilation (60 to 100 breaths per minute) at small tidal volumes (3 to 4 ml./kg.) are used. This allows for a quiet operative field during pulmonary surgery and can be helpful in cases of barotrauma or bronchopleural fistula by minimizing mean airway pressure. Carlon and Howland have recently edited an excellent monograph on the subject.[15]

In addition to providing various modes of ventilation, ventilators must humidify the inspired gases to saturation and provide alarm systems to prevent catastrophic complications. The basic alarms necessary for safe use are outlined as follows:

Low Pressure Disconnect. Alarms when system pressure becomes atmospheric, signifying mechanical disconnection of the ventilator.

Inspiratory Pressure Limit. Alarms when system pressure exceeds a prescribed value during inspiration or during sighs. Most ventilators allow separate establishment of the high pressure limit for normal tidal volumes and sighs.

Low Expired Volume. Alarms when the expired volume does not equal the inspired volume in a volume cycled ventilator. This may be offset to allow for system leak and usually warns of the new onset of a system leak.

The most important alarm is, of course, represented by the personnel who monitor patients on mechanical ventilator support. The most appropriate response to any of these alarms is an immediate and complete evaluation of the ventilator, its connections, and the patient. Should an easily correctable fault or explanation not be immediately forthcoming, the ventilator should be disconnected and manual respiration begun until a complete assessment has been made.

CONTROL OF ARTERIAL BLOOD GASES

The control of respiration with a mechanical ventilator permits manipulations of arterial Po_2, Pco_2 and pH that are not possible in any other setting.

Arterial Pco_2, reflecting alveolar ventilation, can be lowered by increasing minute ventilation, either by increased tidal volume or by increased respiratory rate. Initial settings of a tidal volume of 10 to 15 ml. per kg. at a rate of 8 to 12 breaths per minute usually result in a normal Pco_2. When the Pco_2 is too low and the resulting arterial pH is too high, minute ventilation supplied by the ventilator can be decreased in compensation. When spontaneous patient ventilation causes hypocapnea, sedation and increased ventilator control may be necessary. The addition of dead space to the breathing circuit or the addition of CO_2 to the inspired gases may also be necessary.

The arterial Po_2 can be modified by a variety of maneuvers. Initially, oxygenation can be improved by the administration of oxygen enriched gases. An arterial oxygen saturation greater than 90 per cent is desirable and must be obtained initially even if the Fio_2 must be increased to 1.0. The ability to maintain oxygenation by this means is limited by the toxic nature of oxygen in concentrations higher than atmospheric.

Oxygen toxicity results in a pathologic picture of atelectasis, edema, inflammation, and thickening of alveolar membranes. Bacterial clearance and macrophage function become diminished.[21, 26, 40] The biochemical mechanism of this toxicity appears to be the development of intracellular oxygen radicals and chemically active oxygen metabolites[35] in concentrations exceeding the cellular defense mechanisms. Prevention is the best treatment, but methods to enhance cellular defenses are on the horizon.[19] An additional adverse feature of elevated oxygen concentration is the development of venous admixture because of shunting at the alveolar level owing to atelectasis or edema.[39] At the present time, an absolutely safe level of oxygen supplementation has not been established. It appears that an Fio_2 of 0.4 to 0.5 is well tolerated for prolonged periods.[26] An Fio_2 of 0.6 or greater is hazardous, the hazard increasing directly with increasing oxygen concentration. An Fio_2 of 1.0 should not be maintained for more than 48 hours.[19]

In order to improve arterial oxygenation without excessive oxygen administration, other methods are necessary. The use of PEEP has become fundamental in the therapy of respiratory failure in this regard. PEEP has been shown to reduce oxygen requirements by improving ventilation-perfusion matching and by increasing the FRC toward normal in postoperative patients.[23] PEEP should be increased to the highest levels tolerated that also decrease venous admixture.[29] It should be recognized that the effect of PEEP is nonspecific, that patients have individual responses to its use, and that certain patients will respond to PEEP with an increase in venous admixture. The use of PEEP is limited by dose-related decrease in cardiac output and by barotrauma resulting in pneumothorax. The cardiac output effect has been shown to be related to a decrease in left heart filling secondary to an increase in right ventricular afterload and to direct effects on the right ventricle that are responsive to volume loading.[46]

Extracorporeal membrane oxygenation, either venovenous or venoarterial, has been utilized to support systemic oxygenation while allowing recovery of the injured lung. A prospective study demonstrated that this therapy was no more effective than standard ventilatory support in ARDS.[58] Renewed interest in the treatment of neonatal pulmonary insufficiency by membrane oxygenation has developed with the reporting of improved survival with this modality.[30, 31]

WEANING FROM VENTILATORY SUPPORT

Once pulmonary function has recovered, usually through specific treatment of underlying infections, bronchospasm, or resolution of the constellation of disorders evident in ARDS, support must be discontinued.

Weaning from ventilatory support conceptually begins at the time that it is instituted. Support of nutrition during intubation is imperative, as the respiratory muscles must function at full capacity once the ventilator is discontinued. Once the pathologic process that required support is controlled, the patient should gradually assume more and more responsibility for minute ventilation. This is usually accomplished by gradually decreasing the IMV rate while maintaining approximately 5 cm. of H_2O of PEEP. Minimal support prior to extubation should be 5 cm. of H_2O CPAP or IMV at 2 breaths per minute with 5 cm. H_2O PEEP.[3, 43] Further reductions in support prior to extubation are in reality unwarranted stress tests. The rate of weaning is determined by the patient's response and by serial arterial blood gas determinations. Slow weaning is required when there has been prolonged intubation in order to rehabilitate the respiratory musculature. Theophyllines, as mentioned, can be used to improve diaphragmatic contractility. In difficult situations, the use of pressure support ventilation has allowed successful discontinuation of mechanical ventilation. This modality has many advantages, not the least of which appears to be improved patient comfort.

The cooperation of the patient is essential in the transition to spontaneous ventilation. Occasionally, behavioral modification by a psychotherapist is useful in the chronically supported individual. The final decision to discontinue ventilatory support rests upon the measurement of respiratory mechanics, the measurement of arterial blood gases, and observation of the patient on minimal support.

CONCLUSIONS

The management of the pulmonary system in surgical patients requires careful attention to the physiologic principles outlined in this section. With proper selection of patients and attention to preoperative preparation based on a knowledge of the probable postoperative alterations in pulmonary function, excellent surgical results can be obtained. It should always be remembered that if pulmonary resection has not been performed, the alterations in pulmonary physiology that occur following operation are temporary and reversible with appropriate therapy.

SELECTED REFERENCES

Bates, V. C., Macklem, P. T. and Christie, R. V.: Respiratory Function in Disease: An Introduction to the Integrated Study of the Lung, 2nd ed. Philadelphia, W. B. Saunders Company, 1971.

This is the second edition of a textbook reviewing pulmonary diseases and respiratory physiology. It has an excellent bibliography covering the early research on pulmonary function in disease and gives extensive coverage of the individual pulmonary disease states.

Comroe, J. H., Jr., Forster, R. E. II, Dubois, A. B., Briscoe, W. A., and Carlsen, E.: The Lung: Clinical Physiology and Pulmonary Function Tests, 2nd ed. Chicago, Year Book Medical Publishers, Inc., 1962.
This is a classic text with excellent diagrams and illustrations. It includes the clinical aspects of pulmonary physiology, particularly those bearing on the treatment of acute and chronic disease.

Tisi, G. M.: Pulmonary Physiology in Clinical Medicine, 2nd ed. Baltimore, Williams and Wilkins Company, 1983.
This is the second edition of a fine text on clinical aspects of pulmonary medicine. It contains an excellent description of the primary chronic lung diseases encountered in practice and correlates clinical findings with pulmonary function tests. It has an excellent chapter on preoperative evaluation and an up-to-date bibliography.

REFERENCES

1. Ali, M. K., Mountain, C., Miller, J. M., Johnston, D. A., and Shullenberger, C. C.: Regional pulmonary function before and after pneumonectomy using ^{133}xenon. Chest, 68:288, 1975.
2. American Heart Association Cardiopulmonary Council: Manual for evaluation of lung function by spirometry. Circulation, 65:644A, 1982.
3. Annest, S. J., Gottlieb, M., Paloski, W. H., Stratton, H., Newell, J. C., Dutton, R., and Powers, S. R., Jr.: Detrimental effects of removing end-expiratory pressure prior to endotracheal extubation. Ann. Surg., 191:539, 1980.
4. Aubier, M., De Teroyer, A., Sampson, M., Macklem, P. T., and Roussos, C.: Aminophylline improves diaphragmatic contractility. N. Eng. J. Med., 305:249, 1981.
5. Bartlett, R. H., Gazzaniga, A. B., and Geraghty, T.: Respiratory maneuvers to prevent postoperative pulmonary complications: A critical review. J.A.M.A., 224:1017, 1973.
6. Bates, D. V., Macklem, P. T., and Christie, R. V.: Respiratory Function in Disease: An Introduction to the Integrated Study of the Lung, 2nd ed. Philadelphia, W. B. Saunders Company, 1971.
7. Boyd, A. D., Bernhard, W. N., and Spencer, F. C.: Tracheal intubation and assisted ventilation: I. Tracheal intubation and mechanical ventilation. *In* Sabiston, D. C., Jr., and Spencer, F. C. (Eds.): Gibbon's Surgery of the Chest, 4th ed. Philadelphia, W. B. Saunders Company, 1983.
8. Boyd, A. D., Bernhard, W. N., and Spencer, F. C.: Tracheal intubation and assisted ventilation: II. Mechanical ventilation: Airway pressure therapy. *In* Sabiston, D. C., Jr., and Spencer, F. C. (Eds.): Gibbon's Surgery of the Chest, 4th ed. Philadelphia, W. B. Saunders Company, 1983.
9. Boyd, A. D., Romita, M. D., Conlan, A. A., Fink, S. D., and Spencer, F. C.: A clinical evaluation of cricothyroidotomy. Surg. Gynecol. Obstet., 149:365, 1979.
10. Brantigan, C. O., and Grow, J. B.: Cricothyroidotomy: Elective use in respiratory problems requiring tracheostomy. J. Thorac. Cardiovasc. Surg., 71:72, 1976.
11. Brogden, R. N., Heel, R. C., Speight, T. M., and Avery, G. S.: Beclomethasone dipropionate: A reappraisal of its pharmacodynamic properties and therapeutic efficacy after a decade of use in asthma and rhinitis. Drugs, 28:99, 1984.
12. Bukowskyj, M., Nakatsu, K., and Munt, P. W.: Theophylline reassessed. Ann. Intern. Med., 101:63, 1984.
13. Burrows, B., and Earle, R. H.: Course and prognosis of chronic obstructive lung disease. N. Engl. J. Med., 280:397, 1969.
14. Burrows, B., Knudson, R. J., and Kettel, L. J.: Respiratory insufficiency. Chicago, Year Book Medical Publishers, Inc., 1975.
15. Carlon, C. C., and Howland, W. S.: High-frequency ventilation in intensive care and during surgery. New York, Marcel Dekker, Inc., 1985.
16. Comroe, J. H., Forster, R. E. II, Dubois, A. B., Briscoe, W. A., and Carlsen, E.: The Lung: Clinical Physiology and Pulmonary Function Tests, 2nd ed. Chicago, Year Book Medical Publishers, Inc., 1962.
17. Craig, D. B.: Postoperative recovery of pulmonary function. Anesth. Analg., 60:46, 1981.
18. Cummiskey, J. M., and Popa, V.: Theophyllines—A review. J. Asthma, 21:243, 1984.
19. Deneke, S. M., and Fanburg, B. L.: Normobaric oxygen toxicity of the lung. N. Engl. J. Med., 303:76, 1980.
20. Dubick, M. W., and Wright, B. D.: Comparison of laryngeal pathology following long-term oral and nasal endotracheal intubation. Anesth. Analg., 57:663, 1978.
21. Fisher, A. B., Diamond, S., Mellen, S., and Zubrow, A.: Effect of 48-

and 72-hour oxygen exposure on the rabbit alveolar macrophage. Chest, 66:(Suppl.)4S, 1974.
22. Gross, N. J., and Skorodin, M. S.: Anticholinergic, antimuscarinic bronchodilators. Am. Rev. Respir. Dis., 129:856, 1984.
23. Hammon, J. W., Jr., Wolfe, W. G., Moran, J. F., and Jones, R. H.: The effect of positive end-expiratory pressure on regional ventilation and perfusion in the normal and injured primate lung. J. Thorac. Cardiovasc. Surg., 72:680, 1976.
24. Hodgkin, J. E., Dines, D. E., and Didier, E. P.: Preoperative evaluation of the patient with pulmonary disease. Mayo Clin. Proc., 48:114, 1973.
25. Hoeppner, V. H., Cooper, D. M., Zamel, N., Bryan, A. C., and Levison, H.: Relationship between elastic recoil and closing volume in smokers and nonsmokers. Am. Rev. Respir. Dis. 109:81, 1974.
26. Huber, G. L., Porter, S. L., Burley, S. W., La Force, F. M., and Mason, R. J.: The effect of oxygen toxicity on the inactivation of bacteria by the lung. Chest, 61:(Suppl.)665, 1972.
27. Hyatt, R. E., and Rodarte, J. R.: Closing volume: One man's noise — other men's experiment. Mayo Clin. Proc. 50:17, 1975.
28. Kaplan, H. P., Robinson, F. R., Kapanci, Y., and Weibel, E. R.: Pathogenesis and reversibility of the pulmonary lesions of oxygen toxicity in monkeys: I. Clinical and light microscopic studies. Lab. Invest., 20:94, 1969.
29. Kirby, R. R., Downs, J. B., Civetta, J. M., Modell, J. H., Danenmiller, F. J., Klein, E. F., and Hodges, M.: High level positive end expiratory pressure (PEEP) in acute respiratory insufficiency. Chest, 67:156, 1975.
30. Klein, M. D., Andrews, A. F., Wesley, J. R., Toomasian, J., Nixon, C., Roloff, D., and Bartlett, R. H.: Venovenous perfusion in ECMO for newborn respiratory insufficiency. Ann. Surg., 201:520, 1985.
31. Krummel, R. M., Greenfield, L. J., Kirkpatrick, B. V., Mueller, D. G., Kerkering, K. W., Ormazabal, M., Napolitano, A., and Salzberg, A. M.: Alveolar-arterial oxygen gradients versus the neonatal pulmonary insufficiency index for prediction of mortality in ECMO candidates. J. Pediatr. Surg., 19:380, 1984.
32. Latimer, R. G., Dickman, M., Day, W. C., and Gunn, M. L.: Ventilatory patterns and pulmonary complications after upper abdominal surgery determined by preoperative and postoperative computerized spirometry and blood gas analysis. Am. J. Surg., 122:622, 1971.
33. Lewis, F. R., Schlobohm, R. M., and Thomas, A. N.: Prevention of complications from prolonged intubation. Am. J. Surg., 135:452, 1978.
34. Lumb, P. D.: Perioperative pulmonary physiology. *In* Sabiston, D. C., Jr., and Spencer, F. C. (Eds.): Gibbon's Surgery of the Chest, 4th ed. Philadelphia, W. B. Saunders Company, 1983.
35. McCord, J. M., and Fridovich, I.: The biology and pathology of oxygen radicals. Ann. Intern Med., 89:122, 1978.
36. McPherson, S. P.: Respiratory Therapy Equipment, 2nd ed. St. Louis, C. V. Mosby Co., 1981.
37. Meyers, J. R., Lembeck, L., O'Kane, H., and Baue, A. E.: Changes in functional residual capacity of the lung after operation. Arch. Surg., 110:576, 1975.
38. Mittman, C.: Assessment of operative risk in thoracic surgery. Am. Rev. Respir. Dis., 84:197, 1961.
39. Moran, J. F., Robinson, L. A., Lowe, J. E., and Wolfe, W. G.: Effects of oxygen toxicity on regional ventilation and perfusion in the primate lung. Surgery, 89:575, 1981.
40. Murphy, S. A., Hyams, J. S., Fisher, A. B., and Root, R. K.: Effects of oxygen exposure on the in vitro function of pulmonary alveolar macrophages. J. Clin. Invest., 56:503, 1975.
41. Orringer, M. B.: Endotracheal intubation and tracheostomy. Surg. Clin. North Am., 60:1447, 1980.
42. Pontoppidan, H., Griffin, B., and Lowenstein, E.: Acute Respiratory Failure in the Adult. Boston, Little, Brown and Co., 1973.
43. Quan, S. F., Falltrick, R. T., and Schlobohm, R. M.: Extubation from ambient or expiratory positive airway pressure in adults. Anesthesiology, 55:53, 1981.
44. Shapiro, B. A., et al.: Clinical Application of Respiratory Care, 2nd ed. Chicago, Year Book Medical Publishers, 1979.
45. Shim, C.: Adrenergic agonists and bronchodilator aerosol therapy in asthma. Clin. Chest. Med., 5:659, 1984.
46. Smith, P. K., Tyson, G. S., Jr., Hammon, J. W., Jr., Olsen, C. O., Hopkins, R. A., Maier, G. W., Sabiston, D. C., Jr., and Rankin, J. S.: Cardiovascular effects of ventilation with positive expiratory airway pressure. Ann. Surg., 195:121, 1982.
47. Smith, T. C., Cook, F. D., DeKornfeld, T. J., and Siebecker, K. L.: Pulmonary function in the immediate postoperative period. J. Thorac. Cardiovasc. Surg., 39:788, 1960.
48. Stauffer, J. L., Olson, D. E., and Petty, T. L.: Complications and consequences of endotracheal intubation and tracheostomy. Am. J. Med., 70:65, 1981.
49. Stein, M., and Cassara, E. L.: Preoperative pulmonary evaluation and therapy for surgery patients. J.A.M.A., 211:787, 1970.

50. Stein, M., Koota, G. M., Simon, M., and Frank, H. A.: Pulmonary evaluation of surgical patients. J.A.M.A., *181*:765, 1962.
51. Tisi, G. M.: Preoperative evaluation of pulmonary function: Validity, indications and benefits. Am. Rev. Respir. Dis., *119*:293, 1979.
52. Tisi, G. M.: Pulmonary Physiology in Clinical Medicine, 2nd ed. Baltimore, Williams & Wilkins, 1983.
53. Tucker, D. H., and Sieker, H. O.: The effect of change in body position on lung volumes and intrapulmonary gas mixing in patients with obesity, heart failure and emphysema. Am. Rev. Respir. Dis., *83*:787, 1960.
54. West, J. B.: Ventilation-blood Flow and Gas Exchange, 3rd ed. Philadelphia, J. B. Lippincott Company, 1977.
55. West, J. B.: Respiratory Physiology, 2nd ed. Baltimore, Williams & Wilkins, 1979.
56. Wolfe, W. G.: Preoperative assessment of pulmonary function: Quantitative evaluation of ventilation and blood-gas exchange. *In* Sabiston, D. C., Jr., and Spencer, F. C. (Eds.): Gibbon's Surgery of the Chest, 4th ed. Philadelphia, W. B. Saunders Company, 1983.
57. Wolfe, W. G., Robinson, L. A., Moran, J. F., and Lowe, J. E.: Reversible pulmonary oxygen toxicity in the primate. Ann. Surg., *188*:530, 1978.
58. Zapol, W. M., Snider, M. T., Hill, J. D., Fallat, R. J., Bartlett, R. H., Edmunds, H., Morris, A. J., Peirce, E. C., Thomas, A. N., Proctor, H. J., Drinker, P. A., Pratt, P. C., Bagniewski, A., and Miller, R. G.: Extracorporeal membrane oxygenation in severe acute respiratory failure: A randomized prospective study. J.A.M.A., *242*:2193, 1979.

II

Bronchoscopy

ROSS M. UNGERLEIDER, M.D.
DAVID C. SABISTON, JR., M.D.

With the use of the bronchoscope, the thoracic surgeon is able to obtain a spectacular view of the endobronchial anatomy. This technique provides critical information for diagnosing and evaluating the extent of various chest diseases. In fact, recent advances in technology have enabled bronchoscopy to become so intricately woven into the treatment of diseases of the chest that it is now no longer possible to practice in this field without attaining some mastery of this procedure.

HISTORIC ASPECTS

In 1806, Bozzini designed an endoscopic instrument and utilized a wax candle as a light source. However, it was the development of Edison's miniature electric lamps that led to modern bronchoscopy. The first therapeutic success for the bronchoscopic procedure was provided by Killian, the "father of bronchoscopy," who in 1897 removed an aspirated pork bone from the bronchus of a 63-year-old farmer. Further advances in instrumentation followed, and by the 1900s, an instrument was available with features such as tip illumination and suction. At the forefront of this rapidly advancing field stood Chevalier Jackson, who attracted and trained many students, producing leaders in the field. Jackson's monograph, *Bronchoesophagology*, first published in 1950,[10] is an important work that remains educational reading.

Recent developments with fiberoptics[6, 7, 13] and an interest in early diagnosis of lung cancer led Ikeda to develop the flexible bronchofiberscope, which was eventually introduced in 1967.[8] This instrument transformed bronchoscopy into a procedure that was easily mastered by all physicians and created an explosion of trained bronchoscopists.

CONTEMPORARY BRONCHOSCOPES

Bronchoscopes are available as *rigid*, open tubes or as *flexible*, fiberoptic instruments. The hollow metal tubes

(Fig. 1*A*) are similar to the first bronchoscopes developed. They are inserted transorally in a sedated or anesthetized patient and allow the examiner to view the trachea and mainstem bronchi directly. The view through these tubes is limited by the size of the lumen and is dissipated by the length of the tube. Special telescopes can be passed into these open tubes to enhance the viewing capability. The major advantage of rigid bronchoscopes is that they provide a large, controlled airway that is of particular value in patients with excessive secretions or massive hemoptysis. They also enable passage of large accessory instruments

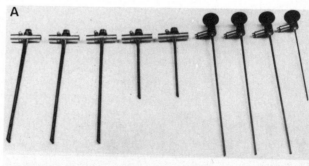

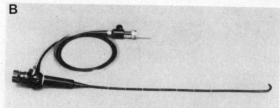

Figure 1. The two types of bronchoscopes. A, Rigid open tubes (five different sizes pictured to the left) with telescope inserts (four are shown to the right) that can enhance viewing ability. B, Flexible fiberoptic bronchoscope. (From de Kock, M. A.: Dynamic Bronchoscopy, New York, Springer-Verlag, 1977; and Oho, K., and Amemiya, R.: Practical Fiberoptic Bronchoscopy, New York, Igaku-Shoin, 1980.)

into the airway for biopsy and especially for extraction of foreign bodies.

The flexible bronchofiberscope (Fig. 1*B*) is a more highly developed and delicate instrument that utilizes the principles of light transmission along special fibers. Its primary advantage is that this instrument is highly maneuverable and, in conjunction with smaller size, can reach areas in the endobronchial tree not accessible with rigid tubes. Because of its size and flexibility, it can be inserted transnasally as well as transorally and is well tolerated by the awake patient with topical anesthesia. The major drawback to the flexible instrument is that, unlike the rigid open tube, it is a "closed" system that does not provide an airway, and the small inner channel is considered by many to be incapable of allowing adequate suction in the face of copious secretions or massive hemoptysis.[14]

TECHNIQUE

Regardless of the type of bronchoscope selected, the patient should be properly prepared for the procedure with nothing by mouth since the previous night and with adequate topical anesthesia applied. The bronchoscopic technique should then follow a routine system so that all parts of the endobronchial anatomy are consistently observed. It is wise to proceed first to the area of disease so that information will be obtained even if the procedure needs to be terminated before its completion. Excellent descriptions of a routine bronchoscopic examination can be found in the literature[7, 12, 13] and should include evaluation of the vocal cords (for movement on phonation and for lesions), the trachea (mucosal pattern, masses, or evidence of

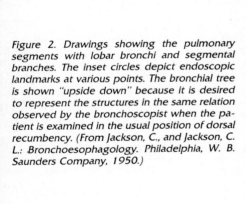

Figure 2. Drawings showing the pulmonary segments with lobar bronchi and segmental branches. The inset circles depict endoscopic landmarks at various points. The bronchial tree is shown "upside down" because it is desired to represent the structures in the same relation observed by the bronchoscopist when the patient is examined in the usual position of dorsal recumbency. (From Jackson, C., and Jackson, C. L.: Bronchoesophagology. Philadelphia, W. B. Saunders Company, 1950.)

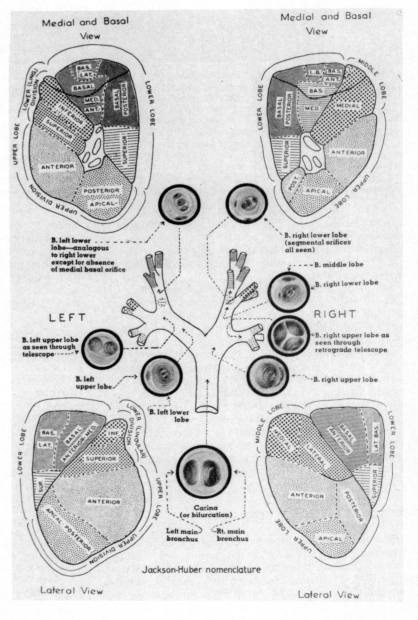

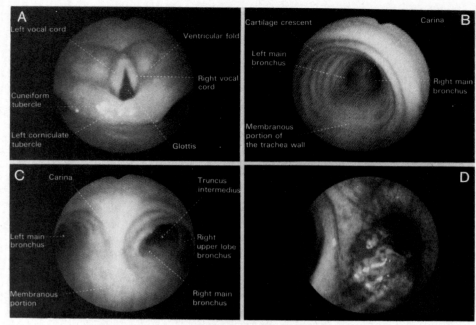

Figure 3. Photographs taken through the bronchoscope at certain important landmarks.

A, The tip of the bronchoscope is poised above the vocal cords. This is the gateway to the tracheobronchial tree. The epiglottis which is anterior (top) must be passed to obtain this view.

B, Upon passing through the cords, the trachea is entered. The posterior membranous portion and anterior cartilaginous rings are helpful for orientation. The carina can be seen in the distance.

C, At the level of the carina, the endoscopist has the choice of pursuing the right or left mainstem bronchus. The bronchus to the right upper lobe usually arises from the right mainstem bronchus just below the carina. The left mainstem bronchus is usually quite long and must be negotiated to visualize its division into left upper and lower lobe branches. (From Oho, K., and Amemiya, R.: Practical Fiberoptic Bronchoscopy. New York, Igaku-Shoin, 1980.)

D, A large tumor arising just below the carina in the right mainstem bronchus. Although not visible on the chest film, this lesion is diagnosed easily by bronchoscopy. (From de Kock, M. A.: Dynamic Bronchoscopy. New York, Springer-Verlag, 1977.)

compression), the carina (which should appear sharp and move freely with respiration), and both mainstem bronchi and their lobar orifices (which are normally free of masses, foreign bodies, compression, inflammation, bleeding, or excessive secretions).

An adequate examination mandates familiarity with endobronchial anatomy. The ability to translate bronchoscopic findings into a reliable and understandable communication of the disease process requires a standard nomenclature. This was first provided by Jackson and Huber in 1943[9] and has been expanded in the era of flexible bronchofiberscopy.[12] It is important to understand the relationship and bronchoscopic appearance of the major lobar and segmental divisions (Fig. 2). Exceptional quality color photographs abound in the literature[3, 12] (Fig. 3), but despite the many atlases available, nothing replaces the experience of actually performing the procedure (or observing through a teaching attachment). The student is urged to view at least one examination from start to finish before embarking on a medical career.

INDICATIONS, USES, AND COMPLICATIONS

The indications for bronchoscopy are shown in Table 1. The use of bronchoscopy in diagnosing and treating pulmonary disease is growing rapidly, and Jackson's statement in 1915 — "In case of doubt as to whether bronchoscopy should be done or not, bronchoscopy should always be done"—remains timely.

Bronchoscopy provides the clinician with the unique

ability to view inside the patient, beyond the sensitivity of x-rays and laboratory tests, and to visually diagnose early cancers or other causes of hemoptysis. The examination of bronchial brush and washing cytology, combined with sputum cytology, transthoracic needle aspiration, and bronchoscopic forceps biopsy, should enable preoperative diagnosis of 95 per cent of pulmonary neoplasms,[11] even when a

TABLE 1. Indications for Bronchoscopy*

Diagnostic Indications	Therapeutic Indications
Cough	Foreign bodies
Hemoptysis	Accumulated secretions
Wheeze	Atelectasis
Atelectasis	Aspiration
Unresolved pneumonia	Lung abscess
Positive cytology	
Abnormal chest x-ray film findings	**Preoperative Evaluation**
Diffuse lung disease	R/o multiple primary tumors
Recurrent nerve paralysis	Metastases
Diaphragmatic paralysis	Bronchiectasis (with bronchography)
Selective bronchography	Assess resectability
Acute inhalation injury	
Immediately after intubation	
During mechanical ventilation	
Before extubation	
After extubation	
Assess local recurrence	
When in doubt	

*After Landa, J. F.: Chest, 73:690, 1978.

lesion is not evident on the chest film.[1] Washings of selective bronchial segments can also be obtained to help isolate the origin of positive cytology. In addition, bronchoscopy is essential in evaluating patients prior to pulmonary resection, with signs such as carinal or mainstem bronchial involvement, vocal cord paralysis, bilateral lesions, tumor location, pulmonary function, or tumor cell type (i.e., small cell) suggesting irresectable disease. The ease and rapidity of flexible bronchoscopy have made it a useful technique in the diagnosis of etiologic agents in pulmonary infections and diffuse interstitial pneumonitis, in the evaluation of the extent of injury in patients with smoke inhalation and burn injury and in the performance of selective bronchography.

Extraction of foreign bodies with the bronchoscope has provided therapeutic benefit for thousands of patients.[1, 4, 10] Many patients with foreign body aspiration cannot provide a history (i.e., small children or comatose patients), and if the foreign body is not radiopaque, the diagnosis as well as treatment requires bronchoscopy. Presentation of cough, wheezing, or hemoptysis, or a chest film showing either atelectasis or hyperlucency of a portion of the lung, may be reason enough to undertake this procedure. The bronchoscope has also proved of particular benefit in treating atelectasis in postoperative patients. In these instances, it can be utilized to aspirate areas in the endobronchial tree selectively that are blocked by secretions or mucous plugs that the patient has been unable to clear with the usual forms of pulmonary toilet. In operating rooms and intensive care units, the bronchoscope can facilitate endobronchial intubation in difficult patients by being used as a visually guided stylet over which an endotracheal tube can be advanced into the proper position.

Advanced technology of the smaller flexible bronchoscopes as well as the special telescope systems to be used with the open tube instruments has opened new vistas in the practice of pediatric endoscopy.[6] Indications are the same as for adults, and the majority of foreign bodies are extracted from the pediatric population.[1, 6, 10] An exciting use of bronchoscopy has been in the diagnosis and preoperative respiratory stabilization of esophageal atresia with tracheoesophageal fistula[5] and in the localization of isolated tracheoesophageal fistulas to help determine whether they can be best approached via a thoracic or cervical incision.

When performed by properly trained individuals, bronchoscopy is an extraordinarily safe procedure. Among 24,521 flexible bronchoscopic procedures,[2] the minor and major complication rates were 0.2 and 0.08 per cent, respectively. Mortality was 0.01 per cent. Most complications relate to premedication or to topical anesthesia and not to the procedure itself. However, a variety of other problems have been reported; these include pneumothorax, bronchospasm, hemorrhage, bronchial perforation, subglottic edema, infections, arrhythmias, and, rarely, cardiopulmonary arrest.[2]

The advent of laser technology has provided a method of palliation of obstructing endobronchial lesions. Working through the bronchoscope, both CO_2 and neodymium-YAG (yttrium-aluminum-garnet) lasers have been successfully employed to relieve obstruction of the trachea or a mainstem bronchus.[15] Both of these lasers have also been effective in controlling bleeding from endobronchial lesions. As new methods of medical technology become available, the bronchoscope promises to be an instrument of the future with applications limited only by the imagination.

SELECTED REFERENCES

Anderson, H. A., and Faber, L. P. (Eds.): Diagnostic and therapeutic applications of the bronchoscope. Chest. *73* (No. 5), May 1978.
   This supplement to Chest *is devoted entirely to bronchoscopy. It features several articles by well-known experts discussing a variety of topics. It provides an excellent overview of the various applications of bronchoscopy.*

Ikeda, S.: Atlas of Flexible Bronchofiberoscopy. Baltimore, University Park Press, 1974.
   As the classic compilation of Ikeda's work that led to the development of the bronchofiberscope, this atlas is usually recommended by all experts in the field. This work not only contains a fine discussion of the principles of fiberoptics but also shows how these principles can enable visualization to fifth-order bronchi. An exceptional work both for its historic value and its value as a thorough atlas.

Jackson, C., and Jackson, C. L.: Bronchoesophagology. Philadelphia, W. B. Saunders Company, 1950.
   Still a classic, this monograph by the "dean of American bronchoscopy" and his son is filled with wisdom regarding the presentation and treatment of foreign body aspiration. In addition, the work covers the experience of the Jackson Clinic with a variety of endoscopic procedures. Although it was written before the advent of fiberoptic technology, it remains an indispensable part of any education in the field of bronchoscopy.

REFERENCES

1. Anderson, H. A., and Faber, L. P. (Guest Eds.): Diagnostic and therapeutic applications of the bronchoscope. Chest, *73*:(No. 5), May 1978.
2. Credle, W. F., Smiddy, J. F., and Elliott, R. C.: Complications of fiberoptic bronchoscopy. Am. Rev. Respir. Dis., *109*:87, 1974.
3. deKock, M. A.: Dynamic Bronchoscopy. New York, Springer-Verlag, 1977.
4. Faber, L. P., Monson, D. O., Amato, J. J., and Jensik, F. J.: Flexible fiberoptic bronchoscopy. Ann. Thorac. Surg., *18*:163, 1973.
5. Filston, H. C., Rankin, J. S., and Grimm, J. J.: Esophageal atresia. Prognostic factors and contribution of preoperative telescopic endoscopy. Ann. Surg., *199*:532, 1984.
6. Gans, S. L.: Pediatric Endoscopy. New York, Grune & Stratton, 1983.
7. Ikeda, S.: Atlas of Flexible Bronchofiberoscopy. Baltimore, University Park Press, 1974.
8. Jackson, C.: Bronchoscopy: past, present, and future. N. Engl. J. Med., *199*:759, 1928.
9. Jackson, C. L., and Huber, J. F.: Correlated applied anatomy of the bronchial tree and lungs with a system of nomenclature. Dis. Chest, *9*:319, 1943.
10. Jackson, C., and Jackson, C. L.: Bronchoesophagology. Philadelphia, W. B. Saunders Company, 1950.
11. Johnston, W. W., and Frable, J. J.: The cytopathology of the respiratory tract. Am. J. Pathol., *84*:372, 1978.
12. Oho, K., and Amemiya, R.: Practical Fiberoptic Bronchoscopy. New York, Igaku-Shoin, 1980.
13. Sackner, M. A.: Bronchofiberscopy. Am. Rev. Respir. Dis., *111*:62, 1975.
14. Taylor, F. H., Evangelist, F. A., and Barham, B. F.: The flexible fiberoptic bronchoscope: Diagnostic tool or medical tool? Ann. Thorac. Surg., *29*:548, 1979.
15. Wolfe, W. G., Cole, P. H., and Sabiston, D. C., Jr.: Experimental and clinical use of the YAG laser in the management of pulmonary neoplasms. Ann. Surg., *199*:526, 1984.

III

Lung Abscess and Fungal Infections

RONALD C. HILL, M.D.
DAVID C. SABISTON, JR., M.D.

LUNG ABSCESS

A lung abscess is defined as a localized area of pulmonary suppurative disease usually preceded by pneumonitis with subsequent cavitation.[1] There are many additional causes of lung abscess, including tuberculosis, mycotic diseases, infected cysts, bronchiectasis, pulmonary infarction, and tumor with either cavitation of the tumor or secondary distal atelectasis.

Etiology

The most common predisposing factor in the development of a lung abscess is *aspiration pneumonitis*. Alcoholism is a common underlying factor with aspiration, although anesthesia, epilepsy, drugs, other neurologic conditions and esophageal disorders have been associated with this complication. Most of these patients have associated poor oral hygiene and dental infections of gingival disease, which lead to the aspiration of highly pathogenic bacteria from the oral cavity.[4]

Clinical Presentation

Patients usually present with cough, fever, pleuritic chest pain, and occasional hemoptysis and weight loss.[4] The diagnosis is based upon the chest film, which usually shows a single cavity greater than 2 cm. in diameter in one lobe or segment (Fig. 1). Because patients usually aspirate in the supine position, most lung abscesses are found in the most dependent portion of the right lung, i.e., the superior basilar segment of the right lower lobe or the posterior segment of the right upper lobe.[3, 4, 13] The right main stem bronchus is shorter, less angulated, and larger than the left, accounting for the majority of abscesses being in the right lung. Anaerobic bacteria are the significant pathogens in most primary lung abscesses as a result of their preponderance in the oral cavity, although aerobic bacteria may be found in lung abscesses and include beta-hemolytic *Streptococcus*, *Pseudomonas*, *Pneumococcus pneumoniae*, *Staphylococcus aureus* (especially in children and debilitated or elderly patients), *Escherichia coli*, and *Klebsiella pneumoniae*.[2, 3]

Management

Evaluation of the patient includes a complete history and physical examination along with a chest x-ray, which usually shows the localized abscess. Sputum should be examined by Gram stain and should be cultured for aerobic, anaerobic, fungal, and tuberculosis organisms. All organisms should be tested for antimicrobial sensitivity. Since most of these abscesses demonstrate air-fluid levels caused by bronchial communication, pulmonary toilet and bronchoscopy may facilitate drainage.

Antimicrobial therapy is the treatment of choice and includes high doses of penicillin to which most of the organisms are usually sensitive. Clindamycin or chloramphenicol may be used to control the anaerobic bacteria.[1]

Surgical intervention is required when there is a failure to resolve the abscess with antimicrobial therapy, suspicion of malignancy, residual cavity greater than 2 cm. despite improvement after 4 to 6 weeks of treatment, recurrent infection, or rupture of the abscess into the pleural cavity with pyopneumothorax. Mortality in an uncomplicated abscess approaches zero, whereas with associated diseases it approaches 30 to 40 per cent.[4] Antibiotic therapy should be continued until constitutional symptoms have resolved and the abscess is shown to be clearing by chest radiographs.

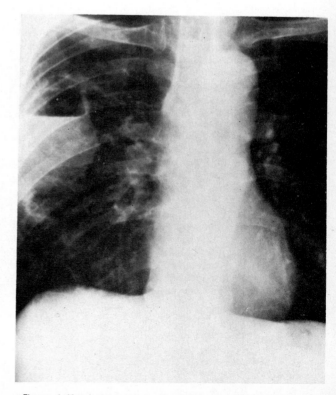

Figure 1. X-ray appearance of a right upper lobe lung abscess.

At this point, oral antibiotics may be instituted until the chest film becomes normal.[1]

FUNGAL INFECTIONS OF THE LUNGS

Surgical therapy for mycotic diseases of the chest may be indicated for several reasons. First, bronchoscopy and biopsy may be necessary to establish a diagnosis. Second, surgical extirpation may be required for pulmonary fungal infections that are not responsive to medical treatment. Third, the surgeon may encounter fungal diseases when operating on isolated pulmonary nodules or tumors. Since most chemotherapeutic agents for the treatment of fungal diseases are toxic, it is important to establish the diagnosis by culture and obtain antimicrobial sensitivities for appropriate treatment.[11]

Histoplasmosis

Histoplasma capsulatum is a soil-based, non-encapsulated fungus that is associated with excrement from birds. It is endemic in the Mississippi and Ohio Valley basins and is usually a benign, pneumonic process that tends toward spontaneous healing. Darling named the organisms, since he found them in histiocytes and thought they were encapsulated protozoa.[9] *H. capsulatum* utilizes the uric acid present in fowl excreta as a source of nitrogen. Other conditions found in the endemic regions that favor fungus growth include a relatively high humidity, aerobic conditions, acidic soil, and warm temperatures. Starlings, blackbirds, chickens, bats, and pigeons are the usual animals associated with the organism. Following inhalation of the organism, the incubation period is 12 to 16 days. Symptoms include fever, chills, headaches, cough, and chest pain.[9] The diagnosis is based on the history together with chest radiographic findings of one or more sites of pneumonitis, enlargement of hilar and mediastinal lymph nodes, and a significant histoplasmin complement fixation titer (greater than 1:32 or a fourfold rise in titer). Culture or histologic proof may occasionally be obtained. Although helpful, skin tests are nondiagnostic.[9]

The histoplasmoma may appear in an otherwise asymptomatic patient as a coin lesion and may be identified by concentric rings of calcification. The lesions may be single or multiple, and they slowly enlarge by development of concentric rings (Fig. 2).[9, 11] Histoplasmosis is treated symptomatically, since it usually resolves spontaneously, although in severe cases the use of amphotericin B may be required. Surgical intervention may be necessary for the persistent cavities and for nonresponsiveness to medical therapy.[11]

The major complication of histoplasmosis is mediastinal granulomata with *fibrosing mediastinitis*, which results from rupture of granulomas, producing intense inflammatory reaction. With healing, a fibrosing mediastinitis develops. As a result, superior vena caval obstruction, together with obstruction of the other major veins in the mediastinum and bronchi, may develop in addition to esophageal compression and traction diverticula of the esophagus. After several months, signs of the superior vena caval syndrome often abate as venous collateral channels develop over the chest and communicate with branches of the inferior vena cava. Some authors believe that large mediastinal granulomas should be excised because there is no evidence that steroid treatment or chemotherapy is efficacious.[6, 11]

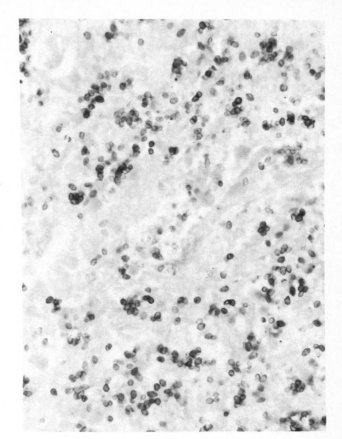

Figure 2. Non-encapsulated yeast (Histoplasma capsulatum) from a histoplasmoma. (Methenamine silver stain, × 680)

North American Blastomycosis

Although blastomycosis is found endemic east of the Mississippi River, it is also found in Africa and the northern part of South America. Soil enriched by bird excreta (chicken and starling guano) provides favorable environmental conditions for growth of the fungus.[16] Clinically, the patient usually presents with findings of a pneumonic infiltrate and a skin lesion, secondary to dissemination from the lung. The chest x-ray commonly shows necrosis and poorly formed granulomas. Diagnosis is made by culturing the organism, *Blastomyces dermatitidis*, from the sputum, and if a skin lesion is present, a biopsy should be obtained (Fig. 3). Prostatic fluid is also an excellent source for the fungus.[16]

Although there are documented cases of spontaneous remission of the disease, most patients require a course of amphotericin B. Even though 2-hydroxystilbamidine is effective, with dissemination to organs other than the skin, amphotericin B is the agent of choice.[16]

Coccidioidomycosis

Coccidioides immitis is a dimorphic fungus found edemic in the southwestern portion of the United States, including the San Joaquin Valley in California, plus Central America, Mexico, and South America. Clinical presentation may range from a relatively mild respiratory disorder associated with red bumps and aching joints—known as "valley fever," "desert rheumatism," or the "bumps"—to

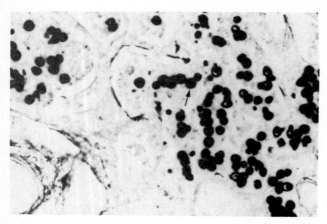

Figure 3. Yeast forms with moderate pleomorphism, identifiable internal structure, and broad-based budding (arrow), characteristic of Blastomyces dermatitidis. Crowding of yeast forms may be confused with multiple budding. (Methenamine silver stain, lung, × 200) (From Pickett, J. P., and Roggli, V. L.: Am. J. Med. Tech., 48:893, 1982.)

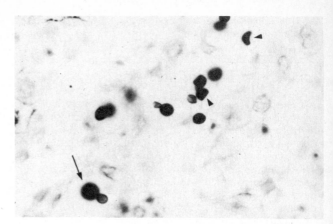

Figure 4. Encapsulated budding yeast forms of Cryptococcus neoformans (arrow) adjacent to Pneumocystis organisms (arrowheads) in lung at autopsy. (Methenamine silver stain, × 800) (From Pickett, J. R., and Roggli, V. L.: Am. J. Med. Tech., 48:893, 1982.)

a virulent, debilitating illness with rapid dissemination and a fatal outcome. Diagnosis is usually made by history and a sensitivity to coccidioidin that usually occurs 3 days to 3 weeks after the onset of symptoms. Erythema nodosum may be associated with coccidioidomycosis and ordinarily portends a good prognosis. The chest x-ray may reveal an infiltrate and miliary nodules with hilar adenopathy.[8]

Although primary pulmonary coccidioidomycosis may resolve spontaneously, amphotericin B remains the drug of choice with dissemination in severely ill patients. Surgical therapy is indicated when patients do not respond to medical treatment or when they present with solitary pulmonary nodules. Persisting cavities 2 cm. or greater may enlarge and rupture, resulting in severe hemoptysis.[8]

Cryptococcosis

Cryptococcus neoformans is a yeast-like fungus found in the soil and associated with pigeon excrement. It is a round, budding yeast with a thick, gelatinous capsule that can be demonstrated easily by mucin-carmine stains or India ink preparation on fresh tissue (Fig. 4; see also Fig. 7).[11]

Patients usually present with a nonspecific pneumonitis, weight loss, fatigability, and a low-grade fever. The chest radiograph usually demonstrates a solitary round lesion. Diagnosis is made by the cultures and histologic preparations. Once diagnosed, extrapulmonary lesions should be sought by examination of the cerebrospinal fluid (CSF) and biopsy of any suspicious bone lesions.[10, 11]

Most patients with cryptococcosis localized to the lung do well with conservative treatment. If there is colonization of the sputum plus normal CSF levels and no evidence of disease elsewhere, nonspecific therapy is indicated. For those who require treatment, amphotericin B and 5-fluorocytosine are the chemotherapeutic agents of choice. If the lesion is a calcified small nodule without infiltrate or pleural reaction and is completely removed surgically, no chemotherapy is required. However, if the lesion is incised or if it is active and disseminated, chemotherapeutic agents should be used prophylactically. Patients who have diabetes mellitus, who are chronically ill, or who receive immuno-

suppressive drugs or steroids should be treated prophylactically as well.[10, 11]

Aspergillosis

There are three hypersensitivity reactions to Aspergillus. First, extrinsic asthma associated with acute bronchospasm is mediated by mast cells, which release Aspergillus-directed IgE antibodies. The second type is extrinsic allergic alveolitis, commonly known as "malt-worker's lung" or "farmer's lung." Clinically, fever and chills develop 4 to 6 hours after exposure and the chest x-ray shows an abnormal diffuse interstitial infiltrate. Biopsy reveals interstitial round cell infiltrates with alveolar septal thickening. These patients have an elevated IgG antibody to the inhalant. The third reaction is allergic bronchopulmonary aspergillosis. Individuals demonstrating this reaction are atopic with an IgG and IgE antibody directed toward the fungus. The

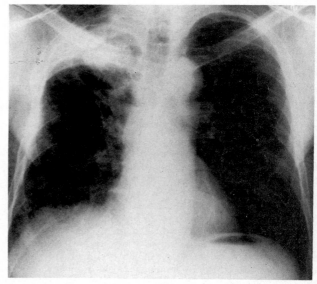

Figure 5. Chest x-ray showing a right upper lobe fungus ball in a patient who presented with hemoptysis.

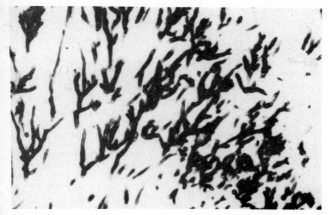

Figure 6. Septate hyphae branching at acute angles (45°) typically seen with invasive aspergillosis. (Methenamine silver stain, lung, × 320) (From Pickett, J. P., and Roggli, V. L.: Am. J. Med. Tech., 48:893, 1982.)

organism colonizes in the patient's airways with continual exposure to the antigen, and the sputum contains golden-brown plugs of viscus material, which can be cultured for *Aspergillus*.[15]

The noninvasive form of pulmonary aspergillosis is usually referred to as the "fungus ball." This is a rounded mass located inside a chronic pulmonary cavity and suggestive of a mycetoma (Fig. 5). Patients usually present with a chronic lung disease predisposing to cavities and hemoptysis and often have a positive serum precipitins to *Aspergillus*. If there are no symptoms, the patient may be treated conservatively. However, symptomatic patients with good pulmonary function warrant surgical removal with prophylactic treatment with amphotericin B. In the high-risk patient, the pulmonary cavity may be drained percutaneously and sodium iodide or amphotericin B may be instilled into the cavity.[15, 18] Invasive pulmonary aspergillosis with vascular invasion is seen in severely immunosuppressed patients, and amphotericin B is the agent of choice. The mortality approaches 80 per cent (Fig. 6).[15]

Miscellaneous Fungal Infections

Mucormycosis. Mucormycosis is caused by fungi belonging to the class *Phycomycetes*. The organisms are broad, nonseptate hyphae that characteristically invade blood vessels, causing thrombosis and infarction. Species of *Mucor* show resistance to amphotericin B in sensitivity studies. Most cases of pulmonary mucormycosis are terminal because of the pre-existing immune-deficient state of the patient and the resistance of the organisms to chemotherapy. Occasionally, infarcted lung tissue may be removed surgically with removal of the source of infection.[11, 14]

Moniliasis. *Candida albicans* is a yeast-like organism responsible for moniliasis. Although the organism is commonly found in the sputum, it can produce extensive bronchopneumonia in the immunosuppressed patient. Surgical intervention is required to make the diagnosis so that amphotericin B may be appropriately instigated.[11]

Sporotrichosis. Sporotrichosis caused by *Sporothrix schenckii* may involve the lungs with the chest x-ray showing upper lobe infiltrates and hilar adenopathy. Combined lung resection and iodides or amphotericin B therapy seem to be most effective for cavitary sporotrichosis.[11, 12]

Monosporosis. *Monosporium apiospermum* resides in the soil and may invade pre-existing pulmonary cavities, creating a fungus ball. Chemotherapy is not effective, but the infection may be treated by local surgical resection.[11]

OTHER LUNG INFECTIONS

Actinomycosis

Actinomycosis, caused by the anaerobic bacterium *Actinomyces israelli*, is associated with abscess and sinus formation. Only if the organism cultured from the sputum of the patient is pathogenic in animals can the assumption be made that the pulmonary infiltrate is caused by *A. israelli*. Penicillin G is the antibiotic of choice for actinomycosis. Surgical therapy includes establishing a diagnosis by biopsy and radical excision of chronic, thick-walled lesions.[18]

Nocardiosis

Nocardia asteroides is a gram-positive bacterium that is a partially acid-fast aerobic actinomycete associated with immunosuppressed patients (Fig. 7). If the lesion is localized, a cure rate approaching 100 per cent can be achieved by resection. If it is diffuse, however, treatment with sulfonamides is preferred.[5, 18]

Pneumocystosis

Caused by the protozoan *Pneumocystis carinii*, pneumocystosis is associated with interstitial plasma cell pneumonia (Fig. 4). It is the most common opportunistic infection associated with the *acquired immune deficiency syndrome* (AIDS).[17] Pathologically, there are areas of parenchymal, interstitial, and mediastinal emphysema with foamy or honeycomb-like material distending the alveoli. The chest x-ray usually shows extensive bilateral pneumonitis with a nodular or granular pattern without hilar adenopathy. Open lung biopsy may be required to establish

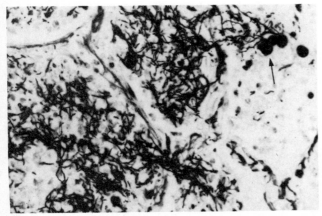

Figure 7. Fine branching filamentous forms of Nocardia *intermixed with occasional large budding yeast forms of* Cryptococcus *(arrow). (Methenamine silver stain, lung, × 320) (From Pickett, J. P., and Roggli, V. L.: Am. J. Med. Tech., 48:893, 1982.)*

the diagnosis, and treatment is with pentamidine isenthionate.[7]

SELECTED REFERENCES

Alexander, J. C., Jr., and Wolfe, W. G.: Lung abscess and empyema of the thorax. Surg. Clin. North Am., *60*:835, 1980.
An excellent resource for the manifestations and treatment of lung abscesses and their complications.

Drutz, D. J., and Catanzaro, A.: State of the art — coccidioidomycosis. Am. Rev. Respir. Dis., *117*:559, 1978.
An extensive review of coccidioidomycosis with aspects of history, ecology, epidemiology, immunology, diagnosis, and treatment.

Goodwin, R. A., Loyd, J. E., Des Prez, R. M.: Histoplasmosis in normal hosts. Medicine, *60*:231, 1981.
An in-depth review of the pathology, clinical presentation, and treatment of histoplasmosis.

Hammon, J. W., Jr., and Prager, R. L.: Surgical management of fungal diseases of the chest. Surg. Clin. North Am., *60*:897, 1980.
A review of the most common fungal pulmonary infestations with details concerning diagnosis and treatment.

Sarosi, G. A., and Davies, S. F.: State of the art—blastomycosis. Am. Rev. Respir. Dis., *120*:911, 1979.
A thorough review of blastomycosis with discussion of the immunology, epidemiology, clinical presentation, diagnosis, and treatments.

REFERENCES

1. Alexander, J. C., Jr., and Wolfe, W. G.: Lung abscess and empyema of the thorax. Surg. Clin. North Am., *60*:835, 1980.
2. Asher, M. I., Spier, S., Beland, M., Coates, A. L., and Beaudry, P. H.: Primary lung abscess in childhood. Am. J. Dis. Child., *136*:491, 1982.
3. Barlett, J. G., Gorbach, S. L., Tally, F. P., and Finegold, S. M.: Bacteriology and treatment of primary lung abscess. Am. Rev. Respir. Dis., *109*:510, 1974.
4. Chidi, C. C., and Mendelsohn, H. J.: Lung abscess. J. Thorac. Cardiovasc. Surg., *68*:168, 1974.
5. Curry, W. A.: Human nocardiosis. Arch. Intern. Med., *140*:818, 1980.
6. Dines, D. E., Payne, W. S., Bernatz, P. E., and Pairolero, P. C.: Mediastinal granuloma and fibrosing mediastinitis. Chest, *75*:320, 1979.
7. Dominy, D. E., and Lucas, R. N.: Pneumocystis carinii infection diagnosed by antemortem lung biopsy. Ann. Thor. Surg., *1*:305, 1965.
8. Drutz, D. J., and Catanzaro, A.: State of the art—coccidioidomycosis. Am. Rev. Respir. Dis., *117*:559, 1978.
9. Goodwin, R. A., Loyd, J. E., and Des Prez, R. M.: Histoplasmosis in normal hosts. Medicine, *60*:231, 1981.
10. Hammerman, K. J., Powell, K. E., Christianson, C. S., Huggin, P. M., Larsh, H. W., Vivas, J. R., and Tosh, F. E.: Pulmonary cryptococcosis: Clinical forms and treatment. Am. Rev. Respir. Dis., *108*:1116, 1973.
11. Hammon, J. W., Jr., and Prager, R. L.: Surgical management of fungal diseases of the chest. Surg. Clin. North Am., *60*:897, 1980.
12. Jay, S. J., Platt, M. R., and Reynolds, R. C.: Primary pulmonary sporotrichosis. Am. Rev. Respir. Dis., *115*:1051, 1977.
13. Johanson, W. G., Jr., and Harris, G. D.: Aspiration pneumonia, anaerobic infections, and lung abscess. Med. Clin. North Am., *64*:385, 1980.
14. Medoff, G., and Kobayashi, G. S.: Pulmonary mucormycosis. N. Engl. J. Med., *286*:86, 1972.
15. Pennington, J. E.: Aspergillus lung disease. Med. Clin. North Am., *64*:475, 1980.
16. Sarosi, G. A., and Davies, S. F.: State of the art—blastomycosis. Am. Rev. Respir. Dis., *120*:911, 1979.
17. Stover, D. E., White, D. A., Romano, P. A., Gellene, R. A., and Robeson, W. A.: Spectrum of pulmonary diseases associated with the acquired immune deficiency syndrome. Am. J. Med., *78*:429, 1985.
18. Takaro, T.: Actinomycetic and fungal infections of the lungs. In Sabiston, D. C., Jr. (Ed.): Davis-Christopher Textbook of Surgery, 12th ed. Philadelphia, W. B. Saunders Company, 1981.

IV

Disorders of the Pleura and Empyema

RONALD C. HILL, M.D.
DAVID C. SABISTON, JR., M.D.

The pleura is a serous membrane that covers the surface of the lung (visceral pleura); another lines the inner surface of the chest wall (parietal pleura). The potential space between the two pleural surfaces (pleural space) becomes evident only when air or fluid is present in the space.[10] This space with its minimal layer of fluid reduces the friction between the lung and chest wall during respiration as well as the movement of fluid through the lymphatics.[16] Although there are sensory nerve endings as well as blood vessels and lymphatics in the parietal pleura, there are no sensory nerve endings in the visceral pleura.[13] During quiet respiration, the intrapleural pressure varies between −2 cm. of water on expiration to −7 cm. of water during inspiration.[13] During coughing, as well as in the Valsalva maneuver with a closed glottis, the intrathoracic pressure may be raised to 200 mm. Hg above atmospheric pressure.[13]

The pleura has been found to produce and reabsorb between 600 to 1000 ml. of fluid per day. Erythrocytes as well may be absorbed by the normal pleura. These normal functions may be altered in disease states and in associated changes in intrapleural, capillary, and/or alveolar pressures.[16]

PLEURAL EFFUSIONS

A pleural effusion is the presence of fluid in the pleural space. These effusions may be either *transudates* or *exudates*, depending on the components of the fluid. Pleural effusions can be found even in the asymptomatic patient and are usually a sign of some underlying disease.[4] Once a pleural effusion is present on chest film, it is estimated that between 300 to 500 ml. of fluid has already accumulated and has been concealed radiologically in the costophrenic sinuses.[4, 16]

Diseases occurring within the chest that may cause pleural effusions include neoplasms, congestive heart failure, pulmonary infections, pulmonary infarcts, sarcoidosis, trauma, and other less common conditions such as Loeffler's syndrome. Pleural effusions may be associated with diseases of the abdomen, and it is felt that the pleural fluid that accumulates has passed from the peritoneal cavity through the lymphatics in the retroperitoneal region, then into the pulmonary and pleural lymphatics. Specific causes include pancreatitis, subdiaphragmatic abscesses, Meigs' syndrome (pleural effusion with an ovarian tumor, usually a fibroma), nephrotic syndromes, and cirrhosis of the liver. Systemic diseases that may be associated with pleural effusions include many of the collagen vascular diseases such as rheumatoid arthritis and lupus erythematosus.

Examination of the fluid can be diagnostic. A thoracentesis is performed, and the chest film should be reviewed with the patient in the upright position to identify the site of the pleural effusion to determine the most appropriate intercostal space for aspiration. Left and right decubitus films may be obtained to differentiate free from loculated pleural fluid. In performance of a thoracentesis, the patient is placed in either the supine or upright position. After the level of dullness to percussion on the correct side is determined, a 14-gauge needle or a plastic catheter can be inserted into the pleural space above the rib in order to avoid laceration of the intercostal bundle, which runs below the rib. The procedure is performed using local anesthesia, and a small amount of fluid should be withdrawn into the syringe to identify the presence and type of fluid. If the tap is for diagnosis, enough fluid is removed for the appropriate studies, the needle is withdrawn, and a chest film is obtained. If the tap is therapeutic, the fluid is withdrawn until no more of it can be obtained; a chest film is then made to be certain that a pneumothorax has not been produced.

The fluid is evaluated first for its appearance and odor. It may be purulent, serous, bloody, or milky. If the specific gravity is 1.016 or less and the protein content is 3.0 gm. per 100 ml. or less, the fluid is a *transudate*; if greater, it is an *exudate*. If the fat content is greater than 400 mg. per 100 ml. the fluid is from the lymphatic system (chyle). An elevated lactic dehydrogenase level in the pleural fluid may be indicative of metastatic neoplastic disease involving the pleura, whereas elevated amylase activity is usually indicative of pancreatitis. A portion of the fluid is sent for bacterial and fungal cultures and cytologic studies. If there is concern about a primary or secondary pleural process causing the effusion, a pleural biopsy may be performed in conjunction with thoracentesis.[4]

PNEUMOTHORAX

Pneumothorax occurs when air enters the potential pleural space and separates the visceral and parietal pleura. The pneumothorax may be *spontaneous*, as when a subpleural bleb, cyst, or bulla ruptures. Other causes include trauma, either by laceration of the lung with a sharp instrument or by rib fractures; ruptured bronchi or trachea; perforated esophagus; or perforation of an abdominal viscus with retroperitoneal dissection of air. Spontaneous pneu-

mothoraces are often seen in emphysematous patients and those with a smoking history, but they may also occur in those who are otherwise apparently normal. Atelectasis with compensatory emphysema is another cause in infants, and if the atelectasis results from hyaline membrane formation, the prognosis is usually poor.[12]

With a pneumothorax, air enters the pleural space on inspiration in the presence of negative intrapleural pressure, whereas during expiration the leak is sealed, creating a ball-valve mechanism. A *tension pneumothorax* occurs when one pleural cavity has completely filled with air and air continues to enter the space, causing a mediastinal shift with distortion of the venae cavae, partial obstruction of systemic venous return, and diminished cardiac output.[9] A patient with a pneumothorax may be asymptomatic or may complain of a sharp, knife-like pain or may have respiratory distress, hypoxemia, and hyperresonance on the side of the pneumothorax. Marked tracheal deviation, subcutaneous emphysema, and cyanosis may be present. The diagnosis is usually made by physical examination and confirmed by chest film. With small *apparent* pneumothoraces, expiration and inspiration films may be helpful in delineating a pneumothorax from a large pulmonary bulla or cyst.

The treatment depends on several factors. In patients who have partial pneumothoraces on one side (less than 50 per cent) and who are asymptomatic, expectant treatment may be indicated with surveillance by serial chest films.[9] Inspiration of oxygen during this time period may accelerate the resolution of the pneumothorax by displacing the nitrogen within the pleural space.[6] If the pneumothorax does not begin to resolve within a matter of hours, treatment should consist of placement of a small plastic catheter[17] or of large tube thoracostomy.

A total pneumothorax should be treated with a tube thoracostomy even if the patient is asymptomatic. A tension pneumothorax is an *emergency* and should be relieved immediately with a chest tube. If this is not readily available, a large-bore needle may be temporarily inserted into the chest in order to alleviate a life-threatening condition.[6,9]

Patients in whom spontaneous pneumothoraces develop can usually be treated nonoperatively with their *first* episode. If the pneumothorax recurs, approximately 60 per cent will recur again unless some therapeutic procedure is performed. An irritative substance such as tetracycline can be injected into the pleural cavity to produce pleurodesis. However, if a large air leak continues or if a recurrence appears, a thoracotomy may be necessary to suture, excise, or ligate the bullous component and abrade the parietal and visceral pleura to create adhesions to allow the lung to re-expand and become adherent to the chest wall. Although pleurectomy has been advocated as a surgical treatment, most surgeons perform pleural abrasion, which is more rapid, involves less blood loss, and is followed by better pulmonary function.[6] Patients on *respirators* in whom a pneumothorax develops should be treated with tube thoracostomy, irrespective of the size of the leak, to prevent a tension pneumothorax.

The drainage system for the chest tube involves a three-bottle principle. The first bottle is a trap for collecting the drainage fluid so that it can be monitored. The second bottle fulfills the function of a one-way valve that permits air to be removed from the chest but prevents it from re-entering the pleural space, especially if the patient is on water seal only. The third bottle regulates the suction on the chest tube. A preferred alternative to the three-bottle system is disposable plastic units — *Pleurevacs*—with one-way valves, which function on the same principle but are safer to use and less likely to be overturned or broken.[9]

Once the pneumothorax has resolved and no air leak or drainage is apparent, the chest tube is removed on a deep inspiration and active Valsalva maneuver to prevent air from re-entering the pleural space. A chest film is then obtained to ensure that the pneumothorax has not recurred.

HEMOTHORAX

The accumulation of blood in the pleural space is termed *hemothorax*; when associated with pneumothorax, it is termed a *hemopneumothorax*. Causes of hemothorax include trauma, malignant effusions, spontaneous pneumothoraces in which adhesions and pulmonary tissue are torn, and thoracic or cardiac surgical procedures.

In patients with sterile hemothoraces, the blood may be reabsorbed with conservative treatment. However, if the hemothorax is infected or associated with air, the chances of reabsorption are reduced and a tube thoracostomy may be required. Following surgical procedures on the thorax, air and blood are usually present and chest tubes are placed at the time of operation. A complication that sometimes follows a hemothorax is a *fibrothorax*, which is the result of defibrination of the intrapleural blood and the distribution of fibrin over the pleural surface, causing a restrictive pulmonary disease ("trapped lung") that may later require surgical decortication.[7, 16]

CHYLOTHORAX

Chylothorax is defined as a pleural effusion that contains fat (greater than 400 mg. per 100 ml.). These are usually associated with neoplastic disease, trauma, or tuberculosis,[4] or they may result from damage to the thoracic duct, which enters the chest from the cisterna chyli in the abdomen and drains into the left subclavian vein.

The treatment of chylothorax is usually conservative initially and includes tube thoracostomy and parenteral hyperalimentation (or enteral feedings with low-fat and low-protein content) to decrease the production of chyle. This may take as long as 6 weeks, but when conservative treatment fails, surgical correction with ligation of the thoracic duct at the site of the leakage is usually effective. Identification of the thoracic duct can be achieved by giving the patient some milk or a fatty meal just prior to surgery so that the chyle can be seen leaking from the injured thoracic duct. When the chylothorax is due to malignancy, surgical correction may not be useful.[16]

EMPYEMA

Empyema in the thorax is defined as an infected pleural effusion (Fig. 1). The purulent material may be localized, or it may involve the entire thoracic cavity. Empyemas have been classified as *exudative, fibropurulent,* or *chronic.* The exudative stage is characterized by a thin, infected pleural fluid. The fibropurulent stage is associated with thicker fluid and fibrin that may begin to organize and extend into a chronic phase in which the peel becomes organized with capillaries and fibroblasts. This may begin as early as 7 to 10 days, or it may not begin until the fourth to sixth week.[1, 2]

Empyema may result from direct extension from a

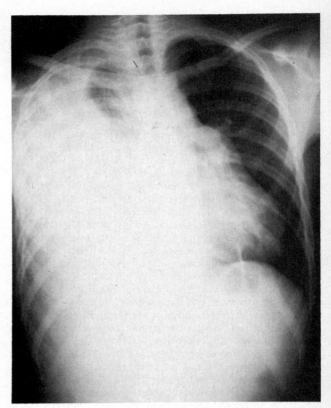

Figure 1. Chest x-ray of a pneumococcal empyema following pneumonia in a 12-year-old male who required decortication.

pneumonic or abscess component or may spread from hematogenous or lymphatic origin. Other causes include rupture of the trachea or bronchi, rupture of the esophagus, subphrenic abscesses, or liver abscesses; or the cause may be iatrogenic from tapping pleural effusions; or there may be a less common cause, such as osteomyelitis.[1] The patient usually presents with generalized symptoms of sepsis, and physical examination shows an acutely ill patient with evidence of a pleural effusion.

Prior to the antibiotic era, the most common organisms found were pneumococci and streptococci. However, because antibiotics have been used more frequently, the more common current organisms are *Staphylococcus aureus* and gram-negative bacteria. Tuberculous empyema is now uncommon because of antibiotic control.[1, 16]

Once a diagnosis of empyema is established by chest x-ray and aspiration of purulent material, treatment involves the control of the primary infection with the appropriate antibiotics and evacuation of the purulent material from the pleural space. If the empyema is in the exudative phase and can be totally evacuated with a large-bore thoracentesis needle, this may be sufficient.[1] In the pediatric patient, repeated aspirations may be required.[15] If the empyema cannot be totally evacuated, or if it is in the fibropurulent or chronic phase, a large tube thoracostomy early in the course of the empyema may be curative.[1, 14]

Again, in the pediatric population, once the pleural space is evacuated, no further accumulation has occurred, and the patient remains asymptomatic, the tube may be removed.[15] In the adult patient, however, it is usually necessary to convert the tube to open drainage after the visceral and parietal pleura have become adherent. A short segment of rib at the inferior border of the cavity is usually resected to ensure adequate drainage.[1] The tube can later be removed gradually as granulation tissue fills the pleural space and the lungs re-expand. A tissue flap (Eloesser) may be created to place over the fistula to achieve closure as well as to enable permanent drainage. This allows the patient to irrigate the cavity on a daily basis to promote granulation of the empyema space.[8, 14]

If the lung becomes entrapped from the chronic empyema, formal decortication is required using a thoracotomy and removal of the thick, fibrous peel from the lung, diaphragm, and mediastinum as well as the pleural surface of the chest wall. Once this is performed and the lung re-expands, the chest is then irrigated and large catheters are placed to remove any air and fluid and to allow the pleural surfaces to adhere.[1] Postpneumonectomy empyema may be treated by the placement of a chest tube with neomycin irrigation until three consecutive cultures are negative, followed by the instillation of neomycin solution and removal of the catheter. If this is not successful, the patient may require an open drainage procedure followed by a thoracoplasty.[1, 5] Tuberculous empyema usually requires combined chemotherapy, drainage procedures, and thoracoplasty.

PLEURAL NEOPLASMS

Pleural neoplasms may be primary or metastatic. The more common pleural metastases usually occur in patients with primary neoplasms of the lung, breast, pancreas, and stomach. These effusions are usually bloody, and cytologic examination of the aspirate is usually diagnostic. Management may be by chemotherapy, hormonal therapy, or radiation.[16] If the patient is symptomatic, the malignant pleural effusion is usually drained by closed tube thoracostomy. Once the drainage has decreased to less than 100 ml. per day, sclerosing agents such as talc, quinacrine, nitrogen mustard, or tetracycline may be used to produce an inflammatory pleuritis to cause adherence of the visceral and parietal pleura and prevent further accumulation of fluid. Once the drainage is less than 100 ml. per day, the chest tube is removed with the anticipation that the parietal and visceral pleura are sealed.

Primary tumors of the pleura may be benign or malignant. The incidence of *primary mesothelioma* is between 0.02 to 0.2 per cent of all autopsies, with a male-to-female ratio of 1:2.[3] It is felt that the benign variety arises from the submesothelial fibroblast and that they have no relationship to asbestos exposure or malignant mesotheliomas. The *benign mesotheliomas* usually arise from the visceral pleura and occur in patients who may be asymptomatic or patients who may have systemic symptoms of clubbing, arthralgias, and fever. These tumors should be excised.[3, 11]

Malignant mesotheliomas arise from a mesothelial cell that has its origin from the mesoderm formed from the ectodermal and entodermal layers. This origin produces three primary types of malignant mesotheliomas: (1) *epithelial*, (2) *mesenchymatous* or *sarcomatous*, and (3) a mixed type. The epithelial type is the most common. Asbestosis is intimately related to the development of malignant mesotheliomas and may give origin to all three types. A latency period of 35 to 40 years may exist from the first exposure to asbestos. Other possible etiologic factors in-

clude radiation, beryllium, hereditary factors, chronic inflammation, and viruses. Although patients usually present with dyspnea and chest pain, other presenting complaints include pleural thickening, nonspecific pleuritis, pneumothorax, dysphagia, Horner's syndrome, recurrent laryngeal nerve paralysis, acute paraplegia, and superior vena cava syndrome.[11]

The diagnosis is usually made by the history, physical examination, and chest film. A high level of hyaluronic acid (greater than 0.8 mg. per ml.) is commonly seen in the pleural exudate. If a cytologic diagnosis cannot be established, pleural biopsies (closed or open) should be obtained.

The treatment of malignant mesothelioma has not been satisfactory. Surgical excision has included extensive operations, such as extrapleural pleuropneumonectomy, including the pericardium and/or diaphragm, and radical decortication. The immediate mortality from these procedures varies from 10 to 18 per cent and the median survival from 7 to 9 months. Chemotherapy with multiple agents appears to have the best effect, with tumor regression in approximately 50 per cent of the patients.[11] Radiation therapy (4000 rads or more) has been shown to yield a median survival of 11 months and is associated with reasonable palliation with reduction of pleural effusion and pain.[11]

SELECTED REFERENCES

Alexander, J. C., Jr., and Wolfe, W. G.: Lung abscesses and empyema of the thorax. Surg. Clin. North Am., *60*:835, 1980.
    An excellent presentation on all aspects of empyema and its treatment.

Carr, D. T., Soule, E. H., and Ellis, F. H., Jr.: Management of pleural effusions. Med. Clin. North Am., *48*:961, 1964.
    A complete review of the diagnostic procedures to be performed to determine the etiology of pleural effusions as well as management.

DeVries, W. C., and Wolfe, W. G.: The management of spontaneous pneumothorax and bullous emphysema. Surg. Clin. North Am., *60*:851, 1980.
    This reference provides the basic fundamental aspects in treating spontaneous pneumothorax.

Fishman, N. H.: Thoracic Drainage: A Manual of Procedures. Chicago, Year Book Medical Publishers, Inc., 1983.
    An excellent reference for the techniques of chest tube placement, the mechanics of controlled suction, and procedures for cardiac tamponade.

REFERENCES

1. Alexander, J. C., Jr., and Wolfe, W. G.: Lung abscess and empyema of the thorax. Surg. Clin. North Am., *60*:835, 1980.
2. American Thoracic Society Subcommittee on Surgery: Management of non-tuberculous empyema. Am. Rev. Respir. Dis., *85*:935, 1962.
3. Borrow, M., Conston, A., Livornese, L. L., and Schalet, N.: Mesothelioma and its association with asbestosis. J.A.M.A., *201*:93, 1967.
4. Carr, D. T., Soule, E. H., and Ellis, F. H., Jr.: Management of pleural effusions. Med. Clin. North Am., *48*:961, 1964.
5. Clagett, O. T., and Geraci, J. E.: A procedure for the management of post-pneumonectomy empyema. J. Thorac. Cardiovasc. Surg., *45*:141, 1963.
6. DeVries, W. C., and Wolfe, W. G.: The management of spontaneous pneumothorax and bullous emphysema. Surg. Clin. North Am., *60*:851, 1980.
7. Drummond, D. S., and Craig, R. H.: Traumatic hemothorax: Complications and management. Am. Surg., *33*:403, 1967.
8. Eloesser, L.: Of an operation for tuberculous empyema. Ann. Thorac. Surg., *8*:355, 1969.
9. Fishman, N. H.: Thoracic Drainage: A Manual of Procedures. Chicago, Year Book Medical Publishers, Inc., 1983.
10. Goss, C. M.: Anatomy of the Human Body by Henry Gray. Philadelphia, Lea & Febiger, 1966.

11. Hillerdal, G.: Malignant mesothelioma 1982: Review of 4710 published cases. Br. J. Dis. Chest, 77:321, 1983.
12. Mills, M., and Baisch, B. F.: Spontaneous pneumothorax. Ann. Thorac. Surg., 1:286, 1965.
13. Passmore, R., and Robson, J. S.: A Comparison to Medical Studies. Philadelphia, F. A. Davis Company, 1968.
14. Starkey, G. W. B., and Ullyot, D. J.: Pleural empyema. Surg. Clin. North Am., 48:507, 1968.
15. Sabiston, D. C., Jr., Hopkins, E. H., Cooke, R. E., and Bennett, I.

L., Jr.: The surgical management of complications of staphylococcal pneumonia in infancy and childhood. J. Thorac. Cardiovasc. Surg., 38:421, 1959.
16. Takaro, T, and Scott, S. M.: The pleura and empyema. In Sabiston, D. C., Jr. (Ed.): Davis-Christopher Textbook of Surgery. Philadelphia, W.B. Saunders Company, 1981.
17. Wayne, M. A., and McSwain, N. E., Jr.: Clinical evaluation of a new device for the treatment of tension pneumothorax. Ann. Surg., 191:760, 1980.

V

Bronchiectasis

RONALD C. HILL, M.D.
DAVID C. SABISTON, JR., M.D.

Bronchiectasis, a suppurative pulmonary disease characterized by dilatation of the bronchi, was first described by Laennec in 1819. He cited the pathologic changes in the bronchial wall and pulmonary parenchyma and noted that the disorder rarely occurred in the upper lobes.[6] Surgical management for bronchiectasis began with drainage of lung abscesses, and other procedures included removal of a lobe, either partial or complete, by scalpel or by the actual cautery. This was followed by the standard complete and partial lobectomies for bronchiectatic lobes.[6] Subsequent investigation revealed that segmental resection was often the surgical procedure of choice.[5]

ETIOLOGY

Bronchiectasis may be either a congenital or acquired disorder (Table 1).[4] The congenital types include bronchiectasis with situs inversus and paranasal sinusitis (Kartagener's syndrome), characterized by defective cilia or ciliary motion in the bronchial mucosa.[2, 3, 10] Hypogammaglobulinemia may be associated with bronchiectasis and is regarded as a predisposing factor in the development of pneumonia in those patients by lowering the immune response.[10] Abnormally thick bronchial secretions are found in patients with cystic fibrosis, which results in the development of mucous plugs and purulent bronchial secretions, ultimately producing bronchiectasis.[3]

Although infections formerly represented the primary cause of acquired bronchiectasis (pertussis, measles, influenza, and bronchial pneumonia), these diseases have largely been brought under control by antibiotics and immunization.[2, 10]

Currently, *intrinsic* obstruction of the bronchi from purulent secretions, mucous plugs, aspiration, foreign bodies, tuberculosis, neoplasms, and chronic lung abscesses are more common causes. *Extrinsic* bases from enlarged lymph nodes, resulting in the *middle lobe syndrome*, and anomalous blood vessels causing bronchial obstruction have become of more importance.

PATHOPHYSIOLOGY

Reid classifies bronchiectasis into three subgroups: (1) *cylindrical*, in which the dilated bronchi have a regular outline without an increase in diameter and end abruptly; (2) *varicose*, with greater dilatation and irregularity, absent peripheral filling, and a bulbous termination; and (3) *saccular* (cystic), demonstrating bronchial dilatation and ballooning, which increases toward the periphery of the lung.[7]

Bronchiectasis is usually located in the basal segments of the lower lobes with involvement of the corresponding middle lobe or lingula as well. The superior segments of the lower lobes are usually free of disease because of the

TABLE 1. Causative Factors of Importance in Development of Bronchiectasis*

Congenital
Congenital cystic bronchiectasis
Selective IgA deficiency
Primary hypogammaglobulinemia
Alpha₁-antitrypsin deficiency
Cystic fibrosis
Congenital deficiency of bronchial cartilage
Kartagener's syndrome: situs inversus, sinusitis, and bronchiectasis
Bronchopulmonary sequestration

Acquired
Infection: bacterial, viral
Bronchial obstruction
Intrinsic: neoplasm, foreign body, mucous plug
Extrinsic: enlarged lymph nodes
"Middle lobe syndrome"
Scarring secondary to tuberculosis
Acquired hypogammaglobulinemia

*From Bolman, R. M., III, and Wolfe, W. G.: Bronchiectasis and bronchopulmonary sequestration. Surg. Clin. North Am., 60:867, 1980.

adequate gravity drainage. When the left basilar segments are diseased, the lingula is involved in 60 to 80 per cent of cases; when the right basilar segments are involved, the right middle lobe is diseased in 45 to 60 per cent. Bronchiectasis occurs bilaterally in approximately 40 per cent of patients.[3]

The gross anatomic manifestations of bronchiectasis include thickened and dilated bronchial walls (occasionally abscesses, pleural perforation, and/or empyema) and intervening lung parenchyma, which demonstrates inflammation and fibrosis.[1, 3] Microscopically, the elastic and muscular laminae of the bronchial walls are replaced with fibrous tissue.[3] The resultant impaired peristaltic activity of the cilia tends to decrease the ability of clearing secretions and debris from the tracheobronchial tree. Abnormal communications between the bronchial and pulmonary arteries may lead to hemoptysis.[1]

DIAGNOSIS AND TREATMENT

The patient with bronchiectasis usually presents with a productive cough and purulent secretions.[2, 10] A foul odor (*fetor oris*), produced by the fetid sputum, is usually present.[2] This occurs less frequently today because of the availability of antibiotic therapy. These patients may also exhibit areas of pneumonitis of the lung parenchyma and hemoptysis. Hemoptysis occurs in about 40 per cent of localized bronchiectatic segments and in some 65 per cent of patients with multisegmental bronchiectasis, and is thought to be secondary to anastomotic communications between the hypertrophied bronchial circulation and the pulmonary vasculature at sites of extensive disease.[1, 9]

On physical examination of the chest, the patient may exhibit dullness to percussion, moist rales, and expiratory rhonchi.[2] The chest film may show areas of atelectasis, cystic spaces, and increased markings in the diseased segments.[2, 10] The definitive diagnosis is made by *bronchography*, which is best performed during the non-acute phase (Fig. 1). If it is done during the acute phase, the delicate anatomy may not be delineated because of the inspissated plugging by secretions.[2, 10] Bronchoscopy should also be performed to delineate the segmental nature of the disease by revealing those segmental bronchi with purulent secretions. Bacterial cultures for anaerobic and aerobic organisms may then be performed for sensitivities and appropriate choice of an antibiotic.[2] Foreign bodies and neoplasms may also be identified if involved in the pathogenesis. Arterial blood gases and pulmonary functions should be obtained in complete assessment, especially if pulmonary resection is being considered.

The treatment of bronchiectasis may be either medical or surgical. Most patients in whom bronchiectasis develops are initially managed with a medical regimen that includes antibiotics and appropriate postural drainage. Bronchoscopy may be used to remove the thick purulent secretions. The avoidance of smoking and polluted air is important, and these patients should also receive pneumococcal and annual influenzal vaccines.[2] Prior to 1941, the mortality for conservative medical treatment ranged between 20 and 50 per cent. In the ensuing years, it has declined to approximately 6 to 9 per cent. During this time, the surgical mortality has fallen from about 10 per cent in 1940 to less than 1 per cent today. Patients who are candidates for surgical therapy are usually those who have failed medical

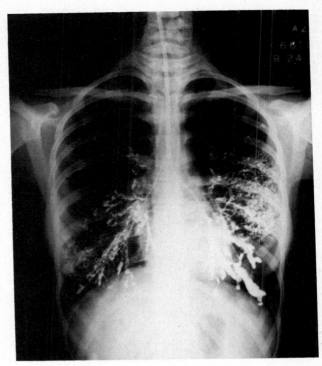

Figure 1. Bronchogram demonstrating cylindrical and saccular bronchiectasis.

management and who have continual recurrent pneumonitis or frequent episodes of hemoptysis.[2]

In a series of 140 patients, 70 with localized disease and 70 with multisegmental disease, an intensive preoperative regimen was initiated directed toward reducing the secretions and clearing of acute infections. Operation was deferred for at least 3 weeks after the bronchographic examination. The aim of the surgical procedure was to eradicate the diseased pulmonary tissue and to conserve as much normal pulmonary tissue as possible. The results indicated that the operative treatment in the localized group frequently provided complete relief. The multisegmental group, however, underwent a more palliative procedure. In the patients with bilateral disease, the side with the more extensive involvement was first approached, and in many such patients the result was quite satisfactory and a resection on the opposite side was not required. Over 80 per cent of the patients with *localized* disease gained relief of respiratory symptoms by resection, 36 per cent of the multisegmental group showed *complete* resolution of symptoms, and 53 per cent were improved.[9] In another series of 99 patients undergoing bilateral pulmonary resections for severe multisegmental bronchiectasis, a good result was obtained in 84 per cent with a mortality of 1.4 per cent and a complication rate of 7 per cent.[4]

Children in whom bronchiectasis develops should be considered for surgical therapy as well. In a recent review, 195 children with bronchiectasis were evaluated; 84 required 96 consecutive pulmonary resections, and 111 patients were followed medically. Of those managed by surgery, 75 per cent were well or much improved, 22 per cent were improved, and 4 per cent were unchanged; of those followed medically, 69 per cent remained largely unchanged and 23 per cent became worse. When partially diseased segments were retained, the slightly altered bronchi deteriorated in the convalescence. Although preservation of lung parenchyma is important, the residual tissue should be as normal as possible. In the young child, diffuse bronchiectasis is quite unstable and such children should be followed until the cause of the disease and its severity have become clearly manifest before pulmonary resection is advocated, generally between the ages of 6 and 12. The data suggested that children with *localized* bronchiectasis should undergo a resection for better prognosis and not be treated conservatively.[11]

SELECTED REFERENCES

Bolman, R. M., III, and Wolfe, W. G.: Bronchiectasis and bronchopulmonary sequestration. Surg. Clin. North Am., *60*:867, 1980.
   An excellent monograph reviewing the pathophysiology and treatment of bronchiectasis and bronchopulmonary sequestration.

Ochsner, A.: The development of pulmonary surgery with special emphasis on carcinoma and bronchiectasis. Am. J. Surg., *135*:732, 1978.
   This is an excellent paper on the history of thoracic surgery with special emphasis on bronchiectasis and carcinoma.

Sealy, W. C., Bradham, R. R., and Young, W. G., Jr.: The surgical treatment of multisegmental localized bronchiectasis. Surg. Gynecol. Obstet., *123*:80, 1966.
   The experience of one clinic with bronchiectasis is reviewed. The results of surgical treatment and the complications of operation are emphasized.

REFERENCES

1. Ackerman, L. V., and Rosai, J.: Surgical Pathology. St. Louis, C. V. Mosby Co., 1974.
2. Bolman, R. M., III, and Wolfe, W. G.: Bronchiectasis and bronchopulmonary sequestration. Surg. Clin. North Am., *60*:867, 1980.
3. Campbell, G. S.: Bronchiectasis. *In* Sabiston D. C., Jr. (Ed.): Davis-Christopher Textbook of Surgery. Philadelphia, W. B. Saunders Company, 1981.
4. George, S. A., Leonardi, H. K., and Overholt, R. H.: Bilateral pulmonary resection for bronchiectasis: A 40-year experience. Ann. Thorac. Surg., *28*:48, 1979.
5. Kent, E. M., and Blades, B.: Surgical anatomy of pulmonary lobes. J. Thorac. Surg., *12*:18, 1942.
6. Ochsner, A.: The development of pulmonary surgery, with special emphasis on carcinoma and bronchiectasis. Am. J. Surg., *135*:732, 1978.
7. Reid, L. M.: Reduction in bronchial subdivision in bronchiectasis. Thorax, *5*:233, 1950.
8. Sanderson, J. M., Kennedy, M. C. S., Johnson, M. F., and Manley, D. C. E.: Bronchiectasis: Results of surgical and conservative management. Thorax, *29*:407, 1974.
9. Sealy, W. C., Bradham, R. R., and Young, W. G., Jr.: The surgical treatment of multisegmental localized bronchiectasis. Surg. Gynecol. Obstet., *123*:80, 1966.
10. Takaro, T.: Lung infections and diffuse interstitial diseases of the lungs. *In* Sabiston, D. C., Jr., and Spencer, F. C. (Eds.): Gibbon's Surgery of the Chest. Philadelphia, W. B. Saunders Company, 1983.
11. Wilson, J. F., and Decker, A. M.: The surgical management of childhood bronchiectasis. Ann. Surg., *195*:354, 1982.

VI

The Surgical Treatment of Pulmonary Tuberculosis

JON F. MORAN, M.D.

The majority of cases of tuberculosis occur in less developed parts of the world, although the incidence has begun to rise again in some urban centers within the United States. The death rate per 100,000 population in the United States has fallen from 200 cases per year in 1900 to one case per year in 1980.[2] The total number of new cases of pulmonary mycobacterial infection in the United States in 1984 was approximately 25,000. With modern antituberculous chemotherapy, less than 2 per cent of these patients will require surgical treatment.

Surgical treatment for pulmonary tuberculosis began in the later part of the nineteenth century using artificially induced pneumothorax to collapse the affected portions of the lung. By the 1920s, paravertebral thoracoplasty was widely used to induce permanent collapse of infected portions of the lung. As pulmonary resectional surgery developed in the 1930s and 1940s, lobectomy and segmental resection techniques were applied to the treatment of localized mycobacterial infections. The discovery of streptomycin in 1944 and the development of other effective chemotherapy for tuberculosis markedly reduced the perioperative morbidity. Modern chemotherapy regimens control tuberculosis so effectively that the need for surgical intervention in pulmonary tuberculosis has become infrequent.

BACTERIOLOGY

The majority of cases of pulmonary tuberculosis are caused by the species of mycobacteria originally isolated by Koch in 1882, *Mycobacterium tuberculosis*. A number of other species have been isolated during the past century. A subgroup known as atypical mycobacteria is an unusual cause of pulmonary infection. In 50 per cent of patients who are referred for surgical therapy of mycobacterial disease, the infecting organism is one of the atypical mycobacteria.

Atypical mycobacteria as a group are much more frequently resistant to standard antituberculous drugs. Runyon divided all the mycobacteria into four groups according to differences in growth rate and pigment production by the growing colonies.[9] *Group I*, the photochromogens, produce a yellow pigment when grown in the light and are slow growing organisms. *Group II*, the scotochromogens, grow slowly and produce yellow pigment when grown in the dark. *Group III*, the nonphotochromogens (including *M. tuberculosis*) grow slowly and produce no pigment even when exposed to light. *Group IV* includes the rapidly growing mycobacteria.

Mycobacterium intracellulare and *Mycobacterium kansasii* are the two atypical organisms most frequently found to cause clinical pulmonary infection. *M. intracellulare* is usually resistant to most antituberculosis drugs *in vitro*. Empiric five- and six-drug long-term chemotherapy, when able to be tolerated, has enabled conversion to sputum-negative status in 60 to 70 per cent of patients with *M. intracellulare* disease.[4] Localized pulmonary disease responds to excisional surgery combined with multiple drug chemotherapy in well over 90 per cent of these patients.[8] *M. kansasii* is common in the midwestern portion of the United States and commonly shows *in vitro* susceptibility to a number of the antituberculous drugs. A two- or three-drug chemotherapy regimen including rifampin is generally successful in more than 95 per cent of patients.[4] Adjunctive surgical therapy will be required in only a small minority of patients with *M. kansasii* pulmonary disease.

DIAGNOSIS

The isolation of mycobacterial organisms from the sputum or lung tissue is necessary to confirm the diagnosis of mycobacterial disease. Mycobacterial cultures require 3 to 6 weeks to grow, and it is often necessary to obtain multiple sputum samples before a positive culture is obtained. An acid-fast (Ziehl-Neelsen) stain allows a rapid presumptive diagnosis if organisms are seen, although there are other rare pulmonary pathogens that will take up this particular stain. With the increasing relative incidence of drug-resistant forms of tuberculosis, accurate culture results with sensitivity testing for all antituberculous agents are particularly important in patients being considered for surgical intervention.

Most patients will be sensitized to the protein fraction of the tubercle bacillus within several weeks following the onset of infection. Intradermal injection of this purified protein fraction (PPD) causes a delayed hypersensitivity reaction with an area of induration at 48 hours. Anergic patients, immunosuppressed individuals, or desperately ill patients with widespread tuberculosis may exhibit false-negative PPD skin tests. The intermediate PPD, five tuberculin units (TU) of Tween 80 Purified Protein Derivative, will be positive (greater than or equal to 10 mm. induration) in at least 90 per cent of cases of tuberculosis.[6]

PATHOLOGY

Pulmonary mycobacterial infection follows inhalation of the acid-fast organism. The bacilli tend to lodge in peripheral locations and cause an exudative alveolitis that proceeds to a caseous necrosis. Enlargement of the hilar lymph nodes occurs secondary to organisms draining into the lymphatics at the hilum of the lung. Generally, healing of the peripheral lesion occurs, leaving a small calcified lung mass and enlarged hilar lymph nodes that form the "primary Ghon complex." This phase is known as primary pulmonary tuberculosis and only rarely progresses directly into post-primary pulmonary tuberculosis.

The majority of clinical tuberculosis is caused by post-primary infection as a result of reactivation of a previously quiescent lesion in middle-age or older individuals. Post-primary pulmonary mycobacterial infection is found in the apical and posterior segments of the upper lobes (85 per cent) or the superior segments of the lower lobes (10 per cent) generally. It begins as a pneumonic infiltrate and progresses to cavitation with caseous necrosis. Microscopically, epithelioid cells with Langhans' giant cells and caseous necrosis are seen. Fibrous reaction occurs around the edge of the lesion. Acid-fast organisms can usually be seen within the lesions. Involved segments of lung contract in the healing process and initially small cavities may fuse to form larger cavities (Fig. 1) with very thick and fibrous walls. Erosion of the cavities into bronchial vessels may cause severe hemoptysis.

Endobronchial tuberculosis may result as the infection spreads, causing swelling and even ulceration of the bronchial mucosa. Secondarily, this may lead to stenosis of a lobar or segmental bronchus. Distal to such a stenosis, bronchiectasis frequently occurs with secondary infection by nontuberculous organisms. The cavities created by tuberculosis may become infected by other bacteria or, more commonly, by fungi, particularly *Aspergillus*, leading to

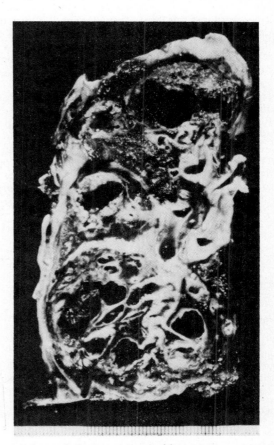

Figure 1. Cut pathologic specimen of the right lung shows total destruction of the lung by pulmonary tuberculosis. Superimposed fungal infection can be seen within the large cavitary lesions of the upper and middle lobes while the lower lobe shows severe bronchiectasis. (From Harrison, L. H., Jr.: Surg. Clin. North Am., 60:883, 1980.)

further destruction of the lung and often severe intermittent hemoptysis. The tubercles tend to be peripheral within the lung, causing an intense pleural reaction with obliteration of the pleural space over the involved segments of the lung. A caseous focus may rupture into the pleural space, resulting in tuberculous empyema or even creating a bronchopleural fistula if the cavity also communicates with the bronchus. The empyema that results frequently contains secondary organisms in addition to mycobacteria.

CHEMOTHERAPY

There are ten common antituberculous agents available in the United States (Table 1). Pulmonary tuberculosis is treated with at least two and sometimes three drugs for treatment periods ranging from 9 to 24 months. Two- and three-drug therapy is used to avoid the emergence of drug-resistant organisms. The most commonly employed chemotherapy regimen at present consists of rifampin and isoniazid (INH) for 9 months. INH and rifampin are bactericidal for both extra- and intracellular acid-fast organisms. If either INH or rifampin cannot be tolerated, streptomycin and pyrazinamide may be substituted, since streptomycin is bactericidal against extracellular acid-fast organisms within tuberculous cavities and pyrazinamide kills intracellular organisms. If ethambutol, a bacteriostatic drug, is used to replace either INH or rifampin, therapy must be continued for 18 to 24 months, and an aminoglycoside, usually streptomycin, is given for the first 1 to 3 months.

The incidence of primary drug resistance in tuberculosis in the United States has risen to nearly 10 per cent.[1] Disease secondary to drug-resistant organisms is selectively referred for surgical intervention, and therefore accurate sensitivity testing and a familiarity with the use of all antituberculous agents[7] are particularly important in the planning of surgical treatment of mycobacterial infections.

Complications of resectional surgery can be reduced if conversion to sputum-negative status occurs prior to operation. Optimal pulmonary toilet, careful selection of the appropriate chemotherapy, and the addition of one or two new drugs during the perioperative period are useful steps for reducing operative complications. If at all possible, patients should always have received 3 to 4 weeks of chemotherapy prior to surgical intervention. For the atypical mycobacteria that exhibit resistance to many or all chemotherapeutic agents, the administration of INH and rifampin and an aminoglycoside perioperatively and the maintenance of the patient on INH and rifampin for a period of 9 to 12 months postoperatively is recommended. Whenever possible, one should select chemotherapeutic agents to which the infecting organism has been proved sensitive.

OPERATIVE TREATMENT

The evolution of chemotherapy for tuberculosis that initially made resectional surgery feasible has now severely curtailed the need and indications for surgical intervention. Surgical treatment is indicated when the expected operative morbidity and mortality are minimal, the prospect for complete control of the infectious disease is excellent, and the period of disability entailed by the surgery is brief. The standard indications for surgical intervention in mycobacterial disease are the following:

1. Persistently positive sputum cultures following 6 months of continuous optimal chemotherapy with two or more drugs. Usually, underlying cavitary disease, bronchiectasis, or bronchial stenosis will be contributing to the failure of the chemotherapeutic regimen.

2. Localized pulmonary disease caused by *M. intracellulare* (or another atypical mycobacteria with broad resistance to chemotherapy).

3. The presence of a mass lesion suspicious for carcinoma of the lung in an area of tuberculous involvement.

4. Massive life-threatening hemoptysis or recurrent severe hemoptysis.

5. A bronchopleural fistula in association with mycobacterial infection that does not respond to tube thoracostomy.

Other situations occasionally call for surgical intervention. Patients severely symptomatic from a destroyed lobe or a bronchiectatic area may benefit from resection. Also, patients with particularly thick-walled cavities who have a

TABLE 1. Antimycobacterial Drugs

Drug	Adult Dosage	Common Side Effects	Comments
Isoniazid (INH)	300 mg./day, PO or IM	Hepatotoxicity, peripheral neuritis	Bactericidal; pyridoxine 50 mg./day as prophylaxis for neuritis
Rifampin (RIF)	600 mg./day, PO	Hepatotoxicity	Bactericidal; colors urine orange; blocks effect of birth control pills
Streptomycin (SM)	1 gm./day, IM	Nephrotoxicity, ototoxicity	Bactericidal
Ethambutol (EMB)	900–1200 mg./day, PO	Optic neuritis, hyperuricemia	Requires periodic eye testing
Pyrazinamide (PZA)	2–3 gm./day, PO in 3–4 divided doses	Hepatotoxicity, hyperuricemia	Combination with aminoglycoside (SM, KM, or CM) is bactericidal
Ethionamide (ETA)	1 gm./day, PO in 3–4 divided doses	Gastrointestinal intolerance, hepatotoxicity	Divided or bedtime dosage may decrease gastrointestinal intolerance
Para-amino salicylic acid (PAS)	12 gm./day, PO in 3 divided doses	Gastrointestinal intolerance, hepatotoxicity	50 per cent incidence of gastrointestinal intolerance
Cycloserine (CS)	1 gm./day, PO in 2 divided doses	Psychosis, depression, seizures	Rarely tolerated; pyridoxine may mitigate side effects
Kanamycin (KM)	1 gm./day, IM	Nephrotoxicity, ototoxicity	Bactericidal
Capreomycin (CM)	1 gm./day, IM	Nephrotoxicity, ototoxicity	Bactericidal

reactivated infection or who are clearly unreliable in complying with prolonged chemotherapy may be best treated by resection of the diseased area. Finally, a patient with a "trapped lung" with limitation of ventilatory capacity following a tuberculous empyema may benefit from decortication allowing full re-expansion of the involved lung. Endobronchial tuberculosis documented by bronchoscopy is a relative contraindication to resectional surgery until it can be cleared by chemotherapy.

Preoperatively, bronchoscopy should be performed to ensure that there is no evidence of endobronchial tuberculosis or unsuspected proximal bronchial stenosis. The use of a double-lumen endotracheal tube can make resections for tuberculosis technically easier while simultaneously protecting the dependent lung from contamination during manipulation of the infected lung. Type of resection is dependent upon the extent of disease and is guided by the principle that all gross evidence of disease should be resected. In patients with known active mycobacterial disease, either a lobectomy or pneumonectomy will usually be necessary. It is occasionally necessary to combine upper lobectomy with wedge excision of the superior segment of the lower lobe to remove all gross disease. Pneumonectomy is rarely indicated except in the setting of a totally destroyed lung. Full re-expansion of the remaining lung tissue is important for avoiding the complications of atelectasis, hemothorax, and apical space problems. Postoperative bronchoscopy may be required to optimize pulmonary toilet and to avoid segmental or lobar atelectasis, since in many of these patients secretions are very thick and tenacious.

Improved anesthetic techniques, better chemotherapy, careful patient selection, and use of stapling devices have all contributed to a steadily decreasing morbidity and mortality for resectional surgery for pulmonary mycobacterial disease. However, at the present time resectional surgery is employed only in a selected group of difficult patients in whom chemotherapy has failed or in those who have a serious complication, such as massive hemoptysis or bronchopleural fistula. Consequently, the mortality rate in various series will vary from zero per cent with minimal morbidity when surgical intervention is elective[8] to 15 per cent when resection is performed as an emergency.[3] The major postoperative complications are pulmonary insufficiency and bronchopleural fistula. The prognosis for long-term survival free of further mycobacterial disease is excellent, with 95 per cent of patients free of disease 5 to 8 years postoperatively.

The most common cause of *massive hemoptysis* continues to be pulmonary tuberculosis.[3] Because pulmonary resection is the most effective way to stop bleeding and to avoid asphyxiation in massive hemoptysis, it is essential to rapidly identify the site of bleeding. An area of cavitation, possibly with an intracavitary fungus ball, is most likely to be the source of the hemorrhage. Mild hemoptysis will ordinarily abate once the patient is sedated with good control of his blood pressure, but brisk hemoptysis should be managed aggressively. Bronchoscopy is performed in the operating room to identify the site of bleeding or to confirm the site of bleeding if an area of cavitary disease has previously been identified. Blockage of the involved bronchus using a Fogarty catheter placed with bronchoscopic guidance can be very helpful in avoiding aspiration of blood into normal areas of lung. When the involved bronchus is blocked or excluded using a double-lumen endotracheal tube, the patient can be turned to the lateral

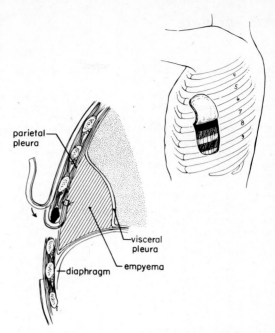

Figure 2. Technique for construction of an Eloesser flap. The flap is based superiorly and the rib at the base of the flap is resected. The flap is turned in to maintain the opening and to give a valvelike action to maintain a negative pressure within the pleural space. (From DeMeester, T. R., and Lafontaine, E.: The pleura. In Sabiston, D. C., Jr., and Spencer, F. C. [Eds.]: Gibbon's Surgery of the Chest, 4th ed. Philadelphia, W. B. Saunders Company, 1983, p. 385.)

thoracotomy position and resection performed expeditiously and safely.

Bronchopulmonary fistula and *empyema* in the patient with tuberculosis are difficult management problems whether they occur spontaneously or in the postoperative setting. Bronchopleural fistula should be managed by tube thoracostomy and adequate chemotherapy. In the early postoperative setting, an immediate attempt at operative reclosure of the stump is indicated. In a late postoperative situation, adequate drainage followed by thoracoplasty to obliterate any residual pleural space is the treatment of choice. In spontaneous bronchopleural fistula, adequate drainage may be followed by resection of the involved lung with decortication of the remaining lung and/or thoracoplasty as necessary.

Spontaneous tuberculous empyema is now rare. Because of the dense pleural reaction, tube thoracostomy will seldom result in full re-expansion of the underlying lung. Decortication may lead to full re-expansion with excellent recovery of pulmonary function. Occasionally, resection of the associated area of pulmonary disease is required as well. If the empyema follows pneumonectomy or is complicated by a bronchopleural fistula with secondary superimposed infection, or if the patient's overall condition is too poor to tolerate a major thoracotomy, open drainage of the pleural space by creation of an Eloesser flap (Fig. 2) provides excellent drainage.[5] Later thoracoplasty with or without decortication will frequently be necessary.

SELECTED REFERENCES

Harrison, L. H., Jr.: Current aspects of surgical management of tuberculosis. Surg. Clin. North Am., *60*:883, 1980.
This chapter contains a concise summary of the modern surgical treatment of tuberculosis.

Lester, W.: Treatment of tuberculosis. *In* Fishman, A. P. (Ed.): Pulmonary Diseases and Disorders. New York, McGraw-Hill, 1980, pp. 1305–1323.
This chapter contains the modern guidelines for medical treatment of tuberculosis.

Myers, J. A.: The Captain of All These Men of Death: Tuberculosis Historical Highlights. St. Louis, Warren H. Green, 1977.
This book contains a review of the impact of tuberculosis over the centuries as well as a very detailed description of the contributions of the past hundred years that brought tuberculosis under control.

Stead, W. W., and Dutt, A. K.: Chemotherapy for tuberculosis today. Am. Rev. Respir. Dis., *125*:94, 1982.
This article outlines the latest developments in short course chemotherapy for tuberculosis as well as retreatment programs and the role of bacteriostatic drugs in therapy.

REFERENCES

1. Carpenter, J. L., Obnibene, A. J., Gorby, E. W., Neimes, R. E., Koch, J. R., and Perkins, W. L.: Antituberculosis drug resistance in South Texas. Am. Rev. Respir. Dis., *128*:1055, 1983.
2. Comstock, G. W.: Epidemiology of tuberculosis. Am. Rev. Respir. Dis., *125*:8, 1982.
3. Conlan, A. A., Hurwitz, S. S., Krige, L., Nicolaou, N., and Pool, R.: Massive hemoptysis. J. Thorac. Cardiovasc. Surg., *85*:120, 1983.
4. Davidson, P. T.: The management of disease with atypical mycobacteria. Clin. Notes Respir. Dis., *18*:3, 1979.
5. Eloesser, L.: Of an operation for tuberculous empyema. Ann. Thorac. Surg., *8*:355, 1969.
6. Glassroth, J., Robins, A. G., and Snider, D. E., Jr.: Tuberculosis in the 1980's. N. Engl. J. Med., *302*:1441, 1980.
7. Lester, W.: Treatment of drug-resistant tuberculosis. DM, April, 1971.
8. Moran, J. F., Alexander, L. G., Staub, E. W., Young, W. G., Jr., and Sealy, W. C.: Long-term results of pulmonary resection for atypical mycobacterial disease. Ann. Thorac. Surg., *35*:597, 1983.
9. Runyon, E. H.: Anonymous mycobacteria and pulmonary disease. Med. Clin. North Am., *43*:273, 1959.

VII

Carcinoma of the Lung

DAVID C. SABISTON, JR., M.D.

During the past several decades, carcinoma of the lung has risen to the rank of first place in incidence of malignant neoplasms in both males and females. It is quite extraordinary that at the turn of the century malignant pulmonary neoplasms were quite rare, but with males initiating the onset of cigarette smoking the incidence continued to increase, so that by 1986 cancer of the lung in females surpassed both that of breast and utero-ovarian neoplasms (Fig. 1). This cancer now accounts for a third of all malignant tumors in males and approximately a fifth in females. In 1933, Graham performed the first successful one-stage pneumonectomy for carcinoma of the lung. The patient was the first to be cured of the disease and lived many years without recurrence.

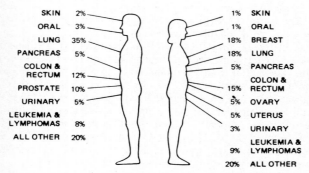

Figure 1. 1985 estimated cancer deaths by site and sex. (From Silverberg, E.: Ca—A Cancer Journal for Clinicians, 35:19, 1985.)

PATHOGENESIS

It is now widely accepted that cigarette smoking is the primary inciting factor in the pathogenesis of carcinoma of the lung. In order to convince patients that they should cease smoking, especially when scientific evidence is needed to cite the cause-and-effect relationship, several points should be emphasized:

1. Polycyclic hydrocarbons (benzpyrenes) are present in significant concentrations in cigarette smoke, and unburned tobacco in the stub of cigarettes contains N'-nitrosonornicotine. Both of these substances are strong carcinogens.[43]

2. When studied in detail at autopsy, the cytologic changes that occur in the lungs of smokers can be followed from the earliest stages of neoplasia of basal cell hyperplasia, to carcinoma *in situ*, and finally to frank carcinoma. It has been shown that independent evaluation of the smoking history of an individual can be correlated quite precisely with the degree of severity of the premalignant and malignant changes found at autopsy. In a fascinating postmortem study of 117 males, the smoking history was carefully documented by one group of workers and another group carefully assessed the entire tracheobronchial tree at autopsy. Each patient in the study was evaluated with more than 200 histologic sections. Of the 117 patients in the study, 34 died of bronchogenic carcinoma and all were smokers. In the remaining 83 patients, it was possible to find a direct correlation of the severity of the premalignant changes with the number of pack-years of cigarette smok-

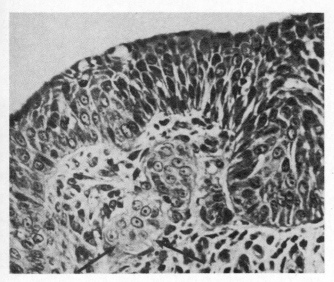

Figure 2. Invasive squamous cell carcinoma from bronchus of dog that has smoked 6210 cigarettes. The arrows indicate the area of invasion (H&E, × 560). (From Hammond, E. C., Auerbach, O., Kirman, D., and Garfinkel, L.: Cancer, 21:78, 1971. By permission of the authors and the American Cancer Society.)

ing. The earliest changes showed basal cell hyperplasia, then epithelial stratification, followed by squamous metaplasia, with progression to carcinoma *in situ*. Finally, frank pulmonary carcinoma was present in the most severe smokers. A combined exposure to asbestos and cigarette smoke is synergistic in carcinogenic effect.[13]

3. On a statistical basis alone it can be shown that cigarette smoking is significant: In nonsmokers the annual incidence of carcinoma of the lung is only 3.4 per 100,000; for those who smoke 10 to 20 cigarettes daily, the figure rises to 59.3 annually; and for those smoking over 40 cigarettes daily, the figure is 217.3. Moreover, if a person ceases smoking, the likelihood of pulmonary cancer decreases appreciably.[11]

4. In animals with a tracheostomy, carcinoma of the lung can be produced experimentally with continuous smoking of cigarettes. Under these circumstances, metaplastic lesions occur in the tracheobronchial epithelium, later followed by appearance of noninvasive carcinoma and finally by frank carcinoma, including metastases to regional lymph nodes.[12] A photomicrograph of a lesion of this type is shown in Figure 2.

5. Finally, in a review of 2668 patients with proven carcinoma of the lung there were only 134 individuals who were validated *nonsmokers* (5 per cent).[19] Clearly, this indicates the strong causal effect of cigarette smoking in this pathogenesis of carcinoma of the lung.

PATHOLOGIC TYPES

One of the most useful classifications for carcinoma of the lung includes the five following types:

1. *Squamous cell carcinoma.* The most common type, with an incidence varying from 40 to 70 per cent of the total lesions. Nearly all of these patients have had a history of cigarette smoking, and there is only a 1 per cent likelihood that such a lesion will occur in a nonsmoker.[3] The cytologic changes merge toward anaplasticity in some neoplasms and become undifferentiated carcinomas. These primary lesions have a tendency to be large and frequently undergo central necrosis.

2. *Undifferentiated carcinoma.* In most series, represents 20 to 30 per cent of the total. These neoplasms have also been designated "oat cell" lesions. They may be either round cell or large cell, or they may take on a typical oat cell appearance. These lesions are highly malignant and are associated with a poor prognosis if untreated.

3. *Adenocarcinoma.* In most series, occurs in 5 to 15 per cent, more often seen peripherally. There is a higher incidence in females. This cell type also has the greatest tendency to metastasize to the liver, brain, bone, and adrenals as well as lymph nodes.

4. *Bronchoalveolar carcinoma.* A very well differentiated neoplasm, the cells representing a hyperplastic variety of the normal alveolar lining. It is associated with the most favorable prognosis of pulmonary cancers.[29] In one series, this type of cancer was resectable in two thirds of the patients at the time of operation, with 5-year survival of 48 per cent.[27]

5. *Giant cell carcinoma.* A variant of bronchogenic adenocarcinoma and an unusually aggressive tumor with bizarre pathologic features, ranging in incidence from 1 to 10 per cent of the total series. It spreads rapidly with metastases, and the pathologic appearance is characteristic.

There are other special types of neoplasms, including *scar carcinomas*, that appear to arise in previous scars caused by other pulmonary diseases.[6] Scarring may be the result of tuberculosis, pneumoconiosis, trauma, infarcts, or other inflammatory lesions. A number of pulmonary *scar tumors* are of the bronchoalveolar type.[38] *Dual primary carcinoma* is of interest and occurs in about 1 per cent of patients. It is generally recognized that a significant interval between the appearance of the two lesions is important in establishing this diagnosis.[37]

Metastases are very frequent with pulmonary neoplasms and often occur early. Common sites for pulmonary metastases are the mediastinal and supraclavicular lymph nodes, adrenals, liver, bones, and brain (Fig. 3). In general, among 100 patients first seen with carcinoma of the lung,

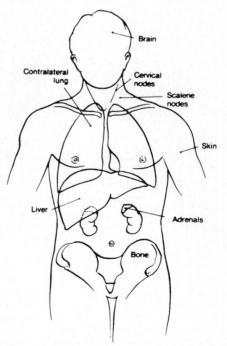

Figure 3. Common sites of metastases from carcinoma of the lung. (From Beahrs, O. H., and Myers, M. H. (Eds.): American Joint Committee on Cancer: Manual for Staging of Cancer, 2nd ed. Philadelphia, J. B. Lippincott Company, 1983.)

50 already have demonstrable evidence of metastases that precludes a curative operation. Of the remaining 50 patients who are appropriate candidates for exploratory thoracotomy, 25 will be found to be inoperable at thoracotomy because of spread of the disease locally within the chest or involvement of the mediastinum, great vessels, and nerves. Cancer in the remaining 25 patients in the original group of 100 is resectable for potential cure, and approximately eight of the original 100 patients are alive after 5 years. Therefore, the *overall* survival for the original 100 patients is approximately 8 per cent. It should be remembered, however, that in some forms of carcinoma of the lung (e.g., lesions in the periphery that are 4 cm. or less in diameter and without metastases) *the 5-year survival is 44 per cent.*[17]

CLINICAL MANIFESTATIONS

A number of patients with carcinoma of the lung are *asymptomatic* at the time of presentation. Diagnosis is suspected by a lesion found on a routine chest film. Among the clinical symptoms that may be present are cough, weight loss, dyspnea, chest pain, hemoptysis, bone pain, clubbing of the fingers, and the presence of the superior vena caval syndrome (Table 1).[15]

The *anatomic* location of the primary tumor is often related to the symptom complex. For example, those tumors around the superior vena cava may obstruct this vessel with appearance of the superior vena caval syndrome (Fig. 4). Metastases to the hilar structures may infiltrate or press upon the recurrent laryngeal nerve, producing hoarseness. If the superior mediastinum is invaded near the cervical sympathetic plexus, *Horner's syndrome* may be present. Erosion of the mucosa in the tracheobronchial tree by the

TABLE 1. Initial Symptoms of 2000 Patients with Bronchogenic Carcinoma*

	VA Lung Cancer Group (1969–1972) (%)
Cough	74
Weight loss	68
Dyspnea	58
Chest pain	49
Hemoptysis	29
Lymphadenopathy	23
Bone pain	25
Hepatomegaly	21
Clubbing	20
Superior vena caval syndrome	4

*From Hyde, L., and Hyde, C. I.: Chest, 65:299, 1974.

tumor causes hemoptysis. Cough is generally the result of bronchial irritation produced by the primary lesion. Metastases may be painful, for example, in osseous spread, or there may be central nervous system manifestations with presence of cerebral metastases. Significant weight loss is highly suggestive of metastases, particularly more than 10 to 15 pounds in a short period.

Endocrinologic Syndromes

There are a number of interesting syndromes associated with bronchogenic carcinoma that produce clinical endocrinopathies, including inappropriate diuresis, hyper-

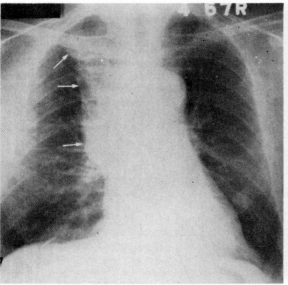
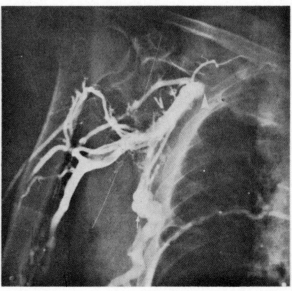

A   B

Figure 4. Bronchogenic carcinoma and superior vena caval obstruction.
A, There is enlargement of the right hilum and widening of the mediastinum on the right (arrows) due to mediastinal extension of a bronchogenic carcinoma. There was clinical evidence of superior vena caval obstruction.
B, Venogram reveals complete blockage of the subclavian vein (arrowhead). There are large dilated and anastomotic channels (arrow) extending between the superior vena cava and subclavian vein. In the presence of such findings, the lesion is inoperable.
(From Teplick, J. G., and Haskin, M. E.: Roentgenologic Diagnosis: A Complement in Radiology to the Beeson and McDermott Textbook of Medicine, Vol. 1, 3rd ed. Philadelphia, W. B. Saunders and Company, 1976.)

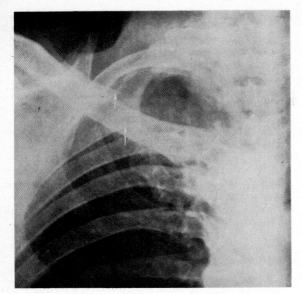

Figure 5. Superior sulcus tumor. The posterior portions of the third and fourth ribs (arrows) have been destroyed. The innocuous-appearing density in the right apex is due to an infiltrating anaplastic carcinoma that has destroyed the ribs. Tumors in the apical sulcus frequently simulate benign pleural thickenings, but rib erosion and the clinical symptoms of intractable shoulder pain and Horner's syndrome should aid in diagnosis. A superior sulcus lesion (Pancoast's tumor) may be either a squamous cell bronchogenic tumor or an anaplastic lesion. (From Teplick, J. G., and Haskin, M. E.: Roentgenologic Diagnosis: A Complement in Radiology to the Beeson and McDermott Textbook of Medicine, Vol. 1, 3rd Ed. Philadelphia, W. B. Saunders Company, 1976.)

calcemia, and the carcinoid syndrome. One of the most common hormonal manifestations is that of *Cushing's syndrome*, which is often associated with small cell carcinomas. *Antidiuretic hormone* (ADH) can be produced, especially from a poorly differentiated tumor or adenocarcinoma, and is associated with clinical signs of mental confusion and can proceed to coma with marked hyponatremia (100 to 120 mEq. per ml.). Such patients can be managed by reduction of fluid intake to less than 1000 ml. a day to maintain a relatively normal level of serum sodium. Bronchogenic tumors may also secrete parathormone, usually arising from squamous cell lesions, producing the manifestations of hypercalcemia and mental confusion. *Hypoglycemia* has been reported with the carcinoid syndrome, and gynecomastia may be associated with excessive gonadotropin production.[31]

In addition, there are other conditions, such as *neuromyopathy*, that occur in about 15 per cent of patients. Cortical cerebellar degeneration as well as degeneration of the spinocerebellar tracts may occur as an effect of bronchiogenic carcinoma with the expected clinical manifestations.

A *Pancoast tumor* is one that arises anatomically in the superior sulcus of the lung (Fig. 5). In this position, the neoplasm can infiltrate the upper mediastinum and involve the brachial plexus and cervical sympathetic nerves. These patients often have pain in the shoulder, arm, and axillae as well as Horner's syndrome.

Physical Findings

Many patients with carcinoma of the lung have few, if any, findings on physical examination. Occasionally, wheez-

ing is heard on auscultation or signs of a pleural effusion are present. Enlarged and hard nodes may be present in the supraclavicular, cervical, and axillary regions, and they should be carefully sought. An enlarged liver usually indicates metastatic disease. Evidence of weight loss and painful joints with pulmonary osteoarthropathy are also signs of distant spread.

ESTABLISHING THE DIAGNOSIS

The chest film represents the primary method for diagnosis of a pulmonary neoplasm. Although a variety of radiographic changes may occur, the presence of a mass, often with an irregular border, unless metastatic, is apparent (Fig. 6). A pleural effusion may be present, particularly if associated with pleural metastases. If the phrenic nerve is involved, the corresponding diaphragm may be paralyzed and elevated. The *isolated* pulmonary lesion, often termed a "coin lesion," is often found on routine chest films. Approximately half of these are malignant neoplasms. Of interest is that cancer of the lung can occasionally be *occult* without any obvious roentgenographic change. In a 10-year study, 54 patients—all of whom were males—were found to have carcinoma of the lung *without* any initial lesions on the chest film.[4] Diagnosis was established by cytologic examination of the sputum, and in each patient the lesion was seen on bronchoscopy. Fortunately, a pulmonary resection could be performed in each of these 54 patients and the 5-year survival was 91 per cent. Therefore, occult cancer of the lung from a radiographic point of view is a very favorable sign of life expectancy.

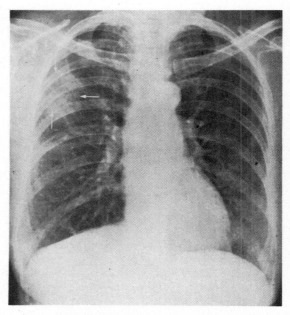

Figure 6. Alveolar cell carcinoma. Chest film in a 55-year-old woman demonstrates an ill-defined density with an indistinct lower border (arrows) in the right upper lobe. The hilar nodes are not enlarged. This picture simulated pneumonitis but proved to be an alveolar cell carcinoma. (From Teplick, J. G., and Haskin, M. E.: Roentgenologic Diagnosis: A Complement in Radiology to the Beeson and McDermott Textbook of Medicine, Vol. 1, 3rd ed. Philadelphia, W. B. Saunders Company, 1976.)

Scanning Techniques

Radioisotope Scanning. This method is useful in examination of the lungs to determine the extent of the neoplastic invasion. For example, if a scan shows a defect larger than the lesion itself, involvement of the regional nodes will be seen in more than three quarters of such patients. When the size of the defect is approximately the same size of the lesion, extension of the process to the mediastinum will be present in less than a quarter of patients.[23] Obstruction of the pulmonary veins by tumor is indicated by reduced perfusion of that anatomic region on the nuclear scan. Scanning techniques are also quite useful in delineating metastases to bone, liver, and brain.

Computed Tomography. Computed tomography (CT) has become a very valuable means of assessing the extent of the lung primary lesion and for intrathoracic involvement of lymph nodes and direct invasion of other structures. Because the adrenal glands are quite commonly involved, the scan should also include this area. In about 40 per cent of patients with bronchogenic carcinoma, there are metastases to the adrenal gland at autopsy.

Magnetic Resonance Imaging. Magnetic resonance imaging (MRI) has been found quite useful in establishing a primary diagnosis and in detecting metastases. With this technique, there is the ability to differentiate mediastinal fat from lymph nodes through its special signals. In some patients, MRI actually has demonstrated lymph nodes that were difficult to recognize on CT scan and the reason is the ease with which vessels and masses can be distinguished by MRI. On the other hand, CT scan may identify *smaller* lymph nodes than MRI. Magnetic resonance imaging also has the potential for detecting replacement of mediastinal fat by metastatic tumor.[7]

Tumor Markers

Certain neoplastic cells release substances corresponding to their normal cell type. In the recent past, specific tumors have been found to produce substances such as calcitonin in the presence of medullary carcinoma of the thyroid. Primary carcinoma of the lung may be associated with tumor markers such as the carcinoembryonic antigen (CEA). Adrenocorticotropic hormone (ACTH) as well as ADH is produced by small cell carcinomas. Cerebrospinal fluid has been analyzed for several unspecific biochemical compounds and neuron-specific enolase seems to be related both to the presence of parenchymal and meningeal metastases.[31, 35] At this time, the markers appear to be of value in isolated clinical settings, although their ultimate role is not yet identified; very likely, they have an important role in the future.[14]

Cytologic Studies

Approximately 50 per cent of patients with primary carcinoma of the lung have an endobronchial lesion that is apparent when biopsy and bronchoscopy are obtained. When a lesion is not seen on bronchoscopy, the bronchus leading to the site of the mass as seen on the chest film can be brushed and also irrigated to obtain a cytologic preparation for diagnosis. In addition, the patient's sputum should be examined on a daily basis for the presence of malignant cells.

Percutaneous Transthoracic Aspiration Needle Biopsy. In the recent past, aspiration needle biopsy has become an unusually valuable method for obtaining cells for diagnosis of bronchogenic carcinoma (Figs. 7 and 8). In one large

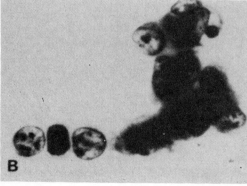

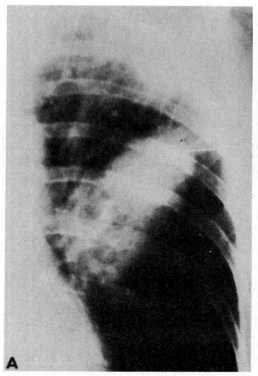

Figure 7. A posterior approach to the lesion is preferred to maintain the patient in a prone position and to avoid stimulating parasympathetic responses, but the most direct route is employed. A, A lateral puncture appeared appropriate to avoid the overlying scapula and breast tissue in this 62-year-old woman's midplane mass. B, Poorly differentiated adenocarcinoma. Cytologically, bronchogenic adenocarcinomas are most characterized by the presence of three-dimensional cell clusters with slight or no intercellular molding. Nuclear chromatin may be finely granular with one large centrally located nucleolus. Lobulations of the nuclear membranes are frequent. Cytoplasmic evidence of secretory activity may be manifested by foaminess and large vacuoles. (Membrane filter. Papanicolaou stain, × 1000) (From Heaston, D. K., et al.: Percutaneous thoracic needle biopsy. In Putman, C. E. (Ed.): Pulmonary Diagnosis: Imaging and Other Techniques. New York, Appleton-Century-Crofts, 1981.)

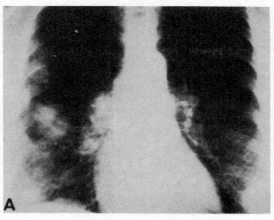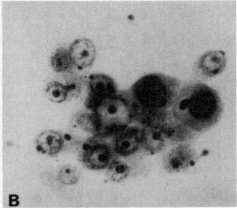

Figure 8. This 61-year-old woman presented with hematuria. Admission chest films disclosed discrete bilateral masses suggesting metastases. Aspiration with a 20-gauge needle confirmed their metastatic origin and the diagnosis of hypernephroma. B, Metastatic hypernephroma. The cytologic picture of this neoplasm metastatic to the lung is one of the most diagnostic ones seen. The cells occur in sheets; cytoplasm is granular; nuclei possess huge central nucleoli frequently surrounded by a halo. (Membrane filter. Papanicolaou stain, × 1000), (From Heaston, D. K., et al.: Percutaneous thoracic needle biopsy. In Putman, C. E. (Ed.): Pulmonary Diagnosis: Imaging and Other Techniques. New York, Appleton-Century-Crofts, 1981.)

series of malignant intrathoracic neoplasms, the needle aspirate demonstrated malignant cells in 96 per cent.[39] False cytologic diagnoses were present in only two patients.

Scalene Node Biopsy. Whenever a palpable lymph node is present, particularly if it is firm or hard, it should be removed under local anesthesia for diagnosis. In one series of 101 consecutive patients with bronchogenic carcinoma thought to be appropriate candidates for pulmonary resection, positive scalene nodes were present in 9 per cent. Most of these were adenocarcinomas.[40]

Mediastinoscopy. A small incision in the suprasternal notch can be made with passage of the mediastinoscope under the sternum and anterior to the trachea. Lymph nodes in the mediastinum can be seen by this technique and biopsies can be obtained. However, the test can be hazardous and rare complications occur, such as serious bleeding, which may be difficult to control because of limited exposure. *Bone marrow* aspirates are quite helpful in providing cytologic confirmation of a radiographic abnormality.[10]

Differential Diagnosis

A number of pulmonary conditions simulate bronchogenic carcinoma—pneumonia, abscess, tuberculosis, histoplasmosis, coccidioidomyocosis, and blastomyocosis. Cultures for routine, anaerobic, acid-fast, and fungal organisms are helpful in excluding other diagnoses. Specific skin test sensitivities should be assessed as well as a radiologic search for metastatic lesions, especially appropriate examination of the liver, adrenals, bones, and brain.

EVIDENCE OF INOPERABILITY

The presence of metastases other than resectable hilar nodes usually indicates an incurable situation. Ominous signs include bloody pleural effusion, phrenic nerve paralysis, vocal cord paralysis, Horner's syndrome, and the superior vena caval syndrome. Obviously metastatic deposits, particularly when confirmed by needle aspiration biopsy, are important in making an absolute and objective diagnosis of inoperability.

THE ISOLATED LESION (COIN LESION)

Frequently, isolated pulmonary nodules present for differential diagnosis and deserve careful investigation because many are malignant neoplasms. In general, a younger individual is likely to have a *benign* lesion (Table 2). If a lesion is followed and does not increase in size, it is more likely to be benign. However, this is a risky course because it is well known that pulmonary lesions that remain static for many years are ultimately found to be carcinomas and often with mediastinal spread or distant metastases. The differential diagnosis of these solitary lesions includes a number of pulmonary granulomas such as tuberculomas, histoplasmomas, blastocytomas, coccidioidomas. Pulmonary metastases may also be present, and such is likely if the lesions are multiple. Certainly, when a metastatic lesion is suspected, a CT scan should be obtained for careful analysis of both lungs. The diagnosis should be confirmed by percutaneous needle biopsy and cytologic examination for selection of appropriate therapy.

TABLE 2. *Incidence of Malignancy in Solitary Pulmonary Nodules Related to Age**

Age	Malignant (%)
35–44	15
45–49	26
50–59	41
60–69	50
70–79	70
Over 80	Approaches 100%

*From Sabiston, D. C., Jr.: Carcinoma of the Lung. *In* Sabiston, D. C., Jr., and Spencer, F. C. (Eds.): Gibbon's Surgery of the Chest, 4th ed. Philadelphia. W. B. Saunders Company, 1983.

MANAGEMENT

Surgical Procedures

When there is no evidence of metastases or of invasion of structures within the thorax, *exploratory thoracotomy* is indicated. This is generally done through a posterolateral thoracotomy through the bed of the fifth or sixth rib. A double-lumen endotracheal tube (Carlens) is useful for collapsing the affected lung, allowing the operation to be conducted in a simpler and safer manner. Moreover, the primary lesion and metastases can be more easily felt in the collapsed than in the expanded lung. A careful search is made for the extent of neoplastic involvement of the lung, pleura, mediastinal nodes, pericardium, heart, and great vessels. Frequently, *local excision* is indicated, particularly when respiratory insufficiency is present preoperatively. An *automatic stapling device* has been useful in achieving hemostasis and preventing air leaks postoperatively. In most patients, *lobectomy* is the operation of choice for bronchogenic carcinoma. If more than one lobe is involved by the neoplasm, a pneumonectomy may be necessary.

The automatic stapling device has become quite popular and represents a distinct technical advance in pulmonary resection (Fig. 9). It permits a very secure bronchial closure with control of both the pulmonary arteries and veins during resection (Fig. 10). It is interesting that both

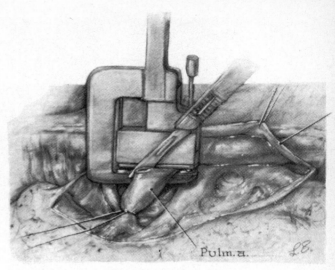

Figure 10. Following distal ligature and proximal stapling, the right pulmonary artery is divided. (From Sabiston, D. C., Jr.: Carcinoma of the lung. In Sabiston, D. C., Jr., and Spencer, F. C. (Eds.): Gibbon's Surgery of the Chest, 4th ed. Philadelphia, W. B. Saunders Company, 1983.)

clinical and experimental studies have demonstrated that bronchial healing is better with metal staples compared with hand-placed sutures.[41]

Radiation Therapy

Radiation therapy is frequently employed in patients with bronchogenic carcinoma. It has been quite useful in prolonging life and in reducing symptoms for those with metastatic lesions in whom pulmonary resection is considered inappropriate. The results of radiation therapy administered as the primary treatment are depicted in Table 3. Those patients with residual tumor lymph nodes or direct involvement of the mediastinal structures, including the great vessels, pericardium, and heart, should also be managed by radiation therapy.

The dosage of radiation recommended varies, but in general 5000 to 6000 rads are given five times weekly for 5 to 6 weeks (180 to 200 rads daily) as a reasonable course. Some radiotherapists prefer a split course of radiation in preference to continuous daily treatments. The split course has the advantage of accommodating a limited tolerance of the lungs for higher dosage of radiation. If this approach is selected, 3000 rads are administered over a 2-week period (300 rads per treatment); this is followed by a 2-week

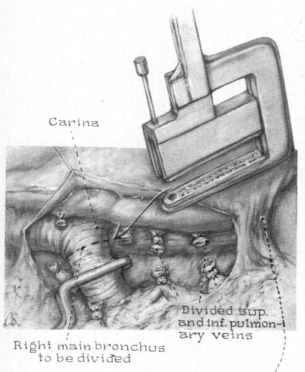

Figure 9. The right main bronchus is dissected and occluded distally. The stapler is placed at the origin of the right main bronchus, and the bronchus is closed. The bronchus is then divided and the specimen removed from the chest. (From Sabiston, D. C., Jr.: Carcinoma of the lung. In Sabiston, D. C., Jr., and Spencer, F. C. (Eds.): Gibbon's Surgery of the Chest, 4th ed. Philadelphia, W. B. Saunders Company, 1983, p. 485.)

TABLE 3. *Results of Radiation Therapy in the Primary Management of Carcinoma of the Lung**

Number of Patients	Radiation Dose	Survival		
		1 yr.	3 yrs.	5 yrs.
93 (Hocker and Guttman, 1944)	4000	22	5	
349 (Holsti, 1969)	5000	38	8	
150 (Guttmann, 1971)	5000–6000	40		2.5
419 (Schumacher, 1978)	5000–7000	62	14	6

*From Sabiston, D. C., Jr.: Carcinoma of the lung. In Sabiston, D. C., Jr., and Spencer, F. C. (Eds.): Gibbon's Surgery of the Chest, 4th ed. Philadelphia, W. B. Saunders Company, 1983.

period of rest, and an additional 2000 rads are given in the 1- to 2-week period.

In current practice, complications of radiation therapy are minimal and include radiation pneumonitis and esophagitis. Both are usually mild and frequently asymptomatic. If pneumonitis does become symptomatic, it is usually associated with fever, mild cough, and, occasionally, slight hemoptysis. Late pulmonary fibrosis may occur, and damage to the spinal cord can be prevented by reducing the amount of radiation over this area.

Chemotherapy

Chemotherapy has been evaluated in a number of studies in the management of metastatic bronchogenic carcinoma. There is general agreement that most patients with small cell carcinoma of the lung are candidates for chemotherapy because the results of surgical resection are dismal.[45] In small cell carcinoma the combination of chemotherapy and radiation improves the results. Cyclophosphamide is considered an effective agent, especially with the addition of vincristine and doxorubicin (Adriamycin).

A response rate has been reported as high as 75 per cent in patients with limited disease. However, with extensive metastatic disease, this response falls to about 40 per cent.[18] It is interesting that *complete* remission has occurred in as many as 41 per cent of patients without extensive disease whereas such a complete remission is achieved in only 14 per cent of those with extensive disease.[21]

Emphasis should be placed upon the fact that the small cell carcinoma of the lung (oat cell) is a diagnosis that is best made by a combination of light microscopy as well as electron microscopy (EM). It is quite possible that a primary bronchogenic carcinoma can be considered small cell in type by light microscopy whereas it may not be possible to confirm this diagnosis by EM in 25 to 40 per cent of patients.[16] Pathognomonic features in the EM section are the *dense core granules* (Fig. 11).

Immunotherapy

Some patients with bronchogenic carcinoma are immunoincompetent, as can be demonstrated by delayed cutaneous hypersensitivity skin testing.[45] Moreover, *in vitro*

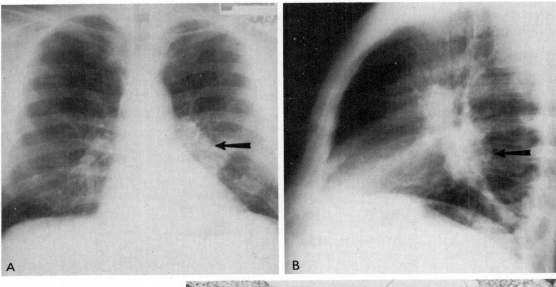

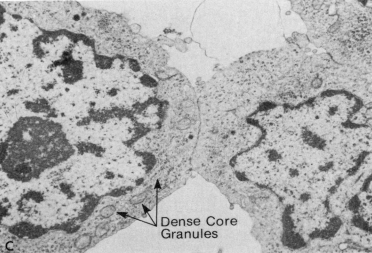

Figure 11. A and B, Posterolateral and lateral chest film of patient with small cell carcinoma of the left hilum (arrow). C, Electron photomicrograph of neoplasm seen in Fig. 11 A and B demonstrating the typical core granules. (From Sabiston, D. C., Jr. (Ed.): The Textbook of Surgery, 13th ed. Philadelphia, W. B. Saunders Company, 1986, p. 2070.)

Dense Core Granules

lymphocyte function also demonstrates this phenomenon.[2] Follow-up of patients with depressed cellular immunity shows a poor clinical prognosis. In patients sensitized to 2,4-dinitrochlorobenzene (DNCB), an antigen to which they have not been previously exposed, cancer patients with solid tumors react much less frequently (64 per cent) than do normal controls (95 per cent). Moreover, the sensitivity to DNCB is associated with a favorable prognosis, whereas in nonreactive patients the prognosis is generally poor.[30]

Immunotherapy has been used in patients with metastatic bronchogenic carcinoma by intrapleural administration of bacille Calmette-Guérin (BCG).[26] Whereas initial reports were favorable, indicating improvement for longterm survival, more recent studies are not confirmatory.[28] Therefore, the role of BCG remains controversial.

Bronchoplastic Procedures

In localized bronchogenic carcinoma, particularly in patients with reduced pulmonary function, it is occasionally appropriate to excise the bronchus involved with reanastomosis to preserve the pulmonary parenchymal tissue for continued function. This procedure is also useful for the resection of benign lesions (including bronchial carcinoids), which, although premalignant, are very frequently cured by bronchoplastic procedures.[22]

In 1932 Pancoast described the "superior sulcus tumor" and provided a description of clinical manifestations that have since become known as *Pancoast syndrome*.[33, 34] This includes the constant and characteristic clinical phenomenon of pain in the eighth cervical and first and second thoracic trunk distribution together with Horner's syndrome. The chest film shows a shadow in the extreme apex as well as frequent presence of rib destruction and often involvement of the vertebrae. This lesion frequently extends into the superior mediastinum. Paulson has studied this lesion extensively and believes that complete resection is

TABLE 4. *Nodal Involvement and Prognosis: Superior Pulmonary Sulcus Carcinomas (1956 to 1977)**

Stage of Involvement	No. of Patients	Survival	
		1 Yr.	3 Yr.
No nodes (T3 N0)	51	38	22
Intersegmental nodes (T3 N1)	1	1	1
Hilar or mediastinal nodes (T3 N1 or N2)	15	2	0
TOTAL	67	41	23

*From Paulson, D. L.: Superior sulcus carcinoma. In Sabiston, D. C., Jr., and Spencer, F. C. (Eds.): Gibbon's Surgery of the Chest, 4th ed. Philadelphia, W. B. Saunders Company, 1983.

at times impossible unless preoperative radiation therapy has been administered. Moreover, it is believed that use of radiation before operation provides improved long-term results (Fig. 12 and Table 4).

Results

The natural history of bronchogenic carcinoma emphasizes its exceedingly poor prognosis. For example, in a series of more than 3800 patients those who were *untreated* had a 1-year mortality of 95 per cent![31] Cell type may have a role in predicting response to therapy, but it is quite variable. Small cell carcinoma (oat cell) was formerly associated with a very poor prognosis, but today chemotherapy has changed the survival time. If a curative resection can be achieved at operation, 5- and 10-year survival rates of 36 and 14 per cent, respectively, have been reported in the recent past.[20] However, among patients *without* nodal metastases, the 5-year survival is 49 per cent and 31 per cent if *only* the hilar nodes are positive. The best prognosis is found in patients with *solitary, peripheral lesions* less than 4 cm. in diameter who have a 45 per cent 5-year survival following resection.[17]

Surgical Management of Pulmonary Metastatic Lesions

Blood-borne pulmonary metastases are quite common and may be isolated (solitary) lesions. For example, malig-

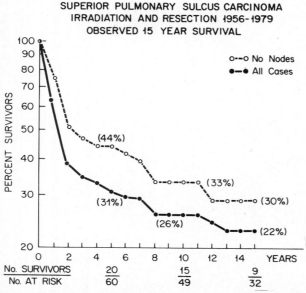

Figure 12. Observed 5-, 10-, 15-year actuarial survival curves of 70 patients after combined treatment from 1956 to 1979 in patients with no lymph nodes involved and all cases including those with nodal involvement. (From Paulson, D. L.: Superior sulcus carcinomas. In Sabiston, D. C., Jr., and Spencer, F. C. (Eds.): Gibbon's Textbook of Surgery, 4th ed. Philadelphia, W. B. Saunders Company, 1983, p. 510.)

TABLE 5. *Frequency of Metastases from Carcinomas to the Lung**

Site of Primary Tumor	No. of Cases	Percentage of Metastases of Lung (%)
Colon/rectum	274	23.4
Kidney	193	16.5
Breast	164	14.0
Testis	142	12.1
Uterus	136	11.6
Head and neck	81	6.9
Melanoma	78	6.7
Bladder	29	2.5
Ovary	13	1.0
Miscellaneous	62	5.3
TOTAL	1172	

*Data collected from Wilkins et al. (1978): Morrow et al. (1980); Brandt and Ehrenhaft (1980); McCormack and Martini (1979); Mountain et al. (1978); and Takita et al. (1981). (From Mark, J. B. D.: In Sabiston, D. C., Jr., and Spencer, F. C. (Eds.): Gibbon's Surgery of the Chest, 4th ed. Philadelphia, W. B. Saunders Company, 1983.)

TABLE 6. *Frequency of Metastases from Sarcomas to the Lung**

Type of Sarcoma	No. of Cases	Percentage of Metastases to Lung (%)
Osteogenic sarcoma	185	37.3
Fibrosarcoma	67	13.5
Synovial sarcoma	63	12.7
Others	181	36.5
TOTAL	496	

*Data collected from Wilkins et al. (1978); Morrow et al. (1980); Brandt and Ehrenhaft (1980); McCormack and Martini (1979); Mountain et al. (1978); and Takita et al. (1981). (From Mark, J. B. D. *In* Sabiston, D. C., Jr., and Spencer, F. C. (Eds.): Gibbon's Surgery of the Chest, 4th ed. Philadelphia, W. B. Saunders Company, 1983.)

nant lesions, such as choriocarcinoma, carcinoma of the kidney, and osteosarcoma of bone, metastasize in approximately 75 per cent. Multiple metastases are also common with primary neoplasms in the thyroid and breast and with melanoma. Single metastatic lesions from the colon and stomach are also relatively common. Endobronchial metastases are rare, but when present they are more likely to be from the kidney or colon.[1] If the lesion is an *isolated* pulmonary metastasis from a primary neoplasm, surgical resection is generally indicated.

In a large series, 663 resections for pulmonary metastases were performed in 448 patients.[24] There were 246 patients with metastatic carcinoma and 202 with metastatic sarcoma. The majority (70 per cent) were managed by wedge pulmonary resection, and the operative mortality was only 1 per cent. This allowed increased effectiveness of chemotherapy for patients with metastatic osteogenic sarcoma and carcinoma of the breast or testes. In children with metastases from osteogenic sarcoma, the prognosis was better when pulmonary resection was accompanied by chemotherapy and irradiation.[9, 44] The frequency of metastases from carcinomas to the lung and various organs in the body is depicted in Table 5. Similarly, the frequency of metastases from sarcomas in the various organs throughout the body to the lung is depicted in Table 6.

Role of Staging Procedures

Several studies have indicated the significance of American Joint Committee system of staging and its role in predicting long-term survival. In other words, occult carcinoma has the most favorable prognosis, followed in order by Stage I invasive carcinoma, without metastases or metastases limited to the ipsilateral hilar region only, which has the next best prognosis. This is followed by Stages II, III, and IV in which there are extensive metastatic lesions (Table 7).

Laser Therapy

Recently, the yttrium-aluminum-garnet (YAG) laser and, to a lesser extent, the carbon dioxide laser have been effectively used in the treatment of malignant lesions of the trachea and bronchi.[25] Essentially, the laser beam causes the tumor to vaporize on contact. The YAG laser is quite effective in nonresectable intrabronchial neoplasms, particularly when there is serious hemorrhage or obstruction of the bronchus causing distal infection.[46]

BENIGN PULMONARY AND BRONCHIAL NEOPLASMS

There are a large number of benign lesions of the lung and tracheobronchial tree, most of which are detectable on appropriate chest films. It has been estimated that these lesions account for as many as 15 per cent of all neoplasms of the lungs and bronchi.[5, 42]

Clinical Manifestations

The majority of benign neoplasms of the lung and bronchi are located peripherally and may be asymptomatic. Those within the tracheobronchial tree are likely to produce symptoms of bronchial obstruction and secondary pneumonitis. Bronchoscopy is quite helpful in demonstrating these tumors and provides an opportunity to obtain a biopsy for histologic diagnosis. For peripheral lesions, brush or irrigation techniques are quite useful.

Types of Benign Neoplasms

There are a wide variety of benign *neoplasms* that occur in the lung and bronchi. The classification cited by

TABLE 7. *Stage Grouping in Carcinoma of the Lung**

Occult Carcinoma	
TXN0M0	An occult carcinoma with bronchopulmonary secretions containing malignant cells but without other evidence of the primary tumor or evidence of metastasis to the regional lymph nodes or distant metastasis
Invasive Carcinoma	
Stage I	
T1N0M0	A tumor that can be classified T1 without any metastasis or with metastasis to the
T1N1M0	lymph nodes in the ipsilateral hilar region only, or a tumor that can be classified
T2N0M0	T2 without any metastasis to nodes or distant metastasis
Stage II	
T2N1M0	A tumor classified as T2 with metastasis to the lymph nodes in the ipsilateral hilar region only
Stage III	
T3 with any N or M	Any tumor more extensive than T2, or any tumor with metastasis to the lymph
N2 with any T or M	nodes in the mediastinum or with distant metastasis
M1 with any T or N	

*Reprinted by permission of the American Joint Committee for Cancer Staging and End Results Reporting, Chicago

Greenfield (Table 8) is quite useful and includes the vast majority of those found clinically.

Tracheal Tumors. Endotracheal benign lesions are uncommon but are approximately the same in number as are malignant lesions of the trachea. In children, malignant tracheal lesions are quite rare. Specific types of neoplasms include papilloma, fibroma, and hemangioma, and the latter are particularly likely to occur in children. Benign lesions may be locally excised or treated by the YAG laser; surgical resection and reanastomosis are required for malignant lesions.[8]

Bronchial Tumors. Benign bronchial tumors are often symptomatic with cough, dyspnea, and hemoptysis as a result of the obstruction they produce. Bronchial adenomas are generally classified into three types: *carcinoid* (70 per cent), *cylindroma* (adenoid cystic adenoma or carcinoma), and *mucoid epidermoid*. The most frequent of these, the carcinoid, originates from the neural crest. They are interesting tumors because in addition to local effects they may also function as endocrine lesions with ectopic hormone production. Bioactive hormones and hormone-like products of carcinoids and small cell carcinoma are shown in Table 9. Bronchial adenomas should be resected by lobectomy or by a bronchoplastic procedure.

Polyps. Polyps of the bronchi also occur as peduncu-

TABLE 8. Benign Tumors of the Lung and Tracheobronchial Tree*

Epithelial Tumors
1. Papilloma
2. Polyps

Mesodermal Tumors
1. Vascular
   a. Angiomas
      1. Hemangioma
      2. Lymphangioma
      3. Hemangioendothelioma
   b. Lymphangiomyomatosis
2. Bronchial tumors
   a. Fibroma
   b. Chondroma, osteochondroma
   c. Lipoma
   d. Granular cell myoblastoma
   e. Leiomyoma
   f. Neurogenic tumors

Developmental or Unknown Origin Tumors
1. Hamartoma
   a. Chondromatous hamartoma
   b. Adenomatous malformation (diffuse hamartoma)
2. Teratoma
3. Chemodectoma
4. Clear cell ("sugar") tumor
5. Thymoma

Inflammatory and Other Pseudotumors
1. Plasma cell granuloma (histiocytoma)
2. Pseudolymphoma
3. Xanthoma
4. Amyloid
5. Tracheobronchopathic osteoplastica

Polypoid Lesions (Bronchial Adenomas)
1. Carcinoid
2. Salivary gland types
   a. Cylindroma
   b. Mixed tumors (pleomorphic)

*From Greenfield, L. J.: Benign tumors of the lung and bronchi. *In* Sabiston, D. C., Jr., and Spencer, F. C. (Eds.): Gibbon's Surgery of the Chest, 4th ed. Philadelphia, W. B. Saunders Company, 1983.

TABLE 9. Bioactive Hormones or "Hormone-like" Products of Carcinoids and Small Cell Carcinoma*

Carcinoid	Small Cell Carcinoma
β-Endorphin	Neurophysin
β-Lipotropin (MSH)	β-Lipotropin
Pro-γ melanotropin-like	
5-Hydroxytryptophan	
5-Hydroxytryptamine	
5-Indoleacetic acid	
Serotonin-like (common)	Serotonin (rare)
Dopamine	
Neuron-specific enolase	
ACTH and big-17-oxyhydroxycorticosterone	Big-ACTH
Corticotropin RF	
Parathormone	Parathormone, usually in other cell types
Calcitonin	Calcitonin
Insulin	Insulin (??)
Glucagon	Glucagon
Vasointestinal peptides	Vasointestinal peptides (rare, gastrin)
Somatostatin RF	
Gonadotropin RF	
Prolactin	Prolactin-like
Oxytocin	Oxytocin (??)
HCT-like	
Chorionic gonadotropin	Human chorionic gonadotropin-usually in other cell types
Growth hormone ?? (RF)	Growth hormone (?)—other cell types placental lactogen
ADH-like	ADH (vasopressin)

*From Pate, J. W.: Bronchial adenoma. *In* Sabiston, D. C., Jr. (Ed.): The Textbook of Surgery, 13th ed. Philadelphia, W. B. Saunders Company, 1986, p. 2055.

Abbreviations: RF = Releasing factor; MSH = melanocyte-stimulating hormone; ACTH = adrenocorticotrophic hormone; ADH = antidiuretic hormone; HCT = human chorionic placental thyrotropin.

lated masses of mucosa. Children are prone to papillomatosis of the larynx, which often involves the trachea and bronchi. These neoplasms are covered with epithelium, which may be either squamous or ciliated. Removal is necessary to maintain an open airway.

Chondroma (Hamartoma). A common pulmonary neoplasm, chondroma usually appears as an asymptomatic coin lesion on the chest film. This lesion may cause bronchial obstruction but is generally associated with few clinical symptoms. Chondromas that occur in the pulmonary parenchyma are best removed by local ("wedge") excision. The automatic stapler is very efficiently used in this type of resection with excellent results.

Other Lesions. Other benign lesions include hemangiomas, lymphangiomas, arteriovenous fistulas, sclerosing hemangiomas, lipomas, fibromas, and osteochondromas. In addition, neurogenic tumors, leiomyoma, and granular cell tumors also occur. Tumors of developmental origin, including some of unknown origin, include the pulmonary blastoma, teratoma, chemodectoma, and lymphoma. In general, local resection is appropriate for these lesions.[36]

SELECTED REFERENCES

Bates, M. (Ed.): Bronchial Carcinoma: An Integrated Approach to Diagnosis and Management. New York, Springer-Verlag, 1984.
   This monograph thoroughly reviews all aspects of bronchogenic carci-

noma, providing detailed updates in the field. The illustrations are outstanding, and the text is easily readable.

Grillo, H. C.: Complications of tracheal reconstruction: Incidence, treatment, and prevention. J. Thorac. Cardiovasc. Surg., 91:322, 1986.
The author reports the largest series of tracheal tumors and reconstruction for post-intubation injury. The results reported are excellent, and the author is an internationally recognized figure in this field. This is a key reference on this subject.

Iglehart, J. D., Wolfe, W. G., Vernon, W. B., Vollmer, R. T., Shelburne, J. D., and Sabiston, D. C., Jr.: Electron microscopy in selection of patients with small cell carcinoma of the lung for medical versus surgical therapy. J. Thorac. Cardiovasc. Surg., 90:351, 1985.
In this review of a series of patients with bronchogenic carcinoma, the lesion was examined both by light and electron microscopy. The latter technique proved to be superior in establishing an objective diagnosis. Emphasis is placed on identification of the dense core granules seen on electron microscopy as being definitive for the diagnosis for small cell ("oat cell") carcinoma of the lung.

Katsuki, H., Shimada, K., Koyama, A., Okita, M., Yamaguchi, Y., and Okamoto, T.: Long-term intermittent adjuvant chemotherapy for primary, resected lung cancer. J. Thorac. Cardiovasc. Surg., 70:590, 1975.
The authors used two chemotherapeutic agents to suppress local and distant recurrences in patients following resection for carcinoma of the lung. Radiotherapy was given postoperatively to patients with known residual disease. A course of long-term, intermittent chemotherapy with mitomycin C and chromomycin A was administered. The results were encouraging and appeared to show a difference between the treated and the untreated groups. However, caution should be taken in interpretation of these results, since it was not a randomized study.

Kirsch, M. M., Dickerman, R., Fayos, J., Lampe, I., Pellegrini, R. V., Gago, O., and Sloan, H.: The value of chest wall resection in the treatment of superior sulcus tumors of the lung. Ann. Thorac. Surg., 15:339, 1973.
These authors differ with Paulson and associates regarding the value of preoperative irradiation followed by extensive surgery in the management of superior sulcus tumors. The conclusions drawn from their data provide the reader with a different point of view.

Macumber, H. H., and Calvin, J. W.: Perfusion lung scan patterns in 100 patients with bronchogenic carcinoma. J. Thorac. Cardiovasc. Surg., 72:299, 1976.
The relationship between size of the perfusion defect as seen by perfusion lung scan and size of the mass as seen in the chest film was correlated with the presence of regional lymph node involvement with tumor in 100 consecutive patients with bronchogenic carcinoma. All patients underwent scanning before open thoracotomy or mediastinotomy, and each had histologic documentation of the disease. The perfusion lung scans were classified into those with (1) perfusion defect larger than the mass lesion, (2) perfusion defect of the same size as the mass lesion, or (3) no focal defect seen. Among patients with a larger perfusion defect, 84 per cent had regional lymph node involvement, whereas among patients in whom a larger defect was not present only 23 per cent had such extension.

Paulson, D. L., and Urschel, H. C., Jr.: Superior sulcus carcinomas. In Sabiston, D. C., Jr., and Spencer, F. C. (Eds.): Gibbon's Surgery of the Chest, 4th ed. Philadelphia, W. B. Saunders Company, 1983.
These authors are advocates for use of preoperative irradiation followed by radical surgery in the treatment of superior sulcus tumors. Their results are excellent but differ from those reported by Kirsh and associates.

REFERENCES

1. Braman, S. S., and Whitcomb, M. E.: Endobronchial metastasis. Arch. Intern. Med., 135:543, 1975.
2. Brugarolas, A., Han, T., Takita, H., and Minowada, J.: Immunologic assays in lung cancer. N.Y. State J. Med., 1:747, 1973.
3. Cohen, S., and Hossain, S-A.: Primary carcinoma of the lung: A review of histologically proved cases. In Fraser, R. G., and Pare, J. A. P. (Eds.): Diagnosis of Diseases of the Chest: An Integrated Study Based on the Abnormal Roentgenogram. Philadelphia, W. B. Saunders Company, 1970.
4. Cortese, D. A., Pairolero, P. C., Bergstralh, E. J., Woolner, L. B., Uhlenhopp, M. A., Piehler, J. M., Sanderson, D. R., Bernatz, P. E., Williams, D. E., Taylor, W. F., Payne, W. S., and Fontana, R. S.: Roentgenographically occult lung cancer: A ten-year experience. J. Thorac. Cardiovasc. Surg., 86:373, 1983.
5. Davis, E. W., Peabody, J. W. H., and Katz, S.: The solitary pulmonary nodule: A ten-year study based on 215 cases. J. Thorac. Cardiovasc. Surg., 32:728, 1956.
6. Friedrich, G.: Periphere Lungenkrebse auf dem Boden pleuranaher Narben. Virchows Arch. Pathol. Anat., 304:230, 1939.
7. Gamsu, G.: Magnetic resonance imaging in lung cancer. Chest, 89:242s, 1986.
8. Grillo, H. C., Zannini, P., and Michelassi, F.: Complications of tracheal reconstruction: Incidence, treatment, and prevention. J. Thorac. Cardiovasc. Surg., 91:322, 1986.
9. Giritsky, A. S., Etcubanas, E., and Mark, J. B. D.: Pulmonary resection in children with metastatic osteogenic sarcoma: Improved survival with surgery, chemotherapy, and irradiation. J. Thorac. Cardiovasc. Surg., 75:354, 1978.
10. Gutierrez, A. C., Vincent, R. G., Sandberg, A. A., Takita, H., and Stanley, K.: Evaluation of sternal bone marrow aspiration for detection of tumor cells in patients with bronchogenic carcinoma. J. Thorac. Cardiovasc. Surg., 77:392, 1979.
11. Hammond, E. C.: Evidence on the effects of giving up cigarette smoking. Am. J. Public Health, 55:682, 1965.
12. Hammond, E. C., Auerbach, O., Kirman, D., and Garfinkel, L.: Effects of cigarette smoking on dogs. Ca., 21:78, 1971.
13. Hammond, E. C., and Selikoff, I. J.: Relation of cigarette smoking to risk of death of asbestos-associated disease among insulation workers in the United States. In Bogovski, P., Gilson, J. C., Timbrell, V., and Wagner, J. C. (Eds.): Biological Effects of Asbestos. Lyon, France, International Agency for Research on Cancer, 1973.
14. Hansen, M., and Pederson, A. G.: Tumor markers in patients with lung cancer. Chest, 89:219s, 1986.
15. Hyde, L., and Hyde, C. I.: Clinical manifestations of lung cancer. Chest, 65:299, 1974.
16. Iglehart, J. D., Wolfe, W. G., Vernon, W. B., Vollmer, R. T., Shelburne, J. D., and Sabiston, D. C., Jr.: Electron microscopy in selection of patients with small cell carcinoma of the lung for medical versus surgical therapy. J. Thorac. Cardiovasc. Surg., 90:351, 1985.
17. Jackman, R. J., Good, C. A., Clagett, O. T., and Woolner, L. B.: Survival rates in peripheral bronchogenic carcinomas up to four centimeters in diameter presenting as solitary pulmonary nodules. J. Thorac. Cardiovasc. Surg., 57:1, 1969.
18. Johnson, R. E., Brereton, H. D., and Kent, C. H.: "Total" therapy for small cell carcinoma of the lung. Ann. Thorac. Surg., 25:510, 1978.
19. Kabat, G. C., and Wynder, E. L.: Lung cancer in nonsmokers. Cancer, 53:1214, 1984.
20. Kirsh, M. M., Rotman, H., Argenta, L., Bove, E., Cimmino, V., Tashian, J., Ferguson, P., and Sloan, H.: Carcinoma of the lung: Results of treatment over ten years. Ann. Thorac. Surg., 21:371, 1976.
21. Livingston, R. B., Moore, T. N., Heilbrun, L., Bottomley, R., Lehane, D., Rivkin, S. E., and Thigpen, T.: Small cell carcinoma of the lung: Combined chemotherapy and radiation. A Southwest Oncology Group study. Ann. Intern. Med., 88:194, 1978.
22. Lowe, J. E., Bridgman, A. H., and Sabiston, D. C., Jr.: The role of benign and malignant pulmonary lesions. J. Thorac. Cardiovasc. Surg., 83:227, 1982.
23. Macumber, H. H., and Calvin, J. W.: Perfusion lung scan patterns in 100 patients with bronchogenic carcinoma. J. Thorac. Cardiovasc. Surg., 72:299, 1976.
24. McCormack, P. M., and Martini, N.: The changing role of surgery for pulmonary metastases. Ann. Thorac. Surg., 28:139, 1979.
25. McElvein, R. B., and Zorn, G.: Treatment of malignant disease in trachea and main-stem bronchi by carbon dioxide laser. J. Thorac. Cardiovasc. Surg., 86:858, 1983.
26. McKneally, M. F., Maver, C., Kausel, H. W., and Alley, R. D.: Regional immunotherapy with intrapleural BCG for lung cancer. J. Thorac. Cardiovasc. Surg., 72:333, 1976.
27. McNamara, J. J., Kinglsey, W. B., Paulson, D. L., Arndt, J. H., Salinas-Izaquirre, S. F., and Urschel, H. C., Jr.: Alveolar cell (bronchiolar) carcinoma of the lung. J. Thorac. Cardiovasc. Surg., 57:648, 1969.
28. Mountain, C. F., and Gail, M. H.: Surgical adjuvant intrapleural BCG treatment for Stage I non-small cell lung cancer: Preliminary report of the National Cancer Institute Lung Cancer Study Group. J. Thorac. Cardiovasc. Surg., 82:649, 1981.
29. Munnell, E. R., Dilling, E., Grantham, R. N., Harkey, M. R., and Mohr, J. A.: Reappraisal of solitary bronchiolar (alveolar cell) carcinoma of the lung. Ann. Thorac. Surg., 25:289, 1978.
30. Olkowski, Z. L., McLaren, J. R., and Mansour, K. A.: Immunocompetence of patients with bronchogenic carcinoma. Ann. Thorac. Surg., 21:546, 1976.
31. Omenn, G. S., and Wilkins, E. W., Jr.: Hormone syndromes associated with bronchogenic carcinoma: Clues to histologic type. J. Thorac. Cardiovasc. Surg., 59:877, 1970.
32. Overholt, R. H., Neptune, W. B., and Ashraf, M. M.: Primary cancer of the lung: A 42-year experience. Ann. Thorac. Surg., 20:511, 1975.
33. Paulson, D. L.: Carcinomas in the superior pulmonary sulcus. J. Thorac. Cardiovasc. Surg., 70:1095, 1975.

34. Paulson, D. L., and Urschel, H. C., Jr.: Superior sulcus carcinomas. *In* Sabiston, D. C., Jr., and Spencer, F. C. (Eds.): Gibbon's Surgery of the Chest, 3rd ed. Philadelphia, W. B. Saunders Company, 1976.

35. Pederson, A. G., Becker, K., Marangos, P., et al.: Bombesin (BM), creatine kinase BB (CK-BB), calcitonin (C), and neuron-specific enolase (NSE) in the cerebrospinal fluid (CSF) as a marker of CNS metastases and meningeal carcinomatosis (MC) in small cell lung cancer (SCLC). Am. Assoc. Cancer Res., 26:146, 1985.

36. Perloff, M., Killen, J. Y., and Wittes, R. E.: Small cell bronchogenic carcinoma. Curr. Probl. Cancer, 4:173, 1986.

37. Razzuk, M. A., Pockey, M., Urschel, H. C., Jr., and Paulson, D. L.: Dual primary bronchogenic carcinoma. Ann. Thorac. Surg., 17:425, 1974.

38. Ripstein, C. G., Spain, D. M., and Bluth, I.: Scar cancer of the lung. J. Thorac. Cardiovasc. Surg., 56:362, 1968.

39. Sagel, S. S., Ferguson, T. B., Forrest, J. V., Roper, C. L., Weldon, C. S., and Clark, R. E.: Percutaneous transthoracic aspiration needle biopsy. Ann. Thorac. Surg., 26:399, 1978.

40. Schatzlein, M. H., McAuliffe, S., Orringer, M. B., and Kirsh, M. M.: Scalene node biopsy in pulmonary carcinoma: When is it indicated? Ann. Thorac. Surg., 31:322, 1981.

41. Scott, R. N., Faraci, R. P., Hough, A., and Chretien, P. B.: Bronchial stump closure techniques following pneumonectomy: A serial comparative study. Ann. Surg., 184:205, 1976.

42. Steele, J. D.: The solitary pulmonary nodule: Report of a cooperative study of resected asymptomatic solitary pulmonary nodules in males. J. Thorac. Cardiovasc. Surg., 46:21, 1963.

43. Tayler, R., and Piper, D. W.: The carcinogenic effect of cigarette smoke: The effect of cigarette smoke on human gastric mucosal cells in organ culture. Cancer, 39:2520, 1977.

44. Telander, R. L., Pairolero, P. C., Pritchard, D. J., Sim, F. H., and Gilchrist, G. S.: Resection of pulmonary metastatic osteogenic sarcoma in children. Surgery, 84:335, 1978.

45. Wells, S. A., Burdick, J. F., Joseph, W. L., Christiansen, C. L., Wolfe, W. G., and Adkins, P. C.: Delayed cutaneous hypersensitivity reactions to tumor cell antigens and to nonspecific antigens: Prognostic significance in patients with lung cancer. J. Thorac. Cardiovasc. Surg., 66:557, 1973.

46. Wolfe, W. G., Cole, P. H., and Sabiston, D. C., Jr.: Experimental and clinical use of the YAG laser in the management of pulmonary neoplasms. Ann. Surg., 199:526, 1984.

VIII

Thoracic Outlet Syndrome

WILLIAM L. HOLMAN, M.D.
DAVID C. SABISTON, JR., M.D.

The thoracic outlet syndrome consists of a group of symptoms produced by the abnormal compression of neural and vascular structures as they enter the cervicoaxillary canal passing to the upper extremity. This syndrome has also been known as the cervical rib syndrome, costoclavicular syndrome, scalenus anticus syndrome, shoulder-girdle syndrome, and cervical brachial compression syndrome. The site of neurovascular compression in thoracic outlet syndrome is at the first rib, and treatment consists either of exercise to strengthen the shoulder girdle and improve posture or of surgical removal of the first rib. Controversy remains concerning the methods for the objective diagnosis of this syndrome and the optimal approach in management.

HISTORIC ASPECTS

Pathologic compression of the neurovascular bundle at the thoracic outlet was initially recognized in association with anomalous cervical ribs,[24] and this finding led to the first successful excision of a cervical rib by Coote in 1861.[5] As reviewed by Keen[10] in 1907, the excision of a cervical rib for thoracic outlet syndrome remained an infrequently performed procedure for nearly 50 years until neurovascular compression across the anatomically normal first rib was recognized and successfully treated by first rib resection.[22] Attention was subsequently drawn to the role of the scalenus anticus muscle in compressing the neurovascular bundle against the first rib, and in 1927 the treatment of thoracic outlet syndrome by division or resection of the anterior scalenus muscle was described.[2, 14, 15] Eventually,

the work of Clagett[4] re-emphasized the primary role of the first rib in thoracic outlet syndrome, and resection of the first rib through a posterior approach became the recommended treatment. In 1966, Roos[20] described the *transaxillary approach* to the first rib. This is now the most commonly employed surgical method of first rib resection.

ANATOMY

The anatomy of the thoracic outlet is displayed in Figure 1. The cervicoaxillary canal is an anatomic designation for the structures that surround the neurovascular bundle as it passes from the thoracic cavity to the upper extremity. Neurovascular compression causing thoracic outlet syndrome occurs most frequently in the proximal cervicoaxillary canal. This proximal portion of the canal consists of the clavicle, first rib, costoclavicular ligament, and the scalenus medius muscle. The scalenus anticus descends within this anatomic region to attach to the first rib and separate the brachial plexus and subclavian artery posteriorly from the subclavian vein anteriorly. Compression of the neurovascular bundle in this limited space can produce a clinical syndrome and can be associated with considerable discomfort. Congenital anomalies causing compression include cervical ribs, enlarged transverse process of the C7 vertebral body, fibrous bands uniting the cervical spine and the ribs, bifid clavicle, and scoliosis or kyphosis of the upper thoracic and lower cervical spine.[6, 17, 18] Poor posture and occupations in which prolonged abduction of the arms is required are common causes of acquired narrowing of

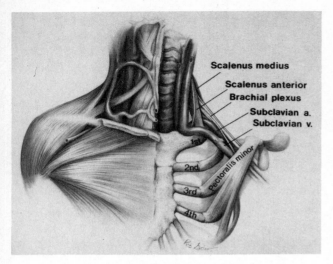

Figure 1. Anatomy of the thoracic outlet.

the proximal cervicoaxillary canal, although whiplash injuries, chest wall trauma, and cervical spondylosis can also produce neurovascular compression.[6] The distal portion of the canal is the axilla; in this region the tendon of the pectoralis minor produces narrowing of the canal, but actual pathologic compression of the neurovascular bundle is very rare.

If the anatomy of the proximal cervicoaxillary canal is approached with a consideration of the multiple factors that can cause pathologic neurovascular compression typical of thoracic outlet syndrome, the central role of the first rib as a primary anatomic structure becomes obvious. Removal of the first rib enlarges the floor of the proximal cervicoaxillary canal and, together with division of the insertion of the scalenus medius and anticus muscles, eliminates the compressive forces on the neural and vascular structures.[6, 11, 17]

SIGNS AND SYMPTOMS

The thoracic outlet syndrome occurs in both sexes and all age groups. The signs and symptoms are the result of varying degrees of compression of the brachial plexus, subclavian artery, and subclavian vein. In approximately 90 per cent of patients with thoracic outlet syndrome, neurologic symptoms are predominant and most frequently consist of pain and paresthesia in an ulnar distribution over the arm and hand. Motor weakness with atrophy of the hypothenar eminence may also be present, but this is rare.[4, 6, 14] The neurologic symptoms are often transient and temporally related to working or sleeping with the arms abducted and the neck extended. Objective physical signs of neural pathology, therefore, may be difficult to elicit upon examination.

Subclavian artery compression occurs in 10 per cent and may lead to coolness, weakness, fatigue, and ischemic pain in the upper extremity. Poststenotic dilation and even aneurysmal formation, Raynaud's phenomenon, and thrombosis can also follow prolonged compression of the artery. Venous compression can cause edema, cyanosis, and swelling in the upper extremity, and thrombosis of the vein can cause an exacerbation of these symptoms until collateral venous drainage develops.

The signs and symptoms of thoracic outlet syndrome are very similar to syndromes produced by other conditions, including cervical disc rupture, cervical spondylosis, bursitis, arthritis, superior pulmonary sulcus (Pancoast's) tumor, and carpal tunnel syndrome. The transient nature of the neurologic signs and the wide range of differential diagnoses emphasize the need for a painstaking history and physical examination before a diagnosis of thoracic outlet syndrome is made.

DIAGNOSIS

A variety of maneuvers have been advocated for detection and diagnosis of the thoracic outlet syndrome. These include the *Adson*[1] *maneuver*, in which pain follows holding a deep breath while extending the neck and rotating the head toward the affected side; the *costoclavicular maneuver*,[7] in which the shoulders are drawn backward and downward, producing discomfort; and the *hyperabduction test*,[25] in which the arm is hyperabducted to 180 degrees. Reproduction of symptoms and obliteration of the radial pulse by these maneuvers are suggestive of thoracic outlet syndrome; however, many asymptomatic individuals may show positive test results.[11, 12, 21] Tenderness produced by pressure over the supraclavicular fossa and reproduction of symptoms by elevation of the arms for 3 minutes have also been used to diagnose thoracic outlet syndrome.[15] Most recently, neural pathology produced by presumed thoracic outlet syndrome has been evaluated by nerve conduction studies.[3, 23]

Nerve conduction velocities are obtained over proximal and distal segments of the ulnar nerve and are determined by the recording of action potentials generated in the hypothenar or first dorsal interosseous muscles following proximal stimulation. Stimulation should be applied in the supraclavicular fossa (Erb's point), in the mid-upper arm, below the elbow and at the wrist.[23] Diminution of velocity in a given segment or increased delay at the wrist is indicative of some pathologic processes, such as compression, neuropathy, and traumatic injury or other neurologic disorders. Decreased velocity across the outlet is consistent with the thoracic outlet syndrome. The matter of accuracy and usefulness of such studies has been controversial, although they are often used.[9, 11, 12, 21] Arteriography of the subclavian vessels is not often used, except when specific pathology (e.g., post-stenotic dilatation or thrombosis) is suspected.[11, 21]

MANAGEMENT

When thoracic outlet syndrome is suspected by history and physical examination, initial treatment usually consists of physical therapy. Such programs are designed to improve posture and strengthen the shoulder girdle, thereby opening the proximal cervicoaxillary canal. Various studies have shown that 2 to 8 weeks of physical therapy is successful in 50 to 90 per cent of patients.[11, 12, 16] If physical therapy fails, further assessment to confirm the diagnosis may be performed, and if it seems indicated, surgical therapy by resection of the first rib can be discussed with the patient.

Resection of the first rib can be performed via the axillary approach[20] or the posterior approach,[4] although supraclavicular and subclavicular approaches have also been described.[8, 13] Resection of the scalenus anticus muscle is still advocated for certain groups of patients with thoracic outlet syndrome[19] but is only rarely performed today. Complications following rib resection are low (3 to 5 per cent) but include pneumothorax, wound hematoma, transient injury to the brachial plexus and long thoracic nerve, and injury to the axillary or subclavian vessels. Among properly selected patients with thoracic outlet syndrome, a good to excellent result will be obtained in 90 to 95 per cent following operation.[4, 6, 11, 12]

SELECTED REFERENCES

Clagett, O. T.: Research and prosearch. J. Thorac. Cardiovasc. Surg., *44*:153, 1962.
  The clinical features of thoracic outlet syndrome and the posterior approach for first rib resection are described. An interesting discourse on the historic development of this procedure is also included.

Kelly, T. R.: Thoracic outlet syndrome: Current concepts of treatment. Ann. Surg., *190*:657, 1979.
  The author presents his personal experience with 304 patients who underwent surgery for thoracic outlet syndrome. The pathophysiology of the syndrome and a flow diagram for the management of patients with thoracic outlet syndrome are described in the text together with data on diagnostic methods and surgical results.

McGough, E. C., Pearce, M. B., and Byrne, J. P.: Management of thoracic outlet syndrome. J. Thorac. Cardiovasc. Surg., *77*:169, 1979.
  In this paper, the authors define the signs and symptoms of thoracic outlet syndrome seen in their group of 1200 patients and data on the results of nonoperative and surgical therapy in this group are presented.

Roos, D. B.: Transaxillary approach for first rib resection to relieve thoracic outlet syndrome. Ann. Surg., *163*:354, 1966.
  The author describes the transaxillary approach for resection of the first rib, which is now the most commonly employed surgical therapy for the treatment of thoracic outlet syndrome.

REFERENCES

1. Adson, A. W.: Surgical treatment for symptoms produced by cervical ribs and the scalenus anticus muscle. Surg. Gynecol. Obstet., *85*:687, 1947.
2. Adson, A. W., and Coffey, J. R.: Cervical ribs: A method of anterior approach for relief of symptoms by division of the scalenus anticus. Ann. Surg., *85*:839, 1927.
3. Caldwell, J. W., Crane, C. R., and Krusen, E. M.: Nerve conduction studies: An aid in the diagnosis of thoracic outlet syndrome. South. Med. J., *64*:210, 1971.
4. Clagett, O. T.: Research and prosearch. J. Thorac. Cardiovasc. Surg., *44*:153, 1962.
5. Coote, H.: Exostosis of the left transverse process of the seventh cervical vertebra, surrounded by blood vessels and nerves: Successful removal. Lancet, *1*:360, 1861.
6. Crawford, F. A.: Thoracic outlet syndrome. Surg. Clin. North Am., *60*:947, 1980.
7. Falconer, M. A., and Li, F. W.: Resection of the first rib in costoclavicular compression of the brachial plexus. Lancet, *1*:59, 1962.
8. Hempel, G. K., Rusher, A. H., Wheeler, C. G., Hunt, D. G., and Bukhari, H. I.: Supraclavicular resection of the first rib for thoracic outlet syndrome. Am. J. Surg., *141*:213, 1981.
9. Jerrett, S. A., Cuzzone, L. J., and Pasternak, B. M.: Thoracic outlet syndrome: Electrophysiologic reappraisal. Arch. Neurol., *41*:960, 1984.
10. Keen, W. W.: The symptomatology, diagnosis and surgical treatment of cervical ribs. Am. J. Med. Sci., *133*:173, 1907.
11. Kelly, T. R.: Thoracic outlet syndrome. Current concepts of treatment. Ann. Surg., *190*:657, 1979.
12. McGough, E. C., Pearce, M. B., and Byrne, J. P.: Management of thoracic outlet syndrome. J. Thorac. Cardiovasc. Surg., 77:169, 1979.
13. Murphy, T. O., Piper, C. A., Kanar, E. A., and McAlexander, R. A.: Subclavicular approach to first rib resection. Am. J. Surg., *139*:634, 1980.
14. Naffziger, H. C., and Grant, W. T.: Neuritis of the brachial plexus mechanical in origin: The scalenus syndrome. Surg. Gynecol. Obstet., *67*:722, 1938.
15. Ochsner, A., Gage, M., and DeBakey, M.: Scalenus anticus (Naffziger) syndrome. Am. J. Surg., *28*:669, 1935.
16. Peet, R. M., Henriksen, J. D., and Anderson, T. P.: Thoracic outlet syndrome: Evaluation of a therapeutic exercise program. Mayo Clin. Proc., *31*:281, 1956.
17. Pollack, E. W.: Surgical anatomy of the thoracic outlet syndrome. Surg. Gynecol. Obstet., *150*:97, 1980.
18. Roos, D. B.: Congenital anomalies associated with thoracic outlet syndrome. Am. J. Surg., *132*:771, 1976.
19. Roos, D. B.: The place for scalenectomy and first-rib resection in thoracic outlet syndrome. Surgery, *92*:1077, 1982.
20. Roos, D. B.: Transaxillary approach for first rib resection to relieve thoracic outlet syndrome. Ann. Surg., *163*:354, 1966.
21. Sadler, T. R., Rainer, W. G., and Twombley, G.: Thoracic outlet compression: Application of positional arteriographic and nerve conduction studies. Am. J. Surg., *130*:704, 1975.
22. Stopford, J. S. B., and Telford, E. D.: Compression of the lower trunk of the brachial plexus by a first dorsal rib. Br. J. Surg., *7*:168, 1919.
23. Urschel, H. C., Razzuk, M. A., Wood, R. E., Parekh, M., and Paulson, D. L.: Objective diagnosis (ulnar nerve conduction velocity) and current therapy for thoracic outlet syndrome. Ann. Thorac. Surg., *12*:608, 1971.
24. Willshire: Supernumerary first rib. Lancet, *2*:633, 1860.
25. Wright, I. S.: The neurovascular syndrome produced by hyperabduction of the arms. Am. Heart J., *29*:1, 1945.

IX

Disorders of the Chest Wall

DAVID C. SABISTON, JR., M.D.

A variety of congenital and acquired lesions involve the chest wall. The malformations amenable to surgical therapy are generally followed by excellent therapeutic and cosmetic results. The results of surgical procedures for benign neoplasms are excellent but somewhat less than optimal with malignant tumors.

CONGENITAL MALFORMATIONS

Pectus Excavatum ("Funnel Chest")

The most frequent of the severe deformities of the chest wall is pectus excavatum. This deformity ranges from

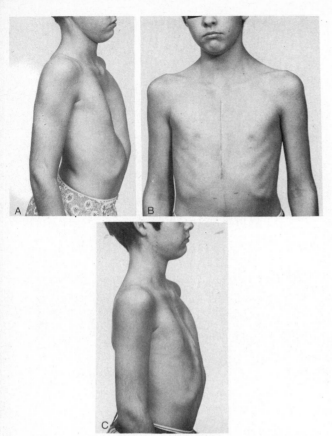

Figure 1. Three views of pectus excavatum. A, Oblique view demonstrating severe pectus deformity. B, Postoperative view illustrating correction of defect. C, Postoperative oblique illustrating correction of defect.

a very mild and barely noticeable disorder to those that are quite severe (Fig. 1). Frequently termed "funnel chest," it is primarily a deformity of the costal cartilages, which curve posteriorly rather than joining the sternum in the normal manner. The sternum is secondarily depressed, thus reducing the distance between the posterior surface of the sternum and the anterior surface of the vertebral column (Fig. 2).[7]

Clinical manifestations may be absent, or there may be varying degrees of respiratory insufficiency, especially with exercise. Few patients with this disorder become competitive athletes and thus have intolerance to exercise. The *cosmetic* effects of this deformity have been appreciable, and the vast majority of children become quite sensitive to this deformity by the time they enter school. Moreover, continuing psychological difficulties persist if the condition is not corrected surgically. Although it has been suggested that spontaneous correction may ensue, this occurs only rarely.

For significant pectus excavatum, surgical correction is generally indicated. The operation involves subperichondrial resection of all the costal cartilages with total separation of the sternum from surrounding structures except for the manubrium. A posterior wedge osteotomy is also performed at the sternomanubrial joint, and the sternum overcorrected with a wedge of cartilage placed in the osteotomy (Fig. 3). This procedure has been developed, refined, and largely advocated by Ravitch and is quite successful.[6]

Pectus Carinatum ("Pigeon Breast")

Pectus carinatum is a less common deformity and is characterized by unusual prominence of the sternum (Fig. 4). The sternum bulges anteriorly as a result of the positions of the costal cartilages. Management of this condition is by resection of the costal cartilages subperichondrially with freeing of the sternum in a manner quite similar to that done for pectus excavatum. The results are generally quite good, and the patient's psychological health usually returns to normal.

Poland's Syndrome

Poland's syndrome consists of variable absence of the costal cartilages, pectoral muscles, and portions of the ribs (Fig. 5).[8] It is a part of a spectrum of anomalies in which syndactylism, absent phalanges, and other anomalies occur. Surgical correction can be achieved in this malformation but is more complicated than pectus excavatum or pectus carinatum.

Sternal Clefts

Sternal clefts are congenital lesions usually obvious at birth. There are three principal types: (1) those involving

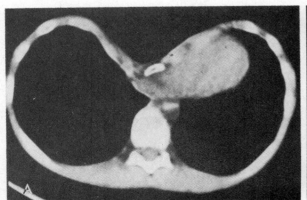
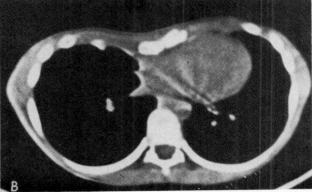

Figure 2. Pectus excavatum CT scan showing (A) the deformation and compression of the heart and (B) striking relief by operation. (From Ravitch, M. M.: In Sabiston, D. C., Jr. (Ed.): Textbook of Surgery, 13th ed. Philadelphia, W. B. Saunders Company, 1986, p. 2082.)

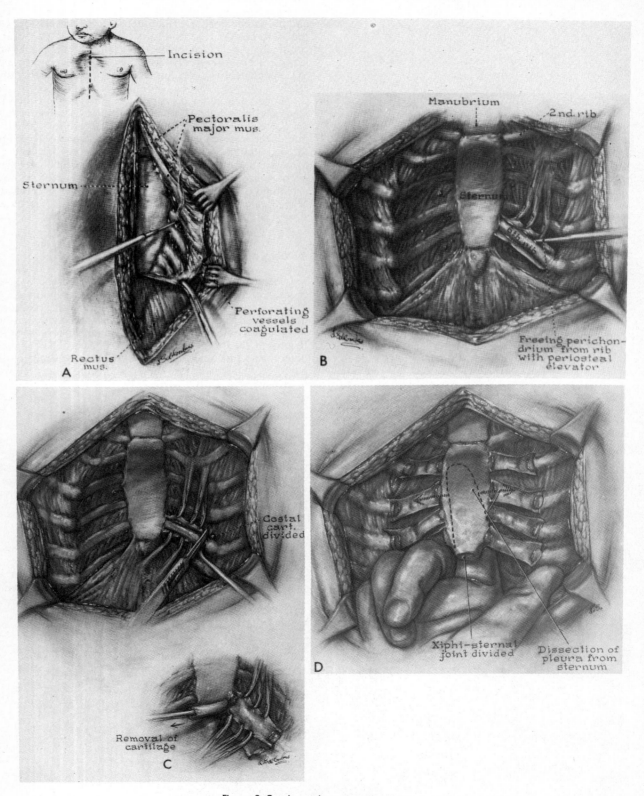

Figure 3. See legend on opposite page

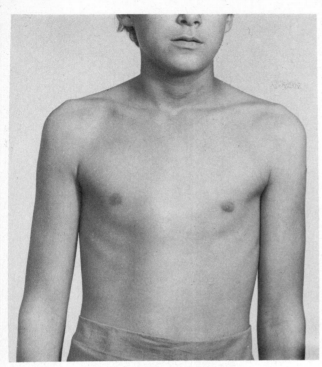

Figure 4. Pectus carinatum.

the manubrium and gladiolus to the third or fourth inter-costal space, (2) distal clefts involving the lower third or half of the sternum, and (3) the complete sternal cleft.

A Type 1 lesion involving the manubrium and upper sternum is shown in Figure 6.[10] This deformity can be effectively corrected by the technique shown in Figures 7, 8, and 9. The distal sternal defect may be associated with ectopia cordis, and an operation may be required in the first few months of life. Both diaphragmatic and pericardial defects are associated with this lesion and can be appropriately closed. *Complete sternal cleft* is rare and may be associated with a ventral abdominal or diaphragmatic defect. Prosthetic material may be required to close these lesions.

NEOPLASMS OF THE STERNUM AND RIBS

There are a variety of benign and malignant neoplasms arising in the chest wall. These neoplasms may be primary in the sternum, ribs, and diaphragm. These lesions may be primary, metastatic, or the result of direct invasion of the chest wall from either a bronchogenic or breast neoplasm. Primary tumors arising in the chest wall account for approximately 8 per cent of all intrinsic bone tumors.[4, 12]

Benign Neoplasms

Some of the more common benign neoplasms of the chest wall include chondromas, osteochondromas, bone cysts, fibrous dysplasia, and eosinophilic granuloma. Some lesions present with the appearance of a mass, at times tender, and show few clinical signs or symptoms to suggest the specific type of neoplasm. The chondroma is the most common benign tumor of the chest wall with most appearing in the ribs and a minority in the sternum. En bloc excision with a 4-cm. margin around the lesion is the appropriate operation. The same type of treatment applies to osteo-chondromas as well as bone cysts and eosinophilic granuloma. In a study of 53 primary chest wall tumors, 26 were benign, with 49 occurring in the ribs and four in the sternum.[9] All the patients with benign neoplasms were treated by excision with no recurrence or mortality. In general, it was not possible to distinguish benign neoplasms from malignant ones occurring in the chest wall *unless* cortical destruction and involvement of soft tissues are visualized. Therefore, in the management of benign as well as malignant lesions, all neoplasms should be considered malignant until proven otherwise and wide excision with a 4-cm. margin is appropriate. In this way, the largest number of patients will become long-term survivors.

Malignant Tumors

In many series, malignant tumors outnumber benign tumors in lesions arising in the chest wall. *Chondrosarcoma* is generally the most common malignant lesion and appears as a lobulated, smooth, firm mass often showing destruction

---

Figure 3. Posterior wedge osteotomy. A, I generally employ a midline incision from the manubrium to the epigastrium. In girls, a concealed submammary incision is satisfactory but more dissection and larger skin flaps are required than in a midline incision; in big girls or women, it does not provide adequate exposure. The patient's head is generally held extended, and the chest is elevated by a folded towel placed longitudinally under the spine. The incision is carried down to the sternum, and flaps of skin, fat, and pectoralis major are reflected as one. The perforating branches of the internal mammary artery can be seen, clamped and coagulated. There is essentially no bleeding. The entire dissection is performed with the needle-tipped electrocautery. (From Ravitch, M. M.: In Shields, T. W.: General Thoracic Surgery. Philadelphia, Lea & Febiger, 1972.)

B, The pectoral muscles have been laid back to expose the deformed cartilages for the entire extent of the deformity. The two lowermost cartilages will generally be exposed by making an oblique incision through the rectus muscle, which is not detached. The cartilages are excised subperichondrially, after the periochondrium has been incised longitudinally for the full extent of the deformity and transversely at either end of the longitudinal incision so that rectangular flaps can be elevated. If the edges of these flaps are seized with multiple fine hemostats, the cartilage can be freed with a delicate elevator such as a Freer. (From Ravitch, M. M.: In Sabiston, D. C., Jr. (Ed.): Davis-Christopher Textbook of Surgery. 10th ed. Philadelphia, W. B. Saunders Company, 1972.)

C, Often, as shown, it is possible to free the cartilage circumferentially, to divide it laterally, elevate it, and divide it from the sternum medially. In other instances, it is easiest to seize the partially freed cartilage with a Kocher clamp and to elevate and transect it in its midportion until the posterior perichondrium is reached and pushed out of the way.

D, The xiphisternal joint has been divided. The operator's finger has been inserted into the mediastinum behind the sternum and slid from side to side, displacing the pleural envelopes laterally.

(C and D from Ravitch, M. M.: Congenital Deformities of the Chest Wall and Their Operative Correction. Philadelphia, W. B. Saunders Company, 1977.)

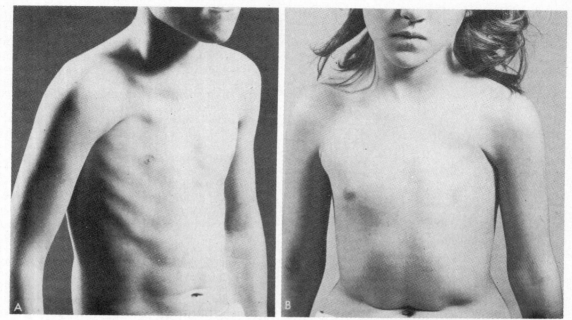

Figure 5. Congenital absence of the costosternal portion of the pectoralis major, on the right side in a boy (A) and on the left side in a girl (B). There was no familial history of such a defect in either one. Note the abnormally high border of the axillary fold, the prominent ribs and the flattening of the chest wall due almost entirely to the absence of the pectoralis major. The breast and nipple in the girl are obviously hypoplastic. The ribs are uninvolved. The hands were normal in both. This probably represents a forme fruste of Poland's syndrome. (From Ravitch, M. M.: Disorders of the sternum and the thoracic wall. In Sabiston, D. C., Jr., and Spencer, F. C. (Eds.): Gibbon's Surgery of the Chest, 4th ed. Philadelphia, W. B. Saunders Company, 1983.)

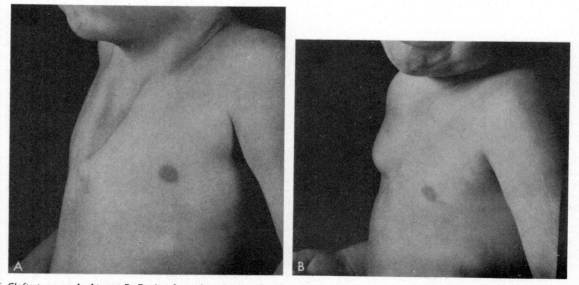

Figure 6. Cleft sternum. A, At rest. B, During forced expiration. Superior clefts of the sternum are variously V- or U-shaped. The appearance of the child as he cries explains the term "ectopia cordis," although the heart is actually not misplaced. In the newborn, defects of this kind can be corrected by direct apposition of the sternal halves. In this child, closure of the defect was made possible by sliding chondrotomies on either side. (From Sabiston, D. C., Jr.: J. Thorac. Surg., 35:118, 1958.)

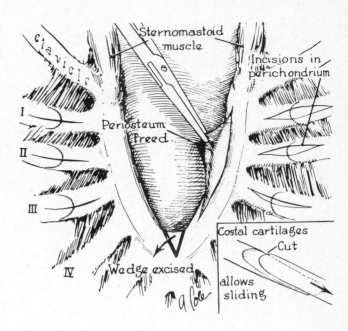

Figure 7. *Illustration of the defect after dissection of the skin flaps. The sternal bands are shown and the periosteum is being freed from the anterior surface. Incisions have been made into the perichondrium of the first, second, third, and fourth costal cartilages. The inset illustrates the incisions in the costal cartilage. (From Sabiston, D. C., Jr.: J. Thorac. Surg., 35:118, 1958.)*

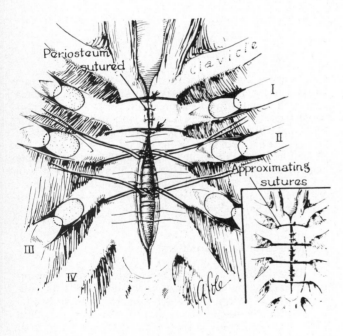

Figure 8. *Illustration showing approximation of sternal bands with encircling sutures following the oblique incisions in the costal cartilages. Multiple fine silk sutures are shown in the periosteal flaps. The inset shows the final appearance. (From Sabiston, D. C., Jr.: J. Thorac. Surg., 35:118, 1958.)*

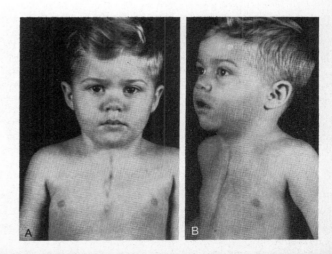

Figure 9. *Correction of sternal cleft.* A, *Postoperative photograph.* B, *Postoperative photograph (oblique).*

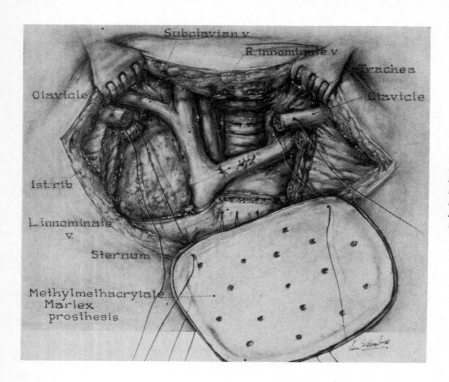

Figure 10. The methyl methacrylate sandwich, between two layers of Marlex, has multiple drill holes to prevent accumulation of fluid and permit ingrowth of granulation tissue. A free margin of Marlex beyond the acrylic facilitates suture fixation to the chest wall.

of cortex on x-ray film. It should be removed by radical en bloc dissection.

Ewing's tumor is best evaluated by chest film and shows evidence of destruction or lysis of bone with a diffuse, expanded bone lesion with little periosteal reaction in some of the patients. Both surgical excision[9] and treatment with radiation and chemotherapy[3] are employed. Lymphomas are also managed primarily by chemotherapy and radiation.

Plasmacytoma also occurs as a primary malignant lesion, and radical excision, with or without radiation, is necessary. Clinical features suggesting that a neoplasm is malignant include recent and rapid increase in size, invasion of surrounding structures, and distant metastases. Although diagnostic biopsy has been reported, most today believe that initial wide excision of the neoplasm is the most appropriate treatment. In a series of 27 malignant primary chest wall tumors, the overall 5-year survival was 33 per cent and the 10-year survival 18 per cent.[9] Other malignant neoplasms include osteogenic sarcoma, neurosarcoma, fibrous sarcoma, liposarcoma, and angioplastic sarcoma.

Metastatic neoplasms arising in other structures may also involve the chest wall by extension through metastases or blood-borne deposits. In general, surgical intervention in such lesions is palliative and should be done only to establish the diagnosis or in the management of otherwise uncontrollable discomfort. Although some neoplasms are amenable to radiotherapy, those that are radioresistant include chondrosarcoma, osteogenic sarcoma, neurosarcoma, fibrosarcoma, liposarcoma, angiosarcoma, and anaplastic neoplasms. The radiosensitive malignant tumors include Ewing's sarcoma, reticulum cell sarcoma, plasma cell myeloma, Hodgkin's disease, and lymphosarcoma.

In one series of 100 patients with chest wall tumors, metastases were present in 32 instances, including 12 from sarcomas, nine from the breast, four from the kidney, three from the lung, three from other genitourinary sources, and

one from the thyroid gland.[3] The value of en bloc resection of the chest wall for patients with bronchogenic carcinoma has been demonstrated.[5] More controversial, however, is radical resection of breast cancer with metastases to the chest wall. Skin ulceration was present in 11 of 14 cases of breast cancer, and these were treated with excision and palliation.[3] Wide radical chest wall resection with immediate reconstruction, including the use of flaps and chest wall muscles as well as omentum and prosthetic materials, e.g., Prolene or polytetrafluoroethylene patch, is effective for many malignant lesions (Fig. 10).

Neoplasms of the Diaphragm

Benign tumors of the diaphragm that have been reported include fibromas, lipomas, mesotheliomas, angiofibromas, and neurogenic tumors. In addition, congenital cysts of the diaphragm occur. Considerably more common have been malignant lesions, primarily metastatic, from neighboring structures such as the esophagus, lung, liver, and colon. Retroperitoneal malignant neoplasms may also extend to the diaphragm. Primary malignant lesions include fibrosarcomas and neurofibrosarcomas. Symptoms may be elusive and the lesions are generally diagnosed by radiography. Computed tomography scans have also become quite useful in the diagnosis of these lesions.

The management of benign lesions is simple excision; for malignant primary lesions, wide removal with replacement by fascia lata or prosthetic material is required. Radiotherapy and chemotherapy are infrequently indicated.[2, 11]

It has been reported that of the primary tumors of the diaphragm the malignant lesions predominate in 60 per cent while the remaining 40 per cent of neoplasms are benign.[1, 13]

SELECTED REFERENCES

Groff, D. B. III, and Adkins, P. C.: Collective review: Chest wall tumors. Ann. Thorac. Surg., *4*:260, 1967.
This is a collective review of a large number of cases of chest wall tumors with descriptions of the various types.

Pairolero, P. C., and Arnold, P. G.: Chest wall tumors: Experience with 100 consecutive patients. J. Thorac. Cardiovasc. Surg., *90*:367, 1985.
A recent update of a 10-year experience of 100 consecutive patients with neoplasms of the chest wall.

REFERENCES

1. Anderson, L. S., and Forrest, J. V.: Tumors of the diaphragm. Roentgenol. Radium Ther. Nucl. Med., *119*:259, 1973.
2. Clagett, O. T., and Johnson, M. A.: Tumors of the diaphragm. Am. J. Surg., *78*:526, 1949.
3. Pairolero, P. C., and Arnold, P. G.: Chest wall tumors: Experience with 100 consecutive patients. J. Thorac. Cardiovasc. Surg., *90*:367, 1985.
4. Pascuzzi, C. A., Dahlin, D. C., and Clagett, O. T.: Primary tumors of the ribs and sternum. Surg. Gynecol. Obstet., *104*:390, 1957.
5. Piehler, J. M., Pairolero, P. C., Weiland, L. H., Offord, K. P., Payne, W. S., and Bernatz, P. E.: Bronchogenic carcinoma with chest wall invasion: Factors affecting survival following en bloc resection. Ann. Thorac. Surg., *34*:684, 1982.
6. Ravitch, M. M.: Congenital Deformities of the Chest Wall and Their Operative Correction. Philadelphia, W. B. Saunders Company, 1977.
7. Ravitch, M. M.: Disorders of the chest wall. *In* Sabiston, D. C., Jr. (Ed.): Textbook of Surgery, 13th ed. Philadelphia, W. B. Saunders Company, 1986.
8. Ravitch, M. M.: Disorders of the sternum and the thoracic wall. *In* Sabiston, D. C., Jr., and Spencer, F. C. (Eds.): Gibbon's Surgery of the Chest, 4th ed. Philadelphia, W. B. Saunders Company, 1983.
9. Sabanathan, S., Salama, F. D., Morgan, W. E., and Harvey, J. A.: Primary chest wall tumors. Ann. Thorac. Surg., *39*:4, 1985.
10. Sabiston, D. C., Jr.: The surgical management of congenital bifid sternum with a partial ectopia cordis. J. Thorac. Surg., *35*:118, 1958.
11. Samson, P. C., and Childress, M. E.: Primary neurofibrosarcoma of the diaphragm. J. Thorac. Surg., *20*:901, 1950.
12. Teitelbaum, S. L.: Twenty years' experience with intrinsic tumors of the bony thorax at a large institution. J. Thorac. Cardiovasc. Surg., *63*:776, 1972.
13. Trivedi, S. A.: Neurolemmoma of the diaphragm causing severe hypertrophic pulmonary osteoarthropathy. Br. J. Tuberculosis, *52*:214, 1958.

THE MEDIASTINUM

45

I

Primary Mediastinal Cysts and Neoplasms

R. DUANE DAVIS, JR., M.D.
DAVID C. SABISTON, JR., M.D.

The mediastinum is an important subdivision of the thorax. It lies between the pleural cavities and contains many important organs and vital structures. Important processes that involve the mediastinum include infection, emphysema, hemorrhage, and a large variety of primary tumors and cysts. Systemic disorders, such as metastatic carcinoma, and many granulomatous diseases also may be manifest by involvement within the mediastinum. Lesions originating primarily in the esophagus, trachea, heart, and great vessels are usually related to the specific organ system involved rather than the mediastinum. Earlier and more accurate diagnosis of mediastinal processes has been made possible by the increasing use of chest roentgenography, computed tomography (CT), radioisotope scanning techniques, and magnetic resonance imaging (MRI) and has improved the success in treating mediastinal lesions. In conjunction with these advances in diagnostic techniques, advances in anesthesia, chemotherapy, immunotherapy, and radiation therapy have increased survival and improved the quality of life.

HISTORIC ASPECTS

Before the advent of endotracheal anesthesia, surgical intervention in the mediastinum was rare owing to the hazards of pneumothorax upon entering the pleural cavity. Bastianelli, a noted Italian surgeon, successfully removed a dermoid cyst from the anterior mediastinum by resecting the manubrium in 1893. In 1897, Milton reported the first sternal splitting approach to the mediastinum when he excised two large caseous lymph nodes from a young Egyptian male with tuberculosis of the sternum.[18] He left the wound open, successfully utilizing a delayed primary closure on the second postoperative day.

With the introduction of endotracheal anesthesia, the transpleural thoracic surgical approach to mediastinal and pulmonary neoplasms was made possible. The classic writings of Harrington in the 1920s and of Heuer and Andrus

in the 1940s describe the early experience in resecting tumors of the thorax and mediastinum.[12, 15] In 1939, Blalock pioneered the surgical treatment of myasthenia gravis, performing a thymectomy in a myasthenic female that resulted in marked improvement in symptoms.[3] More recently, the usage of megavoltage radiation therapy, pioneered by Kaplan, and the increasingly successful utilization of chemotherapeutic agents have greatly improved the prognosis in patients with malignant diseases of the mediastinum, particularly those with lymphomas and germ cell tumors.

ANATOMY

The mediastinum is a subdivision of the thoracic cavity that is bounded laterally by the mediastinal pleura, anteriorly by the sternum, and posteriorly by the vertebral column. It extends from the diaphragm inferiorly to the thoracic inlet superiorly. The mediastinum has classically been compartmentalized into four divisions. The *superior mediastinum* is divided from the inferior mediastinum by a plane extending through the sternal angle to the fourth intervertebral space. The pericardial sac further divides the inferior mediastinum into the *anterior*, *middle*, and *posterior mediastinum*. The use of these artificial subdivisions has been helpful in differentiating lesions within the mediastinum because of the characteristic location of many of the neoplasms within the mediastinum.

Anatomically, the *superior mediastinum* contains the thymus, the upper trachea, the esophagus, and the aortic arch and its branches. The *anterior mediastinum* contains the inferior aspect of the thymus gland as well as adipose, lymphatic, and areolar tissue. *Middle mediastinal contents* include the heart, pericardium, phrenic nerves, tracheal bifurcation, and main bronchi as well as the tracheal and bronchial lymph nodes. Within the *posterior mediastinum* lie the esophagus, the vagus nerve, the sympathetic nervous chain, the thoracic duct, the descending aorta, the azygos

Mediastinum

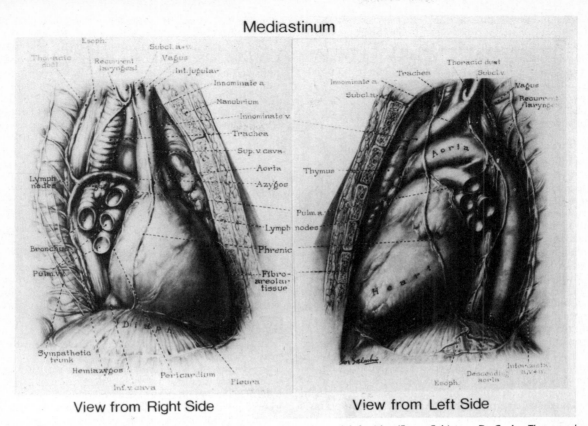

View from Right Side   View from Left Side

Figure 1. Anatomic structures of the medastinum seen from the right and left side. (From Sabiston, D. C., Jr.: The esophagus and mediastinum. In Cooke, R. E. (Ed.): The Biologic Basis of Pediatric Practice. New York, McGraw-Hill Book Company, 1968.)

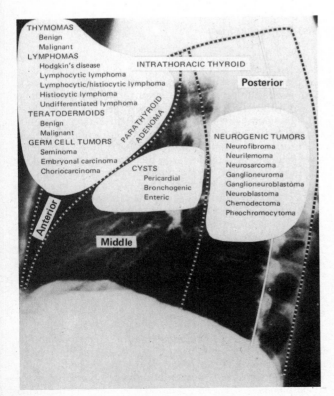

THYMOMAS
  Benign
  Malignant
LYMPHOMAS
  Hodgkin's disease
  Lymphocytic lymphoma
  Lymphocytic/histiocytic lymphoma
  Histiocytic lymphoma
  Undifferentiated lymphoma
TERATODERMOIDS
  Benign
  Malignant
GERM CELL TUMORS
  Seminoma
  Embryonal carcinoma
  Choriocarcinoma

INTRATHORACIC THYROID

Posterior

PARATHYROID ADENOMA

CYSTS
  Pericardial
  Bronchogenic
  Enteric

NEUROGENIC TUMORS
  Neurofibroma
  Neurilemoma
  Neurosarcoma
  Ganglioneuroma
  Ganglioneuroblastoma
  Neuroblastoma
  Chemodectoma
  Pheochromocytoma

Anterior

Middle

figure 2. Lateral chest film divided into three anatomic subdivisions with the most common location of the tumors and cysts.

and hemiazygos systems, and paravertebral lymph nodes as well as areolar tissue (Fig. 1).

Certain lesions cannot be easily categorized using this system of artificial subdivisions. Thymomas or teratodermoid tumors occur in the anterior aspect of the superior mediastinum as well as the anterior mediastinum. Neurogenic tumors occur in the posterior aspect of the superior mediastinum as well as the posterior mediastinum. Thus, another means of subdividing the mediastinum has been proposed that creates three anatomic subdivisions (Fig. 2). The posterior mediastinum is redefined as the mediastinal space posterior to the posterior border of the pericardium. The anterosuperior division contains the anterior aspect of the superior mediastinum as well as the previously defined anterior mediastinum.

MEDIASTINITIS

Acute mediastinitis is a serious and potentially fatal infectious process of the mediastinal space. A number of factors are responsible for the development of acute mediastinitis. These include perforation of the esophagus in either the cervical or thoracic region due to instrumentation, foreign bodies, or penetrating trauma; spontaneous esophageal rupture, including Boerhaave's syndrome; leakage from an esophageal anastomosis; mediastinal extension from an infectious process involving the pleura, pulmonary parenchyma, chest wall, vertebrae, or the neck; and tracheobronchial perforation. An increasing number of cases of mediastinitis occur as postoperative complications of median sternotomy because of the increased use of this surgical approach in the performance of open heart surgery and as access to anterior mediastinal masses. Wound infections following median sternotomy occur with an incidence of approximately 2 per cent, and approximately half of these infections will involve the mediastinum.

Clinical Presentation

The clinical presentation of patients with mediastinitis is usually initiated by fever, leukocytosis, tachycardia, and pain that may be localized to the neck or chest. In cases of esophageal perforation caused by instrumentation, foreign body, or blunt trauma, the most frequent site of perforation is at the level of the cricopharyngeal muscle. The pain therefore is usually referred to the neck and is associated with subcutaneous emphysema. Mediastinitis occurring following median sternotomy may be characterized by a rapid and progressive clinical course, or it may follow a slower course. Risk factors for the development of wound infections postoperatively include a long operative time, prolonged cardiopulmonary bypass time, re-exploration for postoperative bleeding, dehiscence, external cardiac massage, and the postoperative low cardiac output state.

Chronic mediastinitis may be due to a bacterial infection, as in cases following postoperative infection. However, the majority of chronic infections are due to granulomatous diseases such as tuberculosis or fungi. With progressive chronic infection, the granulomatous process within the mediastinal lymph nodes may begin to compress adjacent mediastinal structures, leading to obstruction of the superior vena cava, the trachea, the bronchi, or the esophagus. Surgical excision or bypass may be necessary to relieve symptoms in these patients in addition to the appropriate medical therapy.

Diagnosis

Considering the importance of early diagnosis and evaluation of the extent of involvement, CT scanning has been a great asset in the treatment and diagnosis of postoperative mediastinitis. In a series of patients with postoperative wound complications, it was shown that CT successfully differentiated those cases with retrosternal involvement requiring early surgical intervention from those in which the infection involved only the superficial soft tissues.[16]

Treatment

Treatment of mediastinitis requires correction of the inciting cause. Supportive therapy includes supplemental oxygen and sedation. In addition, the appropriate antimicrobial therapy should be given after culture reports and organism sensitivity are available. Although a few patients will respond to nonoperative management, the majority require thorough débridement of infected and devitalized tissue and surgical drainage. Emphasis should be placed on early diagnosis and surgical intervention. Especially in cases caused by esophageal perforation or tracheobronchial disruption, delays in treatment are associated with a marked increase in mortality and morbidity. In patients with infected sternotomy wounds, the use of closed mediastinal antibiotic irrigation with tube thoracostomy drainage has significantly reduced the mortality associated with postoperative mediastinitis. Recently, the early use of pedicle flaps to obliterate dead space and cover the heart and great vessels following surgical débridement of the involved sternum and infected soft tissue has produced a further reduction in morbidity and mortality. The use of flaps should follow the initial débridement, drainage, and local wound care, and these are mobilized only after the wound is clean. The pectoralis major muscle, the rectus abdominis muscle, or, more rarely, the omentum has been used as tissue flaps.

MEDIASTINAL EMPHYSEMA

Air within the mediastinum produces mediastinal emphysema or pneumomediastinum. The sources of air include the esophagus and tracheobronchial tree. Penetrating wounds or perforations of these structures as well as trauma associated with fractures of ribs or vertebrae are known causes of pneumomediastinum. Positive pressure ventilation and blunt trauma can increase intra-alveolar pressure sufficiently to cause rupture of the alveoli. Subsequent dissection of air along vascular planes into the hilum and the mediastinum results in pneumomediastinum. Pneumoperitoneum may dissect through the diaphragmatic hiatus into the mediastinum.

Spontaneous mediastinal emphysema can also occur, as was initially described by Hamman in 1939.[11] In these patients, the pneumomediastinum is probably preceded by interstitial emphysema caused by a ruptured bleb within the lung parenchyma and is often seen in patients with exacerbation of bronchospastic disease. Air dissects within the bronchial or vascular planes back through the hilar structures into the mediastinum.

Clinical Presentation

The clinical hallmarks of mediastinal emphysema include substernal chest pain, which may radiate to the back, and crepitance in the substernal notch, chest wall, or neck. With increasing pressure, the emphysematous process may spread within the soft tissue planes of the neck, face, chest, and abdomen as well as extend into the retroperitoneum. Hamman described a characteristic crunching over the precordium that is accentuated during systole. This sound has been described as similar to the sound made by walking on snow. Frequently, pneumomediastinum is accompanied by pneumothorax. In cases where sufficient pressure is introduced, the air within the mediastinum may cause compression of venous structures, creating cardiac tamponade. This syndrome is manifested by cyanosis, prominence of neck veins, and dyspnea. Only rarely does sufficient tension develop within the mediastinum to cause circulatory failure. Symptoms of dysphagia may be noted in patients with sufficient pressure to compress the esophagus.

Diagnosis

The diagnosis of pneumomediastinum is confirmed by the presence of air within the tissue planes of the mediastinum, which may be seen on the routine chest film. Frequently air is seen radiographically or is palpated in the tissue planes of the neck, pectoralis muscle, and the upper extremities.

Treatment

Treatment is directed toward correcting the inciting cause. In cases of spontaneous pneumomediastinum, the symptoms usually resolve without intervention. Supportive therapy with supplemental oxygen and sedation as well as careful observation for evidence of progression of symptoms is usually sufficient. Only rarely is surgical decompression of the mediastinum required in cases of pneumomediastinum. A pneumothorax accompanied by mediastinal emphysema requires tube thoracostomy. In patients with pneumomediastinum requiring continuous positive pressure ventilation and high levels of positive end-expiratory pressures, bilateral chest tube placement may be appropriate prophylaxis against the development of a tension pneumothorax.

MEDIASTINAL COMPRESSIVE SYNDROME (SUPERIOR VENA CAVAL SYNDROME)

Obstruction of the superior vena cava may be caused by a number of benign and malignant processes involving the mediastinum. The increased pressure within the venous system drained by the superior vena cava produces the characteristic features of the syndrome: distended neck veins; tissue edema of the head, neck, and upper extremities; dilated collateral veins over the upper extremity; cyanosis; headache; and confusion. With sudden occlusion, the clinical presentation is much more striking. Rapid development of cerebral edema, with subsequent intracranial thrombosis, may occur, resulting in coma or death.

Etiology

The majority of cases of superior vena caval obstruction are caused by malignant processes. Bronchogenic carcinoma, usually of the right upper lobe, is the most frequent cause of this syndrome. Malignant thymomas, primary carcinomas, lymphomas, germ cell tumors, and metastatic tumors are other frequent malignancies causing superior vena caval obstruction.

In less than 25 per cent of cases, benign lesions are the cause. Examples of benign causes of superior vena caval obstruction include mediastinal granulomatous diseases, such as histoplasmosis, idiopathic mediastinal fibrosis, multinodular goiter, pleural calcification, bronchogenic cyst, and thoracic aortic aneurysm. With the increasing use of indwelling central venous catheters, thrombosis secondary to catheter trauma or the presence of a foreign body has been identified more frequently. However, only rarely are these cases associated with this syndrome.

Pathophysiology and Diagnosis

The pathophysiology of the obstruction varies from simple compression to malignant invasion as well as thrombosis of the superior vena cava. CT scanning has been increasingly useful in the diagnosis of this condition, especially with the injection of intravenous contrast media. Venous angiography is less frequently required to confirm the diagnosis, although it does provide more exact identification of the site of obstruction.

Treatment

Malignant processes causing superior vena caval obstruction are usually inoperable at the time of diagnosis. Percutaneous fine-needle biopsy is usually successful in establishing a tissue diagnosis. However, surgical intervention may be necessary for diagnosis. Histologic diagnosis is attempted before the institution of treatment because of the alteration of the histologic appearance following the initial courses of therapy. Radiation therapy and, more frequently, multiagent chemotherapy are the usual means of therapy. In cases of rapid progression of symptoms or with central nervous system symptoms, therapy may be necessary on an emergent basis. Improved results have been obtained in the treatment of lymphomas, thymomas, and germ cell tumors causing superior vena caval obstruction. Even when the obstruction is secondary to bronchogenic carcinoma, decompression of at least a transient nature is usually achieved.

In cases refractory to radiation therapy and chemotherapy, surgical intervention with bypass grafting of the obstructed segment has been performed. Historically, results have been discouraging. However, with the use of autologous grafts and some of the newer prosthetic grafts, improved successes have been reported. Superior vena caval obstruction due to benign diseases usually follows a more benign course marked by clinical regression as collateral channels develop.

Medical therapy with diuretics, salt restriction, and positional maneuvers frequently is successful in alleviating symptoms associated with benign lesions causing superior vena caval obstruction.

HEMORRHAGE

Mediastinal hemorrhage is most frequently caused by traumatic injuries or is seen as a complication of surgical intervention within the mediastinum and thorax. Penetrating wounds of the thorax or cervical region may cause lacerations of major arteries and veins. Blunt trauma to the chest may result in the transection of the aorta, most frequently occurring immediately distal to the origin of the left subclavian artery. Dissecting thoracic aneurysms, iatrogenic laceration of the great vessels during angiography or placement of central arterial or venous lines, hemorrhagic diathesis, anticoagulation therapy, uremia, infection, erosion of tracheostomy tubes into the great vessels, and bleeding from primary tumors or cysts of the mediastinum are less frequent causes of mediastinal hemorrhage. Significant hemorrhage may occur during operations within the thorax and mediastinum, particularly those procedures involving the heart and great vessels. Routine use of large-caliber chest tubes for mediastinal drainage usually prevents development of significant symptoms of mediastinal tamponade.

Spontaneous mediastinal hemorrhage, usually into the superior mediastinum, was first reported by Epstein in 1959.[7] It is thought that this syndrome is due to the rupture of small mediastinal vessels during periods of markedly increased intrathoracic pressure, such as that occurring during coughing or vomiting. Unlike the aforementioned cases, spontaneous mediastinal hemorrhage usually has a benign clinical course with resolution of symptoms without long-term sequelae.

TABLE 1. Primary Mediastinal Tumors and Cysts in 2399 Patients

	Sabiston and Scott 1952	Heimburger and Battersby 1963	Burkell et al. 1969	Fontenelle et al. 1971	Benjamin et al. 1972	Conkle 1972	Rubush et al. 1973	Vidne and Levy 1973	Ovrum and Birkeland 1979	Nandi et al. 1980	Adkins et al. 1984	Parish et al. 1984	Davis and Sabiston 1986	Totals	Incidence (%)
Neurogenic	20	21	13	17	49	8	36	9	19	27	8	212	59	498	21
Thymoma	17	10	12	17	34	11	42	10	10	18	4	206	70	461	19
Lymphoma	11	9	12	16	32	10	14	6	11	4	7	107	56	295	12
Germ cell neoplasm	9	10	3	7	27	2	14	3	5	7	11	99	45	242	10
Primary carcinoma	10	11	0	2	0	10	3	2	9	0	5	25	32	109	5
Mesenchymal tumor	1	4	4	4	24	2	10	4	4	2	0	60	24	143	6
Endocrine tumor	2	8	4	4	24	0	13	2	21	6	2	56	13	155	6
Other	14							1	2	1	1	36		55	2
Cyst															
Pericardial	2	4	4	2	3		10	2	7	2	0	72	37	145	6
Bronchogenic	5	12	9	13	11	0	6	2	0	0	0	54	41	153	6
Enteric	2	5	0	4	1	0	2	1	0	0	0	29	12	56	2
Other	8	3	0	4	4	0	3	3	3	7	0	41	11	87	4
						0									
Total	101	97	61	90	209	43	153	45	91	74	38	997	400	2399	

Mediastinal hemorrhage may present with retrosternal chest pain that can radiate to the back or be accompanied by pain in the cervical region. Dyspnea, venous distention, cyanosis, and ecchymosis extending into the neck occur with increasing accumulation of blood within the mediastinum. With sufficient hemorrhage, mediastinal tamponade may develop. The clinical presentation is that of tachycardia, hypotension, falling urinary output, and equalization of left- and right-sided cardiac filling pressures. Mediastinal tamponade, however, usually develops somewhat more insidiously than pericardial tamponade owing to the larger volume of the mediastinum. Mediastinal tamponade requires prompt surgical decompression. Diagnosis before the development of hemodynamic alterations is the goal. Surgical intervention is directed toward evacuating the accumulated blood and hematoma so as to correct the hemodynamic alterations associated with the tamponade and controlling the underlying source of bleeding.

PRIMARY TUMORS AND CYSTS OF THE MEDIASTINUM

The wide variety of tissues and organ systems present within the mediastinum gives rise to a number of histologically different neoplasms. In addition, numerous lymph nodes are present within the mediastinum and may be involved in a number of systemic diseases, such as metastatic carcinoma, infectious granulomatous disorders, and connective tissue disorders.

Primary tumors and cysts present with a wide variety of clinical signs and symptoms. The natural history of mediastinal tumors and cysts varies from a slow benign growth with minimal symptoms to an aggressive, invasive neoplasm that is widely metastatic and rapidly causes death. Advances in the number of diagnostic techniques and the increasing utilization of routine chest roentgenography have allowed the earlier diagnosis of these tumors. Because surgical excision has been shown to successfully cure both benign and malignant lesions and with the increasingly successful utilization of radiation and multiagent chemotherapy in the treatment of a number of other malignant lesions, observation of a mediastinal mass without an appropriate histologic diagnosis can only rarely be accepted.

Although mediastinal masses are infrequently encountered in routine practice, the apparent increase in their incidence and the ability to provide effective therapy underscore the importance of understanding the clinical characteristics of these primary tumors and cysts. A collected series of 2399 patients demonstrates the relative incidence with which specific neoplasms occur within the mediastinum (Table 1).[2, 5, 8, 14, 20, 23, 25, 33] Although differences in incidence with regard to specific lesions occur between series, it is apparent that certain neoplasms are more frequently diagnosed than others. In addition, most mediastinal neoplasms occur frequently in a characteristic location within the mediastinum.

Lesions of the anterosuperior mediastinum are most likely to be thymic neoplasms, lymphomas, or germ cell tumors. Middle mediastinal lesions are most frequently pericardial or bronchogenic cysts, primary carcinomas, lymphomas, or thymomas. Neurogenic tumors, bronchogenic or enteric cysts, and mesenchymal lesions are the neoplasms found most frequently in the posterior mediastinum (Table 2).

Symptoms

Mediastinal masses may be found in asymptomatic patients on a routine chest film or may cause symptoms

TABLE 2. Usual Location of Mediastinal Tumors and Cysts

Anterosuperior	Middle	Posterior
Thymoma	Lymphoma	Neurogenic tumors
Lymphoma	Carcinoma	Enteric cysts
Germ cell tumors	Pericardial cysts	Bronchogenic cysts
Teratodermoid	Bronchogenic cysts	Mesenchymal
Malignant germ	Enteric cysts	tumors
cell tumors	Mesenchymal	
Carcinoma	tumors	
Thyroid adenoma		
Parathyroid		
adenoma		
Mesenchymal		
tumors		

TABLE 3. Significance of Symptoms in 232 Patients, 1966–1985*

	Number	Benign	Malignant
Asymptomatic†	100	80 (80%)	20 (20%)
Symptomatic	132	49 (37%)	83 (63%)
Total	232	129	103

*At the Duke University Medical Center.
†Lesion found on routine chest film.

due to local mechanical effects secondary to tumor compression or invasion of mediastinal structures. Systemic symptoms may be nonspecific or may constitute a symptom complex that is virtually pathognomonic for a specific neoplasm.

The majority of patients with mediastinal tumors will have symptoms at the time of their initial presentation. Most series report that between 56 and 65 per cent of patients have symptoms at the time of presentation, and those with *malignant* lesions are much more likely to have symptoms at presentation. In a review of patients from Duke University Medical Center, over 90 per cent of patients with malignant lesions presented with symptoms. Patients with benign mediastinal masses had a reduced incidence of symptoms (46 per cent). However, with the increasing use of routine chest roentgenography, a greater portion of mediastinal masses are being seen in patients who are asymptomatic. The presence of symptoms in a patient with a mediastinal mass is of prognostic importance and suggests a higher likelihood of malignant neoplasms. At Duke University Medical Center, patients who presented with a symptomatic mediastinal mass had a malignant neoplasm in 60 per cent of cases, whereas, in those with a mediastinal mass discovered on a routine chest film, 80 per cent of the patients had a benign lesion (Table 3).[28, 29]

Currently, it is apparent that more benign and malignant neoplasms are diagnosed in the asymptomatic stage. In the period prior to 1965 at Duke, asymptomatic mediastinal masses were benign in 95 per cent of cases, whereas 50 per cent of symptomatic lesions were benign.[22] Thus, it also appears that the presence of symptoms currently has a higher correlation with malignancy than was previously observed.

Although vague systemic symptoms of anorexia, weight loss, and increasing fatigue may be the presenting symptoms in a patient with a mediastinal mass, more commonly symptoms are caused by local compression or invasion by the neoplasm of adjacent mediastinal structures (Table 4). Chest pain occurs secondary to compression or invasion of the chest wall or intercostal nerves. Chest pain occurs most frequently with tumors of the anterosuperior mediastinum. Back pain, in a similar fashion, is usually caused by compression or invasion of the posterior chest wall and the intercostal nerves. Compression of the tracheobronchial

tree usually is manifested by symptoms such as dyspnea, cough, recurrent pneumonitis, or, less frequently, stridor. Esophageal involvement may lead to dysphagia or symptoms of obstruction. Involvement of the recurrent laryngeal nerve, the sympathetic chain, or the brachial plexus produces vocal cord paralysis, Horner's syndrome, and Pancoast's syndrome, respectively. Mediastinal tumors causing these symptoms are most frequently localized in the superior mediastinum. Phrenic nerve involvement may cause a paralyzed diaphragm. It must be emphasized that although malignant lesions are more frequently implicated in causing symptoms related to local involvement, benign tumors may also cause similar symptomatology.

Systemic Syndromes

Many mediastinal tumors are capable of producing a variety of hormonal and chemical products (Table 5). Classic examples include hypercalcemia secondary to parathyroid hormone production by mediastinal parathyroid adenomas, Cushing's syndrome caused by ACTH-secreting carcinoid tumors, and arterial hypertension from catecholamine-secreting pheochromocytomas. Some tumors are associated with transient hypoglycemia secondary to production of insulin-like substances that lower serum glucose and usually are associated with normal levels of circulating insulin known as the *Doege-Potter syndrome*. Other symptom complexes associated with mediastinal masses cannot be as easily explained as those caused by hormonal production (Table 6). Osteoarthropathy associated with neurogenic tumors, chest pain associated with alcohol ingestion, and the cyclic *Pel-Ebstein fever* occurring with Hodgkin's disease are examples of disorders, the pathophysiology of which is not well understood. In other systemic syndromes, such as the association of myasthenia gravis, red cell aplasia, and a number of the other syndromes with benign and malignant thymomas, it is felt that an autoimmune mechanism is involved.

Diagnosis

HISTORY AND PHYSICAL EXAMINATION

The patient's history and a careful evaluation of the patient's symptoms frequently will assist in the localization of the tumor and may suggest the probable histologic diagnosis. The physical examination in patients with mediastinal tumors and cysts may frequently reveal positive findings. However, only rarely will a precise diagnosis be obtained by historic information or physical examination alone.

TABLE 4. Clinical Manifestations of Anatomic Invasion or Compression by Primary Lesions of the Mediastinum

Vena caval obstruction	Vocal cord paralysis
Pericardial tamponade	Horner's syndrome
Congestive heart failure	Paralyzed diaphragm
Arrhythmias	Chylothorax and
Acquired pulmonary stenosis	chylopericardium
Tracheal compression	Hemiplegia
Esophageal compression	Pancoast's syndrome

TABLE 5. Systemic Syndromes Caused by Hormonal Production by Mediastinal Neoplasms

Syndrome	Tumor
Hypertension	Pheochromocytoma, chemodectoma, ganglioneuroma, neuroblastoma
Hypercalcemia	Parathyroid, Hodgkin's disease
Hypoglycemia	Mesothelioma, teratoma, fibrosarcoma, neurosarcoma
Thyrotoxicosis	Thyroid
Cushing's disease	Carcinoid
Diarrhea	Ganglioneuroma, neuroblastoma
Gynecomastia	Germ cell tumors

TABLE 6. Systemic Syndromes Associated with Primary Mediastinal Tumors and Cysts

Syndrome	Tumor
Thymoma	Myasthenia gravis
	Pure red blood cell aplasia
	Hypogammaglobulinemia
	Megaesophagus
	Collagen vascular disease
	Dermatomyositis
	Myocarditis
	Malignancy
Lymphoma	Anemia
Neurofibroma	von Recklinghausen's disease
Carcinoid	Cushing's syndrome
Carcinoid, thymoma	Multiple endocrine adenomatosis
Thymoma, neurofibroma, neurilemmoma, mesothelioma	Osteoarthropathy
Enteric cysts	Vertebral anomalies
Hodgkin's disease	Alcohol-induced pain
	Pel-Ebstein fever
Neuroblastoma	Opsomyoclonus
Enteric cysts, neurilemmoma	Peptic ulcer

ROENTGENOGRAPHY

The basis of the diagnostic evaluation is the roentgenographic examination. The standard posteroanterior and lateral chest films are useful in localizing the mass within the mediastinum. Mediastinal neoplasms occur predictably in a particular subdivision of the mediastinum. Plain films may identify the relative density of the mass, whether solid or cystic, and the presence or absence of calcification. Ultrasound has been useful in delineating cystic structures and their location within the mediastinum. Fluoroscopy and barium swallow may further assist in the delineation of the contours of the mass and the relationship to other mediastinal structures, particularly the esophagus and great vessels.

Advances in nuclear medicine have been useful in the diagnosis of a number of tumors. Radioisotopic iodine scanning is useful in differentiating intrathoracic goiters from other superior mediastinal lesions. Gallium and technetium scanning have greatly improved the ability with which parathyroid adenomas are diagnosed and localized. Recently, advances in radiopharmacology have led to the accurate diagnosis of pheochromocytomas and enteric cysts containing gastric mucosa.

MONOCLONAL ANTIBODIES

The development of *monoclonal antibody* technology, with its subsequent application to the development of accurate radioimmunoassays, has been of great utility in the diagnosis of a number of mediastinal neoplasms. Alphafetoprotein and human chorionic gonadotropin measurements are of great importance in the diagnosis and differentiation of germ cell tumors. Hormone-producing tumors of the mediastinum may also be diagnosed using the newer radioimmunoassays. Future application of the monoclonal antibodies may include scanning techniques for a wide range of neoplasms dependent upon specific surface antigens characteristic for a given neoplasm.

COMPUTED TOMOGRAPHY

The greatest advance in the diagnosis and delineation of mediastinal masses in recent years has been the addition of CT scanning to the diagnostic armamentarium of clinicians. Providing an excellent cross-sectional anatomic definition of the mediastinum, CT is able to separate mediastinal masses from other mediastinal structures. Particularly with the use of intravenous contrast material to assist in the delineation of vascular structures, the CT scan is able to differentiate lesions of vascular origin from mediastinal neoplasms. Previously, angiographic studies were frequently needed to differentiate mediastinal masses from a variety of cardiac and aortic processes such as thoracic aneurysms and sinus of Valsalva aneurysms. With recent improvements in resolution, CT has become a much more sensitive diagnostic tool than routine radiographic techniques. It has been useful in the diagnosis of bronchogenic cysts in infants with recurrent infections and thymomas in patients with myasthenia gravis, cases in which plain films had frequently failed to detect any abnormalities. Computed tomography also provides considerable information regarding the relative invasiveness of mediastinal tumors. Differentiation between compression and invasion as manifested by disruption of the mediastinal fat planes can be made by careful examination. Additionally, in recent reports the preoperative diagnosis of a number of lesions, including pericardial cysts, parathyroid adenomas, enteric cysts, and tumors, has been made by CT owing to their characteristic appearances.

MAGNETIC RESONANCE IMAGING

Magnetic resonance imaging has the attractive potential of allowing differentiation of vascular structures from mediastinal masses without the use of contrast material or radiation. In the future, this technique may provide superior information regarding the presence or absence of malignancy within lymph nodes and tumor masses.

BIOPSY

Various invasive techniques for obtaining a tissue diagnosis are currently available. The marked improvement in cytologic techniques has allowed the use of fine-needle aspiration biopsies to be successful in diagnosing three quarters of patients with mediastinal lesions. The technique is especially useful in diagnosing metastatic disease in patients with known primary malignancy elsewhere. The utility of this technique in diagnosing primary tumors of the mediastinum remains to be defined.

In tumors such as lymphomas and germ cell tumors where surgical excision is not of prime importance in their treatment, the optimal therapeutic regimen requires a precise histologic subclassification, which usually cannot be obtained with the amount of specimen provided by the fineneedle biopsy. In these cases, mediastinoscopy has been utilized to evaluate resectability and make a tissue diagnosis. Particularly good results have been obtained with anterosuperior tumors and some middle mediastinal masses. However, it must be emphasized that median sternotomy or posterolateral thoracotomy may be performed with little or no increase in morbidity or mortality when compared with these procedures, and in cases with resectable lesions, surgical excision may be performed at the time of the initial procedure.

DIFFERENTIAL DIAGNOSIS

A number of intrathoracic and extrathoracic lesions may resemble primary mediastinal tumors and cysts. Cardiovascular abnormalities, such as aneurysms of the great vessels or heart, and abnormal vascular patterns occurring in congenital diseases may present as mediastinal masses on the chest film. Abnormalities of the spinal column, such as meningoceles, must be differentiated from posterior mediastinal masses. Lesions such as achalasia, esophageal diverticulum, diaphragmatic herniations, coarctation of the aorta, hiatal hernias, herniations of peritoneal fat, and mediastinitis may also resemble primary tumors and cysts. Through the use of CT and myelography as well as many of the other diagnostic modalities, most of these lesions should be differentiated from primary mediastinal masses prior to operative intervention.

Types of Tumors

NEUROGENIC TUMORS

Neurogenic tumors are the most common neoplasms encountered in the mediastinum, accounting for 21 per cent of all primary tumors and cysts in a collected series (see Table 1). Classically, these tumors arise from either intercostal nerves or the sympathetic ganglia and are usually located in the paravertebral gutter in the posterior mediastinum. Rarely, these tumors may be located in the anterior mediastinum. Although the peak incidence for neurogenic tumors occurs in adults, these tumors compose a high proportion of the mediastinal masses in children, accounting for 31 per cent of the mediastinal neoplasms seen in a collected series of children with primary mediastinal tumors and cysts (Table 7).[9, 10, 13, 24, 31] Approximately 10 to 20 per cent of neurogenic tumors are malignant, with a greater likelihood of malignancy occurring in infancy.

Many neurogenic tumors produce few symptoms and are found on routine chest films. Symptoms are usually the result of pressure on adjacent structures. Chest or back pain is usually the result of tumor compression or invasion of an intercostal nerve or erosion into adjacent bone. Cough and dyspnea are symptoms related to compression of the tracheobronchial tree. When they grow to sufficient size in the posterosuperior mediastinum, these tumors may cause Pancoast's or Horner's syndrome owing to compression of the brachial plexus or cervical sympathetic chain.

Approximately 10 per cent of neurogenic tumors have an intraspinal component and are referred to as "dumbbell tumors" because of the significant paravertebral and intraspinal components that are in continuity via the intervertebral foramen. In 60 per cent of patients with such lesions, symptoms of spinal cord compression are present. However, because a significant number of patients with dumbbell tumors do not provide symptoms indicating an intraspinal component, it is recommended that the evaluation of these masses include CT or vertebral tomography. In those patients with evidence of intervertebral widening, myelography should be performed. Most recent series recommend a one-stage removal of dumbbell tumors using a team approach composed of thoracic surgeons and neurosurgeons.

A number of neurogenic tumors are also capable of producing hormones that result in a variety of systemic syndromes. Catecholamine production by pheochromocytomas and neuroblastomas is associated with the classic syndrome of episodic or sustained hypertension, sweating, headache, and palpitations. Ganglioneuromas and neuroblastomas may produce vasoactive intestinal polypeptide, causing a syndrome composed of abdominal distention and profuse watery diarrhea. Neurosarcomas, through either a primary secretion of insulin or another secondary messenger that stimulates pancreatic release of insulin, have been associated with recurrent hypoglycemic episodes.

Neurilemmomas

Neurilemmomas are the most common neurogenic tumors arising from the Schwann cells of the nerve sheath. Frequently called *schwannomas*, these tumors have a peak incidence between the third and fifth decades. Histologically, neurilemmomas have two characteristic appearances. The Antoni Type A pattern is manifested by an organized architecture with a cellular palisading pattern of growth. The Antoni Type B appearance has a loose reticular pattern. These tumors are grossly well encapsulated and appear as dense, homogeneous, well-circumscribed masses in the paravertebral region of the mediastinum on chest roentgenography.

Neurofibromas

Neurofibromas are formed by a combined proliferation of all the elements of the peripheral nerves. These tumors differ from neurilemmomas in that they are not well encapsulated, and microscopically they are composed of randomly arranged spindle-shaped cells. Both neurilemmomas and neurofibromas may be seen as a manifestation of neurofibromatosis (*von Recklinghausen's disease*). These tumors must be differentiated from meningiomas and meningoceles, both of which may also occur in patients with neurofibromatosis.

Neurosarcomas

In 25 to 30 per cent of neurofibromas or neurilemmomas, malignant degeneration may occur, resulting in the formation of a neurosarcoma. Microscopically, neurosar-

TABLE 7. Relative Frequency of Primary Mediastinal Tumors and Cysts in 518 Children

	Haller et al.	Grosfeld et al.	Whittaker and Lynn	Pokorny and Sherman	Heimburger and Battersby	Boyd and Mitchell	Duke Series	Totals	Incidence (%)
Neurogenic tumor	18	36	37	35	9	41	26	202	39
Lymphoma	9	20	9	27	3	12	13	93	18
Germ cell neoplasm	8	5	21	4	4	5	11	58	11
Primary malignancy	10	0	0	6	0	0	1	17	3
Cysts									
Pericardial	1	0	0	0	0	1	3	5	1
Bronchogenic	4	0	5	11	8	6	14	48	9
Enteric	6	6	7	3	2	0	5	29	6
Other	0	0	2	3	0	11	4	20	4
Mesenchymal tumor	7	1	13	8	6	0	5	40	8
Other							6	6	1
Total	63	68	94	97	32	76	88	518	

comas have the appearance of an extremely cellular spindle cell neoplasm. Except when seen as a manifestation of neurofibromatosis, these tumors are usually found in adults. Owing to the tumor's rapid growth and invasiveness, complete surgical excision is rarely possible, and adjuvant therapies have been unsuccessful in prolonging survival.

Gangliomas

Gangliomas are benign tumors originating from the sympathetic chain and are composed of ganglion cells and neural elements. Occurring more frequently in children than the other neurogenic tumors, these tumors may attain very large size before becoming symptomatic. Grossly, these lesions are well encapsulated with a smooth external surface. On cross-section these tumors will frequently have areas of cystic degeneration. Classically gangliomas have an elongated or triangular appearance on chest film with the broader base pointing toward the mediastinum. These tumors are poorly defined on lateral projection, and they frequently have an indistinct inferior and superior margin.

Ganglioneuroblastomas

Ganglioneuroblastomas are tumors showing an intermediate degree of differentiation between neuroblastomas and ganglioneuromas containing mature and immature ganglion cells. Two different histologic patterns exist as defined by Stout. Composite ganglioneuroblastomas histologically are composed predominantly of tissue containing mature neuroblasts with discrete nodules containing primitive neuroblasts. The diffuse ganglioneuroblastoma contains a diffuse mixture of primitive and well-differentiated neuroblasts. Composite ganglioneuroblastomas have a much greater predisposition to metastasize, with most series reporting an incidence between 65 and 75 per cent.[1] Less than 5 per cent of diffuse pattern ganglioneuroblastomas metastasize. Younger patients and those with an earlier clinical stage tumor have the best prognosis.

Circumscribed noninvasive tumors are defined as Stage I lesions. Stage II lesions are defined as tumors with invasion of adjacent soft tissue without extension across the midline. In Stage I and II disease, a 5-year survival rate of 88 per cent has been reported in one series of 80 patients. Multiagent chemotherapy, which is the basis of treatment for neuroblastomas, may be withheld in the treatment of ganglioneuroblastomas except in Stage III (local invasion across the midline), Stage IV disease (metastatic spread), in patients older than 3 years, or in those patients with tumors that fit the composite histologic pattern.

Neuroblastomas

Neuroblastomas are the least differentiated malignancies derived from the sympathetic nervous system. Although the majority of these tumors occur retroperitoneally in the adrenal location, 10 to 20 per cent occur as primary lesions in the mediastinum. Metastases are often present at the time of diagnosis in the regional lymph nodes, bone, brain, liver, and lung. Neuroblastoma primarily occurs in children, with more than 75 per cent occurring in those under 4 years. Histologically these tumors are composed of small, round, immature cells growing in a rosette pattern. Owing to the aggressive nature of these tumors, neuroblastomas are usually symptomatic at the time of diagnosis. Local mass effects frequently produce symptoms of cough, dysphagia, dyspnea, back pain, and recurrent pulmonary

infections. Hormonal production is not uncommon, as these tumors have been known to produce catecholamines and vasoactive intestinal polypeptides. An unexplained symptom complex of acute cerebellar and truncal ataxia with rapid darting eye movements (dancing eyes), known as the opsoclonus-polymyoclonus syndrome, has been described in association with neuroblastomas. The presumptive etiology of this syndrome is an autoimmune process.

Treatment. A majority of patients with this syndrome will respond to tumor control or corticosteroids. Treatment for neuroblastomas is dependent upon the stage of the disease. Staging is the same as with ganglioneuroblastomas. Surgical excision is adequate for Stage I disease. Radiation therapy is added in cases of Stage II disease. Stage III or IV disease is treated with a combination of surgical debulking, radiation therapy, and multiagent chemotherapy. Children younger than 1 year of age have an excellent prognosis even when found to have widespread disease. However, with increasing age and increasing extent of involvement, the prognosis markedly worsens. Mediastinal neuroblastomas, however, appear to have a better survival rate than those neuroblastomas found elsewhere.

Immunobiology. The immunobiology of neuroblastomas is unique. Cases of spontaneous regression or maturation into ganglioneuromas are well documented. Lymphocytes obtained from patients whose tumors have regressed demonstrate cytotoxicity to neuroblastoma cells *in vitro*, whereas patients who have progression of disease appear to produce blocking factors that are presumably antigen antibody complexes. These factors are capable of inhibiting the cytotoxic activities of the lymphocytes acquired from patients exhibiting tumor regression.

Pheochromocytomas

Mediastinal pheochromocytomas account for less than 1 per cent of all pheochromocytomas, with the majority occurring in the paravertebral sulcus of the posterior mediastinum. However an increasing number of middle mediastinal pheochromocytomas have been found arising from the extra-adrenal chromaffin tissue present in the brachial arch structures, coronary and aortopulmonary paraganglia, the atria, and islands of tissue in the pericardium. Catecholamine production by these tumors produces the classic symptom complex of periodically or sustained hypertension, sweating, palpitations, and headaches. Measurement of elevated urinary or serum catecholamines is usually diagnostic. Extra-adrenal pheochromocytomas usually produce norepinephrine and only rarely epinephrine in contrast to adrenal pheochromocytomas, which usually produce both hormones.

Tumor localization has been greatly assisted by the combined use of CT and [1-131]meta-iodobenzylguanidine (I-131 MIBG) scintigraphy.[27] In 30 per cent of cases a tumor blush may be seen during thoracic arteriography due to the highly vascular nature of these tumors. Differentiation between benign and malignant pheochromocytomas requires that the patient's clinical course be followed. Although 50 per cent of these tumors appear histologically malignant, in only 3 per cent of cases will metastatic disease develop. Alpha-methyl tyramine, a tyrosine hydroxylase inhibitor that blocks the production of catecholamines, is useful in alleviating the symptoms present with metastatic disease. Especially in patients with the multiple endocrine neoplastic syndrome, if removal of an intra-abdominal pheochromocytoma fails to return the patient to a normotensive status, a search for a mediastinal pheochromocytoma should be performed.

Chemodectomas or Nonchromaffin Paragangliomas

Chemodectomas or nonchromaffin paragangliomas arise from chemoreceptor tissues around the aortic arch, pulmonary artery, and vagus nerves. Despite a similar histologic appearance, these tumors are different from pheochromocytomas because of their negative chromaffin reaction. Historically, this was thought to indicate that these tumors were hormonally inactive. However, with the use of radioimmunoassays a minority of these tumors have been found to secrete catecholamines. Like pheochromocytomas, these tumors are determined to be malignant by clinical criteria of invasion or metastic disease. In a review of 35 patients with aortic body tumors, 16 died as a direct result of the tumor or were found to have evidence of metastatic disease.

THYMOMAS

Thymomas are the second most frequent lesions of the mediastinum and the most common found in the antero-superior mediastinum. They represented 20 per cent of the 2400 primary tumors and cysts in the collected series. Rarely found in patients under 20 years of age, thymomas have a peak incidence in the third through fifth decades of life. The roentgenographic appearance ranges from a small, circumscribed lesion to a bulky lobulated density confluent with adjacent mediastinal structures. Thymomas are usually symptomatic at the time of diagnosis. Over 70 per cent of patients at Duke University Medical Center with thymomas had symptoms at the time of presentation. As with other mediastinal masses, thymomas may present with symptoms related to local mass effects, including chest pain, dyspnea, hemoptysis, cough, or symptoms related to superior vena caval obstruction.

Myasthenia Gravis

Thymomas are also frequently associated with systemic syndromes. Myasthenia gravis is the most frequently associated syndrome, occurring in 10 to 50 per cent of patients with thymomas. Myasthenia gravis is characterized clinically by weakness and fatigue of the voluntary muscles. Current theories suggest that the disease is due to an autoimmune process directed against the postsynaptic nicotinic acetylcholine receptors. The incidence with which myasthenia gravis occurs in patients with a thymoma appears to increase with advancing age of the patient. In males over 50 years of age and females over 60 years of age with thymomas, the incidence appears to be greater than 80 per cent.[19] It must be emphasized that many patients with myasthenia gravis do not have thymomas, and the incidence ranges from 10 to 42 per cent. Male patients with myasthenia gravis are approximately 1.8 to 2 times more likely to have a thymoma than females.

It was previously held that myasthenia gravis associated with thymoma portended a poor prognosis. However, with improved anesthesia and medical management, the prognosis appears to be dependent upon the stage of the tumor at the time of diagnosis and is not significantly altered by the presence or absence of coexisting myasthenia gravis.[26]

Since Blalock's pioneering work in 1939, surgical removal of the thymus gland has been a major aspect of treatment of myasthenia gravis. In conjunction with advances in anesthesia, the advent of plasmapheresis, and improving medications, surgical therapy has proved increasingly beneficial. Surgical excision of the thymus in patients both with and without thymomas has proved effective, with reduction in symptoms and a decrease in the need for medical support. In a series of 47 patients undergoing total thymectomy after plasmapheresis, 83 per cent were asymptomatic and 61 per cent required no medication.[21] Use of a median sternotomy approach for extended thymectomy, which includes thymectomy with removal of all anterior mediastinal fat and all ectopic foci of thymic tissue in the mediastinum or neck, has led to improved clinical benefit with fewer recurrences of thymoma. Recurrence of thymoma after use of the transcervical approach for thymectomy is well documented. In addition, extended thymectomy has been shown to achieve significantly better symptomatic improvement than that seen following simple thymectomy.

The pathophysiology of the clinical improvement in patients with myasthenia gravis after thymectomy is not completely understood. The acetylcholine receptor antibody titer is not necessarily decreased following thymectomy and may in fact be increased despite marked improvement in the patient's symptoms.

Other Systemic Syndromes

Other systemic syndromes associated with thymoma include red cell aplasia, Cushing's syndrome, hypogammaglobulinemia, dermatomyositis, systemic lupus erythematosus, rheumatoid arthritis, megaesophagus, and granulomatous myocarditis. Red cell aplasia occurs in 5 per cent of patients with thymomas. In 33 to 50 per cent of adults with red cell aplasia, a thymoma is present.

Histologic Classification

Histologically, thymomas are classified by the predominance of epithelial or lymphocytic cells. Previous classifications into predominantly epithelial, mixed lymphoepithelial, or predominantly lymphocytic cells are arbitrary in that there exists a wide variance of patterns with regard to cellular type within a tumor. More important, a consistent association cannot be made between histologic appearance and biologic behavior or predisposition to the development of any of the associated systemic syndromes. Differentiation between benign and malignant histology requires microscopic or gross evidence of invasion into adjacent mediastinal structures or evidence of metastasis. Most series report that between 15 and 65 per cent of thymomas are benign. These benign tumors are well encapsulated without evidence of invasion into the capsule either grossly or histologically (Stage I). Tumors with pericapsular growth into adjacent mediastinal fat or tissues or invading only the adjacent pleura or pericardium are designated as Stage II. Tumors exhibiting invasive growth into surrounding organs or with the presence of intrathoracic metastasis are classified as Stage III. Extrathoracic metastatic spread is infrequent.

Treatment

Therapy for thymomas is based primarily on surgical excision, when possible, with extended thymectomy in those with well-circumscribed lesions. Complete surgical resection with excision of nonvital contiguous structures is recommended for Stage II tumors. Many thymomas are radiosensitive, and placement of surgical clips to outline the extent of anatomic disease in preparation for postoperative radiotherapy is frequently helpful. Radiation therapy is usually given (3500 to 5000 rads) for Stage II and Stage III tumors. Preoperative radiation therapy is frequently used in the presence of superior vena caval obstruction or with extensive invasion as shown by CT or magnetic resonance imaging. Multiagent chemotherapy has been of little benefit in the treatment of malignant thymomas.

GERM CELL TUMORS

Germ cell tumors are identical histologically to those found in the gonads. However, they are thought to arise from primordial mediastinal germ cells that fail to complete the migration from the urogenital ridge and not as a result of metastatic spread from the gonads. Germ cell tumors are classified as seminomas, embryonal cell carcinomas, choriocarcinomas, yolk sac tumors, teratocarcinomas, and, in the most well-differentiated state, teratodermoid tumors.

Teratomas

Teratomas are neoplasms composed of multiple tissue elements foreign to the area in which they occur. Teratomas are most frequently present in the anterior mediastinum (Fig. 3) found frequently at the level of the pericardial reflection. They made up 9 per cent of the mediastinal neoplasms in the collected series of primary tumors and cysts. Histologically, they are composed of elements derived from the three primitive embryonic layers. *Dermoid cysts* are the simplest histologic form of teratoma. They are composed predominantly of epidermal tissue, including dermal and epidermal glands, hair, and sebaceous material. They are usually found in unilobular but occasionally multilobular cysts. Careful examination of the cyst wall of dermoid tumors usually reveals tissue derived from endodermal and mesodermal layers. The composition of teratomas is more complex. The solid components of the tumor contain well-differentiated elements of bone, cartilage, teeth, muscle connective tissue, fibrous and lymphoid tissue, nerve, thymus, mucous and salivary glands, pancreas, lung, or liver. The peak incidence of diagnosis is in the second and third decades of life. Teratomas occur with equal frequency in both sexes.

Patients with teratomas usually present with symptoms related to local mass effects, such as chest pain, cough, dyspnea, or postobstructive pneumonitis. In cases in which a communication between the tumor and the tracheobronchial tree develops, pathognomonic symptoms of a cough productive of hair or sebaceous material may occur. Hemoptysis or recurrent infections caused by the irritative

effects of the tumor by contiguous spread from a hematogenously infected cyst may develop. Unusual presentations of these tumors include recurrent pericarditis or pericardial tamponade following invasion or rupture into the pericardium. Because of the marked irritative effects of the cyst fluid, rupture into the pleural space may result in respiratory distress. With the increased use of chest films in clinical practice, a greater proportion of these tumors are being discovered while still asymptomatic and of small size. In a series of patients with teratomas seen between 1930 and 1981, 64 per cent of patients were symptomatic at the time of presentation.[17] More recently, 50 per cent of the patients with teratomas seen at the Duke University Medical Center over the past 20 years were symptomatic.

Diagnosis of these tumors may be made on routine chest roentgenography by the finding of well-formed teeth. A predominantly fatty mass with a denser dependent element containing globular calcifications, bone, or teeth and a solid protuberance extending into a cystic cavity are findings by CT scan that are considered specific. Despite characteristic appearances, differentiation between benign and malignant teratomas depends on histologic examination. Therefore, diagnosis and therapy rely on surgical excision. Even partial resection of benign tumors whose size and mediastinal involvement made them irresectable has resulted in resolution of symptoms.

Malignant germ cell tumors arise predominantly in the anterior mediastinum and account for approximately 4 per cent of the primary tumors and cysts in a collective series. Males are much more frequently affected. The peak incidence is in the third and fourth decades of life. Clinically these tumors are usually symptomatic at presentation. Symptoms of chest pain, cough, shortness of breath, or hemoptysis or symptoms indicative of superior vena caval obstruction are most frequent. The chest film usually shows a large anterior mediastinal mass that is often multilobulated. Computed tomography is most useful in defining the extent of involvement and in monitoring results following initiation of therapy. Germ cell tumors metastasize most frequently to the pleura, lung, chest wall, lymph nodes, liver, bone, and retroperitoneum.

Seminomas

Because of the marked radiosensitivity of seminomas, the most important distinction made between germ cell tumors is that between seminomas and non-seminomas.

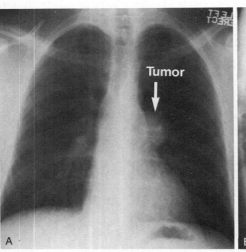
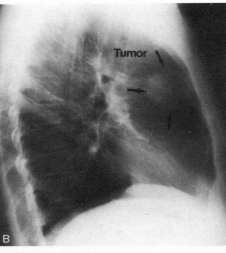

Figure 3. A and B, *Chest films showing teratoma of the anterior mediastinum.*

Seminomas, in addition, tend to remain more indolent and are more frequently localized within the mediastinum without extrathoracic metastatic spread. Only 7 per cent of seminomas produce beta human choriogonadotropin, and, when produced, only low titers can be measured. Seminomas do not produce alpha-fetoprotein. The presence of a measurable amount of alpha-fetoprotein implies a significant non-seminomatous component without the tumor. Patients with seminomas have a relatively good prognosis. With surgical excision or radiation therapy, 5-year survival rates of 75 per cent have been reported. Even with documented recurrences or metastatic disease, the use of cis-platinum–based chemotherapeutic regimens has been successful in effecting disease-free remission in patients with seminomas.[4]

Non-seminomas

Non-seminoma germ cell tumors are more aggressive, with frequent widespread dissemination at the time of diagnosis. These lesions are infrequently radiosensitive. Over 90 per cent of non-seminomas elaborate either beta human choriogonadotropin or alpha-fetoprotein. Historically, patients with non-seminomas have a very poor prognosis. Only 2 of 63 patients reported in the literature between 1964 and 1978 survived longer than 16 months. However, with the use of cis-platinum–based chemotherapeutic regimens the mean survival has increased from 4 to 14 months. Using complete surgical excision after preoperative treatment with a cis-platinum–based multiagent chemotherapeutic regimen, 4 of 12 patients are alive and

well without evidence of disease at 12, 15, 30 and 56 months after surgical excision.[6, 30]

LYMPHOMAS

The mediastinum is frequently involved in cases of disseminated lymphomas, with approximately 40 to 60 per cent of patients having mediastinal involvement sometime during the disease course. Much less frequently is the mediastinum the sole site of disease at the time of diagnosis. Hodgkin's disease, particularly the nodular sclerosing subtype, occurs with sole mediastinal involvement in approximately 5 per cent of cases at the time of diagnosis. Non-Hodgkin's lymphoma may be localized in the mediastinum in 6 per cent of cases. These non-Hodgkin's tumors tend to have a diffuse histologic pattern. The poorly differentiated lymphocytic or diffuse large cell histologic types are the most frequently seen. Non-Hodgkin's lymphomas typically have a more extensive contiguous pattern of spread, involving the pericardium, sternum, chest wall, and pulmonary parenchyma with frequent superior vena caval obstruction. Lymphomas usually are seen on the chest film as large anterosuperior mediastinal or hilar masses (Fig. 4). There is no difference in incidence between the sexes.

Patients with lymphomas of the mediastinum are usually symptomatic at the time of presentation. As with other malignant tumors of the anterior mediastinum, symptoms of cough, shortness of breath, chest pain, hoarseness, and superior vena caval obstruction are those most frequently encountered. In addition, in cases where the lymphomatous process has encased the pulmonary artery, an initial diag-

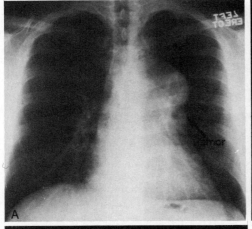
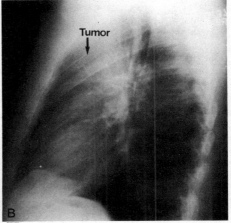
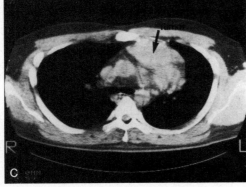

Figure 4. Hodgkin's disease of the anterior mediastinum. A and B, Chest films. C, Computed tomography better delineates the extensive nature of the tumor.

nosis of pulmonary embolism has been made. Pulmonary angiography has been required to make the correct diagnosis. Nonspecific symptoms of fevers and chills, weight loss, and anorexia are frequently described. The cyclic fevers as described by Pel and Ebstein and chest pain following alcohol ingestion are symptoms characteristic of Hodgkin's lymphomas.

Newer multiagent chemotherapeutic regimens and radiation therapy have resulted in marked improvement in patient survival. Currently, the role of surgical intervention is limited to providing adequate tissue for diagnosis and precise histologic subclassification. This subtyping usually requires a larger tumor specimen than can be obtained using needle biopsy techniques.

PRIMARY CARCINOMAS

Primary carcinoma of the mediastinum comprises approximately 3 to 11 per cent of primary mediastinal tumors. In the collected series, primary carcinoma comprised 4 per cent of the lesions. These tumors usually occur in the anterosuperior or middle mediastinum. The histogenesis of primary carcinomas in the mediastinum remains unclear.

It is important to differentiate these tumors from malignant thymomas, germ cell tumors, lymphomas, mediastinal extension from a bronchogenic carcinoma, and metastatic tumor. Metastasis to the mediastinum is usually from malignancies of the lung or esophagus. Metastatic disease from extrathoracic neoplasm is much less frequently encountered. Only 2.3 per cent of 1071 patients with extrathoracic neoplasms developed evidence of hilar or mediastinal lymph node involvement over a 2-year period as determined by serial chest roentgenography. Tumors of the head and neck, genitourinary tract, and breast and malignant melanoma are the most likely to metastasize to the mediastinum. Primary carcinomas of the mediastinum histologically are most frequently the large cell undifferentiated type, although small cell and squamous cell tumors have been described. The increasing use of electron microscopy and immunohistochemical staining may further characterize the origin of some of these tumors.

Although most previous reports have noted a male predominance, over the past 20 years there was an equal sex distribution in those patients diagnosed with primary carcinomas at Duke University Medical Center. The majority of patients are symptomatic at the time of diagnosis. Cough, chest pain, shortness of breath, hoarseness, and dysphagia are commonly described. A large percentage of patients with primary carcinomas have evidence of superior vena caval obstruction. Most primary carcinomas have diffuse spread within the mediastinum or evidence of extrathoracic metastasis, which prevents an effective surgical excision.

Despite the routine use of multiagent chemotherapeutic regimens and radiation therapy, these tumors characteristically pursue a rapidly fatal course. Two of 32 patients at Duke University Medical Center are alive at 6 and 11 years after surgical excision and biopsy with radiation therapy, respectively. A third patient died 7 years after surgical biopsy and radiation therapy of complications secondary to a ruptured aortic abdominal aneurysm. There was no evidence of carcinoma at the time of autopsy.

ENDOCRINE TUMORS

Although substernal thyroid adenoma is common, these lesions are usually attached to the cervical thyroid gland. Truly *intrathoracic thyroid tumors* are quite rare and comprise 1 per cent of all mediastinal masses in the current collected series. Among 17,000 patients undergoing thyroidectomy, only 135 intrathoracic goiters were encountered. These tumors arise from heterotopic thyroid tissue found in the anterior mediastinum, but they also may occur in the middle mediastinum between the trachea and esophagus or in the posterior mediastinum. Intrathoracic goiter must be differentiated from the more common occurrence of a substernal extension of a cervical goiter. Unlike the latter circumstance, mediastinal thyroid tumors usually derive their blood supply from thoracic vessels. However, there may be a demonstrable connection with the cervical thyroid gland.

The peak incidence is in the six and seventh decades of life, and females are more frequently affected than males. Symptoms are usually related to compression of the trachea causing dyspnea, cough, shortness of breath, wheezing, or stridor. In those tumors occurring in the posterior mediastinum, compression of the esophagus usually is manifested by symptoms of dysphagia. Rarely, symptoms related to thyrotoxicosis may cause the patient to seek medical attention. Chest roentgenography is usually not helpful in making the diagnosis. However, the use of the thyroid scan utilizing radioactive iodine is usually diagnostic in cases where functioning thyroid tissue exists. Thyroid scanning should be performed preoperatively in those patients with asymptomatic anterosuperior mediastinal masses to document functioning cervical thyroid tissue and prevent the excision of the sole functioning thyroid tissue.

Histologically most tumors are adenomas; however, intrathoracic carcinomas have occurred. In cases where the intrathoracic thyroid is not causing symptoms and is the only demonstrably functioning thyroid tissue, surgical exploration and excision are not indicated. However, all symptomatic lesions should be excised when possible. Owing to the thoracic derivation of its blood supply, intrathoracic thyroid tumors are better approached via a median sternotomy when the tumor is localized in the anterior mediastinum or a posterolateral thoracotomy when present in the middle or posterior mediastinum. In contrast, most standard substernal extensions of a cervical goiter can be excised using a cervical incision.

PARATHYROID TUMORS

In approximately 10 per cent of cases of hyperfunctioning parathyroid glands, a parathyroid adenoma is found in the mediastinum. In the majority the parathyroid adenoma is located in the anterosuperior aspect of the mediastinum, usually embedded or near the superior pole of the thymus.

The close relation to the thymus is associated with the parathyroid glands' embryogenesis from the third and fourth branchial clefts. The thymus is derived from the third branchial cleft. Thus, those glands derived from that cleft will have a close embryologic relationship to the thymus, explaining their proximity in the mediastinum. Rarely, parathyroid tissues are found in the posterior mediastinum. These glands, however, usually have a vascular pedicle that extends into the cervical region to the thyroid gland.

Manifestations of mediastinal parathyroid adenomas are similar to those found in the neck, including hypercalcemia and a variety of systemic symptoms due to excess parathyroid hormone secretion. Because of their small size, parathyroid lesions are rarely visualized using conventional roentgenography or barium swallow. The use of CT, thallium and technetium scanning, venous angiography with selective sampling, and selective arteriography has greatly improved the ability to localize these tumors preoperatively. Preoperative localization is probably possible in less than 80 per cent.

Most frequently the mediastinal parathyroid adenoma may be excised via a cervical incision at the same time that the neck exploration is undertaken. Parathyroids that have descended further into the mediastinum or in patients who are being re-explored for persistent hyperparathyroidism are better approached using a median sternotomy. Parathyroid cysts are defined as those cysts with parathyroid cells identifiable within the cyst wall. These cysts are only rarely associated with hyperparathyroidism. They are usually larger than parathyroid adenomas and more frequently cause symptoms due to local mass effects. They are also more likely to be seen on routine chest film. Parathyroid carcinomas in the mediastinum have been reported, and these tumors are usually hormonally active.

Carcinoid Tumors

Carcinoid tumors in the mediastinum arise from cells of Kultchitsky found in the thymus. These tumors are routinely found in the anterior mediastinum. Mediastinal carcinoid tumors are much more frequently diagnosed in male patients. Unlike thymomas, these tumors are not associated with myasthenia gravis or red cell aplasia nor do these tumors ever exhibit signs or symptoms consistent with the carcinoid syndrome. However, as tumors derived from the APUD system they may be associated with hormonal production and the multiple endocrine neoplastic syndromes.

Frequently, mediastinal carcinoids have been associated with Cushing's syndrome through the ectopic secretion of ACTH. In a series of 15 patients with mediastinal carcinoids, six had tumors producing ectopic ACTH[32] and five had clinical evidence of Cushing's syndrome. In addition, one of the 15 had Type I multiple endocrine neoplastic syndrome and three others had evidence of possible multiple endocrine neoplastic syndromes. In those tumors without evidence of hormonal production, the neoplasms were large and frequently had extensive local invasion resulting in symptoms of chest pain, dyspnea, or cough or evidence of superior vena caval obstruction. Metastatic spread to mediastinal and cervical lymph nodes, liver, bone, skin, or lungs occurs in the majority of cases. Among the 15 patients, 73 per cent developed metastic spread. Late metastatic spread is not uncommon, as three of the 15 did not exhibit metastases until five, six, and eight years, respectively.

Histologically, these tumors are difficult to differentiate from thymomas or germ cell tumors. The findings of *dense core neurosecretory granules* by electron microscopy or immunohistochemical staining of ACTH confirms the diagnosis of a carcinoid tumor.

Surgical excision is dependent on the extent of local invasion. Radiation therapy and multiagent chemotherapy have been used as adjunctive agents to surgical excision or when surgical excision has not been possible. Unfortunately, consistent benefit from these two modalities has not been documented.

Mesenchymal Tumors

Mediastinal mesenchymal tumors are a diverse group of neoplasms that originate from connective tissues, fat, striatal and smooth muscle, lymph, and blood vessels. The soft tissue masses include lipomas, liposarcomas, fibromatosis, fibrosarcomas, xanthogranulomas, leiomyomas, leiomyosarcomas, benign and malignant mesenchymomas, rhabdomyosarcomas, and mesotheliomas.

Relative to other sites in the body, these are uncommon tumors, composing only 7 per cent of the primary tumors and cysts in the collected series. There is no difference in incidence between sexes. The tumors have a similar histopathologic appearance and follow generally the same clinical course as tumors found elsewhere in the body. Fifty-five per cent of the patients with mesenchymal masses have malignant disease. The symptoms related to local extension are more likely with malignant disease or large benign masses. Surgical excision remains the primary treatment, with little benefit exhibited from the use of various chemotherapy agents or radiation therapy.

Mesenchymal tumors of blood and lymph vessel origin are common in other areas of the body but are exceedingly rare in the mediastinum. The histologic types include capillary, cavernous, and venous hemangiomas, hemangioendotheliomas, hemangiopericytomas, lymphangiomas, and lymphangiomyomas. These tumors are found throughout the mediastinum; however, they are most frequently found in the anterior mediastinum.

The symptoms are usually correlated with the size of the lesion and local invasion. In cases of rapid expansion, as with hemorrhage into these masses, progressive respiratory embarrassment may occur. Rupture of hemangiomas may result in exsanguination or, if the rupture is limited to the mediastinal space, mediastinal tamponade. Capillary, cavernous, and venous hemangiomas are differentiated histologically by the size of the vascular space and the presence of smooth muscle cells within the vascular wall. Hemangioendotheliomas are characterized by proliferation of the endothelial cells inside the reticulum sheath of the capillaries. Hemangiopericytomas, on the other hand, are characterized by proliferation of pericytes around the reticulum sheath of the capillaries. Hemangiopericytomas have the highest incidence of malignancy and usually occur in older patients.

Malignancy has been reported to be between 10 and 30 per cent in vascular tumors, and differentiation between benign and malignant lesions may be difficult. The histologic appearance, number of mitotic figures, and gross appearance of benign and malignant vascular tumors are quite similar. Vascular tumors are not well encapsulated, and even benign tumors may show evidence of local invasion. The incidence of metastatic spread remains low (approximately 3 per cent). The absence of large vessels supplying mediastinal vascular tumors prevents opacification during angiographic studies. Local excision remains the only effective means of therapy, although radiation therapy has been utilized.

Tumors originating from lymph vessels may present as small, discrete lesions or as large cysts of either unilocular or multilocular form. Usually found in the anterior mediastinum, lymphatic tumors appear as rounded or lobulated densities on the chest film. Chylothorax or chylopericardium may be associated. Differentiating tumors of lymph vessel origin from tumors of blood vessel origin is based on indirect evidence, such as the absence of red blood cells within the lumen, the extrusion of chylous fluid from cut tumor surfaces, or the tumor's relationship to documented lymphatic tissue.

The most common histologic entity is the lymphangioma, which has also been called cystic hygroma, lymphatic cyst, and lymphaginous cyst. In the majority of cases, mediastinal lymphangiomas are located in the superior mediastinum as an extension of a cervical lesion. These tumors usually present in childhood and cause symptoms due to obstruction of the trachea, producing stridor, recurrent respiratory tract infections, or tachypnea. The origin of these tumors is unknown. Their growth is by proliferation of endothelium-lined buds that spread along tissue planes. Local ingrowth of vessels and fibrous reaction to these endothelial buds prevent easy surgical removal owing to the lack of well-defined tissue planes. Injection of sclerosing agents or use of radiation therapy has not been of great utility and is not recommended. Lymphangiomyomas or lymphangiopericytomas are rare tumors that present in similar fashion to lymphangiomas with frequent local invasion but without distant metastases.

Extramedullary hematopoiesis occurs in the newborn or the adult. In the adult it occurs as a response to altered hematopoiesis, such as following massive hemolysis, myelofibrosis, spherocytic anemia, or thalassemias. This lesion is composed of hematopoietic tissue usually located in the posterior mediastinum. The extramedullary hematopoietic tissue is readily labeled by the radioisotope-labeled gold, allowing differentiation from other posterior mediastinal masses in patients with known hematologic abnormalities.

OTHER LESIONS

Angiofollicular lymphoid hyperplasia, as described initially by Castleman, is a rare tumor composed of hyperplastic lymphoid tissue with scattered hyalinized centers of lymphoid follicles. These tumors are usually found in the anterior mediastinum and are most frequently asymptomatic. Usually they are detected on a routine chest film. Surgical excision results in cure.

Chondromas are extremely rare tumors arising in the posterior mediastinum. They originate from the remnants of the primitive notochord. Males are affected twice as frequently as females, with the highest incidence occurring in the fifth, sixth, and seventh decades of life. Growing from the intervertebral notochord rest, this tumor may grow toward the prevertebral area, presenting as a posterior mediastinal mass with symptoms of chest pain, cough, or dysphagia. Chondromas may also grow into the spinal cord, producing signs and symptoms of spinal cord compression. Radical surgical excision remains the only effective therapy, although the majority of patients develop distant metastasis. The mean length of survival is approximately 17.5 months from the time of diagnosis.

Types of Cysts

Cysts of the mediastinum comprise approximately 20 per cent of the lesions in the collected series. Cysts may be bronchogenic, pericardial, enteric, thymic, or of an unspecified nature, and more than 75 per cent are asymptomatic. However, it is important to differentiate these lesions from malignant tumors. Also, because of the proximity in which vital structures exist within the mediastinum, even benign cysts may cause significant morbidity with increasing size.

PERICARDIAL CYSTS

Pericardial cysts are the most frequently encountered cysts within the mediastinum, accounting for 6.5 per cent of all lesions and 33 per cent of primary cysts. Most frequently found in the middle and anterior mediastinum,

pericardial cysts classically occur in the cardiophrenic angles. Seventy per cent occur in the *right* cardiophrenic angle and 22 per cent in the left. Embryologically, these cysts are thought to develop either from a failure of fusion of one or more mesenchymal lacunae that coalesce to form the pericardium or as a persistent ventral parietal recess of the pericardial coelom. The pericardial cyst may or may not have a communication with the pericardium. Numerous reports have described the characteristic CT appearance of pericardial cysts. Subsequent needle aspiration or follow-up with serial computed tomograms, rather than surgical excision, has been used to manage these patients. Since they rarely cause symptoms, surgical excision of pericardial cysts is indicated primarily for diagnosis and to differentiate these cysts from malignant lesions.

BRONCHOGENIC CYSTS

Bronchogenic cysts are the second most common cysts in the mediastinum, comprising 5 per cent of primary mediastinal masses and 33 per cent of cysts. They originate as sequestrations from the ventral foregut, which is the antecedent to the tracheobronchial tree. The bronchogenic cyst may lie within the lung parenchyma or the mediastinum. The cyst wall is composed of cartilage, mucous glands, smooth muscle, and fibrous tissue with an inner layer of ciliated respiratory epithelium. When bronchogenic cysts occur in the mediastinum, they are usually located proximal to the trachea or bronchi and may be just posterior to the carina. Rarely, a true communication between the cyst and the tracheobronchial tree exists, in which case an air-fluid level may be seen on the chest film.

Clinical Presentation

Two thirds of patients with bronchogenic cysts are asymptomatic. These cysts may cause severe respiratory compromise by compressing the trachea or the bronchus, and compression of the bronchus may cause bronchial stenosis and recurrent pneumonitis. Since these tumors are sometimes not well seen when occurring below the carina, the routine use of CT has been recommended to evaluate children with recurrent pulmonary infections for a possible bronchogenic cyst. More often, these tumors occur in older children and adults, in whom they may cause symptoms of chest pain, dyspnea, cough, and stridor.

Bronchial cysts are manifested by a smooth density at the carinal level that may be seen to compress the esophagus on barium swallow. Differentiation from hilar structures may be difficult in the occasional symptomatic cyst.

Surgical Excision

Surgical excision is recommended in all cases to provide a definite histologic diagnosis, alleviate symptoms, and prevent the development of associated complications. Malignant degeneration has been reported, as has the recurrence of a bronchial adenoma within the cyst wall.

ENTERIC CYSTS

Enteric cysts (duplication cysts) arise from the posterior division of the primitive foregut, which gives rise to the upper division of the gastrointestinal system. These cysts occur less frequently than bronchogenic cysts and comprise 3 per cent of the mediastinal masses in the collected series. They are also known as inclusion cysts,

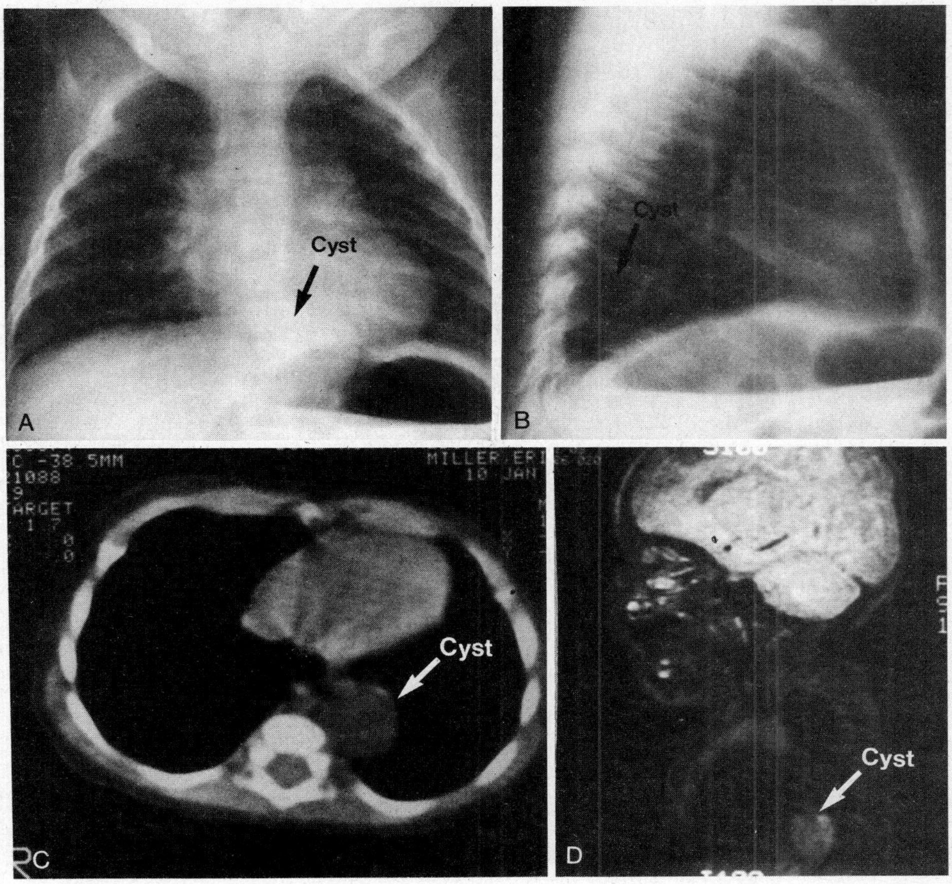

Figure 5. Enteric cyst of the posterior mediastinum. A and B, Chest films. C, Computed tomography demonstrates more clearly the anatomic location of the mass. However, it provides no additional information to differentiate the mass from a neurogenic tumor. D, Magnetic resonance imaging manifests the cystic nature of the mass and its relationship to the esophagus.

gastric cysts, or enterogenous cysts and are most frequently located in the posterior mediastinum, usually adjacent to the esophagus (Fig. 5).

These lesions are composed of smooth muscle with an inner epithelial lining that may be similar to the esophagus, stomach, or intestinal mucosa. When gastric mucosa is present, peptic ulceration with perforation of an esophageal or bronchial lumen may occur, resulting in hemoptysis or hematemesis. Erosion into the lung parenchyma may result in a lung abscess. Gastric mucosa within enteric cysts may be visualized using technetium-99 scanning. Usually, enteric cysts have an attachment to the esophagus, but they may also be embedded within the muscularis.

Symptoms are usually due to compression of the esophagus leading to dysphagia or obstructive symptomatology. Compression of the tracheobronchial tree with symptoms of cough, dyspnea, recurrent pulmonary infections, or chest pain may also result. The majority of enteric cysts are diagnosed in children, who are also more likely to be symptomatic.

When enteric cysts are associated with anomalies of the vertebral column, they are sometimes referred to as *neuroenteric cysts*. These cysts may be connected to the meninges, or, less frequently, a direct communication with the dural space may exist. Vertebral anomalies associated with this syndrome include spina bifida, hemivertebrae, and widened neural canal. CT and myelography are useful in delineating the vertebral deformities, the spinal column, and the possibility of a connection between the dural space and the cysts. The embryogenesis of these tumors seems to be related to the failure of complete separation of the notochord from the primitive gut at the time of embryogenesis, when these two structures are intimately juxtaposed.

Rarely, multiple mediastinal enteric cysts may exist or there may be an association with a duplication of the abdominal portion of the alimentary tract. In the latter case, there may be a transdiaphragmatic connection between abdominal and mediastinal components. Surgical excision is the basis of therapy, providing a definite histologic diagnosis as well as alleviating symptoms and preventing potential complications. In cases of neuroenteric cysts, preoperative evaluation for potential spinal cord involvement is mandatory.

THYMIC CYSTS

Thymic cysts may be inflammatory, neoplastic, or congenital lesions. Congenital cysts are thought to originate from the third branchial cleft and are not usually related to thymomas. These cysts are diagnosed by the presence of thymic tissue within the cyst wall.

NONSPECIFIC CYSTS

Nonspecific cysts include those lesions in which a specific epithelial or mesothelial lining cannot be identified. These lesions may originate in any of the aforementioned cysts by the destruction of the inner epithelial lining by an inflammatory or digestive process. Other etiologies include postinflammatory cysts and hemorrhagic cysts.

REFERENCES

1. Adam, A., and Hochholzer, L.: Ganglioneuroblastoma of the posterior mediastinum: A clinicopathologic review of 80 cases. Cancer, 47:373, 1981.
2. Adkins, R. B., Maples, M. D., and Hainsworth, J.D.: Primary malignant mediastinal tumors. Ann. Thorac. Surg., 38:648, 1984.
3. Blalock, A., Mason, M. F., Morgon, H. J., and Riven, S. S.: Myasthenia gravis and tumors of the thymic region: Report of a case in which tumor was removed. Ann. Surg., 110:544, 1939.
4. Brodeur, G. M., Howarth, C. B., Pratt, C.B., Caces, J., and Hustu, H. O.: Malignant germ cell tumors in 57 children and adolescents. Cancer, 48:1890, 1981.
5. Conkle, D. M., and Adkins, R. B.: Primary malignant tumors of the mediastinum. Ann. Thorac. Surg., 14:553, 1972.
6. Economou, J. S., Trump, D. L., Holmes, E. C., and Eggleston, J. E.: Management of primary cell tumors of the mediastinum. J. Thorac. Cardiovasc. Surg., 83:643, 1982.
7. Epstein, A. M., and Klassen, K. P.: Spontaneous superior mediastinal hemorrhage. J. Thorac. Cardiovasc. Surg., 39:740, 1960.
8. Fontenelle, L. J., Armstrong, R. G., Stanford, W., Lindberg, E. F., and Dooley, B. N.: Asymptomatic mediastinal mass. Arch. Surg., 102:98, 1971.
9. Grosfeld, J. L., Weinberg, M., Kilmann, J. W., and Clatworthy, H. W.: Primary mediastinal neoplasms in infants and children. Ann. Thorac. Surg., 12:179, 1971.
10. Haller, J. A., Mazur, D. O., and Morgan, W. M.: Diagnosis and management of mediastinal masses in children. J. Thorac. Cardiovasc. Surg., 58:385, 1969.
11. Hamman, L.: Spontaneous mediastinal emphysema. Bull. Johns Hopkins Hosp., 64:1, 1939.
12. Harrington, S. W.: Surgical treatment of intrathoracic tumors. Arch. Surg., 19:1679, 1929.
13. Heimburger, I. L., and Battersby, J. S.: Primary mediastinal tumors of childhood. J. Thorac. Cardiovasc. Surg., 50:92, 1965.
14. Heimburger, I. J., Battersby, J. S., and Vellios, F.: Primary neoplasms of the mediastinum. A fifteen-year experience. Arch. Surg., 86:978, 1963.
15. Heuer, G. J., and Andrus, W. D.: The surgery of mediastinal tumors. Am. J. Surg., 50:146, 1940.
16. Koy, H. R., Goodman, L. R., Teplick, S. K., and Mundth, E. D.: Use of computed tomography to assess mediastinal complications after median sternotomy. Ann. Thorac. Surg., 36:706, 1983.
17. Lewis, B. D., Hurt, R. D., Payne, W. S., Farrow, G. M., Knapp, R. H., and Muhm, J. R.: Benign teratomas of the mediastinum. J. Thorac. Cardiovasc. Surg., 86:727, 1983.
18. Milton, H.: Mediastinal surgery. Lancet, 1:872, 1897.
19. Monden, Y., Nakolara, K., Kagotani, K., Fujii, Y., Masooka, A., and Kawashima, Y.: Myasthenia gravis with thymoma: Analysis of and postoperative prognosis for 65 patients with thymomatous myasthenia gravis. Ann. Thorac. Surg., 38:46, 1984.
20. Nandi, P., Wong, K. C., Mok, C. K., and Ong, G. B.: Primary mediastinal tumours. Review of 74 cases. J. R. Coll. Surg. Edinb., 25:460, 1980.
21. Olanow, C. W., Wechsler, A. S., and Roses, A. D.: A prospective study of thymectomy and serum, acetylcholine receptor antibodies in myasthenia gravis. Ann. of Surg., 196:113, 1982.
22. Oldham, H. N., and Sabiston, D. C.: Primary tumors and cysts of the mediastinum. Monogr. Surg. Sci., 4:243, 1967.
23. Parish, J. M., Rosenow, E. C., and Muhm, J. R.: Mediastinal masses. Clues to interpretation of radiologic studies. Postgrad. Med. 76:173, 1984.
24. Pokorny, W. J., and Sherman, J. O.: Mediastinal masses in infants and children: J. Thorac. Cardiovasc. Surg., 68:869, 1974.
25. Rubush, J. L., Gardner, I. R., Boyd, W. C., and Ehrenhaft, J. L.: Mediastinal tumors: Review of 186 cases. J. Thorac. Cardiovasc. Surg., 65:216, 1973.
26. Shamji, F., Pearson, F. G., Todd, T. R. J., Ginsberg, R. J., Ilves, R., and Cooper, J. D.: Results of surgical treatment for thymoma. J. Thorac. Cardiovasc. Surg., 87:43, 1984.
27. Shapiro, B., Sisson, J., Kalff, V., Glowniak, J., Satterlee, W., Glazer, G., Francis, I., Bowers, R., Thompson, N., Orringer, M., Gross, M., and Bierwaltes, W.: The location of middle mediastinal pheochromocytomas. J. Thorac. Cardiovasc. Surg., 87:814, 1984.
28. Silverman, N. A., and Sabiston, D. C.: Mediastinal masses. Surg. Clin. North Am., 60:756, 1980.
29. Silverman, N. A., and Sabiston, D. C.: Primary tumors and cysts of the mediastinum. Curr. Probl. Cancer, 2:1, 1977.
30. Vogelzang, N. J., Raghaven, D., Anderson, R. W., Rosai, J., Levitt, S. H., and Kennedy, B. J.: Mediastinal nonseminomatous germ cell tumors: The role of combined modality therapy. Ann. Thorac. Surg., 33:333, 1982.
31. Whittaker, L. D., and Lynn, H. B.: Mediastinal tumors and cysts in the pediatric patient. Surg. Clin. North Am., 53:893, 1973.
32. Wick, M. R., Bernatz, P. E., Carney, J. A., and Brown, L. R.: Primary mediastinal carcinoid tumors. Am. J. Surg. Pathol., 6:195, 1982.
33. Wychulis, A. R., Payne, W. S., Clagett, O. T., and Woolner, L. B.: Surgical treatment of mediastinal tumors. A 40-year experience. J. Thorac. Cardiovasc. Surg., 62:379, 1971.

II

The Diagnosis and Management of Myasthenia Gravis

W. RANDOLPH CHITWOOD, JR., M.D.

Myasthenia gravis represents a functional impairment of the neuromuscular junction, resulting in weakness and fatigability of voluntary muscles. Specific muscle groups are affected selectively; however, a *generalized* weakness usually occurs. The first description of this disorder was probably that of Sir Thomas Willis (1672).[8] However, the description recognized by most as the classic one was published in 1877 by Wilks of Guy's Hospital.[38] The name "myasthenia gravis pseudoparalytica" was given to this disease by Jolly in 1895.[11] Subsequently, pathologist Weigert

noted the connection between thymic abnormalities and muscle weakness (1901).[36] Remen and Walker independently introduced neostigmine and physostigmine for the treatment of myasthenia gravis in 1932 and 1934, respectively.[26, 35] From patient studies, Walker proposed that impaired neuromuscular transmission was responsible for this debilitating condition. Although Sauerbruch had noted improvement in weakness following a cervical thymectomy for a hypertrophied thymus (1912), Blalock was the first to extirpate a gland deliberately for the treatment of myasthenia gravis (1936).[4, 30] By 1944, Blalock had performed 20 thymectomies for this disorder and found a noticeable improvement in weakness in over 80 per cent of operative survivors.[3] He noted that, following thymectomy, muscular strength often returned later and that myasthenia gravis was not always associated with a thymoma. Pulmonary complications following surgery were even more dreaded in those days as they often resulted in death. Today, both medical and surgical therapy have become safe and effective for treating patients with even the most severe myasthenia gravis.

PATHOPHYSIOLOGY

Muscle contraction following a stimulus results from the interaction of released presynaptic vesicles containing acetylcholine and activation of postsynaptic membrane receptors at the neuromuscular junction (Fig. 1). Normally, this association causes a transient increase in membrane permeability to sodium and potassium ions resulting in electrical depolarization.[5] This triggers many end-plate potentials, leading to an action potential that results in muscular contraction. The amplitude of depolarization relates to the number of acetylcholine packets interacting at postsynaptic receptor sites. Removal of acetylcholine by either diffusion or hydrolysis via acetylcholinesterase normally terminates this neuromuscular activity.

In 1960, Simpson proposed that myasthenia gravis resulted from an abnormal autoimmune response at the neuromuscular junction.[31] Subsequently, Patrick and Lindstrom (1973) found that because of this interaction a reduced number of acetylcholine receptors occurred at the end-plate.[24] Acetylcholine receptor antibodies have been demonstrated in up to 90 per cent of myasthenia patients.[34] These antibodies appear responsible for either complement-dependent lysis of postsynaptic membranes or an increased rate of acetylcholine receptor degradation. Complement C3

and C9 probably play a role in membrane lysis. Receptor blockage by antibody moieties may be additive to this overall decrement in receptor activity. In any event, the synthesis of either acetycholine or receptors does not seem to be affected by myasthenia gravis.[5] Experimentally, myasthenic conditions can be induced by transfer of IgG fractions from affected patients to animals with resultant weakness.[24] Although some clinicians have found a relationship between measured receptor antibody levels and the degree of debilitation, an absolute correlation between improved symptoms and diminution in antibody titer following thymectomy does not always exist.[18, 34] The origins and mechanism of this autoimmune response still remain controversial. Cell-mediated factors may also be important. An additional thymic factor has been implicated as being necessary for this disease to become manifest clinically.[21] Thus, the beneficial effects of plasmapheresis and immunosuppressive drug therapy may emanate either by decreasing receptor antibodies or by altering thymic influences.[19] At present, the quantitative relationship between anti-acetylcholine receptor levels and thymic factors remains unclear. However, recent studies continue to suggest a close association of these in the pathogenesis of myasthenia gravis.

NORMAL ANATOMY AND HISTOLOGY

The lobulated thymus gland arises during the sixth week of gestation and develops primarily from anlage present in the third and fourth pharyngeal pouches. By the eighth week of fetal life, proximity with these embryonic origins is lost with cephalad growth of the head and neck regions. Thymic primordia share their origin with those of the thyroid and parathyroid glands. Epithelial cells proliferate and form solid glandular components by the thirteenth to fourteenth week of gestation.[13] Subsequently, the pyramid-shaped lobes descend and become associated closely to form a common structure in the anterior mediastinum. Thymic lymphocytes then migrate into and populate the gland. At puberty, the gland reaches maximal size, weighing between 40 and 50 gm. When a person is about 50 years of age, involution begins, and fatty infiltration reduces the gland to between 10 and 15 gm. by age 60.[13] Despite the smaller size, the involuted thymus gland has been shown to exhibit significant immunologic activity.[21] Usually, a fibrous capsule persists even in very small involuted glands, aiding in thymectomy in older patients.

Anatomically, two thyrothymic ligaments lie anterior to the trachea in the inferior neck region and widen out in the upper mediastinum to form the normal bilobed gland (Figs. 2 and 3). Thymic tissue generally lies anterior to the innominate vein and pericardium and often is associated closely with pleural and pericardial margins, sometimes making surgical dissection difficult. Masaoka and Jaretzki have shown independently that variations in thymic anatomy are frequent (82 per cent) and may lead to incomplete thymectomy.[10, 14] These anomalies include accessory or discontinuous lobes, an abnormally high superior pole, feathery tissue margins, and ectopic thymus obscured in mediastinal fat. The arterial supply to the thymus arises diffusely from small branches of the inferior thyroid, internal mammary, and pericardiophrenic arteries.[13, 28] In contrast, as shown in Figure 3, discrete thymic veins drain superiorly into the anterior surface of the left innominate system. In about 15 per cent of patients, the thymus will lie posterior to the innominate vein, with thymic veins emptying into the dorsal side of this vessel.[9] Fibers of the vagus nerve

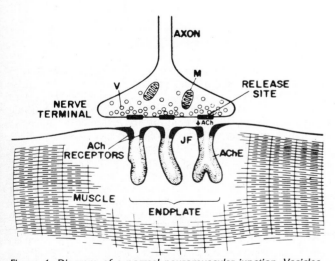

Figure 1. Diagram of a normal neuromuscular junction. Vesicles (V) of acetylcholine (ACh) are formed in the distal presynaptic axon. Following release, they traverse the synaptic space to interact with acetylcholine receptors present in junctional folds (JF) on the muscular end plate. This results in an action potential and muscular contraction. Subsequently, acetylcholinesterase (AChE) hydrolyzes the vesicles, terminating the event. M = Mitochondria. (From Drachman, D. B.: N. Engl. J. Med., 298:136, 1978.)

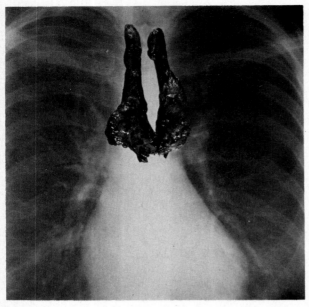

Figure 2. This thymus gland from a myasthenic patient has been superimposed over the superior mediastinal location on the preoperative chest radiograph. Note the tapering superior poles of each lobe.

and cervical sympathetic chain innervate the thymus gland. Small efferent lymphatics drain into mediastinal and lower cervical nodes; however, afferent lymphatics have not been demonstrated.[28]

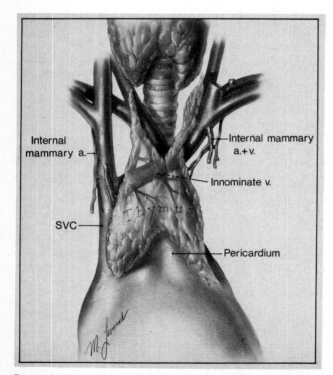

Figure 3. This drawing illustrates the anatomy of the normal thymus gland before involution. The majority of glands are located anterior to the innominate vein and drain via small thymic veins. Inferiorly, the bulk of the gland sweeps onto the anterior pericardial surface. Superiorly, then, each lobe tapers into the neck as thin, poorly defined thyrothymic ligaments. SVC = Superior vena cava.

The fibrous thymic capsule extends into the parenchyma to form interdigitating compartmentalizing septae. The basic cellular architecture consists of individual lobules (0.5 to 2.0 mm. in diameter), each having a definable medulla and cortex.[28] The peripherally located cortex is composed of densely organized lymphocytes known as *thymocytes*. Cortical epithelial cells are interspersed in a reticular pattern and may be difficult to identify without ultrastructural studies. These epithelial components are characterized by indented nuclei with intracytoplasmic tonofilaments. In each lobule the more central medulla is composed of less densely arranged lymphocytes, making staining in this region lighter. Recent studies suggest that medullary T-lymphocytes represent helper T cells, and cortical components are suppressor-cytotoxic cells.[13] Medullary masses of mature epithelial cells form characteristic discrete concentric layers of acidophilic staining material known as *Hassall's corpuscles*. Other less prominent cellular components of the normal thymus gland include histiocytes, eosinophils, acidophilic myoid cells, and argyrophilic elements. Myoid cells are thought to have acetylcholine receptors and may be involved in the autoimmune response of myasthenia gravis.

The thymus gland is the major organ responsible for development and propagation of cell-mediated immunity. A normal maturation pattern for T cell lymphocytes probably occurs within the thymus gland.[13] Immature lymphoblasts are thought to migrate from bone marrow stores to the thymic *cortex*, where the majority acquire suppressor-cytotoxic characteristics. In the medulla, most (75 per cent) immature lymphocytes probably proceed to become inducer (helper) T cells. Additionally, it is thought that medullary thymocytes (15 per cent) are immature thymic blast cells from the thymic cortex. Local epithelial cells may regulate helper T cell activity. Thereafter, thymically matured T cells appear to circulate and exert their influence peripherally. Despite these theories, the exact role of cellular influences of the thymus remains unclear. Thymus hormones circulate and help regulate peripheral lymphocyte differentiation and cellular immunocompetence.

PATHOLOGY AND HISTOPATHOLOGY

Thymic abnormalities are present in approximately 75 per cent of patients who have myasthenia gravis.[28] Follicular or germinal center hyperplasia occurs in 60 to 80 per cent of these patients.[13, 29] Ten to 25 per cent have a demonstrable thymoma, and 30 per cent of those found to have an isolated thymoma will have associated myasthenia gravis.[15, 21, 28] Lymphoid hyperplasia, associated with myasthenia gravis, results in medullary germinal center proliferation.[13] In normal glands, germinal centers are infrequent. This type of lymphoid hyperplasia may be associated with other autoimmune diseases, such as systemic lupus erythematosus, scleroderma, and rheumatoid arthritis. Although some studies have correlated the degree of germinal center hyperplasia in myasthenia gravis with levels of clinical weakness and response to therapy, other investigators have failed to define a clear relationship.[13, 25] At present the stimulus for lymphoid hyperplasia in myasthenia gravis remains unknown.

In most patients, *thymomas* are encapsulated (90 per cent) and can be removed with relative ease. Seventy-five per cent are found in the immediate anterior mediastinum.[28] Invasion of surrounding structures, including the pericardium, pleura, and innominate vein, suggests malignancy.

Thymomas may reach a very large size; however, the average size ranges between 5 and 10 cm. in diameter, with mean weight being 150 gm. Larger thymomas often are composed of spindle or elongated epithelial cells and generally are not associated with myasthenia gravis.[28] When a thymoma is associated with myasthenia gravis, it is often discovered after recognition of the myasthenic condition. Older patients with myasthenia gravis are more likely to have a thymic tumor. Wilkins and Castleman have suggested that the remission of muscular weakness occurs in only 25 per cent of myasthenic patients undergoing thymectomy for a thymoma.[27, 37] Unlike the case of follicular hyperplasia, there is no histologic guide that links a thymic tumor with clinical myasthenia gravis. However, in about 50 per cent of these patients, there are germinal centers in other non-neoplastic areas of the same gland, which may facilitate diagnosis.[1] Thymomas usually consist of septated, soft lobules that resemble lymphoid tissue grossly. Areas of calcification, cystic changes, hemorrhage, and necrosis occur in up to 40 per cent of thymomas.[13]

Histologically, thymomas are composed predominantly of either lymphocytes or epithelial cells, and most have variable mixtures of each cell type. Usually, the lymphocytes are small and mature-appearing. Epithelial cells are round, oval, or spindle-shaped, and may be interspersed as islets, cords, or isolated cells among a field of lymphocytes. Marchevsky and Rosai both point out that most encapsulated thymomas have few atypical cells and that the mitotic rate remains very low.[13, 28] Rosettes of epithelial cells and pseudoglands, composed of cuboidal or flattened spindle cells, are present in up to 20 per cent of thymomas. Myoid cells of the type present in normal glands are very unusual in thymic tumors. Perivascular spaces are formed in almost 55 per cent of thymomas and are composed of flattened epithelial cells surrounding capillaries.[28] These spaces have been helpful in identifying thymomas.[13]

Ultrastructurally, thymomas resemble a normal gland.[13, 28] Epithelial cells have long cytoplasmic processes and form spaces in which darker lymphocytes are found frequently (Fig. 4). Although some series have reported that up to 43 per cent of thymomas in myasthenic patients were malignant, other authors have found very few malignant ones.[20, 32] As mentioned before, the aggressive behavior of these tumors is based on degree of local invasiveness and not the histologic character.[28] Patients with thymoma have fewer remissions and a higher death rate because of respiratory insufficiency.[22, 25]

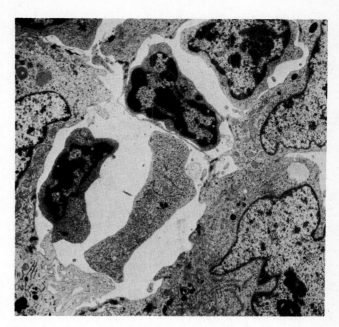

Figure 4. Electron micrograph of a lymphoepithelial thymoma showing dark lymphocytes in spaces lined by epithelial cells (× 2600, original courtesy of Dr. Marchevsky). (From Marchevsky, A. M., and Kaneko, M.: Surgical Pathology of the Mediastinum. New York, Raven Press, 1984.)

genetic predisposition for this disease has been suggested by some authors.

SYMPTOMS AND FINDINGS

The first symptoms usually noted relate to weakness of the extraocular muscles. The levator muscles of the lids and oculomotor muscles are affected together, causing a severe ptosis and strabismus (Cogan's sign). Asymmetric involvement in muscle groups can result in severe diplopia. As mentioned before, in about 15 per cent of patients with myasthenia gravis the disease remains localized to the extraocular muscles. These patients generally are easier to treat and often can be maintained using steroids and anticholinesterase inhibitors. In 40 to 50 per cent of patients, the initial symptoms relate to ocular muscle weakness with subsequent progression to generalized myasthenia.[7, 20] Ultimately 90 per cent of patients have ocular muscle involvement, and of the 85 per cent who develop global symptoms, the majority do so within the first year after diagnosis. The proximal muscles are affected first. Most frequently, symptoms begin in facial regions and proceed caudally in a sequential fashion, with the lower legs and respiratory muscles impaired last. Dysarthria and dysphagia eventually occur in up to 40 per cent of patients.[12] Masseter weakness may cause difficulty in chewing and, when combined with dysphagia, may result in pulmonary aspiration. Classically, the severity of symptoms fluctuates both during the day and with repeated exercise of muscle groups. Usually, muscle strength is rejuvenated partially by rest. It is noteworthy that patients rarely have sensory complaints (10 per cent) and that deep tendon reflexes are not affected by this disease. However, repetitive stimulation of a tendon often tires an involved muscle unit and may cause temporary suspension of the reflex.

CLINICAL AND DIAGNOSTIC CHARACTERISTICS

Myasthenia gravis affects the skeletal musculature, with no functional alterations of either smooth or cardiac muscle fibers. Cranial nerves are involved more frequently; however, weakness may progress and become so severe that respiratory failure ensues. In some patients, the disease remains localized to the extraocular muscles but more frequently becomes generalized (85 per cent). The localized ocular pattern occurs more frequently in males.[7] Myasthenia gravis affects approximately one in 20,000 people and is more common in females (3:2). Symptoms generally occur earlier in females (mean 28 years) than in males (mean 42 years). Usually, the generalized form becomes manifest in females between the ages of 20 and 40; in males it often begins later (30 to 70 years). Localized ocular weakness most often develops between 30 and 50 years of age.[7] A

Death results from either difficulty in clearing respiratory secretions or food aspiration, both of which predispose to pneumonia. At present, the overall mortality for myasthenia gravis is approximately 12.5 per cent, a reduction from 34 per cent prior to 1960. Approximately one fourth of patients will have at least one spontaneous remission in symptoms, which may last up to 5 years. Most of these patients (90 per cent) will have only a single remission. During pregnancy the disease worsens in approximately a third of patients, whereas improvement is noted in a third.[7] Myasthenia gravis usually does not affect gestation or delivery, and termination of the pregnancy rarely is necessary. *Congenital* myasthenia gravis accounts for about 0.2 per cent of those with the adult disease. Usually, this disease occurs in children of non-myasthenic mothers and should be distinguished from *neonatal myasthenia gravis*.[16, 17] The latter condition results in an often severe but transient (18-day, mean) weakness in babies born to myasthenic mothers. This is believed to result from transfer of anti-acetylcholine receptor antibodies across the placenta. Congenital myasthenia gravis has a familial predominance but a slower, less rampant clinical course than that of the adult counterpart.[17] It is of note that in 10 per cent of adults with myasthenia gravis, symptoms of weakness develop in childhood.[7]

Frequently, the diagnosis of myasthenia gravis can be made on the characteristic clinical history, location of involved muscles, and temporal variations in strength. The differential diagnosis should include diseases that are of myopathic or neurogenic origin, including muscular dystrophy, polymyositis, thyrotoxicosis, various encephalopathies, Guillain-Barré syndrome, Eaton-Lambert syndrome, and periodic paralysis, among others. Weakness of muscles innervated by cranial nerves often occurs with brain stem strokes and myasthenia gravis alike; however, the weakness associated with myasthenia gravis is more symmetrical, fluctuates periodically, and is not associated with long tract or sensory findings.[12] Meningeal irritation and amyotrophic lateral sclerosis must be considered also during evaluation of myasthenic patients. Between 4 and 10 per cent of patients have concomitant hyperthyroidism.[7, 12] Either of these diseases may develop first; however, hyperthyroidism generally aggravates myasthenic weakness. Other clearly autoimmune conditions have been reported in concert with myasthenia gravis and include polymyositis, lupus erythematosus, rheumatoid arthritis, idiopathic thrombocytopenia purpura, and chronic thyroiditis.[12]

Pharmacodiagnostic Tests

When myasthenia gravis is suspected clinically, the widely used edrophonium (Tensilon) test can confirm the diagnosis effectively and safely. This short-acting anticholinesterase inhibitor provides a brief increment in muscle strength in about 95 per cent of these patients. Generally, the extraocular muscle group has been observed during this test. Following a test dose to determine hypersensitivity, 10 mg. of edrophonium is given intravenously in triple-blind fashion using either normal saline or nicotinic acid as control agents. Nicotinic acid will produce some of the muscarinic effects of edrophonium without eliciting concomitant muscular potentiation.[20] An immediate improvement in strength of observed muscle groups occurs as a positive response to edrophonium, establishing the diagnosis of myasthenia gravis. Transient side effects such as flushing and sweating occur most of the time. After 5 to 10 minutes, the salutary effects of edrophonium fade and weakness returns. Longer-acting agents such as neostigmine (Prostigmine) also can be used to assess sustained responses to anticholinesterase inhibitors.

Electrodiagnostic Studies

In 1895, Jolly first found that repetitive electrical stimulation of motor nerves in patients with myasthenia gravis resulted in rapid deterioration of contractile function in many involved muscle groups.[12] Normal human muscles retain similar action potentials when their innervating nerves are stimulated up to 40 to 50 times per second. In patients with myasthenia gravis, stimulus rates as low as one per second effect a characteristic decrement in strength. The usual test involves stimulation of the median or ulnar nerve at three per second to five per second for a duration of 2 to 3 seconds. Superficial measurements then are taken from the abductor pollicis brevis and abductor digiti minimi muscles. Comparisons between the first and fifth responses are made, and the percentage difference in these results calculated. A fall in function of greater than 10 per cent is considered diagnostic for myasthenia gravis. Very rapid stimulation (100 per minute) may bring about slowed nerve conduction, which may falsely appear as impaired synaptic neuromuscular dysfunction. With this method, now known as the *Jolly test*, decremental responses have been reported in up to 95 per cent of patients, if three separate muscle groups are evaluated independently; however, other clinicians report the test to be much less sensitive.[5, 20]

The single *fiber electromyogram* was developed by Ekstedt and Stalberg (1960) to measure action potentials of individual fibers in a muscle unit.[7, 12] This technique is believed to be a more sensitive electrophysiologic indicator of myasthenia gravis than the Jolly test. Two separate muscle fibers within the same motor unit are monitored while the single innervating nerve is stimulated repeatedly. Synchronous contractile activity occurs in both fibers as they become entrained. In normal muscles the latency period between the two action potentials, or *neuromuscular jitter*, is small with sequential stimulation. However, with diminished end-plate sensitivity to acetylcholine, single fiber action potentials fail to follow paired nerve stimuli and blocking of one occurs, resulting in an increased jitter response. Single-fiber electromyography shows an abnormal jitter response in up to 95 per cent of myasthenia gravis patients and can be used to follow clinical responses to various therapies.[7, 12, 20] For most accurate testing, multiple studies should be performed on up to 20 individual muscle fibers.

Other Diagnostic Studies

Both *chest radiography* and *mediastinal computed tomography* (CT) provide helpful information in evaluating myasthenic patients for a thymoma. On the posteroanterior (PA) view of the standard chest film, most thymomas present as a well-circumscribed mass extending laterally from the borders of the normal mediastinal shadow (Fig. 5). In addition, calcification may be seen. An anterior mediastinal mass may be delineated more on a lateral view than on PA projection; however, a small thymoma may not be obvious in either projection. Plain film tomography, fluoroscopy, and pneumomediastinography all have been employed in the past. Recently, CT has become the major radiologic modality for the demonstration of mediastinal

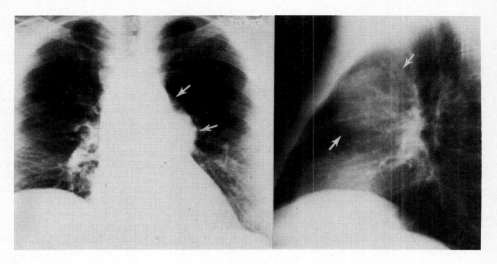

Figure 5. Thymoma. Posteroanterior (left) and lateral (right) radiographs showing a large anterior mediastinal mass (arrows). (Courtesy of Dr. David Godwin, Department of Radiology, Duke University.)

tumors (Fig. 6). Although the boundaries of nearly all thymomas may be defined using this technique, CT scanning does not distinguish this tumor from other mediastinal masses, nor does it predict the malignant potential.

Other *less frequently used diagnostic drug tests* include both generalized and regional tests using curare (d-tubocurarine), which is a postsynaptic blocking agent. When up to a tenth of the dose needed to induce paralysis in a normal patient is given incrementally by the intravenous route to a patient with myasthenia gravis, weakness develops, indicating a positive response. With each administration, the degree of muscular weakness is graded carefully. The test is very sensitive, but involves a definite risk of respiratory impairment. The regional test is safer, as peripherally administered d-tubocurarine is prevented from circulating freely by venous occlusion of the extremity with a blood pressure cuff. When this study is performed in conjunction with electrophysiologic stimulation, the diagnostic accuracy for myasthenia gravis is high.[12] In previous years, *ophthalmologic testing* has been used to evaluate conjugate eye motion, optokinetic nystagmus, and pupillary changes in patients suspected of having myasthenia gravis. Although results of these tests may be helpful, they are used rarely as a primary indicator of this disease.

TREATMENT

Medical Management

At present there is no single therapy for myasthenia gravis. Treatment must be individualized for each patient and for a particular period of an individual's disease course. *Cholinesterase inhibitors* have been the major form of therapy for myasthenia gravis since neostigmine was introduced in 1935.[5] Pyridostigmine bromide (Mestinon) and neostigmine bromide (Prostigmin) are used most commonly today in clinical practice. These drugs affect the neuromuscular junction and prevent degradation of acetylcholine by interaction with cholinesterase. Symptomatic improvement occurs in most patients; however, there is evidence that the ultimate course of the disease is altered significantly by these medications. Muscarinic side effects may become problematic and include gastrointestinal symptoms, anxiety, irritability, increased salivation, and increased bronchial secretions.[12] Cholinergic weakness can result from overmedication and may be difficult clinically to separate from a myasthenic crisis. Following thymectomy, cholinesterase inhibitors also may cause problems related to increased

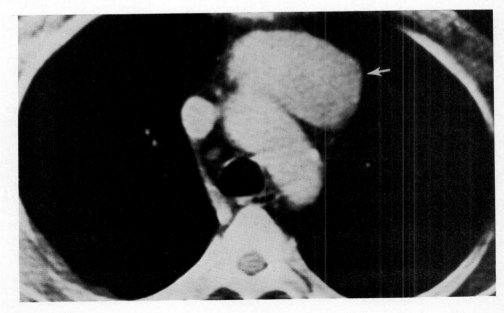

Figure 6. A contrast-enhanced computed tomogram from the patient with the thymoma shown in Figure 5. A homogeneous mass (arrow) is present anterior to the aortic arch. (Courtesy of Dr. David Godwin, Department of Radiology, Duke University.)

pulmonary secretions and to an increased tendency for unsuspected cholinergic crisis.[20]

There was little interest in using *corticosteroids* to treat myasthenia gravis prior to 1970. At present in selected cases, high doses of prednisone are initiated and continued in the hospital over a 2-week period. Close observation is necessary, since worsening of symptoms may occur in about half of these patients.[12] After this initial regimen, alternate-day therapy can be begun at nearly twice the daily dose. Remission occurs in 30 per cent, and a marked improvement in symptoms results in 45 per cent of those treated with steroids. The best responses have been in patients with symptoms of short duration. Some clinicians prefer to use steroids only in patients with ocular disease or those who refuse thymectomy.[20] Many others use these drugs as primary therapy or in combination with immunosuppressive agents; however, the side effects remain significant. Also, patients receiving steroids may be more difficult to manage compared with other treatment modalities. Many individuals will require steroids indefinitely, and significant alterations in muscle strength occur with only minimal changes in dosage.

Immunosuppressive drugs, including azathioprine, methotrexate, cyclophosphamide, and mercaptopurine, have been used successfully to treat myasthenia gravis.[12] Improved strength results in a significant number of patients when immunosuppressive drugs are used alone or in combination with steroid therapy or plasmapheresis. However, the hematologic and gastrointestinal side effects are significant, and often the therapeutic response is delayed markedly. Despite these troublesome factors, immunosuppressive drugs still offer much promise in the treatment of myasthenia gravis.

Recently, plasma exchange, or *plasmapheresis*, has been used widely in preparation for a surgical thymectomy. This modality has provided relief in situations in which traditional therapy has failed.[33] However, the clinical benefits of plasmapheresis are not sustained when it is used as the sole treatment. The technique reduces unwanted circulating humoral antibodies to acetylcholine receptors temporarily, and nearly all patients improve following plasmapheresis. Removal of other plasma components may also contribute to the clinical improvement after treatment. Presently, the complications are related to technical problems alone and not to systemic results of therapy.

In treating patients with myasthenia gravis, familiarity with *drugs that may potentiate their weakness* is imperative.[7] Competitive muscle relaxants, such as d-tubocurarine and pancuronium, as well as depolarizing agents, including succinylcholine, should be used with extreme caution. Also, many aminoglycoside antibiotics produce significant neuromuscular blocking effects, as do some antiarrhythmics (quinidine and procainamide). Many psychotropic medications have an adverse effect on muscular strength in these individuals.[20]

Surgical Management: Thymectomy

EARLY SURGICAL INTERVENTION

Thymectomy has been shown to be a safe and very effective method for treating myasthenia gravis.[21, 25] Today, the surgical complications of the transcervical or transsternal approach are equally very low, with mortality from operation being about 0.5 to 2 per cent. Recently, in many centers thymectomy has become the *primary* form of therapy for the initial treatment of myasthenia gravis.[9, 20, 21] In past years, surgical intervention was reserved for those whom medical treatment had failed or those having complications from medications. Following thymectomy, remission or permanent improvement in generalized weakness has been reported in 80 to 90 per cent of patients.[5, 21, 25] However, up to 20 per cent of patients may have residual ocular symptoms.[21] Usually, these continuing symptoms are controlled with corticosteroids. Although older patients do respond to thymectomy, young individuals show the best results from surgical extirpation. When presenting muscular weakness is localized to ocular muscles, pharmacologic control remains preferable and thymectomy has been delayed. In most cases, ocular myasthenia gravis is controlled satisfactorily with alternate-day corticosteroids. However, when generalized symptoms develop *first* or as a progression of ocular involvement, many clinicians now consider thymectomy early in the clinical course.[21] In many situations, thymectomy has been performed at the initial evaluation following stabilization of muscular weakness. Prolonged management with cholinesterase inhibitors may make surgical treatment more difficult because inadvertent cholinergic weakness can occur during the perioperative period. Thus, these medications should be withdrawn and surgery performed within 72 hours of plasmapheresis.[33] Postoperatively, anticholinesterase medications should not be necessary in most patients. Preoperative plasmapheresis is effective, produces very few side effects, and provides rapid control of generalized weakness.

The malignant potential of a thymoma is a clear indication for surgery, since these tumors cannot be assessed fully without exploration. Some series report a high incidence of malignancy (up to 40 per cent); however, groups who promote early thymectomy have found relatively few malignant thymomas.[21, 23] As mentioned previously, patients with myasthenia gravis who have a thymoma do not respond as well to thymectomy as those who have hyperplastic glands.

SURGICAL TECHNIQUE

Both the transcervical and transmediastinal thymectomy have been advocated. Most surgeons now believe that a more complete operation can be performed with a vertical sternotomy.[21, 25] This is quite important, since recurrent weakness may result with incomplete thymectomy. Moreover, thymomas have been reported as occurring in thymic remnants of patients undergoing thymectomy via the cervical approach.[2]

Incisions preferred for performing a thymectomy are shown in Figure 7. In males, a vertical skin incision is made from the sternal notch to the xiphoid and the sternum is divided in standard fashion using a reciprocating saw. In contrast, maximal cosmesis in females has been provided by a transverse V-shaped incision placed along the superior aspect of both breasts. An inframammary approach is just as effective, and both allow the surgical scar to be hidden by even the briefest clothing. After the initial transverse incision, superior and inferior flaps involving the skin, subcutaneous tissues, and pectoralis muscles are elevated with electrocautery. A nearly bloodless field can be obtained with this technique. Subsequently, the sternal saw can be angled superiorly to hook over the sternal notch to begin the vertical sternotomy. Then the saw should be turned and the incision completed upward from the xiphoid end. After the retractor is opened 5 to 8 cm., excellent mediastinal exposure will be provided (Fig. 8). Subsequently, the inferior border of the thymic fat pad is identified. The dissection is begun inferiorly and proceeds

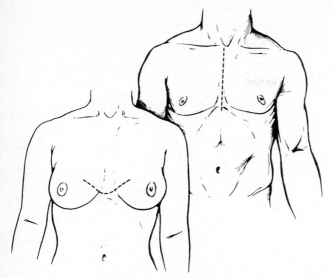

Figure 7. Both of these skin incisions provide adequate exposure to perform a vertical sternotomy for thymectomy. Generally, we have preferred the transverse supramammary incision (left) in female patients because it can be covered completely by clothing.

superiorly, with care taken not to injure the innominate vein. By blunt dissection using an index finger, the thymic capsule can be separated from the adjacent pleura and pericardium with ease. Sharp dissection is not advised because thin tissue planes may be transgressed easily. Occasionally, the cautery may be needed to divide tough

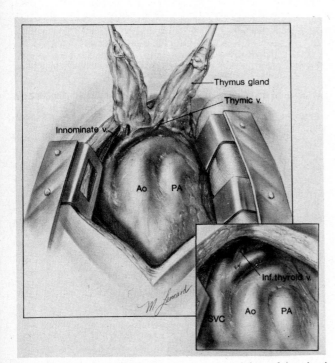

Figure 8. Following a vertical sternotomy, both lobes of the gland are separated from the pericardium and pleura using blunt dissection and the thymic veins are ligated individually. Thereafter, the superior poles of each lobe are usually visible and can be ligated prior to delivery of the gland. Inset, Following removal of the thymus, anatomic relationships in the superior mediastinum can be seen easily. Ao = Aortic indentation in the pericardium; PA = pulmonary artery indentation; SVC = superior vena cava.

fibrous strands attached to the pericardium and to cauterize small vessels. The dissection mobilizes each lobe individually to the level of the innominate vein. Usually, one or two discrete thymic veins are present and can be clipped or ligated. Separate thymic arteries are rare because the diffuse blood supply originates from several vessels. Cephalad to the innominate vein, sharp dissection may become necessary; however, to ensure complete thymectomy, care must be taken not to divide the superior poles until they taper in the neck as thyrothymic ligaments. After complete hemostasis, a single chest drainage tube (#28 Fr.) is placed in the anterior mediastinum and the sternum is reapproximated in the standard fashion with #5 steel wire. When the pleura is entered inadvertently during the dissection, the same tube can be positioned through the mediastinum and into the pleural space for re-expansion of the lung. As shown in Figure 2, a complete thymectomy can be assured if this technique is performed carefully.

Postoperative Management

Previously, the duration of disease, history of associated respiratory disease or failure, the presence of oropharyngeal dysfunction, and preoperative pulmonary vital capacity all have been used to predict postoperative respiratory failure in patients undergoing a transsternal thymectomy.[6] The recent use of plasmapheresis immediately before surgery has decreased the need for prolonged intubation in most centers. Usually, anticholinesterase medications can be withheld following plasmapheresis, decreasing accompanying respiratory secretions. Recent clinical studies have shown that pulmonary vital capacity, negative inspiratory pressure, and positive expiratory pressure correlate strongly with the length of postoperative ventilatory support necessary following thymectomy.[39] Expiratory pressure may be an even better predictor of postoperative respiratory strength than serial vital capacity measurements.

Arterial blood gases should never be used as the sole means of assessing post-thymectomy respiratory function, since clinical deterioration can occur in the presence of relatively good values. Expiratory pressures of greater than 40 cm. of water and vital capacities of at least 15 ml. per kg. have been considered sufficient for extubation. When airways are maintained by careful chest physiotherapy, endotracheal suctioning, and bronchodilators, most patients (80 per cent) can be extubated within 12 to 24 hours of thymectomy.[6] Rarely is tracheostomy necessary. Despite these advances, patients with myasthenia gravis with relatively refractory preoperative weakness may require ventilatory support for several days following surgery.

SELECTED REFERENCES

Blalock, A., Mason, M. F., Morgan, H. J., and Riven, S. S.: Myasthenia gravis and tumors of the thymic region: Report of a case in which the tumor was removed. Ann. Surg., *110*:544, 1939.
Although an association between thymic pathology and myasthenia gravis had been made earlier, Blalock first removed a thymus deliberately to treat this disease. He was encouraged by the response in the young woman described in this paper and subsequently performed 20 additional thymectomies for myasthenia gravis, which he reported in 1944. His review of the literature and understanding of the disease provide excellent reading for students and teachers alike.

Grob, D.: Clinical manifestations of myasthenia gravis. *In* Albuquerque, E. X., and Eldefrawi, A. T. (Eds.): Myasthenia Gravis. New York, Chapman and Hall, 1983.
This chapter is replete with the clinical and historial findings characteristic of myasthenia gravis. Excellent sections are provided on differential diagnosis, pharmacologic testing, and conditions coexisting with myas-

thenia gravis. Other chapters in this book are devoted to the modern immunologic, biochemical, and pathologic understanding of this disease. A comprehensive summary of current medical and surgical therapy is provided in this text.

Jaretzki, A., Bethea, M., Wolff, M., Olarte, M., Lovelace, R. E., Penn, A. S., and Rowland, L. A.: A rational approach to total thymectomy in the treatment of myasthenia gravis. Ann. Thorac. Surg., 24:120, 1977.

A surgical anatomic study of the thymus gland is presented for 22 patients undergoing a transsternal thymectomy for myasthenia gravis. Anatomic variations are presented as detailed drawings. Based on findings of widely variable thymic anatomy, these well-known authors advocate that the transsternal approach may minimize incomplete thymectomy compared with a cervical incision.

Marchevsky, A. M., and Kaneko, M.: Surgical Pathology of the Mediastinum. New York, Raven Press, 1984.

The authors provide a comprehensive guide to pathology of the mediastinum, including thymic, mesenchymal, neurogenic, and lymphatic abnormalities. The majority of the book deals with thymic pathology. Much of the text is devoted to the pathophysiology of specific diseases, including myasthenia gravis. Several sections relate specifically to thymic pathology found in myasthenia gravis and provide detailed electron and light photomicrographs of these changes.

Olanow, C. W., Wechsler, A. S., and Roses, A. D.: A prospective study of thymectomy and serum receptor antibodies in myasthenia gravis. Ann. Surg., 196:113, 1982.

This modern report provides a prospective study of 47 consecutive patients in whom thymectomy was applied as either early or primary therapy for myasthenic weakness. Generalized weakness was improved in all patients with complete resolution in 83 per cent. Younger patients with myasthenia gravis were relieved more often than older patients. The authors emphasize that a lasting improvement in weakness can be obtained by thymectomy without either intervening or subsequent medical therapy. Also, the study suggests that acetylcholine receptor antibody titers may not correlate with the preoperative clinical status or postoperative response to thymectomy and that alteration of other thymic factors may be responsible for this improvement.

REFERENCES

1. Alpert, L. I., Papatestas, A., and Kark, A.: A histological reappraisal of the thymus in myasthenia gravis: A correlative study of thymic pathology and response to thymectomy. Arch. Pathol., 91:55, 1971.
2. Austin, E. H., Olanow, C. W., and Wechsler, A. S.: Thymoma following transcervical thymectomy for myasthenia gravis. Ann. Thorac. Surg., 35:548, 1983.
3. Blalock, A.: Thymectomy in the treatment of myasthenia gravis: Report of twenty cases. J. Thorac. Surg., 13:316, 1944.
4. Blalock, A., Mason, M. F., Morgan, H. J., and Riven, S. S.: Myasthenia gravis and tumors of the thymic region: Report of a case in which the tumor was removed. Ann. Surg., 110:544, 1939.
5. Drachman, D. B.: Myasthenia gravis. N. Engl. J. Med., 298:136 and 186, 1978.
6. Gracey, D. R., Divertie, M. B., Howard, F. M., and Payne, W. S.: Postoperative respiratory care after transsternal thymectomy in myasthenia gravis: A 3-year experience in 53 patients. Chest, 86:67, 1984.
7. Grob, D.: Clinical manifestations of myasthenia gravis. In Albuquerque, E. X., and Eldefrawi, A. T. (Eds.): Myasthenia Gravis. New York, Chapman and Hall, 1983.
8. Guthrie, L. G.: Myasthenia gravis in the seventeenth century. Lancet, 1:330, 1903.
9. Heiser, J. C., Rutherford, R. B., and Ringel, S. P.: Thymectomy for myasthenia gravis: A changing perspective. Arch. Surg., 117:533, 1982.
10. Jaretzki, A., Bethea, M., Wolff, M., Olarte, M. R., Lovelace, R. E., Penn, A. S., and Rowland, L.: A rational approach to total thymectomy in the treatment of myasthenia gravis. Ann. Thorac. Surg., 24:120, 1977.
11. Jolly, F.: Ueber Myasthenia Gravis Pseudoparalytica. Berliner Klin. Wochenschr., 32:1, 1895.
12. Lisak, R. P. and Barachi, R. L.: Myasthenia Gravis. Philadelphia, W. B. Saunders Company, 1982.
13. Marchevsky, A. M., and Kaneko, M.: Surgical Pathology of the Mediastinum. New York, Raven Press, 1984.
14. Masaoka, A., Nagaoka, Y., and Kotake, Y.: Distribution of thymic tissue at the anterior mediastinum: Current procedures in thymectomy. J. Thorac. and Cardiovasc. Surg., 70:747, 1975.
15. Mulder, D. G., Herrmann, C., Keesey, J., and Edwards, H.: Thymectomy for myasthenia gravis. Am. J. Surg., 146:61, 1983.
16. Namba, T., Brown, S. B., and Grob, D.: Neonatal myasthenia gravis: Report of two cases and review of the literature. Pediatrics, 45:488, 1970.
17. Namba, T., Brunner, N. G., and Brown S. B.: Familial myasthenia gravis: Report of 27 cases in 12 families and review of 164 patients in 73 families. Arch. Neurol., 25:49, 1971.
18. Olanow, C. W., and Roses, A. D.: A ChR antibody titer and clinical response to thymectomy in M.G. Neurology (N.Y.), 34:987, 1984.
19. Olanow, C. W., Roses, A. D., and Fay, J. W.: The effect of plasmapheresis on post-thymectomy ocular dysfunction. Can. J. Neurol. Sci., 8:169, 1981.
20. Olanow, C. W., and Wechsler, A. W.: The Surgical Management of Myasthenia Gravis. In Sabiston, D. C., Jr., and Spencer, F. C. (Eds.): Gibbon's Surgery of the Chest, 4th ed. Philadelphia, W. B. Saunders Company, 1983.
21. Olanow, C. W., Wechsler, A. W., and Roses, A. D.: A prospective study of thymectomy and serum acetylcholine receptor antibodies in myasthenia gravis. Ann. Surg., 196:113, 1982.
22. Oosterhuis, H. J.: Observations of the natural history of myasthenia gravis and the effect of thymectomy. Ann. N.Y. Acad. Sci., 377:678, 1981.
23. Paletto, A. E., and Maggi, G.: Thymectomy in the treatment of myasthenia gravis: Results in 320 patients. Int. Surg., 67:13, 1982.
24. Patrick, J., and Lindstrom, J. M.: Autoimmune response to acetylcholine receptor. Science, 180:871, 1973.
25. Penn, A. S., Jaretzki, A., Wolff, M., Chang, H. W., and Tennyson, V.: Thymic abnormalities: Antigen or antibodies? Response to thymectomy in myasthenia gravis. Ann. N.Y. Acad. Sci., 377:786, 1981.
26. Remen, L.: Zur Pathogenese und Therapie der Myasthenia gravis pseudoparalytica. Deutsch z. Nervenheilk., 128:68, 1932.
27. Robinson, C. L.: The role of the thymus for myasthenia gravis. Ann. R. Coll. Surg. Engl., 65:145, 1983.
28. Rosai, J., and Levine, G. D.: Tumors of the thymus. In Atlas of Tumor Pathology (Fascicle 3, Series 2): Washington, D.C., Armed Forces Institute of Pathology, 1976.
29. Rubin, J. W., Ellison, R. G., Moore, H. V., and Pai, G. P.: Thymectomy in myasthenia gravis: The timing of surgery and significance of thymic pathology. Am. Surg., 47:152, 1981.
30. Schumacher, and Roth: Thymektomie bei einem Fall von Morbus Basdowi mit Myasthenie. Mitt. Grenzgeb. Med. Chir., 25:746, 1913.
31. Simpson, J. A.: Myasthenia gravis: A new hypothesis. Scottish Med. J., 5:419, 1960.
32. Slater, G., Papatestas, A., and Genkin, S. G.: Thymomas in patients with myasthenia gravis. Ann. Surg., 188:171, 1978.
33. Spence, P. A., Morin, J. E., and Katz, M.: Role of plasmapheresis in preparing myasthenic patients for thymectomy: Initial results. Can. J. Surg., 27:303, 1984.
34. Vincent, A., Newsom-Davis, J., Newton, P., and Beck, N.: Acetylcholine receptor antibody and clinical response to thymectomy in myasthenia gravis. Neurology (Cleveland), 33:1276, 1983.
35. Walker, M. B.: Treatment of myasthenia gravis with physostigmine. Lancet, 1:1200, 1934.
36. Weigert, C.: Pathologisch-anatomischer Beitrag zur Erb'schen Krankheit (myasthenia gravis). Neurol. Zbl., 20:597, 1901.
37. Wilkins, E. W., and Castleman, B.: Thymoma: A continuing survey at the Massachusetts General Hospital. Ann. Thorac. Surg., 28:252, 1979.
38. Wilks, S.: On cerebritis, hysteria, and bulbar paralysis, as illustrative of arrest of function of the cerebrospinal centres. Guy's Hosp. Rep. (3rd ser.), 22:2, 1877.
39. Younger, D. S., Braun, N. M., Jaretzki, A., Penn, A. S., and Lovelace, R. E.: Myasthenia gravis: Determinants of independent ventilation after transsternal thymectomy. Neurology (N.Y.), 34:336, 1984.

SURGICAL DISORDERS OF THE PERICARDIUM

JOSEPH S. McLAUGHLIN, M.D.

46

In the fourth century B.C., Hippocrates described the pericardium as "a smooth tunic which envelops the heart and contains a small amount of fluid resembling urine." Galen, in the second century A.D., named the structure, identified pericardial inflammation and effusion in animals, and indicated that a similar occurrence might occur in humans. A thousand years passed before Avenzoar in the 12th century described the condition in man. Richard Lower, the brilliant English physician and scientist of the 17th century, described the pathophysiology of pericardial effusion and tamponade, and Riolan in 1649 recommended pericardial aspiration. Lancisi in 1728 and Morgagni in 1761 correlated the clinical and autopsy findings in constrictive pericarditis.

Romero performed the first successful pericardial drainage in 1819, and in 1829, Larrey, Chief Surgeon to Napoleon's Army, performed a pericardial incision to relieve a traumatically induced bloody effusion.

Many others have contributed to our knowledge of disorders of the pericardium. Hope described the friction rub. Kussmaul described distention of the cervical veins and weakening of the pulse during inspiration. The first finding bears his name, and the second he termed "pulsus paradoxus." Pick described ascites (pseudocirrhosis) as a manifestation of pericardial constriction, and Ewart noted the occurrence of dullness below the left scapula in large effusions. Pericardial resection was first performed independently by Rehn and Sauerbruch in 1913.

ANATOMY

The pericardium is a fibrous sac of considerable strength composed of elastic tissue and collagen. The inner layer reflects onto and intimately covers the heart as the visceral pericardium. The serous space produced contains approximately 30 ml. of fluid and provides an essentially frictionless environment for contraction and relaxation of the heart. Laterally, the pericardial sac abuts the pleura, inferiorly the diaphragm, anteriorly the sternum, superiorly the thymus, and posteriorly the carina and esophagus.

Superiorly, the pericardium reflects onto the aorta just proximal to the innominate artery and the main pulmonary artery divides within the sac. The ligamentum arteriosus or ductus arises at the apex of the pulmonary artery and is enclosed by a pericardial reflection. The right pulmonary artery passes behind the aorta and superior vena cava for 3 to 5 cm. prior to exiting the sac and giving rise to its first branch to the upper lobe, whereas the left pulmonary artery almost immediately exits the sac. Both vessels are enveloped by pericardial fibers for a short distance following penetration. The superior vena cava is enclosed in the pericardial sac to the level of the azygos vein. The inferior vena cava penetrates the diaphragm, and only the most proximal portion is within the pericardial sac. The pericardium reflects onto the main pulmonary veins at their origins. A transverse sinus exists behind the aorta and pulmonary artery, and the ligamentous remnant of the left anterior cardinal vein originating from the coronary sinus may be seen coursing on the posterior surface (Marshall's ligament). At times this structure may be patent as a left superior vena cava.

Blood vessels, nerves, and lymphatics course the outer layer of the parietal pericardium within loose adipose tissue covered laterally by the pleural membrane. These structures lie beneath the visceral pericardium (epicardium) on the surface of the heart. The blood supply of the pericardium originates from the internal mammary arteries, and their musculophrenic branches and from the descending thoracic aorta. The nerve supply is from the vagus and phrenic nerves and from branches of the sympathetic trunk. Only the lower portion of the pericardial sac is sensitive to painful stimuli, including distention; the pain is referred to the base of the neck. Although this is the pathway of the phrenic nerve, sympathetic efferents must also be involved, since left stellate ganglion blockade completely relieves such pain.

CLINICAL AND PATHOPHYSIOLOGIC CONSIDERATIONS

The pericardium provides a friction-free environment for the constant motion of the heart and prevents torsion of the heart and the great vessels. Experimental evidence suggests that this structure prevents overdistention of the heart, particularly the right ventricle, and thereby prevents injury to myocardial fibers sensitive to overstretching. In contrast to these findings, patients in whom the pericardium has been removed appear to suffer no significant consequence.[3]

Inflammation of the pericardium results in a number of signs and symptoms that classically herald the disorder.[15] Nonspecific findings of fever, leukocytosis, and general malaise are common. More specific findings include chest pain, a friction rub, pericardial effusion, abnormal jugular venous pulsations, and pulsus paradoxus.

Pain

In acute inflammation of the pericardium, pain is invariably present, but the type and severity vary considerably. In viral, nonspecific, and bacterial pericarditis, pain is often abrupt in onset and sharp in nature. It is usually located substernally, but may radiate widely to the back, neck, and epigastrium. Radiation to the epigastrium may suggest intra-abdominal illness and may further be confused because of upper abdominal muscular tenseness. Pericardial pain may be described as a dull substernal ache or heaviness that radiates to the neck and shoulders but, unlike the pain of myocardial infarction, it rarely spreads to the arms. Patients frequently are more comfortable sitting up and leaning forward.

Friction Rub

The hallmark of pericarditis is a friction rub produced by the rubbing together of the inflamed and roughened serous surfaces of the parietal and visceral pericardium with a sound not unlike that of walking on dry snow. It is usually present in the early stages of the illness prior to the development of significant effusion, but may persist with loculated or posterior effusions. Rubs are best heard to the left of the sternum during inspiration with the patient in the sitting position. The pericardial rub may be present intermittently during the course of illness.

Pericardial Effusion

Inflammation produces an outpouring of fluid into the pericardial sac. The nature of this fluid varies with the etiology of the condition and may be clear or straw-colored (viral or nonspecific pericarditis), turbid or frankly purulent (bacterial and other infectious agents), or grossly bloody (uremia and tumors). Occasionally, chronic effusions high in cholesterol are encountered (cholesterol pericarditis). The effusion has a fluorescent quality, a "gold paint" appearance. Such effusions are common to conditions in which cholesterol turnover is reduced (myxedema), but they also may represent a nonspecific response to a variety of stimuli.[3]

The pericardium has great elastic properties, and if the effusion occurs slowly, large volumes may accumulate without significant compression of the heart. Physical examination of a patient with a large pericardial effusion generally will reveal an increase in venous pressure demonstrated by distention of the cervical veins. The apical impulse is diffuse or absent, and the heart sounds are muffled or distant. However, the heart sounds may be clear and easily heard with posterior or loculated effusions. *Ewart's sign*, or dullness to percussion below the left scapula, may be present, but is unreliable in the presence of left pleural effusion. If cardiac compression is present, the dramatic findings of cardiac tamponade are present.

Cardiac Tamponade

Cardiac tamponade is the syndrome of compression of the heart and produces physiologic and metabolic consequences.[14] This condition has multiple etiologies, but the basic manifestations are the same. The chambers of the compressed heart are unable to receive and, therefore, to pump the quantity of blood required for normal metabolism. Tamponade may be insidious in onset, as with malignancy, or acute and disastrous, as with penetrating trauma. Tamponade results in decreased stroke volume and increased diastolic filling pressure with equalization of right and left atrial pressures. Compensatory sympathetic activity results in tachycardia and increased systemic resistance. As the process worsens, the cardiac output continues to fall and the signs of cardiogenic shock appear.

The clinical manifestations of cardiac tamponade vary with the etiology of the condition and with the rapidity of its progression, but certain physical findings are usually present and include tachycardia, cervical venous distention, narrowed pulse pressure, systolic blood pressure below 100 mm. Hg, and pulsus paradoxus.

Pulsus paradoxus may be defined as a change of greater than 10 mm. Hg in the systolic pressure between inspiration and expiration, the lower pressure being determined during inspiration. This phenomenon should be considered an exaggeration of the usual difference in systolic blood pressure found between the two stages of respiration. Blood return to the right heart normally increases during inspiration as a result of the negative pressure in the thorax. The increase in right ventricular stroke volume is easily accommodated in the expanded pulmonary vascular bed and return to the left heart, and its stroke volume is lessened. This situation is exaggerated when the left ventricle is compressed. This finding may be readily appreciated by arterial palpation and at times may be associated with the complex absence of a palpable pulse during inspiration. A word of caution: Paradoxical pulse may be found in other conditions that may be confused with pericardial tamponade, including constrictive pericarditis, obesity, and obstructive lung disease (asthma or emphysema).

Clinically, cardiac tamponade may evolve slowly, and a rapid evaluation of the etiology may be undertaken prior to definitive therapy. Acute tamponade is an emergency: Appropriate treatment must be immediately instituted if the patient is to survive.

Chronic constrictive pericarditis is the term applied to progressive thickening and contraction of the pericardium with cardiac restriction. The chronically elevated venous pressure and low flow state produce a number of physiologically significant findings. Reduced perfusion of the kidneys results in salt and water retention with an increased blood volume and a further increase in venous pressure. However, the normal physiologic consequence of this series of events—an increase in cardiac output—does not take place because of mechanical restriction of the heart. Diuretics may be effective in reducing the excessive blood volume without reducing cardiac output. This is in contradistinction to the *acute* tamponade state, in which diuretics are contraindicated; reduction in blood volume and venous pressure may further compromise cardiac output.

Ascites may appear with little if any peripheral edema. The increase in hepatoportal venous pressure with resultant enlargement of the liver also may produce significant increases in lymphatic production and venous congestion of the intestinal mucosa. Malabsorption and loss of protein and fat may be significant, and the malabsorptive state may be the predominant presenting symptom complex.

Pericardectomy improves these physiologic abnormalities, but the patient's condition may not return to normal.[11] This lack of response may be due to incomplete pericardectomy or, more often, to reduced myocardial function.[2] It has been postulated that prolonged constriction results in "disuse atrophy," and indeed some patients may improve significantly over time. Unfortunately, some patients worsen, probably from myocardial fibrosis and damage from both the original inflammatory process and the effects of chronic compression.

IMAGING AND ELECTROCARDIOGRAPHIC ASSESSMENT

Radiology

The basic chest roentgenogram may provide important clues to the diagnosis of pericardial disease, but the absence of findings does not necessarily exclude disorders of this structure.[15] In acute pericarditis, the heart shadow may be normal in size and configuration. Small to moderate effusions (less than 200 ml.) are not apparent. With the development of larger effusion, the heart shadow symmetrically increases in size and may take on a "water bottle" shape (Figs. 1 and 2). Because an enlarged heart shadow may represent primary myocardial disease as well as a pericardial effusion, the absence of pulmonary congestion in pericardial constriction may be an important finding.

Echocardiography

Echocardiography has become a standard in cardiac evaluation and is valuable in identifying pericardial effusion and myocardial wall motion abnormalities.[15, 16] Small effusions (less than 50 ml.) can be identified, but exact quantification is difficult. Generally, if the visceral and parietal pericardial echoes do not completely separate, the effusion is small. Complete separation occurs with an effusion of moderate size, and a large effusion results in an echo-free

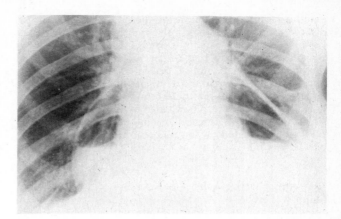

Figure 2. Pericardial effusion following aspiration revealing a moderately thickened pericardial wall in a patient with nonspecific pericarditis.

space both anteriorly and posteriorly (Fig. 3). This modality has been particularly useful in following the progression of effusions in patients with viral and nonspecific pericarditis and following cardiac surgical procedures. An extensive

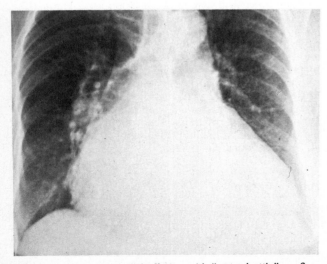

Figure 1. A large pericardial effusion with "water bottle" configuration of the heart shadow.

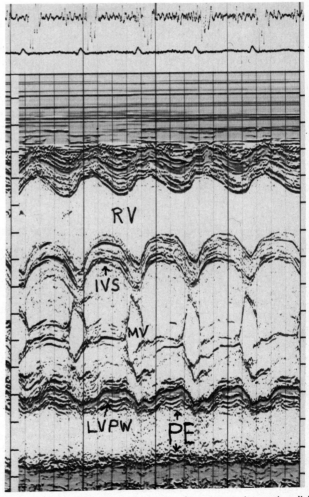

Figure 3. Echocardiogram showing a large posterior pericardial effusion. RV = Right ventricle; IVS = interventricular septum; MV = mitral valve; LVPW = left ventricular posterior wall; PE = pericardial effusion.

amount of literature concerning the nuances of pericardial disorders and chamber and valve function has evolved. For example, echocardiography clearly demonstrates the exaggerated enlargement of the right ventricular chamber and the decreased diameter of the left ventricular chamber during inspiration in cardiac tamponade. However, the difficulty of interpreting these often minimal and overlapping findings detracts somewhat from its clinical usefulness. Certainly, in acute pericardial tamponade the diagnosis is predominantly clinical and valuable time may be lost in performing this study.

Computed Tomography

Computed tomography (CT scanning) is of considerable use in evaluating the pericardium (Figs. 4 and 5). Effusions can be identified, neoplasms can be seen, and the thickness of the pericardium and heart chamber size can be determined with accuracy; when correlated with the clinical findings, CT scanning may confirm the diagnosis of constrictive disorders.

Electrocardiography

Because the pericardium is electrically silent, the commonly seen electrocardiographic (ECG) changes are related to the effect of the disease process on the underlying myocardium. Except in Dressler's syndrome, pericarditis following myocardial infarction, ECG changes rarely indicate the etiology of the pericardial disease, only its presence. In acute pericarditis, changes resulting from pericardial effusion and the current of injury in the superficial myocardium produce changes in the QRS complex and the ST segment.[15] Pericardial effusion may produce low voltage of the QRS complex, and acute pericarditis is usually associated with ST segment elevation without the development of Q waves. Tachycardia is common, and transient atrial fibrillation occurs in a third of patients. An important finding is *electrical alternans*, an abnormality in which

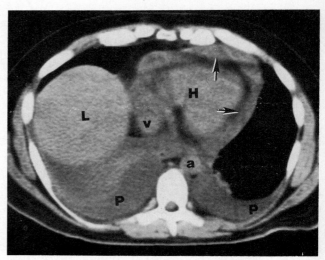

Figure 5. CT scan of the chest at the level of the right hemidiaphragm reveals marked thickening (1.2 cm.) of the pericardium (arrows) with bilateral pleural effusions. Echocardiography demonstrated restricted wall motion and cardiac catheterization pressure changes compatible with constrictive pericarditis. The patient underwent pericardectomy. L = Liver; H = heart; P = pleural effusion; A = descending aorta; V = inferior vena cava.

alternating amplitude of the QRS complex is seen with every other beat and most commonly occurs in pericardial tamponade and at times in constrictive pericarditis. Other conditions which produce this unusual finding are severe myocardial dysfunction, tension pneumothorax, and supraventricular tachycardia.

CONGENITAL ABNORMALITIES

The pericardial cavity begins its development during the third week of embryonic life.[12] Within the mesoderm, a series of spaces appear that soon coalesce to form the intraembryonic coelom. During the second month, the coelom is divided into the pericardial, pleural, and peritoneal cavities. The septum transversum, composed of mesoderm, appears during the third week and rapidly develops to form the central tendon of the diaphragm. The pericardial and pleural cavities are formed by the ingrowth of the pleuropericardial membranes, which are mesenchymal partitions containing the common cardinal veins and phrenic nerves. The right pleuropericardial membrane is larger, probably because of the larger size of the right common cardinal vein, and it divides the right cavity somewhat earlier than the left. Although necessarily simplistic, the foregoing discussion provides a mechanism of explanation for the two most commonly seen congenital anomalies of the pericardium, namely, (1) pericardial cysts and diverticula and (2) pericardial defects.

Pericardial Cysts

It is thought that cysts of the pericardium are remnants of the original lacunar structure of the primitive pericardial coelom. Typically, they are asymptomatic and are discovered on the chest film as smooth masses in the anterior chest at the pericardial phrenic sulcus (Fig. 6). They usually are seen on the right, but they may occur on either side

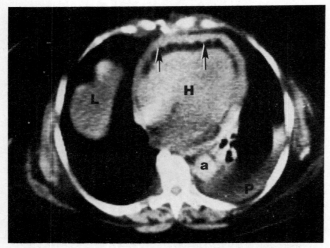

Figure 4. CT scan of the chest at the level of the right hemidiaphragm demonstrating nodular thickening of the pericardium (arrows) with a left pleural effusion. The patient had breast carcinoma, and metastases to the pericardium necessitated pericardial drainage. L = Liver; H = heart; P = pleural effusion; A = descending aorta.

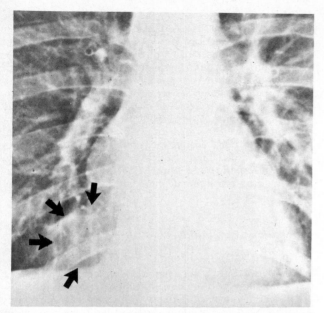

Figure 6. Chest film showing a pericardial cyst. Tomography is helpful in demonstrating the cystic structure of the lesion.

and rarely may be higher in the mediastinum. At times these cysts communicate with the pericardial cavity, forming diverticula. They are fibrous in structure and are lined by mesothelial cells. They are invariably benign, but there are a few anecdotal reports of large cysts producing life-threatening mediastinal compression. Since these cysts may be confused with other potentially more dangerous mediastinal and lung tumors, excision for definitive diagnosis is generally recommended.

Pericardial Defects

Defects of the pericardium may occur because of incomplete development and closure, particularly of the normally thinner and later closing left pleuropericardial membrane, and have been said to occur because of premature atrophy of the left cardinal vein (sinus of Cuvier). Such defects nearly always are seen on the left, usually near the hilum of the lung; right-sided and diaphragmatic defects and total absence are rare. Approximately a third of patients will have other anomalies of the heart or lung.

Small defects (1 to 2 cm.) are asymptomatic and are usually discovered at the time of cardiac surgery or at autopsy. Larger defects and complete absence of the left pericardium rarely are of clinical significance, and most individuals with such defects live normal lives. Cardiac catheterization of patients with large defects usually has demonstrated normal hemodynamics.

Some patients have a history of vague chest discomfort, ascribed but not proven to be due to compression of the coronary arteries by the edge of the defect, partial torsion of the great vessels, and adhesions between the heart and lung through the defect. A systolic murmur is frequently present in patients with large defects or absence of the left pericardium. There are rare reports of herniation and strangulation of the left atrium through moderate-sized defects and sudden death, presumably as a result of torsion of the heart through larger defects.

Radiologic evaluation of the chest may offer clues to the diagnosis. Fullness of the left hilum and irregularity of the left heart border because of left atrial herniation have been described, as has prominence of the pulmonary artery. With absence of the pericardium, the heart may be markedly displaced to the left without deviation of the trachea, and lung tissue may be seen between the aorta and pulmonary artery and between the heart and left hemidiaphragm. Treatment for these disorders is rarely necessary.

PERICARDITIS

Acute Pericarditis

Acute pericarditis is the syndrome characterized by chest pain, a pericardial friction rub, and ECG and other laboratory studies demonstrating pericardial inflammation. It is commonly preceded by an upper respiratory infection. Although presumably infectious and possibly often viral in origin, a specific etiology is uncommonly found, thus the multiplicity of terms: benign, viral, nonspecific, and idiopathic. Other common causes of acute pericarditis include bacterial infection, uremia, postpericardectomy syndrome, and neoplasia.

Nonspecific Pericarditis

Nonspecific pericarditis usually begins with fever, precordial chest pain, and dyspnea. The magnitude and abruptness of these symptoms vary considerably. Some patients are seen with minimal symptoms and findings, and presumably there are patients whose course is so mild that they do not seek medical advice unless late sequelae develop.

The classic presentation of the illness usually is seen in the youthful patient. As many as 60 per cent give a history of respiratory infection in the preceding 3 weeks. Fever and at times chills and diaphoresis accompany the onset of sharp and stabbing substernal pain. The pain may radiate widely and is frequently relieved by sitting up. Breathing and coughing accentuate the pain, and shallow and at times grunting respiration may be present. Dyspnea is an early symptom, but it may worsen with the development of effusion.

Leukocytosis with a relative increase in lymphocytes is commonly found. The chest film may reveal enlargement of the cardiac shadow, and echocardiography may reveal a pericardial effusion. The ECG shows ST segment elevation without the development of Q waves.

The diagnosis is primarily one of exclusion, and myocardial infarction and myocarditis must be considered.[15] A tuberculin skin test and blood cultures are indicated to exclude a bacterial etiology, and fungal serology should be obtained in endemic regions. Rheumatic fever should be excluded by determination of Streptococcus antigens or antistreptococcal antibodies. Collagen disorders including lupus should be considered. Cold agglutinins and heterophils may be required to exclude Mycoplasma and infectious mononucleosis. Viral studies should be obtained when possible and practical. Pericardiocentesis may be required in the diagnosis of bacterial or neoplastic pericarditis and as treatment for persistent large effusions and cardiac tamponade.

Assuming a specific etiology is not determined, the treatment is symptomatic. Generally, nonspecific pericarditis follows a benign and self-limiting course of 2 to 6 weeks. Hospitalization is indicated during the initial period, and aspirin usually relieves the pain; however, at times narcotics are necessary. Corticosteroids produce a dramatic response, but large doses are necessary (prednisone, 60 to 80 mg. per day) and relapse is not uncommon.

Persistent large pericardial effusions may be troublesome and may be discovered in patients without a history of preceding illness. In the latter instance, the problem becomes one of both diagnosis and therapy. The course of such effusions can be followed by periodic echocardiography. If the effusion does not respond to corticosteroids, pericardiocentesis is indicated. At times, because of fibrin formation and loculation, this technique produces unsuccessful results and drainage of the pericardial sac or pericardectomy is necessary.[11]

Pericardial tamponade or the development of constricting pericarditis is unusual in nonspecific pericarditis. However, recurrence is common and it is not unusual to see exacerbations of the process with pain, fever, and recurrence of the friction rub for a year or more. It has been suggested that this sequence is not recurrence of infection but, rather, an immunologic response to serosal injury.

Viral Pericarditis

With the development of more precise means of identification of specific viruses, many cases of pericarditis, previously classified as "nonspecific," can be ascribed to a specific viral agent. Echovirus and adenovirus are among the most common. Identification usually is made serologically by demonstration of a rise in specific antibody titer; however, coxsackievirus and influenza virus have been identified in pericardial fluid culture, and other viruses, including mumps and varicella, have been implicated by association with the classic disease state.

Certain findings are pertinent to the surgeon. Coxsackievirus, influenza virus, and echovirus have been shown to produce severe myocarditis that may result in significant heart damage and heart failure. These viruses may also produce a frankly purulent effusion that leads to fibrosis, calcification, and constriction. Fortunately, this series of events occurs in only 5 per cent of patients. Infectious mononucleosis and other viral disorders have been reported to produce a similar outcome rarely.

Bacterial Pericarditis

Prior to the advent of antibiotics, bacterial infection was a relatively common cause of pericarditis,[8, 13] and the organisms usually responsible were pneumococci and streptococci. With the introduction of penicillin, the overall incidence of this type of infection declined significantly, and staphylococcal and gram-negative infections became predominant. The infection may be blood-borne from osteomyelitis, pneumonia, or other infections. Bacterial endocarditis and myocardial abscess are less common causes. Bacterial pericarditis may occur following cardiothoracic operations or penetrating trauma to the pericardium and by direct extension from contiguous infections above and below the diaphragm.

Clinically, the presentation is influenced and at times obscured by the precipitating illness, particularly if this illness involves the chest and if the patient has been treated with antibiotics. In patients with blood-borne infection, the initial presentation is similar but is usually more dramatic than that seen with viral or nonspecific pericarditis.

Pyogenic infections progress rapidly, and large effusions and early onset of cardiac tamponade are the rule. Chest pain is a prominent feature in only 25 per cent of patients, and friction rubs are appreciated in half the patient population. The diagnosis requires examination of pericardial fluid and may be achieved by pericardiocentesis initially or by performance of subxiphoid pericardial window drainage and biopsy. Treatment of antibiotics alone is followed by a high mortality despite measurable levels of antibiotics in the pericardial fluid. Effective drainage is mandatory, and because pericardial constriction is a common sequela, some authors recommend immediate or early pericardectomy.

Tuberculous Pericarditis

Prior to the introduction of antimicrobial drugs, tuberculous pericarditis was common, occurring in 5 to 10 per cent of patients with pulmonary tuberculosis and responsible for the majority of patients with constrictive pericarditis.[6] This incidence has fallen precipitously, although since culture and tissue diagnosis are difficult even in acute illness, the exact incidence is unknown. Active tuberculous infection of the pericardium when left untreated carries an 85 per cent mortality. With treatment, the mortality is reduced to less than 7 per cent but constriction occurs in approximately 60 per cent.

Although it is evident that tuberculosis may produce constrictive pericarditis, a valid question concerns the incidence of tuberculosis in constrictive pericarditis. Today it is encountered much less frequently than it was prior to antimicrobials. Increasing numbers of patients have no known previous illness to explain the thickened pericardial wall. It is speculated that the initiating tuberculous or viral infection may be so mild that it is unrecognized, yet it sets in motion a series of events leading to pericardial thickening and constriction.

Tuberculous pericarditis is often of insidious onset.[6] In approximately 50 per cent of patients, there are no other evident foci of tuberculous infection, suggesting that infection occurs with the primary and not demonstrable pulmonary infection and reaches the pericardium by hematogenous dissemination, through lymphatic channels or by direct extension from a contiguously involved segment of lung. The disease is slowly progressive with gradual evolution from granulation through an effusive to an absorptive stage, followed by fibrosis and constriction of the pericardium (Fig. 7). The symptoms are usually those of low-grade fever, malaise, and weight loss. Cough and other pulmonary symptoms may be present, although hemoptysis is unusual. In the effusive stage, clinical evidence of effusion may be confirmed by chest film and echocardiogram. When a diagnosis of pericarditis is made, a tuberculous etiology may be difficult to prove and depends upon a high degree of suspicion. The tuberculin skin test findings may be negative, and culture of pericardial fluid and cultures and microscopic examination of pericardial biopsies frequently have been nondiagnostic.

There is evidence that delay in treatment results in a higher incidence of constrictive pericarditis. If tuberculosis is proved or is highly suspected, triple drug therapy is indicated. Isoniazid, ethambutol, and, initially, streptomycin are recommended, but rifampicin (rifampin) may be

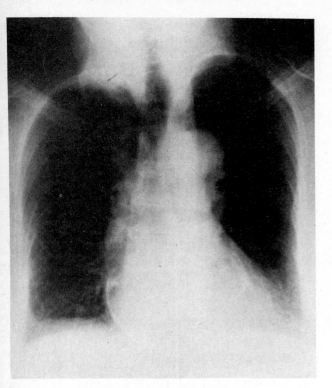

Figure 7. Chest film in a patient with chronic constrictive pericarditis. The heart shadow is not enlarged, and calcium is apparent in the pericardial wall.

substituted for one of the foregoing. Corticosteroids have been recommended for large effusions, and retrospective studies suggest that use of these agents results in a lower incidence of constriction. Because surgical treatment is both diagnostic and therapeutic, pericardial biopsy is indicated. Subxiphoid drainage may be required for large effusions with compressive symptoms. Pericardectomy is indicated for potential and frank constrictive disorders.

Fungal and Other Infectious Forms of Pericarditis

Histoplasmosis, coccidioidomycosis, and blastomycosis may invade the pericardium during the course of systemic disease with their respective organisms (*Histoplasma, Coccidioides, Blastomyces*). Histoplasmosis has been reported to produce both massive effusions and constrictive pericarditis.

The widespread use of antibiotics and immunosuppressive drugs has produced an increase in systemic fungal infection and resultant pericarditis. Narcotics addicts have a high incidence of unusual infections, including systemic fungal infections.

Reports of systemic illness from *Monilia* and *Aspergillus* with myocardial and pericardial involvement should lead to awareness of this possibility. Actinomycosis may involve the pericardium and has been reported to do so in 2 per cent of cases. *Actinomyces* is an anaerobe and generally is found in necrotic and neoplastic conditions of the chest and mediastinum. *Nocardia*, an aerobe, may invade the pericardium from adjacent lung infection, most often in patients with lymphoma or leukemia.

Parasitic disorders of the pericardium are rare in this country. Amebic involvement of the pericardium is usually by direct invasion through the diaphragm from liver abscesses. Echinococcal pericarditis results from rupture of hydatid cysts of the heart.

Uremic Pericarditis

Uremic pericarditis was recognized by Bright in 1836, and since then an incidence up to 50 per cent has been reported in chronic renal failure. The etiology is not clearly understood and may be multifactorial. The incidence is very low in mild renal failure and is reduced with hemodialysis in severe kidney failure (approximately 10 per cent); however, even with adequate dialysis the condition occurs and may be quite troublesome. The symptoms and signs include chest pain, fever, a friction rub, neck vein distention, and at times cardiac tamponade of sudden onset. Treatment initially is ensuring adequacy of dialysis by increasing length and frequency[9], which is successful in 40 per cent of cases. Corticosteroids and indomethacin frequently bring about significant relief. However, despite these measures, in approximately 10 per cent of patients, cardiac constriction develops and pericardectomy is required.

Post-irradiation Pericarditis

Prior to the adoption of modern techniques, pericarditis was a frequent sequela of irradiation therapy to the chest.[10] Pericardial effusion was common in the first year, and constrictive disorders were identified many years following treatment and appeared to be dose-related. The present therapy of Hodgkin's disease—utilizing multiple ports and shielding—has reduced the incidence to 2.5 per cent. Corticosteroids have been recommended for those in whom pericarditis develops, but recurrence is not uncommon following withdrawal of therapy. Pericardiocentesis may be required in effusions producing tamponade, but reaccumulation is common and this procedure is of limited long-term benefit. Pericardectomy has been successful in relieving persistent effusions and is the treatment of choice if evidence of constriction appears.

Neoplastic Pericarditis

The pericardium is involved in approximately 8 per cent of metastatic malignant neoplasms. Statistically, the most common tumors are carcinoma of the lung in males and carcinoma of the breast in females. Melanoma frequently metastasizes to the heart and pericardium, and leukemic and lymphoma involvement is common. Rare primary malignant tumors of the pericardium include mesothelioma and hemangiosarcoma. These tumors generally produce hemorrhagic pericardial effusions and tamponade, and are rapidly fatal. Benign tumors make up somewhat less than half of the primary tumors of the pericardium and are often fibromas or lipomas, usually discovered accidentally. Leukemia and lymphoma may have little functional significance, and the degree of functional impairment by lung and breast tumors is variable.

Treatment is difficult and discouraging. Leukemia, lymphomas, and breast tumors may respond to chemotherapy, and irradiation therapy and carcinoma of the lung may respond to irradiation. Malignant effusions may be temporarily relieved by pericardial drainage.[7] However, the usual situation is one in which the tumor has spread widely and the patient is in desperate condition.

Postmyocardial Infarction Syndrome

Transmural myocardial infarction by definition involves the epicardium, and in a fifth of patients diffuse pericarditis results. A friction rub may be heard in as many as 15 per cent of patients, usually within the first 96 hours following the event. In 1956, Dressler described a group of patients in whom pericarditis developed 2 to 4 weeks following an infarction.[4] The illness is characterized by fever, chest pain, pericardial and pleural effusion, frequently a friction rub, and ECG changes indicative of pericarditis. Evidence exists that this condition finds its etiology in the autoimmune mechanisms, and antiheart antibodies have been described.

Postpericardiotomy Syndrome

Postpericardiotomy syndrome is an interesting and common condition that may occur following any injury of the pericardium, surgical or otherwise.[5] The syndrome includes pericardial inflammation with chest pain, fever, a friction rub and pericardial effusion, pleurisy, and, at times, pulmonary infiltrates and arthralgias. Atrial arrhythmias are common. The syndrome was originally noted following pericardial and cardiac injury, gained prominence as the "postcommissurotomy syndrome" in the 1950s, and has been recognized following catheter perforation of the heart and blunt trauma to the chest. It occurs in as many as 70 per cent, with an average of 30 per cent of patients undergoing cardiac surgery. The etiology is unknown and probably is multifactorial. Injection of blood into the pericardium causes pericarditis, and antiheart antibodies have been demonstrated as having significant rises of antibody titers to viral agents.

Although the condition is usually mild and self-limiting, it may mimic other more serious conditions, including pneumonia, pulmonary embolism, and infection. It is particularly troublesome psychologically in patients who have undergone coronary artery bypass surgery and who experience a recurrence of chest pain.[1]

Treatment depends on the severity of the condition. In mild presentations, only rest and mild analgesia are required. Aspirin, 650 mg. every 4 hours, usually is effective in more severe states, and steroids are indicated if symptoms continue.

TECHNICAL CONSIDERATIONS

Pericardiocentesis

Pericardiocentesis is a procedure associated with definite risks. When possible, it should be performed in an intensive care environment with appropriate monitoring, electrical defibrillation equipment, and cardiovascular drugs and with an operating team available. Most physicians prefer the left perixiphoid approach, since the lung is not in the path of the needle and coronary injury is said to be less common; however, the pericardium may be entered to

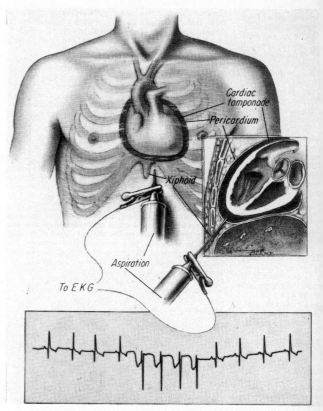

Figure 8. Technique of pericardiocentesis. Negative deflection of the QRS complex indicates contact with the epicardium. (From Ebert, P.: The pericardium. In Sabiston, D. C., and Spencer, F. C. (Eds.): Gibbon's Surgery of the Chest, 4th ed. Philadelphia, W. B. Saunders Company, 1983, p. 996.)

the left of the sternum in the fourth interspace particularly in large effusions (Fig. 8).

The patient is placed upright at a 45-degree angle, and the area is cleansed and draped. Local anesthesia is used for the skin and subcutaneous tissues. A 3-inch short beveled No. 16 or No. 18 needle, attached to an aspirating syringe, is inserted between the xiphoid and left costal margin and is directed superiorly at a 45-degree angle to the abdominal wall toward the midline of the spine. Lead V of the ECG should be attached to the needle when past the skin, and an observer should monitor the ECG. Contact with the myocardium results in marked ST segment elevation. Once the parietal pericardium is perforated and free flow of fluid established, a plastic catheter may be substituted to allow continuous drainage.

Pericardial Biopsy and Drainage

Pericardial biopsy and drainage must be performed in the operating room. Mild sedation with local anesthesia is satisfactory for most adults, but children usually require general anesthesia. The pericardium may be approached through the left anterior chest, at times by resecting the fourth or fifth costal cartilage or by the midline subxiphoid approach. Left thoracotomy has the advantage of superior exposure. The subxiphoid approach avoids pleural contamination and provides excellent drainage.

Pericardectomy

Pericardectomy is indicated in patients with chronic and at times acute inflammation of the pericardium and is the definitive treatment for constrictive pericarditis. Preoperative preparation includes nutritional support, correction of electrolyte and fluid abnormalities, and treatment of congestive heart failure and arrhythmias when present. Antibiotics usually are administered prophylactically and antituberculosis drugs are given where tuberculosis is suspected or proven.

The patient is given a general anesthesia and carefully monitored. A midline sternal splitting incision exposes the pericardium, and dissection should begin over the left ventricle. Generally, a longitudinal incision is made through the parietal pericardium and deepened until the epicardium is encountered. A plane of dissection is developed, and the pericardium is removed from the entire left ventricle; such a plane is essential to avoid injury to the subepicardial vessels, which may produce myocardial infarction. The phrenic nerve should be identified and carefully preserved. The dissection then is directed to the right side, the pericardium is resected from the thinner right ventricle and atrium, and the venae cavae are freed. The diaphragmatic surface of the pericardium is often exceedingly diseased and calcified, and it should be removed as completely as is safe and possible. Hemostasis is obtained, and the sternotomy is closed with chest tube drainage. Postoperative care includes proper management of fluids and electrolytes, blood replacement, control of arrhythmias, and, at times, pharmacologic support of the circulation.

SELECTED REFERENCES

Darsee, J. R., and Braunwald, E.: Diseases of the pericardium. *In* Braunwald, M. D. (Ed.): Heart Disease: A Textbook of Cardiovascular Medicine. Philadelphia, W. B. Saunders Company, 1980.
The authors report a very complete and detailed description of various conditions that affect the pericardium. Included are pathophysiologic, clinical, and laboratory findings. An excellent reference source for students, residents, and practicing physicians.

Fowler, N. O.: Pericardial diseases in key references. Circulation, *63*:1429, 1981.
This source contains more than 200 references relating to all aspects of pericardial disease.

Miller, J. I., Mansour, K. A., and Hatcher, C. R.: Pericardectomy: Current indications, concepts and results in a university center. Ann. Thorac. Surg., *34*:40, 1982.
*This study is an excellent review of current surgical practice. One hundred and two patients underwent pericardectomy in the Emory University Hospitals for a wide variety of pericardial disease. Seventy-six patients had predominant effusive pericardial disease, and 26 patients had con-*strictive pericarditis. A detailed description of each subgroup of patients is given.

Shabetai, R., Mangiardi, L., Bhargava, V., Ross, J., and Higgins, C. B.: The pericardium and cardiac function. Prog. Cardiovasc. Dis., *22*:107, 1979.
This review is conveniently divided into three major areas: (1) normal physiology, (2) the contribution of the pericardium to abnormalities in cardiac function, and (3) effects of disease of the pericardium on cardiac function. Included are studies on experimental animals and humans and an excellent bibliography.

REFERENCES

1. Borkon, A. M., Schaff, H. V., Gardner, T. J., Merrill, W. H., Brawley, R. K., Donahoo, J. S., Watkins, L., Weiss, J. L., and Gott, V. L.: Diagnosis and management of postoperative pericardial effusions and late cardiac tamponade following open heart surgery. Ann. Thorac. Surg., *31*:512, 1981.
2. Culliford, A. T., Lipton, M., and Spencer, F. C.: Operation for chronic constrictive pericarditis: Do the surgical approach and degree of pericardial resection influence the outcome significantly? Ann. Thorac. Surg., *29*:146, 1980.
3. Darsee, J. R., and Braunwald, E.: Diseases of the pericardium. *In* Braunwald, M. D. (Ed.): Heart Disease: A Textbook of Cardiovascular Medicine, Philadelphia, W. B. Saunders Company, 1980.
4. Dressler, W.: The post-myocardial infarction syndrome: A report of forty-four cases. A.M.A. Arch. Intern. Med., *102*:23, 1959.
5. Engle, M. A., McCabe, J. C., Ebert, P. A., and Zabriskie, J.: The post-pericardiotomy syndrome and antiheart antibodies. Circulation, *49*:401, 1974.
6. Hageman, J. H., D'Esopo, N. D., and Glenn, W. W.: Tuberculosis of the pericardium: A long term analysis of 44 proved cases. N. Engl. J. Med., *27*:327, 1964.
7. Hankins, J. R., Satterfield, J. R., Aisner, J., Wiernik, P. H., and McLaughlin, J. S.: Pericardial window for malignant pericardial effusion. Ann. Thorac. Surg., *30*:465, 1980.
8. Klacsmann, P. G., Bulkley, B. H., and Hutchins, G. M.: The changed spectrum of purulent pericarditis: An 86 year autopsy experience in 200 patients. Am. J. Med., *63*:666, 1977.
9. Koopot, R., Zerefos, N. S., Lavender, A. R., and Pifarre, R.: Cardiac tamponade in uremic pericarditis: Surgical approach and management. Am. J. Cardiol., *32*:846, 1973.
10. Martin, R. G., Ruckdeschel, J. C., Chang, P., Byhardt, R., Bouchard, R. J., and Wiernik, P. H.: Radiation related pericarditis. Am. J. Cardiol., *35*:217, 1975.
11. Miller, J. I., Mansour, K. A., and Hatcher, C. R.: Pericardectomy: Current indications, concepts and results in a university center. Ann. Thorac. Surg., *34*:40, 1982.
12. Moore, K. L.: The Developing Human, 3rd ed. Philadelphia, W. B. Saunders Company, 1982.
13. Morgan, R. J., Stephenson, L. W., Woolf, P. K., Edie, R. N., and Edmunds, L. H.: Surgical treatment of purulent pericarditis in children. J. Thorac. Cardiovasc. Surg., *85*:527, 1983.
14. Shabetai, R., Mangiardi, L., Bhargava, V., Ross, J., and Higgins, C. B.: The pericardium and cardiac function. Prog. Cardiovasc. Dis., *22*:107, 1979.
15. Spodick, D. H.: Differential diagnosis of acute pericarditis. Prog. Cardiovasc. Dis. *14*:192, 1971.
16. Tajik, A. J.: Echocardiography in pericardial effusion. Am. J. Med. *63*:29, 1977.

47

I

Cardiopulmonary Resuscitation

J. SCOTT RANKIN, M.D.

Sudden cardiopulmonary arrest is an acute emergency common to all medical specialties, and most physicians should be knowledgeable and proficient in resuscitation techniques. In fact, every physician at some point should gain direct experience in practical courses using dummy models and in supervised clinical emergencies. Although cardiopulmonary resuscitation (CPR), like all scientific subjects, is undergoing a continuous evolution, this chapter will attempt to define the current understanding of this important topic.

HISTORICAL ASPECTS

Cardiopulmonary resuscitation has been practiced since antiquity. References to ancient Hebrew methods exist in the Bible,[20] and Galen described the use of bellows to inflate the lungs of a dead animal.[7] Eighteenth-century physicians standardized techniques for performing mouth-to-mouth ventilation, and in 1786 a surgeon in England, John Sherwin, suggested that "the surgeon should go on inflating the lungs and alternately compressing the sternum."[12] Koenig, professor of surgery at Gottingen, Germany, is credited as the father of external cardiac compression, reporting in 1885 six successful resuscitative efforts in man.[10] Further application of the closed-chest technique was reported by Maas in 1892,[11] and Igelsrud successfully employed direct cardiac massage in 1901.[13] Crile studied adrenaline injections in the treatment of cardiac arrest and later applied his techniques extensively on the battlefields of World War I.[6] In 1947, Beck and associates[1] reported the first successful internal electrical defibrillation, which was followed in 1956 by the development of external cardioversion.[25] In 1960, Kouwenhoven and co-workers[14] initiated the modern era of CPR by combining expired air ventilation, external cardiac massage, and electrical defibrillation in the treatment of cardiac arrest. In 1963, the American Heart Association established the Committee on Cardiopulmonary Resuscitation, which published guidelines for CPR in 1974 and 1980.[16] These reports emphasized the importance of a standardized approach to CPR and stressed the relevance of extensive training at the community level. Initial results of this program clearly demonstrate that large numbers of cardiac arrest victims can be salvaged by early and effective application of CPR followed by transport and appropriate hospital therapy.

PATHOPHYSIOLOGY

Approximately one million individuals experience acute myocardial infarction annually in the United States, and approximately half of this number die each year from ischemic heart disease. It is estimated that over 300,000 of these deaths occur prior to hospital admission, most commonly from ventricular fibrillation. Based on experiences in coronary care units and supervised exercise programs, it is likely that the majority of sudden death victims could be resuscitated at the scene of the arrest with immediate cardiopulmonary support and defibrillation. Therefore, it is essential that a large portion of the public be trained to initiate CPR immediately at arrest and that paramedical systems be organized to respond with a defibrillator within 3 minutes. With this type of training, over 40 per cent of out-of-hospital arrest victims with documented ventricular fibrillation can be resuscitated,[2, 4, 9] and it is estimated that 100,000 lives could be saved annually by providing effective CPR at the site of arrest.

The most common cause of sudden, unexpected cardiac arrest is *ventricular fibrillation* associated with ischemic heart disease.[2] Fibrillation may occur as the end result of acute cardiac decompensation during myocardial infarction, or it may be a primary electrical event occurring coincident with coronary thrombosis or reversible imbalances in coronary blood flow. Early resuscitation in the last category may be associated with little permanent damage, and even in patients with coronary thrombosis, successful resuscitation now can be followed by definitive therapy such as streptokinase thrombolysis, coronary balloon angioplasty, or coronary artery bypass grafting.[8, 18, 19, 23] Recently developed methods for treating acute ischemic heart disease make successful resuscitation more important than ever. In addition, efforts now are being turned to identifying patients with ischemic heart disease who are at risk for sudden death and applying appropriate therapy at an earlier stage.[2] Other primary cardiac causes of sudden arrest, such as ventricular tachycardia or fibrillation associated with left ventricular aneurysms or Wolff-Parkinson-White syndrome, also can be treated on a routine basis with a high degree of success.[5]

The next most common cause of sudden cardiac arrest is *inadequate ventilation or pulmonary gas exchange*. The resultant hypoxia, hypercarbia, and systemic acidosis produce an acute deterioration of cardiac function and ventricular fibrillation. Many such conditions are encountered in daily practice, such as with suffocation, drowning, drug overdosage, foreign body aspiration, electrocution, or hypoventilation from primary pulmonary or neurologic disease. Early recognition of the etiology is essential so that ventilatory support can be provided before progression to cardiac arrest. In fact, no hospitalized patient under direct medical observation should ever progress from having acute ventilatory failure to cardiac arrest. With adequate monitoring of (1) ventilatory patterns, (2) work of breathing, (3) mental alertness, and (4) arterial blood gases, respiratory support should be initiated before cardiac decompensation occurs. In the case of foreign body aspiration, a high index of suspicion and alert diagnosis can lead to early dislodgment of the obstruction by one of several methods.

The final general etiologies of cardiopulmonary arrest are metabolic disorders. Hyperkalemia leading to ventricular fibrillation or asystole is associated with a very low rate of recovery and is best treated by prevention. When the serum potassium approaches 6.0 mg. per 100 ml. or the rate of increase in serum potassium is rapid, aggressive initial therapy with intravenous glucose (25 gm.) and insulin (20 microns) or sodium bicarbonate (44 mEq.) is indicated. At that point, the situation can be assessed further, the cause corrected, and long-term ion exchange resins, e.g., sodium polystyrene sulfonate (Kayexalate), or dialysis initiated. Other metabolic disturbances such as hypocalcemia or metabolic acidosis are more rarely associated with cardiac arrest, but also should be effectively treated at an early stage before they result in circulatory standstill.

Independent of the specific causative factor, cardiopulmonary arrest is manifested by ineffective cardiac output and arterial blood pressure. Cessation of oxygenated blood flow to the body is associated with rapidly progressing tissue hypoxia and metabolic acidosis. Because of high metabolic demands, the central nervous system is most vulnerable to circulatory arrest and can tolerate no more than 5 to 7 minutes of normothermic ischemia before permanent neurologic injury ensues. After longer periods of arrest, successful resuscitation may result in recovery of other organs, but return of central nervous system (CNS) function is unlikely. Thus, the ultimate limitation to successful resuscitation is preservation of neurologic integrity.

DIAGNOSIS

The diagnosis of cardiac arrest should be entertained whenever a previously alert patient collapses or becomes unconscious. The first step in approaching the problem is documenting total loss of consciousness. In addition, complete arrest usually is accompanied in initial phases by tonic muscular movements and rolling back of the eyes. Although agonal respiratory motion occurs transiently, spontaneous breathing soon stops if the arrest sequence progresses untreated. In a mechanically ventilated patient, thoracic motion and breath sounds obviously persist after cardiac arrest and respiratory movements are of little help. If there is a question of ventilator malfunction, the patient should be removed from the respirator and manually ventilated with 100 per cent oxygen.

The presumptive diagnosis of cardiac arrest is made by loss of a previously palpable central arterial pulse. Either the carotid or femoral artery is adequate to establish the diagnosis, and in monitored patients, loss of the electrocardiogram or arterial pressure waveform is confirmatory. Occasionally, patients continue to have a cardiac rhythm, even though the pulse is absent and the systolic blood pressure is less than 60 mm. Hg. In this case, resuscitation should be initiated because of ineffective circulatory performance. *One warning is in order.* On more than one occasion, resuscitation has been instituted because electrocardiographic leads became disconnected or for other erroneous reasons. This should never occur if each patient is initially approached slowly and thoughtfully. A period of at least 15 seconds of careful diagnostic data collection is prudent in most cases, including the documentation of absent pulses. In emergency situations, the tendency always is to proceed with haste; however, a short initial evaluation is not detrimental and the potentially harmful complications of an unnecessary resuscitation can be avoided. This is especially important in postoperative cardiac surgical patients in whom chest compression can produce sternal disruption, suture line hemorrhage, or perforation of the ventricles by artificial valves. Conversely, if there is a firm indication of arrested circulation, one should not hesitate to begin resuscitation while further evaluation is pursued. Coincident with beginning resuscitation, a call for help is given because effective CPR requires the coordinated efforts of multiple individuals.

RESUSCITATION METHODS

As defined by the subcommittee on Emergency Cardiac Care of the American Heart Association,[16] cardiopulmonary resuscitation can be divided into two phases: (1) Basic Life Support, and (2) Advanced Life Support. During inpatient resuscitation, the phases are not distinct because aspects from both proceed simultaneously. For the sake of clarity, however, each will be discussed individually as if applied sequentially.

Basic Life Support

VENTILATION

After the diagnosis of cardiac arrest is made, efforts are directed toward maintaining cardiopulmonary function and flow of oxygenated blood to the body. If evidence exists of isolated airway obstruction, such as produced by laryngeal meat impaction, a combination of back blows and abdominal manual thrusts frequently can dislodge the impaction.[16] Otherwise, the patient is placed supine in the hospital bed or on the ground. With a complete cardiopulmonary arrest, the mouth is opened and inspected; any foreign objects such as dentures or chewing gum are re-moved. The airway is established by extending the neck and tilting the victim's head backward. If difficulty is encountered in opening the airway, the jaw can be extended by applying forward pressure at the mandibular angles. Ventilation then is begun with a valved mask system, taking care to maintain an airtight seal around the face. If a mask is not available, mouth-to-mouth breathing is employed while occluding the patient's nostrils with one hand. With either technique, respirations should be maintained at 12 to 15 breaths per minute. Ventilatory pressure should be great enough to raise the chest and to produce satisfactory breath sounds. However, care should be taken not to ventilate so forcefully as to distend the stomach; gastric dilatation can produce vomiting, aspiration, and long-term pulmonary complications. It should be emphasized that mask ventilation is *entirely satisfactory* in most cases, and intubation should not be attempted until ventilation first has been re-established with a mask and until trained personnel are available. Unsuccessful attempts at intubation can negatively influence the outcome or directly injure the patient by lacerating the pharynx or vocal cords.

Endotracheal intubation in a semiconscious patient is generally performed nasally, and this method is preferred if ventilatory efforts are still present. In a patient with cardiac arrest, intubation is always performed orally with the aid of a laryngoscope.[3] The blade of the laryngoscope is inserted into the mouth while the instrument is held delicately (Fig. 1A). With gentle forward pressure, the blade is advanced in the midline until the epiglottis comes into view (Fig. 1B). At this time, the laryngoscope is passed further until the tip lies behind the epiglottis, and the entire tongue and mandible are elevated by an upward and forward movement of the laryngoscope (Fig. 1C). Excessive force or a prying motion never should be used. The glottis and vocal cords then should come clearly into view just beyond the tip of the blade. It is often helpful to have a suction catheter available to clear obscuring secretions. With the endotracheal balloon deflated, the tube is passed *gently* through the vocal cords into the upper trachea (Fig. 1D). Care is taken to advance the tube only 2 to 3 inches beyond the vocal cords so as not to intubate the right main

stem bronchus. The endotracheal balloon is inflated until an airtight seal with the trachea is obtained, and the patient is ventilated manually throughout the resuscitation at 12 breaths per minute with 100 per cent oxygen, if available. Bilateral thoracic breath sounds are confirmed by auscultation. Mechanical ventilation is begun only after restoration of stable cardiovascular function.

CIRCULATION

Before chest compression is begun in a patient with documented cardiac arrest, a precordial thump is delivered in the hope of restoring cardiac rhythm. If this is unsuccessful, circulatory support is initiated with external cardiac massage. The patient is placed in the horizontal position. A board or other rigid surface is positioned behind the back to provide support. The heel of one hand is placed over the other, and force is applied rhythmically over the lower sternum (Fig. 2). The arms are locked to transmit the full momentum of the upper body to the patient.

Although the topic of external chest compression is somewhat controversial at present, recent research has clarified many issues.[15] First, systemic blood flow during CPR seems to be generated by two mechanisms: (1) a *direct* transmission of compression force to the heart through the chest wall, and (2) an indirect transmission of

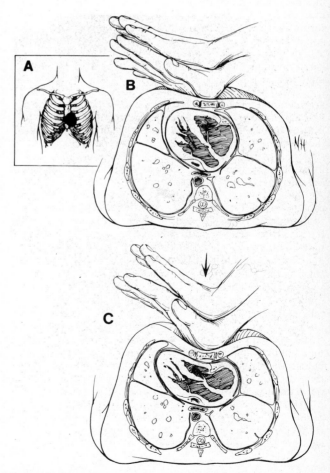

Figure 2. Manual compression is performed over the lower sternum (A). The position of the hands on the sternum is shown (B). External cardiac massage is performed with high-velocity compressions of moderate force and brief duration (C).

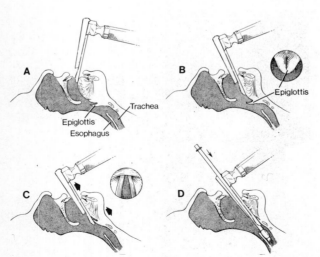

Figure 1. Standard technique of laryngoscopic endotracheal intubation. A, The laryngoscope is inserted into the mouth. B, The blade is advanced to expose the vocal cords. C and D, The trachea is intubated. (From Collins, V. J.: Principles of Anesthesiology. Philadelphia, Lea & Febiger, 1976.[3])

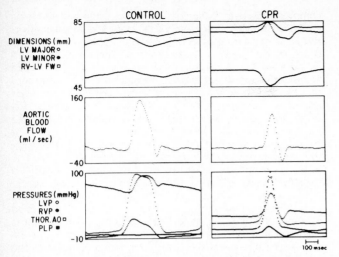

Figure 3. Digital measurements of left ventricular dimensions, aortic blood flow, and cardiac chamber pressures during control (left panels) and during cardiopulmonary resuscitation (CPR) in the arrested state (right panels). (From Maier, G. W., et al.: Circulation, 70:86, 1984.[15])

force mediated through an increase in intrathoracic pressure.[21] Both mechanisms are operative in most situations, but manual external chest compression seems to utilize the direct component primarily. To illustrate the physiology of external chest compression, measurements of ventricular dimensions, aortic blood flow, and cardiac chamber pressures from an anesthetized dog are shown in Figure 3 in the control state (left panel) and during CPR with an arrested circulation (right panel). Several important principles are evident. First, a flattening of ventricular shape is observed with external massage, consistent with direct chamber compression. Second, peak aortic flow velocity and stroke volume, compared with control, are reduced significantly during CPR. Finally, peak ventricular and aortic pressures approach normal values with external compression but diastolic and mean aortic perfusion pressures remain low because of reduced cardiac output. In other experiments, it has been shown that the best values for stroke volume are obtained with compressions of high velocity, moderate force, and brief duration (high-impulse CPR). Further interesting data are illustrated in Figure 4. When compression rate is increased, ventricular filling is not impaired but in fact remains maximal because of

ineffective chamber emptying provided by external compression. Moreover, with increasing compression rate, stroke volume remains constant so that cardiac output and diastolic aortic pressure are significantly improved. Coronary blood flow occurs primarily during noncompression or diastolic periods and falls to zero or even slightly negative values throughout compression. This finding reflects another example of a vascular waterfall phenomenon, where pressure generated in the ventricular cavity acts as a resistance to coronary blood flow through the ventricular wall. Because of this fact, compression should not be prolonged but should be brief to provide sufficient diastolic time for coronary perfusion. Increasing the rate of manual compression (Fig. 5) improves overall cardiac output, aortic perfusion pressure, and coronary blood flow velocity.[24] However, diastolic perfusion time declines linearly with increasing rate so that total coronary blood flow is optimized at a manual compression rate of 120 per minute. The values for coronary blood flow observed with this technique are the best ever reported during CPR. Improved coronary perfusion is one major advantage of high-impulse, rapid compression and is especially important in providing the best possible conditions for quick defibrillation.

When rapid manual compression with the high-impulse technique is compared with other types of CPR (Fig. 6), the manual method produces significantly better cardiac output, brachiocephalic blood flow, and total coronary perfusion.[17] Although similar quantitative measurements are currently impossible in man, clinical assessment of this method in our practice over the past 3 years has been extremely favorable. Thus, available data suggest that sternal compression during CPR should be of *high velocity*, *moderate force*, and *brief duration*. A compression rate of *120 per minute* has been shown to optimize cardiac output and coronary blood flow. High-impulse techniques introduce a fatigue factor for the resuscitator, and with in-hospital arrests, frequent changes of personnel are required. In current practice, ventilations are interspersed randomly at 12 to 15 breaths per minute.

When cardiac arrest occurs in the community with only one witness, single-rescuer CPR can be performed after a call for help is made. With the single-rescuer method, it is more difficult to optimize resuscitation factors because the same person performs mouth-to-mouth ventilation and external cardiac massage. Sternal compression proceeds at a rate of 80 per minute, and after each five compressions, two breaths are interposed by the rescuer during a brief pause in compressions. Needless to say, this method is not ideal and should be used only as a last resort. Finally, it

Figure 4. Effects of increasing the rate of manual chest compression on cardiac physiologic variables during CPR. With increasing compression rate, cardiac filling was not impaired, stroke volume remained constant, and cardiac output increased significantly while diastolic aortic pressure and coronary blood flow were well maintained. (From Maier, G. W., et al.: Circulation 70:86, 1984.[15])

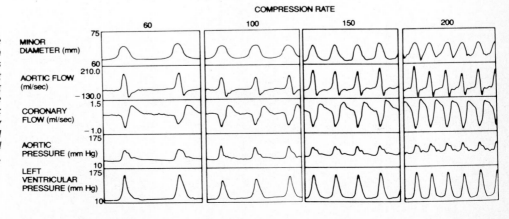

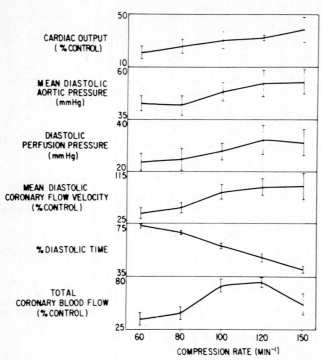

compression. If facilities are available, open-chest cardiac massage should be attempted if external massage is ineffective or if a question of pericardial tamponade exists. It has been shown in several studies that cardiac output and diastolic aortic perfusion pressure are better with open techniques, and direct cardiac massage is still a useful tool that has a definite place in clinical practice. Open methods are used commonly when arrest occurs after cardiac surgery, when quick access to the heart is available through the sternotomy incision. In other situations, the left anterior chest is entered surgically after brief application of antiseptic solution and a rib retractor is inserted (Fig. 7). The heart is compressed directly by squeezing the ventricles with the hands; a pericardiotomy is not always necessary. Ventricular emptying is more complete with open massage, so that a compression rate of 60 to 80 per minute is utilized to allow adequate diastolic filling. Finally, defibrillation is accomplished by direct application of paddles to the heart, and if resuscitation is successful, the patient is taken to the operating room for chest closure. There is a surprisingly low incidence of thoracic infection with this technique, and little is lost by converting to the open-chest method for the patient in whom closed resuscitation is otherwise not progressing well.

Figure 5. With increasing rate of compression, cardiac output and aortic diastolic pressure were progressively augmented, but diastolic perfusion time decreased. As a result, coronary blood flow was optimized at a compression rate of 120 per minute. (Courtesy of J. Alan Wolfe, M.D.[24])

should be emphasized that external cardiac massage is relatively ineffective, providing only 25 to 40 per cent of the normal cardiac output, even under the best of conditions. Therefore, the primary goal of every resuscitation should be the restoration of normal cardiac function as soon as possible.

In occasional hospitalized arrest victims, effective circulatory dynamics cannot be achieved with external chest

Advanced Life Support

Because of the low cardiac output attainable with CPR, efforts are directed toward restoring intrinsic cardiac function as soon as possible. The senior physician or the most experienced person takes charge of coordinating the care. As the resuscitation continues, an electrocardiogram (ECG) is obtained to document the cardiac rhythm. In most cases, the paddles of the defibrillator also serve as electrocardiographic chest electrodes and the rhythm can be assessed initially without other equipment. If ventricular tachycardia or fibrillation is observed, an immediate attempt at cardioversion is made using a maximal energy setting of 400 joules. The direct current countershock across the chest simultaneously depolarizes all myocardial cells and interrupts re-entry phenomena or totally disorganized electrical

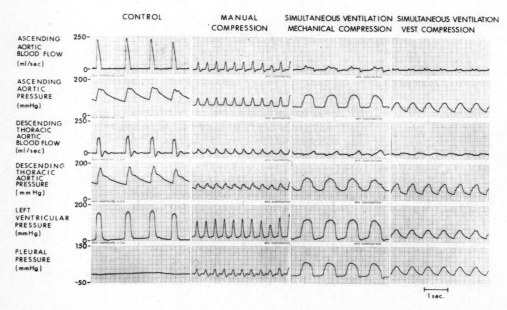

Figure 6. In the intact dog model, total cardiac output and brachiocephalic blood flow were significantly better with high-impulse manual compression compared with other methods of CPR. (Courtesy of Joseph R. Newton, M.D.[17])

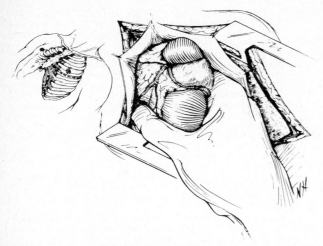

Figure 7. Open cardiac massage is performed through a short left anterior thoracotomy. The ventricles are compressed directly with the hands at 60 to 80 per minute.

activity. After repolarization, pacemaker activity of the sinus node resumes and a coherent wavefront of depolarization spreads over the heart. Most defibrillators have two hand-held paddles that are applied to the right of the upper sternum and lateral to the nipple in the left anterior axillary line. To maximize the current transmitted to the heart, a low-impedance gel is applied to increase conductivity at the paddle-skin interface. Occasionally, placing one defibrillator paddle behind the back improves the efficacy of cardioversion. Chest compression should be discontinued for no more than 5 to 10 seconds during diagnosis or defibrillation. To decrease the chance of an inadvertent electrical shock, all personnel should stand well away from the patient during defibrillation. If initial attempts are unsuccessful, CPR is continued and further interventions to improve cardioversion are initiated. During long resuscitations or after defibrillation, a standard ECG monitor also should be employed.

Venous access is obtained by inserting a large-bore plastic catheter into the subclavian or femoral vein; large antecubital veins also can be used. If central or pulmonary artery lines are present, drugs are administered through them to diminish the transit time to the coronary circulation. Because of the transit time, 10 to 20 seconds of CPR are provided after drug administration before further cardioversions are attempted. Periodically, CPR is discontinued briefly to assess changes in electrocardiographic rhythm and hemodynamics.

Restoration of coronary blood flow by CPR and correction of myocardial hypoxia or acidosis often improves the coarseness of fibrillation and make successful cardioversion more likely. As a routine, sodium bicarbonate is administered intravenously to correct metabolic acidosis. Arterial blood gases are drawn frequently to evaluate the adequacy of bicarbonate therapy as well as arterial gas exchange. Intravenous or intracardiac cardiotonic drugs such as calcium chloride and epinephrine may improve the success of defibrillation. Both drugs produce arterial vasoconstriction, which increases arterial blood pressure at a given cardiac output and thereby improves coronary blood flow. If ventricular tachycardia or fibrillation persists, intravenous antiarrhythmic agents may be helpful. Intravenous lidocaine and/or pronestyl are used as first-line drugs; in especially refractory cases, bretylium may be required.

Detailed dosages and protocols for drug therapy have been formulated by McIntvre and Parker[16] and by Safar.[22]

If cardiac arrest occurs during induction of anesthesia for noncardiac operations, resuscitation is accomplished (using open-chest techniques if necessary) and the operation is terminated. The patient is transferred to an intensive care unit, where hemodynamics are monitored by a thermodilution Swan-Ganz catheter to measure pulmonary capillary wedge pressure and cardiac output. When the patient is stabilized, cardiologic consultation is obtained and coronary arteriography is considered. When cardiac arrest occurs during anesthetic induction for cardiac procedures, the operation is initiated immediately and the patient is placed rapidly on cardiopulmonary bypass, which in many ways is the ultimate resuscitation technique. Similarly, if arrest occurs after the conclusion of a cardiac operation, bypass is reinstituted as quickly as possible. When circulatory function has been stabilized by the bypass circuit, the cause of the problem is investigated and further therapy initiated accordingly.

RESULTS

The two most important factors determining the success of resuscitation are (1) the severity and reversibility of the patient's underlying disease and (2) the time from arrest to defibrillation. With improved intensive-care monitoring of high-risk patients with myocardial infarction, and with more rapid response times for defibrillation, the incidence of in-hospital sudden death from cardiac electrical events is now extremely low. In the general hospital population, approximately half of the patients sustaining sudden cardiac arrest can be resuscitated and half of these survive to discharge. Likewise, paramedical response times for outpatient arrests have improved and the combination of extensive public education in immediate bystander CPR and excellent response times have enhanced resuscitation rates. With paramedical response times averaging 2.9 minutes in the Seattle program, 60 per cent of out-of-hospital victims of cardiac arrest now can be resuscitated and transported to the hospital for further evaluation; half of this group survive to discharge.[2] Hospital management after admission is designed to diagnose and treat the underlying cause of the arrest. If ischemic heart disease is suspected, cardiac catheterization is indicated, and for patients with coronary obstruction the options of coronary thrombolysis, balloon angioplasty, and coronary bypass grafting offer excellent prospects for long-term survival.

External cardiac massage is associated with a significant incidence of costochondral fractures that worsen with lengthening time of resuscitation. Occasionally, a flail sternal segment is produced that can interfere with subsequent ventilatory function. Lacerations of the liver, spleen, or lung also can occur. In patients after cardiac surgery, vascular suture line disruption and perforation of the ventricular myocardium by prosthetic valves are significant risks. In victims of cardiac arrest, however, these risks have to be incurred if the patient is to be saved. Experienced personnel can minimize complications somewhat by exercising care with external chest massage. As shown experimentally,[15] additional stroke volume is not generated by using excessive force; thus, compressions should be performed with brief, high-velocity strokes and only *moderate* compression force. Finally, adequate training and proficiency with other techniques such as central line placement and intubation should minimize the well-known complications of these procedures.

Because of ineffective maintenance of circulatory dynamics with CPR, the chance of resuscitation diminishes directly with time after arrest. Therefore, as stated previously, the goal of resuscitation should be to restore the patient's own cardiac function as quickly as possible. As the time of arrest increases, progressive and generalized ischemic injury occurs throughout the body, resulting in permanent organ dysfunction and worsening vasodilatation. As systemic arterial resistance deteriorates, the aortic blood pressure attainable with CPR also decreases, resulting in worsening of coronary blood flow and cerebral perfusion. As a general rule, persistent cardiac arrest after 1 hour of full CPR is unlikely to be reversible and resuscitation should be discontinued at that point. In summary, CPR has evolved into a highly technical and effective form of therapy for sudden cardiopulmonary arrest. With acquisition of additional knowledge in future years, and with better physician and community training, results should improve even further.

SELECTED REFERENCES

Cobb, L. A., Werner, J. A., and Trobaugh, G. B.: Sudden cardiac death: I. Experience with out-of-hospital resuscitation: II. Outcome of resuscitation, management, and future directions. Mod. Concepts Cardiovasc. Dis., *49*:31, 1980.
This paper presents a good review of an extensive clinical experience with CPR by leaders in the field. Detailed information about current results of CPR is given, along with recommendations for future development.

Kouwenhoven, W. B., Jude, J. R., and Knickerbocker, G. G.: Closed chest cardiac massage. J.A.M.A., *173*:1064, 1960.
This historic reference initiated the modern era of cardiopulmonary resuscitation. The history of CPR to that date, as well as the original experimental data on closed chest cardiac massage, is given. The methods of artificial ventilation, external chest compression, and external defibrillation were combined in 5 patients and reported for the first time. This is a landmark paper and is highly recommended.

Maier, G. W., Tyson, G. S., Jr., Olsen, C. O., Kernstine, K. H., Davis, J. W., Conn, E. H., Sabiston, D. C., Jr., and Rankin, J. S.: The physiology of external cardiac massage: High impulse cardiopulmonary resuscitation. Circulation, *70*:86, 1984.
This recent manuscript considers in detail the physiology of closed chest cardiac massage. Instrumented dog models were utilized to investigate ventricular dynamics, cardiac output, and coronary blood flow during a variety of different compression techniques. In this study, the method of "high-impulse" chest compression was developed.

McIntyre, K. M., and Parker, M. R.: Standards and guidelines for cardiopulmonary resuscitation (CPR) and emergency cardiac care (ECC). J.A.M.A., *244*:453, 1980.
This publication is an important reference on current topics in CPR. Detailed information about CPR techniques, as well as exact dosage schedules for pharmacologic therapy, is presented. Every physician should be familiar with this paper.

REFERENCES

 1. Beck, C. S., Pritchard, W. H., and Feil, H. S.: Ventricular fibrillation abolished by electric shock. J.A.M.A., *135*:985, 1947.

 2. Cobb, L. A., Werner, J. A., and Trobaugh, G. B.: Sudden cardiac death: I. Experience with out-of-hospital resuscitation. II. Outcome of resuscitation, management, and future directions. Mod. Concepts Cardiovasc. Dis., *49*:31, 1980.

 3. Collins, V. J.: Endotracheal anesthesia: II. Technical considerations. *In* Principles of Anesthesiology. Philadelphia, Lea & Febiger, 1976.

 4. Copley, D. P., Mantle, J. A., Rogers, W. J., Russell, R. O., Jr., and Rackley, C. E.: Improved outcome for prehospital cardiopulmonary collapse with resuscitation by bystanders. Circulation, *56*:901, 1977.

 5. Cox, J. L.: Surgical management of cardiac arrhythmias. *In* Sabiston, D. C., Jr, and Spencer, F. C. (Eds.): Gibbon's Surgery of the Chest, 4th ed. Philadelphia, W. B. Saunders Company, 1983.

 6. Crile, G.: Anemia and resuscitation: An experimental and clinical research. New York, Daniel Appleton and Co., 1914.

 7. DeBard M. L.: The history of cardiopulmonary resuscitation. Ann. Emerg. Med., *9*:273, 1980.

 8. DeWood, M. A., Spores, J., Notske, R. N., Lang, H. T., Shields, J. P., Simpson, C. S., Rudy, L. W., and Grunwald, R.: Medical and surgical management of myocardial infarction. Am. J. Cardiol., *44*:1356, 1979.

 9. Eisenberg, M. S., Gergner, L., and Hallstrom, A.: Cardiac resuscitation in the community: Importance of rapid provision and implication for program planning. J.A.M.A., *241*:1905, 1979.

10. Jude, J. R., Kouwenhoven, W. B., and Knickerbocker, G. S.: Cardiac arrest. J.A.M.A., *128*:1063, 1961.

11. Jude, J. R., Kouwenhoven, W. B., and Knickerbocker, G. S.: External cardiac resuscitation. Monogr. Surg. Sci., *1*:59, 1964.

12. Julian, D. G.: Cardiac resuscitation in the eighteenth century. Heart Lung, *4*:46, 1975.

13. Keen, W. W.: Case of total laryngectomy (unsuccessful) and a case of abdominal hysterectomy (successful) in both of which massage of the heart for chloroform collapse was employed, with notes on 25 other cases of cardiac massage. Therapy Gazette, *28*:217, 1904.

14. Kouwenhoven, W. B., Jude, J. R., and Knickerbocker, G. S.: Closed chest cardiac massage. J.A.M.A., *173*:1064, 1960.

15. Maier, G. W., Tyson, G. S., Jr., Olsen, C. O., Kernstine, K. H., Davis, J. W., Conn, E. H., Sabiston, D. C., Jr., and Rankin, J. S.: The physiology of external cardiac massage: High impulse cardiopulmonary resuscitation. Circulation, *70*:86, 1984.

16. McIntyre, K. M. and Parker, M. R.: Standards and guidelines for cardiopulmonary resuscitation (CPR) and emergency cardiac care (ECC). J.A.M.A., *244*:453, 1980.

17. Newton, J. R., Glower, D. D., Wolfe, J. A., Tyson, G. S., Spratt, J. A., and Rankin, J. S.: Quantitative comparison of several methods of external cardiac massage. J. Am. Coll., *3*:596, 1984.

18. Phillips, S. J., Zeff, R. H., Kongtahworn, C., Skinner, J. R., Iannone, L., Brown, T. M., Wickemeyer, W., and Gordon, D. F.: Surgery for evolving myocardial infarction. J.A.M.A., *248*:1325, 1982.

19. Rentrop, P., Blanke, H., Karsch, K. R., Kaiser, H., Kostering, H., and Leitz, K.: Selective intracoronary thrombolysis in acute myocardial infarction and unstable angina pectoris. Circulation, *63*:307, 1981.

20. Rosen, Z., and Davidson, J. T.: Respiratory resuscitation in ancient Hebrew sources. Anesthes. Analg., *51*:502, 1972.

21. Rudikoff, M. T., Maughan, W. L., Effron, M., Freund, P., and Weisfeldt, M. L.: Mechanisms of blood flow during cardiopulmonary resuscitation. Circulation, *61*:345, 1980.

22. Safar, P.: Advances in Cardiopulmonary Resuscitation. New York, Springer-Verlag, 1977.

23. Stack, R. S., Phillips, H. R., III, Grierson, D. S., Behar, V. S., Kong, Y., Peter, R. H., Swain, J. L., and Greenfield, J. C., Jr.: Functional improvement of jeopardized myocardium following intracoronary streptokinase infusion in acute myocardial infarction. J. Clin. Invest., *72*:84, 1983.

24. Wolfe, J. A., Maier, G. W., Tyson, G. S., Newton, J. R., Glower, D. D., and Rankin, J. S.: Determinants of coronary blood flow during external cardiac massage. Circulation, 68 (Suppl. III):941, 1983.

25. Zoll, P. M., Paul, M. H., Linenthal, A. J., Norman, L. R., and Gibson, W.: The effects of external electric currents on the heart: Control of cardiac rhythm and induction and termination of cardiac arrhythmias. Circulation, *14*:745, 1956.

Patent Ductus Arteriosus, Coarctation of the Aorta, Aortopulmonary Window, and Anomalies of the Aortic Arch

J. WILLIAM GAYNOR, M.D.
DAVID C. SABISTON, JR., M.D.

PATENT DUCTUS ARTERIOSUS

Nature is neither lazy nor devoid of foresight. Having given the matter thought, she knew in advance that the lung of the fetus, a lung still contained in the uterus and in the process of formation and spared continual motion, does not require the same arrangements of a perfected lung endowed with motion. She has, therefore, anastomosed the pulmonary artery to the aorta. . . .

Galen[88]

Harvey demonstrated the role of the ductus arteriosus in the fetal circulation in 1628. During the 19th century the morbidity associated with patent ductus arteriosus (PDA) was recognized, and Gibson described the characteristic murmur.[39] In 1907, Munro proposed surgical correction by ligating or crushing the ductus[81]; surgical intervention was attempted unsuccessfully by Graybiel and colleagues, in 1937, in a patient with bacterial endocarditis.[41] Gross successfully ligated a patent ductus arteriosus, in 1938, initiating the modern era.[47] An increased incidence of patent ductus arteriosus in premature infants was reported by Burnard[15a] in 1959, and in 1963 Powell[85a] and DeCancq[30a] independently treated premature infants by ligating a PDA.

Embryology and Pathologic Anatomy

The fetal ductus arteriosus is derived from the sixth aortic arch and normally extends from the main or left pulmonary artery to the descending aorta just distal to the origin of the left subclavian artery. The length of the ductus is usually 5 to 10 mm., but is variable, and the diameter ranges from a few millimeters to 1 to 2 cm. The aortic orifice is usually larger than the pulmonary orifice. Rarely the ductus may be on the right side, bilateral, or completely absent. In utero blood ejected by the right ventricle flows almost exclusively through the ductus to the lower extremities and placenta, bypassing the high-resistance pulmonary circulation.

Closure of the ductus occurs at birth during the transition from the fetal to the adult circulation. The lungs expand with the first breath, decreasing the pulmonary vascular resistance, which results in increased pulmonary blood flow and arterial oxygen concentration. In the normal full-term neonate functional closure of the ductus occurs within the first 10 to 15 hours of life. This occurs after constriction of the smooth muscle layer, which causes the apposition of intimal cushions in the wall of the ductus. Closure is mediated by a variety of substances that constrict or dilate ductal smooth muscle. The rising oxygen arterial tension causes constriction of the muscle fibers in the wall of the ductus. Prostaglandins of the E series dilate the ductus and therefore the lower concentrations after birth potentiate closure. Anatomic closure by fibrosis is usually complete by 2 to 3 weeks postnatally and produces the ligamentum arteriosum, which connects the pulmonary artery and the aorta. Closure is complete in 88 per cent of newborns by 8 weeks of life.[20]

Delayed closure of the ductus is termed *prolonged patency* and failure of closure results in *persistent patency*. Final closure may occur at any age but is uncommon after age 6 months. Intermittent closure and reopening of the ductus may also occur. Persistent patency of the ductus may occur as an isolated lesion or may be associated with a variety of other congenital defects. In infants with complex congenital heart disease, pulmonary or systemic blood flow may be dependent on patency of the ductus and the infants may experience sudden decompensation as the ductus closes. Infusion of prostaglandins to dilate the ductus often results in dramatic improvement and allows stabilization prior to surgical intervention.

Prolonged or persistent patency of the ductus results in a left-to-right shunt of blood with pulmonary congestion and left ventricular volume overload. The magnitude of the shunt depends mainly on the size of the ductus; however, with a large nonrestrictive ductus the level of pulmonary vascular resistance is important in determining the severity of shunting. Shunting occurs throughout systole and diastole, resulting in diastolic hypotension and possibly impaired perfusion of the brain, lower extremities, and abdominal organs. ST-T wave changes suggestive of subendocardial ischemia have been reported in infants with patent ductus arteriosus.[110a] Myocardial dysfunction may result and lead to worsening left ventricular failure.

Incidence, Mortality, and Morbidity

Isolated patent ductus arteriosus occurs in approximately 1 in 2500 to 5000 live births. The incidence increases markedly with prematurity and with decreasing birth weight.[62] The incidence may be greater than 80 per cent in infants weighing less than 1000 gm., although a recent report suggests the incidence may be much lower in a standard population.[36] The increased incidence with prematurity is related to several factors, including decreased smooth muscle in the ductal wall and diminished responsiveness of the ductal smooth muscle to oxygen. Persistent patency of the ductus occurs more commonly in females than in males with a 2:1 ratio. Genetic factors may be involved and there is an association with maternal rubella. The prenatal administration of betamethasone may decrease the incidence of PDA as well as increase surfactant production.[24]

Patent ductus arteriosus is not a benign entity, although prolonged survival occurs. The mortality of untreated infants with PDA may be as high as 30 per cent. In a classic series, Abbott reported an average age at death of 24 years.[17] Campbell calculated that 42 per cent of patients with untreated PDA are dead by age 45.[17] In the preantibiotic era bacterial endocarditis was a common cause of death of patients with PDA. Affected individuals surviving to adulthood may develop congestive heart failure or pulmonary hypertension with reverse shunting through the ductus. Premature infants with patent ductus arteriosus often have associated problems of prematurity, which may be aggravated by the left-to-right shunting and abnormal hemodynamics; these include respiratory distress syndrome,[23] necrotizing enterocolitis, and intraventricular hemorrhage. Congestive heart failure often results and may respond poorly to medical management. The incidence of long-term sequelae of prematurity such as bronchopulmonary dysplasia may be increased by the presence of a PDA. Young children with persistent patency of the ductus may show growth retardation. Aneurysmal dilatation and rupture may occur in infants or adults, although this complication is rare.[61] Infants with a large PDA often develop severe pulmonary hypertension at an early age. Calcification is often seen in older patients and may complicate surgical repair.

Clinical Manifestations and Diagnosis

The signs and symptoms of patent ductus arteriosus depend on the size of the ductus, the pulmonary vascular resistance, the age at presentation, and associated anomalies. Full-term infants usually do not become symptomatic until the pulmonary vascular resistance falls at 6 to 8 weeks of life. Because premature infants have less smooth muscle in the pulmonary arterioles, vascular resistance will decrease earlier and symptoms may develop in the first week of life.

A large hemodynamically significant PDA usually presents in infancy with congestive heart failure. The infants are irritable, tachycardiac, and tachypneic and take feedings poorly. Physical examination reveals evidence of a hyperdynamic circulation with a hyperactive precordium and bounding peripheral pulses. The systolic blood pressure is usually normal, but diastolic hypotension is often present because of the large left-to-right shunt.

Auscultation reveals a systolic or continuous murmur, which is often termed a *machinery murmur*. This is heard best in the pulmonic area and radiates toward the middle third of the clavicle. The classic description of the murmur was provided by Gibson:

. . . a murmur which may be regarded as almost pathognomonic. Beginning distinctly after the first sound, it accompanies the latter part of that sound, occupies the short pause, accompanies the second sound, which may be accentuated in the pulmonary area, or may be, and often is, doubled, and finally dies away during the long pause.[39]

Absence of the characteristic murmur does not, however, exclude the presence of a patent ductus arteriosus. A middiastolic apical rumble may result from increased flow across the mitral valve. If cardiac failure is present, a gallop may be heard. Hepatomegaly is frequently present. Cyanosis is not present in uncomplicated isolated PDA.

The diagnosis of PDA often can be made noninvasively and the physical examination alone may be almost diagnostic. The chest x-ray usually shows cardiomegaly and, if cardiac failure is present, pulmonary congestion is seen. In older infants, children, and adults, the electrocardiogram (ECG) may show left ventricular hypertrophy. Two-dimensional echocardiography demonstrates the ductus and other associated anomalies. The left atrial and aortic root dimensions can be measured and if their ratio is greater than 1.4 or 1.5, a left-to-right shunt is likely.[103] However, the ratio may be normal in infants with PDA who have experienced fluid restriction and have been treated with diuretics. Contrast echocardiography with agitated saline may demonstrate the shunt,[112] and Doppler echocardiography can document abnormal aortic flow patterns and allow estimation of the magnitude of ductal flow.[102] Echocardiography can provide evidence of significant left-to-right shunting before it has become clinically apparent. Retrograde aortography to visualize the PDA may be performed in infants with an umbilical artery catheter. Formal cardiac catheterization usually is not required in children and young adults with classic findings and should be reserved for older patients or those with atypical findings, the possibility of associated anomalies, or pulmonary hypertension.

Patients with a moderate-sized PDA may remain asymptomatic until the second or third decade of life when left ventricular failure occurs. The earliest symptom is usually dyspnea on exertion followed by signs and symptoms of worsening congestive heart failure. Auscultation will reveal the typical murmur. The ECG and chest x-ray may show evidence of left ventricular enlargement. A small PDA usually causes no symptoms or growth retardation. A systolic or continuous murmur is present. The ECG and chest x-ray usually appear normal.

Management

The presence of a persistent patent ductus arteriosus is sufficient indication for surgical closure. In symptomatic patients closure should be undertaken when the diagnosis is made. In asymptomatic patients, intervention can be postponed if desired but should be performed in the preschool years. Older patients should have the ductus closed when the diagnosis is made. However, if severe pulmonary hypertension has occurred with reversal of the ductal shunt, closure is associated with a higher mortality and may not improve symptoms.

SURGICAL PROCEDURES

Gross initially used simple ligation to interrupt the patent ductus.[47] However, because of early problems with recanalization he pioneered division as the therapy of

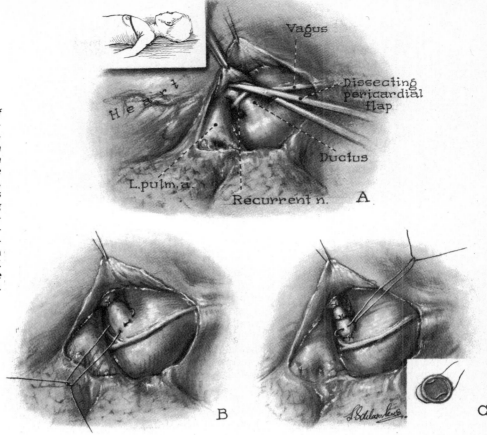

Figure 1. Operative treatment of ductus arteriosus by ligation. Incision is anterolateral in the third interspace. In females the incision circles beneath the breast. Elevation of pericardial lappet exposes the ductus. A purse-string suture, which does not enter the lumen, is placed at each end, and perforating mattress sutures are placed in between. The ductus should be obliterated over an 8- to 10-mm. distance. (From Bahnson, H. T.: In Sabiston, D. C., Jr., and Spencer, F. C. (Eds.): Gibbon's Surgery of the Chest, 3rd ed. Philadelphia, W. B. Saunders Company, 1976.)

choice.[42] Blalock suggested ligation with multiple transfixion sutures as the preferable method.[11] In children, either division or multiple suture–ligation of the ductus is appropriate. Simple ligation is usually performed in neonates due to simplicity and rare, if any, recurrences. In the large ductus (10 mm. or greater) or with pulmonary hypertension, division is indicated.

The operation is performed through either a left anterior or posterior thoracotomy. The lung is retracted and an incision is made in the pleura overlying the pulmonary artery between the phrenic and vagus nerves. The ductus is exposed, with care being taken to avoid damage to the recurrent laryngeal nerve. After the ductus has been mobilized, it may be closed by multiple suture–ligation (Fig. 1) or by division and closure (Fig. 2). If division is planned, vascular clamps are placed across the ductus and it is then divided. Closure of each end is accomplished with two rows of non-absorbable suture. If the ductus is particularly short and wide, it may be necessary to cross-clamp the aorta above and below the ductus as in a coarctation repair. The pulmonary end of the ductus is clamped and the ductus is divided, leaving a sufficient margin for closure. The opening in the aorta is closed, and the cross-clamps are removed. A calcified ductus in older patients is a difficult surgical problem. A variety of techniques utilizing cardiopulmonary bypass and closure from within the aorta or pulmonary artery are useful.

NONOPERATIVE THERAPY

In recent years there has been increasing interest in the *nonoperative* closure of PDA in high-risk patients. Porstmann, in 1966, successfully used a transcatheter technique to block the PDA with an Ivalon plug,[85] and Rashkind, in 1979, utilized a double-umbrella device inserted via a right-sided catheter to close the ductus.[89] These techniques are potentially useful in patients who are poor surgical candidates. However, these procedures are still experimental, the long-term results are not known, and the exact role in the management of PDA has not been determined. Nonsurgical closure is rarely recommended at present.

TREATMENT OF PREMATURE INFANTS

Premature infants face a multitude of problems, including immature lungs and hyaline membrane disease. These infants often require mechanical ventilation and oxygen therapy. There is an increased incidence of PDA in these infants, which correlates with increasing prematurity and decreasing birth weight. The additional burden on the heart and lungs imposed by the left-to-right shunting may be poorly tolerated. The increased pulmonary blood flow causes increased pulmonary arterial pressures, decreased lung compliance, hypercarbia, and hypoxia, often necessi-

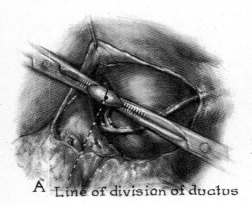 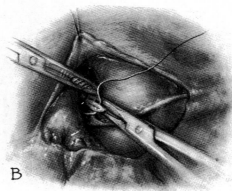

A Line of division of ductus B

Figure 2. Treatment of ductus arteriosus by division. Anterolateral third interspace incision is used with exposure as for ligation. A thin occluding clamp is placed at each end and the ductus is divided. Pressing the clamp against the pulmonary artery or aorta after division reduces likelihood of slipping. Suture of ductus is by a continuous mattress suture adjacent to clamp, followed by whipstitch back-up over the free edge. Suture of the pulmonary artery is easier when done from the patient's right side. (From Bahnson, H. T.: In Sabiston, D. C., Jr., and Spencer, F. C. (Eds.): Gibbon's Surgery of the Chest, 3rd ed. Philadelphia, W. B. Saunders Company, 1976.)

tating prolonged mechanical ventilation. This, in turn, may result in an increased incidence of bronchopulmonary dysplasia and retrolental fibroplasia. The abnormal hemodynamics may potentiate other problems of prematurity such as necrotizing enterocolitis and intraventricular hemorrhage. At times, it is difficult to differentiate the effects of a PDA from the underlying lung disease. If the lung disease is severe, ligation of the patent ductus may result in little or no improvement. A hemodynamically significant PDA is suggested by the presence of a hyperactive precordium, a continuous murmur, and bounding pulses. The chest x-ray usually shows cardiomegaly, pulmonary congestion, and the changes of hyaline membrane disease. Echocardiography may be useful in determining the presence of a significant left-to-right shunt in these patients.

Management of PDA in the premature infant is controversial because the ductus may close as the child matures. There is an increased incidence of PDA in neonatal units that do not restrict fluid.[7] Some infants can be managed satisfactorily with fluid restriction and diuretics. Anemia worsens the heart failure and transfusion of packed red blood cells is indicated to maintain the hematocrit near 45 per cent. Digitalis is rarely used in these infants as there is little evidence of therapeutic benefit and a high incidence of toxicity.[9]

In some infants conservative therapy will fail. In a child with evidence of left-to-right shunting, the persistence of congestive heart failure, the need for continuing mechanical ventilation, and the inability to receive adequate nutrition as a result of fluid restriction are indications for further intervention. Two therapeutic options exist at this point.[78] Pharmacologic closure can be attempted with prostaglandin inhibitors such as indomethacin.[35, 38, 54] Final closure may be achieved in greater than 70 per cent of infants, although the ductus may reopen transiently in some children. The success of therapy with indomethacin is related to the birth weight and the age of the infant. Side effects of indomethacin include renal dysfunction, hyponatremia, impaired platelet function, gastrointestinal hemorrhage, and displacement of bilirubin from protein-binding sites. No adverse long-term sequelae of successful indomethacin therapy have been identified.[84] Surgical closure can be used if indomethacin is contraindicated or the ductus fails to close. In some centers, surgery is the primary therapy if conservative medical therapy is ineffective. Simple ligation is the usual procedure, although hemaclips have been used

successfully to close the ductus.[2] Several authors have advocated closure of the ductus in the neonatal intensive care unit to avoid transporting critically ill neonates to the operating theater.[56]

In recent years there has been a trend toward earlier intervention in premature infants. There is evidence that early closure can decrease the need for mechanical ventilation, possibly decrease complications such as bronchopulmonary dysplasia and necrotizing enterocolitis, and shorten the duration of hospitalization. One study showed improved results with prophylactic administration of indomethacin to premature infants in the first days of life even before there was evidence of a left-to-right shunt.[71]

Results

Surgical closure of isolated PDA has become a safe procedure. Operative mortality approaches zero even for critically ill neonates. In premature infants, hospital mortality and long-term results depend mainly on associated lung disease and the degree of prematurity. Mortality is high and long-term results are poorer in older patients with a calcified ductus. The mortality is highest in patients with severe pulmonary hypertension and reverse shunting. Most patients with PDA become functionally normal with a normal life expectancy after closure.

COARCTATION OF THE AORTA

Coarctation is derived from the Latin coarctatio (a drawing or pressing together). Coarctation of the aorta refers to a narrowing that diminishes the lumen and produces an obstruction to the flow of blood. The lesion may be a definite localized obstruction or may be a diffusely narrowed segment, which is termed tubular hypoplasia. Localized coarctation of the aorta and tubular hypoplasia may occur separately or may coexist. Isolated coarctation may occur at any site in the aorta, but the most common location by far is at the site of the insertion of the ductus (or ligamentum) arteriosus. Externally the aorta appears to be sharply indented or constricted; internally the obstructing diaphragm on the posterior wall (located preductally, postductally, or paraductally) is usually more marked than is apparent by external appearance. The "shelf" consists of an infolding of the aortic media with a ridge of intimal hyperplasia. Tubular hypoplasia most often occurs in the aortic *isthmus* (the segment of aorta between the left subclavian artery and the insertion of the ductus arteriosus). Localized coarctation of the aorta and tubular hypoplasia are part of a spectrum of disorders varying from pseudo-coarctation[37] (a kinking or buckling of the aorta without producing obstruction to flow) to, rarely, complete interruption of the aorta. Aortic atresia occurs when the lumen is totally obliterated with a fibrous connection remaining between the proximal and distal segments.

The first accurate description of coarctation of the aorta was by Paris in 1791.[83] Earlier Meckel (1750)[58] and Morgagni (1760) had reported finding aortic narrowing at autopsy.[79] Throughout the 19th century coarctation of the aorta was considered a rare disorder. Legrand in 1835[67] made the first premortem diagnosis of obstruction of the thoracic aorta, and in 1903 Bonnet published an extensive review and distinguished between preductal coarctation (infantile) and postductal coarctation (adult).[14] In 1928 Abbott collected 200 cases of coarctation in patients over the age of 2.[1] This landmark report stimulated much interest in the disorder and, in 1944, Blalock and Park proposed anastomosis of the left subclavian artery to the descending aorta to bypass the obstruction.[12] In the same year Crafoord and Nylin performed the first surgical correction with resection of the coarctation and end-to-end anastomosis.[29] Gross and colleagues independently performed this procedure in 1945.[43]

The etiology of coarctation of the aorta and tubular hypoplasia is controversial.[55, 93] Genetic factors may play a role as there are reports of familial occurrences and 15 to 36 per cent of patients with Turner's syndrome have a coarctation. There is also an increased incidence of aortic arch anomalies, especially interrupted arch, in patients with DiGeorge's syndrome.

Coarctation of the aorta accounts for 5 to 10 per cent of congenital heart disease, the incidence is 1 per 3000 to 4000 autopsies,[89a] and it is the fourth most common congenital heart defect.[36a] Males are affected more often with isolated coarctation, but there is no sex difference in patients with more complex lesions. Several anomalies occur commonly in patients with coarctation of the aorta: bicuspid aortic valve, ventricular septal defect, patent ductus arteriosus, and a variety of mitral valve disorders.[19] Coarctation may also coexist with more complex intracardiac defects. Patients with severe associated defects tend to have tubular hypoplasia rather than isolated coarctation.

Clinical Manifestations

The age of presentation and the mode of presentation are largely dependent on the location of the coarctation and the associated anomalies. When the obstruction is preductal, there is an increased incidence of other cardiac defects and the patients usually have congestive heart failure in infancy. Preductal coarctation usually consists of tubular hypoplasia terminating in an obstructing shelf. Paraductal and postductal coarctation are usually isolated obstructions with a low incidence of associated defects. Preductal coarctation was considered by Bonnet to be the infantile form because of its usual presentation in infancy. However, the terms "infantile" and "adult" are inappropriate descriptions of preductal and postductal coarctation because patients with the "infantile" form can survive to adulthood and some patients with the "adult" type develop clinical manifestations in infancy.

Preductal coarctation or even interruption of the aortic arch may not seriously alter the normal fetal circulation and therefore does not provide a stimulus to the development of collateral circulation. Such infants may appear normal at birth and may have palpable femoral pulses. Symptoms usually develop several days after birth when the pulmonary vascular resistance decreases and the ductus arteriosus is closing. The infant becomes irritable, is tachypneic, and has little interest in feeding. Differential cyanosis may be present between the upper and lower extremities. A systolic murmur may be noted over the left precordium and posteriorly between the scapulae with a posterior diastolic murmur. Although the blood pressure is difficult to accurately record in neonates, moderate upper extremity hypertension and an arm-leg systolic pressure gradient are usually present. These findings may be absent in critically ill infants with a low cardiac output. In severe obstruction or complete aortic interruption and a patent ductus arteriosus, a pulmonary artery pulse may be felt in the femoral arteries and obscure the diagnosis. In the neonate, there are no signs of collateral circulation as this becomes clinically manifest only later.

Older children and adults often have unexplained hypertension or complications of hypertension and some may be entirely asymptomatic for many years and lead an active life. Presenting complaints include headache, epistaxis, visual disturbances, and exertional dyspnea. Some patients present with a cerebrovascular accident, aortic rupture, dissecting aneurysm, or bacterial endocarditis. Many cases are discovered during evaluation of hypertension or by the presence of a murmur on routine examination.

Diagnosis

The diagnosis of coarctation usually can be made clinically and depends on evidence of obstruction to blood flow in the thoracic aorta. The findings include hypertension, a systolic pressure gradient between the arm and leg, a systolic murmur heard over the left precordium and posteriorly between the scapulae, diminished or absent femoral pulses with a delayed upstroke, and evidence of collateral circulation in older children and adults. An anterior diastolic murmur may indicate aortic regurgitation caused by a bicuspid aortic valve. The blood pressure must be obtained in both arms as the orifice of either subclavian artery may be involved in the coarctation or distal to the obstruction. The collateral circulation involves branches of the subclavian arteries, including the internal mammary, vertebral, thyrocervical, and costocervical arteries. These vessels anastomose with intercostals and other arteries below the obstruction. Enlarged collateral vessels may often be seen or palpated in the infrascapular region. Aneurysmal dilatation of the intercostal arteries can occur and complicate surgical reconstruction. Post-stenotic dilatation of the descending aorta is common and an aneurysm of the ascending or descending aorta may rarely occur.

Other confirmatory tests may be helpful in evaluation of possible complications and associated cardiac defects. In infancy the electrocardiogram may show right, left, or biventricular hypertrophy. In older children and adults it may appear normal or show evidence of left ventricular hypertrophy, often with a "strain" pattern. The chest film is usually quite helpful, demonstrating cardiomegaly with left ventricular hypertrophy. In infants with heart failure, extreme cardiomegaly and pulmonary congestion may be present. Rib notching caused by the enlarged, tortuous

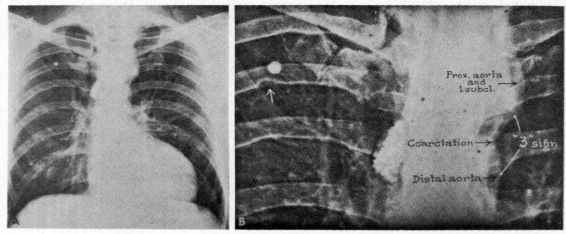

Figure 3. Roentgenologic signs, which are diagnostic but not always present in coarctation, include notching of the ribs and the "3" sign caused by the dilated proximal segment and left subclavian artery, by the constricted area, and by post-stenotic dilatation. A, Note rounded lower left cardiac border, indicating left ventricular enlargement. B, Enlargement from A showing notching of rib (adjacent to calcified lesion) and "3" sign. (From Bahnson, H. T.: In Sabiston, D. C. Jr., and Spencer, F. C. (Eds.): Gibbon's Surgery of the Chest, 3rd ed. Philadelphia, W. B. Saunders Company, 1976.)

intercostal vessels is pathognomonic and was first described by Meckel in 1827.[76] Rosler in 1928[19a] and Railsback and Dock in 1929[87] emphasized the presence of rib "notching" roentgenographically (Fig. 3A). These erosions may be unilateral if the orifice of the left subclavian artery is narrowed by the coarctation or arises distal to the obstruction, or if there is anomalous origin of the right subclavian artery distal to the coarctation. Absence of rib notching in older patients may indicate a poor collateral circulation. The "3" sign may be present, consisting of proximal enlargement of the aorta, aortic constriction, and post-stenotic dilatation (Fig. 3B).

Angiocardiography remains the most objective means of demonstrating the coarctation, providing evidence of the location and extent of narrowing, the involvement of the great vessels, and the extent of collateral circulation. The pressure gradient can be measured and associated cardiac defects can be evaluated by cardiac catheterization.

Newer methods of noninvasive imaging also provide valuable information. Two-dimensional and Doppler echocardiography demonstrate the site of obstruction, suggest or exclude associated anomalies, and provide an estimate of the arterial pressure gradient.[74, 102] Computed tomography (CT), digital subtraction angiography, and magnetic resonance imaging (MRI) are also helpful and can be used postoperatively to assess the result (Fig. 4).[4]

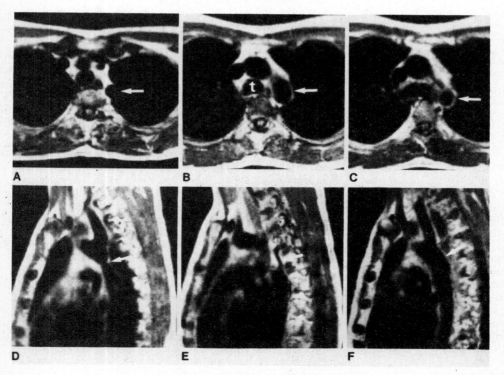

Figure 4. Magnetic resonance images.

A, Transaxial section above arch. Dilated left subclavian artery (arrow).

B, More caudal section. Posterior aortic arch immediately proximal to coarctation (arrow). t = trachea.

C, 1 cm. below B. Reduction in caliber of descending aorta (arrow).

D, Parasagittal section. Coarctation distal to dilated left subclavian artery (arrow). Diaphragm-like stricture is better appreciated than on transaxial sections.

E, Parasagittal section through distal descending aorta. Dilated collateral artery (arrow).

F, Postoperative parasagittal section. Widely patent lumen at previous site of coarctation.

(From Amparo, E. G., Higgins, C. B., and Shafton, E. P.: A.J.R., 143:1192, 1984.[4])

Natural History

The natural history of untreated coarctation of the aorta depends on the age at presentation and associated anomalies. Symptomatic infants have a high mortality, depending on the severity of the coarctation and the presence of associated defects.[16, 52, 53] Some symptomatic children with isolated coarctation survive with medical therapy alone. Interestingly, complete interruption of the aorta without associated defects, although rare, appears to be a favorable lesion as clinical manifestations do not occur until later childhood or in adult life. This is apparently because of the development of an extensive collateral circulation *in utero*.

Patients surviving until adulthood have a markedly decreased life expectancy.[18] In the pre-antibiotic and pre–surgical correction era, Abbott found the average age at death to be 32 years. The presence of coarctation, however, does not preclude a long life, and the oldest patient reported with this lesion lived to the age of 92 years. The most common causes of death are cerebrovascular accidents, bacterial endocarditis, aortic rupture, and congestive heart failure.[1, 18] There is an increased incidence of intracranial aneurysms in patients with coarctation. The advent of surgical therapy significantly increased the life expectancy of patients with coarctation, although there remains an increased incidence of premature death.

The pathogenesis of hypertension in coarctation is multifactorial and the most prominent causes appear to be mechanical and renal factors. Scott and Bahnson showed that the hypertension in experimental coarctation could be eliminated by transplanting one kidney to the neck (proximal to the obstruction) with contralateral nephrectomy.[98] Renal blood flow is usually normal in patients with coarctation and studies of the renin-angiotensin system have yielded conflicting results.[3, 110] Other factors that appear to be involved include abnormal rigidity of the prestenotic aorta, altered baroreceptor function, and increased sympathetic nervous activity.[101, 110]

Management

Nonsurgical therapy has only a small role in the management of patients with coarctation and the presence of coarctation is generally sufficient indication for surgical correction. The major questions are the timing and method of repair. Symptomatic infants usually will require intervention, although a few will improve with medical treatment of congestive heart failure and can then undergo elective surgical correction. A major advance in the treatment of critically ill neonates with coarctation and interrupted arch has been the introduction of prostaglandin E_1 therapy.[25] Prostaglandin E_1 can reopen and maintain patency of the ductus arteriosus in many neonates and allows perfusion of lower body and correction of the severe metabolic acidosis that is often present. Stabilization of these severely ill patients enables surgical correction to be accomplished under more optimal conditions with decreased mortality.

The timing of elective repair of coarctation of the aorta is perhaps the most important determinant of surgical results. Repair in late childhood or adulthood,[82] although providing relief of some symptoms, has an increased incidence of persistent hypertension and its associated morbidity. Repair in infancy using the classic method of resection and end-to-end anastomosis has a high incidence (up to 60 per cent) of residual or recurrent stenosis. Alternative techniques have been developed to allow repair earlier with fewer recoarctations. The current trend is for elective repair at an early age. Some authors think repair should be undertaken at the time of diagnosis in symptomatic and asymptomatic infants to prevent development of complications[16]; others prefer elective repair at the age of 1 to 6 years to decrease the recoarctation rate.

Surgical Procedures

The classic method of repair is resection of the area of obstruction with primary end-to-end anastomosis (Fig. 5). This is performed through a left thoracotomy. An incision is made in the pleura overlying the coarctation. The proximal aorta, left subclavian artery, area of coarctation, and the ligamentum (or ductus) arteriosum are dissected first, avoiding damage to the recurrent laryngeal nerve. Abbott's artery, an anomalous branch sometimes originating from the isthmus, may be present and should be ligated and divided. The ductus or ligamentum is divided, which greatly increases the mobility of the aorta. Care must be taken not to injure any enlarged intercostal arteries during the dissection. It may be necessary to divide these, but it is preferable to preserve all collaterals. The aorta is cross-clamped proximally and distally and the area of constriction is excised. To obtain an optimal result, it is absolutely necessary to resect the entire constricted segment and construct the anastomosis without tension (Fig. 6). In patients with tubular hypoplasia it may be necessary to insert a graft. Gross first used aortic homografts to bridge the gap. Others have utilized prosthetic interposition grafts. Initial repairs were done with a continuous silk suture. An unacceptable rate of restenosis resulted, probably because

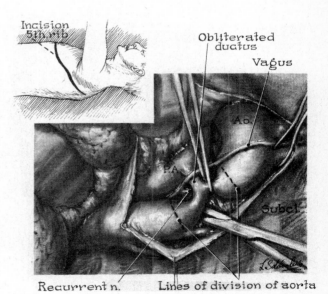

Figure 5. Operative exposure for resection of coarctation of the aorta is through the bed of the fifth rib. The entire rib is removed from neck to cartilage. The constricted segment is usually held medially by an obliterated ductus, division of which allows considerable mobility. The coarctation is held forward to facilitate dissection posteriorly. Large intercostal arteries must be carefully avoided. Division of the aorta should be through a point of normal diameter. (From Bahnson, H. T.: In Sabiston, D. C., Jr., and Spencer, F. C. (Eds.): Gibbon's Surgery of the Chest, 3rd ed. Philadelphia, W. B. Saunders Company, 1976.)

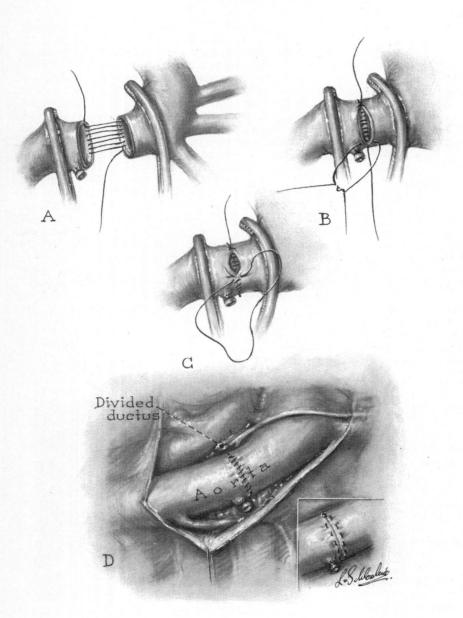

Figure 6. Anastomosis following excision of coarctation. (A) An everting mattress suture is placed over about one third of the posterior row before the vessels are approximated and the suture is pulled up (B). (C) The anastomosis is completed with continuous over-and-over suture. Inset in D shows the everting mattress suture sometimes used. In children, interrupted mattress sutures are used for the entire anterior row. (From Bahnson, H. T.: In Sabiston, D. C., Jr., and Spencer, F. C. (Eds.): Gibbon's Surgery of the Chest, 3rd ed. Philadelphia, W. B. Saunders Company, 1976.)

of failure of the anastomosis to grow. Currently many surgeons use interrupted sutures, fine non-absorbable monofilament sutures (polypropylene), or fine absorbable monofilament sutures (polydioxanone)[81a] to improve results. Several recent series suggest that resection and end-to-end anastomosis can be performed, even in neonates, with low mortality and a less than 10 per cent recoarctation rate.[64]

Because of early unsatisfactory results, especially in infants, other techniques were introduced. In 1957, Voss-schulte introduced the *prosthetic patch onlay graft technique* (Fig. 7).[108] This involves incising the area of constriction longitudinally then utilizing a patch of Dacron or, more recently, Gore-tex to enlarge the lumen. Theoretically growth of the posterior wall is possible with this procedure. This approach is especially useful in patients with a long narrowed segment and in those requiring reoperation for restenosis. Advantages include decreased dissection, less need for sacrifice of collaterals, and decreased cross-clamp time. The operative mortality in critically ill neonates is lower than with the classic operation. There is a low incidence of recoarctation and persistent hypertension. Several groups have used the technique with excellent results.[94, 111] Criticisms include the use of prosthetic material and an increased incidence of the formation of aneurysms and pseudoaneurysms.[8, 22, 53a]

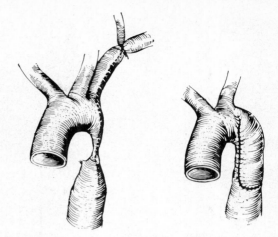

Figure 8. The operative technique of repair of coarctation with a subclavian flap. (From Waldhausen, J. A., and Nahrwold, D. L.: J. Thorac. Cardiovasc. Surg., 51:532, 1966.)

The *subclavian flap aortoplasty* was introduced by Waldhausen in 1966 (Fig. 8).[109] The left subclavian artery is dissected free and ligated at its first branch. The vertebral artery is often ligated to prevent a subclavian steal phenomenon. A longitudinal incision is made through the region of coarctation and continued onto the subclavian artery, creating a flap. The posterior obstructing shelf is resected and the flap of subclavian artery is turned down to enlarge the constriction. Advantages of this technique are decreased dissection, increased growth as there is no circumferential suture line, and avoidance of prosthetic material. As with the prosthetic patch onlay graft technique, there is decreased aortic occlusion time and decreased mortality. There is a generally lower incidence of recoarctation, although in young neonates the rate of early recoarctation may be as great as 20 per cent.[26, 77, 96] There is also concern over the sacrifice of the major vascular supply to the left arm. Although no major sequelae have been reported, there is evidence of decreased length and mass of the extremity.[107]

A variety of other techniques have been used to correct coarctation. These include the Blalock-Park anastomosis, prosthetic tube interposition graft, and ascending aorta–to–descending aorta bypass grafts. These may be useful in patients with difficult anatomy or those requiring reoperation. Recently percutaneous transluminal balloon angioplasty[66, 68] has been used to manage patients with coarctation (Fig. 9). Balloon angioplasty has been particularly successful in patients with recoarctation. Aneurysmal dilatation has been reported after balloon angioplasty of native coarctations.[69] The long-term results are unknown and the role in the management of coarctation is unclear.

The optimal management of defects occurring with coarctation of the aorta has not been determined. Surgical mortality is lowest in patients with isolated coarctation, increasing if there is a ventricular septal defect, and increasing markedly if there are associated complex anomalies. In the past, the pulmonary artery was often banded at the time of repair of the coarctation in infants with a nonrestrictive ventricular septal defect. Currently some advocate repair of the coarctation alone; then, if the congestive heart failure does not resolve, the septal defect is closed at a second operation.[39, 52, 59] In many children the ventricular septal defect decreases in size or closes after coarctation repair. Children with complex anomalies may improve sufficiently after coarctation repair to allow elective repair

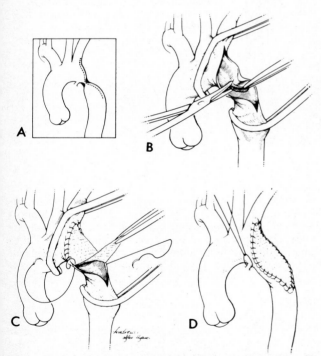

Figure 7. Coarctation of the aorta (aortoplasty with patch graft).

A, The usually posterolateral fourth intercostal space incision is used, and the distal aortic arch, ligamentum, and distal aorta are mobilized.

B, The proximal clamp should be applied high on the subclavian artery and the distal clamp well below the coarcted area. Intercostal arteries should be individually occluded. This permits a longitudinal incision that extends along the subclavian artery above and for a distance distally. A veil of tissue is often present at the site of coarctation, and this should be excised.

C and D, Usually a preclotted patch of knitted double velour Dacron is used, but in small infants (in whom the clotting factors may not be adequate) or in a patient under heparinization for intracardiac surgery, the tightly woven Dacron fabric is preferred.

(From Cooley, D. A.: Techniques in Cardiac Surgery, 2nd ed. Philadelphia, W. B. Saunders Company, 1984.)

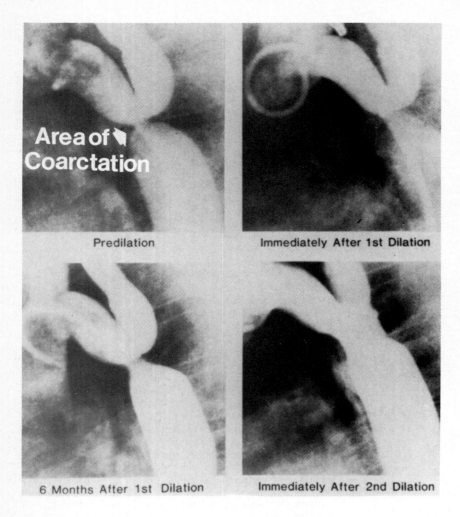

Predilation

Immediately After 1st Dilation

6 Months After 1st Dilation

Immediately After 2nd Dilation

Figure 9. Aortic coarctation in a patient with a 6-year-old surgical correction with an end-to-end anastomosis.

A, Before percutaneous transluminal angioplasty (PTA), the diameter of the aorta at the stenosis was 2.3 mm. with an associated pressure gradient of 67 mm. Hg.

B, After initial dilatation using an 8-mm. balloon, the lumen diameter increased to 5.4 mm., but the pressure gradient remained elevated at 49 mm. Hg.

C, Six months after initial dilatation, the vessel lumen measured 5.2 mm. and the pressure gradient had fallen to 28 mm. Hg.

D, After repeat angioplasty using a 12-mm. balloon, the vessel diameter measured 9.3 mm. and the pressure gradient had fallen to 8 mm. Hg. At follow-up 3 months later, the gradient across the coarctation was zero.

(From Locke, J. E., Bass, J. L., Amplatz, K., et al.: Circulation, 68:114, 1983.)

or palliation of the associated defects at a later date. Some authors advocate a one-stage repair of the coarctation and other defects.

Complications

Several problems may develop in the postoperative period. Paradoxical elevation of the blood pressure to greater than preoperative levels may occur, apparently caused by increased catecholamine levels and elevated renin levels.[91] Paradoxical hypertension may lead to the post-coarctectomy syndrome.[106] This syndrome was first reported by Sealy in 1953.[100] Up to 20 per cent of patients will experience some abdominal pain and distention postoperatively. The syndrome appears to be due to mesenteric ischemia possibly related to elevated renin levels and leads to gangrenous changes, but is rarely seen today. The postcoarctectomy syndrome may be prevented by aggressive therapy of postoperative hypertension. Many drugs have been used successfully to control the postoperative hypertension, including sodium nitroprusside, methyldopa, propranolol, and reserpine.

A dreaded complication of coarctation repair is paraplegia, which occurs in 0.5 to 1.0 per cent of patients.[15] It may be related to poor collaterals, anomalous origin of the right subclavian artery, distal hypotension during the period of aortic cross-clamping, reoperation, or hyperthermia during surgery.[30] Several authors have recommended monitoring distal pressure and using partial cardiac bypass or shunts if the distal pressure is less than 50 mm. Hg.[57, 65] Other complications include hemorrhage, chylothorax, recurrent nerve paralysis, and suture line thrombosis.

Results

The results of surgical correction depend on the age at repair, the type of repair used, and the associated anomalies. Operative mortality in neonates has decreased to 5 to 10 per cent and is lower in older patients. It is extremely low in patients with isolated coarctation and no associated anomalies. In patients who undergo resection and end-to-end anastomosis in infancy, the rate of recoarctation may be as high as 60 per cent. There is a decreased incidence of recurrent coarctation with the subclavian patch aortoplasty and the prosthetic patch graft repair. Recent series indicate that resection and end-to-end anastomosis, even in neonates, compare favorably to other methods in terms of mortality and recoarctation.[16, 64, 111]

Recoarctation usually manifests as persistent hypertension or arm-leg pressure gradient. The arm-leg gradient should be checked in the immediate postoperative period to differentiate residual stenosis due to an inadequate repair from true recoarctation. The causes of recoarctation include failure of growth of the anastomosis, inadequate resection of the narrowed segment, residual abnormal ductal tissue, and suture line thrombosis. Exercise testing with measurement of the arm-leg gradient should be done to evaluate postoperative patients.[34, 72] Many patients who are normotensive at rest without an arm-leg gradient will develop severe hypertension and a gradient after exercise. They may have a significant restenosis. The long-term consequences of the exercise-induced hypertension are unknown, but it may adversely affect the prognosis.

Reoperation is indicated if significant hypertension or other symptoms occur and a pressure gradient can be demonstrated. Reoperation is more difficult because of scarring from initial surgery and there is an increased morbidity and mortality. In patients who have undergone previous resection and end-to-end anastomosis, subclavian flap aortoplasty or prosthetic patch onlay grafting are good methods for repair of the recoarctation.

Some patients who have received a technically excellent repair may not have complete resolution of the elevated blood pressure.[73] The etiology of this persistent hypertension is unclear, but it is related to the age at repair and the duration of the preoperative hypertension. Follow-up of surgical patients indicates that they may not be rendered entirely normal. There is evidence of abnormal left ventricular function despite relief of the obstruction.[60] There appears to be an increased incidence of atherosclerotic cardiovascular disease and premature cardiac death.[73] Aortic stenosis or regurgitation due to a bicuspid aortic valve may develop and necessitate valve replacement. As has been emphasized, the long-term prognosis of many patients is determined mainly by the associated anomalies.

AORTOPULMONARY WINDOW

Aortopulmonary window is a rare congenital heart defect, first reported by Elliotson in 1830, which results from abnormal septation of the truncus arteriosus into the aorta and pulmonary artery.[33] It is also termed *aortopulmonary fistula* or *aortic septal defect*. The lesion is a communication between the aorta and the pulmonary artery, varying in size from a few millimeters to 2 to 3 cm., which may be found either immediately above the valve rings or more distally (Fig. 10).[80, 90, 99] A related lesion is anomalous origin of the right pulmonary artery from the aorta.[10, 50] Anomalous origin of either coronary artery from the pulmonary trunk near the defect may be present and complicate repair. Many patients have associated cardiac defects, including patent ductus arteriosus, ventricular septal defects, and aortic arch hypoplasia.[105]

Aortopulmonary window allows a left-to-right shunt of blood, resulting in pulmonary hypertension, left ventricular volume overload, and congestive heart failure.[32] Patients usually have congestive heart failure in infancy. Physical examination reveals a hyperactive precordium with a systolic or continuous murmur. The chest x-ray shows cardiomegaly and pulmonary congestion. Differential diagnosis includes patent ductus arteriosus, truncus arteriosus, and ventricular septal defect with aortic insufficiency. Cardiac catheterization should be done to confirm the diagnosis, delineate the anatomy, and evaluate associated anomalies.

Surgical correction should be undertaken soon after the diagnosis is made to prevent the development of irreversible pulmonary vascular changes. Gross successfully ligated an aortopulmonary window in 1948[46] and Scott and Sabiston divided an aortopulmonary window using a closed technique in 1953.[99] Since the advent of cardiopulmonary bypass, several techniques have been used successfully: division, transpulmonary closure, and transaortic closure. The preferred method is transaortic closure using direct suture for small defects and patch closure for large defects.[21] This approach allows clear definition of the anatomy of the right pulmonary artery and the coronary arteries. Operative mortality varies from 0 to 50 per cent. The long-term results of repair of isolated aortopulmonary window without pulmonary hypertension are good; however, associated anomalies and pulmonary vascular disease adversely affect survival.

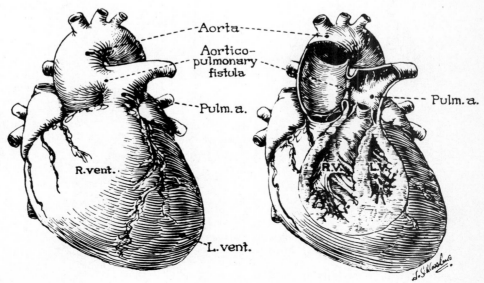

Figure 10. Aortopulmonary window. The size of the fistula and its relation to the semilunar valves are variable. (From Scott, H. W., Jr., and Sabiston, D. C., Jr.: J. Thorac. Surg., 25:26, 1953.)

Aorta

Aortico-pulmonary fistula

Pulm. a.

Pulm. a.

R. vent.

R.V.   L.V.

L. vent.

ANOMALIES OF THE AORTIC ARCH

The aorta, pulmonary artery, and other great vessels are derived from six paired aortic arches. During fetal development segments of these arches either grow or regress to produce the adult anatomy. Failure of a segment to grow or regress normally produces an anomaly of the aortic arch or great vessels. Many of these anomalies cause no symptoms; a few, however, constrict the trachea or esophagus and are termed *vascular rings*. Persistent double aortic arch was described in 1737 by Hommel. In 1794, Bayford reported a patient with severe dysphagia and an aberrant right subclavian artery.[6] Gross in 1945 successfully divided a double aortic arch and an aberrant right subclavian artery.[44, 45]

Clinical Manifestations

The natural history of vascular rings is obscured by the wide spectrum of anomalies and the range of symptoms. Many affected infants have dysphagia, respiratory distress, stridor, repeated pulmonary infections, vomiting, or failure to thrive. Fatal obstruction of the trachea can occur. However, children with mild symptoms may improve markedly as they grow. Many patients with these anomalies are totally asymptomatic.

A variety of lesions can produce tracheal or esophageal compromise.[48] Most common is the double aortic arch, which results from persistence of both the left and the right fourth aortic arches, forming a ring around the trachea and esophagus (Fig. 11*A*). The left subclavian and carotid arteries usually arise from the anterior arch, whereas the right-sided vessels arise from the posterior arch. The anterior arch is usually smaller than the posterior arch and may have an atretic segment (Fig. 12). If the right fourth arch persists while the left regresses, a right aortic arch is produced. In patients with a right aortic arch, a retroesophageal segment and a left descending aorta may be present or, more commonly, a right-sided descending aorta is found.[63] The great vessels may arise in mirror-image fashion or an aberrant left subclavian artery may originate as the last vessel from the arch or from an aortic diverticulum. The ductus (or ligamentum) arteriosus is usually left-sided with a right aortic arch. Vascular rings with a right aortic arch are possible if there is mirror-image branching with a left ligamentum arteriosum, if an aberrant left subclavian artery with a retroesophageal course is present, or if a retroesophageal segment of the arch with a left descending aorta and left ligamentum arteriosum is present.

A vascular ring may occur with a normal left arch and aberrant origin of the right subclavian artery as the last branch of the arch. This vessel courses retroesophageally and may cause significant dysphagia. Rarely abnormal origin of the innominate artery causes anterior tracheal

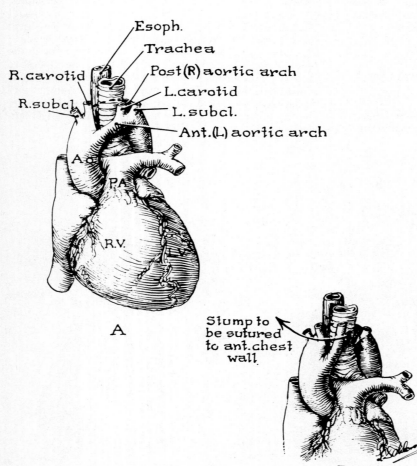

Esoph.
Trachea
Post (R) aortic arch
R. carotid
L. carotid
R. subcl
L. subcl.
Ant. (L) aortic arch

A.
P.A.
R.V.
L.V.

A

Stump to be sutured to ant. chest wall

B

Figure 11. Double aortic arch. A, The larger channel is usually posterior and on the right. Branches of the arch arise independently. In almost all instances the descending thoracic aortic is on the left as shown. B, Point of division of the smaller arch is selected to preserve circulation to the branches. The left common carotid artery is then tacked to the anterior chest wall to further relieve tracheal compression. (From Bahnson, H. T.: In Sabiston, D. C., Jr., and Spencer, F. C. (Eds.): Gibbon's Surgery of the Chest, 3rd ed. Philadelphia, W. B. Saunders Company, 1976.)

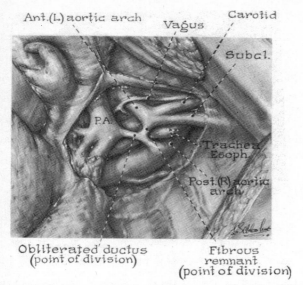

Ant.(L) aortic arch   Vagus   Carotid

Subcl.

P.A.

Trachea Esoph.

Post.(R) aortic arch

Obliterated ductus   Fibrous
(point of division)   remnant
                          (point of division)

Figure 12. Operative view of tracheal ring completed by obliter-ated remnant of distal left arch and ligamentum arteriosum. After complete exposure of the vascular components, the proper point of division of the ligaments can easily be determined. (From Bahnson, H. T.: In Sabiston, D. C., Jr., and Spencer, F. C. (Eds.): Gibbon's Surgery of the Chest, 3rd ed. Philadelphia, W. B. Saunders Company, 1976.)

compression and produces respiratory symptoms. A variety of other developmental anomalies have been reported as rare causes of vascular rings.

A lesion that causes similar symptoms is the vascular sling or *pulmonary artery sling*.[95] The left pulmonary artery arises from the right pulmonary artery, passes over the right mainstem bronchus, and travels between the trachea and esophagus. Hyperinflation of the right lung, respiratory distress, and repeated pulmonary infections may occur. Pulmonary artery sling is associated with a high incidence of anomalies of the tracheobronchial tree, including hypoplasia of the distal trachea with complete cartilaginous rings.

Vascular rings should be suspected in any child with stridor, dysphagia, frequent respiratory infections, or diffi-

cult feeding. Anomalies that become symptomatic almost always present by age 6 months. Hyperextension of the neck may reduce the constriction and marked respiratory distress may occur if the neck is flexed. Respiratory symptoms may be exacerbated by feeding. The physical findings are otherwise nonspecific. The plain chest x-ray may be normal, may show pneumonia, or may show compression of the air-filled trachea. The barium esophagogram is a valuable study. The combination of posterior compression of the esophagus on barium swallow and anterior tracheal compression is almost pathognomonic for vascular ring (Fig. 13). The level and angle of compression will usually permit exact diagnosis of the vessels involved. The esophagogram is normal in a patient with aberrant origin of the innominate artery. Cardiac catheterization will delineate the anatomy of vascular rings clearly. Although some vascular rings can be divided without preoperative catheterization, misdiagnosis can occasionally occur. Many centers routinely perform catheterization in all patients with suspected vascular rings.

Surgical Management

Surgical management is designed to divide the vascular ring and relieve the constriction.[92] As the long-term prognosis of medical therapy is poor in patients with marked symptoms, surgical intervention should be undertaken at the time of diagnosis. Adequate exposure is an absolute necessity. Most vascular rings can be safely divided through a left thoracotomy; however, a few anomalies do require approach through a right thoracotomy.

In patients with a double aortic arch, division of the smaller arch should be performed to relieve symptoms. The anterior or left arch is often the smallest and can be divided at its junction with the descending aorta so that the left carotid and subclavian arteries arise from the ascending aorta. The ligamentum arteriosum is also divided and the constricting vessels are dissected away from the trachea and esophagus. The end of the left arch may be suspended from the posterior surface of the sternum to further free the trachea and esophagus (see Fig. 11*B*). If a right aortic arch with retroesophageal segment and left descending aorta or

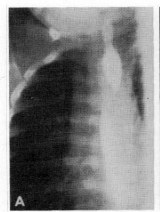
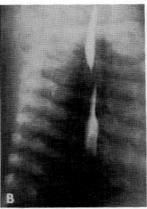
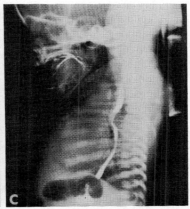

Figure 13. Roentgenograms of vascular ring. A and B, Double aortic arch. The location and direction of esophageal compression suggest a larger posterior arch coursing from above downward but with anterior compression also. C, Obstruction from remnant of left fourth arch and obliterated ductus as shown in Figure 12. (From Bahnson, H. T.: In Sabiston, D. C., Jr., and Spencer, F. C. (Eds.): Gibbon's Surgery of the Chest, 3rd ed. Philadelphia, W. B. Saunders Company, 1976.)

a right arch with mirror-image branching is present, division of the left ligamentum arteriosum will relieve the obstruction.

If an aberrant subclavian artery is present, it can be safely divided to relieve the constriction. An anomalous innominate artery can be dissected free and suspended from the sternum to free the trachea and esophagus. If a pulmonary artery sling is present, the left pulmonary artery should be divided and reanastomosed to the main pulmonary artery anterior to the trachea.

Results

Operation usually results in marked improvement, although complete resolution of symptoms may take several months. This is especially true in patients with pulmonary artery slings and abnormalities of the tracheobronchial tree. Operative mortality is related primarily to underlying problems with the trachea or bronchi. Postoperatively, special attention must be given to respiratory care. The long-term progress for patients after division of isolated vascular rings is excellent.

SELECTED REFERENCES

Abbott, M. E.: Coarctation of the aorta of the adult type, II. A statistical study and historical retrospect of 200 recorded cases, with autopsy, of stenosis or obliteration of the descending arch in subjects above the age of two years. Am. Heart J., *3*:574, 1928.
A classic series reporting the medical history, physical examination, and natural history of patients with coarctation of the aorta.

Gross, R. E., and Hubbard, J. P.: Surgical ligation of a patent ductus arteriosus. J.A.M.A., *112*:729, 1939.
A landmark paper reporting the first successful surgical therapy of congenital heart disease.

Schuster, S. R., and Gross, R. E.: Surgery for coarctation of the aorta: A review of 500 cases. J. Thorac. Cardiovasc. Surg., *43*:54, 1962.
A report by Gross, a pioneer in cardiac surgery, of his extensive experience with coarctation of the aorta.

REFERENCES

1. Abbott, M. E.: Coarctation of the aorta of the adult type, II. A statistical study and historical restrospect of 200 recorded cases, with autopsy, of stenosis or obliteration of the descending arch in subjects above the age of two years. Am. Heart J., *3*:574, 1928.
2. Adzick, N. S., Harrison, M. R., and deLorimier, A. A.: Surgical clip ligation of patent ductus arteriosus in premature infants. J. Pediatr. Surg., *21*:158, 1986.
3. Alpert, B. S., Bain, H. H., Balfe, J. W., Kidd, B. S. L., and Olley, P. M.: Role of the renin-angiotensin-aldosterone system in hypertensive children with coarctation of the aorta. Am. J. Cardiol., *43*:828, 1979.
4. Amparo, E. G., Higgins, C. B., and Shafton, E. P.: Demonstration of coarctation of the aorta by magnetic resonance imaging. A. J. R., *143*:1192, 1984.
5. Arciniegas, E., Hakimi, M., Hertzler, J. H., Farooki, Z. Q., and Green, E. W.: Surgical management of congenital vascular rings. J. Thorac. Cardiovasc. Surg., *77*:721, 1979.
6. Bayford, D., and Hulme, H.: An account of a singular case of obstructed deglutition. Article XXIV. *In* Memoirs of the Medical Society of London, Vol. 11. London, 1794, p. 275.
7. Bell, E. F., Warburton, D., Stonestreet, B. S., and Oh, W.: Effect of fluid administration on the development of symptomatic patent ductus arteriosus and congestive heart failure in premature infants. N. Engl. J. Med., *302*:598, 1980.
8. Bergdahl, L., and Ljungqvist, A.: Long-term results after repair of coarctation of the aorta by patch grafting. J. Thorac. Cardiovasc. Surg., *80*:177, 1980.
9. Berman, W., Jr., Dubynsky, O., Whitman, V., Friedman, Z., Maisels, M. J., and Musselman, J.: Digoxin therapy in low-birth-weight infants with patent ductus arteriosus. J. Pediatr., *93*:652, 1978.
10. Berry, T. E., Bharati, S., Muster, A. J., Idriss, F. S., Santucci, B., Lev, M., and Paul, M. H.: Distal aortopulmonary septal defect, aortic origin of the right pulmonary artery, intact ventricular septum, patent ductus arteriosus and hypoplasia of the aortic isthmus: A newly recognized syndrome. Am. J. Cardiol., *42*:108, 1982.
10a. Binet, J. P., and Langlois, J.: Aortic arch anomalies in children and infants. J. Thorac. Cardiovasc. Surg., *73*:248, 1977.
11. Blalock, A.: Operative closure of the patent ductus arteriosus. Surg. Gynecol. Obstet., *82*:113, 1946.
12. Blalock, A., and Park, E. A.: The surgical treatment of experimental coarctation (atresia) of the aorta. Ann. Surg., *119*:445, 1944.
13. Blieden, L. C., and Moller, J. H.: Aorticopulmonary septal defect: An experience with 17 patients. Br. Heart J., *36*:630, 1974.
14. Bonnet, L. M.: Sur la lesion dite stenose congenitale de l'aorte dans la region de l'isthme. Rev. Med. Paris, *23*:108, 255, 335, 418, 481, 1903.
15. Brewer, L. A., III, Fosburg, R. G., Mulder, G. A., and Verska, J. J.: Spinal cord complications following surgery for coarctation of the aorta. A study of 66 cases. J. Thorac. Cardiovasc. Surg., *64*:368, 1972.
15a. Burnard, E. D.: Discussion on the significance of continuous murmurs in the first few days of life. Proc. Roy. Soc. Med., *52*:77, 1959.
16. Campbell, D. B., Waldhausen, J. A., Pierce, W. S., Fripp, R., and Whitman, V.: Should elective repair of coarctation of the aorta be done in infancy? J. Thorac. Cardiovasc. Surg., *88*:929, 1984.
17. Campbell, M.: Natural history of persistent ductus arteriosus. Br. Heart J., *30*:4, 1968.
18. Campbell, M.: Natural history of coarctation of the aorta. Br. Heart J., *32*:633, 1970.
19. Celano, V., Pieroni, D. R., Morera, J. A., Roland, J. M., and Gingell, R. L.: Two-dimensional echocardiographic examination of mitral valve abnormalities associated with coarctation of the aorta. Circulation, *69*:924, 1984.
19a. Christensen, N. A.: Coarctation of the aorta: Historical review. Proc. Staff Meet. Mayo Clin., *23*:322, 1948.
20. Christie, A.: Normal closing time of the foramen ovale and ductus arteriosus: An anatomic and statistical study. Am. J. Dis. Child., *40*:323, 1930.
21. Clarke, C. P., and Richardson, J. P.: The management of aortopulmonary window: Advantages of transaortic closure with a Dacron patch. J. Thorac. Cardiovasc. Surg., *72*:48, 1976.
22. Clarkson, P. M., Brandt, P. W. T., Barratt-Boyes, B. G., Rutherford, J. D., Kerr, A. R., and Neutze, J. M.: Prosthetic repair of coarctation of the aorta with particular reference to Dacron onlay patch grafts and late aneurysm formation. Am. J. Cardiol., *56*:342, 1985.
23. Clyman, R.: The role of the patent ductus arteriosus in respiratory distress syndrome. Semin. Perinatol., *8*:293, 1984.
24. Clyman, R. I., Ballard, P. L., Sniderman, S., Ballard, R. A., Roth, R., Heymann, M. A., and Granberg, J. P.: Prenatal administration of betamethasone for prevention of patent ductus arteriosus. J. Pediatr., *98*:123, 1981.
25. Clyman, R. I., and Heymann, M. A.: Pharmacology of the ductus arteriosus. Pediatr. Clin. North Am., *28*:77, 1981.
26. Cobanoglu, A., Teply, J. F., Grunkemeier, G. L., Sunderland, C. O., and Starr, A.: Coarctation of the aorta in patients younger than three months: A critique of the subclavian flap operation. J. Thorac. Cardiovasc. Surg., *89*:128, 1985.
27. Cooley, D. A., McNamara, D. G., and Latson, J. R.: Aorticopulmonary septal defect: Diagnosis and surgical treatment. Surgery, *42*:101, 1957.
28. Cooper, R. S., Ritter, S. B., and Golinko, R. J.: Balloon dilatation angioplasty: Nonsurgical management of coarctation of the aorta. Circulation, *70*:903, 1984.
29. Crafoord, C., and Nylin, G.: Congenital coarctation of the aorta and its surgical treatment. J. Thorac. Surg., *14*:347, 1945.
30. Crawford, F. A., Jr., and Sade, R. M.: Spinal cord injury associated with hyperthermia during aortic coarctation repair. J. Thorac. Cardiovasc. Surg., *87*:616, 1984.
30a. Decanq, H. G.: Repair of patent ductus arteriosus in a 1417 gm. infant. Am. J. Dis. Child, *106*:402, 1963.
31. Deverall, P. B., Lincoln, J. C. R., Aberdeen, E., Bonham-Carter, R. E., and Waterston, D.: Aortopulmonary window. J. Thorac. Cardiovasc. Surg., *57*:479, 1969.
32. Doty, D. B., Richardson, J. V., Falkovsky, G. E., Gordonova, M. I., and Burakovsky, V. I.: Aortopulmonary septal defect: Hemodynamics, angiography, and operation. Ann. Thorac. Surg., *32*:244, 1981.
33. Elliotson: Case of malformation of the pulmonary artery and aorta. Lancet, *1*:247, 1830.
34. Freed, M. D., Rocchini, A., Rosenthal, A., Nadas, A. S., and Castaneda, A. R.: Exercise-induced hypertension after surgical repair of coarctation of the aorta. Am. J. Cardiol., *43*:253, 1979.

35. Friedman, W. F., Hirschklau, M. J., Printz, M. P., Pitlick, P. T., and Kirkpatrick, S. E.: Pharmacologic closure of patent ductus arteriosus in the premature infant. N. Engl. J. Med., *295*:526, 1976.

36. Furzan, J. A., Reisch, J., Tyson, J. E., Laird, P., and Rosenfeld, C. R.: Incidence and risk factors for symptomatic patent ductus arteriosus among inborn very-low-birth-weight infants. Early Hum. Dev., *12*:39, 1985.

36a. Fyler, D. C., et al.: Report of the New England infant cardiac program. Pediatrics, *65*:375, 1980.

37. Gay, W. A., Jr., and Young, W. G., Jr.: Pseudocoarctation of the aorta. A reappraisal. J. Thorac. Cardiovasc. Surg., *58*:739, 1969.

38. Gersony, W. M., Peckham, G. J., Ellison, R. C., Miettinen, O. S., and Nadas, A. S.: Effects of indomethacin in premature infants with patent ductus arteriosus: Results of a national collaborative study. J. Pediatr., *102*:895, 1983.

39. Gibson, G. A.: Clinical lectures on circulatory affections. Lecture I. Persistence of the arterial duct and its diagnosis. Edinburgh Med. J., *8*:1, 1900.

40. Goldman, S., Hernandez, J., and Papps, G.: Results of surgical treatment of coarctation of the aorta in the critically ill neonate. J. Thorac. Cardiovasc. Surg., *91*:732, 1986.

41. Graybiel, A., Strieder, J. W., and Boyer, N. H.: An attempt to obliterate the patent ductus arteriosus in a patient with subacute bacterial endarteritis. Am. Heart J., *15*:621, 1938.

42. Gross, R. E.: Complete surgical division of the patent ductus arteriosus. A report of fourteen successful cases. Surg. Gynecol. Obstet., *78*:36, 1944.

43. Gross, R. E.: Surgical correction for coarctation of the aorta. Surgery, *18*:673, 1945.

44. Gross, R. E.: Surgical relief for tracheal obstruction from a vascular ring. N. Engl. J. Med., *233*:586, 1945.

45. Gross, R. E.: Surgical treatment for dysphagia lusoria. Ann. Surg., *124*:532, 1946.

46. Gross, R. E.: Surgical closure of an aortic septal defect. Circulation, *5*:858, 1952.

47. Gross, R. E., and Hubbard, J. P.: Surgical ligation of a patent ductus arteriosus. J.A.M.A., *112*:729, 1939.

48. Gross, R. E., and Neuhauser, E. B. D.: Compression of the trachea or esophagus by vascular anomalies. Surgical therapy in 40 cases. Pediatrics, *7*:69, 1951.

49. Gross, R. E., and Ware, P. F.: The surgical significance of aortic arch anomalies. Surg. Gynecol. Obstet., *83*:435, 1946.

50. Gula, G., Chew, C., Radley-Smith, R., and Yacoub, M.: Anomalous origin of the right pulmonary artery from the ascending aorta associated with aortopulmonary window. Thorax, *33*:265, 1978.

51. Hamilton, W. F., and Abbott, M. E.: Coarctation of the aorta of the adult type. I. Complete obliteration of the descending arch at insertion of the ductus in a boy of fourteen; bicuspid aortic valve; impending rupture of the aorta; cerebral death. Am. Heart J., *3*:381, 1928.

52. Hammon, J. W., Jr., Graham, T. P., Jr., Boucek, R. J., Jr., and Bender, H. W., Jr.: Operative repair of coarctation of the aorta in infancy: Results with and without ventricular septal defect. Am. J. Cardiol., *55*:1555, 1985.

53. Harlan, J. L., Doty, D. B., Brandt, B., III, and Ehrenhaft, J. L.: Coarctation of the aorta in infants. J. Thorac. Cardiovasc. Surg., *88*:1012, 1984.

53a. Hehrlein, F. W., Mulch, J., Rautenburg, H. W., Schlepper, M., and Schled, H. H.: Incidence and pathogenesis of late aneurysms after patch graft aortoplasty for coarctation. J. Thorac. Cardiovasc. Surg., *92*:226, 1986.

54. Heymann, M. A., Rudolph, A. M., and Silverman, N. H.: Closure of the ductus arteriosus in premature infants by inhibition of prostaglandin synthesis. N. Engl. J. Med., *295*:530, 1976.

55. Ho, S. Y., and Anderson, R. H.: Coarctation, tubular hypoplasia, and the ductus venosus. Histological study of 35 specimens. Br. Heart J., *41*:268, 1979.

56. Hubbard, C., Rucker, R. W., Realyvasquez, F., et al.: Ligation of the patent ductus arteriosus in newborn respiratory failure. J. Pediatr. Surg., *21*:3, 1986.

57. Hughes, R. K., and Reemtsma, K.: Correction of coarctation of the aorta: Manometric determination of safety during test occlusion. J. Thorac. Cardiovasc. Surg., *62*:31, 1971.

58. Jarcho, S.: Coarctation of the aorta (Meckel, 1750; Paris, 1791). Am. J. Cardiol., *7*:844, 1961.

58a. Jung, J. Y., Almond, C. H., Saab, S. B., and Lababidi, Z.: Surgical repair of right aortic arch with aberrant left subclavian artery and left ligamentum arteriosum. J. Thorac. Cardiovasc. Surg., *75*:237, 1978.

59. Kamau, P., Miles, V., Toews, W., et al.: Surgical repair of coarctation of the aorta in infants less than six months of age. Including the question of pulmonary artery banding. J. Thorac. Cardiovasc. Surg., *81*:171, 1981.

60. Kimball, B. P., Shurvell, B. L., Houle, S., Fulop, J. C., Rakowski, H., and McLaughlin, P. R.: Persistent ventricular adaptations in postoperative coarctation of the aorta. J. Am. Coll. Cardiol., *8*:172, 1986.

61. Kirks, D. R., McCook, T. A., Serwer, G. A., and Oldham, H. N., Jr.: Aneurysm of the ductus arteriosus in the neonate. A.J.R., *134*:573, 1980.

62. Kitterman, J. A., Edmunds, L. H., Jr., Gregory, G. A., Heymann, M. A., Tooley, W. H., and Rudolph, A. M.: Patent ductus arteriosus in premature infants. Incidence, relation to pulmonary disease and management. N. Engl. J. Med., *287*:473, 1972.

63. Knight, L., and Edwards, J. E.: Right aortic arch: Types and associated cardiac anomalies. Circulation, *50*:1047, 1974.

64. Korfer, R., Meyer, H., Kleikamp, G., and Bircks, W.: Early and late results after resection and end-to-end anastomosis of coarctation of the thoracic aorta in early infancy. J. Thorac. Cardiovasc. Surg., *89*:616, 1985.

65. Krieger, K. H., and Spencer, F. C.: Is paraplegia after repair of coarctation of the aorta due principally to distal hypotension during aortic cross-clamping? Surgery, 97:2, 1985.

66. Lababidi, Z. A., Daskalopoulos, D. A., and Stoeckle, H., Jr.: Transluminal balloon coarctation angioplasty: Experience with 27 patients. Am. J. Cardiol., *54*:1288, 1984.

67. Legrand, A.: Stenosis of the aorta: Diagnosis and treatment of this disease followed by a case of cured aneurysm of the heart. Ann. Med. Physiol., *24*:298, 451, 608, 1833.

68. Lock, J. E., Bass, J. L., Amplatz, K., Fuhrman, B. P., and Castaneda-Zuniga, W.: Balloon dilatation of aortic coarctations in infants and children. Circulation, *68*:109, 1983.

69. Lock, J. E., Keane, J. F., and Fellows, K. E.: The use of catheter intervention procedures for congenital heart disease. J. Am. Coll. Cardiol., 7:1420, 1986.

70. Luisi, S. V., Ashraf, M. H., Gula, G., Radley-Smith, R., and Yacoub, M.: Anomalous origin of the right coronary artery with aortopulmonary window: Functional and surgical considerations. Thorax, *35*:446, 1980.

71. Mahony, L., Carnero, V., Brett, C., Heymann, M. A., and Clyman, R. I.: Prophylactic indomethacin therapy for patent ductus arteriosus in very-low-birth-weight infants. N. Engl. J. Med., *306*:506, 1982.

72. Markel, H., Rocchini, A. P., Beekman, R. H., Martin, J., Palmisano, J., Moorehead, C., and Rosenthal, A.: Exercise-induced hypertension after repair of coarctation of the aorta: Arm versus leg exercise. J. Am. Coll. Cardiol., *8*:165, 1986.

73. Maron, B. J., Humphries, J. O., Rowe, R. D., and Mellits, E. D.: Prognosis of surgically corrected coarctation of the aorta: A 20-year postoperative appraisal. Circulation, *47*:119, 1973.

73a. Marvin, W. J., Mahoney, L. T., and Rose, E. F.: Pathologic sequelae of balloon dilatation angioplasty for unoperated coarctation of the aorta. J. Am. Coll. Cardiol., 7:117A, 1986.

74. Marx, G. R., and Allen H. D.: Accuracy and pitfalls of Doppler evaluation of the pressure gradient in aortic coarctation. J. Am. Coll. Cardiol., 7:1379, 1986.

75. McFaul, R., Millard, P., and Nowicki, E.: Vascular rings necessitating right thoracotomy. J. Thorac. Cardiovasc. Surg., *82*:306, 1981.

76. Meckel, A.: Verschliessung der Aorta am vierten Brustwirbel. Arch. F. Anat. Physiol. Leipzig, 1827, p. 345.

77. Metzdorff, M. T., Cobanoglu, A., Grunkemeier, G. L., Sunderland, C. O., and Starr, A.: Influence of age at operation on late results with subclavian flap aortoplasty. J. Thorac. Cardiovasc. Surg., *89*:235, 1985.

78. Mikhail, M., Lee, W., Toews, W., Synhorst, D. P., Hawes, C. R., Hernandez, J., Lockhart, C., Whitfield, J., and Pappas, G.: Surgical and medical experience with 734 premature infants with patent ductus arteriosus. J. Thorac. Cardiovasc. Surg., *83*:349, 1982.

79. Morgagni, J. P.: De Sedibus et Causis Morborum. Epistle XVII. Article VI, 1760.

80. Mori, A., Ando, M., Takao, A., Ishikawa, H., and Imai, Y.: Distal type of aortopulmonary window. Report of 4 cases. Br. Heart J., *40*:681, 1978.

81. Munro, J. C.: Ligation of the ductus arteriosus. Ann. Surg., *46*:335, 1907.

81a. Myers, J. L., Campbell, D. B., and Waldhausen, J. A.: The use of absorbable monofilament polydioxanone suture in pediatric cardiovascular operations. J. Thorac. Cardiovasc. Surg., *92*:771, 1986.

82. Ostermiller, W. E., Jr., Somerndike, J. M., Hunter, J. A., Dye, W. S., Javid, H., Najafi, H., and Julian, O. C.: Coarctation of the aorta in adult patients. J. Thorac. Cardiovasc. Surg., *61*:125, 1971.

83. Paris, M.: Detrecissiment considerable de l'aorte pectorale observe a l'Hotel de Paris. J. Chir. Desault, *2*:107, 1791.

84. Peckham, G. J., Miettinen, O. S., Ellison, R. C., Kraybill, E. N., Gersony, W. M., Zierler, S., and Nadas, A. S.: Clinical course to

1 year of age in premature infants with patent ductus arteriosus: Results of a multicenter randomized trial of indomethacin. J. Pediatr., *105*:285, 1984.

85. Portsmann, W., Wierny, L., Warnke, H., Gerstberger, G., and Romaniuk, P. A.: Catheter closure of patent ductus arteriosus: 62 cases treated without thoracotomy. Radiol. Clin. North Am., *9*:203, 1971.

85a. Powell, M. L.: Patent ductus arteriosus in premature infants. Med. J. Aust., *2*:58, 1963.

86. Putnam, T. C., and Gross, R. E.: Surgical management of aortopulmonary fenestration. Surgery, *59*:727, 1966.

87. Railsback, O. C., and Dock, W.: Erosion of the ribs due to stenosis of the isthmus (coarctation) of the aorta. Radiology, *12*:58, 1929.

88. Rashkind, W. J.: Pediatric cardiology: A brief historical perspective. Pediatr. Cardiol., *1*:63, 1979.

89. Rashkind, W. J., and Cuaso, C. C.: Transcatheter closure of patent ductus arteriosus: Successful use in a 3.5-kilogram infant. Pediatr. Cardiol., *1*:3, 1979.

89a. Reifenstein, G. H., Levine, S. A., and Gross, R. E.: Coarctation of the aorta: A review of 104 autopsied cases of the "adult type," 2 years of age or older. Am. Heart J., *33*:146, 1947.

90. Richardson, J. V., Doty, D. B., Rossi, N. P., and Ehrenhaft, J. L.: The spectrum of anomalies of aortopulmonary septation. J. Thorac. Cardiovasc. Surg., *78*:21, 1979.

91. Rocchini, A. P., Rosenthal, A., Barger, A. C., Castaneda. A. R., and Nadas, A. S.: Pathogenesis of paradoxical hypertension after coarctation resection. Circulation, *54*:382, 1976.

92. Roesler, M., De Leval, M., Chrispin, A., and Stark, J.: Surgical management of vascular ring. Ann. Surg., *197*:139, 1983.

93. Rudolph, A. M., Heymann, M. A., and Spitznas, U.: Hemodynamic considerations in the development of narrowing of the aorta. Am. J. Cardiol., *30*:514, 1972.

94. Sade, R. M., Crawford, F. A., Hohn, A. R., Riopel, D. A., and Taylor, A. B.: Growth of the aorta after prosthetic patch aortoplasty for coarctation in infants. Ann. Thorac. Surg., *38*:21, 1984.

95. Sade, R. M., Rosenthal, A., Fellows, K., and Castaneda, A. R.: Pulmonary artery sling. J. Thorac. Cardiovasc. Surg., *69*:333, 1975.

96. Sanchez, G. R., Balsara, R. K., Dunn, J. M., Mehta, A. V., and O'Riordan, A. C.: Recurrent obstruction after subclavian flap repair of coarctation of the aorta in infants. Can it be predicted or prevented? J. Thorac. Cardiovasc. Surg., *91*:738, 1986.

97. Schuster, S. R., and Gross, R. E.: Surgery for coarctation of the aorta: A review of 500 cases. J. Thorac. Cardiovasc. Surg., *43*:54, 1962.

98. Scott, H. W., Jr., and Bahnson, H. T.: Evidence for a renal factor in the hypertension of experimental coarctation of the aorta. Surgery, *30*:206, 1951.

99. Scott, H. W., Jr., and Sabiston, D. C., Jr.: Surgical treatment for congenital aorticopulmonary fistula: Experimental and clinical aspects. J. Thorac. Surg., *25*:26, 1953.

100. Sealy, W. C., Harris, J. S., Young, W. G., Jr., and Callaway, H. A., Jr.: Paradoxical hypertension following resection of coarctation of aorta. Surgery, *42*:135, 1957.

101. Sehested, J., Baandrup, U., and Mikkelsen, E.: Different reactivity and structure of the prestenotic and poststenotic aorta in human coarctation: Implications for baroreceptor function. Circulation, *65*:1060, 1982.

102. Serwer, G. A., Armstrong, B. E., and Anderson, P. A. W.: Continuous wave Doppler ultrasonographic quantitation of patent ductus arteriosus flow. J. Pediatr., *100*:297, 1982.

103. Silverman, N. H., Lewis, A. B., Heymann, M. A., and Rudolph, A. M.: Echocardiographic assessment of ductus arteriosus shunt in premature infants. Circulation, *50*:821, 1974.

104. Smallhorn, J. F., Anderson, R. H., and Macartney, F. J.: Two dimensional echocardiographic assessment of communications between ascending aorta and pulmonary trunk or individual pulmonary arteries. Br. Heart J., *47*:563, 1982.

105. Tabak, C., Moskowitz, W., Wagner, H., Weinberg, P., and Edmunds, L. H., Jr.: Aortopulmonary window and aortic isthmic hypoplasia: Operative management in newborn infants. J. Thorac. Cardiovasc. Surg., *86*:273, 1983.

106. Tawes, R. L., Jr., Bull, J. C., and Roe, B. B.: Hypertension and abdominal pain after resection of aortic coarctation. Ann. Surg., *171*:409, 1970.

107. Todd, P. J., Dangerfield, P. H., Hamilton, D. I., and Wilkinson, J. L.: Late effects on the left upper limb of subclavian flap aortoplasty. J. Thorac. Cardiovasc. Surg., *85*:678, 1983.

108. Vossschulte, K.: Surgical correction of coarctation of the aorta by an "isthmusplastic" operation. Thorax, *16*:338, 1961.

109. Waldhausen, J. A., and Nahrwold, D. L.: Repair of coarctation of the aorta with a subclavian flap. J. Thorac. Cardiovasc. Surg., *51*:532, 1966.

110. Warren, J., Smith, R. S., and Naik, R. B.: Inappropriate renin secretion and abnormal cardiovascular reflexes in coarctation of the aorta. Br. Heart J., *45*:733, 1981.

110a. Way, G. L., Pierce, J. R., Wolfe, R. R., McGrath, R., Wiggins, J., and Merenstein, G. B.: ST depression suggesting subendocardial ischemia in neonates with respiratory distress syndrome and patent ductus arteriosus. J. Pediatr., *95*:609, 1979.

111. Yee, E. S., Turley, K., Soifer, S., and Ebert, P. A.: Synthetic patch aortoplasty: A simplified approach for coarctation in repairs during early infancy and thereafter. Am. J. Surg., *148*:240, 1984.

112. Zednikova, M., Baylen, B. G., Yoshida, Y., and Emmanouilides, G. C.: Precordial contrast echocardiographic detection of patent ductus arteriosus in small preterm infants. Pediatr. Cardiol., *2*:271, 1982.

III

Atrial Septal Defect, Ostium Primum Defect, and Atrioventricular Canal

GARY K. LOFLAND, M.D.
DAVID C. SABISTON, JR., M.D.

The first anatomic details of cardiac septal defects were described in 1875 by Rokitansky.[25] Atrial septal defect has the distinction of being the first true cardiac lesion corrected using open heart surgery and was reported in 1948.[21] Prior to cardiopulmonary bypass, the techniques utilized for attempted closure included external invagination,[6] ligation of the defect,[21] and open blind suture through a blood-filled rubber well sutured to the right atrium.[13] Twenty years after beginning his research, Gibbon was the first to successfully use cardiopulmonary bypass, and the modern era of open heart surgery was launched with closure of an atrial septal defect under direct visualization.[11]

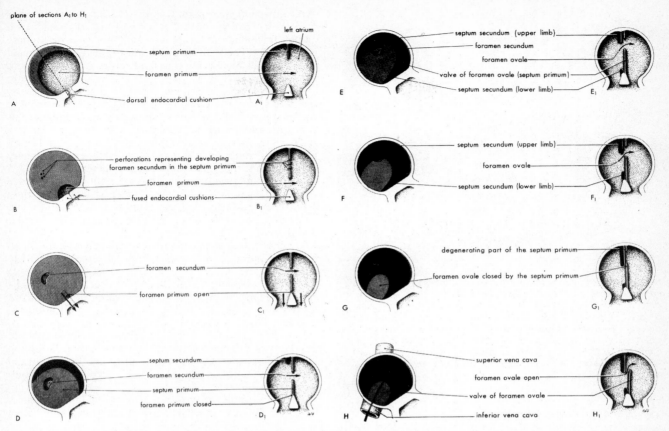

Figure 1. Schematic illustration of partitioning of the interatrial septum. The entire sequence (A through H) occurs at between 25 and 35 days of fetal development. (From Moore, K. L.: The Developing Human: Clinically Oriented Embryology, 3rd ed. Philadelphia, W. B. Saunders Company, 1982.)

Atrial septal defect is recognized as the fifth most common congenital cardiac anomaly, occurring in 1 in 13,500 children under the age of 14 years.[16] It accounts for 7 per cent of all congenital anomalies in individuals under the age of 20, and it is the most common cardiac defect detected in individuals over 20 years of age.[10]

The precise etiology of atrial septal defect is unknown, with evidence supporting both genetic and environmental influences. The increased incidence in mongolism,[1] Ellis-van Creveld syndrome,[12] Marfan's syndrome, Ehlers-Danlos syndrome,[31] and Turner's syndrome[23] supports genetic predispositions. However, the lack of association of most defects with known hereditary abnormalities, the high incidence of associated defects of other structures developing embryologically simultaneously with the atrial septum, and the lack of concordance of cardiac defects in identical twins all favor as yet undetermined environmental influences. Two known cardiac mutagens are maternal rubella infections and the ingestion of thalidomide during the first trimester of pregnancy.

With a knowledge of the embryologic development and *partitioning* of the interatrial septum, one can understand the anatomic location and pathophysiology of the various types of atrial septal defects (Fig. 1).[20] Partitioning of the interatrial septum begins around the 25th day of fetal development and is essentially complete by the 35th day. During the fourth week, bulges of mesenchymal tissue called *atrioventricular endocardial cushions* form on the dorsal and ventral walls of the atrioventricular canal. Dur-

ing the fifth week, the actively growing cushions approach each other and fuse, forming the septum of the atrioventricular canal and dividing the canal into right and left components. As this is occurring, the primitive right and left atria are being divided by the formation and fusion of two septa, the *septum primum* and the *septum secundum*. The septum primum also fuses with the endocardial cushions.

During its growth, the septum secundum forms an incomplete partition and leaves an opening (the *foramen ovale*). The remaining part of this septum primum forms the valve of the foramen ovale. Incomplete fusion of the primitive endocardial cushions produces an atrioventricular canal defect. Incomplete fusion of the septum primum with the endocardial cushions produces a secundum atrial septal defect. Incomplete growth or fusion of the septum secundum and the septum primum produces a patent foramen ovale. Finally, incomplete fusion of the sinus venosus with the caudal wall of the right atrium produces a sinus venosus defect. The anatomic locations of each of these defects in the embryologically mature heart are illustrated in Figure 2. Within the total spectrum of atrial septal defects, roughly half are secundum defects, one fourth are atrioventricular canal defects, and one fifth are ostium primum defects. A patent and hemodynamically insignificant foramen ovale is extremely common and is estimated to occur in as many as one third of all adults. A sinus venosus defect is less common. Any type of atrial septal defect may occur in combination with other cardiac defects.

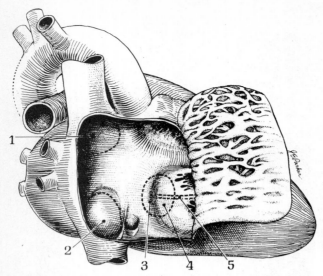

Figure 2. Schematic illustration of the usual location of interatrial septal defects. 1, Sinus venosus defect. 2, Ostium secundum defect. 3, Ostium primum defect. 4, Atrioventricular (A-V) canal defect. 5, Cleft mitral valve seen in A-V canal and ostium primum defects. (From Waldhausen, J. A., and Tyers, G. F.: Atrial septal defects, ostium primum defects, and atrioventricular canals. In Sabiston, D. C., Jr. (Ed.): Davis-Christopher Textbook of Surgery, 12th ed. Philadelphia, W. B. Saunders Company, 1981.)

OSTIUM SECUNDUM DEFECTS

Around the 30th day of fetal life, a defect appears in the ostium primum known as the *ostium secundum*. It normally closes within several days by the growth of the septum secundum and fusion of the septum secundum with the septum primum. An ostium secundum defect may vary in size from several millimeters to several centimeters. A secundum defect may also exist as multiple fenestrations or may involve most of the atrial septum. Rarely, a secundum defect may occur so low in the atrium that the right pulmonary vein empties into what becomes the inferior vena cava. One or more pulmonary veins, usually on the right side, may enter the right atrium *anomalously*.[26]

The pathophysiology of ostium secundum defects is a left-to-right shunt. In the normal heart, there is a positive pressure difference that exists between the two atria, a difference related to atrial filling, timing of atrial contraction, and ventricular compliance. In small to moderate defects, this is abolished and the magnitude of the shunt is determined largely by the compliance of the ventricles. At birth the thickness of the two ventricles is relatively equal. With reduction in pulmonary artery pressure, however, the right ventricle gradually becomes considerably thinner and is more compliant than the left ventricle. This leads to an increase in flow across the atrial septal defect into the right ventricle, resulting in an increase in pulmonary blood flow.

As pulmonary hypertension develops in later life, there is a reversal of the left-to-right shunt. Even in normal subjects there may be an instantaneous reversal of the flow across a patent foramen ovale, which can be detected by cineangiography and indicator dilution curves. This is due in part to streaming of blood from the inferior vena cava across the defect. In patients without pulmonary hypertension, where there is a fixed right-to-left shunt, the instantaneous shunting is hemodynamically insignificant. How-

ever, this phenomenon may permit venous emboli to enter the systemic circulation and emerge clinically as paradoxical emboli involving the cerebral, renal, visceral, or extremity circulation.[29] The left-to-right shunt may be quite large and may result in blood flow that is as much as three or more times the systemic flow.

Children with moderate shunts may have few if any symptoms, and the diagnosis is frequently made during a routine physical examination.[30] Examination usually reveals a healthy child with an accentuated first heart sound, a right ventricular lift, and a split-second heart sound in all phases of respiration. With the development of pulmonary hypertension, the second heart sound increases. The electrocardiogram reveals an incomplete right bundle branch block and a prominent T wave. The chest film shows right atrial and ventricular enlargement; a normal left atrium, ventricle, and aorta; and an increase in pulmonary vascular markings.

Echocardiography has proved extremely useful in evaluation of patients with suspected atrial septal defects. By measuring the size of the right ventricle and assessing motion of the interventricular septum, echocardiography can distinguish between ventricular septal defects, patent ductus arteriosus, and atrial septal defects.[9] In addition, microcavitation studies may demonstrate the direction of the shunting across the defect. Cardiac catheterization and oxygen measurements show a step-up in oxygen saturation in the right atrium. Injection of contrast into the left atrium may also demonstrate the direction of the shunt and pulmonary recirculation.

The prognosis of patients with secundum defects is based largely upon the magnitude of the shunt. The defect

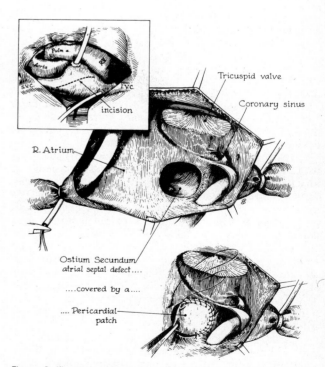

Figure 3. Illustration of closure of an ostium secundum type atrial septal defect. Small defects may be closed primarily, but larger defects require patch closure. (From Waldhausen, J. A., and Tyers, G. F.: Atrial septal defects, ostium primum defects, and atrioventricular canals. In Sabiston, D. C., Jr. (Ed.): Davis-Christopher Textbook of Surgery, 12th ed. Philadelphia, W. B. Saunders Company, 1981.)

may be extremely insidious, and survival into the seventh and eighth decades is not uncommon.[27] Most patients have a few symptoms during infancy and childhood, but in an occasional patient with a very large defect, congestive heart failure will develop, necessitating an aggressive approach.[8] The development of pulmonary hypertension is a serious prognostic finding, and surgical correction is directed toward prevention of this occurrence.

The indication for operation is the presence of a shunt resulting in pulmonary blood flow at least 1.5 times systemic flow without severe pulmonary vascular disease. The optimal time for repair is before the child starts school or between 5 and 8 years.

The operative correction of secundum defect is illustrated in Figure 3. Small defects can be closed with continuous suture of the margins of the defect. Larger defects may require closure with a prosthetic patch. A variety of plastic materials have been employed for such closure, but pericardium is preferred. Moderate hypothermia is also employed. Inspection of the interior of the atrium is carefully made for anomalous pulmonary venous drainage, which can easily be corrected by appropriate tailoring of the repair. The operative mortality of repair is quite low and is less than 2 per cent in all series.[19] Operative mortality increases in direct proportion to the degree of pulmonary hypertension. Attempts to close the defect in patients in whom pulmonary vascular resistance approaches systemic have proven either largely unsuccessful in altering the degree of hypertension or fatal.

SINUS VENOSUS DEFECTS

Sinus venosus defects develop as a result of incomplete fusion of the posterior-superior portion of the interatrial septum with the sinus venosus. This results in a high defect overlying the superior vena cava. Frequently, a portion of the venous drainage of the right upper and middle lobes is incorporated into the defect, resulting in partial anomalous pulmonary venous drainage.

Although anatomically different, the pathophysiology, clinical presentation, diagnostic features, natural history, and indications for operation are identical for sinus venosus defects and ostium secundum defects.

Repair usually requires a patch to direct the anomalous pulmonary venous drainage into the left atrium (Fig. 4). Results of surgery are excellent and comparable to the results expected with repair of ostium secundum defects.

OSTIUM PRIMUM DEFECT

Incomplete fusion of the septum primum with the endocardial cushions produces an ostium primum defect. Although there is no ventricular septal component, there is variable involvement of the mitral valve, usually resulting in a cleft leaflet. The pathophysiology of this lesion is a left-to-right shunt, which is usually large and dependent upon the size of the defect and the ventricular compliance. There is also mitral insufficiency, resulting in regurgitant jets into both atria.

Clinical manifestations include fatigue, dyspnea, failure to thrive, and congestive heart failure. Physical examination reveals both right and left ventricular lifts. A prominent pulmonic flow murmur and wide fixed splitting of the second heart sound are present. The electrocardiogram is diagnos-

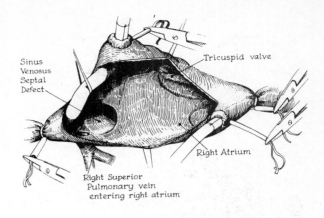

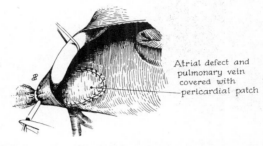

Figure 4. Schematic illustration of closure of a sinus venosus–type atrial septal defect. Note that patch closure of the defect must accommodate the right superior pulmonary vein entering the right atrium. (From Waldhausen, J. A., and Tyers, G. F.: Atrial septal defects, ostium primum defects, and atrioventricular canals. In Sabiston, D. C., Jr. (Ed.): Davis-Christopher Textbook of Surgery, 12th ed. Philadelphia, W. B. Saunders Company, 1981.)

tic with left axis deviation, prominent P waves indicating atrial enlargement, and a prolonged P-R interval. The chest film reveals cardiac enlargement and increased pulmonary vasculature.

Two-dimensional echocardiography has proved extremely useful with delineation of both atrial and ventricular septae. Valve leaflet attachments and ostium primum defects can be easily distinguished from atrioventricular canal defects. Cardiac catheterization demonstrates an oxygen step-up from the vena cava to the right atrium. The left ventricular angiogram is diagnostic, demonstrating a characteristic "goose neck" deformity of the ventricular outflow tract together with mitral regurgitation.

The natural history of uncorrected ostium primum defects is dismal, and the median age of death was approximately 3 years in one series.[2, 10] Although older patients have been reported, survival is unusual beyond the age of 40. Dysrhythmias are common and are a poor prognostic sign. They occur more frequently with increasing age.

Because of the poor prognosis of untreated ostium primum defect and the excellent results of operation, presence of the lesion is indication for surgical correction. Repair is accomplished using cardiopulmonary bypass, hypothermia, and either induced fibrillation or cold potassium cardioplegia. The technique of repair is depicted in Figure 5.

ATRIOVENTRICULAR CANAL DEFECTS

Incomplete growth and fusion of the primitive endocardial cushions result in a defect with both atrial septal

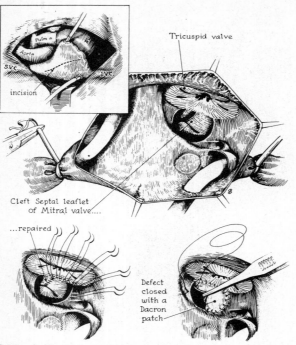

Figure 5. Illustration of steps in the closure of an ostium primum–type atrial septal defect. Note repair of cleft mitral valve followed by patch closure of the atrial septal defect. (From Waldhausen, J. A., and Tyers, G. F.: Atrial septal defects, ostium primum defects, and atrioventricular canals. In Sabiston, D. C., Jr. (Ed.): Davis-Christopher Textbook of Surgery, 12th ed. Philadelphia, W. B. Saunders Company, 1981.)

and ventricular septal components.[22] The degree of pathophysiologic change is determined by several factors: (1) size of the ventricular septal defect, (2) degree of atrioventricular valve insufficiency, (3) level of pulmonary hypertension, and (4) size of the atrial septal defect.[5] Associated defects such as pulmonic stenosis, tetralogy of Fallot, or patent ductus may also affect the hemodynamics.[4, 30]

A large left-to-right shunt is usually present, and pulmonary hypertension results from the increased pulmonary blood flow, with dissipation of kinetic energy across the pulmonary vascular bed. In addition to elevated right-sided pressures, there is also left atrial pressure elevation because of atrioventricular valve incompetence. This pressure elevation may produce cyanosis, which does not necessarily reflect high pulmonary vascular resistance and therefore does not signify inoperability.

This entity manifests itself very early in infancy and presents as failure to thrive, repeated respiratory infections, and congestive heart failure. On physical examination, the infants are thin, dyspneic, and exhibit marked precordial activity with a prominent thrill. Cyanosis may be present in about 15 per cent. The following combination of murmurs are audible: (1) split first heart sound due to pulmonary hypertension, (2) holosystolic murmur along the left sternal border from the ventricular septal defect, (3) a high-pitched murmur from mitral insufficiency at the apex, and (4) mid-diastolic flow murmur across the common atrioventricular valve.

Radiographically, four-chamber cardiac enlargement is seen with markedly increased pulmonary vasculature. Two-dimensional echocardiography has proved to be a useful adjunct in evaluating patients with suspected atrioventricular canal defects. This modality allows visualization of

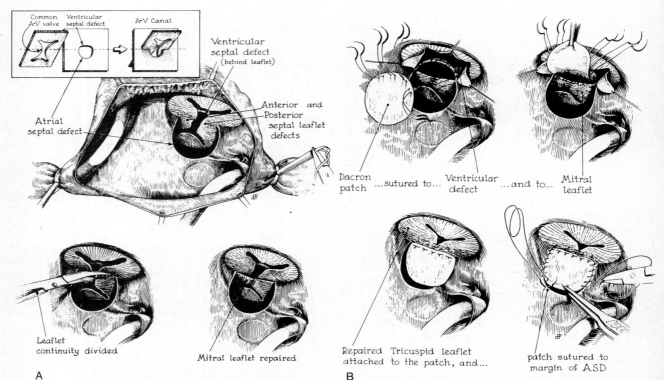

Figure 6. Illustration of closure of a complete atrioventricular canal defect. Note repair of both the cleft mitral and tricuspid valves (A), followed by patch closure of the atrioventricular defect (B). (From Waldhausen, J. A., and Tyers, G. F.: Atrial septal defects, ostium primum defects, and atrioventricular canals. In Sabiston, D. C., Jr. (Ed.): Davis-Christopher Textbook of Surgery, 12th ed. Philadelphia, W. B. Saunders Company, 1981.)

septal and valvular components.[14] Cardiac catheterization demonstrates an oxygen step-up in the right atrium and right ventricle and pulmonary to systemic blood flow ratios that are usually greater than 1. Most patients have significant pulmonary hypertension defined as greater than 75 per cent of systemic systolic pressure. Angiocardiography demonstrates a long, narrow ventricular outflow tract with a scalloped right margin. Frequently, a notch in the mitral valve is visualized.

The life span is markedly shortened, with survival beyond 2 years being rare.[15] If associated defects coexist, median survival is 4 months. Therefore, the indication for operation is the presence of the lesion and surgical results are extremely satisfactory in long-term follow-up.[2, 17, 24] The goal of surgical correction is prevention of irreversible pulmonary hypertension.[18] Pulmonary artery banding to control hypertension was formerly advocated; currently, however, total correction in early infancy is much preferred.[3, 7] Cardiopulmonary bypass is employed, with either surface or core cooling, combined with ventricular fibrillation or cold potassium cardioplegia. The operative repair is depicted in Figure 6.

The most frequent complication of this procedure is complete heart block, but the incidence of this problem has been substantially reduced in recent years.[28] Because of the complexity of the lesion and the condition of the patient, perioperative mortality is approximately 20 per cent, but long-term survival with successful surgical correction is excellent.

SELECTED REFERENCES

Keith, J. D., Rowe, R. D., and Vlad, P.: Heart Disease in Infancy and Childhood, 3rd ed. New York, Macmillan Company, 1978.
This textbook of pediatric cardiology is a definitive and authoritative text by a group of eminent authors. It provides an in-depth review of the medical and diagnostic aspects of congenital heart disease.

Spencer, F. C.: Atrial septal defect, anomalous pulmonary veins, and atrioventricular canal. *In* Sabiston, D. C., Jr., and Spencer, F. C. (Eds.): Gibbon's Surgery of the Chest, 4th ed. Philadelphia, W. B. Saunders Company, 1983.
This definitive chapter by a highly respected surgeon provides an excellent review of the surgical approach to these conditions.

Waldhausen, J. A., and Tyers, G. F.: Atrial septal defects, ostium primum defects, and atrioventricular canals. *In* Sabiston, D. C., Jr. (Ed.): Davis-Christopher Textbook of Surgery, 12th ed. Philadelphia, W. B. Saunders Company, 1981.
This chapter in a major textbook of surgery details the clinical presentation and management of patients with these conditions and is an excellent single reference source.

REFERENCES

1. Berg, J. M., Crome, L., and France, N. E.: Congenital cardiac malformations in mongolism. Br. Heart J., *22*:331, 1960.
2. Berger, T. J., Blackstone, E. H., Kirklin, J. W., Bargeron, L. M., Jr., Hazelrig, J. B., and Turner, M. E., Jr.: Survival and probability of cure without and with operation in complete atrioventricular canal. Ann. Thorac. Surg., *27*:104, 1979.
3. Berger, T. J., Kirklin, J. W., Blackstone, E. H., Pacifico, A. D., and Kouchoukos, N. T.: Primary repair of complete atrioventricular canal in patients less than 2 years old. Am. J. Cardiol., *41*:906, 1978.
4. Bharati, S., Kirklin, J. W., McAllister, H. A., Jr., and Lev, M.: The surgical anatomy of common atrioventricular orifice associated with tetralogy of Fallot, double outlet right ventricle and complete regular transposition. Circulation, *61*:1142, 1980.
5. Bharati, S., Lev, M., McAllister, H. A., Jr., and Kirklin, J. W.: Surgical anatomy of the atrioventricular valve in the intermediate type of common atrioventricular orifice. J. Thorac. Cardiovasc. Surg., *79*:884, 1980.
6. Cohn, R.: An experimental method for the closure of interauricular septal defects in dogs. Am. Heart J., *33*:453, 1947.
7. Culpepper, W., Kolff, J., Lin, C. Y., Vitullo, D., Lamberti, J., Arcilla, R. A., and Replogle, R.: Complete common atrioventricular canal in infancy—surgical repair and postoperative hemodynamics. Circulation, *58*:550, 1978.
8. Bull, C., Deanfield, J., de Leval, M., Stark, J., Taylor, J. F. N., and Macartney, J. F.: Correction of isolated secundum atrial septal defect in infancy. Arch. Dis. Child., *56*:784, 1981.
9. Diamond, M. A., Dillon, J. C., Haine, C. L., Chang, S., and Feigenbaum, H.: Echocardiographic features of atrial septal defect. Circulation, *243*:129, 1971.
10. Fontana, R. W., and Edwards, J. E.: Congenital Cardiac Disease: A Review of 357 Cases Studied Pathologically. Philadelphia, W. B. Saunders Company, 1962.
11. Gibbon, J. H., Jr.: Application of a mechanical heart and lung apparatus to cardiac surgery. Minn. Med., *37*:171, 1954.
12. Giknis, F. L.: Single atrium and the Ellis-van Creveld syndrome. J. Pediatr., *62*:558, 1963.
13. Gross, R. E., Watkins, E., Jr., Pomeranz, A. A., and Goldsmith, E. L.: A method for surgical closure of interauricular septal defects. Surg. Gynecol. Obstet., *96*:1, 1953.
14. Hagler, D. J., Tajik, A. J., Seward, J. B., Mair, D. D., and Ritter, D. G.: Real-time wide-angle sector echocardiography. Atrioventricular canal defects. Circulation, *59*:140, 1979.
15. Hynes, J. K., Tajik, A. J., Seward, J. B., Fuster, V., Ritter, D. G., Brandenburg, R. O., Puga, F. J., Danielson, G. K., and McGoon, D. C.: Partial atrioventricular canal defect in adults. Am. J. Cardiol., *47*:466, 1981.
16. Keith, J. D., Rowe, R. D., and Vlad, P.: Heart Disease in Infancy and Childhood. New York, Macmillan Company, 1978.
17. Kirklin, J. W., and Blackstone, E. H.: Management of the infant with complete atrioventricular canal. J. Thorac. Cardiovasc. Surg., *78*:32, 1979.
18. McCabe, J. C., Engle, M. A., Gay, W. A., Jr., and Ebert, P. A.: Surgical treatment of endocardial cushion defects. Am. J. Cardiol., *39*:72, 1977.
19. Meyers, R. A., Korfhagen, J. C., Covitz, W., and Kaplan, S.: Long-term follow-up study after closure of secundum atrial septal defect in children: An echocardiographic study. Am. J. Cardiol., *50*:143, 1982.
20. Moore, K. L.: The Developing Human. Clinically Oriented Embryology, 3rd ed. Philadelphia, W. B. Saunders Company, 1982.
21. Murray, G.: Closure of defects in cardiac septa. Ann. Surg., *128*:843, 1948.
22. Piccoli, G. P., Wilkinson, J. L., Macartney, F. J., Gerlis, L. M., and Anderson, R. H.: Morphology and classification of complete atrioventricular defects. Br. Heart J., *42*:633, 1979.
23. Rainier-Pope, C. R., Cunningham, R. D., Nadas, A. S., and Crigler, J. F.: Cardiovascular malformation in Turner's syndrome. Pediatrics, *33*:919, 1964.
24. Rastelli, G. C., Ongley, P. A., Kirklin, J. W., and McGoon, D. C.: Surgical repair of the complete form of persistent common atrioventricular canal. J. Thorac. Cardiovasc. Surg., *55*:299, 1968.
25. Rokitansky, C. F.: Die Defekte der Scheidewande des Herzens. Vienna, Braumuller, 1875.
26. Spencer, F. C.: Atrial septal defect, anomalous pulmonary veins, and atrioventricular canal. *In* Sabiston, D. C., Jr., and Spencer, F. C. (Eds.): Gibbon's Surgery of the Chest, 4th ed. Philadelphia, W. B. Saunders Company, 1983.
27. Sutton, M. G. St. J., Tajik, A. J., and McGoon, D. C.: Atrial septal defect in patients ages 60 years or older: Operative results and long-term postoperative follow-up. Circulation, *64*:402, 1981.
28. Thiene, G., Wenink, A. C. G., Frescura, C., Wilkinson, J. L., Gallucci, V., Ho, S. Y., Mazzucco, A., and Anderson, R. R.: Surgical anatomy and pathology of the conduction tissues in atrioventricular defects. J. Thorac. Cardiovasc. Surg., *82*:928, 1981.
29. Thompson, J., and Evans, W.: Paradoxical embolism. Q. J. Med., *23*:135, 1930.
30. Waldhausen, J. A., and Tyers, F. O.: Atrial septal defects, ostium primum defects, and atrioventricular canals. *In* Sabiston, D. C., Jr. (Ed.): Textbook of Surgery, 12th ed. Philadelphia, W. B. Saunders Company, 1981.
31. Wendet, V. E., Keech, M. K., Read, R. C., Bustue, A. R., and Bianchi, F. A.: Cardiovascular features of Marfan's syndrome: Family studies. Circulation, *32*(Suppl. 2):218, 1965.

IV

Disorders of Pulmonary Venous Return: Total Anomalous Pulmonary Venous Connection

ERLE H. AUSTIN, M.D.
DAVID C. SABISTON, JR., M.D.

Total anomalous pulmonary venous connection (TAPVC) occurs in 1 to 2 per cent of all cardiac malformations.[9] In this anomaly, the pulmonary veins do not join the left atrium but return saturated blood to the right side of the heart via connections into the right atrium or into its tributaries. The only inlet of blood into the left atrium is through a communication in the interatrial septum. Patients with the anomaly commonly present as critically ill infants requiring urgent evaluation and prompt surgical intervention.

HISTORICAL ASPECTS

Wilson was the first to give a pathologic description of TAPVC in 1798.[26] Clinical interest in this entity was renewed in 1942, when Brody reviewed 102 cases of anomalous pulmonary venous drainage, of which 37 were TAPVC.[2] The premortem diagnosis of this disorder became possible with the advent of cardiac catheterization.[8] In 1951 Muller described successful palliation of a patient with TAPVC using a closed technique of anastomosing the left pulmonary vein to the left atrial appendage.[15] The first successful corrections of TAPVC were performed by Kirklin in 1954 using the atrial well technique[4] and by Lewis in 1955 using moderate hypothermia and venous inflow occlusion.[14] Subsequent successful repairs were performed using cardiopulmonary bypass.[4, 5] Despite these early successes, the surgical mortality for TAPVC remained high throughout the 1960s and early 1970s, especially in infants. Recent improvements in preoperative evaluation and management as well as the increased use of hypothermic circulatory arrest have significantly reduced the risk of operation for this complex heart defect.

EMBRYOLOGY AND PATHOLOGIC ANATOMY

The lung develops as an outpouching of the foregut, and its venous plexus arises as part of the splanchnic venous system separate from the primitive heart. The pulmonary venous plexus initially connects with the cardinal and umbilicovitteline veins. These connections normally involute as the pulmonary venous plexus coalesces with the posterior region of the left atrium. Failure of these primitive connections to absorb produces anomalous communications between the pulmonary veins and the systemic venous system. Failure of the pulmonary venous plexus to unite with the

atrial portion of the heart results in TAPVC, and the route of pulmonary venous drainage is determined by the primordial pulmonary venous connections that persist.[16]

The classification of TAPVC is based on the anatomic level of the resultant anomalous venous connection[6]:

1. *Type I (supracardiac type).* The common pulmonary vein drains by means of an anomalous left vertical vein into the left innominate vein (Fig. 1A). This left vertical vein represents a persistent remnant of the left cardinal vein. A less common form connects directly into the right superior vena cava. The supracardiac type is the most common form of TAPVC representing 50 per cent of the cases in most series.[7]

2. *Type II (intracardiac type).* In the next most common type, comprising approximately 25 per cent of the

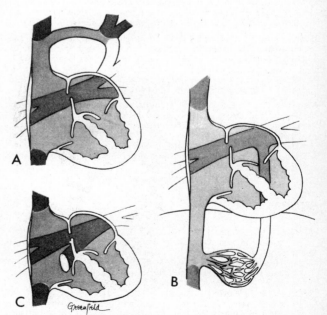

Figure 1. Types of total anomalous pulmonary venous connection (TAPVC). A, Supracardiac type with vertical vein joining innominate vein. B, Infracardiac type with drainage through diaphragm into the portal venous system. C, Intracardiac type with connection to coronary sinus. (From Norwood, W. I., and Castaneda, A. R.: Disorders of pulmonary venous return. In Sabiston, D. C., Jr. (Ed.): Textbook of Surgery: The Biological Basis of Modern Surgical Practice, 13th ed. Philadelphia, W. B. Saunders Company, 1986, p. 2207.)

cases, the anomalous pulmonary drainage occurs at the level of the heart either directly into the right atrium or, more commonly, through the coronary sinus (Fig. 1C). Such a connection arises when the left common cardinal vein atrophies cephalad to its junction with the pulmonary veins and persists proximally where it becomes the coronary sinus.

3. *Type III (infracardiac type)*. Drainage of the pulmonary veins is by means of a persistent connection with the umbilicovitteline venous system. This connection, encountered in 20 to 25 per cent of TAPVC patients, occurs as a common trunk that passes through the diaphragm and joins the portal vein at the level of the sinus venosus (Fig. 1B).

4. *Type IV (mixed type)*. The remaining patients, less than 5 per cent, demonstrate independent connections at two or more levels.

The type of interatrial communication that exists and the potential presence of anatomic pulmonary venous obstruction are important factors affecting the pathophysiology and natural history of this anomaly. A patent foramen ovale occurs in approximately 75 per cent of patients. The remaining 25 per cent exhibit a secundum type of atrial septal defect. Pulmonary venous obstruction occurs most commonly at the site where the anomalous pulmonary venous connection joins the systemic venous system. All patients with infracardiac TAPVC and as many as 50 per cent of patients with the supracardiac type have some degree of pulmonary venous obstruction.[7, 12]

PATHOPHYSIOLOGY AND NATURAL HISTORY

In TAPVC, all of the oxygenated pulmonary venous blood mixes with the desaturated systemic venous blood in the right atrium. Some of this mixed blood passes into the right ventricle and is circulated back to the lungs. The remaining portion crosses the interatrial septum to support the systemic circulation. The relative volumes that flow into the pulmonary and systemic circulations are determined by the presence and degree of pulmonary venous obstruction and the size of the interatrial communication. These factors affect the severity of the circulatory derangement and the resultant natural history.

In the absence of pulmonary venous obstruction, pulmonary blood flow is increased and a large volume of oxygenated blood returns to the right atrium. The oxygen saturation of the right atrial and thus systemic arterial blood is relatively high in these patients (usually greater than 80 per cent), and cyanosis is usually mild or unnoticed. The large left-to-right shunt produces enlargement of the right ventricle and pulmonary artery in addition to right ventricular hypertrophy. If flow into the left atrium is restricted by a small patent foramen ovale, adequate systemic circulation is achieved by an excessive load on the right side of the heart. A large atrial septal defect permits easy egress of blood into the systemic circuit and requires less work from the right ventricle.

When pulmonary venous obstruction is present, the increased hydrostatic pressure is transmitted to the pulmonary capillary bed, causing transudation of fluid into the lung parenchyma and increased pulmonary arterial pressure and resistance. Blood flow through the lungs is less, and the smaller proportion of oxygenated blood returning to the right atrium causes significant systemic arterial desaturation. The presence of a nonrestrictive atrial septal defect does not diminish the severity of the cyanosis, but may lessen the right ventricular overload. The combination of

pulmonary venous obstruction and a patent foramen ovale results in severe cyanosis, intractable congestive heart failure, and early death. These variations in pathophysiologic patterns explain the variations in clinical presentation from the rare noncyanotic adult with minimal disability to the more common cyanotic neonate who without surgical intervention dies in the first weeks of life.

Infants without pulmonary venous obstruction are usually tachypneic at birth but may not appear cyanotic. The presence of heart disease is often not considered until the child fails to thrive during the first 1 or 2 months of life and re-evaluation reveals a precordial bulge, a hyperactive heart, and hepatomegaly. Congestive heart failure becomes progressively worse, and without surgical therapy 75 per cent will die before the age of 1 year.[3, 7, 13] Those patients who survive beyond 1 year usually have an atrial septal defect, in contrast to a patent foramen ovale. If the defect is large enough, the pathophysiology and natural history may resemble that seen in isolated atrial septal defects with survival into early adulthood.

Patients with pulmonary venous obstruction present with intense cyanosis soon after birth, and tachypnea and hepatomegaly may be marked. The course is usually stormy, with death from pulmonary edema or anoxia. In the absence of surgical treatment, the median survival for this group is only 3 weeks in contrast to a median survival of 3 months for the group without pulmonary venous obstruction.[7] The high prevalence of patent foramen ovales and pulmonary venous obstruction in the overall TAPVC group necessitates surgical intervention in early infancy in the majority of patients. Prior to the availability of successful surgical correction, 90 per cent of TAPVC patients were dead by 1 year of age.[13]

DIAGNOSIS

TAPVC should be suspected in any infant with tachypnea and precordial bulging. Cyanosis may not be clinically apparent in the first weeks of life, but by the second or third month cyanosis, a cardiac murmur (usually of pulmonary flow origin), and signs of congestive heart failure are noted. Failure to thrive is the most common presentation in infants diagnosed after 3 months of life.[19] The combination of mild cyanosis, cardiomegaly with increased pulmonary vascularity, and electrocardiographic evidence of right atrial and right ventricular hypertrophy indicates the presence of TAPVC without pulmonary venous obstruction. TAPVC with pulmonary venous obstruction is clinically diagnosed soon after birth by the presence of marked cyanosis, normal heart size, and congestive failure.

The definitive diagnosis of TAPVC is accomplished by cardiac catheterization. TAPVC is the only congenital cardiac malformation in which the oxygen saturation of the right atrium is equal to that of the systemic arteries.[22] Once the presence of TAPVC is confirmed by catheterization, contrast cineangiography is employed to demonstrate the location of the anomalous connection. Recent advances in two-dimensional echocardiography indicate that this technique may soon supplant the need for catheterization in determining the presence and type of TAPVC.[20, 21]

SURGICAL MANAGEMENT

Operative correction of TAPVC requires anastomosis of the common pulmonary venous channel to the left

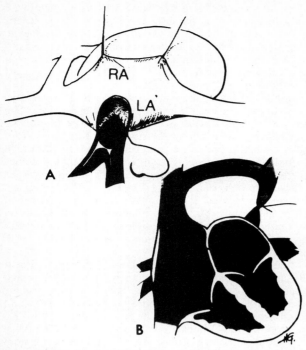

Figure 2. Repair of supracardiac type TAPVC. A, Exposure for anastomosing the common horizontal pulmonary vein to the left atrium. B, The completed repair following ligation of the anomalous vertical vein and closure of the interatrial communication. (From Norwood, W. I., and Castaneda, A. R.: Disorders of pulmonary venous return. In Sabiston, D. C., Jr. (Ed.): Textbook of Surgery: The Biological Basis of Modern Surgical Practice, 13th ed. Philadelphia, W. B. Saunders Company, 1986, p. 2209.)

atrium, obliteration of the anomalous venous connection, and closure of the interatrial communication (Fig. 2). All types of TAPVC are approached via a median sternotomy. To achieve a widely patent and accurate anastomosis in neonates and infants, most surgeons currently employ the technique of deep hypothermia and circulatory arrest.[1, 11, 18, 23, 25] With this method, the infant's body temperature is cooled to 20°C. using cardiopulmonary bypass. When this temperature is reached, bypass is discontinued and a quiet, bloodless field is achieved. The anomalous connection is ligated, the common pulmonary vein and the posterior wall of the left atrium are incised, and a wide anastomosis is created between these two structures. The interatrial communication is closed through a separate incision in the right atrium. The heart is then refilled with blood, cardiopulmonary bypass is resumed, and the infant is rewarmed to 37°C. Repair of infracardiac TAPVC is similar to that depicted in Figure 2 for the supracardiac type, except that the vertical vein is divided at the diaphragm and the proximal portion is opened longitudinally for incorporation in a patulous anastomosis to the left atrium.[17] Patients with the intracardiac type of TAPVC can be repaired via the right atrium by opening the coronary sinus into the left atrium and closing the ostium of the coronary sinus.[24] In all patients, left and right atrial catheters are placed at the time of operation to allow careful postoperative monitoring.

SURGICAL RESULTS

The earliest surgical successes with TAPVC were in patients over 1 year of age. By 1970 the operative mortality in this group was between 5 and 15 per cent.[9, 27] The mortality in infants younger than 1 year of age, however, was in excess of 50 per cent.[27] Since 1970 and the introduction of techniques of hypothermic circulatory arrest, the operative mortality in infants has decreased to approximately 25 per cent.[11, 17] Mortality as low as 9 per cent has been reported,[17] but infants with infracardiac TAPVC continue to have the highest mortality.[23]

The prognosis for patients who survive operation is good,[10, 25] and follow-up of 49 patients at the Mayo Clinic revealed that 48 were surviving from 1 to 14 years in good clinical condition.[10] When late problems arise, they are primarily related to residual stenosis at the anastomosis or pulmonary vascular obstructive disease.

SELECTED REFERENCES

Burroughs, J. T., and Edwards, J. E.: Total anomalous pulmonary venous connection. Am. Heart. J., 59:913, 1960.
    A thorough analysis of TAPVC written at the time when surgical repair first became possible.

Katz, N. M., Kirklin, J. W., and Pacifico, A. D.: Concepts and practices in surgery for total anomalous pulmonary venous connection. Ann. Thorac. Surg., 25:479, 1978.
    A comprehensive review discussing refinements in surgical techniques and determinants of outcome.

REFERENCES

1. Bailey, L. L., Takeuchi, Y., Williams, W. G., Trusler, G. A., and Mustard, W. T.: Surgical management of congenital cardiovascular anomalies with the use of profound hypothermia and circulatory arrest: Analysis of 180 consecutive cases. J. Thorac. Cardiovasc. Surg., 71:485, 1976.
2. Brody, H.: Drainage of the pulmonary veins into the right side of the heart. Arch. Pathol., 33:221, 1942.
3. Burroughs, J. T., and Edwards, J. E.: Total anomalous pulmonary venous connection. Am. Heart J., 59:913, 1960.
4. Burroughs, J. T., and Kirklin, J. W.: Complete surgical correction of total anomalous pulmonary venous connection: Report of three cases. Staff Meet. Mayo Clin., 31:182, 1956.
5. Cooley, D. A., and Ochsner, A., Jr.: Correction of total anomalous pulmonary venous connection. Surgery, 42:1014, 1957.
6. Darling, R. C., Rothney, W. B., and Craig, J. M.: Total pulmonary venous drainage into the right side of the heart. Lab. Invest., 6:44, 1957.
7. Delisle, G., Ando, M., Calder, A. L., Zuberbuhler, J. R., Rochenmacher, S., Alday, L. E., Mangini, O., Van Praagh, S., and Van Praagh, R.: Total anomalous pulmonary venous connection: Report of 93 autopsied cases with emphasis on diagnostic and surgical considerations. Am. Heart J., 91:99, 1976.
8. Friedlich, A., Bing, R. J., and Blount, S. G., Jr.: Physiological studies in congenital heart disease: IX. Circulatory dynamics in the anomalies of venous return to the heart including pulmonary arteriovenous fistula. Bull. Hopkins Hosp., 86:20, 1950.
9. Gomes, M. M. R., Feldt, R. H., McGoon, D. C., and Danielson, G. K.: Total anomalous pulmonary venous connection: Surgical considerations and results of operation. J. Thorac. Cardiovasc. Surg., 60:116, 1970.
10. Gomes, M. M. R., Feldt, R. H., McGoon, D. C., and Danielson, G. K.: Long-term results following correction of total anomalous pulmonary venous connection. J. Thorac. Cardiovasc. Surg., 61:253, 1971.
11. Katz, N. M., Kirklin, J. W., and Pacifico, A. D.: Concepts and practices in surgery for total anomalous pulmonary venous connection. Ann. Thorac. Surg., 25:479, 1978.
12. Kauffman, S. L., Ores, C. N., and Anderson, D. H.: Two cases of total anomalous pulmonary venous return of the supracardiac type with stenosis simulating infradiaphragmatic drainage. Circulation, 25:376, 1962.
13. Keith, J. D., Rowe, R. D., Vlad P., and O'Hanley, J. H.: Complete anomalous pulmonary venous drainage. Am. J. Med., 16:23, 1954.
14. Lewis, F. J., Varco, R. L., Taufic, M., and Niazi, S. A.: Direct vision repair of triatrial heart and total anomalous pulmonary venous drainage. Surg. Gynecol. Obstet., 102:713, 1956.

15. Muller, W. H., Jr.: The surgical treatment of transposition of the pulmonary veins. Ann. Surg., *134*:683, 1951.

16. Neill, C. A.: Development of the pulmonary veins: With reference to the embryology of anomalies of pulmonary venous return. Pediatrics, *18*:880, 1956.

17. Norwood, W. I., and Castaneda, A. R.: Disorders of pulmonary venous return. *In* Sabiston, D. C., Jr. (Ed.): Textbook of Surgery: The Biological Basis of Modern Surgical Practice, 13th ed. Philadelphia, W. B. Saunders Company, 1986, p. 2206.

18. Norwood, W. I., Hougen, T. J., and Castaneda, A. R.: Total anomalous pulmonary venous connection: Surgical considerations. Cardiovasc. Clin. *11*:353, 1981.

19. Rowe, R. D.: Anomalies of venous return. *In* Keith, J. D., Rowe, R. D., and Vlad, P. (Eds.): Heart Disease in Infancy and Childhood, 3rd ed. New York, Macmillan, 1978, p. 566.

20. Skovranek, J., Tuma, S., Urbancova, D., and Samanek, M.: Range-gated pulsed Doppler echocardiographic diagnosis of supracardiac total anomalous pulmonary venous drainage. Circulation, *61*:841, 1980.

21. Snider, A. R., Silverman, N. H., Turley, K., and Ebert, P. A.: Evaluation of infradiaphragmatic total anomalous pulmonary ve-

nous connection with two-dimensional echocardiography. Circulation, *66*:1129, 1982.

22. Taussig, H. B.: Congenital Malformations of the Heart. New York, The Commonwealth Fund, 1947, p. 309.

23. Turley, K., Tucker, W. Y., Ullyot, D. J., and Ebert, P. A.: Total anomalous pulmonary venous connection in infancy: Influence of age and type of lesion. Am. J. Cardiol., *45*:92, 1980.

24. Van Praagh, R., Harken, A. H., Delisle, G., Ando, M., and Gross, R. E.: Total anomalous pulmonary venous drainage to the coronary sinus: A revised procedure for its correction. J. Thorac. Cardiovasc. Surg., *64*:132, 1972.

25. Whight, C. M., Barratt-Boyes, B. G., Calder, A. L., Neutze, J. M., and Brandt, P. W. T.: Total anomalous pulmonary venous connection. Long-term results following repair in infancy. J. Thorac. Cardiovasc. Surg., *75*:52, 1978.

26. Wilson, J.: A description of a very unusual formation of the human heart. Phil. Trans. R. Soc. Lond., *88*:346, 1798.

27. Wukasch, D. C., Deutsch, M., Reul, G. J., Hallman, G. L., and Cooley, D. A.: Total anomalous pulmonary venous return. Ann. Thorac. Surg., *19*:622, 1975.

V

Ventricular Septal Defects

GARY K. LOFLAND, M.D.
DAVID C. SABISTON, JR., M.D.

The clinical signs and pathologic anatomy of ventricular septal defects were carefully described by Roger in 1879. With the development of cardiac catheterization, the precise definition of the hemodynamic alterations produced by these defects was delineated. Along with atrial septal defect, ventricular septal defect was one of the first congenital cardiac lesions to be attacked surgically, and, like atrial septal defect, ingenious attempts were made to correct ventricular septal defects prior to the development of cardiopulmonary bypass. In 1954, Lillehei and colleagues repaired ventricular septal defects using controlled cross-circulation with an adult human functioning as the oxygenator.[22] Six of the eight patients survived, with three of the survivors being in the first year of life. In 1956, DuShane and co-workers reported a series of 20 patients with large ventricular septal defects who had undergone repair using cardiopulmonary bypass.[9] With improvement in perfusion and myocardial preservation techniques, numerous investigators reported success with progressively sicker and younger infants.[1, 2]

Isolated ventricular septal defect is the most common congenital cardiac lesion, accounting for 30 to 40 per cent of all congenital lesions at birth.[13, 15] Anatomically, ventricular septal defects may occur anywhere in the interventricular septum. Excluding those occurring in association with other congenital anomalies, such as transposition of the great vessels, corrected transposition or atrioventricular canal, ventricular septal defects can be divided into four general anatomic types[17, 27] (Fig. 1):

1. *Supracristal or subarterial ventricular septal defects* are high defects and lie beneath the central portion of the right coronary cusp. From the right ventricular aspect, they are located in the outlet portion or infundibulum of the right ventricle immediately beneath the pulmonary valve.

2. *High or perimembranous ventricular septal defects* are the most common types and are usually located immediately under the aortic valve in the region of the membranous septum.

3. *Atrioventricular canal-type defects* are located beneath the septal leaflet of the tricuspid valve and are similar to those found in complete atrioventricular canal defect. They more closely resemble perimembranous defects extending into the inlet septum.[19]

4. *Muscular-type defects* may be located anywhere in the interventricular septum. They are completely surrounded by muscle, may be multiple, and may occur in association with any of the other three types of ventricular septal defects. Multiple defects behave pathophysiologically and hemodynamically as a single large defect. An important anatomic aspect to consider in closing a ventricular septal defect is the location of the bundle of His. This is especially important in perimembranous or atrioventricular canal type defects and less so in supracristal or muscular defects. Ventricular septal defects have a tendency to close *spontaneously*, and this fact must be considered when operation is being contemplated.[4, 14, 15] This explains the infrequency with which large ventricular septal defects are encountered in adults. The graphically inverse relationship between the probability of spontaneous closure of a ventricular septal defect and the age of the patient is shown in Figure 2.

In many instances of ventricular septal defects, the defect is very small and there are few, if any, symptoms. It

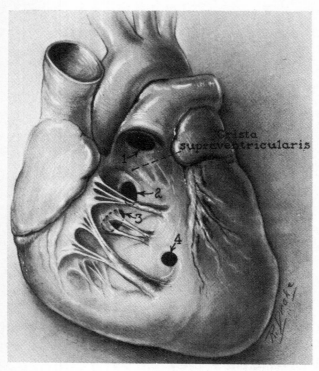

Figure 1. Common locations of ventricular septal defects. 1, Supracristal (subarterial) defect. 2, High (perimembranous) defect. 3, Atrioventricular canal type defect. 4, Muscular type defect. The perimembranous type defect is the most common type. (From Kirklin, J. W., Harshbarger, H. G., Donald, D. E., and Edwards, J. E.: J. Thorac. Surg., 33:45, 1957.)

The direction and magnitude of shunts in patients with ventricular septal defects depend upon the size of the defect and the difference in pressure between the ventricles during systole and diastole.[19] When the defect is small, it offers considerable resistance to flow and only a large pressure difference, as that occurring in middle to late systole, results in significant flow. When the defect is large, it offers little resistance to flow and relatively smaller pressure differences may result in significant flow across the defect. Other factors may influence the degree of shunting, such as compliance of the two ventricles and the presence of asynchronous contraction. The defect may also vary in size and shape during various phases of the cardiac cycle.[20, 28]

Right ventricular compliance increases early in neonatal life; this has a tendency to show increased left to right shunting. This increase results in an increase in pulmonary blood flow, which predisposes to pulmonary hypertension. Pulmonary vascular disease and pulmonary hypertension develop as a direct result of large ventricular septal defects, and the hemodynamic state of these patients is determined by the pulmonary vascular resistance. Pulmonary vascular resistance is expressed numerically in resistance units, normalized to body surface area (BSA):

$$\frac{\text{mean pulmonary artery pressure} - \text{mean left atrial pressure}}{\text{cardiac output/body surface area}}$$

Although the absolute value for pulmonary vascular resistance is important, the ratio between pulmonary and systemic vascular resistance is of equal significance. When the pulmonary-systemic ratio is between 0.45 and 0.75, pulmonary blood flow is moderately elevated relative to systemic flow. When the resistance ratio is greater than 0.75, flow across the defect is bidirectional or right to left and pulmonary blood flow is equal to or less than systemic blood flow.

Normal individuals are able to accommodate a fourfold increase in pulmonary blood flow without a significant increase in pulmonary artery pressure. The increase in pulmonary artery pressure and pulmonary vascular resistance in patients with ventricular septal defects is associated with a change in small arteries and arterioles in the lungs, which has been well documented histologically.[11, 12, 29]

In patients with moderate elevation of pulmonary vascular resistance, pulmonary vascular walls are thickened as a result of medial hypertrophy and intimal fibrosis. With further elevation in pulmonary pressures, the intimal fibrosis and proliferation are more pronounced,[19] with actual occlusion of the muscular arteries and arterioles.[11] Although infants with large defects may present with congestive heart failure early, patients with large defects generally do not present with symptoms until 6 to 12 weeks of age. It is during this period of neonatal growth that pulmonary vascular resistance is falling, allowing for an increase in left to right shunting and a sharp increase in pulmonary blood flow. It is also at this time that infants with large defects will present with tachypnea, failure to thrive, pneumonia, and severe cardiac failure.

Patients with small defects, however, may remain asymptomatic. Children with moderate-sized defects may present with growth failure, and some exercise intolerance and not the striking presentation of those patients with large defects. Thus, the clinical presentation of patients with large ventricular septal defects is a function of the degree of left to right shunting, which is directly related to the size of the defect (Table 1).

Patients with markedly elevated pulmonary vascular resistance and right to left shunting across the defect

is estimated that only 10 to 20 per cent of the patients with ventricular septal defects have defects large enough to incur serious difficulties. Infants with large ventricular septal defects have moderate elevation of pulmonary vascular resistance because of persistence of thickening of the media in the small pulmonary arteries present in the normal fetus.[19, 29] Pulmonary vascular resistance declines, however, early in neonatal life, and as resistance declines, flow generally increases and symptoms develop.

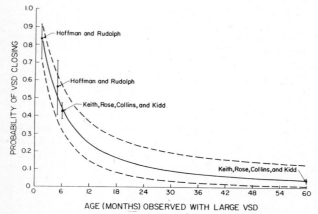

Figure 2. Probability of spontaneous closure of a large ventricular septal defect compared with age at which patient is observed, with dotted lines enclosing 70 per cent confidence limits. (From Blackstone, E. H., Kirklin, J. W., Bradley, E. L., DuShane, J. W., and Appelbaum, A.: J. Thorac. Cardiovasc. Surg., 72:661, 1976.)

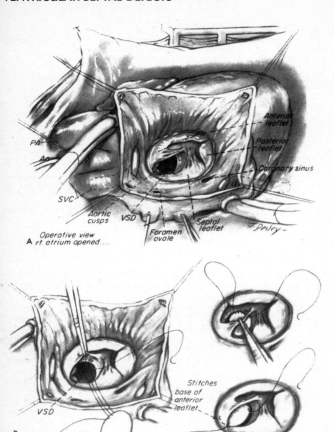

PA—
Ao—
SVC—

Anterior leaflet
Posterior leaflet
Coronary sinus
Aortic cusps
VSD
Foramen ovale
Septal leaflet
Pesley

Operative view
A rt. atrium opened....

VSD
B
Patch
Stitches base of anterior leaflet

Figure 3. Illustration of operative repair of perimembranous ventricular septal defect through a right atrial approach. (From Kirklin, J. W., Pacifico, A. D., Kirklin, J. K., and Bargeron, L. M., Jr.: Surgical treatment of ventricular septal defect. In Sabiston, D. C., Jr., and Spencer, F. C. (Eds.): Gibbon's Surgery of the Chest, 4th ed. Philadelphia, W. B. Saunders Company, 1983.)

(Eisenmenger's complex) are cyanotic, polycythemic, and severely limited in their activities.[19]

Physical examination of patients with large ventricular septal defects reveals growth failure, loss of subcutaneous fat, tachypnea, and subcostal retraction. Jugular venous distention may be present, even when an infant is held upright. Usually, a prominent precordial thrill and loud murmur are present in the third to fifth left intercostal space. There may be accentuation and splitting of the second heart sound. The liver is usually enlarged, and peripheral pulses may be weak.

Patients with small ventricular septal defects may show no precordial hyperactivity and only a systolic murmur. Patients with high pulmonary vascular resistance may have a bidirectional shunt, and a systolic murmur may be faint or absent. They may have no left ventricular enlargement or heave, but they virtually always have right ventricular prominence.

Electrocardiography has proved to be extremely useful in evaluation and follow-up of ventricular septal defects. Patients with small defects may have an entirely normal electrocardiogram (ECG). When the defect is slightly larger, the increase in left ventricular stroke volume is manifested by an increase in R wave voltage and peaked T waves in the left precordial leads. When the shunt is even larger, a pattern of mild right ventricular overload may be seen, manifested by an RSR' pattern in the V_1 lead. Further

approximation of shunt size and estimates of pulmonary vascular resistance can be made by examining the configuration of the QRS complex and by gauging axial deviation. Electrocardiography supplements the physical findings and chest film. When all three are considered, accurate approximation of shunt size and pulmonary vascular resistance can be made.

Cardiac catheterization is indicated in all patients in whom the history, physical examination, chest roentgenograms, and ECG suggest a ventricular septal defect. Catheterization is performed primarily to provide accurate determinations of pulmonary and systemic flows and resistances. It is also helpful in defining associated lesions.[21]

The decision to perform surgical correction is based upon the knowledge of the natural history of similar groups of patients with untreated defects.[5] Infants with large defects, congestive failure, growth failure, repeated infections, or evidence of increasing pulmonary vascular disease warrant surgical correction. All patients with large defects should undergo elective repair before the age of 2 years. Those in whom aortic valve insufficiency develops should also undergo expeditious closure. Patients with small- to moderate-sized defects may experience spontaneous closure, but this becomes increasingly unlikely after the age of 10 to 12 years.

Patients in whom the pulmonary to systemic resistance ratio is greater than 0.9 should not undergo closure. If this ratio is between 0.75 and 0.9, operation may be advised, but with full recognition of a possible unsatisfactory long-term result.[3, 8, 9] The presence of pulmonary hypertension is not a contraindication if the pulmonary to systemic resistance ratio is 0.75 or less.[10, 19]

Surgical repair is accomplished through a median sternotomy utilizing total cardiopulmonary bypass. Hypothermia with either induced fibrillation or cold potassium cardioplegia is usual. These defects may be repaired through either a transatrial or transventricular approach, with the atrial approach being preferred to avoid diminished right ventricular function. A ventriculotomy may be utilized if the defect is of the supracristal (subaortic) type or if there is concomitant pulmonary valvular or infundibular stenosis. Through an atrial approach, exposure of the defect is obtained by merely retracting the chordae and leaflets of the tricuspid valve.[17] If the defect cannot be clearly defined, the ventricular approach can then be used.[23] Details of closure are illustrated in Figure 3.[18] Small defects may be

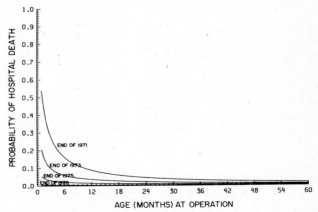

Figure 4. Probability of hospital death after repair of a single large ventral septal defect. Note the steady decline from 1971 to 1979. (From Rizzoli, G., Blackstone, E. H., Kirklin, J. W., Pacifico, A. D., and Bargeron, L. M., Jr.: J. Thorac. Cardiovasc. Surg., 80:494, 1980.)

TABLE 1. Categorization of Patients with Ventricular Septal Defects*

Size of Defect	Pulmonary Arterial Hypertension		Pulmonary Blood Flow		Pulmonary Vascular Disease		Resistance Units
	Degree	P_p/P_s	Magnitude of Increase	Q_p/Q_s	Severity	R_p/R_s	
Small	None	<0.25	Mild	<1.4	None	<0.25	<5
	None	<0.25	Moderate	1.4–1.8	None	<0.25	<5
Large	Mild	0.25–0.45	Large	>1.8	Mild	<0.25	5–7
	Moderate	0.45–0.75	Large	>1.8	Mild	<0.25	5–7
	Severe	>0.75	Large	>1.8	Mild	0.25–0.45	5–7
			Moderate	1.4–1.8	Moderate	0.45–0.75	8–10
			Small	<1.4	Severe	>0.75	>10

*From Kouchoukos, N. T., and Kirklin, J. W.: Ventricular septal defects. *In* Sabiston, D. C., Jr. (Ed.): Davis-Christopher Textbook of Surgery, 12th ed. Philadelphia, W. B. Saunders Company, 1981.

Abbreviations: Pp/Ps = Ratio between peak pressure in pulmonary and systemic arteries; Qp/Qs = ratio between pulmonary and systemic flow; Rp/Rs = ratio between pulmonary and systemic vascular resistance.

closed by direct suture, but large defects require synthetic patch closure, either with Dacron or Teflon.[6, 16] Care must be taken at all times during closure to avoid injury to the mitral and aortic valves and the conduction system, as well as the prevention of air embolism.

Complications of operation include heart block and incomplete repair. The incidence of both of these has declined steadily with improved operative techniques and should be well below 1 per cent for heart block and 10 per cent for incomplete repair. Likewise, the overall operative mortality is now extremely low (Fig. 4).[26] Results of treatment are a reflection of the preoperative condition of the patient and degree of pulmonary vascular disease.[25] Patients with little to moderate elevation of pulmonary vascular resistance have an excellent prognosis. Patients with severe pulmonary vascular resistance elevation preoperatively have a high incidence of unsatisfactory results. The results are especially favorable when the defect is repaired during the first 2 years of life.[2, 7]

SELECTED REFERENCES

Barratt-Boyes, B. G., Neutze, J. M., Clarkson, P. M., Shardey, G. C., and Brandt, P. W. T.: Repair of ventricular septal defect in the first two years of life using profound hypothermia-circulatory arrest techniques. Ann. Surg., *184*:376, 1976.
This is a classic paper describing the primary repair of ventricular septal defect in a very young group of patients. It has had a great impact worldwide on cardiac surgery.

Hoffman, J. I. E., and Rudolph, A. M.: The natural history of ventricular septal defects in infancy. Am. J. Cardiol., *16*:634, 1965.
A classic paper by two eminent authors who followed 62 infants with ventricular septal defects. This series provides a rational basis for surgical management of these infants.

Kouchouchos, N. T., and Kirklin, J. W.: Ventricular septal defects. *In* Sabiston, D. C., Jr. (Ed.): Davis-Christopher Textbook of Surgery, 12th ed. Philadelphia, W. B. Saunders Company, 1981.
This excellent chapter describes in detail the anatomy and pathophysiology of ventricular septal defects and is a superb reference.

REFERENCES

1. Barratt-Boyes, B. G., Neutze, J. M., Clarkson, P. M., Shardey, G. C., and Brandt, P. W. T.: Repair of ventricular septal defect in the first two years of life using profound hypothermia-circulatory arrest techniques. Ann. Surg., *184*:376, 1976.
2. Blackstone, E. H., Kirklin, J. W., Bradley, E. W., DuShane, J. W., and Appelbaum, A.: Optimal age and results in repair of large ventricular septal defects. J. Thorac. Cardiovasc. Surg., *72*:661, 1976.
3. Cartmill, T. B., DuShane, J. W., McGoon, D. C., and Kirklin, J. W.: Results of repair of ventricular septal defect. J. Thorac. Cardiovasc. Surg., *52*:486, 1966.
4. Collins, G., Calder, L., Rose, V., Kidd, L., and Keith, J.: Ventricular septal defect: Clinical and hemodynamic changes in the first five years of life. Am. Heart J., *84*:695, 1972.
5. Corone, P., Doyon, F., Gaudeau, S., Guerin, F., Vernant, P., Ducam, H., Rumeau-Rouquette, C., and Gaudeul, P.: Natural history of ventricular septal defect: A study involving 790 cases. Circulation, *55*:908, 1977.
6. Doty, D. B., and McGoon, D. C.: Closure of perimembranous ventricular septal defect. J. Thorac. Cardiovasc. Surg., *85*:781, 1983.
7. DuShane, J. W., and Kirklin, J. W.: Late results of the repair of ventricular septal defect on pulmonary vascular disease. *In* Kirklin, J. W. (Ed.): Advances in Cardiovascular Surgery. New York, Grune & Stratton, 1973.
8. DuShane, J. W., and Kirklin, J. W.: Selection for surgery of patients with ventricular septal defect and pulmonary hypertension. Circulation, *21*:13, 1960.
9. DuShane, J. W., Kirklin, J. W., Patrick, R. T., Donald, D. E., Terry, H. R., Jr., Burchett, H. B., and Wood, E. H.: Ventricular septal defects with pulmonary hypertension: Surgical treatment by means of a mechanical pump-oxygenator. J. A. M. A., *160*:950, 1956.
10. Friedli, B., Kidd, B. S. L., Mustard, W. T., and Keith, J. D.: Ventricular septal defect with increased pulmonary vascular resistance. Am. J. Cardiol., *33*:403, 1974.
11. Heath, D., and Edwards, J. E.: The pathology of hypertension pulmonary vascular disease: A description of six grades of structural changes in the pulmonary arteries with special references to congenital cardiac septal defects. Circulation, *18*:533, 1958.
12. Heath, D., Helmholz, H. F., Jr., Burchell, H. B., DuShane, J. W., and Edwards, J. E.: Graded pulmonary vascular changes and hemodynamic findings in cases of atrial and ventricular septal defect and patent ductus arteriosus. Circulation, *18*:1155, 1958.
13. Hoffman, J. I. E.: Natural history of congenital heart disease: Problems in its assessment with special reference to ventricular septal defect. Circulation, *37*:97, 1968.
14. Hoffman, J. I. E., and Rudolph, A. M.: The natural history of ventricular septal defects in infancy. Am. J. Cardiol., *16*:634, 1965.
15. Hoffman, J. I. E., and Rudolph, A. M.: The natural history of isolated ventricular septal defect with special reference to selection of patients for surgery. Adv. Pediatr., *17*:57, 1970.
16. Kirklin, J. K., Castaneda, A. R., Keane, J. F., Fellows, K. E., and Norwood, W. I.: Surgical management of multiple ventricular septal defects. J. Thorac. Cardiovasc. Surg., *80*:485, 1980.
17. Kirklin, J. W., Harshbarger, H. G., Donald, D. E., and Edwards J. E.: Surgical correction of ventricular septal defect: Anatomic and technical considerations. J. Thorac. Surg., *33*:45, 1957.
18. Kirklin, J. W., Pacifico, A. D., Kirklin, J. K., and Bargeron, L. M., Jr.: Surgical treatment of ventricular septal defect. *In* Sabiston, D. C., Jr., and Spencer, F. C. (Eds.): Gibbon's Surgery of the Chest, 4th ed. Philadelphia, W. B. Saunders Company, 1983.
19. Kouchoukos, N. T., and Kirklin, J. W.: Ventricular septal defects. *In* Sabiston, D. C., Jr. (Ed.): Davis-Christopher Textbook of Surgery, 12th ed. Philadelphia, W. B. Saunders Company, 1981.
20. Levin, A. R., Spach, M. S., Canent, R. V., Jr., Boineau, J. P., Clapp, M. P., Jain, V., and Barr, R. C.: Intracardiac pressure-flow dynamics in isolated ventricular septal defects. Circulation, *35*:430, 1967.
21. Lillehei, C. W., Anderson, R. C., Eliot, R. S., Wany, Y., and Ferlic,

22. Lillehei, C. W., Cohen, M., Warden, H. E., Ziegler, N. R., and Varco, R. L.: The results of direct vision closure of ventricular septal defects in eight patients by means of controlled cross circulation. Surg. Gynecol. Obstet., *101*:446, 1955.

23. Lincoln, C., Jamieson, S., Joseph, M., Shinebourne, E., and Anderson, R. H.: Transatrial repair of ventricular septal defects with reference to their anatomic classification. J. Thorac. Cardiovasc. Surg., 74:183, 1977.

24. Oh, K. S., Park, S. C., Galvis, A. G., Young, L. W., Neches, W. H., and Zuberbuhler, J. R.: Pulmonary hyperinflation in ventricular septal defect. J. Thorac. Cardiovasc. Surg., 76:706, 1978.

25. Rein, J. G., Freed, M. D., Norwood, W. I., and Castaneda, A. R.: Early and late results of closure of ventricular septal defect in infancy. Ann. Thorac. Surg., 24:19, 1977.

26. Rizzoli, G., Blackstone, E. H., Kirklin, J. W., Pacifico, A. D., and Bargeron, L. M.: Incremental risk factors in hospital mortality rate after repair of ventricular septal defect. J. Thorac. Cardiovasc. Surg., 80:494, 1980.

27. Soto, B., Becker, A. E., Moulaert, A. J., Lie, J. T., and Anderson, R. H.: Classification of ventricular septal defects. Br. Heart J., *43*:332, 1980.

28. Vincent, R. N., Lang, P., Chipman, C. W., and Castaneda, A. R.: Assessment of hemodynamic status in the intensive care unit immediately after closure of ventricular septal defect. Am. J. Cardiol., *55*:526, 1985.

29. Wagenvoort, C. A., Neufeld, H. N., DuShane, J. W., and Edwards, J. E.: The pulmonary arterial tree in ventricular septal defect. A quantitative study of anatomic features in fetuses, infants and children. Circulation, *23*:740, 1961.

VI

The Tetralogy of Fallot

DAVID C. SABISTON, JR., M.D.

One of the most frequent of the more serious congenital heart conditions accompanied by cyanosis is the tetralogy of Fallot. The anatomic variations in this malformation extend from minimal malformations to serious and life-threatening defects. Most infants with this condition develop symptoms during the first 6 weeks of life. Fortunately, in the vast majority of patients it is a correctable lesion and current results of surgical treatment are excellent.

HISTORICAL ASPECTS

This malformation was described by several authors prior to the report of Fallot in 1888, which described the clinical and pathologic aspects of this congenital lesion.[11] His name is associated with this anomaly because he was the first to describe the clinical manifestations and to emphasize that a diagnosis could be made during life.

In a landmark surgical achievement in 1944, Blalock performed the first operation for tetralogy of Fallot by creation of a subclavian-pulmonary anastomosis.[2] This procedure dramatically relieved the cyanosis and severe respiratory insufficiency of these infants and children and heralded the onset of modern cardiac surgery. With the advent of cardiopulmonary bypass, complete correction became possible and was achieved by Lillehei in 1955.[7]

ANATOMIC FEATURES

Although Fallot emphasized *four* primary anatomic defects in these hearts, including pulmonary stenosis, ventricular septal defect (VSD), dextroposition of the aorta, and hypertrophy of the right ventricle, it is now recognized that the *two most important* malformations are (1) obstruction of the right ventricular outflow tract (which is nearly always in the infundibular position) and (2) a ventricular septal defect. The overriding aorta is the result of the location of the VSD. The pulmonary valve may also be stenotic (15 to 20 per cent).

CLINICAL MANIFESTATIONS

The systemic manifestations of this disorder are dependent on the severity of individual malformations, which ranges widely. For example, when the infundibular stenosis is minimal and the predominant shunt is left to right, the patient may be nearly asymptomatic; this has been termed a *pink tetralogy*. Although these patients may not appear cyanotic, nearly all have slight oxygen desaturation in the systemic arterial blood. A severe variant of this lesion is *pulmonary atresia* in which there is no communication between the right ventricle and the pulmonary artery. Such infants exhibit symptoms quite early in life and usually require an emergency surgical procedure.

There are a number of variations and subtypes of the tetralogy of Fallot.[5] A diagrammatic illustration of the tetralogy of Fallot together with the cardiac pressures and arterial oxygen saturations is depicted in Figure 1.[12]

DIAGNOSIS

The diagnosis of tetralogy of Fallot is initially suspected from the physical examination. The primary feature is the presence of cyanosis, particularly with crying or exercise. It is interesting that in most patients cyanosis is *not* present

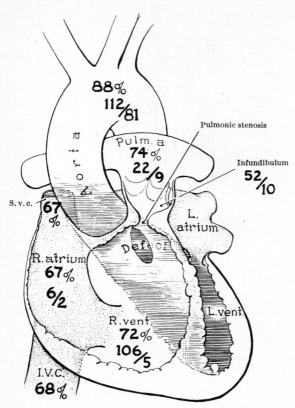

Figure 1. Diagram of results obtained at cardiac catheterization in patient with tetralogy of Fallot. This patient has a relatively high arterial oxygen saturation and represents one of the less severe anatomic types. Values of oxygen are expressed as percentage of saturation. The pressures are given in millimeters of mercury. (From Sabiston, D. C., Jr., and Blalock, A.: The tetralogy of Fallot, tricuspid atresia, transposition of the great vessels, and associated disorders. In Derra, E. (Ed.): Encyclopedia of Thoracic Surgery. Heidelberg, Springer-Verlag, 1959.)

at birth, probably because of the persistence of the patent ductus arteriosus; but as the ductus closes, cyanosis and dyspnea appear. Moreover, a characteristic feature of this malformation is that when affected children are dyspneic they squat until their dyspnea is relieved. This *squatting* position has considerable diagnostic significance for the tetralogy of Fallot. In the more severe forms such as pulmonary atresia, symptoms usually appear at birth with severe respiratory insufficiency and cyanosis.

The physical examination shows the presence of cyanosis of the lips and nail beds. The child is usually smaller than normal for the age and clubbing of the fingers and toes (hypertrophic pulmonary osteoarthropathy) may appear later. On palpation of the chest, a thrill is present anteriorly, with a harsh systolic murmur audible over the pulmonary area and along the left sternal border.

The chest film usually shows diminished vascular markings in the lungs and an absence of prominence of the pulmonary artery. Later the classic "boot-shaped" heart appears (Fig. 2), which is a characteristic feature of the chest film in tetralogy of Fallot.[10]

Examination of the blood shows an elevation in hemoglobin level and hematocrit and the latter may rise as high as 90 per cent. The erythrocyte count is elevated. The oxygen saturation in the systemic arterial blood is variable depending on the severity of the malformation, but usually ranges between 65 and 70 per cent. However, in the most

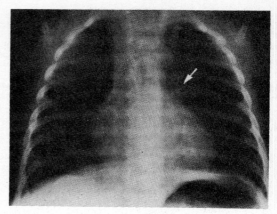

Figure 2. Chest film of infant with tetralogy of Fallot. Note diminished vascular markings in the lungs and reduced prominence of the pulmonary artery shadow. (From Sabiston, D. C., Jr.: Tetralogy of Fallot. In Sabiston, D. C., Jr., and Spencer, F. C. (Eds.): Gibbon's Surgery of the Chest, 4th ed. Philadelphia, W. B. Saunders Company, 1983.)

severe forms, the oxygen saturation in the arterial blood, particularly during exercise, can fall as low as 25 per cent. The platelet count and total fibrinogen level may be slightly diminished, occasionally associated with prolonged prothrombin coagulation times.

The electrocardiogram (ECG) is often characteristic, showing right ventricular hypertrophy on the standard leads, which is most consistently found in unipolar leads. Tall and peaked T waves are present together with reversal of the RS ratio with a normal PR interval and QRS duration. If right ventricular hypertrophy is not suggested by the ECG, a diagnosis of tetralogy should be seriously questioned. Ultrasound has also been of use in the diagnosis of tetralogy with emphasis on the type of VSD and the degree and extent of hypertrophy.[8] Angiocardiograms are usually diagnostic and demonstrate the site and size of the VSD as well as the extent of obstruction of the pulmonary outflow tract and the presence of pulmonic valvular stenosis. Arteriography may demonstrate anomalies of the coronary circulation and the most common is origin of the anterior descending coronary from the right coronary artery. In addition, a single coronary orifice arising from the aorta is seen, and this has an incidence of about 4 per cent.[3] The angiocardiogram is usually quite definitive as depicted in Figure 3.[6] Moreover, angiocardiography is quite helpful in selecting those infants who are candidates for total correction using extracorporeal circulation as distinct from those with small pulmonary arteries who are generally best treated with a systemic pulmonary anastomosis as the first procedure to enlarge the pulmonary arteries with further correction later (Fig. 4).

INDICATIONS FOR OPERATION

The vast majority of patients with tetralogy of Fallot are candidates for operative correction. Generally, a total corrective procedure can be performed and should be done preferably between the ages of 3 and 5 years and before the child enters school.[4] However, in the more severe forms, particularly with pulmonary atresia and with marked hypoplasia of the pulmonary arteries, earlier operation is usually indicated and a systemic-pulmonary anastomosis may be preferred, especially if dilatation of the small

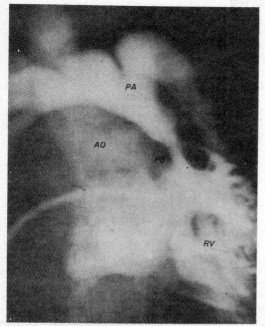

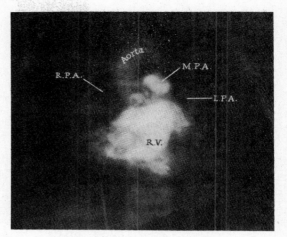

Figure 4. Angiocardiogram of infant with tetralogy of Fallot in whom the pulmonary arteries are small. An anastomotic operation was performed because of serious symptoms. The infant greatly benefited from the procedure. Evidence has been presented that enlargement of the right and left pulmonary arteries is produced by a systemic pulmonary anastomosis in these patients. (From Sabiston, D. C., Jr.: Tetralogy of Fallot. In Sabiston, D. C., Jr., and Spencer, F. C. (Eds.): Gibbon's Surgery of the Chest, 4th ed. Philadelphia, W. B. Saunders Company, 1983.)

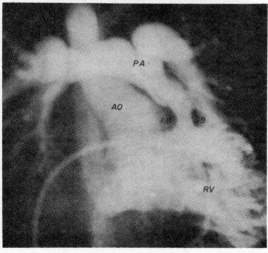

Figure 3. Obstruction of the infundibulum. A, Frame made in systole. B, Frame made in diastole. The negative shadows of the hypertrophied parietal (PB) and septal (SB) bands are particularly well demonstrated. The pulmonary valve appears domed, and at operation was bicuspid, but not stenotic. The aorta (AO) is opacified by this right ventricular injection and its diameter is three times that of the pulmonary artery. The underdevelopment of the infundibulum of the right ventricle, a basic characteristic of the tetralogy of Fallot, is apparent in this angiocardiogram. RV = Right ventricle; PA = pulmonary artery. (From Kirklin, J. W., and Karp, R. B.: The Tetralogy of Fallot from a Surgical Viewpoint. Philadelphia, W. B. Saunders Company, 1970.)

anastomosis (Blalock-Taussig) is an excellent operation (Fig. 5),[1] and has recently been revised with the substitution of a graft between the subclavian artery and the pulmonary artery, particularly on the left side where the subclavian makes an unfavorable angle when reflected downward toward the pulmonary artery. This anastomosis is usually made with a Gore-Tex graft as shown in Figure 6.

An alternative procedure used in the past is anastomosis of the descending aorta to the left pulmonary artery (Potts operation),[9] but this has largely been discontinued because the anastomosis continues to grow with development of pulmonary hypertension and congestive heart failure. Similarly, anastomosis of the right pulmonary artery to the ascending aorta (Waterston operation)[13] continues to

pulmonary arteries is desired before total correction is attempted. However, corrective procedures can be performed in young infants in selected instances.

SURGICAL PROCEDURES

Systemic-pulmonary anastomoses are palliative procedures and are usually reserved for infants who are not suitable for total correction. The subclavian-pulmonary

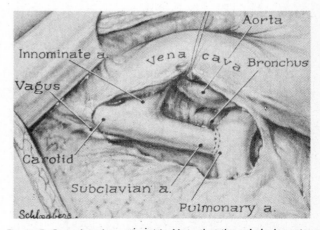

Figure 5. Completed anastomosis. Note that the subclavian artery at its origin from the innominate artery is circular. When the anastomosis is performed between the subclavian branch of the aorta and the pulmonary artery, there is usually a kink (oval shape) of the left subclavian artery at its origin; this diminishes the blood flow through the anastomosis. (From Blalock, A.: Surg. Gynecol. Obstet., 87:385, 1948.)

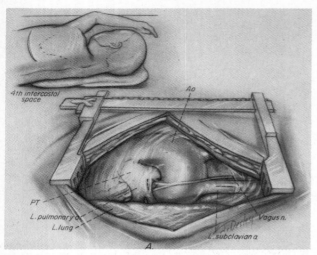

Figure 6. The classic left Gore-Tex interposition shunt (left aortic arch). A, Exposure and sites of incision (dashed lines) in pulmonary and subclavian arteries. (From Kirklin, J. W., and Barratt-Boyes, B. G.: Cardiac Surgery: Morphology, Diagnostic Criteria, Natural History, Techniques, Results, and Indications. New York, John Wiley & Sons, 1986.)

enlarge and is more difficult to reconstruct at the time of total correction.

Open correction of tetralogy of Fallot with extracorporeal circulation is the procedure of choice whenever feasible. The procedure is performed through a median sternotomy with opening of the pericardium and careful inspection of the coronary arteries to exclude anomalies.

The main pulmonary artery and its branches have been well demonstrated by angiography prior to operation and these are reassessed. The patient is attached to cardiopulmonary bypass, potassium cardioplegia is usually used with general and topical hypothermia, and intracardiac correction of the VSD generally is achieved with a plastic patch. The excess infundibular muscle creating the obstruction to the outflow tract is excised. The pertinent points are illustrated in Figure 7. An alternate approach through an atriotomy rather than a ventriculotomy is depicted in Figure 8.

RESULTS

The results following operations for tetralogy of Fallot are quite good. Although procedures used to palliate those infants with seriously malformed hearts do not yield optimal results, nevertheless following a second (corrective) operation, these children also respond favorably. The corrective procedure can be done with a minimal mortality (about 5 per cent). Serious postoperative complications include the rare occurrence of heart block during closure of the VSD, congestive heart failure due to a poor or failing right ventricle, and right ventricular hypertension if the infundibular pulmonary arterial stenosis is not sufficiently relieved. However, modern postoperative care in cardiac units with multiple continuous monitoring systems and administration of inotropic and other cardiotonic agents as well as maintenance of appropriate fluid balance and the use of diuretics allow the vast majority of these children to recover normally.

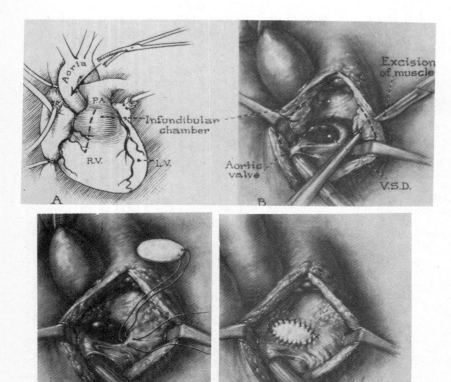

Figure 7. Steps in the total correction of the tetralogy of Fallot.

A, Note infundibular chamber and normal distribution of coronary vessels. The superior and inferior venae cavae are separately cannulated. The left atrium is decompressed by a catheter in the left atrial appendage.

B, Marked infundibular stenosis is present in the outflow tract of the right ventricle. The pulmonary valve is normal. The interventricular defect is of the standard type. Through the defect, the cusps of the aortic valve are easily visualized. The aorta is temporarily occluded to prevent reflux of blood that would obscure the operative field in the region of the ventricular septal defect.

C, The placement of the initial suture in the ventricular septal defect border. Intermittent aortic occlusion is employed.

D, Completion of placement of ventricular prosthesis.

(From Sabiston, D. C., Jr.: Tetralogy of Fallot. In Sabiston, D. C., Jr., and Spencer, F. C. (Eds.): Gibbon's Surgery of the Chest, 4th ed. Philadelphia, W. B. Saunders Company, 1983.)

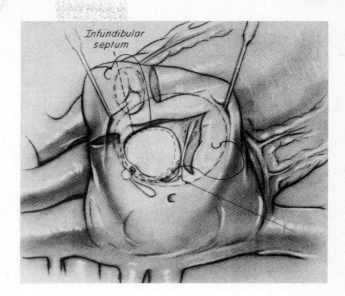

Figure 8. In this drawing, the ventricular septal defect in a patient with tetralogy of Fallot is being closed with a plastic patch using an approach through the right atrium rather than through the right ventricle. (From Kirklin, J. W., and Barratt-Boyes, G. B.: Cardiac Surgery: Morphology, Diagnostic Criteria, Natural History, Techniques, Results, and Indications. New York, John Wiley & Sons, 1986.)

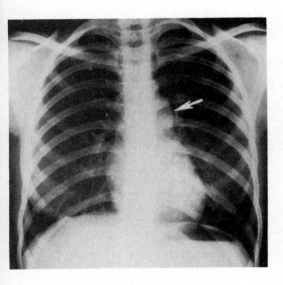

Figure 9. Chest film of patient with isolated valvular pulmonary stenosis, demonstrating typical appearance of dilatation of the pulmonary artery. (From Sabiston, D. C., Jr.: Tetralogy of Fallot. In Sabiston, D. C., Jr., and Spencer, F. C. (Eds.): Gibbon's Surgery of the Chest, 4th ed. Philadelphia, W. B. Saunders Company, 1983.)

Figure 10. Illustration of open correction of pulmonary valvular stenosis employing extracorporeal circulation. A, An incision is made in the main pulmonary artery, exposing the dome-shaped pulmonary valve. B, Radial incisions are made in each of the fused commissures, with complete opening of the valve. (From Sabiston, D. C., Jr.: Tetralogy of Fallot. In Sabiston, D. C., Jr., and Spencer, F. C. (Eds.): Gibbon's Surgery of the Chest, 4th ed. Philadelphia, W. B. Saunders Company, 1983.)

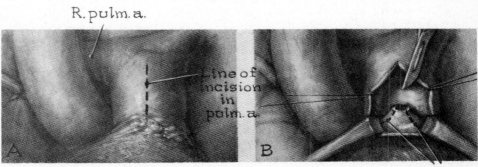

PULMONARY VALVULAR STENOSIS WITH INTACT VENTRICULAR SEPTUM

Pulmonary valvular stenosis may occur in the presence of an intact ventricular septum and without hypertrophy of the outflow tract of the right ventricle. Symptoms in these patients are generally less pronounced, although the stenosis may be quite severe and create an emergency in infancy, making operation necessary. Cyanosis may or may not be present in the early stages, but usually develops later, particularly in the presence of an atrial septal defect (trilogy of Fallot). A prominent thrill and murmur are noted over the precordium, particularly along the left sternal border. The chest film usually shows evidence of an enlarged pulmonary artery due to post-stenotic dilatation (Fig. 9). Correction is straightforward using cardiopulmonary bypass with opening of the pulmonary artery and division of the stenotic pulmonary valvar commissures (Fig. 10).

Open correction of the pulmonary valvar stenosis achieves excellent results and recurrence of the condition is rare. Rarely, isolated infundibular stenosis of the right ventricle occurs, with symptoms similar to those of valvar stenosis. Under these circumstances, the hypertrophied right ventricular tissue, which is obstructing outflow of blood from the right ventricle to the pulmonary artery, can be resected using extracorporeal circulation. Again, excellent results are obtained.

SELECTED REFERENCES

Blalock, A., and Taussig, H. B.: Surgical treatment of malformations of the heart in which there is pulmonary stenosis or pulmonary atresia. J.A.M.A., *128*:189, 1945.
In this paper, Blalock's first three operations for creation of a systemic-pulmonary artery anastomosis are reported. The first patient, a 15-month-old infant with severe cyanosis, had a history of multiple episodes of loss of consciousness. An anastomosis of the left subclavian artery to the left pulmonary artery was made, and the clinical improvement was striking. Two additional patients with successful results are also described. It is of interest that Blalock refers to earlier experimental work in which subclavian-pulmonary anastomoses were performed in the dog in an effort to produce pulmonary hypertension. Although these experiments did not succeed in producing an elevated pulmonary arterial pressure, the operation was subsequently used for an entirely different purpose. This procedure was the first of many additional cardiac surgical advances.

Chopra, P. S., Levy, J. M., Dacumos, G. C., Jr., Berkoff, H. A., Loring, L. L., and Kahn, D. R.: The Blalock-Taussig operation—the procedure of choice in the hypoxic infant with tetralogy of Fallot. Ann. Thorac. Surg., *22*:235, 1976.
These authors advocate systemic pulmonary anastomosis (Blalock) as the ideal procedure in the infant. It is their belief that a better long-term result is obtained by using a preliminary shunt followed by open correction than by performing the definitive procedure with extracorporeal circulation as the initial operation.

Kirklin, J. W., and Barratt-Bayes, B. G.: Cardiac Surgery. Morphology, Diagnostic Criteria, Natural History, Techniques, Results, and Indications. New York, John Wiley & Sons, 1986.
This is a classic monograph edited by two world authorities in the field of surgical correction of congenital heart disease. It is an exceedingly valuable reference and it is highly recommended to students as an authoritative source.

Lillehei, C. W., Cohen, M., Warden, H. E., Read, R. C., Aust, J. B., DeWall, R. A., and Varco, R.: Vision intracardiac surgical correction of the tetralogy of Fallot, pentalogy of Fallot, and pulmonary atresia defects. Ann. Surg., *142*:418, 1955.
In this paper the original descriptions for surgical correction of the tetralogy of Fallot are provided. The paper is a classic one in the

development of surgical techniques for complete correction of this malformation.

Sabiston, D. C., Jr.: Role of the Blalock-Taussig operation in the hypoxic infant with tetralogy of Fallot (editorial). Ann. Thorac. Surg., *22*:303, 1976.
In this editorial, the use of an initial systemic-to-pulmonary shunt procedure is contrasted with total correction of the tetralogy of Fallot in infancy. The reasoning advanced by the advocates of each of these methods is discussed in detail.

Sabiston, D. C., Jr., Cornell, W. P., Criley, J. M., Neill, C. A., Ross, R. S., and Bahnson, H. T.: The diagnosis and surgical correction of total obstruction of the right ventricle. J. Thorac. Cardiovasc. Surg., *48*: 577, 1964.
In this paper, the most severe of the forms of tetralogy of Fallot, those with complete obliteration of the outflow tract of the right ventricle, and its communication with the pulmonary artery, are described together with the details of operative correction and results. It is interesting that in these patients who have no communication between the right ventricle and pulmonary artery and, following correction, have total pulmonary insufficiency, the subsequent course is generally surprisingly good. In other words, pulmonary valvular insufficiency can be well tolerated.

Taussig, H. B.: Tetralogy of Fallot: Early history and late results. Neuhauser Lecture. A.J.R., *133*:423, 1979.
This is a classic and updated reference written by a distinguished pediatric cardiologist. She summarizes the early and late results of the Blalock-Taussig operation in a large series of patients. In addition, an excellent historical review of the subject is included.

Tucker, W. Y., Turley, K., Ullyot, D. J., and Ebert, P. A.: Management of symptomatic tetralogy of Fallot in the first year of life. J. Thorac. Cardiovasc. Surg., *78*:494, 1979.
A series of patients is presented in whom correction of symptomatic tetralogy of Fallot in the first year was recommended with excellent results.

REFERENCES

1. Blalock, A.: Surgical procedures employed and anatomical variations encountered in the treatment of congenital pulmonic stenosis. Surg. Gynecol. Obstet., *87*:385, 1948.
2. Blalock, A., and Taussig, H. B.: The surgical treatment of malformation of the heart in which there is pulmonary stenosis or pulmonary atresia. J.A.M.A., *128*:189, 1945.
3. Dabizzi, R. P., Caprioli, G., Aiazzi, L., Castelli, C., Baldrighi, G., Parenzan, L., and Baldrighi, V.: Distribution and anomalies of coronary arteries in tetralogy of Fallot. Circulation, *61*:95, 1980.
4. Dobell, A. R. C., Charrette, E. P., and Chughtai, M. S.: Correction of tetralogy in the young child. J. Thorac. Cardiovasc. Surg., *55*:70, 1968.
5. Kirklin, J. W., and Barratt-Boyes, B. G.: Cardiac Surgery. Morphology, Diagnostic Criteria, Natural History, Techniques, Results, and Indications. New York, John Wiley & Sons, 1986.
6. Kirklin, J. W., and Karp, R. B.: The Tetralogy of Fallot from a Surgical Viewpoint. Philadelphia, W. B. Saunders Company, 1970.
7. Lillehei, C. W., Cohen, M., Warden, H. E., Read, R. C., Aust, J. B., DeWall, R. A., and Varco, R. L.: Vision intracardiac surgical correction of the tetralogy of Fallot, pentalogy of Fallot, and pulmonary atresia defects. Ann. Surg., *142*:418, 1955.
8. Morris, D. C., Felner, J. M., Schlant, R. C., and Franch, R. H.: Echocardiographic diagnosis of tetralogy of Fallot. Am. J. Cardiol., *36*:908, 1975.
9. Potts, W. J., Smith, S., and Gibson, S.: Anastomosis of the aorta to a pulmonary artery for certain types of congenital heart disease. J.A.M.A., *132*:629, 1946.
10. Sabiston, D. C., Jr.: Tetralogy of Fallot. *In* Sabiston, D. C., Jr., and Spencer, F. C. (Eds.): Gibbon's Surgery of the Chest, 4th ed. Philadelphia, W. B. Saunders Company, 1983.
11. Sabiston, D. C., Jr.: The tetralogy of Fallot. *In* Sabiston, D. C., Jr.: Texbook of Surgery, 13th ed. Philadelphia, W. B. Saunders Company, 1986.
12. Sabiston, D. C., Jr., and Blalock, A.: The tetralogy of Fallot, tricuspid atresia, transposition of the great vessels, and associated disorders. *In* Derra, E. (Ed.): Encyclopedia of Thoracic Surgery. Heidelberg, Springer-Verlag, 1959.
13. Waterston, D. J.: Treatment of Fallot's tetralogy in children under 1 year of age. Rozhl. Chir., *41*:181, 1962.

VII

Double Outlet Right Ventricle

ROSS M. UNGERLEIDER, M.D.
DAVID C. SABISTON, JR., M.D.

Rather than being a specific entity with a predictable clinical presentation, double outlet right ventricle (DORV) defines a type of ventriculoarterial connection that may have a variety of characteristics. To meet the requirements that define this entity, the whole of one and more than 50 per cent of the other great vessel must originate from the morphologic right ventricle.[8, 12] Double outlet right ventricle accounts for approximately 1 per cent of cardiac defects in children with congenital heart disease.[11] The defect is probably caused by malalignment of the septum that ordinarily separates the right and left ventricular outflow tracts.[6] Although a number of anatomic studies[6, 8, 10, 18, 24] have addressed the specific defects that probably create and define DORV, the important concept is the fact that both great vessels originate from the right ventricle. A ventricular septal defect (to vent left ventricular blood into the circulation) is present in nearly all patients, and it is the location of this ventricular septal defect (VSD), in relationship to the great vessels that largely influences the physiology of the lesion, its clinical course, and the recommended repair. An additional factor that influences the prognosis is the association of other cardiac anomalies. Although the incidence of chromosomal and other noncardiac abnormalities is only 12.5 per cent, the association of DORV with other cardiovascular defects can be as high as 85 per cent.[17, 25] Cardiovascular defects usually include subpulmonic or subaortic stenosis, coarctation of the aorta, total anomalous pulmonary venous connection, atrioventricular valve, and coronary artery or endocardial cushion anomalies.[8, 17, 19, 20, 25]

ANATOMIC TYPES

The four most common locations of the VSD in relation to the great arteries in DORV are shown in Figure 1. A VSD located in the subaortic, doubly committed or uncommitted position (Fig. 1A, C, and D, respectively) is usually associated with the clinical features of an isolated VSD with a large left to right shunt. This is potentiated by low pulmonary artery resistance, compared with systemic resistance, and in these children there is an unfortunate tendency for the changes of pulmonary vascular obstruction to develop at an early age,[9, 16, 20] probably secondary to the high flow at high pressure that is generated across the pulmonary vascular bed. This can be termed an *Eisenmenger type* of DORV.[19]

A VSD in any of the locations just described can be associated with pulmonary stenosis that decreases the amount of left to right shunting and produces the clinical characteristics of tetralogy of Fallot (TOF) (Fallot-type of DORV).[19] Because of the similarity, some authors[12] consider this particular type of DORV to be a TOF unless as much as 90 per cent of the aorta arises from the right ventricle. However, others[6] do not regard TOF and DORV as mutually exclusive, and they define TOF as a form of DORV with a specific anatomic placement of the infundibular septum. In this respect, nomenclature of congenital heart lesions can result in overlap that leads to confusion, and this emphasizes the importance of understanding the patterns (rather than the names) of congenital lesions as they relate to physiology and to options for correction.[19, 23, 24]

One of the more fascinating types of DORV (Fig. 1B) occurs when the VSD is located in the subpulmonic position. This condition was described by Taussig and Bing in 1949[22] and thus bears their names as an eponym. In this presentation of DORV, there is streaming of systemic venous blood (unsaturated) into the aorta and of pulmonary venous blood from the left ventricle (oxygenated) into the pulmonary artery. Right ventricular pressure equals systemic pressure, and this increases flow and pressure in the pulmonary artery bed. The physiology of this presentation is identical to that of transposition of the great vessels with large VSD (TGA type of DORV),[19] and such pediatric patients are at a great risk for the early development of pulmonary vascular disease. The Taussig-Bing DORV is commonly associated with subaortic stenosis, which increases pulmonary blood flow and exacerbates the seriousness of the lesion.[25]

CLINICAL PRESENTATION AND DIAGNOSIS

In view of the wide variety of anatomic lesions that constitute the spectrum of DORV, the clinical presentation is highly variable. Those patients with subaortic VSDs and no pulmonary stenosis may present in congestive heart failure and may have a history of recurrent pulmonary infections. Pulmonary stenosis, coupled with a subaortic VSD, may lead to a more benign clinical course with varying degrees of cyanosis (depending on the severity of the pulmonary stenosis), providing a pattern that suggests the diagnosis of tetralogy of Fallot. These children may have a history of dyspnea on exertion, and parents may describe squatting behavior employed by these children after exercise. Patients with subpulmonic VSDs are usually cyanotic and are difficult to distinguish from those with TGA. The large VSD potentiates the development of pulmonary vascular changes, and children with DORV who have no protection from pulmonary stenosis usually experience a more rapidly deteriorating clinical course with the development of severe pulmonary vascular disease at an early age.[20]

The diagnosis is best made using high-quality angiograms, with separate injections of the right and left ventricle

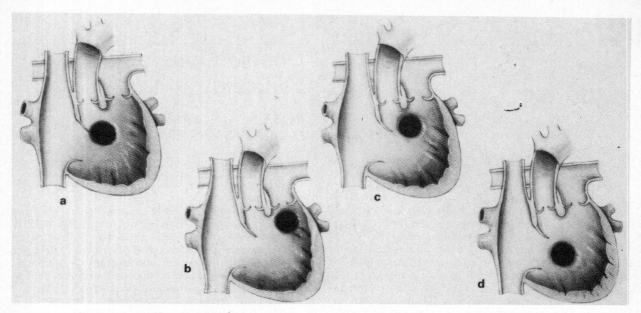

Figure 1. Anatomic types of double outlet right ventricle as determined by location of ventricular septal defect. A, Subaortic. B, Subpulmonary (Taussig-Bing). C, Doubly committed. D, Uncommitted. (From Stark, J.: Double-outlet ventricles. In Stark, J., and de Leval, M. (Eds.): Surgery for Congenital Heart Defects. New York, Grune & Stratton, 1983.)

to demonstrate the interventricular septum, the origin of both great vessels, and the location of the VSD. In addition, other cardiovascular anomalies are sought. Catheterization pressures in the various cardiac chambers as well as oxygen saturation of blood obtained from these chambers is helpful in understanding the physiologic characteristics of each presentation. The use of two-dimensional ultrasound in achieving an accurate noninvasive diagnosis of this entity has been reported.[12]

SURGICAL MANAGEMENT

In an anatomic study of 63 hearts with DORV,[24] it was determined that 23 hearts (36.5 per cent) were inoperable as a result of the extent of their anatomic aberrancy. This group of hearts had associated lesions such as straddling valves, multiple septal defects, left ventricular hypoplasia, or other combinations of complex lesions that made the possibility of successful operation unlikely. In an autopsy series of 50 hearts with DORV,[19] 26 were found to be so severely abnormal that surgical correction could not have been performed. Despite these discouraging figures, DORV is often a correctable lesion that can be associated with a good prognosis.[7, 9, 19, 20]

Repair was first successfully accomplished by Kirklin in 1956[12]; since then, advances in technology and the approach to some of the more complex presentations of DORV have allowed correction of lesions within the entire spectrum of this malformation.

Surgical repair requires cardiopulmonary bypass; in infants deep hypothermia with circulatory arrest may be desired, but the procedure can also be performed with moderate hypothermia and cardioplegia.[19] The goal of repair is to separate the systemic and pulmonary circulations, and this is accomplished by a variety of intra- and extracardiac baffles and conduits, depending on the nature of the lesion.

The most common presentation is a subaortic VSD with or without pulmonary stenosis (Fig. 2)[13]; fortunately, this is one of the easiest lesions to repair. An intracardiac baffle is constructed and sewn over the VSD and aortic outflow tract in such a way as to channel all left ventricular outflow through the VSD and into the aorta, thus restoring normal ventriculoarterial concordance. Since there is a tendency for pulmonary vascular disease to develop in these children at an early age, complete repair is recommended by age 1 to 2 years. A large VSD in a child who is not a candidate for complete repair can be managed with banding the pulmonary artery to decrease the flow and pressure to this circuit.

For those undergoing total correction, a small VSD (less than the size of the aortic anulus) requires enlargement prior to patching.[7, 20] The geometry of this patch is critical[10, 12, 19] and must be designed to prevent obstruction to flow in either the systemic or pulmonary circuit. Late left ventricular outflow obstruction from such a patch has occurred.[4, 19] Although some have suggested placing this interventricular baffle through a right atrial approach,[5] most surgeons utilize the right ventricular approach shown in Figure 2. If pulmonary stenosis cannot be relieved by valvotomy or by infundibular resection, or if it appears that the interventricular baffle will encroach too much on the right ventricular outflow tract, the right ventriculotomy may be closed with a transanular patch or with a valved conduit that will direct blood from the right ventricle to the pulmonary artery distal to the site of stenosis. A valved conduit rather than a transanular patch is probably more useful in patients with some element of pulmonary hypertension.[20] An evaluation of preoperative angiograms permits an ingenious method of predicting the need for a valved conduit.[1] In these patients, it may be preferable to wait until the age of 3 to 5 years to allow for more growth before placing a conduit. This enables selection of a larger conduit and provides a larger chest cavity in which it can be positioned. For this group of children, who usually have severe pulmonary stenosis, an initial systemic to pulmonary artery

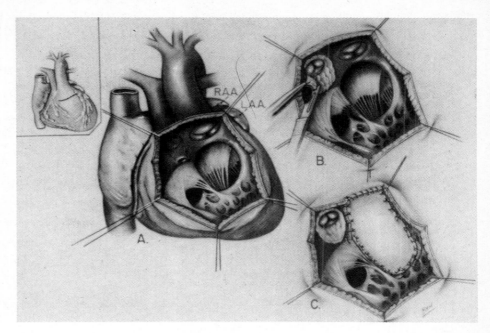

Figure 2. Double outlet right ventricle with large subaortic ventricular septal defect (VSD) and subpulmonic stenosis.

A, *Exposure via right ventriculotomy (inset). Mitral valve can be seen through VSD.*

B, *Resection of subvalvular pulmonary stenosis.*

C, *Patch over VSD directing left ventricular blood into aorta. The right ventriculotomy can be closed primarily if the pulmonary stenosis is relieved. Other options for repairing the pulmonary outflow tract include a transanular patch or a valved conduit from the ventricle to the distal pulmonary artery depending on specific defects encountered (see text).*

(A–C from Pacifico, A. D., Kirklin, J. W., and Bargeron, L. M.: Complex congenital malformations: Surgical treatment of double outlet right ventricle and double outlet left ventricle. In Kirklin, J. W. (Ed.): Advances in Cardiovascular Surgery. New York, Grune & Stratton, 1973.)

shunt will provide for growth of the pulmonary arteries and prepare the patient for a future operation to correct the DORV and place the RV to PA conduit.

Patients with DORV and a subpulmonary VSD (Taussig-Bing anomaly) often require a somewhat different approach. The anatomy of the lesion is usually such that the pulmonary artery is posterior to the aorta, and it is impossible to place an intracardiac baffle from the VSD to the aorta that excludes the pulmonary artery. A number of alternative options are available, one being conversion of this lesion (which resembles TGA) into a true transposition by closing the VSD with a patch that places the pulmonary artery on the left ventricular side with the aorta remaining on the right ventricular side. The lesion can then be repaired with any of the techniques utilized to repair a simple transposition. These include repair at the atrial level (Mustard or Senning)[9, 12, 19] or at the ventricular level (arterial switch with or without coronary artery translocation).[3, 9, 14, 16] If pulmonary artery stenosis is present, none of these repairs may be desirable. In this situation, there are two other options. One is to baffle the left ventricular flow through the VSD into the aorta, and to close the proximal pulmonary artery. A conduit can then be utilized to direct right ventricular blood to the distal pulmonary artery (the Rastelli repair for transposition with subpulmonic stenosis).[19] The second option is to perform a modified Fontan procedure by closing the tricuspid anulus and proximal pulmonary artery. The right atrium is then connected to the distal pulmonary artery. This may be useful in patients with straddling atrioventricular valves or with tricuspid stenosis and DORV. As in patients with subaortic VSDs, patients in this group who may require placement of a conduit should be managed by banding of the pulmonary artery and/or systemic to pulmonary artery shunts until they are old enough and big enough to enable selection of a more appropriate conduit size. It has been observed that

infants with DORV and a subpulmonary VSD who require palliative surgery in the first months of life require a combination of banding and shunting, since banding alone will not relieve the severe hypoxia.[12]

Intraoperative mapping of the conduction system can aid in preventing heart block.[21] The greatest immediate postoperative problems include heart failure, arrhythmias, and bleeding.[7] Hemolysis from the baffle has been reported and usually disappears within 6 weeks after the surface of the baffle endothelializes.[15] Operative mortality ranges from 35 to 45 per cent[9, 19, 20] and is related to the type of lesion and the presence of compounding variables such as pulmonary stenosis.[9] For those children surviving repair, long-term follow-up shows an 86 per cent survivorship (over 7 years) for uncomplicated DORV, but only a 38 per cent (over 6 years) survivorship for those with the Taussig-Bing anomaly.[20] Pulmonary vascular disease has a major role in late death.[9, 20]

Finally, it should be emphasized that variations of this anomaly exist, such as *double outlet left ventricle*[2] and DORV with atrioventricular discordance (ventricular inversion).[21] The physiologic aspects of these anomalies parallel those of DORV and methods of repair employ many of the same concepts.

SELECTED REFERENCES

McGoon, D. C.: Origin of both great vessels from the right ventricle. Surg. Clin. North Am., *41*:1113, 1961.
    A still timely description of double outlet right ventricle and its treatment by an individual who has had an undeniable effect on the practice of congenital heart surgery as it exists today.

Pacifico, A. D.: Double outlet right ventricle. *In* Sabiston, D. C., Jr. (Ed.): Davis-Christopher Textbook of Surgery, 12th ed. Philadelphia, W. B. Saunders Company, 1981.
    A well-written and comprehensive overview by an experienced and knowledgeable author.

REFERENCES

1. Blackstone, E. H., Kirklin, J. W., Bertranou, E. G., Labrosse, C. J., Soto, B., and Bargeron, L. M., Jr.: Preoperative prediction from cineangiograms of postrepair right ventricular pressure in tetralogy of Fallot. J. Thorac. Cardiovasc. Surg., *78*:542, 1979.
2. Brandt, P. W. T., Calder, A. L., Barratt-Boyes, B. G., and Neutze, J. M.: Double outlet left ventricle: Morphology, cineangiocardiographic diagnosis and surgical treatment. Am. J. Cardiol., *38*:897, 1976.
3. Ceithaml, E. L., Puga, F. J., Danielson, G. K., McGoon, D. C., and Ritter, D. S.: Results of the Damus-Stansel-Kaye procedure for transposition of the great arteries and for double-outlet right ventricle with subpulmonary ventricular septal defect. Ann. Thorac. Surg., *38*:433, 1984.
4. Chaitman, B. R., Grondin, C. M., Theroux, P., and Bourassa, M. G.: Late development of left ventricular outflow tract obstruction after repair of double-outlet right ventricle. J. Thorac. Cardiovasc. Surg., *72*:265, 1976.
5. Cherian, K. M., John, T. A., and Abraham, K. A.: Transatrial correction of origin of both great vessels from right ventricle with pulmonary hypertension. J. Thorac. Cardiovasc. Surg., *84*:783, 1982.
6. Edwards, W. D.: Double-outlet right ventricle and tetralogy of Fallot. Two distinct but not mutually exclusive entities. J. Thorac. Cardiovasc. Surg., *82*:418, 1981.
7. Judson, J. P., Danielson, G. K., Puga, F. J., Mair, D. D., and McGoon, D. C.: Double-outlet right ventricle: Surgical results 1970–1980. J. Thorac. Cardiovasc. Surg., *85*:32, 1983.
8. Lev, M., Bharati, S., Meng, C. C. L., Liberthson, R. R., Paul, M. H., and Idriss, F.: A concept of double-outlet right ventricle. J. Thorac. Cardiovasc. Surg., *64*:271, 1972.
9. Mazzucco, A., Faggian, G., Stellin, G., Bortolotti, U., Livi, U., Rizzoli, G., and Gallucci, V.: Surgical management of double-outlet right ventricle. J. Cardiovasc. Surg., *90*:29, 1985.
10. McGoon, D. C.: Origin of both great vessels from the right ventricle. Surg. Clin. North Am., *41*:1113, 1961.
11. Mitchell, S. C., Korones, S. B., and Berendes, H. W.: Congenital heart disease in 56,109 births: Incidence and natural history. Circulation, *43*:323, 1971.
12. Pacifico, A. D.: Double outlet right ventricle. *In* Sabiston, D. C., Jr. (Ed.): Davis-Christopher Textbook of Surgery, 12th ed. Philadelphia, W. B. Saunders Company, 1981.
13. Pacifico, A. D., Kirklin, J. W., and Bargeron, L. M.: Complex congenital malformations: Surgical treatment of double outlet right ventricle and double outlet left ventricle. *In* Kirklin, J. W. (Ed.): Advances in Cardiovascular Surgery. New York, Grune & Stratton, 1973.
14. Quaegebeur, J. M.: The optimal repair for the Taussig-Bing heart. J. Thorac. Cardiovasc. Surg., *85*:276, 1983.
15. Singh, A., Letsky, E. A., and Stark, J.: Hemolysis following correction of double-outlet right ventricle. J. Thorac. Cardiovasc. Surg., *71*:226, 1976.
16. Smith, E. E. J., Pucci, J. J., Walesby, R. K., Oakley, C. M., and Sapsford, R. N.: A new technique for correction of the Taussig-Bing anomaly. J. Thorac. Cardiovasc. Surg., *83*:901, 1982.
17. Sondheimer, H. M., Freedom, R. M., and Olley, P. M.: Double outlet right ventricle: Clinical spectrum and prognosis. Am. J. Cardiol., *39*:709, 1977.
18. Sridaromont, S., Ritter, D. G., Feldt, R. H., Davis, G. D., and Edwards, J. E.: Double-outlet right ventricle. Anatomic and angiocardiographic correlations. Mayo Clin. Proc., *53*:555, 1978.
19. Stark, J., and de Leval, M. (Eds.): Surgery for Congenital Heart Defects. London, Grune & Stratton, 1983.
20. Stewart, R. W., Kirklin, J. W., Pacifico, A. D., Blackstone, E. H., and Bargeron, L. M., Jr.: Repair of double-outlet right ventricle: An analysis of 62 cases. J. Thorac. Cardiovasc. Surg., *78*:502, 1979.
21. Tabry, I. F., McGoon, D. C., Danielson, G. K., Wallace, R. B., Davis, Z., and Maloney, J. D.: Surgical management of double-outlet right ventricle associated with atrioventricular discordance. J. Thorac. Cardiovasc. Surg., *76*:336, 1978.
22. Taussig, H. B., and Bing, J. F.: Complete transposition of the aorta and a levoposition of the pulmonary artery: Clinical, physiological, and pathological findings. Am. Heart J., *37*:551, 1949.
23. Tynan, M. J., Becker, A. E., Macartney, F. J., Jimenez, M. Q., Shinebourne, E. A, and Anderson, R. H.: Nomenclature and classification of congenital heart disease. Br. Heart J., *41*:544, 1979.
24. Wilcox, B. R., Ho, S. Y., Macartney, F. J., Becker, A. E., Gerlis, L. M., and Anderson, R. H.: Surgical anatomy of double-outlet right ventricle with situs solitus and atrioventricular concordance. J. Thorac. Cardiovasc. Surg., *82*:405, 1981.
25. Zamora, R., Moller, J. H., and Edwards, J. E.: Double-outlet right ventricle. Anatomic types and associated anomalies. Chest, *68*:672, 1975.

VIII

Tricuspid Atresia

JAMES D. SINK, M.D.
DAVID C. SABISTON, JR., M.D.

Tricuspid atresia is a congenital malformation characterized by the absence of a direct communication between the right atrium and right ventricle, varying degrees of underdevelopment of the right ventricle, and an atrial septal defect. The lesion is classified according to its associated anomalies such as transposition of the great vessels, obstruction of pulmonary blood flow, and the size of the ventricular septal defect. Tricuspid atresia is uncommon, constituting 1 to 5 per cent of all congenital heart defects, and is the third most common anomaly producing cyanosis following tetralogy of Fallot and transposition of the great arteries (TGA).

With 70 per cent of patients with tricuspid atresia experiencing decreased pulmonary blood flow, the most common clinical presentation is cyanosis.[8] While squatting occurs rarely, clubbing is present in most patients over 2 years of age. Dyspnea may be quite striking and is directly related to the degree of hypoxia. In those patients without pulmonary outflow tract obstruction, increased pulmonary blood flow is usually present, and these patients present most commonly with evidence of congestive heart failure. While the appearance of the chest film is extremely variable,[11] left axis deviation on the electrocardiogram (ECG) is found in the great majority of patients.[3] Left axis deviation seen in a cyanotic infant should incite a strong suspicion of tricuspid atresia. The diagnosis is made by cardiac angiography. Contrast media injected into the right atrium passes into in the left atrium, the left ventricle, and finally into the great vessels.

Both palliative and corrective procedures are available.

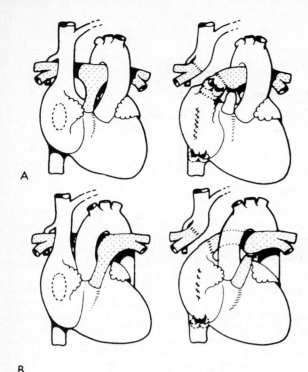

A

B

Figure 1. Fontan's operation. A, The operation consists of the construction of an end-to-side superior vena cava to right pulmonary artery anastomosis and an anastomosis between the right atrial appendage and the proximal stump of the right pulmonary artery, with interposition of a segment of aortic allograft with intact valve. On cardiopulmonary bypass, the right atrium is opened, the interatrial communication closed, and a pulmonary valve allograft inserted into the inferior vena cava. The main pulmonary artery is ligated and bypass is discontinued. The last step of the procedure is division of the superior vena cava below the pulmonary anastomosis and suture closure of the two ends. B, In one patient, the same procedure was performed, but no allograft was used at the atrium to pulmonary artery anastomosis. (From Fontan, F., and Baudet, E.: Thorax, 26:240, 1971.)

The most common indication for palliation is cyanosis, which is seen in those patients with decreased pulmonary blood flow. Increased pulmonary blood flow can be achieved with a subclavian artery to pulmonary artery shunt (Blalock-Taussig[2]), with an aorta to pulmonary artery shunt (Potts,[9] Waterston[10]), or a superior vena cava to pulmonary artery shunt (Glenn[7]). Each type has distinctive advantages and disadvantages related to technical and physiologic considerations. A Blalock-Taussig type of subclavian artery to pulmonary artery shunt is probably the procedure of choice in infants requiring a shunt in the first few weeks of life.

Surgical correction of tricuspid atresia was made possible by the realization that a ventricle is not necessary to maintain adequate pulmonary circulation, and Fontan and Baudet[5] reported the first successful corrective procedure

for tricuspid atresia in 1971. The atrial septal defect was closed and the systemic venous return was diverted to the lungs through a valve containing conduit connecting the right atrium to the pulmonary artery. The superior vena cava was anastomosed to the right pulmonary artery, and a valve was placed at the junction of the right atrium and inferior vena cava to prevent reflux of blood into the inferior vena cava with atrial systole (Fig. 1).

Modifications of the original Fontan procedure have continued, and in recent years techniques have become popular that avoid all prosthetic material and have no valves in the right side of the circulation.[4] Others have suggested that the subpulmonary ventricular chamber, when adequate, should be utilized.[1]

Results of corrective procedures in patients meeting Fontan's original criteria have been encouraging. Clinically, most patients do well despite higher than normal right heart filling pressures and a relatively fixed stroke volume. Good results have also been demonstrated in patients who do not meet Fontan's criteria, but there is an increased operative risk.[6]

SELECTED REFERENCES

Fontan, F., Deville C., Quaegebeur, J., Ottenkamp, J., Sourdille, N., Choussat, A., and Brom, G. A.: Repair of tricuspid atresia in 100 patients. J. Thorac. Cardiovasc. Surg., *85*:647, 1983.

This report concerns 100 consecutive patients undergoing surgical repair of tricuspid atresia since 1968. The overall hospital mortality was 12 per cent, with a late mortality of 6 per cent. No hospital deaths in the last 26 patients were reported. The functional status and postoperative catheterization data are discussed.

REFERENCES

1. Bjork, V. O., Olin, C. L., Bjarke, B. B., and Thoren, C. A.: Right atrial—right ventricular anastomosis for correction of tricuspid atresia. J. Thorac. Cardiovasc. Surg., 77:452, 1979.
2. Blalock, A., and Taussig, H. B.: The surgical treatment of malformations of the heart in which there is pulmonary stenosis or pulmonary atresia. J.A.M.A., *128*:189, 1945.
3. Camboa, R., Gersony, W. M., and Nadas, A. S.: The electrocardiogram in tricuspid and pulmonary atresia with intact ventricular septum. Circulation, *34*:24, 1966.
4. Doty, D. B., Marvin, W. J., Jr., and Lauer, R. M.: Modified Fontan procedure: Methods to achieve direct anastomosis of right atrium to pulmonary artery. J. Thorac. Cardiovasc. Surg., *81*:470, 1981.
5. Fontan, F., and Baudet, E.: Surgical repair of tricuspid atresia. Thorax, *26*:240, 1971.
6. Gale, A. W., Danielson, G. K., McGoon, D. C., Wallace, R. B., and Mair, D. D.: Fontan procedure for tricuspid atresia. Circulation, *62*:91, 1980.
7. Glenn, W. W. L.: Circulatory bypass of the right side of the heart: IV. Shunt between superior vena cava and distal right pulmonary artery—report of a clinical application. N. Engl. J. Med., *259*:117, 1958.
8. Keith, J. D., Rowe, R. D., and Vlad, P.: Heart Disease in Infancy and Childhood, 3rd ed. New York, Macmillan Company, 1979.
9. Potts, W. J., Smith, S., and Gibson, S.: Anastomosis of the aorta to a pulmonary artery. J.A.M.A., *132*:627, 1946.
10. Waterston, D. J.: The treatment of Fallot's tetralogy in children under one year of age. Rozhl. Chir., *41*:181, 1962 (in Czech).
11. Wittenborg, M. H., Neuhauser, E. B. D., and Sprunt, W. H.: Roentgenographic findings in congenital tricuspid atresia with hypoplasia of the right ventricle. Am. J. Roentgenol., *66*:712, 1951.

IX

Truncus Arteriosus

JAMES D. SINK, M.D.
DAVID C. SABISTON, JR., M.D.

HISTORICAL ASPECTS

Persistent truncus arteriosus is a congenital cardiac deformity characterized by the presence of a single arterial trunk that arises from the base of both ventricles by way of a semilunar valve, by a high ventricular septal defect, and by pulmonary arteries originating from the truncus. The truncus provides the orifices of the coronary and pulmonary arteries and continues as the ascending aorta. This anomaly is uncommon, constituting between 1 and 4 per cent of congenital cardiac defects in autopsy series. Taruffi[12] first described the pathologic anatomy of persistent truncus arteriosus in 1875. In 1949, Collett and Edwards[3] proposed a classification, which is the basis for surgical classification today. McGoon and co-workers[10] reported the first successful repair of truncus arteriosus in 1968. With minor modifications, this is the technique currently used for definitive repair of this malformation.

ANATOMY AND CLASSIFICATION

The classification of Collett and Edwards is based on the origin of the pulmonary arteries (Fig. 1). In Type I, the pulmonary arteries arise from a common pulmonary trunk that originates from the truncus. In Type II, the right and left truncus arteries arise closely together from the dorsal wall of the truncus arteriosus. In Type III, the right and left pulmonary arteries arise separately from the lateral aspect of the truncus, and in Type IV, the proximal pulmonary arteries are absent and pulmonary blood flow originates from the bronchial arteries. In the series of Collett and Edwards, Types I and II make up 76 per cent

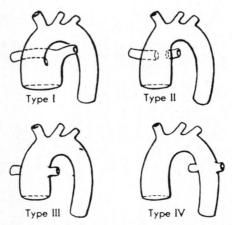

Figure 1. Anatomic types of truncus arteriosus. Collett and Edwards' classification. (From Keith, J. D., Rowe, R. D., and Vlad, P.: Heart Disease in Infancy and Childhood. New York, Macmillan Company, 1958, p. 521. By permission.)

of the cases and Type III, 13 per cent. Type IV should more appropriately be considered *pulmonary atresia* with a ventricular septal defect.

Although the truncal valve usually has three cusps, it may have from two to six cusps. In one series, truncal valve incompetence was severe in 6 per cent, moderate in 31 per cent, and absent or minimal in 63 per cent.[4] Congenital absence of one of the pulmonary arteries has been reported, as have associated patent ductus arteriosus, persistent left superior vena cava, right-sided aortic arch, and atrial septal defect. As in any condition in which there is increased pulmonary arterial blood flow and pressure, the pathologic changes associated with pulmonary vascular obstructive disease may be present. Some patients may survive to middle age, but most die within the first year of life. In autopsy series, the median age of death has been reported to be between a few weeks to 6 months, with most patients dying in infancy from congestive heart failure.[1, 6, 13.]

DIAGNOSIS

There may be little evidence of cardiac disease present during the first few weeks of life because of the normally increased pulmonary vascular resistance present during this time. As the pulmonary vascular resistance decreases and pulmonary blood flow increases, symptoms of congestive heart failure, including tachypnea, tachycardia, excessive sweating, and poor feeding, may occur. Early cyanosis is not usually apparent unless stenosis at the origin of one or both pulmonary arteries is present. There is, however, some arterial desaturation present because mixing of the systemic and pulmonary venous blood occurs in the common truncus. Patients who survive infancy usually become progressively cyanotic and pulmonary blood flow decreases concomitant with increasing pulmonary vascular resistance. In infants with severe truncal valvar incompetence, symptoms of congestive heart failure may appear during the early neonatal period. The physical findings in patients with truncus arteriosus usually include a systolic thrill along the left sternal border. The increased pulmonary blood flow may result in a third heart sound as well as an apical middiastolic murmur. A decrescendo diastolic murmur indicates the presence of truncal valve incompetence. The electrocardiogram (ECG), although not distinctive, usually shows biventricular hypertrophy. The chest film often shows biventricular enlargement and increased pulmonary vascular markings. A right-sided aortic arch in the absence of cyanosis is suggestive of the diagnosis of truncus arteriosus.

While two-dimensional echocardiography is useful in identifying the anatomic features of truncus arteriosus,[7] right and left heart catheterization and angiography are necessary to provide precise anatomic and hemodynamic data. Angiographic studies define the origins, sizes, and distribution of the pulmonary arteries. Both pulmonary arteries should be catheterized to obtain the pressure and oxygen content for calculation of pulmonary vascular resistance. The competency of the truncal valve should be assessed by a truncal root injection.

INDICATIONS FOR OPERATION

Infants with intractable congestive heart failure must be operated upon regardless of age. In those infants who are well maintained with medical therapy, elective corrective operation should be performed at about 6 months of age because pulmonary vascular obstructive disease may develop prior to 1 year. Patients with a pulmonary vascular resistance greater than 8 units/M[2] have a better prognosis without operation.[9] For those patients with a single pulmonary artery, however, operability can be determined by the calculated resistance divided by two.[8]

TREATMENT

Medical therapy is limited to supportive treatment for congestive heart failure and prophylaxis against infective endocarditis. Operative intervention is necessary if the unfavorable natural history is to be improved. Pulmonary artery banding to reduce pulmonary blood flow, control congestive heart failure, and limit the progression of pulmonary vascular obstructive disease in patients with large left to right shunts was first proposed by Muller and Dammann in 1952.[11] This procedure has been applied in patients with truncus arteriosus, and although the mortality has been high, successful palliation has been achieved in some patients.[2]

The physiologic correction of truncus arteriosus was described by McGoon and associates[10] and Weldon and

Cameron in 1968.[14] The operation is performed through a median sternotomy utilizing cardiopulmonary bypass and moderate hypothermia (Fig. 2). The aorta is cross-clamped, and the pulmonary arteries are separated from the truncus. In Types I and II, the arteries are separated as a single segment. Following excision of the pulmonary arteries, the resulting truncal defect is closed. An incision is then made in the right ventricle avoiding injury to the coronary arteries. The aortic cross-clamp is temporarily released and the competency of the truncal valve is assessed. If truncal valve incompetency is severe, the operation may need to include replacement of the valve. A patch is used to close the ventricular septal defect, and a valved conduit is then used to establish continuity between the right ventricle and pulmonary arteries. This conduit should be as large as possible in order to avoid a gradient across the conduit and to delay development of a gradient as the patient grows.

RESULTS

In a series of 167 patients with Types I and II truncus arteriosus undergoing repair between 1965 and 1982, there was a 28.7 per cent overall hospital mortality rate with a 70 per cent operative mortality for patients under the age of 2 years.[4] Late follow-up of hospital survivors revealed 5- and 10-year survival rates of 84.4 per cent and 68.8 per cent, respectively. Among the patients surviving at the end of the follow-up period, 66 per cent were New York Heart Association (NYHA) Class I, 31 per cent in Class II, and 3 per cent in Class III.

In another recent series of 100 consecutive patients operated upon under 6 months of age, the hospital mortality rate was 11 per cent.[5] There were three late deaths, one from bacterial endocarditis and two from causes unrelated to the cardiac condition. None of the survivors has shown

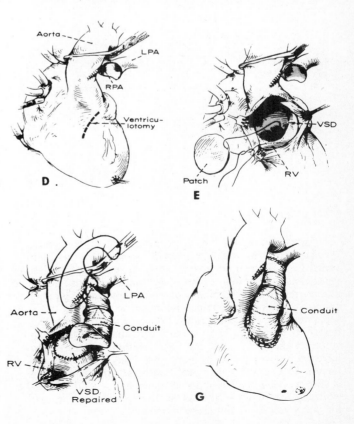

Figure 2. Surgical repair.
A, Cardiopulmonary bypass, left ventricle vented at apex, aorta cross-clamped. B, Origin of pulmonary arteries excised from truncus. C, Closure of defect in truncus. (From Wallace, R. B., et al.: J. Thorac. Cardiovasc. Surg., 57:95, 1966. By permission of C. V. Mosby Company.)
D, Incision made high in right ventricle. E, Ventricular septal defect closed with Teflon patch. F, Dacron graft with porcine valve sutured to pulmonary arteries. G, Proximal end of graft anastomosed to right ventricle. (LPA, left pulmonary artery; RPA, right pulmonary artery; VSD, ventricular septal defect; RV, right ventricle.) (Modified from Wallace, R. B.: Truncus arteriosus. In Sabiston, D. C., Jr., and Spencer, F. C. (Eds.): Gibbon's Surgery of the Chest, 3rd ed. Philadelphia, W. B. Saunders Company, 1976.)

evidence of pulmonary vascular obstructive disease in the follow-up period. Fifty-five of the survivors have required conduit replacement, which has been performed without mortality. This remarkable series has established complete repair in infancy as the procedure of choice for patients with truncus arteriosus.

SELECTED REFERENCES

Di Donato, R. M., Fyfe, D. A., Puga, F. J., Danielson, G. K., Ritter, D. G., Edwards, W. D., and McGoon, D. C.: Fifteen year experience with surgical repair of truncus arteriosus. J. Thorac. Cardiovasc. Surg., 89:414, 1985.

These authors reviewed the Mayo Clinic experience with 167 patients operated on for truncus arteriosus from 1965 until March 1982. There were 48 hospital deaths for a hospital mortality of 28.7 per cent. Long-term survival at 5 and 10 years was 84.4 per cent and 68.8 per cent, respectively. Thirty-six patients required reoperation, 32 had replacement of an obstructed valved conduit, and 9 required truncal valve replacement. Of the 90 surviving patients, 66 per cent were in functional NYHA Class I, 31 per cent in Class II, and 3 per cent in Class III.

Ebert, P. A., Turley, K., Stranger, P., Hoffman, J. I. E., Heymann, M. A., and Rudolph, A. M.: Surgical treatment of truncus arteriosus in the first 6 months of life. Ann. Surg., 200:415, 1984.

In this paper 100 patients undergoing physiologic correction of truncus arteriosus prior to 6 months of age at the University of California, San Francisco, are reported. The mortality was 11 per cent. Of the 86 long-term survivors, 55 have required conduit change as a result of body growth or pseudointima obstruction of the conduit. No mortality was reported at the time of conduit change, and no patients showed evidence of pulmonary vascular disease during the follow-up period. This series clearly documents the efficacy of repair of truncus arteriosus in infancy.

REFERENCES

1. Bharati, S., McAllister, H. A., Jr., Rosenquist, G. C., Miller, R. A., Tatooles, C. J., and Lev, M.: The surgical anatomy of truncus arteriosus communis. J. Thorac. Cardiovasc. Surg., 67:501, 1974.

2. Ciaravella, J. M., Jr., McGoon, D. C., Danielson, G. K., Wallace, R. B., Mair, D. D., and Ilstrup, D. M.: Experience with the extracardiac conduit. J. Thorac. Cardiovasc. Surg., 78:920, 1979.

3. Collett, R. W., and Edwards, J. E.: Persistent truncus arteriosus: A classification according to anatomic types. Surg. Clin. North Am., 29:1245, 1949.

4. Di Donato, R. M., Fyfe, D. A., Puga, F. J., Danielson, G. K., Ritter, D. G., Edwards, W. D., and McGoon, D. C.: Fifteen-year experience with surgical repair of truncus arteriosus. J. Thorac. Cardiovasc. Surg., 89:414, 1985.

5. Ebert, P. A., Turley, K., Stranger, P., Hoffman, J. I. E., Heymann, M. A., and Rudolph, A. M.: Surgical treatment of truncus arteriosus in the first 6 months of life. Ann. Surg., 200:451, 1984.

6. Fontana, R. S., and Edwards, J. E.: Congenital Cardiac Disease: A Review of 357 Cases Studied Pathologically. Philadelphia, W. B. Saunders Company, 1962, p. 95.

7. Hagler, D. J., Tajik, A. J., Seward, J. B., Mair, D. D., and Ritter, D. G.: Wide-angle two-dimensional echocardiographic profiles of conotruncal abnormalities. Mayo Clinic. Proc., 55:73, 1980.

8. Mair, D. D., Ritter, D. G., Danielson, G. K., Wallace, R. B., and McGoon, D. C.: Truncus arteriosus with unilateral absence of a pulmonary artery: Criteria for operability and surgical result. Circulation, 55:641, 1977.

9. Mair, D. D., Ritter, D. G., Davis, G. D., Wallace, R. B., Danielson, G. K., and McGoon, D. C.: Selection of patients with truncus arteriosus for surgical correction: Anatomic and hemodynamic considerations. Circulation, 49:144, 1974.

10. McGoon, D. C., Rastelli, G. C., and Ongley, P. A.: An operation for the correction of truncus arteriosus, J.A.M.A., 205:69, 1968.

11. Muller, W. H., Jr., and Dammann, J. F., Jr.: The treatment of certain congenital malformations of the heart by the creation of pulmonic stenosis to reduce pulmonary hypertension and excessive pulmonary blood flow: A preliminary report. Surg. Gynecol. Obstet., 95:213, 1952.

12. Taruffi, C.: Sulle malattie congenite e sulle anomalie del cuore. Mem. Soc. Med. Chir. Bologna., 8:215, 1875.

13. Van Praagh, R., and Van Praagh, S.: The anatomy of common aortico-pulmonary trunk (truncus arteriosus communis) and its embryologic implications: A study of 57 necropsy cases. Am. J. Cardiol., 16:406, 1965.

14. Weldon, C. S., and Cameron, J. L.: Correction of persistent truncus arteriosus. J. Cardiovasc. Surg., 9:463, 1968.

Transposition of the Great Arteries

JAMES D. SINK, M.D.
DAVID C. SABISTON, JR., M.D.

Transposition of the great arteries is a congenital cardiac defect in which the aorta arises from the right ventricle and the pulmonary artery arises from the left ventricle. As a result, cyanosis is usually obvious shortly after birth. To survive, mixing of blood between the parallel systemic and venous circulations must occur via an atrial septal defect, patent ductus arteriosus, or ventricular septal defect. If untreated, most infants with this condition succumb by the end of the first year. Methods of correction have been developed over many years and by many investigators. Although the surgical treatment for this anomaly is still evolving, the surgeon currently has several options which have proved successful in treating a condition that for many years was considered uncorrectable.

HISTORY

Transposition of the great arteries was noted as an anatomic variant in 1672 by Steno, in 1761 by Morgagni, and in 1779 by Bailey. The first clinical recognition of this anomaly in life was not reported until 1932 by Fanconi,[5] and the first palliative operation was performed in 1950 when Blalock and Hanlon[2] described an ingenious technique for creating an atrial septal defect to increase mixing of blood between the systemic and pulmonary circulations.

Attempted repair of transposition of the great arteries was first reported in 1954. Mustard and co-workers[9] described a technique for switching the great arteries plus one coronary artery, but they were unsuccessful. A technique for complete repair by redirecting venous inflow at the atrial level was first suggested by Albert[1] in 1955. After unsuccessful attempts by various groups, Senning[13] reported the first successful intra-atrial repair in 1959. Although the Senning procedure was employed with success, the mortality remained high. In 1964, Mustard[10] described a technique of excising the atrial septum and placing a pericardial baffle within the atrium to direct superior and inferior vena caval blood to the pulmonary ventricle and oxygenated pulmonary venous blood to the systemic ventricle. This procedure was reproducible and relatively safe and stimulated a widespread interest in the surgical repair of transposition of the great arteries.

In 1976, Jatene[8] reported success in switching the great arteries with reimplantation of the coronary arteries in patients with transposition. This procedure was initially associated with a high mortality, but recent success with the arterial switch technique in infants has resulted in renewed interest in this procedure.[4]

ANATOMY

In complete transposition of the great arteries, the aorta usually arises anteriorly from the anatomic right ventricle, and the pulmonary artery arises from the anatomic left ventricle. The pulmonary artery usually lies posterior and to the left of the aorta. Common associated anomalies include patent ductus arteriosus, patent foramen ovale, ventricular septal defect, and left ventricular outflow tract obstruction. About 70 per cent of patients have an intact ventricular septum without left ventricular outflow tract obstruction, a small patent foramen ovale, and a small patent ductus arteriosus. Transposition of the great arteries comprises approximately 9 per cent of cases of cyanotic congenital heart disease and is a leading cause of death resulting from congenital heart disease in early life.

PATHOPHYSIOLOGY

In transposition of the great arteries, the systemic venous blood is pumped into the aorta while the pulmonary venous blood is returned to the pulmonary arteries. The pulmonary and systemic circulations are separate and parallel rather than being in series, as is the normal situation. Survival is therefore dependent on mixing between the parallel circulations. The more associated anomalies, such as ventricular septal defect, atrial septal defect, and patent ductus arteriosus, the greater the mixing of blood between the two circulations. When these anomalies are absent, mixing is limited and cyanosis is severe. In those patients with a large associated ventricular septal defect or patent ductus arteriosus, congestive heart failure may be prominent and difficult to manage medically. Patients with a ventricular septal defect and left ventricular outflow tract obstruction have a natural history similar to patients with tetralogy of Fallot. As the left ventricular outflow tract obstruction increases in severity, polycythemia and cyanosis may progress.

Pulmonary vascular obstructive disease is seen in most children with transposition of the great arteries older than 2 years of age, and intimal fibrosis has been noted as early as 1 month. The histologic findings do not, however, completely agree with hemodynamic measurements because many patients do not have evidence of increased pulmonary vascular resistance. A decrease in pulmonary vascular resistance is observed in many cases following correction.

CLINICAL FEATURES

There is a definite sex predominance, with two-thirds of cases involving transposition occurring in males. The birth weight is usually normal or above normal, but growth and development are retarded. In patients with transposition registered in the New England Regional Infant Cardiac Program, 9 per cent had extracardiac anomalies, although the majority were minor.

As the majority of patients show evidence of inadequate circulatory mixing, these infants usually present in the first week of age with cyanosis. The cyanosis of transposition is persistent and fails to respond to increased oxygen concentrations. When cyanosis appears later than 1 week of age or when it is less intent, there is usually significant intracirculatory shunting through a large ventricular septal defect or patent ductus arteriosus. If a patent ductus is responsible for decreased cyanosis, ductal closure can lead to rapid deteriorization. Clubbing of the fingers is common after 6 months of age, but squatting is rarely seen. Hypoxia from inadequate circulatory mixing with metabolic acidosis can result in anoxic spells characterized by prolonged dyspnea and increased cyanosis. Signs and symptoms of congestive heart failure are common at about 1 month of age and include dyspnea, cardiomegaly, hepatomegaly, pulmonary rales, and, occasionally, peripheral edema.

Physical findings usually include an overactive heart with a prominent left peristernal lift. Most patients, including those in whom the ventricular septum is intact, have a systolic ejection murmur along the left sternal border. The second heart sound is single and usually loud owing to the closeness of the aorta to the chest wall. A diastolic gallop is a common finding, and an apical diastolic murmur may be associated with a ventricular septal defect. Pulmonary valvular stenosis is associated with a left peristernal crescendo-decrescendo murmur.

The chest film usually shows cardiomegaly, an egg-shaped cardiac configuration, a narrow superior mediastinum, and pulmonary plethora. Although the heart size may be normal in the first several weeks of life, cardiac enlargement is soon evident in almost all patients with transposition of the great arteries. The electrocardiogram (ECG) usually demonstrates a sinus tachycardia, right atrial hypertrophy, right ventricular hypertrophy, and right axis deviation. Since right ventricular hypertrophy is characteristic in the newborn, the ECG in early infancy may appear normal. ST-T wave changes are sometimes present and may reflect myocardial ischemia in the severely cyanotic patient.

MANAGEMENT

Most infants with transposition of the great arteries become cyanotic within the first 1 to 2 weeks of life. The diagnosis is usually suspected from the physical findings, ECG and chest film, and can be confirmed by two-dimensional echocardiography.[7]

Cardiac catheterization should be performed to confirm the diagnosis and to define the anatomy. The presence or absence of a ventricular septal defect or left ventricular outflow tract obstruction should be determined. Once the diagnosis is confirmed, a balloon atrial septostomy is usually indicated, as described by Rashkind.[11] A balloon-tipped catheter is passed from the right atrium into the left atrium via the foramen ovale, and the balloon is then inflated with 1 to 3 ml. of contrast material and vigorously withdrawn across the atrial septum to enlarge the foramen ovale. As a result, there is increased mixing of the venous and systemic blood at the atrial level. Balloon atrial septostomy is recognized as an excellent palliative procedure in the infant and can be repeated if necessary.

PALLIATIVE PROCEDURES

Prior to development of balloon atrial septostomy, surgical atrial septectomy was performed to increase systemic and pulmonary venous mixing. The original procedure described by Blalock and Hanlon[2] in 1950 remains the palliative surgical procedure of choice. With improvement in operative techniques and perioperative care, elective repair is now done at an earlier age and most surgeons recommend a corrective procedure when the palliation of the balloon atrial septostomy fails. Therefore, palliative atrial septectomy is seldom performed today.

VENTRICULAR SEPTAL DEFECTS

In patients with a large ventricular septal defect and systemic pressures within the left ventricle, there is a danger of pulmonary vascular obstructive disease developing. In the past, pulmonary artery banding was the recommended treatment for these infants, but today early repair is preferred. High pulmonary artery pressures must not be allowed to persist beyond the first several months of life to prevent the development of irreversible pulmonary vascular changes.

LEFT VENTRICULAR OUTFLOW TRACT OBSTRUCTION

Left ventricular outflow tract obstruction in patients with transposition of the great arteries can be difficult to correct surgically. If a ventricular septal defect is not present, an intra-atrial baffle repair can be performed and the left ventricular outflow tract obstruction approached through the pulmonary artery. Because it is the left ventricle that pumps blood past the obstruction, however, this situation is usually well tolerated. Subsequent procedures to relieve left ventricular outflow tract obstruction may be required as the child becomes older.

If left ventricular outflow tract obstruction is severe, construction of a systemic to pulmonary artery shunt and an atrial septectomy provide the best palliation. A conduit between the left ventricle and pulmonary artery may be required at the time of repair with an intra-atrial baffle procedure. If a ventricular septal defect is present with severe left ventricular outflow tract obstruction, a systemic to pulmonary artery shunt is indicated until a repair can be performed. If the ventricular septal defect is large and the left ventricular outflow tract obstruction cannot be relieved, the *Rastelli*[12] *operation* is the best approach (Fig. 1) and is best performed after the age of 5. This operation involves directing the left ventricular output through the ventricular septal defect into the aorta and placing a valved conduit between the right ventricle and pulmonary artery.

TOTAL CORRECTION

A variety of procedures are available for surgical correction of transposition of the great arteries, with anatomy having the largest influence on the choice of procedures. As mentioned, the Rastelli procedure can be used in patients with transposition of the great arteries, ventricular septal defect, and left ventricular outflow tract obstruction. Intra-atrial repair is performed most commonly for transposition of the great arteries, with two primary operations being available.

Senning[13] in 1959 developed a technique for diverting venous inflow at the atrial level. By realignment of incised atrial tissue, two large intra-atrial channels are developed to cross the systemic and pulmonary venous return (Fig. 2). Although this technique was originally unpopular because of technical difficulty, the Senning procedure is becoming the procedure of choice for repair of simple transposition of the great arteries. A lower incidence of atrial arrhythmias and superior vena caval obstruction has been reported with this repair than with the *Mustard procedure*.

Mustard[10] described an operation for the intra-atrial repair of transposition of the great arteries in 1964 (Fig. 3). In this procedure, the atrial septum is completely excised and pericardium is used to form an intra-atrial baffle directing pulmonary venous blood into the right ventricle and systemic venous blood into the left ventricle. A low operative mortality and excellent results have been reported with this procedure.

As the basic problem in transposition of the great arteries is the abnormal connection of the ventricles and great arteries, it is not surprising that some of the earliest attempts in surgical correction of this anomaly involved repositioning of the transposed arteries over the appropriate ventricle. These attempts were abandoned in favor of the Mustard and Senning procedures until 1976, when Jatene[8] described the successful relocation of the great arteries in a patient with transposition of the great arteries and a ventricular septal defect. The coronary arteries, likewise, must be transferred to provide the heart with oxygenated blood (Fig. 4). The transfer of the coronary arteries with a "button" of tissue at the orifice makes the procedure technically challenging. With the arterial switch procedure, the left ventricle must support the systemic circulation. In transposition, the left ventricular muscle mass regresses or fails to grow with the normal drop in pulmonary artery pressure after birth. To be successful, therefore, the arterial repair must be limited to those patients in whom the left ventricle has adjusted to a greater work load due to a ventricular septal defect, a patent ductus arteriosus, or pulmonary artery banding. Because all infants are born with elevated pulmonary artery pressure, the left ventricle at birth is capable of supporting the systemic circulation. Recently, success has been reported when the arterial switch procedure is performed within the first month of life in patients with transposition of the great arteries and an intact ventricular septum.[4] Although the long-term results of this procedure are not yet available, and the operative mortality is higher than with the Mustard or Senning procedures, it may emerge as the procedure of choice in certain anatomic situations.

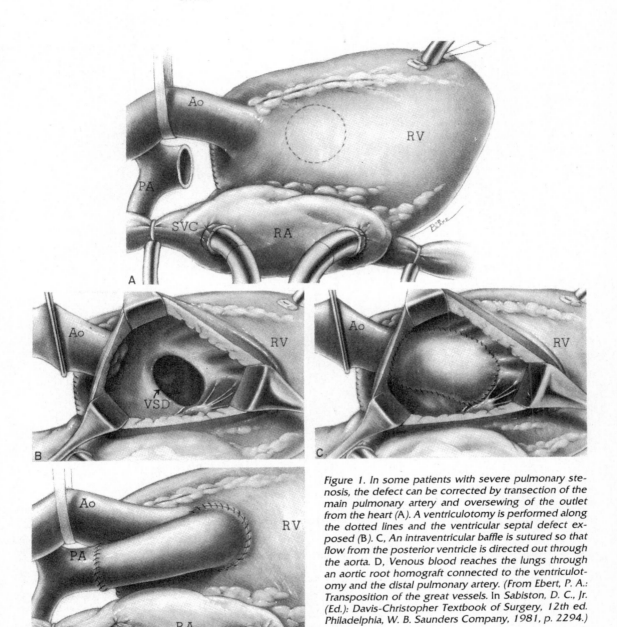

Figure 1. In some patients with severe pulmonary stenosis, the defect can be corrected by transection of the main pulmonary artery and oversewing of the outlet from the heart (A). A ventriculotomy is performed along the dotted lines and the ventricular septal defect exposed (B). C, An intraventricular baffle is sutured so that flow from the posterior ventricle is directed out through the aorta. D, Venous blood reaches the lungs through an aortic root homograft connected to the ventriculotomy and the distal pulmonary artery. (From Ebert, P. A.: Transposition of the great vessels. In Sabiston, D. C., Jr. (Ed.): Davis-Christopher Textbook of Surgery, 12th ed. Philadelphia, W. B. Saunders Company, 1981, p. 2294.)

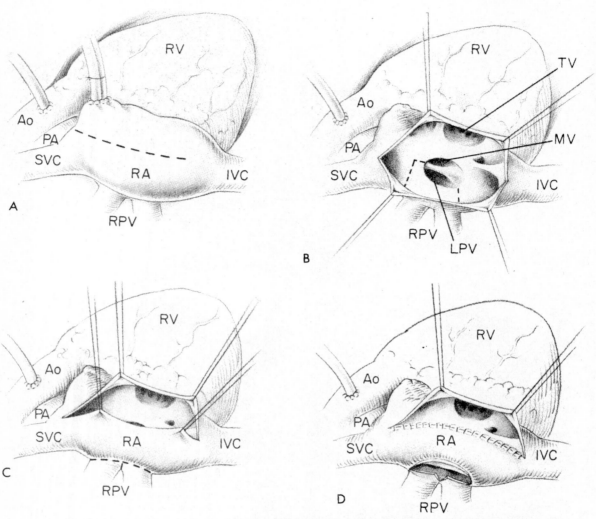

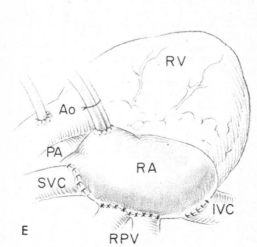

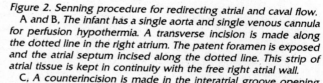

Figure 2. Senning procedure for redirecting atrial and caval flow.

A and B, The infant has a single aorta and single venous cannula for perfusion hypothermia. A transverse incision is made along the dotted line in the right atrium. The patent foramen is exposed and the atrial septum incised along the dotted line. This strip of atrial tissue is kept in continuity with the free right atrial wall.

C, A counterincision is made in the interatrial groove opening at the junction of the right pulmonary vein to the left atrium. This frees the entire flap of the atrial tissue.

D, The remnant of atrial septum is sutured across the floor of the left atrium above the left pulmonary veins. The anterior wall of the free atrial flap is then sutured across the medial portion of the atrial septum. This allows the vena cava to pass behind this flap into the left ventricle. E, This shows the completed operation, in which the free anterior wall of the atrial septum is sutured to the left atrium just above the right pulmonary veins. Interrupted sutures are placed in this area to allow growth. The cannulas are reinserted and the infant rewarmed by cardiopulmonary bypass.

(From Ebert, P. A.: Transposition of the great vessels. In Sabiston, D. C., Jr. (Ed.): Davis-Christopher Textbook of Surgery, 12th ed. Philadelphia, W. B. Saunders Company, 1981, p. 2295.)

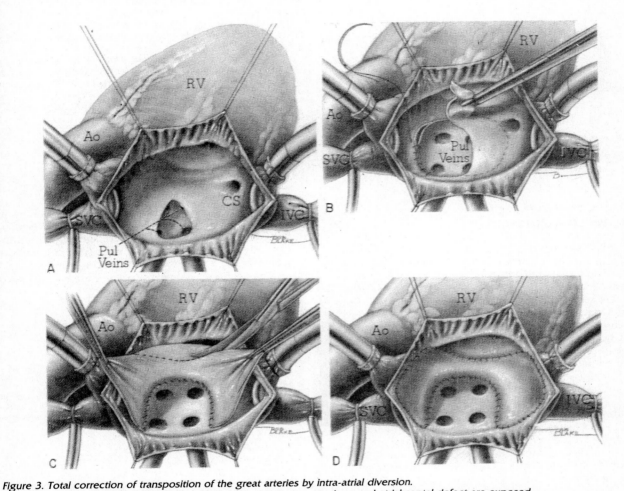

Figure 3. Total correction of transposition of the great arteries by intra-atrial diversion.
   A, The right atrium is opened, so that the atrial septum, coronary sinus, and atrial septal defect are exposed.
   B, The atrial septum is excised. If the excision extends outside the heart in the interatrial groove, it is repaired by direct suture.
   C, The pericardial or prosthetic patch is fashioned around the pulmonary veins and trimmed to fit the atrium. D, To complete repair, the baffle is sutured around the caval orifices and to the remnant of tissue across the top of the ventricular septum. Caval blood is now diverted posteriorly into the left ventricle, while pulmonary venous blood enters the right ventricle and then the aorta. (From Ebert, P. A.: Transposition of the great vessels. In Sabiston, D. C., Jr. (Ed.): Davis-Christopher Textbook of Surgery, 12th ed. Philadelphia, W. B. Saunders Company, 1981, p. 2296.)

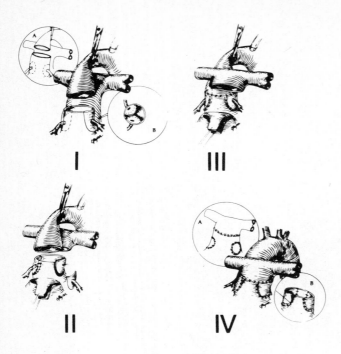

Figure 4.

I, The aorta is transected and the left and right coronary arteries are excised using (A) either a button of aortic wall or (B) a segment of aortic wall extending from the rim of the aorta.

II, An equivalent segment of pulmonary arterial wall (previously marked) is excised, and the coronary arteries are sutured to the pulmonary artery.

III, The distal pulmonary artery is brought anterior to the ascending aorta, and the proximal pulmonary artery is anastomosed to the distal aorta.

IV, The sites of coronary artery explantation are repaired using either (A) a patch of Gore-Tex or (B) a segment of pericardium. Finally, the proximal aorta is sutured to the distal pulmonary artery.

(From Castaneda, A. R., et al.: Ann. Thoracic Surg., 38:438, 1984.)

OPERATIVE COMPLICATIONS

Cardiac arrhythmias after operative correction of transposition of the great arteries are quite common. In most series, 65 to 75 per cent of patients are reported to have sinus rhythm after either a Mustard of Senning repair, with the others being, for the most part, in a nodal rhythm. The nodal rhythm is generally well tolerated. In the Mustard procedure, atrial contraction adds little to the cardiac output because of the large noncontracting baffle. Atrial contraction may make a more significant contribution to cardiac output with the Senning repair because the entire construction is with atrial tissue.[3] Atrial tachycardia or flutter in the postoperative period may be difficult to control.

Superior vena caval obstruction occurs occasionally and is more commonly seen after the Mustard than after the Senning procedure. Partial superior vena caval obstruction is usually well tolerated, but reconstruction may be necessary if symptoms of superior vena caval obstruction occur.[3] Pulmonary venous obstruction is a less common but more serious complication of the Mustard procedure and has been reported as a cause of late death following repair.[14]

Some degree of congestive heart failure is often seen in the immediate postoperative period, as evidenced by pulmonary congestion and pleural effusion. This can usually be easily controlled by judicious use of fluids, diuretics, and digoxin. The heart is especially sensitive to any space-occupying lesions immediately after correction of transposition of the great arteries, and therefore the mediastinum must be well drained. Low-grade tamponade can impair filling of the systemic ventricle and lead to decreased cardiac output.

RESULTS OF OPERATION

Repair of transposition of the great arteries with intact ventricular septum with either the Mustard or Senning procedures is associated with a 90 to 95 per cent survival.

Patients enjoy relatively unlimited activity postoperatively with normal oxygen saturations. The incidence of postoperative arrhythmias remains of concern and decreased contractility of the right ventricle has been seen in a number of patients.[6] The ability of the right ventricle and tricuspid valve to function at systemic pressures over a prolonged time remains unknown.

SELECTED REFERENCES

Brom, A. G.: The Senning I procedure. *In* Moulton, A. L. (Ed.): Congenital Heart Surgery: Current Techniques and Controversies. Pasadena, Calif., Appleton Davies, 1984, pp. 16–24.
Brom was principally responsible for reviving the Senning procedure in the 1970s. In this excellent review, the surgical technique, as well as the results at the University of Leiden, is presented. Included is an interesting discussion of the Senning versus Mustard procedures.

Trusler, G. A., and Freedom, R. M.: Transposition of the great arteries: I. The Mustard Procedure. *In* Sabiston, D. C., Jr., and Spencer, F. C. (Eds.): Gibbon's Surgery of the Chest, 4th ed. Philadelphia, W. B. Saunders Company, 1983, pp. 1126–1150.
An excellent review by one of the major proponents of the Mustard procedure. Techniques and indications as well as results and postoperative complications are discussed.

Yacoub, M.: Anatomic correction of transposition of the great arteries at the arterial level. *In* Sabiston, D. C., Jr., and Spencer, F. C. (Eds.): Gibbon's Surgery of the Chest, 4th ed. Philadelphia, W. B. Saunders Company, 1983, pp. 1156–1171.
Dr. Yacoub has been a proponent of and major contributor to the development of the anatomic correction of transposition of the great arteries. In this excellent review, the preparation of the left ventricle, operative techniques, results, and follow-up are presented.

REFERENCES

1. Albert, H. M.: Surgical correction of transposition of the great vessels. Surg. Forum, 5:74, 1955.
2. Blalock, A., and Hanlon, C. R.: The surgical treatment of complete transposition of the aorta and pulmonary artery. Surg. Gynecol. Obstet., 90:1, 1950.
3. Brom, A. G.: The Senning I procedure. *In* Moulton, A. L. (Ed.): Congenital Heart Surgery: Current Techniques and Controversies. Pasadena, Calif., Appleton Davies, Inc., 1984, pp. 16–24.

4. Castaneda, A. R., Norwood, W. I., Jonas, R. A., Colon, S. D., Sanders, S. P., and Lang, P.: Transposition of the great arteries and intact ventricular septum: Anatomic repair in the neonates. Ann. Thorac. Surg., *38*:438, 1984.

5. Fanconi, G.: Die Transposition der grossen Gefuse (das charakteristische Rontgenbild). Arch. Kinderheilk., *95*:202, 1932.

6. Hagler, D. J., Ritter, D. G., Mair, D. D., Tajik, A. J., Seward, J. B., Fulton, R. E., and Retiman, E. L.: Right and left ventricular function after the Mustard procedure in transposition of the great arteries. Am. J. Cardiol., *44*:276, 1979.

7. Houston, A. B., Gregory, N. L., and Coleman, E. N.: Echocardiographic identification of aorta and main pulmonary artery in complete transposition. Br. Heart J., *40*:377, 1978.

8. Jatene, A. D., Fontes, V. F., Paulista, P. P., Souza, L. C. B., Neger, F., Galantier, M., and Sousa, J. E. M. R.: Anatomic correction of transposition of the great vessels. J. Thorac. Cardiovasc. Surg., *72*:364, 1976.

9. Mustard, W. T., Chute, A. L., Keith, J. D., Sireck, A., Rowe, R. D.,

and Vlad, P.: A surgical approach to transposition of the great vessels with extracorporeal circuit. Surgery, *36*:39, 1954.

10. Mustard, W. T., Keith, J. D., Trusler, G. A., Fowler, R., and Kidd, L.: The surgical management of transposition of the great vessels. J. Thorac. Cardiovasc. Surg., *48*:953, 1964.

11. Rashkind, W. J., and Miller, W. W.: Transposition of the great arteries: Results of palliation by balloon atrioseptostomy in 31 patients. Circulation, *38*:453, 1968.

12. Rastelli, G. C., Wallace, R. B., and Ongley, P. A.: Complete repair of transposition of the great arteries with pulmonary stenosis: A review and report of a case corrected by using a new surgical technique. Circulation, *39*:83, 1969.

13. Senning, A.: Surgical correction of transposition of the great vessels. Surgery, *45*:966, 1959.

14. Trusler, G. A.: The Mustard procedure: Still a valid approach. *In* Moulton, A. L. (Ed.): Congenital Heart Surgery: Current Techniques and Controversies. Pasadena, Calif., Appleton Davies, Inc., 1984, pp. 3–11.

XI

Congenital Aortic Stenosis

ROSS M. UNGERLEIDER, M.D.
DAVID C. SABISTON, JR., M.D.

Congenital aortic stenosis may be caused by a spectrum of lesions that obstruct the flow of blood from the left ventricle (LV) into the aorta. Aortic stenosis may be of congenital origin in 3 to 10 per cent of cases[22, 24, 25, 29] and is frequently associated (8 to 30 per cent of patients)[2, 21, 29] with a variety of other cardiovascular anomalies, including coarctation of the aorta, patent ductus arteriosus, endocardial fibroelastosis, ventricular septal defects, pulmonary stenosis, and mitral stenosis.[29] The site of congenital obstruction is classified anatomically as *valvular, subvalvular,* or *supravalvular* (Fig. 1). A fourth form, caused by hypertrophy of the interventricular muscular septum, presents a unique variety of subvalvular obstruction that varies physiologically from the other forms of stenotic lesions and is therefore considered a separate entity. Although these lesions usually occur separately, patients can present with combinations of the anatomic varieties[24] and *left ventricular outflow tract obstruction* (LVOTO) is perhaps a more descriptive term for this spectrum of congenital anomalies.

HISTORICAL ASPECTS

Stenosis of the aortic valve was described as early as 1646 by Riverius,[24] but the congenital etiology of this form of stenosis was not appreciated for another two centuries. In 1842, Chevers described discrete subaortic stenosis.[8] In 1844, Paget described obstruction from congenitally bicuspid aortic valves, and 42 years later Osler described a patient with endocarditis occurring on a bicuspid aortic valve.[24] The clinical effect of these lesions was mentioned by Thursfield and Scott in 1913, when they described sudden death in a 14-year-old boy with subaortic stenosis. In that

same year, Tuffier first successfully dilated a calcific aortic valve.[24] In 1950, Bailey performed successful dilatation of the aortic valve, and in 1955, Swan and Kortz performed the first open aortic valvotomy using hypothermia.[24] Since the advent of extracorporeal circulation, and the first aortic valvotomy by Lillihei[13] using this approach in 1958, the treatment of the spectrum of lesions causing LVOTO has expanded rapidly.

NATURAL HISTORY, CLINICAL PRESENTATION, AND DIAGNOSIS

Aortic valvar stenosis may occur at any age from the infant to the elderly. In most patients it is a progressive problem that tends to worsen with growth.[1, 11] Few patients survive to the sixth decade without serious, unfavorable signs or symptoms developing, and those who are initially asymptomatic should be followed routinely because the untreated mortality can be 60 per cent or more by the age of 40.[5, 11] Infants who present with symptoms have a 23 per cent mortality if untreated in the first year of life, and the mean age of death for patients with untreated lesions is 35 years.[5]

The primary symptoms attributable to LV outflow tract obstruction are expected from increasing ventricular work. As the systolic pressure gradient across the outflow tract increases, flow can be maintained only by increasing LV pressure. The LV muscle undergoes concentric hypertrophy, and this alters myocardial mechanics. This larger muscle mass creates greater systolic wall tension, which increases myocardial oxygen consumption or, in other

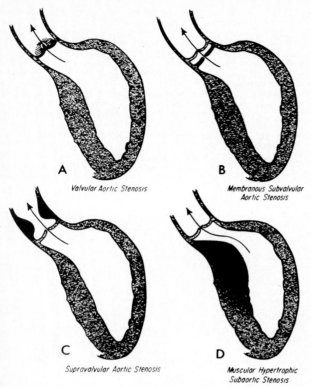

A *Valvular Aortic Stenosis*

B *Membranous Subvalvular Aortic Stenosis*

C *Supravalvular Aortic Stenosis*

D *Muscular Hypertrophic Subaortic Stenosis*

Figure 1. Diagrammatic representation of the location of lesions causing left ventricular outflow tract obstruction. (From Oldham, H. N., Jr.: Congenital aortic stenosis. In Sabiston, D. C., Jr. (Ed.): Davis-Christopher Textbook of Surgery: The Biologic Basis of Modern Surgical Practice, 12th ed. Philadelphia, W. B. Saunders Company, 1981.)

terms, increases the amount of oxygen necessary to adequately meet the metabolic demands of the myocardium. Unfortunately, the hypertrophied left ventricle is also somewhat stiffer than the normal ventricle (less compliant) and the end-diastolic pressure necessary to adequately volume load the ventricular chamber is increased. This higher end-diastolic pressure occurs during the time the myocardium receives its coronary blood flow and probably prevents an adequate supply to the subendocardial layer. This produces ischemia because oxygen demand is increasing but supply is decreasing, and this is the reason that severe stenosis eventually leads to heart failure. With the exception of infants with significant stenosis in the first year of life, 70 per cent of children with congenital aortic stenosis are entirely asymptomatic and develop normally.[25] The discovery of a heart murmur is the usual reason for referral.[25] If the pressure gradient between the left ventricle and the aorta is less than 50 mm. Hg, and the aortic valve orifice size is greater than 0.7 cm.[2] per m.[2] of body surface area, the heart can usually adapt to its increased demands without clinical evidence of failure.[24] Nevertheless, it must be recognized that exercise necessitates an increase in the cardiac output and, therefore, the flow per minute across the obstruction. This augments the severity of the lesion and demonstrates that the measured gradient must be correlated to the cardiac index in order to have a reasonable degree of accuracy regarding its severity. The inability to increase forward flow to meet the metabolic demands of the body explains why most patients experience initial symptoms with exercise as fatigue, dyspnea on exertion, angina (ischemic pain), or effort syncope. As the stenosis becomes

more severe with growth,[11] these symptoms may become more prominent and are thought to reflect hemodynamically severe obstruction, which requires appropriate treatment to prevent death.[12]

A major issue is the proper time for therapeutic intervention, and periodic re-evaluation of children with suspicious murmurs is advised.[3, 11, 12] These children may show little more than a harsh systolic ejection murmur most prominent over the second right intercostal space radiating to the neck and often associated with a thrill. As many as 22 per cent of patients may have a diastolic murmur of aortic insufficiency,[3] and there may also be a precordial lift. A number of criteria have been evaluated as indicators of more severe obstruction,[3, 12] since these children would be at greater risk. Symptoms rarely occur, except with severe stenosis. In addition, a systolic precordial thrill usually suggests a gradient greater than 30 mm. Hg.[12] Likewise, narrowing of the peripheral pulse pressure (indicative of obstructed forward flow) suggests a severe stenosis. It is now well recognized that the chest film may be normal despite significant stenosis.[12] Aortic valves rarely calcify until the fourth decade[5, 24] but the presence of calcification in this location is evidence of an abnormal aortic valve. Although an electrocardiographic (ECG) pattern of LV strain (ST segment and T wave abnormalities) often suggests advanced disease, this correlation is not absolute and children have died suddenly from aortic stenosis with a previously documented normal ECG.[3, 12, 24]

When significant stenosis is suspected, the diagnosis can be established by cardiac ultrasound, radionuclide angiography, or cardiac catheterization.[24] Although advanced modes of echocardiography[24] and radionuclide angiography[24] may assist in localizing the site of the stenosis and provide information regarding LV performance and the gradient, for the majority of patients these modalities do not provide the accurate data available from catheterization and are perhaps best reserved for screening patients for catheterization.[8, 24] There have been some recent studies in infants relying only on echocardiography prior to operation with good results.[27] For older patients, however, cardiac catheterization is still used most frequently to confirm the type and degree of the stenosis as well as to rule out associated lesions. Withdrawal of the catheter from the left ventricle into the ascending aorta can provide critical pressure measurements delineating the area of obstruction, as well as quantitating the gradient across it at a given cardiac index. Excellent examples of these are nicely reproduced in the literature.[24]

INDICATIONS FOR OPERATION AND TREATMENT

Infants in congestive heart failure who respond poorly to medical management require operation.[13] Older children and young adults with severe stenosis should also undergo surgical correction because they have a higher risk of sudden death.[3, 8, 12, 13, 24, 25] It is generally accepted that a peak systolic gradient across the obstruction of 50 to 75 mm. Hg during normal cardiac output, or a valve surface area of less than 0.5 cm.[2] per m.[2] body surface area, constitutes parameters appropriate for operation. It is felt by some that subvalvular stenosis necessitates earlier repair (i.e., gradient of 44 mm. Hg) to prevent progression of the lesion to a subaortic fibromuscular tunnel that can be more difficult to repair later.[8, 23, 24]

The modern operative approach to patients with LVOTO is via a median sternotomy utilizing cardiopulmonary bypass, moderate hypothermia, and cold cardioplegia. This provides for a myocardium that is flaccid to enable easy repair of difficult lesions as well as supplying an element of protection to the heart that permits the surgeon to take the time necessary to perform the best possible procedure while the remainder of the body is still perfused with oxygenated blood. Some groups have advocated repair of valvular aortic stenosis in infants under venous occlusion[8, 27] where both cavae are occluded, thus emptying the heart and obliterating cardiac output. This allows for opening of the aorta, proximal to a cross clamp, and quick repair of the lesion, but during this time neither the body nor the heart receives any blood flow and repair must be accurately performed in less than 2 to 3 minutes. This technique has been criticized by others experienced in this procedure.[18] In certain, special instances, closed dilation of aortic stenosis has been performed employing either a dilator introduced through the LV apex[29] or an angioplasty balloon introduced via the femoral artery.[30] Overall, however, the usual procedures are best performed with cardiopulmonary bypass.

Valvular Stenosis

In the majority of cases (70 per cent), LVOTO is caused by *valvular* lesions[14, 22, 24] and usually entails thickening of the valve leaflets and some degree of fusion of the commissures. This results in valves that appear bicuspid, unicuspid, or, rarely, quadricuspid (Fig. 2). Bicuspid valves occur in 1 per cent of human hearts,[26] and although they may function normally,[26] many calcify and become stenotic in later life. These valves are abnormal because of commissural fusion, while the valve annulus and coronary arteries are normal. There is no surgical procedure that can restore a stenotic valve to a completely normal one, and the goal of operation is to relieve the stenosis. This is usually performed by an incision separating the fused commissures. It is important to restrict this incision so that it does not extend to the anulus because in such a situation the support mechanism of the leaflet could be destroyed resulting in aortic insufficiency. This goal is more easily accomplished in some anomalies than in others, and along with the relief of obstruction, some element of aortic insufficiency will usually be created. Although infants may tolerate aortic regurgitation better than the previous stenosis, the diastolic pressure after the valvotomy should remain greater than 60 mm. Hg.[13] Since these valves remain abnormal after relief of the stenosis, valvotomy is a palliative procedure and parents should be informed that as many as one third of these children may require a second operation within 10 years.[1, 9, 28] If the immediate goal of relief from LVOTO is achieved, the children can continue to develop until such a time that their increased size permits placement of an adult-sized aortic valve prosthesis if such is necessary. The smallest available prosthesis (17 mm.) may be smaller than desirable, but if immediate results of valvotomy are poor, *anular enlarging procedures* can be used to allow insertion of an adult-sized prosthetic valve into the LV outflow tract.[15, 18] Unfortunately, because of the association of endocardial fibroelastosis with aortic valve stenosis, the success of even the best procedures has been limited[8] and mortality in the infant has been reported between 9 and 33 per cent.[16, 17] Older children respond better, but because of the palliative nature of this procedure they may eventually require valve replacement.

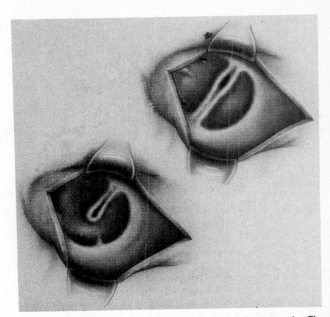

Figure 2. Two lesions typical of valvular aortic stenosis. The uppermost valve is unicuspid. The commissure may be located in any of the three possible normal locations for a valve commissure. Abortive commissures or raphes may be present. Repair is usually achieved by incision of the commissure toward the aortic anulus. Incision in the opposite direction, into the leaflet, could result in overwhelming aortic regurgitation. The lower valve depicted is bicuspid. The coronary arteries may arise on the same or opposite side of the commissure. A raphe may be present between the coronary arteries when they are on the same side of the commissure. When a bicuspid valve is stenotic, there is usually a small eccentric opening on one side of the commissure and correction involves incision in the fused portion of the commissure to enlarge this opening. Incisions should not be made in the rudimentary raphes. (From de Leval, M.: Left ventricular outflow tract obstruction. In Stark, J., and de Leval, M. (Eds.): Surgery for Congenital Heart Defects. New York, Grune & Stratton, 1983.)

Subvalvular Stenosis

Stenosis of the left ventricular outflow tract below the aortic valve is next most common in frequency (8 to 20 per cent).[8] It presents as either a thin, discrete membrane located anteriorly immediately below the aortic valve (Fig. 3) or, less commonly, as a diffuse fibromuscular "tunnel" beneath the aortic leaflets. Correction of the membranous form necessitates an incision in the aorta, retraction of the usually normal aortic valve leaflets, and careful resection of the membrane, with care being taken not to injure the conduction system or the anterior leaflet of the mitral valve, which is usually subjacent to the lesion (Fig. 3). It is felt that early resection may prevent progression to the more severe fibromuscular variety.[24] Repair of LVOTO caused by the more diffuse, fibromuscular lesions may be amenable to resection of enough of the obstructing tissue to relieve the stenosis, although there is an increased danger of damaging the integrity of the interventricular septum, the mitral valve or the conduction system. Some obstructions cannot be safely relieved by resection of tissue and require more complicated procedures such as aortoventriculoplasty (which produces enlargement of the aortic anulus and interventricular septum)[8, 15] or implantation of a valved

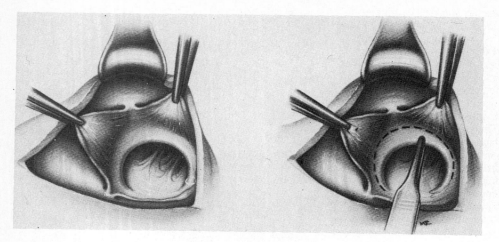

Figure 3. Example of discrete, membranous subaortic stenosis. The aortic valve leaflets are reflected and a dashed line demonstrates a suggested incision for resection. Care must be taken to avoid the anterior leaflet of the mitral valve that is immediately subjacent to lesion. (From de Leval, M.: Left ventricular outflow tract obstruction. In Stark, J., and de Leval, M. (Eds.): Surgery for Congenital Heart Defects. New York, Grune & Stratton, 1983.)

conduit between the left ventricle and the aorta, thus bypassing the normal outflow tract.[8]

A variant of subaortic stenosis is created by asymmetric septal hypertrophy. It has been well described by Braunwald and Morrow and is termed *idiopathic hypertrophic subaortic stenosis*.[4, 20] Unlike the other forms of fixed LVOTO, this appears to be a dynamic obstruction created by variable interference from the hypertrophied septum to outflow, depending on the contractile state of the heart and the LV systolic volume. This obstruction is increased by inotropic agents, by diminished blood volume, by the Valsalva maneuver, or by nitroglycerin.[4] The gradient is reduced by propranolol or adrenergic blockage, by increased blood volume, or by general anesthesia.[24] These patients can be treated medically with propranolol, or they may be managed surgically by myectomy with excision of a portion of the hypertrophied septum (through the aortic valve). A surgical approach is indicated when the patient remains symptomatic despite appropriate medical management.[20]

Supravalvular Stenosis

A relatively uncommon form of LVOTO, supravalvular stenosis, is also found in *localized* and *diffuse* forms.[8] A

peculiar syndrome consisting of supravalvular aortic stenosis in conjunction with mental retardation and "elfin"-like facies (Williams' syndrome)[7, 31] is now often recognized, but the stenosis can also occur as an isolated entity. The lesion is in reality a coarctation of the ascending aorta with varying degrees of intimal hyperplasia.[6] Correction of the discrete lesion is best performed by insertion of a patch of synthetic polyester (Dacron) over the stenotic region, thus relieving the obstruction without jeopardizing the coronary ostia (Fig. 4).[8, 10] The diffuse form presents a more difficult problem and was previously felt to be inoperable.[2] However, success can be achieved in some with a patch to enlarge the involved aorta[10] or by valved conduits sutured between the left ventricle and the descending aorta.[8, 14]

RESULTS

In the evaluation of any procedure on young patients for congenital lesions, it is crucial to assess the long-term benefits of the surgical intervention. The complications of LVOTO include sudden death, subacute bacterial endocarditis (SBE), and heart failure (from chronic LV systolic overload or aortic insufficiency). Most procedures performed on infants or young children are palliative, with the intent being to relieve the stenosis and reduce the chance of early death. Many such patients (with valvular lesions) will eventually require valve replacement, which, it is hoped, can be performed after they have had a chance to become larger.

The risk of sudden death in untreated patients has been estimated at 0.9 per cent per annum.[5] Those with more severe lesions, as evidenced by symptoms, pertinent physical findings, or objective pressure data, appear to be at greatest risk for sudden death.[3, 5, 12] Valvotomy does not eliminate this risk, but it does reduce it to an estimated 0.29 per cent per annum.[28]

Subacute bacterial endocarditis is always a risk in the presence of turbulence across abnormal anatomy. Without operation, approximately 3.1 episodes of SBE will occur for every 1000 patient years with aortic stenosis, or—put in other terms—there is a 1.4 per cent chance of endocarditis in the first 30 years of life. This incidence is increased after operation with a 7.4 per cent risk of SBE in the first 30 years of life.[28]

Although the chance of heart failure from systolic overload is effectively reduced by an adequate procedure,

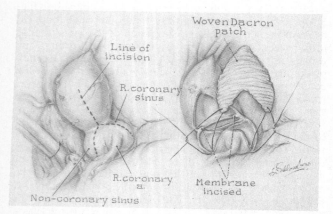

Figure 4. Discrete supravalvular aortic stenosis may present like a coarctation of the ascending aorta. This lesion can be repaired with an inverted Y patch that straddles the right coronary artery and prevents constriction at the aortic root.

the incidence of aortic insufficiency probably triples in patients with primarily valvular lesions from 11 per cent preoperatively to 30 to 40 per cent postoperatively.[28] Twenty per cent of these patients may by symptomatic.

Despite these figures, it seems clear that the survival of patients with *significant* stenotic lesions is enhanced by surgery.[28] However, because the procedures for valvular aortic stenosis are palliative and result in increased risk of SBE and aortic regurgitation, they should probably be performed only for children with severe lesions who have the higher likelihood of experiencing sudden death.[25] Correction of subvalvular forms of LVOTO can lead to a better long-term result—depending on the nature of the lesion—but stenosis can still occur again.[23] The palliative nature of these procedures necessitates proper timing and patient selection so that the current clinical condition is not replaced by new problems of equal or greater concern.

SELECTED REFERENCES

Campbell, M.: The natural history of congenital aortic stenosis. Br. Heart J., *30*:514, 1968.
An excellent description that is critical in helping to determine plans for therapy.

Oldham, H. N., Jr.: Congenital aortic stenosis. *In* Sabiston, D. C., Jr. (Ed.): Davis-Christopher Textbook of Surgery, 12th ed. Philadelphia, W. B. Saunders Company, 1981.
A superb overview of the causes and physiologic effects of the various forms of left ventricular outflow tract obstruction.

REFERENCES

1. Ankeney, J. L., Tzena, T. S., and Liebman, J.: Surgical therapy for congenital aortic valvular stenosis. J. Thorac. Cardiovasc. Surg., *85*:41, 1983.
2. Bernhard, W. F., Keane, J. F., Fellows, K. E., et al.: Progress and problems in the surgical management of congenital aortic stenosis. J. Thorac. Cardiovasc. Surg., *66*:404, 1973.
3. Braunwald, E., Goldblatt, A., Aygen, M. M., et al.: Congenital aortic stenosis: I. Clinical and hemodynamic findings in 100 patients. Morrow, A. G., Goldblatt, A., and Braunwald, E.: II. Surgical treatment and results of operation. Circulation, *27*:426, 1963.
4. Braunwald, E., Oldham, H. N., Ross, J., et al.: The circulatory response of patients with idiopathic hypertrophic subaortic stenosis to nitroglycerin and to the Valsalva maneuver. Circulation, *29*:422, 1964.
5. Campbell, M.: The natural history of congenital aortic stenosis. Br. Heart J., *30*:514, 1968.
6. Cooley, D. A., Beall, A. C., Hallman, G. L., and Bricker, D. L.: Obstructive lesions of the left ventricular outflow tract. Circulation, *31*:612, 1965.
7. Cornell, W. P., Elkins, R. C., Criley, J. M., and Sabiston, D. C., Jr.: Supravalvular aortic stenosis. J. Thorac. Cardiovasc. Surg., *51*:484, 1966.
8. de Leval, M.: Left ventricular outflow tract obstruction. *In* Stark, J., and de Leval, M. (Eds.): Surgery for Congenital Heart Defects. New York, Grune & Stratton, 1983.
9. Dobell, A. R. C., Bloss, R. S., Gibbons, J. E., and Collins, G. F.: Congenital valvular aortic stenosis. J. Thorac. Cardiovasc. Surg., *81*:916, 1981.
10. Doty, D. B., Polansky, D. B., and Jenson, C. B.: Supravalvular aortic stenosis: Repair by extended aortoplasty. J. Thorac. Cardiovasc. Surg., *74*:362, 1977.
11. El-Said, G., Galioto, F. M., Mullins, C. E., et al.: Natural hemodynamic history of congenital aortic stenosis in childhood. Am. J. Cardiol., *30*:6, 1972.
12. Glew, R. H., Varghese, P. J., Krovetz, L. J., et al.: Sudden death in congenital aortic stenosis: A review of eight cases with an evaluation of premonitory clinical features. Am. Heart J., *78*:615, 1969.
13. Hallman, G. L., and Cooley, D. A.: Congenital aortic stenosis. *In* Sabiston, D. C., Jr., and Spencer F. C. (Eds.): Gibbon's Surgery of the Chest, 4th ed. Philadelphia, W. B. Saunders Company, 1983, pp. 1109–1115.
14. Keane, J. F., Fellows, K. E., Lafarge, C. G., et al.: The surgical management of discrete and diffuse supravalvular aortic stenosis. Circulation, *54*:112, 1976.
15. Konno, S., Yasuharu, I., Yoshinau, I., et al.: A new method for prosthetic valve replacement in congenital aortic stenosis associated with hypoplasia of the aortic valve ring. J. Thorac. Cardiovasc. Surg., *70*:909, 1975.
16. Kugler, J. C., Campbell, E., Vargo, T. A., et al.: Results of aortic valvotomy in infants with isolated aortic valvular stenosis. J. Thorac. Cardiovasc. Surg., *78*:553, 1979.
17. Messina, L. M., Turley, K., Stanger, P., et al.: Successful aortic valvotomy for severe congenital valvular aortic stenosis in the newborn infant. J. Thorac. Cardiovasc. Surg., *88*:92, 1984.
18. Misbach, G. A., Turley, K., Ullyot, D. J., and Ebert, P. A.: Left ventricular outflow enlargement by the Konno procedure. J. Thorac. Cardiovasc. Surg., *84*:696, 1982.
19. Mitchell, S. C., Korones, S. B., and Berendes, H. W.: Congenital heart disease in 56,109 births. Circulation, *43*:323, 1971.
20. Morrow, A. G., Reitz, B. A., Epstein, S. E., et al.: Operative treatment in hypertrophic subaortic stenosis: Techniques and the results of pre- and postoperative assessments in 83 patients. Circulation, *52*:88, 1975.
21. Mulder, D. G., Katz, R. D., Moss, A. J., et al.: The surgical treatment of congenital aortic stenosis. J. Thorac. Cardiovasc. Surg., *88*:786, 1968.
22. Nadas, A. S., and Fyler, D.: Pediatric Cardiology. Philadelphia, W. B. Saunders Company, 1972.
23. Newfeld, E. A., Muster, A. J., and Paul, M. H.: Discrete subvalvular aortic stenosis in childhood: Study of 51 patients. Am. J. Cardiol., *38*:53, 1976.
24. Oldham, H. N., Jr.: Congenital aortic stenosis. *In* Sabiston, D. C., Jr. (Ed.): Davis-Christopher Textbook of Surgery: The Biologic Basis of Modern Surgical Practice, 12th ed. Philadelphia, W. B. Saunders Company, 1981, pp. 2301–2311.
25. Olley, P. M., Bloom, K. R., and Rowe, R. D.: Aortic stenosis: Valvular, subaortic, and supravalvular. *In* Keith, J. D., Rowe, R. D., and Vlad, P. (Eds.): Heart Disease in Infancy and Childhood, 3rd ed. New York, Macmillan Publishing Company, 1978, pp. 698–727.
26. Roberts, W. C.: The congenitally biscupid aortic valve: A study of 85 autopsy cases. Am. J. Cardiol., *26*:72, 1970.
27. Sink, J. D., Smallhorn, J. F., Macartney, F. J., et al.: Management of critical aortic stenosis in infancy. J. Thorac. Cardiovasc. Surg., *87*:82, 1984.
28. Stewart, J. R., Paton, B. C., Blount, S. G., et al.: Congenital aortic stenosis: Ten to 22 years after valvulotomy. Arch. Surg., *113*:1248, 1978.
29. Trinkle, J. K., Norton, J. B., Richardson, J. D., et al.: Closed aortic valvotomy and simultaneous correction of associated anomalies in infants. J. Thorac. Cardiovasc. Surg., *69*:758, 1975.
30. Walls, J. T., Lababidi, Z., Curtis, J. J., et al.: Assessment of percutaneous balloon pulmonary and aortic valvuloplasty. J. Thorac. Cardiovasc. Surg., *88*:352, 1984.
31. Williams, J. C. P., Barrett-Boyes, B. G., and Lowe, J. B.: Supravalvular aortic stenosis. Circulation, *26*:1311, 1961.

XII

1 • PHYSIOLOGIC DETERMINANTS OF CORONARY BLOOD FLOW, CARDIAC METABOLISM, AND INTRAOPERATIVE MYOCARDIAL PROTECTION

DAVID C. SABISTON, JR., M.D.

Coronary artery disease, primarily due to atherosclerosis, remains the single most common cause of death in the United States and most of the countries of the Western world. Myocardial ischemia due to coronary arterial stenosis manifests in two major ways. *Angina pectoris* is a symptom complex in which exercise or emotion triggers an episode of chest pain. This may progress to spontaneous pain at rest as the disease becomes more severe. A second mode of presentation is *acute myocardial infarction* with little if any forewarning.

Attention has been called to the epidemic nature of coronary artery disease in the civilized world; routine autopsies on young United States military casualties in both the Korean and the Vietnam conflicts showed that 77 per cent had gross evidence of coronary atherosclerosis and 10 per cent showed advanced disease with occlusion at a level of 70 per cent or more of one of the major coronary arteries.[10] Moreover, these observations have been confirmed in community studies noting lesions varying from 24 per cent obstruction to complete occlusion in three fourths of the population.[45] Thus, there is little doubt that coronary atherosclerosis, and its attendant complication of myocardial ischemia, is widespread in this country and abroad. Despite its frequency today, it is paradoxical that a diagnosis of acute myocardial infarction *before* death was not made until 1912 when Herrick reported the first patient.[22] Fortunately, most patients with symptomatic coronary artery disease can now be managed either by coronary artery bypass grafts (CABG) or, in selected patients, by percutaneous balloon dilatation of the obstructing lesions.

ANATOMIC ASPECTS

The first two branches of the aorta are the right and left coronary arteries. The left coronary artery is approximately 1 cm. in length and gives rise to the anterior descending and circumflex branches (Fig. 1).[12] The anterior descending supplies the anterolateral wall of the left ventricle and provides approximately two thirds of the blood supply to the interventricular septum. The right coronary artery supplies the right ventricle, as well as a portion of the posterior ventricle, because the right coronary ends in the posterior descending coronary artery in most instances (Fig. 2).[12] Arteriograms that demonstrate lesions in the left coronary artery are shown in Figure 3.[33] In 10 per cent of patients, the posterior descending artery has its origin from the distal groove portion of the circumflex artery.

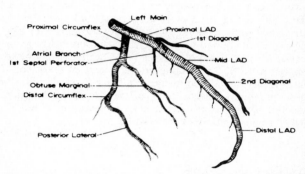

Figure 1. Normal left coronary artery anatomy seen from a right anterior oblique orientation. (From Franch, R. H., et al.: Techniques of cardiac catheterization including coronary arteriography. In Hurst, J. W. (Ed.): The Heart, 5th ed. New York, McGraw-Hill Book Company, 1982.)

The term *coronary artery dominance* can be misleading unless the definition is thoroughly understood. The concept was promoted on the basis that the right or left coronary artery was predominant depending on which artery crossed the crux of the heart, in the region of the posterior surface of the heart where all four chambers intersect. Therefore, if a large posterior descending branch arose from the right coronary and supplied the posterior-inferior septum and part of the left ventricle, the term *right predominant* was applied. However, if this vessel was supplied by the left coronary artery, it is termed a *left predominant* heart. At times both contribute and this is termed a *balanced* coronary circulation.

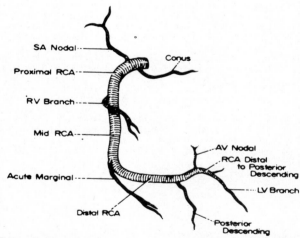

Figure 2. Normal right coronary artery anatomy seen from a left anterior oblique orientation. (From Franch, R. H., et al.: Techniques of cardiac catheterization including coronary arteriography. In Hurst, J. W. (Ed.): The Heart, 5th ed. New York, McGraw-Hill Book Company, 1982.)

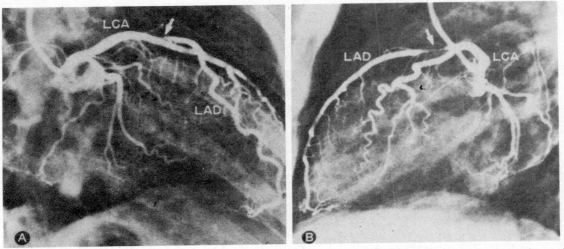

Figure 3. A, *Right anterior oblique angiogram of the left coronary artery. A severe stenosis of the proximal left anterior descending artery (arrow) is almost completely obscured by overlapping branches. B, Left lateral view of the same artery shows the stenosis (arrow) clearly. LAD = Left anterior descending artery. LCA = Left circumflex artery. (From Mitchell, W.: Clinical angiographic description of the coronary artery anatomy. In Boucek, R. J., et al. (Eds.): Coronary Artery Disease. Baltimore, Williams & Wilkins, 1984.)*

There is a distinct pattern of anatomic location of atherosclerotic coronary lesions. Generally, a "significant" stenosis represents a 50 per cent or greater lesion, whereas other authors use 75 per cent as the criterion for stenosis. Quite clearly, a 75 per cent or greater stenosis is associated with a poorer long-term prognosis than is a 50 per cent lesion.[20]

The most common sites of lesions in both the right and the left coronary arteries are shown in Figure 4.[21] A coronary arteriogram demonstrating specific branches of both the anterior descending and the circumflex coronary arteries is depicted in Figure 5.[34] A lesion of the right coronary artery together with its branches is shown in Figure 5C.

CLINICAL MANIFESTATIONS OF MYOCARDIAL ISCHEMIA

Myocardial ischemia is usually caused by a primary atherosclerotic lesion in the coronary arteries. However, it must be remembered that other conditions can also reduce coronary blood flow, including aortic stenosis, aortic insufficiency, syphilitic coronary ostial stenosis, hypertension, embolism, other forms of arteritis, and congenital malformations of the coronary arteries.[2] Patients with angina pectoris usually complain of substernal discomfort and describe it as a choking, pressure sensation, or tightness

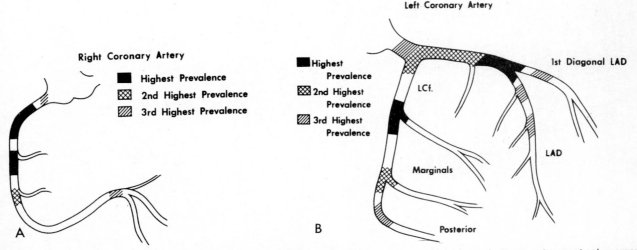

Figure 4. Distribution of atherosclerotic lesions in the right (A) and left (B) coronary arteries. Note the predilection for proximal segments and branch points. (Reprinted by permission from Herman, M. V., et al.: Pathophysiology of ischemic heart disease. In Levine, H. J. (Ed.): Clinical Cardiovascular Physiology. New York, Grune & Stratton, 1976.)

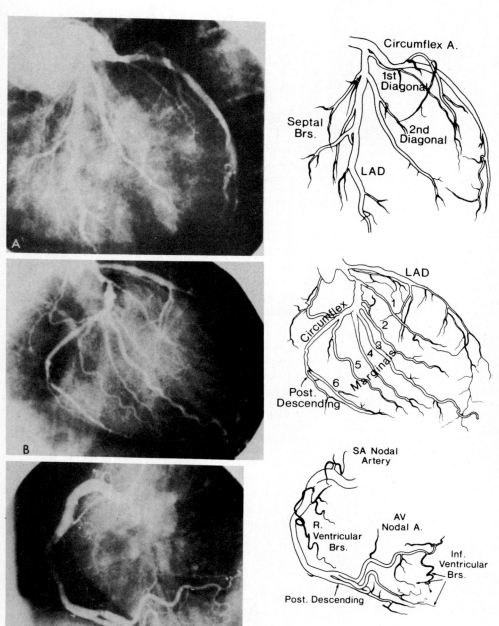

Figure 5. A, The left anterior descending coronary artery (LAD) and its diagonals are demonstrated in this left anterior oblique projection. Further slight rotation may be necessary to make the first diagonal completely visible. B, Circumflex marginal branches are best seen in the right anterior oblique projection. Seven branches of the circumflex coronary artery are visible, with collateral circulation from the third marginal artery to the occluded left anterior descending artery. C, The right coronary artery inscribes a C into the left anterior oblique view as seen here. The artery distal to the posterior descending is well visualized. (From Ochsner, J. L., and Mills, N. L.: Coronary Artery Surgery. Philadelphia, Lea & Febiger, 1978.)

that is quite unpleasant. Exercise usually accentuates the symptoms as do emotional disturbances.

The results of physical examination are unremarkable. The electrocardiogram (ECG) at rest is normal in approximately half the patients. Changes include the presence of an inverted T wave, especially ST segment and T wave changes that occur during the course of an anginal episode. ST segment depression is a particularly reliable sign and, if not present at rest, may be elicited by an exercise stress test. Exercise electrocardiography is quite useful, but false-negative responses occur in patients with clinically suspected coronary disease. Contrariwise, *false-positive* responses are frequent in asymptomatic patients.[3]

Radionuclide angiocardiography is useful in the evaluation of coronary artery disease. Both thallium perfusion scintigraphy and radionuclide measurements of ventricular function during rest and exercise contribute considerably to the diagnosis and severity of myocardial ischemia. Patients with a normal thallium-201 study have been shown to have an excellent prognosis in contrast to those with multiple severe defects who have a high incidence of untoward cardiac events.[4, 13] It has been clearly demonstrated in a large number of patients treated medically for coronary disease that the exercise ejection fraction is an important variable in predicting ultimate survival as well as freedom from myocardial infarction.[36] Patients with an ejection fraction greater than 50 per cent during exercise had a low incidence of either myocardial infarction or death. Complications as well as death were more likely to occur in those patients with an exercise ejection fraction less than 50 per cent.

TABLE 1. Normal Hemodynamic Values (Recumbent Adults)*

Pressure Site	Systolic (mm. Hg)	Diastolic (mm. Hg)	Mean (mm. Hg)
Right atrium	—	—	0–8
Right ventricle	5–30	0–8	—
Pulmonary artery	15–30	5–15	10–18
Pulmonary artery wedge	—	—	1–12
Left ventricle	90–140	2–12	—
Aorta	90–140	60–90	70–105

Fick Cardiac Output Parameter	Normal Range
AV O$_2$ difference	3.0–5.5 vol.%†
O$_2$ consumption	140–390 ml./min.
O$_2$ consumption index	110–150 ml./min./m.^{2}
Cardiac output	3.5–8.5 L./min.
Cardiac index	2.5–4.5 L./min./m.^{2}

*From Mark, D. B., Califf, R. M., Stack, R. S., and Phillips, H. R.: Cardiac catheterization. *In* Sabiston, D. C., Jr. (Ed.): Textbook of Surgery, 13th ed. Philadelphia, W. B. Saunders Company, 1986.

†To convert to milliliters per liter, multiply by 10.

Abbreviation: AV = Arteriovenous.

Development of a new multicrystal camera (Scinticor) makes possible the acquisition of multiple simultaneous views of the heart during a single radionuclide transit. It is an astonishing instrument, is quite compact, achieves count rates greater than 800,000 counts per second, and can portray several different views during a single period of exercise.[23] This is a portable instrument and can be used to determine pulmonary blood flow as well. A study of single-pass radionuclide angiocardiography before and after coronary artery bypass grafting (CABG) shows the positive effect of the grafts on relief of myocardial ischemia (Fig. 6).[26]

In assessing ventricular function, hemodynamic values are of considerable importance and normal values are listed in Table 1.[32]

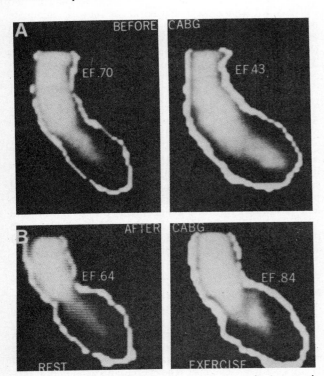

Figure 6. End-diastolic perimeters and end-systolic image obtained in a patient with myocardial ischemia at rest and during exercise before (A) and after (B) bypass grafting to three coronary arteries. The typical ischemic response to exercise with cardiac dilatation and a decrease in ejection fractions from 0.70 and 0.43 is abolished by successful revascularization, which improved left ventricular function during exercise. (From Jones, R. H., Rerych, S. K., Newman, G. E., et al.: World J. Surg., 2:811, 1978.)

CANDIDATES FOR SURGICAL THERAPY

Many patients with chronic stable myocardial ischemia can be managed by appropriate pharmacologic therapy including nitroglycerin, beta-blockers, and calcium antagonists. The decision to perform operation is made jointly by the cardiologist and the cardiac surgeon and is based primarily on the patient's symptoms, severity of the coronary lesions on coronary arteriography, and the status of left ventricular performance. In addition, the patient's wishes must frequently be respected as some individuals want to proceed immediately to operative therapy to avoid prolonged pharmacologic therapy as well as to prevent anxiety concerning an unheralded acute myocardial infarction. In general, medical therapy is recommended for single vessel disease if longevity is the primary consideration.[5, 30] However, there are definite indications for operating on single vessel disease and such surgery frequently entails coronary balloon angioplasty. In general, revascularization is recommended for patients with double and triple coronary arterial involvement, including all those with *left main* coronary artery lesions. The latter are particularly significant and affected patients are often considered to be urgently in need of operation because of the poor and unpredictable prognosis. Much evidence now indicates that CABG increases longevity as well as providing distinct symptomatic improvement.[24]

Patients with *unstable* angina characterized by progressive ischemic chest pain of sufficient severity to cause the presence of acute myocardial infarction, particularly if initiated at rest, usually have associated transient ECG changes. Thus, if beta-blocking agents, intravenous nitrates, the calcium channel-blocking agents are not successful, cardiac catheterization should be done forthwith to determine suitability for either balloon angioplasty or CABG. The National Institutes of Health cooperative study of patients with unstable angina showed that management was far from ideal in those patients randomly assigned to medical treatment because many subsequently required surgery.[42]

In the recent past, increased attention was given to patients with *acute evolving myocardial infarction* because they are often in urgent need of myocardial revascularization. This can be first achieved by coronary catheterization and angiography together with thrombolytic therapy, followed by a coronary balloon angioplasty. If these are not successful, immediate CABG should be performed. Improvements in coronary balloon angioplasty have increased the success rate of this approach in management of such patients. The surgical mortality in these patients with acute evolving myocardial infarction is now quite satisfactory unless the patient has experienced a period of prolonged cardiogenic shock.[35]

MYOCARDIAL METABOLISM

The heart is the most metabolically active of any organ in the body. Its oxygen consumption is great, approximately 80 ml. per 100 gm. of heart per minute.[41] The oxygen consumption of other organs of the body is depicted in Figure 7.[15] The average coronary arteriovenous difference is approximately 11 ml. per 100 ml. of blood (range 10.3 to 12.5 ml.).[15] The coronary venous P_{O_2} is in the range of 20 mm. Hg. These data clearly emphasize the high oxygen utilization of the myocardium. It is interesting that maximal blood flow in coronary arteries occurs in *diastole* because ventricular systole *impedes* coronary flow and decreases it by muscular contraction of the ventricle. The factors that control coronary blood flow are depicted in Figure 8,[15] and a more complete description of coronary blood flow physiology is provided elsewhere.[44]

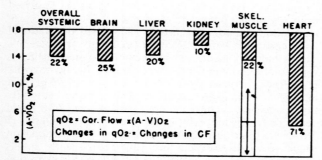

Figure 7. Systemic and regional arteriovenous oxygen extraction. qO_2 = Oxygen consumption per minute. Exercising skeletal muscle extracts an increasing but varying amount of oxygen during effort (arrow). Oxygen extraction by cardiac muscle remains relatively constant and exceeds that of other organs. (From Gorlin, R.: Br. Heart J. (Suppl.) 33:9, 1971.)

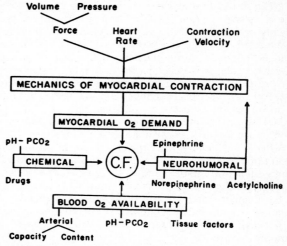

Figure 8. Factors regulating coronary flow (C.F.) These factors can be subdivided into those affecting myocardial oxygen requirements (above), those affecting oxygen availability per unit flow (below), and those acting directly on the arteriole. Neurohumoral factors can affect coronary flow not only through primary vasomotion but also through altered oxygen demand. Likewise, pH can affect both arteriolar resistance and oxygen availability. (From Gorlin, R.: Br. Heart J. (Suppl.) 33:9, 1971.)

It has long been recognized that the heart has a limited capacity for *anaerobic* metabolism. If there is adequate oxygen, glucose is converted to pyruvate with production of adenosine triphosphate (ATP) in the tricarboxylic acid (Krebs') cycle. Lactate is converted to pyruvate and oxidative phosphorylation of the latter is greatly slowed with reduced oxygen supply.

SURGICAL APPROACHES

For years surgeons have directed considerable attention toward revascularization of the myocardium. However, it was not until the introduction of CABG in 1962 that a successful means of increasing coronary blood flow could be achieved[43] (Fig. 9). Much credit must be given Johnson[25] and Favaloro[11] for their independent efforts in the late 1960s in making CABG a popular and much practiced procedure. Specfic details of the development of surgical approaches to myocardial ischemia are available.[43]

PERCUTANEOUS TRANSLUMINAL CORONARY ANGIOPLASTY

In 1977, Gruntzig was the first to perform percutaneous coronary angioplasty (PTCA) successfully.[18] Since then the role of PTCA has increased dramatically in the management of myocardial ischemia. The percutaneous femoral approach is usually used and several coronary arteriogram views are obtained after passage of the catheter into the coronary orifice. The balloon catheter is then advanced along the guiding catheter, with the latter directed across the area of stenosis and into the distal coronary artery. Contrast injections through the guiding wire confirm the location. When the guide wire is placed, the balloon cath-

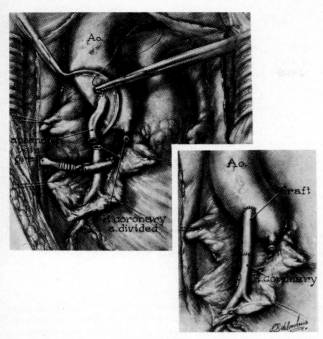

Figure 9. Illustration of use of the first saphenous vein autograft anastomosed from the ascending aorta to the right coronary artery for proximal coronary arterial occlusion in 1962. (From Sabiston, D. C., Jr.: Johns Hopkins Med. J., 134:314, 1974.)

TABLE 2. Composition of Modified St. Thomas' Cardioplegic Solution*†

Constituent	Concentration
Sodium chloride	110.0 mM./liter
Potassium chloride	16.0 mM./liter
Magnesium chloride	16.0 mM./liter
Calcium chloride	1.2 mM./liter
Sodium bicarbonate	10.0 mM./liter
Procainamide	50.0 mg./liter
Sodium heparin	1000.0 U/liter
Human serum albumin	12.5 gm./liter

*From Sabiston, D. C., Jr.: The coronary circulation. *In* Sabiston, D. C., Jr. (Ed.): Textbook of Surgery, 13th ed. W. B. Saunders Company, 1986.

†Obtained as Plegisol from Abbott Laboratories, Inc.

eter is passed over it until radiopaque markers on the balloon are seen in appropriate position at the site of stenosis. The balloon is then inflated with radiopaque contrast media to a pressure of 4 to 10 atmospheres for 20 to 60 seconds to dilate the artery. Successful dilatation is defined by the National Heart, Lung and Blood Institute Registry as a *20 per cent increase in luminal diameter*. Although major complications can occur with this technique, they have become infrequent as experience has been gained. Serious problems include death (usually less than 1 per cent), nonfatal myocardial infarction (5 per cent), and the need for emergency CABG (5 to 6 per cent). In addition, intracoronary *thrombolysis* can be achieved by the administration of appropriate enzymes when demonstrable thrombi are present in the coronary arteries. This technique has been successful, especially since the introduction recently of tissue plasminogen activator (TPA), which has greatly reduced the toxic reactions to enzymatic therapy.[14] This is a recombinant human tissue–type plasminogen activator, which largely eliminates problems associated with hypersensitivity.

MYOCARDIAL PROTECTION

J. Scott Rankin, M.D. ● David C. Sabiston, Jr., M.D.

The sharp reduction in surgical mortality for coronary artery bypass grafts has been the result of many advances, including those in technique, anesthesia, cardiac pharmacologic agents, and monitoring. However, the improvement generally regarded as the most important has been in myocardial protection during the period of ischemia needed to perform the best technical coronary arterial anastomoses in a bloodless field. This has been primarily due to the use of topical hypothermia and potassium cardioplegia. In addition, generalized hypothermia is used in most patients, reducing the total body temperature to approximately 24 to 28°C. Topical hypothermia is perhaps the most important single aspect of preservation because it greatly reduces myocardial metabolism (when the temperature is in the range of 8 to 10°C.) for the entire period of ischemia. The potassium cardioplegic solution varies with individual preference but generally contains 16 to 30 mEq. of potassium per liter and additional components are often added. One commercially available solution is St. Thomas' solution (Table 2). An initial injection into the root of the aorta with the distal aorta occluded such that the cardioplegic solution enters the coronary arteries is given in the amount of approximately 1200 ml., with additional 200 to 300 ml. being administered every 30 to 45 minutes while the heart is ischemic. During this period the heart is kept cold by introduction of topical cold saline or ice slush temperature in the range of 4°C. The purpose of the potassium is to place the heart in complete diastolic arrest such that all myocardial fibers are relaxed with no work being done and with minimal oxygen being consumed at this low temperature.

CORONARY ARTERY BYPASS GRAFT

Preoperative Preparation

The goals and general principles of the operation as well as the common or serious complications should be explained to the patient and family prior to operation. Aspirin should be discontinued for approximately 2 weeks prior to operation to prevent bleeding. Dipyridamole is administered preoperatively and, together with aspirin, is given postoperatively to improve the patency of the bypass grafts.[8] Most agents being administered for angina pectoris, including beta-blockers, calcium-blockers, isosorbide dinitrate, and nitroglycerin, should be continued until the time of operation. If further medication is needed, intravenous infusion of nitroglycerin can be helpful.

Surgical Procedures

The obstructed coronary arteries are generally bypassed with a combination of internal mammary artery grafts and reversed saphenous vein grafts. The procedure is conducted with extracorporeal circulation and cold potassium cardioplegia. In general, those coronary arteries with a luminal diameter of 1.5 mm. or greater and have a

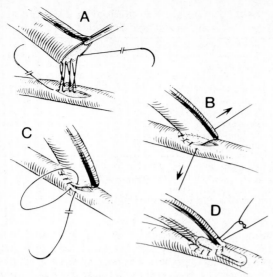

Figure 10. *A standard method for distal vein graft anastomosis using a running suture technique. (From Sabiston, D. C., Jr.: The coronary circulation. In Sabiston, D. C., Jr. (Ed.): Textbook of Surgery, 13th ed. Philadelphia, W. B. Saunders Company, 1986.)*

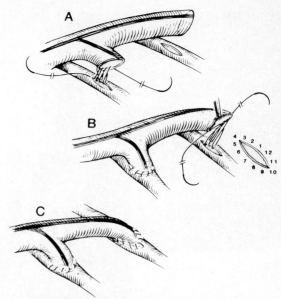

Figure 12. *A method for performing natural Y sequential vein grafts. (From Sabiston, D. C., Jr.: The coronary circulation. In Sabiston, D. C., Jr. (Ed.): Textbook of Surgery, 13th ed. Philadelphia, W. B. Saunders Company, 1986.)*

more than 50 per cent stenotic lesion are selected for bypass. If a major vessel appears to be completely occluded on the arteriogram, it may not necessarily be occluded at the time of operation and may be explored for the possibility of a lumen. In general, an average of four grafts are currently being placed in each patient undergoing revascularization. Quite clearly, the internal mammary artery graft is preferred because of its superiority in long-term patency. Recent evidence indicates that the 10-year patency of internal mammary artery grafts is approximately 85 per cent or more, whereas the saphenous vein bypass grafts are patent at 10 years in approximately 40 per cent. Therefore,

a combination of these two grafts is usually done. Bilateral mammary dissection is often performed and sequential anastomoses with the internal mammary arteries are achievable. This technique can also be used with saphenous vein grafts. The standard method for saphenous graft anastomosis is depicted in Figure 10. The method for a proximal anastomosis of the saphenous vein is shown in Figure 11. In addition, Y sequential grafts can be placed by using branches of veins as depicted in Figure 12. A method for sequential vein graft anastomosis using the diamond technique is depicted in Figure 13.

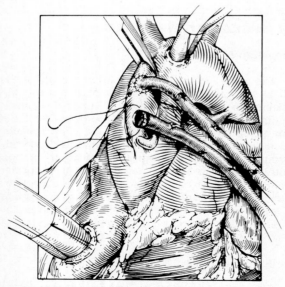

Figure 11. *Method for performing proximal saphenous vein anastomoses to the aorta. A portion of the aorta is excluded using a partial occlusion clamp, and the vein grafts are anastomosed to circular aortotomies with running 6-0 polypropylene sutures. (Modified from Ochsner, J. L., and Mills, N. L.: Coronary Artery Surgery. Philadelphia, Lea & Febiger, 1978.)*

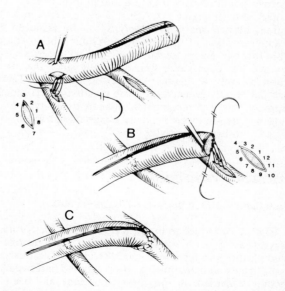

Figure 13. *A method for sequential vein graft anastomoses using the diamond technique. (From Sabiston, D. C., Jr.: The coronary circulation. In Sabiston, D. C., Jr. (Ed.): Textbook of Surgery, 13th ed. Philadelphia, W. B. Saunders Company, 1986.)*

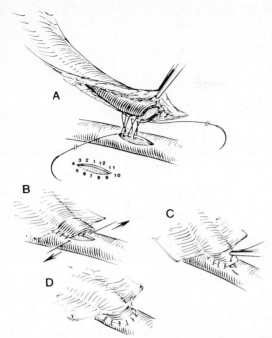

Figure 14. A running suture technique for constructing distal internal mammary artery anastomoses. (From Sabiston, D. C., Jr.: The coronary circulation. In Sabiston, D. C., Jr. (Ed.): Textbook of Surgery, 13th ed. Philadelphia, W. B. Saunders Company, 1986.)

In most patients, both internal mammary arteries can be used for grafts and these are dissected with wide pedicles with electrocautery from the chest wall. Spasm can be prevented by topical application of papaverine. The distal anastomoses are particularly important and demand meticulous technique (as depicted in Figure 14 for construction of an internal mammary artery–to–coronary artery anastomosis). A method for performing sequential internal mammary bypass grafts is shown in Figure 15. The success of these anastomoses is indicated by an *in situ* left internal mammary arteriogram (Fig. 16). Increased attention is focused on the use of the internal mammary arteries in view of their marked superiority for long-term patency.[31, 37, 38, 46]

Using appropriate techniques, the operative mortality for elective CABG is generally 1 to 2 per cent and in some series is less. For emergency CABG or in those patients with cardiac lesions in addition to coronary stenosis, the mortality is higher.

Postoperative Management

Careful assessment of each postoperative patient following CABG is essential. Precipitous changes may occur that require instant correction and therefore all patients should be placed in a special care unit with the constant attendance of skilled personnel. This factor has allowed the most severely ill to be selected for surgical therapy. Careful monitoring of a variety of parameters, including systemic arterial pressure, venous pressure, continuous ECG, urinary output, appropriate determinations of Po_2, Pco_2, and pH, is important. Cardiac function should be repeatedly assessed in those patients requiring it with measurements of cardiac output and registration of pulmonary capillary wedge pressure. These can be provided by a thermodilution Swan-Ganz catheter, which is left in place in all seriously

ill patients. Body weight is another excellent predictor of fluid loss or overload and should be determined daily.

A serious postoperative complication is *low cardiac output* which is generally seen in patients with poor left ventricular function. This is a preoperative problem and/or a result of inadequate myocardial protection during operation. Incidence of this complication has been greatly reduced with the advent of topical hypothermia and potassium cardioplegia.

The aortic pressure may need manipulation in the event of persistent low cardiac output despite adequate filling pressure. Thus, a continuous infusion of sodium nitroprusside provides a safe and reproducible afterload reduction because it acts directly on vascular smooth muscle to produce vasodilatation independent of the sympathetic nervous system. Infusion rates up to 10 μg. per kg. per minute may be used to reduce the aortic pressure to an optimal level. In the presence of a continuing low cardiac index, dopamine has become increasingly important in treatment because it enhances myocardial contractility and has a minimal effect on heart rate. Moreover, it tends to produce less cardiac irritability and increases renal blood flow. This agent may be continuously administered intravenously at rates of 5 to 20 μg. per kg. per minute. Epinephrine can be effective, but must be used carefully because it causes peripheral vasoconstriction and increased ventricular irritability. It should be used cautiously in continuous intravenous doses of 0.03 to 0.12 μg. per kg. per minute.

Cardiac tamponade is another postoperative complication that must be carefully monitored. The characteristic findings include low cardiac output, elevated central venous pressure, and low arterial pressure. The chest film may show a wide mediastinal shadow and an echocardiogram

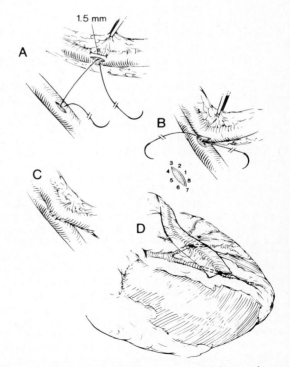

Figure 15. A method for performing sequential internal mammary bypass grafts. (From Sabiston, D. C., Jr.: The coronary circulation. In Sabiston, D. C., Jr. (Ed.): Textbook of Surgery, 13th ed. Philadelphia, W. B. Saunders Company, 1986.)

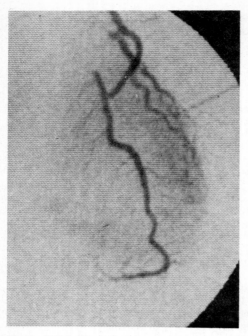

Figure 16. A digital subtraction arteriogram of an in situ *left internal mammary graft to the diagonal and left anterior descending coronary arteries. (From Sabiston, D. C., Jr.: The coronary circulation.* In *Sabiston, D. C., Jr. (Ed.): Textbook of Surgery, 13th ed. W. B. Saunders Company, 1986.)*

may show the clot around the heart. If blood loss continues from chest tubes at 100 ml. an hour or more for a period of 5 hours, reoperation and evacuation of the blood and clots should be considered. If the low cardiac output syndrome persists despite all standard therapy, the insertion of an intra-aortic balloon pump should be considered and can be lifesaving.[28]

Congestive heart failure may cause low cardiac output, particularly in patients with poor ventricular function, and may necessitate the use of appropriate diuretics such as furosemide and ethacrynic acid. The resulting diuresis is associated frequently with urinary losses of potassium, sodium, chloride, and ammonium ions and requires close surveillance and replacement. In this situation, digoxin is usually indicated and administered (0.5 mg. intravenously). It should be effective within 30 to 60 minutes and the initial dose should be followed by 0.25 mg. intravenously at 3- to 4-hour intervals over approximately 9 to 12 hours.

Dysrhythmias are common following cardiac surgical procedures, and sinus tachycardia is the most frequent, being caused by hypovolemia, congestive heart failure, anxiety, and fever. Therapy is directed toward the inciting cause. *Atrial dysrhythmias* are also common; the most frequent are atrial premature beats, which are seldom of clinical significance. However, if troublesome, they respond to administration of propranolol. Atrial flutter, the more significant dysrhythmia, can be controlled by quinidine, procainamide, or verapamil. Temporary pacing wires are generally applied at operation and atrial flutter can easily be diagnosed and often converted to sinus rhythm by pacing the atrium at rates of 300 to 350 beats per minute until the atrium is captured.[48] Intravenous procainamide also is likely to be effective. *Paroxysmal atrial tachycardia* can usually be converted by massage of the carotid sinus with a return to sinus rhythm. If this fails, intravenous edrophonium chloride (Tensilon) should be administered (5 to 10 mg.).

Rapid intravenous digoxin or verapamil infusion is also likely to be successful. If all other methods fail, electrical cardioversion can be performed. *Nodal rhythms* are among the most serious and difficult therapeutic problems among the postoperative dysrhythmias. They may signify myocardial injury or digitalis toxicity and it is essential to eliminate any underlying causes such as acidosis, hypoxemia, and hypokalemia.

Lidocaine or propranolol can be successful in controlling the *tachycardia*. Electrocardioversion is usually hazardous, especially in the presence of excess digitalis. If the dysrhythmia produces hemodynamic problems, atrial capture by an atrial pacemaker with gradual reduction of the pacing rate to a level sufficient to suppress the nodal ectopic pacemaker is indicated. Ordinarily, both atrial and ventricular pacing wires would have been left in place at the time of operation, and it is possible to perform temporary AV sequential pacing as a nodal rhythm develops. This provides an atrial contribution to cardiac output, which appears to be particularly helpful in the immediate postoperative period.

Premature ventricular contractions (PVCs) occur frequently following operation and generally are of little consequence unless they occur at rates of more than three or four per minute. Multifocal beats, coupled beats, and ectopic beats that occur near the peak of the T waves of the preceding QRS complex are more dangerous. PVCs have many predisposing factors, including acidosis, hypokalemia, hypoxemia, and myocardial ischemia. It has been noted that inadequate positioning of the tip of a Swan-Ganz monitoring catheter can be a cause; if the tip is just beyond the pulmonary valve, the right bundle is often stimulated, resulting in PVCs. Floating the catheter tip into correct position in the right pulmonary artery causes disappearance of the rhythm. If the arrhythmia persists, lidocaine should be administered (100 mg. initially, followed by continuous intravenous infusion of 1 to 4 mg. per minute). If this is unsuccessful, procainamide, bretylium tosylate, propranolol, disopyramide, or quinidine may be useful in suppressing ectopic activity.

Ventricular tachycardia is a serious arrhythmia and should be treated immediately with intravenous lidocaine (100 mg.). If the blood pressure cannot be maintained, external cardiac massage should be instituted and plans made for immediate tracheal intubation and attachment to mechanical ventilation with 100 per cent oxygen. At this point, electrocardioversion is in order and is usually successful in converting the ventricular tachycardia.

Postoperative hypertension is much more frequent in current practice owing in large part to better myocardial preservation. This allows the catecholamines, which are secreted in greater than normal amounts postoperatively, to act on a relatively normal myocardium and therefore produce hypertension This complication is best managed by judicious administration of nitroprusside intravenously.

Perioperative myocardial infarction is a complication that occurs in 3 to 5 per cent of patients and can be responsible for hypotension and cardiac conduction defects. Generally such infarcts are limited and do not cause serious problems. Moreover, many would not be recognized were it not for changes occurring in routine electrocardiograms as they are usually accompanied by minimal if any clinical manifestations. However, quite significant infarction *can* occur, especially in the presence of graft occlusion.

Respiratory insufficiency following many CABG procedures should be observed carefully and appropriate respiratory assistance should be given when indicated.

Postoperative infections such as pneumonitis, wound infection, urinary tract infection, and mediastinitis should be borne in mind. Bacterial endocarditis is a serious problem, particularly with valve replacement, but fortunately is quite rare. Prophylactic antibiotics, such as cephalosporin (1 gm. every 6 hours), are generally administered just before and for 2 to 5 days after cardiac surgical procedures.

One of the most serious complications of CABG is *postoperative mediastinitis*, which occurs in about 1 per cent of patients. Formerly this infection was often fatal, but increased diagnostic sensitivity and institution of appropriate treatment either by open drainage or by catheter instillation of antibiotics have reduced the morbidity and mortality. If conservative measures are not successful, the assistance of a plastic surgeon in rotating various flaps to the mediastinum after it has been widely opened and drained has been quite successful.[27]

Pericarditis is a frequent postoperative complication and is manifested by chest pain, fever, and tachycardia. Dysrhythmias also accompany this complication. In general, pericarditis responds to dexamethasone (5 mg. intravenously) followed by oral indomethacin for 10 days with tapering toward the end. If this is ineffective, oral corticosteroids (prednisone) can be given on a tapering schedule.

Finally, *psychiatric disorders* including delirium following cardiopulmonary bypass occur but seem less common after CABG than after other cardiac procedures. In many instances, the original cardiac status together with the severity of the physical illness and complexity of the procedure combine to be influential factors in the pathogenesis of the postcardiotomy delirium.[9]

Results

Following CABG, complete relief of pain occurs in more than two thirds of all patients and the remainder have only minor discomfort usually requiring minimal medication.

It has now been thoroughly established that changes in ventricular performance can be demonstrated with improved myocardial contractility. Left ventricular function is more effective and cardiac output is greater, with decreased diastolic volume and improved left ventricular wall motion. Each of these has been demonstrated postoperatively.[39, 40] Moreover, these improvements in ventricular function have been shown as early as 1 week postoperatively by exercise using single-pass radioisotope angiocardiography.[1]

Further confirmation of the improvement in ventricular function following operation is shown by the postoperative changes that occur in the ECG. The stress test, frequently used to assess the status of ventricular performance, shows positive changes and improvement in more than two thirds of patients, with conversion of the preoperative ischemic exercise ECG test results to normal.

It should be emphasized to all patients that the progression of coronary atherosclerosis *continues* after CABG because the operation does not *prevent* the pathogenesis of the basic disease. Thus, patients should be urged to cease smoking, to maintain normal weight, and to remain on an appropriate diet.

The patency of the bypass grafts has been a subject of considerable interest. In one series, a 2-week patency rate was 92 per cent and a 1-year patency was 86 per cent with an attrition rate of later closure at 2 per cent annually, which was probably in the range of most series.[6, 7] However, intimal fibrosis occurs in vein grafts and may cause late obstruction[6] as well as fibrous endarteritis.[47] In a recent study, saphenous vein patency at 10 years was 53 per cent, whereas internal mammary artery (IMA) patency in the same series was 84 per cent.[17] In addition, of the patent vein grafts, 44 per cent exhibited gross atherosclerotic lesions. These are nearly always in saphenous vein grafts, whereas they rarely occur in internal mammary artery grafts. In a recent series of 207 patients, an overall postoperative graft patency of 94 per cent was found in the first postoperative year utilizing the techniques for the anastomosis illustrated in this chapter. There were 841 total grafts (503 vein grafts and 338 IMA grafts) with 91 per cent vein patency rate and 99 per cent IMA patency.[38] Thus, IMA grafts are preferred whenever possible. Several studies indicate that the incidence of myocardial infarction and return of angina is significantly reduced following CABG.[19, 29] Thus, positive effects of operation are now achieved in the vast majority of patients, including relief of anginal pain, improvement in ventricular function, a high patency rate in the grafts (especially in the IMA grafts), and a reduced incidence of recurrent myocardial infarction.

SELECTED REFERENCES

Blumgart, H. L., Schlesinger, M. J., and David, D.: Studies on the relation of clinical manifestations of angina pectoris, coronary thrombosis and myocardial infarction to the pathologic findings with particular reference to significance of collateral circulation. Am. Heart J., *19*:1, 1940.
   A classic reference describing the site and incidence of occlusions of the coronary circulation owing to atherosclerotic lesions.

Herrick, J. B.: Clinical features of sudden obstruction of the coronary arteries. J.A.M.A., *59*:2015, 1912.
   The first report of a premortem diagnosis of coronary occlusion. In this patient a severe left coronary lesion was accompanied by a thrombus producing an acute myocardial infarction. This article is a classic.

Jurkiewicz, M. J., Bostwick, J., III, Hester, T. R., Bishop, J. B., and Craven, J.: Infected median sternotomy wound—successful treatment by muscle flaps. Ann. Surg., *190*:738, 1980.
   A key reference on the management of mediastinitis by muscle flaps. The use of this technique has made a considerable difference in the mortality in a number of patients with this serious complication.

Rerych, S. K., Scholz, P. M., Newman, G. E., Sabiston, D. C., Jr., and Jones, R. H.: Cardiac function at rest and during exercise in normals and in patients with coronary heart disease: Evaluation by radionuclide angiocardiography. Ann. Surg., *187*:449, 1978.
   This article concerns the response of the heart to exercise in normal patients and in those with coronary artery disease. In this paper the highest recorded cardiac output ever demonstrated is discussed. The patient, a world-class athlete who was a Silver Medalist in the Montreal Olympics, had a cardiac output of 57 liters per minute during peak exercise.

Sabiston, D. C., Jr.: The coronary circulation. The William F. Rienhoff, Jr. Lecture. Johns Hopkins Med. J., *134*:314, 1974.
   Physiologic aspects of the coronary circulation, together with a description of the first use of a saphenous vein for a coronary bypass, are reviewed.

REFERENCES

1. Austin, E. H., Oldham, H. N., Jr., Sabiston, D. C., Jr., and Jones, R. H.: Early assessment of rest and exercise left ventricular function following coronary artery surgery. Ann. Thorac. Surg., *35*:159, 1983.
2. Blumgart, H. L., Pitt, B., Zoll, P. M., and Freiman, D. G.: Anatomic factors influencing the location of coronary occlusions and development of collateral coronary circulation (Henry Ford Hospital International Symposium). *In* James, T. N., and Keyes, J. W. (Eds.): The Etiology of Myocardial Infarction. Boston, Little, Brown & Company, 1963.
3. Borer, J. S., Brensike, J. F., Redwood, D. R., Itscoitz, S. B., Passamani, E. R., Stone, N. J., Richardson, J. M., Levy, R. I., and Epstein, S. E.: Limitations of the electrocardiographic response to

exercise in predicting coronary-artery disease. N. Engl. J. Med., *293*:367, 1975.

4. Brown, K. A., Boucher, C. A., Okada, R. D., Newell, J., Strauss, H. W., and Pohost, G. M.: The prognostic value of serial exercise thallium-201 imaging in patients presenting for evaluation of chest pain: Comparison to contrast angiography, exercise electrocardiography and clinical data. Am. J. Cardiol., *49*:967, 1981.

5. Califf, R. M., Tomabechi, Y., Lee, K. L., Phillips, H. R., Pryor, D. B., Harrell, F. E., Jr., Harris, P. J., Peter, R. H., Behar, V. S., Kong, Y. S., and Rosati, R. A.: Outcome in one-vessel coronary artery disease. Circulation, *67*:283, 1983.

6. Campeau, L., Crochet, D., Lesperance, J., Bourassa, M. G., and Grondin, C. M.: Postoperative changes in aortocoronary saphenous vein grafts revisited. Angiographic studies at two weeks and at one year in two series of consecutive patients. Circulation, *52*:369, 1975.

7. Campeau, L., Lesperance, J., Corbara, F., Hermann, J., Grondin, C. M., and Bourassa, M. G.: Aortocoronary saphenous vein bypass graft changes 5–7 years after surgery. Circulation, *58*(Suppl. 1):170, 1978.

8. Chesebro, J. H., Fuster, V., Elveback, L. R., et al.: Effect of dipyridamole and aspirin on late vein-graft patency after coronary bypass operations. N. Engl. J. Med., *310*:209, 1984.

9. Dubin, W. R., Field, H. L., and Gasfriend, D. R.: Postcardiotomy delirium: A critical review. J. Thorac. Cardiovasc. Surg., *77*:586, 1979.

10. Enos, W. F., Holmes, R. H., and Beyer, J.: Coronary disease among United States soldiers killed in action in Korea. Preliminary report. J.A.M.A., *152*:1090, 1953.

11. Favaloro, R. G., Effler, D. B., and Groves, L. K.: Severe segmental obstruction of the left main coronary artery and its divisions: Surgical treatment by the saphenous vein graft technic. J. Thorac. Cardiovasc. Surg., *60*:469, 1970.

12. Franch, R. H., et al.: Techniques of cardiac catheterization including coronary arteriography. *In* Hurst, J. W. (Ed.): The Heart, 5th ed. New York, McGraw-Hill Book Company, 1982.

13. Gibson, R. S., Watson, D. D., Craddock, G. B., Crampton, R. S., Kaiser, D. L., Denny, M. J., and Beller, G. A.: Prediction of cardiac events after uncomplicated myocardial infarction: A prospective study comparing predischarge exercise thallium-201 scintigraphy and coronary angiography. Circulation, *68*:321, 1983.

14. Gold, H. K., Fallon, J. T., Yasuda, T., Leinbach, R. C., Khaw, B. A., Newell, B. A., Guerrero, J. L., Vislosky, F. M., Hoyng, C. F., Grossbard, E., and Collen, D.: Coronary thrombolysis with recombinant human tissue–type plasminogen activator. Circulation, *70*:700, 1984.

15. Gorlin, R.: Regulation of coronary blood flow. Br. Heart J., *33*:9, 1971.

16. Grondin, C. M., Meere, C., Castonguay, Y., Lepage, G., and Grondin, P.: Progressive and late obstruction of an aortocoronary venous bypass graft. Circulation, *43*:689, 1971.

17. Grondin, C. M., Campeau, L., Lesperance, J., Enjalbert, M., and Bourassa, M. G.: Comparison of late changes in internal mammary artery and saphenous vein grafts in two consecutive series of patients 10 years after operation. Circulation, *70* (Suppl. 1):I-208, 1984.

18. Gruntzig, A.: Transluminal dilatation of coronary-artery stenosis. Lancet, *1*:263, 1978.

19. Hammermeister, K. E., DeRouen, R. A., and Dodge, H. T.: Variables predictive of survival in patients with coronary disease. Selection by univariate and multivariate analyses from the clinical, electrocardiographic, exercise, arteriographic, and quantitative angiographic evaluations. Circulation, *59*:421, 1979.

20. Harris, P. J., Behar, V. S., Conley, M. J., Harrell, F. E., Lee, K. L., Peter, R. H., Kong, Y., and Rosati, R. A.: The prognostic significance of 50% coronary stenosis in medically treated patients with coronary artery disease. Circulation, *62*:240, 1980.

21. Herman, M. V., et al.: Pathophysiology of ischemic heart disease. *In* Levine, H. J. (Ed.): Clinical Cardiovascular Physiology. New York, Grune & Stratton, 1976.

22. Herrick, J. B.: Clinical features of sudden obstruction of the coronary arteries. J.A.M.A., *59*:2015, 1912.

23. Heyda, D. W., and Jones, R. H.: A new digital gamma camera. (Abstract) J. Nucl. Med., *25*:P22, 1984.

24. Hurst, J. W., King, S. B., III, Logue, R. B., Hatcher, C. R., et al.: Value of coronary bypass surgery. Controversies in cardiology: Part 1. Am. J. Cardiol., *42*:308, 1978.

25. Johnson, W. D., Flemma, R. J., Lepley, D., Jr., and Ellison, E. H.: Extended treatment of severe coronary artery disease: A total surgical approach. Ann. Surg., *170*:460, 1969.

26. Jones, R. H., Rerych, S. K., Newman, G. E., Scholz, P. M., Howe, R., Oldham, H. N., Goodrich, J. K., and Sabiston, D. C., Jr.: Noninvasive radionuclide procedures for diagnosis and management of myocardial ischemia. World J. Surg., *2*:811, 1978.

27. Jurkiewicz, M. J., Bostwick, J., III, Hester, T. R., Bishop, J. B., and Craven, J.: Infected median sternotomy wound—successful treatment by muscle flaps. Ann. Surg., *191*:738, 1980.

28. Kaiser, G. C., Marco, J. D., Barner, H. B., Codd, J. E., Laks, H., and Willman, V. L.: Intraaortic balloon assistance. Ann. Thorac. Surg., *21*:487, 1976.

29. Kloster, F. E., Kremakau, E. L., Ritzmann, L. W., Rahimtoola, S. H., Rosch, J., and Kanarek, P. H.: Coronary bypass for stable angina—a prospective randomized study. N. Engl. J. Med., *300*:149, 1979.

30. Kouchoukos, N. T., Oberman, A., Russell, R. O., Jr., and Jones, W. B.: Surgical versus medical treatment of occlusive disease confined to the left anterior descending coronary artery. Am. J. Cardiol., *35*:836, 1975.

31. Lytle, B. W., Cosgrove, D. M., Saltus, G. L., Taylor, P. C., and Loop, F. D.: Multivessel coronary revascularization without saphenous vein: Long-term results of bilateral internal mammary artery grafting. Ann. Thorac. Surg., *36*:542, 1983.

32. Mark, D. B., Califf, R. L. M., Stack, R. S., and Phillips, H. R.: Cardiac catheterization. *In* Sabiston, D. C., Jr. (Ed.): Textbook of Surgery, 13th ed. Philadelphia, W. B. Saunders Company, 1986.

33. Mitchell, W.: Clinical angiographic description of the coronary artery anatomy. *In* Boucek, R. J., et al. (Eds.): Coronary Artery Disease. Baltimore, Williams & Wilkins, 1984.

34. Ochsner, J. L., and Mills, N. L.: Coronary Artery Surgery. Philadelphia, Lea & Febiger, 1978.

35. Oyamadi, A., and Queen, F. V.: Spontaneous rupture of the interventricular septum following acute myocardial infarction with some clinicopathological observations on survival in 5 cases. Presented at Pan Pacific Pathology Congress, Tripler U.S. Army Hospital, 1961.

36. Pryor, D. B., Harrell, F. E., Jr., Lee, K. L., Rosati, R. A., Coleman, R. E., Cobb, F. R., Califf, R. M., and Jones, R. H.: Prognostic indicators from radionuclide angiography in medically treated patients with coronary artery disease. Am. J. Cardiol., *53*:18, 1984.

37. Puig, L. B., Neto, F. L., Rati, M., Ramires, J. A. F., da Luz, P. L., Pileggi, F., and Jatene, A. D.: A technique of anastomosis of the right internal mammary artery to the circumflex artery and its branches. Ann. Thorac. Surg., *38*:533, 1984.

38. Rankin, J. S., Newman, G. E., Bashore, T. M., Muhlbaier, L. H., Tyson, G. S., Jr., Ferguson, T. B., Jr., Reves, J. G., and Sabiston, D. C., Jr.: Clinical and angiographic assessment of complex mammary artery bypass grafting. J. Thorac. Cardiovasc. Surg., *92*:832, 1986.

39. Rankin, J. S., Newman, G. E., Muhlbaier, L. H., Behar, V. S., Fedor, J. M., and Sabiston, D. C., Jr.: Effects of coronary revascularization on left ventricular function in ischemic heart disease. J. Thorac. Cardiovasc. Surg., *90*:818, 1985.

40. Rerych, S. K., Scholz, P. M., Newman, G. E., Sabiston, D. C., Jr., and Jones, R. H.: Cardiac function at rest and during exercise in normals and in patients with coronary heart disease: Evaluation by radionuclide angiocardiography. Ann. Surg., *187*:449, 1978.

41. Rowe, G. G., Castillo, C. A., Maxwell, G. M., and Crumpton, C. W.: Comparison of systemic and coronary hemodynamics in the normal human male and female. Circ. Res., *7*:728, 1959.

42. Russell, R. O., Jr., Resnekov, L., Wolk, M., Rosati, R. A., et al.: Unstable angina pectoris: National cooperative study group to compare surgical and medical therapy: II. In-hospital experience and initial follow-up results in patients with one, two and three vessel disease. Am. J. Cardiol., *42*:839, 1978.

43. Sabiston, D. C., Jr.: The coronary circulation. The William F. Rienhoff, Jr. Lecture. Johns Hopkins Med. J., *134*:314, 1974.

44. Sabiston, D. C., Jr. (Ed.): Textbook of Surgery, 13th ed. Philadelphia, W. B. Saunders Company, 1986.

45. Spiekerman, R. E., Brandenburg, J. T., Achor, R. W. P., and Edwards, J. E.: The spectrum of coronary artery disease in a community of 30,000. A clinico-pathologic study. Circulation, *25*:57, 1962.

46. Tector, A. J., and Schmahl, T. M.: Techniques for multiple internal mammary artery grafts. Ann. Thorac Surg., *38*:281, 1984.

47. Vlodaver, A., and Edwards, J. E.: Pathologic changes in aortic-coronary arterial saphenous vein grafts. Circulation, *44*:719, 1971.

48. Waldo, A. L., and MacLean, W. A. H.: Diagnosis and Treatment of Cardiac Arrhythmias Following Open Heart Surgery. Emphasis on the Use of Atrial and Ventricular Epicardial Wire Electrodes. Mount Kisco, N.Y., Futura Publishing Co., 1980, p. 59.

2 · VENTRICULAR ANEURYSM

ROBERT B. PEYTON, M.D.
DAVID C. SABISTON, JR., M.D.

A ventricular aneurysm is a "thinned out transmural scar that has completely lost its trabecular pattern . . . always clearly delineated from the surrounding muscle."[16]

The majority of cardiac aneurysms involve the left ventricle and are the result of myocardial infarction. However, cardiac aneurysms caused by trauma,[4] infection,[26] and congenital defects[6] have been described. The prognosis of patients with an untreated left ventricular aneurysm is poor.[20, 23, 28] With the development of successful techniques of cardiopulmonary bypass, resection of ventricular aneurysms can be accomplished with low mortality and has resulted in improved ventricular function and survival in patients with ventricular aneurysm.[15, 21, 22, 25, 30]

CLINICAL MANIFESTATIONS

Following myocardial infarction, a left ventricular aneurysm develops in 5 to 35 per cent of patients.[1, 18] Three basic pathologic phenomena occur that lead to the clinical manifestations associated with left ventricular aneurysm.

The most common symptom in patients with a ventricular aneurysm is congestive heart failure with associated angina. The infarcted ventricular muscle is replaced with fibrous tissue, causing paradoxical systolic wall motion. According to LaPlace's law, enlargement of the ventricular cavity results in greater tension at the ventricular wall. This imposes increased wall stress upon the nonaneurysmal myocardial fibers, increasing systolic shortening and thus myocardial oxygen uptake. When an aneurysm involves more than 25 per cent of the ventricular surface, myocardial fiber shortening limits are exceeded. Therefore, the ventricle dilates and stiffens, stroke volume decreases, end-diastolic pressure increases, and congestive heart failure ensues.[9, 13]

Recurrent ventricular tachycardia is a well-recognized complication in patients with ventricular aneurysm. The thin wall of a left ventricular aneurysm and the adjacent jeopardized border are composed of a mixture of viable myocardium, necrotic muscle, and fibrous tissue. The electrophysiologic properties of conduction and refractoriness in these tissues predispose these patients to re-entrant ventricular tachyarrhythmias.[9, 10, 12]

The less common symptom of systemic emboli is produced by a combination of mechanisms.[24] Stasis of blood in the ventricular aneurysm promotes thrombus formation and transmural or subendocardial infarction transforms the smooth endocardium into a microscopically rough surface that encourages formation of thrombi.[9] Despite the high prevalence of mural thrombi, clinical episodes of thromboembolism have been reported with a frequency of 5 per cent.[29]

Several physical signs, such as enlargement of transverse cardiac fullness, forceful cardiac impulse at the apex, and a ventricular gallop are indicators of left ventricular aneurysms. The chest film may show an enlargement in the area of the left ventricle, and smaller aneurysms may be undetected. Noninvasive procedures, including cardiac fluoroscopy, two-dimensional ultrasound, and radionuclide cineangiography, are helpful in identifying the presence and severity of ventricular aneurysms. The diagnosis of left ventricular aneurysm is confirmed by cineangiography, which outlines the location, the size, the presence of thrombus, and the expansile nature of the aneurysm. The majority of ventricular aneurysms are located in the apical and anterior portions of the heart. Selective coronary arteriography is always performed to assess the extent of coronary artery disease, and the left anterior descending artery is the most commonly involved coronary artery.[8]

TREATMENT

The current accepted indications for left ventricular aneurysmectomy with or without associated coronary surgery are as follows:

1. Angina in association with congestive heart failure.
2. Angina with bypassable multivessel coronary artery disease.
3. Congestive heart failure.
4. Recurrent systemic arterial emboli.
5. Ventricular tachyarrhythmias refractory to medical management.
6. Multivessel coronary artery disease and a large ventricular aneurysm in an asymptomatic patient.[19]

Rupture of a *chronic* ventricular aneurysm is rare. During the *acute* phase of an evolving infarct, ventricular rupture occurs in 10 per cent of patients dying of myocardial infarction.[31] The risk associated with surgical intervention during this phase is prohibitively high. Therefore, avoidance of possible ventricular rupture for acute and chronic left ventricular aneurysm is not routinely considered an indication for operation.

Repair of a ventricular aneurysm was first reported by Beck in 1944.[2] He attempted surgical correction by reinforcing the aneurysm with fascia lata to reduce expansile pulsation and prevent rupture. Likoff and Bailey in 1954[14] successfully resected a left ventricular aneurysm by placing a vascular clamp at its base, excising the aneurysm, and plicating the ventricle below the clamp. Cooley and associates, in 1959,[5] first resected a ventricular aneurysm using *cardiopulmonary bypass*, which is the technique used today.

The operation is performed through a midline sternotomy incision, and cardiopulmonary bypass is initiated. Delineation of the thin-walled aneurysm is facilitated by left ventricular venting via the right superior pulmonary vein. Manipulation of the heart should be done with extreme care in order to prevent dislodgment of any mural thrombi. Because simultaneous coronary revascularization and aneurysmectomy are now advocated, potassium cardioplegia and external cardiac cooling are administered at the time of the aortic cross-clamping. This not only provides a motionless, bloodless field but excellent myocardial protection.

The steps in excising the aneurysm are depicted in Figure 1. The aneurysm usually presents as an oval or elliptical "dimple," and the initial incision should be along the long axis of the aneurysmal scar.[19] The mural thrombus should be carefully and completely removed, and the aneurysmal scar can be excised, leaving a rim of fibrous tissue (5 to 10 mm.). After completion of all distal coronary anastomoses, the ventriculotomy is closed with interrupted horizontal mattress sutures through strips of Teflon placed on either side of the incision. The sutures are tied and the suture line is reinforced by a simple continuous suture. All air is evacuated from the left side of the heart, the aortic cross-clamp is removed, and the proximal coronary anastomosis is completed.[8]

RESULTS

The operative mortality for elective excision of left ventricular aneurysm is reported to be less than 10 per cent.[3, 11] In several studies symptomatic relief and improved ventricular function have occurred following left ventricular aneurysmectomy.[7, 22] Substantial progress has been made in

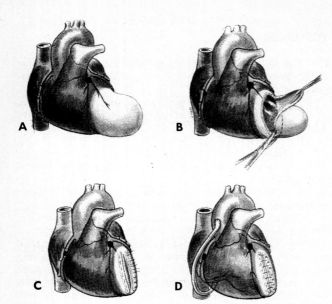

Figure 1. A, *An apical-anterior ventricular aneurysm that has resulted from occlusion of the left anterior descending coronary artery. There is also significant occlusive disease of the right coronary artery.* B, *The aneurysm is opened and resected, leaving a 5- to 10-mm rim of scar tissue.* C, *The ventricle is closed using sutures over Teflon pledgets.* D, *The right coronary artery is bypassed using autologous saphenous vein. (From Gay, W. A., Jr.: Ventricular aneurysm.* In *Sabiston, D. C., Jr. (Ed.): Davis-Christopher Textbook of Surgery, 12th ed. Philadelphia, W. B. Saunders Company, 1981, p. 2337.)*

the surgical management of ventricular tachyarrhythmias, and intraoperative electrophysiologic studies, cryoablation, and directed endocardial excision have proved to be effective in preventing recurrence of life-threatening arrhythmias.[10, 12, 17]

Long-term survival following aneurysmectomy and coronary bypass grafting appear dependent on preoperative ventricular function and complete revascularization at the time of surgery.[1, 3, 15, 21, 22, 25, 30] Most series report a 60 to 80 per cent survival of 4 to 5 years, a marked improvement over the annual mortality of 13 to 15 per cent in patients treated medically.[20, 27, 28]

SELECTED REFERENCES

Jatene, A. D.: Left ventricular aneurysmectomy: Resection or reconstruction. J. Thorac. Cardiovasc. Surg., *89*:321, 1985.
  In this series, there was a 4.3 per cent hospital mortality in 508 patients following resection and reconstruction of left ventricular aneurysms with a Dacron patch. Emphasis is placed upon the importance of ventricular geometry following aneurysmectomy, and a new concept of the surgical management of left ventricular aneurysms is presented.

Schlichter, J., Hellerstein, H. K., and Katz, L. N.: Aneurysm of the heart: A correlative study of 102 proved cases. Medicine, *33*:43, 1954.
  This series is the classic reference concerning the natural history of cardiac aneurysms. One hundred and two postmortem cases of ventricular aneurysm are reviewed in detail. This was the first study to document the substantial mortality associated with left ventricular aneurysm.

REFERENCES

1. Barratt-Boyes, B. G., White, H. D., Agnew, T. M., Pemberton, J. R., and Wild, C. J.: The results of surgical treatment of left ventricular aneurysms. J. Thorac. Cardiovasc. Surg., *87*:87, 1984.
2. Beck, C. S.: Operation for aneurysm of the heart. Ann. Surg., *120*:34, 1944.
3. Burton, N. A., Stinson, E. B., Oyer, P., and Shumway, N. E.: Left ventricular aneurysm: Preoperative risk factors and long term postoperative results. J. Thorac. Cardiovasc. Surg., *77*:65, 1979.
4. Candell, J., Valle, V., Paya, J., Cortadellas, J., Esplugas, E., and Ruis, J.: Post-traumatic coronary occlusion and early left ventricular aneurysm. Am. Heart J. *97*:509, 1979.
5. Cooley, D. A., Collins, H. A., Morris, G. C., and Chapman, D. W.: Ventricular aneurysm after myocardial infarction: Surgical excision with the use of temporary cardiopulmonary bypass. J. A. M. A., *167*:557, 1958.
6. Flemma, R. J., Marx, L., Litwin, S. B., and Gallen, W. J.: Left ventricular aneurysmectomy in a child. Ann. Thorac. Surg., *19*:457, 1975.
7. Froehlich, R. T., Falsetti, H. L., Doty, D. B., and Marcus, M. L.: Prospective study of surgery for left ventricular aneurysm. Am. J. Cardiol., *45*:923, 1980.
8. Gay, W. A.: Ventricular aneurysms. *In* Sabiston, D. C., Jr. (Ed.): Textbook of Surgery. The Biologic Basis of Modern Surgical Practice. Philadelphia, W. B. Saunders Company, 1985, p. 2335.
9. Harken, A. H.: Left ventricular aneurysm. *In* Sabiston, D. C., Jr., and Spencer, F. C. (Eds.): Surgery of the Chest. Philadelphia, W. B. Saunders Company, 1983, p. 1480.
10. Harken, A. H., Horowitz, L. N., and Josephson, M. E.: The surgical treatment of ventricular tachycardia. Ann. Thorac. Surg., *30*:499, 1980.
11. Jatene, A. D.: Left ventricular aneurysmectomy: Resection or reconstruction. J. Thorac. Cardiovasc. Surg., *89*:321, 1985.
12. Kastor, J. A., Horowitz, L. N., Harken, A. H., and Josephson, M. E.: Clinical electrophysiology of ventricular tachycardia. N. Engl. J. Med., *304*:1004, 1981.
13. Klein, M. D., Herman, M. V., and Gorlin, R. A.: A hemodynamic study of left ventricular aneurysm. Circulation, *35*:614, 1967.
14. Likoff, W., and Bailey, C. P.: Ventriculoplasty: Excision of myocardial aneurysm. J. A. M. A., *158*:915, 1955.
15. Loop, F. D., and Cosgrove, D. M.: Results of ventricular aneurysmectomy. Am. J. Surg., *141*:684, 1981.
16. Loop, F. D., Effler, D. B., Navia, J. A., Sheldon, W. C., and Groves, L. K.: Aneurysms of the left ventricle: Survival and results of a ten-year surgical experience. Ann. Surg., *178*:399, 1973.
17. Martin, J., Untereker, W. J., Harken, A. H., Horowitz, L. N., and Josephson, M. E.: Aneurysmectomy and endocardial resection for ventricular tachycardia: Favorable hemodynamic and anti-arrhythmic results in patients with global left ventricular dysfunction. Am. Heart J., *103*:960, 1982.
18. Meizlish, J. L., Berger, H. J., Plankey, M., Errico, D., Levy, W., and Zaret, B. L.: Functional left ventricular aneurysm formation after acute anterior transmural myocardial infarction: Incidence, natural history, and prognostic implications. N. Engl. J. Med., *311*:1001, 1984.
19. Mundth, E. D.: Left ventricular aneurysmectomy. *In* Cohn, L. H. (Ed.): Cardiac/Thoracic Surgery. Mount Kisco, N. Y., Futura Publishing Co., 1979.
20. Nagle, R. E., and Williams, D. O.: Natural history of ventricular aneurysm without surgical treatment. Br. Heart. J., *36*:1037, 1974.
21. Novick, R. J., Stefaniszyn, H. J., Morin, J. E., Symes, J. F., Sniderman, A. D., Dobell, A. R.: Surgery for postinfarction left ventricular aneurysm: Prognosis and long-term follow-up. Can. J. Surg., *27*:161, 1984.
22. Olearchyk, A. S., Lemole, G. M., and Spagna, P. M.: Left ventricular aneurysm: Ten years' experience in surgical treatment of 244 cases. Improved clinical status, hemodynamics and long-term longevity. J. Thorac. Cardiovasc. Surg., *88*:544, 1984.
23. Proudfit, W. L., Bruschke, A. V., and Sones, F. M., Jr.: Natural history of obstructive coronary artery disease: Ten year study of 601 nonsurgical cases. Prog. Cardiovasc. Dis., *21*:53, 1978.
24. Reeder, G. S., Longyel, M., Tajik, A. J., Seward, J. B., Smith, H. C., and Danielson, G. K.: Mural thrombus in left ventricular aneurysm: Incidence, role of angiography, and relation between anticoagulation and embolization. Mayo. Clin. Proc., *56*:77, 1981.
25. Rittenhouse, E. A., Sauvage, L. R., Mansfield, P. B., Smith, J. D., Davis, C. C., Hall, D. G., and O'Brien, M. A.: Results of combined left ventricular aneurysmectomy and coronary artery bypass: 1974 to 1980. Am. J. Surg., *143*:575, 1982.
26. Sapsford, R. N., Fitchett, D. H., Tarin, D., and Anderson, R. H.: Aneurysms of left ventricle secondary to bacterial endocarditis. J. Thorac. Cardiovasc. Surg., *78*:79, 1979.
27. Schattenberg, T. T., Guiliani, E. R., Campion, B. C., and Danielson, K. J.: Post-infarction ventricular aneurysm. Mayo Clin. Proc., *45*:13, 1970.
28. Schlichter, J., Hellerstein, H. K., and Katz, L. N.: Aneurysm of the heart: A correlative study of 102 proved cases. Medicine, *33*:43, 1954.
29. Simpson, M. T., Oberman, A., Kouchoukos, N. T., and Rogers, W. J.: Prevalence of mural thrombi and systemic embolization with

left ventricular aneurysm: Effect of anticoagulation therapy. Chest, 77:463, 1980.

30. Skinner, J. R., Rasak, C., Kongtahworn, C., Phillips, S. J., Zeff, R. H., Toon, R. S., and Solomon, V. B.: Natural history of surgically treated ventricular aneurysm. Ann. Thorac Surg., 38:42, 1984.

31. Vlodaver, Z., Coe, J. I., and Edwards, J. E.: True and false left ventricular aneurysms: Propensity for the latter to rupture. Circulation, 51:567, 1975.

3 • CARDIAC TRANSPLANTATION: THE TOTAL ARTIFICIAL HEART

DAVID C. SABISTON, JR., M.D.

Cardiac transplantation has become increasingly successful in recent years and is being performed more widely than ever. Much of the improvement in survival has been the result of several important factors, including (1) better management of graft rejection as well as improvements in myocardial preservation, (2) reduction in the interval between harvesting the heart from the donor and placement in the recipient, (3) improved technical aspects of surgical implantation of the heart, and (4) better use of pharmacologic support of the circulation postoperatively. This subject is considered in detail in Chapter 15 on Transplantation.

Despite the many advances made in cardiac surgery in the recent past, there remain a number of patients with *end-stage cardiac disease* for whom neither medical nor surgical therapy is effective. Although cardiac transplantation is the preferred approach under these circumstances, it is not always feasible. For such patients, the totally implantable artificial heart has stimulated the imagination and industry of a number of workers. The National Institutes of Health and other agencies have supported basic and clinical research in this field, and the role of the clinical use of the implantable heart is being explored in selected patients. There have been modest improvements in the device, and it is being implanted in a few terminal patients while donor hearts for transplantation are being awaited.

Landmarks in the development of the implantable heart began with the suggestion of Legallois in 1813 that life could be maintained indefinitely if an appropriate artificial pumping mechanism could be devised. Several workers constructed pump-oxygenators in the last century, and Lindbergh and Carrel demonstrated experimentally the basis of total body perfusion with an artificial pump-oxygenator in 1935. In 1953, Gibbon was the first to use an artificial heart-lung machine successfully for closure of an intracardiac defect. Since then, many workers have approached the entire subject with many innovative concepts and achievements.

During the past 15 years, several mechanical devices have been used to substitute for a failing heart at the end of an operative procedure when cardiopulmonary bypass could not safely be discontinued. However, such patients usually lived for only a matter of days. Jarvik is deserving of much credit, together with Kolff and co-workers, for the design of an improved artificial heart. The Jarvik-7 has been successfully implanted into a series of patients with long-term survival (up to 620 days). This unit is constructed of polyurethane and is pneumatically powered by cable from a heart driver, which is connected both to electric power and compressed air. The unit was tested quite thoroughly in a large series of experimental animals prior to use in man.[2] The Jarvik-7 artificial heart was first successfully implanted for long-term use by DeVries and associates in 1982, and the patient lived 112 days. The primary indication for the use of the totally implantable mechanical heart at this time is to permit terminally ill patients with congestive heart failure who are suitable candidates for transplantation to live until an appropriate donor can be obtained. In view of the risk involved as well as the limitations of the ultimate results of these devices, it is apparent that the patient should be *terminally ill* as a prime indication for use of a mechanical heart.

SURGICAL TECHNIQUE

The heart is excised with oversewing of the coronary sinus, and connections are made to the natural atria achieved by atrial cuffs fabricated of Dacron and attached by a quick-connect cuff. Anastomoses are then made to the pulmonary artery and aorta. The left ventricle is snapped into position followed by the right ventricle (Figs. 1 and 2).

There have been a number of postoperative complications associated with mechanical cardiac implants, including bleeding and the necessity for re-exploration, hemolytic anemia, renal insufficiency, pulmonary insufficiency, infection in the urinary tract and in wounds, device failure, and disseminated intravascular coagulation. At this time, one of the prime and most feared complications is multiple emboli, especially those to the brain with resultant cerebrovascular accidents.

RESULTS

At the end of 1985, 11 total artificial hearts had been implanted with survival ranging from several days to nearly

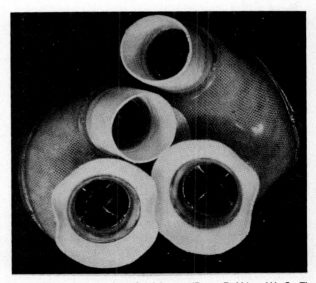

Figure 1. Jarvik-7 total artificial heart. (From DeVries, W. C.: The total artificial heart. In Sabiston, D. C., Jr. (Ed.): Textbook of Surgery, 13th ed. Philadelphia, W. B. Saunders Company, 1986, p. 2482.)

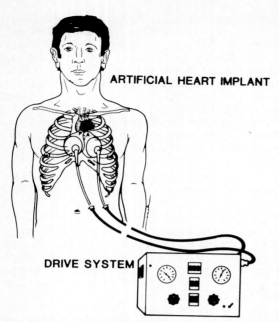

ARTIFICIAL HEART IMPLANT

DRIVE SYSTEM

Figure 2. Artificial heart and drive system. (From DeVries, W. C.: The total artificial heart. In *Sabiston, D. C., Jr. (Ed.): Textbook of Surgery, 13th ed. Philadelphia, W. B. Saunders Company, 1986, p. 2482.)*

2 years.[3] There is general consensus that the *limited* success and especially the proven *need* for a totally artificial heart are such that work should be continued and these units implanted in suitable patients by those with a committed

interest in the field. The practical, philosophical, and ethical as well as medical implications of the entire subject are obvious, and individual assessment is needed in each patient being considered as a candidate.

SELECTED REFERENCES

Anderson, F. L., DeVries, W. C., Anderson, J. L., and Joyce, L. D.: Evaluation of total artificial heart performance in man. Am. J. Cardiol., *54*:394, 1984.
  The cardiodynamics of the artificial heart are reviewed in this publication by authors closely associated with the problem.

DeBakey, M. E.: Mechanical circulatory support: Current status. Am. J. Cardiol. 27:1, 1971.
  This is an early summary of the initial progress in mechanical circulatory support.

Yared, S. F., Johnson, G. S., and DeVries, W. C.: Results of artificial heart implantation in man. Transplant. Proc., *18* (Suppl. 2):69, 1986.
  A summary of artificial heart implantation in man through 1985. Each patient is reviewed with pertinent data.

REFERENCES

1. DeVries, W. C.: The total artificial heart. *In* Sabiston, D. C., Jr. (Ed.): Textbook of Surgery, 13th ed. Philadelphia, W. B. Saunders Company, 1986.
2. Jarvik, R. K.: Recent successes with total replacement of the heart. *In* Hwang, N. H. C., Gross, D. R., and Patel, D. J. (Eds.): Quantitative Cardiovascular Studies: Clinical and Research Applications of Engineering Principles. Baltimore, University Park Press, 1979, p. 751.
3. Yared, S. F., Johnson, G. S., and DeVries, W. C.: Results of artificial heart implantation in man. Transplant. Proc., *18* (Suppl. 2):69, 1986.

XIII

Congenital Lesions of the Coronary Arteries

DAVID C. SABISTON, JR., M.D.

Since the introduction of selective coronary arteriography by Sones in 1959, the number of congenital coronary arterial malformations diagnosed during life has increased dramatically. Many patients formerly followed for unexplained cardiac murmurs, often with symptoms and complications, now undergo coronary arteriography with the establishment of a precise anatomic diagnosis. In view of the natural history of most of these congenital malformations, surgical correction is generally indicated and should be performed electively before the onset of troublesome symptoms and serious complications.

CONGENITAL CORONARY ARTERIAL FISTULAS

In 1865, Krause described the first coronary arterial fistula,[11] and in a survey 286 patients with this disorder were found in the literature.[12] Although it had been previously thought by many that the majority of these patients were asymptomatic, in our experience in 30 patients with this disorder 55 per cent were symptomatic at the time of presentation. The symptoms are caused by the left-to-right cardiac shunt and most commonly consist of dyspnea (particularly on exertion), congestive heart failure, angina pectoris, and subacute bacterial endocarditis.

The physical findings in patients with coronary arterial fistulas generally consist of a continuous murmur over the site of the abnormal communication. The differential diagnosis usually includes a patent ductus arteriosus, aortic-pulmonary window, and fistulas of the sinus of Valsalva. Ventricular septal defects, particularly those associated with aortic insufficiency, may also produce a similar murmur. The same is true of pulmonary arteriovenous malformations as well as fistulas of systemic vessels such as subclavian and internal mammary artery fistulas connecting to the veins of the chest wall or to the lung.[14]

Among the 30 patients seen, 19 were female and 11 male with an age range between 6 weeks and 76 years. The right coronary artery was the origin of the fistula in 11 patients, the left anterior descending in 9, the left circumflex in 3, the right coronary plus the left anterior descending in 4, and the left main coronary in 1; another unusual patient had origin of the fistulas from the right, anterior descending, and circumflex coronary arteries. These fistulas drained into the pulmonary artery in 16 patients, into the right ventricle in 7, into the right atrium in 6, and into the left atrium in 1 patient. These findings were first demonstrated by coronary arteriography and confirmed at the time of surgical correction. It is interesting that the youngest patient (5 weeks) and the oldest (76 years) both had severe congestive heart failure requiring urgent operation. Both recovered uneventfully and remain well (Figs. 1 through 6).

Early in the series, the majority of patients had closure of their fistulas without extracorporeal circulation,[14] whereas more recently extracorporeal circulation has been employed in most patients. Of 24 patients managed surgically among the total group of 30, there have been no operative deaths.[13]

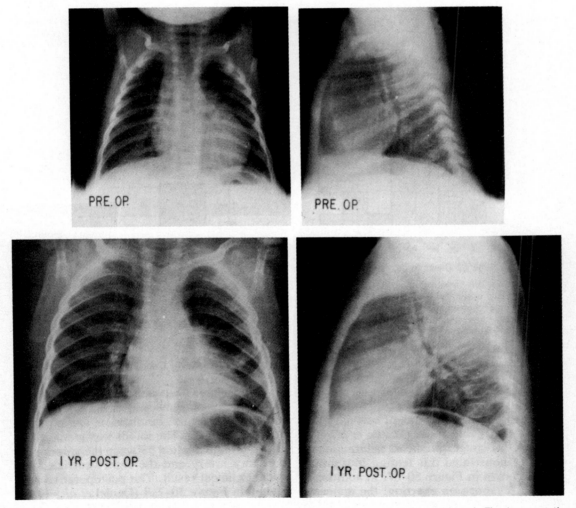

Figure 1. Preoperative chest films of an infant with a coronary artery fistula at 5 weeks of age (above). The interpretation included biventricular enlargement, left atrial enlargement, and increased pulmonary vasculature. Chest films one year after operation show decrease in cardiomegaly (below). (From Daniel, T. M., Graham, T. P., and Sabiston, D. C., Jr.: Surgery, 67:985, 1970.)

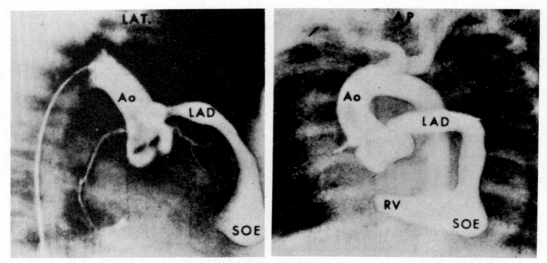

Figure 2. *Ascending aortogram (lateral and anteroposterior views) in a 6-week-old infant who had severe congestive heart failure. The aortogram shows a left coronary artery–right ventricular fistula. Ao = Aorta; LAD = left anterior descending coronary artery; SOE = site of entry of the fistula into the right ventricle; RV = incompletely opacified right ventricle. (From Daniel, T. M., Graham, T. P., and Sabiston, D. C., Jr.: Surgery, 67:985, 1970.)*

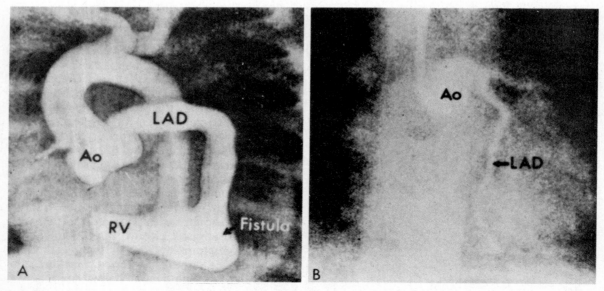

Figure 3. *A, Preoperative aortogram of patient in Figure 2. B, Repeat aortogram one year following successful surgical obliteration of the fistula. The left anterior descending coronary artery (LAD) has returned to normal size. (From Daniel, T. M., Graham, T. P., and Sabiston, D. C., Jr.: Surgery, 67:985, 1970.)*

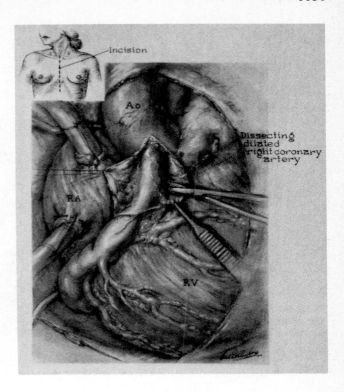

Figure 4. Right coronary–to–right atrial congenital coronary fistula as seen at operation in a 76-year-old female who had severe congestive heart failure. Through a median sternotomy, the patient was placed on cardiopulmonary bypass with separate venous return cannulas placed in the superior and inferior venae cavae. (From Lowe, J. E., and Sabiston, D. C., Jr.: Congenital coronary malformations. In Cohn, L. (Ed.): Modern Technics in Surgery, Cardiac-Thoracic Surgery. Mt. Kisco, N.Y., Futura Publishing Co., 1981.)

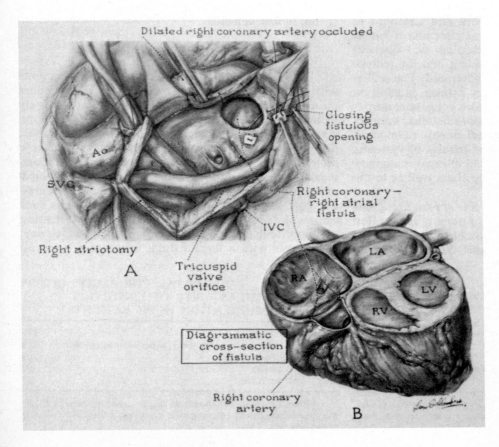

Figure 5. Tapes are secured around the superior and inferior venae cavae to eliminate venous return to the right atrium. The heart is then fibrillated and the right atrium is opened. The large fistulous opening is identified and closed using interrupted non-absorbable pledgeted sutures (A). The site of entry into the right coronary fistula is shown in B. (From Lowe, J. E., and Sabiston, D. C., Jr.: Congenital coronary malformations. In Cohn, L. (Ed.): Modern Technics in Surgery, Cardiac-Thoracic Surgery. Mt. Kisco, N.Y., Futura Publishing Co., 1981.)

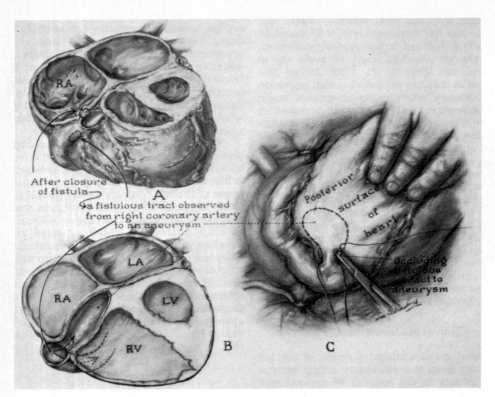

Figure 6. After closure of the site of entry into the right atrium, a second fistulous tract was found entering an aneurysm over the posterior surface of the heart (A and B). This fistulous tract was closed using multiple transfixion sutures (C). (From Lowe, J. E., and Sabiston, D. C., Jr.: Congenital coronary malformations. In Cohn, L. (Ed.): Modern Technics in Surgery, Cardiac-Thoracic Surgery. Mt. Kisco, N.Y., Futura Publishing Co., 1981.)

CONGENITAL ORIGIN OF THE LEFT CORONARY ARTERY FROM THE PULMONARY ARTERY

Abbott described a patient whose left coronary artery arose from the pulmonary artery in her classic monograph published in 1908.[1] Her report was followed in 1911 by that of Abrikossoff, who described a 5-month-old infant dying of congestive heart failure with a left ventricular aneurysm associated with origin of the left coronary artery from the pulmonary artery.[2] The electrocardiographic changes were described by Bland and associates in an infant with this malformation in 1933, and they demonstrated for the first time that a diagnosis could be made in life.[3] Keith, the noted pediatric cardiologist, estimated that 95 per cent of infants born with this malformation die within the first year of life unless surgical correction is undertaken.[10] Therefore, it is apparent that the majority of patients with this congenital malformation develop symptoms during infancy, although a small number may appear normal until several years of life or older. In fact, there are examples of patients who lived for many years before appearance of clinical symptoms.[15]

The physiologic changes associated with this malformation were originally attributed to the fact that myocardial ischemia was produced by perfusion of the left coronary arterial system with poorly oxygenated blood because the vessel arose from the pulmonary artery and that the pressure within the left coronary artery was quite low. However, this theory was dispelled when it was shown that blood flow in the left coronary artery is actually *reversed* and that blood in this vessel originates from collaterals from the *right* coronary artery and then passes into the left coronary and flows *retrograde* into the pulmonary artery. This is

easily demonstrated by coronary arteriography (Fig. 7). Thus, the left ventricular myocardium is deprived of much needed oxygen because most of the blood in the anterior descending and circumflex branches drains needlessly into the pulmonary artery and actually represents a coronary arteriovenous fistula. Moreover, selective injection of the right coronary artery with contrast medium demonstrates the collateral vessels with direct filling of the left coronary system and drainage of the contrast medium into the pulmonary artery.

Thirty-six patients with origin of the left coronary artery from the ventricular artery were studied (21 females and 15 males). The ages ranged from 1 month to 61 years, the latter presenting with severe congestive heart failure. Among the 36 patients, 19 had severe congestive heart failure, 5 had angina pectoris, and 2 infants exhibited failure to thrive. In 9 patients, the evaluation was the result of the finding of a cardiac murmur of uncertain cause associated with cardiomegaly and/or unexplained dyspnea. The 10 patients who were not operated on died within several hours to several months following diagnosis. Of the 26 patients undergoing surgical correction, 14 were operated on early for this condition and had simple ligation of the vessel at its origin (Fig. 8)[18] with 5 operative deaths. Most of these 13 infants had acute myocardial infarction as the indication for operation. Seven patients were managed with coronary artery bypass graft by ligation and division of the left coronary artery at its origin and anastomosis to a saphenous vein graft end-to-end from the ascending aorta (Fig. 9). One infant with myocardial infarction was treated by ligation of the left coronary artery at its origin and anastomosis end-to-end with the left subclavian artery (Fig. 10). Two patients early in the series were treated with de-epicardialization and are long-time survivors.[17] Thus, of the

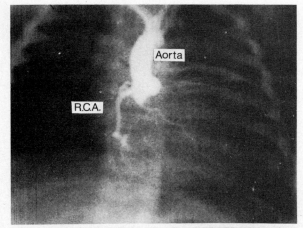

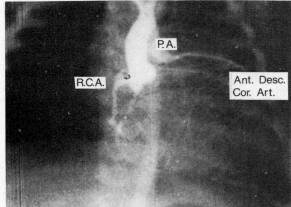

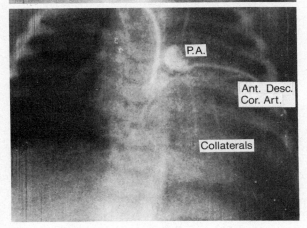

Figure 7. Several cine frames taken from a series illustrating coronary arterial filling during aortography. A, Filling of the right coronary artery (R.C.A.) as it arises normally from the aorta. Note that its size is somewhat greater than normal. B, Filling of the branches of the left coronary artery through collaterals from the right coronary artery. C, Filling of the pulmonary artery (P.A.) by retrograde flow from the left coronary artery. (From Sabiston, D. C., Jr., and Orme, S. K.: J. Cardiovasc. Surg., 9:543, 1968.)

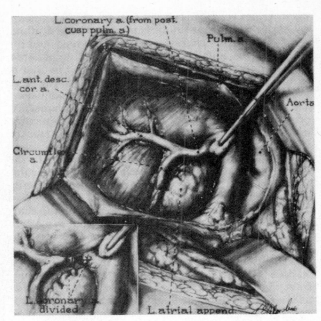

Figure 8. Congenital origin of the left coronary artery from the posterior sinus of Valsalva of the pulmonary artery. The origin of the left coronary from the pulmonary artery is carefully dissected, then occluded at its origin with suture ligatures, and divided (inset). (From Sabiston, D. C., Jr., Ross, R. S., Criley, J. M., et al.: Ann Surg., 157:908, 1963.)

ORIGIN OF THE RIGHT CORONARY ARTERY FROM THE PULMONARY ARTERY

It is fortunate that when the right coronary artery arises from the pulmonary artery there are few signs or symptoms. In fact, the first description of this condition originated incidentally from dissections in two cadavers by Brooks in 1886.[5] He noted markedly dilated collaterals joining the anomalous right coronary artery with the left coronary artery and correctly predicted that during life the flow in the right coronary artery originated from collateral branches from the left coronary and that blood in the right coronary flowed retrograde into the pulmonary artery.

Among 17 patients collected in the literature by Tingelstad, the condition was found in individuals ranging in age from 17 to 90 years.[19] The lesion may have been associated with death in but two instances, one being a 17-year-old female patient who died suddenly and at autopsy showed complete occlusion of the left coronary artery by a thrombus and left ventricular infarction. The other patient, aged 55 years, had angina and congestive heart failure.

Although symptoms are rare and the natural history is benign, it may lead in some instances to sudden death. Thus consideration should be given to the operative procedure reported in one patient with this disorder in whom the right coronary artery was anastomosed directly to the aorta using a cuff of pulmonary artery tissue at the origin for the anastomosis.[19]

It is also interesting that five infants have been reported in whom *both* coronary arteries arose from the pulmonary artery. The survival time was obviously quite short in these patients and ranged from 9 hours to 5 months, with the exception of one child who lived to the age of 7 years

26 patients undergoing an operative procedure 18 are alive and well, including all those patients with coronary artery bypass procedures or direct anastomosis of the left subclavian artery to the left coronary artery, which are the procedures of choice.

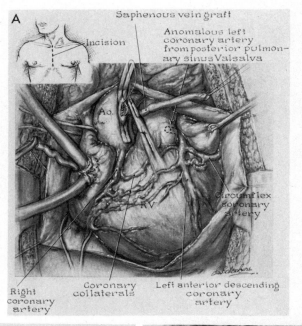

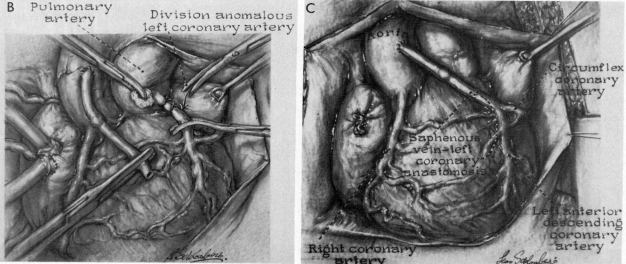

Figure 9. A, Congenital origin of the left coronary from the pulmonary artery can also be managed by division of the left coronary artery at its site of origin and reconstruction of two-coronary system using a saphenous vein graft. Through a median sternotomy, and with the patient on cardiopulmonary bypass, the saphenous vein graft is attached to the ascending aorta using a partial occluding clamp. B, The left coronary artery is then divided at its site of origin from the pulmonary artery. C, The saphenous vein graft is then anastomosed in end-to-end fashion to the left coronary artery using interrupted 7-0 non-absorbable sutures. (From Lowe, J. E., and Sabiston, D. C., Jr.: South. Med. J., 75:1508, 1982.)

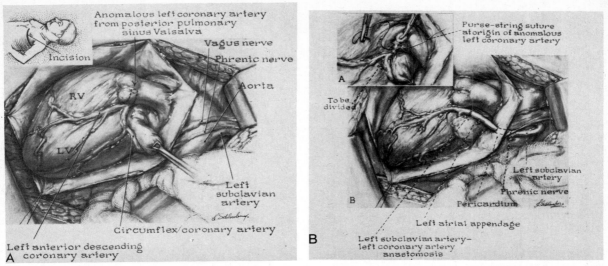

Figure 10. A, Congenital origin of the left coronary artery from the pulmonary artery. Through a left anterior third interspace thoracotomy, the left coronary artery is occluded at its site of origin with suture ligatures and then is divided. B, The left subclavian artery is then anastomosed to the left coronary artery in end-to-end fashion using interrupted 7-0 non-absorbable sutures. (From Lowe, J. E., and Sabiston, D. C., Jr.: South. Med. J., 75:1508, 1982.)

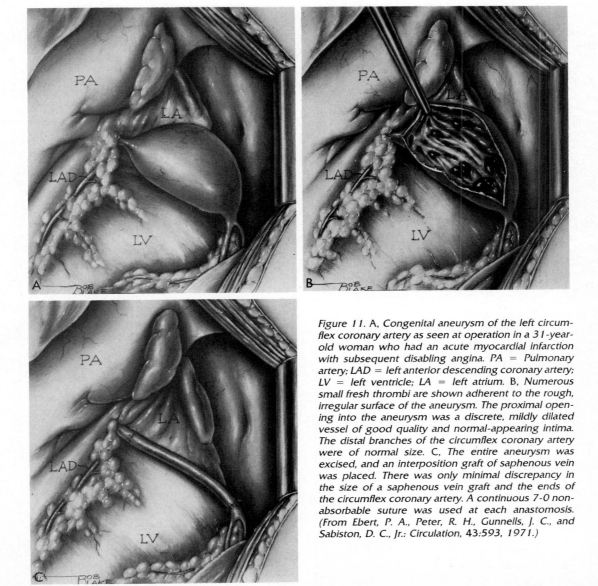

Figure 11. A, Congenital aneurysm of the left circumflex coronary artery as seen at operation in a 31-year-old woman who had an acute myocardial infarction with subsequent disabling angina. PA = Pulmonary artery; LAD = left anterior descending coronary artery; LV = left ventricle; LA = left atrium. B, Numerous small fresh thrombi are shown adherent to the rough, irregular surface of the aneurysm. The proximal opening into the aneurysm was a discrete, mildly dilated vessel of good quality and normal-appearing intima. The distal branches of the circumflex coronary artery were of normal size. C, The entire aneurysm was excised, and an interposition graft of saphenous vein was placed. There was only minimal discrepancy in the size of a saphenous vein graft and the ends of the circumflex coronary artery. A continuous 7-0 non-absorbable suture was used at each anastomosis. (From Ebert, P. A., Peter, R. H., Gunnells, J. C., and Sabiston, D. C., Jr.: Circulation, 43:593, 1971.)

because of the presence of an interventricular septal defect with pulmonary hypertension and congenital mitral stenosis. Under these circumstances, the pressure in the pulmonary artery was sufficient to force blood into the myocardial capillary bed.

CONGENITAL ANEURYSMS OF THE CORONARY ARTERIES

Since the first report by Bougon in 1812 of an aneurysm of the coronary artery,[4] these lesions have been reported from infancy to adult life.[6] Nevertheless, *congenital* lesions account for only 15 per cent of coronary arterial aneurysms, whereas atherosclerosis, mycotic aneurysms, syphilis, rheumatic heart disease, and other disorders cause the vast majority.[7]

If a congenital aneurysm occurs, it is likely to be the site of an intramural thrombus, which can then serve as a source of emboli to the distal coronary circulation. For this reason, this condition is preferentially managed by excision of the aneurysm with replacement of a saphenous vein autograft (Fig. 11).[8]

FUSION OF THE LEFT AORTIC CUSP TO THE AORTIC WALL WITH OCCLUSION OF THE LEFT CORONARY OSTIUM

A rare but fascinating lesion has been termed fusion of the left aortic cusp to the aortic wall with occlusion of the left coronary ostium. In this condition, the distal left coronary is quite normal and the patient develops massive collaterals from the right coronary to the left coronary, which supplies the ventricular myocardium until such time as symptoms appear.[20]

Congenital ostial membrane of the left main coronary artery at its origin has also been described and treatment is excision of the obstructing membrane.[9]

SELECTED REFERENCES

Daniel, T. M., Graham, T. P., and Sabiston, D. C., Jr.: Coronary artery–right ventricular fistula with congestive heart failure: Surgical correction in the neonatal period. Surgery, *67*:985, 1970.
In this review, almost 200 patients with coronary arteriovenous fistulas are reported. The incidence of congestive heart failure was 14 per cent. Approximately half of all patients with isolated arteriovenous fistulas were symptomatic. The age of onset of dyspnea, congestive heart failure, bacterial endocarditis, and angina pectoris are reviewed.

Lowe, J. E., and Sabiston, D. C., Jr.: Congenital coronary malformations. *In* Cohn, L. (Ed.): Modern Technics in Surgery, Cardiac-Thoracic Surgery. Mt. Kisco, New York, Futura Publishing Company, 1981.
This review presents the surgical techniques used to correct congenital coronary artery fistulas, anomalous origin of the left or right coronary artery from the pulmonary artery, and congenital coronary artery aneurysms. The details of the preoperative evaluation, anesthetic management, and postoperative care are also reviewed.

REFERENCES

1. Abbott, M. E.: Congenital cardiac disease. *In* Osler, W. (Ed.): Modern Medicine, Vol. 4. Philadelphia, Lea & Febiger, 1908.
2. Abrikossoff, A.: Aneurysma des liken Herzventrikels mit abnormer Abgangsstelle der linken Koronarterie von der Pulmonalis bei einem funfmonatlichen Kinde. Virchows Arch. (Pathol. Anat.), *203*:413, 1911.
3. Bland, E. F., White, P. D., and Garland, J.: Congenital anomalies of coronary arteries: Report of an unusual case associated with cardiac hypertrophy. Am. Heart J., *8*:787, 1933.
4. Bougon: Bibl. Med., *37*:183, 1812. Cited by Packard, M., and Wechsler, H. F.: Aneurysm of the coronary arteries. Arch. Intern. Med., *43*:1, 1929.
5. Brooks, H. St. J.: Two cases of an abnormal coronary artery of the heart arising from the pulmonary artery. J. Anat. Physiol., *20*:26, 1886.
6. Crocker, D. W., Sobin, S., and Thomas, W. C.: Aneurysms of the coronary arteries. Report of three cases in infants and review of the literature. Am. J. Pathol., *33*:819, 1957.
7. Daoud, A. S., Pankin, D., Tulgan, H., and Florentin, R. A.: Aneurysms of the coronary artery. Am. J. Cardiol., *11*:228, 1963.
8. Ebert, P. A., Peter, R. H., Gunnells, J. C., and Sabiston, D. C., Jr.: Resecting and grafting of coronary artery aneurysm. Circulation, *43*:593, 1971.
9. Josa, M., Danielson, G. K., Weidman, W. H., and Edwards, W. D.: Congenital ostial membrane of left main coronary artery. J. Thorac. Cardiovasc. Surg., *81*:338, 1981.
10. Keith, J. D.: The anomalous origin of the left coronary artery from the pulmonary artery. Br. Heart J., *21*:149, 1959.
11. Krause, W.: Ueber den Ursprung einer accessorischen Arterie coronaria cordis aus der arterie pulmonalis. Zeitsch. rationelle Med., *24*:225, 1865.
12. Lowe, J. E., Oldham, H. N., Jr., and Sabiston, D. C., Jr.: Surgical management of congenital coronary artery fistulas. Ann. Surg., *194*:371, 1981.
13. Lowe, J. E., and Sabiston, D. C., Jr.: Surgical correction of congenital malformations of the coronary circulation. South. Med. J., *75*:1508, 1982.
14. Robinson, L. A., and Sabiston, D. C., Jr.: Syndrome of congenital internal mammary-to-pulmonary arteriovenous fistula associated with mitral valve prolapse. Arch. Surg., *116*:1265, 1981.
15. Sabiston, D. C., Jr., Floyd, W. L., and McIntosh, H. D.: Anomalous origin of the left coronary artery from the pulmonary artery in adults. Arch. Surg., *97*:963, 1968.
16. Sabiston, D. C., Jr., Neill, C. A., and Taussig, H. B.: The direction of blood flow in anomalous left coronary artery arising from the pulmonary artery. Circulation, *22*:591, 1960.
17. Sabiston, D. C., Jr., and Orme, S. K.: Congenital origin of the left coronary artery from the pulmonary artery. J. Thorac. Cardiovasc. Surg., *9*:543, 1968.
18. Sabiston, D. C., Jr., Ross, R. S., Criley, J. M., et al.: Surgical management of congenital lesions of the coronary circulation. Ann. Surg., *157*:908, 1963.
19. Tingelstad, J. B., Lower, R. R., and Eldredge, W. J.: Anomalous origin of the right coronary artery from the main pulmonary artery. Am. J. Cardiol., *30*:670, 1972.
20. Waxman, M. B., Kong, Y., Behar, V. S., Sabiston, D. C., Jr., and Morris, J. J., Jr.: Fusion of the left aortic cusp to the aortic wall with occlusion of the left coronary ostium, and aortic stenosis and insufficiency. Circulation, *41*:849, 1970.

XIV

Acquired Diseases of the Aortic Valve

J. MARK WILLIAMS, M.D.
DAVID C. SABISTON, JR., M.D.

ANATOMY AND FUNCTION

The aortic valve consists of three equal-sized leaflets attached to the root of the aorta. The root of the aorta bulges outward behind each leaflet, forming a sinus of Valsalva. The coronary arteries normally arise in the upper third of the sinuses. Left ventricular ejection occurs when left ventricular pressure exceeds aortic pressure. The forward pressure gradient ceases during the first half of systole, and thereafter flow is maintained by a mass acceleration effect. Valve closure is accomplished by reversal of aortic flow and approximation of the free edges of the leaflets.[41]

Eighty per cent or more of coronary artery blood flow occurs during diastole. Diastolic blood flow is enhanced by low ventricular intramural pressures. Low diastolic aortic pressure, high ventricular intramural pressure, high ventricular cavitary pressures, and short diastolic intervals decrease coronary arterial blood flow.

AORTIC STENOSIS

Etiology and Pathology

Rheumatic Aortic Stenosis. Rheumatic fever is an inflammatory disease that is a delayed sequela of pharyngeal infection by group A streptococci. All layers of the heart (epicardium, myocardium, and endocardium) may be involved in the inflammatory process. Endocardial involvement may result in swelling, edema, and deformity of valve leaflets. Resolution of inflammation occurs with fibrous thickening, contracture, and by a tendency for fusion of adjacent cusps at commissures. With progressive thickening and fusion of one cusp to another, the valve becomes stenotic (Fig. 1A).[31]

Calcific Aortic Stenosis. Calcific aortic stenosis occurs primarily in bicuspid valves (Fig. 1B). The bicuspid valve may be congenital or acquired from previous episodes of rheumatic disease. The congenital bicuspid valve is more common than the acquired valve by a ratio of 4:1.[32] Valves that undergo progressive calcification and result in aortic stenosis are usually competent and are not associated with other valve lesions.[33] A "wear and tear" theory of origin postulates a gradual progression of fibrous thickening and calcification as a result of improper contact between two unequal leaflets of a malformed bicuspid valve.[13] Tricuspid valves with minimally unequal but misaligned cusps may undergo the same process (Fig. 1C).[32] Turbulent flow with secondary hemolysis, adenosine diphosphate (ADP) release, platelet aggregation, and microthrombic formation may also contribute to formation of nodular calcific deposits on the surface of the valve leaflets.[39]

Physiology

Gradual reduction in effective orifice size results in a systolic pressure gradient between the left ventricular chamber and ascending aorta. Compensatory myocardial hypertrophy and an increase in ventricular mass are required to maintain stroke volumes in the presence of the transvalvular gradient. Maintenance of stroke volume also requires prolongation of the duration of systole, resulting in decreased coronary perfusion time. Prolonged pressure overload leads to depression of the contractile state of the ventricular myocardium.[11] Chamber dilatation then occurs in order to maintain stroke volume and forward cardiac output. Eventually, progressive chamber dilatation reduces ejection fraction, and marked elevation of end-diastolic pressure ensues.

Clinical Manifestations

Characteristic clinical manifestations include chest pain, syncope, and congestive heart failure. Angina may occur in the absence of coronary artery disease when the increased myocardial oxygen demands of hypertrophied myocardium exceed oxygen availability. Decreased diastolic perfusion time, increased left ventricular end-diastolic pressures, and increased intramural pressures have been implicated as possible causes of diminished endocardial coronary artery blood flow and oxygen availability. Effort syncope has been related to arrythmias and to an exercise-induced reduction in peripheral resistance that diminishes diastolic perfusion pressure and further reduces coronary blood flow to the left ventricular myocardium.[15, 36] Congestive failure is related to loss of contractile reserve, chamber dilatation, and rising left ventricular end-diastolic pressures.

Indications for Surgery

Development of symptoms in patients with aortic stenosis is associated with a poor long-term prognosis.[30] *Chest pain* reduces life expectancy to an average of 5 years, and *syncope* is generally associated with 3 to 4 years of survival. The onset of *congestive failure* reduces survival to an average of only 2 years. Two or more symptoms together significantly shorten survival. Thus, development of symptoms is an indication for valve replacement in patients with aortic stenosis. Cardiac catheterization usually demon-

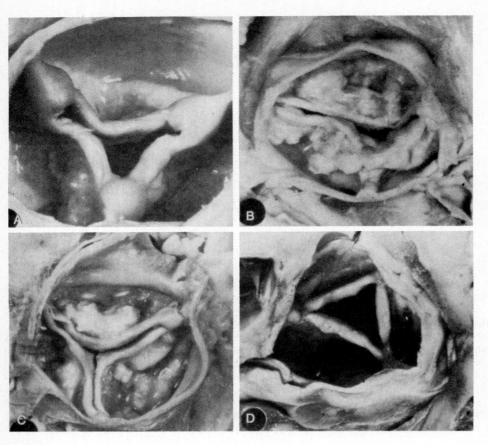

Figure 1. A, Rheumatic aortic stenosis with fusion of commissures and thickening of cusps. B, Calcific aortic stenosis in a congenital bicuspid valve. C, Calcific aortic stenosis in a tricuspid valve. D, Rheumatic aortic insufficiency. Thickened and shortened cusps are unable to close with diastole. (From Edwards, J. E.: Pathology of acquired diseases of the heart. Semin. Roentgenol., 14:108, 1979.)

strates a severe pressure gradient and a reduction in orifice area to 0.8 cm.[2] or less.

AORTIC INSUFFICIENCY

Etiology and Pathology

Intrinsic Diseases of the Valve. Rheumatic fever results in an insufficient valve when cusps undergo fibrous thickening and contracture (Fig. 1D). If fusion of commissures occurs, a combination of insufficiency and stenosis may occur.[13] Bacterial endocarditis may result in incompetence from destruction of cusp attachments or perforation of leaflets. Congenitally bicuspid valves are most often involved, although virulent organisms may infect previously normal valves. Less common causes of aortic insufficiency include connective tissue disorders,[31] prolapse of one cusp of a congenitally bicuspid valve,[5] and traumatic disruption of an aortic cusp.[10]

Diseases of the Ascending Aorta. Several conditions result in insufficiency by causing dilatation of the aortic root and secondary failure of free valve cusp coaptation during diastole. Cystic medial necrosis with subsequent secondary aortic root dilatation and aortic valvular insufficiency are seen in association with connective tissue disorders and with Marfan's syndrome. Formerly, syphilis was a common cause[21] but is rarely seen today.

Intimal tears in patients with cystic medial necrosis or severe hypertension cause dissection of the media of the aorta. If retrograde dissection occurs to the level of the aortic root, the valve cusp support apparatus may be involved, causing valve leaflet prolapse and acute aortic insufficiency.[34]

Physiology

The incompetent aortic valve produces an increase in ventricular volume with each diastole. The regurgitant volume is dependent on the area of valve incompetence, the pressure gradient across the valve, and the duration of diastole.[4] In chronic aortic insufficiency, stroke volume is increased in order to maintain forward output within normal ranges. Compensatory ventricular dilatation and hypertrophy follow to maintain forward stroke volume in the presence of gradually increasing regurgitant fraction. Eventually, myocardial contractile factors may decline, causing reduction in the capacity for augmenting stroke volume and a corresponding increase in end-diastolic volume. Increased end-systolic volume and a decreased end-diastolic compliance eventually produce a progressive increase in left ventricular filling pressures. The volume overload state is well tolerated when it occurs chronically. In contrast, acute aortic insufficiency causes sudden increases in left ventricular pressure in a chamber unable to dilate acutely. Acute pulmonary venous hypertension and pulmonary edema then ensue.

Clinical Manifestations

Patients with slowly progressive aortic insufficiency may remain asymptomatic for years. With reduction in myocardial contractile factors and with rising left ventricular filling pressures, symptoms become manifest. The onset of dyspnea, fatigue, orthopnea, and paroxysmal nocturnal dyspnea are usually insidious. Nocturnal chest pain and atypical chest pain are infrequently noted.[20] Although hemodynamically significant aortic insufficiency is tolerated well for many years, rapid deterioration may occur after the onset of symptoms. Patients developing congestive failure often die within 2 years. Average survival after the development of angina is 5 years.[30]

Indications for Operation

All patients with symptomatic aortic insufficiency are candidates for valve replacement. However, progression of ventricular dysfunction has occurred in some patients who have undergone valve replacement for symptomatic aortic insufficiency.[23] There is, therefore, an interest in identification of the patient who has not lost cardiac reserve at the time of valve replacement. The long asymptomatic latent period of aortic insufficiency has made identification of the ideal timing of operation difficult. Current parameters being evaluated include echocardiographic determination of left ventricular end-systolic dimension and per cent fractional shortening as well as the failure of exercise to augment or maintain ejection fraction.[2, 9, 24]

Aortic insufficiency associated with bacterial endocarditis is managed medically with appropriate antibiotic therapy. If hemodynamic deterioration occurs or if persistent bacteremia is present, valve replacement should be undertaken.[8]

Operative Treatment

Operations for aortic valve replacement are performed through a median sternotomy. Cardiopulmonary bypass is established by cannulation of the ascending aorta or femoral artery for arterial inflow, and venous return to the oxygenator and bypass pump is achieved by right atrial cannulation. The ascending aorta is clamped and an aortotomy made at the base of the aorta in order to expose the aortic valve. During the period of aortic occlusion, the myocardium is not perfused and is thus at risk for ischemic injury and cell death. Myocardial protection and preservation is accomplished by a combination of potassium induced asystolic arrest and hypothermia. Solutions of potassium-containing cold crystalloid or blood cardioplegia are infused into the aortic root after the ascending aorta has been clamped. Alternatively, the solutions may be directly infused into the coronary ostia after the aortotomy is made. Topical hypothermia is also employed by continuously surrounding the heart with iced saline and slush.

The diseased valve is excised and a prosthetic valve is sewn into the aortic anulus, usually with interrupted sutures (Fig. 2). Two general classifications of prosthetic valves are available. *Tissue* valves are composed of gluteraldehyde fixed tissue (aortic homograft, porcine aortic valve, or bovine pericardium) mounted on a stent. *Mechanical* valves consist of metallic frames with movable balls, discs, or hinged poppets. Although mechanical valves have the advantage of longevity and low valve-related failure rates, they are uniformly thrombogenic and require systemic anticoagulation. Tissue valves, although minimally thrombogenic, show a significant incidence of wear-related valve failure with time. In addition, tissue valves undergo pre-

mature calcification in children and in adults younger than 30 years of age.[19]

Patients with acute aortic insufficiency from aortic dissection may avoid valve replacement if the pre-existing valve is anatomically normal. Resuspension of the valve commissures allows for normal closure during diastole.[28] A prosthetic conduit is usually required for replacement of the dissected ascending aorta. A valve with a conduit may be required in patients with aortic insufficiency from aneurysmal dilatation of the aortic root and ascending aorta.[1]

Results of Surgery

Evaluation of operative results must include operative mortality, complications of operations, complications of the prosthetic valve, long-term survival, and functional improvement. These must be compared and contrasted with the natural history of the specific patient involved.

In a series of 1479 operations for aortic valve replacement, independent determinants of operative mortality were advanced New York Heart Association (NYHA) functional class, renal dysfunction, physiologic subgroup (stenosis, regurgitation, or stenosis/regurgitation), atrial fibrillation, and advanced age.[37] The overall operative mortality was 7 per cent. In one series of 1117 patients with mechanical aortic valve replacements followed for up to 20 years, the late mortality rate was 4.7 per cent per year.[40] Thromboembolic and hemorrhagic complications were seen at a rate of 4 per cent per year,[17, 37] and endocarditis occurred at a rate of 1 per cent per year.

Tissue valves have been implanted with similar operative mortality, late mortality, and rates of endocarditis.[25] Thromboembolic episodes are significantly less common, however, with rates of 1 per cent per year.[3, 7, 18] Failure rates from tissue valve calcific degeneration and late leaflet tears range from 1 to 2 per cent per year.[29, 35] Failure rates in children and young adults are significantly higher, ranging from 8 to 12 per cent per year.[12, 19]

IDIOPATHIC HYPERTROPHIC SUBAORTIC STENOSIS

Pathology

Idiopathic hypertrophic subaortic stenosis (IHSS) is a condition characterized by hypertrophy of the left ventricle and its outflow tract. The hypertrophy is frequently asymmetric with greater involvement of the septum. Microscopic examination reveals generalized disorganization of muscle bundles along with increased interstitial connective tissue.[14]

Physiology

A variable systolic pressure gradient is demonstrated at cardiac catheterization on pullback from the left ventricular apex to the infundibulum. The degree of obstruction is determined by contraction of septal myocardium and by systolic displacement of the anterior leaflet of the mitral valve. Factors increasing the degree of obstruction are those associated with increased inotropic state or with increased fractional shortening of myocardium. Thus, inotropic agonists, reduction in ventricular end-diastolic volume, and decreasing afterload will augment the degree of outflow obstruction. Conversely, decreasing inotropy, increased end-diastolic volume, and augmented afterload will cause reduction in the systolic pressure gradient.[14]

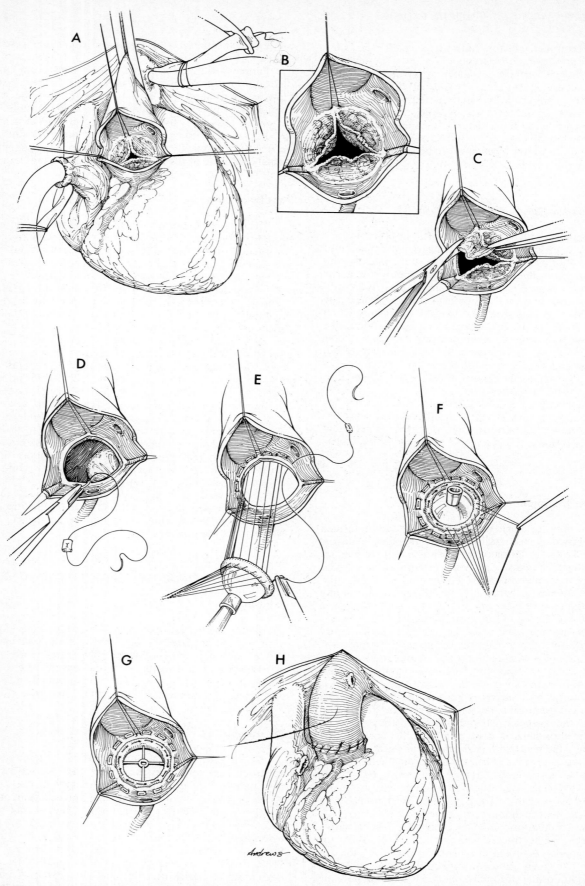

Figure 2. The standard aortic valve replacement. (From Cooley, D. A.: Techniques in Cardiac Surgery, 2nd ed. Philadelphia, W. B. Saunders Company, 1984, p. 179.)

Clinical Features

This disorder occurs in both sexes with a male-to-female distribution of 2:1. A large number of patients provide a familial history.[6] The age of presentation is variable, and IHSS has been described from infancy to the eighth decade. The most common presenting symptoms are effort dyspnea, angina pectoris, presyncope, syncope, and palpitations. Older patients tend to be more symptomatic.[38]

The diagnosis is suggested by bedside maneuvers that affect the degree of obstruction and thus alter the associated systolic murmur. The diagnosis is confirmed by echocardiographic determination of asymmetric septal hypertrophy and abnormal systolic anterior movement of the anterior mitral valve leaflet.[22] Cardiac catheterization is required to quantitate the resting pressure gradient, as well as to assess the degree of increase in gradient with provocative maneuvers.

The natural history of patients with IHSS is variable. Frank and Braunwald[16] suggested a relatively benign clinical course, although 25 per cent of their patients deteriorated or died. A sudden death rate of up to 3.4 per cent per year has been reported. There have been no reliable clinical criteria to predict those at risk for sudden death, as the problem occurs in patients at almost any age, in either sex, and regardless of whether or not symptoms have been present.[38]

Treatment

Propranolol is effective in reducing the effort induced outflow tract obstruction by reducing the inotropic state of the myocardium. Although symptomatic improvement occurs in many patients, disease progression and sudden death occur in patients treated with propranolol as well as in those untreated.[27]

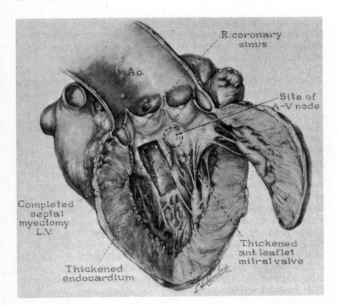

Figure 3. The appearance of the resected area of the septum and its relation to the aortic valve leaflets are shown semidiagrammatically. Also illustrated is the area of the conduction tissue, which must be avoided in performing the procedure. (From Crosby, I. K., and Muller, W. H., Jr.: Acquired disease of the aortic valve. In Sabiston, D. C., Jr., and Spencer, F. C. (Eds.): Gibson's Surgery of the Chest, 4th ed. Philadelphia, W. B. Saunders Company, 1983, p. 1301.)

The role of surgical correction in the management of patients with IHSS is controversial. Operation is usually reserved for those patients with severe symptoms or high resting gradients. The most successful approach involves resection of a portion of the septal myocardium in the obstructed outflow tract (Fig. 3). In a series of 124 patients,[26] the operative mortality was 8 per cent and survivors reported significant improvement in symptoms. A reduction in outflow tract obstruction at rest could be demonstrated. However, operation did not entirely prevent persistent (6 per cent) or recurrent (6 per cent) severe functional limitation. The late death rate related to cardiomyopathy was 1.8 per cent per year. The threat of sudden death was not relieved, as 6 of the 11 late deaths were sudden. However, no preoperative or postoperative clinical, hemodynamic, or electrocardiographic parameter could predict those patients at risk for late postoperative death or poor long-term symptomatic result.

SELECTED REFERENCES

Cohn, L. H., and Gallucci, V. (Eds.): Cardiac Bioprostheses: Proceedings of the Second International Symposium. New York, Yorke Medical Books, 1982.
This is a collection of papers on the hemodynamics, the short- and long-term clinical results, the risks of thromboembolism, and the problems of bioprosthetic engineering.

McKenna, W. J., and Goodwin, J. F.: The natural history of hypertrophic cardiomyopathy. *In* Current Problems in Cardiology. Chicago, Year Book Medical Publishers, 1981.
A comprehensive review of the natural history and a comparison of the reported operative and nonoperative treatment.

Tepley, J. F., Grunkemeier, G. L., Sutherland, H. D., Lambert, L. E., Johnson, V. A., and Starr, A.: The ultimate prognosis after valve replacement: An assessment at 20 years. *Ann. Thorac. Surg.,* 32:111–119, 1981.
This report of 1117 patients undergoing isolated aortic valve replacement provides an excellent analysis of the long-term operative results.

REFERENCES

1. Bentall, H., and DeBono, A.: A technique for complete revascularization of the ascending aorta. Thorax, 23:338, 1968.
2. Bonow, R. O., Rosing, D. R., McIntosh, C. L., Jones, M., Maron, B. J., Lan, G., Lakators, E., Bacharach, S. L., Green, M. V., and Epstein, S. E.: The natural history of asymptomatic patients with aortic regurgitation and normal left ventricular function. Circulation, 68:509, 1983.
3. Brais, M. P., Bedard, J. P., Goldstein, W., Kashal, A., and Keon, W. J.: Ionescu-Shiley pericardial xenografts: Follow-up of up to six years. Ann. Thorac. Surg., 39:105, 1985.
4. Brawley, R. K., and Morrow, A. G.: Direct determination of aortic blood flow in patients with aortic regurgitation: Effects of alterations in heart rate, increased ventricular preload and afterload, and isoproterenol. Circulation, 35:32, 1967.
5. Carter, J. B., Sethi, S., Lee, G. B., and Edwards, J. E.: Prolapse of semilunar cusps as causes of aortic insufficiency. Circulation, 43:922, 1971.
6. Clark, C. E., Henry, W. L., and Epstein, S. E.: Familial prevalence and genetic transmission of idiopathic hypertrophic subaortic stenosis. N. Engl. J. Med., 289:709, 1973.
7. Cohn, L. H., and Gallucci, V. (Eds.): Cardiac Bioprostheses: Proceedings of the Second International Symposium. New York, Yorke Medical Books, 1982.
8. Cukingham, R. A., Casey, J. S., Wittig, J. H., and Cimochowski, G. E.: Early valve replacement in active infective endocarditis: Results and late survival. J. Thorac. Cardiovasc. Surg., 85:163, 1983.
9. Daniel, W. G., Hood, W. P., Anette, S., Hausmann, D., Nellessen, V., Oelert, H., and Lichtlen, P. R.: Chronic aortic regurgitation: Reassessment of the prognostic value of preoperative left ventricular end-systolic dimension and fractional shortening. Circulation, 71:669, 1985.

10. Devineni, R., and McKenzie, F. N.: Avulsion of a normal valve cusp due to blunt chest trauma. J. Trauma, *24*:910, 1984.

11. Dodge, H. T., and Baxley, W. A.: Left ventricular volume and mass and their significance in heart disease. Am. J. Cardiol., *23*:528, 1969.

12. Dunn, J. M.: Porcine valve durability in children. Ann. Thorac. Surg., *32*:357, 1981.

13. Edwards, J. E.: Pathology of acquired valvular disease of the heart. Semin. Roentgenol., *14*:96, 1979.

14. Epstein, S. E., Henry, W. L., Clark, C. E., et al.: Asymmetric septal hypertrophy. Ann. Intern. Med., *81*:650, 1974.

15. Flamm, M. D., Braiff, B. A., Kimball, R., and Hancock, E. W.: Mechanism of effort syncope in aortic stenosis. Circulation, *36* (Suppl. 2): II-109, 1967.

16. Frank, S., and Braunwald, E.: Idiopathic hypertrophic subaortic stenosis: Clinical analysis of 126 patients with emphasis on the natural history. Circulation, *37*:759, 1968.

17. Fuster, V., Pumphrey, C. W., McGoon, M. D., Cheselbro, J. H., Pluth, J. R., and McGoon, D. C.: Systemic thromboembolism in mitral and aortic Starr-Edwards prostheses. Circulation, *66* (Suppl. 2):II–157, 1982.

18. Gallo, I., Ruiz, B., and Duran, C. M. G.: Five to eight year follow-up of patients with the Hancock cardiac bioprosthesis. J. Thorac. Cardiovasc. Surg., *86*:897, 1983.

19. Geha, A. S., Laks, H., Stansel, H. C., Cornhill, J. F., Kelman, J. W., Buckley, M. J., and Roberts, W. C.: Late failure of porcine valve heterografts in children. J. Thorac. Cardiovasc. Surg., *78*:351, 1979.

20. Goldschlager, N., Pfeifer, J., Cohn, K., Popper, R., and Selzer, A.: The natural history of aortic regurgitation: A clinical and hemodynamic study. Am. J. Med., *54*:577, 1973.

21. Heggtreit, H. A.: Syphilitic aortitis, a clinicopathologic autopsy study of 100 cases. Circulation, *29*:346, 1964.

22. Henry, W. L., Clark, C. E., and Epstein, S. E.: Asymmetric septal hypertrophy (ASH): Echocardiographic identification of the pathognomonic anatomic abnormality of IHSS. Circulation, *47*:225, 1973.

23. Henry, W. L., Bonow, R. O., Borer, J. S., Ware, J. H., Kent, K. M., Redwood, D. R., McIntosh, C. L., Morrow, A. G., and Epstein, S. E.: Observations on the optimum time for operative intervention for aortic regurgitation: I. Evaluation of the results of aortic valve replacement in symptomatic patients. Circulation, *61*:471, 1980.

24. Henry, W. L., Bonow, R. O., Rosing, D. R., and Epstein, S. E.: Observations on the optimum time for operative intervention for aortic regurgitation: II. Serial echocardiographic evaluation of asymptomatic patients. Circulation, *61*:484, 1980.

25. Magilligan, D. J., Lewis, J. W., Tilley, B., and Peterson, E.: The porcine valve: Twelve years later. J. Thorac. Cardiovasc. Surg., *89*:499, 1985.

26. Maron, J., Merrell, W. H., Freier, P. A., Kent, K. M., Epstein, S. E., and Morrow, A. G.: Long-term clinical course and symptomatic status of patients after operation for hypertrophic subaortic stenosis. Circulation, *57*:1205, 1978.

27. McKenna, W. J., and Goodwin, J. F.: The natural history of hypertrophic cardiomyopathy. *In* Current Problems in Cardiology. Chicago, Year Book Medical Publishers, 1981.

28. Najafi, H., Dye, W. S., Hunter, J. A., Golden, M. D., and Julian, O. C.: Acute aortic regurgitation secondary to aortic dissection: Surgical management without valve replacement. Ann. Surg., *14*:474, 1972.

29. Pomar, J. L., Bosch, X., Chaitman, B. R., Pelletier, C., and Grondin, C. M.: Late tears in leaflets of porcine bioprostheses in adults. Ann. Thorac. Surg., *37*:78, 1984.

30. Rapaport, E.: Natural history of aortic and mitral valve disease. Am. J. Cardiol., *35*:221, 1975.

31. Roberts, W. C., Kehoe, J. A., Carpenter, D. F., and Golden, A.: Cardiovascular valvular lesions in rheumatoid arthritis. Arch. Intern. Med., *122*:141, 1968.

32. Roberts, W. C.: Anatomically isolated aortic valvular disease: The case against it being of rheumatic etiology. Am. J. Med., *49*:151, 1970.

33. Roberts, W. C.: The structure of the aortic valve in clinically isolated aortic stenosis: An autopsy study of 162 patients over 15 years of age. Circulation, *42*:91, 1970.

34. Roberts, W. C.: Aortic dissection: anatomy, consequences, and causes. Am. Heart J., *101*:195, 1981.

35. Schoen, F. J., Collins, J. J., and Cohn, L. L.: Long-term failure rates and morphologic correlations in porcine bioprosthetic heart valves. Am. J. Cardiol., *51*:957, 1983.

36. Schwartz, L. D., Goldfischer, J., Sprague, G. L., and Schwartz, S. P.: Syncope and sudden death in aortic stenosis. Am. J. Cardiol., *23*:647, 1969.

37. Scott, W. C., Miller, D. C., Haverich, A., Dawkins, K., Mitchell, R. S., Jamieson, S. W., Oyer, P. E., Stinson, E. B., Baldwin, J. C., and Shumway, N. E.: Determinants of operative mortality for patients undergoing aortic valve replacement: Discriminant analysis of 1,479 operations. J. Thorac. Cardiovasc. Surg., *89*:400, 1985.

38. Shah, P. M., Adelman, A. G., Wigle, E. D., Gobel, F. L., Burchell, H. B., Hardarson, T., Currel, R., de la Calzada, C., Oakley, C. M., and Goodwin, J. F.: The natural (and unnatural) history of hypertrophic obstructive cardiomyopathy. Circ. Res., *35*(Suppl. 2):II–179, 1974.

39. Stein, P. D., Sabbah, H. N., and Pitha, J. V.: Continuing process of calcific aortic stenosis: Role of microthrombi and turbulent flow. Am. J. Cardiol., *39*:159, 1977.

40. Teply, J. F., Grunkemeier, G. L., Sutherland, H. D., Lambert, L. E., Johnson, V. A., and Starr, A.: The ultimate prognosis after valve replacement: An assessment at twenty years. Ann. Thorac. Surg., *32*:111, 1981.

41. Thubrikar, M., Nolan, S. P., Bosher, L. D., and Deck, J. D.: The cyclic changes and structure of the base of the aortic valve. Am. Heart J., *99*:217, 1980.

XV

Acquired Mitral and Tricuspid Valvular Disease

PETER VAN TRIGT, M.D.
DAVID C. SABISTON, JR., M.D.

HISTORICAL ASPECTS

Surgical correction of mitral stenosis was first suggested in 1902 by Brunton.[11] Although his suggestion was rebuked, this stimulated considerable interest in the pathophysiology and surgical treatment of valvular heart disease. In 1923,

Cutler and Levine reported an operation on a 12-year-old girl with severe mitral stenosis.[15] The result was unsatisfactory because resection of portions of the valve produced severe mitral regurgitation. In 1925, Souttar described a digital mitral commissurotomy through the left atrial appendage.[65] Although a favorable result was achieved, no significant progress was made over the next two decades.

During this interval, the technique of cardiac catheterization was developed and added greatly to the knowledge of valvular heart disease.[25] In 1947, Bailey[4] and Harken[36] and later Brock successfully performed closed digital commissurotomy for mitral stenosis and established the procedure as an acceptable surgical approach.

Only after the development of cardiopulmonary bypass was effective surgical treatment of mitral regurgitation developed. In 1960, Starr and Edwards introduced the mechanical prosthesis, which provided a consistently successful surgical procedure for patients with both mitral stenosis and insufficiency.[68] In the subsequent years, numerous mechanical and bioprosthetic tissue valves have been designed and evaluated.

ANATOMY AND PHYSIOLOGY

Although the mitral valve is quadricuspid during early embryogenesis, the commissural cusps regress and two leaflets are present in adults—the large "sail-like" anterior leaflet and the smaller posterior, or mural, leaflet. The two commissures do not divide the leaflet tissue completely to the valve anulus. The anterior leaflet has a greater base-to-margin length, but because the posterior leaflet has a greater amount of anular attachment[68] the surface area of each leaflet is nearly equal. The leaflets are trapezoidal and are attached by chordae tendineae to the papillary muscles, which arise from the endocardial surface of the ventricular chamber. Each leaflet is attached to both the anterior and posterior papillary muscles by the thin fibrous chordae, which fan out along the leaflet margin as well as along the ventricular surface of the leaflets.[58]

The blood supply to the papillary muscles is provided by distal branches of the coronary arteries.[16] The anterolateral papillary muscle is supplied by branches of the left anterior descending system. The posteromedial papillary muscle is usually supplied by posterolateral branches of the right coronary artery or, in the case of left coronary dominance, by posterolateral branches of the circumflex coronary artery.

In almost all hearts, the papillary muscle is an accurate guide to the corresponding commissure, even in a severely deformed rheumatic valve.[20] The point of coaptation of the two leaflets is not the free edge, but is located on the atrial surface a short distance toward the anulus.

The anatomy of the tricuspid valve apparatus is similar, except that *three* leaflets are present: anterior, posterior, and septal. The largest leaflet is usually the anterior, the posterior being the smallest. The papillary muscles of the tricuspid valve tend to be multiple, but can be categorized into three groups: (1) *anterior* (arising from right ventricular free wall), (2) *inferior* (arising from the inferior aspect of the interventricular septum), and (3) *septal* (arising from the high septum). Similar to the mitral valve, each papillary muscle component contributes chordae to multiple leaflets.[45]

Functionally, the atrioventricular valves allow free flow of blood from atria to ventricles during ventricular diastole and prevent regurgitation of blood into the atria during systole. This is achieved through a coordinated contraction pattern of myocardium and papillary muscles during the cardiac cycle. When left ventricular pressure falls during isovolumic relaxation and becomes lower than that of the full atrium, the valve opens and rapid filling of diastole occurs. The majority of diastolic filling occurs during this phase. Early transmitral flow is the result of a pressure gradient across the valve as well as active forces related to myocardial relaxation.[76]

During ventricular systole after closure of the atrioventricular valves, valve competence is aided by active motions of the valve anulus and papillary muscles. The anular area shows significant changes during the cardiac cycle and decreases by one third from end-diastole to mid-systole.[64] Active shortening of circumferential myocardial fibers around the anulus reduces valve orifice area during systole and contributes to valvular competence. The papillary muscles contract during systole and shorten the subvalvular apparatus to compensate for contraction of the ventricular walls. Intact chordae and normal papillary muscle function are necessary for proper leaflet closure. Regardless of the presence of intact leaflets, competence of the mitral valve is lost in the presence of anular dilatation, chordal disruption, or papillary muscle dysfunction.

MITRAL STENOSIS

Etiology and Pathology

The predominant cause of mitral stenosis is rheumatic fever, although a history of one or more attacks of acute rheumatic fever is present in only half of patients with mitral stenosis. For unknown reasons, the lesion is much more common in females. Mitral stenosis on a rheumatic basis can be associated with an atrial septal defect (Lutembacher's syndrome). Isolated mitral stenosis occurs in approximately 40 per cent of all patients with rheumatic valvular heart disease. Because of the widespread effective prophylaxis of rheumatic fever for the past several decades, the frequency of mitral stenosis has declined markedly. Congenital mitral stenosis is rare,[62] being observed almost exclusively in infants and children. Other rare causes of mitral stenosis include malignant carcinoid, systemic lupus erythematosus, and endomyocardial fibrosis.[32]

Rheumatic valvulitis results in a number of pathologic changes that contribute to narrowing of the mitral orifice. The process is progressive, with pathologic changes occurring over a number of years following the initial attack of rheumatic fever. The exudative-degenerative phase lasts 2 to 3 weeks, followed by development of the characteristic histologic lesion of rheumatic fever, the Aschoff body. The proliferative and healing phase then begins and lasts several years. Aschoff bodies may persist in surgical biopsies of the atrial appendage several years after the resolution of rheumatic fever.

Most patients remain asymptomatic in a latent phase for two decades before the onset of symptoms.[74, 75] Fusion of the valve leaflets at the commissures is the most common result of rheumatic inflammation, occurring alone in 30 per cent of involved valves. The endocardial surface ulcerates where the two leaflets normally coapt in systole. The valve leaflets become thickened, calcified, and rigid, with the ingrowth of fibrous tissue. Concomitantly, the chordae tendineae may become thickened, retracted, and fused, with displacement of the valve into the left ventricular chamber. These combined processes result in a rigid narrowed mitral valve that is funnel-shaped and with an orifice frequently described as a "fish-mouth" (Fig. 1). The degree of pathologic change is important in determining surgical approach. If commissural fusion alone is present, excellent results can be obtained by commissurotomy. More commonly, extensive fibrosis and calcification with leaflet retraction and fusion of the chordae require mitral valve replacement.

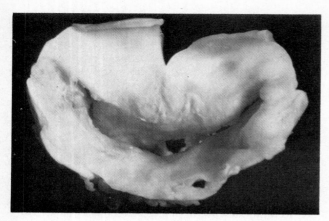

Figure 1. Excised mitral valve showing characteristic pathologic changes of rheumatic mitral stenosis producing in a "fish-mouth" configuration of the orifice. (From Becker, A. E., and Anderson, R. H.: Cardiac Pathology. New York, Raven Press, 1982.)

Pathophysiology

The normal adult mitral valve has a cross-sectional area between 4 cm.^{2} and 6 cm.^{2} Significant hemodynamic changes associated with onset of symptoms do not occur until the cross-sectional area is reduced to below 2.0 to 2.5 cm.^{2} Patients with a cross-sectional valve area of 1.5 to 2.0 cm.^{2} usually are symptomatic on moderate exertion (New York Heart Association Class II), and if the area is reduced to 1.0 to 1.5 cm.^{2}, these symptoms become more severe. When valve cross-sectional area falls below 1.0 cm.^{2}, patients are significantly disabled and symptomatic at rest (Class IV). An opening near 0.5 cm.^{2} is about the smallest size consistent with life.

Three significant physiologic alterations are associated with mitral stenosis: (1) left atrial hypertension, (2) reduction in cardiac output, and (3) increase in pulmonary vascular resistance. As obstruction to mitral flow develops, an elevation in left atrial pressure above the normal range (10 to 12 mm. Hg) is initially seen with dilatation of the left atrial chamber. The degree of elevation of left atrial pressure is dependent on the cross-sectional area of the mitral orifice, the cardiac output, and the length of diastole as determined by heart rate. At cardiac catheterization, elevation of left atrial pressure to levels of 15 to 20 mm. Hg is commonly seen in moderate to severe mitral stenosis. If mean left atrial pressure exceeds 30 mm. Hg, transudation of fluid into pulmonary interstitial tissues results and pulmonary edema may develop, dependent on the transport capacity of the pulmonary lymphatics. The elevation in left atrial pressure is transmitted to raise pulmonary venous and capillary pressure, and this results in exertional dyspnea as well as in other symptoms of pulmonary congestion, including orthopnea, cough, hemoptysis, and paroxysmal nocturnal dyspnea. The first bouts of dyspnea in patients with mitral stenosis are usually precipitated by exercise, emotional stress, infection, or atrial fibrillation, all of which increase the rate of blood flow delivered to the stenotic mitral orifice and further elevate left atrial pressure.[55]

Because of the reduced mitral valve orifice, a restriction in cardiac output at a low level results. This leads to symptoms of fatigue, exercise intolerance, and muscular wasting associated with cardiac cachexia. Patients with severe mitral stenosis may live for many years with a sedentary existence.

The delayed pathophysiologic effects of long-standing left atrial hypertension are directed against the pulmonary vasculature and right ventricle.[18] Along with congestion of the pulmonary vessels and thickening of the alveolar capillaries, intimal hypertrophy of the arterioles and veins is also observed. In advanced cases, medial thickening and fibrosis are common. Pulmonary hypertension progresses with time as the result of two mechanisms: (1) retrograde transmission of left atrial hypertension to the pulmonary vasculature and (2) a reactive increase in pulmonary vascular resistance. There is a great deal of variation among individual patients in the degree of increase in pulmonary vascular resistance. Fortunately, in the majority of patients, the elevated pulmonary vascular resistance either greatly decreases or completely resolves following operation, unlike the situation in congenital heart disease—when elevated pulmonary vascular resistance is often irreversible. Pulmonary hypertension causes right ventricular hypertrophy, and myocardial protection of the right ventricle is important at the time of operation on a patient with mitral stenosis. In pure mitral stenosis, the left ventricle remains non-enlarged and left ventricular dysfunction does not contribute to the pathophysiology of the disease.

Other clinical abnormalities that result from mitral stenosis include the development of chronic atrial fibrillation and systemic embolization. The exact cause of atrial fibrillation is unknown, but it may be a result of atrial dilatation and alterations in normal atrial conduction patterns.[70] Atrial contraction augments ventricular filling significantly in mitral stenosis so that when atrial fibrillation occurs, left atrial pressure increases and cardiac output is reduced by approximately 20 per cent. Thrombi develop in the dilated atrium, which may be limited to the atrial appendage, or laminate the entire wall. These thrombi develop in 15 to 20 per cent of patients with mitral stenosis and may embolize to the systemic circulation in a random manner. Embolization is most common soon after the development of atrial fibrillation.[1, 5]

Diagnosis

The characteristic symptom of mitral stenosis is dyspnea, largely the result of reduced pulmonary vascular compliance. Several other symptoms occur secondary to recurrent pulmonary congestion. These include orthopnea, paroxysmal nocturnal dyspnea, hemoptysis, easy fatigability, and episodes of frank pulmonary edema. Eventually right ventricular failure appears and is reflected by venous distention, hepatic enlargement, and peripheral edema. These symptoms may be intensified by functional tricuspid insufficiency.

On physical examination the patient characteristically appears thin and frail, with muscular wasting typical of chronic illness. A reddish blush of the cheeks and peripheral cyanosis may be present; these symptoms are secondary to low cardiac output and low flow through peripheral capillary beds. Bibasilar rales are frequently present on auscultation. Jugular venous pulsations may be prominent secondary to fluid overload or with secondary tricuspid regurgitation. Peripheral edema and hepatic enlargement may be present.

On examination of the heart, cardiac size is usually normal, with a normal or slightly reduced apical impulse. If pulmonary hypertension has produced right ventricular hypertrophy, a forceful impulse may be palpable over the right parasternal area. Auscultation characteristically yields an apical diastolic rumble, an increased first heart sound,

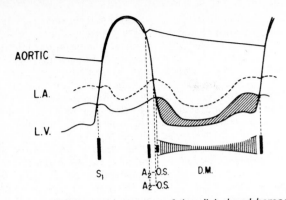

AORTIC

L.A.

L.V.

S_1 A_2-O.S.   D.M.
         A_2-O.S.

Figure 2. Schematic representation of the clinical and hemodynamic features of mitral stenosis. The dotted line shows the difference between moderate and severe stenosis; when the stenosis is severe, the opening snap occurs earlier.

and an opening snap (Fig. 2). These are sufficiently characteristic to establish the diagnosis with an accuracy approaching almost 100 per cent on physical examination alone. Calcifications or severé thickening of the leaflets may reduce the amplitude of S_1 later in the course of the disease. An *opening snap* (OS) of the mitral valve, heard best at the apex, is common and appears to result from sudden tension on the leaflets by the chordae after the cusps complete their initial opening. The presence of an OS indicates leaflet pliability and is absent in the valve with rigid, calcified, immobile leaflets. The opening snap follows S_2 by 40 to 120 msec., with a shorter interval indicating more severe mitral stenosis (Fig. 2). The low-pitched apical diastolic rumble is best heard at the apex and is produced by blood flowing through the stenotic orifice. The murmur begins immediately after the OS, and its duration is directly related to the severity of valve obstruction. It should be remembered that left atrial myxoma may produce auscultatory findings quite comparable with those in rheumatic mitral valvar stenosis.

The electrocardiogram (ECG) is seldom an accurate guide as to the severity of mitral stenosis. Left atrial enlargement will be reflected by a broad, notched P wave in lead II, the so-called P mitrale. In later stages of the disease, atrial fibrillation and right ventricular hypertrophy are seen. The QRS axis in the frontal plane often correlates with the severity of valve obstruction and with the level of pulmonary vascular resistance. According to Braunwald,[9] an axis greater than 60 degrees generally indicates that the valve area is less than 1.3 cm.[2]

The chest roentgenogram will reveal several abnormalities in mitral stenosis. The cardiac silhouette in the frontal projection may be normal, with the exception of left atrial enlargement. This finding is usually evident on the lateral and left anterior oblique views. The classic radiographic signs of left atrial enlargement include prominence of the left atrial appendage, elevation of the left main stem bronchus, round double density through the central shadow of the heart on the frontal projection, and posterior extension of the left atrium on the lateral projection. Engorged pulmonary veins can be prominent, especially in the distribution to the upper lobes (cephalization of pulmonary blood flow). In severe mitral stenosis associated with pulmonary hypertension, right ventricular hypertrophy and enlargement of the main pulmonary arteries will be present. Interstitial edema is manifested as Kerley B lines, short, dense, horizontal lines most commonly seen in the costophrenic angles.[16]

Cardiac catheterization is required for mitral stenosis to be assessed precisely and is preferred in most patients considered for surgical therapy. It also provides simultaneous information on the presence of mitral regurgitation, aortic valve disease, and coronary artery disease. The transvalvular gradient across the mitral valve is obtained by transseptal cannulation of the left atrium and retrograde cannulation of the left ventricle through the aorta, across the aortic valve. A diastolic pressure gradient across the mitral valve is usually 10 to 20 mm. Hg in patients with severe stenosis. Because left atrial pressure depends on several factors, including cardiac output and heart rate as well as the degree of stenosis, the most precise measurement is mathematical calculation of the cross-sectional area of the valve. The calculation, according to the Gorlin formula, takes into account the mean diastolic mitral gradient and average diastolic mitral flow. Estimation of orifice area is subject to some error at low flow rates or in the presence of valvular regurgitation. Hence, it is important to realize that catheterization findings are supplemental, and the entire clinical setting must be evaluated when making therapeutic decisions.

Indications for Operation

Justification for an aggressive surgical approach to mitral stenosis is based on the natural history of the disease. It appears that after a relatively asymptomatic latent period of 10 to 20 years after an episode of rheumatic fever, the condition of most patients will progress from a functional (Class II) status to total disability (Class IV) in 5 to 10 years. This deterioration occurs rapidly in up to half of the affected patients, commonly as a result of the onset of atrial fibrillation or systemic embolization.[61] In the presurgical era, Olesen found a 62 per cent 5-year and 38 per cent 10-year survival among patients with Class III symptoms, but only a 15 per cent 5-year survival in patients with Class IV functional impairment.[50] Congestive failure was responsible for death in 62 per cent, 22 per cent died from thromboembolic complications, and 8 per cent from infectious endocarditis. These data indicate that, although patients with mitral stenosis remain initially asymptomatic for several years, once serious symptoms develop the disease rapidly progresses to death. Operation should not be delayed until Class IV symptoms develop. In patients with less severe symptoms (Class II), cardiac catheterization should be performed and valve cross-sectional area calculated. If mitral orifice size is less than 1.0 cm.[2] per m.[2] of body surface area, operation should generally be recommended. Available data support early application of surgical therapy to patients with mitral stenosis, with Roberts concluding that the natural history of mitral stenosis ranks second only to aortic stenosis in terms of mortality from all forms of valvular heart disease.[59]

Surgical Therapy

Three basically different operative approaches are available for the treatment of rheumatic mitral stenosis: (1) closed mitral commissurotomy, (2) open mitral commissurotomy (performed under direct vision on cardiopulmonary bypass), and (3) mitral valve replacement.

OPEN VERSUS CLOSED COMMISSUROTOMY

Closed mitral commissurotomy is reserved for the patient with predominant mitral stenosis and little mitral regurgitation, without evidence of atrial thrombus, and without serious valvular calcification.[14] The presence of an opening snap is favorable, for it indicates the leaflets are still pliable. The operation is performed through a left posterolateral thoracotomy, with exposure of the left groin in the event the femoral vessels need to be cannulated, and cardiopulmonary bypass is ready on a standby basis. After placement of a pursestring suture in the appendage, the surgeon places a finger through the pursestring into the atrium. The presence of thrombus is carefully assessed, and if regurgitation is minimal and there is little valvular calcification, the surgeon proceeds with placement of a transventricular dilator.[31] The tip of the dilator is passed through the mitral valve and palpated by the operator, then opened to a preset length of 3.0 to 3.5 cm. This produces a division of the fused commissures, and with a finger the surgeon can assess the adequacy of relief of stenosis and any induced mitral regurgitation.

Desired goals include minimal mitral regurgitation and low transvalvular gradients (4 mm. Hg) measured at the conclusion of the procedure. The closed approach should be converted to an open procedure if the surgeon is unable to perform an adequate commissurotomy or if there is significant left atrial thrombus with a high risk of embolization during surgical manipulation.

One advantage of the closed approach is that a median sternotomy and cardiopulmonary bypass can be avoided; also, this is a shorter and simpler procedure and the valve can be assessed in the working heart. Disadvantages include the risk of hemorrhage from an atrial tear, systemic emboli, mitral regurgitation, and inadequate commissurotomy.

Most surgeons prefer to perform a *direct-vision commissurotomy*,[35, 60] although the procedure was first devised for less optimal valves or for complications following closed procedures.[2] Most series indicate that closed and open procedures are associated with an equivalent mortality and that the effectiveness of the procedure is enhanced using an open approach. Improved hemodynamic results associated with the open procedure also may reflect a selection factor at the time of operation by which more severely diseased valves can be recognized and selected for valve replacement, thereby reserving commissurotomy for those valves with favorable potential for good long-term results.

Open commissurotomy is performed through a median sternotomy with cardiopulmonary bypass and cardioplegic arrest (Fig. 3). The left atrium is exposed through the interatrial groove. The commissures are opened with a scalpel, with the incisions being designed to stop short of the valve anulus. Subvalvular chordal fusion should be released if possible. After the commissurotomy is completed, valve competence is assessed by injection of saline into the ventricle[13, 39] or by induction of aortic insufficiency after removal of the aortic cross-clamp.[34]

It should be recognized that mitral commissurotomy, whether open or closed, is a palliative rather than a curative procedure and does not yield a normal valve, but one that resembles its status perhaps 10 years previously. Most patients obtain immediate improvement in symptoms, and many maintain clinical improvement for 10 to 15 years, at which time mitral valve replacement may become necessary.

MITRAL VALVE REPLACEMENT

The surgical approach for mitral valve replacement is usually through a median sternotomy, although a right anterior thoracotomy provides adequate exposure as well. After arterial and venous return cannulae are placed, bypass is initiated, and the body temperature is reduced to 32° C. The aorta is cross-clamped as cold potassium cardioplegia is delivered into the root of the aorta to perfuse the coronary arteries. The left atrium is opened and the valve is circumferentially excised, leaving a small rim of leaflet tissue attached to the anulus. Care is taken not to cut through the anulus, especially posteriorly along the mural leaflet, which can result in an atrioventricular disconnection and myocardial rupture.[17] Detached chordae must be removed to avoid interference with motion of the prosthetic valve (Fig. 4).

Valve sutures are placed using a horizontal mattress suture technique with subanular pledgets. Sutures are carefully placed in the anular tissue and not beyond, so as to avoid injury to the circumflex coronary artery, the aortic valve, and the conduction system. Careful spacing of the sutures, together with extra support of the subanular pledgets, has reduced the incidence of paravalvular leaks and

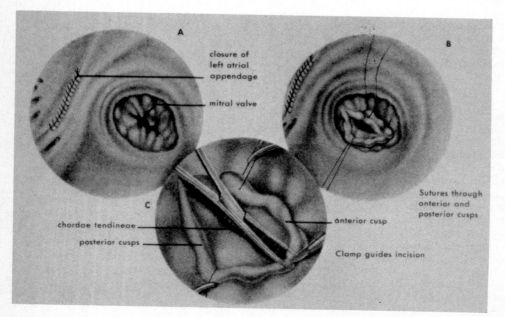

closure of
left atrial
appendage

mitral valve

chordae tendineae

posterior cusps

Sutures through
anterior and
posterior cusps

anterior cusp

Clamp guides incision

Figure 3. Technique of open mitral commissurotomy. A, Closure of left atrial appendage. B, Exposure of valve with horizontal traction on sutures. C, Incision made along the commissures. (From Sabiston, D. C., Jr., and Spencer, F. C. (Eds.): Gibbon's Surgery of the Chest. 4th ed. Philadelphia, W. B. Saunders Company, 1983, p. 1233.)

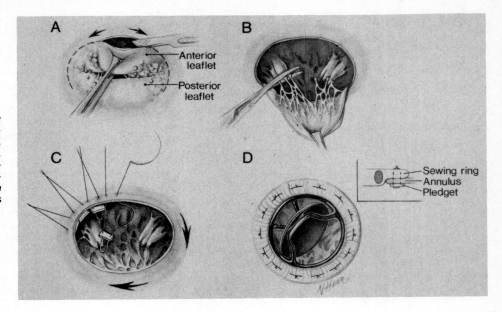

Figure 4. Technique for mitral valve replacement. A, Excision of the leaflets. B, Division of the chordae, leaving the papillary muscles intact. C, Placement of horizontal pledgeted mattress sutures. D, Bjork-Shiley valve seated in the anulus, with position of subanular pledgets shown in the inset.

primary valve dehiscence.[40, 49] A Foley catheter is placed across the mechanical valve during atriotomy closure to maintain mitral incompetence and evacuate air from the left side of the heart. Once the valve is inserted, the heart is not removed from the pericardium again to reduce the risk of atrioventricular dehiscence or ventricular perforation.

A variety of prosthetic valves are available for valve replacement, and they can be generally classified as either *bioprosthetic* or *mechanical*.

Bioprosthetic Valves

As a group, bioprosthetic mitral valves (Fig. 5) (Carpentier-Edwards and Hancock being porcine tissue valves, Ionescu-Shiley being made of bovine pericardium) have low thromboembolic rates, do not require coumadin anticoagulation, and may have marginal flow characteristics with significant transvalvular gradients in small sizes.

The main concern with tissue valves is durability. Degeneration of leaflet tissue with calcification and structural failure results in valve dysfunction, often within a 7- to 10-year period with porcine heterografts.[24, 29, 67] The rate of valve failure is higher in the mitral than the aortic position because of higher stresses associated with valve closure.[8] The issue of valve durability becomes more significant as increasing numbers of patients with valve failure are returning for reoperation. Tissue valves are generally not recommended for patients under 30 years of age because of a well-demonstrated accelerated rate of calcific degeneration in such patients.[23, 28] Young females desiring children may choose a tissue valve to reduce complications of anticoagulation during pregnancy, recognizing that another valve replacement may eventually be needed.[33] In addition, patients with contraindications to coumadin anticoagulation are candidates for tissue valves.

Mechanical Valves

Current mechanical valves (Starr-Edwards, Bjork-Shiley, St. Jude, Medtronic-Hall) offer better durability and more predictable performance than tissue valves (Fig. 6).

All adult patients require anticoagulation with coumadin. However, this is associated with bleeding complications and a mortality of approximately 1 per cent per year.[33] Even with adequate anticoagulation, the thromboembolic complication rate for current mechanical valves approaches 2 to 5 per cent per patient year.[19] With low-profile valves, late obstruction of the disc or leaflets may occur from various causes.[37, 72] In children or small adults, the Bjork-Shiley or St. Jude valve is often employed because of excellent flow characteristics in small sizes.[30, 73] The Starr-Edwards valve, the best evaluated prosthetic valve and that with the longest follow-up, should not be used in extremely small left ventricles (such as with mitral stenosis) because the ball and cage may obstruct left ventricular outflow.

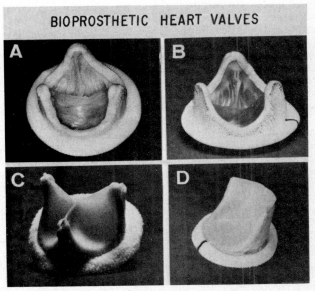

Figure 5. Commonly used bioprosthetic mitral valves. A, Hancock porcine valve. B, Carpentier-Edwards porcine valve. C, Ionescu-Shiley bovine pericardium valve. D, Meadox-Gabbay unicusp pericardial valve (undergoing clinical trials).

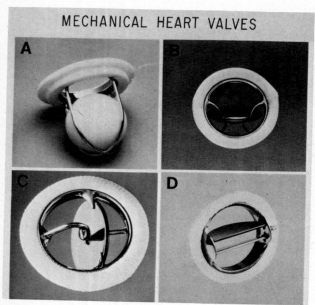

Figure 6. Commonly used mechanical heart valves for mitral replacement. A, Starr-Edwards model 6120. B, Bjork-Shiley convexoconcave mitral prosthesis. C, Medtronic-Hall valve. D, St. Jude medical valve.

Postoperative Care

Low cardiac output from cardiac failure can occur in patients undergoing surgery for mitral valve disease and is usually associated with long-standing mitral stenosis with pulmonary hypertension. Right ventricular dysfunction is most commonly seen after correction of mitral stenosis, but the left ventricle may also be involved.

Proper management requires placement of catheters for measurement of central venous pressure and left atrial pressure, with careful attention given to the primary determinants of cardiac output, i.e., (1) *preload* (filling pressures); (2) *afterload* (peripheral or pulmonary vascular resistance), (3) *heart rate* (which may be managed with atrial and ventricular pacing wires), and (4) *contractility* (which can be augmented with dopamine or epinephrine as needed). Other potential problems less commonly seen after mitral valve replacement include ventricular ectopy, respiratory failure, renal failure, peripheral emboli, valvular infection, and hemorrhage, all of which are approached according to the standard principles of postoperative care.

Patients with tissue valves are generally given the anticoagulants aspirin and dipyridamole, independent of cardiac rhythm. In adult patients with mechanical valves, coumadin is generally begun on the fourth or fifth postoperative day and is continued indefinitely to maintain the prothrombin ratio between 1.7 and 2.0. Digoxin and diuretics are continued postoperatively, and fluid restriction is necessary because the tendency to retain fluid in these patients persists for weeks or months. Antibiotics are given prophylactically preoperatively and are generally continued for 2 to 3 days after surgery.

Surgical Results

The operative risk of mitral procedures primarily depends on the severity of the disease preoperatively, with operative mortality varying between 1 and 5 per cent in most series. Other factors that adversely influence outcome include severe pulmonary hypertension and right ventricular failure. Elevated pulmonary vascular resistance usually decreases after commissurotomy or valve replacement,[22] although persistent pulmonary hypertension is observed in some patients with end-stage valve disease, emphysema, or previous pulmonary emboli.[71] The improved early survival rates reflect improvements in the area of operative techniques and myocardial preservation rather than improvements in valve design. Excellent long-term valve function and patient survival have been reported for both bioprosthetic and mechanical valves. Oyer and associates reported a series of 1407 patients receiving Hancock bioprostheses between 1971 and 1979.[51] The probability of freedom from valve failure 5 years after mitral valve replacement was 95 per cent. In 1979, Bjork and Henze reviewed an experience with 1800 Bjork-Shiley valves over a 10-year period. The 5-year survival after mitral replacement was 66 per cent, with a 1.3 per cent per year frequency of valve thrombosis.[7]

MITRAL REGURGITATION

Etiology and Pathology

Mitral regurgitation results from an abnormality of any one of the components of the mitral valve apparatus—the leaflets, the chordae tendineae, the mitral anulus, or the papillary muscles. The most common cause of mitral regurgitation requiring operation is rheumatic valvulitis, accounting for 35 to 45 per cent of cases. The rheumatic process results in a shortening, rigidity, deformity, and retraction of one or both cusps, as well as shortening and fusion of the chordae and papillary muscles. Varying degrees of valvular stenosis may occur in association with mitral regurgitation. Obstruction of the mitral leaflets can also result from endocarditis and rarely from trauma.

Idiopathic calcification of the mitral anulus can occur in the elderly and can cause mitral regurgitation by interfering with the normal sphincteric action of the anulus during ventricular systole. This process can be accelerated in the presence of hypertension, diabetes, aortic stenosis, and some connective tissue disorders.[26] Abnormalities of the chordae tendineae are important causes of mitral regurgitation, and chordal rupture can result from infectious endocarditis, rheumatic fever, trauma, or myxomatous degeneration. In most patients, a specific cause for chordal rupture is not apparent but does produce acute mitral regurgitation.

The mitral prolapse syndrome (Barlow's syndrome, "midsystolic click" syndrome, and "floppy mitral valve") is a common, but variable syndrome resulting from myxomatous degeneration of the valve leaflets and chordae tendineae (Fig. 7).[56] This syndrome occurs in 5 to 10 per cent of the general population and is felt to have a strong hereditary component transmitted as an autosomal dominant trait.[57] Progressive and clinically significant mitral regurgitation develops in approximately 15 per cent of these patients and, when severe, mitral valve replacement is indicated.[47]

Disease of the ventricular papillary muscles frequently causes mitral regurgitation. Because the papillary muscles are perfused by the terminal portion of the coronary arterial system, they are especially vulnerable to ischemia. The posteromedial papillary muscle is most prone to ischemia because it is supplied by the distal right coronary system with little arterial collateral support. A variation in severity of regurgitation exists, from transient mitral insufficiency

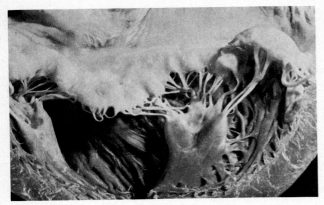

Figure 7. Appearance of the mitral valve in mitral valve prolapse with overshoot of the posterior leaflet. (From Becker, A. E., and Anderson, R. H.: Cardiac Pathology. New York, Raven Press, 1982.)

associated with episodes of angina to severe acute pulmonary edema associated with myocardial infarction and papillary muscle necrosis (frank rupture of the papillary muscle being rare).[48] Chronic ischemia can also lead to generalized ventricular dilatation with enlargement of the anulus and subsequent mitral regurgitation.[27]

Pathophysiology

The basic pathophysiologic alteration is elevation of left atrial pressure as blood passes retrograde through the incompetent mitral valve during ventricular systole. This extra blood is then returned as an added volume load to the left ventricle during diastole. Because the regurgitant mitral orifice is parallel with the aortic valve, the resistance to left ventricular ejection is reduced in mitral regurgitation. Thus at any level of preload, mitral regurgitation reduces the tension developed by the left ventricular myocardium, which explains how the left ventricle can adapt so well to the increased volume load imposed by chronic mitral regurgitation. This reduction in left ventricular tension accounts for why patients with mitral regurgitation can sustain large regurgitant volumes for prolonged periods, while maintaining forward cardiac output at normal levels for several years. Although the left ventricle can initially compensate for mitral regurgitation by emptying more completely,[66] as regurgitation persists and pump efficiency declines,[66] left ventricular function deteriorates and left ventricular end-diastolic volume progressively increases. Cardiomegaly due to left ventricular eccentric hypertrophy is associated with chronic mitral regurgitation, unlike pure mitral stenosis, which does not cause left ventricular enlargement.

An increase in pulmonary vascular resistance develops more slowly than in pure mitral stenosis, because of the intermittent nature of left atrial hypertension. In addition, atrial thrombosis is less common in mitral regurgitation owing to the absence of stasis of blood in the left atrium.

Clinical Features

The time interval between the episode of rheumatic fever and development of symptoms is usually longer than in mitral stenosis, as patients remain fairly asymptomatic until the left ventricle begins to fail.[21] The more important symptoms that develop include dyspnea on exertion, easy fatigability, and at times palpitations. The sudden worsening of symptoms in a patient with chronic regurgitation should suggest the presence of bacterial endocarditis or ruptured chordae tendineae. The development of atrial fibrillation is common in severe cases, but does not affect the course as adversely as in patients with mitral stenosis, because the arrhythmia does not cause as great an increase in left atrial pressure.

Physical examination findings include a peripheral arterial pulse that is small in volume, but has a rapid upstroke. The cardiac impulse is hyperdynamic and displaced to the left. On auscultation a holosystolic murmur, heard best at the apex, begins shortly after a soft S_1 and continues beyond A_2. The murmur of chronic regurgitation is usually of constant intensity, blowing, and high-pitched in character. There is little correlation between the intensity of the murmur and severity of the regurgitation. In mitral valve prolapse, the murmur is usually later in systole and is accompanied by a mid-systolic click caused by a sudden systolic prolapse of the leaflets back into the left atrium.[52]

The electrocardiogram (ECG) reveals left ventricular hypertrophy and left atrial enlargement in chronic cases. The chest film displays an enlarged left atrium, which is associated with a dilated left ventricular chamber. Changes in the lung fields are less prominent in mitral regurgitation than in mitral stenosis, but pulmonary congestion with Kerley B lines is frequently seen with acute mitral regurgitation.

Cardiac catheterization best quantitates the degree of mitral insufficiency by revealing the amount of dye refluxed from left ventricle to atrium during systole. The left atrial pressure tracing displays prominent V waves. The ejection fraction calculated from the ventriculogram may be normal or slightly elevated in the compensated state, owing to retrograde ejection into the low resistance left atrium. Therefore, a moderately reduced value (ejection fraction of 40 to 50 per cent) generally indicates severe impairment of contractility.[63] An elevated left ventricular end-systolic volume (greater than 30 ml. per m.²) has been correlated with high perioperative mortality and a persistent reduction in left ventricular function postoperatively.[53]

Operative Indications

Patients with significant mitral regurgitation can function for years with only minimal symptoms on medical management. However, symptoms alone are an unreliable guide to the timing of surgical intervention, and factors such as progressive cardiomegaly or pulmonary hypertension need to be considered. Operation should not be delayed until Class IV is reached, because of higher operative mortality and depressed long-term survival in these severely disabled patients.[44]

Surgical Therapy

The surgical correction of mitral regurgitation includes a valve repair (valvuloplasty, anuloplasty) or prosthetic valve replacement. Although conservative procedures utilizing newer techniques of valve reconstruction are gaining popularity, the standard procedure for the treatment of mitral regurgitation under most circumstances is mitral valve replacement. The technical considerations, types of

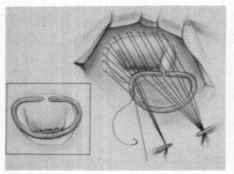 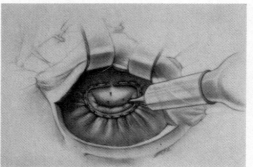

A   B

Figure 8. Technique of mitral anuloplasty utilizing the Carpentier ring. A, Placement of sutures. B, Testing the competence of the repaired valve. (From Carpentier, A.: J. Thorac. Cardiovasc. Surg., 86:323, 1983.)

valve substitutes, and postoperative problems are similar to those in mitral valve replacement for mitral stenosis (see above).

Mitral valve repair is most commonly performed for regurgitation caused by anular dilatation, chordal rupture, or papillary muscle dysfunction or, more rarely, for leaflet prolapse. The most popular techniques have been developed and advocated by Carpentier and associates.[12] The valve is approached as for an open commissurotomy with assistance of extracorporeal circulation. Anular reduction and remodeling is a component of most repairs. A Carpentier prosthetic ring, which is matched to the size of the anterior leaflet, is used, as the dilatation of the anulus usually involves the free wall of the left ventricle. The ring is sutured to the anulus and accomplishes a reduction in anular circumference as well as restoration of the normal shape of the orifice to provide normal leaflet coaptation (Fig. 8). In patients with ruptured chordae, especially those to the posterior leaflet, quadrangular resection of the flail leaflet combined with ring anuloplasty can restore valve competence.

Operative Results

In most series, operative mortality for isolated mitral valve replacement averages 2 to 5 per cent, but depends in part on the preoperative symptomatic status as well as secondary myocardial and pulmonary effects.[42] For patients with Class IV lesions, the mortality approaches 15 per cent, and procedures for ischemic mitral regurgitation in association with coronary artery revascularization are associated with an even higher risk. As in mitral stenosis, pulmonary hypertension usually resolves after a successful operation for mitral regurgitation. Symptoms of congestive failure also generally subside, and up to 95 per cent of operative survivors improve to Class I or II. Symptomatic improvement in patients in Class IV, although less uniform, can still be dramatic.

TRICUSPID VALVE DISEASE

Etiology and Pathology

Tricuspid stenosis is almost always rheumatic in origin and generally accompanies mitral valve disease. Tricuspid stenosis is present at autopsy in 14 per cent of patients with rheumatic heart disease.[41] The pathologic changes of rheu-

matic tricuspid stenosis resemble those of mitral stenosis, with fusion of the cusp edges and shortening and fusion of the chordae tendineae. Other causes of tricuspid stenosis are unusual and include right atrial tumors, tricuspid atresia, and the carcinoid syndrome.[38]

Tricuspid regurgitation is most commonly caused by a functional defect due to dilatation of the right ventricle and the tricuspid valve anulus, leaving the leaflets and chordae intact. Causes of functional tricuspid insufficiency include mitral valve disease, primary pulmonary hypertension, cor pulmonale, and right ventricular infarction. In all patients, tricuspid regurgitation indicates the presence of, as well as further aggravates, right ventricular failure. Disease processes that can affect the tricuspid valve directly and cause regurgitation include congenital heart disease (Ebstein's anomaly), papillary muscle rupture, infective endocarditis, trauma, and the carcinoid syndrome. Both tricuspid stenosis and insufficiency result in right atrial hypertension, systemic venous engorgement with peripheral edema, and hepatic congestion. The process contributes to low cardiac output. A mean diastolic gradient exceeding 5 mm. Hg will elevate mean right atrial pressures to levels that will cause systemic venous congestion with resulting fluid retention, edema, and debility.

Clinical Diagnosis

The diagnosis of tricuspid valve disease is often easily overlooked. The symptoms of tricuspid valve disease parallel those resulting from right heart failure due to mitral valve disease. The low cardiac output causes fatigue, and patients complain of discomfort due to hepatomegaly, ascites, and anasarca. Absence of symptoms of pulmonary congestion in a patient with clinically evident mitral stenosis suggests the presence of tricuspid stenosis.

Inspection of the neck veins is an important aspect of the diagnosis of tricuspid valve disease. In the presence of a stenotic valve and under conditions of sinus rhythm, the A wave is tall and sharp and is associated with a slow Y descent, indicative of abnormal early rapid filling. With tricuspid regurgitation, the jugular V wave is pronounced. A tricuspid opening snap may be present, which follows the mitral OS. Tricuspid murmurs are similar to those heard in mitral valve disease, but are located along the left lower sternal border; tricuspid murmurs are greatly augmented by inspiration.

The chest film and ECG show enlargement of the right side of the heart, but do not differentiate primary tricuspid disease from changes secondary to pulmonary hypertension caused by mitral valve disease. At catheterization the diagnosis of tricuspid stenosis is established by measuring the diastolic gradient between atrium and ventricle. A mean diastolic gradient of 5 mm. Hg is significant and will cause symptoms and reduce cardiac output. With serious tricuspid regurgitation, the right atrial pressure tracing reveals a prominent V wave, and cineangiography shows reflux of dye into the atrium after injection into the ventricle. An important surgical maneuver at the time of mitral valve operations is palpation of the tricuspid valve through the right atrium prior to cardiopulmonary bypass, to confirm or exclude the presence and severity of tricuspid disease.

Indications for Operation

The decision to correct functional tricuspid regurgitation is best made after correction of the left-sided lesions at operation. Some think that correction of mitral valve disease, followed by regression of pulmonary hypertension, decreases the degree of tricuspid regurgitation to insignificant levels.[69] However, severe functional tricuspid regurgitation should be managed operatively using tricuspid anuloplasty, as persistent tricuspid insufficiency will reduce cardiac output and jeopardize the patient's opportunity for recovery after mitral valve replacement.

For patients with infective endocarditis of the tricuspid valve due to gram negative organisms (usually heroin addicts), total excision of the valve without replacement has been shown to be effective in eradicating infection,[3] with later valve replacement in those displaying low cardiac output and high venous pressures. In most patients, prosthetic valve replacement is avoided because of the risk of later prosthetic valve endocarditis due to persistent drug use.

Surgical Therapy

TRICUSPID VALVE REPLACEMENT

In patients with significant organic tricuspid valve disease, valve replacement is indicated. The procedure is performed with techniques similar to those applied to mitral valve replacement, with care to avoid the right coronary artery and bundle of His. Bioprostheses are preferable to mechanical valves in the tricuspid position, owing to thrombotic problems associated with mechanical valves. Bioprosthetic durability is thought to be enhanced in the tricuspid position, because of decreased stress associated with lower right ventricular pressure.

TRICUSPID ANULOPLASTY

Tricuspid anuloplasty for functional tricuspid regurgitation is being done more commonly at the time of mitral valve replacement or repair, as persistent uncorrected tricuspid regurgitation is associated with early postoperative complications and later postoperative morbidity. Tricuspid repair is usually performed during the reperfusion period of cardiopulmonary bypass to reduce ischemic time. The tricuspid valve is approached via a right atriotomy. Competence of the valve can be re-established with either the Carpentier ring or DeVega anuloplasty (a semicircular pursestring suture placed around the anulus, sparing the septal leaflet).[54] Recent evidence suggests the Carpentier technique may be superior,[56] although the DeVega technique has the advantage of simplicity and requires less time to perform.

Operative Results

Patients undergoing tricuspid valve procedures are usually at a late stage of multivalve disease and require more complicated, prolonged procedures. The presence of pulmonary hypertension increases postoperative morbidity and usually results in prolonged respiratory support. Low cardiac output, arrhythmias, and renal failure occur in a relatively high incidence. Because of the presence of multiple valve problems with secondary pulmonary and myocardial effects, the late mortality in this group is higher than in those undergoing isolated mitral valve replacement.

SELECTED REFERENCES

Arbula, A., and Asfaw, I.: Tricuspid valvulectomy without prosthetic replacement: Ten years of clinical experience. J. Thorac. Cardiovasc. Surg., 82:684, 1981.
This is a review of 61 patients (intravenous drug abusers) undergoing tricuspid valvulectomy for intractable infective endocarditis. The vast majority tolerated the procedure well, with only 11 requiring subsequent prosthetic valve insertion.

Bjork, V. D., and Henze, A.: Ten years experience with the Bjork-Shiley tilting disc valve. J. Thorac. Cardiovasc. Surg., 78:331, 1979.
A decade of experience with the tilting disc valve in over 1800 patients is reported with an evaluation of the valve's performance.

Carpentier, A.: Cardiac valve surgery—the "French correction." J. Thorac. Cardiovasc. Surg., 86:323, 1983.
The author summarizes the techniques of mitral valve reconstruction, including use of the flexible ring, which is gaining popularity as an alternative to prosthetic valve replacement.

Oyer, P. E., Miller, D. C., Stinson, E. B., et al.: Clinical durability of the Hancock porcine bioprosthetic valve. J. Thorac. Cardiovasc. Surg., 80:824, 1980.
The extensive Stanford experience with the Hancock valve in over 1400 patients is reported, with a 95 per cent probability of freedom from failure at 6 years in the mitral position.

Teply, J. F., Grunkemeier, G. L., Sutherland, N. D., Lambert, L. E., Johnson, V. A., and Starr, A.: The ultimate prognosis after valve replacement: An assessment at twenty years. Ann. Thorac. Surg., 32:111, 1981.
The first mitral valve prosthesis was placed by Starr in 1961. This paper summarizes the author's 20-year experience with over 2000 patients undergoing prosthetic valve replacement with the ball-cage valve.

REFERENCES

1. Abernathy, W. S., and Willis, P. W.: Thromboembolic complications of rheumatic heart disease. Cardiovasc. Clin., 5:131, 1973.
2. Ankeney, J. L.: Indications for closed or open-heart surgery for mitral stenosis: Review of 153 operated cases. Ann. Thorac. Surg., 3:339, 1967.
3. Arbula, A., and Asfaw, I.: Tricuspid valvulectomy without prosthetic replacement: Ten years of clinical experience. J. Thorac. Cardiovasc. Surg., 82:684, 1981.
4. Bailey, C. P.: The surgical treatment of mitral valve stenosis (mitral commissurotomy). Dis. Chest., 15:377, 1949.
5. Bannister, R. G.: The risks of deferring valvulotomy in patients with moderate mitral stenosis. Lancet, 2:239, 1960.
6. Barlow, J. B., and Pocock, W. A.: The problem of non-ejection systolic clicks and associated mitral systolic murmurs: Emphasis on the billowing mitral leaflet. Am. Heart J., 90:636, 1975.
7. Bjork, V. D., and Henze, A.: Ten years experience with the Bjork-Shiley tilting disc valve. J. Thorac. Cardiovasc. Surg., 78:331, 1979.
8. Bolooki, H., Mallon, S., Kaiser, G. A., Thurer, R. J., and Kieval, J.: Failure of Hancock xenograft valve: Importance of valve position. Ann. Thorac. Surg., 36:246, 1983.
9. Braunwald, E.: Valvular heart disease. *In* Braunwald, E. (Ed.): Heart Disease: A Textbook of Cardiovascular Medicine, 2nd ed. Philadelphia, W. B. Saunders Company, 1984.
10. Brock, R. C., and Campbell, M.: Discussion on surgery of the heart and great vessels. Proc. R. Soc. Med., 44:995, 1951.
11. Brunton, L.: Preliminary note on the possibility of treating mitral stenosis by surgical methods. Lancet, 1:332, 1902.
12. Carpentier, A.: Cardiac valve surgery—the "French correction." J. Thorac. Cardiovasc. Surg., 86:323, 1983.

13. Carpentier, A.: Valve reconstruction in mitral valve incompetence. *In* Duran, C., Angell, W. W., Johnson, A. A., and Oury, J. H., (Eds.): Recent Progress in Mitral Valve Disease. London, Butterworth, 1984.

14. Commerford, P. J., Hastie, T., and Beck, W.: Closed mitral valvulotomy: Actuarial analysis of results of 654 patients over 12 years and analysis of pre-operative predictors of long-term survival. Ann. Thorac. Surg., *33*:473, 1982.

15. Cutler, E. C., and Levine, S. A.: Cardiotomy and valvulotomy for mitral stenosis. Boston Med. Surg. J., *188*:1023, 1923.

16. Dale, J. E., and Albert, J. S.: Valvular Heart Diseases. Boston, Little, Brown & Company, 1981.

17. Devineri, R., and McKenzie, F. N.: Type I left ventricular rupture after mitral valve replacement. J. Thorac. Cardiovasc. Surg., *86*:742, 1983.

18. Dubin, A. A., March, H. W., Cohn, K., and Selzer, A.: Longitudinal hemodynamic and clinical study of mitral stenosis. Circulation, *64*:381, 1971.

19. Edmunds, L. H., Jr.: Thromboembolic complications of current cardiac valvular prostheses. Ann. Thorac. Surg., *34*:96, 1982.

20. Ellis, F. H., Jr.: Surgery for Acquired Mitral Valve Disease. Philadelphia, W. B. Saunders Company, 1967.

21. Ellis, J. B., and Ramirez, A.: The clinical course of patients with severe rheumatic mitral insufficiency. Am. Heart J., *78*:406, 1969.

22. Faltz, B. D., Hessel, E. A., and Juey, T. D.: The early course of pulmonary artery hypertension in patients undergoing valve replacement. J. Thorac. Cardiovasc. Surg., *88*:238, 1984.

23. Fiddler, G. I., Gerlis, L. M., Walter, D. R., Scott, U., and Williams, G. J.: Calcification of glutaraldehyde-preserved porcine and bovine xenografts in children. Ann. Thorac. Surg., *35*:237, 1983.

24. Fishbein, M. C., Levy, R. J., Ferrans, V. J., Dearden, L. C., et al.: Calcification of cardiac valve bioprostheses. J. Thorac. Cardiovasc. Surg., *83*:602, 1982.

25. Forssmann, W.: Uber kontrast darste llung der hohler des laberden richter herzens und der lunger schlagader. Munch. Med. Wochenschr., *78*:439, 1931.

26. Fulkerson, P. K., Beaver, B. M., Avseon, J. C., and Graber, H. L.: Calcification of the mitral annulus: Etiology, clinical associations, complications and therapy. Am. J. Med., *66*:967, 1979.

27. Gahl, K., Sutton, R., Pearson, M., et al: Mitral regurgitation in coronary heart disease. Br. Heart J., *39*:13, 1977.

28. Galioto, F. M., Jr., Midgley, F. M., Kapur, S., Perry, L. W., Watson, D. C., et al.: Early failures of Ionescu-Shiley bioprosthesis after mitral valve replacement in children. J. Thorac. Cardiovasc. Surg., *83*:306, 1982.

29. Gallo, I., Ruiz, B., Nistalf, F., and Duran, C. M.: Degeneration in porcine bioprosthetic cardiac valves: Incidence of primary tissue failures among 938 bioprostheses at risk. Am. J. Cardiol., *53*:1061, 1984.

30. Gardner, T. J., Roland, J. M. A., Neill, C. A., and Donahoo, J. J.: Valve replacement in children: A fifteen year perspective. J. Thorac. Cardiovasc. Surg., *83*:178, 1982.

31. Gerbode, F.: Transventricular mitral valvulotomy. Circulation, *21*:563, 1963.

32. Gonzalez-Lavin, L., Friedman, L. P., Hooker, P., and McFadden, P. M.: Endomyocardial fibrosis: Diagnosis and treatment. Am. Heart J., *105*:699, 1983.

33. Gonzalez-Lavin, L., Tardon, D. P., Chi, S., Blair, T. C., et al.: The risk of thromboembolism and hemorrhage following mitral valve replacement. J. Thorac. Cardiovasc. Surg., *87*:340, 1984.

34. Halseth, W. L., Elliott, D. P., and Walker, E. L.: Simplified operative technique to test mitral valve repair. J. Thorac. Cardiovasc. Surg., *80*:792, 1980.

35. Halseth, W. L., Elliott, D. P., Walker, E. L., and Smith, E. A.: Open mitral commissurotomy: A modern re-evaluation. J. Thorac. Cardiovasc. Surg., *80*:842, 1980.

36. Harken, D. E., Ellis, L. B., Ware, P. F., and Norman, L. R.: The surgical treatment of mitral stenosis. N. Engl. J. Med., *239*:802, 1948.

37. Jackson, G. M., Wolf, P. L., and Blour, C. M.: Malfunction of mitral Bjork-Shiley prosthetic valve due to septal interference. Am. Heart J., *104*:158, 1982.

38. Kay, J. H.: Eleven year follow-up after tricuspid valve replacement and pulmonic valvulotomy in the carcinoid syndrome. Am. J. Cardiol., *53*:651, 1984.

39. King, H., Csicsko, J., and Leshnower, A.: Intraoperative assessment of mitral valve following reconstructive procedures. Ann. Thorac. Surg., *29*:81, 1980.

40. Kirsh, M. M., and Sloan, H.: Technique of mitral valve replacement. Ann. Thorac. Surg., *30*:490, 1980.

41. Kitchin, A., and Turner, R.: Diagnosis and treatment of tricuspid stenosis. Br. Heart J., *26*:354, 1964.

42. Leply, D., Jr., Flemma, R. J., Muller, D. C., Motl, M., Anderson,

A. J., and Weirauch, E.: Long-term follow-up of the Bjork-Shiley prosthetic valve used in the mitral position. Ann. Thorac. Surg., *30*:164, 1980.

43. Limet, R., and Grondin, C. M.: Cardiac valve prosthesis, anticoagulation, and pregnancy. Ann. Thorac. Surg., *23*:337, 1977.

44. Marshall, W. G., Jr., Kouchoukos, N. T., Kays, R. B., and Williams, J. B.: Late results after mitral valve replacement with the Bjork-Shiley and porcine prostheses. J. Thorac. Cardiovasc. Surg., *85*:902, 1983.

45. McAlpine, W. A.: Heart and Coronary Arteries: An Anatomical Atlas for Clinical Diagnosis, Radiological Investigation, and Surgical Treatment. New York, Springer-Verlag, 1975.

46. Melhem, R. E., Dunbar, J. D., and Booth, R. W.: B lines of Kerley and left atrial size in mitral valve disease. Radiology, *76*:65, 1961.

47. Mills, P., Rose, J., Hollingsworth, J., Amara, I., and Craig, E.: Long-term prognosis of mitral valve prolapse. N. Engl. J. Med., *297*:13, 1977.

48. Morrow, A. G., Cohen, L. S., Roberts, W. C., Braunwald, N. S., and Braunwald, E.: Severe mitral regurgitation following acute myocardial infarction and ruptured papillary muscle. Circulation, *37* (Suppl. II):124, 1968.

49. Newton, J. R., Glower, D. D., Davis, J. W., and Rankin, J. S.: Evaluation of suture techniques for mitral valve replacement. J. Thorac. Cardiovasc. Surg., *88*:248, 1984.

50. Olesen, K. H.: The natural history of 271 patients with mitral stenosis under medical treatment. Br. Heart J., *24*:349, 1962.

51. Oyer, P. E., Stinson, E. B., Reitz, B. A., Miller, D. C., et al.: Long-term evaluation of the porcine homograft bioprosthesis. J. Thorac. Cardiovasc. Surg., *78*:343, 1979.

52. Perloff, J. K.: Evolving concepts of mitral-valve prolapse. N. Engl. J. Med., *307*:369, 1982.

53. Peterson, C. R., Herr, R., Crissen, R. V., Starr, A., Bristow, D., and Griswald, H. E.: The failure of hemodynamic improvement after valve replacement surgery. Ann. Intern. Med., *66*:1, 1967.

54. Rabago, G., DeVega, N. G., Castillon, L., et al.: The new DeVega technique in tricuspid annuloplasty. J. Thorac. Cardiovasc. Surg., *21*:231, 1980.

55. Reichek, N., Shelburne, J. C., and Perloff, J. R.: Clinical aspects of rheumatic valvular disease. Prog. Cardiovasc. Dis., *15*:491, 1973.

56. Rivera, R., Duran, E., and Ajuria, M.: Carpentier's flexible ring versus DeVega's annuloplasty: A prospective randomized study. J. Thorac. Cardiovasc. Surg., *89*:196, 1985.

57. Rizzon, P., Biasco, G., Brindice, G., and Mauro, F.: Familial syndrome of midsystolic click and late systolic murmur. Br. Heart J., *35*:245, 1973.

58. Roberts, W. C.: Morphologic features of the normal and abnormal mitral valve. Am. J. Cardiol., *51*:1005, 1983.

59. Roberts, W. C., and Perloff, J. K.: Mitral valvular disease: A clinicopathologic survey of conditions causing the mitral valve to function abnormally. Ann. Intern. Med., *77*:939, 1972.

60. Roe, B. B., Edmunds, L. H., Jr., Fishman, N. H., and Hutchinson, J. C.: Open mitral valvuloplasty. Ann. Thorac. Surg., *12*:483, 1971.

61. Rowe, J. C., Bland, E. F., Sprague, H. B., and White, P. D.: The course of mitral stenosis without surgery: Ten and twenty year perspectives. Ann. Intern. Med., *52*:741, 1960.

62. Ruckman, R. N., and Van Praagh, R.: Anatomic types of congenital mitral stenosis: Report of 49 autopsy cases with consideration of diagnosis and surgical implications. Am. J. Cardiol., *42*:592, 1979.

63. Schuler, G., Peterson, K. L., Johnson, A., Francis, G., et al.: Temporal response of left ventricular performance to mitral valve surgery. Circulation, *59*:1218, 1979.

64. Shah, P. M., and Tei, C.: Functional anatomy of the mitral valve and annulus in man. *In* Duran, C., Angell, W. W., Johnson, A. D., and Oury, J. H. (eds.): Recent Progress in Mitral Valve Disease. London, Butterworth, 1984.

65. Souttar, H. J.: Surgical treatment of mitral stenosis. Br. Med. J., *2*:603, 1925.

66. Spratt, J. A., Olsen, C. O., Tyson, G. S., Jr., Glower, D. D., Jr., Davis, J. W., and Rankin, J. S.: Experimental mitral regurgitation: Physiologic effects of correction on left ventricular dynamics. J. Thorac. Cardiovasc. Surg., *86*:479, 1983.

67. Spray, T. L., and Roberts, W. C.: Structural changes in porcine xenografts used as substitute cardiac valves: Gross and histologic observations in 51 glutaraldehyde-preserved Hancock valves in 41 patients. Am. J. Cardiol., *40*:319, 1977.

68. Starr, A., and Edwards, M. L.: Mitral replacement: Clinical experience with a ball-valve prosthesis. Ann. Surg., *154*:726, 1961.

69. Starr, A., Herr, R., and Wood, J.: Tricuspid replacement for acquired valve disease. Surg. Gynecol. Obstet., *122*:1295, 1966.

70. Unverferth, D. V., Fentel, R. H., Unverferth, B. J., and Leier, C. V.: Atrial fibrillation in mitral stenosis: Histologic, hemodynamic and metabolic factors. Int. J. Cardiol., *5*:143, 1984.

71. Walston, A., Peter, R. H., Morris, J. J., Kong, V. H., and Behar,

V. S.: Clinical implications of pulmonary hypertension in mitral stenosis. Am. J. Cardiol., 32:650, 1973.

72. Williams, D. B., Pluth, J. R., and Onszulak, T. A.: Extrinsic obstruction of the Bjork-Shiley valve in the mitral position. Ann. Thorac. Surg., 32:58, 1981.

73. Williams, W. G., Pollock, J. C., Geiss, D. M., Trusler, G. A., and Fowler, R. S.: Experience with aortic and mitral valve replacement in children. J. Thorac. Cardiovasc. Surg., 81:326, 1981.

74. Wood, P.: An appreciation of mitral stenosis, Part I: Clinical features. Br. Med. J., 1:1051, 1954.

75. Wood, P.: An appreciation of mitral stenosis, Part II: Investigations and results. Br. Med. J., 1:1113, 1954.

76. Yellin, E. L., Yoran, C., and Frater, R. W. M.: Physiology of mitral valve flow. In Duran, C., Angell, W. W., Johnson, A. D., and Oury, J. H. (eds.): Recent Progress in Mitral Valve Disease. London, Butterworth, 1984.

XVI

Ebstein's Anomaly

ROBERT N. JONES, M.D.
DAVID C. SABISTON, JR., M.D.

A specific cardiac malformation that primarily involves the tricuspid valve and the right ventricle was described by Ebstein in 1866.[5] The *septal* and *posterior* leaflets of the tricuspid valve are attached distally to the right ventricular wall and septum rather than to the tricuspid anulus[9] (Fig. 1). The anterior cusp *is* attached to the anulus but is large and "sail-like." The distally displaced septal and posterior leaflets partition the right ventricle into two segments, (1) a proximal "atrialized" chamber and (2) a small distal chamber. Cardiac conduction abnormalities are frequent because of the presence of a Kent bundle or other pathway. In 1958, a surgical approach was initiated to treat this anomaly with plication of the atrialized ventricle both to eliminate it and to transpose the leaflets to a more normal position, thus reducing the size of the tricuspid anulus.[10] With modifications this continues to be an acceptable approach.[4, 8, 11] The abnormal tricuspid valve was replaced with a prosthesis in 1963[1] and this technique has been emphasized in recent series.[2, 16]

ANATOMY

Distal displacement and malattachment of the tricuspid valve leaflets are the essential features of this anomaly,[17] and the displaced valve produces a partition between the proximal and distal right ventricles. The malformed valve may be incompetent, stenotic, or, rarely, imperforate. The proximal part of the right ventricle functionally becomes a part of the right atrium. The walls of the atrialized ventricle are thin and frequently dilated. The tricuspid anulus is dilated, and interatrial communications in the form of an atrial septal defect or a patent foramen are usually present.

PATHOPHYSIOLOGY

Although the hemodynamic defects in Ebstein's anomaly are not completely understood,[12] diminished pulmonary blood flow is a primary problem. The tricuspid valve may functionally range from insufficient to stenotic, and symp-

toms may result from obstruction between the atrialized ventricle and distal chamber. With the presence of increased pulmonary vascular resistance during infancy, neonates with tricuspid valve insufficiency may develop heart failure and intense cyanosis from a right-to-left shunt. As the early pulmonary arterial pressure diminishes, the right-to-left shunt and symptoms of congestive heart failure and cyanosis ameliorate. Arrhythmias due to a Kent bundle or other aberrant pathways frequently occur and may constitute the reason for operative intervention.[13] The presence of an

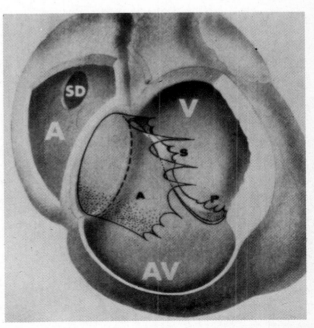

Figure 1. Portions of right atrium and right ventricle are cut away, revealing "sail-like" anterior leaflet (A) and small, displaced septal (S) and posterior (P) leaflet. SD = Septal defect; A = right atrium; V = right ventricle; AV = atrialized ventricle. (From Hardy, K. L., and Roe, B. R.: J. Thorac. Cardiovasc. Surg., 58:553, 1969.)

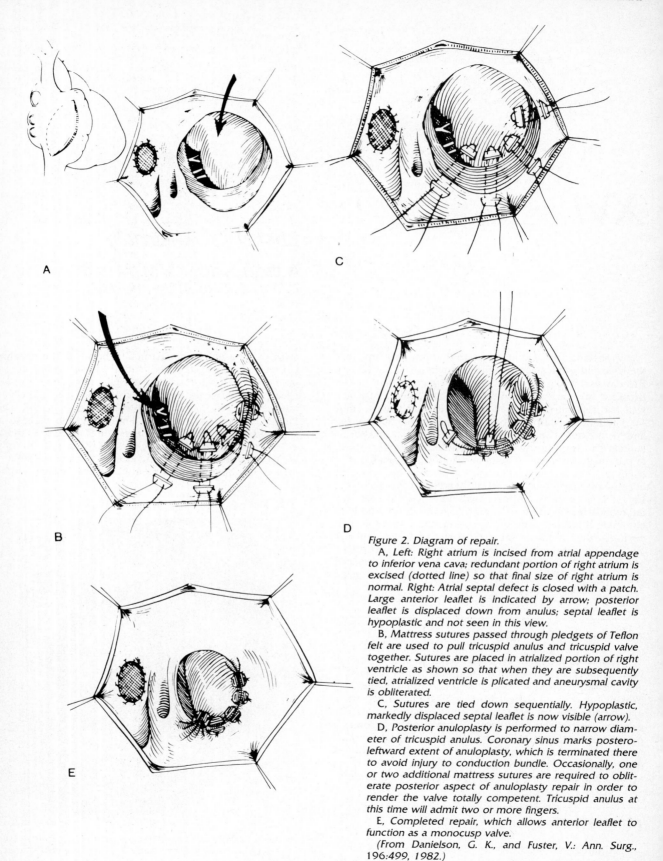

Figure 2. Diagram of repair.

A, Left: Right atrium is incised from atrial appendage to inferior vena cava; redundant portion of right atrium is excised (dotted line) so that final size of right atrium is normal. Right: Atrial septal defect is closed with a patch. Large anterior leaflet is indicated by arrow; posterior leaflet is displaced down from anulus; septal leaflet is hypoplastic and not seen in this view.

B, Mattress sutures passed through pledgets of Teflon felt are used to pull tricuspid anulus and tricuspid valve together. Sutures are placed in atrialized portion of right ventricle as shown so that when they are subsequently tied, atrialized ventricle is plicated and aneurysmal cavity is obliterated.

C, Sutures are tied down sequentially. Hypoplastic, markedly displaced septal leaflet is now visible (arrow).

D, Posterior anuloplasty is performed to narrow diameter of tricuspid anulus. Coronary sinus marks postero-leftward extent of anuloplasty, which is terminated there to avoid injury to conduction bundle. Occasionally, one or two additional mattress sutures are required to obliterate posterior aspect of anuloplasty repair in order to render the valve totally competent. Tricuspid anulus at this time will admit two or more fingers.

E, Completed repair, which allows anterior leaflet to function as a monocusp valve.

(From Danielson, G. K., and Fuster, V.: Ann. Surg., 196:499, 1982.)

atrial septal defect or patent foramen ovale may result in paradoxical embolization.

CLINICAL FEATURES AND DIAGNOSIS

Less than 5 per cent of patients with this rare disease live beyond the age of 50 years; however, 60 per cent in New York Heart Association Class I or II who survive infancy and enter adulthood may live comfortably.[15] Symptoms are related to the degree and nature of malformation of the tricuspid valve, the presence of an atrial septal defect, and impairment of right ventricular function. In patients surviving the neonatal period, the most common symptoms are dyspnea and cyanosis.[7] The physical findings include possible cyanosis and a variety of abnormal auscultatory findings over the right heart; S_2 is widely split and the intensity of the various sounds is influenced by the phases of respiration. The systolic murmur of tricuspid regurgitation is best heard along the left sternal border.

The chest film usually shows the heart to be enlarged and balloon-shaped. The increase in cardiac size is primarily due to right atrial enlargement. Angiocardiography is usually diagnostic. During monitoring of pressures and electrical potentials in right heart catheterization, the pressure wave changes from a ventricular to an atrial pattern; yet right ventricular electrical potentials persist. Echocardiography is also helpful and may delineate the size of the distal right ventricle and the degree of tethering of the anterior tricuspid leaflet. This may be of considerable value in deciding whether tricuspid valve replacement or reconstruction is most appropriate.[6, 14]

SURGICAL MANAGEMENT

Although patients with Ebstein's anomaly in Class I or II are generally treated medically, indications for surgical intervention include deterioration with a shift to Class III or IV. This is usually accompanied by the development of severe cyanosis, progressive increase in cardiac size, emboli, and disabling or life-threatening arrhythmias.[2] The operative approach is directed toward movement of the tricuspid valve into the correct anatomic position, elimination of tricuspid stenosis or regurgitation, closure of the interatrial septal defect, removal of any right ventricular outflow tract obstruction, and improvement in the functional capacity of the right ventricle.[3] The two main surgical approaches for managing Ebstein's anomaly are (1) tricuspid valve replacement (with or without ventricular plication) or (2) plastic reconstruction of the tricuspid valve.

Surgical excision of the tricuspid valve and replacement with a competent prosthesis removes any obstruction that may exist between the atrialized right ventricle and the more distal right ventricular chamber and simultaneously eliminates tricuspid regurgitation. Several series with long-term follow-up report excellent results with the use of valve replacement, and the type of valves used has ranged from porcine heterografts to a variety of mechanical valves.[2, 3, 16] During the insertion of the valves, care must be taken to avoid injuring the atrioventricular node. Consequently, the suture line is usually placed *above* the coronary sinus so that it drains distal to the valve.

Concern over the long-term use of a prosthetic valve, particularly in children, and the opinion that repair of the malformed valve offers acceptable hemodynamic results have led some to adopt reconstructive procedures to correct this anomaly.[6] The basis of the repair is the creation of a monocusp valve of the anterior tricuspid leaflet. In addition, part of the right atrial wall is excised to reduce its size, and the diameter of the tricuspid anulus is narrowed by performing a posterior anuloplasty (Fig. 2).[4] In some patients, such a procedure is not possible because of deficiencies of the anterior leaflet or its attachment to the right ventricular wall. This notwithstanding, 81 per cent of one large series of patients with Ebstein's anomaly were treated with such a reconstruction.[4]

In summary, patients who develop compromising symptoms should usually undergo surgical treatment with expectation of acceptable results. Further time is required before the basic controversy concerning valve reconstruction or replacement as the preferred technique is resolved.

SELECTED REFERENCE

Danielson, G. K., and Fuster, V.: Surgical repair of Ebstein's anomaly. Ann. Surg., *196*:499, 1982.
 This is a good review of the surgical management of Ebstein's anomaly and presents the advantages of tricuspid valvular reconstruction.

REFERENCES

1. Barnard, C. N., and Schire, V.: Surgical correction of Ebstein's malformation with prosthetic tricuspid valve. Surgery, *54*:302, 1963.
2. Behl, T. R., and Blesovsky, A.: Ebstein's anomaly: Sixteen years experience with valve replacement without plication of the right ventricle. Thorax, *39*:8, 1984.
3. Bove, E. L., and Kirsh, M. M.: Valve replacement for Ebstein's anomaly of the tricuspid valve. J. Thorac. Cardiovasc. Surg., *78*:229, 1979.
4. Danielson, G. K.: Ebstein's anomaly: Editorial comments and personal observations. Ann. Thorac. Surg., *34*:396, 1982.
5. Danielson, G. K., and Fuster, V.: Surgical repair of Ebstein's anomaly. Ann. Surg., *196*:499, 1982.
6. Ebstein, W.: Uber einen sehr seltenen Fall von insufficienz der Valvula tricuspidalis, bedingt durch eine angeborene hochgradige Missbildung derselben. Arch. Anat. Physiol., *33*:238, 1866.
7. Giuliani, E. R., Fuster, V., Brandenburg, R. O., and Mair, D. D.: Ebstein's anomaly: The clinical features and natural history of Ebstein's anomaly of the tricuspid valve. Mayo Clin. Proc., *54*:163, 1979.
8. Hardy, K. L., May, I. A., Webster, C. A., and Kimball, K. G.: Ebstein's anomaly: A functional concept and successful definitive repair. J. Thorac. Cardiovasc. Surg., *48*:927, 1964.
9. Hardy, K. L., and Roe, B. R.: Ebstein's anomaly. Further experience with definitive repair. J. Thorac. Cardiovasc. Surg., *58*:553, 1969.
10. Hunter, S. W., and Lillehei, C. W.: Ebstein's malformation of the tricuspid valve: A study of a case together with suggestions of a new form of surgical therapy. Dis. Chest, *33*:297, 1958.
11. Schmidt-Habelmann, P., Meisner, H., Struck, E., and Sebening, F.: Results of valvuloplasty for Ebstein's anomaly. Thorac. Cardiovasc. Surg., *29*:155, 1981.
12. Sealy, W. C.: The cause of hemodynamic disturbances in Ebstein's anomaly based on observations at operation. Ann. Thorac. Surg., *27*:536, 1979.
13. Sealy, W. C., Gallagher, J. J., Pritchett, E. L., and Wallace, A. G.: Surgical treatment of tachyarrhythmias in patients with both Ebstein's anomaly and a Kent bundle. J. Thorac. Cardiovasc. Surg., *75*:847, 1978.
14. Shiina, A., Seward, J. B., Tajik, A. J., Hagler, D. J., and Danielson, G. K.: Two-dimensional echocardiographic-surgical correlation in Ebstein's anomaly: Preoperative determination of patients requiring tricuspid valve plication vs replacement. Circulation, *68*:534, 1983.
15. Watson, H.: Natural history of Ebstein's anomaly of tricuspid valve in childhood and adolescence: An international cooperative study of 505 cases. Br. Heart J., *36*:417, 1974.
16. Westaby, S., Karp, R. B., Kirklin, J. W., Waldo, A. L., and Blackstone, E. H.: Surgical treatment in Ebstein's malformation. Ann. Thorac. Surg., *38*:388, 1982.
17. Zuberbuhler, J. R., Allwork, S. P., and Anderson, R. H.: The spectrum of Ebstein's anomaly of the tricuspid valve. J. Thorac. Cardiovasc. Surg., *77*:202, 1979.

XVII

Surgical Treatment of Cardiac Arrhythmias

JAMES E. LOWE, M.D.

In pioneering work in 1967, Durrer first used intraoperative epicardial mapping showing direct electrophysiologic evidence of ventricular pre-excitation through an accessory atrioventricular connection in the Wolff-Parkinson-White (WPW) syndrome.[5] The following year Sealy successfully divided an accessory pathway in a patient with medically refractory paroxysmal atrial tachycardia secondary to the WPW syndrome.[2] Many new surgical approaches have since been developed to treat patients with a variety of disabling supraventricular and ventricular dysrhythmias.[3] In addition to the WPW syndrome, defects currently capable of being treated by electrophysiologically directed operations include supraventricular tachycardia due to concealed accessory atrioventricular (AV) connections, AV node re-entry tachycardia, ectopic atrial tachycardia, selected cases of atrial flutter-fibrillation, and, most recently, medically refractory inappropriate sinus tachycardia.[15, 28] Certain patients with ischemic and non-ischemic ventricular tachycardia are also candidates for surgery. Based on the excellent surgical results that have been achieved and an increased awareness of the role of tachyarrhythmias in the sudden death syndrome, it is anticipated that increasing numbers of patients will be referred for electrophysiologically guided operative procedures in the future.

PATIENT SELECTION

In the past most patients with supraventricular and ventricular dysrhythmias were referred for operation only when it became apparent that medical treatment was ineffective or poorly tolerated. However, in view of the excellent surgical results that have been achieved in the treatment of a variety of dysrhythmias, increasing numbers of patients are referred for surgery much earlier following diagnosis. Considering the safety and gratifying long-term results obtained in patients with both supraventricular and ventricular dysrhythmias it has become apparent that early operative intervention is often preferable to chronic pharmacologic therapy.

Patients with supraventricular arrhythmias due to one of the pre-excitation syndromes, concealed AV connections, an ectopic atrial focus, or inappropriate medically refractory sinus tachycardia are low-risk candidates with an operative mortality in the range of 1 to 2 per cent. In contrast, patients with intractable ventricular tachycardia usually have severe coronary artery disease commonly associated with a left ventricular aneurysm or cardiomyopathy and have an increased surgical risk because of compromised ventricular function. The operative mortality in this group is in the range of 7 to 16 per cent; however, with mortality approaching 100 per cent in medically refractory patients, surgery offers gratifying results.[3]

PREOPERATIVE EVALUATION

Patients considered candidates for surgical treatment of arrhythmias undergo a thorough preoperative electrophysiology catheter study to localize the site of origin of the dysrhythmia.[10] Patients with refractory supraventricular tachycardia due to the WPW syndrome, concealed accessory connections that conduct only retrograde, enhanced AV node conduction, AV node re-entry, Mahaim fibers, and inappropriate sinus tachycardia undergo a detailed mapping study, which is conducted by placing catheters high in the right atrium, coronary sinus, and right ventricular apex and adjacent to the bundle of His (Fig. 1). Common types of accessory atrioventricular connections are depicted in Figure 2. The normal cardiac conduction activation sequence and position of the His bundle electrogram are shown in Figure 2A. An accessory connection, which bypasses the AV node and results in shortening of the A-H and A-V intervals but no change in the H-V interval, is shown in Figure 2B. This type of accessory pathway is referred to as enhanced AV node conduction; if refractory to medical therapy it requires surgical cryoablation of both the accessory pathway and the His bundle or endocardial catheter ablation of the His bundle because they usually cannot be separated anatomically.[9, 21] A Mahaim fiber connecting the His bundle to the septal myocardium is shown in Figure 2C. This type of connection results in a normal A-V interval because the conducted impulse is

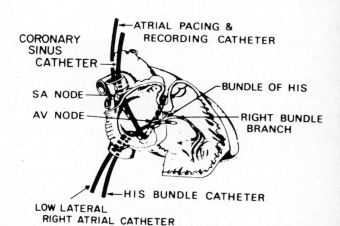

Figure 1. Position of intracardiac electrode catheters during preoperative electrophysiologic study. There are two right atrial electrodes, one near the region of the S-A node and one in the low lateral portion of the right atrium. The coronary sinus catheter is quadripolar, thus allowing four separate sites of the posterior left atrium to be recorded simultaneously. A right ventricular catheter electrode is usually positioned into the right ventricular apex. (From Cox, J. L.: Curr. Probl. Cardiol., 8:8, 1983.)

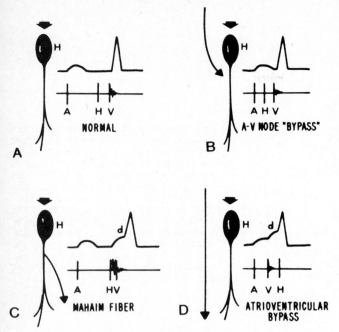

Figure 2. Types of accessory pathways. The electrocardiogram, His bundle electrogram, and schematic of the conducting pathways associated with a normal conduction system (A), an atrioventricular node bypass (B), a Mahaim fiber (C), and complete atrioventricular bypass (D). A = Atrial electrogram; H = His bundle electrogram; V = ventricular electrogram; d = delta wave. (From Gallagher, J. J., et al.: Med. Clin. North Am., 60:101, 1976.)

not affected until after it exits the AV node. However, as shown, the H-V interval is shortened because the impulse can travel through the Mahaim fiber to the septal myocardium, resulting in pre-excitation and a delta wave. A complete atrioventricular bypass tract exists in the WPW syndrome as shown in Figure 2D. This causes a conducted electrical impulse traveling antegrade down the normal conduction system, resulting in a normal A-H interval, as well as antegrade down the accessory atrioventricular conduction, resulting in a markedly shortened A-V interval. This type of accessory connection produces pre-excitation of ventricular myocardium at the site of insertion of the pathway and subsequent short P-R interval, delta wave, and wide QRS complex (characteristic of the WPW syndrome). Following recording of electrograms during sinus rhythm, programmed electrical stimulation of the atrium is performed to induce reciprocating tachycardia. Using a variety of recording techniques and insertion of premature ventricular stimuli, the type of arrhythmia can further be characterized. In addition to identifying the type of supraventricular dysrhythmia, an important goal of catheter mapping is precise localization.[10]

Patients with medically refractory ventricular tachycardia undergo preoperative endocardial catheter mapping to confirm that the arrhythmia is ventricular rather than supraventricular in origin; to demonstrate that it can be induced and terminated by programmed electrical stimulation techniques, which confirms that it is a re-entrant arrhythmia; and finally to localize its site of origin.[3] In general, automatic ventricular tachyarrhythmias are not amenable to operative treatment.[3] However, a large number of ventricular tachyarrhythmias associated with prior myocardial infarction and left ventricular aneurysms are re-entrant in origin and can be eliminated with surgery.[11]

SURGICAL TREATMENT OF SUPRAVENTRICULAR ARRHYTHMIAS

Although disabling tachycardia caused by the WPW syndrome represents the most common supraventricular dysrhythmia that is surgically treatable, a variety of other supraventricular tachycardias are amenable to operation.

Wolff-Parkinson-White Syndrome

Surgical treatment of the WPW syndrome is possible because an abnormal anatomic connection exists between the atrium and ventricle, which is capable of conducting cardiac impulses. These accessory AV connections may occur at any point around the anulus fibrosus on either side of the heart, except over the portion of the anterior mitral valve anulus between the right and left fibrous trigones (Fig. 3). Based on anatomic location, accessory atrioventricular connections resulting in the WPW syndrome are classified as left free wall, right free wall, anterior septal, or posterior septal. Regardless of the location of the accessory pathway, the defect is approached through a median sternotomy. A detailed intraoperative mapping procedure is done to confirm the exact location of the suspected connection and to determine if additional accessory pathways exist. Often, induced tachycardia results in hemodynamic instability and cardiopulmonary bypass is required to complete the intraoperative mapping procedure.

Arterial perfusion is accomplished by cannulation of the ascending aorta. For right-sided pathways, the superior vena cava is cannulated via the right atrial appendage and the inferior vena cava is cannulated through the right femoral vein. In the past, the heart was arrested with cold potassium cardioplegic solution for the dissection of all accessory atrioventricular connections.[3] However, at present cardioplegic arrest is employed only for left-sided pathways. Dissection to eliminate right-sided accessory atrioventricular connections, including those located in the posterior septal space, can be performed with the heart in sinus rhythm from within the right atrium. Prior to opening the right atrium, the heart is briefly fibrillated if a patent foramen ovale or atrial septal defect is suspected. Following closure of the patent foramen ovale or atrial septal defect, the heart is defibrillated and the procedure is then completed with the patient in sinus rhythm and with systemic temperature maintained at normothermia. The area of the anulus fibrosus associated with the site of the accessory AV connection is identified and a supra-anular incision is placed 2 mm. above the tricuspid valve anulus, exposing the fat pad containing the right coronary artery and vein. Usually, the incision is extended 2 to 3 cm. on each side of the previously determined location of the accessory pathway. The AV groove fat pad containing the coronary vessels is dissected free from the top of the external wall of the ventricle to the level of the ventricular epicardial reflection throughout the extent of the supra-anular incision. All fibromuscular bands (accessory connections) and small vessels are divided as they attach to the ventricle. After completion of the AV groove dissection, a sharp nerve hook is used to divide any remaining fibers connecting the atrium and ventricle along the tricuspid valve anulus. The supra-anular incision is then closed using a continuous suture of 4-0 Prolene.

Division of left free wall pathways is accomplished by cannulating the superior vena cava through the right atrial appendage and inferior vena cava through a separate purse-

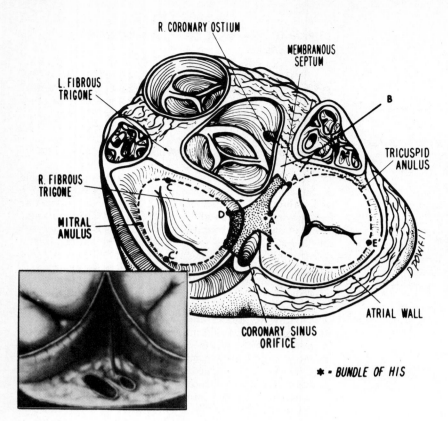

R. CORONARY OSTIUM

MEMBRANOUS
SEPTUM

L. FIBROUS
TRIGONE

B

TRICUSPID
ANULUS

R. FIBROUS
TRIGONE

MITRAL
ANULUS

A

D

A'

C'

E

E'

ATRIAL WALL

CORONARY SINUS
ORIFICE

* = BUNDLE OF HIS

Figure 3. Superior view of the heart with the atria dissected away to demonstrate the extent of various supraanular incisions used to interrupt accessory pathways. Right anterior septal or anterior free-wall pathways occur between points A and E. Right posterior freewall pathways occur between points E and E. Left freewall pathways occur between points C and just to the right of C. Septal pathways may be anywhere within the heavy stippled area. Inset, dissection of the pyramidal space above the posterior ventricular septum to interrupt septal accessory pathways. (From Cox, J. L.: Curr. Probl. Cardiol., 8:8, 1983.)

string suture placed over the inferior body of the right atrium (Fig. 4). The interatrial groove between the right and left atria is then exposed in a manner identical to the approach taken for mitral valve replacement. The myocardium is then cooled to 27° C. and the heart is arrested using cold potassium cardioplegic solution. A left atriotomy is performed to expose the mitral valve. Generally, patients with left free wall pathways undergo the same surgical dissection regardless of the precise location of the pathway. A supra-anular incision is placed 2 mm. above the posterior mitral valve anulus extending from the left fibrous trigone to the posterior interventricular septum. The AV groove fat pad is entered and the atrium is disconnected from the top of the posterior left ventricle throughout the length of the supra-anular incision. This plane of dissection is extended to the epicardial reflection of the posterior left ventricle. A sharp nerve hook is used to transect any remaining fibers connecting the atrium to the ventricle along the posterior mitral valve anulus, and the supra-anular incision is closed with a continuous 4-0 Prolene suture followed by closure of the atrium.[3]

The most difficult accessory atrioventricular connections to interrupt surgically are those located posteriorly in the region of the crux referred to as posterior septal space.[23] A right atriotomy is performed with the heart normally perfused and maintained at normothermia on cardiopulmonary bypass. The His bundle is identified using a handheld mapping probe. Following identification of the His bundle, a supra-anular incision is begun just posterior to the site of the His bundle and extended in a counterclockwise fashion onto the posterior right atrial free wall from within the atrium. A plane of dissection is established between the fat pad and the top of the posterior interventricular septum.[3, 23] In the past, this dissection was performed with cardioplegic arrest, but recently it has been

found that this dissection can be safely accomplished with the heart beating. The dissection is extended deep into the posterior pyramidal space overlying the posterior interventricular septum (Fig. 3, inset). The dissection is continued medially until the mitral valve anulus is visualized and posteriorly to the epicardial reflection of the ventricle at the crux of the heart. After completion of the dissection, the supra-anular incision is closed with a continuous suture of 4-0 Prolene.

An alternative approach for the elimination of accessory pathways in the Wolff-Parkinson-White syndrome is a modification of the original epicardial approach devised by Sealy.[24] Guiraudon and colleagues have advocated the use of cryolesions to the exposed atrial-anular region of the heart after retraction of the AV groove fat pad.[12] This operative approach can be applied externally, but care must be taken to avoid injury to the anular ring and closely adjacent coronary arteries. However, the endocardial approach to divide accessory AV connections is recommended because of its proven success (98 per cent) and low mortality (less than 1 per cent) and because over 20 per cent of the patients in our recent series have had multiple pathways. In addition, a significant number of patients have also required concomitant cardiac surgical procedures, such as repair of defects associated with Ebstein's anomaly, closure of atrial septal defect, or patent foramen ovale repair as well as revascularization procedures.

Paroxysmal Supraventricular Tachycardia Due to Concealed Accessory Atrioventricular Connection

Patients with paroxysmal supraventricular tachycardia (PSVT) due to a concealed accessory atrioventricular connection have a pathway that conducts in the retrograde

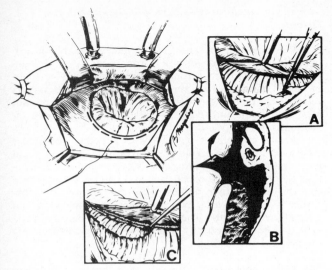

Figure 4. Operative procedure for correcting left free wall pathways. To the left and above is the left atrial cavity exposed by an incision in the right side of the left atrium. The suture in the atrium marks the external site of the pathway's entry into the left atrium. The extent of the incision is shown by the dotted line. The superior vena cava is to the left with the left fibrous trigone marked as a solid black ellipse-shaped disc on the left. The black ellipse on the right is the right fibrous trigone.

Inset A, which is the exposure after the atrial incision is made, demonstrates the ventricular summit below. The nerve hook is shown dividing the fibers connecting the sulcus fat to the myocardium.

Inset B, Extent of the dissection of the sulcus fat from the atrium and the ventricle.

Inset C, The last step when, with a small sharp nerve hook, all the superficial fibers of the ventricular myocardium are divided as they enter the anulus fibrosus.

(From Sealy, W. C., and Gallagher, J. J.: J. Thorac. Cardiovasc. Surg., 81:698, 1981.)

(ventricular to atrial) direction only and are approached surgically in identical manner to patients with WPW syndrome. Because these concealed accessory AV pathways function only in the retrograde direction, no delta wave is present on the ECG during normal sinus rhythm and ventricular epicardial mapping is of no value. Therefore, retrograde atrial mapping is performed during induced reciprocating tachycardia or during ventricular pacing to identify the site of atrial insertion of the accessory pathway.[3] The surgical dissection is then accomplished as described for the Wolff-Parkinson-White syndrome.

Paroxysmal Supraventricular Tachycardia Due to Atrioventricular Node Re-entry

In the recent past, the only operative treatment available for patients with medically refractory AV node re-entry tachycardia was elective cryoablation of the bundle of His followed by permanent pacemaker insertion. Surgical ablation of the His bundle is performed on cardiopulmonary bypass through a right atriotomy.[22] A hand-held exploring electrode is positioned over the membranous portion of the interatrial septum to identify the His bundle electrogram. When the His bundle is accurately located, the electrode is replaced with a cryoprobe. The tip of the cryoprobe can be cooled internally with nitrous oxide. The cryoprobe temperature is lowered to 0° C., at which time atrioventric-

ular conduction should cease. The area is then allowed to rewarm and AV conduction returns. This temporary cooling and rewarming confirms that the tip of the cryoprobe is overlying the His bundle. The temperature of the probe is then lowered to −60° C. for 2 to 3 minutes, resulting in destruction of the His bundle and permanent atrioventricular block. In 1981, a closed-chest technique was described for permanent His bundle ablation utilizing 200 to 500 joules delivered through a transvenous catheter adjacent to the His bundle.[9, 21] The catheter technique has essentially replaced cryoablation of the His bundle for the treatment of medically refractory AV node re-entry tachycardia because it does not require an operative procedure.

Because both His bundle cryoablation and His catheter ablation require permanent pacemaker insertion, Holman and associates developed a new surgical technique for the treatment of AV node re-entry using discrete cryolesions applied around the borders of the AV node in an effort to alter the functional characteristics of the AV node and its input pathways.[14] As many as nine separate 4-mm. cryolesions are placed around the vicinity of the His bundle and AV node. Each small cryolesion is applied until temporary AV block occurs or permanent prolongation of the A-H interval develops. In selected patients, it appears that AV node re-entry tachycardia can be treated without complete destruction of the normal cardiac conduction system.[3]

Ectopic (Automatic) Atrial Tachycardia

Patients with ectopic atrial tachycardia develop supraventricular dysrhythmias due to an ectopic focus in the atrium. These arrhythmias occur as a result of automatic activity, and the clinically observed dysrhythmias cannot be induced by standard programmed electrical stimulation techniques because it does not result from re-entry. If the site of the automatic focus can be identified during the preoperative catheter study and the intraoperative study, this area can be ablated surgically, excised, or surgically isolated.[3] However, if the focus cannot be precisely located but is thought to originate from the left atrium, a left atrial isolation procedure can be used to electrically disconnect the left atrium from the remaining heart.[27] This procedure confines the ectopic automatic activity to the left atrium and thereby prevents it from being transmitted through the normal cardiac conduction system. This allows the remaining portion of the heart to continue in sinus rhythm regardless of whether or not ectopic activity is present in the isolated left atrium. In 1982, this procedure was successfully performed by Cox in a 39-year-old female patient with medically refractory supraventricular tachycardia resulting from an ectopic automatic focus arising in the left atrium.[3]

Atrial Flutter-Fibrillation

Occasional patients with atrial flutter-fibrillation and a rapid ventricular response are refractory to all medical therapy. In such patients, discrete cryosurgery around the borders of the AV node may be capable of controlling the ventricular response rate to atrial flutter or fibrillation. Experimental studies have shown that discrete cryolesions can induce permanent prolongation of the A-H interval without causing complete heart block.[14] Based on these experimental observations, in the future discrete cryosurgical techniques may be successful in controlling ventricular response rate in selected patients with medically refractory atrial flutter-fibrillation.[2]

Chronic atrial fibrillation is found in approximately 60 per cent of all patients undergoing isolated mitral valve replacement.[20] There is no evidence that these arrhythmias originate preferentially in the left atrium. However, in the future if it is found that patients with left atrial hypertrophy and a normal right atrium have atrial fibrillation originating in left atrial muscle, the left atrial isolation procedure performed at the time of mitral valve surgery may be capable of confining fibrillation to the left atrium.[3, 27]

Medically Refractory Inappropriate Sinus Tachycardia

Self-limiting episodes of acute sinus tachycardia are an appropriate physiologic response to exercise, emotion, certain drugs, or acute illness. Chronic sinus tachycardia has been associated with hyperthyroidism, pheochromocytoma, decompensated cardiac or pulmonary disease, malignancy, and chronic infection. Chronic sinus tachycardia has only rarely been reported in otherwise healthy individuals.

Recently, three female patients (ages 20, 36, and 30 years) were referred for electrophysiologic evaluation of medically refractory, disabling episodes of inappropriate sinus tachycardia. None of these patients had any known underlying illnesses and all had undergone extensive evaluations to eliminate hyperthyroidism, pheochromocytoma, underlying malignancy, or abnormal autonomic response. Each patient experienced frequent disabling episodes of inappropriate sinus tachycardia, resulting in presyncope or frank syncope. All patients had previously received without success a variety of pharmacologic agents. Each patient underwent an extensive preoperative electrophysiology study, which revealed sinus tachycardia and, in one patient, asymptomatic Wolff-Parkinson-White syndrome. Because these patients were refractory to medical therapy and totally disabled by their sinus tachycardia, each underwent intraoperative mapping while on cardiopulmonary bypass to determine the area of earliest atrial activation. This area corresponded anatomically to the region of the sinoatrial node and was widely excised in each patient; the right atrial defect was repaired using a pericardial patch. Each patient developed a lower atrial pacemaker within hours following sinoatrial node excision and did not require permanent pacemaker insertion. These three patients are the first to undergo complete excision of the sinoatrial node for medically refractory disabling sinus tachycardia.[15] Although the etiology of this syndrome remains unknown, it can be successfully managed by this new surgical approach.

Prior to this operative approach, Guiraudon and colleagues treated a similar patient using a sinoatrial node isolation procedure. A circumferential incision was made through the midportion of the right atrium, disconnecting the sinoatrial node and upper right atrium from the remainder of the right atrium. This operative approach was also successful in eliminating inappropriate sinus tachycardia but required placement of a permanent pacemaker.[28]

SURGICAL TREATMENT OF VENTRICULAR TACHYARRHYTHMIAS

Ventricular dysrhythmias that can be surgically treated are divided into those associated with ischemic heart disease and those unrelated to ischemic heart disease.

Ventricular Tachycardias Due to Ischemic Heart Disease

Ventricular tachycardia associated with ischemia can occur in patients with critical coronary stenoses who develop ventricular tachycardia with exertion or with episodes of angina. This has been termed "effort induced or angina related ventricular tachycardia."[4] These patients do not have aneurysms and require only standard myocardial revascularization procedures.

Another group of patients with ischemic ventricular tachycardia have suffered a prior myocardial infarction and have ventricular tachycardia associated with a left ventricular aneurysm. There is experimental and clinical evidence that the site of origin of this re-entrant ventricular tachycardia is at the border zone between the aneurysm and normal myocardium.[11] These patients can be cured of their ventricular tachycardia by removing, ablating, or isolating the discrete site of origin.

In the past, occasional patients were cured of ventricular tachycardia when subjected to a variety of different operative procedures. None of these procedures was directed by electrophysiologic mapping procedures and therefore they are referred to as nondirected operations. In general, these nondirected procedures were associated with a high operative mortality and a low overall success rate (Table 1). These poor results led to the development of electrophysiological guidance to identify the exact site of origin of ventricular tachycardia. The first successful directed operation for ischemic ventricular tachycardia was performed by Oldham in 1973.[8] At the time of this procedure, epicardial mapping was first used to identify the site of origin of ventricular tachycardia in a patient with a left ventricular aneurysm. The area of origin was excised followed by resection and repair of the aneurysm. This patient remains alive and has had no further ventricular tachycardia.

The first operation that gained widespread application was the encircling endocardial ventriculotomy (EEV) procedure introduced by Guiraudon and associates in 1978.[11] This operation was based on the observation that ventricular tachycardia in conjunction with previous myocardial infarction and a left ventricular aneurysm is associated with a re-entrant circuit in the borderzone between dead and viable myocardium. Therefore, a standard left ventricular aneurysmectomy that leaves this borderzone intact will not result in cure of ventricular tachycardia. In the EEV operation, an endocardial incision is placed above the junction of endocardial fibrosis and normal endocardium and is extended around the entire base of the aneurysm or

TABLE 1. Results of Nondirected Operations for Ischemic Ventricular Tachycardia*

Procedure	Patients	Operative Mortality (%)	Failure (%)	Success (%)
Sympathectomy	12	25	17	58
CABG	37	27	27	46
Resection	95	24	17	59
CABG and resection	27	41	4	55
TOTAL	171	27%	17%	56%

*From Cox, J. L.: Curr. Probl. Cardiol., 8(4), 1983.

Abbreviations: CABG = Coronary artery bypass grafting; resection = myocardial infarctectomy or aneurysmectomy.

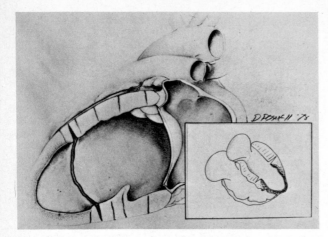

Figure 5. The encircling endocardial ventriculotomy is indeed circular and completely surrounds the diseased zone at the edge of the endocardial fibrosis. Inset, Depth of the ventriculotomy in the septum and in the free wall of the ventricle. (From Guiraudon, G., Fontaine, G., Frank, R., et al: Ann. Thorac. Surg., 26:438, 1978.)

origin of the arrhythmia guided by electrophysiologic mapping.[13] In 1982, Moran and co-workers suggested that the endocardial resection procedure should be extended (extended ERP) to remove all visible scar tissue.[17] An extended endocardial resection procedure is currently performed at our center in patients with anterior apical or inferior apical aneurysms associated with re-entrant ventricular tachycardia.

A more difficult subgroup of patients with ischemic ventricular tachycardia are those in whom dysrhythmia originates high on the interventricular septum or closely adjacent to the mitral valve anulus. These patients can be treated with discrete cryoablation with or without partial encircling endocardial ventriculotomy.[3, 11] The results achieved in 302 patients treated with directed surgical procedures for ventricular tachycardia associated with aneurysms are summarized in Table 2. At the present time, the overall operative mortality rate is 10 per cent (range 7 to 16 per cent) and the overall success rate is 84 per cent.[1, 6, 18, 19, 26] These are impressive results in view of the near 100 per cent mortality that occurs in medically refractory patients.

Ventricular Tachyarrhythmias Unrelated to Ischemic Heart Disease

A number of patients have been shown to have ventricular tachycardia due to nonischemic cardiomyopathy. The majority of these patients have been found to have diffuse dilatation of both ventricles with widespread patchy myocardial fibrosis. These tachyarrhythmias frequently arise in the right ventricle and can be treated by surgical isolation of the right ventricle or cryoablation of the site of origin of the arrhythmia. A particularly interesting subgroup of patients with non-ischemic ventricular tachycardia was reported in 1978 by Fontaine who described a previously unrecognized form of cardiomyopathy localized

infarction (Fig. 5). Only the subepicardial myocardium and subepicardial blood vessels are spared. The incision is then closed from within the ventricle. This procedure was effective in eliminating ventricular tachycardia but was associated with a substantial operative mortality because of its detrimental effects on left ventricular function.[25]

In 1979, Harken and colleagues introduced the endocardial resection procedure (ERP) (Fig. 6).[13] This procedure ablates the arrhythmogenic region identified by endocardial mapping through excision of subendocardial scar tissue as it joins normal myocardium at the borderzone of the aneurysm. The operation as originally described removes 2 to 4 cm. of subendocardial fibrosis surrounding the area of

Figure 6. Operative drawing revealing a left ventricular aneurysmectomy with edges held open. A large flap of endocardium is peeled off the septum in order to obliterate the arrhythmia origin. (From Harken, A. H., Josephson, M. E., and Horowitz, L. N.: Ann. Surg., 190:456, 1979.)

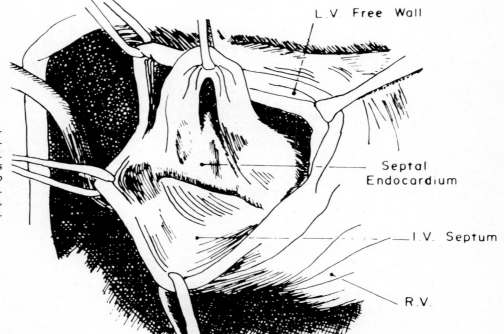

L.V. Free Wall

Septal Endocardium

I.V. Septum

R.V.

TABLE 2. *In-Hospital Results of Directed Surgical Procedures for Ventricular Tachycardia Associated with Aneurysms*

Procedure	Patients	Operative Mortality	Failure	Success
EEV				
Guiraudon et al.[11]	27	15% (4)	8% (2)	78%
Ostermeyer et al.[19]	12	8% (1)	0	92%
Partial EEV				
Ostermeyer et al.[19]	28	7% (2)	8% (2)	85%
ERP				
Harken et al.[13]	107	9% (10)	7% (7)	84%
EERP				
Moran et al.[17]	94	9% (8)	9% (8)	83%
Lowe et al.[15]	15	7% (1)	7% (1)	87%
Mixed EEV/ERP				
Brodman et al.[1]	19	16%	11% (2)	77%
TOTAL	302	10% (29)	7% (22)	84% (254)

Abbreviations: EEV = Encircling endocardial ventriculotomy; ERP = endocardial resection procedure; EERP = extended endocardial resection procedure.

to the right ventricle and associated with ventricular tachycardia.[7] He applied the term *arrhythmogenic right ventricular dysplasia* to describe this entity. The etiology of the syndrome is unknown but it is characterized by a transmural infiltration of fatty tissue, resulting in thinning and aneurysmal bulging of the apical basilar and posterior regions of the right ventricle. Depending on the site of origin of the arrhythmia in the right ventricle, it can be treated by an ablative procedure or a complete right ventricular disconnection procedure.[3]

In addition to arrhythmogenic right ventricular dysplasia, rare causes of non-ischemic ventricular tachycardia have been cured surgically in patients with cardiac sarcoidosis, Purkinje cell tumors, and benign cardiac tumors such as rhabdomyomas and in those with postoperative cardiac scars following repair of tetralogy of Fallot or following apical venting of the left ventricle. The majority of these patients can be treated successfully by electrophysiologically guided excision or cryoablation of the site of origin of ventricular tachycardia.

ANTITACHYCARDIA DEVICES

Several pacing techniques have been used successfully to terminate dysrhythmias. These include competitive or underdrive pacing, burst pacing, overdrive pacing, and critically timed premature stimuli.[16] The major limitation to the widespread use of antitachycardia pacemakers in the treatment of serious ventricular arrhythmias has been the potential for arrhythmia acceleration or ventricular fibrillation. Therefore, extensive preimplant testing is required to document the efficacy and safety of a chosen pacing technique. In view of the extremely effective operative procedures available for a variety of supraventricular and ventricular dysrhythmias, antitachycardia devices such as the automatic internal cardioverter-defibrillator are currently used to treat only patients who cannot benefit from an electrophysiologically guided procedure. The majority of such patients have ventricular tachycardia with multiple sites of origin or have automatic ventricular tachycardia or primary ventricular fibrillation. Patients with these disorders who remain medically refractory are candidates for implantation of a device such as the automatic internal

cardioverter-defibrillator. This device is capable of delivering single shocks of 20 to 25 joules in response to ventricular tachycardia or ventricular fibrillation. Although these devices remain in the investigational stage, it is likely that they will gain more widespread use in the treatment of refractory arrhythmias and may ultimately provide back-up for other pacing techniques incorporated into a single totally implantable device. It should be underscored, however, that antitachycardia pacing and implantation of automatic internal cardioverter-defibrillators should be reserved for patients who are not candidates for an electrophysiologically guided surgical procedure.

SELECTED REFERENCES

Cobb, F. R., Blumenschein, S. D., Sealy, W. C., et al.: Successful surgical treatment of the bundle of Kent in a patient with Wolff-Parkinson-White syndrome. Circulation, 38:1018, 1968.
This manuscript reports the first successful surgical treatment of a cardiac arrhythmia, which was performed by Sealy in 1968. The patient was a 32-year old fisherman from the coast of North Carolina with medically refractory paroxysmal atrial tachycardia secondary to the Wolff-Parkinson-White syndrome. Sealy successfully divided the accessory atrioventricular connection and this landmark procedure was the first electrophysiologically guided operation.

Cox, J. L.: Surgery for cardiac arrhythmias. Curr. Probl. Cardiol., 8(4), 1983.
This excellent monograph is an authoritative evaluation of the current status of the surgical treatment of a variety of dysrhythmias. The preoperative evaluation and operative procedures available for both supraventricular and ventricular dysrhythmias are described in detail and an outstanding number of references are provided.

Guiraudon, G., Fontaine, G., Frank, R., et al.: Encircling endocardial ventriculotomy: A new surgical treatment for life-threatening ventricular tachycardia resistant to medical treatment following myocardial infarction. Ann. Thorac. Surg., 26:438, 1978.
The encircling endocardial ventriculotomy procedure was the first widespread electrophysiologically guided operation that was successful in treating re-entrant ventricular tachycardia. This operation was based on experimental and clinical evidence showing that the site of origin of re-entrant ventricular tachycardia is at the borderzone between the aneurysm and normal myocardium. Partial encircling ventriculotomy procedures are now used to treat patients with ventricular tachycardia associated with aneurysms arising near the base of the heart.

Harken, A. H., Josephson, M. E., and Horowitz, L. N.: Surgical endocardial resection for the treatment of malignant ventricular tachycardia. Ann. Surg., 190:456, 1979.
Harken and associates have acquired the largest experience in treating patients with ischemic ventricular tachycardia associated with left ventricular aneurysms. This manuscript introduced the endocardial resection procedure, which removes the site of origin for re-entrant ventricular tachycardia. This operation and its modifications are still the most widely used in the treatment of ischemic ventricular tachycardia.

Moran, J. M., Kehoe, R. F., Loeb, J. M., et al.: Extended endocardial resection for the treatment of ventricular tachycardia and ventricular fibrillation. Ann. Thorac. Surg., 34:538, 1982.
Moran and associates recommend that all visible scar be removed from the endocardium to treat patients with ischemic ventricular tachycardia associated with ventricular aneurysms. The extended endocardial resection procedure is highly effective and presently is the operation of choice for patients with anterior apical or inferior apical aneurysms associated with re-entrant ventricular tachycardia.

REFERENCES

1. Brodman, R., Fisher, J. D., Johnston, D. R., et al.: Results of electrophysiologically guided operations for drug-resistant recurrent ventricular tachycardia and ventricular fibrillation due to coronary artery disease. J. Thorac. Cardiovasc. Surg., 87:431, 1984.
2. Cobb, F. R., Blumenschein, S. D., Sealy, W. C., et al.: Successful surgical interruption of the bundle of Kent in a patient with Wolff-Parkinson-White syndrome. Circulation, 38:1018, 1968.
3. Cox, J. L.: Surgery for cardiac arrhythmias. Curr. Probl. Cardiol., 8(4), 1983.

4. Cox, J. L., Woodruff, W. W., III, and Lowe, J. E.: The surgical treatment of exercise-induced or angina-associated ventricular tachyarrhythmias. (Submitted for publication)

5. Durrer, D., and Roos, J. T.: Epicardial excitation of the ventricles in a patient with Wolff-Parkinson-White syndrome. Circulation, *38*:1018, 1968.

6. Fontaine, G.: Surgery for ventricular tachycardia. The view from Paris, Int. J. Cardiol., *1*:351, 1982.

7. Fontaine, G., Guiraudon, G., and Frank, R.: Management of chronic ventricular tachycardia. *In* Narula, O. S. (Ed.): Innovations in Diagnosis and Management of Cardiac Arrhythmias. Baltimore, Williams & Wilkins, 1979.

8. Gallagher, J. J., Oldham, H. N., Wallace, A. G., et al.: Ventricular aneurysm with ventricular tachycardia: Report of a case with epicardial mapping and successful resection. Am. J. Cardiol., *35*:696, 1975.

9. Gallagher, J. J., Svenson, R. H., Kasell, J. H., et al.: Catheter technique for closed chest ablation of the atrioventricular conduction system in man. Read before the 31st Annual Scientific Session, American College of Cardiology, Atlanta, Ga., April 28, 1982.

10. Gallagher, J. J., Svenson, R. H., Sealy, W. C., et al.: The Wolff-Parkinson-White syndrome and the preexcitation dysrhythmias: Medical and surgical management. Med. Clin. North Am., *60*:101, 1976.

11. Guiraudon, G., Fontaine, G., Frank, R., et al.: Encircling endocardial ventriculotomy: A new surgical treatment for life-threatening ventricular tachycardias resistant to medical treatment following myocardial infarction. Ann. Thorac. Surg., *26*:438, 1978.

12. Guiraudon, G. M., Klein, G. J., Gulamhusein, S., et al.: Surgical repair of Wolff-Parkinson-White syndrome: A new closed-heart technique.

13. Harken, A. H., Josephson, M. E., and Horowitz, L. N.: Surgical endocardial resection for the treatment of malignant ventricular tachycardia. Ann. Surg., *190*:456, 1979.

14. Holman, W. L., Ikeshita, M., Lease, J. G., et al.: Elective prolongation of atrioventricular conduction by multiple discrete cryolesions. A new technique for the treatment of paroxysmal supraventricular tachycardia. J. Thorac. Cardiovasc. Surg., *84*:554, 1982.

15. Lowe, J. E., Sabiston, D. C., Jr.: The surgical management of cardiac arrhythmias. J. Appl. Cardiol., *1*:1, 1986.

16. Lowe, J. E., and German, L. D.: Cardiac pacemakers. *In* Sabiston, D. C., Jr. (Ed.): Textbook of Surgery, 13th ed. Philadelphia, W. B. Saunders Company, 1986.

17. Moran, J. M., Kehoe, R. F., Loeb, J. M., et al.: Extended endocardial resection for the treatment of ventricular tachycardia and ventricular fibrillation. Ann. Thorac. Surg., *34*:538, 1982.

18. Moran, J. M., Kehoe, R. F., Loeb, J. M., et al.: Operative therapy of malignant ventricular rhythm disturbances. Ann. Surg., *198*:479, 1983.

19. Ostermeyer, J., Breithardt, G., Borggrefe, M., et al.: Surgical treatment of ventricular tachycardias: Complete versus partial encircling endocardial ventriculotomy. J. Thorac. Cardiovasc. Surg., *87*:517, 1984.

20. Salomon, N., Stinson, E., Randall, B., et al.: Patient related risk factors as predictors of results following isolated mitral valve replacement. Ann. Thorac. Surg., *24*:519, 1977.

21. Scheinman, M., Morady, F., Hess, D., et al.: Transvenous catheter technique for induction of damage to the atrioventricular junction in man. Read before the 31st Annual Scientific Session, American College of Cardiology, Atlanta, Ga., April 28, 1982.

22. Sealy, W. C., Gallagher, J. J., and Kasell, J. H.: His bundle interruption for control of inappropriate ventricular responses to atrial arrhythmias. Ann. Thorac. Surg., *32*:429, 1981.

23. Sealy, W. C., and Mikat, E. M.: Anatomical problems with identification and interruption of posterior septal Kent bundles. Ann. Thorac. Surg., *36*:584, 1983.

24. Sealy, W. C., and Wallace, A. G.: Surgical treatment of Wolff-Parkinson-White syndrome. J. Thorac. Cardiovasc. Surg., *68*:757, 1974.

25. Ungerleider, R. M., Holman, W. L., Calcagno, D., et al.: Encircling endocardial ventriculotomy for refractory ischemic ventricular tachycardia. III. Effects on regional left ventricular function. J. Thorac. Cardiovasc. Surg., *83*:857, 1982.

26. Wetstein, L., Michelson, E. L., Moore, E. N., et al.: Surgical therapy for ventricular tachyarrhythmias. Surg. Gynecol. Obstet., *157*:487, 1983.

27. Williams, J. M., Ungerleider, R. M., Lofland, G. K., et al.: Left atrial isolation. A new technique for the treatment of supraventricular arrhythmias. J. Thorac. Cardiovasc. Surg., *80*:373, 1980.

28. Yee, R., Guiraudon, G. M., Gardner, M. J., et al.: Refractory paroxysmal sinus tachycardia: management by subtotal right atrial exclusion. J. Am. Coll. Cardiol., *3*:400, 1984.

XVIII

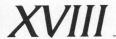

Cardiac Neoplasms

RALPH J. DAMIANO, JR., M.D.
DAVID C. SABISTON, JR., M.D.

Cardiac neoplasms are rare and until recently were seldom diagnosed during life. Following Columbo's description of cardiac tumors in 1559,[9] over three centuries passed before Barnes and associates reported the first clinical premortem diagnosis of a primary cardiac neoplasm.[1] Surgical removal was first successfully performed in 1951.[33] In the last two decades, the development of modern cardiac noninvasive diagnostic techniques and advances in cardiac surgery have had a significant impact on the prognosis of many primary cardiac tumors. Both echocardiography and radionuclide angiocardiography have proved reliable, noninvasive methods, which enable the clinician to diagnose and surgically cure many benign lesions that previously were found only at autopsy.[37, 45, 48, 49]

INCIDENCE AND CLINICAL PRESENTATION

The autopsy incidence of primary cardiac tumors varies between 0.002 and 0.03 per cent.[34, 48, 54] Myxoma is the most common, constituting 25 per cent of all tumors of the heart and pericardium and 40 per cent of all benign tumors (Table 1). Rhabdomyoma is the most common neoplasm in children. In infants less than 1 year of age, rhabdomyomas and teratomas account for over 75 per cent of all cardiac tumors. Malignant tumors constitute 25 per cent of all primary neoplasms, with sarcomas being most frequent. Overall, malignant tumors in children are rare and account for less than 10 per cent of all pediatric neoplasms.[34]

TABLE 1. Neoplasms of the Heart and Pericardium

Type	Number	Percentage
Benign		
Myxoma	130	29.3
Lipoma	45	10.1
Papillary fibroelastoma	42	9.5
Rhabdomyoma	36	8.1
Fibroma	17	3.8
Hemangioma	15	3.4
Teratoma	14	3.2
Mesothelioma of the AV node	12	2.7
Granular cell tumor	3	0.7
Neurofibroma	3	0.7
Lymphangioma	2	0.5
SUBTOTAL	319	72
Malignant		
Angiosarcoma	39	8.8
Rhabdomyosarcoma	26	5.8
Mesothelioma	19	4.2
Fibrosarcoma	14	3.2
Malignant lymphoma	7	1.6
Extraskeletal osteosarcoma	5	1.1
Neurogenic sarcoma	4	0.9
Malignant teratoma	4	0.9
Thymoma	4	0.9
Leiomyosarcoma	1	0.2
Liposarcoma	1	0.2
Synovial sarcoma	1	0.2
SUBTOTAL	125	28
TOTAL	444	100

From McAllister, H. A., Jr., and Fenoglio, J. J., Jr.: Tumors of the cardiovascular system. *In* Atlas of Tumor Pathology, Fasc. 15, 2nd Series. Washington, D.C., Armed Forces Institute of Pathology, 1978.

Secondary metastatic tumors involving the heart are 20 to 40 times more common than primary tumors and should be considered in any patient with a malignant lesion who develops symptoms of cardiovascular disease.[21, 40] In large necropsy series of patients with malignant neoplasms, as many as 21 per cent have secondary cardiac involvement.[21, 49]

It is estimated that only 5 to 10 per cent of all cardiac neoplasms produce symptoms.[20] This is due to both the slow growth of the tumors and the relative resistance of the myocardium and fibrous skeleton of the heart to tumor invasion. In patients with symptoms, the clinical presentations are myriad and can simulate many other forms of cardiac disease. Cardiac tumors produce symptoms by obstruction, local invasion, emboli, or systemic effects.[4, 23] Intracavitary tumors may cause valvular or cavitary obstruction. Valvular obstruction causes murmurs of valvular stenosis or regurgitation and later leads to syncope, angina, or congestive heart failure. Obstruction to ventricular outflow or inflow can resemble cardiomyopathy, and may lead to congestive heart failure with pulmonary or peripheral edema. Similarly, local tumor invasion can result in myocardial or valvular dysfunction and cardiac pain. In occasional individuals, involvement of the conduction system can lead to the development of recurrent arrhythmias, heart block, or Stokes-Adams attacks.

Tumor emboli are also an important source of morbidity and mortality in patients with cardiac neoplasms. Both systemic emboli from left-sided tumors and pulmonary emboli from those on the right side of the heart have been reported and can cause varying symptoms. There are rare instances of emboli to or extrinsic compression of the coronary arteries, which have resulted in ischemic cardiac pain.[26]

Finally, cardiac tumors can cause numerous systemic and hematologic symptoms. These include fever, malaise, arthralgia, skin lesions, weight loss, elevated erythrocyte sedimentation rate, hyperglobulinemia, polymyositis, hepatic dysfunction, and Raynaud's phenomenon.[23, 24, 48] Hematologic abnormalities associated with cardiac tumors include hemolytic anemia, polycythemia, leukocytosis, thrombocytosis, and thrombocytopenia.

DIAGNOSIS

The diagnosis of cardiac tumors can be difficult because symptoms can simulate more common cardiac abnormalities, including rheumatic valvular disease, ischemic coronary disease, idiopathic cardiomyopathy, and even bacterial endocarditis. Thus, astute clinical suspicion is required. Electrocardiographic (ECG) and conventional radiographic findings are often absent or nondiagnostic. Two-dimensional and M-mode echocardiography have become the most useful and accurate techniques for the premortem diagnosis of these lesions[12, 13, 32, 43] (Fig. 1). Greater than 95 per cent of patients examined with echocardiography exhibit findings suggestive of cardiac tumors. Two-dimensional echocardiographic examination provides substantial advantages over conventional M-mode techniques because all four chambers can be visualized and tumor size, point of attachment, and mobility can be better assessed.[12] Radionuclide studies also have been utilized to identify intracavitary and myocardial tumors.[37] Although this technique lacks the resolution of echocardiography, it has yielded information concerning the presence of tumors when other methods have failed. Computerized tomography (CT) is being used to diagnose cardiac tumors more frequently.[17, 25] ECG-gated computed tomography and nuclear magnetic resonance imaging (MRI) are likely to be useful for defining both local invasion and extracardiac extension of tumors, while at the same time eliminating the motion artefact that hampers conventional computed tomography.

Cardiac catheterization, although an extremely accurate means of diagnosis, is no longer necessary because of the availability of safe, reliable, noninvasive diagnostic techniques.[3, 43, 46, 51] Patients are thus not subjected to the risk of tumor embolization with intracardiac manipulation during catheterization.[6] However, there are several indications for angiocardiography in patients with cardiac tumors,[4] including a tumor not identified by noninvasive methods, malignant tumors, and the likelihood of coexisting cardiac lesions.

BENIGN TUMORS

Myxoma

Myxomas are the most common benign tumors of the heart.[34] Although they have been reported from ages 3 to 83 years, they most commonly occur in patients aged 30 to 60 years. Women are affected two to three times more frequently than men. Seventy-five per cent of myxomas are located in the left atrium, 20 per cent occur in the right atrium, and the remainder are equally distributed between the two ventricles. In 5 per cent of cases, the myxomas are multiple.

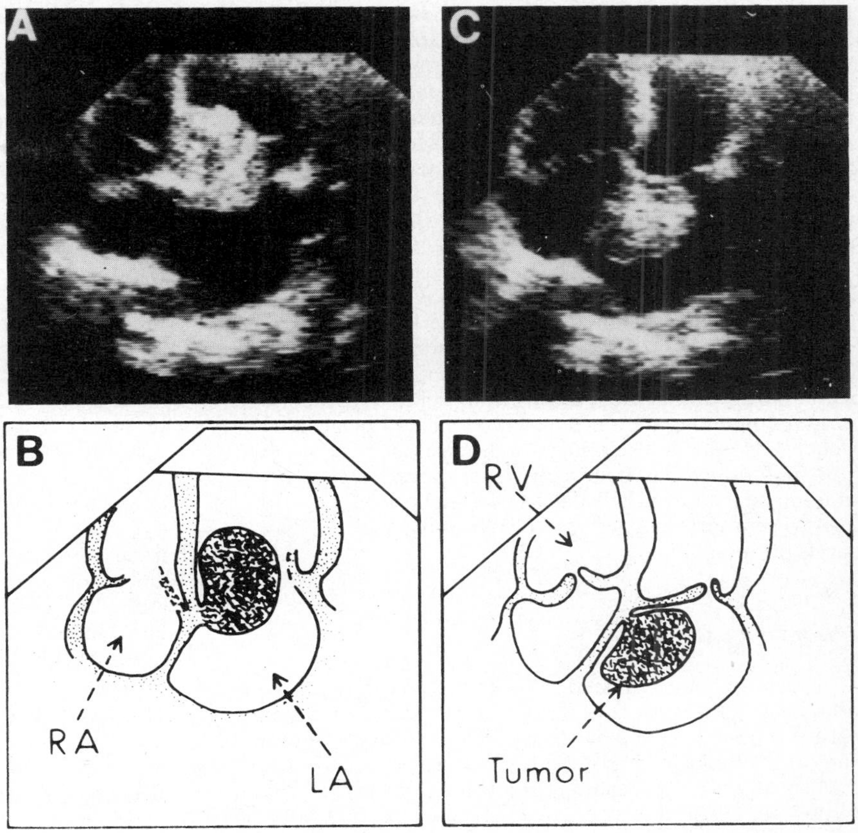

Figure 1. Two-dimensional echocardiogram demonstrating a left atrial myxoma. Prolapse of the myxoma into the left ventricle during distole (A, B) and return into the atrium (LA) during systole (C, D) is clearly documented. (From Silverman, N. A., and Sabiston, D. C., Jr. Cardiac neoplasms. In Sabiston, D. C., Jr. (Ed.): Textbook of Surgery, 13th ed. Philadelphia, W. B. Saunders Company, 1986, p. 2406.)

Myxomas are endocardial tumors that are pedunculated, gelatinous, and polypoid in nature; they usually vary in size from 4 to 8 cm. but have been reported as large as 15 cm. In 90 per cent of patients, the tumor is attached to the atrial septum usually in the region of the fossa ovalis. Other less common sites include the posterior atrial wall, the anterior wall, and atrial appendage.[34] In the ventricles, myxomas usually originate on the lateral free walls. Microscopically, they appear as a myxoid matrix composed of acid mucopolysaccharide within which are polygonal cells with scant eosinophilic cytoplasm. These polyhedral cells have small round or oval nuclei and are pathognomonic. Although some authors have supported a thrombotic origin of cardiac myxomas,[44] most evidence confirms that these tumors are true neoplasms.[34, 41] They can undergo malignant degeneration, and systemic metastases, although rare, have been documented.[41]

The size, location, and pedunculated nature of myxomas explain their varying modes of presentation. Ball-valve blockage of the atrioventricular (AV) valves is common, with over 40 per cent of patients having signs and symptoms of mitral valve disease.[4] Symptoms, murmurs, and arterial blood pressure often vary with positional changes and on different examinations. In some patients, an opening snap, or "tumor plop," is present on auscultation. This is generated by either tension on the tumor stalk or the impact of the tumor on the endocardial surface. Systemic emboli occur in up to 50 per cent of patients. They most commonly involve the central nervous system; however, embolization to the coronary arteries, renal arteries, aortic bifurcation, and lower extremities has been reported.[6, 26] Unexplained systemic emboli in a young person in normal sinus rhythm should suggest an intracavitary tumor and these patients should be screened with echocardiography. Moreover, all surgically removed arterial emboli should be examined histologically because this may establish the diagnosis of a cardiac tumor.

Right atrial tumors can produce signs and symptoms of right-sided heart failure by obstructing either tricuspid valve outflow or vena caval return.[4, 54] The clinical presentation can often be confused with that of constrictive pericarditis, cardiomyopathy, carcinoid heart disease, pulmonary stenosis, or tricuspid valve disease. Moreover, they may embolize to the pulmonary arteries and cause dyspnea, cough, and chest pain. Arrhythmias, particularly right bundle branch block, atrial flutter, or fibrillation accompanied by abnormally peaked T waves on the ECG are frequently seen in patients with right-sided myxomas. Often, these patients are diagnosed as having Ebstein's anomaly because of the presence of apparent tricuspid valve uisease and associated arrhythmias. Left ventricular myxomas may simulate either aortic stenosis or hypertrophic obstructive cardiomyopathy.[35] These patients have an extremely high incidence of systemic embolization. Right ventricular myxomas have a predilection for the young and produce right ventricular outflow obstruction.[5] Constitutional symptoms may predominate in some patients, particularly those with left atrial myxomas. In these instances, the differential diagnosis includes bacterial endocarditis, collagen vascular disease, occult malignancy, or infection.

Rhabdomyoma

Rhabdomyoma occurs in as many as 20 per cent of all patients with benign tumors and is the most common tumor in childhood.[14, 34] It is associated with tuberous sclerosis in 50 per cent of cases.[18, 28] These tumors are usually multiple and occur with equal frequency in both ventricles. In 50 per cent of patients, the tumor extends into the ventricular cavity. Patients usually have symptoms referable to obstruction of ventricular inflow or outflow or recurrent ventricular tachyarrhythmias. In one series, 60 per cent of patients had arrhythmias and the association between myocardial tumors and ventricular tachycardia in children is an important one to recognize.[42]

In gross appearance, rhabdomyomas are well-circumscribed (but not encapsulated) and yellow-gray. They may grow to 20 mm. in diameter and can be located anywhere in the myocardium. Histologically, rhadomyoma cells are large and filled with glycogen. Classic "spider cells" are seen, with centrally or eccentrically placed cytoplasmic masses containing the nucleus and elongated projectiles of slender myofibrils extending to the periphery. Prognosis with this tumor has been considered poor because of its multiplicity, poor encapsulation, and deep location. However, recent series suggest improved survival with aggressive surgical therapy.[42]

Fibromas

Fibromas are connective tissue tumors derived from fibroblasts. They are the second most common primary cardiac tumor in the pediatric age group, although fibromas can occur at all ages and in both sexes. They are most often solitary and usually located in the ventricular myocardium, frequently in the interventricular septum. The majority of these tumors encroach on or invade the conduction system and patients often experience arrhythmias or sudden death. Grossly, these are large, firm, sharply demarcated, gray-white tumors, often with areas of central calcification and/or necrosis. Histologic examination reveals fibromas to be non-encapsulated tumors consisting of hyalinized fibrous tissue that interdigitates with surrounding myocardium. The prognosis for these tumors is excellent if they are completely excised.[42, 53] Traditionally, septal tumors have been considered inoperable; however, even these can be successfully excised and cured in some instances.[42]

Mesotheliomas

Mesotheliomas are lethal tumors that are located in the atrial septum in the region of the atrioventricular node, occurring most commonly in adult females. These patients have complete or partial heart block or sudden death. Other benign tumors of the heart include lipomas, hemangiomas, teratomas, neurofibromas, lymphangiomas, hamartomas, and granular cell tumors (see Table 1). Papillary fibroelastomas and simple cysts are found specifically on the cardiac valves but rarely cause hemodynamic impairment.

Management of Benign Tumors

All cardiac tumors are potentially fatal as a result of cavitary or valvular obstruction, embolization, or arrhythmias. Thus, once a primary tumor is diagnosed, operative excision is the treatment of choice. Except for rare pericardial and epicardial tumors, the operative approach employs extracorporeal circulation, cardioplegic arrest, and removal of the tumor under direct vision. Great care must be taken to avoid tumor dislodgment or embolization. Atrial myxomas are resected through an atriotomy and complete excision includes the entire tumor, stalk, and a margin of normal atrial tissue around the point of attachment[48] (Fig. 2). This margin is important in preventing local recurrence.[11, 13, 48] Septal defects created by excision can be repaired primarily or with a patch. Ventricular myxomas can be removed through a ventriculotomy, an atriotomy, or an aortotomy with retraction of the aortic valve. The latter is the most common approach to left ventricular tumors. Special surgical considerations in removing ventricular tumors include preservation of adequate myocardial function, maintenance of proper AV valve function, and preservation of the conduction system. However, extensive resections often necessitate valve replacement and/or implantation of a pacemaker.[30] Cardiac transplantation also presents a reasonable alternative for otherwise unresectable tumors.

The modern surgical treatment of benign cardiac tumors can be performed with little if any operative mortality.[7, 30, 42, 48] Postoperative complications, besides supraventricular tachyarrhythmias, are infrequent and include heart block, low output syndrome, or valvular dysfunction.[2, 42] If the resection is complete, prognosis is excellent with long-term survival and infrequent recurrence.[13, 42, 46, 51] Partial resection may even provide excellent short-term results with some tumors.[42] Long-term postoperative follow-up with serial echocardiography is essential in all patients.

MALIGNANT TUMORS

The most common malignant tumors are sarcomas; angiosarcoma and rhabdomyosarcoma being the most frequent[34] (see Table 1). Histologic subdivision is largely academic because prognosis is uniformly grave.[38] Angiosarcomas most commonly originate in the right atrium and occur particularly in young adult males. These patients have clinical findings of right-sided heart failure or pericardial disease. Rhabdomyosarcomas, the second most common primary malignant cardiac tumor, are often multiple and originate with equal frequency in the left and right ventricles. The pericardium is involved in 50 per cent of patients, usually by direct tumor extension. All sarcomas grow rapidly to involve all layers of the heart, invade adjacent structures, and metastasize widely.[47] Metastases most commonly occur in the lungs and mediastinal lymph nodes. Characteristic signs and symptoms include progressive congestive heart failure, syncope, chest pain, fever, dyspnea, cardiomegaly, cardiac murmurs, embolic phenomena, and arrhythmias. Sudden death or vena caval obstruction has been described. Other primary malignant cardiac tumors include lymphoma, plasmacytoma, and malignant teratoma. All of these tumors have similar presentations and poor prognoses.

Most primary malignant cardiac tumors are unresectable or metastatic at the time of diagnosis. The major objective of operation is often to establish the diagnosis and exclude the possibility of a benign tumor. Multimodal therapy is usually ineffective. However, in isolated instances, palliation of symptoms or prolonged survival may be achieved with various combinations of aggressive surgical resection, chemotherapy, and radiation therapy.[15, 34, 47, 52] A collective review of 28 patients undergoing surgical resection revealed a mean survival of 14 months with no 5-year survivors.[38] Postoperative radiation therapy increased mean survival to 19.8 months but chemotherapy did not appear beneficial.

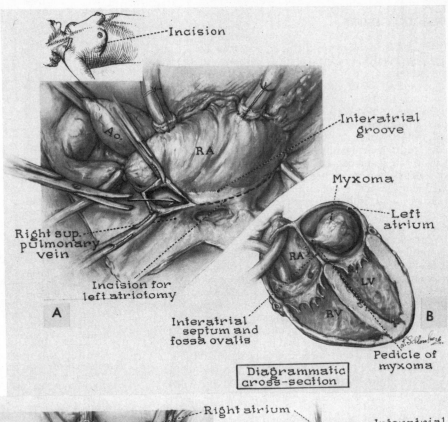

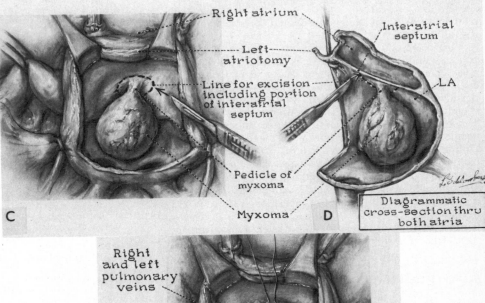

Figure 2. Surgical technique for removal of a left atrial myxoma.

A, B, The aorta is cross-clamped, and cardioplegic arrest is induced. A left atriotomy is performed.

C, The myxoma is exposed, and a portion of the atrial septum is excised at the attachment of the pedicle.

D, The atrial defect created by the excision is closed primarily. Large defects require patch closure for the atrial repair. For large, broad-based tumors attached to the atrial septum, exposure is often better via a right atrial approach.

(From Silverman, N. A., and Sabiston, D. C., Jr.: Cardiac neolasms. In Sabiston, D. C., Jr. (Ed.): Textbook of Surgery, 13th ed. Philadelphia, W. B. Saunders Company, 1986, p. 2410.)

METASTATIC TUMORS

Metastatic carcinoma of the heart occurs in 2 to 21 per cent of patients dying of malignancies, although it is rarely diagnosed during life.[21, 49] The most frequent primary carcinomas are those of lung and breast. Leukemia, lymphoma, and melanoma have a special predilection for metastasizing to the heart, being found in up to 64 per cent of cases at necropsy.[16, 21]

Metastases reach the heart by direct intrathoracic extension, retrograde lymphatic spread, or hematogenous spread. In rare instances, carcinoma can reach the heart by direct venous extension, especially with renal cell carcinoma and hepatoma, which extend up the inferior vena cava into the right atrium. Cardiac metastatic tumor growth is usually solid, small, and multiple and can occur anywhere in the heart or conduction system.

Approximately 10 to 13 per cent of cardiac metastases are symptomatic.[34, 49] Clinical presentation depends on the predominance of pericardial, myocardial, or endocardial involvement. Pericardial metastases exhibit effusion, tamponade, or constriction. Endocardial metastases cause obstructive symptoms or valvular dysfunction, whereas myocardial metastases often result in either congestive heart failure or arrhythmias. Myocardial infarction can be caused by external compression, transmural replacement with solid tumor, or tumor emboli. Cardiac manifestations of metastatic disease include (1) unexplained rapid cardiac enlargement, (2) symptoms of cardiac decompensation, (3) congestive heart failure, and (4) arrhythmias.[4] Although none is specific, the presence of one or more of these findings in patients with known malignancy should raise the clinician's suspicion.

Echocardiography, radionuclide angiocardiography, and computed tomography have been helpful in the diagnosis of metastatic lesions.[17, 19, 50] The goal of therapy for cardiac metastases is palliation, relief of symptoms, and, if possible, arrest of tumor growth. Radiation therapy and/or chemotherapy have shown short-term benefit in alleviating symptoms in selected patients.[8, 31] Pericardiocentesis and needle aspiration can often obviate the need for surgery by both establishing a tissue diagnosis and decompressing malignant effusions.[29] When this fails, open surgical drainage by the subxiphoid or transthoracic approach is a viable and often lifesaving alternative.[22, 36] Although surgery plays a minor role in the treatment of metastatic disease, it may be indicated for tumor debulking and resection. This is particularly true for indolent, radioresistant tumors and for right atrial extensions of renal tumors.[39]

SELECTED REFERENCES

Bloor, C. M., and O'Rourke, R. A.: Cardiac tumors: Clinical presentations and pathologic correlations. Curr. Probl. Cardiol., 9(6):1, 1984.
This superb, up-to-date review of cardiac tumors clearly describes the various clinical presentations and the modern diagnostic findings. The numerous illustrations and figures are particularly helpful. An extensive bibliography is provided.

McAllister, H. A., Jr., and Fenoglio, J. J.: Tumors of the cardiovascular system. In Atlas of Tumor Pathology, Fasc. 15, 2nd Series. Washington, D.C., Armed Forces Institute of Pathology, 1978.
This monograph reviews the extensive experience of the Armed Forces Institute of Pathology with 533 tumors and cysts of the heart and pericardium. The beautifully written and illustrated text contains a wealth of clinical and pathologic information about cardiac neoplasms.

Silverman, N. A.: Primary cardiac tumors. Ann. Surg., 191:127, 1980.
This is an excellent overview of primary cardiac tumors and provides an excellent summary of their history, incidence, clinical presentation, and diagnosis. A surgical series is presented and documents the excellent results that can be obtained in treating cardiac tumors with modern surgical techniques and strict attention to the avoidance of perioperative tumor embolization.

Sutton, M. G. St. J., Mercier, L-A., Giuliani, E. R., and Lie, J. T.: Atrial myxomas: A review of clinical experience with 40 patients. Mayo Clin. Proc., 55:371, 1980.
This report represents the largest series of atrial myxomas, the most common tumor of the heart, from a single institution. The importance of echocardiography in establishing the diagnosis is emphasized. The complete patient follow-up demonstrates that operation can be performed with low mortality with excellent long-term results and a low recurrence rate.

REFERENCES

1. Barnes, A. R., Beaver, D. C., and Snell, A. M.: Primary sarcoma of the heart: Report of a case with electrocardiographic and pathological studies. Am. Heart J., 9:480, 1934.
2. Bateman, T. M., Gray, R. T., Raymond, M. J., Chaux, A., Czer, L. S. C., and Matloff, J. M.: Arrhythmias and conduction disturbances following cardiac operation for the removal of left atrial myxomas. J. Thorac. Cardiovasc. Surg., 86:601, 1983.
3. Bini, R. M., Westaby, S., Bargeron, L. M., Jr., Pacifico, A. D., and Kirklin, J. W.: Investigation and management of primary cardiac tumors in infants and children. J. Am. Coll. Cardiol., 2:351, 1983.
4. Bloor, C. M., and O'Rourke, R. A.: Cardiac tumors: Clinical presentations and pathologic correlations. Curr. Probl. Cardiol., 9(6):1, 1984.
5. Bortolotti, V., Mazzucco, A., Valfre, C., et al.: Right ventricular myxoma: Review of the literature and report of two patients. Ann. Thorac. Surg., 33:277, 1982.
6. Bulkley, B. H., and Hutchins, G. M.: Atrial myxomas: A fifty year review. Am. Heart J., 97:639, 1979.
7. Castaneda, A. R., and Varco, R. L.: Tumors of the heart: Surgical considerations. Am. J. Cardiol., 21:357, 1968.
8. Chan, W. C., Freiman, A. H., Carstens, P. M. B., et al.: Radiation therapy of cardiac and pericardial metastases. Radiology, 114:701, 1975.
9. Colombo, R.: De Re Anatomica. Venice, Typopr. Nicolai Benalicquae Publisher, 1559, Lib XV, p. 259.
10. Crafoord, C.: Case report. In International Symposium Cardiovascular Surgery. Detroit, Henry Ford Hospital, 1955, p. 202.
11. Dang, C. R., and Hurley, E. J.: Contralateral recurrent myxoma of the heart. Ann. Thorac. Surg., 21:59, 1976.
12. Depace, N. L., Soulen, R. L., Kotler, M. N., and Mintz, G. S.: Two-dimensional echocardiographic detection of intra-atrial masses. Am. J. Cardiol., 48:954, 1981.
13. Donahoo, J. S., Weiss, J. L., Gardner, T. J., Fortvin, N. J., and Brawley, R. K.: Current management of atrial myxoma with emphasis on a new diagnostic technique. Ann. Surg., 189:763, 1979.
14. Foster, E. D., Spooner, E. W., Farina, M. A., Shaher, R. M., and Alley, R. D.: Cardiac rhabdomyoma in the neonate: Surgical management. Ann. Thorac. Surg., 37:249, 1984.
15. Garfein, O. B.: Lymphosarcoma of the right atrium: Angiographic and hemodynamic documentation of response to chemotherapy. Arch. Intern. Med., 135:325, 1975.
16. Glancy, D. L., and Roberts, W. C.: The heart in malignant melanoma: A study of 70 autopsy cases. Am. J. Cardiol., 21:555, 1968.
17. Godwin, J. D., Axel, J., Adams, J. R., et al.: Computed tomography: A new method for diagnosing tumor of the heart. Circulation, 63:448, 1981.
18. Goyer, R. A., and Bowden, D. H.: Endocardial fibroelastosis associated with glycogen tumors of the heart and tuberous sclerosis. Am. Heart J., 64:539, 1962.
19. Grenadier, E., Lima, C. O., Barron, J. V., et al.: Two-dimensional echocardiography for evaluation of metastatic cardiac tumors in pediatric patients. Am. Heart J., 107:122, 1984.
20. Griffiths, G. D.: A review of primary tumors of the heart. Progr. Cardiovasc. Dis., 7:465, 1965.
21. Hanfling, S. M.: Metastatic cancer of the heart: Review of the literature and report of 127 cases. Circulation, 22:474, 1960.
22. Hankins, J. R., Satterfield, J. R., Aiser, S., Wiernik, P. M., and McLaughlin, J. S.: Pericardial window for malignant pericardial effusions. Ann. Thorac. Surg., 30:465, 1980.
23. Harvey, W. P.: Clinical aspects of cardiac tumors. Am. J. Cardiol., 21:328, 1968.
24. Hattler, B. G., Jr., Fuchs, J. C. A., Cosson, R., and Sabiston, D. C., Jr.: Atrial myxoma: An evaluation of clinical and laboratory manifestations. Ann. Thorac. Surg., 10:65, 1970.
25. Hildago, H., Korobkin, M., Breiman, R. S., and Kisslo, J. R.: CT of intracardiac tumor. Am. J. Radiol., 137:608, 1981.

26. Isner, J. M., Falcone, M. W., Virmani, R., and Roberts, W. C.: Cardiac sarcoma causing ASH and simulating coronary heart disease. Am. J. Med., 66:1025, 1979.

27. James, T. N., and Galakhov, I.: De Subitaneis Mortibus XXVI. Fatal electrical instability of the heart associated with benign congenital polycystic tumor of the atrioventricular node. Circulation, 56:667, 1977.

28. Kidder, L. A.: Congenital glycogenic tumors of the heart. Arch. Pathol. Lab. Med., 49:55, 1950.

29. Krikorian, J. C., and Hancock, E. W.: Pericardiocentesis. Am. J. Med., 65:808, 1978.

30. Larrieu, A. J., Jamieson, W. R. E., Tyers, G. F. O., et al: Primary cardiac tumors: Experience with 25 cases. J. Thorac. Cardiovasc. Surg., 83:339, 1982.

31. Magovern, G. J., Yusuf, M. F., Liebler, G. A., et al.: The surgical resection and chemotherapy of metastatic osteogenic sarcoma of the right ventricle. Ann. Thorac. Surg., 29:76, 1980.

32. Marx, G. R., Bierman, F. Z., Matthews, E., and Williams, R.: Two-dimensional echocardiographic diagnosis of intra-cardiac masses in infancy. J. Am. Coll. Cardiol., 3:827, 1984.

33. Maurer, E. R.: Successful removal of tumor of the heart. J. Thorac. Surg., 23:479, 1952.

34. McAllister, H. A., Jr., and Fenoglio, J. J.: Tumors of the cardiovascular system. In Atlas of Tumor Pathology, Fasc. 15, 2nd Series. Washington, D. C., Armed Forces Institute of Pathology, 1978.

35. Meller, J., Teichholz, L. E., Pichard, A. D., Matta, R., and Herman, M. V.: Left ventricular myxoma: Echocardiographic diagnosis and review of the literature. Am. J. Med., 63:816, 1977.

36. Miller, J. I., Mansour, K. A., and Hatcher, C. R.: Pericardiectomy: Current indications, concepts, and result in a university center. Ann. Thorac. Surg., 34:40, 1982.

37. Pitcher, D., Wainwright, R., Brennand-Roper, D., et al.: Cardiac tumors: Non-invasive detection and assessment by gated-blood pool radionuclide imaging. Br. Heart J., 44:143, 1980.

38. Poole, G. V., Jr., Meredith, J. W., Breyer, R. H., and Mills, S. A.: Surgical implications in malignant cardiac disease. Ann. Thorac. Surg., 36:484, 1983.

39. Prager, R. L., Dean, R., and Turner, B.: Surgical approach to intra-cardiac renal cell carcinoma. Ann. Thorac. Surg., 33:74, 1982.

40. Prichard, R. W.: Tumors of the heart: Review of the subject and report of one hundred and fifty cases. Arch. Pathol. 51:98, 1951.

41. Read, R. C., White, H. J., Murphy, M. L., Williams, D., Sun, C. N., and Flanagan, W. H.: The malignant potential of left atrial myxoma. J. Thorac. Cardiovasc. Surg., 68:857, 1974.

42. Reece, I. J., Cooley, D. A., Frazier, O. H., et al: Cardiac tumors: Clinical spectrum and prognosis of lesions other than classical benign myxoma in 20 patients. J. Thorac. Cardiovasc. Surg., 88:439, 1984.

43. Salcedo, E. E., Adams, K. V., Lever, H. M., and Gill, C. C.: Echocardiographic findings in 25 patients with left atrial myxoma. J. Am. Coll. Cardiol., 1:1162, 1983.

44. Salyer, W. R., Page, D. L., and Hutchins, G. M.: The development of cardiac myxomas and papillary endocardial lesions from mural thrombus. Am. Heart J., 89:4, 1975.

45. Schattenberg, T. T.: Echocardiographic diagnosis of left atrial myxoma. Mayo Clin. Proc., 43:620, 1968.

46. Semb, B. K. H.: Surgical considerations in the treatment of cardiac myxoma. J. Thorac. Cardiovasc. Surg., 87:251, 1984.

47. Shackell, M., Mitko, A., Williams, P. L., and Sutton, G. C.: Angiosarcoma of the heart. Br. Heart J., 41:498, 1979.

48. Silverman, N. A.: Primary cardiac tumors. Ann. Surg., 191:127, 1980.

49. Stark, R. M., Perloff, J. K., Glick, J. H., Hirshfield, J. W., Jr., and Devereux, R. B.: Clinical recognition and management of cardiac metastatic disease. Am. J. Med., 63:653, 1977.

50. Steiner, R. M., Bull, M. I., Kumpel, F., et al.: The diagnosis of intracardiac metastasis of colon carcinoma by radioisotopic and roentgenographic studies. Am. J. Cardiol., 26:300, 1970.

51. Sutton, M. G. St. J., Mercier, L-A., Giuliani, E. R., and Lie, J. T.: Atrial myxomas: A review of clinical experience in 40 patients. Mayo Clin. Proc., 55:371, 1980.

52. Terry, L. N., and Kilgerman, M. M.: Pericardial and myocardial involvement by lymphomas and leukemias: The role of radiotherapy. Cancer, 25:1003, 1970.

53. Williams, D. B., Danielson, G. K., McGoon, D. C., Feldt, R. H., and Edwards, W. D.: Cardiac fibroma: Long-term survival after excision. J. Thorac. Cardiovasc. Surg., 84:230, 1982.

54. Wold, L. E., and Lie, J. T.: Cardiac myxoma: A clinicopathologic profile. Am. J. Pathol., 101:219, 1980.

XIX

Cardiac Pacemakers

JAMES E. LOWE, M.D.
LAWRENCE D. GERMAN, M.D.

Although cardiac electrostimulation began in the mid-18th century with the use of currents from the Leyden jar or voltaic pile to stimulate cardiac muscle in animals and to attempt resuscitation of execution victims, the modern artificial cardiac pacemaker is a device largely perfected over the past 25 years.[17] It is clearly evident that the implantable pacemaker is one of the greatest contributions of modern medicine to the prolongation and improvement in human life. The exact number of individuals with an artificial pacemaker is unknown. However, estimates indicate that approximately 500,000 are living with pacemakers in this country and each year another 100,000 or more patients will require permanent pacemakers in the United States.[20] Approximately 1.5 to 2 million pacemakers have been implanted worldwide over the past 20 years.[4]

INDICATIONS FOR PACEMAKER THERAPY

The implantation of a permanent cardiac pacemaker commits the physician and patient to a lifetime of follow-up care as well as exposure to the possible complications of pacing. In the early 1960s, following the introduction of the completely implantable pacing system, the major indication for pacemaker therapy was complete heart block associated with presyncope or syncope. However, during the past several years indications for implantation of permanent pacemakers have changed. Although complete heart block remains a definite indication for pacing, the majority of permanent pacemakers are implanted in patients with the sick sinus syndrome. In many patients with this syndrome, there are coexisting conduction disturbances including atrioventricular (AV) block and/or fascicular block. When the decision is made that a patient is a candidate for a permanent pacemaker, the type and mode of the pacemaker most suitable for the patient must be determined. Factors involved in selecting an appropriate pacing system include the patient's age, general condition, underlying heart disease, and the characteristics of the dysrhythmia being treated. Oftentimes, particularly in older patients, a conventional ventricular inhibited demand pacemaker is adequate for daily activity. On the other hand, in young and active individuals, an atrial synchronized pacemaker allows a changing heart rate according to varying physiologic demands, such as with exercise. Dual-chamber pacing is also indicated in those who have demonstrated that the atrial component to cardiac filling is essential for adequate cardiac output. At present, the general trend is toward the use of more dual-chamber pacemakers with multiprogrammable capability so that various pacing parameters can be adjusted noninvasively over time as the patient's need for pacing changes.

As with temporary pacing, there are differing views regarding the indications for permanent cardiac pacing. Most, however, would agree with the indications for permanent pacing recently reported in detail by Chung and outlined in Table 1.[4]

Sick Sinus Syndrome and Brady-tachyarrhythmia Syndrome. Pharmacologic therapy alone is often ineffective in patients with the sick sinus syndrome and permanent pacing is indicated in those who remain symptomatic because of bradycardia. The most common manifestation of the sick sinus syndrome is marked sinus bradycardia associated with intermittent sinus arrest or sinoatrial block and episodes of AV junctional escape rhythm.[4] In more advanced forms of the sick sinus syndrome, chronic atrial fibrillation may develop and may be associated with a slow ventricular rate secondary to advanced AV block. An additional group of patients develop various atrial tachyarrhythmias in association with the sick sinus syndrome. These components of the sick sinus syndrome are referred to as the *brady-tachyarrhythmia syndrome*, which is a common end result of far advanced sick sinus syndrome.

In many patients, a ventricular inhibited demand pacemaker is adequate therapy. However, in those in whom the atrial contribution to cardiac output is essential, dual-chamber pacing should be utilized. Atrial arrhythmias can occasionally be suppressed by atrial pacing. In patients with the brady-tachyarrhythmia syndrome, one or more antiarrhythmic agents are frequently required in addition to permanent pacemaker therapy.[4]

Mobitz Type II Atrioventricular Block. It is generally recommended that permanent pacing is indicated for patients with Mobitz Type II AV block associated with a wide QRS complex, regardless of whether the patient is symp-

tomatic or not. It has been documented that Mobitz Type II AV block frequently leads to advanced AV block.[4]

Complete Atrioventricular Block. Before pacemaker therapy became clinically available, 50 per cent of those with complete heart block died within one year.[12] Complete heart block is frequently caused by sclerodegenerative disease of the cardiac skeleton or of the conduction system itself and is often preceded by the development of bifascicular blocks such as right bundle branch block with left or right axis deviation and left bundle branch block. Therefore, most would agree that complete AV block represents a definite indication for permanent cardiac pacing. In addition to sclerodegenerative disease, ischemic myocardial injury, infiltrative cardiomyopathies, Chagas' disease, trauma, and cardiac surgery represent other causes of acquired complete AV block. Permanent pacing is usually recommended for surgically induced complete heart block lasting more than one week following operation.[4] Generally, complete AV block associated with acute anterior wall myocardial infarction is irreversible and also will require permanent pacemaker implantation.[4] Conversely, complete atrioventricular block following a diaphragmatic myocardial infarction is usually reversible and may require only temporary pacing. In general, permanent pacing is recommended in all myocardial infarction patients when complete AV block persists more than 2 to 3 weeks.

Symptomatic Bilateral Bundle Branch Block. Bilateral bundle branch block includes both bifascicular and trifascicular blocks and usually signifies extensive conduction system pathology. When bilateral bundle branch block causes symptoms, there is often intermittent occurrence of bradyarrhythmias secondary to episodes of advanced or complete trifascicular block. Types of bilateral bundle branch block that may become symptomatic include right bundle branch block and left anterior or posterior hemiblock with or without first-degree AV block. Permanent pacing should be considered in symptomatic patients with bifascicular block with marked first-degree atrioventricular block manifested by a P–R interval of 280 msec. or greater or prolonged H–V intervals of 100 msec. or more. In those with documented episodes of complete AV block associated with incomplete bilateral bundle branch block, implantation of a permanent pacemaker should be an urgent consideration. The majority of this group can be treated with demand ventricular pacing. However, dual-chambered pacing is preferred in those in whom the atrial contribution to cardiac output is considered essential.

Bifascicular or Incomplete Trifascicular Block with Intermittent Complete Atrioventricular Block Following Acute Myocardial Infarction. Recent evidence suggests that the potential risk of sudden death within 6 months following acute myocardial infarction is increased in patients with bifascicular or incomplete trifascicular block associated with intermittent complete AV block during the peri-infarction period.[4] Therefore, it is now recommended that this group of patients be considered candidates for permanent pacemaker implantation prior to discharge from the hospital following their infarction.

Carotid Sinus Syncope. A permanent pacemaker may be indicated in patients with carotid sinus syncope or near syncope when a vasodepressor component can be excluded.

Recurrent Drug-Resistant Tachyarrhythmias Improved by Temporary Pacing. Occasional patients with tachyarrhythmias, particularly paroxysmal ventricular tachycardia, can be successfully managed by temporary pacing. In those who respond, permanent pacing techniques can be considered as part of their therapy. In view of the excellent surgical results obtained in patients with the Wolff-Parkin-

TABLE 1. *Indications for Permanent Pacing*

- Sick sinus syndrome and brady-tachyarrhythmia syndrome
- Mobitz Type II AV block (symptomatic)
- Complete AV block
- Symptomatic bilateral bundle branch block
- Bifascicular or incomplete trifascicular block with intermittent complete AV block following acute myocardial infarction
- Carotid sinus syncope (selected patients)
- Recurrent drug-resistant tachyarrhythmias improved by temporary pacing
- Intractable low cardiac output syndrome benefited by temporary pacing

son-White syndrome and ventricular tachycardia associated with left ventricular aneurysms and micro–re-entry, surgery should be considered as primary therapy.[17] However, in those who have ectopic arrhythmias not amenable to surgery, a variety of antitachycardia pacing techniques appear promising.[17]

Intractable Congestive Heart Failure and Cerebral or Renal Insufficiency Benefited by Temporary Pacing. As described earlier, the condition of occasional patients with refractory congestive heart failure and decreased perfusion causing cerebral or renal insufficiency may be improved by increasing the heart rate with temporary pacing. If temporary pacing is effective under these conditions and long-term therapy is indicated, permanent pacing should be considered.[4] The overwhelming majority of these patients require atrial contraction to improve cardiac output. Therefore, atrial pacing, atrial-synchronous pacing, or bifocal demand pacing is usually indicated in this select subgroup. The exact mode of pacing chosen depends on the presence or absence of underlying conduction disturbances.

PACEMAKER COMPONENTS

The Impulse Generator

An implantable cardiac pacemaker consists of an impulse generator, lead wire, and electrode (Fig. 1). The impulse generator itself contains a power source or battery, hybrid circuits, and a lead connector (Fig. 2). All of these components are housed in a hermetically sealed metal container. The size and weight of the impulse generator depend on the size of the battery and the number of electronic components. Impulse generators are usually housed in rectangular or oval packages with rounded edges and weigh between 32 and 135 gm.[24]

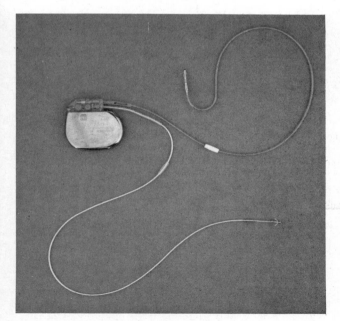

Figure 1. The modern implantable cardiac pacemaker consists of an impulse generator, lead wire, and electrode. A bipolar, dual-chambered impulse generator (Symbios 7006, Medtronic, Inc.) is shown connected to an atrial J tined lead (Medtronic, Inc., model 4512) and a ventricular tined lead (Medtronic, Inc., model 4002). Devices such as the system shown represent the current state of the art in pacemaker technology.

POWER SOURCES

The modern power cell or battery is composed of an anode, a cathode, and an electrolyte. The power cell is generally named for the materials used in the anode and cathode, for example, lithium-iodine. Current solid state cells have a dry, crystalline electrolyte between the anode and cathode. Electrical current is produced by ionization of the anode, which results in the migration of positively charged metallic ions through the electrolyte toward the cathode. Electrons are left behind on the anode, which becomes negatively charged relative to the cathode. When the anode and cathode are connected by a conductive pathway, a flow of electrons or electrical current passes from the anode to the cathode. The higher the resistance in the conductor, the slower the flow of electrons and the longer the power cell will last. In the modern lithium-iodine power cell, the migrating or positively charged lithium ions combine with iodine from the cathode to form a lithium-iodine electrolyte barrier.[25] The majority of currently available lithium powered pacemakers contain a single power cell, unlike the original mercury-zinc generators, which were powered by multiple-cell batteries.

PACEMAKER ELECTRONICS

The first implantable pacemakers contained individual or discrete components, including resistors, capacitors, diodes, transistors, reed switches, and wire coils for induction. These individual components were mounted on or between printed circuit boards. A major advance in pacemaker electronics has been the development of "hybrid" circuits. Hybrid technology allows all components of the circuit, including semiconductors, resistors, and capacitors, to be diffused into a substrate to produce a monolithic silicon chip. The major advantage of the single chip circuit is its small size. At present, custom, digital, silicon, large-scale integrated circuits are used in virtually all multiprogrammable pacemakers and may include as many as 40,000 transistors on a 4 mm.[2] wafer.[25] This technology combined with the improved lithium power source has allowed modern multiprogrammable pacemakers to be much smaller, lighter, and more reliable than earlier simpler pacemakers.

The lithium powered pacemaker containing a custom integrated circuit design is exceptionally reliable and capable of providing both multiprogrammable and physiologic pacing functions. However, its capacity for monitoring and data processing is limited.[25] Single-chip microcomputers are available, although high current drain and software limitations have prevented their widespread use in pacemakers. Future pacemakers will most likely utilize low-current-drain, custom microcomputers consisting of a central processing unit, a memory unit, and an input-output circuit.[1] Pacemakers containing microcomputers will be capable of monitoring a variety of physiologic changes to control on-line pacemaker function. Physiologic changes that may be monitorable include energy threshold needs and cardiac output requirements as determined by on-line measurement of pH and P_{O_2}.[17] Furthermore, future microcomputer-based pacemakers may be able to automatically select an appropriate pacing technique for the control of a variety of dysrhythmias.[17]

The Lead-Electrode

A pacemaker lead is an insulated wire used to connect the impulse generator to the heart. The electrode is the

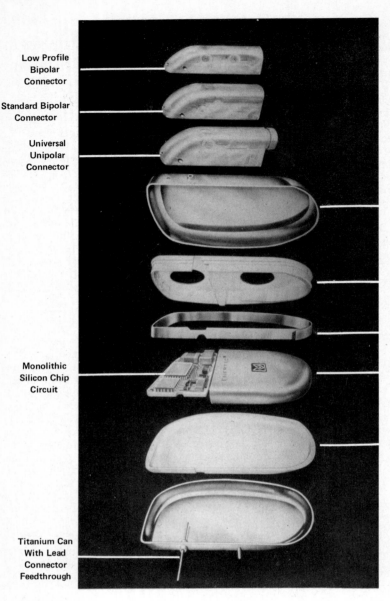

Low Profile
Bipolar
Connector

Standard Bipolar
Connector

Universal
Unipolar
Connector

Monolithic
Silicon Chip
Circuit

Titanium Can
With Lead
Connector
Feedthrough

Lead
Connector
Options

Titanium
Can

Polypropylene
Cup

Titanium
Weld Ring

Lithium Iodine
Battery

Polypropylene
Cup

Figure 2. Exploded view of a modern multiprogrammable impulse generator. As shown, a variety of lead connectors are available to accept a variety of epicardial and transvenous leads. The battery and pacemaker electronics are enclosed in a titanium metal case. Hybrid circuit technology allows all components of the circuit, including semiconductors, resistors, and capacitors, to be diffused into a substrate to produce what is called a monolithic silicon chip. As shown, the major advantage of the silicon chip circuit is its extremely small size. This technology, combined with the improved lithium power source, has allowed modern multiprogrammable pacemakers to be much smaller, lighter, and more reliable than earlier pacemakers. (Courtesy of Paul Craven, Joe Hitselberger, and Gene Boone, Medtronic, Inc.)

uninsulated, electrically active metal tip in contact with the myocardium (Fig. 1). The lead-electrode system in a demand pacemaker has two equally important functions in that (1) it carries the electrical stimulus from the impulse generator to the myocardium and (2) it transmits an endocardial electrogram from the heart to the pacemaker.[25] In unipolar systems, only the cathode is in the heart and the indifferent electrode, or anode, which is a part of the metallic pacemaker case, is in soft tissue. In a bipolar system, a double wire runs from the pacemaker to the heart, with the two electrodes being separated by approximately 1 cm. within the heart. The lead wire is most often a continuous helical coil or braided wire, which is resistant to fracture caused by repeated flexion. Carbon leads as well as multistrand leads made of combinations of metals such as nickel alloy and silver are under evaluation in Europe and in the United States. It is hoped that these new leads will offer improved flexibility and lower resistance, which will result in decreased energy consumption. In the recent past, the lead was most commonly insulated with silicone rubber. Recently, however, polyurethane in-

sulation has been introduced because of its greater elasticity and tensile strength, which allow lead diameter to be reduced with improved durability. Furthermore, polyurethane has a smoother surface, which improves handling characteristics during multilead placement and reduces the risk of venous thrombosis.

The uninsulated electrically active metal tip of the lead in contact with the myocardium is the electrode. This exposed tip is most commonly made of platinum, iridium, or nickel alloys. Platinum-iridium electrodes are the most common and may be porous or solid.

There are two general types of lead-electrode systems; the most common are those passed transvenously to embed within the subendocardium of the right atrium or right ventricle. The second group are those placed transthoracically, which are directly attached to the myocardium of any chamber. These leads have been referred to as epicardial leads, but this is a misnomer because they are actually embedded within the myocardium and not just the epicardium. Transthoracic leads are used primarily in small infants and children; after repeated failure of the transvenous approach; and when the chest is already open, such as following cardiac surgical procedures. Generally, transvenous lead-electrode systems are preferred because of their improved long-term thresholds and decreased incidence of electrode displacement and lead fracture.

Transvenous systems are termed *active* or *passive*. Passive leads have a small flanged expansion just proximal to the exposed distal electrode, or short, flexible tines (Fig. 3A). These tined leads are designed to catch beneath trabeculae and reduce the incidence of dislodgment, which should be less than 5 per cent.[6] Active leads are designed for insertion into large, smooth-walled ventricular cavities as well as for placement in the atrial appendage. Active leads contain barbs, hooks, jaws, arrowheads, or, most commonly, sharpened screws, which are remotely activated and retractable[25] (Fig. 3B). Polyurethane-coated tined leads are preferred for routine transvenous ventricular pacing and sharp corkscrew-type screw-in electrodes are recommended for placement in the right atrium or the right ventricle under adverse circumstances when the rate of dislodgment is increased. Leads designed primarily for placement in the atrial appendage via the transvenous route differ from ventricular leads in that, when the stylette is withdrawn, they assume a J shape, which allows them to be positioned well up into the atrial appendage (see Fig. 1).

As mentioned earlier, pacemaker lead-electrode systems are either bipolar or unipolar. Possible advantages of a unipolar system include a more simple connection, a decreased failure rate for both the pacemaker and electrode, slightly decreased energy requirements, lower risk of pacemaker-induced fibrillation, improved detection of sensing signals, and decreased risk of anodal corrosion.[25] Advantages of bipolar pacing include reduced risk of skeletal muscle stimulation, lower susceptibility to electromagnetic interference, elimination of pacemaker suppression by skeletal myopotentials, decreased risk of "cross-talk" between atrial and ventricular stimuli, and increased sensing selectivity.[25] The advantages and disadvantages of unipolar and bipolar pacing should be considered when selecting the most appropriate pacemaker for a given patient.

To a certain extent, decreasing the electrode tip size results in lower thresholds, both at the time of implantation as well as during continuous use. However, better sensing function is directly related to electrode area and is adversely affected by small electrode size.[11] Therefore, the typical electrode surface tip area should range from 12 to 20 mm.[2] to achieve a compromise between pacing and sensing efficiency.[25] It is hoped that porous-tipped electrodes will improve sensing function for a given size because the interstices will increase the sensing area without increasing overall electrode area size and subsequent stimulation energy requirements (Fig. 3A).

OPERATIVE TECHNIQUES

Implantation of a permanent impulse generator and lead-electrode system should be performed in an operating room equipped with a fluoroscopic unit or in a cardiac catheterization laboratory where sterile procedures can be performed. A variety of impulse generators and lead-electrodes as well as a pacing system analyzer should be readily available. Most commonly, the pacemaker lead-electrode is passed transvenously under local anesthesia to embed within the subendocardium of the right atrium or right ventricle. Transthoracic leads are used primarily in small infants and children, after repeated failure of the transvenous approach, and following cardiac surgery when a permanent pacemaker is indicated. In general, for elective permanent pacemakers, transvenous leads are preferred because of their improved long-term thresholds and decreased incidence of electrode displacement and lead fracture.

Preoperatively, patients receive a therapeutic dose of an antistaphylococcal antibiotic based on the proven beneficial effects of prophylactic antibiotic administration in general for thoracic surgical procedures. Antibiotics are discontinued 24 hours postoperatively. Regardless of the planned approach for implantation, the entire anterior chest from the chin to the umbilicus should be prepared and draped as a sterile field. This wide field of preparation allows conversion from one transvenous approach to another and permits a limited anterior thoracotomy to be performed without interruption of the procedure. Even when general anesthesia is not anticipated, an anesthesiol-

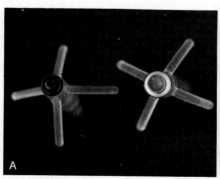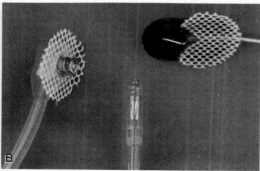

Figure 3. Types of pacemaker leads.

  A, Examples of transvenous passive leads. These tined leads are designed to catch beneath trabeculae and reduce the incidence of dislodgment. They can be used in both the right atrium and the right ventricle. Shown on the left is a tined lead with a polished platinum electrode tip (Medtronic, Inc., model 6971). Shown on the right is a platinum-iridium target tip electrode (Medtronic, Inc., model 4011). It appears that target tip electrodes have improved sensing function, since the interstices increase the sensing area without increasing overall electrode size and subsequent energy stimulation requirements for pacing.

  B, Active leads contain barbs, hooks, or screws. Shown on the left is a three-turn epicardial screw-in lead (Medtronic, Inc., model 6917). In the center, a transvenous endocardial screw-in lead is shown. The screw can be remotely activated or retracted. The lead is shown with the screw activated (Medtronic, Inc., model 6957). On the far right, an epicardial fishhook lead is shown (Medtronic, Inc., model 4951). We have found that the fishhook lead provides improved pacing and sensing thresholds in both the atrial and ventricular epicardial positions.

ogist should be available on a stand-by basis because of the potential for life-threatening dysrhythmias and the occasional necessity of anterior thoracotomy for either lead placement or cardiac tamponade due to perforation.

Based on the work of Langergren and Johansson[15] in Sweden and by Furman and Schwedel[7] and Chardak and associates[3] in the United States, the transvenous approach under local anesthesia is now used in over 90 per cent of patients requiring pacemakers. The venous anatomy of the anterior chest wall is particularly well suited for implantation of pacing leads (Fig. 4). Generally, the pacemaker pocket is placed over the anterior chest beneath the junction of the inner and middle thirds of the clavicle on the patient's nondominant side. The cephalic or subclavian veins are the preferred venous approaches for lead introduction. Implantation through the external or internal jugular veins requires a separate neck incision and the lead must be tunneled over or under the clavicle to reach the pacemaker pocket and generator. Passing the lead over the clavicle predisposes to skin erosion and tunneling beneath the clavicle increases the risk of hemorrhage from vascular injury.

An oblique incision on the anterior chest wall inferior to the deltopectoral groove provides excellent exposure to the cephalic vein and also allows introducer cannulation of the subclavian vein. The pacemaker pocket should be as far medial as is comfortable for the patient and made only slightly larger than the impulse generator so that the chance

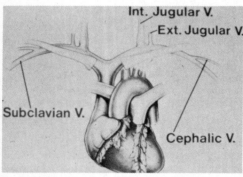

Figure 4. Anatomy for preferred venous approaches. Any vein in the neck, chest, or shoulder may be used for a permanent transvenous lead, but it is preferable to expose the vein through the same incision used for making the pocket. In order of preference, acceptable veins are as follows:

1. Cephalic vein, a tributary of the subclavian vein. It lies in the deltopectoral groove and is usually big enough to admit a lead up to 7 or 8 French. In 10 per cent of patients, it is quite delicate and may not be usable. It is occasionally absent.

2. Subclavian vein or tributary. If the cephalic vein cannot be used, it is always possible to expose another tributary of the subclavian or the subclavian vein itself through the same incision by freeing the pectoralis major from its lateral origin from the inferior surface of the clavicle. The subclavian vein is now commonly used as the primary choice for lead insertion with introducer techniques.

3. External jugular vein. This is usually the most prominent visible vein in the neck, although it may be absent in 10 per cent of patients. Because of the necessity of tunneling the electrode over or under the clavicle, with an increased incidence of fracture and erosion, this is a poor choice for permanent pacing.

4. Internal jugular vein. This is also a poor choice, except if there are purulent infections at every other potential site, or if an unusually large electrode is required as for an implantable defibrillator.

(From Parsonnet, V.: Implantation of Transvenous Pacemakers. Tarpon Springs, Fla., Tampa Tracings, 1972.)

of migration laterally, which tends to follow the curvature of the chest wall, is minimized. Small arterial and venous bleeders are ligated or electrocoagulated to avoid postoperative hematoma formation. The pacemaker generator packet should be just superficial to the pectoralis major in thick-chested individuals or beneath the premuscular fascia or muscle itself in thin-chested patients.

Following cannulation of the cephalic or subclavian vein, a gentle twisting motion is used to introduce the lead-electrode system into the right atrium. The guide wire is then exchanged for one with a J tip, which allows the lead to be passed across the tricuspid valve. The lead is then advanced across the pulmonary valve to confirm that the right ventricle has been cannulated and not the coronary sinus. The lead is then withdrawn into the cavity of the right ventricle and the curved guide wire is replaced with a straight wire. The lead is then gradually withdrawn until the electrode falls and points toward the apex of the right ventricle. The guide wire is then withdrawn a few millimeters and the lead is gently maneuvered to lodge the pacing and sensing electrode beneath right ventricular trabeculae. If a dual-chamber procedure is planned, ventricular lead placement is first accomplished, followed by placement of an atrial J lead, which is designed to lodge in the right atrial appendage. If stable positioning of an atrial J lead cannot be accomplished, an endocardial screw-in lead is placed into the wall of the right atrium. Following transvenous positioning and testing of thresholds, the lead is anchored at the fascial or venous exit site to prevent dislodgment. After testing of the impulse generator, the lead-electrode system is connected to the impulse generator, which is then positioned in its pocket. Finally, the wound is irrigated with a dilute bacitracin-saline solution and closed in layers using absorbable suture.

Permanent transthoracic leads can be placed through either a small left anterior thoracotomy or subxiphoid mediastinotomy. Generally, sutureless screw-in or hook leads are used and tunneled beneath the costal margin to the pacemaker pocket, which is created over the left upper quadrant of the abdomen well above the belt line or occasionally placed retroperitoneally in either lower quadrant in small infants (Fig. 5). The electrode is placed by opening the pericardium and identifying a fat-free area on the anterior, lateral, or posterior aspect of the left ventricle. The electrode should not be placed too close to the apex of the heart because of its thinness and because increased motion in this area may cause electrode dislodgment or lead fracture. Furthermore, the electrode should not be placed in myocardium adjacent to the pericardial course of the phrenic nerve; this can result in diaphragmatic pacing.

EVALUATION OF PACEMAKER FUNCTION

A thorough evaluation of pacing threshold energy requirements, atrial and ventricular endocardial electrograms, and impulse generator parameters should be performed at the time of initial pacemaker implantation as well as at the time of replacement.[17]

A pacing system analyzer provided by the pacemaker's manufacturer is capable of simulating the function of a given pacemaker's output and sensing circuits (Fig. 6) and is also capable of evaluating the integrity of the impulse generator itself. In addition, the pacing system analyzer is used to evaluate pacemaker rate, interval, pulse width, voltage, current, sensitivity, refractory period, and AV interval in dual-chamber devices.[17] After complete testing

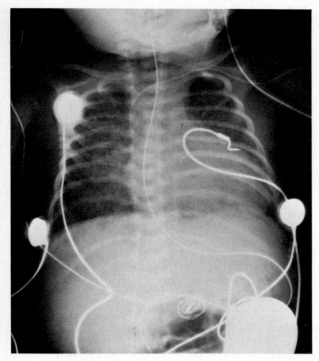

Figure 5. Chest film of a 36-hour-old infant born with congenital complete heart block. A fishhook lead-electrode (Medtronic, Inc., model 4951) was embedded over the lateral aspect of the left ventricle. The lead was then tunneled beneath the musculature of the anterior abdominal wall down to the left lower quadrant. A left lower quadrant incision was made, and the anterior abdominal wall musculature was split. The peritoneum was identified and swept down and medially in order to create a retroperitoneal pacemaker pocket. The lead was connected to a Pacesetter Programalith III unipolar impulse generator. The majority of children who require pacemakers will not require a retroperitoneal pocket in view of the small size of current impulse generators. However, in the extremely small infant, it is occasionally necessary to place the impulse generator in a retroperitoneal position. To our knowledge, this particular patient is the youngest ever to receive a permanent pacemaker.

sensitivity, refractory period, and AV interval in dual-chamber devices.[17] After complete testing of threshold energy requirements, atrial and ventricular endocardial signals, and pacemaker parameters, high-voltage settings are used to detect diaphragmatic or phrenic nerve stimulation, which will require lead repositioning. Deep breathing and coughing exercises are also performed to determine if electrode dislodgment can occur before securing the pacemaker leads and implanting the generator.

PHYSIOLOGICAL ASPECTS OF PACING

Pacing Modes

Perhaps the most dramatic example of the expansion of pacemaker technology is the number of variations in the way the heart can be paced. The way in which an impulse generator functions is referred to as the pacing mode. An accurate description of pacing mode must convey not only the chamber of the heart that is being paced, but also the chamber sensed by the pacemaker and the way in which the pacemaker responds to sensed activity. Simple descrip-

tive terms, such as ventricular demand pacemaker, sufficed well for single-chamber devices but have become more awkward as the complexity of pacemakers has increased. Devices that pace and sense both atrial and ventricular activity are now frequently implanted. To meet the need for a uniform method of describing pacemaker function, the Inter-society Commission for Heart Disease Resources (ICHD) recommended a three-letter code that succinctly and accurately describes various pacing modes[21] (Table 2).

The ICHD code uses the letters A and V for atrium and ventricle. The letter D stands for dual, indicating both chambers or, when indicating a mode of response, more than one mode. The two traditional response modes to sensed activity, either inhibition or initiation, are indicated by I and T. When there is no function or response possible, the letter O is used. In the three-letter code system, the first letter designates the chamber(s) paced, the second letter the chamber(s) sensed, and the third letter the mode of response of the pacemaker to sensed activity. Thus, a pacemaker that paces only the ventricle, senses ventricular activity when intrinsic beats are present, and responds to the sensed activity by inhibiting its output (the well-known ventricular demand pacemaker) is designated VVI. An asynchronous ventricular pacemaker that does not sense

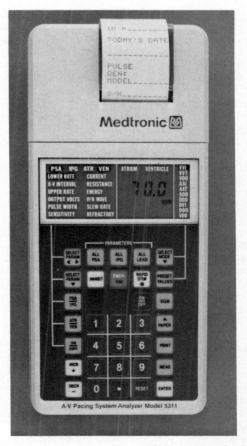

Figure 6. A pacing system analyzer (PSA) simulates the function of the pacemakers output and sensing circuits and is also capable of evaluating the integrity of the impulse generator itself. A thorough evaluation of pacing threshold energy requirements, atrial and ventricular endocardial electrograms, and impulse generator parameters should be made at the time of initial pacemaker implantation as well as at the time of generator or lead electrode replacement.

TABLE 2. Pacing Modes

Position	1 Chamber Paced	2 Chamber Sensed	3 Mode of Response	4 Programmability	5 Antitachycardia Features
	A—atrium V—ventricle D—dual	A—atrium V—ventricle O—none D—dual	I—inhibited T—triggered O—none D—dual* R—reverse	P—programmable M—multiprogrammable O—nonprogrammable	B—burst S—scanning extrastimulus E—externally triggered N—normal rate competition O—none

*Atrial triggered, ventricular inhibited.

but paces at a constant rate regardless of intrinsic cardiac rhythm would be designated VOO (the ventricle is paced, neither chamber is sensed, and there is therefore no response mode to sensed events). In the case of the standard AV sequential pacemaker in which both atrium and ventricle are paced, but only ventricular activity is sensed, the designation is DVI. The letter R in the third position stands for reverse, and denotes a mode of response in which pacemaker function is initiated in response to a rapid intrinsic rate and is inhibited at slower rates. This is an antitachycardia feature, which will be more commonly used in future devices.

The three-letter ICHD code has a tremendous advantage in describing not only a certain pacemaker, but also a variety of possible modes of function incorporated into a single programmable pacemaker. The magnet mode of a pacemaker may also be described. This is the test mode in which a pacemaker functions when the internal reed switch is closed by the external application of a strong magnet. Thus, a VVI pacemaker will generally function in the VOO (asynchronous) mode when an external magnet is applied. Likewise, a sophisticated DDD pacemaker may be programmed to function in one of many modes, including DVI, VVI, AAI, AOO, and VDD.

With the advent of multiprogrammability, defined as the ability to noninvasively change three or more pacing parameters, and the addition of antitachycardia features to implantable pacemakers, a revision of the three-letter ICHD code was introduced.[22] This system adds a fourth and fifth letter to denote programmability and antitachycardia capabilities, respectively (Table 2). In this system, the letter P in the fourth position indicates the ability to program one or two parameters, and the letter M denotes multiprogrammability. An O in the fourth position would indicate a nonprogrammable pacemaker. In the fifth position, a variety of antitachycardia functions may be indicated, including B for burst, N for normal rate competition, S for scanning, and E for external triggering.

Programmability

Programmability is defined as the ability to permanently and noninvasively change one or more of the operating characteristics of an implanted pacemaker. The advantages of being able to modify pacemaker function following implantation have long been apparent. Early devices were made with the capability of changing rate by means of a transcutaneous needle that turned a potentiometer in the pacemaker. Noninvasive programming was originally made possible through the use of an external magnet that activated a switch inside the pacemaker, changing its rate in incremental steps.

Today, virtually all pacemakers implanted have at least one programmable function. The utility of programmability

in terms of avoiding reoperation for pacing system malfunction and of improving patient tolerance of the pacemaker has been documented and there are essentially no indications for the implantation of nonprogrammable pacemakers. Simple programmability usually includes the capacity to change rate, pulse width, mode (usually from inhibited to asynchronous), and refractory period. The ability to change many parameters is referred to as *multiprogrammability*.

COMPLICATIONS

Complications of pacemakers can be divided into four categories: (1) immediate surgical complications, (2) wound problems, (3) delayed complications, and (4) pacemaker malfunctions (Table 3). Fortunately, these complications are relatively uncommon, making pacemaker insertion an exceptionally safe procedure when performed properly.

Immediate Surgical Complications

Perhaps the safest way of inserting a permanent transvenous lead-electrode system is via the cephalic vein. The risk of pneumothorax, vascular injury, air embolism, and air entrapment within the pacing pocket are increased when the subclavian vein access route is chosen. Air entrapment

TABLE 3. Pacemaker Complications

Immediate Surgical Complications	Delayed Complications
Pneumothorax	Venous thrombosis
Vascular injury	Pulmonary embolism
Air embolism	Twiddler's syndrome
Cardiac perforation	Constrictive pericarditis
Tamponade	Tricuspid insufficiency
Lead-electrode dislodgment	Pacemaker syndrome
Neural injury—phrenic, recurrent laryngeal	
Air entrapment in pocket	

Wound Problems	Pacemaker Malfunctions
Hematoma	Radiation damage
Infection	Runaway pacemaker
Skin erosion	Pacemaker-induced
Migration of impulse generator	ventricular fibrillation
Skeletal muscle stimulation	Irregular pacing
	Failure of sensing
	Failure of capture
	Electrode fracture
	Knotting of lead
	Inhibition of pacemaker by skeletal myopotentials
	Electromagnetic interference

within the pacemaker pocket (caused by pneumothorax with subcutaneous emphysema or air entrapped during pacemaker pocket closure) can result in pacemaker failure in unipolar systems due to insulation of the unipolar anodal plate (indifferent electrode) from the subcutaneous tissue.[10, 14, 16] Neural injury to both the phrenic and the recurrent laryngeal nerves has been reported when the lead-electrode system is introduced through the internal jugular vein.[5] Regardless of the venous access route chosen, cardiac perforation can occur but fortunately only rarely leads to hemopericardium and tamponade. A final complication is immediate electrode dislodgment. The risk of this complication can be reduced by performing provocative maneuvers at the time of initial implantation, such as coughing and deep breathing. Interestingly, transvenous electrode dislodgment problems have not been significantly increased in patients with congenitally corrected transposition of the great vessels, although this would have been expected because of the decreased trabeculation of the embryologic left ventricle, which is where the pacing lead lies.

Wound Problems

Perhaps the most common wound problem associated with permanent pacemaker implantation is a hematoma. This complication is preventable with strict attention to hemostasis during operation. In patients who require impulse generator change, the pacemaker pocket should be debrided of excess pseudocapsule to prevent the formation of a sterile seroma. Fortunately, wound infection is a rare problem and can be prevented by meticulous operative technique and the appropriate use of prophylactic antibiotics. In general, however, when infection occurs, the entire pacing system (including the impulse generator and lead-electrode system) should be removed, the patient should be treated with appropriate intravenous antibiotics, and a temporary pacemaker should be used for an interim period. When infection has cleared completely, a new pacemaker system should be implanted via another access site. Skin erosion by either the impulse generator or lead can be prevented by proper positioning of pacemaker hardware deep within the subcutaneous tissues or beneath the fascia of the pectoralis major muscle itself. It should be noted that unipolar impulse generators can cause muscle stimulation if placed immediately adjacent to skeletal muscle. However, bipolar impulse generators can be placed in the subcutaneous tissue or beneath muscle. Migration of the impulse generator most commonly occurs in infraclavicular pacemaker pockets. Migration tends to follow the curvature of the chest wall and the impulse generator tends to migrate laterally. This can be prevented by creating an anterior-medial pocket just large enough to house the impulse generator and lead. In susceptible individuals, the impulse generator can be further secured to the chest wall to prevent migration.

Delayed Complications

Unusual delayed complications are uncommon and those associated with transvenous pacemakers include thrombosis of the superior vena cava with resultant superior vena caval syndrome, axillary vein thrombosis with upper extremity edema, cerebral venous sinus thrombosis, and right atrial and right ventricular thrombosis.[2, 9] Pulmonary thromboembolism has also been recognized as a rare but lethal complication, most often occurring in those with low cardiac output and underlying right atrial or right ventricular thrombi.[13] Constrictive pericarditis has been reported in patients who have received both transvenous and transthoracic electrodes. Tricuspid insufficiency is rare, is usually asymptomatic, and is caused by either lead placement or lead removal.[8, 19] Electrode dislodgment and lead fracture can result from unconscious or habitual "twiddling" of the impulse generator (Fig. 7). Twiddler's syndrome has been reported most commonly in patients with transvenous pacing systems but has also been noted in those with transmediastinal pacing systems.[23] Finally, several reports have suggested that permanent pacemaker implantation with the impulse generator lying over the infraclavicular area is associated with an increased risk of breast carcinoma in female patients. However, based on information recently reported by Magilligan and Isshak, the appearance of breast cancer in women with pacemakers is probably coincidental and not related to materials, electrochemical stimulation, or chronic trauma.[18]

Pacemaker Malfunctions

Improvements in biomedical engineering have led to exceptionally durable and reliable permanent pacemakers. However, random failures still occur and underscore the necessity of appropriate long-term patient follow-up. Pacemaker malfunctions are secondary to alterations of the preset pacing rate (acceleration or slowing), irregular pacing, failure of sensing, failure of cardiac capture or depolarization, and various combinations of these events.

Sudden acceleration of pacing rate has been referred

Figure 7. Abdominal films. A, Film one year after initial implant shows normal relationship between wires and impulse generator. B, Film two years later shows rotation of impulse generator 180 degrees and that wires close to generator are twisted. C, Six months after implantation of new impulse generator, additional twisting is evident.

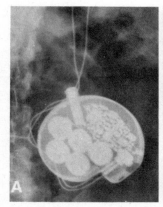
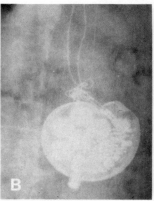
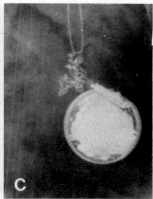

to as *runaway pacemaker*. Runaway pacemaker results in pacemaker-induced ventricular tachycardia. This complication was most often a manifestation of malfunction of fixed rate devices. Fortunately, the runaway pacemaker has been rarely encountered, because demand ventricular pacemakers have gradually replaced fixed rate models. In the far advanced runaway pacemaker syndrome, ventricular fibrillation may occur and lead to sudden death. The runaway pacemaker is a medical emergency that should be treated by immediate replacement with a new impulse generator.

Slowing of the pacing rate is a much more common manifestation of pacemaker malfunction in modern demand impulse generators. Irregular pacing usually indicates an advanced form of malfunction and may be associated with acceleration or slowing of the pacing rate. Failure of sensing can occur as an isolated finding but is commonly associated with failure of cardiac capture. Failure of sensing (when the sensing circuit does not work properly) causes a demand unit to function as a fixed rate pacemaker. Failure of cardiac capture may be complete but is usually intermittent. The most common cause of failure of capture is malposition of the pacemaker electrode or lead fracture. Electrode displacement may be observed at any time but most often occurs within the first month following implantation.[4] Late causes of failure of capture include fibrosis around the pacemaker electrode, advancement of underlying heart disease, severe hyperkalemia or hypokalemia, and drug toxicity, especially with quinidine and procainamide.[4] If none of the above factors is present, the pacemaker impulse generator is most likely malfunctioning.

Ventricular fibrillation can occur during insertion, especially when ventricular fibrillation thresholds are low, such as in those with acute myocardial infarction. Ventricular fibrillation is uncommon today because the R on T phenomenon should not occur in a properly functioning demand pacemaker.

Inhibition of demand pacemakers by musculoskeletal potentials is always a possibility when unipolar pacing systems are utilized. Inhibition of bipolar demand pacemakers by noncardiac muscle potentials, however, is a relatively uncommon phenomenon. Transient inhibition of unipolar pacemakers may also result from active contraction of the diaphragm, such as that created by deep inspiration, straining, and coughing.

Previously, it was thought that ionizing radiation did not have any adverse affect on the function of impulse generators. Recent reports, however, suggest that ionizing radiation can result in malfunction of new-generation programmable pacemakers. There appears to be no deleterious effect from diagnostic x-ray exposure, but radiation for therapeutic purposes can cause permanent malfunction of susceptible programmable devices. The mode of failure cannot be predicted.

The demand pacemaker is much less likely to create ventricular fibrillation than is the fixed rate pacemaker, but it is more susceptible to interference by various electromagnetic sources, including commercial radar, defribrillators, microwave ovens, electrocautery, electrical motors, and malfunctioning television sets.

Recently, a complex of symptoms caused by pacemaker insertion has been recognized. This syndrome has been referred to as the *pacemaker syndrome* and is characterized by vertigo, light-headedness, syncope, and hypotension occurring after implantation of a ventricular pacemaker. The cause has been attributed to a decrease in cardiac output occurring during ventricular pacing due to loss of the atrial contribution to ventricular end-diastolic volume. Pacemaker syndrome is most likely to occur in patients who require the atrial contribution to cardiac output. Usually, the symptoms can be relieved by placement of a dual-chamber pacing system, which allows for more physiologic pacing if lowering the demand pacing rate is ineffectual.

SELECTED REFERENCES

Chung, E. K. (Ed.): Artificial Cardiac Pacing: Practical Approach, 2nd ed. Baltimore, Williams & Wilkins, 1984.
The pathophysiology of conduction system disorders and the indications and techniques of cardiac pacing are discussed in detail in this excellent text. Each section is concise and well written, and an outstanding number of references are provided at the end of each chapter.

Lowe, J. E., and German, L. D.: Cardiac pacemakers. *In* Sabiston, D. C., Jr. (Ed.): Textbook of Surgery, 13th ed. Philadelphia, W. B. Saunders Company , 1986.
An extensive overview of cardiac pacemaker therapy is provided in this review. The history of cardiac pacing, indications for temporary and permanent pacing, insertion techniques, and the physiology of pacing are reviewed in detail. A total of 130 references are provided.

Parsonnet, V., Furman, S., Smyth, N. P., and Bilitch, M.: Optimal resources for implantable cardiac pacemakers: Pacemaker study group of the Inter-society Commission for Heart Disease Resources. Circulation, 68:226A, 1983.
The first section of this report describes the types of pacemakers currently available, how they function, and how they can be modified through noninvasive programming. Recommendations are then given for a modified and updated version of the widely accepted ICHD code for identification of pacing modes. The final section of this report summarizes the role of physicians, pacemaker manufacturers, and the FDA in the area of complex dual-chamber, multiprogrammable pacemakers.

Tyers, G. F. O., and Brownlee, R. R.: Power pulse generators, electrodes, and longevity. Prog. Cardiovasc. Dis., 23:421, 1981.
This comprehensive review details the development of pacemaker power sources and the relative merits of different power cells available. Electrode selection, programmability, and dual-chambered modes of pacing are also discussed in detail. Pacemaker electronics and power cell chemistry are thoroughly reviewed and explained in nontechnical terms.

REFERENCES

1. Barold, S. S., and Mugica, J.: The Third Decade of Cardiac Pacing: Advances in Technology and Clinical Applications. Mount Kisco, N. Y., Futura, 1982.
2. Branson, J. A.: Radiology of cardiac pacemakers and their complications with three cases of superior vena caval obstruction. Australas. Radiol., 22:125, 1978.
3. Chardak, W. M., Gage, A. A., Federico, A. J., et al.: Five years' clinical experience with an implanted pacemaker. An appraisal. Surgery, 58:915, 1965.
4. Chung, E. K.: Artificial Cardiac Pacing: Practical Approach, 2nd ed. Baltimore, Williams & Wilkins, 1984.
5. Dieter, R. A., Jr., Asselmeier, G. H., Hamouda, F., Kuzycz, G. B., and McCray, R. M.: Neural complications of transvenous pacemaker implantation: Hoarseness and diaphragmatic paralysis: Case Reports. Milit. Med., 146:647, 1981.
6. Furman, S., Pannizzo, F., and Campo, I.: Comparison of active and passive leads for endocardial pacing—II. P.A.C.E., 4:78, 1981.
7. Furman, S., and Schwedel, J. B.: An intracardiac pacemaker for Stokes-Adams seizures. N. Engl. J. Med., 261:943, 1959.
8. Gibson, T. C., Davidson, R. C., and DeSilvey, D. L.: Presumptive tricuspid valve malfunction induced by a pacemaker lead: A case report and review of the literature. P.A.C.E., 3:88, 1980.
9. Girard, D. E., Reuler, J. B., Mayer, B. S., Nardone, D. A., and Jendrzejewski, J.: Cerebral venous sinus thrombosis due to indwelling transvenous pacemaker catheter. Arch. Neurol., 37:113, 1980.
10. Hearne, S. F., and Maloney, J. D.: Pacemaker system failure secondary to air entrapment within the pulse generator pocket: A complication of subclavian venipuncture for lead placement. Chest, 82:651, 1982.
11. Hughes, H. C., Jr., Brownlee, R. R., and Tyers, G. F.: Failure of demand pacing with small surface area electrodes. Circulation, 54:128, 1976.
12. Johansson, B. W.: Longevity in complete heart block. Ann. N.Y. Acad. Sci., 167:1031, 1969.

13. Kinney, E. L., Allen, R. P., Weidner, W. A., Pierce, W. S., Leaman, D. M., and Zelis, R. F.: Recurrent pulmonary emboli secondary to right atrial thrombus around a permanent pacing catheter: A case report and review of the literature. P.A.C.E., 2:196, 1979.

14. Kreis, D. J., Jr., Licalzi, L., and Shaw, R. K.: Air entrapment as a cause of transient cardiac pacemaker malfunction. P.A.C.E., 2:641, 1979.

15. Lagergren, H., and Johansson, L.: Intracardiac stimulation for complete heart block. Acta Chir. Scand., 125:562, 1963.

16. Lasala, A. F., Fieldman, A., Diana, D. J., and Humphrey, C. B.: Gas pocket causing pacemaker malfunction. P.A.C.E., 2:183, 1979.

17. Lowe, J. E., and German, L. D.: Cardiac pacemakers. In Sabiston, D. C., Jr. (Ed.): Textbook of Surgery, 13th ed. Philadelphia, W. B. Saunders Company, 1986.

18. Magilligan, D. J., Jr., and Isshak, G.: Carcinoma of the breast in a pacemaker pocket. Simple recurrence or oncotaxis? P.A.C.E., 3:220, 1980.

19. Ong, L. S., Barold, S. S., Craver, W. L., Falkoff, M. D., and Heinle, R. A.: Partial avulsion of the tricuspid valve by tined pacing electrode. Am. Heart J., 102:798, 1981.

20. Parsonnet, V., Bernstein, A. D., and Norman, J. C.: Dual-chamber pacing for cardiac arrhythmias: Controversies in cloning the conduction system. Tex. Heart Inst. J., 11:208, 1984.

21. Parsonnet, V., Furman, S., and Smyth, N. P. D.: Implantable cardiac pacemakers status report and resource guideline. Circulation, 50:A21, 1974.

22. Parsonnet, V., Furman, S., Smyth, N. P., and Bilitch, M.: Optimal resources for implantable cardiac pacemakers: Pacemaker study group of the Inter-society Commission for Heart Disease Resources. Circulation, 68:226A, 1983.

23. Rodan, B. A., Lowe, J. E., and Chen, J. T. T.: Abdominal twiddler's syndrome. Am. J. Roentgenol., 131:1084, 1978.

24. Samet, P., and El-Sherif, N.: Cardiac Pacing, 2nd ed. New York, Grune & Stratton, 1980, pp. 631–643.

25. Tyers, G. F. O., and Brownlee, R. R.: Power pulse generators, electrodes, and longevity. Prog. Cardiovasc. Dis., 23:421, 1981.

XX

Management of the Surgical Patient with Cardiac Disease

T. BRUCE FERGUSON, JR., M.D.
DAVID C. SABISTON, JR., M.D.

Patients with a history of significant cardiac disease who are undergoing surgical procedures require careful preoperative preparation and close surveillance during and after operation. Their management is based on a thorough understanding of physiologic principles and pharmacologic interventions to maintain cardiovascular homeostasis. Clinical pharmacology has progressed to the point that specific drugs can now alter virtually any parameter of cardiac physiology. This chapter concerns the pharmacology of the cardiovascular system in the perioperative surgical patient.

CLINICAL PHYSIOLOGY

Postoperative cardiac performance is assessed by (1) evaluation of *clinical signs*, including peripheral pulses, capillary refill, and skin temperature; (2) *hemodynamic measurements*, including central venous, systemic, and pulmonary arterial pressures; and (3) *measurement of cardiac output*.[2] A cardiac index (stroke volume times heart rate divided by body surface area) of 2 liters per minute per m.[2] is considered adequate.[8] Based on these measurements, the following determinants of cardiac function are controlled to optimize cardiac performance: heart rate, afterload, preload, and contractility.[7]

Afterload is the impedance to ventricular emptying that results from increasing arteriolar resistance. In the postoperative patient, this is most often due to hypertension. A greater afterload increases the work of the heart, and thus myocardial oxygen consumption, during the critical period during and following operations.

Preload is the volume of blood available to fill the ventricles during diastole. On the basis of the Frank-Starling relationship, preload determines cardiac performance at the myocardial level on a beat-to-beat basis. The status of the peripheral venous capacitance and pulmonary arterial systems plays a major role in determining preload.

Contractility describes the vigor with which the heart contracts during each beat. It is largely determined by the level of endogenous or exogenous catecholamines acting on the cardiovascular system. The contractile state of the heart can be increased only with a concomitant increase in myocardial oxygen consumption.

Autonomic receptors on the heart, lungs, kidneys, and vascular smooth muscle are classified as alpha (or excitatory) and beta (or inhibitory) according to their response to catecholamine stimulation.[9] The vessels that create arteriolar resistance (afterload) and venous capacitance (preload) contain alpha- and beta-receptors, as do myocardial (contractility) and conduction (heart rate) tissues in the heart. Specific agonist and antagonist drugs can alter all four aspects of myocardial function by interaction at these vascular receptor sites (Table 1).

THE PERIPHERAL CARDIOVASCULAR SYSTEM

In the perioperative patient, it is useful to group the venous and arteriolar vascular beds, the lungs, and the kidneys as one system involved in the regulation of intravascular volume. Pharmacologic agents that affect the peripheral cardiovascular system are listed in Table 2.

TABLE 1. Receptor Pharmacology of the Cardiovascular System

Effector Organ	Receptor Type	Agonist	Antagonist

Cardiac
  Conduction
  Myocardium
	Beta-1
	  Heart rate
	  Contractility
		Isoproterenol
		Epinephrine
		Dopamine
		Dobutamine
		Norepinephrine
			Propranolol
			Atenolol
			Metaprolol
			Esmolol

Arterioles	Alpha-1, alpha-2 (vasoconstrictor)	Norepinephrine Epinephrine Dopamine Phenylephrine	Prazocin Phentolamine
	Beta-2 (vasodilator)	Isoproterenol Dopamine Dobutamine Epinephrine	Propranolol
Pulmonary	Beta-2 (bronchodilator)	Terbutaline Metaproterenol Isoproterenol Epinephrine	Propranolol
Renal	Dopaminergic (vasodilator)	Dopamine	

Vasodilating Agents[3, 4]

Peripheral vasodilator agents are used perioperatively to control hypertension and to optimize cardiac performance by altering afterload and preload.

Sodium nitroprusside is given intravenously; a hemodynamic response is noted rapidly following administration or termination of the drug. It acts on both the arteriolar and venous systems, augmenting stroke volume by increasing preload and decreasing afterload by alpha-blockade at the arteriolar level. It is metabolized to thiocyanate, which can be toxic at high levels.

Chlorpromazine, a phenothiazine, is a quick-acting (within 15 minutes) vasodilator useful in the treatment of acute postoperative hypertension. Its action is due to a combination of central and peripheral alpha-blockade effects.

Hydralazine is a fast-acting agent that causes arteriolar and venous dilatation in 15 to 30 minutes following intramuscular (IM) or intravenous (IV) administration. It is also thought to have a positive inotropic effect, causing a significant increase in cardiac output with a relatively small drop in filling pressure. It causes a reflex tachycardia, which may be harmful.

Prazocin is a direct antagonist of the vascular alpha-1 receptor. It dilates both the arteriolar and the venous peripheral systems and is useful in weaning patients from nitroprusside.

Phentolamine temporarily blocks both alpha-1 and alpha-2 receptors and is used as an arteriolar vasodilator. Its primary indications are for hypertensive crises and during anesthesia for pheochromocytoma surgery.

Nitrates are antianginal agents, and in addition have systemic vasodilating properties. A major effect is pulmonary vasodilatation, and thus they are useful in patients with pulmonary congestion.

Vasoconstrictive Agents[16]

Phenylephrine is a rapid-acting arteriolar and venous vasoconstrictor. This effect is mediated by alpha-1 stimulation. It is used primarily to increase peripheral vascular resistance in postoperative cardiac patients.

Angiotensin II Inhibitors[17]

Captopril inhibits the formation of angiotensin II, a potent vasoconstrictor. Used as an afterload reducing agent in the treatment of heart failure, it has been shown to increase myocardial oxygen demand to a lesser degree than either prazocin or hydralazine. It has been successfully used to control hypertension in postoperative coronary bypass patients with residual myocardial dysfunction, acting to increase forward cardiac output with minimal increase in oxygen demand.

Diuretics[1]

In the postoperative patient, diuretics are used to decrease total body water, thereby acting to decrease preload.

Furosemide is a rapid-acting loop diuretic, with an effect lasting 2 to 3 hours following intravenous injection. Its action is kaliuretic, and potassium must be rigorously replaced in the postoperative patient to prevent arrhythmias. Following cardiac surgical procedures, it is used to remove excess fluid accumulated as a result of cardiopulmonary bypass. It is also a pulmonary vasodilator and is effective in acute pulmonary edema.

Ethacrynic acid is also a loop agent, usually reserved for patients not responding to initial diuretic therapy.

Metolazone is an oral thiazide diuretic, given in combination with intravenous loop agents to stimulate diuresis in patients developing acute renal failure postoperatively.

Pulmonary Bronchodilators[15]

Because the pulmonary vasculature is innervated with alpha- and beta-adrenoreceptors, agents used to treat bronchoconstriction in the immediate postoperative period can have significant cardiac effects.

Metaproterenol is a beta-2 agonist bronchodilator used as an aerosolized inhaler for bronchial constriction (wheezing). Cardiovascular side effects including tachycardia can be minimized by adjusting the dosage.

Aminophylline is an intravenous xanthine dilator and

TABLE 2. Pharmacologic Agents That Affect the
Cardiovascular System

The Peripheral Cardiovascular System
A. Vasodilator agents
  1. Sodium nitroprusside
  2. Chlorpromazine
  3. Hydralazine
  4. Prazocin
  5. Phentolamine
  6. Nitrates
B. Vasoconstrictor agents
  Phenylephrine
C. Angiotensin II inhibitors
  Captopril
D. Diuretics
  1. Furosemide
  2. Ethacrynic acid
  3. Metolazone
E. Pulmonary bronchodilators
  1. Metaproterenol
  2. Aminophylline

The Central Cardiovascular System
A. Vascular component
  1. Nitrates
  2. Beta-adrenergic receptor blocking agents
  3. Calcium channel-blocking agents
B. Functional component
  1. Cardiac glycosides
  2. Adrenoreceptor agonists
    a. Dopamine
    b. Dobutamine
    c. Isoproterenol
    d. Epinephrine
    e. Norepinephrine
  3. Calcium chloride or gluconate
  4. Cardiac assist device: intra-aortic balloon pump
C. Electrophysiologic aspects
  1. Supraventricular arrhythmias
    a. Bradycardia
      (1) Atropine
      (2) Isoproterenol
      (3) Temporary pacing
    b. Sinus tachycardia
      (1) Propranolol
      (2) Neostigmine
    c. Atrial fibrillation/flutter
      (1) Digoxin
      (2) Propranolol
      (3) Verapamil
      (4) Procainamide
      (5) Quinidine
  2. Ventricular arrhythmias
    Ventricular premature complexes, tachycardia
      (1) Lidocaine
      (2) Bretylium
      (3) Quinidine
      (4) Procainamide

the drug for initial treatment of significant postoperative bronchoconstriction. Cardiac side effects include tachycardia, decreased coronary blood flow, and increased myocardial oxygen extraction.

THE CENTRAL CARDIOVASCULAR SYSTEM

The heart itself constitutes the central cardiovascular system, which can be separated into vascular, functional, and electrophysiologic components. Optimal care of surgical patients requires knowledge of the multiple pharmacologic agents that affect each component (Table 2).

Vascular Component

Myocardial ischemia results when oxygen demand exceeds oxygen supply, usually because of limitations of coronary blood flow. Surgical procedures constitute a significant stress in patients with cardiac disease, and proper management of antianginal medication is essential. Most patients undergoing coronary artery bypass graft (CABG) procedures have been maintained on a combination of nitrates, beta-blockers, and calcium antagonists.

Nitrates. *Nitroglycerin* causes relaxation of all types of smooth muscle of the vascular system. Relief of angina with nitroglycerin results from decreased wall tension due to decreased ventricular volume (preload) and intraventricular pressure. This results in a decreased myocardial oxygen requirement. Patients with coronary disease should be maintained on intravenous nitroglycerin during the perioperative period for control of angina.

Beta-Adrenergic Receptor Blocking Agents.[12] *Beta-antagonists* block the principal beta-receptor site on the heart. Diminished heart rate, blood pressure, and contractility, together with an increased diastolic perfusion time, are the result, all of which decrease myocardial oxygen requirements. Rebound effects from abrupt withdrawal of the drug should be avoided.

Calcium-Channel Blocking Agents.[6] *Nifedipine, verapamil,* and *diltiazem* inhibit the slow inward current, are potent coronary vasodilators, and diminish myocardial oxygen consumption. Nifedipine is the drug of choice for vasospastic angina.

Functional Component

Myocardial contractility can be altered in the perioperative period by two types of agents, the *digitalis glycosides* and *beta-1 receptor agonists*.

Cardiac Glycosides.[13] Digitalis is the only oral inotropic drug available for routine use. The inhibition of the Na/K ATPase pump at the sarcolemmal level is thought to increase cytosolic calcium concentration and thereby increase the contractile state. Maintenance of postoperative therapeutic drug levels is important for patients with cardiac disease undergoing noncardiac surgery.

Adrenoreceptor Agonists.[11, 14] Across the pharmacologic spectrum, the sympathomimetic amines directly affect all four adrenoreceptor sites. These agents should be used only when it becomes necessary to support the failing circulation, because they uniformly increase myocardial oxygen consumption.

Dopamine is a catecholamine agent with a broad action spectrum. In low doses, it acts on beta-1 receptors of the heart producing positive chronotropic and inotropic responses. At medium doses beta-2 receptors in the periphery are stimulated, producing vasodilatation, but with high doses vasoconstriction occurs, with stimulation of peripheral alpha-1 receptors. At low doses, specific dopamine receptors in the renal vascular bed are stimulated to increase renal blood flow and diuresis.

Dobutamine is a synthetic analog of dopamine and produces a relatively stronger inotropic than chronotropic response. Conversion from dopamine to dobutamine may circumvent dopamine-induced tachycardia.

Isoproterenol acts on the cardiac beta-1 and peripheral beta-2 receptors, causing vasodilatation, tachycardia, and increased contractile force. However, myocardial oxygen consumption *increases* out of proportion to the increase in contractility, limiting the drug's effectiveness. It is used for right-sided heart failure and for the drug's chronotropic effect in patients with sustained sinus bradycardia.

Epinephrine acts on all receptor sites at relatively low concentrations, increasing contractility and causing alpha-mediated vasoconstriction. Medium-dose epinephrine is useful in patients with inadequate peripheral vascular tone and near-adequate myocardial function. It is combined with dopamine to treat significant postoperative myocardial failure. During cardiac arrest, intracardiac epinephrine produces immediate positive inotropic effects on the failed circulation.

Norepinephrine acts predominantly on the alpha-receptors in the periphery and the beta-1 receptors on the heart. The increase in peripheral resistance causes a significant increase in myocardial oxygen consumption without augmentation of cardiac output, however. Its use is usually limited to patients with refractory cardiovascular collapse.

Calcium. Calcium ion concentration within the myocytes is probably the final common pathway of positive inotropic stimulation of the heart. Intravenous injection of calcium chloride or gluconate causes a positive inotropic response without increasing ventricular irritability or altering peripheral vascular tone.

Cardiac Assist Devices. The *intra-aortic balloon pump* is used to treat medically uncontrollable angina in preoperative patients scheduled for CABG and to facilitate discontinuation of cardiopulmonary bypass (CPB) in patients who are difficult or impossible to wean from CPB without such assistance. The pumping mechanism augments diastolic coronary perfusion and diminishes afterload with each beat.[10]

Electrophysiologic Aspects

Arrhythmias in the perioperative surgical patient can be caused by multiple factors, including underlying cardiac disease, induction and reversal of anesthesia, electrolyte imbalance, and hypoxia. Each of these factors must be considered, and corrected if present, whenever supraventricular and ventricular arrhythmias appear in postoperative patients.[18]

SUPRAVENTRICULAR ARRHYTHMIAS

Bradycardia. Bradycardia due to excessive vagal parasympathetic input to the sinoatrial (SA) node can be treated with atropine, isoproterenol, or pacing by epicardial, esophageal, or transcutaneous leads in patients following surgical procedures.

Sinus Tachycardia. This increases myocardial oxygen requirements, and the rapid rate may be slowed by careful propranolol infusion or by neostigmine, an anticholinesterase agent.

Atrial Fibrillation. Atrial fibrillation occurs in as many as 35 per cent of patients undergoing open heart procedures and in a number of patients with underlying cardiac disease who are undergoing general surgical procedures. Treatment depends on the degree of associated hemodynamic instability.

Digoxin slows conduction through the AV node, probably because of parasympathetic stimulation. Digitalization will usually slow the ventricular response, without additional antiarrhythmic agents. Correction of hypokalemia and hypoxia is important, because both conditions can exacerbate digitalis toxicity.

Intravenous *propranolol* acutely slows conduction through the AV node and suppresses atrial ectopic foci.

Bradycardia and cardiodepression are important deleterious side effects of such therapy. Beta-blockade is useful in cases of supraventricular tachycardia secondary to digitalis toxicity.

Intravenous *verapamil* will convert rapid fibrillation to sinus rhythm in 10 to 15 per cent of patients by inhibiting calcium-mediated conduction in AV node tissue. It has no effect on ventricular arrhythmias. Concomitant propranolol therapy or digitalis toxicity are absolute contraindications to intravenous verapamil therapy, because complete heart block can occur.

Procainamide acts on both atrial and ventricular arrhythmias. In atrial fibrillation, it acts to suppress atrial ectopy once conversion to sinus rhythm has occurred. The *N*-acetyl metabolite also has antiarrhythmic properties, and serum levels of both drugs should be monitored.

Quinidine, the prototype Class I antiarrhythmic agent, is used to suppress atrial and ventricular ectopy and to maintain sinus rhythm following chemical or electrical cardioversion.

Atrial Flutter. The mechanism of flutter differs from that of fibrillation, but the treatment is similar. In cardiac patients who have temporary pacing wires in place, rapid atrial pacing will often entrain the atrial focus, with conversion to a sinus rhythm. Atrial fibrillation does not respond to rapid atrial pacing. In both fibrillation and flutter, synchronized electrical cardioversion is used when significant hemodynamic instability is present.

VENTRICULAR ARRHYTHMIAS

All patients exhibiting ventricular ectopy in the perioperative period should be aggressively treated with lidocaine, until suppression occurs. As mentioned, intravenous procainamide can also be used; however, for patients with persistent ectopy, oral suppressive therapy with quinidine or procainamide may be necessary.

Bretylium is effective in managing ventricular fibrillation refractory to lidocaine and to electrical defibrillation, and its use is limited to refractory arrhythmias present during cardiac arrest.

Tachycardia or fibrillation is immediately treated by defibrillation.

CLINICAL THERAPY

A rational plan for evaluating and treating cardiac system dysfunction in the perioperative period is depicted in Figure 1. Aberrations in each of the major determinants of cardiac output, that is, heart rate, preload, afterload, and contractility, are illustrated for each clinical situation.

Bradycardia should be treated with atropine, with isoproterenol, or, when feasible, with temporary pacing to augment cardiac output. Hypertension is treated by afterload reduction. Restoration of adequate preload with volume replacement with blood products or colloid constitutes the initial therapy for hypotension. Carefully planned peripheral vasoconstriction may be necessary to augment peripheral vascular resistance. Addition of afterload reduction to a volume-restored vascular space decreases the resistance to ventricular outflow and thus overall cardiac work. Using this combination of rate augmentation, volume replacement, and afterload reduction, an adequate cardiac output can be achieved in most patients with minimal increase in myocardial oxygen consumption.

With adequate cardiac output, excess extravascular

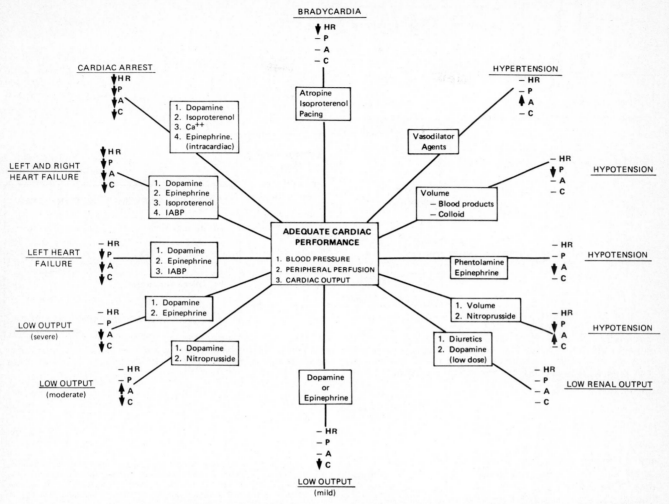

Figure 1. Algorithm for diagnosis and treatment of perioperative cardiac system dysfunction. Aberrations in the four major determinants of cardiac function (heart rate, preload, afterload, and contractility) are on the outside of the circle. The major interventions necessary to restore adequate cardiac function are shown for each clinical situation. HR = Heart rate; P = preload; A = afterload; C = contractility.

volume can be drawn into the vascular space and diuresis can be stimulated with diuretics or with low-dose dopamine acting on receptors in the kidney.

Despite the above measures, however, adequate cardiac performance cannot be achieved in some patients. Addition of sympathomimetic amines is then indicated to augment contractility and to assure perfusion of peripheral organ systems. All of these agents increase the work of the heart, and thus augment myocardial oxygen consumption, and therefore should be used judiciously. Dopamine is usually the first agent of choice, alone or in combination with nitroprusside, for afterload reduction. If performance is still inadequate despite mid-range doses of dopamine, a second agent, usually epinephrine, is added. The failing left ventricle can be additionally supported by insertion of the intra-aortic balloon pump. Isoproterenol can be added to support the right side of the circulation.

The use of sympathomimetic amines and the balloon pump, in addition to continued optimization of preload and afterload, usually provides sufficient cardiac output to perfuse other major organ systems in even very sick postoperative surgical patients.

Similarly, an outline of the treatment of postoperative arrhythmias is depicted in Figure 2. Atrial fibrillation is treated initially by correction of possible etiologic conditions. A rapid ventricular response is controlled with digitalization, and conversion to sinus rhythm can be attempted with intravenous propranolol or verapamil in patients who are hemodynamically stable. Procainamide can be added to maintain sinus rhythm once conversion has occurred. The same sequence is used for atrial flutter, with the added option of rapid atrial pacing in postoperative cardiac patients. Immediate control and suppression of ventricular premature complexes and tachycardia are obtained with intravenous lidocaine, procainamide, or bretylium. Long-term suppression with quinidine or procainamide is sometimes required. Heart block in cardiac patients can be treated with temporary atrioventricular sequential pacing. Hemodynamic instability due to atrial or ventricular dysrhythmias is immediately treated with cardioversion or defibrillation.

Once the acute postoperative phase has passed, patients can be gently weaned from cardiovascular system support and antiarrhythmic therapy in most cases. If con-

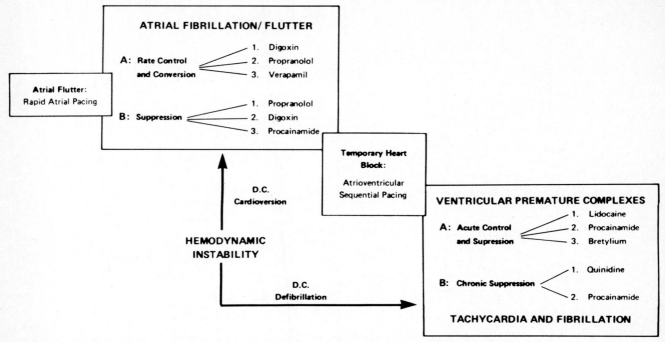

Figure 2. Algorithm for diagnosis and treatment of postoperative arrhythmias. Hemodynamic instability with either supraventricular or ventricular arrhythmias requires cardioversion or defibrillation. Postoperative cardiac patients may be AV sequentially paced for heart block, or rapid atrially paced for entrainment of atrial flutter.

tinued support or therapy is necessary, conversion to oral agents can be easily accomplished during this weaning phase. Often, these oral agents can be discontinued by the time of the first or second postoperative visit, when the patient has fully recovered from the effects of operation. A thorough understanding of these principles can facilitate management of the cardiovascular system in surgical patients to ensure minimal morbidity and maximal recovery of cardiac function postoperatively.

SELECTED REFERENCES

Katz, A. M.: Physiology of the Heart. New York, Raven Press, 1977.
This outstanding text, written for medical students, begins with the fundamentals of cardiac anatomy, physiology, and biochemistry and concludes with a discussion of valvular and ischemic heart disease. The major concepts in the current understanding of cardiac mechanics, contractility, and electrophysiology are thoroughly yet clearly presented. As a text for students seeking a unifying explanation of cardiac physiology, it is excellent.

Opie, L. H.: The Heart—Physiology, Metabolism, Pharmacology and Therapy. London, Grune & Stratton, 1985.
This recent text is an expansion of a six-part series by Opie entitled "Drugs and the heart," published in The Lancet in 1980. It is comprehensive with chapters on nearly every aspect of the cardiovascular system in both normal and abnormal states. With a number of clear illustrations and excellent references, it is an updated reference for students, residents, and physicians alike.

Waldo, A. L., and MacLean, W. A. H.: Diagnosis and Treatment of Cardiac Arrhythmias Following Open Heart Surgery. Mt. Kisco, N.Y., Futura Publishing Company, 1980.
This monograph, subtitled "Emphasis on the Use of Atrial and Ventricular Epicardial Wire Electrodes," firmly established the efficacy of this method in managing postoperative arrhythmias following nearly all cardiac operations. Written by two highly regarded electrophysiologists

and based on an extensive patient population, the text covers all aspects of the diagnosis and treatment of supraventricular, nodal, and ventricular arrhythmias as they occur following open heart surgery. An excellent discussion of the anatomic aspects of cardiac conduction and electrophysiology is also included.

REFERENCES

1. Bastron, R. D.: Diuretics. *In* Kaplan, J. E.: Cardiac Anesthesia, Vol. 2, Cardiovascular Pharmacology. New York, Grune & Stratton, 1983, pp. 325–341.
2. Behrendt, D. M., and Austen, W. G.: Patient Care in Cardiac Surgery. Boston, Little, Brown & Company, 1980.
3. Chaterjee, K., and Potts, T. A.: Physiologic and pharmacologic basis for the use of vasodilators in heart failure. *In* Wilkerson, R. D.: Cardiac Pharmacology. New York, Academic Press, 1981, pp. 150–201.
4. Culliford, A. T., and Sherrin, R.: Post-operative care. *In* Sabiston, D. C., Jr., and Spencer, F. C.: Gibbon's Surgery of the Chest, 4th ed. Philadelphia, W. B. Saunders Company, 1983, pp. 155–181.
5. Curling, P. E., and Kaplan, J. E.: Indications and uses of intravenous nitroglycerin during cardiac surgery. Angiology, *33*:302, 1982.
6. Epstein, S. E., Rosing, D. R., and Conti, C. R. (Eds.): Symposium on calcium-channel blockers: Present status and future directions. Am. J. Cardiol., *55*(3), 1985.
7. Katz, A. M.: Physiology of the Heart. New York, Raven Press, 1977.
8. Kortz, W. A., and Lumb, P. A.: Surgical Intensive Care: A Practical Guide. Chicago, Year Book Medical Publishers, Inc., 1984.
9. Mayer, S. E.: Neurohumoral transmission and the autonomic nervous system. *In* Goodman, L. S., and Gilman, A.: The Pharmacologic Basis of Therapeutics. New York, Macmillan Publishing Company, 1982, pp. 56–90.
10. Mundth, E. D.: The coronary circulation. 6. Assisted circulation. *In* Sabiston, D. C., Jr., and Spencer, F. C. (Eds.): Gibbon's Surgery of the Chest, 4th ed. Philadelphia, W. B. Saunders Company, 1983, pp. 1490–1515.
11. Neville, W. E., and Deiter, R. A.: The adult cardiac patient. *In* Neville, W. E. (Ed.): Intensive Care of the Surgical Cardiopulmonary

Patient. Chicago, Year Book Medical Publishers, Inc., 1982, pp. 140–159.

12. Oka, H., Frishman, W., and Becker, W.: Clinical pharmacology of the new beta-adrenergic blocking drugs. Part 10. Beta-adrenoreceptor blockade and coronary artery surgery. Am. Heart J., 99:255, 1980.

13. Opie, L. H.: Drugs and the heart. V. Digitalis and sympathomimetic stimulants. Lancet, 1:912, 1980.

14. Opie, L. H.: Arrhythmias and antiarrhythmics. In Opie, L. H.: The Heart—Physiology, Metabolism, Pharmacology and Therapy. London, Grune & Stratton, 1985, pp. 314–337.

15. Plummer, A. L.: Bronchodilator drugs and the cardiac patient. In

Kaplan, J. E. (Ed.): Cardiac Anesthesia, Vol. 2, Cardiovascular Pharmacology. New York, Grune & Stratton, 1983, pp. 409–451.

16. Rackley, C. E., Russell, R. O., Mantle, J. A., and Rogers, W. J.: Cardiogenic shock. In Rackley, C. E. (Ed.): Critical Care Cardiology. Philadelphia, F. A. Davis Co., 1981, pp. 15–24.

17. Vidt, D. G., Bruno, E. L., and Fouad, F. M.: Captopril. N. Engl. J. Med., 306:214, 1982.

18. Waldo, A. L., and MacLean, W. A. H.: Diagnosis and Treatment of Cardiac Arrhythmias Following Open Heart Surgery. Mt. Kisco, N.Y., Futura Publishing Company, 1980.

Cardiopulmonary Bypass for Cardiac Surgery

CRAIG O. OLSEN, M.D.
DAVID C. SABISTON, JR., M.D.

HISTORICAL PERSPECTIVE

The development of the technique to temporarily replace the pumping action of the heart and the gaseous exchange of the lungs by a mechanical device attached to the vascular system of the patient is fascinating. The concept of an extracorporeal circulation was first originated by LeGallois in 1812, and the first artificial oxygenation of blood is credited to Ludwig in 1869. The first report of an isolated organ perfusion system using a blood film spread on a rotating cylinder was by Frey and Grubber in 1885.[14] The pioneering experimental work of Gibbon in the 1930s advanced cardiopulmonary bypass (CPB) from a laboratory dream into the reality of clinical application. In 1953, Gibbon performed the first successful cardiac operation (correction of an atrial septal defect in a young female) in which the patient was totally supported by CPB using a disc oxygenator.[8] By 1956, the disposable bubble oxygenator was developed by DeWall[6] and the first clinical application of a membrane oxygenator was reported.[3] The field of open heart surgery has expanded because of CPB and has steadily and rapidly grown from the first success in 1953 to more than 200,000 operations per year in 1986 in the United States alone.

THE PUMP-OXYGENATOR APPARATUS

The basic circuit employed for CPB is depicted in Figure 1. The circuit receives venous blood from the body, oxygenates the blood while allowing elimination of carbon dioxide, and pumps it back into the arterial system. In addition to these basic functions, provisions are made for intracardiac suction and scavenging of blood, filtration of organic and inorganic particulate emboli, prevention of air bubbles, maintenance of sterility, and control of temperature.

Venous Reservoir. A reservoir is usually present and is positioned to provide adequate siphonage of blood by gravity. This provides storage of excess volume and allows escape of any air bubbles returning with the venous blood.

Oxygenator. Two types of oxygenators are predominantly used in current clinical practice: the bubble oxygenator and the membrane oxygenator. In the *bubble oxygenator*, oxygen is bubbled through the blood and gas exchange occurs at the direct blood-gas interface.[11] Three per cent carbon dioxide is added to prevent respiratory alkalosis, and the gas mixture is passed through a microporous filter to prevent bacterial contamination. Silicone antifoaming agents are used to burst the microbubbles, thus preventing air emboli and allowing the gas to escape from the oxygenator through exhaust portals. Bubble oxygenators are compact, disposable, economical, and relatively safe for the duration of perfusion necessary for most cardiac operations.

In the *membrane oxygenator* a semipermeable membrane is partitioned between moving layers of blood and gas. The rate of gas transfer across the membrane depends on the special characteristics of the membrane, the formation of a boundary layer phenomenon, and the partial pressure differences of the diffusing gases across the membrane.[11] The major advantage of the membrane oxygenator is the absence of the direct blood-gas interface with reduction in the resultant red blood cell hemolysis, blood protein denaturation, and formation of microemboli. There appear to be no clear clinical differences between the membrane and bubble oxygenators for perfusions of 2 hours or less in duration.[9] In perfusions longer than 2 hours, use of the membrane oxygenator results in less trauma to blood components with potentially better preservation of the perfused tissues. The major disadvantages include increased cost and complexity of most membrane oxygenator systems.

Heat Exchanger. This apparatus controls the perfusate temperature to achieve systemic cooling and rewarming during CPB. Most exchangers function by circulating heated or cooled water through conduits in juxtaposition to the

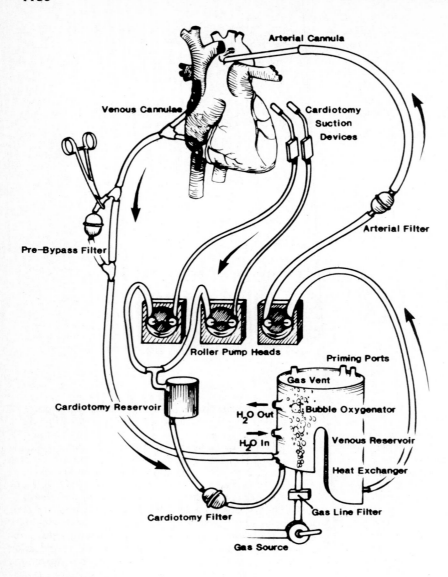

Figure 1. Diagrammatic representation of cardiopulmonary bypass circuit connected to the vascular system of a patient with arterial inflow into the ascending aorta and venous return from bicaval cannulae in the right atrium. See text for explanation of component parts.

blood in the bypass circuit. To avoid blood injury and gaseous microemboli formation, the temperature difference between blood and water should not exceed 14°C. and at no time should the water temperature exceed 42°C. during rewarming.[16]

Pumps. The arterial pump is usually a roller pump originally described by DeBakey in 1934.[5] The adjustable pumping head is set prior to each perfusion to be slightly nonocclusive to avoid excessive blood trauma and spallation of the roller tubing.[16] Although this pump design is simple, accurate, and reliable, the resultant nonpulsatile blood flow is nonphysiologic and may cause increased vasomotor tone and peripheral vascular resistance during prolonged use. Pulsatile perfusion is achieved by a variety of mechanisms and results in a more physiologic flow pattern, which has been demonstrated to have beneficial effects on the end organs but has the drawback of adding increased complexity to the bypass system.[10, 16]

Filters. Embolization of gas and particulate emboli is a constant hazard of CPB. The pump-oxygenator priming solution should be recirculated and filtered through 20- to 40-µm. pore filters to remove foreign particles prior to CPB. Similar filters are placed in the bypass circuit between

the arterial pump and the patient during CPB and significantly reduce the number of microemboli perfused to the patient.[11, 16]

Cardiotomy Suction. Several suction lines may be used to return blood shed into the operative field to the oxygenator for recirculation to the patient. The suction on these lines may be individually regulated by the adjustable pump heads and should be set at the minimal necessary rate to avoid excessive shear forces that result in trauma to the blood elements.[11, 16] The blood returned by the cardiotomy suction devices is collected in a reservoir where gaseous and solid particulate microemboli are removed prior to returning the blood to the oxygenator for oxygenation and recirculation to the patient. The cardiotomy suction system is the largest single source of solid particulate emboli in the pump-oxygenator system.

TECHNIQUE OF PERFUSION

Following proper surgical exposure and adequate hemostasis, the patient is systemically anticoagulated with heparin. Activated clotting times of greater than 8 minutes ensure adequate heparinization and prevent fibrin formation.[11]

Arterial Cannulation. The ascending aorta is generally employed for the arterial inflow cannula. Under special circumstances when aortic cannulation is not appropriate, the common femoral artery may be used. The arterial cannula is connected to the arterial perfusion line in such a way as to exclude or remove any air bubbles and the line and cannula are secured to ensure unobstructive flow from the pump-oxygenator into the cannulated artery.

Venous Cannulation. For most cardiac operations in infants and children, two angled, cage-tipped venous cannulae are inserted directly into each vena cava, particularly if the operation involves entering the right atrium or right ventricle. A single right atrial cannula may be used if the operation involves procedures performed through the left atrium, left ventricle, or ascending aorta. In adults, two venous cannulae are employed when working in the right atrium. For coronary bypass grafting and mitral or aortic valve operations, a single, large, two-stage cavoatrial cannula with openings in the inferior vena cava and right atrium may be used. This cannula provides more efficient drainage of the right atrium than bicaval cannulae and has the added advantage of easier insertion through a single right atrial incision.[2] The venous cannula or cannulae are connected to the venous drainage line of the pump-oxygenator circuit.

Venting. To decompress the heart, a suction line may be placed directly into the right side of the left atrium or via the right superior pulmonary vein and positioned across the mitral valve to lie in the left ventricle. Ventricular venting improves surgical exposure of intracardiac structures during valve or congenital heart procedures. Because ventricular venting may introduce air into the ventricle, causing embolization, some surgeons use an aortic needle or cannula for venting after infusion of cardioplegic solution.[16]

Pump-Oxygenator Priming Fluids. During the early days of CPB, whole blood or blood products were used to prime the pump-oxygenator system. Open heart surgery was limited by difficulty in procuring fresh blood, especially for patients with rare blood types. Currently, the priming volume for most adult pump-oxygenator systems is 1500 to 2000 ml. of an isotonic dextrose-saline solution containing balanced electrolytes to which oncotic agents (low-molecular-weight dextran, mannitol, hydroxyethyl starch, or albumin) are added to help maintain plasma colloid oncotic pressure and preserve renal function during CPB. If the resultant hematocrit is too low, banked CPD blood along with calcium, heparin, and buffer may be added to the pump-oxygenator system.[11, 17]

Intraoperative phlebotomy with hemodilution prior to initiation of CPB and autologous transfusion at the conclusion of bypass has been demonstrated to significantly reduce the need for heterologous blood transfusions in patients undergoing open heart surgery.[4]

EXTERNALLY CONTROLLED VARIABLES

Perfusion Flow Rate. During total CPB at normothermia, with flow rates at or less than 1.6 liters per minute per m.[2] lactic acidosis regularly occurs.[7] The optimal flow rate remains controversial; no absolute criteria exist for safe flow rates at any specific temperature. The perfusion flow rate is adequate when the entire microcirculation is

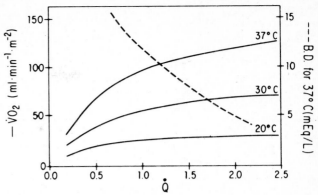

Figure 2. Relationship of oxygen consumption (V_{O_2}) to perfusion flow rate (Q) during cardiopulmonary bypass at various perfusion temperatures (solid lines). Hypothermia decreased the (V_{O_2}) requirement such that the maximum Q required to perfuse the microcirculation at near normal tissue oxygen levels is reduced. The relationship of base deficit (B. D.) to Q is shown at normothermia (broken line). Hypothermia shifts this relationship to the left. (Modified from Ionescu, M. I.: Techniques in Extracorporeal Circulation. London, Butterworth, 1981[11]; Kirklin, J. W., et al.: In Sabiston, D. C., Jr., and Spencer, F. C.: Gibbon's Surgery of the Chest. Philadelphia, W. B. Saunders Company, 1983, p. 909.[13])

perfused at flows such that near-normal tissue-oxygen levels are maintained. At lower body temperatures, the amount of flow required to achieve this is less. During hypothermic CPB, maximal perfusion of the microcirculation probably occurs near the asymptote of the temperature-specific curve relating flow to oxygen consumption as shown in Figure 2.[7, 12]

Perfusate Temperature. Hypothermic perfusion is utilized for most cardiac operations and provides an element of safety against hypoxia. For example, hypothermia nearly doubles the tolerance time of cerebral ischemia for each 5°C. of cooling.[15] At normothermia, the brain tolerates from 4 to 5 minutes of ischemia before irreversible cellular damage occurs. This is increased to 20 minutes at 22°C. and 75 minutes at 10°C. (Fig. 3). During hypothermia, there are significant changes in pH as well as other metabolic alterations; these appear to correct spontaneously on rewarming with no residual effect.

Hematocrit. Numerous factors affect the hematocrit during cardiac procedures, including the amounts of blood and fluids administered before and during CPB, the amount of blood loss, the amount and composition of the initial volume of the pump-oxygenator circuit, and transcapillary movement of fluid from the intravascular to the extravascular space and into urine volume.[11] During CPB, the hematocrit is deliberately lowered (hemodilution) because the resultant reduction in blood viscosity and lower shear rates allow better perfusion of the microcirculation and less red cell hemolysis, especially under hypothermic conditions. Thus a hematocrit of 25 per cent is desirable during moderate hypothermic perfusion (26 to 32°C.) and one of 20 per cent is preferable during profound hypothermic perfusion (16 to 22°C.).[11, 15] During the rewarming phase of CPB, oxygen demands are increased and a higher hematocrit (greater than 30 per cent) is desirable. Nomograms exist for calculating the resultant mixed patient-machine hematocrit that occurs during CPB.[13]

Systemic and Venous Pressures. Systemic venous pressure during CPB is directly proportional to perfusion flow rate, blood viscosity, and venous line suction and inversely

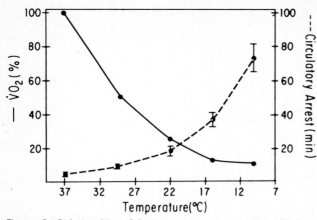

Figure 3. Relationship of brain oxygen consumption (V_{O_2}) to perfusion temperature (solid line) and the period of safe cerebral ischemia (circulatory arrest) tolerated at various perfusion temperatures (broken line). (Modified from Utley, J. R., and Ashleigh, E. A.: Pathophysiology and Techniques of Cardiopulmonary Bypass, Vol. 1. Baltimore, Williams and Wilkins, 1981.)

proportional to venous cannula and line size. Because there is no apparent physiologic advantage in an elevated central systemic venous pressure during CPB, it is kept as near zero as possible. This may be achieved by selecting an adequately large venous cannula with venous drainage lines that are larger than the smallest diameter of the venous cannula and ensuring maximal gravity drainage (at least 30 to 50 cm.) between the patient's chest and the venous reservoir.[16] Reduction in perfusion flow rate, hemodilution to decrease blood viscosity, and gentle suction on the venous lines are other factors favoring a low systemic venous pressure.

Elevations of the pulmonary venous pressure during CPB result in pulmonary edema by increasing extravascular lung water. Pulmonary venous pressure should be kept near zero at all times and any elevation during operation should be kept transient to avoid the complication of pulmonary edema.[16]

PATHOPHYSIOLOGY OF CARDIOPULMONARY BYPASS

Safe CPB may be characterized by the absence of functional or structural tissue and organ damage following perfusion. The vast majority of patients undergoing CPB have no significantly apparent ill effects, but occasionally some have severe multiorgan dysfunction. Certain factors are known to increase the risks associated with CPB and include (1) duration of bypass beyond 2 hours, with a sharp increase after 3 hours; (2) young age, less than 3 to 6 months; and (3) advanced age, especially in the presence of pre-existing renal dysfunction.[13] An understanding of the abnormal physiologic effects of CPB is necessary to appreciate its limitations and ensure maximal safety for the majority of patients who undergo open heart procedures.

Fluid and Electrolytes

Weight gains of 6 to 7 kg. during CPB are not uncommon and are caused primarily by an increase in the extracellular fluid space that may persist for 7 to 10 days postoperatively. Hemodilution has been determined to be the main source of fluid retention during CPB; it causes a fall in plasma proteins that results in a decreased plasma colloid oncotic pressure.[15] Other contributing factors include diminished blood viscosity, diminished oxygen-carrying capacity, and vasodilatation. Decreased blood viscosity from hemodilution increases tissue blood flow, especially to the myocardium, outer renal cortex, cerebral cortex, spleen, and intestine, and is another potent cause of tissue edema. The increased extravascular fluid volume results in an increased interstitial fluid pressure and decreased plasma volume. Total body water and sodium are increased, though there is usually a mild hyponatremia and hypokalemia until the extravascular fluid volume is mobilized and excreted by the kidneys.

Blood

Denaturation of both the formed and the unformed blood elements remains one of the major limiting factors in the development of improved techniques in CPB (Fig. 4). Shear forces generated by the roller pumps, cardiotomy suction device, and cavitation around the distal end of the arterial cannula cause increased leukocyte disruption and dysfunction, which persists for several days following bypass.[15] Lymphocyte function, including that of both B and T cells, is also depressed.

The amount of free plasma hemoglobin is a measure of red blood cell hemolysis induced by the pump-oxygenator system and is increased by prolonged CPB, increased use of intracardiac suction devices, and use of bubble oxygenators.[11] A decreased erythrocyte survival time following CPB results in a progressive loss of red cell mass during the first 4 postoperative days.

Probably the greatest damage during CPB results from exposure of the blood elements to nonphysiologic surfaces, the most critical of which occur in the oxygenator where the largest proportion of blood is deliberately exposed to the boundary layer (either a gas bubble or an artificial semipermeable membrane) for gas exchange.[13] The proportion of blood in the boundary layer is relatively small in the rest of the bypass system. The effect of this exposure promotes platelet aggregation with resultant platelet emboli, thrombocytopenia, and platelet dysfunction during as well as following CPB. The blood proteins (albumin, lipoproteins, and immunoglobulins) are denatured, resulting in fatty microemboli and erythrocyte clumping. The blood proteins composing the complex interrelated humoral amplification system (coagulation, fibrinolytic, complement, and kallikrein cascades) are activated by the abnormal, nonphysiologic surfaces of the pump-oxygenator system and initiate a whole body "inflammatory" response. Activation of the coagulation cascade results in progressive consumption of clotting factors despite adequate heparinization. Activation of the kallikrein cascade causes production of bradykinin, which increases vascular permeability and vasoconstriction. Because bradykinin is metabolized mainly in the lungs, exclusion of the pulmonary circulation during CPB sustains the elevated circulating bradykinin levels.[11, 15] The glycoproteins constituting the complement system may be activated via interaction with antigen-antibody complexes or via an alternative pathway when blood is exposed to the nonphysiologic surfaces of the pump-oxygenator system. During CPB, complement levels fall and the complement degradation products C3a and C5a are elaborated. These anaphylatoxins promote vasoconstriction

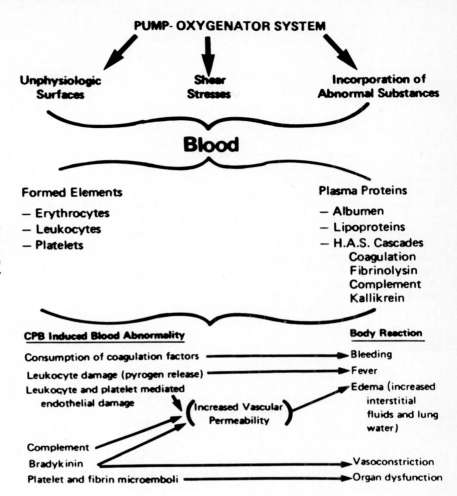

Figure 4. Schematic representation of the damaging effects of cardiopulmonary bypass related to the exposure of blood to the bypass circuit. H.A.S. = Humeral amplification system. (Modified from Kirklin[12, 13] and Utley and Ashleigh.[15])

and increase capillary permeability. They bind to neutrophils, which are then deposited in the lungs, as well as other organs, where lysosomal enzyme release produces further endothelial cell damage. Serum levels of C3a and C5a remain elevated for several hours following CPB, are proportional in elevation to the duration of bypass, and may contribute significantly to coagulation and microcirculatory dysfunction involving multiple organ systems following bypass.[13]

The incorporation of microemboli (both organic and inorganic) from the priming solutions and pump-oxygenator system may activate the humoral amplification system, as well as causing organ damage by embolization.

Central Nervous System

Cerebral dysfunction remains a hazard to patients undergoing CPB and may be the result of either inadequate perfusion or embolization. The cerebral effects of CPB may be minor or transient (in as many as 25 per cent of patients) or they may be major and permanent (in 1 to 2 per cent of patients).[1, 11]

The autoregulatory properties of the cerebral circulatory system maintain normal cerebral blood flow throughout a wide range of cerebral arterial perfusion pressures until the mean arterial pressure falls below 50 mm. Hg at normothermia. In experimental animals hypothermia re-

duces the cerebral metabolic rate (see Fig. 3) and does not alter autoregulation until the brain temperature falls to 13°C. Because carbon dioxide is a potent cerebral vasodilator, current methods of CPB maintain carbon dioxide at normal levels during hypothermia to maintain cerebral blood flow near normal levels. Hypothermia may be used as an adjunct to cerebral protection during CPB and permits reduction in both pressure and flow without any impairment to cerebral function.[15] Although the importance of maintaining an adequate perfusion pressure during CPB has been reported, there is disagreement about which perfusion pressure is adequate. Patients with cerebrovascular disease or other neurologic disorders may have impaired cerebral circulatory autoregulation and are at increased risk of postoperative CNS dysfunction. Higher perfusion pressures may be required for such individuals during CPB.

Most central nervous system (CNS) dysfunction is manifested as delirium or disorientation and disappears in 1 to 4 weeks. This reversible syndrome is probably due to microbubble embolization and is correlated with duration of bypass using bubble oxygenators.[1] Membrane oxygenators and microbubble filters minimize the incidence and severity of this syndrome. Major CNS damage is usually due to particulate embolism or hypotension superimposed on atherosclerosis. Adequate filtration of the arterial inflow blood with microporous filters and adequate perfusion pressures largely eliminate this problem. Factors that may increase the risk of major CNS damage include advanced patient age, valvular heart disease (particularly aortic lesions), history of cerebrovascular disease, and prolonged CPB times.[1]

Lungs

Pulmonary dysfunction following CPB can best be characterized by excessive capillary fluid filtration related to capillary endothelial damage resulting from complement release and activation of the coagulation cascade.[16] Hemodilution with a reduction in the plasma colloidal osmotic pressure and elevation of the capillary hydrostatic pressure (pulmonary venous pressure) during bypass also contribute to postperfusion pulmonary edema. Factors that may lessen pulmonary complications of CPB include static inflation of the lungs during bypass to prevent alveolar collapse, reduction in the amount of transfused blood, minimizing blood trauma or prolonged bypass times, effective left heart decompression during bypass, careful control of the cardiac filling pressures and afterload postoperatively, and effective use of pulmonary physiotherapy and ventilatory support postoperatively to maintain pulmonary function.

Kidney

Renal dysfunction is relatively common following CPB and some degree of failure may occur in 1 to 13 per cent of patients. This is usually a result of acute tubular necrosis, which is reversible. Severe forms of renal failure requiring dialysis following CPB have a significantly high mortality. Factors that affect perioperative renal function include preoperative renal disease, nephrotoxic drugs, hemolysis, renal ischemia, microemboli, and postoperative cardiac function. Successful perioperative management of renal failure depends on recognition of the preoperative and intraoperative risk factors; optimal management of operative interventions; early detection of renal failure; use of appropriate osmotic, diuretic, and vasoactive drugs; and selective use of peritoneal dialysis or hemodialysis in severe renal failure.[15]

WITHDRAWAL FROM PERFUSION

Following completion of the cardiac operation, the patient is systemically rewarmed by increasing the pump flow rate from 2.0 to 2.5 liters per minute per m.[2] and raising the temperature of the water in the heat exchanger. Reperfusion of the heart is established and air is evacuated from the cardiac chambers and aortic root by various maneuvers.[11, 16] When the cardiac action is vigorous and the core body temperature reaches 36 to 37°C., CPB is discontinued by progressive occlusion of the venous return and reduction of the pump arterial flow rate, allowing the heart to take over the circulation again. The venous and arterial cannulae are removed and the systemic heparinization is reversed with protamine, using activated clotting times to calculate the appropriate dose.[13]

SELECTED REFERENCES

Nelson, R. M.: Era of extracorporeal respiration. Surgery, *78*:685, 1975.
This review presents the development of the technique of cardiopulmonary bypass since the first concept of extracorporeal oxygenation.

Gibbon, J. H., Jr.: Application of a mechanical heart and lung apparatus to cardiac surgery. Minn. Med., *37*:171, 1954.
This classic reviews the first successful clinical use of CPB and provides details of the basic mechanical and physiologic aspects of extracorporeal circulation.

Utley, J. R., and Ashleigh, E. A.: Pathophysiology and Techniques of Cardiopulmonary Bypass, Vol. I. Baltimore, Williams and Wilkins, 1981; Utley, J. R., and Betleski, R.: Pathophysiology and Techniques of Cardiopulmonary Bypass, Vol. II, 1983.
This reference thoroughly summarizes the aspects of CPB unifying the basic, clinical, and applied sciences relating to extracorporeal circulation and includes a discussion of most of the practical problems related to postperfusion syndromes. It is an excellent course for the reader desiring an in-depth discussion of CPB.

REFERENCES

1. Aberg, T., and Kihlgren, M.: Cerebral protection during open-heart surgery. Thorax, *32*:525, 1977.
2. Bennett, E. V., Fewel, J. G., Ybarra, J., Grover, F. L., and Trinkle, J. K.: Comparison of flow differences among venous cannulas. Ann. Thorac. Surg., *36*:59, 1983.
3. Clowes, G. H. A., Jr., Hopkins, A. L., and Neville, W. E.: An artificial lung dependent upon diffusion of oxygen and carbon dioxide through plastic membranes. J. Thorac. Cardiovasc. Surg., *32*:630, 1956.
4. Cohn, L. H., Fosberg, A. M., Anderson, W. P., and Collins, J. J.: The effects of phlebotomy, hemodilution and autologous transfusion on systemic oxygenation and whole blood utilization in open-heart surgery. Chest, *68*:283, 1975.
5. DeBakey, M. E.: Simple continuous flow blood transfusion instrument. New Orleans Med. Surg. J., *87*:386, 1934.
6. DeWall, R. A., Warden, H. E., Gott, V. L., Read, R. C., Varco, R. L., and Lillehei, C. W.: Total body perfusion for open cardiotomy utilizing the bubble oxygenator. J. Thorac. Cardiovasc. Surg., *32*:591, 1956.
7. Fox, L. S., Blackstone, E. H., Kirklin, J. W., Stewart, R. W., and Samuelson, P. N.: Relationship of whole oxygen consumption to perfusion flow rate during hypothermic cardiopulmonary bypass. J. Thorac. Cardiovasc. Surg., *83*:239, 1982.
8. Gibbon, J. H., Jr.: Application of a mechanical heart and lung apparatus to cardiac surgery. Minn. Med., *37*:171, 1954.
9. Hessel, E. A., II, Johnson, D. D., Ivey, T. D., and Miller, D. W., Jr.: Membrane versus bubble oxygenator for cardiac operations. J. Thorac. Cardiovasc. Surg., *80*:111, 1980.
10. Hickey, P. R., Buckley, M. J., and Philbin, D. M.: Pulsatile and nonpulsatile cardiopulmonary bypass: Review of a counterproductive controversy. Ann. Thorac. Surg., *36*:720, 1983.
11. Ionescu, M. I.: Techniques in Extracorporeal Circulation. London, Butterworth, 1981.
12. Kirklin, J. W., Kirklin, J. K., and Lell, W. A.: Cardiopulmonary bypass for cardiac surgery. *In* Sabiston, D. C., Jr., and Spencer, F. C. (Eds.): Gibbon's Surgery of the Chest, 4th ed. Philadelphia, W. B. Saunders Company, 1983, p. 909.
13. Kirklin, J. K., Westaby, S., Blackstone, E. H., Kirklin, J. W., Chenoweth, D. E., and Pacifico, A. D.: Complement and the damaging effects of cardiopulmonary bypass. J. Thorac. Cardiovasc. Surg., *86*:845, 1983.
14. Nelson, R. M.: Era of extracorporeal respiration. Surgery, *78*:685, 1975.
15. Utley, J. R., and Ashleigh, E. A.: Pathophysiology and Techniques of Cardiopulmonary Bypass, Vol I. Baltimore, Williams & Wilkins, 1981.
16. Utley, J. R., and Betleski, R.: Pathophysiology and Techniques of Cardiopulmonary Bypass, Vol. II. Baltimore, Williams & Wilkins, 1983.
17. Verska, J. J., Ludington, L. G., and Brewer, L. A.: A comparative study of cardiopulmonary bypass with nonblood and blood prime. Ann. Thorac. Surg., *18*:72, 1974.

XXII

Arteriovenous Fistula

H. KIM LYERLY, M.D.
DAVID C. SABISTON, JR., M.D.

There are few disorders in clinical medicine that have the ability to produce as many pathophysiologic changes throughout the entire body as does an arteriovenous fistula. The changes are most prominent in large fistulas in which enormous amounts of arterial blood pass directly into the venous circulation but are present to some extent in most of these lesions. A number of important physiologic changes occur in an attempt to *compensate* for this circulatory abnormality.

In 1758, William Hunter first recognized that an *arteriovenous* aneurysm was characterized not only by the aneurysm but also by a direct communication between the involved artery and the accompanying vein.[3] Prior to this observation, such lesions had been interpreted as simple aneurysms, whereas Hunter designated these as "aneurysm by anastomosis" and placed emphasis upon the communication between the two vascular systems. Early surgical attempts to correct these lesions consisted primarily of ligation of the involved artery *proximal* to the fistula.[5] Whereas the threat of rupture of a classic arterial aneurysm might be diminished by ligating the arterial proximally, this approach in the presence of an arteriovenous fistula is apt to end disastrously because it is quite likely to be followed by gangrene of the extremity. This can result because the blood reaching the distal extremity by arterial collaterals is apt to drain retrograde through the fistula directly into the venous system, thus depriving the limb of adequate distal arterial blood flow. The first successful treatment of an arteriovenous fistula was proximal and distal ligation of both the artery and the vein.[23] This corrected the fistula and was not followed by peripheral vascular insufficiency of the limb due to the large number of arterial collaterals that had formed as a result of the fistula.

PATHOPHYSIOLOGY AND DIAGNOSIS

The pathophysiologic changes that follow a direct communication between the arterial and venous systems are classically demonstrated by the presence of a *thrill* over the site of the lesion, especially if it is located near the surface. On auscultation, a *bruit* is audible, continuing throughout most or all of the cardiac cycle. An aneurysm, or arterial and venous dilatation, is usually present. Enlarged veins are also present, either subcutaneously or apparent on angiography, in the more deeply located fistulas. These may also be demonstrated by ultrasonic determination.[35] The *magnitude* of systemic symptoms is generally related to the size of the fistula and its proximity to the heart. These changes are maximal in a *large* artery. Under these circumstances, much blood flows through the fistula because the venous side offers very little peripheral resistance. With large shunts directly into the venous circulation, a sequence of changes occurs that is directly related to the volume of blood passing through the fistula

The *cardiac output* increases, the heart rate increases, and the diastolic arterial pressure diminishes, usually with an increase in systolic pressure. The cardiac and pulmonary pressures also change with increases in ventricular end-diastolic pressures, elevated right and left atrial pressures, and increased pulmonary wedge pressure (Table 1). The blood and plasma volumes each increase in an effort to compensate for the increased volume of blood in the venous circulation. Moreover, with high cardiac output the heart increases in size, particularly the atrial and ventricular cavities, and ultimately cardiac hypertrophy results. Large fistulas may ultimately lead to congestive heart failure, and if the fistula is acute with a large volume of flow through it, the heart may not be able to compensate adequately with resultant pulmonary edema and death. It is interesting that experimental and clinical studies have indicated that digitalis preparations are largely ineffective in the management of high-output cardiac failure.[31] All of these features can be dramatically illustrated in experimental animals in whom large fistulas are created and physiologic measurements determined.[29]

In 1875, Nicoladoni described a patient with an arteriovenous fistula in whom compression of the fistula (with cessation of flow through it) caused a decrease in the pulse rate from 96 to 64 per minute.[22] This phenomenon was described by Branham in 1890 with obliteration of the pulse in a patient with acquired femoral arteriovenous fistula.[4] The famed Rudolph Matas termed this the "Branham bradycardiac reaction," and it has since borne that name.[12]

Physiologic changes occurring in the circulation with an arteriovenous fistula are most marked in the presence of a large fistula. These changes may be minimal to absent with a small fistula. Late manifestations of a large fistula include congestive heart failure, pulmonary edema, and death in untreated patients.

In the presence of a high cardiac output due to the

TABLE 1. Manifestations of Arteriovenous Fistula

		Systemic	
Pulse rate	↑	Diastolic arterial pressure	↓
Cardiac output	↑	Peripheral resistance	↓
Blood volume	↑		
Cardiac size	↑		

Local
Thrill
Continuous murmur
Increased arterial collaterals
Aneurysmal formation
Diminished pulse rate with occlusion

Physiologic changes occurring in the circulation with an arteriovenous fistula are most marked in the presence of a large fistula. These changes may be minimal to absent with a small fistula. Late manifestations of a large fistula include congestive heart failure, pulmonary edema, and death in untreated patients.

fistula, the oxygen saturation of the mixed venous blood in the right heart is greatly increased because much of the blood bypasses the capillary bed. The central venous pressure is usually increased. Of considerable importance is the *anatomic site* of the fistula in the systemic circulation because the diameter of the involved vessel is of crucial importance. For example, much more blood will flow through a fistula of a given size from an artery with a large diameter than from one with a smaller diameter. It has been shown experimentally that small aortic fistulas can produce severe symptoms when the shunts are located near the heart, for example, between the ascending aorta and the pulmonary artery or the superior vena cava contrasted with similar more distal shunts such as between the abdominal aorta and the vena cava or the iliac or femoral vessels.[30]

Significant structural changes in the vascular wall are also created by hemodynamic disturbances associated with arteriovenous fistulas. In large fistulas, the venous wall becomes very thin, closely simulating the sac of a false aneurysm. In small fistulas, the vein may become thickened and assume the appearance of an artery. Thrombi are also apt to form in and around these fistulas and may harbor organisms.

Arteriovenous fistulas may be associated with the development of bacterial endocarditis. In fact, the first patient ever cured of a chronic bloodstream infection (*Streptococcus*) prior to the introduction of antibiotics was managed by surgical closure of an iliac artery-iliac vein arteriovenous fistula. Following closure, the bloodstream infection disappeared, and the patient was cured.[27] Until that time all such illnesses had ended fatally.

LOCAL EFFECTS OF ARTERIOVENOUS FISTULAS

An *aneurysmal dilatation* is usually present at the site of the fistula involving both the artery and the vein. This is produced by the turbulence that occurs in the presence of the high to low pressure interface within the fistula. In response to the *low distal* arterial pressure beyond the site of the fistula, an extensive *collateral circulation* develops connecting the arteries arising above the fistula with those below. The vessels become greatly dilated and tortuous and deliver considerable blood to the distal extremity as a result of a marked pressure gradient. This collateral circulation can become massive and often results in an increase in temperature in both skin and muscle. When fistulas occur in an extremity, a limb may have *increased length,* a fact that has been confirmed by both experimental[15] and clinical observations.[14] The explanation for this increased bone growth is probably the result of the increase by 1 or 2 degrees C. in the local temperature.

TYPES OF ARTERIOVENOUS FISTULAS

The two major types of arteriovenous fistulas are *congenital* and *acquired.* Among congenital fistulas, the terms cirsoid aneurysms and cavernous angiomata have also been used. These lesions are generally the result of failure of differentiation of the common embryologic anlage into artery and vein because both arteries and veins differentiate from a common capillary plexus in embryologic development. Thus, as arteries and veins differentiate, a multitude of communications exist between them, and these may persist into adult life.

Congenital arteriovenous fistulas of the extremities are quite common,[37] especially those involving the legs, and varicose veins often result. Cavernous hemangiomas may involve a considerable part of the extremity and produce serious cosmetic and physiologic problems. Congenital arteriovenous fistulas have been reported in all organs in the body and are frequently difficult to manage. While surgical therapy has a role in specific types, some of these lesions are too extensive for appropriate surgical excision, and palliative surgical procedures are reserved to control disabling ulceration and infection or life-threatening hemorrhage. Alternative techniques of nonsurgical closure include selective intra-arterial embolization of autologous clot, wire, coil, plastic materials, or transcatheter coagulation.[17, 19, 25, 26] Each of these techniques has been reported as successful in closing some of the large fistulas that would be difficult if not impossible to manage surgically. Other types of therapy include injection of sclerosing solutions or irradiation. In one series of patients seen over a 10-year period, congenital arteriovenous fistulas represented 77 per cent, whereas 23 per cent were acquired (Table 2).[9] Some congenital fistulas are difficult to understand embryologically, such as those between the internal mammary artery and the pulmonary vessels.[28] Although such shunts may be small, closure of these lesions is nevertheless recommended owing to potential complications.

Congenital *pulmonary* arteriovenous aneurysms are common and are frequently multiple. They are usually seen as well-circumscribed lesions on the chest film and if large may be accompanied by cyanosis due to right-to-left shunting. The symptoms include exertional dyspnea, easy fatigability, cyanosis, and clubbing of the fingers.[21] About 10 to 15 per cent occur in children. Complications of these lesions include cerebrovascular accidents, brain abscess, hemoptysis, and intrapleural rupture.[38] A continuous bruit with systolic accentuation during sleep inspiration is heard in about two thirds of patients. Pulmonary arteriography confirms the diagnosis. Hereditary telangiectasis (Rendu-Osler-Weber disease) is quite common and may be familial in origin. These patients also have a tendency to develop additional fistulas with the passage of time.

The management of pulmonary arteriovenous fistulas is primarily surgical, and because only the lesion itself need be removed, most can be managed by either local or wedge resection. In the presence of bilateral fistulas, the side with the major involvement is usually treated and the remaining lung approached only as necessary. Some patients have also been managed by selective arterial embolization.[36] Penetrating pulmonary injuries can also produce this type of arteriovenous fistula, which should be surgically corrected.[34]

TABLE 2. Ten-Year Experience in Incidence of Congenital and Acquired Arteriovenous Fistula*

	Congenital	Acquired
AV fistulas of the extremities	80	17
Aorta–inferior vena cava fistulas	0	7
Pulmonary AV fistulas	47	0
Renal AV fistulas	0	6
AV fistulas of the portal system	0	1
AV fistulas of the neck and face	11	4
Pelvic AV fistulas	1	5
AV fistulas of the chest wall	0	2
Total	139	42

*Adapted from Gomes, M. M. R., and Bernatz, P. E.: Mayo Clin. Proc., *45*:81, 1970.

Acquired fistulas are most frequently seen in the extremities and are often secondary to penetrating trauma with accompanying varices, edema, and pigmentation. Vascular insufficiency of the digits and ulceration may also be present in the more severe forms. A palpable *thrill* is usually present at the site of the fistula, as is an audible coarse machinery-like bruit. The extremity is generally warmer than the control, and compression of the fistula usually results in a diminished heart rate and an increase in diastolic arterial pressure.

Iatrogenic fistulas have been described as a result of a variety of surgical procedures including operations on the kidney and intervertebral discs. Iatrogenic fistulas following thyroid surgery, coronary artery bypass grafting, distal splenorenal shunts, small bowel resection, and pelvic surgery have been described.[7, 8, 10, 24, 39] Central venous catheterization and percutaneous transhepatic variceal embolization for bleeding varices have also been complicated by arteriovenous fistulas.[2, 11] Renal arteriovenous fistulas after nephrectomy are usually large communications, and high cardiac failure is not uncommon.[20] All such fistulas should be surgically closed. Intervertebral disc procedures may also be associated with fistulas in the iliac vessels or aortic-calvic fistulas.[16] Atherosclerosis in the wall of aneurysms can also erode into accompanying veins, the prominent example being that of an aortocaval fistula from an abdominal aneurysm. Such a lesion may place the patient precipitously in congestive heart failure and require emergent surgical correction.

In current practice, the most common *acquired* arteriovenous fistula is that associated with vascular *access* to permit renal dialysis in the management of renal insufficiency. Problems associated with this type of fistula are discussed in Chapter 19. Arteriovenous fistulas have also been surgically constructed to increase blood flow and patency through vascular anastomoses such as those used in venous reconstruction and limb salvage procedures.[6, 18]

MANAGEMENT

Since most arteriovenous fistulas are actually or potentially symptomatic, closure of the communication is generally recommended. In congenital forms, excision of diffuse malformations may not be possible. The site of the fistula should always be carefully localized by arteriography, and the ideal surgical management is direct closure of the fistula with restoration of arterial and venous continuity. When this is not possible, quadripolar ligation is acceptable when there is sufficient arterial collateral circulation to adequately supply the tissues distally.[3] However, in the majority of patients it is possible to close the fistula without any distal ischemia or need for subsequent amputation.[1] Selective intra-arterial embolization is also a useful technique for treating these lesions, as previously mentioned. Rarely, a small fistula may close spontaneously as was reported in 5 of 245 patients surveyed in World War II.[32]

SELECTED REFERENCES

Gomes, M. M. R., and Bernatz, P. E.: Arteriovenous fistulas: A review and ten-year appearance at the Mayo Clinic. Mayo Clin. Proc., *45*:81, 1970.
This article reports a large series of patients with congenital and acquired arteriovenous fistulas over a 10-year period at the Mayo Clinic. It is a valuable reference work and provides data on the large numbers of specific types of these lesions.

Holman, E.: Abnormal Arteriovenous Communications. Springfield, Ill., Charles C Thomas, 1968.
This monograph is a world classic and an often-cited authoritative reference on the entire subject of arteriovenous fistulas. All aspects of these lesions are considered from both the experimental and clinical viewpoints. This work deservedly won its author the Samuel D. Gross Prize.

REFERENCES

1. Beall, A. C., Jr., Diethrich, E. B., Morris, G. C., Jr., and DeBakey, M. E.: Surgical management of vascular trauma. Surg. Clin. North Am., *46*:1001, 1966.
2. Bedell, J. E., Keller, F. S., and Rosch, J.: Iatrogenic intrahepatic arterial-portal fistula. Radiology, *151*:79, 1984.
3. Bramman F.: Das arteriell-venous Aneurysma. Arch. Klin. Chir., *33*:1, 1886.
4. Branham, H. H.: Aneurismal varix of the femoral artery and vein following a gunshot wound. Int. J. Surg., *3*:250, 1890.
5. Breschet, G.: Memoire sur les aneurysmes. Mem. Acad. Roy. Med. (Paris), *3*:101, 1883.
6. Dardik, H., Sussman, B., Ibrahim, I. M., Kahn, M., Svoboda, J. J., Mendes, D., and Dardik, I.: Distal arteriovenous fistula as an adjunct to maintaining arterial and graft patency for limb salvage. Surgery, *94*:478, 1983.
7. Decker, D. G., Fish, C. R., and Juergens, J. L.: Arteriovenous fistulas of the female pelvis. A diagnostic problem. Obstet. Gynecol., *31*:799, 1968.
8. Diehl, J. T., and Beven, E. G.: Arteriovenous fistulas of the mesenteric vessels. Report of a case and review of the literature. J. Cardiovasc. Surg., *23*:334, 1982.
9. Gomes, M. M. R., and Bernatz, P. E.: Arteriovenous fistulas: A review and ten-year experience at the Mayo Clinic. Mayo Clin. Proc., *45*:81, 1970.
10. Gonzalez, E. M., Garcia, I. G., Blanch, G. G., Garcia, I. L., and Gonzalez, J. S.: Left gastric artiovenous fistula after selective distal splenorenal shunt. Surgery, *93*:510, 1983.
11. Hansbrough, J. F., Narrod, J. A., and Rutherford, R.: Arteriovenous fistulas following central venous catheterization. Intensive Care Med., *9*:287, 1983.
12. Holman, E.: Abnormal Arteriovenous Communications. Springfield, Ill, Charles C Thomas, 1968.
13. Hunter, W.: The history of an aneurysm of the aorta, with some remarks on aneurysms in general. Med. Observ. Inquir., *1*:323, 1757.
14. Janes, J. M., and Jennings, W. K., Jr.: Effect of induced arteriovenous fistula on leg length: 10-year observations. Mayo Clin. Proc., *36*:1, 1961.
15. Janes, J. M., and Musgrove, J. E.: Effect of induced arteriovenous fistula on growth of bone: An experimental study. Surg. Clin. North Am., *30*:1191, 1950.
16. Jarstfer, B. S., and Rich, N. M.: The challenge of arteriovenous fistula formation following disk surgery: A collective review. J. Trauma, *16*:726, 1976.
17. Kerber, C. W., Freeny, P. C., Cromwell, L., et al.: Cyanoacrylate occlusion of a renal arteriovenous fistula. Am. J. Roentgenol., *128*:663, 1977.
18. Levin, P. M., Rich, N. M., Hutton J. E., Barker, W. F., and Zeller, J. A.: A role of arteriovenous shunts in venous reconstruction. Am. J. Surg., *122*:183, 1971.
19. McAlister, D. S., Johnsrude, I., Miller, M. M., Clapp, J., and Thompson, W. M.: Occlusion of acquired renal arteriovenous fistula with transcatheter electrocoagulation. Am. J. Roentgenol. *132*:998, 1979.
20. McCutcheon, F. B., and Hara, M.: Arteriovenous fistula following nephrectomy. J Cardiovasc. Surg., *8*:253, 1967.
21. Moyer, J. H., Glantz, G., and Brest, A. N.: Pulmonary arteriovenous fistulas. Physiologic and clinical considerations. Am. J. Med., *32*:417, 1962.
22. Nicoladoni, C.: Phlebacteriectasie der rechten oberen Extremitat. Arch. Klin. Chir., *18*:252, 1975.
23. Norris, G. W.: Varicose aneurism at the bend of the arm: Ligature of the artery above and below the sac; secondary hemorrhages with a return of the aneurismal thrill on the tenth day; cure. Am. J. Med. Sci., *5*:27, 1843.
24. Przybojewski, J. Z.: Iatrogenic aortocoronary vein fistula. S. Afr. Med. J., *62*:908, 1982.
25. Ramchandani, P., Goldenberg, N. J., Soulen, R. L., and White, R. L., Jr.: Isobutyl 2-cyanoacrylate embolization of hepatoportal fistula. Am. J. Roentgenol., *140*:137, 1983.
26. Ricketts, R. R., Finck, E., and Yellin, A. E.: Management of major

arteriovenous fistulas by arteriographic techniques. Arch. Surg., *113*:1153, 1978.

27. Rienhoff, W. F., Jr., and Hamman, L.: Subacute *Streptococcus viridans* septicemia cured by the excision of an arteriovenous aneurysm of the external iliac artery vein. Ann. Surg., *102*:905, 1935.

28. Robinson, L. A., and Sabiston, D. C., Jr.: Syndrome of congenital internal mammary-to-pulmonary arteriovenous fistula associated with mitral valve prolapse. Arch. Surg., *116*:1265, 1981.

29. Sabiston, D. C., Jr., Theilen, E. O., and Gregg, D. E.: Physiologic studies in experimental high output cardiac failure produced by aortic-caval fistula. Surg. Forum, *6*:233, 1956.

30. Scott, H. W., Jr., and Sabiston, D. C., Jr.: Surgical treatment for congenital aorticopulmonary fistula. J. Thorac. Surg., *25*:26, 1953.

31. Shadle, O. W., Ferguson, T. B., Sabiston, D. C., Jr., and Gregg, D. E.: The hemodynamic response to lanatoside C of dogs with experimental aortic-caval fistulas. J. Clin. Invest., *36*:335, 1957.

32. Shumacker, H. B.: Arterial aneurysms and arteriovenous fistulas. Spontaneous cures. *In* Elkin, D. C., and DeBakey, M. E. (Eds.): Surgery in World War II: Vascular Surgery. Washington, D.C. Office of the Surgeon General, Department of Army, 1955.

33. Sumner, D. S.: Arteriovenous fisstula. Physiology and pathological anatomy. *In* Strandness, D. E., Jr. (Ed.): Collateral Circulation in Clinical Surgery. Philadelphia, W. B. Saunders Company, 1969.

34. Symbas, P. N., Goldman, M., Erbesfeld, M. H., and Vlasis, S. E.: Pulmonary arteriovenous fistula, pulmonary artery aneurysm, and other vascular changes of the lung from penetrating trauma. Ann. Surg., *191*:336, 1980.

35. Tafreshi, M., Steinbaum, S., Scarlett, K., and Alexander, L. L.: Ultrasonic demonstration of arteriovenous fistulas. J. Clin. Ultrasound, *12*:299, 1984.

36. Taylor, B. G., Cockerill, E. M., Manfredi, F., and Klatte, E. C.: Therapeutic embolization of the pulmonary artery in pulmonary arteriovenous fistula. Am. J. Med., *64*:360, 1978.

37. Tice, D. A., Clauss, R. H., Keirle, A. M., and Reed, G. E.: Congenital arteriovenous fistulae of the extremities: Observations concerning treatment. Arch. Surg., *86*:460, 1963.

38. Waldhausen, J. A., and Shumacker, H. B., Jr.: Pulmonary arteriovenous fistulae. Heart Bull., *14*:57, 1963.

39. Webster, M. W.: Arteriovenous fistula following thyroidectomy. J. Cardiovasc. Surg., *23*:515, 1982.

NORMAL VALUES

REX B. CONN, M.D.

48

INTRODUCTION

The quantitative procedures carried out in a clinical laboratory represent measurements of substances normally present within rather narrow ranges of concentration. In order to use such data, we must know the values to be expected in a normal individual and what is considered a significant deviation from normal. Actually, there can be no sharp dividing line between abnormal and normal values, since there is a gradual transition during any pathological process from what is clearly normal to what is clearly a pathological condition.

In medicine, it is a logical impossibility to define normality, and the term "reference values" has replaced the earlier term "normal values." Reference values are derived from statistical studies on subjects believed to have no condition that might affect the measurements under consideration. The traditional and most widely used statistical approach is to carry out the measurement on a large group of subjects and to set the reference limits at the mean value plus or minus two standard deviations. Since values obtained for many measurements are not Gaussian in distribution, additional steps are frequently used in calculation of the reference ranges. The important consideration is that the reference ranges derived by these statistical methods contain only 95 per cent of the reference population. Thus, a value slightly outside the reference range might be due either to chance distribution or to an underlying pathological process.

A single reference range for all individuals may be inadequate for some clinical measurements. Values obtained on presumably normal persons may vary because of age, sex, body build, race, environment, and state of gastrointestinal absorption. A universal caveat in the use of reference values is that for many procedures the reference range will vary with the method used. This is particularly true for enzyme measurements and measurements based upon immunochemical principles.

THE INTERNATIONAL SYSTEM OF UNITS FOR LABORATORY MEASUREMENTS (LE SYSTÈME INTERNATIONAL D'UNITÉS)

An extensive modification of the metric system has been adopted by clinical laboratories in many countries. This adaptation is the International System of Units (Le

TABLE 1. Base Units

Property	Base Unit	Symbol
Length	metre	m
Mass	kilogram	kg
Amount of substance	mole	mol
Time	second	s
Thermodynamic temperature	kelvin	K
Electric current	ampere	A
Luminous intensity	candela	cd

Système International d'Unités), usually abbreviated S.I. Units. Whereas the metric system utilizes the centimeter, the gram, and the second as base units, the International System uses the meter, the kilogram, and the second as well as four other base units.

The International System is a coherent approach to all types of measurement that utilizes seven dimensionally independent base quantities: mass, length, time, thermodynamic temperature, electric current, luminous intensity, and amount of substance. Each of these quantities is expressed in a clearly defined *base unit* (Table 1).

Two or more base units may be combined to provide *derived units* (Table 2) for expressing other measurements such as mass concentration (kilograms per cubic meter) and velocity (meters per second). Standardized prefixes (Table 3) for base and derived units are used to express fractions or multiples of the base units so that any measurement can be expressed in a value between 0.001 and 1000.

Medical Applications

The most profound change in laboratory reports will result from expressing concentration as amount per volume

TABLE 2. Derived Units

Derived Property	Derived Unit	Symbol
Area	square metre	m^2
Volume	cubic metre	m^3
	litre	l
Mass concentration	kilogram/cubic metre	kg/m^3
	gram/litre	g/l
Substance concentration	mole/cubic metre	mol/m^3
	mole/litre	mol/l ·
Temperature	degree Celsius	C = K − 273.15

TABLE 3. Standard Prefixes

Prefix	Multiplication Factor	Symbol
atto	10^{-18}	a
femto	10^{-15}	f
pico	10^{-12}	p
nano	10^{-9}	n
micro	10^{-6}	μ
milli	10^{-3}	m
centi	10^{-2}	c
deci	10^{-1}	d
deca	10^{1}	da
hecto	10^{2}	h
kilo	10^{3}	k
mega	10^{6}	M
giga	10^{9}	G
tera	10^{12}	T

(moles per liter) rather than mass per volume (milligrams per 100 milliliters). The advantages of the former expression can be seen in the following:

Conventional Units

    1.0 gram of hemoglobin
        Combines with 1.37 ml of oxygen
        Contains 3.4 mg of iron
        Forms 34.9 mg of bilirubin

S.I. Units

    1.0 mmol of hemoglobin
        Combines with 4.0 mmol of oxygen
        Contains 4.0 mmol of iron
        Forms 4.0 mmol of bilirubin

Chemical relationships between lactic acid and pyruvic acid and the glucose from which both are derived, as well as the relationship between bilirubin and the binding capacity of albumin, are other examples of chemical relationships that will be clarified by using the new system.

There are a number of laboratory and other medical measurements for which the S.I. Units appear to offer little advantage, and some that are disadvantageous because the change would require replacement or revision of instruments such as the sphygmomanometer. The cubic meter is the derived unit for volume; however, it is inappropriately large for medical measurements, and the liter has been retained. Thermodynamic temperature expressed in kelvins is not more informative for medical measurements. Since the Celsius degree is the same as the kelvin degree, the Celsius scale is used. Celsius rather than centigrade is the preferred term.

Selection of units for expressing enzyme activity presents certain difficulties. Literally dozens of different units have been used in expressing enzyme activity, and interlaboratory comparison of enzyme results is impossible unless the assay system is precisely defined. In 1964, the International Union of Biochemistry attempted to remedy the situation by proposing the International Unit for enzymes. This unit was defined as the amount of enzyme that will catalyze the conversion of 1 micromole of substrate per minute under standard conditions. Difficulties remain, however, as enzyme activity is affected by the temperature,

pH, the type and amount of substrate, the presence of inhibitors, and other factors. Enzyme activity can be expressed in S.I. Units, and the katal has been proposed to express activities of all catalysts, including enzymes. The katal is that amount of enzyme that catalyzes a reaction rate of 1 mole per second. Thus, adoption of the katal as the unit of enzyme activity would provide no more information than is obtained when results are expressed in International Units.

Hydrogen ion concentration in blood is customarily expressed as pH, but in S.I. Units it would be expressed in nanomoles per liter. It appears unlikely that the very useful pH scale will be discarded.

Pressure measures, such as blood pressure and partial pressures of blood gases, would be expressed in S.I. Units using the pascal, a unit that can be derived from the base units for mass, length, and time. This change probably will not be adopted in the early phases of the conversion to S.I. Units. Similarly, a proposed change in expressing osmolality in terms of the depression of freezing point is inappropriate, because osmolality may be calculated from vapor pressure as well as freezing point measurement.

Conventions

A number of conventions have been adopted to standardize usage of S.I. Units:

1. No periods are used after the symbol for a unit (kg not kg.), and it remains unchanged when used in the plural (70 kg not 70 kgs).

2. A half space rather than a comma is used to divide large numbers into groups of three (e.g., 5 400 000 not 5,400,000).

3. Compound prefixes should be avoided (nanometer not millimicrometer).

4. Multiples and submultiples are used in steps of 10^3 or 10^{-3}.

5. The degree sign for the temperature scales is omitted (38 C not 38°C).

6. The preferred spelling is metre not meter, litre not liter.

7. Report of a measurement should include information on the system, the component, the kind of quantity, the numerical value, and the unit. For example: *System,* serum. *Component,* glucose. *Kind of quantity,* substance concentration. *Value,* 5.10. *Unit,* mmol/l.

8. The name of the component should be unambiguous; for example, "serum bilirubin" might refer to unconjugated bilirubin or to total bilirubin. For acids and bases, the maximally ionized form is used in naming the component; for example, lactate or urate rather than lactic acid or uric acid.

Tables of Reference Values

Tables accompanying this article indicate "normal values" for most of the commonly performed laboratory tests. The title of the tables has been changed from the "normal values" of previous years to "reference values" to conform to current usage. The reference value is given in conventional units, and the value in S.I. Units is calculated from these figures. Notes (page 1207) provide additional information.

Reference Values in Hematology

	Conventional Units		S.I. Units		Notes
Acid hemolysis test (Ham)	No hemolysis		No hemolysis		
Alkaline phosphatase, leukocyte	Total score 14–100		Total score 14–100		
Carboxyhemoglobin	Up to 5% of total		0.05 of total		a
Cell counts					
Erythrocytes					
Males	4.6–6.2 million/cu mm		$4.6–6.2 \times 10^{12}/l$		
Females	4.2–5.4 million/cu mm		$4.2–5.4 \times 10^{12}/l$		
Children (varies with age)	4.5–5.1 million/cu mm		$4.5–5.1 \times 10^{12}/l$		
Leukocytes					
Total	4500–11,000/cu mm		$4.5–11.0 \times 10^{9}/l$		
Differential	*Percentage*	*Absolute*			
Myelocytes	0	0/cu mm	0/1		b
Band neutrophils	3–5	150–400/cu mm	$150–400 \times 10^{6}/l$		
Segmented neutrophils	54–62	3000–5800/cu mm	$3000–5800 \times 10^{6}/l$		
Lymphocytes	25–33	1500–3000/cu mm	$1500–3000 \times 10^{6}/l$		
Monocytes	3–7	300–500/cu mm	$300–500 \times 10^{6}/l$		
Eosinophils	1–3	50–250/cu mm	$50–250 \times 10^{6}/l$		
Basophils	0–0.75	15–50/cu mm	$15–50 \times 10^{6}/l$		
Platelets	150,000–350,000/cu mm		$150–350 \times 10^{9}/l$		
Reticulocytes	25,000–75,000/cu mm		$25–75 \times 10^{9}/l$		b
	0.5–1.5% of erythrocytes				

Bone marrow, differential cell count ·

	Range	*Average*	*Range*	*Average*	
Myeloblasts	0.3–5.0%	2.0%	0.003–0.05	0.02	a
Promyelocytes	1.0–8.0%	5.0%	0.01–0.08	0.05	
Myelocytes: Neutrophilic	5.0–19.0%	12.0%	0.05–0.19	0.12	
Eosinophilic	0.5–3.0%	1.5%	0.005–0.03	0.015	
Basophilic	0.0–0.5%	0.3%	0.00–0.005	0.003	
Metamyelocytes	13.0–32.0%	22.0%	0.13–0.32	0.22	
Polymorphonuclear neutrophils	7.0–30.0%	20.0%	0.07–0.30	0.20	
Polymorphonuclear eosinophils	0.5–4.0%	2.0%	0.005–0.04	0.02	
Polymorphonuclear basophils	0.0–0.7%	0.2%	0.00–0.007	0.002	
Lymphocytes	3.0–17.0%	10.0%	0.03–0.17	0.10	
Plasma cells	0.0–2.0%	0.4%	0.00–0.02	0.004	
Monocytes	0.5–5.0%	2.0%	0.005–0.05	0.02	
Reticulum cells	0.1–2.0%	0.2%	0.001–0.02	0.002	
Megakaryocytes	0.3–3.0%	0.4%	0.003–0.03	0.004	
Pronormoblasts	1.0–8.0%	4.0%	0.01–0.08	0.04	
Normoblasts	7.0–32.0%	18.0%	0.07–0.32	0.18	

Coagulation tests				Notes
Antithrombin III (synthetic substrate)	80–120% of normal		0.8–1.2 of normal	
Bleeding time (Duke)	1–5 min		1–5 min	
Bleeding time (Ivy)	Less than 5 min		Less than 5 min	
Bleeding time (template)	2.5–9.5 min		2.5–9.5 min	
Clot retraction, qualitative	Begins in 30–60 min		Begins in 30–60 min	
	Complete in 24 hrs		Complete in 24 h	
Coagulation time (Lee-White)	5–15 min (glass tubes)		5–15 min (glass tubes)	
	19–60 min (siliconized tubes)		19–60 min (siliconized tubes)	
Euglobulin lysis time	2–6 hr at 37°		2–6 h at 37 C	
Factor VIII and other coagulation factors	50–150% of normal		0.50–1.5 of normal	a
Fibrin split products (Thrombo-Wellco test)	Less than 10 mcg/ml		Less than 10 mg/l	
Fibrinogen	200–400 mg/dl		5.9–11.7 μmol/l	c
Fibrinolysins	0		0	
Partial thromboplastin time, activated (APTT)	20–35 sec		20–35 sec	
Prothrombin consumption	Over 80% consumed in 1 hr		Over 0.80 consumed in 1 h	a
Prothrombin content	100% (calculated from prothrombin time)		1.0 (calculated from prothrombin time)	a
Prothrombin time (one stage)	12.0–14.0 sec		12.0–14.0 sec	
Tourniquet test	Ten or fewer petechiae in a 2.5 cm circle after 5 min		Ten or fewer petechiae in a 2.5 cm circle after 5 min	
Cold hemolysin test (Donath-Landsteiner)	No hemolysis		No hemolysis	
Coombs' test				
Direct	Negative		Negative	
Indirect	Negative		Negative	

Table continued on following page

Reference Values in Hematology (*Continued*)

	Conventional Units	S.I. Units	Notes
Corpuscular values of erythrocytes (values are for adults; in children, values vary with age)			
MCH (mean corpuscular hemoglobin)	27–31 picogm	0.42–0.48 fmol	d
MCV (mean corpuscular volume)	80–96 cu micra	80–96 fl	
MCHC (mean corpuscular hemoglobin concentration)	32–36%	0.32–0.36	a
Haptoglobin (as hemoglobin binding capacity)	100–200 mg/dl	16–31 μmol/l	d
Hematocrit			
Males	40–54 ml/dl	0.40–0.54	a
Females	37–47 ml/dl	0.37–0.47	
Newborn	49–54 ml/dl	0.49–0.54	
Children (varies with age)	35–49 ml/dl	0.35–0.49	
Hemoglobin			
Males	14.0–18.0 grams/dl	2.17–2.79 mmol/l	d
Females	12.0–16.0 grams/dl	1.86–2.48 mmol/l	
Newborn	16.5–19.5 grams/dl	2.56–3.02 mmol/l	
Children (varies with age)	11.2–16.5 grams/dl	1.74–2.56 mmol/l	
Hemoglobin, fetal	Less than 1% of total	Less than 0.01 of total	a
Hemoglobin A_{1c}	3–5% of total	0.03–0.05 of total	a
Hemoglobin A_2	1.5–3.0% of total	0.015–0.03 of total	a
Hemoglobin, plasma	0–5.0 mg/dl	0–0.8 μmol/l	d
Methemoglobin	30–130 mg/dl	4.7–20 μmol/l	e
Osmotic fragility of erythrocytes	Begins in 0.45–0.39% NaCl	Begins in 77–67 mmol/NaCl	
	Complete in 0.33–0.30% NaCl	Complete in 56–51 mmol/l NaCl	
Sedimentation rate			
Wintrobe: Males	0–5 mm in 1 hr	0–5 mm/h	
Females	0–15 mm in 1 hr	0–15 mm/h	
Westergren: Male	0–15 mm in 1 hr	0–15 mm/h	
Females	0–20 mm in 1 hr	0–20 mm/h	
(May be slightly higher in children and during pregnancy)			

Reference Values for Blood, Plasma, and Serum
(For some procedures the reference values may vary depending upon the method used)

	Conventional Units	S.I. Units	Notes
Acetoacetate plus acetone, serum			
Qualitative	Negative	Negative	
Quantitative	0.3–2.0 mg/dl	3–20 mg/l	
Adrenocorticotropin (ACTH), plasma			
6 AM	10–80 picogm/ml	10–80 ng/l	
6 PM	Less than 50 picogm/ml	Less than 50 ng/l	
Alanine aminotransferase, *see* Transaminase			
Aldolase, serum	0–11 milliunits/ml (30°)	0–11 units/l (30 C)	f
Aldosterone			
Adult, supine	3–10 nanogm/dl	0.08–0.3 nmol/l	
standing			
male	6–22 nanogm/dl	0.17–0.61 nmol/l	
female	5–30 nanogm/dl	0.14–0.8 nmol/l	
Alpha amino nitrogen, serum	3.0–5.5 mg/dl	2.1–3.9 mmol/l	
Ammonia (nitrogen), plasma	15–49 mcg/dl	11–35 μmol/l	
Amylase, serum	25–125 milliunits/ml	25–125 units/l	
Anion gap	8–16 mEq/liter	8–16 mmol/l	
Ascorbic acid, blood	0.4–1.5 mg/dl	23–85 μmol/l	
Aspartate aminotransferase, *see* Transaminase			
Base excess, blood	0 ± 2 mEq/liter	0 ± 2 mmol/l	
Bicarbonate, serum	23–29 mEq/liter	23–29 mmol/l	
Bile acids, serum	0.3–3.0 mg/dl	3.0–30.0 mg/l	
Bilirubin, serum			
Direct	0.1–0.4 mg/dl	1.7–6.8 μmol/l	
Indirect	0.2–0.7 mg/dl (Total minus direct)	3.4–12 μmol/l (Total minus direct)	
Total	0.3–1.1 mg/dl	5.1–19 μmol/l	a

Table continued on opposite page

Reference Values for Blood, Plasma, and Serum (*Continued*)
(For some procedures the reference values may vary depending upon the method used)

Calcium, serum	4.5–5.5 mEq/liter	2.25–2.75 mmol/l
	9.0–11.0 mg/dl	
	(Slightly higher in children)	(Slightly higher in children)
	(Varies with protein concentration)	(Varies with protein concentration)
Calcium, ionized, serum	2.1–2.6 mEq/liter	1.05–1.30 mmol/l
	4.25–5.25 mg/dl	
Carbon dioxide content, serum		
Adults	24–30 mEq/liter	24–30 mmol/l
Infants	20–28 mEq/liter	20–28 mmol/l
Carbon dioxide tension (P_{CO_2}), blood	35–45 mm Hg	35–45 mm Hg g
Carotene, serum	40–200 mcg/dl	0.74–3.72 µmol/l
Ceruloplasmin, serum	23–44 mg/dl	230–440 mg/l h
Chloride, serum	96–106 mEq/liter	96–106 mmol/l
Cholesterol, serum		
Total	150–250 mg/dl	3.9–6.5 mmol/l
Esters	68–76% of total cholesterol	0.68–0.76 of total cholesterol a
Cholinesterase		
Serum	0.5–1.3 pH units	0.5–1.3 pH units f
Erythrocytes	0.5–1.0 pH unit	0.5–1.0 pH unit f
Copper, serum		
Males	70–140 mcg/dl	11–22 µmol/l
Females	85–155 mcg/dl	13–24 µmol/l
Cortisol, plasma		
8 AM	6–23 mcg/dl	170–635 nmol/l
4 PM	3–15 mcg/dl	82–413 nmol/l
10 PM	Less than 50% of 8 AM value	Less than 0.5 of 8 AM value
Creatine, serum	0.2–0.8 mg/dl	15–61 µmol/l
Creatine kinase, serum (CK, CPK)		
Males	12–80 milliunits/ml (30°)	12–80 units/l (30 C) f
	55–170 milliunits/ml (37°)	55–170 units/l (37 C) f
Females	10–55 milliunits/ml (30°)	10–55 units/l (30 C) f
	30–135 milliunits/ml (37°)	30–135 units/l (37 C) f
Creatine kinase isoenzymes, serum		
CK-MM	Present	Present
CK-MB	Absent	Absent
CK-BB	Absent	Absent
Creatinine, serum	0.6–1.2 mg/dl	53–106 µmol/l
Cryoglobulins, serum	0	0
Fatty acids, total, serum	190–420 mg/dl	7–15 mmol/l i
nonesterified, serum	8–25 mg/dl	0.30–0.90 mmol/l
Ferritin, serum	20–200 nanogm/ml	20–200 µg/l
Fibrinogen, plasma	200–400 mg/100 ml	5.9–11.7 µmol/l c
Folate, serum	1.8–9.0 nanogm/ml	4.1–20.4 nmol/l
Erythrocytes	150–450 nanogm/ml	340–1020 nmol/l
Follicle-stimulating hormone (FSH), plasma		
Males	4–25 milliunits/ml (I.U.)	4–25 IU/l
Females	4–30 milliunits/ml (I.U.)	4–30 IU/l
Postmenopausal	40–250 milliunits/ml (I.U.)	40–250 IU/l
Gamma glutamyltransferase		
Males	6–32 milliunits/ml (30°)	6–32 units/l (30 C) f
Females	4–18 milliunits/ml (30°)	4–18 units/l (30 C) f
Gastrin, serum	0–200 picogm/ml	0–200 ng/l
Glucose (fasting)		
Blood	60–100 mg/dl	3.33–5.55 mmol/l
Plasma or serum	70–115 mg/dl	3.89–6.38 mmol/l
Growth hormone, serum	0–10 nanogm/ml	0–10 µg/l
Haptoglobin, serum	100–200 mg/dl	16–31 µmol/l d
	(As hemoglobin binding capacity)	(As hemoglobin binding capacity)
Hydroxybutyric dehydrogenase, serum (HBD)	0–180 milliunits/ml (30°)	0–180 units/l (30 C) f
17-Hydroxycorticosteroids, plasma	8–18 mcg/dl	0.22–0.50 µmol/l j
Immunoglobulins, serum		
IgG	550–1900 mg/dl	5.5–19.0 g/l
IgA	60–333 mg/dl	0.60–3.3 g/l
IgM	45–145 mg/dl	0.45–1.5 g/l
IgD	0.5–3.0 mg/dl	5–30 mg/l
IgE	<500 nanogm/ml	<500 µg/l
	(Varies with age in children)	(Varies with age in children)
Insulin, plasma (fasting)	5–25 microunits/ml	36–179 pmol/l

Table continued on following page

Reference Values for Blood, Plasma, and Serum (*Continued*)
(For some procedures the reference values may vary depending upon the method used)

	Conventional Units	S.I. Units	Notes
Iodine, protein bound, serum	3.5–8.0 mcg/dl	0.28–0.63 μmol/l	k
Iron, serum	75–175 mcg/dl	13–31 μmol/l	
Iron binding capacity, serum			
Total	250–410 mcg/dl	45–73 μmol/l	
Saturation	20–55%	0.20–0.55	a
Lactate, blood, venous	4.5–19.8 mg/dl	0.5–2.2 mmol/l	
arterial	4.5–14.4 mg/dl	0.5–1.6 mmol/l	
Lactate dehydrogenase, serum (LD,	45–90 milliunits/ml (I.U.) (30°)	45–90 units/1 (30 C)	f
LDH)	100–190 milliunits/ml (37°)	100–190 milliunits/ml (37 C)	
LDH_1	22–37% of total	0.22–0.37 of total	
LDH_2	30–46% of total	0.30–0.46 of total	a
LDH_3	14–29% of total	0.14–0.29 of total	
LDH_4	5–11% of total	0.05–0.11 of total	
LDH_5	2–11% of total	0.02–0.11 of total	
Leucine aminopeptidase, serum	14–40 milliunits/ml (30°)	14–40 units/l (30 C)	f
Lipase, serum	0–1.5 units (Cherry-Crandall)	0–1.5 units (Cherry-Crandall)	f
Lipids, total, serum	450–850 mg/dl	4.5–8.5 g/l	m
Lipoprotein cholesterol, serum			
LDL cholesterol	60–180 mg/dl	600–1800 mg/l	
HDL cholesterol	30–80 mg/dl	300–800 mg/l	
Luteinizing hormone (LH), serum			
Males	6–18 milliunits/ml (I.U.)	6–18 IU/l	
Females, premenopausal	5–22 milliunits/ml (I.U.)	5–22 IU/l	
midcycle	3 times baseline	3 times baseline	
postmenopausal	Greater than 30 milliunits/ml (I.U.)	Greater than 30 IU/l	
Magnesium, serum	1.5–2.5 mEq/liter	0.75–1.25 mmol/l	
	1.8–3.0 mg/dl		
Nitrogen, nonprotein, serum	15–35 mg/dl	10.7–25.0 mmol/l	
5′-Nucleotidase, serum	3.5–12.7 milliunits/ml (37°)	3.5–12.7 units/l (37 C)	f
Osmolality, serum	285–295 mOsm/kg serum water	285–295 mmol/kg serum water	n
Oxygen, blood			
Capacity	16–24 vol % (varies with hemoglobin)	7.14–10.7 mmol/l (varies with hemoglobin)	o
Content Arterial	15–23 vol %	6.69–10.3 mmol/l	o
Venous	10–16 vol %	4.46–7.14 mmol/l	o
Saturation Arterial	94–100% of capacity	0.94–1.00 of capacity	a
Venous	60–85% of capacity	0.60–0.85 of capacity	a
Tension, PO_2 Arterial	75–100 mm Hg	75–100 mm Hg	g
P_{50}, blood	26–27 mm Hg	26–27 mm Hg	g
pH, arterial, blood	7.35–7.45	7.35–7.45	p
Phenylalanine, serum	Less than 3 mg/dl	Less than 0.18 mmol/l	
Phosphatase, acid serum	0.11–0.60 milliunit/ml (37°)	0.11–0.60 units/l	f
	(Roy, Brower, Hayden)		
Phosphatase, alkaline, serum (ALP)	20–90 milliunits/ml (30°)	20–90 units/l (30 C)	f
	(Values are higher in children)	(Values are higher in children)	
Phosphate, inorganic, serum			
Adults	3.0–4.5 mg/dl	1.0–1.5 mmol/l	
Children	4.0–7.0 mg/dl	1.3–2.3 mmol/l	
Phospholipids, serum	6–12 mg/dl	1.9–3.9 mmol/l	
	(As lipid phosphorus)	(As lipid phosphorus)	
Potassium, serum	3.5–5.0 mEq/liter	3.5–5.0 mmol/l	
Prolactin, serum			
Males	1–20 nanogm/ml	1–20 μg/l	
Females	1–25 nanogm/ml	1–25 μg/l	
Protein, serum			
Total	6.0–8.0 grams/dl	60–80 g/l	m
Albumin	3.5–5.5 grams/dl	35–55 g/l	q
	52–68% of total	0.52–0.68 of total	a
Globulin			
$Alpha_1$	0.2–0.4 gram/dl	2–4 g/l	m
	2–5% of total	0.02–0.05 of total	a
$Alpha_2$	0.5–0.9 gram/dl	5–9 g/l	m
	7–14% of total	0.07–0.14 of total	a
Beta	0.6–1.1 grams/dl	6–11 g/l	m
	9–15% of total	0.09–0.15 of total	a
Gamma	0.7–1.7 grams/dl	7–17 g/l	m
	11–21% of total	0.11–0.21 of total	a
Protoporphyrin, erythrocyte	27–61 mcg/dl packed RBC	0.48–1.09 μmol/l packed RBC	
Pyruvate, blood	0.3–0.9 mg/dl	0.03–0.10 mmol/l	

Table continued on opposite page

Reference Values for Blood, Plasma, and Serum (*Continued*)
(For some procedures the reference values may vary depending upon the method used)

	Conventional Units	S.I. Units	Notes
Sodium, serum	136–145 mEq/liter	136–145 mmol/l	
Sulfates, inorganic, serum	0.8–1.2 mg/dl	83–125 μmol/l	
Testosterone, plasma			
Males	275–875 nanogm/dl	9.5–30 nmol/l	
Females	23–75 nanogm/dl	0.8–2.6 nmol/l	
Pregnant	38–190 nanogm/dl	1.3–6.6 nmol/l	
Thyroid-stimulating hormone (TSH), serum	0–7 microunits/ml	0–7 milliunits/l	
Thyroxine, free, serum	1.0–2.1 nanogm/dl	13–27 pmol/l	
Thyroxine (T₄), serum	4.4–9.9 mcg/dl	57–128 nmol/l	
Thyroxine binding globulin (TBG), serum (as thyroxine)	10–26 mcg/dl	129–335 nmol/l	
Thyroxine iodine, serum	2.9–6.4 mcg/dl	229–504 nmol/l	k
Transaminase, serum			
SGOT (aspartate aminotransferase, AST)	8–20 milliunits/ml (30°) 7–40 milliunits/ml (37°)	8–20 units/l (30 C) 7–40 units/l (37 C)	
SGPT (alanine aminotransferase, ALT)	8–20 milliunits/ml (30°) 5–35 milliunits/ml (37°)	8–20 units/l (30 C) 5–35 units/l (37 C)	f f
Triglycerides, serum	40–150 mg/dl	0.4–1.5 g/l 0.45–1.71 mmol/l	r
Triiodothyronine (T₃), serum	150–250 nanogm/dl	2.3–3.9 nmol/l	
Triiodothyronine (T₃) uptake, resin (T₃RU)	25–38% uptake	0.25–0.38 uptake	a
Urate, serum			
Males	2.5–8.0 mg/dl	0.15–0.48 mmol/l	
Females	1.5–7.0 mg/dl	0.09–0.42 mmol/l	
Urea			
Blood	21–43 mg/dl	3.5–7.3 mmol/l	
Plasma or serum	24–49 mg/dl	4.0–8.3 mmol/l	
Urea nitrogen			
Blood	10–20 mg/dl	7.1–14.3 mmol/l	k
Plasma or serum	11–23 mg/dl	7.9–16.4 mmol/l	
Viscosity, serum	1.4–1.8 times water	1.4–1.8 times water	
Vitamin A, serum	20–80 mcg/dl	0.70–2.8 μmol/l	
Vitamin B₁₂, serum	180–900 picogm/ml	133–664 pmol/l	

Reference Values for Urine
(For some procedures the reference values may vary depending upon the method used)

	Conventional Units	S.I. Units	Notes
Acetone and acetoacetate, qualitative	Negative	Negative	
Albumin			
Qualitative	Negative	Negative	
Quantitative	10–100 mg/24 hrs	10–100 mg/24 h 0.15–1.5 μmol/24 h	q
Aldosterone	3–20 mcg/24 hrs	8.3–55 nmol/24 h	
Alpha amino nitrogen	50–200 mg/24 hrs	3.6–14.3 mmol/24 h	
Ammonia nitrogen	20–70 mEq/24 hrs	20–70 mmol/24 h	
Amylase	1–17 units/hr	1–17 units/h	f
Amylase/creatinine clearance ratio	1–4%	0.01–0.04	
Bilirubin, qualitative	Negative	Negative	
Calcium			
Low Ca diet	Less than 150 mg/24 hrs	Less than 3.8 mmol/24 h	
Usual diet	Less than 250 mg/24 hrs	Less than 6.3 mmol/24 h	
Catecholamines			
Epinephrine	Less than 10 mcg/24 hrs	Less than 55 nmol/24 h	
Norepinephrine	Less than 100 mcg/24 hrs	Less than 590 nmol/24 h	
Total free catecholamines	4–126 mcg/24 hrs	24–745 nmol/24 h	s
Total metanephrines	0.1–1.6 mg/24 hrs	0.5–8.1 μmol/24 h	t
Chloride	110–250 mEq/24 hrs (Varies with intake)	110–250 mmol/24 h (Varies with intake)	
Chorionic gonadotropin	0	0	
Copper	0–50 mcg/24 hrs	0–0.80 μmol/24 h	

Table continued on following page

Reference Values for Urine (*Continued*)
(For some procedures the reference values may vary depending upon the method used)

	Conventional Units	S.I. Units	Notes
Cortisol, free	10–100 mcg/24 hrs	27.6–276 mmol/24 h	
Creatine			
Males	0–40 mg/24 hrs	0–0.30 mmol/24 h	
Females	0–100 mg/24 hrs	0–0.76 mmol/24 h	
	(Higher in children and during pregnancy)	(Higher in children and during pregnancy)	
Creatinine	15–25 mg/kg body weight/24 hrs	0.13–0.22 mmol·kg⁻¹body weight/24 h	
Creatinine clearance			
Males	110–150 ml/min	110–150 ml/min	
Females	105–132 ml/min	105–132 ml/min	
	(1.73 sq meter surface area)	(1.73 m² surface area)	
Cystine or cysteine, qualitative	Negative	Negative	
Dehydroepiandrosterone	Less than 15% of total 17-ketosteroids	Less than 0.15 of total 17-ketosteroids	a
Males	0.2–2.0 mg/24 hrs	0.7–6.9 μm/24 h	
Females	0.2–1.8 mg/24 hrs	0.7–6.2 μm/24 h	
Delta aminolevulinic acid	1.3–7.0 mg/24 hrs	10–53 μmol/24 h	
Estrogens			
Males			
Estrone	3–8 μg/24 hrs	11–30 nmol/24 h	
Estradiol	0–6 μg/24 hrs	0–22 nmol/24 h	
Estriol	1–11 μg/24 hrs	3–38 nmol/24 h	
Total	4–25 μg/24 hrs	14–90 nmol/24 h	u
Females			
Estrone	4–31 μg/24 hrs	15–115 nmol/24 h	
Estradiol	0–14 μg/24 hrs	0–51 nmol/24 h	
Estriol	0–72 μg/24 hrs	0–250 nmol/24 h	
Total	5–100 μg/24 hrs	18–360 nmol/24 h	u
	(Markedly increased during pregnancy)	(Markedly increased during pregnancy)	
Glucose (as reducing substance)	Less than 250 mg/24 hrs	Less than 250 mg/24 h	
Hemoglobin and myoglobin, qualitative	Negative	Negative	
Homogentisic acid, qualitative	Negative	Negative	
17-Hydroxycorticosteroids			
Males	3–9 mg/24 hrs	8.3–25 μmol/24 h	j
Females	2–8 mg/24 hrs	5.5–22 μmol/24 h	
5-Hydroxyindoleacetic acid			
Qualitative	Negative	Negative	
Quantitative	Less than 9 mg/24 hrs	Less than 47 μmol/24 h	
17-Ketosteroids			
Males	6–18 mg/24 hrs	21–62 μmol/24 h	l
Females	4–13 mg/24 hrs	14–45 μmol/24 h	
	(Varies with age)	(Varies with age)	
Magnesium	6.0–8.5 mEq/24 hrs	3.0–4.3 mmol/24 h	
Metanephrines (see Catecholamines)			
Osmolality	38–1400 mOsm/kg water	38–1400 mmol/kg water	n
pH	4.6–8.0, average 6.0	4.6–8.0, average 6.0	p
	(Depends on diet)	(Depends on diet)	
Phenolsulfonphthalein excretion (PSP)	25% or more in 15 min	0.25 or more in 15 min	a
	40% or more in 30 min	0.40 or more in 30 min	
	55% or more in 2 hrs	0.55 or more in 2 h	
	(After injection of 1 ml PSP intravenously)	(After injection of 1 ml PSP intravenously)	
Phenylpyruvic acid, qualitative	Negative	Negative	
Phosphorus	0.9–1.3 gram/24 hrs	29–42 mmol/24 h	
Porphobilinogen			
Qualitative	Negative	Negative	
Quantitative	0–0.2 mg/dl	0–0.9 μmol/l	
	Less than 2.0 mg/24 hrs	Less than 9 μmol/24 h	
Porphyrins			
Coproporphyrin	50–250 mcg/24 hrs	77–380 nmol/24 h	
Uroporphyrin	10–30 mcg/24 hrs	12–36 nmol/24 h	
Potassium	25–100 mEq/24 hrs	25–100 mmol/24 h	
	(Varies with intake)	(Varies with intake)	
Pregnanediol			
Males	0.4–1.4 mg/24 hrs	1.2–4.4 μmol/24 h	
Females			
Proliferative phase	0.5–1.5 mg/24 hrs	1.6–4.7 μmol/24 h	
Luteal phase	2.0–7.0 mg/24 hrs	6.2–22 μmol/24 h	
Postmenopausal phase	0.2–1.0 mg/24 hrs	0.6–3.1 μmol/24 h	

Table continued on opposite page

Reference Values for Urine (*Continued*)
(For some procedures the reference values may vary depending upon the method used)

	Conventional Units	S.I. Units	Notes
Pregnanetriol	Less than 2.5 mg/24 hrs in adults	Less than 7.4 μmol/24 h in adults	
Protein			
Qualitative	Negative	Negative	
Quantitative	10–150 mg/24 hrs	10–150 mg/24 h	m
Sodium	130–260 mEq/24 hrs	130–260 mmol/24 h	
	(Varies with intake)	(Varies with intake)	
Specific gravity	1.003–1.030	1.003–1.030	
Titratable acidity	20–40 mEq/24 hrs	20–40 mmol/24 h	
Urate	200–500 mg/24 hrs	1.2–3.0 mmol/24 h	
	(With normal diet)	(With normal diet)	
Urobilinogen	Up to 1.0 Ehrlich unit/2 hrs	Up to 1.0 Ehrlich unit/2 h	
	(1–3 PM)	(1–3 PM)	
	0–4.0 mg/24 hrs	0–6.8 μmol/24 h	
Vanillylmandelic acid (VMA)	1–8 mg/24 hrs	5–40 μmol/24 h	
(4-hydroxy-3-methoxymandelic acid)			

Reference Values for Therapeutic Drug Monitoring

Drug	Therapeutic Range	Toxic Levels	Proprietary Names
Antibiotics			
Amikacin, serum	15–25 mcg/ml	Peak: >35 mcg/ml	Amikin
		Trough: >5–8 mcg/ml	
Chloramphenicol, serum	10–20 mcg/ml	>25 mcg/ml	Chloromycetin
Gentamicin, serum	5–10 mcg/ml	Peak: >12 mcg/ml	Garamycin
		Trough: >2 mcg/ml	
Tobramycin, serum	5–10 mcg/ml	Peak: >12 mcg/ml	Nebcin
		Trough: >2 mcg/ml	
Anticonvulsants			
Carbamazepine, serum	5–12 mcg/ml	>12 mcg/ml	Tegretol
Ethosuximide, serum	40–100 mcg/ml	>100 mcg/ml	Zarontin
Phenobarbital, serum	10–30 mcg/ml	Vary widely because of developed tolerance	
Phenytoin, serum (diphenylhydantoin)	10–20 mcg/ml	>20 mcg/ml	Dilantin
Primidone, serum	5–12 mcg/ml	>15 mcg/ml	Mysoline
Valproic acid, serum	50–100 mcg/ml	>100 mcg/ml	Depakene
Analgesics			
Acetaminophen, serum	10–20 mcg/ml	>250 mcg/ml	Tylenol
			Datril
Salicylate, serum	100–250 mcg/ml	>300 mcg/ml	
Bronchodilator			
Theophylline (aminophylline)	10–20 mcg/ml	>20 mcg/ml	
Cardiovascular drugs			
Digitoxin, serum	15–25 nanogm/ml (Specimen obtained 12–24 hrs after last dose)	>25 nanogm/ml	Crystodigin
Digoxin, serum	0.8–2 nanogm/ml (Specimen obtained 12–24 hrs after last dose)	>2.4 nanogm/ml	Lanoxin
Disopyramide, serum	2–5 mcg/ml	>5 mcg/ml	Norpace
Lidocaine, serum	1.5–5 mcg/ml	>5 nanogm/ml	Anestacon
			Xylocaine
Procainamide, serum	4–10 mcg/ml	>16 mcg/ml	Pronestyl
	*10–30 mcg/ml (*Procainamide + *N*-Acetyl Procainamide)	*>30 mcg/ml	
Propranolol, serum	50–100 nanogm/ml	Variable	Inderal
Quinidine, serum	2–5 mcg/ml	>10 mcg/ml	Cardioquin
			Quinaglute
			Quinidex
			Quinora

Table continued on following page

Reference Values for Therapeutic Drug Monitoring (*Continued*)

Drug	Therapeutic Range	Toxic Levels	Proprietary Names
Psychopharmacologic drugs			
Amitriptyline, serum	*120–150 nanogm/ml (*Amitriptyline + Nortriptyline)	*>500 nanogm/ml	Amitril Elavil Endep Etralon Limbitrol Triavil
Desipramine, serum	*150–300 nanogm/ml (*Desipramine + Imipramine)	*>500 nanogm/ml	Norpramin Pertofrane
Imipramine, serum	*150–300 nanogm/ml (*Imipramine + Desipramine)	*>500 nanogm/ml	Antipress Imavate Janimine Presamine Tofranil
Lithium, serum	0.8–1.2 mEq/liter (Specimen obtained 12 hrs after last dose)	>2.0 mEq/liter	Lithobid Lithotabs
Nortriptyline, serum	50–150 nanogm/ml	>500 nanogm/ml	Aventyl Pamelor

Reference Values in Toxicology

	Conventional Units	S.I. Units	Notes
Arsenic, blood	3.5–7.2 mcg/dl	0.47–0.96 μmol/l	
Arsenic, urine	Less than 100 mcg/24 hrs	Less than 1.3 μmol/24 h	
Bromides, serum	0 Toxic levels: Above 17 mmol/l	0 Toxic levels: Above 17 mmol/l	
Carbon monoxide, blood	Up to 5% saturation Symptoms occur with 20% saturation	Up to 0.05 saturation Symptoms occur with 0.20 saturation	a
Ethanol, blood	Less than 0.005%	Less than 1 mmol/l	
Marked intoxication	0.3–0.4%	65–87 mmol/l	
Alcoholic stupor	0.4–0.5% mcg/dl	87–109 mmol/l	
Coma	Above 0.5%	Above 109 mmol/l	
Lead, blood	0–40 mcg/dl	0–2 μmol/l	
Lead, urine	Less than 100 mcg/24 hrs	Less than 0.48 μmol/24 h	
Mercury, urine	Less than 100 mcg/24 hrs	Less than 50 nmol/24 h	

Reference Values for Cerebrospinal Fluid

	Conventional Units	S.I. Units	Notes
Cells	Fewer than 5/cu mm; all mononuclear	Fewer than 5/μl; all mononuclear	
Chloride	120–130 mEq/liter (20 mEq/liter higher than serum)	120–130 mmol/l (20 mmol/l higher than serum)	
Electrophoresis	Predominantly albumin	Predominantly albumin	
Glucose	50–75 mg/dl (20 mg/dl less than serum)	2.8–4.2 mmol/l (1.1 mmol/l less than serum)	
IgG			
Children under 14	Less than 8% of total protein	Less than 0.08 of total protein	a,m
Adults	Less than 14% of total protein	Less than 0.14 of total protein	
Pressure	70–180 mm water	70–180 mm water	g
Protein, total	15–45 mg/dl (Higher, up to 70 mg/dl, in elderly adults and children)	0.150–0.450 g/l (Higher, up to 0.70 g/l, in elderly adults and children)	m

Reference Values for Gastric Analysis

	Conventional Units	S.I. Units	Notes
Basal gastric secretion (1 hour)			
Concentration	(Mean ± 1 S.D.)	(Mean ± 1 S.D.)	
Males	25.8 ± 1.8 mEq/liter	25.8 ± 1.8 mmol/l	
Females	20.3 ± 3.0 mEq/liter	20.3 ± 3.0 mmol/l	

Table continued on opposite page

Reference Values for Gastric Analysis (*Continued*)

	Conventional Units	S.I. Units	Notes
Output	(Mean ± 1 S.D.)	(Mean ± 1 S.D.)	
Males	2.57 ± 0.16 mEq/hr	2.57 ± 0.16 mmol/h	
Females	1.61 ± 0.18 mEq/hr	1.61 ± 0.18 mmol/h	
After histamine stimulation			
Normal	Mean output 11.8 mEq/hr	Mean output 11.8 mmol/h	
Duodenal ulcer	Mean output 15.2 mEq/hr	Mean output 15.2 mmol/h	
After maximal histamine stimulation			
Normal	Mean output 22.6 mEq/hr	Mean output 22.6 mmol/h	
Duodenal ulcer	Mean output 44.6 mEq/hr	Mean output 44.6 mmol/h	
Diagnex blue (Squibb):			
Anacidity	0–0.3 mg in 2 hrs	0–0.3 mg in 2 h	
Doubtful	0.3–0.6 mg in 2 hrs	0.3–0.6 mg in 2 h	
Normal	Greater than 0.6 mg in 2 hrs	Greater than 0.6 mg in 2 h	
Volume, fasting stomach content	50–100 ml	50–100 ml	
Emptying time	3–6 hrs	3–6 h	
Color	Opalescent or colorless	Opalescent or colorless	
Specific gravity	1.006–1.009	1.006–1.009	
pH (adults)	0.9–1.5	0.9–1.5	p

Gastrointestinal Absorption Tests

	Conventional Units	S.I. Units
D-Xylose absorption test	After an 8 hour fast, 10 ml/kg body weight of a 0.05 solution of D-xylose is given by mouth. Nothing further by mouth is given until the test has been completed. All urine voided during the following 5 hours is pooled, and blood samples are taken at 0, 60, and 120 minutes. Normally 0.26 (range 0.16–0.33) of ingested xylose is excreted within 5 hours, and the serum xylose reaches a level between 25 and 40 mg/100 dl after 1 hour and is maintained at this level for another 60 minutes.	No change
Vitamin A absorption	A fasting blood specimen is obtained and 200,000 units of vitamin A in oil is given by mouth. Serum vitamin A level should rise to twice fasting level in 3 to 5 hours.	No change

Reference Values for Feces

	Conventional Units	S.I. Units	Notes
Bulk	100–200 grams/24 hrs	100–200 g/24 h	
Dry matter	23–32 grams/24 hrs	23–32 g/24 h	
Fat, total	Less than 6.0 grams/24 hrs	Less than 6.0 g/24 h	
Nitrogen, total	Less than 2.0 grams/24 hrs	Less than 2.0 g/24 h	
Urobilinogen	40–280 mg/24 hrs	40–280 mg/24 h	
Water	Approximately 65%	Approximately 0.65	a

Reference Values for Immunologic Procedures

	Conventional Units
Lymphocyte subsets	
T cells	60–85%
B cells	1–20%
T-helper cells	35–60%
T-suppressor cells	15–30%
T-H/S ratio	1.5–2.5
Complement	
C3	85–175 mg/dl
C4	15–45 mg/dl
CH_{50}	25–55 H_{50} units/ml
Tumor markers	
Carcinoembryonic antigen (CEA)	
(Roche)	Less than 5 nanogm/ml
(Abbott)	Less than 4.1 nanogm/ml
Alpha-fetoprotein (AFP)	Less than 10–30 nanogm/ml (depends on method)

Reference Values for Semen Analysis

	Conventional Units	S.I. Units	Notes
Volume	2–5 ml; usually 3–4 ml	2–5 ml; usually 3–4 ml	
Liquefaction	Complete in 15 min	Complete in 15 min	
pH	7.2–8.0; average 7.8	7.2–8.0; average 7.8	p
Leukocytes	Occasional or absent	Occasional or absent	
Count	60–150 million/ml	60–150 million/ml	
	Below 60 million/ml is abnormal	Below 60 million/ml is abnormal	
Motility	80% or more motile	0.80 or more motile	a
Morphology	80–90% normal forms	0.80–0.90 normal forms	a

Oral Glucose Tolerance Test

The oral glucose tolerance test (OGTT) may be unnecessary if the fasting plasma glucose concentration is elevated (venous plasma ≥140 mg/dl or 7.8 mmol/l) on two occasions. The OGTT should be carried out only on patients who are ambulatory and otherwise healthy and who are known not to be taking agents that elevate the plasma glucose (see reference 9). The test should be conducted in the morning after at least 3 days of unrestricted diet (≥150 grams of carbohydrate) and physical activity. The subject should have fasted for at least 10 hours but no more than 16 hours. Water is permitted during the test period; however, the subject should remain seated and should not smoke throughout the test.

The dose of glucose administered should be 75 grams (1.75 grams per kg of ideal body weight, up to a maximum of 75 grams for children). Commercial preparations containing a suitable carbohydrate load are acceptable. If criteria for gestational diabetes are used, a dose of 100 grams of glucose is required.

A fasting blood sample should be collected, after which the glucose dose is taken within 5 minutes. Blood samples should be collected at 30 minute intervals for 2 hours (for gestational diabetes, fasting 1, 2 and 3 hours). The following diagnostic criteria have been recommended by the National Diabetes Data Group:

Normal OGTT in Nonpregnant Adults
Fasting venous plasma glucose <115 mg/dl (6.4 mmol/l); ½ h, 1 h, and 1½ h OGTT venous plasma glucose <200 mg/dl (11.1 mmol/l); 2 h OGTT venous plasma glucose <140 mg/dl (7.8 mmol/l)

Diabetes Mellitus in Nonpregnant Adults
Both the 2 hour sample *and* some other sample taken between administration of the 75 gram glucose dose and 2 hours later must show a venous plasma glucose ≥200 mg/dl (11.1 mmol/l)

Impaired Glucose Tolerance in Nonpregnant Adults
Three criteria must be met: Fasting venous plasma glucose <140 mg/dl (7.8 mmol/l); ½ h, 1 h, or 1½ h OGTT value ≥200 mg/dl (11.1 mmol/l); 2 h OGTT venous plasma glucose between 140 and 200 mg/dl (7.8 and 11.1 mmol/l)

Gestational Diabetes
Two or more of the following values after a 100 gram oral glucose challenge must be met or exceeded:
(values are for venous plasma glucose)

Fasting	105 mg/dl	5.8 mmol/l
1h	190 mg/dl	10.6 mmol/l
2h	165 mg/dl	9.2 mmol/l
3h	145 mg/dl	8.1 mmol/l

NOTES

a. Percentage is expressed as a decimal fraction.

b. Percentage may be expressed as a decimal fraction; however, when the result expressed is itself a variable fraction of another variable, the absolute value is more meaningful. There is no reason, other than custom, for expressing reticulocyte counts and differential leukocyte counts in percentages or decimal fractions rather than in absolute numbers.

c. Molecular weight of fibrinogen = 341,000 daltons.

d. Molecular weight of hemoglobin = 64,500 daltons. Because of disagreement as to whether the monomer or tetramer of hemoglobin should be used in the conversion, it has been recommended that the conventional grams per deciliter be retained. The tetramer is used in the table; values given should be multiplied by 4 to obtain concentration of the monomer.

e. Molecular weight of methemoglobin = 64,500 daltons. See note d above.

f. Enzyme units have not been changed in these tables because the proposed enzyme unit, the katal, has not been universally adopted (1 International Unit = 16.7 nkat).

g. It has been proposed that pressure be expressed in the pascal (1 mm Hg = 0.133 kPa); however, this convention has not been universally accepted.

h. Molecular weight of ceruloplasmin = 151,000 daltons.

i. "Fatty acids" includes a mixture of different aliphatic acids of varying molecular weight. A mean molecular weight of 284 daltons has been assumed in calculating the conversion factor.

j. Based upon molecular weight of cortisol 362.47 daltons.

k. The practice of expressing concentration of an organic molecule in terms of one of its constituent elements originated when measurements included a heterogeneous class of compounds (nonprotein nitrogenous compounds, iodine-containing compounds bound to serum proteins). It was carried over to expressing measurements of specific substances (urea, thyroxine), but the practice should be discarded. For iodine and nitrogen 1 mole is taken as the monoatomic form, although they occur as diatomic molecules.

l. Based upon molecular weight of dehydroepiandrosterone 288.41 daltons.

m. Weight per volume is retained as the unit because of the heterogeneous nature of the material measured.

n. The proposal that osmolality be reported as freezing point depression using the millikelvin as the unit has not been received with universal enthusiasm. The milliosmole is not an S.I. unit, and the unit used here is the millimole.

o. Volumes per cent might be converted to a decimal fraction; however, this would not permit direct correlation with hemoglobin content, which is possible when oxygen content and capacity are expressed in molar quantities. One millimole of hemoglobin combines with 4 millimoles of oxygen.

p. Hydrogen ion concentration in S.I. units would be expressed in nanomoles per liter; however, this change has not received general approval. Conversion can be calculated as antilog ($-$pH).

q. Albumin is expressed in grams per liter to be consistent with units used for other proteins. Concentration of albumin may be expressed in mmol/l also, an expression that permits assessment of binding capacity of albumin for substances such as bilirubin. Molecular weight of albumin is 65,000 daltons.

r. Most techniques for quantitating triglycerides measure the glycerol moiety, and the total mass is calculated using an average molecular weight. The factor given assumes a mean molecular weight of 875 daltons for triglycerides.

s. Calculated as norepinephrine, molecular weight 169.18 daltons.

t. Calculated as metanephrine, molecular weight 197.23 daltons.

u. Conversion factor calculated from molecular weights of estrone, estradiol, and estriol in proportions of 2:1:2.

REFERENCES

1. AMA Drug Evaluations, 5th ed. Chicago, American Medical Association, 1983.
2. AMA Council on Scientific Affairs: J.A.M.A. *253*:2552, 1985.
3. Gilman, A. G., Goodman, L. S.: Goodman and Gilman's The Pharmacological Basis of Therapeutics, 7th ed. New York, Macmillan, 1985.
4. Henry, J. B.: Clinical Diagnosis and Management by Laboratory Methods, 17th ed. Philadelphia, W. B. Saunders Company, 1984.
5. Henry, R. J., Cannon, D. C., and Winkleman, J. W.: Clinical Chemistry—Principles and Techniques, 2nd ed. New York, Harper & Row, 1974.
6. International Committee for Standardization in Hematology, International Federation of Clinical Chemistry and World Association of Pathology Societies: Clin. Chem. *19*:135, 1973.
7. Lundberg, G. D., Iverson, C., and Radulescu, G.: J.A.M.A. *255*:2247, 1986.
8. Miale, J. B.: Laboratory Medicine—Hematology, 6th ed. St. Louis, C. V. Mosby, 1982.
9. National Diabetes Data Group: Diabetes *28*:1039, 1979.
10. Page, C. H., and Vigoureux, P.: The International System of Units (S.I.). U.S. Department of Commerce, National Bureau of Standards, Special Publication 330, 1974.
11. Physicians' Desk Reference, 40th ed. Oradell, N.J., Medical Economics Company, 1986.
12. Scully, R. E., McNeely, B. U., and Mark, E. J.: N. Engl. J. Med. *314*:39, 1986.
13. Tietz, N. W.: Clinical Guide to Laboratory Tests. Philadelphia, W. B. Saunders Company, 1983.
14. Tietz, N. W.: Textbook of Clinical Chemistry: Philadelphia, W. B. Saunders Company, 1986.
15. Williams, W. J., Beutler, E., Erslev, A. J., and Lichtman, M. A.: Hematology, 3rd ed. New York, McGraw-Hill Book Company, 1983.

Some of the values have been established by the Clinical Pathology Laboratories, Emory University Hospital, Atlanta, Georgia, and have not been published elsewhere.

Note: Page numbers in *italics* refer to illustrations; page numbers followed by (t) refer to tables.

Abdomen, abscess in, 154, 157, *204*, 204–205, *205*
  acute, 388–404. See also *Abdominal pain.*
  air in, 392, *392*
  anastomotic breakdown in, 205
  mass in, in children, 679–681
  pain in. See *Abdominal pain.*
  sepsis in, 153–154, 204–205
    changed mental status as sign of, 203
    treatment of, antimicrobials in, 157, 157(t)
      drainage in, 154, 157, 204–205, *205*
  surgery of, dehiscence of wound after, 120
  trauma to, 189–195
    diagnosis of, 189–191
      angiography in, 190–191
      computed tomography in, 190, *190*
      peritoneal lavage in, 183, 189
      radionuclide scanning after, 190
  wall of, congenital defects of, 671–672
Abdominal aorta, aneurysm of, 401–402
Abdominal esophagus, 363, 364
Abdominal pain, 388–404
  causes of, 389(t), 393(t), 393–404
    diagnosis of, 388–393
      auscultation in, 389
      Cullen's sign in, 391
      iliopsoas test in, 391, *391*
      inspection in, 389
      laboratory tests in, 393
      Murphy's sign in, 391
      obturator test in, 391, *391*
      palpation in, 389–390
      patient history in, 388–389
      pelvic examination in, 391
      percussion in, 390
      physical examination in, 389–391
      radiography in, 392, *392*
      rectal examination in, 391
      Rovsing's sign in, 391, *391*
    location of pain in relation to, *390*
      gut origin of involved organs and, 388, *389*
  Crohn's disease and, 444, 481
  in female patients, 388, 395, 402–403
  in male patients, 395, 403–404
  pancreatitis and, 398, 602, 604, 605
Abdominoperineal resection, of rectum, for cancer, 492–494, *493*, 494(t)
ABO cross-matching, before transplantation, 229
Abortion, radio- or chemotherapy as indication for, 325
  septic, 403
Abscess, amebic, 504, 523–524, *524*
  complications of, 523, *525*
  anorectal, 507, *508*
  Bartholin's gland, 813
  breast, 302, *302*

Abscess (*Continued*)
  interloop, 205
  intra-abdominal, 154, 157, *204*, 204–205, *205*
  intraperitoneal, 154, 204–205
  liver, 154, 521–524, *522*
    amebic, 504, 523–524, *524*
      complications of, 523, *525*
    pyogenic, 521(t), 521–524
  lung, 984, *984*
  pancreatic, 607
  parapharyngeal, 699
  perinephric, 834
  peritonsillar, 699
  pyogenic, of liver, 521(t), 521–523
  retropharyngeal, 699
  splenic, 630–631
  subhepatic, 204, 205
  subphrenic, 204
    drainage of, 204–205, *205*
  surgical treatment of, 153
  visceral, 154, 205
Absorbable sutures, 136, 137
Absorption, 433–435
  disorders of. See *Malabsorption.*
Absorption tests, 1205(t)
Acalculous cholecystitis, 565
Accelerated rejection, 228
Accessory conducting pathways, 1156–1157, *1157*
  surgery for, 1156–1162, *1158, 1159, 1161*
    intracardiac electrode catheter study preceding, *1156*
Accessory spleens, 616, 630
Acetabulum, fracture of, 762
Acetylcholine receptor antibodies, in myasthenia gravis, 1037
Achalasia, *374*, 374–376, *375*
Acid-base balance, 53–54
  disorders of, 57(t), 57–60, 65
    compensatory responses to, 55–57, 57(t)
    treatment of, 65
Acid-base nomogram, *56*
Acid injury, to esophagus, 368, 678–679
Acidosis, 57(t), 59–60
  metabolic, 57(t), 60, 60(t), 65
    treatment of, 65
  respiratory, 57(t), 59(t), 59–60
Acoustic neuroma, 694
Acquired immune deficiency syndrome (AIDS), 173–177, 174(t)
  Kaposi's sarcoma in, 177, 800
  opportunistic infections in, 176(t), 176–177, 987
  pathogen causing, 173, 270
    antibodies to, 175
      tests for, 173, 175(t)
    tests for, 173, 175(t)
  pediatric cases of, standards for differential diagnosis of, 174(t)

Acquired immune deficiency syndrome (AIDS) (*Continued*)
  symptom complex related to (ARC), 173, 174(t)
  transfusion-transmitted, 94, 175
Acromegaly, 353
Actinomycosis, 166
  of lung, 987
Activated partial thromboplastin time, 88–89
Acupuncture, 114
Acute disorders. See specific conditions, e.g., *Pancreatitis, acute.*
Addison's disease, 360
Adenocarcinoma, of appendix, 467
  of breast, 309, 313. See also *Breast cancer.*
  of colon. See *Colorectal cancer.*
  of endometrium, 816–817
  of lung, 999, *1002*
  of pancreas, *599*, 609
  of small intestine, Crohn's disease and, 445
  of stomach, 423–424
Adenohypophysis, hormones secreted by, 351–352
  excess of, 353–354
  hypothalamic hormones affecting, 352(t)
  precursor(s) of, *352*
  tumors of, 353–354
Adenoiditis, 699
Adenoma, ACTH-secreting, 353, 356–358
  laboratory findings in patients with, 357(t)
  adrenal, 356–358
    CT findings in, 356, *356*
    laboratory findings in patients with, 357(t)
  bronchial, 1008
  endocrine-active, 353–354
  endocrine-inactive, 353
  gallbladder, 575
  gastrin-secreting, 417–418, 449, 610(t), 611
  glucagon-secreting, 610(t), 611
  growth hormone–secreting, 353
  hepatocellular, 544, *544*
  insulin-secreting, 610(t), 611
  islet cell, 610(t), 610–612
  liver, 544, *544*
  parathyroid, 342, 345, *345*, 346, *347*
    in mediastinum, 1032–1033
  pituitary, 353–354
    extension of, diaphragma sellae and, 350
  prolactin-secreting, 354
  prostate, 841–842
  somatostatin-secreting, 610(t), 612
  thyroid, intrathoracic, 1032
  vasoactive intestinal polypeptide–secreting, 449, 610(t), 612

Adenomatoid malformation of lung, 663
Adenomatous polyp, of colon, and colorectal cancer, 485
of stomach, 423
Adenomyosis, 816
Adenosine triphosphate, production of, *14*
Adhesion, platelet, 82–83
Adhesive tape, in surgery, 137, *137*
Adoptive immunotherapy, for cancer, 283
Adrenal(s), *354*, 354
carcinoma of, 358–359
hormones secreted by, 355
deficiency of, 72, 360
excess of, 356–361
resection of, for aldosteronism, 359
for Cushing's syndrome, 358
for pheochromocytoma, 361
in treatment of prostate cancer, 844
tumors of, 356–358, 360–361
CT findings in, 356, *356*
laboratory findings in patients with, 357(t)
Adrenal cortex, 354, *355*
hormones secreted by, 355
deficiency of, 72, 360
excess of, 356–359
Adrenal insufficiency, 72, 360
Adrenal medulla, hormones secreted by, 355
excess of, 72, 360–361
Adrenalectomy, for aldosteronism, 359
for Cushing's syndrome, 358
for pheochromocytoma, 361
in treatment of prostate cancer, 844
medical, for Cushing's syndrome, 358
in treatment of breast cancer, 324
Adrenergic agonists, for bronchospasm, 975
Adrenocorticotropic hormone, 38, 351
secretion of, by pituitary, 351
by tumor, 353, 356–358, 357(t)
excessive, 353, 356–358, 357(t)
Adrenogenital syndrome, 359–360
Adson maneuver, 1011
Adult respiratory distress syndrome, 25, *26*, 210
mechanical ventilation for, 211
postoperative, 210
Advanced life support, 1058–1059
Advancement flap, in reconstructive surgery, after radical neck dissection for cancer, *726*, 729
Adventitia, vascular, 80
Aerobic bacteria, gastrointestinal, 144(t)
antimicrobials effective against, 157(t)
Aerobic bacterial infection, necrotizing, of soft tissue, 159(t)
surgical, 145(t)–146(t), 146. See also *Bacterial infection, surgical.*
Aerodigestive tract, 707, 711, *711*
epithelium of, 708, *709*, 711
injury-induced changes in, 708
premalignant to malignant, 710. See also *Head and neck cancer.*
Afferent loop syndrome, 419
Afferent neurologic pathways, 97
Afterload, 18, 1179
Aganglionic megacolon, 668, *668*
Aggregation, of platelets, 79, 80(t), 82, 83
laboratory tests of, 88, *88*
Agitation, postoperative, 202
Agnogenic myeloid metaplasia, 629
AIDS (acquired immune deficiency syndrome). See *Acquired immune deficiency syndrome (AIDS).*
AIDS-related complex (ARC), 173, 174(t)

Air, in abdomen, 392, *392*
in biliary tract, 558
in mediastinum, 1022–1023
in peritoneum, due to gastric perforation, 670
in newborn, 670, *670*
in pleural space, 989–990
in newborn, 661, *661*
in trauma patients, 181
in portal vein, 392, *392*
Air contrast barium enema, in examination of colon, 475
Air exchange, emergency assessment of, 181
trauma compromising, 181–182
Airway, artificial, emergency use of, 181
cancer compromising, radiation therapy for, 275
emergency management of, 181, 976
in CPR, 1056
hemangioma compromising, in newborn, 658
intubation of, 976, 976(t)
Airway obstruction, relief of, 181
Albumin, serum levels of, as index of nutritional status, 102, 103(t)
synthesis of, in liver, 518
Alcohol abuse, and acute pancreatitis, 601
and delirium tremens, 203
and smoking, as risk factors in cancer, of head and neck, 706
of larynx, *706*
management of surgical patients with history of, 74
Aldosterone, 37, 355
hypersecretion of, 359
Aldosteronism, 359
Alkali injury, to esophagus, 367–368, 678–679
Alkaline reflux gastritis, after gastrectomy, 420
Alkalosis, 57(t), 57–59
metabolic, 57(t), 58–59, 59(t), 65
treatment of, 65
respiratory, 57(t), 58
Alkylating agents, in cancer chemotherapy, 278
Allen test, of arteries of wrist, 741
Allergic rhinitis, 696
Alpha-fetoprotein, 281
in hepatoma, 281
Alpha granules, of platelets, 82
Alpha toxin, 158
Alveolar membrane, hyalinization of, 25, *26*
Alveolar ventilation, 55, *55*
Amastia, 290
Amaurosis fugax, as sign of carotid artery disease, 894, 920–923
Ambiguous genitalia, 812–813, 854
in newborn, 674
Ambulation, in treatment of atelectasis, 208
Amebiasis, 504, 523–524, *524*
complications of, 523, *525*
Amenorrhea, 821
Amino acids, in parenteral nutrition, 24–25, 104
metabolism of, in liver, 518
Amino-amide and amino-ester local anesthetics, 114
Aminoglutethimide, medical adrenalectomy with, in treatment of breast cancer, 324
Aminophylline, 1180

Ampulla of Vater, carcinoma of, 578–579, *579*
inflammation of, 583
Amputation injury, of hand, 752–753, *754*
reimplantation following, *265*
Amylase, 593
elevated serum levels of, 602
Amylase-creatinine clearance ratio, in acute pancreatitis, 603
Anaerobic bacteria, gastrointestinal, 144(t)
antimicrobials effective against, 157(t)
Anaerobic bacterial infection, necrotizing, of soft tissue, 159(t), 162
surgical, 145(t)–146(t), 146. See also *Bacterial infection, surgical.*
Anal sphincter, *505*
resection of, for anal fissure, 507, *507*
Analgesia, 110
refrigeration, 115
Analgesics, 1203(t)
in management of burns, 127
in treatment of atelectasis, 208
Anaplastic carcinoma, of thyroid, 338
Anastomosis, intra-abdominal, breakdown of, 205
of vessels involved in acute trauma, 197
Anastomotic stapling, in bronchial closure, 1004, *1004*
in gastric surgery for obesity, *428*
in intestinal surgery, *493*
in transection of esophagus, *535*
Anatomic dead space, in lung, 973
Anatomical studies, Vesalius's contributions to, 1
Androgen(s), 355
blocking of, in treatment of prostate cancer, 844
excess of, in women, 822–823
Anemia, after gastrectomy, 421, 448
hemolytic, 625–628
splenectomy for, 625–626
in Crohn's disease, 444–445
sickle cell, 627
preparation of surgical patients with, 66
transfusion for, in surgical patients, 66
Anergy, 102
and surgical infection, 68
Anesthesia, 109–116
and dependence on mechanical ventilation, 210
and hepatitis, 216
cardiac arrest during, 1059
complications of, 116
conditions contraindicating, 116
development of, 2
electrical, 115
failure to awaken from, 202
general, 110–113
inhalation, 111–112
intravenous, 110–111
local, 114
monitoring during, 115
neuromuscular blocking agents in, 112–113
premedication and, 109–110
preoperative preparation and, 109
regional (nerve block), 113–114
sequelae of, 116
visit with patient after, 116
visit with patient before, 110
Aneurysm(s), *861*, 904–908, 906(t), *907*
abdominal aortic, 401–402
and peripheral arterial occlusion, 900
carotid artery, 866

Aneurysm(s) (*Continued*)
  coronary artery, congenital, *1135*, 1136
  false, of hand, 742
  intracranial, 865–866, *867*
  left ventricular, 1125
    surgery for, 1125–1126, *1126*
  peripheral artery, hemodynamics of, 891–892
  splenic artery, 630
  ventricular tachycardia associated with, results of directed surgical treatment of, 1162(t)
Angiocardiography, in diagnosis of tetralogy of Fallot, 1090, *1091*
  radionuclide, 1117, *1117*
Angiodysplasia, colonic, 502–503
Angiofibroma, juvenile, of nasopharynx, 700
Angiofollicular lymphoid hyperplasia, 1034
Angiography, as aid to diagnosis, of cancer of pancreas, 598–599, *599*
  of trauma to abdomen, 190–191
  digital subtraction, 861–862
  spleen on, 620, *621*
Angioma, of brain, 866–867
  of spinal cord, 868–869
Angiomyolipoma, of kidney, 833
Angioplasty, balloon, for chronic arterial occlusive disease, 911
  for coarctation of aorta, 1069, *1070*
  for myocardial ischemia, 1118–1119
Angiosarcoma, 800
Angiotensin, 38, 355, 836, 928
Angiotensin II inhibition, by captopril, 1180
Animal bite, of hand, 751
Ankle, fracture of, 766–767, *767*
Ann Arbor classification, in staging of lymphoma, 632(t)
Annular pancreas, 600
Anomalous pulmonary venous connection, *1082*, 1082–1083
  surgery for, 1084, *1084*
Anorchia, 850
Anorectum, *505*
  disorders of, 504, 506–510
    in Crohn's disease, 445
Anorexia, postoperative, 218
Anovulation, androgen excess and, 822–823
Antacid, in prophylaxis against stress ulcers, 417
Anterior cervical lymph nodes, 715
Anterior cord syndrome, 872–873
Anterior pituitary, hormones secreted by, 351–352
  excess of, 353–354
  hypothalamic hormones affecting, 352(t)
  precursor(s)of, *352*
  tumors of, 353–354
Anterior resection, of rectum, for cancer, 492–494, *493*, 494(t)
Antibiotic(s). See *Antimicrobial(s)*.
Antibody (antibodies), acetylcholine receptor, in myasthenia gravis, 1037
  antidonor/anti-idiotypic, induction of tolerance with, 233
  monoclonal, 282
    in detection of antigens, 226
    in detection of mediastinal tumors, 1026
    in suppression of transplant rejection, 232, 238
    in treatment of cancer, 282

Antibody (antibodies) (*Continued*)
  to hepatitis antigens, 165, 170(t), *172*
  to HTLV-III/LAV antigen, 175
    tests for, 173, 175(t)
  to T cells, in reversal of transplant rejection, 232
  to tumor antigens, 281, 282
Antibody-dependent cell-mediated cytotoxicity, in rejection, 228
Anticholinergic(s), for bronchospasm, 975
Anticoagulant, lupus, 89
Anticoagulant therapy, for deep venous thrombosis, 942
  in prophylaxis against stroke, 924, 925
  management of surgical patients receiving, 65
Anticonvulsant(s), 1203(t)
  for seizure disorders, in surgical patients, 74
Antidiuretic hormone, 38, 352
  for bleeding esophageal varices, 529, 530(t)
  secretion of, inappropriate, 49, 215
Antidonor antibody, induction of tolerance with, 233
Antigen(s), carcinoembryonic, 281
  in cancer, of colon, 281, 495
  cell surface, 224
  detection of, monoclonal antibodies in, 226
  donor vs. recipient, transplantation based on minimal disparity in, 230
  hepatitis, 165, 170(t), *172*
    antibodies to, 165, 170(t), *172*
  histocompatibility, 224, *225*, 225(t)
  HLA, 224, *225*, 225(t)
    Class I, 224, *225*, 225(t)
    Class II, 224, *225*, 225(t)
      dendritic cells as source of, 226
    pre-transplant typing for match of, 230, 238
  HLA-DR, pre-transplant typing for match of, 231
  HTLV-III/LAV, antibodies to, 173, 175, 175(t)
    tests for, 173, 175(t)
  induction of tolerance with, 233
  oncofetal, 281
  T4, 226
  T8, 226
  tolerance to, 232–234
  transplantation, tumor-specific, 281
  tumor, 281
    antibodies to, 281, 282
Anti-idiotypic antibody, induction of tolerance with, 233
Antilymphocyte globulin, in reversal of transplant rejection, 232, 238
Antimetabolites, in cancer chemotherapy, 278
Antimicrobial(s), and *Clostridium difficile*–associated colitis, 161–162, 503–504
  cephalosporin, 157(t)
    cost of, 157(t)
  colonic flora–inhibiting, 157, 157(t), 476(t)
  for abscess, of liver, 523
  for cholangitis, 570
  for Crohn's disease, 483
  for gas gangrene, 159
  for intra-abdominal sepsis, 157, 157(t)
  for pneumonia, 209
  for surgical infection, 153, 154(t), 155(t)
  in cancer chemotherapy, 278

Antimicrobial(s) (*Continued*)
  in prophylaxis against surgical infection, 68, 120, 150–152
    in procedures not usually requiring coverage, 151(t)
  ototoxic, 694
  toxicity of, 156(t), 1203(t)
Antimuscarinics, for bronchospasm, 975
Antimycobacterial drugs, 996, 996(t)
Antiplatelet therapy, in prophylaxis against stroke, 924, 925
Antireflux surgery, 380–381, *381*
  in children, 675
Antisepsis, 132–134
  early advocates of, 141
  intestinal, 68, 475–476
  iodine in, 132, *133*
Antiseptic, preoperative showering with, as means of reducing postsurgical infection, 149
Antishock garment, 182–183
Antitachycardia devices, 1162
Antithrombin III, heparin interaction with, 85, *86*
Antithymocyte globulin, in reversal of transplant rejection, 232
Antitoxin, clostridial, problems with use of, in cases of gas gangrene, 159
Antivenom, for snake bite, 199
Antrectomy, for peptic ulcer, 413
Anuria, 44
Anus. See also *Anorectum*.
  abscess of, 507
  cancer of, 508, *509*, 510
  fissures of, 506
    treatment of, 506–507, *507*
  imperforate, 668–669, *669*
  pruritus of, 510
  resection of, for cancer, 510
  squamous cell carcinoma of, 508, 510
Anxiety, postoperative, 202
Aorta, abdominal, aneurysm of, 401–402
  ascending, diseases of, 1138
  coarctation of, 1064–1067, *1066*
    percutaneous transluminal balloon angioplasty for, 1069, *1070*
    surgery for, 1067–1069, 1067–1071
      recurrence after, 1070–1071
  thoracic, transection of, radiographic findings in, 189
  trauma to, 189
Aortic arch, double, and vascular ring, 661, *661*, *1072*, 1072–1074, *1073*
Aortic cusp, left, fusion of, to aortic wall, with occlusion of left coronary ostium, 1136
Aortic valve, 1137
  inadequate functioning (insufficiency) of, *1138*, 1138–1139
    treatment of, by replacement with prosthetic valve, 1139, *1140*
  replacement of, with prosthesis, 1139, *1140*
  stenosis of, acquired, 1137, *1138*
    congenital, 1109–1113, *1110–1112*
Aortoplasty with patch graft, for coarctation of aorta, 1069, *1069*
Aortopulmonary window, 1071, *1071*
Apathy, in cancer patients, after surgery, 203
Aperistalsis, esophageal, in scleroderma, 376, *376*
Apert's syndrome, 877
Apical lymph node group, 291, *292*
Apoplexy, pituitary, 353

Appendectomy, for inflammation, *465*, 465–466
Appendix. See *Vermiform appendix.*
ARC (AIDS-related complex), 173, 174(t)
Area of body surface, region-specific surface areas as percentage of, 124–125
  age-related changes in, *124*, 125
  estimation of extent of burn based on, 124
Arginine test, 597
Arm, fractures of, 749, 758–761
  trauma to, 186
Arrhythmia(s), accessory conducting pathways and, 1156–1157, *1157*
  as complication of coronary artery bypass graft, 1122
  peri- and postoperative, management of, 1182–1183, *1184*
  surgical treatment of, 1156–1162, *1158, 1159, 1161*
    directed vs. nondirected, 1160(t), 1162(t)
    intracardiac electrode catheter study preceding, *1156*
Arrhythmogenic right ventricular dysplasia, 1162
Arterial blood gases, control of, by mechanical ventilation, 978
  in evaluation of pulmonary function, *970*, 970–971
Arterial cannulation, in cardiopulmonary bypass, 1187
Arteriography, as aid to diagnosis, of arterial trauma, 197
  of cancer of pancreas, 598–599, *599*
  of pulmonary embolism, 957, *958*, 959(t), *960*
  as aid to evaluation of urogenital system, 833
  in carotid artery disease, 923–924
  in chronic occlusive vascular disease, 910
  peripheral, 897–898, *898*
Arterioles, receptor pharmacology of, 1180(t)
Arteriovenous fistula, 1191–1193
  of hand, 742
  splenic, 630
Arteriovenous malformations, in brain, 866–868
Arteriovenous shunt, in hemodialysis, 213, *214*
Arteritis, 912–915
Artery (arteries). See also specific arteries, e.g., *Renal artery.*
  aneurysm of, 904–908, 906(t), *907*
    hemodynamics of, 891–892
  embolism of, 92, 898–903, *902*
  inflammatory disease of, 912–915
  occlusive disease of, chronic, 908–912, *913*
  peripheral, *888*
    aneurysm of, hemodynamics of, 891–892
    disease of, classification of, 887–889, *889*
      diagnosis of, 892–898
      hemodynamics of, 889–892, *890*
      management of, 898, *899*
      vs. deep venous thrombosis, 900–901
  reconstruction of, for chronic occlusive disease, 911
  thrombosis of, 82, 898–903, *902*
  trauma to, 196–199, 903–904, *904*

Arthritis, 789–790
  of hand, 751
  pyogenic, 786–787
Arthrodesis, for arthritis, 790
Arthroplasty, for arthritis, 790
Artificial airway, emergency use of, 181
Artificial heart, *1127*, 1127–1128, *1128*
Ascending aorta, diseases of, 1138
Ascites, 546
  chylous, 638
  pancreatic, 607–608, *608*
  shunt procedures in treatment of, 546–547, *547*
Asepsis, 132–134
  iodine in, 132, *133*
Aspergilloma, 167
Aspergillosis, 167, 986–987, *987*
Aspirated foreign body, as cause of respiratory emergency in child, 674
Aspiration, in diagnosis of cancer, 269
  of lung, *1002*, 1002–1003, *1003*
  of amebic abscess, of liver, 524
  of cells, from breast, 298–299
    from thyroid, *332*, 332–333
  of cyst, of breast, 298, *300*
Aspiration pneumonitis, 984
Aspirin, anti-platelet effect of, *88*, 90
Asplenia, 621
Astrocytoma, 864
Atelectasis, *208*, 208–209
  postoperative, 70, 208–209
    fever due to, 202
Atherosclerosis, and chronic occlusive disease, 908
  and extracranial cerebrovascular disease, 919
  and peripheral arterial occlusion, 899–900
  coronary artery, 1114, 1115, *1115*
    after heart transplantation, 258
  renal, 836
Atlas, fracture of, 185, 769, *769*
Atracurium, 113
Atresia, anal, 668–669, *669*
  biliary, 579–580, 673–674
    surgery for, *581, 673*, 673–674, *674*
  choanal, 657, 695
  duodenal, 664, *664*
  ear canal, 691
  esophageal, 659, *659*, 660
  intestinal, 665
    correction of, 665, *667*
  tricuspid, 1098
    surgery for, 1099, *1099*
  vaginal, 680
Atrial flutter-fibrillation, drugs for, 1182, 1183
  surgical treatment of, 1159
Atrial septum, defects of, 1076–1081, *1078*
  development and partitioning of, 1077, *1077*
Atrial tachycardia, ectopic, surgical treatment of, 1159
  paroxysmal, as complication of coronary artery bypass graft, 1122
Atrioventricular block, pacemaker for, 1170
Atrioventricular canal defects, *1078*, 1079–1081
  surgery for, *1080*, 1081
Atrioventricular valves, 1143
Atrium, myxoma of, 1164, 1165, *1165*
  surgery for, *1167*

Atropine, for bronchospasm, 975
Atypical hyperplasia/dysplasia, 710
Atypical mycobacteria, 994–995
Auscultation, in diagnosis of cause of abdominal pain, 389
  mitral regurgitation on, 1149
  mitral stenosis on, 1145
  signs of obstruction of small intestine on, 438
Autoclave, instrument sterilization with, 133
Autoimmune hemolytic anemia, 628
Autotransplantation, 261–268
Avascular necrosis, of capital femoral epiphysis, *778*, 778–779, *779*
  of lunate, 749
Awakening (recovery) from anesthesia, impaired, 202
Axilla, palpation of, in diagnosis of breast cancer, 295, *296*
Axillary lymph nodes, 291
  breast cancer involving, 309
    physical examination for, 295, *296*
    treatment of, 317
Axillary vein(s), 290, *291*
Axillary vein lymphatics, 291, *292*
Axis, fracture of, 185
Axonotmesis, 873
Azathioprine, 231–232
  in suppression of transplant rejection, 232
  infection in heart transplant patients treated with, 257, *258*
Azotemia, postrenal, postoperative, 44, 214
  prerenal, 44
    polyuric, 47
    postoperative, 211–212
    vs. renal azotemia, 45, 45(t), 213(t)
  renal. See *Renal failure, acute.*

Bacteria, colonic, antimicrobials effective against, 157, 157(t), 476(t)
  gastrointestinal, 143, 144(t)
  in stool, *476*
Bacterial infection, defense mechanisms against, 142
  defects in, 142–143
  in AIDS, 176(t)
  necrotizing, of soft tissue, 159(t)
  surgical, 141–165
    antimicrobial prophylaxis against, 150–152
    antimicrobial treatment of, 153, 154(t), 155(t)
    diagnosis of, 147–148
    microbiology of, 143, 145(t)–146(t), 146–147
    surgical treatment of, 153
    wound in, 148–150
  tissue susceptibility to, 142
  virulence of pathogen in, 142
Bacterial overgrowth, in blind loop syndrome, 449
Bacterial pericarditis, 1050
Bacteroides fragilis, antimicrobial prophylaxis against infection by, in colon surgery, 152
Balance sense, 687
  disturbances in, 690
  organs of, 687, *688*
Balanitis, 845

Balanoposthitis, 845
Balkan nephropathy, 837
Balloon insertion techniques, as means of
    treatment, of biliary stricture, 574
    of bleeding esophageal varices, 530–531,
        531
    of chronic arterial occlusive disease, 911
    of coarctation of aorta, 1069, *1070*
    of myocardial ischemia, 1118–1119
Bankhardt lesion, 758
Barium contrast studies, as aid to diagno-
        sis, of colon cancer, 490
    of Crohn's disease, 445, 481, *482*
    of diverticulitis, 498, *498, 499*
    of duodenal ulcer, 411, *412*
    of ischemic colitis, 502, *502*
    in examination of colon, 475
Barlow test, for congenital hip dislocation,
        776, *776*
Barotrauma, middle and inner ear involve-
        ment in, 693–694
Bartholin's gland, abscess of, 813
Basal cell carcinoma, *795,* 795–796
    of external ear, 691
Basement membrane, 792
Basic life support, 1055–1058
Bassini, Edoardo, 6, *6*
Bassini operation, for inguinal hernia, 639,
        641, *643–644*
B cell, 226
BCG, for cancer, 282
Bell's palsy, 693
Belsey Mark IV operation, 381, *381*
Bench surgery, 266
Bennett's fracture, *748*
Bent inner tube sign, in sigmoid volvulus,
        500, *500*
Beta-adrenergic blocking agents, 1181
    for hyperthyroidism, 333
Beta-streptococcal infection, and gangrene,
        163
Bicarbonate, pancreatic secretion of, 593
    renal reabsorption of, arterial PCO_2 and,
        56, *56*
Bifascicular block, pacemaker for, 1170
Bile, 553–554, *556*
    composition of, 554
    drainage of, percutaneous transhepatic
        catheterization in, 560, *561*
    Gram staining of, 152
    leak of, jaundice due to, 218
        postoperative, 217–218, *218*
    lipids in, 554
    loss of, fluids replacing, 42
    production of, 517, 553–554, *555*
        effects of shock on, 16
    T-tube drainage of, obstruction due to,
        217, *217*
Bile duct(s), 516, 551, *552.* See also *Biliary
        tract.*
    carcinoma of, 539, *539,* 577–578, *578*
    common, 587
        cyst of, 580–582, *581,* 682, *683*
        in relation to pancreatic duct, *589*
        obstruction of, by T-tube, *217*
        stones in, 565–568, *566*
            management of, 566–568, *567*
        surgery of, with resection of biliary
            stricture, 574, *574*
        trauma to, 195
    contrast studies of, 560, *560,* 599–
        600
    endoscopy in delineation of, 560, *560,*
        584

Bile duct(s) (*Continued*)
    inflammation of, 569–573
        acute, 569–570
        pyogenic, recurrent, 572–573
        sclerosing, 570–572, *572*
    tumors of, 539, 575, 577, 578
Bile salts, 433, 554
Biliary colic, 562
Biliary dyskinesia, 582
Biliary-enteric fistula, 568–569
Biliary tract, 551. See also *Bile duct(s).*
    air in, 558
    anatomy of, 551, *552,* 553
    anomalies of, 553, *553,* 579–582
    atresia of, 579–580, 673–674
        surgery for, *581,* 673, 673–674, *674*
    bile leak from, jaundice due to, 218
        postoperative, 217–218, *218*
    blood vessels supplying, 553
    cells of, 551
    cystic dilatation of, 580–582, 682
    development of, 551
    disease of, aids to diagnosis of, 558–561
        and acute pancreatitis, 601
        and malabsorption, 449
    function of, 553–556
    hemorrhage into, 535–537, *536,* 583
    lymphatics of, 553
    nerves supplying, 553
    obstruction of, by T-tube, 217, *217*
        jaundice due to, 217
        postoperative, 217
    stricture of, 573
        balloon dilatation of, 574
        surgery for, *574,* 574–575, *575*
    surgery of, antimicrobial prophylaxis
            against infection in, 152
        complications of, 217–218
        for acute pancreatitis, 604
        stricture formation after, 573
    trauma to, 195
    surgical, 218
Bilirubin, 215
    elevated serum levels of, 558
    metabolism of, 519, 554, *555,* 556
Billroth, Theodor, 3, *4, 6*
Billroth I anastomosis, after gastrectomy
        for peptic ulcer, *413*
Billroth II anastomosis, after gastrectomy
        for peptic ulcer, *413*
    afferent loop syndrome as complication
        of, 419
Biopsy, in diagnosis of cancer, 268–269
    of esophagus, 367(t)
    of lung, *1002,* 1002–1003, *1003*
    in diagnosis of lymphoma, 631
    of breast, 298–300, *299*
        in mammary cancer, 269, 299, 315
    of liver, 528, 561
    of mediastinal tumors, 1026
    of pericardium, 1052
    of scalene lymph nodes, in lung cancer,
        1003
    of thyroid, *332,* 332–333
Bites, 199, 751
B-K mole syndrome, 797
Bladder, 828
    calculi in, 836–837
    distention of, in children, 680
    dysfunction of, postoperative, 74
    exstrophy of, 837
    inflammation of, 840
        infection-related, postoperative, 164
        specimen collection in, 146

Bladder (*Continued*)
    neurogenic, 839–840
    reflux from, 837
    resection of, for cancer, 838–839
    trauma to, 196
Blalock, Alfred, 5, *5*
Blalock-Taussig shunt, in management of
        tricuspid atresia, 1099
Blastomycosis, 166–167, 985, *986*
Bleeding. See *Hemorrhage.*
Bleeding time, 88
Blind loop syndrome, *449,* 449–450
Blood, collection of specimen of, in diag-
        nosis of infection, 147
    in examination for signs of hormone-
        secreting pancreatic tumors, 600
    denaturation of, in cardiopulmonary by-
        pass, 1188, *1189*
    fecal, testing for, in diagnosis of colorec-
        tal cancer, 490
    in pleural space, 990
    laboratory reference values for, 1197(t)–
        1201(t)
    therapeutic use of, 93
Blood dyscrasias, splenectomy for, 625(t),
        625–630
Blood loss. See *Hemorrhage.*
Blood pressure, measurement of, in man-
        agement of trauma, 182
    in peripheral artery disease, 895
Blood volume, 31
    in newborn, 656
    restitution of, *47,* 47–48
Blunt trauma, to chest, 188–189
Bochdalek hernia, *661,* 661–662
    repair of, 662, *662*
Body fluid dynamics. See *Fluid* entries.
Body surface area, region-specific surface
        areas as percentage of, 124–125
    age-related changes in, *124,* 125
    estimation of extent of burn based on,
        124
Boerhaave's syndrome, 422
Bohr effect, 15
Bone. See also specific bones, e.g., *Femur.*
    cancer metastatic to, 789
        radiation therapy for, 275
    infection of, 785–787
    radionuclide scanning of, in breast can-
        cer, 309
    tumors of, 787–789, 788(t)
Bone graft, 264
    in reconstructive surgery, after radical
        neck dissection for cancer, 729
Bone marrow, suppression of, cancer che-
        motherapy and, 279
Bone marrow graft, 266
Boutonnière deformity, 746–747, *747*
Bowen's disease, 795, 846
Brachial plexus, compression of, 915–916,
        1011
    injury of, 873
Brachiocephalic vessels, exposure of, 198
Brachycephaly, 877
Brachytherapy, 272
Bradycardia, 1182
Brady-tachyarrhythmia syndrome, pace-
        maker for, 1170
Brain, *857,* 857–858, *858*
    arteriovenous malformations in, 866–868
    bleeding in, 185, 868
        and stroke, 920
    cancer metastatic to, radiation therapy
        for, 275

Brain (*Continued*)
  effects of cardiopulmonary bypass on, 1189
  effects of shock on, 17–18
  infection of, 885–886
  trauma to, 184–185
  tumors of, 862–863, *863*
Brain death, 235, 235(t)
  and organ donation for transplantation, 235
Breakdown, anastomotic, intra-abdominal, 205
Breast, abscess of, 302, *302*
  absence of, 290
  adenocarcinoma of, 309, 313. See also *Breast cancer.*
  anatomy of, 289, *289*
  anomalies of, 290
  bacterial infection of, 301–302
  benign disease of, 300–304
  biopsy of, 298–300, *299*
    in mammary cancer, 269, 299, 315
  blood vessels supplying, 290, *291*
  cancer of. See *Breast cancer.*
  carcinoma of, *298*, 311–314, 312(t), *312–314.* See also *Breast cancer.*
    in male patient, 325
  changes in, after menopause, 289, *294*, 294–295
    during pregnancy, 294, *294*
    in adolescence, 292, 294, *294*
    with lactation, 294, *294*
  colloid carcinoma (mucinous adenocarcinoma) of, 313
  comedocarcinoma of, 313, *313*
  cyst of, 300
    milk-filled, 301
    needle aspiration of, 298, *300*
  cystic disease of, 300–301
  cystosarcoma phyllodes of, 304, 315
  discharge from nipple of, 302–303
  ductal carcinoma of, 312, *312*, 322
  ectasia of ducts of, 304
  embryonic and fetal development of, 288
    milk line in, 288, *288*, 290
  enlargement of, in male patient, 301
  epidermoid carcinoma of, 314
  examination of, in diagnosis of mammary cancer, 295–296, *296*
  fat necrosis of, 304
  fibroadenoma of, 303, *303*
  fibrocystic disease of, 300–301
  giant fibroadenoma (giant intracanalicular myxoma) of, 303–304
  granular cell myoblastoma of, 304
  hyperplasia of, atypical, and risk of mammary cancer, 306, 306(t), *307*
  infection of, 301–302
  infiltrating ductal carcinoma (scirrhous carcinoma) of, 312, *312*
    xeroradiographic findings in, *298*
  inflammation of, cystic, 300–301
    infection and, 301–302
    plasma cell infiltration and, 304
  inflammatory carcinoma of, 314, *314*, 319
    xeroradiographic findings in, 297, *298*
  intraductal papilloma of, 304
  lobular carcinoma of, 313–314, *314*, 322
  lymphatics of, 290–291, *291*, *292*
    cancer involving, 309
      prognosis with, 312(t)
      treatment of, 316–317
  malignant disease of. See *Breast cancer.*
  medullary carcinoma of, 312–313
  mucinous adenocarcinoma of, 313

Breast (*Continued*)
  needle aspiration of cells or cyst fluid from, 298–299, *300*
  nerves supplying, 290
  neuroendocrine influences on, *293*
  noninfiltrating ductal carcinoma of, 312, 322
  nonproliferative disease of, 300–301
  Paget's disease of, 296, 311
  palpation of, in diagnosis of mammary cancer, 295–296, *296*
  papillary carcinoma of, 313
  plasma cell infiltration of, 304
  proliferative disease of, 300–301
    and risk of mammary cancer, 306, 306(t)
  radiography of, as aid to diagnosis, of cancer, 297, *298*, 307
    benefits vs. risks of, 307
  resection of, for cancer, *316*, 316–322
    as prophylactic measure, 320
    results of, *318–319*, 318–321, 319(t), *321–322*
    with follow-up reconstructive surgery, 320
  sarcoma of, 314–315
  self-examination of, in diagnosis of mammary cancer, 296
  supernumerary, 290
  surgical reconstruction of, after mastectomy for cancer, 320
  trauma to, and fat necrosis, 304
  tuberculoma of, 302
  tubular carcinoma of, 313
  tumors of, benign, 303–304
    malignant. See *Breast cancer.*
Breast cancer, 304–325
  aminoglutethimide for, 324
  axillary lymph node involvement in, 309
    physical examination for, 295, *296*
    treatment of, 317
  breast biopsy in, 269, 299, 315
  chemotherapy for, 280, 322–325
    abortion in patient treated with, 325
  Columbia classification of, 309(t)
  computed tomography in, 309
  diagnosis of, mammography in, 297, *298*, 307
    patient history in, 295
    physical examination in, 295–296, *296*
    thermography in, 297
    ultrasonography in, 297
  epidemiology of, 304–307
  estrogen receptor activity in, 323
  extended simple mastectomy for, 317
  familial, 305
  histologic criteria applied to, 308
  in lactating patient, 325
  in male patient, 325
  in pregnant patient, 325
  lymph node involvement in, 309
    and prognosis, 312(t)
    treatment of, 316–317
  mastectomy for, *316*, 316–322
    prophylactic, 320
    reconstructive surgery after, 320
    results of, *318–319*, 318–321, 319(t), *321–322*
  metastasis of, 291, 308, 309, 311(t)
  microcalcifications in, 297, *298*
  minimal, 321
    treatment of, 322
  modified radical mastectomy for, *316*
  mortality rate in, 304, *305*
    among untreated patients, 307

Breast cancer (*Continued*)
  natural history of, 307–306
  peau d'orange in, 295, *295*, 312
  progesterone receptor activity in, 323
  prognosis in, carcinoma type and, 312(t)
    lymph node involvement and, 312(t)
    severity of lesion and, 307(t), 308
  quadrantectomy-axillary dissection-radiotherapy for, results of, 318, *318–319*
  radiation therapy for, 274, 317–321
    abortion in patient treated with, 325
    results of, *318–319*, 318–321, 319(t), *321–322*
  radical mastectomy for, 317
    results of, 318, *318–319*, 320, 321, *321–322*
  radionuclide bone scanning in, 309
  recurrence of, 318–320
  risk of, age at first pregnancy and, 306
    age at menopause and, 306
    atypical mammary hyperplasia and, 306, 306(t), *307*
    cancer at other sites and, 305
    dietary fat and, 305
    estrogen exposure and, 306
    genetic factors and, 305
    infertility and, 306
    oophorectomy and reduction of, 306
    proliferative disease and, 306, 306(t)
    radiation exposure and, 306–307
  segmental mastectomy for, results of, 319, 319(t)
  severity of, and prognosis, 307(t), 308
  staging of, 308–309, 309(t)–311(t)
  tamoxifen for, 323
  TNM staging of, 310(t)–311(t)
  total mastectomy for, results of, 319(t), 321, *321–322*
  treatment of, 315–325
    recurrence after, 318–320
  tylectomy for, 317–318
  types of, 311–315, *312–314*
    and prognosis, 312(t)
Breathing, assisted, in CPR, 1056
Breslow classification, of melanoma, 285
Bretylium, 1182
Bricker ileal conduit, in urinary diversion, after cystectomy, 839
Brittle diabetes mellitus, 605
Bronchial closure, stapler in, 1004, *1004*
Bronchiectasis, 992(t), 992–994, *993*
Bronchitis, 973–974
Bronchodilators, 1180, 1181(t)
Bronchogenic carcinoma, 998–1007. See also *Lung(s), carcinoma of.*
Bronchogenic cyst, 1034
Bronchoplasty, for lung tumors, 1006
Bronchoscopy, *980*, 980–983, *982*, 982(t)
Bronchospasm, 975–976
Bronchus, closure of, stapler in, 1004, *1004*
  disruption of, 187
  endoscopy of, *980*, 980–983, *982*, 982(t)
  foreign body impaction in, 705
  polyps of, 1008
  rupture of, 187
  tumors of, 1008
Brooke formula, for fluid resuscitation, of burn patients, 126
Brown-Sequard syndrome, 873
Bruit, carotid, asymptomatic, 922
  in peripheral artery disease, 895, *896*
Brunner's glands, 431
Brush cytology, in diagnosis of esophageal carcinoma, 367(t)
BT-PABA test, 596

Bubble oxygenator, in cardiopulmonary bypass, 1185
Buccal mucosa, carcinoma of, 731
Budd-Chiari syndrome, 527, 544–545, *545*
Buerger's disease, *893*, 912–915
Bundle branch block, pacemaker for, 1170
Burn(s), 122–131
   chemical, 128–129
      of esophagus, 367–369, *368*, 678–679
   degree of, in relation to affected skin
      layers, 123, *123*, 124
   electrical, 128
   epidemiology of, 122
   estimation of surface area of, rule of
      nines in, 124–125
   facial, 125
   fat metabolism in patients with, 102(t)
   full-thickness, 123
   glucose metabolism in patients with,
      101(t)
   hand, 125
   healing of, 125, 129
      contractures and hypertrophic scarring
         after, 130–131
   in children, 122, 126
   infection of, 128
   management of, 124–128
      analgesics in, 127
      escharotomy in, 127, *127*
      excision in, 130
      first aid in, 124
      fluid resuscitation in, 125–126, *126*
      history of, 122
      in emergency room, 124
      irrigation in, 128–129
      mafenide acetate in, 127
      silver nitrate in, 127
      silver sulfadiazine in, 127
      skin grafts in, 130, 262
   metabolic response to, 123–124
   paralytic ileus in patients with, 126
   partial-thickness, 123
   pathophysiology of, 122–123
   respiratory tract, 129
   stress ulcers in patients with, 126
Bypass surgery. See specific procedures,
   e.g., *Coronary artery bypass graft.*

Cadaver organs, 234–237, 236(t)
   agencies for procurement of, 235
   availability of, 234
   donor and, 235(t), 235–236
   donor-recipient matching with, 231
   preservation of, 236
   removal procedure for, 237, *237*
Caffey's sign, in Legg-Calve-Perthes disease, *778*, 778–779
Calcaneus, fracture of, 767–768
Calcific aortic stenosis, 1137, *1138*
Calcification, in cancer of breast, 297, *298*
   pancreatic, *392*
Calcitonin, tumor secreting, 337, *337*
Calcium, abnormal serum levels of. See
   Hypercalcemia and *Hypocalcemia.*
   absorption of, in small intestine, 435
   infusion of, induction of cardiac stimulation with, 1182
      pancreatic hormone secretion in response to, 598
   metabolism of, 341
Calcium-channel blocking agents, 1181
Cancer, 268–287, 710
   airway compression by, radiation therapy
      for, 275

Cancer (*Continued*)
   chemotherapy for. See *Chemotherapy.*
   diagnosis of, 268
      biopsy in, 268–269
   etiology of, 270–271, 707, *707*
      chemotherapy agents in, 280
      diethylstilbestrol exposure in, 822
   hydatidiform, 824
   immunotherapy for, 282–283, 720, 722,
      1006
   in AIDS, 177
   in children, 679–684
   incidence of, by sex, *305*
      by site, *305*
   metastasis of, radiation therapy for, 275
      surgery for, 286–287
   mortality rate in, by sex, *305, 998*
      by site, *305, 998*
   of adrenal gland, 358–359
   of anus, 508, *509*, 510
   of bile duct, 539, 577–578
   of bladder, 837–839, *838*
   of bone, 789
   of breast. See *Breast cancer.*
   of buccal mucosa, 731
   of chest wall, 1015, 1018
   of colon. See *Colorectal cancer.*
   of diaphragm, 1018
   of endometrium, 816–817
   of esophagus, 384–386
   of external ear, 691
   of fallopian tube, 819
   of gallbladder, 575–577
   of glottis, 704, 733
   of hard palate, 731
   of head and neck. See *Head and neck
      cancer.*
   of heart, 1164(t), 1166, 1168
   of hypopharynx, 700, 732
   of ileum, 451(t)
   of jejunum, 451(t)
   of kidney, 834–836, *835*
   of larynx, 704, 733
      smoking and alcohol use as risk factors
         in, *706*
   of lip, 730
   of liver, 496, 537–543, 684
   of lung, 998–1007
   of lymph nodes, 268
   of mediastinum, 1024–1034
   of nasopharynx, 700, 733
   of neck. See *Head and neck cancer.*
   of nose, 698–699, 734
   of oral cavity, *708*, 730–731
   of oropharynx, 700
   of ovary, 818–819
      in children, 680
   of palate, 731, 732
   of pancreas, 584, 598–599, *599*, 609–610
   of paranasal sinus, 698–699, 734
   of penis, 846–847
   of pericardium, 1051–1052, 1164(t)
   of pharynx, 700, 731–732
      radiosensitivity of, *723*
      staging of, *721*
   of pleura, 991
   of prostate, 843–844
   of rectum. See *Colorectal cancer.*
   of rib, 1015, 1018
   of salivary glands, 734
   of small intestine, 451(t), 452–453
      Crohn's disease and, 445
   of soft palate, 732
   of spleen, 630
   of sternum, 1015, 1018
   of subglottis, 704, 733

Cancer (*Continued*)
   of supraglottis, 704, 733
   of testis, 851–853
   of thyroid gland, 336(t), 336–338
   of tongue, 731, 732
   of tonsil, 732
   of urethra, 849
   of vagina, 815
   of vulva, 814
   prevention of, 268
   radiation therapy for. See *Radiation therapy.*
   radiosensitivity of, 272–274, *273*
   recurrence of, tests for, 270(t)
   resistance to, immune response and, 281
   spinal cord compression by, radiation
      therapy for, 275
   staging of, 271. See also *TNM staging of
      cancer.*
   superior vena caval obstruction by, *1000*,
      1023
      radiation therapy for, 275
   surgery for, 269. See also specific resections and under tumor types and tissue sites.
      at sites of metastases, 286–287
      debulking, 269
      no-touch, 269
      psychological effects of, 203
      radiation therapy with, 275
      reconstruction after, 269, 320, *726–727*, 728–730
   tests for recurrence of, 270(t)
   treatment of, 269, 273–283. See also specific modalities, e.g., *Chemotherapy.*
      at sites of metastases, 275, 286–287
      follow-up after, 270(t)
      monoclonal antibodies in, 282
      palliative, 269, 275
      recurrence after, tests for, 270(t)
   tumor antigens in, 281
Candidiasis, 167
   in AIDS, 176
   vaginal, 814
Cannulation, in cardiopulmonary bypass,
   1187
Capillary, fluid movement across, 34, 635,
   635
   glomerular, pressure effects on, *39*
Capital femoral epiphysis, avascular necrosis of, *778*, 778–779, *779*
   slipped, *780*, 780–781
Captopril, 1180
Carbohydrate, digestion of, 411, 432
   ingestion of, and hypoglycemia, 419
   malabsorption of, 447
   metabolism of, in liver, 519
Carbon dioxide, in pulmonary function,
   972–973, *973*
   partial pressure of, 207
Carbon monoxide poisoning, 129
Carcinoembryonic antigen, 281
   in cancer of colon, 281, 495
Carcinogenesis, 270–271, 707, *707*
Carcinoid, *453*, 453–455, 466–467, 610(t),
   612
   hormones and hormone-like products secreted by, 1008(t)
   in mediastinum, 1033
   of lung, 1008
Carcinoid syndrome, 454–455, 610(t), 612
   5-hydroxytryptamine metabolism in, 454,
      454
Carcinoma, anaplastic, of thyroid, 338
   basal cell, *795*, 795–796
      of external ear, 691

Carcinoma (*Continued*)
  bronchogenic, 998–1007. See also
    Lung(s), carcinoma of.
  colloid, of breast, 313
  ductal, of breast, 312, *312*, 322
  epidermoid, of breast, 314
  follicular, of thyroid, 337
  hepatocellular, *537*, 537–539, 684
    alpha-fetoprotein in, 281
    viral hepatitis and, 171
  Hürthle cell, 337
  inflammatory, of breast, 297, *298*, 314,
    314, 319
  lobular, of breast, 313–314, *314*, 322
  medullary, of breast, 312–313
    of thyroid, 337–338
  metastasis of, to lung, *1003*, 1006(t)
  mucoepidermoid, of parotid gland, 734
  of adrenal gland, 358–359
  of ampulla of Vater, 578–579, *579*
  of anus, 508, 510
  of bile duct, 539, *539*, 577–578, *578*
  of bladder, 837–839, *838*
  of bone, 789
  of breast, *298*, 311–314, 312(t), *312–314*.
    See also *Breast cancer.*
    in male patient, 325
  of buccal mucosa, 731
  of endometrium, 816–817
  of esophagus, 384–386
    endoscopy in diagnosis of, 367(t)
    staging of, 384, 384(t)
    treatment of, *385*, 385(t), 385–386, *386*
  of external ear, 691
  of gallbladder, 575–577
  of glottis, 704, 733
  of hard palate, 731
  of head and neck. See *Head and neck
    cancer.*
  of hypopharynx, 700, 732
  of kidney, 834–836, *835*
  of larynx, 704, 733
  of lip, 730
  of liver, *537*, 537–539, 684
    alpha-fetoprotein in, 281
    viral hepatitis and, 171
  of lung, 998–1007
  of mediastinum, 1032
  of nasopharynx, 700, 733
  of neck. See *Head and neck cancer.*
  of nose, 698–699, 734
  of oral cavity, *708*, 730–731
  of oropharynx, 700
  of palate, 731, 732
  of pancreas, 584, *599*, 609
  of paranasal sinus, 698–699, 734
  of parotid gland, 734
  of pharynx, 700, 731–732
  of prostate, 843–844
  of salivary gland, 734
  of soft palate, 732
  of stomach, at site of gastrectomy stump,
    420
  of subglottis, 704, 733
  of supraglottis, 704, 733
  of testis, 851–853, *852*
  of thyroid, 336(t), 336–338
  of tongue, 731, 732
    radiosensitivity of, *723*
  of tonsil, 732
  of urethra, 849
  papillary, of breast, 313
    of thyroid, 336–337
  scirrhous, of breast, *298*, 312, *312*
  small cell, hormones and hormone-like
    products secreted by, 1008(t)

Carcinoma (*Continued*)
  squamous cell, 710, 715–716, 795, *795*
    of anus, 508, 510
    of esophagus, 384
    of external ear, 691
    of head and neck. See *Head and neck
      cancer.*
    of lung. See *Lung(s), carcinoma of.*
    of nose and paranasal sinuses, 698–699
  tubular, of breast, 313
  verrucous, 710
Carcinoma in situ, 710
Cardiac arrest, 1054–1055
  anesthesia and, 1059
  perioperative, management of, *1183*
Cardiac arrhythmia(s), accessory conduct-
    ing pathways and, 1156–1157, *1157*
  as complication of coronary artery bypass
    graft, 1122
  peri- and postoperative, management of,
    1182–1183, *1184*
  surgical treatment of, 1156–1162, *1158,
    1159, 1161*
    directed vs. nondirected, 1160(t),
      1162(t)
    intracardiac electrode catheter study
      preceding, *1156*
Cardiac compression, direct (open-chest),
    1058, *1059*
  external, in CPR, *1056*, 1056–1058
    animal model studies of effects of,
      1057, *1057, 1058*
Cardiac output, effect of, on PO_2, 207
  low, as complication of coronary artery
    bypass graft, 1121
    perioperative, management of, *1183*
Cardiac pacemaker(s). See *Pacemaker(s).*
Cardiac pacing system analyzer, 1174, *1175*
Cardiac tamponade, 182, 188, 1046
  as complication of coronary artery bypass
    graft, 1121–1122
Cardiogenic shock, 18–19
Cardioplegic solution, 1119, 1119(t)
Cardiopulmonary bypass, 1185–1190
  apparatus used in, 1185–1186, *1186*
  denaturation of blood in, 1188, *1189*
  effects of hypothermia during perfusion
    in, 1187, *1187, 1188*
Cardiopulmonary resuscitation, 1054–1060
Cardiothoracic surgery, development of, 8–
    9
Cardiotomy suction, in cardiopulmonary
    bypass, 1186
Cardiovascular drugs, 1059, 1180(t), 1180–
    1183, 1181(t), 1203(t)
Cardiovascular system. See also *Heart.*
  disease of, and risk of compromised car-
    diac function, in surgical patient, 69,
    69(t)
    management of surgical patient with,
      69–70, 1179–1184
  function of, as index of fluid balance, 43
  receptor pharmacology of, 1180(t)
Cardioversion, in CPR, 1058–1059
Caroli's disease, 524, 582
Carotid artery, aneurysm of, 866
  disease of, manifestations of, 920–922
  surgery of, for occlusive disease, 924–925
Carotid bruit, asymptomatic, 922
Carotid sinus syncope, pacemaker for,
    1170
Carpal tunnel syndrome, 744
  vs. thoracic outlet compression syn-
    drome, 915
Carpentier ring, and mitral anuloplasty,
    1150, *1150*

Carrel, Alexis, *8*
  contributions of, to vascular surgery, 8
Carrier, of viral hepatitis, 165, 171
Cartilage, tumor of, 787–789, 788(t)
Cartilage graft, 264
Cataract, as complication of electrical in-
    jury, 128
Catecholamine(s), changes in secretion of,
    in response to stress, 97(t)
Catecholamine-secreting tumor, 360–361
Catgut sutures, 136
Catheter, intravascular, sepsis associated
    with, 105–106, 165
  pulmonary artery, in measurement of left
    atrial filling pressure, 115
Catheter electrodes, intracardiac placement
    of, in candidates for surgical correction
    of arrhythmia, *1156*
Catheterization, nephrostomy, for calculous
    disease, 837
Catterall classification, of Legg-Calvé-
    Perthes disease, 779, *779*
Caustic injury, 128–129
  to esophagus, 367–369, *368*, 678–679
Cauterization, 135–136
  of cancer, of rectum, 497
Cavernous hemangioma, of liver, 544
Cavitron ultrasonic surgical aspiration de-
    vice, 520, *520*
Cecal volvulus, *392*, 501, *501*
Cell cycle, 276, *277*
Cell-mediated cytotoxicity, antibody-de-
    pendent, in rejection, 228
Cell surface antigens, 224
Cellular atypia, 710
Cellular hypoperfusion, in shock, 12, *13*
Cellulitis, clostridial, 159(t)
  necrotizing, synergistic, 159(t), 162
Central axillary lymph node group, 291,
    292
Central cardiovascular system, drugs affect-
    ing, 1181(t), 1181–1182
Central cord syndrome, 873
Central nervous system, infection of, 885–
    886
  injury of, 869–873
  radiography of, 859–862, *860, 861*
Cephalic (vagal) stage, of gastric acid se-
    cretion, 408
Cephalic vein, as site for insertion of pace-
    maker lead, *1174*
Cephalosporins, 157(t)
  cost of, 157(t)
Cerebral hemispheres, functions of, *858*,
    858–859
Cerebral hemorrhage, 868
Cerebral ischemia, 868
Cerebrospinal fluid, 857
  in sella turcica, 354
  laboratory analysis of, reference values
    for, 1204(t)
Cerebrovascular disease, 865–868
  extracranial, 918–927
  surgical patients with, 73–74
Cerebrovascular ischemia, 868
  transient, 918–927
Cervical disc syndrome, vs. thoracic outlet
    compression syndrome, 915
Cervical esophagus, 363, 364
  trauma to, 187
Cervical lymph nodes, anterior, 715
Cervical spine, dislocation of, 769–770,
    770
  fractures of, 185, 768–770
  myelopathy of, 879
  radiculopathy of, 878–879, 879(t)

Cervical spine (*Continued*)
trauma to, CT examination for, 186
emergency search for, 181, 185
radiographic examination for, 185
Cervix uteri, 805
examination of, 810–811
mucoid discharge from, 815
tumor of, 815–816
Chance fracture, 771, *771*
Charles procedure, in management of lymphedema, 637
Chemical cautery, 136
Chemical cocarcinogenesis, 707, *707*
Chemical injury, 128–129
to esophagus, 367–369, *368*, 678–679
Chemical sterilization of surgical instruments, 133
Chemodectoma, mediastinal, 1029
Chemotherapy, for cancer, 276–281
adjuvant, 280–281
assays for prediction of effectiveness of, 281
biologic basis of, 276
combination regimens used in, 280, 280(t)
mechanisms of action of agents used in, *277*, 277(t), 277–278
of brain, 862
of breast, 280, 322–325
of head and neck, 722
of liver, 539
secondary to malignant disease at other site, 287, *541*, 541–542, *542*
of lung, 1005
of prostate, 844
radiation therapy with, 276
sensitivity of lesions and lesion sites to, 279(t)
standards for assessment of response to, 278(t)
toxicity of, 279–280
for Cushing's syndrome, 358
for Hodgkin's disease, 274
for lymphoma, 632, 632(t)
for sarcoma, 284
for trophoblastic cancer, 824
Chenodeoxycholate, limited effectiveness of gallstone treatment with, 557
Chest, blunt trauma to, 188–189
infection in, postoperative, 205–206
movement of flail segment of, 181–182
penetrating wounds of, 188
trauma to, 188–189
and mediastinal hemorrhage, 1023
complications of, 181–182
wall of, disorders of, 1012–1013, *1013*, 1015, *1015*, *1016*, 1018
surgery for, 1013, *1014*, 1015, *1017*, 1018, *1018*
fixation of prosthetic materials to, *1018*
Child(ren). See also *Newborn*.
abdominal mass lesions in, 679–681
abuse of, 678
AIDS in, standards for differential diagnosis of, 174(t)
appendicitis in, 395, 463, 676
bladder distention in, 680
bleeding esophageal varices in, 535
bronchiectasis in, 993–994
burns in, 122, 126
cancer in, 679–684
chemical burn of esophagus in, 678–679
choledochal cyst in, 581, 582, 682, *683*
cystic hygroma in, 638, *638*, 658, *658*
enteric cysts in, 684

Child(ren) (*Continued*)
foreign body aspiration in, 674
fractures in, 757
gastroesophageal reflux in, 675–676
heart lesions in. See specific anomalies, e.g., *Ventricular septal defect(s)*.
hernias in, 678
hypertrophic pyloric stenosis in, 674–675
surgery for, 675, *675*
imperforate hymen in, 680
intussusception in, 676
reduction of, 676, *677*
kidney lesions in, 679–680, 834–836
laryngotracheal papillomatosis in, 703
liver transplantation in, 674
liver tumors in, 542–543, *543*, 682, *683*, 684
lymphedema in, 636
mediastinal tumors and cysts in, 1027(t)
nasopharyngeal angiofibroma in, 700
neuroblastoma in, 681, *682*, 1028
ovarian tumors in, 680, *680*
polyposis of colon in, 487
portal hypertension in, 535
rhabdomyosarcoma in, 680–681
splenic trauma in, management of, 195
surgery in, 674–684
teratoma in, 658, *680*, 681–682, *682*
tracheostomy in, *658*
trauma in, 678
tumors in, 542–543, 658, 679–684, 834–836, 1027(t)
vaginal atresia in, 680
Child abuse, 678
Chin lift, in relief of airway obstruction, 181
Chlamydia trachomatis infection, venereal, 846
Chloride, absorption of, in small intestine, 434
Chlorpromazine, 1180
Choanal atresia, 657, 695
Cholangiocarcinoma, 539, *539*, 577–578, *578*
Cholangiography, transhepatic, percutaneous, 560, *560*, 584, 599–600
Cholangiohepatitis, Oriental, 572–573
Cholangiopancreatography, 560, *560*, 584, 599, *599*
Cholangitis, 569–573
acute, 569–570
pyogenic, recurrent, 572–573
sclerosing, 570–572, *572*
Cholecystectomy. See *Gallbladder, resection of*.
Cholecystitis. See *Gallbladder, inflammation of*.
Cholecystography, oral, 558, *559*
Cholecystokinin, secretion of, after meal stimulus, *410*
Choledochal anastomosis to intestinal or biliary tract segment, with resection of biliary stricture, 574, *574*
Choledochal cyst, 580–582, *581*, 682, *683*
Choledocholithiasis, 565–568, *566*
management of, 566–568, *567*
Cholelithiasis. See *Gallstone(s)*.
Cholestasis, 72, *586*
liver biopsy in diagnosis of, 561
ultrasonographic findings in, 560, *586*
Cholesteatoma, 692
Cholesterol, elevated serum levels of, intestinal bypass for, 459–460
Cholesterol stones, 556–557
Cholestyramine, for diarrhea, after vagotomy, 420

Cholinesterase inhibitors, for myasthenia gravis, 1041
Chondroma, mediastinal, 1034
of lung, 1008
Chondrosarcoma, 1015
Chordotomy, for chronic pain, 884
Choriocarcinoma, 824
of testis, 852–853
Chronic disorders. See specific conditions, e.g., *Pancreatitis, chronic*.
Chyle, 638
Chylothorax, 990
Chylous ascites, 638
Chymopapain, 881
Cigarette smoking, and cancer, of head and neck, 706
of larynx, *706*
of lung, 998–999, *999*
and impaired lung function, in surgical patient, 70
and occlusive arterial disease, 910
Cimetidine, in prophylaxis against stress ulcers, 417
Circulatory status, emergency assessment of, 182
Circulatory support, in CPR, 1056–1058
Circumcision, 845
Cirrhosis. See *Liver, cirrhosis of*.
Cis-platinum, 278
Clark microstaging, of melanoma, 285, *285*
Class I HLA antigens, 224, *225*, 225(t)
Class II HLA antigens, 224, *225*, 225(t)
dendritic cells as source of, 226
Claudication, in chronic occlusive arterial disease, 908
in peripheral artery disease, 892
Clean surgical procedures, antimicrobial prophylaxis against infection in, 150–151
Clean wounds, 148
incised, healing of, 118
Clean-contaminated wounds, 148
Cleft sternum, 1013, 1015, *1016*
surgery for, *1017*
Clonal deletion, and tolerance, 233
Clonogenic assay, of tumor inhibition by chemotherapy agents, 281
Closed head injury, 184–185
Closed mitral commissurotomy, 1145–1146
Closed-loop obstruction, of small intestine, 437
Clostridial antitoxin, problems with use of, in cases of gas gangrene, 159
Clostridial cellulitis, 159(t)
Clostridial infections, 157–162, 159(t)
Clostridial myonecrosis, 157–159, 159(t)
radiographic findings in, *158*
Clostridium difficile–associated colitis, 161–162, 503–504
Closure, of wound. See *Wound closure*.
Clubfoot, *781*, 781–782, *782*
Coagulants, in surgery, 136
Coagulation, 79, 83–85
Coagulation cascade, 84, *84*
Coagulation factors, 83–85, 84(t)
Coagulopathy, 221
intravascular, disseminated, 26–27, 27(t), 90–91, *91*, 221
in chronic occlusive arterial disease, 909
Coarctation of aorta, 1064–1067, *1066*
percutaneous transluminal balloon angioplasty for, 1069, *1070*
surgery for, *1067–1069*, 1067–1071
recurrence after, 1070–1071

Cobb angle, in evaluation of scoliosis, 773, 774
Cobblestoning, of colon, in Crohn's disease, 481, 482
Cocarcinogenesis, 707, 707
Coccidioidomycosis, 167, 985–986
Cochlear duct, 689
Coffee bean sign, in strangulated small intestine, 441
Cold agglutinin syndrome, 628
Cold storage, of cadaver organs for transplantation, 236
Colectomy, 476
    antimicrobial prophylaxis against infection in, 150, 152
    for cancer, 492, 492, 493
    localization of ureters before, 475
Colic, biliary, 562
Colitis, 477–485
    Clostridium difficile–associated, 161–162, 503–504
    Crohn's disease and, 480–483, 483(t)
    hemorrhage in, 484
    ischemic, 502, 502
    perforation of colon in, 484
    postoperative, 219
    pseudomembranous, 161–162, 503–504
        postoperative, 219
    radiation-induced, 503
    surgery for, 484–485
    ulcerative, 477–480, 479
        and colorectal cancer, 484, 484, 485, 489
        and toxic dilatation of colon, 479
        vs. Crohn's disease, 477, 483(t)
Collagen, 117
Colles fracture, 749
Collis gastroplasty, 382
Colloid carcinoma (mucinous adenocarcinoma), of breast, 313
Colloid osmotic pressure, 34
Colon, 471
    adenocarcinoma of. See Colorectal cancer.
    aganglionic, 668, 668
    amebiasis of, 504
    anatomy of, 471–472, 471–473, 474
    angiodysplasia of, 502–503
    bacteria endogenous to, 143, 144(t)
        antimicrobials effective against, 157, 157(t), 476(t)
    barium contrast studies of, 475
    blood vessels supplying, 471–472, 473
        sliding inguinal hernia and, 651
    cancer of, 487–497. See also Colorectal cancer.
    cobblestone appearance of, in Crohn's disease, 481, 482
    Crohn's disease involving, 480–483, 482, 483(t)
        vs. ulcerative colitis, 477, 483(t)
    dilatation of, aganglionosis and, 668, 668
        ulcerative colitis and, 479
    diverticula of, 395–396, 497–499, 498, 499
    endoscopy of, 475
        as aid to diagnosis, of cancer, 490
        in reduction of volvulus, 500
        in removal of polyps, 486
    haustra of, radiographic appearance of, in cases of obstruction, 440
    hemorrhage from, colitis and, 484
        diverticulitis and, 497, 499
    inflammation of. See Colitis.

Colon (Continued)
    ischemia of, and inflammation, 502, 502
        following repair of aneurysm, 907
    lymphatics of, 472, 473
    motility of, 474
    nerves supplying, 474
    obstruction of, 399–400, 437
        cancer and, 494
        radiographic findings in, 438, 440, 441
        volvulus and, 500, 501
    perforation of, cancer and, 494
        colitis and, 484
        diverticulitis and, 499
    physiology of, 474
    polyps of, 485–487, 486, 486(t)
        and colorectal cancer, 485, 489
    resection of, 476
        antimicrobial prophylaxis against infection in, 150, 152
        for cancer, 492, 492, 493
        localization of ureters before, 475
    strangulation of, volvulus and, 500, 501
    surgery of, 476–477. See also Colostomy.
        for colitis, 484–485
        preparation for, 68, 475(t), 475–476
    toxic dilatation of, ulcerative colitis and, 479
    trauma to, 192–193
    ulcer of, amebiasis and, 504
        inflammatory, 477–480, 479
            and colorectal cancer, 484, 484, 485
            and toxic dilatation of colon, 479
            vs. Crohn's disease, 477, 483(t)
    vascular malformations of, 502–503
    volvulus of, 500, 500–501, 501
Colon cut-off sign, in acute pancreatitis, 398, 598
Colonoscopy, 475
    as aid to diagnosis, of cancer, 490
    in reduction of volvulus, 500
    in removal of polyps, 486
Colorectal cancer, 487–497
    abdominoperineal vs. anterior resection of, 492–494, 493, 494(t)
    and obstruction of colon, 494
    and perforation of colon, 494
    and tumor invasion of adjacent organ, 494–495
    carcinoembryonic antigen in, 281, 495
    colectomy for, 492, 492, 493
    diagnosis of, 490
    epidemiology of, 488–489
    etiology of, 487–488
    metastasis of, 496
        to liver, 339–342, 496
    prognosis in, 489–490
        patient age and, 496
        tumor stage and, 491, 491(t)
    recurrence of, after treatment, 495
        at site of suture line, 495
    risk factor(s) for, 488(t), 488–489
        polyps of colon as, 485, 489
        ulcerative colitis as, 484, 484, 485, 489
    signs and symptoms of, 490
    staging of, 490–491, 491
    treatment of, 491–497
        in cases of colonic obstruction or perforation, 494
        in cases of tumor invasion of adjacent organ, 495
        palliative, 496
        recurrence after, 495
            at site of suture line, 495
        second-look operation after, 495
    tumor types in, 489(t)

Colostomy, 476–477, 477
    for diverticulitis complicated by perforation, 499
    for trauma, to colon, 193
        to rectum, 193
    hernia through, 652–653
    replacement of fluid losses from, 42
Colporrhaphy, for incontinence, 820
Columbia classification of cancer, of breast, 309(t)
Coma, hepatic, 545–546
Coma scale, 869(t)
Combination chemotherapy regimens, 280, 280(t)
Comedocarcinoma, 313, 313
Commissurotomy, mitral, 1145–1146, 1146
Common bile duct, 587
    cysts of, 580–582, 581, 682, 683
    in relation to pancreatic duct, 589
    obstruction of, by T-tube, 217
    stones in, 565–568, 566
        management of, 566–568, 567
    surgery of, with resection of biliary stricture, 574, 574
    trauma to, 195
Community-acquired infection, 141
Compartment syndrome, after forearm fracture, 761
Composite grafts, 265
    in reimplantation of hand, 265
Compression garments, in management of lymphedema, 637
Computed tomography, as aid to diagnosis, of intrahepatic hematoma, 190
    of liver abscess, 522, 522
    of pericardial disease, 1048, 1048
    of surgical infection, 147
    of trauma, to abdomen, 190, 190
        to brain, 184
        to cervical spine, 186
        to head, 184, 185
    of tumor, of adrenal, 356, 356
        of mediastinum, 1026, 1041
        of pituitary, 353
    biliary tract on, 560
    central nervous system on, 860, 861
    in breast cancer, 309
    in stereotactic neurosurgery, 881
    pancreas on, 598, 598
    peripheral arterial system on, 897, 897
    spleen on, 620
    urogenital system on, 832–833
Concussion, 185
Conducting pathways, accessory, 1156–1157, 1157
    surgery for, 1156–1162, 1158, 1159, 1161
        intracardiac electrode catheter study preceding, 1156
Conductive hearing loss, 689
Condyloma acuminatum, 510, 864
Congestive heart failure, 64
    as complication of coronary artery bypass graft, 1122
    pacemaker for, 1171
Conn's syndrome, 359
Connective tissue, 117
Consciousness level, as index of fluid balance, 43
    estimation of, in management of trauma, 182, 184
    in postoperative period, 201(t), 202–203
Constipation, postoperative, 219
Constrictive pericarditis, 1046, 1051
Constrictor muscles of pharynx, 713

Contaminated wounds, 148
Continence, fecal, 474
  urinary, 831
    loss of, 831, 839–840
      inadequate pelvic support and, *819*, 819–820
Contraceptives, hepatocellular adenomas in patients using, 544
Contractility, of heart, 18, 1179
Contraction, of wound, 119
Contracture, of wound, 119
  in cases of burns, 130–131
Controlled hypotension, 112
Contusion, myocardial, 189
Cooper's ligaments, in structural support of breast, 289, *289*
Coronary artery (arteries), aneurysms of, congenital, *1135*, 1136
  atherosclerosis of, 1114, 1115, *1115*
    after heart transplantation, 258
  congenital lesions of, 1128–1136
  factors regulating blood flow in, *1118*
  fistulas of, 1128–1129, *1129–1131*
    surgery for, *1131*, *1132*
  left, 1114, *1114*, *1116*
    atherosclerosis of, *1115*
    originating from pulmonary artery, 1132, *1133*
      surgery for, 1132, *1134*, *1135*
    ostium of, occlusion of, fusion of left aortic cusp to aortic wall and, 1136
    stenosis of, *1115*
  right, 1114, *1114*, *1116*
    atherosclerosis of, *1115*
    originating from pulmonary artery, 1133
Coronary artery bypass graft, 1119–1123, *1120*, *1121*
  candidates for, 1117–1118
  complications of, 1121–1123
  early work in, 1118, *1119*
  mammary artery in, 1120, 1121, *1121*, *1122*, 1123, *1123*
  protection of myocardium in, cardioplegic solution and, 1119, 1119(t)
  results of, *1117*, 1123
  saphenous vein in, *1119*, 1120, *1120*, 1123
Coronary vein, occlusion of, in control of bleeding esophageal varices, 531
Corpus cavernosum, fibrosis of, 845–846
Corrosive injury, 128–129
  to esophagus, 367–369, *368*, 678–679
Corticosteroids, complication(s) associated with, 243
  acute pancreatitis as, 602
  effects of, on wound healing, 119
  for bronchospasm, 975
  for Crohn's disease, 483
  for myasthenia gravis, 1042
  in suppression of transplant rejection, 231
  use of, in surgical patient, 72
Cortisol, 38, 355
  hypersecretion of, 353, 356–358, 357(t)
  signs of, 356, 356(t)
Corynebacterium parvum, as immunotherapeutic anti-cancer agent, 282
Costoclavicular maneuver, 1011
Cotrel-Dubousset instrumentation, for scoliosis, 775, *775*
Coughing, in treatment of atelectasis, 208
Coumarin, for pulmonary embolism, 949
Countercurrent mechanism, of concentrating urine, *40*
Countershock, in CPR, 1058–1059

Craniocerebral injury, 869–871
Craniopharyngioma, 354
Craniosynostosis, 877
Cranium, congenital abnormalities of, 876–878
Cricopharyngeal myotomy, for oropharyngeal dysphagia, 373, *373*
Cricothyroidotomy, 976
  in emergency establishment of airway, 181
Crohn's disease, 442–446, 480–483, *482*
  and carcinoma of small intestine, 445
  intestinal fistulas in, 481, *482*
  signs of, on barium contrast studies, 445, 481, *482*
  vs. ulcerative colitis, 477, 483(t)
Cronkhite-Canada syndrome, 487
Crouzon's syndrome, 877
Cryoprecipitate, 93–94
Cryotherapy, 115
  for hemorrhoids, 506
Cryococcosis, 167, 986, *986*
Cryptorchidism, 851
  and infertility, 853
Cubital tunnel syndrome, 744–745
Cullen's sign, in diagnosis of cause of abdominal pain, 391
Cupulolithiasis, 695
Curare, 113
Curling's ulcer, in burn patients, 126
Cushing's disease, 353, 356, 357(t)
Cushing's syndrome, 353, 356(t), 356–358, 357(t)
Cyclosporine, 232
  in suppression of rejection, 232, 238
    of heart, 256
    of kidney, 243
    of liver, 247, 248, 249
  infection in heart transplant patients treated with, 257, 258
Cylindrical bronchiectasis, 992
Cyst(s), Bartholin's gland, 813
  biliary tract dilatation by, 580–582, 682
  breast, 300
    needle aspiration of, 298, *300*
  bronchogenic, 1034
  common bile duct, 580–582, *581*, 682, *683*
  dermoid, 1030
  echinococcal, of liver, 525, 525–527, *526*
    of spleen, 630
  enteric, 684, *684*, 1034–1035, *1035*
  epidermal, 794
  epidermoid, of hand, 752
  hydatid, of liver, *525*, 525–527, *526*
    of spleen, 630
  infra-auricular, 691
  kidney, 679, 833
  liver, 524–527, *525*, *526*
    in children, 682
  lung, congenital, 663
  mediastinal, 1024(t), 1034–1035, *1035*
    in children, 1027(t)
    sites of, *1021*, 1024, 1024(t)
  neuroenteric, 876, 1035
  pericardial, 1034, 1048–1049, *1049*
  pilonidal, 510–511, 800–801
  pre-auricular, 691
  seminal vesicle, 844
  spleen, *620*, 630
  thymus, 1035
  thyroglossal duct, 327, *328*
  Tornwaldt's, 701
  urachal, 684
  wolffian duct remnants and, 812
Cystadenocarcinoma, of pancreas, 609

Cystadenoma, of liver, 525
  of pancreas, 609
Cystectomy, for cancer, 838–839
Cystic artery, 553
  anomalies of, 553, *553*
Cystic duct, 551
  anomalies of, 553, *553*
Cystic fibrosis, meconium ileus in, 665
Cystic hygroma, 638, *638*, 658, *658*
  mediastinal, 1033–1034
Cystic mastitis, 300–301
Cystic teratoma, of ovary, *680*
Cystitis, 840
  infection-related, specimen collection in, 164
  postoperative, 164
Cystocele, 819, *819*
Cystography, 831
Cystosarcoma phyllodes, 304, 315
Cytology, exfoliative, in gynecologic examination, 810
Cytomegalovirus infection, in AIDS, 176
Cytotoxic drugs, effects of, on wound healing, 119
Cytotoxic T cell, 226
Cytotoxicity, cell-mediated, antibody-dependent, in rejection, 228

Dacarbazine, 278
Danazol, for cystic disease of breast, 301
Davy, Humphrey, nitrous oxide experiments performed by, 2
De Humani Corporis Fabrica, 1
De Quervain's stenosing tenosynovitis, 750
Dead space, in lung, 973
Deafness, 687, 689
  drugs causing, 694
  noise-induced, 693
  sudden, 695
  tests for, 689–690
Debulking, of malignant tumor, 269
Decompression, of gastrointestal tract, 441
  of volvulus, 501
Deep breathing, in treatment of atelectasis, 208
Deep venous thrombosis, 91, 92, 945, *946*
  prophylaxis against, in surgical patients, 66, 66–67
  vs. peripheral artery disease, 900–901
Defecation, 474
Defibrillation, in CPR, 1058–1059
Deglutition, 365
  difficulty in, 371(t), 371–373
    achalasia and, 374
    esophageal carcinoma and, 384
    treatment of, 373, *373*
Dehiscence, of abdominal wound, 120
Dehydration, 50–51
Delayed menarche, 808
Delayed primary closure, of wound, 120
Delirium, after coronary artery bypass surgery, 1123
Delirium tremens, 203
Delta hepatitis, 169, 170, 170(t)
Denaturation of blood, in cardiopulmonary bypass, 1188, *1189*
Dendritic cell, 226
  in rejection, 226, 227, *227*
Dental disease, in patients with head and neck cancer, 719
Denver shunt, *547*
Depolarizing muscle relaxants, 113
Depression, in cancer patients, after surgery, 203

Depressor muscles of mandible, 712
Dermal sinus tract, 875–876
Dermatofibroma, 798, *798*
Dermatofibrosarcoma protuberans, 799
Dermatome, cutting of donor skin with, in split-thickness grafting, 130
Dermis, 117, 792, *793*
Dermoid cyst, 1030
Detorsion, of volvulus, 501
Detoxification, by liver, 519
   effects of shock on, 17
Devascularization, of esophagus, for portal hypertension, 534
Dexamethasone suppression test, 357
Dextran, in prophylaxis against deep venous thrombosis, in surgical patients, 67
Diabetes mellitus, brittle, 605
   insulin-induced hypoglycemia in, 202
   pancreas transplant for, 249–250
   peripheral artery disease in, 893
   preparation for surgery in patients with, 71
Dialysis, 213–214
   for acute renal failure, 213, 214
Diaphragm, Bochdalek defect of, *661*, 661–662
   repair of, 662, *662*
   eventration of, in newborn, 662
   hernia through, in newborn, *661*, 661–662, *662*
   rupture of, 191
   tumors of, 1018
Diaphragma sellae, 350
Diaphysis, fracture of, 757
Diarrhea, *Clostridium difficile*–associated, 161, 162
   in Crohn's disease, 444
   postoperative, 219
   postvagotomy, 420, 448
   replacement of fluids lost in, 42
Diastematomyelia, 876
Diet, as aid to management, of Crohn's disease, 482
   of hemorrhoids, 506
   of obesity, 427
   fat in, and risk of cancer, of breast, 305
      of colon, 488
Diethylstilbestrol, teratogenetic effects of, 821–822
Diffuse goiter, 331
Digestion, 410–411, 431–433
   carbohydrate, 411, 432
   fat, 411, 433, *433*
   neurohumoral events in, *409*
   protein, 410, 431–432
Digitalis preparations, 1181, 1182
Digital subtraction angiography, 861–862
Dilution principle, 29, *30*
Dimethadione test, 596
Dinitrochlorobenzine, for cancer, 282
Diphosphonates, for hypercalcemia, 344
Direct (open-chest) cardiac massage, 1058, *1059*
Direct inguinal hernia, 640, 641, *641*
Dirty wounds, 148
Disorientation, postoperative, 202, 203
Dissection, 134–135
Disseminated intravascular coagulopathy, 26–27, 27(t), 90–91, *91*, 221
   in chronic arterial occlusive disease, 909
Distributive shock, 23
Diuretic(s), cardiovascular effects of, 1180
   for ascites, 546
   for cirrhosis, 64

Diverticulum, colonic, 395–396, 497–499, *498*, *499*
   duodenal, 422, 455–456, *456*, 583
   epiphrenic, *378*, 378–379
   esophageal, *372*, *373*, *378*, 378–379
   hypopharyngeal, 701
   Meckel's, *457*, 457–458, *467*, 467–470, *468*, 676, *678*
      surgery for, 458, *469*, 469–470
   pharyngoesophageal, *372*
   resection of, *373*
   small intestine, 455–458
   Zenker's, *372*
   resection of, *373*
Dizziness, 690
Dobutamine, 1181
Donor site, in split-thickness skin grafting, with dermatomes, 130
Donor-specific transfusions, pre-transplant, 234, 238
Dopamine, 1181
Doppler ultrasonography, as aid to diagnosis, of peripheral artery disease, *896*, 896–897, *897*
   of venous disorders, 935–936, *936*
Dorsal hernia, 654
Double aortic arch and vascular ring, 661, *661*, *1072*, 1072–1074, *1073*
Double-barrel colostomy, 477
Double bubble sign, in duodenal atresia, *664*
Double outlet right ventricle, 1095–1096, *1096*
   surgery for, 1096–1097, *1097*
Double Roux-en-Y portojejunostomy, for biliary atresia, *581*
Dragsted hypothesis, on formation of gastric ulcer, 415
Drain, 138–140, *139*
   Penrose, 139, *139*
   risk of infection with, *138*, 150
   suction, *139*, 139–140
   sump, *139*, 140
   T-tube, obstruction of biliary tract by, 217, *217*
Drainage, of abscess, 153
   in abdomen, 154, 157, 204–205, *205*
   of anorectum, 507
   of pancreas, 607
   of bile, by percutaneous transhepatic catheterization, 560, *561*
   of fistula contents, 140
   of infected wound, 120
   of pancreatic ascites, 608, *608*
   of pancreatic pseudocyst, 607
   of pericardium, 1052
   of tuberculous empyema, with construction of Eloesser flap, 997, *997*
Drug monitoring, laboratory reference values for, 1203(t)–1204(t)
Dry heat, instrument sterilization with, 133
Ductal carcinoma, of breast, 312, *312*, 322
Ductus arteriosus, patent, 1061–1062
   in premature infants, 1063–1064
   surgery for, 1062–1063, *1063*, *1064*
Dukes staging of cancer, of colon, 490–491, *491*
Dumbbell tumor, 681, *682*
Dumping syndrome, 418–419
Duodenum, 406, 429
   anatomy of, 406–407, *407*, 429, *430*
   atresia of, 664, *664*
   blood vessels supplying, 407, 430
   cancer of, 451(t)
   diverticulum of, 422, 455–456, *456*, 583

Duodenum (*Continued*)
   hematoma in, obstruction of small intestine by, 192
   obstruction of, in newborn, 664
   surgery of, antimicrobial prophylaxis against infection in, 151–152
   trauma to, 191–192
      treatment of, 192, *192*
   tumors of, 451(t)
   ulcer of, 411–412, *412*
      hemorrhage from, 412
         surgery for, 414
      perforation of, 397, 412
         surgery for, 397–398, 414
      recurrence of, after surgery, 418
      surgery for, 413–414, *414*
         in cases of hemorrhage, 414
         in cases of perforation, 397–398, 414
         infection after, 151
         recurrence after, 418
Dupuytren's disease, 742
Dysfibrinogenemia, 91
Dyshormonogenesis, 331
Dyskinesia, biliary, 582
Dysphagia, achalasia and, 374
   esophageal carcinoma and, 384
   oropharyngeal, 371(t), 371–373
      treatment of, 373, *373*
Dysplastic nevus, 797
Dysuria, 831

Ear, 686
   disorders of, 690–695
   historical aspects of study of, 686
   lop deformity of, 690
   middle, *688*
   pain in, 687
      as sign of head and neck cancer, 717–718
   swimming-related infection and inflammation of, 691
Eardrum, 686, *687*, 688
Early postprandial dumping, 418–419
Early satiety, after gastrectomy, 420
Ebstein's anomaly, 1153, *1153*, 1155
   repair of, *1154*, 1155
Echinococcosis, of liver, *525*, 525–527, *526*
   of spleen, 630
Echocardiography, cardiac tumors on, 1164, *1165*
   pericardial effusion on, 1047, *1047*
   signs of pulmonary embolism on, 948, *951*
Ectasia, mammary duct, 304
Ecthyma gangrenosum, 163
Ectopic ACTH syndrome, 356, 357(t), 358
Ectopic atrial tachycardia, surgical treatment of, 1159
Ectopic kidney, 833
Ectopic pancreas, 600
Ectopic pregnancy, 402, 823
Ectopic spleen, 630
Ectopic ureter, 837
Edema, 635
Edrophonium test, for myasthenia gravis, 1040
Efferent loop obstruction, after gastrectomy and restoration of GI continuity, 420
Efferent neurologic pathways, *97*
Effusion, pericardial, 1046, *1047*
   pleural, 988–989
      blood in, 990

Effusion (*Continued*)
  pleural, chyle in, 990
    pancreatic fluid in, 608
    pus in, 206, *990*, 990–991
    tuberculous, Eloesser flap in drainage of, 997, *997*
Ehrlich, Paul, 7, *7*
Eighth cranial nerve, tumors of, 694
Einhorn chemotherapy regimen (PVB regimen), 280
Ejaculatory dysfunction, 848
  after repair of aneurysm, 907
Electrical anesthesia, 115
Electrical burns, 128
Electrocardiography, in diagnosis of pericardial disease, 1048
Electrocautery, 135–136
Electrocoagulation, for cancer of rectum, 497
Electrode, of pacemaker, 1171–1173, *1173*
Electrode catheters, intracardiac placement of, in candidates for surgical correction of arrhythmia, *1156*
Electroencephalography, 861
Electrolyte(s), 54
  absorption of, in small intestine, 414–415
  in body fluids, 32–33, 33(t), 42(t), 63(t)
  in intravenous solutions, 41(t), 63(t)
Electrolyte balance, 35, 35(t)
  and management of surgical patients, 64
  disorders of. See specific conditions, e.g., *Hypercalcemia.*
Electrolyte replacement therapy. See *Fluid replacement therapy.*
Electromyography, 861
  single-fiber, in diagnosis of myasthenia gravis, 1040
Electrosurgery, and cauterization, 135–136
  in treatment of rectal cancer, 497
Electrosurgical incision, risk of infection associated with, *135*
Elevator muscles of mandible, 712
Elliptocytosis, hereditary, 628
Eloesser flap, in drainage of tuberculous empyema, 997, *997*
Embolism, arterial, 92, 898–903, *902*
  cerebral, and ischemic stroke, 920
  fat, 954–955
    as complication of fracture, 756
  pulmonary. See *Pulmonary embolism.*
  retinal, as sign of vascular disease, 894, 920–923
Embolization, of coronary vein, in treatment of bleeding esophageal varices, 531
  of hepatic vessels, in treatment of hemobilia, 536
Emergency room care, of burn patients, 124
Emission tomography, 860
Emphysema, 974
  lobar, congenital, 663, *663*
  mediastinal, 1022–1023
Emphysematous cholecystitis, *559*, 564
Empty sella syndrome, 354
Empyema, *990*, 990–991
  of gallbladder, 565
  postoperative, 206
  tuberculous, Eloesser flap in drainage of, 997, *997*
Emulsification, 411
Encephalocele, 696, 876–877, *877*
Encephalopathy, hepatic, 545–546
Enchondroma, of hand, 752

Encircling endocardial ventriculotomy, for ventricular tachycardia, 1160–1161, *1161*
End colostomy, 477
End-to-end anastomosis stapler, in transection of esophagus, *535*
End-to-side portacaval shunt, for portal hypertension, 533
Endarterectomy, carotid, for occlusive disease, 924–925
Endocardial resection procedure, for ventricular tachycardia, 1161, *1161*
Endocardial ventriculotomy, for ventricular tachycardia, 1160–1161, *1161*
Endocrine glands, autotransplantation of, 265
Endocrine-active tumors, 353–354
Endocrine-inactive tumors, 353
Endocrinopathy, bronchogenic carcinoma and, 1001
  management of surgical patient with, 71–72
Endogenous contamination, of wound, 120, 148
Endolymph, 687
Endolymphatic hydrops, 694
Endometrioma, 818
Endometriosis, 403
Endometrium, 806, *806*
  adenocarcinoma of, 816–817
  evaluation of, 811
  hyperplasia of, 816
  polyp of, 816
Endorphins, 352
Endoscopic retrograde cholangiopancreatography, 560, *560*, 584, 599, *599*
Endoscopic sclerotherapy, for bleeding esophageal varices, *531*, 531–532, *532*
Endoscopy, in delineation of pancreatic and biliary duct anatomy, 560, *560*, 584, 599, *599*
  of bronchi, *980*, 980–983, *982*, 982(t)
  of colon, 475
    as aid to diagnosis, of cancer, 490
    in reduction of volvulus, 500
    in removal of polyps, 486
  of esophagus, 366
    as aid to diagnosis, of achalasia, 375
      of inflammation, 367
      of tumor, 367, 367(t)
    perforation caused by, 367, 369, 369(t)
  of larynx, and endotracheal intubation, 1056, *1056*
  of peritoneal cavity, in gynecologic examination, 811
Endothelial cells, vascular, 80–81
  metabolism of membrane phospholipids in, *81*
Endothelial seeding, of prosthesis, 264
Endotracheal intubation, laryngoscopy and, 1056, *1056*
Endotoxemia, *16*
Enema, barium, in diagnosis of colon cancer, 490
  in examination of colon, 475
Energy balance, changes in, in response to stress, 100(t)
Energy substrates, cellular metabolism and, 13, *13*
  effects of shock on, 12–17, 23–24
  in parenteral nutrition, 104
Enflurane, 112
Enkephalins, 352
Entamoeba histolytica infection (amebiasis), 504, 523–524, *524*

Entamoeba histolytica infection (amebiasis) (*Continued*)
  complications of, 523, *525*
Enteral nutrition, 67, 107(t), 107–108
Enteric cyst, 684, *684*, 1034–1035, *1035*
Enteritis, regional. See *Crohn's disease.*
Enteritis necroticans, 161
Enterocele, 820, *820*
Enterocolitis, Hirschsprung's disease and, 668
  necrotizing, in newborn, 670–671, *671*
Enterohepatic circulation, 517, 554, *555*
Enterokinase, 410
Entrapment neuropathy, of hand and wrist, 744–745
Enuresis, 831
Envenomation, snake, 199
Enzymes, hepatic, 518
  pancreatic, 593–594
    tests of secretion of, 595–596, 596(t)
Ependymoma, 864
Epidermis, 117, 791–792, *793*
  tumors of, *794*, 794–796, *795*
Epidermoid carcinoma, of breast, 314
Epidermoid cyst, of hand, 752
Epididymis, 850
  inflammation of, 404, 850
  tumors of, 850
Epididymitis, 404, 850
Epidural hematoma, 185, 871, *872*, 920
Epigastric hernia, 652
Epiglottitis, 703
Epilation, preoperative, postoperative infection risk associated with, 149
Epilepsy, 882–883
  drugs for, 1203(t)
  management of surgical patients with, 74
Epinephrine, 355
  cardiovascular effects of, 1182
Epiphrenic diverticulum, *378*, 378–379
Epispadias, 848
Epistaxis, 698
  control of, 698, *698*
  nasal septal vasculature and, *697*, 698
Epithelialization, in wound healing, 118
Epithelium, aerodigestive tract, 708, *709*, 711
  injury-induced changes in, 708
  premalignant to malignant, 710. See also *Head and neck cancer.*
Erosion, hemorrhagic, of stomach, 221, 415–417, *416*
Erythema, necrolytic, migratory, in patients with glucagonoma, 611
Erythrocytes, in spleen, 615–616
  transfusion of, 93
Erythroplakia, 710
Erythroplasia, of penis, 846
Erythropoietic porphyria, 628
Escharotomy, in management of burns, 127, *127*
Escherichia coli, antimicrobial prophylaxis against infection by, in colon surgery, 152
Esophagectomy, for cancer, 385
Esophagitis, endoscopy in diagnosis of, 367
  reflux. See *Gastroesophageal reflux.*
Esophagoscopy, 366
  as aid to diagnosis, of achalasia, 375
    of inflammation, 367
    of tumor, 367, 367(t)
  perforation caused by, 367, 369, 369(t)
Esophagus, 363
  abdominal, 363, 364
  achalasia of, *374*, 374–376, *375*
  anatomy of, *363*, 363–364, *364*, *367*

Esophagus (*Continued*)
atresia of, 659, *659, 660*
carcinoma of, 384–386
endoscopy in diagnosis of, 367(t)
staging of, 384, 384(t)
treatment of, *385,* 385(t), 385–386, *386*
caustic injury to, 367–369, *368,* 678–679
cervical, 363, 364
trauma to, 187
coordination disorders of, diverticula
and, 378
devascularization of, for portal hypertension, 534
diverticulum of, *372, 373, 378,* 378–379
endoscopy of, 366
as aid to diagnosis, of achalasia, 375
of inflammation, 367
of tumor, 367, 367(t)
perforation caused by, 367, 369, 369(t)
foreign body impaction in, 369, 705
hypermotility disorders of, 376–378, *377*
hypomotility disorders of, 374–376, *375,*
376
in scleroderma, 376, *376*
inflammation of, endoscopy in diagnosis
of, 367
reflux and. See *Gastroesophageal re-*
flux.
leiomyoma of, 383
lower sphincter function in, 365, *366*
abnormal, 374–378, *375–378*
and gastroesophageal reflux, 379
motor disorders of, 374–378
manometric findings in, 375–378, *375–*
378
radiographic findings in, *374,* 375, 376,
376, 377, 377
perforation of, 369(t), 369–371, *370, 371*
by endoscope, 367, 369, 369(t)
external trauma and, 187–188, 369
peristalsis in, 365, *366*
absence of, in scleroderma, 376, *376*
physiology of, 364–365
polyps of, 383
resection of, for cancer, 385
spasm of, diffuse, 376–378, *377*
sphincter function in, 365, *365, 366*
abnormal, 374–378, *375–378*
and dysphagia, 372
and gastroesophageal reflux, 379
squamous cell carcinoma of, 384
stricture of, 381–382
caustic injury and, *368*
structural lesions of, and dysphagia,
371(t), 372, 384
thoracic, 363, 364
trauma to, 187
transection of, end-to-end anastomosis
stapler in, *535*
for portal hypertension, 534
tumors of, 382–386, 383(t)
endoscopy in diagnosis of, 367, 367(t)
upper sphincter function in, 365, *365*
abnormal, and dysphagia, 372
varices of, hemorrhage from, 528, 529
in children, 535
treatment of, 529–532, 530(t), *530–*
532
vomiting causing injury to, 369, 421, 422
Estrogen, exposure to, and risk of breast
cancer, 306
in treatment of prostate cancer, 844
ovarian production of, neurohumoral influences on, 292
replacement of, after menopause, 809

Estrogen receptor activity, in breast cancer,
323
Ethacrynic acid, 1180
Eventration of diaphragm, in newborn, 662
Evoked potentials, 861
Evolving myocardial infarction, 1118
Ewing's sarcoma, 1018
Excision, tangential, of burns, 130
to muscle fascia, in management of
burns, 130
Exercise, as aid to management, of chronic
arterial occlusive disease, 910
Exfoliative cytology, in gynecologic exami-
nation, 810
Exogenous contamination, of wound, 120,
148
Expansion of skin, 262, *264*
Exploratory surgery, in abdominal trauma,
189
Exstrophy of bladder, 837
Extended simple mastectomy, for cancer,
317
External cardiac compression, in CPR,
1056, 1056–1058
animal model studies of effects of,
1057, *1057, 1058*
External ear, disorders of, 690–691
External hemorrhoids, 504
External jugular vein, as site for insertion
of pacemaker lead, *1174*
External mammary lymph node group, 291,
292
Extracellular water, 31–32
Extracorporeal circulation, 1185–1190
Extramedullary hematopoiesis, 629
Extremity, lower, torsional deformities
of, *783,* 783–785, *784*
trauma to, 186
fracture injuries in, 763–768
vascular injuries in, 198–199
upper, trauma to, 186
fracture injuries in, 749, 758–761
Extrinsic pathway, in coagulation cascade,
84, *84*
Eye, signs of carotid artery disease in, 894,
920–923

Facial burns, 125
Facial lymph nodes, 715
Facial nerve, peripheral, paralysis of, 693
Fallopian tube, 806–807
cancer of, 819
inflammation of, 819
Fallot's tetralogy, 1089–1090, *1090*
angiocardiographic findings in, 1090,
1091
radiographic findings in, 1090, *1090*
surgery for, 1091–1092, *1091–1093*
False aneurysm, of hand, 742
Familial breast cancer, 305
Familial polyposis of colon, 486
Fasciitis, necrotizing, 159(t), 162–163
Fasciotomy, indications for, 198
Fat, as component of body weight, vs. total
body water, 31, *31*
changes in metabolism of, in response to
stress, 99, 101(t), 102(t)
digestion of, 411, 433, *433*
fecal, excess of, after stomach surgery,
421
laboratory findings associated with,
597(t)

Fat (*Continued*)
fecal, tests for, 447, 596
in diet, and risk of cancer, of breast, 305
of colon, 488
malabsorption of, 447
Fat embolism, 954–955
as complication of fracture, 756
Fat necrosis, of breast, 304
Fecal continence, 474
Feces, bacteria in, *476*
blood in, testing for, in diagnosis of colorectal cancer, 490
fat in, excess of, after stomach surgery,
421
laboratory findings associated with,
597(t)
tests for, 447, 596
laboratory analysis of, 475
reference values for, 1205(t)
Felon, 750
Femoral artery, trauma to, femoral fracture
and, 198–199
Femoral hernia, 648, *648, 649*
repair of, 648, *649, 650*
Femoral vein, thrombosis of, 941–942
Femoropopliteal bypass, for occlusive arterial disease, 911
Femur, capital epiphysis of, avascular necrosis of, *778,* 778–779, *779*
slipped, *780,* 780–781
fracture of, 763–765, *763–765*
arterial trauma with, 198–199
Fetus, ultrasonographic detection of abnormalities in, 655
Fever, fluid replacement required in, 43
in Crohn's disease, 444
intraoperative, 147(t)
postoperative, 147, 147(t), 201(t), 201–
202, 204
Fibrillation, atrial, drugs for, 1182, 1183
surgical treatment of, 1159
Fibrin, formation of, 85, *86*
disorders of, 90–91
Fibrinogen assays, 89, 937
Fibrinolysis, 86–87, *87*
disorders of, 91
in chronic pulmonary embolism, 966
Fibroadenoma, of breast, 303–304, *303*
Fibrocystic disease of breast, 300–301
Fibroma, of heart, 1166
of skin, 798, *798*
of small intestine, 452
Fibromuscular dysplasia, in extracranial
cerebrovascular disease, 919
Fibrosis, pancreatic, chronic inflammation
and, 604
penile, 845–846
pulmonary, cancer chemotherapy and,
279
submucous, 710
Fibrous histiocytoma, 789, 799
Fibula, fracture of, 766–767, *767*
Field cancerization, 707
Filters, in cardiopulmonary bypass, 1186
Finger, 737, *738*
boutonniere deformity of, 746–747, *747*
contraction of, in Dupuytren's disease,
742
dislocation of, 748
fractures of, *747,* 747–748, *748*
mallet, 746
range of motion of, *739*
vasoconstriction in, 916–918
Fingertip, *750*
amputation injury of, 752, *752*

Fingertip (*Continued*)
  infection of, 750
First aid, for burns, 124
First intention healing, 118
First rib, resection of, for thoracic outlet
    syndrome, 1010, 1011
First-degree burns, 123, 124
First-order kinetics, in cancer chemother-
    apy, 276
Fissure, anal, 506
  treatment of, 506–507, 507
Fistula, anorectal, 507–508, 508
  in Crohn's disease, 445
  treatment of, 508, 509
  arteriovenous, 1191–1193
    of hand, 742
    splenic, 630
  biliary-enteric, 568–569
  coronary arterial, 1128–1129, 1129–1131
    surgery for, 1131, 1132
  drainage of contents of, 140
  gastrointestinal, parenteral nutrition in
    patients with, 106(t)
  in Crohn's disease, 481
  in diverticulitis, 498, 499, 499
  left coronary artery-right ventricular,
    1130
  right coronary artery-right atrial, 1131
  tracheoesophageal, 659, 659, 660
Flail chest, 181–182
Flap(s), Eloesser, in drainage of tubercu-
    lous empyema, 997, 997
  in reconstructive surgery, after radical
    neck dissection for cancer, 726, 727,
    729–730
  musculocutaneous, 262, 262, 263
Flexor digitorum tendons, testing of, 740,
    740
Fluid absorption, in small intestine, 414
Fluid balance, 35, 35(t)
  effects of cardiopulmonary bypass on,
    1188
  indices of, 43
Fluid distribution, 29, 31(t), 31–32
  measurement of, 29, 30
Fluid loss, 35, 35(t)
  in excess of salt, 50–51
Fluid movement, 33–34, 635, 635
Fluid replacement therapy, 40–43, 48, 63
  electrolyte content of solutions used in,
    41(t), 63(t)
  in burn patients, 125–126, 126
  in newborn, 656
  management of prerenal azotemia with,
    212
  solutions for treatment of shock in, 22(t)
Flushing, in carcinoid syndrome, 455
Flutter, atrial, drugs for, 1182, 1183
  surgical treatment of, 1159
Focal nodular hyperplasia, of liver, 543,
    543–544
Follicle-stimulating hormone, 352
  in menstrual cycle, 808, 808
Follicular carcinoma, of thyroid, 337
Fontan operation, for tricuspid atresia,
    1099, 1099
Food poisoning, clostridial, 161
Foot, fracture of, 767–768
  madura, 166
Foot care, in management of occlusive ar-
    terial disease, 911
Foreign body, in peripheral arterial embo-
    lism, 900
Foreign body aspiration, 674

Foreign body impaction, in bronchus, 705
  in ear, 691
  in esophagus, 369, 705
  in larynx, 704–705
  in lung, bronchoscopic treatment of, 983
  in nose, 698
  in pharynx, 701
  in trachea, 705
Foreskin, nonretractable, 844–845
Fracture(s), 755–757
  Chance, 771, 771
  Colles, 749
  fat embolism as complication of, 756
  Galeazzi, 761
  healing of, 757
  immobilization for, 756
  in children, 757
  Jefferson, 185, 769, 769
  Monteggia, 761
  of acetabulum, 762
  of ankle, 766–767, 767
  of atlas, 185, 769, 769
  of axis, 185
  of calcaneus, 767–768
  of cervical vertebra, 185, 768–770
  of diaphysis, 757
  of femur, 763–765, 763–765
    and arterial trauma, 198–199
  of fibula, 766–767, 767
  of finger, 747, 747–748, 748
  of hand, 747–749, 747–749
  of hip, 763, 763–764, 764
  of humerus, 758, 758–759
  of malleolus, 767, 767
  of nose, 697
  of odontoid, 769, 769
  of olecranon, 760
  of patella, 765
  of pelvis, 762, 763
  of radius, 749, 760–761
  of rib(s), and flail chest, 181
  of scaphoid, 748, 749
  of skull, 184, 185, 870–871
  of spine, 768–771, 769, 771, 872
  of talus, 768
  of temporal bone, 693
  of thoracolumbar spine, 770–771, 771
  of tibia, 765, 766
    external fixation of, 766, 766
  of ulna, 749, 760, 761
  open, 756–757
  Piedmont, 761
  reduction of, 756
Free flaps, in reconstructive surgery, after
    radical neck dissection for cancer, 727,
    730
Frequency discrimination, 686
Fresh blood, therapeutic use of, 93
Fresh frozen plasma, therapeutic use of, 93
Friction rub, in pericarditis, 1046
Frozen fresh plasma, therapeutic use of, 93
FUDR chemotherapy regimen, for liver
    cancer, secondary to malignant disease
    at other site, 541, 542
Full-thickness burns, 123
Full-thickness skin graft, 798
Fulminant hepatitis, 171
Fundoplication, 381, 381
  for gastroesophageal reflux in children,
    675
Fungal infection, 166–167
  and pericarditis, 1051
  in AIDS, 176, 176(t)
  of lung, 985–987, 985–987

Fungus ball, 167
Funnel chest (pectus excavatum), 1012–
    1013, 1013
  surgery for, 1013, 1014
Furosemide, for fluid excess, 1180
  for hypercalcemia, 344
Furuncle, of external ear, 691

Galactocele, 301
Galeazzi fracture, 761
Galeazzi's sign, in congenital hip disloca-
    tion, 776, 777
Gallamine, 113
Gallbladder, 551
  adenoma of, 575
  anomalies of, 553, 553
  carcinoma of, 575–577
  empyema of, 565
  imaging of, 558–561, 559, 561
  inflammation of, 561–565
    acalculous, 565
    acute, 396, 562–565
      radionuclide scanning in, 396, 561,
        561
    chronic, 561–562
    emphysematous, 559, 564
  perforation of, 565
  porcelain, 559
  resection of, antimicrobial prophylaxis
      against infection in, 152
    for acute inflammation, 397, 564
    for cancer, 576
    for chronic inflammation, 562
    symptoms of biliary tract disease after,
      583
  trauma to, 195
  tumors of, 575–577
Gallstone(s), 392, 396, 556–557
  and acute cholecystitis, 563
  and acute pancreatitis, 568, 601
  epidemiology of, 556
  formation of, 556–557
  imaging of, 558, 559, 559
  limited effects of chenodeoxycholate on,
    557
  obstruction of small intestine by, 568,
    569, 569
  silent, 557
Gallstone ileus, 568, 569, 569
Gamekeeper's thumb, 748
Ganglioma, mediastinal, 1028
Ganglion, of hand, 752
Ganglioneuroblastoma, mediastinal, 1028
Gangrene, beta-streptococcal infection and,
    163
  gaseous, 157–159, 159(t)
    radiographic findings in, 158
  in chronic arterial occlusive disease, 909
  in peripheral artery disease, 893
  of scrotum, 849
Gardner's syndrome, 452, 486, 487
Gas gangrene, 157–159, 159(t)
  radiographic findings in, 158
Gastrectomy, carcinoma at stump site after,
    420
  complications of, 418–421, 448
  for adenocarcinoma, 424
  for peptic ulcer, 413, 415
    with follow-up restoration of GI conti-
      nuity, 413, 413
  for Zollinger-Ellison syndrome, 418

Gastric acid, laboratory analysis of, reference values for, 1205(t)
  secretion of, 408–409, *409*
    in peptic ulcer disease, 411
    in Zollinger-Ellison syndrome, 417, 418
Gastric analysis, laboratory reference values for, 1205(t)
Gastric bypass, for obesity, 428
Gastric emptying, 410
  rapid, after gastrectomy, 418–419
Gastric partitioning, for obesity, 428, *428*
Gastric phase, of stomach acid secretion, 408–409
Gastrin, 408–409
  secretion of, after meal stimulus, *410*
    excessive, 417–418, 449, 610(t), 611
Gastrinoma, 417–418, 449, 610(t), 611
Gastritis, hemorrhagic, 221, 415–417, *416*
  reflux, after gastrectomy, 420
Gastroduodenostomy, after gastrectomy for peptic ulcer, *413*
Gastroesophageal reflux, 379–381
  and dysphagia, 372
  in children, 675–676
  treatment of, 380–381, *381*
Gastroileal reflex, 435
Gastrointestinal absorption tests, 1205(t)
Gastrointestinal distress, chemotherapy and, 279
  radiation therapy and, 275
Gastrointestinal emergencies, in newborn, 663–671
Gastrointestinal tract, autotransplantation of tissues or organs of, 266
  bacteria endogenous to, 143, 144(t)
    antimicrobials effective against, 157(t)
  carcinoid of, *453*, 453–455, 466–467
  dysfunction of, postoperative, 218–221
  energy metabolism in, effects of shock on, 13–14
  fistulas of, parenteral nutrition in patients with, 106(t)
  hemorrhage from, in newborn, 671
  lactate production in, in shock, 14, *14*
  secretions of, *414*
    electrolyte content of, 42(t), 63(t)
  surgery of, complications of, 221
  tube decompression of, 441
Gastrojejunostomy, after gastrectomy for peptic ulcer, *413*
  afferent loop syndrome as complication of, 419
Gastrojejunostomy and pyloric exclusion, for duodenal trauma, 192, *192*
Gastropexy, posterior, 381, *381*
Gastroplasty, Collis technique of, *382*
  for obesity, 428
Gastroschisis, *671*, 671–672
  closure of, 672, *673*
Gaucher's disease, 625
General anesthesia, 110–113
  inhalational, 111–112
  intravenous, 110–111
  neuromuscular blocking agents in, 112–113
Generalized lymphadenopathy, progressive, 173
Genioglossus muscle, 712
Genitalia. See also specific structures.
  ambiguous, 812–813, 854
    in newborn, 674
  female, anatomy of, 803–807, *804*, *805*
    blood vessels supplying, 804, *804*

Genitalia (*Continued*)
  female, cancer of, radiation therapy for, 274
    sites of, *814*
    congenital abnormalities of, 811–813, *812*
    embryology of, 802–803, *803*
    examination of, 809–811
    intersex disorders of, 812–813
    lymphatics of, 804
    nerves supplying, 804
    physiology of, *807*, 807–809, *809*
  male, anatomy of, 828–830
    cancer of, radiation therapy for, 274
    intersex disorders of, 813, 854
Genitourinary tract, 826, *827*
  calculi in, 404, 836–837
  disorders of, referral of pain from, *404*
  imaging of, 831–833, *832*
  infection of, 146, 164, 403
  toxic effects of chemotherapy agents on, 280
  trauma to, 195–196
Geriatric patient, appendicitis in, 395, 463
  breast changes in, *289*, *294*, 294–295
    hypertrophic, 301
  colorectal cancer treatment in, 496
Geriatric surgical patient, psychiatric disturbances in, 203
Germ cell tumor, 680
  of mediastinum, 1030–1031
Giant cell arteritis, 912–914
Giant cell tumor, of hand, 752
Giant intracanalicular myxoma (giant fibroadenoma), of breast, 303–304
Giant splenomegaly, 624
Giantism, 353
Gibbs-Donnan equilibrium, 33, *33*
Gingiva, 711
Glanzmann's thrombasthenia, 83
Glasgow coma scale, 869(t)
Glomerular capillary, pressure effects in, *39*
Glomerular filtration, autoregulation of, 46, *46*
Glomus tumor, 692
Glottis, 702
  cancer of, 704, 733
  trauma to, 186
Glucagon, 594
  metabolism of, 594–595
  secretion of, 595
Glucagonoma, 610(t), 611
Glucose, diminished serum levels of, carbohydrate ingestion and, 419
  insulin-induced, in diabetes mellitus, 202
  in parenteral nutrition, 24, 104
  infusion of, effects of, 101, 102(t)
  production of, 23, *23*, *24*
    changes in, in response to stress, 16, 23–24, 97, 99, 101(t)
  sodium as cofactor in transport of, *432*
Glucose-alanine cycle, *101*
Glucose tolerance test, 596–597, 597(t), 1206(t)
Goiter, 331
  diffuse, 331
  multinodular, 331–332
Gonadal dysgenesis, mixed, 854
Gonadotropins, in menstrual cycle, 808
Gonorrhea, 403, 820, 848–849
Goodsall's rule, 508, *508*
Goretex graft, in correction of tetralogy of Fallot, 1091, *1092*
Graft(s), 261

Graft(s) (*Continued*)
  autologous, 261–268
  bone, 264
    in reconstructive surgery, after radical neck dissection for cancer, 729
  bone marrow, 266
  cartilage, 264
  composite, 265
    in reimplantation of hand, *265*
  coronary artery bypass. See *Coronary artery bypass graft.*
  Goretex, in correction of tetralogy of Fallot, 1091, *1092*
  H (interposition H), for portal hypertension, 533, *533*
  hair, 263
  in surgery for coarctation of aorta, 1067, 1069, *1069*
  muscle, 264
  musculoskeletal, 264, 264(t)
  nerve, 264–265
  pancreatic, in pancreas transplant, 250, *251*, *252*
  pedicle, 261, 262, *262*
  skin, 262, 262(t), *798*
    after excision of lymphedematous tissue, 637, *637*
    for burns, 130, 262
    full-thickness, *798*
    in reconstructive surgery, after radical neck dissection for cancer, 729
    meshed, for burns, 130
    split-thickness, 262
      donor site in, cutting of, with dermatomes, 130
      for burns, 130
      in reconstructive surgery, after radical neck dissection for cancer, 729
  vascular, 263–264
    for vessel trauma, 197
    indications for, 263(t)
Graft versus host disease, in animal recipients of small bowel transplant, 261
Gram staining, of bile, 152
Granular cell myoblastoma, of breast, 304
Granulation tissue, in wound healing, 119
Granuloma, in Crohn's disease, 442
Granuloma inguinale, 846
Graves' disease (hyperthyroidism), 71–72, 330, 333(t), 333–334
Great artery transposition, 1102–1103
  surgery for, 1104, *1105–1108*, 1108
    historical aspects of, 1102–1103
Groin, anatomy of, 640, *640*, *642*
Growth hormone, 351
  tumor secreting, 353
Growth hormone–inhibiting factor (somatostatin), 351, 595
  for bleeding esophageal varices, 529
  tumor secreting, 610(t), 612
Gynecology, 802
Gynecomastia, 301

H graft, for portal hypertension, 533, *533*
H2 receptor, of parietal cells, 408
Haemophilus infection, vaginal, 814
Hair transplantation, 263
Halothane, 112
Halsted, William, *4*
  as advocate of minimal tissue handling, 134
  contributions of, to surgical training, 3–5

Halsted (Halsted-Ferguson) operation, for inguinal hernia, 639, *645–646*
Halsted radical mastectomy, for cancer, results of, 318, *318–319*
Hand, 737, *738*
  amputation injury of, *752, 752–753, 754*
    reimplantation following, *265*
  arteries of, occlusive disease of, 743
  arthritis of, 751
  burns of, 125
  circulation in, 741
  enchondroma of, 752
  entrapment neuropathy of, 744–745
  epidermoid cyst of, 752
  fractures of, 747–749, *747–749*
  infection of, 750–751
  nerves of, 737–740, *739, 740*
    injury of, 743–745
    testing of, 740
  range of motion of, *738*
  skin injury of, 741
  surgery of, anesthesia in, 741
    preparation for, 741
  surgical incisions on, 741, *742*
  tendons of, *745*
    surgical repair of, 745–747, *746*
    testing of, 740, *740*
  tumors of, 752
  vascular injury of, 742
Hangman's fracture, 769
Hard palate, tumors of, 731
Harrington rod, for scoliosis, 775
Harvey, William, *2*
  contributions of, to study of circulation, 1
Haustra of colon, radiographic appearance of, in cases of obstruction, *440*
Head, trauma to, 184–185, 869–871
Head and neck cancer, 706–707, 710, 715–730
  approach to patient with, 717–720
  as locoregional disease, 716
  chemotherapy for, 722
  dental disease in patients with, 719
  epidemiology of, 706
  etiology of, 706–707
  extracapsular spread of, 716
  gastrointestinal disease in patients with, 719
  imaging studies in, 719
  immune deficiency in patients with, 719, 720
  immunotherapy for, 720, 722
  lung disease in patients with, 719
  metastasis of, 716
  natural course of, 715–717
  patient history in, 717
  physical examination in, *718*, 718–719
  prognosis in, 716–717
  radiation therapy for, 274, 722–724
    side effects of, 275, 724
    vs. surgical treatment, 724
  recurrence of, 716, *717*
  smoking as etiologic agent in, 706
    alcohol use and, 706
  staging of, 720
  surgery for, 724–725, *726–727, 727–728*
    collection of tumor specimen in, *725*
    complications of, 728
    margin of normal tissue to be excised in, 725
    reconstruction after, *726–727*, 728–730
    use of prostheses after, 730
    vs. radiation therapy, 724

Head and neck cancer (*Continued*)
  synchronous tumor formation in, 707
    field cancerization and, 707
  treatment of, 720, 722–730
Head and neck examination, for cancer, *718*, 718–719
Healing. See *Wound healing.*
Health status/performance scales, 63(t), 279(t)
Hearing, 686
Hearing loss, 687, 689
  drugs causing, 694
  noise-induced, 693
  sudden, 695
  tests for, 689–690
Heart, artificial, *1127*, 1127–1128, *1128*
  cancer metastatic to, 1168
  chemotherapeutic agents toxic to, 279
  contractility of, 18, 1179
  direct (open-chest) compression of, 1058, *1059*
  disease of, and peripheral arterial embolism, 899
    and risk of compromised cardiac function, in surgical patient, 69, 69(t)
    management of surgical patient with, 69–70, 1179–1184
  external compression of, in CPR, *1056*, 1056–1058
    animal model studies of effects of, 1057, *1057, 1058*
  failure of, congestive, 64
    as complication of coronary artery bypass graft, 1122
    pacemaker for, 1171
    perioperative, management of, *1183*
  fibroma of, 1166
  malformations of. See specific defects, e.g., *Ventricular septal defect(s).*
  mesothelioma of, 1166
  metabolism in, 1118
    effects of shock on, 17
  myxoma of, 1164–1165, *1165*
    surgery for, 1166, *1167*
  output of, and PO$_2$, 207
    low, as complication of coronary artery bypass graft, 1121
    perioperative, management of, *1183*
  oxygen extraction by, *1118*
  perioperative dysfunction of, management of, *1183*
  receptor pharmacology of, 1180(t)
  rhabdomyoma of, 1165–1166
  sarcoma of, 1166
  surgery of, cardiopulmonary bypass in, 1185–1190
  transplantation of, 253–259
    after earlier heart transplant, 258, 258(t)
    artificial heart as alternative to, 1127
    care after, 256
    coronary artery atherosclerosis after, 258
    cost of, 259
    donor in, 254
    early developments in, 253
    heterotopic, 253
    immunosuppression in, 256
    infection after, 257–258, *258*
    procedure for, 254, *255*
    recipient in, 253–254
    rejection of, 257, *257*
      acute, 229
    results of, 258, *259*, 259(t)

Heart (*Continued*)
  trauma to, 188, 189
  tumors of, 1163–1168, 1164(t)
    echocardiographic findings in, 1164, *1165*
Heart failure, congestive, 64
  as complication of coronary artery bypass graft, 1122
  pacemaker for, 1171
  perioperative, management of, *1183*
Heat exchanger, in cardiopulmonary bypass, 1185–1186
Helper T cell, 226
Hemangioblastoma, 864
Hemangioma, *799*, 799–800, *800*
  airway obstruction by, in newborn, 658
  in mediastinum, 1033
  of liver, 544, 684
  of small intestine, 452
Hematocrit, effects of cardiopulmonary bypass on, 1187
Hematology, laboratory reference values in, 1197(t)–1198(t)
Hematoma, complicating wound healing, 119, 120
  duodenal, obstruction of small intestine by, 192
  epidural, 185, 871, *872*, 920
  hepatic, CT findings in, *190*
  pinnal, 691
  subdural, 185, 871, *872*, 920
Hematopoiesis, extramedullary, 629
Hematuria, 831
Hemobilia, 535–537, *536*, 583
Hemodialysis, 213
  arteriovenous shunt in, 213, *214*
  for acute renal failure, 213
Hemodynamic norms, 18(t), 889–890, 1117(t)
  deviation from, arterial aneurysm and, 891–892
    arterial obstruction and, *890*, 890–891, *891*
Hemoglobin, combination of oxygen with, *970*, 970–971
Hemolysis, and jaundice, 216
  in reaction to transfusion, 94, 216
  postoperative, 216
Hemolytic anemia, 625–628
  splenectomy for, 625–626
Hemophilia, 90
Hemoptysis, tuberculosis and, 997
Hemorrhage, 182
  from colon, in colitis, 484
    in diverticulitis, 497, 499
  from esophageal varices, 528, 529
    in children, 535
    treatment of, 529–532, 530(t), *530–532*
  from gastrointestinal tract, in newborn, 671
  from hand, 742
  from liver, in abdominal trauma, 193–194
    from Mallory-Weiss tears, 421
  from nose, 698
    control of, 698, *698*
    sites of, *697*, 698
  from peptic ulcer, 412
    surgery for, 414, 415
  from small intestine, in patients with Meckel's diverticulum, 457
  from stress ulcer, 221, 415–417, *416*
  into biliary tract, 535–537, *536*, 583
  into mediastinum, 1023–1024
  intracerebral, 185, 868

Hemorrhage (*Continued*)
  intracerebral, and stroke, 920
  intracranial, trauma and, 184, 185
  intraventricular, 185
  massive, management of, 92–93
  meningeal, 184, 185
  pathophysiologic consequences of, 92
  subarachnoid, 185, 865(t), 865–866
    and stroke, 920
Hemorrhagic gastritis, acute, 221, 415–417,
    416
Hemorrhoid(s), 504, *505*, 506
Hemorrhoidectomy, 506
Hemostasis, 79–87, 80(t)
  anatomic basis of, 79–82, 80(t)
  biochemistry of, 79, 80(t), 82–87
  disorders of, 80(t), 89–92
    and hypercoagulability, 946,
      946(t), *947*, 948(t), 949(t)
  laboratory tests for, 65, 87(t), 87–89
  surgical patients with, 65
  in surgery, 135–136
  physiology of, 82–87
  plug formation in, 81–82
Hemothorax, 990
Heparin, antithrombin III interaction with,
    85, *86*
  in prophylaxis against deep venous
    thrombosis, in surgical patients, 66
  in prophylaxis against pulmonary embo-
    lism, 949
  in treatment of pulmonary embolism, 949
Hepatectomy, 520
  Cavitron ultrasonic surgical aspiration
    device in, 520, *520*
  course after, 520–521
  for cancer, 538–539
    in children, 543
    secondary to malignant disease at
      other site, 286, 496, 540–541
  in transplantation, 246–247, *247*
  with cholangiojejunostomy to Roux-en-Y
    limb, in repair of biliary stricture, 575
Hepatic artery, 514–515, *515*
  ligation of, in treatment of liver cancer,
    539, 542
Hepatic coma, 545–546
Hepatic encephalopathy, 545–546
Hepatic enzymes, 518
Hepatic portoenterostomy, for biliary atre-
    sia, 673, *673, 674*
Hepatic transplantation. See *Liver, trans-
    plantation of.*
Hepatic vein, 513, *514*, 515, *515*
  obstruction of, 527, 544–545
Hepaticojejunostomy to Roux-en-Y limb,
    with transhepatic biliary stent, in re-
    pair of biliary stricture,
    574, *575*
Hepatitis, anesthesia-induced, 216
  viral, 165–166, 169–173, 170(t)
    and hepatoma, 171
    carriers of, 165, 171
    clinical manifestations of, 171
    epidemiology of, 169–171
    fulminant, 171
    pathogenesis of, 171
      etiologic agents in, 169, 170(t)
    postoperative, 216–217
    prevention of spread of, 165–166, 171–
      173, 172(t), 173(t)
    progressive, chronic, 171
    transfusion-transmitted, 94, 170–171
Hepatitis antigens and antibodies, 165,
    170(t), *172*

Hepatitis B immune globulin, 166, 172(t)
Hepatitis B vaccine, 166, 172(t), 172–173,
    173(t)
Hepatobiliary tract. See *Bile duct(s)* and
    Biliary tract.
Hepatoblastoma, 542–543, *543*, *683*, 684
Hepatocellular adenoma, 544, *544*
Hepatocellular carcinoma, *537*, 537–539,
    684
  alpha-fetoprotein in, 281
  viral hepatitis and, 171
Hepatocytes, 516, *516, 517*
  changes in, in shock, *17*
Hepatoma, *537*, 537–539, 684
  alpha-fetoprotein in, 281
  viral hepatitis and, 171
Hereditary elliptocytosis, 628
Hereditary spherocytosis, 626
  splenectomy for, 626
Hermaphroditism, 812–813, 854
Hernia, 639
  Bochdalek, *661*, 661–662
    repair of, 662, *662*
  diaphragmatic, in newborn, *661*, 661–
    662, *662*
  dorsal, 654
  epigastric, 652
  femoral, 648, *648, 649*
    repair of, 648, *649, 650*
  hiatal, 382, *383*
  historical aspects of treatment of, 6, 639
  in children, 678
  incarcerated (irreducible), 651–652
  incisional, 650, *651*
  inguinal, 639–641
    bilateral, 648
    clinical manifestations of, 640
    direct, 640, 641, *641*
    examination for, 641, *641*
    groin anatomy and, 640, *640, 642*
    in children, 678
    indirect, 639, 641, *641*
    repair of, 641, 642–647, 645
      complications of, 645, 648, 648(t)
    sliding, 651
      and blood supply to colon, *651*
  Littre's, 653
  lumbar, 654
  obturator, 653–654
  parastomal, 652–653
  perineal, 654
  Richter's, 653, *653*
  sciatic, 654
  Spigelian, 653
  strangulated, 651–652
  umbilical, 648, 650
    repair of, *650*
  ventral, 650
Herpes progenitalis, 846
Herpes virus infection, vulvar, 813
Herpetic whitlow, 751
Heterotopic heart transplantation, 253
Hiatal hernia, 382, *383*
Hibernoma, 799
Hidradenitis suppurativa, 801
  of vulva, 813
Hill posterior gastropexy, 381, *381*
Hill-Sachs' lesion, 758
Hip, congenital dislocation of, 775–777
  Barlow test for, 776, *776*
  Galeazzi's sign in, 776, *777*
  Ortolani test for, 776, *776*
  Pavlik harness for, 776–777, *777*
  fracture of, *763*, 763–764, *764*
  rotation of, 783

Hirschsprung's disease, 668, *668*
Histiocytoma, fibrous, 789, 799
Histocompatibility antigens, 224, *225*,
    225(t)
Histoplasmosis, 167, 985, *985*
HLA antigen, 224, *225*, 225(t)
  Class I, 224, *225*, 225(t)
  Class II, 224, *225*, 225(t)
    dendritic cells as source of, 226
    pre-transplant typing for match of, 230,
      238
HLA-DR antigen, pre-transplant typing for
    match of, 231
Hodgkin's disease, 274, 631(t), 631–632,
    1031, *1031*
Hofmeister modification, of Billroth II
    anastomosis, *413*
Hollander test, 418
Homans' sign, 934
Homeostasis, 10–11
Hormone receptor activity, in breast can-
    cer, 323
Hormone receptor blockers, in cancer che-
    motherapy, 278
Horseshoe kidney, 833
Hospital-acquired infection, 141
  in surgical patient, *148*, 163–165, 209
Hospitalization, preoperative, duration of,
    and risk of infection, 149
Host defense mechanisms, 142
  defects and abnormalities in, 142–143
HTLV-III infection. See *Immune defi-
    ciency, acquired.*
Huggins, Charles, 7, *7*
Human bite, of hand, 751
Human T lymphotrophic virus type III in-
    fection. See *Immune deficiency, ac-
    quired.*
Humerus, fracture of, *758*, 758–759
Hunter, John, 2
  advocacy of experimental method by, 2
Hürthle cell carcinoma, 337
Hyalinization, of alveolar membrane, 25,
    26
Hydatid cyst, of liver, *525*, 525–527, *526*
  of spleen, 630
Hydatidiform mole, 824
Hydralazine, 1180
Hydrocele, 849–850
Hydrocephalus, 877–878
Hydrogen ion concentration, 54–55, *55*
Hydronephrosis, 679
Hydrops, endolymphatic, 694
Hydrostatic pressure, 34
Hydrothorax, 608
Hydroxytryptamine metabolism, in carci-
    noid syndrome, 454, *454*
Hygroma, cystic, 638, *638, 658, 658*
  in mediastinum, 1033–1034
Hymen, imperforate, 680
Hyperabduction test, 1011
Hyperacute rejection, 228
  avoidance of, 229–230
Hyperaldosteronism, 359
Hyperamylasemia, 602
Hyperbaric oxygen, for gas gangrene,
    159
Hyperbilirubinemia, 558
Hypercalcemia, 341–342, 342(t)
  causes of, 342(t)
    tests used in investigation of, 344(t)
  in hyperparathyroidism, 340–344, 346,
    347
  treatment of, 344
    in surgical patients, 65

Hypercholesterolemia, intestinal bypass for, 459–460

Hypercoagulability, and pulmonary embolism, 945–946, 946(t), *947*, 948(t), 949(t)

Hypercortisolism, 353, 356–358, 357(t)
  signs of, 356, 356(t)

Hypergastrinemia, 417–418, 449, 610(t), 611

Hyperinflation of lung, in newborn, 663

Hyperinsulinism, in newborn, due to islet cell hyperplasia, 611

Hyperkalemia, 45, 52(t), 52–53
  management of surgical patients with, 64

Hyperkeratosis, 708

Hyperlipidemia, in acute pancreatitis, 602

Hypermotility, esophageal, 376–378, *377*

Hypernatremia, 45, 50–51, 64

Hypernephroma, 834, *835*
  metastasis of, to lung, *1003*

Hyperparathyroidism, 342–347
  clinical recognition of, historical aspects of, 340
  hypercalcemia in, 340–344, 346, 347
  treatment of, 344–347
    hypocalcemia after, 346, 348, 349
    hypoparathyroidism after, 348, 349

Hyperplastic polyp, of stomach, 423

Hyperprolactinemia, 303, 354

Hypersplenism, 623(t), 624

Hypertension, as complication of coronary artery bypass graft, 1122
  perioperative, management of, *1183*
  portal, *527*, 527–535
    bleeding esophageal varices in patients with, 529
      treatment of, 529–532, 530(t), *530–532*
    in children, 535
    pathophysiology of, 528, *528*
    surgery for, 533–534, *533–535*
  renovascular, 836, 927–929, *929*

Hyperthyroidism, 330, 333–334, 334(t)
  management of surgical patient with, 71–72

Hypertriglyceridemia, in acute pancreatitis, 602

Hypertrophic pyloric stenosis, 674–675
  surgery for, 675, *675*

Hypertrophic scar, 798
  formation of, after healing of burns, 130–131

Hypertrophic subaortic stenosis, idiopathic, 1112, 1139, 1141
  surgery for, 1141, *1141*

Hypnosis, 114

Hypocalcemia, after parathyroidectomy, 346, 348, 349
  after surgery, 203
  causes of, 348(t)

Hypoglycemia, insulin-induced, in diabetes mellitus, 202
  reactive, 419

Hypokalemia, 45, 51–52, 52(t)
  management of surgical patients with, 64

Hypomotility, esophageal, 374–376, *375*, *376*

Hyponatremia, 45, 48–50, 64

Hypoparathyroidism, 348, 349

Hypoperfusion, cellular, in shock, 12, *13*

Hypopharynx, 699
  carcinoma of, 700, 732
  diverticulum of, 701

Hypophysectomy, for Cushing's syndrome, 353, 358

Hypophysectomy (*Continued*)
  in treatment of prostate cancer, 844

Hypophysis. See *Pituitary*.

Hypospadias, 848

Hyposplenism, 621

Hypotension. See also *Hypovolemia*.
  controlled, 112
  in trauma patient, 182–183
  perioperative, management of, *1183*

Hypothalamus, 350
  effects of hormones of, on pituitary hormones, 352(t)

Hypothermia, regional, 115

Hypothermic perfusion, in cardiopulmonary bypass, 1187, *1187*, *1188*
  in preservation of cadaver organs for transplantation, 236

Hypothyroidism, 330

Hypovolemia, compensatory responses to, 46–47
  management of, 63
    in trauma patient, 182
  treatment of. See *Fluid replacement therapy*.

Hypovolemic shock, 19–20

ICHD code, for pacing modes, 1175–1176, 1176(t)

ICU (intensive care unit), as environment disturbing to patient's mental status, 203

Idiopathic diffuse esophageal spasm, 376–378, *377*

Idiopathic hypertrophic subaortic stenosis, 1112, 1139, 1141
  surgery for, 1141, *1141*

Idiopathic thrombocytopenic purpura, 629

Idiotype, 233
  antibody to, induction of tolerance with, 233

Ileal bypass, for hypercholesterolemia, 459–460

Ileal conduit, in urinary diversion, after cystectomy, 839

Ileostomy, *477*
  replacement of fluid losses from, 42

Ileum, 429
  cancer of, 451(t)
  cystic duplication of, *684*
  tumors of, 451(t)

Ileus, gallstones and, 568, 569, *569*
  meconium and, 665, *667*, 668
  paralytic, 219–220, *220*, 436
    in burn patients, 126
    postoperative, 219
    treatment of, 442
    vs. mechanical small bowel obstruction, 219

Iliofemoral thrombosis, 941–942

Iliopsoas test, in diagnosis of cause of abdominal pain, 391, *391*

Immobilization, for fracture, 756

Immune deficiency, acquired, 173–177, 174(t)
  Kaposi's sarcoma in, 177, 800
  opportunistic infections in, 176(t), 176–177, 987
  pathogen causing, 173, 270
    antibodies to, 175
      tests for, 173, 175(t)
    tests for, 173, 175(t)
  pediatric cases of, standards for differential diagnosis of, 174(t)

Immune deficiency (*Continued*)
  acquired, symptom complex related to (ARC), 173, 174(t)
    transfusion-transmitted, 94, 175
  patient susceptibility to, 221–222
    and cancer, of head and neck, 719, 720
      of lung, 1005–1006

Immune globulin, hepatitis B, 166, 172(t)
  tetanus, 160–161, 199

Immune response, and cancer resistance, 281

Immune thrombocytopenic purpura, 89, 629

Immune tolerance, 232–234
  attempts at induction of, in preparation for transplantation, 234

Immunization, against hepatitis, 166, 172(t), 172–173, 173(t)
  against tetanus, 160(t), 160–161, 199

Immunologic enhancement, 233

Immunology, laboratory reference values in, 1205(t)

Immunosuppression, cancer chemotherapy and, 279

Immunosuppressive(s), 231–232
  for myasthenia gravis, 1042
  in prevention of rejection, 231–232, 237, 238
    of heart, 256
    of heart and lungs, 257
    of kidney, 243
    of liver, 247, 248, 249
    of lungs, 257, 260
    of pancreas, 251
  sites of action of, *232*
  tumor development in patients treated with, 243

Immunotherapy, for cancer, 282–283
  of head and neck, 720, 722
  of lung, 1006

Imperforate anus, 668–669, *669*

Imperforate hymen, 680

Implantation of pacemaker, 1173–1174, *1174*
  complications of, 1176(t), 1176–1177
  in infant, 1174, *1175*

Impotence, 847–848

Impulse generator, of pacemaker, 1171, *1172*

Inappropriate secretion of antidiuretic hormone, 49, 215

Inappropriate sinus tachycardia, surgical treatment of, 1160

Incarcerated (irreducible) hernia, 651–652

Incised clean wound, healing of, 118

Incision, surgical, 134
  risk of infection associated with, 134, *134*, *135*

Incisional hernia, 650, *651*

Incontinence, urinary, 831
  loss of pelvic support and, *819*, 819–820
  neurogenic, 839–840
  stress, 840

Indirect inguinal hernia, 639, 641, *641*

Inducer T cell, 226

Infants. See *Child(ren)* and *Newborn*.

Infarction, myocardial, as complication of coronary artery bypass graft, 1122
  evolving, 1118
  pericarditis following, 1052
  splenic, 630

Infection(s). See also *Sepsis*.
  after transplantation, of heart, 257–258, *258*

Infection(s) (*Continued*)
   after transplantation, of kidney, 242
      of liver, 248–249
   community-acquired, 141
   defense mechanisms against, 142
      defects in, 142–143
   diagnosis of, anaerobe and aerobe identi-
      fication in, 146
      specimen collection in, 146–147
   in AIDS, 176(t), 176–177, 987
   in premature infants, 657
   necrotizing, of soft tissue, 157–159,
      159(t), 162–163
   nosocomial, 141
      in surgical patient, *148*, 163–165, 209
   surgical, 68, 141–167, 203–206, 222
      anergy and, 68
      antimicrobial prophylaxis against, 68,
         120, 150–152
         procedures not requiring, 151(t)
      antimicrobial treatment of, 153, 154(t),
         155(t)
      bacteria causing, 143, 145(t)–146(t),
         146–165
      diagnosis of, 147–148, 203–204
         CT scanning in, *147*
         ultrasonography in, *148*
      fever as sign of, 147, 147(t), 201, 202,
         204
      incisions and, 134, *134*, *135*
      microbiology of, 143, 145(t)–146(t),
         146–147
      nosocomial, *148*, 163–165, 209
      surgical treatment of, 153
      wound closure materials and, *137*,
         138(t)
      wound in, 148–150, *149*, 149(t)
   theories of, historical aspects of, 141
   tissue susceptibility to, 142
   transfusion-transmitted, 94, 170–171, 175
   virulence of pathogen in, 142
   wound, 120, 142
      burns and, 128
      surgery and, 148–150, *149*, 149(t)
Inferior constrictor muscle, of pharynx, 713
Inferior vena cava, surgery of, for pulmo-
      nary embolism, 951–952, *952*, 952(t),
      953, 953(t)
Infertility, 821, 853
   as risk factor for breast cancer, 306
   cancer chemotherapy and, 280
Infiltrating ductal carcinoma (scirrhous car-
      cinoma), of breast, *298*, 312, *312*
Inflammation, in wound healing, 118
Inflammatory carcinoma, of breast, 297,
      298, 314, *314*, 319
Infracardiac anomalous pulmonary venous
      connection, *1082*, 1083
Infusaid pump, *541*
Inguinal hernia, 639–641
   bilateral, 648
   clinical manifestations of, 640
   direct, 640, 641, *641*
   examination for, 641, *641*
   groin anatomy and, 640, *640*, *642*
   in children, 678
   indirect, 639, 641, *641*
   repair of, 641, *642–647*, 645
      complications of, 645, 648, 648(t)
   sliding, 651
      and blood supply to colon, *651*
INH (isoniazid), for mycobacterial infec-
      tions, 996, 996(t)
Inhalation anesthesia, 111–112
Inhalation injury, 129

Injury. See *Trauma* and particular types of
      injury, and see under specific sites.
Inner ear, disorders of, 693–695
Instrument sterilization, 133
Insufficiency, aortic, *1138*, 1138–1139
      treatment of, by replacement with
         prosthetic valve, 1139, *1140*
   mitral, 1148–1149
      treatment of, 1149–1150, *1150*
   tricuspid valve, 1150
Insulin, 594
   metabolism of, 594
   preoperative use of, in diabetic patients,
      71
   secretion of, 594
      excessive, in newborn, due to islet cell
         hyperplasia, 611
      tests of, 597
Insulin-induced hypoglycemia, in diabetes
      mellitus, 202
Insulinoma, 610(t), 611
Intensive care unit (ICU), as environment
      disturbing to patient's mental status,
      203
Interatrial septum, defects of, 1076–1081,
      1078
   development and partitioning of, 1077,
      1077
Intercostal veins, 290, *291*
Intercostobrachial nerve, 290
Interleukin-1, 226
Interleukin-2, 226, 227
   in immunotherapy for cancer, 283
Interloop abscess, 205
Intermittent mandatory ventilation, 977
   for adult respiratory distress syndrome,
      211
Internal hemorrhoids, 504
Internal jugular vein, as site for insertion of
      pacemaker lead, *1174*
Internal mammary veins, 290, *291*
International system of units (S.I. units),
      1195(t), 1195–1196, 1196(t)
Interposition H graft, for portal hyperten-
      sion, 533, *533*
Interrupted sutures, 135
Intersexuality, 812–813, 853–854
Interstitial fluid, 31–32, 635
Interval cholecystectomy, for acute inflam-
      mation, 564
Intestinal anastomosis, stapling and, *493*
Intestinal antisepsis, 68, 475–476
Intestinal bypass, 459–460
   for hypercholesterolemia, 459–460
   for obesity, 428, 459
Intestinal phase, of gastric acid secretion,
      409
Intestine. See also *Colon* and *Small intes-
      tine.*
   atresia of, 665
      correction of, 665, *667*
   clostridial infection of, 161–162
   fistulas of, in Crohn's disease, 481
   ischemia of, mesenteric vascular insuffi-
      ciency and, 400–401, 401(t), 929–931,
      931
   malrotation of, 665
      correction of, 665, *666*
   obstruction of, 399–400
      and vomiting, 438
      in newborn, 663–665, *664*, *666–669*,
         668–669
      radiographic findings in, 438, *439*, *440*,
         441
   perforation of, in newborn, 669–670

Intestine (*Continued*)
   radiation injury to, 458, 503
   rotation of, *665*
      abnormal, 665
         correction of, 665, *666*
Intestino-intestinal inhibitory reflex, 435
Intima, vascular, 80
Intolerance, lactose, after gastrectomy, 421
Intra-abdominal anastomotic breakdown,
      205
Intra-abdominal pressure, increased, and
      acute renal failure, 215
Intra-abdominal sepsis, 153–154, 204–205
   changed mental status as sign of, 203
   treatment of, antimicrobials in, 157,
      157(t)
   drainage in, 154, 157, 204–205, *205*
Intra-abdominal trauma, 189–195
   diagnosis of, 189–191
      angiography in, 190–191
      computed tomography in, 190, *190*
      peritoneal lavage in, 183, 189
      radionuclide scanning after, 190
Intra-aortic balloon pump, 1182
Intracanalicular myxoma, giant, of breast,
      303–304
Intracardiac anomalous pulmonary venous
      connection, *1082*, 1082–1083
Intracardiac electrode catheters, placement
      of, in candidates for surgical correction
      of arrhythmia, *1156*
Intracellular killing, abnormal, 143
Intracellular water, 32
Intracerebral hemorrhage, 185, 868
   and stroke, 920
Intracranial aneurysm, 865–866
Intracranial hemorrhage, trauma and, 184,
      185
Intracranial pressure, 857
   control of, in head injury, 870
   increased, brain tumors and, 862–863
      perioperative, 859
      trauma and, 184
Intraductal papilloma, of breast, 304
Intramedullary nail, for femoral fracture,
      765
In-transit metastases, after surgical excision
      of melanoma, 286
Intraperitoneal abscess, 154, 204–205
Intrapulmonary shunt, 25, *26*, 207, *207*
Intrathoracic infection, postoperative, 205–
      206
Intrathoracic thyroid tumors, 1032
Intravascular catheter-related sepsis, 105–
      106, 165
Intravascular coagulopathy, disseminated,
      26–27, 27(t), 90–91, *91*, 221
   in chronic occlusive arterial disease,
      909
Intravascular volume depletion, 63
Intravenous anesthesia, 110–111
Intravenous antimicrobials, in prophylaxis
      against surgical infection, 150
Intravenous fluid replacement therapy. See
      Fluid replacement therapy.
Intravenous glucose tolerance test, 597
Intraventricular hemorrhage, 185
Intrinsic pathway, in coagulation cascade,
      84, *84*, 85
Intubation, endotracheal, laryngoscopy
      and, 1056, *1056*
Intussusception, 676
   in patients with Meckel's diverticulum,
      458, *467*, 468, *469*
   rectal, 510, *511*

Intussusception (*Continued*)
  reduction of, 676, *677*
Inverted Y irradiation field, *632*
Iodine, in antisepsis, 132, *133*
Iodine isotopes, tests of thyroid uptake of, 330
  treatment of hyperthyroidism with, 333–334
Ionizing radiation. See *Radiation.*
Iron, absorption of, in small intestine, 434
Irreducible (incarcerated) hernia, 651–652
Irrigation, in management of burns, 128–129
Ischemia, and acute pancreatitis, 602
  and rest pain, in chronic occlusive arterial disease, 908–909
  and ulceration, in chronic occlusive arterial disease, 909
  in peripheral arterial disease, 892–893
  cerebrovascular, 868
    transient, 918–927
  colonic, following repair of aneurysm, 907
    inflammation with, 502, *502*
  intestinal, mesenteric vascular insufficiency and, 400–401, 401(t), 929–931, *931*
  myocardial, 1115, 1117
    coronary artery bypass graft for, 1119–1121, *1120, 1121*
      candidates for, 1117–1118
      complications of, 1121–1123
      protection of myocardium in, cardioplegic solution and, 1119, 1119(t)
      results of, *1117*, 1123
    percutaneous transluminal balloon angioplasty for, 1118–1119
    ventricular tachycardia in, 1160
      surgery for, 1160–1161, *1161*
      nondirected, 1160(t)
Ischemic colitis, 502, *502*
Islet cells, pancreatic, 592, *592*
  hyperplasia of, 610
  transplantation of, 252
    autologous, 265
  tumors of, 610(t), 610–612
Isoflurane, 112
Isolation, of patients with hepatitis, 166
Isoniazid (INH), for mycobacterial infections, 996, 996(t)
Isoproterenol, 1181

Jaundice, 519–520, 584, *585*
  in newborn, 673
  obstructive, 584–586, *585, 586*
  postoperative, 201(t), 215(t), 215–218
Jaw thrust, in relief of airway obstruction, 181
Jefferson fracture, 185, 769, *769*
Jejunal bypass, for obesity, 428
Jejunoileal bypass, *459*
  for obesity, 459
Jejunum, 429
  tumors of, 451(t)
Joint(s), infection of, 790
  inflammation of, 789–790
    hand involvement in, 751
    pyogenic, 786–787
Joint fusion, in treatment of arthritis, 790
Joint replacement, in treatment of arthritis, 790
Jolly test, for myasthenia gravis, 1040

Jugular vein, as site for insertion of pacemaker lead, *1174*
Jugulodigastric lymph nodes, 715
Juvenile angiofibroma, of nasopharynx, 700
Juvenile laryngotracheal papillomatosis, 703
Juvenile polyposis of colon, 487

Kaposi's sarcoma, in AIDS, 177, 800
Karnofsky performance scale, 279(t)
Kasai procedure, for biliary atresia, 580, 673
Keloid, 120, *797, 797*–798
Keratin pearls, 710
Keratoacanthoma, 795, *795*
Keratosis, 708
  seborrheic, 794, *794*
Kidney(s), 826
  agenesis of, 833
  angiomyolipoma of, 833
  aplasia of, 833
  bicarbonate reabsorption by, arterial PCO_2 and, 56, *56*
  blood flow in, autoregulation of, 46, *46*
    effect of hypovolemia on, 47
  cancer of, 834–836, *835*
  cyst of, 679, 833
  disease of, management of surgical patient with, 74
    osteodystrophy in, *348*
    recurrent, after transplantation, 239(t)
    surgical infection in patients with, antimicrobials for, 153, 154(t)
  ectopic, 833
  failure of, 63
    acute, 25–26, 44
      parenteral nutrition in management of, 105, 105(t)
      postoperative, 212–214
      vs. prerenal azotemia, 45, 45(t), 213(t)
    and pericarditis, 1051
    as complication of cardiopulmonary bypass, 1190
    postoperative, 211–215
  filtration by, autoregulation of, 46, *46*
  function of, 46
    effects of shock on, 15
  glomerular capillaries of, pressure effects in, *39*
  horseshoe, 833
  hypoplasia of, 833
  infection-related inflammation of, postoperative, 164
  multicystic, 679, 833
  nephrons of, 38, *38*, 39, *39*
  neuroendocrine control of, 35–40
  pain in, 830
  polycystic, 679, 833
  resection of, for cancer, 834
    in transplantation, 240, *240, 241*
  solute reabsorption by, 39(t), 39–40
  surgical approaches to, 826–828
  transplantation of, 237–243
    care after, 241
    complications of, 242
    donor in, 239–240
    early developments in, 237
    favorable factors in, 243(t)
    hypothermic pulsatile perfusion of donor organ in, 236
    immunosuppression in, 243
    infection after, 242

Kidney(s) (*Continued*)
  transplantation of, nephrectomy in, 240, *240, 241*
    pancreatitis following, 602
    preparation for, 239
    procedure for, 241, *242*
    recipient in, 238–239
    rejection of, 242
      accelerated, 228
      acute, 229, *229*
      chronic, 229, *230*
      hyperacute, 228
      initiation of immune response in, *227, 228*
      testing for possible potentiators of, 229–231
    renal diseases recurring after, 239(t)
    results of, 243, *243*
  trauma to, 195–196
  tumors of, in children, 679–680, *680*, 834–836
  urine dilution by, impairment of, and hyponatremia, 49
  vasculature of, disease of, 836, 927–928
    midline approach to, *196*
    trauma to, 196
  Wilms' tumor of, 679–680, *680*, 834–836
Kidney stones, *836*, 836–837
Kienböck's disease, 749
Killer cells, lymphokine-activated, in immunotherapy for cancer, 283
Kimray-Greenfield device, for pulmonary embolism, 951–952, 953(t)
Klatskin tumors, 539
Kneecap, fracture of, 765
Kocher, Theodor, 3, *4*
  contributions of, to thyroid surgery, 6
Kock pouch, in urinary diversion after cystectomy, 839
Küntscher nail, 765
Kupffer's cells, 517

Labia, 804
Laboratory reference values, 1195–1196, 1197(t)–1206(t)
Labyrinthitis, 693
Lactate production, shock and, 14, *14*
Lactation, breast cancer occurring during time of, 325
  changes in breast associated with, 294, *294*
Lactose intolerance, after gastrectomy, 421
Ladd's procedure, in correction of intestinal malrotation, 665, *666*
Landsteiner, Karl, contributions of, to hematology, 7–8
Laparoscopy, in gynecologic examination, 811
Laparotomy, in staging of lymphoma, 633
Laryngectomy, for cancer, 704, 733
Laryngocele, 704
Laryngoscopy, and endotracheal intubation, 1056, *1056*
Laryngotracheal papillomatosis, 703
Laryngotracheal separation, 186
Laryngotracheobronchitis, 703
Laryngotracheoesophageal cleft, 659
Laryngotracheomalacia, 659, 703
Larynx, *701*, 701–702, 713–714
  cancer of, 704, 733
    smoking and alcohol use as risk factors in, *706*

Larynx (*Continued*)
  endoscopy of, and endotracheal intubation, 1056, *1056*
  foreign body impaction in, 704–705
  malformations of, 703
  muscles of, 701, *702*
  obstruction of, in newborn, 658–659
  resection of, for cancer, 704, 733
  trauma to, 186, 703–704
  tumors of, 704, 733
Laser, hemostasis with, 136
  in treatment of bronchial lesions, 983
  in treatment of cancer of lung, 1007
Laser incision, risk of infection associated with, *135*
Late postprandial dumping, 419
Lateral pectoral nerve, 290
Lathyrism, 118
LAV infection. See *Immune deficiency, acquired.*
Lavage, peritoneal, for acute pancreatitis, 604
    in management of trauma, 183
    in suspected cases of intra-abdominal trauma, 183, 189
LaVeen shunt, for ascites, 547
Lead electrode, of pacemaker, 1171–1173, *1173*
Left aortic cusp, fusion of, to aortic wall, with occlusion of left coronary ostium, 1136
Left atrial filling pressure, pulmonary artery catheter in measurement of, 115
Left atrium, myxoma of, 1164, 1165, *1165*
  surgery for, *1167*
Left coronary artery, 1114, *1114, 1116*
  atherosclerosis of, *1115*
  originating from pulmonary artery, 1132, *1133*
    surgery for, 1132, *1134, 1135*
  stenosis of, *1115*
Left coronary ostium, occlusion of, fusion of left aortic cusp to aortic wall and, 1136
Left hepatic lobectomy, 520
  with cholangiojejunostomy to Roux-en-Y limb, in repair of biliary stricture, *575*
Left lateral hepatic segmentectomy, 520
Left ventricle, aneurysm of, 1125
  surgery for, 1125–1126, *1126*
  obstruction of outflow from, congenital, 1109–1110, *1110*
    surgery for, 1110–1112
  in tetralogy of Fallot, 1103, 1104
Leg, torsional deformities of, *783,* 783–785, *784*
  trauma to, 186
    fracture injuries in, 763–768
    vascular injuries in, 198–199
Legg-Calvé-Perthes disease, *778,* 778–779, *779*
Leiomyoma, of esophagus, 383
  of small intestine, 452
  of stomach, 423
  of uterus, *817,* 817–818
Leiomyosarcoma, of small intestine, 452
Lentigo maligna melanoma, 285
Leukagglutinin reaction, to transfusion, 94
Leukemia, myeloid, chronic, splenectomy for, 630
  transfusion for, in surgical patients, 66
Leukoplakia, 708, 710, 794
Levamisole, therapeutic uses of, 282
Level of consciousness, as index of fluid balance, 43

Level of consciousness (*Continued*)
  estimation of, in management of trauma, 182, 184
  in postoperative period, 201(t), 202–203
Lewis procedure, in treatment of esophageal carcinoma, 385–386, *386*
Life support, basic and advanced, 1055–1059
Ligament, injury of, 755
Lingual thyroid, 327
Linitis plastica, 423
Linton procedure, for postphlebitic ulceration, 943, *943*
Lip(s), 711
  carcinoma of, 730
Lipase, 593
Lipid(s), biliary, 554
  elevated serum levels of, in acute pancreatitis, 602
  metabolism of, in liver, 518–519
Lipolysis, 433
Lipoma, 799
  of small intestine, 452
Lipomeningocele, 876
Lister, Joseph, *2*
  contribution of, to antiseptic surgery, 2, 141
Lithotripsy, 837
Littre's hernia, 653
Liver, 513
  abscess of, 154, 521–524, *522*
    amebic, 504, 523–524, *524*
      complications of, 523, *525*
    pyogenic, 521(t), 521–523
  albumin synthesis in, 518
  amebiasis of, 504, 523–524, *524*
    complications of, 523, *525*
  amino acid metabolism in, 518
  anatomy of, 246, 513–517, *514–517,* 551
  artery of, 514–515, *515*
    ligation of, in treatment of hepatic cancer, 539, 542
  bile ducts of, 516
  bile production by, 517, 554
    effects of shock on, 16
  bilirubin metabolism in, 519
  biopsy of, 528, 561
  bleeding from, in abdominal trauma, 193–194
  cancer metastatic to, 496, 539–542
    chemotherapy for, 287, *541,* 541–542, *542*
    prognosis in, in untreated cases, 540, *540*
    radiation therapy for, 275, 542
    surgery for, 286, 540–541
    transplantation for, 542
    treatment of, 286–287, 540–542
      hepatic artery ligation in, 542
  carbohydrate metabolism in, 519
  carcinoma of, *537,* 537–539, 684
    alpha-fetoprotein in, 281
    viral hepatitis and, 171
  cells of, *516,* 516–517, *517*
    changes in, in shock, *17*
  cirrhosis of, 527, 528, 529, 625
    and portal hypertension, 527
    bleeding esophageal varices in patients with, 528, 529
      treatment of, 529–532, 530(t), *530–532*
    development of venous collateral channels in, *515*
    risk of operative mortality in patients with, 73, 73(t)

Liver (*Continued*)
  cirrhosis of, treatment of, diuretics in, 64
  cysts of, 524–527, *525, 526*
    in children, 682
  detoxification in, 519
    effects of shock on, 17
  disease of, in patients with head and neck cancer, 719
    malabsorption in, 449
    surgery in patients with, 73
    transplantation for, 245, 245(t)
    unfavorable prognostic factors in, 246(t)
  dysfunction of, and encephalopathy or coma, 545–546
    and jaundice, 216
    following shock, 16–17, *17,* 216
    following surgery, 216
    surgical infection in patients with, antimicrobials for, 153, 154(t)
  echinococcosis of, *525,* 525–527, *526*
  effects of shock on, 16–17, *17,* 216
  embolization of vessels of, in treatment of hemobilia, 536
  enzyme production in, 518
  failure of, fulminant, 546
    parenteral nutrition in management of, 105
  focal nodular hyperplasia of, *543,* 543–544
  gross anatomy of, 513–516, *514, 515*
  hemangioma of, 544, 684
  hematoma in, CT findings in, *190*
  inflammation of, anesthesia-induced, 216
    viral infection and. See *Viral hepatitis.*
  lipid metabolism in, 518–519
  metabolism in, 518–519
    effects of shock on, 16
  microscopic anatomy of, *516,* 516–517, *517*
  physiology of, 517–519
  protein synthesis in, 518
    effects of shock on, 17
  pyogenic abscess of, 521(t), 521–523
  resection of, 520
    Cavitron ultrasonic surgical aspiration device in, 520, *520*
    course after, 520–521
    for cancer, 538–539
      in children, 543
      secondary to malignant disease at other site, 286, 496, 540–541
    in transplantation, 246–247, *247*
    with cholangiojejunostomy to Roux-en-Y limb, in repair of biliary stricture, *575*
  sinusoids of, 516, *516*
  transplantation of, 244–249, 245(t)
    care after, 247–248
    complications of, 248–249
    donor in, 245
    early developments in, 244
    for cancer, 542
    hepatectomy in, 246–247, *247*
    immunosuppression in, 247, 248, 249
    in children, 674
    indications for, 245, 245(t)
    infection after, 248–249
    procedure for, 247, *248*
    recipient in, 245
    rejection of, 248
    results of, 249
    resuscitation after, 247
  trauma to, 193–194

Liver (*Continued*)
trauma to, and hemobilia, 535
tumors of, 537–544
in children, 542–543, *543*, 682, *683*, 684
veins of, 513, *514*, 515, *515*
obstruction of, 527, 544–545
vitamin metabolism in, 519
Lobar emphysema, congenital, 663, *663*
Lobular carcinoma, 313–314, *314*, 322
Local anesthesia, 114
Long thoracic nerve, 290
Long, Crawford, use of ether anesthesia by, 2
Long-chain triglycerides, digestion of, *433*
Longmire procedure, for biliary stricture, *575*
Loop colostomy, *477*
Loop obstruction, after gastrectomy and restoration of GI continuity, 419–420
Lop ear, 690
Loven reflex, 12
Lower esophageal sphincter, function of, 365, *366*
abnormal, 374–378, *375–378*
and gastroesophageal reflux, 379
Lower extremity, torsional deformities of, *783*, 783–785, *784*
trauma to, 186
fracture injuries in, 763–768
vascular injuries in, 198–199
Lumbar hernia, 654
Lumbar spine, fracture of, 770–771
radiculopathy of, 880–881
Lunate, avascular necrosis of, 749
dislocation of, 749
Lundh test, 596
Lung(s), abscess of, 984, *984*
adenocarcinoma of, 999, *1002*
cancer metastatic to, *1003*, 1006(t), 1006–1007, 1007(t)
surgery for, 286, 1007
carcinoid of, 1008
carcinoma metastatic to, *1003*, 1006(t)
carcinoma of, 998–1007
aids to diagnosis of, 1001–1003
biopsy findings in, *1002*, 1002–1003, *1003*
chemotherapy for, 1005
cigarette smoking and, 998–999, *999*
endocrinopathies in patients with, 1001
hormone-secreting, 1001
immune deficiency in patients with, 1005–1006
inoperable cases of, 1003
laser therapy for, 1007
metastasis of, *999*, 999–1000
and inoperability, 1003
obstruction of subclavian vein by, *1000*
prognosis in, 1006
radiation therapy for, 274, 1004(t), 1004–1005
radiographic findings in, 1001, *1001*
small cell, 1005, *1005*
solitary nodule (coin lesion) as, 1003, 1003(t)
staging of, 1007(t)
superior sulcus as site of, 1001, *1001*, 1006, *1006*, 1006(t)
superior vena cava syndrome in patients with, *1000*
surgery for, 1004, 1006
symptoms and signs of, 1000(t), 1000–1001
chondroma of, 1008

Lung(s) (*Continued*)
coin lesion of, 1003, 1003(t)
cystic adenomatoid malformation of, 663
dead space in, 973
diffusion capacity of, impaired, 973
endoscopy of, *980*, 980–983, *982*, 982(t)
fibrosis of, cancer chemotherapy and, 279
foreign body in, bronchoscopic treatment of, 983
function of, 206–207
assessment of, 969–973, *970–974*
conditions compromising, in patients with head and neck cancer, 719
in surgical patients, 71, 974
postoperative, 206–211
effects of shock on, 15–16
effects of surgery on, 70, 974
cardiopulmonary bypass and, 1190
tests of, preoperative, 70, 71
hyperinflation of, in newborn, 663
hypernephroma metastatic to, *1003*
infection of, and pneumonia. See *Pneumonia.*
fungal, 985–987, *985–987*
specimen collection in, 147
inhalation injury of, 129
nodule of, 1003, 1003(t)
obstructive disease of, chronic, 973–974
spirometric findings in, 207
perfusion of, 971–973, *971–973*
polyps of, 1008
receptor pharmacology of, 1180(t)
resection of, for bronchiectasis, 993
for cancer, 1004
secondary to malignant disease at other site, 286, 496, 1007
for tuberculosis, 997
restrictive disease of, 974
spirometric findings in, 207
sarcoma metastatic to, 1007(t)
shunting in, 25, *26*, 207, *207*
small cell carcinoma of, 1005, *1005*
solitary nodule of, 1003, 1003(t)
space-occupying lesions of, in newborn, 663
superior sulcus of, carcinoma in, 1001, *1001*, 1006, *1006*, 1006(t)
surfactant production by, 15
transplantation of, 259–260
care after, 256, 260
donor in, 254, 259
early developments in, 253, 259
immunosuppression in, 257, 260
procedure for, 260, *260*
recipient in, 253–254, 260
rejection of, 257
results of, 260
tuberculosis of, 994–997, *995*
and pericarditis, 1050–1051
drug therapy for, 996, 996(t)
surgery for, 994, 996–997
vasculature of, embolism in. See *Pulmonary embolism.*
ventilation of, 55, *55*, 971–973, *971–973*
interpretation of PCO₂ as index of, 207
Lung capacity, 969–970, *970*
Lung volume, *70*, 207, 969–970, *970*
Lupus anticoagulant, 89
Luque instrumentation, for scoliosis, 775
Luteinizing hormone, 352
Luteinizing hormone–releasing hormone, in treatment of prostate cancer, 844
Lymph, flow of, 635
Lymph node(s), 634
axillary, 291

Lymph node(s) (*Continued*)
axillary, breast cancer involving, 309
physical examination for, 295, *296*
treatment of, 317
breast cancer involving, 309
and prognosis, 312(t)
treatment of, 316–317
cancer involving, 268
cervical, anterior, 715
facial, 715
jugulodigastric, 715
midjugular, 715
occipital, 714
postauricular, 715
scalene, biopsy of, in lung cancer, 1003
submandibular, 715
submental, 715
Lymphadenectomy, lymphedema secondary to, 637
with surgical excision of melanoma, 286
Lymphadenopathy syndrome, 173
Lymphadenopathy-associated virus infection. See *Immune deficiency, acquired.*
Lymphangiography, 636
Lymphangioma, 638, *638*, 658, *658*
mediastinal, 1033–1034
Lymphangiosarcoma, 638, 800
Lymphatics, 634
anatomy of, 634
breast, 290–291, *291*, *292*
cancer involving, 309
prognosis with, 312(t)
treatment of, 316–317
colonic, 472, *473*
congenital malformations and tumors of, 638, 658, 1033–1034
hepatobiliary, 553
historical aspects of study of, 634
hyperplasia of, 636, *637*
hypoplasia of, 636, *636*
microsurgical repair of, 638
neck, 714–715, *715*
pancreatic, 590, *591*
physiology of, 635
Lymphedema, 635–638
Lymphocele, in kidney transplant recipient, 242
Lymphocyte(s), donor vs. recipient, pre-transplant assay for reactivity of, 230–231
in peripheral blood, 227(t)
Lymphocytotoxic cross-matching, before transplantation, 230
Lymphogranuloma venereum, 510, 846
Lymphoid hyperplasia, angiofollicular, 1034
Lymphokine-activated killer cells, in immunotherapy for cancer, 283
Lymphoma, 631–633, *632*, 632(t)
in AIDS, 177
non-Hodgkin's, 631–632
treatment of, 274
of mediastinum, 1031–1032
of small intestine, 452
of stomach, 424
of thyroid, 338

Macrophage(s), 226
in rejection, 226, 227, *228*
Madura foot, 166
Mafenide acetate, for burns, 127
Magnetic resonance imaging, in brain trauma, 184
in lung cancer, 1002

Magnetic resonance imaging (*Continued*)
  of coarctation of aorta, *1066*
  of nervous system, 860–861
Magnocellular neurons, 350
Malabsorption, 446–447, 447(t)
  after resection, of small intestine, 450
    of stomach, 448
  in blind loop syndrome, 449–450
  in Crohn's disease, 444
  in hepatobiliary disease, 449
  in pancreatic disorders, 448–449
Male breast lesions, 301, 325
Male sexual/reproductive dysfunction, 847–848, 853, 909
Malleolus, fracture of, 767, *767*
Mallet finger, 746
Mallory-Weiss tears, 421–422
Malnutrition, 67
  assessment of, 102, 103(t), 104
  in patients with head and neck cancer, 719
Malocclusion, 712
Malrotation of intestine, 665
  correction of, 665, *666*
Mammary artery, in coronary artery bypass graft, 1120, 1121, *1121, 1122*, 1123, *1123*
Mammary carcinoma. See *Breast cancer.*
Mammary duct, ectasia of, 304
Mammary gland. See *Breast.*
Mammography, in diagnosis of cancer, 297, *298*, 307
  risks vs. benefits of, 307
Manchester staging of cancer, 308
Mandatory ventilation, intermittent, 977
  for adult respiratory distress syndrome, 211
Mandible, 711
  hypoplasia of, 657
Mandibular muscles, 712
Manometry, in esophageal motor disorders, 375–378, *375–378*
  in gastroesophageal reflux, 380
Mantle irradiation field, *632*
Manual external cardiac compression, in CPR, *1056*, 1056–1058
  animal model studies of effects of, 1057, *1057, 1058*
Marrow, suppression of, cancer chemotherapy and, 279
Marrow graft, 266
Marsupialization, of pancreas, in treatment of pancreatic abscess, 607
Mask ventilation, in CPR, 1056
Mastectomy, for cancer, *316*, 316–322
  as prophylactic measure, 320
  results of, *318–319*, 318–321, 319(t), *321–322*
  with follow-up reconstructive surgery, 320
Mastitis, cystic, 300–301
  infection and, 301–302
  plasma cell, 304
Mastoiditis, 692
Matas, Rudolph, 8, *8*
Maxilla, 712
Maxillary sinusitis, 697
McDowell, Ephraim, *6*
  contributions of, to surgery, 6
McVay operation, for inguinal hernia, 639, 645, *647*
Meatus, urethral, malposition of, 848
Mechanical heart valve prostheses, 1139, 1147, *1148*
Mechanical ventilation, 976–978

Mechanical ventilation (*Continued*)
  criteria for cessation of, 210
  for respiratory distress, 211, 976(t), 976–978
  prolonged posotoperative dependence on, 210
Meckel's diverticulum, *457*, 457–458, *467*, 467–470, *468*, 676, *678*
  surgery for, 458, *469*, 469–470
Meconium ileus, 665, *667*, 668
Meconium peritonitis, *664*, 669
Meconium plug syndrome, 668
Media, vascular, 80
Medial pectoral nerve, 290
Median nerve, 737, *739, 740*
  compression of, 744
Mediastinal tamponade, 1024
Mediastinitis, 1021–1022
  as complication of coronary artery bypass graft, 1123
  postoperative, 206
Mediastinum, 1020
  air in, 1022–1023
  anatomy of, 1020–1021, *1021*
  cysts of, 1024(t), 1034–1035, *1035*
    in children, 1027(t)
    sites of, *1021*, 1024, 1024(t)
  enteric cyst in, 1034–1035, *1035*
  hemorrhage into, 1023–1024
  Hodgkin's disease of, 1031, *1031*
  inflammation of, 1021–1022
    as complication of coronary artery bypass graft, 1123
    postoperative, 206
  superior vena caval compression in, 1023
    cancer causing, *1000*, 1023
      radiation therapy for, 275
  surgery of, historical aspects of, 1020
  teratoma of, 1030, *1030*
  tumors of, 1024(t), 1024–1034, *1030, 1031*
    in children, 1027(t)
    signs and symptoms of, 1025, 1025(t), 1026(t)
      prognostic significance of, 1025, 1025(t)
    sites of, *1021*, 1024, 1024(t)
Medical adrenalectomy, for Cushing's syndrome, 358
  in treatment of breast cancer, 324
Medium-chain triglycerides, 433
Medullary carcinoma, of breast, 312–313
  of thyroid, 337–338
Megacolon, aganglionic, 668, *668*
  toxic, ulcerative colitis and, 479
Megaloblastic anemia, after gastrectomy, 448
Megalymphatics, 636
Megavoltage radiation, 272
Melanoma, 284–286, 797, *797*
  Breslow classification of, 285
  Clark microstaging of, 285, *285*
  lentigo maligna, 285
  nodular, 285
  radial growth of, 285
  superficial spreading, 285
  surgical excision of, 286
    in-transit metastases after, 286
    lymphadenectomy with, 286
    satellitosis after, 286
  vertical growth of, 285
Membrane oxygenator, 1185
Menarche, delayed, 808
Menetrier's disease, 422
Meniere's disease, 694

Meningeal hemorrhage, 184, 185
Meningioma, 864
Meningocele, 696, 875
Menopause, 809
  and changes in breast tissue, 289, *294*, 294–295
  and risk of breast cancer, 306
Menstrual cycle, *808*, 808–809
Menstruation, absence of, 821
Mental status, abnormalities of, in postoperative period, 201(t), 202–203
  as index of fluid balance, 43
  estimation of, in management of trauma, 182, 184
Meperidine, for pain of acute pancreatitis, 604
Mesenchymal tumors, of mediastinum, 1033–1034
Mesenteric vascular insufficiency, 400–401, 401(t), 929–931, *931*
Mesenteric vein, thrombosis of, 929–930
Meshed skin grafts, for burns, 130
Mesonephric duct, 803, *803*
  remnants of, 812
Mesothelioma, 991
  of heart, 1166
Metabolic acidosis, 57(t), 60, 60(t), 65
  treatment of, 65
Metabolic alkalosis, 57(t), 58(t), 58–59, 65
  treatment of, 65
Metabolism, abnormal, in newborn, 656
  burn injury and, 123–124
  effect of parenteral nutrition on, 106(t)
  hereditary disorders of, liver transplant for, 245(t)
  in liver, 518–519
  in myocardium, 1118
  shock and, 12–17, 23–24
  stress and, 23–24, 96–97, 99, 99(t)–102(t)
Metaproterenol, 1180
Metatarsal bones, fracture of, 768
Metatarsus adductus, *784*, 784–785
Metocurine, 113
Metolazone, 1180
Metronidazole, for amebic abscess of liver, 524
Metyrapone test, 357
Micelles, 411, 433
Microcalcification, in cancer of breast, 297, *298*
Micrognathia, 657
Microstaging, of melanoma, 285, *285*
Middle constrictor muscle, of pharynx, 713
Middle ear, *688*
  disorders of, 691–693
Midgut volvulus, 665
  relief of, *666*
Midjugular lymph nodes, 715
Migratory necrolytic erythema, in patients with glucagonoma, 611
Milk line, in breast development, 288, *288*, 290
Mineral substrates, 25
Minimum alveolar concentration, as index of potency of inhaled anesthetics, 111
Mithramycin, for hypercalcemia, 344
Mitral anuloplasty, Carpentier ring and, 1150, *1150*
Mitral commissurotomy, closed, 1145–1146
  open, 1146, *1146*
Mitral valve, 1143
  in prolapse syndrome, *1149*
  inadequate functioning (insufficiency) of, 1148–1149
    treatment of, 1149–1150, *1150*

Mitral valve (*Continued*)
 prolapse of, 1148
  appearance of valve in, *1149*
 stenosis of, 1143–1145, *1144, 1145*
  treatment of, 1145, 1148
   by closed commissurotomy, 1145–
    1146
   by open commissurotomy, 1146,
    1146
   by replacement of valve with pros-
    thesis, 1146–1147, *1147, 1148*
  historical aspects of, 1142–1143
Mittelschmerz, 403
Mixed gonadal dysgenesis, 854
Mixed lymphocyte culture, before transplantation, 230–231
Mobin-Uddin device, in treatment of pulmonary embolism, 951–952, 953(t)
Mobitz Type II atrioventricular block,
  pacemaker for, 1170
Modified Brooke formula, for fluid resuscitation, of burn patients, 126
Modified radical mastectomy, for cancer,
  316
Mole, *796,* 796–797
 hydatidiform, 824
Mondor's disease, 302
Monoclonal antibodies, 282
 in detection of antigens, 226
 in detection of mediastinal tumors, 1026
 in suppression of transplant rejection,
  232, 238
 in treatment of cancer, 282
Monofilament sutures, 137
Monteggia fracture, 761
MOPP chemotherapy regimen, 280
Morbid obesity, 427
 surgery for, 428, *428,* 459
Morton, William, *3*
 use of ether anesthesia by, 2
Mouth-to-mouth ventilation, in CPR,
  1056
Movement disorders, 882
Mucinous adenocarcinoma, of breast, 313
Mucocele, of appendix, 467
Mucoepidermoid carcinoma, of parotid
  gland, 734
Mucosal prolapse, rectal, 510, *511*
Müllerian duct, 803, *803*
 defective fusion of, 811–812, *812*
Multicystic kidney disease, 679, 833
Multifilament polyester sutures, 137
Multinodular goiter, 331–332
Multiple endocrine neoplasia I (Wermer's
  syndrome), 342, 417–418
Multiple endocrine neoplasia II, 342
Multiple myeloma, 789
Multiple organ failure, postoperative, 221–
  222, *222*
Murphy's sign, in diagnosis of cause of ab-
  dominal pain, 391
Muscle, appearance of, in gas gangrene,
  158
 laryngeal, 701, *702*
 mandibular, 712
 pharyngeal, 713
Muscle cell, effect of shock on energy metabolism in, 13
Muscle graft, 264
Muscle relaxants, 112–113
 and postoperative dependence on mechanical ventilation, 210
Musculoocutaneous flap, 262, *262, 263*
 in reconstructive surgery, after radical
  neck dissection for cancer, 726, 727,
  729–730

Musculoskeletal graft, 264, 264(t)
Musculoskeletal system, 736. See also specific sites.
 trauma to, 755–757
Mustard procedure, for transposition of
  great arteries, 1104, *1107*
 complications of, 1108
Mutagens, chemotherapy agents as, 280
Myasthenia gravis, 1029, 1036–1041
 management of surgical patients with, 74
 medical treatment of, 1041–1042
 thymectomy for, 1042–1043, *1043*
 thymoma and, 1029, 1038–1039
Mycetoma, 166
Mycobacterium intracellulare infection, 995
 in AIDS, 176(t), 177
Mycobacterium kansasii infection, 995
Mycobacterium tuberculosis infection, in
  AIDS, 177
 of bone, 787
 of breast, 302
 of joints, 787
 of lung, 994–997, *995*
  and pericarditis, 1050–1051
  drug therapy for, 996, 996(t)
  surgery for, 994, 996–997
 of prostate, 841
Mycotic infection, 166–167
 and pericarditis, 1051
 in AIDS, 176, 176(t)
 of lung, 985–987, *985–987*
Myelography, 860, *860*
Myeloid leukemia, chronic, splenectomy
  for, 630
Myeloid metaplasia, agnogenic, 629
Myeloma, multiple, 789
Myelomeningocele, *874,* 874–875
Myelopathy, cervical, 879
Myeloproliferative disease, 626
Myelosuppression, cancer chemotherapy
  and, 279
Myelotomy, for chronic pain, 884
Myoblastoma, granular cell, of breast, 304
Myocardium, contusion of, 189
 infarction of, as complication of coronary
  artery bypass graft, 1122
  evolving, 1118
  pericarditis following, 1052
 ischemia of, 1115, 1117
  coronary artery bypass graft for,
   1119–1121, *1120, 1121*
   candidates for, 1117–1118
   complications of, 1121–1123
   protection of myocardium in, cardi-
    oplegic solution and, 1119, 1119(t)
   results of, *1117,* 1123
  percutaneous transluminal balloon angioplasty for, 1118–1119
  ventricular tachycardia in, 1160
   surgery for, 1160–1161, *1161*
    nondirected, 1160(t)
 metabolic activity of, 1118
Myochosis, in diverticulitis, 395
Myoglobinuria, and acute renal failure, 215
 in patients with electrical burns, 128
Myometrium, sarcoma of, 818
Myonecrosis, clostridial, 157–159, 159(t)
 radiographic findings in, *158*
Myopathy, and dysphagia, 371(t), 371–372
 management of surgical patients with, 74
Myositis, streptococcal, 159(t), 162
Myotomy, cricopharyngeal, for oropharyngeal dysphagia, 373, *373*
Myxoma, of breast, 303–304
 of heart, 1164–1165, *1165*
  surgery for, 1166, *1167*

Nail, intramedullary, for femoral fracture,
  765
 Küntscher, 765
 Zickel, 764, *764*
Nasal septum, deformities of, 697
 sites of bleeding from, *697,* 698
Nasal turbinates, 695, *696*
Nasopharynx, 699, 714
 carcinoma of, 700, 733
 juvenile angiofibroma of, 700
 Tornwaldt's cyst of, 701
Natural killer cell, 226
Natural sutures, 136
Nausea, postoperative, 218
Nebulizer, risk of pneumonia with use of,
  163–164
Neck, *329,* 714–715
 anatomic triangles of, *715*
 cancer of. See *Head and neck cancer.*
 lymphatic drainage of, 714–715, *715*
 muscles of, 714
 surgery of, dysphagia after, 372
 teratoma of, 658
 trauma to, esophageal injury in, 187–188
  laryngotracheal injury in, 186–187, 703
  vascular injury in, 198
  vertebral injury in, 181, 185–186
  zone-based management of vascular injury in, 198
Neck dissection, for cancer, 725, *726,* 727–
  728
Necrolytic erythema, migratory, in patients
  with glucagonoma, 611
Necrosis, avascular, of capital epiphysis of
  femur, *778,* 778–779, *779*
 of lunate, 749
 fat, of breast, 304
 in peripheral artery disease, 892–893
Necrotizing cellulitis, synergistic, 159(t),
  162
Necrotizing enterocolitis, in newborn, 670–
  671, *671*
Necrotizing fasciitis, 159(t), 162–163
Necrotizing infections, of soft tissue, 157–
  159, 159(t), 162–163
Needle aspiration, in diagnosis of cancer,
  269
 of lung, *1002,* 1002–1003, *1003*
 of amebic abscess, of liver, 524
 of cells, from breast, 298–299
  from thyroid, *332,* 332–333
 of cyst, of breast, 298, *300*
Neisseria gonorrhoeae infection, 403, 820,
  848–849
Nelson's syndrome, 358
Neostigmine bromide, for myasthenia
  gravis, 1041
Nephrectomy, for cancer, 834
 in transplantation, 240, *240, 241*
Nephroblastoma, 679–680, *680,* 834–836
Nephron(s), 38, *38,* 39, *39*
Nephropathy, Balkan, 837
Nerve(s), of hand, injury of, 743–745
 peripheral, 743, *743*
Nerve block anesthesia, 113–114
Nerve conduction velocities, 861
Nerve graft, 264–265
Nervous system, 856–858
 central, infection of, 885–886
  injury of, 869–873
  radiography of, 859–862, *860, 861*
 congenital abnormalities of, *874,* 874–
  878, *877*
 disorders of, and dysphagia, 371, 371(t)
 assessment of, 858–862
 localization of, 858–859

Nervous system (*Continued*)
  peripheral, injury of, 873–874
Nesidioblastosis, 610–611
Neural tube, defective closure of, 874–877
Neurapraxia, 873
Neurilemmoma, mediastinal, 1027
Neuroblastoma, 681, 681(t), *682,* 1028
Neuroendocrine system, afferent pathways of, 97
  efferent pathways of, 97
  renal mechanisms controlled by, 35–40
  response of, to stress, 10–11, *11, 46,* 96–97, *98*
Neuroenteric cyst, 876, 1035
Neurofibroma, 799, *799*
  mediastinal, 1027
Neurofibromatosis, 799
Neurogenic bladder, 839–840
Neurogenic tumor, of mediastinum, 1027–1029
Neurohypophysis, hormones secreted by, 352
Neuroleptanalgesia, 111
Neuroleptanesthesia, 111
Neurologic evaluation, in management of trauma, 182, 183, 184
Neuroma, acoustic, 694
Neuromuscular blocking agents, 112–113
  and prolonged postoperative dependence, on mechanical ventilation, 210
Neuromuscular junction, 1037, *1037*
Neuronitis, vestibular, 694–695
Neurosarcoma, mediastinal, 1027–1028
Neurosurgery, functional, 880
  stereotactic, 881–882
Neurotmesis, 873
Neurotoxins, chemotherapy agents as, 280
Neutrophil, 142
  abnormal chemotaxis affecting, 143
Nevus, dysplastic, 797
  nevocellular, *796,* 796–797
Newborn. See also *Child(ren).*
  abdominal wall defects in, 671–672
  ambiguous genitalia in, 674
  biliary atresia in, 579–580, 673–674
    surgery for, *581, 673,* 673–674, *674*
  blood volume in, 656
  choanal atresia in, 657, 695
  cystic disease of lung in, 663
  diaphragmatic eventration in, 662
  diaphragmatic hernia in, *661,* 661–662, *662*
  duodenal obstruction in, 664
  esophageal atresia in, 659, *659, 660*
  fluid replacement therapy in, 656
  gastric obstruction in, 663
    hypertrophic pyloric stenosis and, 674–675
  gastric perforation in, 670
  gastrointestinal bleeding in, 671
  gastrointestinal emergencies in, 663–671
  gastroschisis in, *671,* 671–672
    closure of, 672, *673*
  heart lesions in. See specific anomalies, e.g., *Vascular ring and double aortic arch.*
  hemangioma and airway obstruction in, 658
  hip dislocation in, 775–777, *776, 777*
  Hirschsprung's disease in, 668, *668*
  hyperinsulinism in, islet cell hyperplasia and, 611
  imperforate anus in, 668–669, *669*
  implantation of pacemaker in, 1174, *1175*

Newborn (*Continued*)
  intestinal atresia in, 665
    correction of, 665, *667*
  intestinal malrotation in, 665
    correction of, 665, *666*
  intestinal obstruction in, 663–665, *664, 666–669, 668–669*
  intestinal perforation in, 669–670
  jaundice in, 673
  laryngeal obstruction in, 658–659
  lobar emphysema in, 663, *663*
  meconium ileus in, 665, *667,* 668
  meconium peritonitis in, *664,* 669
  meconium plug syndrome in, 668
  metabolic derangements in, 656
  micrognathia in, 657
  necrotizing enterocolitis in, 670–671, *671*
  omphalocele in, 671, *672*
    syndromes associated with, 672, 672(t)
  parenteral nutrition in, 656–657, *657*
  pneumatosis intestinalis in, 670, *671*
  pneumoperitoneum in, 670, *670*
  respiration and oxygen demand in, 655
  respiratory emergencies in, 657–663
  space-occupying lesions of lung in, 663
  special considerations in management of, 656
  surgical emergencies in, 655–674
  tension pneumothorax in, 661, *661*
  thermoregulation in, 656
  tracheal obstruction in, 658–659
  tracheoesophageal fistula in, 659, *659, 660*
  tracheostomy in, *658*
  transfusion in, 656
Nipple(s), discharge from, 302–303
  embryonic and fetal development of, 288
  examination of, in diagnosis of mammary cancer, 295–296
  supernumerary, 290
Nissen fundoplication, 381, *381*
  for gastroesophageal reflux in children, 675
Nitrates, cardiovascular effects of, 1180, 1181
Nitrogen, in parenteral nutrition, 104
  loss of, in response to stress, 100(t)
Nitroglycerin, 1181
Nitroprusside, 1180
Nitrous oxide, 111
Nocardiosis, 166, 987, *987*
Nocturia, 831
Nodular hyperplasia, of liver, *543,* 543–544
Nodular melanoma, 285
Nodule, thyroid, 331
Noise-induced hearing loss, 693
Non-A, non-B hepatitis, 169, 170, 170(t)
Non-Hodgkin's lymphoma, 274, 631–632
Non-seminoma germ cell tumors, of mediastinum, 1031
Nonabsorbable sutures, 136, 137
Nonchromaffin paraganglioma, mediastinal, 1029
Nondepolarizing muscle relaxants, 113
Noninfiltrating ductal carcinoma, of breast, 312, 322
Nonproliferative breast disease, 300–301
Norepinephrine, 1182
Normal laboratory values, 1195–1196, 1197(t)–1206(t)
Nose, 695, 714
  bleeding from, 698
    control of, 698, *698*
    septal vasculature and, *697,* 698

Nose (*Continued*)
  fracture of, 697
  inflammation of mucosa of, 696
  malformations of, 695–696
  surgery of, historical aspects of, 695
  tumors of, 698–699, 734
Nosocomial infection, 141
  in surgical patient, *148,* 163–165, 209
No-touch approach, to removal of malignant tumor, 269
Nutrition, enteral, 67, 107(t), 107–108
  parenteral, 67, 104–107
    complications of, 105–106, 106(t), 216
    in newborn, 656–657, *657*
    indications for, 105, 222
    metabolic response to, 106(t)
    results of, 106(t), 106–107, 107(t)
    substrates in, 24–25, 104
Nutritional status, assessment of, 102, 103(t), 104
Nutritional support, 104–107
  in newborn, 656–657, *657*
  preoperative, 67
Nystagmus, 690

Obesity, 427
  surgery for, 428, *428,* 459
Obstructive jaundice, 584–586, *585, 586*
Obstructive pulmonary disease, 973–974
  spirometric findings in, 207
Obturator hernia, 653–654
Obturator test, in diagnosis of cause of abdominal pain, 391, *391*
Occipital lymph nodes, 714
Ochsner-Mahorner test, 935
Odontoid, fracture of, 769, *769*
Olecranon, fracture of, 760
Oliguria, 44–45, 45(t)
Omphalocele, 671, *672*
  syndromes associated with, 672, 672(t)
Omphalomesenteric duct, persistence of, 457, 467, *468,* 676, *678*
Oncofetal antigens, 281
Oncology, 268–287. See also *Cancer.*
Oncotic pressure, 34
One-rescuer CPR, 1057
Oophorectomy, and reduced risk of breast cancer, 306
Open biopsy, of breast, 299, *299*
Open cardiac massage, 1058, *1059*
Open fracture, 756–757
Open mitral commissurotomy, 1146, *1146*
Open pneumothorax, 181
Operating team antisepsis, 132–133
Operative pancreatography, 600, *600*
Opsonization, 142
  abnormal, 143
Oral antimicrobials, in prophylaxis against surgical infection, 150
Oral cavity, 711–712
  cancer of, *708,* 730–731
  squamous epithelium of, *709*
Oral cholecystography, 558, *559*
Oral contraceptives, hepatocellular adenomas in patients using, 544
Oral glucose tolerance test, 596–597, 597(t), 1206(t)
Oral vestibule, 711
Orchiectomy, in treatment of prostate cancer, 844
Orchitis, 851

Organ failure, multiple, postoperative, 221–222, *222*

Organ of Zuckerandl, 360

Oriental cholangiohepatitis, 572–573

Oropharyngeal dysphagia, 371(t), 371–373
  treatment of, 373, *373*

Oropharynx, 699, 713
  carcinoma of, 700

Orthokeratosis, 708

Ortolani test, for congenital hip dislocation, 776, *776*

Osmolality, *33*, 33–34

Osmolarity, 33

Osmosis, *33*, 33–34

Osteoarthritis, of hand, 751

Osteodystrophy, renal, *348*

Osteomyelitis, 785–786
  tuberculous, 787

Osteosarcoma, 799

Osteotomy, *1014*
  for arthritis, 790

Ostium primum defect, *1078*, 1079
  surgery for, *1080*

Ostium secundum defects, *1078*, 1078–1079
  surgery for, *1078*, 1079

Otalgia, 687
  as sign of head and neck cancer, 717–718

Otitis externa, 691

Otitis media, 691–692

Otolaryngology, 686–705

Otosclerosis, 692

Ototoxic drugs, 694

Ovarian arteries, 804, *804*

Ovary, 807
  cancer of, 818–819
    in children, 680
  cystic teratoma of, *680*
  hormone production by, 807, *807*
    neurohumoral influences on, 292
  removal of, and reduced risk of breast cancer, 306
  tumors of, in children, 680, *680*

Oxygen, hyperbaric, for gas gangrene, 159
  in pulmonary function, *970*, 970–973, *973*
  partial pressure of, 206–207
  toxicity of, 978

Oxygenation, effect of, on wound healing, 119

Oxygenator, in cardiopulmonary bypass, 1185

Oxygen demand, in newborn, 655

Oxygen extraction, *1118*

Oxytocin, 352

PABA test, 596

Pacemaker(s), 1171–1173, *1171–1173*
  antitachycardia, 1162, 1170–1171
  complications associated with, 1176(t), 1176–1178, *1177*
  evaluation of function of, 1174–1175, *1175*
  implantation of, 1173–1174, *1174*
    complications of, 1176(t), 1176–1177
    in infant, 1174, *1175*
  indications for, 1169–1171, 1170(t)
  malfunction of, 1177–1178
  modes of pacing provided by, 1175–1176, 1176(t)
  programmability of, 1176

Pacing system analyzer, 1174, *1175*

Pack(s), surgical, 136

Packed red cells, therapeutic use of, 93

Paget's disease, 296, 311

Pain. See also site-specific entries.
  neural pathways of, 883–884
  neurosurgery for, 884–885
  rest, in peripheral artery disease, 892

Palate, 713
  carcinoma of, 731, 732

Palm, surgical incisions on, 741, *742*

Palpation, in physical examination of trauma patient, 182, 183
  of abdomen, in diagnosis of appendicitis, 462
    in diagnosis of cause of abdominal pain, 389–390
  of breast and axillae, in diagnosis of mammary cancer, 295–296, *296*
  of enlarged spleen, 620
  of groin, in examination for hernia, 641, *641*
  of pulse, in assessment of peripheral artery disease, 895, *896*
    in examination for arterial trauma, 197
    in trauma patient, 182

Pancoast tumor, 1001, *1001*, 1006, *1006*, 1006(t)

Pancreas, 587
  abscess of, 607
  acini of, 591, *591*
  adenocarcinoma of, *599*, 609
  anatomy of, *587–591*, 587–592
  annular, 600
  anomalies of, 600–601
  arteries supplying, 589, *589*
  autotransplantation of, 265
  bicarbonate secretion by, 593
  calcification of, *392*
  cancer of, 584, 609–610
    angiographic findings in, 598–599, *599*
  carcinoma of, 584, *599*, 609
  CT studies of, 598, *598*
  cystadenocarcinoma of, 609
  cystadenoma of, 609
  development of, 589, *589*
  disorders of, malabsorption in, 448–449
  ectopic, 600
  endocrine, 592
    function of, 594–595
      tests of, 596–598, 597(t)
    tumors of, 610(t), 610–612
  enzyme secretion by, 593–594
    tests of, 595–596, 596(t)
  exocrine, 591–592
    function of, 592–594
      tests of, 595–596, 596(t)
    tumors of, 608–610
  fibrosis of, chronic inflammation and, 604
  function of, 592–595
    tests of, 595–598, 596(t), 597(t)
  hormone secretion by, 592, 594–595
    excess of, 610(t), 610–612
      venous blood sampling for signs of, 600
    tests of, 596–598, 597(t)
  imaging of, 598–600, *598–600*
  inflammation of. See *Pancreatitis.*
  islet cells of, 592, *592*
    hyperplasia of, 610
    transplantation of, 252
      autologous, 265
    tumors of, 610(t), 610–612
  lymphatics of, 590, *591*
  marsupialization of, in treatment of pancreatic abscess, 607
  nerves supplying, 591
  pseudocyst of, 606–607
  replacement of fluid losses from, 42

Pancreas (*Continued*)
  resection of, for cancer, 609
    for chronic inflammation, 605–606, *606*
    for trauma, 194
  segmental graft of, in pancreas transplant, 250, *251*
  surgery of, contrast radiography in, 600, *600*
    for chronic inflammation, 605–606, *606*
    for pancreatic insufficiency, 449
  tests for disorders of, 595–598, 596(t), 597(t)
  transplantation of, 249–252
    autologous, 265
    care after, 251
    complications of, 251
    donor in, 250
    early developments in, 249
    immunosuppression in, 251
    pancreaticoduodenal graft in, 250, *251*, *252*
    procedure for, 250, *251*, *252*
    recipient in, 249–250
    rejection of, 251
    results of, 252
    spleen transplant in, 250, *251*
    thrombosis after, 250, 251
  trauma to, 194
  tumors of, 608–612, 610(t)
    sampling of venous blood for signs of, 600
  ultrasonographic studies of, 598
  venous drainage of, 590, *590*
    sampling of blood from, 600

Pancreas divisum, 600–601

Pancreatectomy, for cancer, 609
  for chronic inflammation, 605–606, *606*
  for trauma, 194

Pancreatic ascites, 607–608, *608*

Pancreatic duct, *588*, 588–589, *589*
  endoscopy in delineation of, 599, *599*
  fluid leak from, 607–608, *608*
  obstruction of, and acute pancreatitis, *601*
  operative contrast radiography of, 600, *600*
  trauma to, diagnosis of, 194

Pancreatic enzymes, 593–594
  tests of secretion of, 595–596, 596(t)

Pancreatic insufficiency, 448–449

Pancreatic polypeptide, 595
  secretion of, after meal stimulus, *410*
  by tumor, 610(t), 612

Pancreaticoduodenal graft, in pancreas transplant, 250, *251*, *252*

Pancreaticojejunostomy, *609*
  for chronic pancreatitis, 605, *606*
  in drainage of pancreatic fluid, *608*

Pancreatitis, 601–606
  abdominal pain in, 398, 602, 604, 605
  abscess in, 607
  acute, 398–399, 601–604
    gallstones and, 568, 601
    obstruction of pancreatic duct and, *601*
    parenteral nutrition in patients with, 107(t)
    patient's appearance in, *398*
    unfavorable prognosis and outcome in, 399(t), *603*, 603(t)
  chronic, 604–606
    surgery for, 605–606, *606*
  pseudocyst in, 606–607
  radiographic findings in, 398, 598

Pancreatography, operative, 600, *600*

Pancuronium, 113

Papanicolaou test, 810
Papillary carcinoma, of breast, 313
  of thyroid, 336–337
Papilloma, intraductal, of breast, 304
  laryngotracheal, 703
  nasal, 698
Papillomatosis, 708
Paracentesis, in treatment of ascites, 546
Paraganglioma, nonchromaffin, of medias-
  tinum, 1029
Parakeratosis, 708
Paralysis, peripheral facial nerve, 693
Paralytic ileus, 219–220, *220*, 436
  in burn patients, 126
  postoperative, 219
  treatment of, 442
  vs. mechanical small bowel obstruction,
  219
Paramesonephric duct, 803, *803*
  defective fusion of, 811–812, *812*
Paranasal sinuses, 695, *696*, 714
  inflammation of, 696–697
  tumors of, 698–699, 734
Parapharyngeal abscess, 699
Paraphimosis, 845
Parastomal hernia, 652–653
Parathyroid, 340
  anatomy of, 340–341, *346*
  autotransplantation of, 265, 348
  discovery and recognition of role of, 340
  hyperplasia of, 342, 345, 346
  resection of, for hyperparathyroidism,
  345–346
    historical aspects of, 340
    hypocalcemia after, 346, 348, 349
    hypoparathyroidism after, 348, 349
  transplantation of, autologous, 265, 348
  tumor of, 342, 345, *345*, 346, *347*
    in mediastinum, 1032–1033
Parathyroid hormone, 341
  and calcium metabolism, 341
  excessive secretion of, 342–347
    clinical recognition of, historical as-
    pects of, 340
    hypercalcemia in, 340–344, 346, 347
    treatment of, 344–347
      hypocalcemia after, 346, 348, 349
      hypoparathyroidism after, 348, 349
  insufficient secretion of, 348, 349
Parathyroidectomy, for hyperparathyroidism, 345–346
  historical aspects of, 340
  hypocalcemia after, 346, 348, 349
  hypoparathyroidism after, 348, 349
Paré, Ambroise, *2*
  contributions of, to surgery, 1–2
Parenteral antimicrobials, in prophylaxis
  against surgical infection, 150
Parenteral nutrition, 67, 104–107
  complications of, 105–106, 106(t)
  in newborn, 656–657, *657*
  metabolic response to, 106(t)
  results of, 106(t), 106–107, 107(t)
  substrates in, 24–25, 104
Parietal cell, 406, 408
  in peptic ulcer disease, 411
Parietal cell vagotomy, for peptic ulcer, 414
Parkland formula, for fluid resuscitation, of
  burn patients, 126
Paronychia, 750
Paroxysmal atrial tachycardia, as complication of coronary artery bypass graft,
  1122
Paroxysmal supraventricular tachycardia,
  surgical treatment of, 1158–1159

Partial-thickness burns, 123
Parvicellular neurons, 350
Pasteur, Louis, contributions of, to study of
  disease, 2
Patella, fracture of, 765
Patent ductus arteriosus, 1061–1062
  in premature infants, 1063–1064
  surgery for, 1062–1063, *1063*, *1064*
Patient performance/physical status scales,
  63(t), 279(t)
Pavlik harness, for congenital hip disloca-
  tion, 776–777, *777*
Peau d'orange, in breast cancer, 295, *295*,
  312
Pectin, for dumping syndrome, 419
Pectoral nerves, 290
Pectoralis major muscle, congenital absence
  of costosternal portion of, *1016*
Pectus carinatum (pigeon breast), 1013,
  1015
Pectus excavatum (funnel chest), 1012–
  1013, *1013*
  surgery for, 1013, *1014*
Pediatric surgery, 655–684
Pedicle graft, 261, 262, *262*
Pelty's syndrome, 625
Pelvic examination, in diagnosis of cause of
  abdominal pain, 391
Pelvic inflammatory disease, 403, 820–821
Pelvis, fracture of, 762, *763*
Penetrating wound, of chest, 188
Penile prosthesis, 847
Penis, 829
  cancer of, 846–847
  disorders of, 844–848
Penrose drain, 139, *139*
Pepsinogen, 408
Peptic stricture, of esophagus, 381–382
Peptic ulcer, 411–415
  at site of Meckel's diverticulum, 457, 468
  hemorrhage from, 412
    surgery for, 414, 415
  parietal cells and acid secretion in, 411
  perforation of, 397, 412
    surgery for, 397–398, 414, 415
  recurrence of, after surgery, 418
  surgery for, 413–415, *414*
    in cases of hemorrhage, 414, 415
    in cases of perforation, 397–398, 414,
    415
    infection after, 151
    recurrence after, 418
Percussion, in diagnosis of cause of abdominal pain, 390
Percutaneous transhepatic biliary drainage,
  560, *561*
Percutaneous transhepatic cholangiography,
  560, *560*, 584, 599–600
Percutaneous transhepatic coronary vein
  occlusion, in control of bleeding
  esophageal varices, 531
Percutaneous transhepatic venous sampling,
  600
Percutaneous transluminal balloon angioplasty, for coarctation of aorta, 1069,
  1070
  for myocardial ischemia, 1118–1119
Percutaneous transthoracic aspiration
  needle biopsy, in diagnosis of lung
  cancer, *1002*, 1002–1003, *1003*
Perforation, appendiceal, inflammation
  and, 464
  cholecystic, 565
  colonic, cancer and, 494
    colitis and, 484

Perforation (*Continued*)
  colonic, diverticulitis and, 499
  esophageal, 369(t), 369–371, *370*, *371*
    endoscope and, 367, 369, 369(t)
    external trauma and, 187–188, 369
  gastric, and pneumoperitoneum, *670*
    in newborn, 670
  intestinal, in newborn, 669–670
  peptic ulcer, 397, 412
    surgery for, 397–398, 414, 415
  small intestine, after surgery, 205
Performance/physical status scales, 63(t),
  279(t)
Perfusion, in cardiopulmonary bypass, 1187
  effects of hypothermia during, 1187,
  1187, *1188*
  withdrawal from, 1190
Perfusion of lung, 971–973, *971–973*
Pericardectomy, 1047, 1053
Pericardial effusion, 1046, *1047*
Pericardiocentesis, 182, 188, 1052, *1052*
Pericarditis, 1046, 1049–1052
  as complication of coronary artery bypass
  graft, 1123
  constrictive, 1046, *1051*
Pericardium, 1045
  biopsy of, 1052
  congenital abnormalities of, 1034, 1048–
  1049, *1049*
  cysts of, 1034, 1048–1049, *1049*
  defects of, 1049
  drainage of, 1052
  inflammation of, 1046, 1049–1052
    as complication of coronary artery by-
    pass graft, 1123
    with constriction, 1046, *1051*
  pain of inflammation in, 1046
  resection of, 1047, 1053
  trauma to, pericarditis following, 1052
  tumors of, 1051–1052, 1164(t)
Perichondritis, of pinna, 691
Perineal hernia, 654
Perineum, female, 805
Peripheral cardiovascular system, 1179
  drugs affecting, 1180, 1181(t)
Peripheral facial nerve paralysis, 693
Peripheral nerves, 743, *743*
Peripheral nervous system, injury of, 873–
  874
Peripheral parenteral nutrition, 107
Peristalsis, esophageal, 365, *366*
  loss of, in scleroderma, 376, *376*
Peritoneal dialysis, 214
  for acute renal failure, 214
Peritoneal fat lines, fluid obscuring, 392,
  392
Peritoneal lavage, for acute pancreatitis,
  604
  in management of trauma, 183
  in suspected cases of intra-abdominal
  trauma, 183, 189
Peritoneoscopy, in gynecologic examina-
  tion, 811
Peritoneovenous shunt, for ascites, 547
Peritoneum, air in, gastric perforation and,
  670
  in newborn, 670, *670*
Peritonitis, 154
  meconium and, *664*, 669
  postoperative, 205
Peritonsillar abscess, 699
Peutz-Jeghers syndrome, 452, 487, *487*
Peyer's patches, 431
Peyronie's disease, 845–846
Phagocytosis, 142

Phagocytosis (*Continued*)
   defects in, 142–143
Pharyngitis, 699
   and abscess formation, 699
Pharyngoesophageal diverticulum, *372*
   resection of, *373*
Pharynx, 699, 713
   cancer of, radiosensitivity of, *723*
      staging of, *721*
   carcinoma of, 700, 731–732
   constrictor muscles of, 713
   foreign body impaction in, 701
   inflammation of, 699
   in swallowing, 365
   squamous epithelium of, *709*
   tumors of, 700, 731–732
Phenacetin abuse, and urinary tract disease, 837
Phentolamine, 1180
Phenylephrine, 1180
Pheochromocytoma, 72, 360–361
   mediastinal, 1028
Phimosis, 844–845
Phlebitis, 941
   and intravascular catheter-related sepsis, 165
   venous insufficiency after, 942–943, *943*
Phlegmasia, 941
Phospholipid metabolism, in endothelial cells and platelets, *81*
Physical status/performance scales, 63(t), 279(t)
Physiologic dead space, in lung, 973
Piedmont fracture, 761
Pigeon breast (pectus carinatum), 1013, *1015*
Pigment stones, 557
Pilonidal sinus (cyst), 510–511, 800–801
Pinna, absence of, 690
   hematoma of, 691
   perichondritis of, 691
   protrusion of, 690
Pituitary, 350, *350*, *351*
   blood vessels supplying, 350, *351*
   hormones secreted by, 351–352
      excess of, 353–354
      hypothalamic hormones affecting, 352(t)
      precursor(s) of, *352*
   resection of, for Cushing's syndrome, 353, 358
      in treatment of prostate cancer, 844
   tumors of, 353–354
      extension of, diaphragma sellae and, 350
Pituitary apoplexy, 353
Plagiocephaly, 877
Plasma, fresh frozen, therapeutic use of, 93
   laboratory reference values for, 1197(t)–1201(t)
Plasma cell mastitis, 304
Plasma protein restitution, in restitution of blood volume, 48
Plasma volume, 31
Plasmacytoma, 1018
Plasmapheresis, for myasthenia gravis, 1042
Plasminogen activator, 81, 87
Plate fixation, of femoral shaft fracture, 765
Platelet(s), 81–82, *82*
   adhesion of, 82–83
   aggregation of, 79, 80(t), 82, 83
      laboratory tests of, 88, *88*
   alpha granules of, 82
   effect of aspirin on, *88*, 90

Platelet(s) (*Continued*)
   metabolism of membrane phospholipids in, *81*
   transfusion of, 90, 93
Platelet disorders, 89–90, 626
Platelet-derived growth factor, in wound healing, 118
cis-Platinum, 278
Plethysmography, in assessment of peripheral artery disease, 896
   in diagnosis of venous disorders, 936–937
Pleura, 988
   tumors of, 991
Pleural effusion, 988–989
   blood in, 990
   chyle in, 990
   pancreatic fluid in, 608
   pus in, 206, *990*, 990–991
   tuberculous, Eloesser flap in drainage of, 997, *997*
Pleural space, air in, 989–990
   in newborn, 661, *661*
   in trauma patients, 181
   blood in, 990
   chyle in, 990
   pancreatic fluid in, 608
   pus in, *990*, 990–991
      postoperative, 206
   tuberculous effusion in, Eloesser flap in drainage of, 997, *997*
Plug, hemostatic, formation of, 81–82
Pneumatic antishock garment, 182–183
Pneumatosis intestinalis, in newborn, 670, *671*
Pneumobilia, 558
Pneumocystis carinii infection, and pneumonia, in AIDS, 176, 987
Pneumomediastinum, 1022–1023
Pneumonectomy. See *Lung(s), resection of.*
Pneumonia, nosocomial, 163–164, 209
   fever due to, 202
   Pneumocystis carinii infection and, in AIDS, 176, 987
   radiographic findings in, 209
   specimen collection in, 147, 209
Pneumonitis, aspiration, 984
Pneumoperitoneum, gastric perforation and, *670*
   in newborn, 670, *670*
Pneumothorax, 989–990
   in newborn, 661, *661*
   in trauma patients, 181
   open, 181
   tension, 181
      in newborn, 661, *661*
Poisoning, carbon monoxide, 129
   food-borne, clostridial, 161
   laboratory determination of, reference values for, 1204(t)
Poland's syndrome, 1013, *1016*
Polyamide sutures, 137
Polycystic kidney disease, 679, 833
Polycythemia, preparation of surgical patients with, 66
Polyester sutures, 137
Polyp(s), adenomatous, of colon, and colorectal cancer, 485
   of stomach, 423
   hyperplastic, of stomach, 423
   of bronchi, 1008
   of colon, 485–487, *486*, 486(t)
      and colorectal cancer, 485, 489
   of endometrium, 816
   of esophagus, 383

Polyp(s) (*Continued*)
   of small intestine, 452
   of stomach, 423
Polyposis of colon, familial, 486
   juvenile, 487
Polypropylene sutures, 137
Polyuria, 43–44, 831
Polyuric prerenal azotemia, 47
Popliteal artery, trauma to, femoral fracture and, 199
Porcelain gallbladder, *559*
Porphyria erythropoietica, 628
Port wine stain, 799–800
Portacaval shunt, for ascites, 546
   for bleeding esophageal varices, 532
   for portal hypertension, 533, *533*
Portal hypertension, *527*, 527–535
   bleeding esophageal varices in patients with, 529
      treatment of, 529–532, 530(t), *530–532*
   in children, 535
   pathophysiology of, 528, *528*
   surgery for, 533–534, *533–535*
Portal vein, 513, *514*, *515*
   air in, 392, *392*
Portosystemic shunt, for portal hypertension, 533
Positional vertigo, benign, 695
Positive end-expiratory pressure, 977, 978
   for adult respiratory distress syndrome, 211
Postauricular lymph nodes, 715
Postcholecystectomy syndrome, 583
Postcoarctectomy syndrome, 1070
Posterior anuloplasty, in repair of Ebstein's anomaly, *1154*
Posterior gastropexy, 381, *381*
Posterior pituitary, hormones secreted by, 352
Posterior wedge osteotomy, *1014*
Posterolateral diaphragmatic defect of Bochdalek, *661*, 661–662
   repair of, 662, *662*
Postgastrectomy syndromes, 418–421, 448
Post-myocardial infarction syndrome, 1052
Postpericardiotomy syndrome, 1052
Postphlebitic syndrome, 92, 942–943, *943*
Postprandial dumping, 418–419
Postrenal azotemia, postoperative, 44, 214
Post-transfusion purpura, 94
Postvagotomy diarrhea, 420, 448
Potassium, absorption of, in small intestine, 434
   diminished serum levels of, 45, 51–52, 52(t)
      management of surgical patients with, 64
   elevated serum levels of, 45, 52(t), 52–53
      management of surgical patients with, 64
Prazocin, 1180
Precocious puberty, in females, 807–808
Prednisone, for myasthenia gravis, 1042
Pregnancy, appendicitis during, 463–464
   breast cancer in, 325
   changes in breast during, 294, *294*
   detection of, 811
   ectopic, 402, 823
   first, and risk of breast cancer, 306
   hyperthyroidism during, 334
   in patient over 30 or under 18, and risk of breast cancer, 306
   surgery during, 823–824

Preload, 18, 1179
Premature infant, infection in, 657
  patent ductus arteriosus in, 1063–1064
Premature ventricular contractions, as complication of coronary artery bypass
  graft, 1122
  postoperative, management of, *1184*
Premedication, and anesthesia, 109–110
Prerenal azotemia, 44
  polyuric, 47
  postoperative, 211–212
  vs. renal azotemia, 45, 45(t), 213(t)
Presbycusis, 694
Preservation, of cadaver organs for trans-
  plantation, 236
Priapism, 845
Primary wound closure, delayed, 120
  in reconstructive surgery, after radical
    neck dissection for cancer, 729
Priming fluids, pump-oxygenator, in cardio-
  pulmonary bypass, 1187
Procainamide, 1182
Proctitis, ulcerative, 480
Proctocolectomy, *476*
Progesterone, neurohumoral influences on
  ovarian production of, 292
Progesterone receptor activity, in breast
  cancer, 323
Prognostic Nutritional Index, 104
Progressive generalized lymphadenopathy,
  173
Progressive hepatitis, chronic, 171
Prolactin, 351–352
  elevated serum levels of, 303, 354
Prolactinoma, 354
Prolapse, mitral valve, 1148
  appearance of valve in, *1149*
  rectal, 510, *511*
  uterine, 820, *820*
Proliferative breast disease, 300–301
  and risk of mammary cancer, 306, 306(t)
Pronator teres syndrome, 744
Propranolol, for bleeding esophageal varices, 530, *530*
  for supraventricular arrhythmias, 1182
Prostacyclin, 80
Prostaglandins, in prophylaxis against stress
  ulcers, 417
Prostate, 829
  cancer of, 843–844
  congenital anomalies of, 840
  hypertrophy of, benign, 841–842
  inflammation of, 840–841
  resection of, for benign hypetrophy, *842*,
    842–843
  for cancer, *843*, 843–844
Prostatectomy, for benign hypetrophy, *842*,
  842–843
  for cancer, *843*, 843–844
Prostatitis, 840–841
Prosthesis, aortic valve, 1139, *1140*
  endothelial seeding of, 264
  fixation of, to chest wall, *1018*
  joint, 790
  mitral valve, 1147, *1147*, *1148*
  penile, 847
  tricuspid valve, 1151, 1155
  use of, after surgery for head and neck
    cancer, 730
Protease, 593
Protein, changes in metabolism of, in response to stress, 17, 97, 100(t)
  digestion of, 410, 431–432
  malabsorption of, 447

Protein (*Continued*)
  serum levels of, as index of nutritional
    status, 102, 103(t)
  synthesis of, in liver, 518
    inhibition of, in cancer chemotherapy,
      278
  shock and, 17
Protein C, 81, 92
Protein S, 92
Protozoal infection, in AIDS, 176(t)
Pruritus ani, 510
Pseudocyst, pancreatic, 606–607
Pseudoepitheliomatous hyperplasia, 708
Pseudohermaphroditism, 812–813, 853–854
Pseudomembranous colitis, 161–162, 503–
  504
  postoperative, 219
Pseudomycotic infections, 166
Pseudo-obstruction, of small intestine, 436
Psychiatric disturbances, postoperative, 203
Psychopharmacologic drugs, 1204(t)
Puberty, in females, 807–808
  and breast development, 292, *294*
  precocious, 807–808
Pulmonary artery, left coronary artery originating from, 1132, *1133*
  surgery for, 1132, *1134*, *1135*
  right coronary artery originating from,
    1133
Pulmonary artery catheter, in measurement
  of left atrial filling pressure, 115
Pulmonary embolism, 92
  clinical presentation in chronic cases of,
    956(t), 956–957, 957(t)
  coumarin for, 949
  diagnosis of, 947–949, 949(t), 951(t)
  fat, 954–955
  heparin for, 949
  laboratory evaluation of, 948–949, 949(t)
  pathogenesis of, 945–946, *946*, 946(t)
  physiologic responses to, 947
  prevention of, 66, *66*, 951
  radiographic findings in, 949, *950*, 957,
    957, *958*, 959(t), *960*
  surgery for, 951–954, 952(t), *952–954*,
    953(t), 957–964, *962–966*
  thrombolytics for, 949–951
Pulmonary fibrosis, cancer chemotherapy
  and, 279
Pulmonary tuberculosis, 994–997, *995*
  and pericarditis, 1050–1051
  drug therapy for, 996, 996(t)
  surgery for, 994, 996–997
Pulmonary valve, stenosis of, in tetralogy
  of Fallot, 1089
  isolated, *1093*, 1094
Pulmonary vascular resistance, 1086
Pulmonary venous connection, anomalous,
  1082, 1082–1083
  surgery for, 1084, *1084*
Pulmonary venous pressure, in cardiopulmonary bypass, 1188
Pulsatile perfusion, hypothermic, in preservation of cadaver organs for transplantation, 236
Pulse, deficits in, in chronic arterial occlusive disease, 910
  palpation of, in assessment of peripheral
    artery disease, 895, *896*
    in examination for arterial trauma, 197
    in trauma patient, 182
Pulse pressure, evaluation of, in management of trauma, 182
Pulsus paradoxus, 1046

Pump-oxygenator apparatus, in cardiopulmonary bypass, 1185–1186, *1186*
  priming fluids used with, 1187
Punch graft method of hair transplantation,
  263
Purpura, post-transfusion, 94
  thrombocytopenic, 89, 629
Pus, in inflamed gallbladder, 565
  in pleural space, *990*, 990–991
  after surgery, 206
PVB chemotherapy regimen, 280
Pyelogram, 831–832, *832*
Pyelonephritis, postoperative, 164
  xanthogranulomatous, 833–834
Pyloric exclusion and gastrojejunostomy,
  for duodenal trauma, 192, *192*
Pyloric stenosis, hypertrophic, 674–675
  surgery for, 675, *675*
Pyloromyotomy, for hypertrophic pyloric
  stenosis, *675*
Pyloroplasty, as drainage procedure with
  vagotomy for peptic ulcer, 413, *414*
Pyogenic abscess, of liver, 521(t), 521–523
Pyogenic arthritis, 786–787
Pyogenic cholangitis, recurrent, 572–573
Pyridostigmine bromide, for myasthenia
  gravis, 1041
Pyruvate kinase deficiency, 628
Pyuria, 831

Quadrantectomy-axillary dissection-radiotherapy, for breast cancer, results of,
  318, *318–319*
Queyrat's erythroplasia, 846
Quinidine, 1182

Radial artery, 741
  occlusive disease of, 743
Radial nerve, *739*, 740, *740*
Radiation, 271–272
  megavoltage, 272
  side effect(s) of, 272–273, 275, 724
    cystitis as, 840
    intestinal injury as, 458, 503
    pericarditis as, 1051
    risk of breast cancer associated with,
      306–307
    teratogenesis as, 325
    thyroid cancer as, 336
  tissue response to, 272–273, *273*, 275,
    724
  tumor response to, 272–274, *273*
Radiation therapy, 271–272
  beam arrangement in, 272
  beam penetration in, 272, 272(t)
  for cancer, 273–276
    at sites of metastases, 275
    chemotherapy with, 276
    in emergencies, 275
    of anus, 510
    of bladder, 839
    of bone, secondary to malignant dis-
      ease at other site, 275
    of brain, 862
      secondary to malignant disease at
        other site, 275
    of breast, 274, 317–321
      results of, *318–319*, 318–321, 319(t),
        321–322
    of gastrointestinal tract, 274

Radiation therapy (*Continued*)
  for cancer, of genital tract, 274
    of head and neck, 274, 722–724
      side effects of, 275, 724
      vs. surgical treatment, 724
    of larynx, 704, 733
    of liver, secondary to malignant disease at other site, 275, 542
    of lung, 274, 1004(t), 1004–1005
    of nasopharynx, 733
    of prostate, 844
    surgery with, 275
  for Cushing's syndrome, 358
  for Hodgkin's disease, 274
  for lymphoma, 632, *632*
  for sarcoma, 284
  short-distance, 272
  side effect(s) of. See *Radiation, side effect(s) of.*
  skin-sparing, 272, 272(t)
Radical mastectomy, for cancer, 317
  results of, 318, *318–319*, 320, 321, *321–322*
  modified, for cancer, *316*
Radical neck dissection, for cancer, 725, *726*, *727–728*
Radiculopathy, cervical, 878–879, 879(t)
  lumbar, 880–881
Radiography, as aid to diagnosis, of appendicitis, 463
  of cancer, of breast, 297, *298*, 307
    of lung, 1001, *1001*
  of cause of abdominal pain, 392, *392*
  of cecal volvulus, 501, *501*
  of coarctation of aorta, 1066, *1066*
  of esophageal atresia, 659, *660*
  of esophageal motor disorders, *374*, *375*, *376*, 376, 377, *377*
  of gallbladder disorders, 558, *559*
  of gas gangrene (clostridial myonecrosis), *158*
  of gastroesophageal reflux, 380
  of intestinal obstruction, 438, *439*, *440*, 441
    in newborn, 663, *664*
  of mediastinal tumors, 1026
  of mitral stenosis, 1145
  of pancreatitis, 398, 598
  of pericardial effusion, 1047, *1047*
  of pneumonia, 209
  of pulmonary embolism, 949, *950*, 957, *957*, *958*, 959(t), *960*
  of sigmoid volvulus, 500, *500*
  of tetralogy of Fallot, 1090, *1090*
  of thymoma, 1040, *1041*
  of tracheoesophageal fistula, 659, *660*
  of trauma, to cervical spine, 185
    to thoracic aorta, 189
  breast, as aid to diagnosis, of cancer, 297, *298*, 307
    benefits vs. risks of, 307
  chest, preoperative, 70
  historical aspects of, 3
  operative, pancreatic duct on, 600, *600*
Radioiodine, tests of thyroid uptake of, 330
  treatment of hyperthyroidism with, 333–334
Radionuclide angiocardiography, 1117, *1117*
Radionuclide scanning, after abdominal trauma, 190
  in acute cholecystitis, 396, 561, *561*
  in Cushing's syndrome, 358
  in lung cancer, 1002
  in pheochromocytoma, 361

Radionuclide scanning (*Continued*)
  of bone, in breast cancer, 309
  of spleen, 621, *621*
  of thyroid, 330
Radius, fracture of, 749, 760–761
Ramstedt-Fredet operation, for hypertrophic pyloric stenosis, *675*
Ranson's criteria, for prognosis in acute pancreatitis, 399(t), 603, 603(t)
Rastelli operation, for outlet tract obstruction, in transposition of great arteries, 1104, *1105*
Ravdin, Isadore, 5, *5*
Raynaud's syndrome, 743, 916–918
Reactive hypoglycemia, 419
Receptive relaxation, of stomach, 410
Receptor activity, in breast cancer, 323
Receptor blockers, in cancer chemotherapy, 278
Reconstructive surgery, after operations for cancer, 269
  of breast, 320
  of head and neck, *726–727*, *728–730*
Recovery (awakening) from anesthesia, impaired, 202
Rectal continence, 474
Rectocele, *819*, 820
Rectum. See also *Anorectum.*
  abscess of, 507
  cancer of. See also *Colorectal cancer.*
    anterior vs. abdominoperineal resection of, 492–494, *493*, 494(t)
    cauterization of, 497
  examination of, in diagnosis of cause of abdominal pain, 391
  inflammation of, ulcerative, 480
  intussusception of, 510, *511*
  prolapse of, 510, *511*
  resection of, for cancer, 492–494, *493*, 494(t)
  trauma to, 192–193
Recurrent pyogenic cholangitis, 572–573
Red blood cells, in spleen, 615–616
  transfusion of, 93
Reduction of fracture, 756
Reflux, gastroesophageal, 379–381
  and dysphagia, 372
  in children, 675–676
  treatment of, 380–381, *381*
  vesicoureteral, 837
Reflux esophagitis. See *Reflux, gastroesophageal.*
Reflux gastritis, after gastrectomy, 420
Refrigeration analgesia, 115
Regional anesthesia, 113–114
Regional enteritis. See *Crohn's disease.*
Regional hypothermia, 115
Regurgitation, aortic, *1138*, 1138–1139
  treatment of, by replacement of aortic valve, 1139, *1140*
  mitral, 1148–1149
    treatment of, 1149–1150, *1150*
  tricuspid valve, 1150
Rejection, 228–229
  accelerated, 228
  acute, 228–229
  antibody-dependent cell-mediated cytotoxicity in, 228
  cell surface antigens in, 224
  chronic, 229
  dendritic cells in, 226, 227, *227*
  hyperacute, 228
    avoidance of, 229–230
  induction of tolerance in circumvention of, 234

Rejection (*Continued*)
  initiation of immune response in, 227, *227*, *228*
  macrophages in, 226, 227, *228*
  of heart, 257, *257*
  of heart and lung, 257
  of kidney, 242
  of liver, 248
  of lung, 257
  of pancreas, 251
  suppression of, 231–232, 237, 238
  T cells in, 225, 226, 227
  testing for possible potentiators of, 229–231
Renal artery, lesions of, and hypertension, 836, 927–928
Renal azotemia. See *Renal failure, acute.*
Renal blood flow, autoregulation of, 46, *46*
  effect of hypovolemia on, 47
Renal failure, 63
  acute, 44
    parenteral nutrition in management of, 105, 105(t)
    postoperative, 212–214
    vs. prerenal azotemia, 45, 45(t), 213(t)
  and pericarditis, 1051
  as complication of cardiopulmonary bypass, 1190
  postoperative, 211–215
Renal medulla, cystic disease of, 833
Renal osteodystrophy, *348*
Renal pedicle, midline approach to, *196*
Renal pelvis, infection-related inflammation of, postoperative, 164
  obstruction of ureteral junction with, 833
  tumors of, 837
Renal transplantation. See *Transplantation, kidney.*
Renal vasculature, trauma to, 196
Renal vein, thrombosis of, 679
Renin, 37–38, 355, 836, 927–928
Renovascular hypertension, 836, 927–929, *929*
Reptilase time, 89
Respiration, in newborn, 655
  conditions compromising, 657–663
Respiratory acidosis, 57(t), 59(t), 59–60
Respiratory alkalosis, 57(t), 58
Respiratory distress, 210
  airway management in, 976
  mechanical ventilation for, 211, 976(t), 976–978
  postoperative, 210
Respiratory emergencies, in newborn, 657–663
Respiratory tract, trauma to, 186–187
  fire-related, 129
Rest pain, in peripheral artery disease, 892
Restrictive pulmonary disease, 974
  spirometric findings in, 207
Resuscitation, after liver transplantation, 247
  cardiopulmonary, 1054–1060
  of trauma patient, 182
Retina, emboli in, as sign of vascular disease, 894, 920–923
Retrograde cholangiopancreatography, 560, *560*, 584, 599, *599*
Retropectoral lymphatics, 291
Retropharyngeal abscess, 699
Rhabdomyoma, of heart, 1165–1166
Rhabdomyosarcoma, 680–681
Rheumatic fever, and aortic insufficiency, 1138, *1138*
  and aortic stenosis, 1137, *1138*

Rheumatic fever (*Continued*)
  and mitral regurgitation, 1148
  and mitral stenosis, 1143, *1144*
  and tricuspid stenosis, 1150
Rheumatoid arthritis, of hand, 751
Rhinitis, 696
Rhinosinusitis, 696
Rhizotomy, for chronic pain, 884
Rhoads, Jonathan, 5, *5*
Rib(s), first, resection of, for thoracic out-
    let syndrome, 1010, 1011
  fractures of, and flail chest, 181
  notching of, as roentgenographic sign of
    coarctation of aorta, 1066, *1066*
  tumors of, 1015, 1018
Richter's hernia, 653, *653*
Rifampin, for mycobacterial infections,
    996, 996(t)
Right coronary artery, 1114, *1114*, *1116*
  atherosclerosis of, *1115*
  originating from pulmonary artery, 1133
Right hepatic lobectomy, 520
Right hepatic trisegmentectomy, 520
Right ventricle, double outlet, 1095–1096,
    1096
  surgery for, 1096–1097, *1097*
  dysplasia of, arrhythmogenic, 1162
  in Ebstein's anomaly, 1153
Rigler's sign, in perforation of duodenal
    ulcer, 412
Rinne test, for hearing loss, 689
Röntgen, Wilhelm, 3, *3*
Rotter's nodes, breast cancer treatment in-
    volving, 317
Roux-en-Y pancreaticojejunostomy, in
    drainage of pancreatic fluid, *608*
Rovsing's sign, in diagnosis of cause of ab-
    dominal pain, 391, *391*
Rubber band ligation, of hemorrhoids, 506
Rugger-jersey spine, in renal osteodystro-
    phy, *348*
Rule of nines, in estimation of surface area
    of burns, 124–125
Rupture, of aneurysm of abdominal aorta,
    402
  of bronchus, 187
  of diaphragm, 191
  of spleen, 631
Rye classification, of Hodgkin's disease,
    631(t)

Saccular bronchiectasis, 992
Sacrococcygeal teratoma, 682, *682*, 876
Saddle bag sign, *670*
Salivary glands, 712
  tumors of, 734
Salpingitis, 819
Salt conservation, 46–47
Salt intoxication, 51
Saphenous vein, 933
  in coronary artery bypass graft, *1119*,
    1120, *1120*, 1123
  stripping of, for varicosity, 939–940, *940*
Sarcoidosis, 625
Sarcoma, 283–284
  Ewing's, 1018
  Kaposi's, in AIDS, 177, 800
  metastasis of, to lung, 1007(t)
  of breast, 314–315
  of heart, 1166
  of myometrium, 818
  of soft tissue, 283–284
    treatment of, 284, *284*
  treatment of, 284, *284*

Satellitosis, after surgical excision of mela-
    noma, 286
Scalene lymph node biopsy, in lung cancer,
    1003
Scalp, laceration of, 870
Scalpel incision, risk of infection associated
    with, *135*
Scaphocephaly, 877
Scaphoid, fracture of, 748, *749*
Scapular lymph node group, 291, *292*
Scar, formation of, in wound healing, 118
  hypertrophic, 798
    formation of, after healing of burns,
      130–131
Schistosomiasis, bladder cancer associated
    with, 838
Schoemaker modification, of Billroth I
    anastomosis, *413*
Schwabach test, for hearing loss, 689–690
Schwannoma, 864
  mediastinal, 1027
Sciatic hernia, 654
Scirrhous carcinoma, of breast, *298*, 312,
    312
Scleroderma, esophagus in, 376, *376*
Sclerosing cholangitis, 570–572, *572*
Sclerotherapy, for bleeding esophageal var-
    ices, *531*, 531–532, *532*
  for hemorrhoids, 506
  for varicose veins, 939, 940
Scoliosis, 772–775, *773–775*
  braces for, 774
  Cotrel-Dubousset instrumentation for,
    775, *775*
  evaluation of, Cobb angle in, 773, *774*
  Luque instrumentation for, 775
Scrotum, 829–830
  gangrene of, 849
  herniation into, 640
  hydrocele in, 849–850
  tumors of, 849
Seborrheic keratosis, 794, *794*
Second-degree burns, 123, 124
Second intention healing, 119
Secretin, 409
  secretion of, after meal stimulus, *410*
Secretin test, 595–596, 596(t)
Seeding, endothelial, of prosthesis, 264
Segmental mastectomy, for cancer, results
    of, 319, 319(t)
Segmental pancreatic graft, in pancreas
    transplant, 250, *251*
Seizure disorders, 882–883
  drugs for, 1203(t)
  management of surgical patients with, 74
Selective vagotomy, for peptic ulcer, 414
Self-examination of breast, in diagnosis of
    mammary cancer, 296
Sella turcica, cerebrospinal fluid in, 354
Semen analysis, laboratory reference values
    for, 1206(t)
Semicircular canals, 687, *688*
Seminal vesicle, 829
  cyst of, 844
  inflammation of, 844
Seminoma, 852
  mediastinal, 1030–1031
Semmelweis, Ignaz, contributions of, to an-
    tiseptic surgery, 141
Sengstaken-Blakemore tube, in balloon
    tamponade, for bleeding esophageal
    varices, 531, *531*
Senning procedure, for transposition of
    great arteries, 1104, *1106*
  complications of, 1108
Sensorineural deafness, 689

Sentinel loop sign, in acute pancreatitis,
    398, 598
Sepsis. See also *Infection(s)*.
  after abortion, 403
  after splenectomy, 621
  effects of, on wound healing, 119
  fat metabolism in, 101(t)
  glucose production in, 102(t)
  in premature infants, 657
  intra-abdominal, 153–154, 204–205
    changed mental status as sign of, 203
    treatment of, antimicrobials in, 157,
      157(t)
      drainage in, 154, 157, 204–205, *205*
  intravascular catheter-related, 105–106,
    165
  parenteral nutrition in management of,
    105
  urea production in, 102(t)
Septic abortion, 403
Septic shock, 20–23, 21(t), 22(t)
Serotonin, tumor secreting, 610(t), 612
Serum, laboratory reference values for,
    1197(t)–1201(t)
Sexual dysfunction, male, 847–848, 907
Sexually transmitted disease, 510, 846
Shaving, preoperative, postoperative infec-
    tion risk associated with, 133, 149
Shock, 11–12, *12*
  cardiogenic, 18–19
  cellular hypoperfusion in, 12, *13*
  complications of, 25–27
  distributive, 23
  effects of, on energy substrates, 12–17,
    23–24
  hypovolemic, 19–20
    management of, 63
      in trauma patients, 182
  lactate production by GI tract in, 14, *14*
  liver dysfunction following, 16–17, *17*, 216
  neuroendocrine response to, *11*, *46*
  septic, 20–23, 21(t), 22(t)
  spinal, 872
Short bowel syndrome, 450
Shoulder, dislocation of, 758
Shouldice operation, for inguinal hernia,
    639, 645
Shunt, intrapulmonary, 25, *26*, 207, *207*
Shunt construction, arteriovenous, in he-
    modialysis, 213, *214*
  Blalock-Taussig, 1099
  Denver, 547
  for ascites, 546–547, *547*
  for bleeding esophageal varices, 532
  for portal hypertension, *533*, 533–534,
    534
  LaVeen, for ascites, 547
  peritoneovenous, for ascites, 547
  portacaval, for ascites, 546
    for bleeding esophageal varices, 532
    for portal hypertension, 533, *533*
  splenorenal, 534, *534*
    for bleeding esophageal varices, 532
    for portal hypertension, 534
  subclavian artery–to–pulmonary artery,
    in management of tricuspid atresia,
    1099
Sickle cell disease, 627
  preparation of surgical patient with, 66
Sick sinus syndrome, pacemaker for, 1170
Side-to-side portacaval shunt, for portal hy-
    pertension, 533
Sigmoid sinus, *692*
Sigmoid volvulus, *500*, 500–501
Sigmoidoscopy, 475
  in reduction of volvulus, 500

Silk sutures, 136
Silver nitrate, for burns, 127
Silver sulfadiazine, for burns, 127
Simple mastectomy, extended, for cancer, 317
Single-fiber electromyography, in diagnosis of myasthenia gravis, 1040
Single-rescuer CPR, 1057
Sinus tachycardia, drugs for, 1182
  surgical treatment of, 1160
Sinus venosus defects, *1078*, 1079
  surgery for, *1079*
Sinusitis, 697
Sinusoids, hepatic, 516, *516*
Skier's thumb, 748
Skin, 117, 791–792, *793*
  antiseptics used on, 132
  cancer of, 284–286
    immunotherapy for, 282
  excision of, in management of lymphedema, 637
  expansion of, 262, *264*
  layers of, 117
    degree of burn injury in relation to, 123, *123*, 124
  of hand, injury of, 741–742
  radiation penetration of, 272, 272(t), 275
  radiotherapy dose sparing, 272, 272(t)
  tumors of, 794–799, *794–799*
Skin cells, effects of shock on energy metabolism in, 14
Skin expansion, 262, *264*
Skin flaps, in reconstructive surgery, after radical neck dissection for cancer, 729
Skin graft(s), 262, 262(t), *798*
  after excision of lymphedematous tissue, 637, *637*
  for burns, 130, 262
  full-thickness, *798*
  in reconstructive surgery, after radical neck dissection for cancer, 729
  meshed, for burns, 130
  split-thickness, 262
    donor site in, cutting of, with dermatomes, 130
    for burns, 130
    in reconstructive surgery, after radical neck dissection for cancer, 729
Skin perfusion, as index of fluid balance, 43
Skull, congenital abnormalities of, 876–878
  fracture of, 184, 185, 880–881
Sliding inguinal hernia, 651
  and blood supply to colon, *651*
Small cell carcinoma, hormones and hormone-like products secreted by, 1008(t)
Small intestine, 429
  absorption in, 433–435
    disorders of. See *Malabsorption.*
  adenocarcinoma of, Crohn's disease and, 445
  anatomy of, 429–431, *431*
  blood vessels supplying, 430
  bypass of segments of, 459–460
    for hypercholesterolemia, 459–460
    for obesity, 428, 459
  cancer of, 451(t), 452–453
    Crohn's disease and, 445
  carcinoid of, *453*, 453–454
  closed-loop obstruction of, 437
  digestion in, 410–411, 431–433
  diverticula of, 455–458
  fibroma of, 452
  gross anatomy of, 429–430
  hemangioma of, 452

Small intestine (*Continued*)
  hemorrhage from, in patients with Meckel's diverticulum, 457
  leiomyoma of, 452
  leiomyosarcoma of, 452
  lipoma of, 452
  lymphoma of, 452
  microanatomy of, 430–431, *431*
  motility of, 435
  necrosis of, clostridial infection and, 161
  obstruction of, 399–400, 436–442
    by duodenal hematoma, 192
    by gallstone, 568, 569, *569*
    in patients with Meckel's diverticulum, 458, *467*, 468
    postoperative, *220*, 220–221
    radiographic findings in, 438, *439*, *440*, 441
    surgery for, 442
    tube decompression of GI tract for, 441
    vs. paralytic ileus, 219
  perforation of, postoperative, 205
  polyps of, 452
  pseudo-obstruction of, 436
  radiation injury to, 458
  resection of, for carcinoid, 455
    for Crohn's disease, 446
    for radiation injury, 458–459
    in treatment of Meckel's diverticulum, 458, *469*, 469–470
    malabsorption after, 450
  strangulation of, 437
    coffee bean sign in, 441
  transplantation of, 260–261
  trauma to, 191
  tumors of, 450–455, 451(t)
  valvulae conniventes of, radiographic appearance of, in cases of obstruction, *440*
  villi of, 431, *431*
Small stomach syndrome, 420
Smoking, and cancer, of head and neck, 706
  of larynx, *706*
  of lung, 998–999, *999*
  and impaired lung function, in surgical patient, 70
  and occlusive arterial disease, 910
Snake envenomation, 199
Sodium, absorption of, in small intestine, 434
  as cofactor in transport of glucose, *432*
  diminished serum levels of, 45, 48–50, 64
  elevated serum levels of, 45, 50–51, 64
Sodium nitroprusside, 1180
Soft palate, 713
  carcinoma of, 732
Soft tissue, effect of radiation on, 275
  necrotizing infections of, 157–159, 159(t), 162–163
  sarcoma of, 283–284
    treatment of, *284*, 284
Solute reabsorption, by kidneys, 39(t), 39–40
Somatostatin, 351, 595
  for bleeding esophageal varices, 529
  tumor secreting, 610(t), 612
Somatotropin, 351
  tumor secreting, 353
Somnolence, postoperative, 202, 203
Space of Disse, 516
Spasm, esophageal, diffuse, 376–378, *377*
Spermatic cord, 830
Spherocytosis, hereditary, 626
  splenectomy for, 626

Sphincter, anal, *505*
  resection of, for anal fissure, 507, *507*
  esophageal, function of, 365, *365*, *366*
    abnormal, 374–378, *375–378*
      and dysphagia, 372
      and gastroesophageal reflux, 379
Sphincter of Oddi, lesions of, 582, 583
Spigelian hernia, 653
Spina bifida cystica, *874*, 874–875
Spinal cord, 859
  cancer compressing, radiation therapy for, 275
  surgery of, for chronic pain, 884–885
  tumors of, 863–865, *864*
  vascular disease involving, 868–869
Spinal shock, 872
Spine, 878
  cervical, degenerative disease of, 878–879, 879(t)
    dislocation of, 769–770, *770*
    fractures of, 185, 768–770
    trauma to, CT examination for, 186
      emergency search for, 181, 185
      radiographic examination for, 185
  congenital abnormalities of, *874*, 874–876
  curvature of, 772–775, *773–775*
  degenerative disease of, 878–881
  dysraphic, 875
  fractures of, 768–771, *769*, *771*, 872
  infection of, 886
  rugger-jersey appearance of, in renal osteodystrophy, *348*
  thoracolumbar, degenerative disease of, 879–881
    fractures of, 770–771, *771*
  trauma to, 871–873
  tumors of, 863–865
Spirometry, 207, 969–970, *970*
  in evaluation of surgical patient, 71
Spleen, 616
  abscess of, 630–631
  absence of, 621
  accessory, 616, 630
  anatomy of, 616, *617–619*, 619
  blood vessels supplying, 616, 619, *619*
    lesions of, 630
  cancer of, 630
  cyst of, *620*, 630
  development of, 616, *618*
  ectopic, 630
  enlargement of, 620, 623–624
    giant, 624
  erythrocytes in, 615–616
  function of, 615(t), 615–616
    assessment of, 620
    disorders of, 621, 623(t), 624
  imaging of, 620, *620*, *621*
  infarction of, 630
  marginal zone of, 619
  red pulp of, 619
  resection of. See *Splenectomy.*
  rupture of, 631
  transplantation of, in pancreas transplant, 250, *251*
  trauma to, 195
  tumors of, 630
  white pulp of, 619
Splenectomy, *622*, 622–623
  effects of, 621–623
  for trauma, 195
  historical aspects of, 615
  indications for, 624–630, 625(t)
    limited, 623
    sepsis after, 621
Splenic arteriovenous fistula, 630

Splenic artery, 619
  aneurysm of, 630
Splenic pulp, 619
Splenomegaly, 620, 623–624
  giant, 624
Splenorenal shunt, 534, *534*
  for bleeding esophageal varices, 532, *532*
  for portal hypertension, 534
Splenosis, 630
Split-thickness skin graft, 262
  donor site in, cutting of, with derma-
    tomes, 130
  for burns, 130
  in reconstructive surgery, after radical
    neck dissection for cancer, 729
Squamous cell carcinoma, 710, 715–716,
    795, *795*
  of anus, 508, 510
  of esophagus, 384
  of external ear, 691
  of head and neck. See *Head and neck
    cancer.*
  of lung. See *Lung(s), carcinoma of.*
  of nose and paranasal sinuses, 698–699
Squamous epithelium, 708, *709*
Squatting, by patients with tetralogy of Fal-
    lot, 1090
St. Thomas' cardioplegic solution, 1119(t)
Staging, of cancer, 271. See also *TNM stag-
    ing of cancer.*
  of lymphoma, 632(t)
  of neuroblastoma, 681(t)
Staging laparotomy, in evaluation of lym-
    phoma, 633
Stainless steel scalpel incision, risk of infec-
    tion associated with, *135*
Stainless steel wire sutures, 136
Staples, 137–138, 138(t)
Stapling, and anastomosis, in closure of
    bronchi, 1004, *1004*
  in gastric surgery for obesity, *428*
  in intestinal surgery, *493*
  in transection of esophagus, *535*
Starling equilibrium, *34*
Starling hypothesis, 34
Stasis, and ulceration, 934, *935*
  and venous thrombosis, 945
Status epilepticus, 883
Steam heat, instrument sterilization with,
    133
Steatorrhea, after stomach surgery, 421
  laboratory findings in, 597(t)
Stem cell assay, of tumor inhibition by che-
    motherapy agents, 281
Stenosis, aortic, acquired, 1137, *1138*
  congenital, 1109–1113, *1110–1112*
  left coronary artery, *1115*
  mitral, 1143–1145, *1144, 1145*
    treatment of, 1145, 1148
      by closed commissurotomy, 1145–
        1146
      by open commissurotomy, 1146,
        1146
      by replacement of valve with pros-
        thesis, 1146–1147, *1147, 1148*
      historical aspects of, 1142–1143
  pulmonary, in tetralogy of Fallot, 1089
    with intact ventricular septum, *1093,*
      1094
  pyloric, hypertrophic, 674–675
    surgery for, 675, *675*
  subaortic, 1111–1112
    hypertrophic, idiopathic, 1112, 1139,
      1141
      surgery for, 1141, *1141*

Stenosis (*Continued*)
  subglottic, 659
  supravalvular (supra-aortic), 1112, *1112*
  tricuspid, 1150
Sterility, cancer chemotherapy and, 280
Sterilization of surgical instruments, 133
Sternal clefts, 1013, 1015, *1016*
  surgery for, *1017*
Sternum, tumors of, 1015, 1018
Steroid(s), complication(s) associated with,
    243
  acute pancreatitis as, 602
  effects of, on wound healing, 119
  for bronchospasm, 975
  for Crohn's disease, 483
  for myasthenia gravis, 1042
  in suppression of transplant rejection,
    231
  use of, in surgical patient, 72
Steroid receptor activity, in breast cancer,
    323
Stomach, 406
  acid secretion by, 408–409, *409*
    in peptic ulcer disease, 411
    in Zollinger-Ellison syndrome, 417,
      418
    laboratory analysis of, reference values
      for, 1205(t)
  adenocarcinoma of, 423–424
  anatomy of, 406–407, *407*
  blood vessels supplying, 407, *407, 408*
  carcinoma of, at stump of gastrectomy
    site, 420
  cells of, 406, *409*
    parietal, 406, 408
      in peptic ulcer disease, 411
  dilatation of, acute, after surgery, 422
  emptying of, 410
    rapid, after gastrectomy, 418–419
  inflammation of, hemorrhagic, 221,
    415–417, *416*
    postgastrectomy reflux and, 420
  laboratory analysis of, reference values
    for, 1200(t)–1201(t)
  leiomyoma of, 423
  lymphoma of, 424
  microflora of, and risk of infection after
    gastric surgery, 151
  mucosa of, hypertrophy of, 422
  nerves supplying, 407, *413*
  obstruction of, in newborn, 663
    with hypertrophic pyloric stenosis,
      674–675
  partitioning of, for obesity, 428, *428*
  perforation of, and pneumoperitoneum,
    670
    in newborn, 670
  pH of contents of, 409
  physiology of, 408–411
  polyps of, 423
  receptive relaxation of, 410
  replacement of fluid losses from, 42
  resection of, carcinoma at stump site
    after, 420
    complications of, 418–421, 448
    for adenocarcinoma, 424
    for peptic ulcer, 413, 415
      with follow-up restoration of GI
        continuity, 413, *413*
    for Zollinger-Ellison syndrome, 418
  stapling of, for obesity, *428*
  surgery of, antimicrobial prophylaxis
    against infection in, 151–152
    in antireflux operations, 381, *381*
    steatorrhea after, 421

Stomach (*Continued*)
  tears of, vomiting and, 421
  trauma to, 191
  tumors of, 423–424
  ulcer of, peptic, 415
    surgery for, 415
      infection after, 151
    stress-induced, 221, 415–417, *416*
Stool. See *Feces.*
Storage, of cadaver organs for transplanta-
    tion, 236
Storage pool disease, 89
Strangulated hernia, 651–652
Streptococcal infection, and gangrene, 163
  and myositis, 159(t), 162
Streptokinase, 87
  therapeutic uses of, 942
Stress, metabolic response to, 96–97, 99,
    99(t)–102(t)
  glucose production in, 16, 23–24, 97,
    99, 101(t)
  parenteral nutrition and, 106(t)
  neuroendocrine response to, 10–11, *11,
    46,* 96–97, *98*
Stress incontinence, 840
Stress ulcer, 221, 415–417, *416*
  in burn patients, 126
Stricture, biliary, 573
  balloon dilatation of, 574
    surgery for, *574,* 574–575, *575*
  esophageal, 381–382
    caustic injury and, *368*
    peptic, of esophagus, 381–382
  urethral, 848, *849*
Stroke, diagnostic studies after, 924
  epidemiology of, 918–919
  hemorrhagic, 920
  ischemic, 920
  management of, 924–925, *926*
  prognosis after, 925
  symptoms of, 920–921
Subaortic stenosis, 1111–1112, *1112*
  hypertrophic, idiopathic, 1112, 1139,
    1141
    surgery for, 1141, *1141*
Subarachnoid hemorrhage, 185, 865(t),
    865–866
  and stroke, 920
Subclavian artery, compression of, 915–
    916, 1011
  trauma to, 198
Subclavian artery–to–pulmonary artery
    shunt, in management of tricuspid
    atresia, 1099
Subclavian flap aortoplasty, for coarctation
    of aorta, 1069, *1069*
Subclavian steal syndrome, 921–922
Subclavian vein, as site for insertion of
    pacemaker lead, *1174*
  obstruction of, bronchogenic carcinoma
    and, *1000*
Subclavicular lymph node group, 291, *292*
Subcutaneous tissue, 117
  excision of, in management of lymph-
    edema, 637, 638
Subdural hematoma, 185, 871, *872,* 920
Subglottis, 702
  cancer of, 704, 733
  stenosis of, 659
Subhepatic abscess, 204, 205
Submandibular lymph nodes, 715
Submental lymph nodes, 715
Submucous fibrosis, 710
Subphrenic abscess, 204
  drainage of, 204–205, *205*

Subscapular lymph node group, 291, *292*
Subtotal gastrectomy, for peptic ulcer, 413
　with follow-up restoration of GI conti-
　　nuity, 413, *413*
Subtotal thyroidectomy, 334
Succinylcholine, 113
Sucralfate, in prophylaxis against stress ul-
　cers, 417
Suction drain, *139*, 139–140
Suction lines, in cardiopulmonary bypass,
　1186
Sudden deafness, 695
Sugiura procedure, EEA stapler in, *535*
　for portal hypertension, 534
Sulfasalazine, for Crohn's disease, 482
Sump drain, *139*, 140
Sundowning, 203
Superficial spreading melanoma, 285
Superficial thoracoepigastric vein, thrombo-
　sis and inflammation of, 302
Superior constrictor muscle, of pharynx,
　713
Superior sulcus of lung, carcinoma in, 1001,
　1001, 1006, *1006*, 1006(t)
Superior vena cava, cancer obstructing,
　1000, 1023
　radiation therapy for, 275
Supernumerary breasts, 290
Supernumerary nipples, 290
Suppressor factors, and tolerance, 233
Suppressor T cell, 226
　and tolerance, 233
Supra-aortic stenosis, 1112, *1112*
Supracardiac anomalous pulmonary venous
　connection, 1082, *1082*
　surgery for, *1084*
Supraglottis, 701
　carcinoma of, 704, 733
　trauma to, 186
Supravalvular (supra-aortic) stenosis, 1112,
　1112
Supraventricular arrhythmias, drugs for,
　1182
　surgical treatment of, 1157–1160
Surface area of body, region-specific sur-
　　face areas as percentage of, 124–125
　age-related changes in, *124*, 125
　estimation of extent of burn based on,
　　124
Surfactant, 15
Surgery, 134–140
　adhesive tape in, 137, *137*
　advances in, 1–9, 7(t)
　anesthesiologist's role in, 109–110, 115,
　　116
　antimicrobial prophylaxis against infec-
　　tion in, 150–152
　arrhythmias after, management of, *1184*
　asepsis in, 132–134
　　iodine and, 132, *133*
　atelectasis after, 70, 208–209
　　fever due to, 202
　bench, 266
　bladder dysfunction after, 74
　cadaveric organ removal, for transplanta-
　　tion, 237, *237*
　cardiac dysfunction during, management
　　of, *1183*
　cautery in, 135–136
　clean, antimicrobial prophylaxis against
　　infection in, 150–151
　coagulants in, 136
　complication(s) of, 201(t), 201–222
　　atelectasis as, 70, 208–209

Surgery (*Continued*)
　fever as, 147, 147(t), 201(t), 201–202,
　　204
　gastrointestinal dysfunction as, 218–
　　221
　infection as. See *Surgical infection(s)*.
　jaundice as, 201(t), 215(t), 215–218
　mental status abnormalities as, 201(t),
　　202–203
　multiple organ failure as, 221–222, *222*
　renal failure as, 211–215
development of training programs in, 3–5
dissection in, 134–135
drains in, 138–140, *139*
　risk of infection with, *138*, 150
duration of, and risk of infection, 149
exploratory, in abdominal trauma, 189
fever after, 147, 147(t), 201(t), 201–202,
　204
fever during, 147(t)
gastric dilatation after, 422
gastrointestinal dysfunction after, 218–
　221
hemostasis in, 135–136
history of, 1–9, 7(t)
hospitalization before, and risk of infec-
　tion, 149
in newborn, infants, and children, 655–
　684
in pregnant patients, 823–824
in presence of active remote infection,
　risks of, 150
incisions in, 134
　risk of infection associated with, 134,
　　134, *135*
increased intracranial pressure during,
　859
infection in. See *Surgical infection(s)*.
jaundice after, 201(t), 215(t), 215–218
mental status abnormalities after, 201(t),
　202–203
milestones in development of, 1–9, 7(t)
multiple organ failure after, 221–222, *222*
nitrogen losses associated with, 100(t)
operating team antisepsis in, 132–133
packs in, 136
pancreatitis after, 602
pediatric, 655–684
pioneers in, 1–2, 7(t)
preparation for, 62–75, 75(t)
　acid-base disturbances and, 65
　adrenal insufficiency and, 72
　alcohol abuse and, 74
　anesthesiologist's role in, 109–110
　anticoagulant use and, 65
　cardiovascular disease and, 69(t), 69–
　　70
　cerebrovascular disease and, 73–74
　cleansing of patient's skin in, 132
　colonic operations and, 68, 475(t),
　　475–476
　communication with patient in, 62
　coronary artery bypass graft and, 1119
　diabetes mellitus and, 71
　electrolyte imbalance and, 64–65
　endocrine disorders and, 71–72
　fluid replacement therapy in, 63
　hand operations and, 741
　hyperthyroidism and, 71–72
　instrument sterilization in, 133
　liver disease and, 73
　malnutrition and, 67
　myopathy and, 74
　nutritional support in, 67

Surgery (*Continued*)
　preparation for, pheochromocytoma and,
　　72
　postoperative infection risk associated
　　with, 133, 149
　prophylaxis against deep venous
　　thrombosis in, *66*, 66–67
　prophylaxis against infection in, 68,
　　120, 150–152
　prophylaxis against pulmonary embo-
　　lism in, 66, *66*
　pulmonary problems and, 71, 974
　renal disease and, 74
　risk estimation in, 62–63
　splenectomy and, 622
　tests for disorders of hemostasis in, 65
　tests of pulmonary function in, 70, 71
　transfusions in, 66
　vascular trauma and, 197
pulmonary effects of, 70, 974
reconstructive, after operations for can-
　cer, 269
　of breast, 320
　of head and neck, *726–727*, 728–730
renal failure after, 211–215
risk(s) of, estimation of, 62–63
sources of contamination in, 132–134
staples in, 137–138, 138(t)
sterilization of instruments to be used in,
　133
sutures in, 135, 136, 137
　risk of infection associated with, *137*,
　　138(t)
sinus tract formation at site of, 120
training programs in, 3–5
Surgical aspiration device, ultrasonic, 520,
　520
Surgical drains, 138–140, *139*
　risk of infection with, *138*, 150
Surgical exploration, in abdominal trauma,
　189
Surgical infection(s), 68, 141–167, 203–206,
　222
　anergy and, 68
　antimicrobial prophylaxis against, 68,
　　120, 150–152
　　procedures not requiring, 151(t)
　antimicrobial treatment of, 153, 154(t),
　　155(t)
　bacteria causing, 143, 145(t)–146(t),
　　146–165
　diagnosis of, 147–148, 203–204
　　CT scanning in, *147*
　　ultrasonography in, *148*
　fever as sign of, 147, 147(t), 201, 202,
　　204
　incisions and, 134, *134*, *135*
　microbiology of, 143, 145(t)–146(t),
　　146–147
　nosocomial, *148*, 163–165, 209
　surgical treatment of, 153
　wound closure materials and, *137*, 138(t)
　wound in, 148–150, *149*, 149(t)
Surgical oncology, 268–287. See also *Can-
　cer*.
Surgical reconstruction, after operations for
　　cancer, 269
　of breast, 320
　of head and neck, *726–727*, 728–730
Surgical wound, 148
　infection of, 148–150, *149*, 149(t)
Suture(s), 135, 136, 137
　risk of infection associated with, *137*,
　　138(t)

Suture(s) (*Continued*)
  sinus tract formation at site of, 120
Swallowing, 365
  difficulty in, 371(t), 371–373
    achalasia and, 374
    esophageal carcinoma and, 384
    treatment of, 373, *373*
Swan-Ganz catheter, in measurement of
    left atrial filling pressure, 115
Sweating, fluid replacement requirements
    associated with, 43
Swimmer's ear, 691
Sympathectomy, for Raynaud's syndrome,
    918
Symptomatic idiopathic diffuse esophageal
    spasm, 376–378, *377*
Syndrome of inappropriate ADH secretion,
    49, 215
Synergistic necrotizing cellulitis, 159(t), 162
Synovectomy, for arthritis, 789
Synthetic sutures, 136–137
Syphilis, 846
Syringomyelia, 876
Systemic venous pressure, effects of car-
    diopulmonary bypass on, 1187–1188

T cell(s), 225–226
  and tolerance, 233
  antibodies to, in reversal of transplant
    rejection, 232
  in peripheral blood, 227(t)
  in rejection, 225, 226, 227
  thymic, 1038
T-tube drain, obstruction of biliary tract
    by, 217, *217*
T4 antigen, 226
T8 antigen, 226
Tachycardia, as complication of coronary
    artery bypass graft, 1122
  drugs for, 1182
  pacemaker for, 1162, 1170–1171
  surgical treatment of, 1158–1162, *1161*
    directed vs. nondirected, 1160(t),
    1162(t)
Takayasu's arteritis, 912–915
Talipes equinovarus, *781*, 781–782, *782*
Talus, fracture of, 768
Tamoxifen, for breast cancer, 323
Tamponade, balloon, for bleeding esopha-
    geal varices, 530–531, *531*
  cardiac, 182, 188, 1046
    as complication of coronary artery by-
    pass graft, 1121–1122
  mediastinal, 1024
Tangential excision, of burns, 130
Tape (adhesive tape), in surgery, 137, *137*
Tarsal bones, fracture of, 768
Telangiectasia, in brain, 866
Teletherapy, 272
Temporal arteritis, 912–914
Temporal bone, fracture of, 693
Temporary colostomy, 476
Tendon(s) of hand, *745*
  surgical repair of, 745–747, *746*
  testing of, 740, *740*
Tendon sheath of hand, giant cell tumor of,
    752
  inflammation of, 749, 750
Tensile strength of wound, development of,
    118, *118*
Tension pneumothorax, 181
  in newborn, 661, *661*

Teratogens, chemotherapy agents as, 280
Teratoma, 681–682
  cystic, of ovary, *680*
  mediastinal, 1030, *1030*
  neck, 658
  sacrococcygeal, 682, *682*, 876
  testicular, 852
Testis, 830
  absence of, 850
  cancer of, 851–853, *852*
  inflammation of, 851
  resection of, in treatment of prostate
    cancer, 844
  torsion of, 404, 851, *851*
  undescended, 851
    and infertility, 853
Tetanus, 159–161, 160(t)
  prophylaxis against, 160(t), 160–161, 199
Tetanus immune globulin, 160–161, 199
Tetanus toxoid, 160–161, 199
Tetralogy of Fallot, 1089–1090, *1090*
  angiocardiographic findings in, 1090,
    1091
  radiographic findings in, 1090, *1090*
  surgery for, 1091–1092, *1091–1093*
Thalassemia, 627–628
Thalomotomy, for chronic pain, 885
Theophylline, for bronchospasm, 975
Therapeutic drug monitoring, laboratory
    reference values for, 1203(t)–1204(t)
Thermography, in diagnosis of breast can-
    cer, 297
Thermoregulation, in newborn, 656
Third-degree burns, 123, 124
Third space losses, 35, 42
Thoracic aorta, transection of, radiographic
    findings in, 189
Thoracic esophagus, 363, 364
  trauma to, 187
Thoracic outlet, anatomy of, 1010–1011,
    1011
Thoracic outlet compression syndrome,
    915–916, 1010–1012
Thoracic spine, disorders of, 879–880
  fractures of, 770–771
Thoracodorsal nerve, 290
Thoracoepigastric vein, superficial, throm-
    bosis and inflammation of, 302
Thoracotomy, in management of chest
    trauma, 188
Thorax. See *Chest.*
Three (3) sign, in coarctation of aorta, *1066*
Thrombasthenia, Glanzmann's, 83
Thrombin, formation of, *84*, 84–85, *85*
  disorders of, 90
Thrombin time, 89
Thromboangiitis obliterans, *893*, 912–915
Thrombocytopenia, 89–90, 626, 629
Thrombolytics, 949–951
Thrombomodulin, 81
Thrombophlebitis, 941
  venous insufficiency after, 942–944, *943*
Thromboplastin (tissue factor), 80–81
Thrombosis, 91–92
  arterial, 82, 898–903, *902*
  as complication of pancreas transplant,
    250, 251
  cerebral, and ischemic stroke, 920
  hemorrhoidal, 504
  iliofemoral, 941–942
  mesenteric vein, 929–930
  renal vein, 679
  thoracoepigastric vein, with inflamma-
    tion, 302
  ulnar artery, 741

Thrombosis (*Continued*)
  venous, 82
    deep, 91, 92, 945, *946*
      prophylaxis against, in surgical
        patients, *66*, 66–67
      vs. peripheral artery disease, 900–
        901
Thumb, Barrett's fracture of, 748
  gamekeeper's, 748
  osteoarthritis of, 751
  skier's, 748
Thumbprinting sign, in ischemic colitis,
    502, *502*
Thymectomy, for myasthenia gravis, 1042–
    1043, *1043*
Thymic cyst, 1035
Thymoma, 1029, *1039*, 1040, *1041*
  and myasthenia gravis, 1029, 1038–1039
Thymus, 1037–1038, *1038*
  resection of, for myasthenia gravis, 1042–
    1043, *1043*
Thyroglossal duct cyst, 327, *328*
Thyroid, 327
  anatomy of, 327–328, *329*
  anomalies of, 327
  cancer metastatic to, 338
  cancer of, 336(t), 336–338
  development of, 327
  enlargement of, 331
    diffuse, 331
    multinodular, 331–332
    nodular (single nodule), 331
  fine-needle aspiration biopsy of, *332*,
    332–333
  function of, 329, *330*
    tests of, 330
  hormones produced by, 329–330, *330*
    defects in, 331
    hypersecretion of, 71–72, 330, 333(t),
      333–334
    hyposecretion of, 330
  inflammation of, 331
  intrathoracic, tumors of, 1032
  lingual, 327
  resection of. See *Thyroidectomy.*
Thyroidectomy, 334, *335*, 336
  complications of, 336
  for cancer, 336, 337
  for hyperthyroidism, 334
  Kocher's work in, 6
Thyroid hormones, 329–330, *330*
  defects in synthesis of, 331
  hypersecretion of, 71–72, 330, 333–334,
    334(t)
  hyposecretion of, 330
Thyroiditis, 331
Thyroid-stimulating hormone, 330, 352
Thyroid storm, 71–72
Thyrotoxicosis (hyperthyroidism), 71–72,
    330, 333(t), 333–334
Thyrotropin-releasing hormone, effects of,
    330
Thyroxine, 329, *330*. See also *Thyroid hor-
    mones.*
Tibia, fracture of, *765*, 766
  external fixation of, 766, *766*
  internal torsion of, 784
Timing of antimicrobial administration, in
    prophylaxis against surgical infection,
    150
Tinnitus, 690
Tissue factor (thromboplastin), 80–81
Tissue heart valve prostheses, 1139, 1147,
    1147
Tissue plasminogen activator, 81, 87

TNM staging of cancer, 271, 271(t)
  of breast, 310(t)–311(t)
  of esophagus, 384, 384(t)
  of head and neck, 720
  of lung, 1007(t)
  of pharynx, *721*
Toe, fracture of, 768
  vasoconstriction in, 916–918
Tolbutamide response test, 597
Tolerance, 232–234
  attempts at induction of, in preparation
    for transplantation, 234
Tomography, computed, as aid to diagno-
      sis, of hepatic abscess, 522, *522*
      of intrahepatic hematoma, *190*
      of mediastinal tumors, 1026, *1041*
      of pericardial disease, 1048, *1048*
      of surgical infection, *147*
      of trauma, to abdomen, 190, *190*
        to brain, 184
        to cervical spine, 186
        to head, 184, 185
      of tumor, of adrenal, 356, *356*
        of pituitary, 353
    biliary tract on, 560
    central nervous system on, 860, *861*
    in breast cancer, 309
    in lung cancer, 1002
    in stereotactic neurosurgery, *881*
    pancreas on, 598, *598*
    peripheral arterial system on, 897, *897*
    spleen on, 620
    urogenital system on, 832–833
  emission, 860
Tongue, 712
  airway obstruction by, relief of, 181
  carcinoma of, 731, 732
    radiosensitivity of, *723*
  ectopic thyroid tissue in, 327
Tongue flap, in reconstructive surgery,
      after radical neck dissection for cancer,
      726, 729
Tonsil, carcinoma of, 732
Tonsillitis, 699
Tornwaldt's cyst, 701
Torsion, of testicle, 404, 851, *851*
Torsional deformities of leg, *783, 783–784,
      784*
Total anomalous pulmonary venous con-
      nection, *1082,* 1082–1083
  surgery for, 1084, *1084*
Total blood volume, 31
Total body surface area, region-specific sur-
      face areas as percentage of, 124–125
    age-related changes in, *124,* 125
    estimation of extent of burn based on,
      124
Total body water, 29, *31,* 31, 31(t)
Total fundoplication, 381, *381*
Total mastectomy, for cancer, results of,
      319(t), 321, *321–322*
Total nodal irradiation field, 632, *632*
Total parenteral nutrition. See *Parenteral
      nutrition.*
Total thyroidectomy, 336
Toxic megacolon, ulcerative colitis and, 479
Toxicology, reference values in, 1204(t)
Toxoid, tetanus, 160–161, 199
Trace element requirements, 104(t)
Trachea, foreign body impaction in, 705
  obstruction of, in newborn, 658–659
  trauma to, 187
  tumors of, 1008
Tracheobronchial disruption, 187
Tracheoesophageal fistula, 659, *659, 660*

Tracheostomy, 704, 976, *977*
  in children, *658*
Tractotomy, medullary, for chronic pain,
      884–885
Transcapillary refill phase, in restitution of
      blood volume, 47–48
Transected thoracic aorta, radiographic
      findings in, 189
Transferrin, serum levels of, as index of
      nutritional status, 102, 103(t)
Transfusion, 92–94
  acute renal failure in reaction to, 215
  AIDS transmitted by, 94, 175
  as aid to management of massive bleed-
      ing, 92–93
  complications of, 94
  donor-specific, pre-transplant, 234, 238
  for anemia, in surgical patients, 66
  for leukemia, in surgical patients, 66
  hemolytic reaction to, 94, 216
  hepatitis transmitted by, 94, 170–171
  historical aspects of, 7–8
  in newborn, 656
  infections transmitted by, 94, 170–171,
      175
  leukagglutinin reaction to, 94
  platelet, 90, 93
  preoperative, 66
  pre-transplant, 234, 238
  purpura following, 94
  red blood cell, 93
Transhepatic biliary drainage, 560, *561*
Transhepatic cholangiography, percuta-
      neous, 560, *560,* 584, 599–600
Transhepatic coronary vein occlusion, in
      control of bleeding esophageal varices,
      531
Transhepatic venous sampling, 600
Transient ischemic attacks, 918–927
Transluminal balloon angioplasty, for
      coarctation of aorta, 1069, *1070*
  for myocardial ischemia, 1118–1119
Transpectoral lymphatics, 290
Transplantation, 224–266
  autologous, 261–268
  cadaver organs in, 234–237, 236(t)
    agencies for procurement of, 235
    availability of, 234
    donor and, 235(t), 235–236
    donor-recipient matching with, 231
    preservation of, 236
    removal procedure for, 237, *237*
  candidates awaiting, 234(t)
  endocrine gland, autologous, 265
  gastrointestinal tissue, 266
  hair, 263
  heart, 253–259
    after earlier heart transplant, 258,
      258(t)
    artificial heart as alternative to, 1127
    care after, 256
    coronary artery atherosclerosis after,
      258
    cost of, 259
    donor in, 254
    early developments in, 253
    heterotopic, 253
    immunosuppression in, 256
    infection after, 257–258, *258*
    procedure for, 254, *255*
    recipient in, 253–254
    rejection of, 257, *257*
      acute, 229
    results of, 258, *259,* 259(t)
  heart and lung, 253–259

Transplantation (*Continued*)
  heart and lung, care after, 256
    donor in, 254
    early developments in, 253
    immunosuppression in, 257
    procedure for, *255,* 256
    recipient in, 253–254
    rejection of, 257
  historical aspects of, 9, 237, 244, 249,
      253, 259
  immunobiology of, 224–234
  immunosuppression in, 231–232, 237, 238
  kidney, 237–243
    care after, 241
    complications of, 242
    donor in, 239–240
    early developments in, 237
    favorable factors in, 243(t)
    hypothermic pulsatile perfusion of do-
      nor organ in, 236
    immunosuppression in, 243
    infection after, 242
    nephrectomy in, 240, *240, 241*
    pancreatitis following, 602
    preparation for, 239
    procedure for, 241, *242*
    recipient in, 238–239
    rejection of, 242
      accelerated, 228
      acute, 229, *229*
      chronic, 229, *230*
      hyperacute, 228
      initiation of immune response in,
        227, 228
      testing for possible potentiators of,
        229–231
    renal diseases recurring after, 239(t)
    results of, 243, *243*
  liver, 244–249, 245(t)
    care after, 247–248
    complications of, 248–249
    donor in, 245
    early developments in, 244
    for cancer, 542
    hepatectomy in, 246–247, *247*
    immunosuppression in, 247, 248, 249
    in children, 674
    indications for, 245, 245(t)
    infection after, 248–249
    procedure for, 247, *248*
    recipient in, 245
    rejection of, 248
    results of, 249
    resuscitation after, 247
  lung, 259–260
    care after, 256, 260
    donor in, 254, 259
    early developments in, 253, 259
    immunosuppression in, 257, 260
    procedure for, 260, *260*
    recipient in, 253–254, 260
    rejection of, 257
    results of, 260
  pancreas, 249–252
    autologous, 265
    care after, 251
    complications of, 251
    donor in, 250
    early developments in, 249
    immunosuppression in, 251
    pancreaticoduodenal graft in, 250, *251,
      252*
    procedure for, 250, *251, 252*
    recipient in, 249–250
    rejection of, 251

Transplantation (*Continued*)
pancreas, results of, 252
spleen transplant in, 250, *251*
thrombosis after, 250, 251
pancreatic islet cell, 252
autologous, 265
parathyroid, 265, 348
preparation for, 229–234, 237–238
ABO cross-matching in, 229
cadaver organs and donor-recipient matching in, 231
donor selection for antigenic match with recipient in, 230
donor-specific transfusions in, 234, 238
induction of tolerance in, 234
lymphocytotoxic cross-matching in, 230
mixed lymphocyte culture in, 230–231
transfusions in, 234, 238
typing for donor-recipient HLA antigen match in, 230, 238
typing for donor-recipient HLA-DR antigen match in, 231
rejection of, 228–229
accelerated, 228
acute, 228–229
antibody-dependent cell-mediated cytotoxicity in, 228
cell surface antigens in, 224
chronic, 229
dendritic cells in, 226, 227, *227*
hyperacute, 228
avoidance of, 229–230
induction of tolerance in circumvention of, 234
initiation of immune response in, 227, *227*, *228*
macrophages in, 226, 227, *228*
suppression of, 231–232, 237, 238
T cells in, 225, 226, 227
testing for possible potentiators of, 229–231
small intestine, 260–261
spleen, in pancreas transplant, 250, *251*
Transplantation antigens, tumor-specific, 281
Transposition of great arteries, 1102–1103
surgery for, 1104, *1105–1108*, 1108
historical aspects of, 1102–1103
Transsexualism, 854
Transthoracic aspiration needle biopsy, in diagnosis of lung cancer, *1002*, 1002–1003, *1003*
Trauma. See also particular types and under specific sites.
in children, 678
management of, 180–199
assessment of cervical spine in, 181, 185
control of hypotension in, 182–183
correction of hypovolemia in, 182
determination of adequacy of air exchange in, 181
establishment of airway in, 181
estimation of consciousness level in, 182, 184
measurement of blood pressure in, 182
neurologic evaluation in, 182, 183, 184
palpation of pulse in, 182
peritoneal lavage in, 183
physical examination in, 182, 183
resuscitation in, 182
neuroendocrine response to, *46*, 96–97
Trendelenburg, Friedrich, 3, *4*
Trendelenburg test, 934–935
Treponema pallidum infection, 846
Trichoepithelioma, 794

Trichomonas infection, vaginal, 814
Tricuspid anuloplasty, 1151
Tricuspid atresia, 1098
surgery for, 1099, *1099*
Tricuspid valve, 1143
disease of, 1150–1151
in Ebstein's anomaly, 1153, *1154*, 1155
prosthetic, 1151, 1155
Trifascicular block, incomplete, pacemaker for, 1170
Triglyceride, elevated serum levels of, in acute pancreatitis, 602
long-chain, digestion of, *433*
medium-chain, 433
Triiodothyronine, 329, 330, *330*. See also *Thyroid hormones.*
Triolein breath test, 596
Trismus, 712
Trophoblastic tumors, 824
Truncal vagotomy, for peptic ulcer, 413
Truncus arteriosus, 1100, *1100*
surgery for, *1101*, 1101–1102
Tube decompression, of gastrointestinal tract, 441
Tuberculoma, of breast, 302
Tuberculosis, in AIDS, 177
of bone, 787
of breast, 302
of joints, 787
of lung, 994–997, *995*
and pericarditis, 1050–1051
drug therapy for, 996, 996(t)
surgery for, 994, 996–997
of prostate, 841
Tuberculous empyema, Eloesser flap in drainage of, 997, *997*
Tuberculous pericarditis, 1050–1051
Tubocurarine test, for myasthenia gravis, 1041
Tubular carcinoma, of breast, 313
Tumor(s), ACTH-secreting, 353, 356–358
laboratory findings in patients with, 357(t)
calcitonin-secreting, 337, *337*
carcinoid. See *Carcinoid.*
catecholamine-secreting, 72, 360–361
development of, in patients treated with immunosuppressives, 243
dumbbell, 681, *682*
endocrine-active, 353–354
endocrine-inactive, 353
fibrous, 787–789, 788(t)
gastrin-secreting, 417–418, 449, 610(t), 611
germ cell, 680
of mediastinum, 1030–1031
giant cell, of hand, 752
glomus, 692
glucagon-secreting, 610(t), 611
growth hormone–secreting, 353
in children, 542–543, 658, 679–684, 834–836, 1027(t)
insulin-secreting, 610(t), 611
Klatskin, 539
mesenchymal, of mediastinum, 1033–1034
neurogenic, of mediastinum, 1027–1029
of adrenal gland, 72, 356–358, 360–361
CT findings in, 356, *356*
laboratory findings in patients with, 357(t)
of appendix, 466–467
of bile duct, 539, 575, 577, 578
of bladder, 837–839
of bone, 787–789, 788(t)
of brain, 862–863, *863*

Tumor(s) (*Continued*)
of breast, 303–325. See also *Breast cancer.*
of bronchus, 1008
of buccal mucosa, 731
of cartilage, 787–789, 788(t)
of cervix, 815–816
of chest wall, 1015, 1018
of diaphragm, 1018
of duodenum, 451(t)
of eighth cranial nerve, 694
of endometrium, 816–817
of epididymis, 850
of esophagus, 382–386, 383(t)
endoscopy in diagnosis of, 367, 367(t)
of external ear, 691
of gallbladder, 575–577
of glottis, 704, 733
of hand, 752
of hard palate, 731
of head and neck. See *Head and neck cancer.*
of heart, 1163–1168, 1164(t)
echocardiographic findings in, 1164, *1165*
of hypopharynx, 700, 732
of ileum, 451(t)
of islet cells, 610(t), 610–612
of jejunum, 451(t)
of kidney, 834–836
in children, 679–680, *680*, 834–836
of larynx, 704, 733
of lip, 730
of liver, 537–544
in children, 542–543, *543*, 682, *683*, 684
of lung, 998–1008, 1008(t)
of lymphatics, 638, 658, 1033–1034
of mediastinum, 1024(t), 1024–1034, *1030*, *1031*
in children, 1027(t)
signs and symptoms of, 1025, 1025(t), 1026(t)
prognostic significance of, 1025, 1025(t)
sites of, *1021*, 1024, 1024(t)
of middle ear, 692
of nasopharynx, 700, 733
of neck. See *Head and neck cancer.*
of nose, 698–699, 734
of oral cavity, *708*, 730–731
of oropharynx, 700
of ovary, 818–819
in children, 680, *680*
of palate, 731, 732
of pancreas, 608–612, 610(t)
sampling of venous blood for signs of, 600
of paranasal sinus, 698–699, 734
of parathyroid gland, 342, 345, *345*, 346, *347*
in mediastinum, 1032–1033
of penis, 846–847
of pericardium, 1051–1052, 1164(t)
of pharynx, 700, 731–732
of pituitary, 353–354
extension of, diaphragma sellae and, 350
of pleura, 991
of renal pelvis, 837
of rib, 1015, 1018
of salivary gland, 734
of scrotum, 849
of skin, 794–799, *794–799*
of small intestine, 450–455, 451(t)
of soft palate, 732

Tumor(s) (*Continued*)
of spermatic cord, 850
of spine, 863–865
of spleen, 630
of sternum, 1015, 1018
of stomach, 423–424
of subglottis, 704, 733
of supraglottis, 704, 733
of testis, 851–853, *852*
of thymus, 1029, *1039*, 1040, *1041*
and myasthenia gravis, 1029, 1038–1039
of thyroid, 336(t), 336–338
intrathoracic, 1032
of tongue, 731, 732
of tonsil, 732
of trachea, 1008
of ureter, 837
of vagina, 815
of vulva, 814
Pancoast, 1001, *1001*, 1006, *1006*, 1006(t)
pancreatic polypeptide-secreting, 610(t), 612
prolactin-secreting, 354
serotonin-secreting, 610(t), 612
somatostatin-secreting, 610(t), 612
trophoblastic, 824
vasoactive intestinal polypeptide–secreting, 449, 610(t), 612
Wilms', 679–680, *680*, 834–836
yolk sac, of testis, 852
Tumor antigens, 281
antibodies to, 281, 282
Tumor-associated antigens, 281
Tumor markers, in lung cancer, 1002
Tumor-Node-Metastasis staging of cancer.
See *TNM staging of cancer.*
Tumor-specific transplantation antigens, 281
Tuning fork tests, for hearing loss, 689–690
Turcot syndrome, 487
Twiddler's syndrome, in patients with cardiac pacemakers, 1177
Tylectomy, for breast cancer, 317–318
Tympanic membrane, 686, *687*, *688*

Ulcer, colonic, amebiasis and, 504
inflammatory, 477–480, *479*
and colorectal cancer, 484, *484*, *485*, 489
and toxic dilatation of colon, 479
vs. Crohn's disease, 477, 483(t)
Curling's, 126
duodenal, 411–412, *412*
hemorrhage from, 412
surgery for, 414
perforation of, 397, 412
surgery for, 397–398, 414
recurrence of, after surgery, 418
surgery for, 413–414, *414*
in cases of hemorrhage, 414
in cases of perforation, 397–398, 414
infection after, 151
recurrence after, 418
gastric, 415
stress-induced, 221, 415–417, *416*
surgery for, 415
infection after, 151
ischemic, in chronic occlusive arterial disease, 909
in peripheral arterial disease, 892–893
peptic, 411–415
at site of Meckel's diverticulum, 457, 468

Ulcer (*Continued*)
peptic, hemorrhage from, 412
surgery for, 414, 415
parietal cells and acid secretion in, 411
perforation of, 397, 412
surgery for, 397–398, 414, 415
recurrence of, after surgery, 418
surgery for, 413–415, *414*
in cases of hemorrhage, 414, 415
in cases of perforation, 397–398, 414, 415
infection after, 151
recurrence after, 418
postphlebitic, 943, *943*
rectal, inflammatory, 480
stasis, 934, *935*
stress, 221, 415–417, *416*
in burn patients, 126
Ulcerative colitis, 477–480, *479*
and colorectal cancer, 484, *484*, *485*, 489
and toxic dilatation of colon, 479
vs. Crohn's disease, 477, 483(t)
Ulcerative proctitis, 480
Ulna, fracture of, 749, 760, 761
Ulnar artery, 741
thrombosis of, 743
Ulnar nerve, 737–740, *739*, *740*
compression of, 744–745
Ulnar tunnel syndrome, 745
Ultrasonic surgical aspiration device, 520, *520*
Ultrasonography, as aid to diagnosis, of cancer of breast, 297
of cholestasis, 560
of fetal abnormalities, 655
of gallstones, 559, *559*
of surgical infection, *148*
cardiac, pericardial effusion on, 1047, *1047*
signs of pulmonary embolism on, 948, *951*
tumors on, 1164, *1165*
Doppler, in peripheral artery disease, 896, 896–897, *897*
in venous disorders, 935–936, *936*
in evaluation of urogenital tract, 832
in gynecologic examination, 811
pancreas on, 598
spleen on, 620, *620*
Umbilical hernia, 648, 650
repair of, *650*
Undescended testis, 851
and infertility, 853
Upper esophageal sphincter, function of, 365, *365*
abnormal, and dysphagia, 372
Upper extremity, fractures of, 749, 758–761
trauma to, 186
Urachus, persistent, 684, 837
Urea, production of, effect of glucose infusion on, 102(t)
Uremia, and pericarditis, 1051
Ureter(s), 828
calculi in, 836–837
ectopic, 837
localization of, before colectomy, 475
obstruction of, at site of junction with renal pelvis, 833
following repair of aneurysm, 906
reflux into, 837
trauma to, 196
tumors of, 837
Ureterocele, 837
Ureteropelvic junction, obstruction of, 833
Urethra, 828–829, *829*

Urethra (*Continued*)
calculi in, 836–837
cancer of, 849
inflammation of, 848–849
meatus of, malposition of, 848
stricture of, 848, *849*
trauma to, 196
valves of, 848
Urethritis, 848–849
Urethrogram, retrograde, 832, *832*
Urgency, urinary, 831
Urinary continence, 831
Urinary incontinence, 831
loss of pelvic support and, *819*, 819–820
neurogenic, 839–840
stress, 840
Urine, blood in, 831
concentration of, countercurrent mechanism of, *40*
impaired dilution of, and hyponatremia, 49
laboratory reference values for, 1201(t)–1203(t)
obstruction of flow of, 214
output of, as index of fluid balance, 43
Urinoma, in kidney transplant recipient, 242
Urobilinogen, 215
Urogenital tract, 826, *827*
calculi in, 404, 836–837
disorders of, referral of pain from, *404*
imaging of, 831–833, *832*
infection of, 146, 164, 403
toxic effects of chemotherapy agents on, 280
trauma to, 195–196
Urokinase, 87
Urolithiasis, 404, 836–837
Uterine artery, 804, *804*
Uterus, 805–806
disorders of, 816–817
prolapse of, 820, *820*

Vaccine, hepatitis B, 166, 172(t), 172–173, 173(t)
Vagina, 805
atresia of, 680
cancer of, 815
discharge from, evaluation of, 810
infection of, 814
Vagotomy, diarrhea after, 420, 448
dumping after, 418
for duodenal ulcer, 413–414, *414*
for gastric ulcer, 415
Vagus nerve(s), 407, *413*
excitation of, and gastric acid secretion, 408
Valvulae conniventes, radiographic appearance of, in obstruction of small intestine, *440*
Varicocele, 850
Varicose bronchiectasis, 992
Varicose veins, 937–940
Varix (varices), esophageal, hemorrhage from, 528, 529
in children, 535
treatment of, 529–532, 530(t), *530–532*
Vascular graft, 263–264
for vessel lesions, 197
indications for, 263(t)
Vascular insufficiency, and acute pancreatitis, 602
Vascular malformations of colon, 502–503

Vascular ring and double aortic arch, 661, *661*, *1072*, 1072–1074, *1073*
Vascular surgery, development of, 8
Vascular trauma, 196–199
Vasculature, adventitia of, 80
  endothelial cells of, 80–81
    metabolism of membrane phospholipids in, *81*
  intima of, 80
  media of, 80
  trauma to, 196–199
Vasculitis, and acute pancreatitis, 602
Vasoactive intestinal polypeptide, tumor secreting, 449, 610(t), 612
Vasoconstriction, digital, 916–918
  phenylephrine and, 1180
Vasodilators, 1180, 1181(t)
  for chronic occlusive arterial disease, 911
Vasomotor rhinitis, 696
Vasopressin, 38, 352
  for bleeding esophageal varices, 529, 530(t)
  secretion of, inappropriate, 49, 215
Vasospasm, of hand, 743
Vecuronium, 113
Vein(s), 933–934, *934*. See also specific veins.
  disorders of, diagnosis of, 934–937, *936*, *937*
  inflammation of, 941
    and intravascular catheter-related sepsis, 165
    venous insufficiency after, 942–943, *943*
  stripping of, for varicosity, 939–940, *940*
  trauma to, 196–198
  varicose, 937–940
Velopharyngeal insufficiency, 701
Vena cava, inferior, surgery of, for pulmonary embolism, 951–952, *952*, 952(t), *953*, 953(t)
  superior, cancer obstructing, *1000*, 1023
    radiation therapy for, 275
Venereal disease, 510, 846
Venereal wart, 510, 846
Venography, 937, *938*
Venous blood reservoir, in cardiopulmonary bypass, 1185
Venous blood sampling, for signs of hormone-secreting pancreatic tumors, 600
Venous cannulation, in cardiopulmonary bypass, 1187
Venous insufficiency, postphlebitic, 942–944, *943*
Venous pressures, pulmonary and systemic, effects of cardiopulmonary bypass on, 1187–1188
Venous thrombosis, 82
  deep, 91, 92, 945, *946*
    prophylaxis against, in surgical patients, 66, 66–67
    vs. peripheral artery disease, 900–901
Ventilation, mask, in CPR, 1056
  mechanical, 976–978
    criteria for cessation of, 210
    for respiratory distress, 211, 976(t), 976–978
    prolonged postoperative dependence on, 210
  mouth-to-mouth, in CPR, 1056
Ventilation-perfusion of lung, 55, *55*, 971–973, *971–973*
  interpretation of PCO₂ as index of, 207
Venting, in cardiopulmonary bypass, 1187

Ventral hernia, 650
Ventricle(s) of brain, bleeding in, 185
Ventricle(s) of heart, left, aneurysm of, 1125
  surgery for, 1125–1126, *1126*
  obstruction of outflow from, congenital, 1109–1110, *1110*
    surgery for, 1110–1112
  in tetralogy of Fallot, 1103, 1104
  right, double outlet, 1095–1096, *1096*
    surgery for, 1096–1097, *1097*
  dysplasia of, arrhythmogenic, 1162
  in Ebstein's anomaly, 1153
Ventricular septal defect(s), 1085–1088, *1086*, 1088(t)
  and double outlet right ventricle, 1095–1097, *1096*, *1097*
  in tetralogy of Fallot, 1089
    correction of, *1092*, *1093*
  in transposition of great arteries, 1103, 1104
  repair of, 1087, *1087*
    probability of death after, *1087*
  spontaneous closure of, *1085*
    probability of, *1086*
Ventricular tachycardia, as complication of coronary artery bypass graft, 1122
  drugs for, 1182
  pacemaker for, 1162, 1170–1171
  surgical treatment of, 1160–1162, *1161*
    directed vs. nondirected, 1160(t), 1162(t)
Ventriculotomy, endocardial, for ventricular tachycardia, 1160–1161, *1161*
Verapamil, 1182
Vermiform appendix, 461
  adenocarcinoma of, 467
  carcinoid of, 466–467
  inflammation of, 393–395, *394*, 461–466
    differential diagnosis of, 395, 463
    in children, 395, 463, 676
    in elderly, 395, 463
    in pregnant patients, 463–464
    surgery for, *465*, 465–466
  mucocele of, 467
  perforation of, inflammation and, 464
  resection of, for inflammation, *465*, 465–466
  tumors of, 466–467
Verner-Morrison syndrome, 610(t), 612
Verruca, 794
Verruca acuminata (venereal wart), 510, 846
Verrucous carcinoma, 710
Vertebra. See *Spine*.
Vertebral basilar insufficiency, 921
Vertigo, 690
  positional, benign, 695
Vesalius, Andreas, *1*
  contributions of, to study of anatomy, 1
Vesicoureteral reflux, 837
Vestibular neuronitis, 694–695
Vestibular system, 687, *688*
  disorders of, 690
Villus, of small intestine, 431, *431*
Viral hepatitis, 165–166, 169–173, 170(t)
  and hepatoma, 171
  carriers of, 165, 171
  clinical manifestations of, 171
  epidemiology of, 169–171
  fulminant, 171
  pathogenesis of, 171
  pathogens causing, 169, 170(t)

Viral hepatitis (*Continued*)
  postoperative, 216–217
  prevention of spread of, 165–166, 171–173, 172(t), 173(t)
  progressive, chronic, 171
  transfusion-transmitted, 94, 170–171
Viral hepatitis antigens and antibodies, 165, 170(t), *172*
Viral infection, and acute pancreatitis, 602
  and pericarditis, 1050
  in AIDS, 176, 176(t)
Virilization, androgen excess and, 822
Visceral abscesses, 154, 205
Vitamin(s), in parenteral nutrition, 25
  metabolism of, in liver, 519
  requirements for, 105(t)
Vitamin C deficiency, effect of, on wound healing, 119
Vitamin D, and calcium metabolism, 341
Vitamin K deficiency, 83, 90
  replacement therapy for, 90
Voice strain, and vocal cord lesions, 703
Volvulus, cecal, *392*, 501, *501*
  midgut, 665
    relief of, *666*
  sigmoid, *500*, 500–501
Vomiting, and injury to esophagus, 369, 421, 422
  in afferent loop syndrome, 419
  intestinal obstruction and, 438
  postoperative, 218
von Langenbeck, Bernhard, *3*
  contributions of, to surgical training, 3
von Recklinghausen's disease, 799
von Willebrand's disease, 90
VP-16, 278
Vulva, 804, *805*
  cancer of, 814
  inflammation of, 813
Vulvitis, 813

Wallerian degeneration, 743
Wangensteen, Owen, 5, *5*
Warm autoimmune hemolytic anemia, 628
Warren, John C., use of ether anesthesia by, 2
Wart, 794
  venereal, 510, 846
Water (body fluid) dynamics. See *Fluid* entries.
Water-bottle-shaped heart shadow, pericardial effusion and, *1047*
Watery diarrhea/hypokalemia/achlorhydria syndrome, 610(t), 612
Web space infection, 750
Weber test, for hearing loss, 689
Wedge osteotomy, *1014*
Weight, as index of fluid balance, 43
  water component of, *98*
    changes in, in response to stress, 97, *99*
  vs. fat component, 31, *31*
Weight loss, as index of nutritional status, 102, 103(t)
  in Crohn's disease, 444
Wen, 794
Wermer's syndrome (multiple endocrine neoplasia I), 342, 417–418
Whitlow, herpetic, 751
Whole blood, therapeutic use of, 93
Wilms' tumor, 679–680, *680*, 834–836

Wolffian duct, 803, *803*
  remnants of, 812
Wolff-Parkinson-White syndrome, surgical
    treatment of, 1157–1158, *1158*, *1159*
Wound, abdominal, dehiscence of, 120
  clean, 148
    incised, healing of, 118
  clean-contaminated, 148
  closure of. See *Wound closure*.
  complications of, 120
  contaminated, 148
  contraction of, 119
  contracture of, 119
    burns and, 130–131
  dehiscence of, 120
  development of tensile strength of, 118,
    118
  dirty, 148
  healing of. See *Wound healing*.
  infection of, 120, 142
    burns and, 128
    surgery and, 148–150, *149*, 149(t)

Wound (*Continued*)
  pacemaker implantation, 1177
  penetrating, of chest, 188
  surgical, 148
    infection of, 148–150, *149*, 149(t)
  with tissue loss, healing of, 119
Wound closure, after appendectomy, 466
  and wound healing, 119
  in reconstructive surgery, after radical
    neck dissection for cancer, 729
  materials used in, 136–138
    risk of infection associated with, *137*,
      138(t)
  primary, delayed, 120
Wound healing, 117–121
  after burns, 125, 129
    with subsequent contracture and hy-
      pertrophic scar formation, 130–131
  after fracture, 757
  by first intention, 118
  by second intention, 119
  factors impairing, 119, 120

Wound healing (*Continued*)
  historical aspects of study of, 117

Xanthogranulomatous pyelonephritis, 833–
    834
Xanthoma, 800
  of hand, 752
Xeromammography, 297, *298*

Yolk sac tumor, of testis, 852
Yttrium-aluminum-garnet laser therapy, for
    lung cancer, 1007

Zenker's diverticulum, *372*
  resection of, *373*
Zickel nail, 764, *764*
Zinc, in wound healing, 119
Zollinger-Ellison syndrome, 417–418, 449,
    610(t), 611